New Learning Solutions

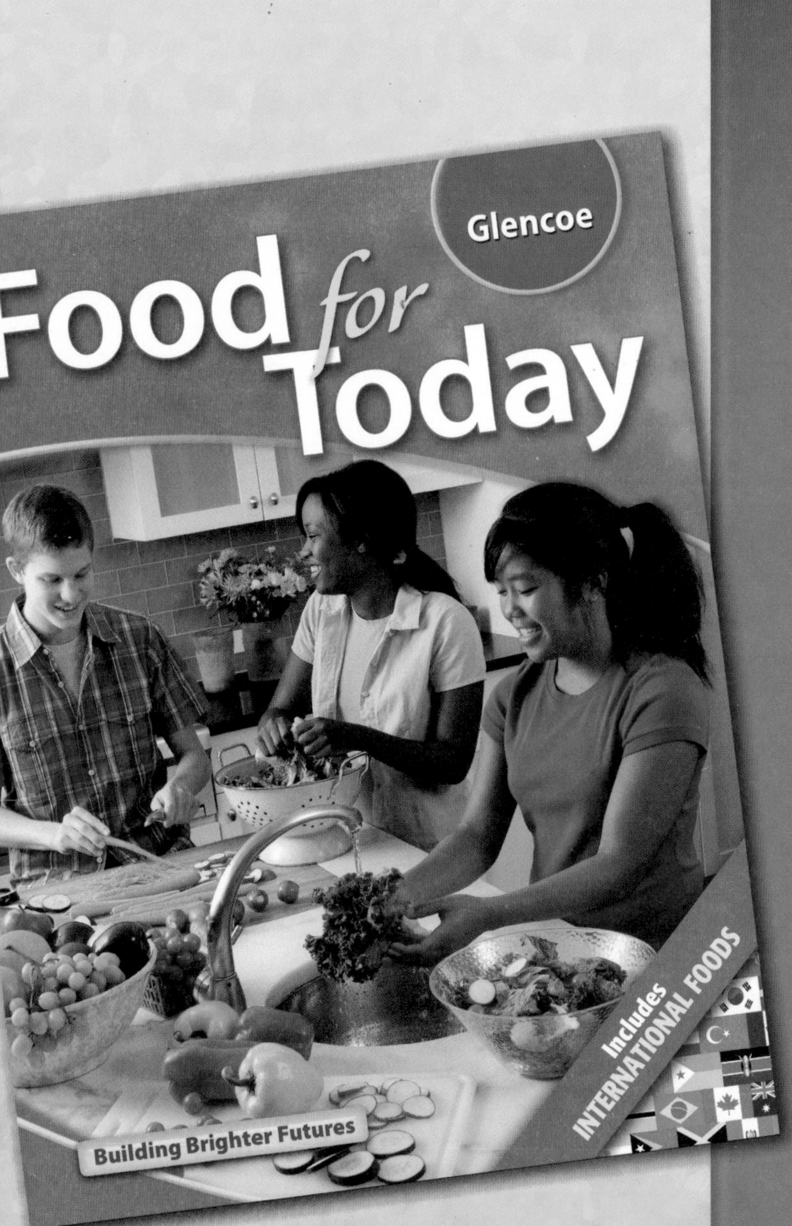

Improve Academic Performance
- National Academic Standards
- Academic Vocabulary
- Reading Guides
- Writing Tips and Activities
- Math and Science Activities
- Standardized Test Practice

Connect to the Real World
- Be a Smart Consumer
- Discover International Foods
- Explore Careers in Food

Hands-On Learning
- Interpersonal and Collaborative Skills Support FCCLA
- Project-Based Learning
- Food Labs
- Light and Healthy Recipes
- How-To Activities
- Unit Thematic Projects

Online Resources
- Online Student Edition
- Graphic Organizers
- Evaluation Rubrics
- English Glossary/Spanish Glosario

Log on to the *Food for Today* Online Learning Center at **glencoe.com**

Food *for* Today

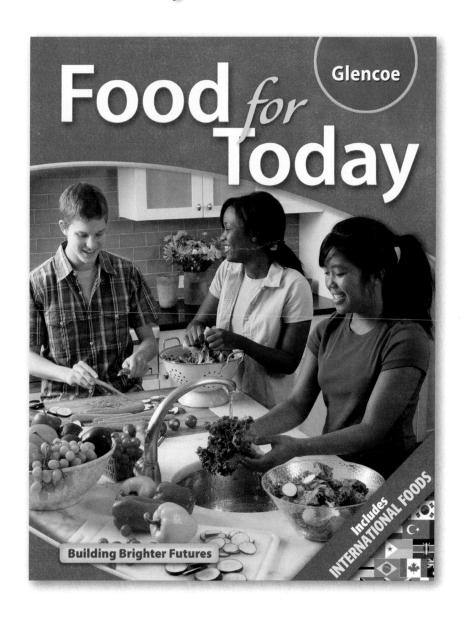

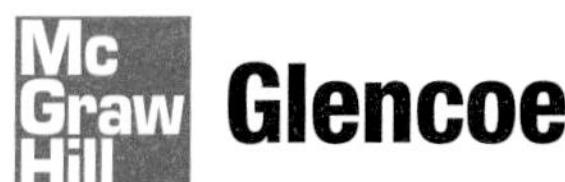

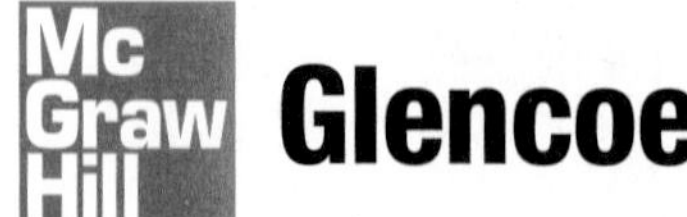

The McGraw·Hill Companies

Printed in the United States of America.

Send all inquiries to:
Glencoe/McGraw-Hill
21600 Oxnard Street, Suite 500
Woodland Hills, CA 91367

ISBN: 978-0-07-888366-8 (Student Edition)
MHID: 0-07-888366-0 (Student Edition)
ISBN: 978-0-07-888450-4 (Teacher Wraparound Edition)
MHID: 0-07-888450-0 (Teacher Wraparound Edition)

2 3 4 5 6 7 8 9 043/071 15 14 13 12 11 10 09

Reviewers

Reviewers

Sabrina Bennett
Family and Consumer Sciences Teacher
Madison County High School
Danielsville, Georgia

Yvonne Britt-Miller
Family and Consumer Sciences Teacher
Hanahan High School
Hanahan, South Carolina

Veronica J. Campbell
Family and Consumer Sciences Teacher
Clintonville High School
Clintonville, Wisconsin

Joyce Glenn
Family and Consumer Sciences Teacher
Nettleton High School
Jonesboro, Arkansas

Dr. Roxie Godfrey
Family and Consumer Sciences Teacher
Mount Vernon High School
Alexandria, Virginia

Carole Havelick
Family and Consumer Sciences Teacher
Lakewood High School
Lake, Colorado

Paula Wright Long
Family and Consumer Sciences Teacher
J.O. Johnson High School
Huntsville, Alabama

Shirley Eddie Moore
Family and Consumer Sciences Teacher
Amory Vocational Center
Amory, Missouri

Val Moses-Shaw
Family and Consumer Sciences Teacher
Downers Grove South High School
Downers Grove, Illinois

Kimberley M. Myers, M. Ed., NBPTS
Family and Consumer Sciences Teacher
Aynor High School
Aynor, South Carolina

Holly P. Nix
Family and Consumer Sciences Teacher
Blacksburg High School
Blacksburg, South Carolina

Vickie Pollard
Family and Consumer Sciences Teacher
Palmetto High School
Williamston, South Carolina

Lynne G. Pritchett
Family and Consumer Sciences Teacher
Gilmer High School
Ellijay, Georgia

Marvelyn Smith
Family and Consumer Sciences Teacher
North Oconee High School
Bogart, Georgia

Ginnie Tate
Family and Consumer Sciences Teacher
East Forsyth High School
Kernersville, North Carolina

Margaret E. Trione
Family and Consumer Sciences Teacher
Daphne High School
Daphne, Alabama

Jennifer Wede
Family and Consumer Sciences Teacher
Carrington High School
Carrington, North Dakota

Anita L. Wilham
Family and Consumer Sciences Teacher
Greenwood Community High School
Greenwood, Indiana

Billie Wilson
Family and Consumer Sciences Teacher
Rosman High School
Rosman, North Carolina

Technical Reviewers

Chef Billie Denunzio, CCE
Director, Institute of Culinary Arts
Eastside High School
Gainesville, Florida

Scavenger Hunt

Food For Today contains a wealth of information. The trick is to know where to look to find all of the information in the book. Use this Scavenger Hunt to preview the text and help you get the most out of this book.

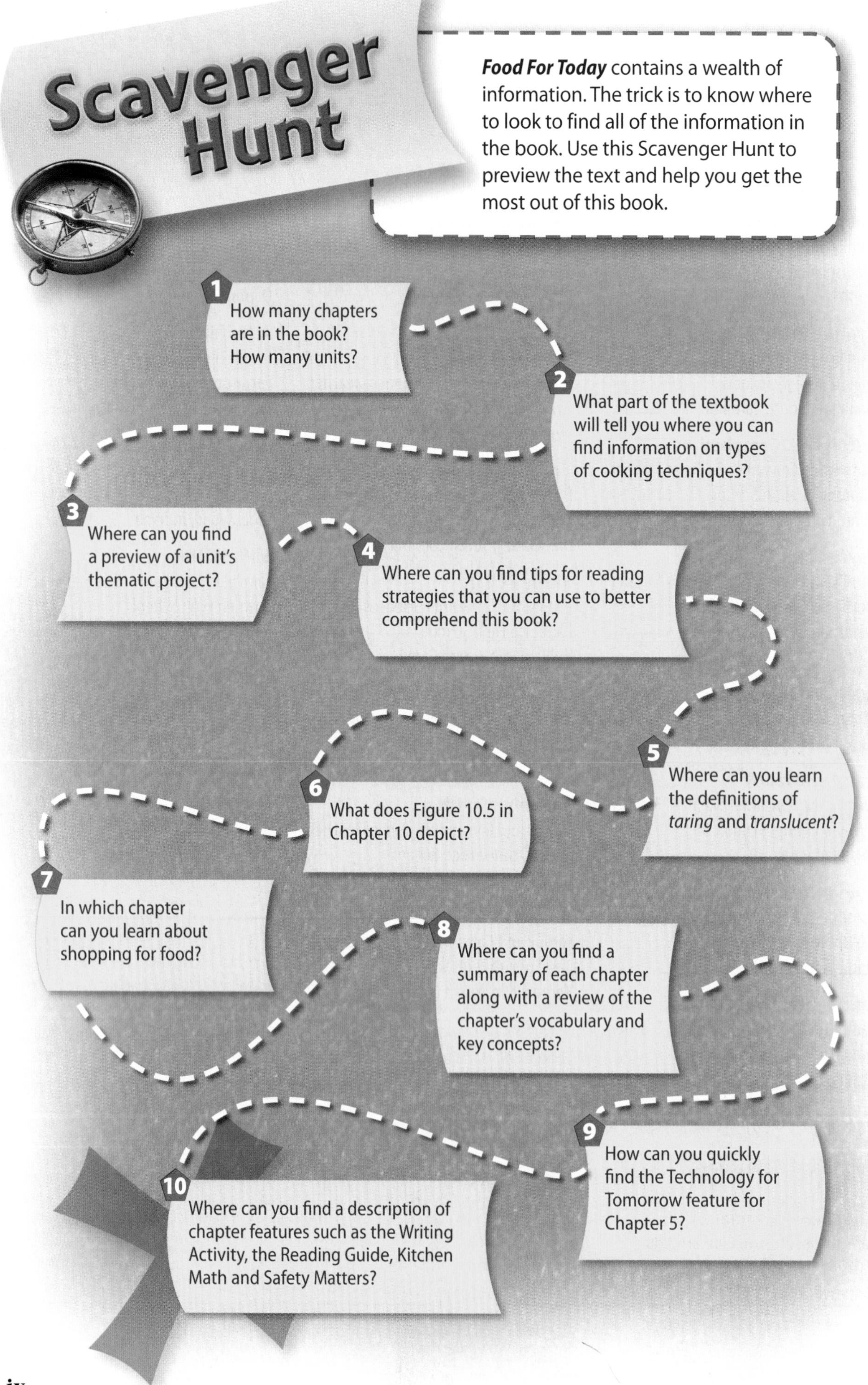

1 How many chapters are in the book? How many units?
2 What part of the textbook will tell you where you can find information on types of cooking techniques?
3 Where can you find a preview of a unit's thematic project?
4 Where can you find tips for reading strategies that you can use to better comprehend this book?
5 Where can you learn the definitions of *taring* and *translucent*?
6 What does Figure 10.5 in Chapter 10 depict?
7 In which chapter can you learn about shopping for food?
8 Where can you find a summary of each chapter along with a review of the chapter's vocabulary and key concepts?
9 How can you quickly find the Technology for Tomorrow feature for Chapter 5?
10 Where can you find a description of chapter features such as the Writing Activity, the Reading Guide, Kitchen Math and Safety Matters?

Table of Contents

Reading Strategies
Look for these reading strategies in each chapter:

- Before You Read
- Graphic Organizer
- Reading Check
- After You Read

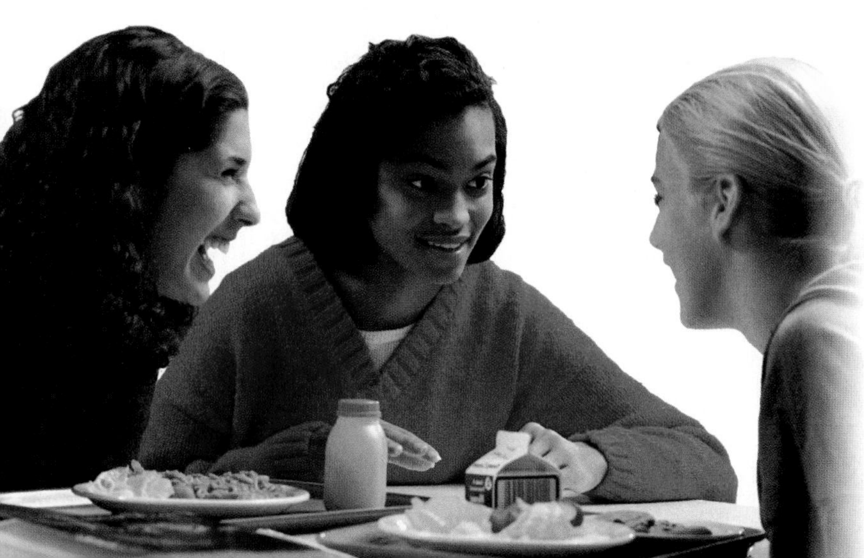

Table of Contents

UNIT 2 Nutrition Basics 56

UNIT 3 Health and Wellness 130

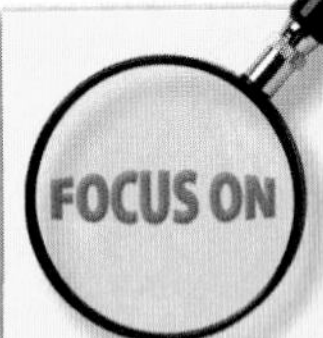

Academic Success
To help you succeed in your classes and on tests, look for these academic skills:

- Reading Guides
- Writing Tips
- Kitchen Math
- Science in Action
- Technology for Tomorrow

UNIT 4 Food Decisions 192

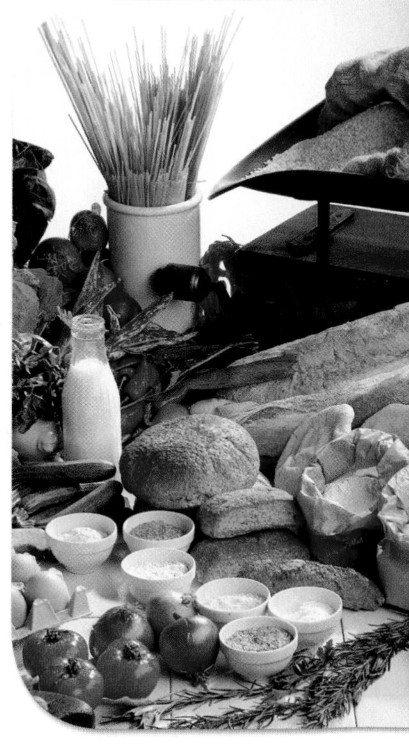

UNIT 5 Kitchen Basics 276

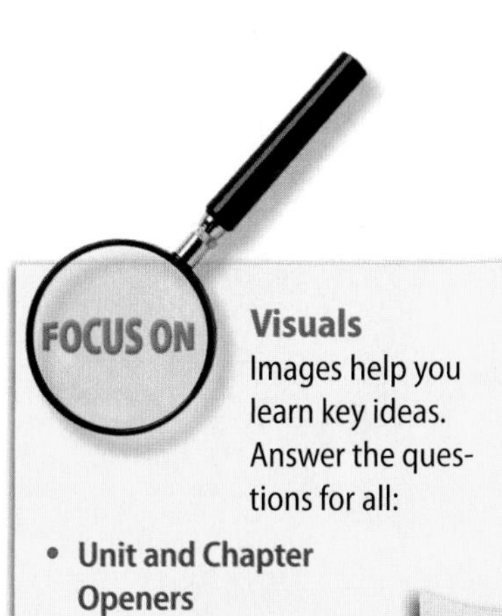

Visuals
Images help you learn key ideas. Answer the questions for all:

- Unit and Chapter Openers
- Photos and Captions
- Figures and Tables

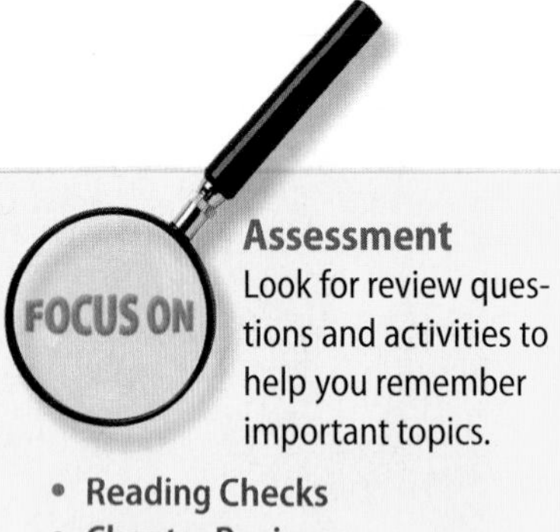
FOCUS ON
Assessment
Look for review questions and activities to help you remember important topics.
• Reading Checks
• Chapter Reviews
• Unit Thematic Projects

UNIT 6 The Art of Cooking 354

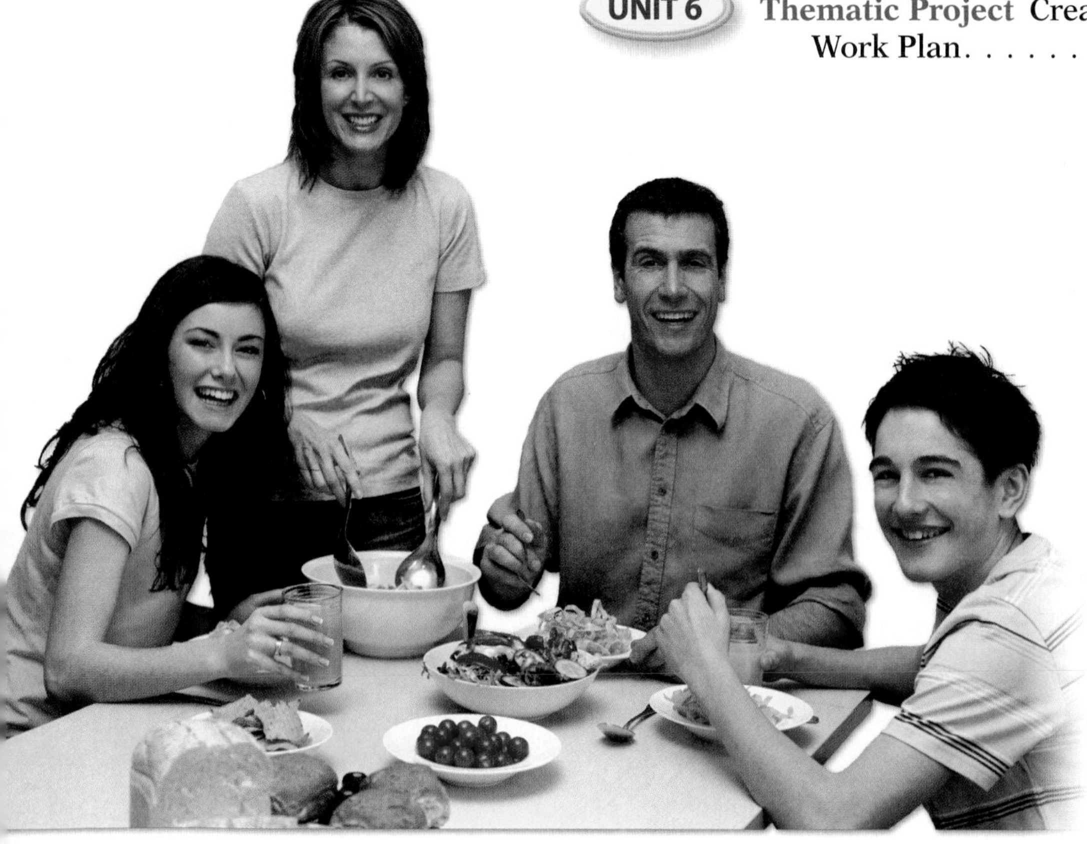

Table of Contents

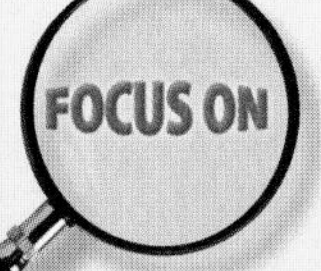

FOCUS ON Project-Based Learning
Projects throughout this book can help you use your skills in real-life situations:

- Real-World scenarios
- Step-by-step instructions
- Independent and group activities

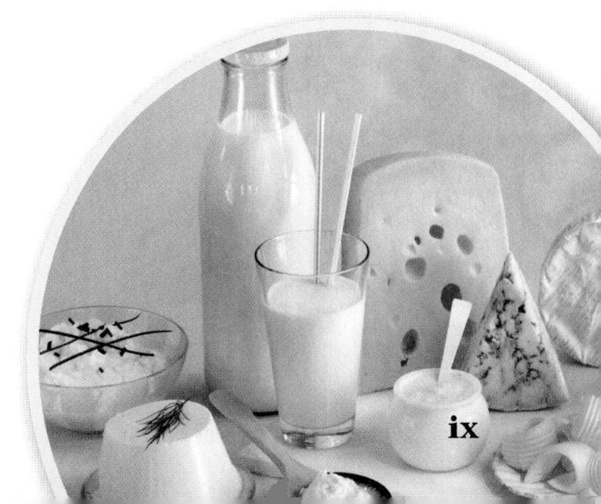

Table of Contents

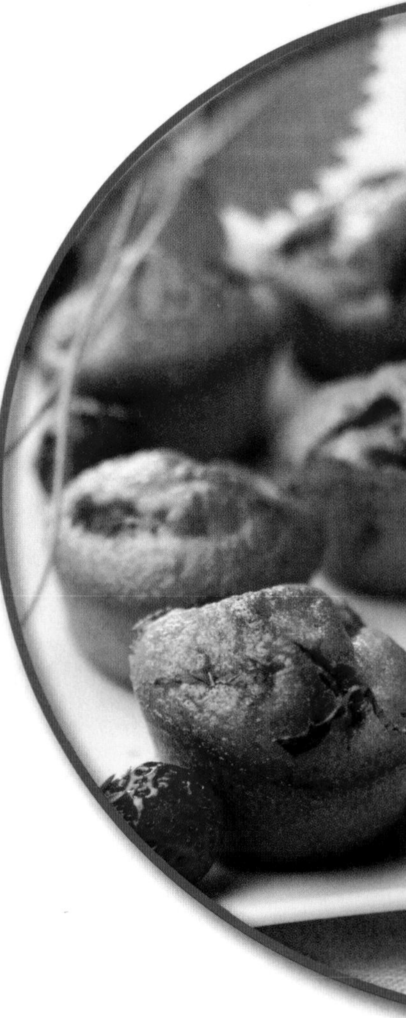

FOCUS ON **Online Resources**
Look for the online icon and go to the book's Online Learning Center at **glencoe.com** for:

- Graphic Organizers
- Practice Tests
- Evaluation Rubrics
- Career Resources
- Additional Activities

Features Table of Contents

Academic Skills for Life!

How do you calculate a tip? Does your food budget need tightening? Why might butter be a better choice than margarine? How does yeast work? These academic features will help you find the answers to these questions.

Kitchen Math

Science in Action

Make Smart Consumer Decisions

How can you determine the right products and services to buy? How can you get the best price? You want the most value for your money. To become a smart shopper, you need to realize that each purchase requires making the right choice when many factors are involved.

Be a *Smart Consumer*

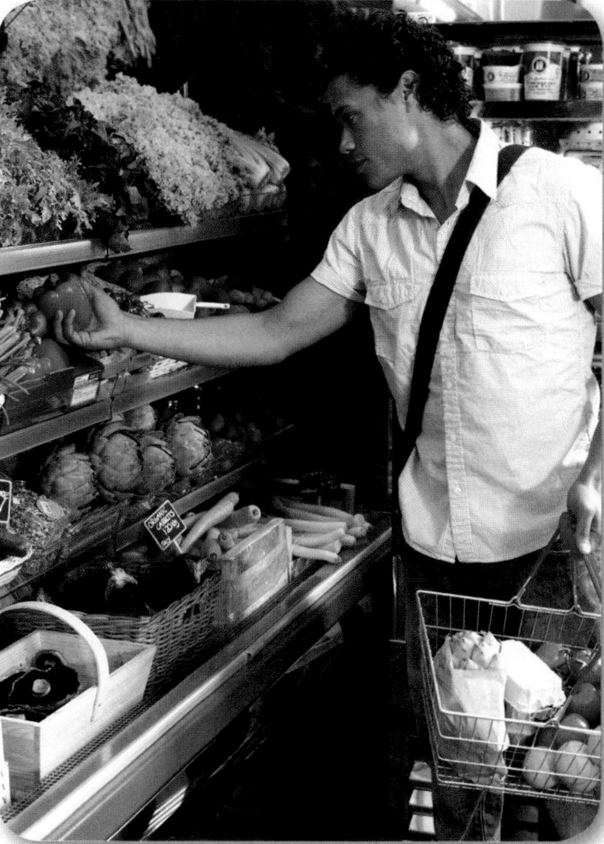

Tasty, Healthful Recipes

Either in the foods lab or home kitchen, you need opportunities to put what you have learned about food and cooking into practice. These recipes will let you practice your kitchen skills.

Light and Healthy Recipe

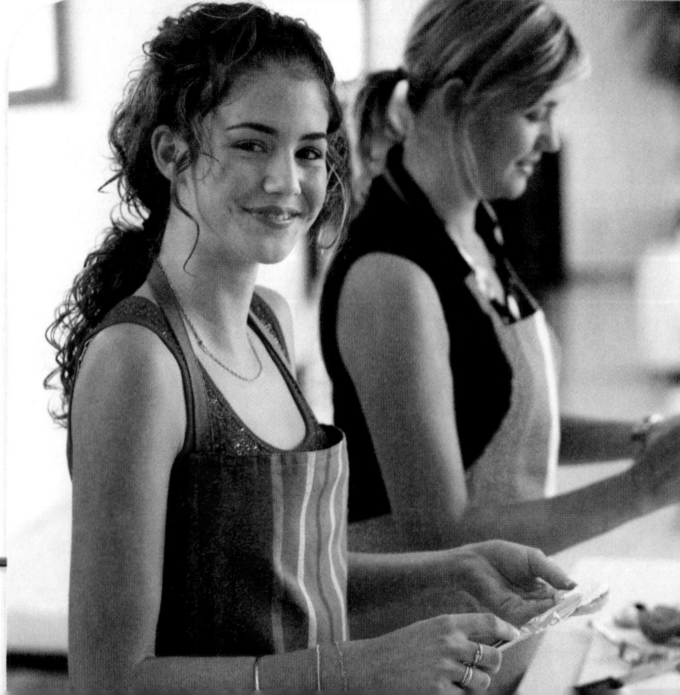

Learn What Makes a Meal Nutritious

Forming good eating habits is important throughout your entire lifespan. These features will give you an understanding of how to make good decisions about food.

Nutrition Check

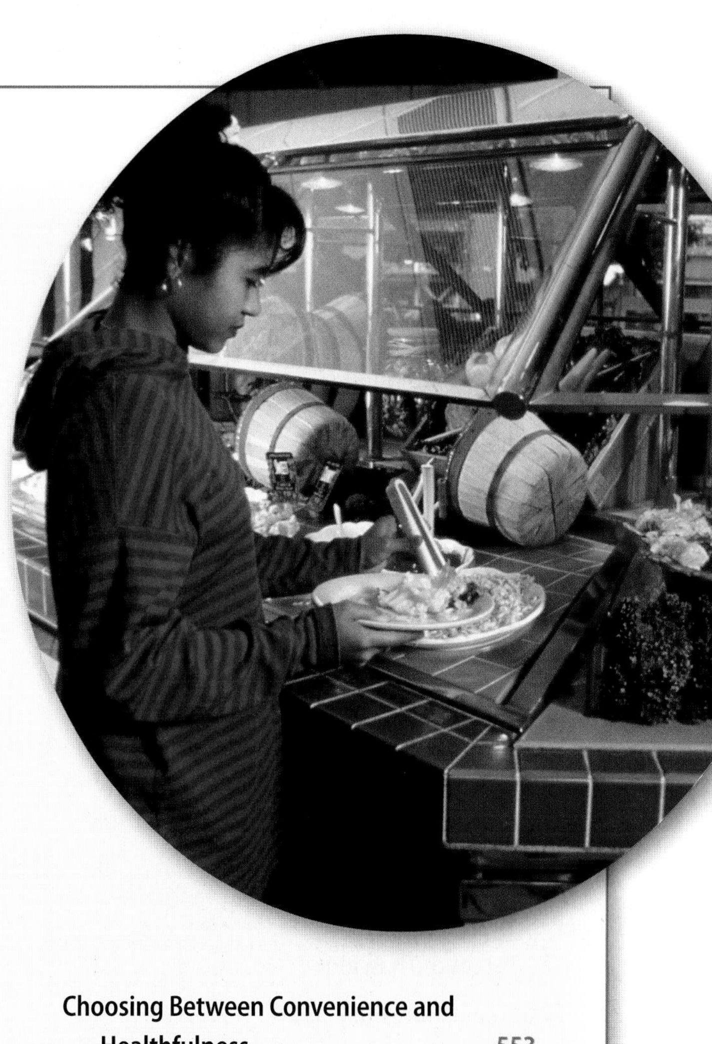

Features Table of Contents

Safety and Technology

The kitchen can be a dangerous place if proper rules are not followed. These features teach you how to work safely to avoid cross-contamination and foodborne illnesses. Science and technology have brought many developments to the kitchen. Knowing how to use technology and being able to make smart choices when purchasing appliances are important skills.

SAFETY MATTERS

TECHNOLOGY FOR TOMORROW

What Do You Want to Be?

The world of food is a gateway to many different careers. These features allow you to learn about many different food-oriented careers and the skills and education you will need to get them.

Careers in Food

To the Student

Begin the Unit

Discover the World of Food For Today

Successful readers first set a purpose for reading. *Food For Today* teaches skills you need to make healthful food choices, prepare nutritious and attractive meals, and bring activity into your daily life. Think about why you are reading this book. Use the unit opener to help you set a reading purpose and understand what you will learn in each unit. Consider how you might be able to use what you learn in your own life.

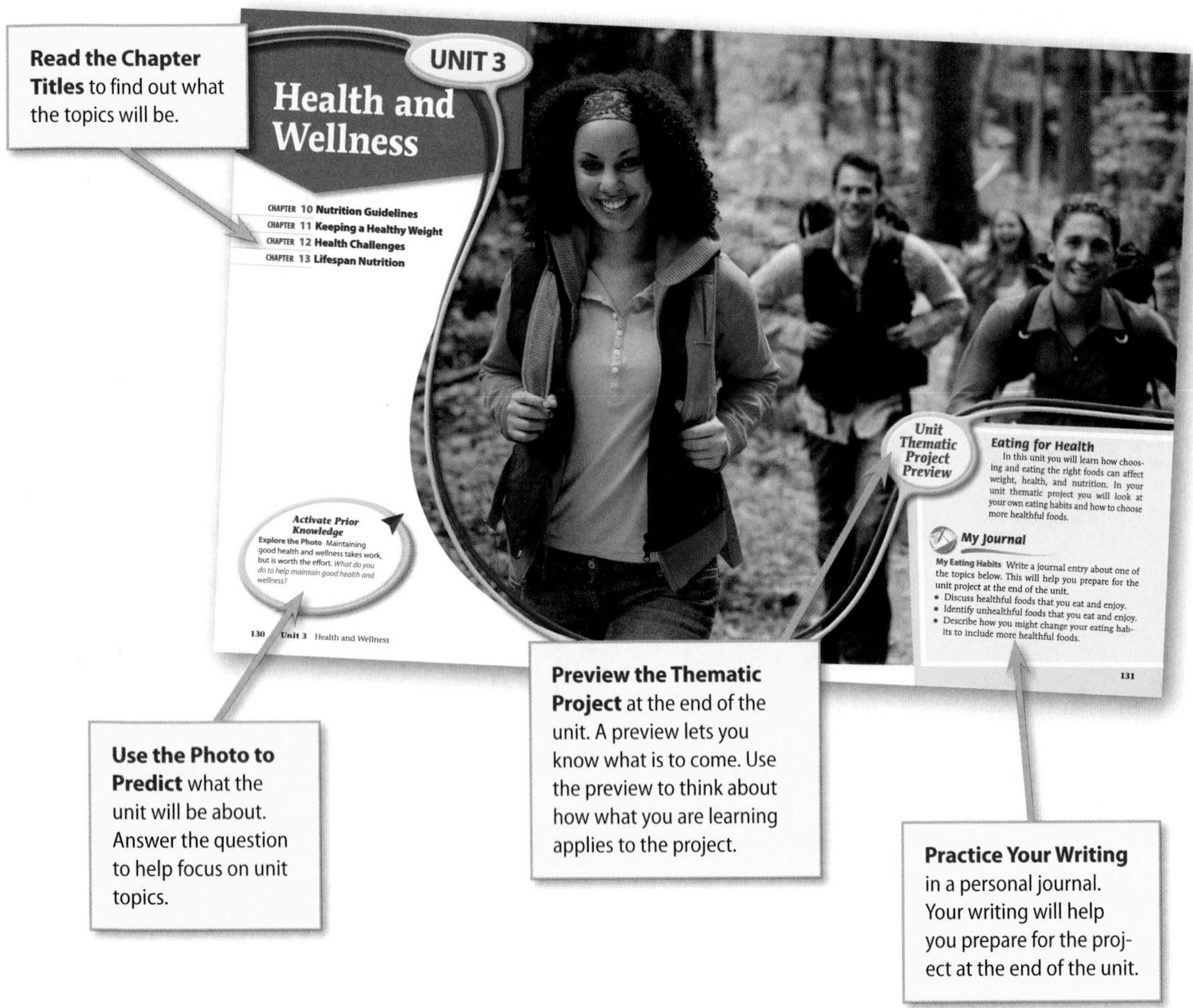

Read the Chapter Titles to find out what the topics will be.
UNIT 3
Health and Wellness
CHAPTER 10 Nutrition Guidelines
CHAPTER 11 Keeping a Healthy Weight
CHAPTER 12 Health Challenges
CHAPTER 13 Lifespan Nutrition
Activate Prior Knowledge
Explore the Photo Maintaining good health and wellness takes work, but is worth the effort. *What do you do to help maintain good health and wellness?*
130 Unit 3 Health and Wellness
Unit Thematic Project Preview
Eating for Health
In this unit you will learn how choosing and eating the right foods can affect weight, health, and nutrition. In your unit thematic project you will look at your own eating habits and how to choose more healthful foods.
My Journal
My Eating Habits Write a journal entry about one of the topics below. This will help you prepare for the unit project at the end of the unit.
• Discuss healthful foods that you eat and enjoy.
• Identify unhealthful foods that you eat and enjoy.
• Describe how you might change your eating habits to include more healthful foods.
131
Use the Photo to Predict what the unit will be about. Answer the question to help focus on unit topics.
Preview the Thematic Project at the end of the unit. A preview lets you know what is to come. Use the preview to think about how what you are learning applies to the project.
Practice Your Writing in a personal journal. Your writing will help you prepare for the project at the end of the unit.

Close the Unit

What Did You Learn About Food For Today?

Every unit ends with a Thematic Project that lets you explore an important issue from the unit. To complete each project, you will make decisions, do research, connect to your community, create a visual, and present your project.

Read the Project Assignment and numbered steps. The assignment explains what you will need to do.

Follow the Project Checklist to make sure that you have done everything you need to complete your thematic project.

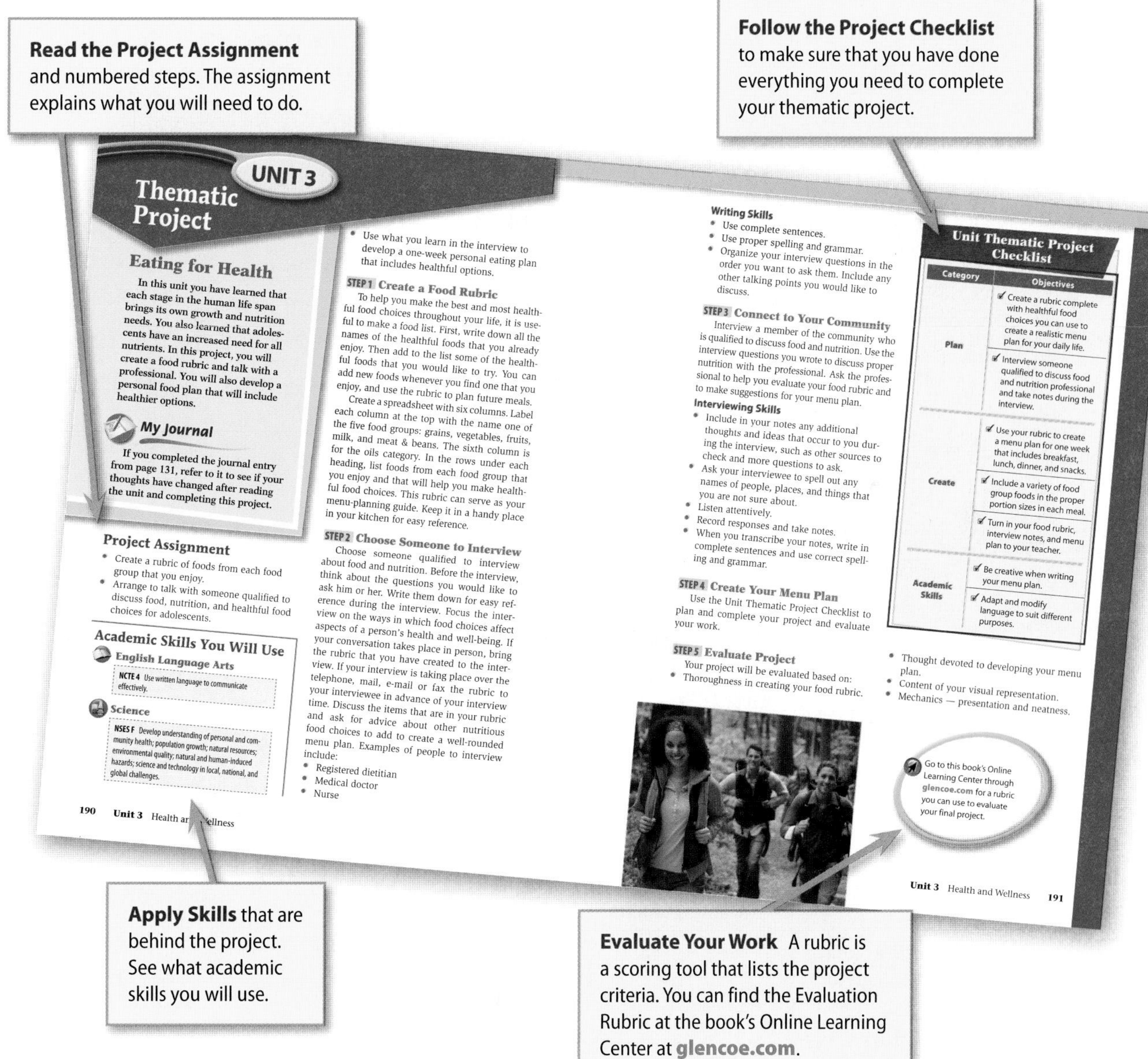

UNIT 3

Thematic Project

Eating for Health

In this unit you have learned that each stage in the human life span brings its own growth and nutrition needs. You also learned that adolescents have an increased need for all nutrients. In this project, you will create a food rubric and talk with a professional. You will also develop a personal food plan that will include healthier options.

My Journal

If you completed the journal entry from page 131, refer to it to see if your thoughts have changed after reading the unit and completing this project.

Project Assignment

- Create a rubric of foods from each food group that you enjoy.
- Arrange to talk with someone qualified to discuss food, nutrition, and healthful food choices for adolescents.
- Use what you learn in the interview to develop a one-week personal eating plan that includes healthful options.

Academic Skills You Will Use

English Language Arts

NCTE 4 Use written language to communicate effectively.

Science

NSES F Develop understanding of personal and community health; population growth; natural resources; environmental quality; natural and human-induced hazards; science and technology in local, national, and global challenges.

STEP 1 Create a Food Rubric

To help you make the best and most healthful food choices throughout your life, it is useful to make a food list. First, write down all the names of the healthful foods that you already enjoy. Then add to the list some of the healthful foods that you would like to try. You can add new foods whenever you find one that you enjoy, and use the rubric to plan future meals.

Create a spreadsheet with six columns. Label each column at the top with the name one of the five food groups: grains, vegetables, fruits, milk, and meat & beans. The sixth column is for the oils category. In the rows under each heading, list foods from each food group that you enjoy and that will help you make healthful food choices. This rubric can serve as your menu-planning guide. Keep it in a handy place in your kitchen for easy reference.

STEP 2 Choose Someone to Interview

Choose someone qualified to interview about food and nutrition. Before the interview, think about the questions you would like to ask him or her. Write them down for easy reference during the interview. Focus the interview on the ways in which food choices affect aspects of a person's health and well-being. If your conversation takes place in person, bring the rubric that you have created to the interview. If your interview is taking place over the telephone, mail, e-mail or fax the rubric to your interviewee in advance of your interview time. Discuss the items that are in your rubric and ask for advice about other nutritious food choices to add to create a well-rounded menu plan. Examples of people to interview include:

- Registered dietitian
- Medical doctor
- Nurse

Writing Skills

- Use complete sentences.
- Use proper spelling and grammar.
- Organize your interview questions in the order you want to ask them. Include any other talking points you would like to discuss.

STEP 3 Connect to Your Community

Interview a member of the community who is qualified to discuss food and nutrition. Use the interview questions you wrote to discuss proper nutrition with the professional. Ask the professional to help you evaluate your food rubric and to make suggestions for your menu plan.

Interviewing Skills

- Include in your notes any additional thoughts and ideas that occur to you during the interview, such as other sources to check and more questions to ask.
- Ask your interviewee to spell out any names of people, places, and things that you are not sure about.
- Listen attentively.
- Record responses and take notes.
- When you transcribe your notes, write in complete sentences and use correct spelling and grammar.

STEP 4 Create Your Menu Plan

Use the Unit Thematic Project Checklist to plan and complete your project and evaluate your work.

STEP 5 Evaluate Project

Your project will be evaluated based on:

- Thoroughness in creating your food rubric.
- Thought devoted to developing your menu plan.
- Content of your visual representation.
- Mechanics — presentation and neatness.

Unit Thematic Project Checklist

Category	Objectives
Plan	Create a rubric complete with healthful food choices you can use to create a realistic menu plan for your daily life.
	Interview someone qualified to discuss food and nutrition professional and take notes during the interview.
Create	Use your rubric to create a menu plan for one week that includes breakfast, lunch, dinner, and snacks.
	Include a variety of food group foods in the proper portion sizes in each meal.
	Turn in your food rubric, interview notes, and menu plan to your teacher.
Academic Skills	Be creative when writing your menu plan.
	Adapt and modify language to suit different purposes.

Go to this book's Online Learning Center through glencoe.com for a rubric you can use to evaluate your final project.

190 Unit 3 Health and Wellness

Unit 3 Health and Wellness 191

Apply Skills that are behind the project. See what academic skills you will use.

Evaluate Your Work A rubric is a scoring tool that lists the project criteria. You can find the Evaluation Rubric at the book's Online Learning Center at **glencoe.com**.

To the Student

Begin the Chapter

What is the Chapter All About?

Use the activities in the opener to help you connect what you already know to chapter topics. Think about the people, places, and events in your own life. Are there any similarities with those in your textbook?

Preview the Chapter to note the key ideas you will learn. Keep these in mind as you read the chapter.

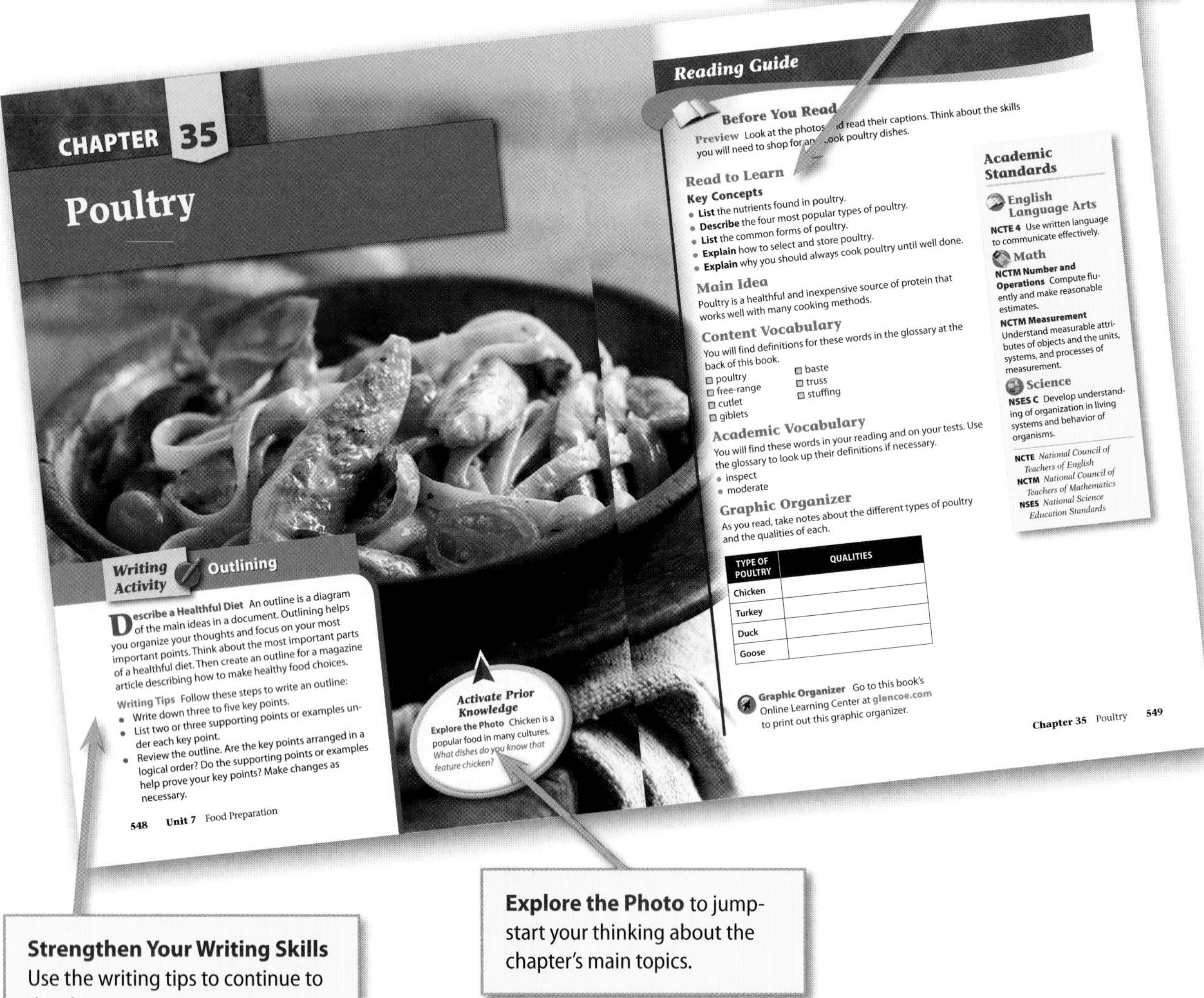

CHAPTER 35

Poultry

Writing Activity — Outlining

Describe a Healthful Diet An outline is a diagram of the main ideas in a document. Outlining helps you organize your thoughts and focus on your most important points. Think about the most important parts of a healthful diet. Then create an outline for a magazine article describing how to make healthy food choices.

Writing Tips Follow these steps to write an outline:
- Write down three to five key points.
- List two or three supporting points or examples under each key point.
- Review the outline. Are the key points arranged in a logical order? Do the supporting points or examples help prove your key points? Make changes as necessary.

Activate Prior Knowledge

Explore the Photo Chicken is a popular food in many cultures. *What dishes do you know that feature chicken?*

548 Unit 7 Food Preparation

Reading Guide

Before You Read

Preview Look at the photos and read their captions. Think about the skills you will need to shop for and cook poultry dishes.

Read to Learn

Key Concepts
- **List** the nutrients found in poultry.
- **Describe** the four most popular types of poultry.
- **List** the common forms of poultry.
- **Explain** how to select and store poultry.
- **Explain** why you should always cook poultry until well done.

Main Idea

Poultry is a healthful and inexpensive source of protein that works well with many cooking methods.

Content Vocabulary

You will find definitions for these words in the glossary at the back of this book.
- poultry
- free-range
- cutlet
- giblets
- baste
- truss
- stuffing

Academic Vocabulary

You will find these words in your reading and on your tests. Use the glossary to look up their definitions if necessary.
- inspect
- moderate

Graphic Organizer

As you read, take notes about the different types of poultry and the qualities of each.

TYPE OF POULTRY	QUALITIES
Chicken	
Turkey	
Duck	
Goose	

Graphic Organizer Go to this book's Online Learning Center at glencoe.com to print out this graphic organizer.

Academic Standards

English Language Arts
NCTE 4 Use written language to communicate effectively.

Math
NCTM Number and Operations Compute fluently and make reasonable estimates.
NCTM Measurement Understand measurable attributes of objects and the units, systems, and processes of measurement.

Science
NSES C Develop understanding of organization in living systems and behavior of organisms.

NCTE *National Council of Teachers of English*
NCTM *National Council of Teachers of Mathematics*
NSES *National Science Education Standards*

Chapter 35 Poultry 549

Explore the Photo to jump-start your thinking about the chapter's main topics.

Strengthen Your Writing Skills Use the writing tips to continue to develop your writing.

Review the Chapter

Make Sure You Know and Understand the Concepts

Every unit ends with a Thematic Project that lets you explore an important issue from the unit. To complete each project, you will make decisions, do research, connect to your community, create a visual, and present your project.

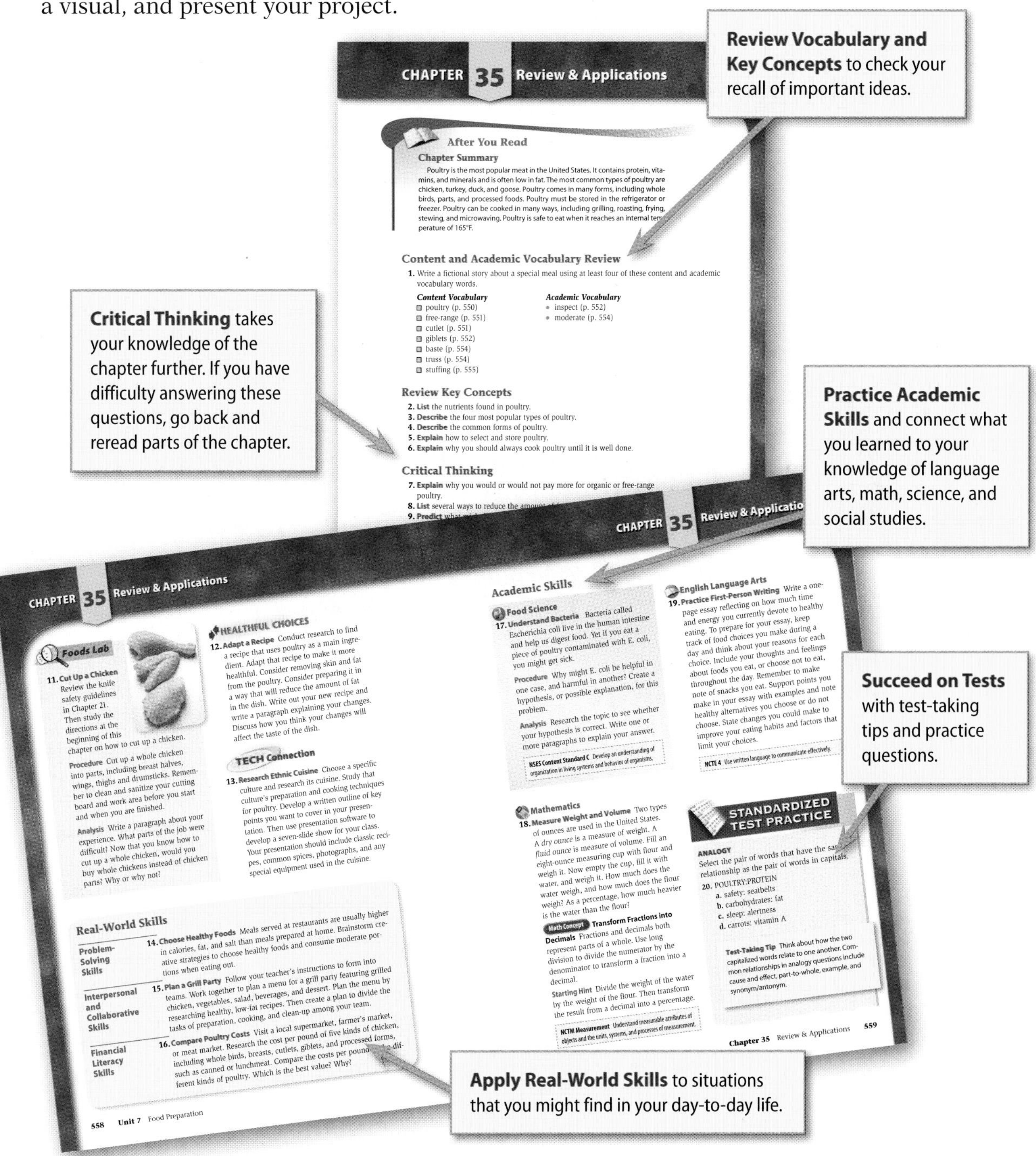

Review Vocabulary and Key Concepts to check your recall of important ideas.

Critical Thinking takes your knowledge of the chapter further. If you have difficulty answering these questions, go back and reread parts of the chapter.

Practice Academic Skills and connect what you learned to your knowledge of language arts, math, science, and social studies.

Succeed on Tests with test-taking tips and practice questions.

Apply Real-World Skills to situations that you might find in your day-to-day life.

To the Student

As You Read

Use Reading Strategies and Visuals to Study Effectively

In addition to the reading guide at the beginning of each chapter, there are reading strategies to help you comprehend the text.

Skim the Headings to help identify the main idea and supporting details.

Examine Visuals to reinforce content. Answer the questions so you can better discuss topics in the chapter.

Reading Checks let you pause to respond to what you have read.

Where to Shop

Just like preparing food, shopping for food is a skill. Practicing this skill helps you to save time, choose the best quality food, and get the best value for your money. You have many choices in buying food. Food stores go by many names, but they fall into two basic types: supermarkets and specialty stores such as food cooperatives and farmers' markets.

Supermarkets

Supermarkets are popular, all-purpose stores that account for about 75 percent of all grocery sales. Most supermarkets are part of a regional or nationwide chain, which gives them the buying power to offer competitive prices. Large supermarkets may stock 50,000 items—all kinds of food and drinks, as well as paper products, cleaning supplies, pet items, and health and beauty aids. Many supermarkets have their own bakeries, butcher shops, and take-out food departments. Local banks may operate a small banking center inside. Supermarkets have different variations that emphasize low prices or convenience.

Supercenters Supercenters are huge stores that combine a supermarket with other types of shops in one building. They may include a full-service pharmacy, a hair salon, a vision center, or a department store.

Warehouse Stores Warehouse stores are large stores with low prices. Warehouse stores usually offer limited customer service. They sell basic food items, like canned goods and bread, in bulk. Shoppers bag or box their own groceries when checking out, using their own bags or spare store boxes. Larger "super warehouse" stores have separate food departments.

Warehouse Clubs Warehouse clubs, or wholesale clubs, are large stores that require an annual membership fee. Members can buy a large variety of food items at low prices, but usually in extra-large quantities only—four-pound bags of tortilla chips and one-gallon jugs of salsa, for example. Some stores carry gourmet items, along with clothing, housewares, and small appliances.

Health Food Supermarkets Health food supermarkets carry only natural foods. A **natural food** is a food that has been minimally processed and has few additives such as dyes and added sugars. Health food supermarkets are sometimes called natural food stores. Health food supermarkets offer many vegetarian foods, including various grains, beans, and

Bulk Foods

Buying food from bulk bins saves money and let you choose exactly the amount you need. Check freshness before you buy. *Where should you look for bulk bins in a supermarket?*

238 **Unit 4** Food Decisions

Using an Oven Thermometer

An oven thermometer tells you whether food has reached a safe temperature. The tip of the probe should reach the thickest part of the meat, without touching the bone. *At what temperature is poultry fully cooked?*

Roasting Poultry

Whole birds are usually cooked by roasting. Turkey, duck, and goose are best roasted. Whole broiler-fryer or roaster chickens also roast well.

Clean the bird and season the cavity with salt, pepper, herbs, and spices. You can insert carrots, onions, celery, or other aromatic vegetables for extra flavor. Many cooks then truss birds before roasting. To **truss** is to hold a roast together with twine or skewers. This makes it easier to handle and more attractive to serve. **Figure 35.7** shows an uncooked chicken trussed with twine.

Turn the chicken and baste it with oil or melted butter to keep it moist. To **baste** is to pour or brush melted fat, cooking juices, or other liquid over food as it cooks. Continue broiling until the chicken is browned and crisp. Test for doneness with an instant-read thermometer. About two minutes before the chicken is done, you can add flavor by applying a sweetened sauce such as barbecue sauce or sweet-and-sour sauce.

Grilling Poultry

Poultry tastes great grilled. To grill a broiler-fryer chicken, first cut the chicken into halves, quarters, or pieces. Brush the grill grate lightly with oil to keep the chicken from sticking. Place the chicken skin-side up on the grate and brush it with oil or melted butter. Grill the chicken over **moderate**, or less than extreme, heat until the outside is browned and the inside is well-done. Turn the pieces often to avoid burning or overcooking the outside before the inside is done. Brush the chicken with oil or melted butter. As always, test pieces for doneness with an instant-read thermometer.

You can marinate poultry before grilling to add flavor or make kebabs by threading cubes of meat and vegetables onto skewers. You can also add flavor by brushing on a sweetened sauce during the last few minutes of cooking.

✓ **Reading Check** Why is it important to brush the grill with oil before grilling chicken?

Kitchen Math

Calculate Roasting Time

At 325° F, an unstuffed turkey needs to roast one minute for every ounce of total weight. How many hours will you need to roast a 12-pound turkey? Round your answer down to a whole number. You round down because when the turkey gets within an hour of being done, you'll check it with a quick-read thermometer.

Math Concept **Multi-Step Problems** This is a multi-step problem since you have make two computations. Think through each step before beginning.

Starting Hint: Remember that there are 16 ounces in a pound. The turkey you need to roast weighs 12 pounds. Multiply 16 times 12. This will give you the number of minutes required and you can divide that number by 60, to get your answer in hours.

Math Appendix For math help, go to the Math Appendix at the back of the book.

NCTM Number and Operations Compute fluently and make reasonable estimates.

554 **Unit 7** Food Preparation

Study with Features

Skills You Can Really Use at School and in Life!

As you read, look for feature boxes throughout each chapter. These features build skills that relate to other academic subjects and prepare you for life on your own.

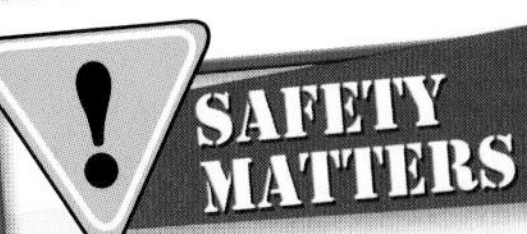

Dull, But Dangerous

Imagine you are teaching a group of young students how to safely cut vegetables. To keep them from cutting themselves, would you provide them with dull knives? Actually, a dull knife is more dangerous than a sharp knife. Why? You have to use more force to cut with a dull knife, which makes it more likely to slip. A dull knife applied to the skin with great force can do harm. A sharp blade, in contrast, cuts with less effort, and is less likely to slip. Keep knives sharp by using a sharpening stone or by having them professionally sharpened. A sharpening steel keeps a blade straight.

What Would You Do? In your foods lab, you notice one of your peers trying to forcefully cut a tomato with a dull knife. "Gee," she says, "this knife works slowly, but at least I won't cut myself." What would you do?

Be a Smart Consumer

The Costs of Convenience

Because their menu items are priced low, fast food restaurants appear to be the least expensive option for dining out. Choosing fast food, however, is costly in other ways. Firstly, it costs time. Have you ever spent fifteen minutes in line at a drive-through waiting to order your so-called "convenient" food? Getting to a fast food restaurant, and idling at a drive-through, costs gas, which in turn poses a cost to the environment. Finally, choosing fast food, which tends to be high in fat and cholesterol and low in nutrients, can cost you your most valuable asset of all: your health.

Challenge Brainstorm other ways besides fast food that you can obtain and eat healthful food in fewer than 20 minutes for 10 dollars or less.

Learn How to Be Kitchen Smart Use consumer and safety tips to make yourself more productive in the kitchen.

Learn the Secrets of Science
The secret is that it can be easy! You can use scientific principles and concepts in your everyday activities. Investigate and analyze the world around you with these basic skills.

Science in Action

Explaining Dark and Light Meat

Why do chickens and turkeys have light and dark meat? The color depends on the amount of exercise a bird's muscles get. Muscles that work hard use more oxygen. The oxygen is stored in a reddish pigment called myoglobin.

Procedure Conduct research about myoglobin. More myoglobin makes darker meat. Age also affects the amount of myoglobin in poultry. All the meat on a Rock Cornish game hen is light colored because it is too young to have had much exercise. A free range chicken has darker meat because it gets more exercise than a chicken that is not free to roam a farm. Ducks have much more fat than chickens because they live in water and need the fat to keep warm. Since a duck not only walks but flies while carrying extra weight, it must work its muscles harder. That causes darker meat.

Analysis Given what you have learned about myoglobin, write a paragraph to explain why the leg meat from a turkey is among the darkest of poultry meat.

NSES C Develop understanding of matter, energy, and organization in living systems; and behavior of organisms.

Kitchen Math

Calculate Roasting Time

At 325° F, an unstuffed turkey needs to roast one minute for every ounce of total weight. How many hours will you need to roast a 12-pound turkey? Round your answer down to a whole number. You round down because when the turkey gets within an hour of being done, you'll check it with a quick-read thermometer.

Math Concept **Multi-Step Problems** This is a multi-step problem since you have make two computations. Think through each step before beginning.

Starting Hint: Remember that there are 16 ounces in a pound. The turkey you need to roast weighs 12 pounds. Multiply 16 times 12. This will give you the number of minutes required and you can divide that number by 60, to get your answer in hours.

Math Appendix For math help, go to the Math Appendix at the back of the book.

NCTM Number and Operations Compute fluently and make reasonable estimates.

Make Math Simple
You use math every day—even if it is just measuring flour to make a recipe. See how to use starting hints to break down math problems and solve them step by step.

Features (continued)

Learn About New Technology in the food industry. Learn the ins and outs of new development.

TECHNOLOGY FOR TOMORROW

Safe Substitutes

People with food allergies must be very careful to avoid even the tiniest amount of problem foods. Fortunately, science and technology have made it possible for food makers to create safe substitutes for some allergenic foods. For example, people with lactose intolerance can substitute lactose-reduced or lactose-free products. Lactose-free milk is made by adding lactase to the milk. Lactase is an enzyme that breaks down lactose into glucose and galactose, digestable sugars. This process removes 70-100 percent of the lactose. In all other aspects, the lactose-free milk is nutritionally the same as regular milk. .

Investigate Research a safe substitute for a food that can cause allergies or intolerance in people. Discover how the substitute is produced, which food or foods it can replace, and its nutritional benefits.

NCSS VIII A Science, Technology, and Society Identify and describe both current and historical examples of the interaction and interdependence of science, technology, and society in a variety of cultural settings.

Learn How to Stay Healthy Nutrition Checks let you consider options and learn how to make smart food choices.

Nutrition Check

Choosing Between Convenience and Healthfulness

Convenience foods made from poultry are tasty. They also are quick and easy to prepare, but they may not be the most healthful choice. A turkey hot dog and a skinless chicken breast each have about 120 calories, but the hot dog can have 530 mg of sodium. That's 10 times what you will find in the average chicken breast. Also, a hot dog can get 70 percent of its calories from fat. Read the nutrition facts to see whether convenience foods are a good deal for your health.

Think About It Under what circumstances might you choose the hot dog over the skinless chicken breast? When would the chicken breast be the best choice? What factors besides healthfulness might weigh in your decision?

Light and Healthy Recipe

Baked Chicken Nuggets with Baked Sweet Potato "Fries"

Ingredients

Chicken Nuggets

1 pound	chicken breast, cut into bite-size cubes
½ cup	ground bran flakes cereal
1½ cups	ground corn flakes cereal
1 cup	lowfat buttermilk
½ tsp	salt
⅛ tsp	black pepper
⅛ tsp	paprika
⅛ tsp	cayenne

Sweet Potato Fries

2 cups	sweet potato, cut into steak fry-sized rectangles
2 Tbsp.	vegetable oil

These chicken nuggets are made with whole chicken breast pieces and bran flakes. They are baked rather than fried.

Directions

1. Put chicken and milk into a sealable plastic bag, mix well and refrigerate for 15–30 minutes.
2. Toss the sweet potatoes in a mixing bowl with the oil and salt and pepper. Lay out on a sheet tray and bake in a 375°F oven for 25–30 minutes.
3. Mix cereals together with paprika and cayenne. Roll chicken pieces in the ground cereal to coat. Place the chicken in a lightly oiled baking pan and bake in a 375°F oven for 20–25 minutes.

Make It A Meal

Serve with steamed vegetables.

Yield 4 servings

Nutrition Analysis per Serving

Calories	363
Total fat	10 g
Saturated fat	1 g
Cholesterol	68 mg
Sodium	541 mg
Carbohydrate	39
Dietary fiber	5 g
Sugars	10 g
Protein	31 g

Nutrition in Recipes helps you learn what foods provide needed nutrients.

Features (continued)

Think About Your Future

What do you want to be? Get profiles of real-world workers to understand more about your career options. Think about what skills you would need to explore various career paths.

Learn from Professionals Hear from real people who share their on-the-job stories.

Careers in Food

Denise Tryner
Fitness Consultant

Q: What is the difference between a fitness consultant and a fitness instructor?

A: I started off as an instructor, teaching classes at a health club. A consultant covers the whole ball instead of just part of it – physical fitness, nutrition, healthy habits. So now I teach classes, do personal training one-on-one – actually groups of four or five people at a time – and nutrition counseling and coaching.

Q: What is your personal philosophy on diet and nutrition?

A: Everything in moderation. You don't have to deprive yourself in order to reach your end goal. Eat healthy, exercise every day, and anything is possible.

Q: Do you go to clients or do they come to you?

A: Both. I go to clients' offices and homes, or sometimes meet at a park. And I also have the basement of my home so they can come to me in my studio.

"Motivating someone to push his or her body to its limit is exhilarating."
— Denise Tryner
Professional Fitness Consultant – Denver, *CO*

Education and Training
Certification in personal training and group fitness training is available through the American Council on Exercise.

Qualities and Skills
Patience, understanding, and a passion to motivate and inspire people to reach their personal goals.

Related Career Opportunities
Physical therapists also help people figure out what's going on with their bodies and help them make changes to reach their goals.

Explore Needed Skills See what skills you would need to have a similar career.

To the Student

Online Learning Center

Use the Internet to Extend Your Learning

Follow these steps to access the textbook resources at *Food for Today* Online Learning Center.

Online Learning Center Icon Look for this icon throughout the text that directs you to the book's Online Learning Center for more activities and information.

Graphic Organizer Go to this book's Online Learning Center at **glencoe.com** to print out this graphic organizer.

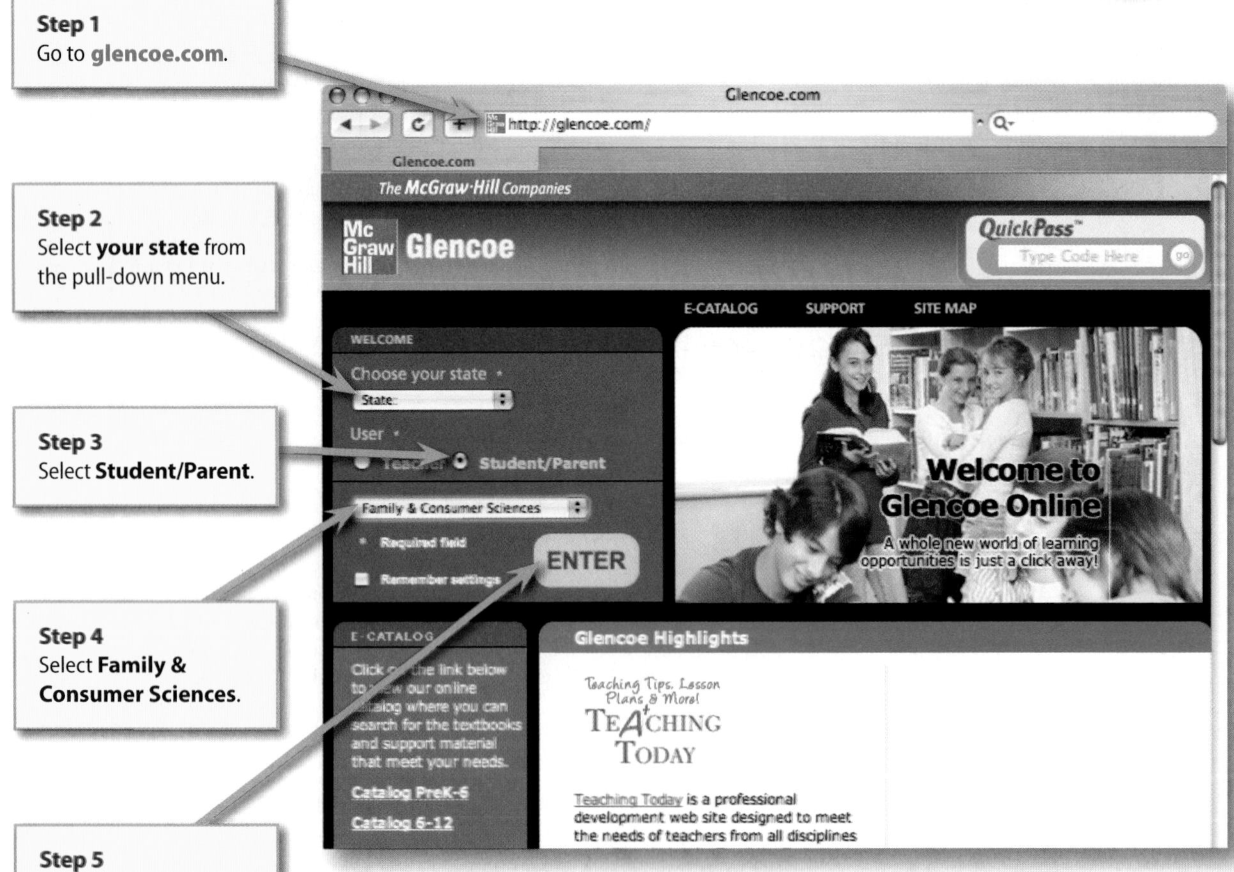

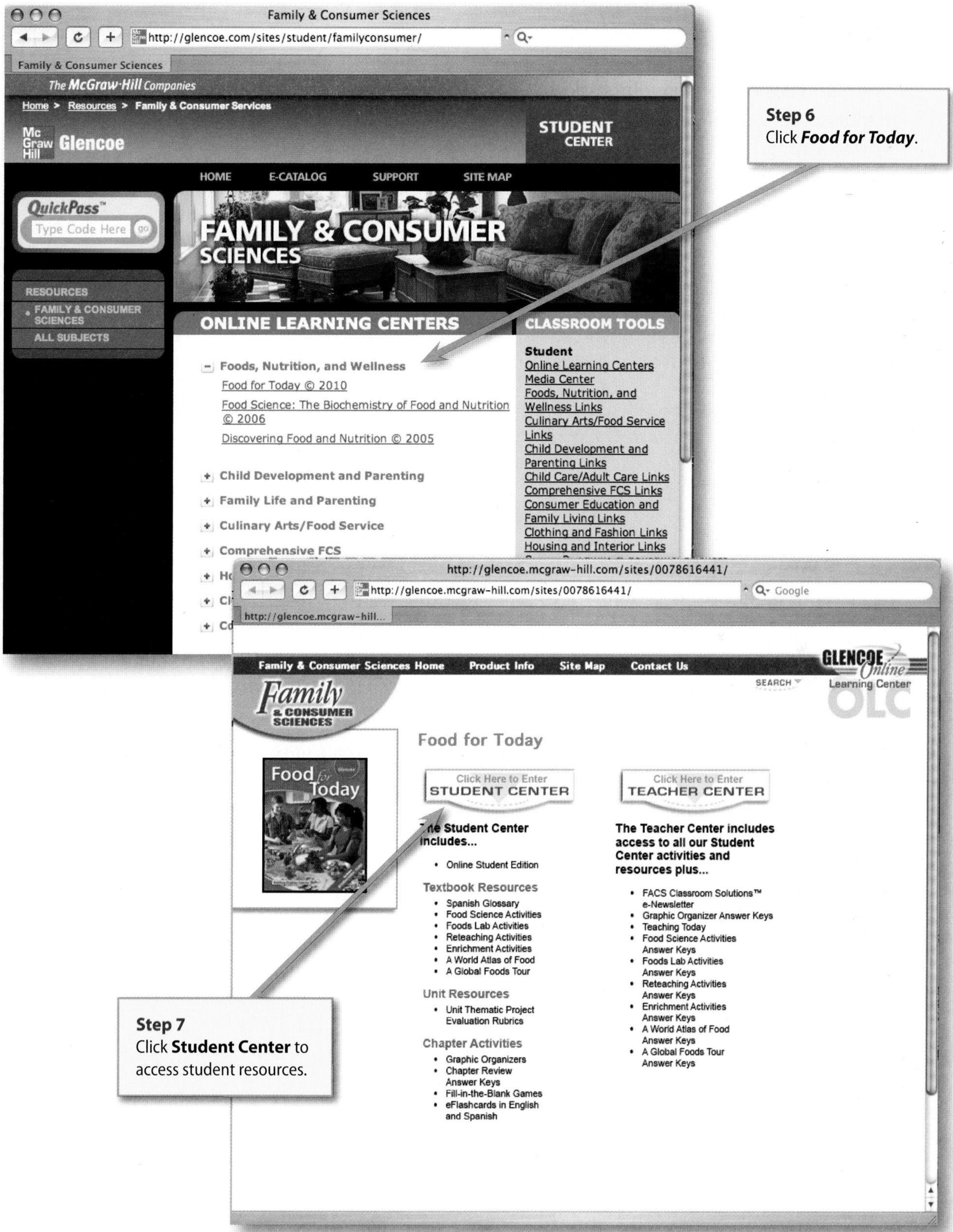

Family & Consumer Sciences
http://glencoe.com/sites/student/familyconsumer/
The McGraw-Hill Companies
Home > Resources > Family & Consumer Services
Glencoe
STUDENT CENTER
HOME
E-CATALOG
SUPPORT
SITE MAP
QuickPass
Type Code Here
FAMILY & CONSUMER SCIENCES
RESOURCES
FAMILY & CONSUMER SCIENCES
ALL SUBJECTS
ONLINE LEARNING CENTERS
Foods, Nutrition, and Wellness
Food for Today © 2010
Food Science: The Biochemistry of Food and Nutrition © 2006
Discovering Food and Nutrition © 2005
Child Development and Parenting
Family Life and Parenting
Culinary Arts/Food Service
Comprehensive FCS
CLASSROOM TOOLS
Student
Online Learning Centers
Media Center
Foods, Nutrition, and Wellness Links
Culinary Arts/Food Service Links
Child Development and Parenting Links
Child Care/Adult Care Links
Comprehensive FCS Links
Consumer Education and Family Living Links
Clothing and Fashion Links
Housing and Interior Links
Step 6
Click *Food for Today*.
http://glencoe.mcgraw-hill.com/sites/0078616441/
Family & Consumer Sciences Home
Product Info
Site Map
Contact Us
GLENCOE Online Learning Center
SEARCH
Food for Today
Click Here to Enter STUDENT CENTER
Click Here to Enter TEACHER CENTER
The Student Center includes...
Online Student Edition
Textbook Resources
Spanish Glossary
Food Science Activities
Foods Lab Activities
Reteaching Activities
Enrichment Activities
A World Atlas of Food
A Global Foods Tour
Unit Resources
Unit Thematic Project Evaluation Rubrics
Chapter Activities
Graphic Organizers
Chapter Review Answer Keys
Fill-in-the-Blank Games
eFlashcards in English and Spanish
The Teacher Center includes access to all our Student Center activities and resources plus...
FACS Classroom Solutions™ e-Newsletter
Graphic Organizer Answer Keys
Teaching Today
Food Science Activities Answer Keys
Foods Lab Activities Answer Keys
Reteaching Activities Answer Keys
Enrichment Activities Answer Keys
A World Atlas of Food Answer Keys
A Global Foods Tour Answer Keys
Step 7
Click **Student Center** to access student resources.

National Academic Standards

Prepare for Academic Success!

By improving your academic skills, you improve your ability to learn and achieve success now and in the future. It also improves your chances of landing a high-skill, high-wage job. The features and assessments in *Food for Today* provide many opportunities for you to strengthen your academic skills.

Academic Standards Look for this box throughout the text to know what academic skills you are learning.

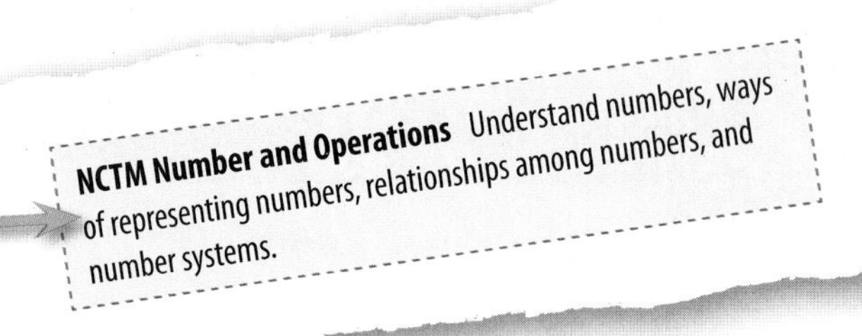

NCTM Number and Operations Understand numbers, ways of representing numbers, relationships among numbers, and number systems.

National English Language Arts Standards

To help incorporate literacy skills (reading, writing, listening, and speaking) into *Food for Today,* each section contains a listing of the language arts skills covered. These skills have been developed into standards by the *National Council of Teachers of English and International Reading Association.*

- Read texts to acquire new information.
- Read literature to build an understanding of the human experience.
- Apply strategies to interpret texts.
- Use written language to communicate effectively.
- Use different writing process elements to communicate effectively.
- Conduct research and gather, evaluate, and synthesize data to communicate discoveries.
- Use information resources to gather information and create and communicate knowledge.
- Develop an understanding of diversity in language use across cultures.
- Participate as members of literacy communities.
- Use language to accomplish individual purposes.

National Math Standards

You also have opportunities to practice math skills indicated by standards developed by the *National Council of Teachers of Mathematics.**

- Algebra
- Data Analysis and Probability
- Geometry
- Measurement
- Number and Operations
- Problem Solving

**Standards are listed with permission of the* National Council of Teachers of Mathematics (NCTM). NCTM *does not endorse the content or validity of these alignments*.

National Science Standards

The *National Science Education Standards* outline these science skills that you can practice in this text.

- Science as Inquiry
- Physical Science
- Life Science
- Earth and Space Science
- Science and Technology
- Science in Personal and Social Perspectives
- History and Nature of Science

National Social Studies Standards

The *National Council for the Social Studies* is another organization that provides standards to help guide your studies. Activities in this text relate to these standards.

- Culture
- Time, Continuity, and Change
- People, Places, and Environments
- Individual Development and Identity
- Individuals, Groups, and Institutions
- Power, Authority, and Governance
- Production, Distribution, and Consumption
- Science, Technology, and Society
- Global Connections
- Civic Ideals and Practices

Reading Skills Handbook

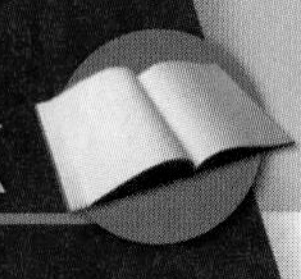

Reading: What's in It for You?

What role does reading play in your life? The possibilities are countless. Are you on a sports team? Perhaps you like to read about the latest news and statistics in sports or find out about new training techniques. Are you looking for a new dish to serve your family? You might be looking for advice about nutrition, cooking techniques, or information about ingredients. Are you enrolled in an English class, an algebra class, or a business class? Then your assignments require a lot of reading.

Improving or Fine-Tuning Your Reading Skills Will:

- Improve your grades.
- Allow you to read faster and more efficiently.
- Improve your study skills.
- Help you remember more information accurately.
- Improve your writing.

The Reading Process

Good reading skills build on one another, overlap, and spiral around in much the same way that a winding staircase goes around and around while leading you to a higher place. This handbook is designed to help you find and use the tools you will need **before, during,** and **after** reading.

Strategies You Can Use

- Identify, understand, and learn new words.
- Understand why you read.
- Take a quick look at the whole text.
- Try to predict what you are about to read.
- Take breaks while you read and ask yourself questions about the text.
- Take notes.
- Keep thinking about what will come next.
- Summarize.

Vocabulary Development

Word identification and vocabulary skills are the building blocks of the reading and writing processes. By learning to use a variety of strategies to build your word skills and vocabulary, you will become a stronger reader.

Use Context to Determine Meaning

The best way to expand and extend your vocabulary is to read widely, listen carefully, and participate in a rich variety of discussions. When reading on your own, though, you can often figure out the meanings of new words by looking at their **context,** or the other words and sentences that surround them.

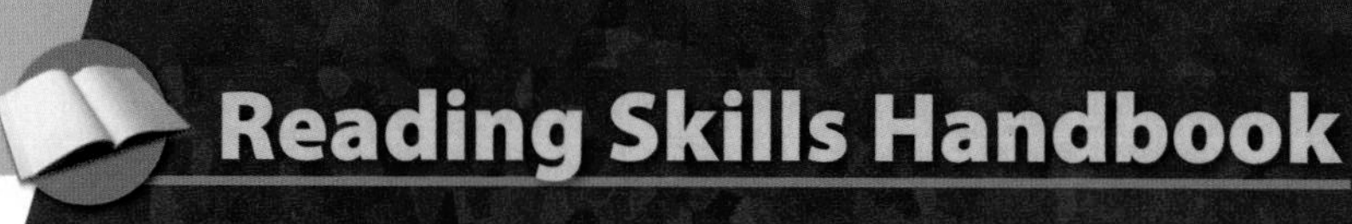

Tips for Using Context

Look for clues like these:

- A synonym or an explanation of the unknown word in the sentence:
  Elise's shop specialized in millinery, or hats for women.
- A reference to what the word is or is not like:
  An archaeologist, like a historian, deals with the past.
- A general topic associated with the word:
  The cooking teacher discussed the best way to braise meat.
- A description or action associated with the word:
  He used the shovel to dig up the garden.

Predict a Possible Meaning

Another way to determine the meaning of a word is to take the word apart. If you understand the meaning of the **base,** or **root,** part of a word, and also know the meanings of key syllables added either to the beginning or end of the base word, you can usually figure out what the word means.

Word Origins Since Latin, Greek, and Anglo-Saxon roots are the basis for much of our English vocabulary, having some background in languages can be a useful vocabulary tool. For example, *astronomy* comes from the Greek root *astro,* which means relating to the stars. *Stellar* also has a meaning referring to stars, but its origin is Latin. Knowing root words in other languages can help you determine meanings, derivations, and spellings in English.

Prefixes and Suffixes A prefix is a word part that can be added to the beginning of a word. For example, the prefix *semi* means half or partial, so *semicircle* means half a circle. A suffix is a word part that can be added to the end of a word. Adding a suffix often changes a word from one part of speech to another.

Using Dictionaries A dictionary provides the meaning or meanings of a word. Look at the sample dictionary entry on the next page to see what other information it provides.

Thesauruses and Specialized Reference Books A thesaurus provides synonyms and often antonyms. It is a useful tool to expand your vocabulary. Remember to check the exact definition of the listed words in a dictionary before you use a thesaurus. Specialized dictionaries such as *Barron's Dictionary of Business Terms* or *Black's Law Dictionary* list terms and expressions that are not commonly included in a general dictionary. You can also use online dictionaries.

Glossaries Many textbooks and technical works contain condensed dictionaries that provide an alphabetical listing of words used in the text and their specific definitions.

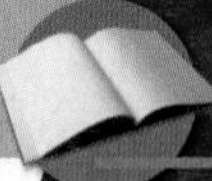

Reading Skills Handbook

Dictionary Entry

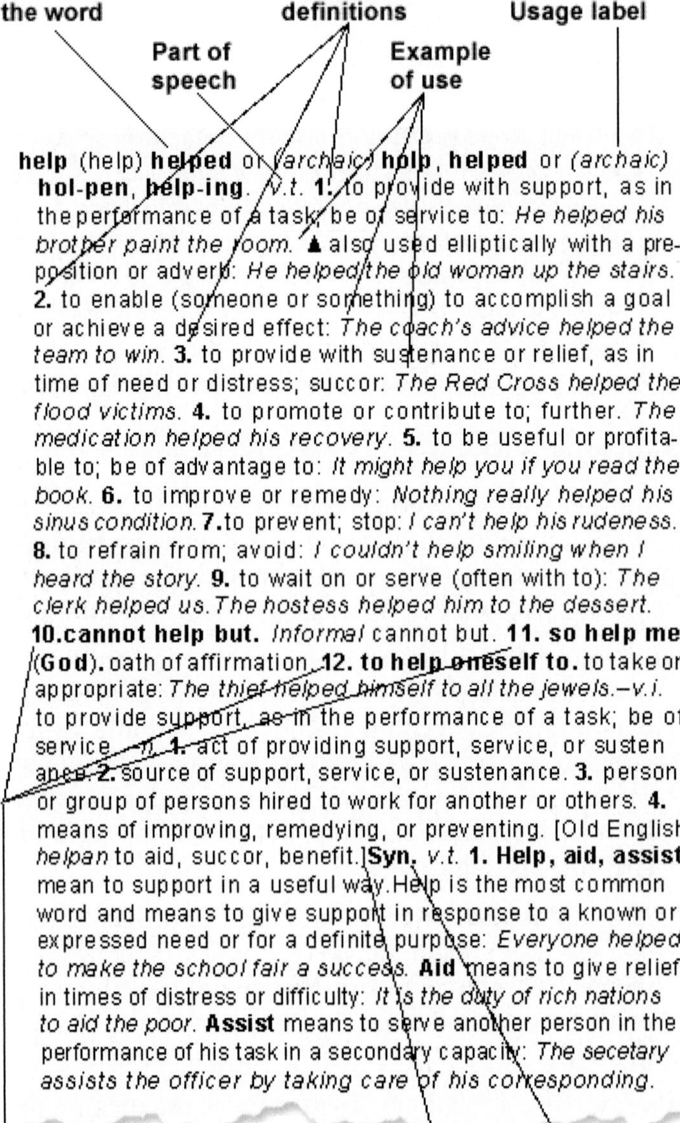

help (help) **helped** or *(archaic)* **holp**, **helped** or *(archaic)* **hol-pen**, **help-ing**. *v.t.* **1.** to provide with support, as in the performance of a task; be of service to: *He helped his brother paint the room.* ▲ also used elliptically with a preposition or adverb: *He helped the old woman up the stairs.* **2.** to enable (someone or something) to accomplish a goal or achieve a desired effect: *The coach's advice helped the team to win.* **3.** to provide with sustenance or relief, as in time of need or distress; succor: *The Red Cross helped the flood victims.* **4.** to promote or contribute to; further. *The medication helped his recovery.* **5.** to be useful or profitable to; be of advantage to: *It might help you if you read the book.* **6.** to improve or remedy: *Nothing really helped his sinus condition.* **7.** to prevent; stop: *I can't help his rudeness.* **8.** to refrain from; avoid: *I couldn't help smiling when I heard the story.* **9.** to wait on or serve (often with to): *The clerk helped us. The hostess helped him to the dessert.* **10. cannot help but.** *Informal* cannot but. **11. so help me (God).** oath of affirmation. **12. to help oneself to.** to take or appropriate: *The thief helped himself to all the jewels.*–*v.i.* to provide support, as in the performance of a task; be of service. –*n.* **1.** act of providing support, service, or susten ance. **2.** source of support, service, or sustenance. **3.** person or group of persons hired to work for another or others. **4.** means of improving, remedying, or preventing. [Old English *helpan* to aid, succor, benefit.] **Syn.** *v.t.* **1. Help, aid, assist** mean to support in a useful way. Help is the most common word and means to give support in response to a known or expressed need or for a definite purpose: *Everyone helped to make the school fair a success.* **Aid** means to give relief in times of distress or difficulty: *It is the duty of rich nations to aid the poor.* **Assist** means to serve another person in the performance of his task in a secondary capacity: *The secetary assists the officer by taking care of his corresponding.*

Recognize Word Meanings Across Subjects Have you learned a new word in one class and then noticed it in your reading for other subjects? The word might not mean exactly the same thing in each class, but you can use the meaning you already know to help you understand what it means in another subject area. For example:

Math Each digit represents a different place **value**.

Health Your **values** can guide you in making healthful decisions.

Economics The **value** of a product is measured in its cost.

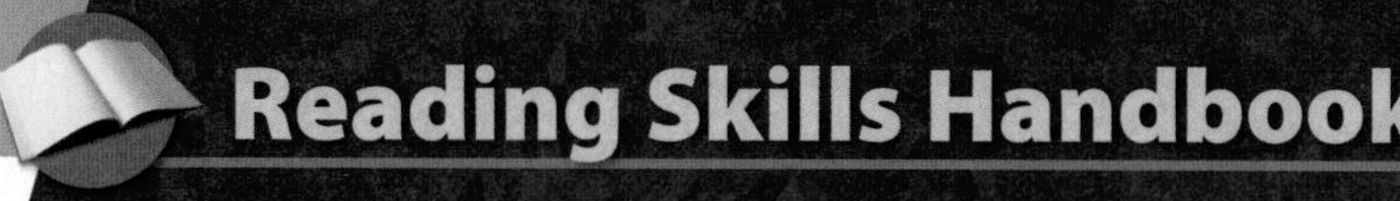

Understanding What You Read

Reading comprehension means understanding—deriving meaning from—what you have read. Using a variety of strategies can help you improve your comprehension and make reading more interesting and more fun.

Read for a Reason

To get the greatest benefit from your reading, **establish a purpose for reading.** In school, you have many reasons for reading, such as:

- to learn and understand new information.
- to find specific information.
- to review before a test.
- to complete an assignment.
- to prepare (research) before you write.

As your reading skills improve, you will notice that you apply different strategies to fit the different purposes for reading. For example, if you are reading for entertainment, you might read quickly, but if you are reading to gather information or follow directions, you might read more slowly, take notes, construct a graphic organizer, or reread sections of text.

Draw on Personal Background

Drawing on personal background may also be called activating prior knowledge. Before you start reading a text, ask yourself questions like these:

- What have I heard or read about this topic?
- Do I have any personal experience relating to this topic?

Using a KWL Chart A KWL chart is a good device for organizing information you gather before, during, and after reading. In the first column, list what you already **know,** then list what you **want** to know in the middle column. Use the third column when you review and assess what you **learned.** You can also add more columns to record places where you found information and places where you can look for more information.

K (What I already know)	W (What I want to know)	L (What I have learned)

Adjust Your Reading Speed Your reading speed is a key factor in how well you understand what you are reading. You will need to adjust your speed depending on your reading purpose.

Scanning means running your eyes quickly over the material to look for words or phrases. Scan when you need a specific piece of information.

Skimming means reading a passage quickly to find its main idea or to get an overview. Skim a text when you preview to determine what the material is about.

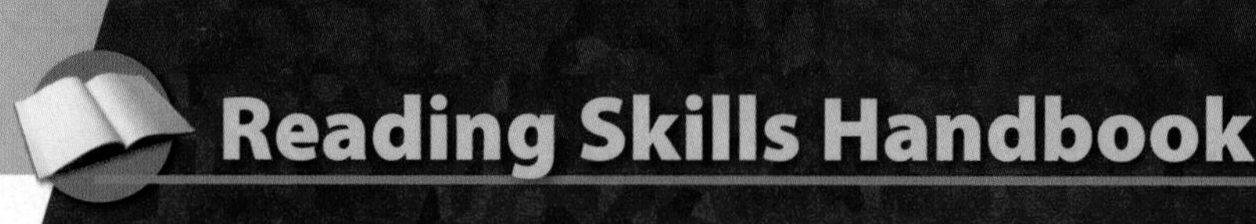

Reading for detail involves careful reading while paying attention to text structure and monitoring your understanding. Read for detail when you are learning concepts, following complicated directions, or preparing to analyze a text.

Techniques to Understand and Remember What You Read

Preview

Before beginning a selection, it is helpful to **preview** what you are about to read.

Previewing Strategies

- Read the title, headings, and subheadings of the selection.
- Look at the illustrations and notice how the text is organized.
- Skim the selection: Take a glance at the whole thing.
- Decide what the main idea might be.
- Predict what a selection will be about.

Predict

Have you ever read a mystery, decided who committed the crime, and then changed your mind as more clues were revealed? You were adjusting your predictions. Did you smile when you found out that you guessed who committed the crime? You were verifying your predictions.

As you read, make educated guesses about story events and outcomes; that is, **make predictions** before and during reading. This will help you focus your attention on the text and will improve your understanding.

Determine the Main Idea

When you look for the **main idea**, you are looking for the most important statement in a text. Depending on what kind of text you are reading, the main idea can be located at the very beginning (news stories in a newspaper or a magazine) or at the end (scientific research document). Ask yourself the following questions:

- What is each sentence about?
- Is there one sentence that is more important than all the others?
- What idea do details support or point out?

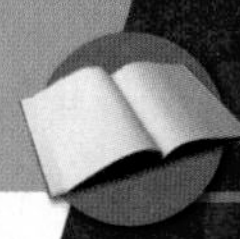

Reading Skills Handbook

Take Notes

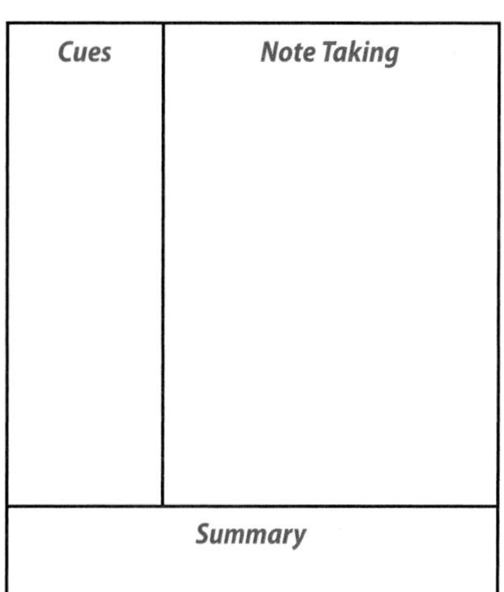

Cornell Note-Taking System There are many methods for note taking. The **Cornell Note-Taking System** is a well-known method that can help you organize what you read. To the right is a note-taking activity based on the Cornell Note-Taking System.

Graphic Organizers Using a graphic organizer to retell content in a visual representation will help you remember and retain content. You might make a **chart** or **diagram,** organizing what you have read. Here are some examples of graphic organizers:

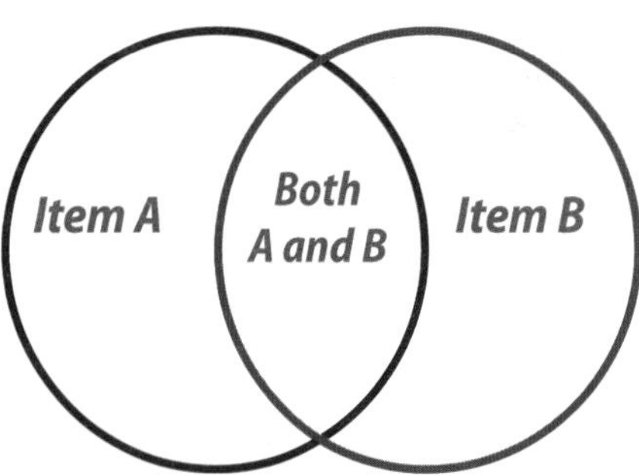

Venn Diagrams When mapping out a compare-and-contrast text structure, you can use a Venn diagram. The outer portions of the circles will show how two characters, ideas, or items contrast, or are different, and the overlapping part will compare two things, or show how they are similar.

Flow Charts To help you track the sequence of events, or cause and effect, use a flow chart. Arrange ideas or events in their logical, sequential order. Then, draw arrows between your ideas to indicate how one idea or event flows into another.

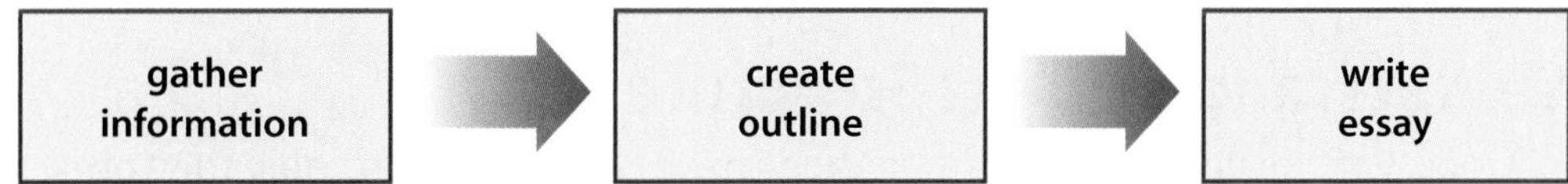

Visualize

Try to form a mental picture of scenes, characters, and events as you read. Use the details and descriptions the author gives you. If you can **visualize** what you read, it will be more interesting and you will remember it better.

Question

Ask yourself questions about the text while you read. Ask yourself about the importance of the sentences, how they relate to one another, if you understand what you just read, and what you think is going to come next.

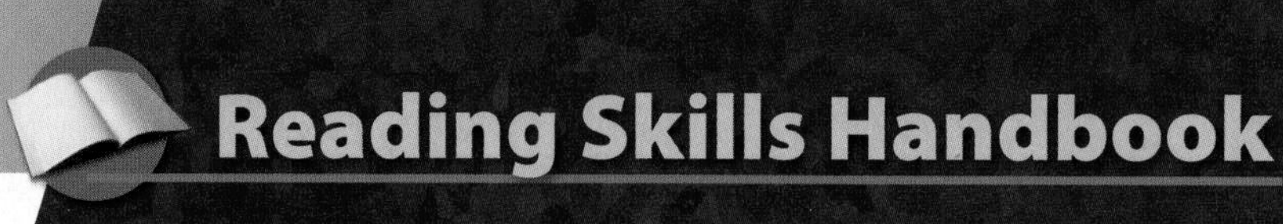

Clarify

If you feel you do not understand meaning (through questioning), try these techniques:

What to Do When You Do Not Understand

- Reread confusing parts of the text.
- Diagram (chart) relationships between chunks of text, ideas, and sentences.
- Look up unfamiliar words.
- Talk out the text to yourself.
- Read the passage once more.

Review

Take time to stop and review what you have read. Use your note-taking tools (graphic organizers or Cornell notes charts). Also, review and consider your KWL chart.

Monitor Your Comprehension

Continue to check your understanding by using the following two strategies:

Summarize Pause and tell yourself the main ideas of the text and the key supporting details. Try to answer the following questions: Who? What? When? Where? Why? How?

Paraphrase Pause, close the book, and try to retell what you have just read in your own words. It might help to pretend you are explaining the text to someone who has not read it and does not know the material.

Understanding Text Structure

Good writers do not just put together sentences and paragraphs, they organize their writing with a specific purpose in mind. That organization is called text structure. When you understand and follow the structure of a text, it is easier to remember the information you are reading. There are many ways text may be structured. Watch for **signal words**. They will help you follow the text's organization. (Also, remember to use these techniques when you write.)

Compare and Contrast

This structure shows similarities and differences between people, things, and ideas. This is often used to demonstrate that things that seem alike are really different, or vice versa.

Signal words: similarly, more, less, on the one hand/on the other hand, in contrast, but, however

Cause and Effect

Writers use the cause-and-effect structure to explore the reasons for something happening and to examine the results or consequences of events.

Signal words: so, because, as a result, therefore, for the following reasons

Problem and Solution

When they organize text around the question how?, writers state a problem and suggest solutions.

Signal words: how, help, problem, obstruction, overcome, difficulty, need, attempt, have to, must

Sequence

Sequencing tells you in which order to consider thoughts or facts. Examples of sequencing are:

Chronological order refers to the order in which events take place.

Signal words: first, next, then, finally

Spatial order describes the organization of things in space (to describe a room, for example).

Signal words: above, below, behind, next to

Order of importance lists things or thoughts from the most important to the least important (or the other way around).

Signal words: principal, central, main, important, fundamental

Reading for Meaning

It is important to think about what you are reading to get the most information out of a text, to understand the consequences of what the text says, to remember the content, and to form your own opinion about what the content means.

Interpret

Interpreting is asking yourself, "What is the writer really saying?" and then using what you already know to answer that question.

Infer

Writers do not always state exactly everything they want you to understand. By providing clues and details, they sometimes imply certain information. To **infer** involves using your reason and experience to develop the idea on your own, based on what an author implies, or suggests. What is most important when drawing inferences is to be sure that you have accurately based your guesses on supporting details from the text. If you cannot point to a place in the selection to help back up your inference, you may need to rethink your guess.

Draw Conclusions

A conclusion is a general statement you can make and explain with reasoning, or with supporting details from a text. If you read a story describing a sport where five players bounce a ball and throw it through a high hoop, you may conclude that the sport is basketball.

Analyze

To understand persuasive nonfiction (a text that discusses facts and opinions to arrive at a conclusion), you need to analyze statements and examples to see if they support the main idea. To understand an informational text (a text, such as a textbook, that gives you information, not opinions), you need to keep track of how the ideas are organized to find the main points.

Hint: Use your graphic organizers and notes charts.

Distinguish Between Facts and Opinions

This is one of the most important reading skills you can learn. A fact is a statement that can be proven. An opinion is what the writer believes. A writer may support opinions with facts, but an opinion cannot be proven. For example:

Fact: California produces fruit and other agricultural products.

Opinion: California produces the best fruit and other agricultural products.

Evaluate

Would you take seriously an article on nuclear fission if you knew it was written by a comedic actor? If you need to rely on accurate information, you need to find out who wrote what you are reading and why. Where did the writer get information? Is the information one-sided? Can you verify the information?

Reading for Research

You will need to **read actively** to research a topic. You might also need to generate an interesting, relevant, and researchable **question** on your own and locate appropriate print and nonprint information from a wide variety of sources. Then, you will need to **categorize** that information, evaluate it, and **organize** it in a new way to produce a research project for a specific audience. Finally, **draw conclusions** about your original research question. These conclusions may lead you to other areas for further inquiry.

Locate Appropriate Print and Nonprint Information

In your research, try to use a variety of sources. Because different sources present information in different ways, your research project will be more interesting and balanced when you read a variety of sources.

Literature and Textbooks These texts include any book used as a basis for instruction or a source of information.

Book Indices A book index, or a bibliography, is an alphabetical listing of books. Some book indices list books on specific subjects; others are more general. Other indices list a variety of topics or resources.

Periodicals Magazines and journals are issued at regular intervals, such as weekly or monthly. One way to locate information in magazines is to use the *Readers' Guide to Periodical Literature*. This guide is available in print form in most libraries.

Technical Manuals A manual is a guide or handbook intended to give instruction on how to perform a task or operate something. A vehicle owner's manual might give information on how to operate and service a car.

Reference Books Reference books include encyclopedias and almanacs, and are used to locate specific pieces of information.

Electronic Encyclopedias, Databases, and the Internet There are many ways to locate extensive information using your computer. Infotrac, for instance, acts as an online readers' guide. CD encyclopedias can provide easy access to all subjects.

Organize and Convert Information

As you gather information from different sources, taking careful notes, you will need to think about how to **synthesize** the information—that is, convert it into a unified whole, as well as how to change it into a form your audience will easily understand and that will meet your assignment guidelines.

1. First, ask yourself what you want your audience to know.
2. Then, think about a pattern of organization, a structure that will best show your main ideas. You might ask yourself the following questions:
   - When comparing items or ideas, what graphic aids can I use?
   - When showing the reasons something happened and the effects of certain actions, what text structure would be best?
   - How can I briefly and clearly show important information to my audience?
   - Would an illustration or even a cartoon help to make a certain point?

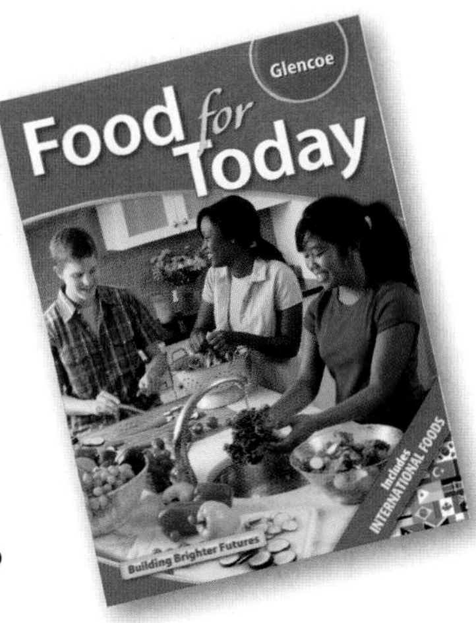

How to Use Technology

Introduction

Technology affects your life in almost every way, both at home and at work. Computers can do wonderful things. They are a path to the libraries of the world. They enhance and enrich your life. You can find the answers to many of your questions on the Internet, often as quickly as the click of your mouse. However, they can also be misused. Knowing some simple guidelines will help you use technology in a safe and secure way.

Practice Safe Surfing!

The Internet can also be a dangerous place. Although there are many Web sites you can freely and safely visit, many others are ones you want to avoid. Before you sign on to any site or visit a chat room, there are several things to consider:

- **Know to whom you are giving the information.** Check that the URL in your browser matches the domain you intended to visit and that you have not been redirected to another site.
- **Never give personal information of any sort** to someone you meet on a Web site or in a chat room, including your name, gender, age, or contact information.
- **Think about why you are giving the information.** For example, if a parent orders something online to be delivered, he or she will need to give an address. But you should never give out your Social Security number, your birth date, or your mother's maiden name without adult consent.
- **Check with a parent or other trusted adult** if you are still unsure whether it is safe to give the information.

Tips for Using the Internet for Research

The Internet is probably the single most important tool for research since the creation of the public library. There is so much information to access on the Internet that it can be difficult to know where to begin.

A good place to start is with a search engine, such as Google. Google is an automated piece of software that searches the Web looking for information. By typing your topic into the search bar, the search engine looks for sites that contain the words you type. You may get many more sites than you expect. Here are some ways to get better results:

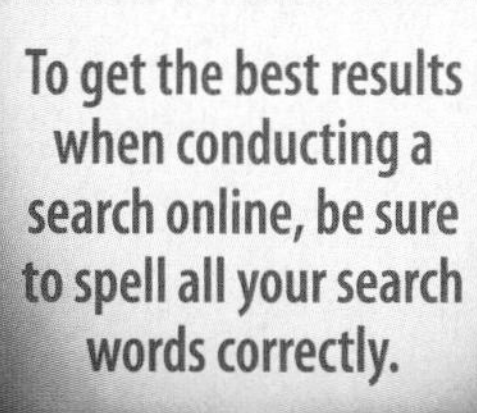

To get the best results when conducting a search online, be sure to spell all your search words correctly.

- **Place quotes around your topic,** for example, "sports medicine." This will allow you to find the sites where that exact phrase appears.
- **Use NEAR.** Typing *sports NEAR medicine* will return sites that contain both words and have the two words close to each other.
- **Exclude unwanted results.** Simply use a hyphen to indicate the words you do not want, for example, "sports medicine"–baseball.
- **Watch out for advertisements.** If you are using Google, know that the links on the right-hand side of the page, or sometimes at the top in color, are paid links. They may or may not be worth exploring.
- **Check for relevance.** Google displays a few lines of text from each page and shows your search phrase in bold. Check to see if the site is appropriate for your work.
- **Look for news.** After you have entered your search phrase and have looked at the results, click on a *News* link on the page. This will show you recent stories about your topic.
- **Try again!** If you have made an extensive search and not found what you want, start a new search with a different set of words.
- **Check other sources.** Combine your Internet search with traditional research tools, such as books and magazines.

How to Evaluate Web Sites

Even though there is a ton of information available online, much of this information can be deceptive and misleading, and often incorrect. The books in your library and classroom have been evaluated by scholars and experts. There is no such oversight on the Web. Learning to evaluate Web sites will make you a more savvy surfer and enable you to gather the information you need quickly and easily. When you are trying to decide whether a Web site provides trustworthy information, consider the following:

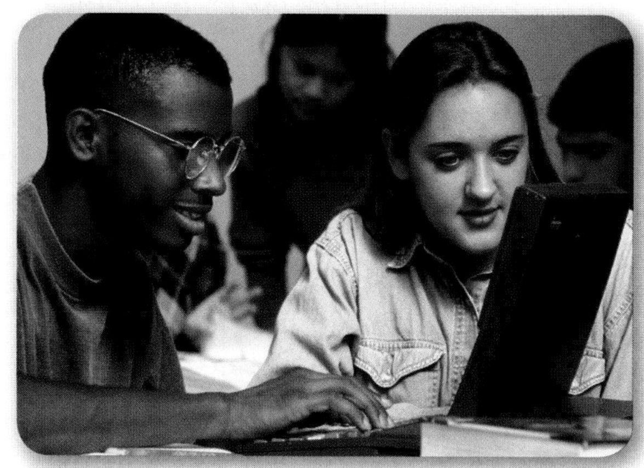

- **First, ask, "Who is the author?"** Once you have the name of the author, do a quick Web search to see what else the author has written. Search online for books he or she has written. This information will help you consider whether the person is credible.
- **Look at the group offering the information.** Be wary if it is trying to sell a product or service. Look for impartial organizations to provide unbiased information.
- **Look for Web sites that provide sources for each of their facts,** just as you do when you write a term paper. Also, look for clues that the information was written by someone knowledgeable. Spelling and grammatical errors are warning signs that the information may not be accurate.
- **Check for the date the article was written and when it was last updated.** The more recent the article, the more likely it will be accurate.
- **Finally, when using information from a Web site, treat it as you would treat print information.** Anyone can post information on a Web site. Never use information that you cannot verify with another source.

Plagiarism

Using your computer in an ethical manner is simple if you follow certain guidelines. Plagiarism is the act of taking someone else's ideas and passing them off as your own. It does not matter if it is just one or two phrases or an entire paper. Be on guard against falling into the trap of cutting and pasting. This makes plagiarism all too easy.

It is acceptable to quote sources in your work, but you must make sure to identify those sources and give them proper credit. Also, some Web sites do not allow you to quote from them. Be sure to check each site or resource you are quoting to make sure you are allowed to use the material. Remember to cite your sources properly.

Copyright

A copyright protects someone who creates an original work. This can be a single sentence, a book, a play, or a piece of music. If you create it, you are the owner. Copyright protection is provided by the Copyright Act of 1976, a federal statute.

If you want to use a portion of a copyrighted work in your own work, you need to obtain permission from the copyright holder. That might be a publisher of a book, an author, an organization, or an estate. Most publishers are willing to grant permission to individuals for educational purposes. If you want to reproduce information you found on the Web, contact the Webmaster or author of the article to request permission.

Once a work's copyright has expired, it is considered to be in the public domain and anyone can reprint it as he or she pleases. Remember the following tips:

- ✧ **What is copyrighted?** All forms of original expression published in the United States since 1923.
- ✧ **Can I copy from the Internet?** Copying information from the Internet is a serious breach of copyright. Check the site's *Terms of Use* to see what you can and cannot do.
- ✧ **Can I edit copyrighted work?** You cannot change copyrighted material, that is, make "derivative works" based on existing material, without permission of the copyright holder.

Student Organizations

What Is a Student Organization?

A student organization is a group or association of students that is formed around activities, such as:

- Family and consumer sciences
- Student government
- Community service
- Social clubs
- Honor societies
- Multicultural alliances
- Technology education
- Artists and performers
- Politics
- Sports teams
- Professional career development

A student organization is usually required to follow a set of rules and regulations that apply equally to all student organizations at a particular school.

Why Should You Get Involved?

Being an active part of a student organization opens a variety of experiences to you. Many student clubs are part of a national network of students and professionals, which provides the chance to connect to a wider variety of students and opportunities.

What's In It for You?

Participation in student organizations can contribute to a more enriching learning experience. Here are some ways you can benefit:

- Gain leadership qualities and skills that make you more marketable to employers and universities.
- Demonstrate the ability to appreciate someone else's point of view.
- Interact with professionals to learn about their different industries.
- Explore your creative interests, share ideas, and collaborate with others.
- Take risks, build confidence, and grow creatively.
- Learn valuable skills while speaking or performing in front of an audience.
- Make a difference in your life and the lives of those around you.
- Learn the importance of civic responsibility and involvement.
- Build relationships with instructors, advisors, students, and other members of the community who share similar backgrounds/world views.

Find and Join a Student Organization!

Take a close look at the organizations offered at your school or within your community. Are there any organizations that interest you? Talk to your teachers, guidance counselors, or a parent or guardian. Usually, posters or flyers for a variety of clubs and groups can be found on your school's Message Board or Web site. Try to locate more information about the organizations that meet your needs. Then, think about how these organizations can help you gain valuable skills you can use at school, at work, and in your community.

What Is FCCLA?

Family, Career and Community Leaders of America is a nonprofit national career and technical student organization for young men and women in Family and Consumer Sciences education in public and private schools through grade 12. Everyone is part of a family, and FCCLA is the only national Career and Technical Student Organization with the family as its central focus. Since 1945, FCCLA members have been making a difference in their families, careers, and communities by addressing important personal, work, and societal issues through Family and Consumer Sciences education.

STAR Events Program

STAR Events (Students Taking Action with Recognition) are competitive events in which members are recognized for proficiency and achievement in chapter and individual projects, leadership skills, and occupational preparation. FCCLA provides opportunities for you to participate at local, state, and national levels.

What Are the Purposes of FCCLA?

1. Provide opportunities for personal development and preparation for adult life.
2. Strengthen the function of the family as a basic unit of society.
3. Encourage democracy through cooperative action in the home and community.
4. Encourage individual and group involvement in helping achieve global cooperation and harmony.
5. Promote greater understanding between youth and adults.
6. Provide opportunities for making decisions and for assuming responsibilities.
7. Prepare for the multiple roles of men and women in today's society.
8. Promote family and consumer sciences and related occupations.

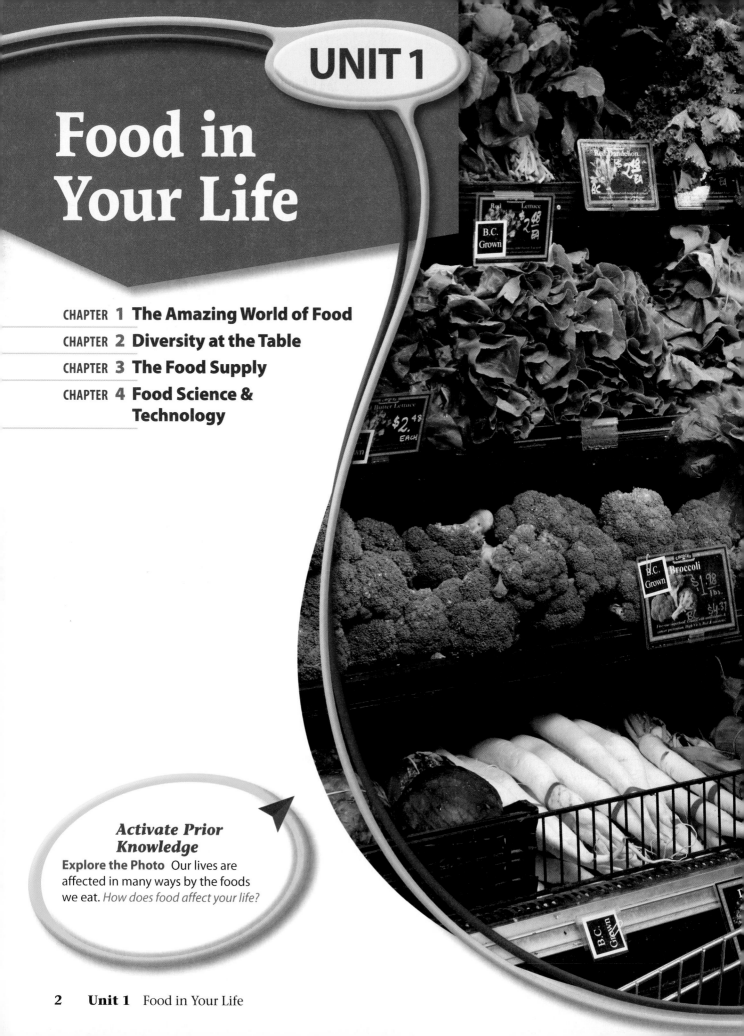

UNIT 1

Food in Your Life

Activate Prior Knowledge

Explore the Photo Our lives are affected in many ways by the foods we eat. *How does food affect your life?*

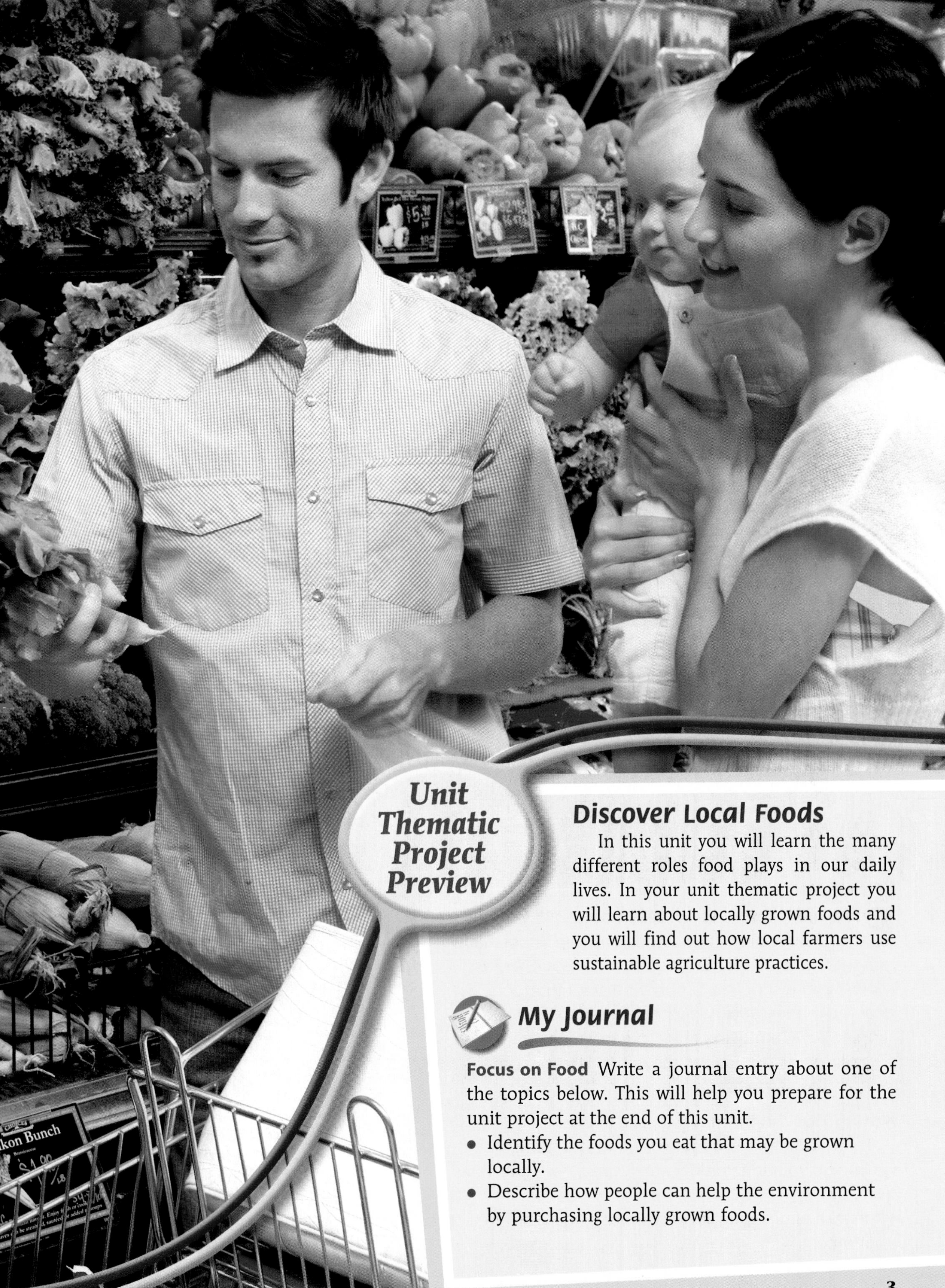

Unit Thematic Project Preview

Discover Local Foods

In this unit you will learn the many different roles food plays in our daily lives. In your unit thematic project you will learn about locally grown foods and you will find out how local farmers use sustainable agriculture practices.

My Journal

Focus on Food Write a journal entry about one of the topics below. This will help you prepare for the unit project at the end of this unit.

- Identify the foods you eat that may be grown locally.
- Describe how people can help the environment by purchasing locally grown foods.

CHAPTER 1

The Amazing World of Food

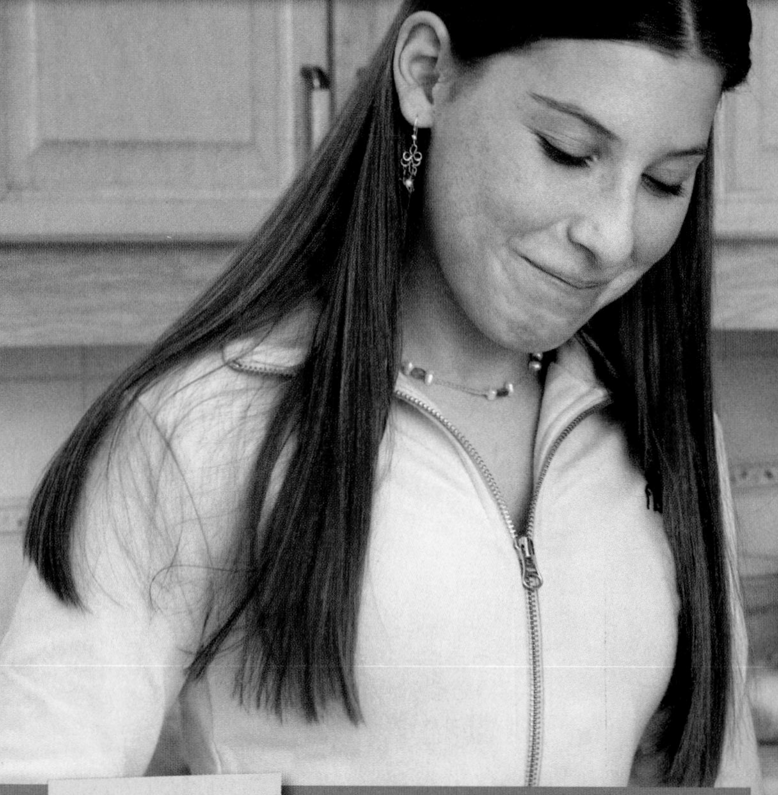

Writing Activity 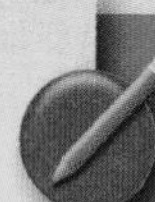 Freewriting

Food and Happiness For ten minutes, write about the relationship between food and happiness. Allow your writing to be spontaneous. Spontaneous means impulsive or instinctive. Simply write your thoughts, ideas, memories, or experiences relating to food and happiness. Do not worry about organization, grammar, or spelling. The purpose of freewriting is to explore a topic and generate ideas.

Writing Tips Follow these steps to freewrite.

- Try to write for ten minutes without stopping.
- Turn off your inner editor and let your thoughts flow freely.
- Instead of planning, let each word or idea lead to another.

Activate Prior Knowledge

Explore the Photo Food and life are strongly connected. *What is one specific, positive effect that food has had on your life?*

Reading Guide

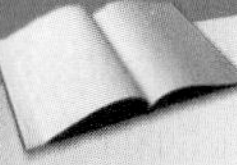

Before You Read

Preview Look at the photos and figure and read their captions. Think about the many ways that food plays a role in your life.

Read to Learn

Key Concepts

- **Explain** what makes food powerful.
- **Describe** the role of science in food.
- **Summarize** the ways that food provides pleasure.
- **Describe** the skills you can build as you learn about food.

Main Idea

Food is a life-sustaining source of nutrients and pleasure that affects many different aspects of life.

Content Vocabulary

You will find definitions for these words in the glossary at the back of this book.

- ☐ nutrient
- ☐ nutrition
- ☐ wellness
- ☐ hospitality
- ☐ comfort foods
- ☐ stress hormone
- ☐ palate
- ☐ self-esteem
- ☐ critical thinking
- ☐ verbal communication
- ☐ nonverbal communication
- ☐ leadership
- ☐ management

Academic Vocabulary

You will find these words in your reading and on your tests. Use the glossary to look up their definitions if necessary.

- career
- organization

Graphic Organizer

As you read, use a web diagram like the one below to organize notes about six aspects of life that are positively affected by food.

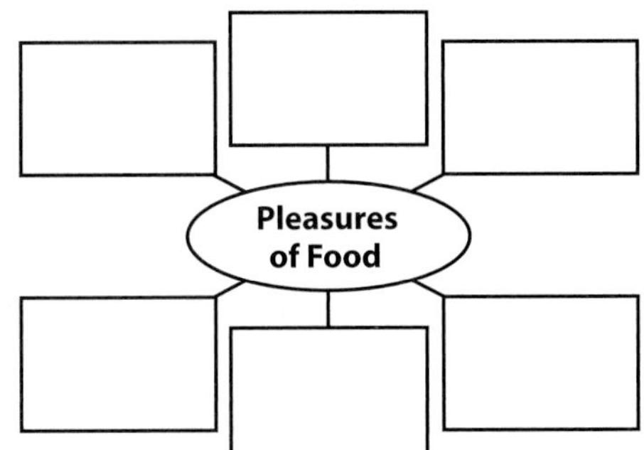

Graphic Organizer Go to this book's Online Learning Center at **glencoe.com** to print out this graphic organizer.

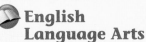

Academic Standards

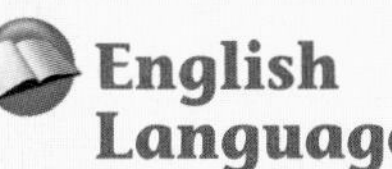

English Language Arts

NCTE 4 Use written language to communicate effectively.

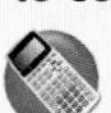

Mathematics

NCTM Number and Operations Compute fluently and make reasonable estimates.

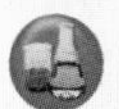

Science

NSES A Develop abilities necessary to do scientific inquiry, understandings about scientific inquiry.

NSES G Develop an understanding of science as a human endeavor.

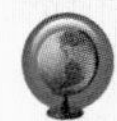

Social Studies

NCSS VIII B Science, Technology, and Society Make judgments about how science and technology can transform the physical world and human society.

NCTE *National Council of Teachers of English*
NCTM *National Council of Teachers of Mathematics*
NSES *National Science Education Standards*
NCSS *National Council for the Social Studies*

The Power of Food

The incredible story of food begins with its power to help keep you alive and healthy. Food is essential for survival. Food affects the quality of your life, too. It can bring enjoyment and closeness with family and friends. Good food choices help you stay well physically, mentally, and emotionally.

Nutrition and Wellness

Food is made of many different life-sustaining chemicals. Digestion releases these chemicals, which are known as nutrients. A **nutrient** is a chemical substance, such as protein, carbohydrate, fat, or fiber, that your body needs to function, grow, repair itself, and create energy.

There is a branch of science called nutrition. **Nutrition** is the study of nutrients and how the body uses them. The word *nutrition* can also mean the combination of nutrients in a person's diet. When you choose foods that provide all the nutrients you need, you have good nutrition.

Food has a powerful effect on health. Healthy food choices promote wellness. **Wellness** is good health and positive well-being. It includes physical, mental, and emotional health. It is reflected in both attitudes and behavior. When you practice wellness, you take active steps to stay at your peak of good health.

Four key behaviors for wellness are:

- Making positive food choices.
- Staying physically active.
- Managing difficult feelings and emotions.
- Staying free of alcohol and other drugs.

Practicing wellness is not a guarantee against sickness. It is a way to achieve the highest level of health possible for you. You can adopt healthy attitudes and behaviors no matter what your physical, mental, or emotional challenges are. Everyone has the potential for health.

✓ Reading Check **Explain** What are four key behaviors for wellness?

The Role of Science in Food

What difference does it make whether you eat french fries and milkshakes every day or only once in a while? It makes a big difference, and science can tell you why.

Thanks to science it is known exactly what chemicals are in different foods and how your body processes them. Science tells you what nutrients do in your body and how nutrients work together. Science also tells you why eating too many foods high in sugar, fat, or sodium can damage your health.

Science plays a big role in the kitchen, too. Why does yeast dough have to be kneaded? How can you keep a sliced apple from turning brown? Science has answers to questions like these. Your cooking skills and confidence improve when you understand kitchen science. Science also helps ensure a healthy food supply in these areas:

- **Agriculture** Farmers use science to increase the food supply and grow top-quality food.

Food and Fun

Sharing a meal with family and friends is one way food brings enjoyment. *What are some other ways food creates enjoyment?*

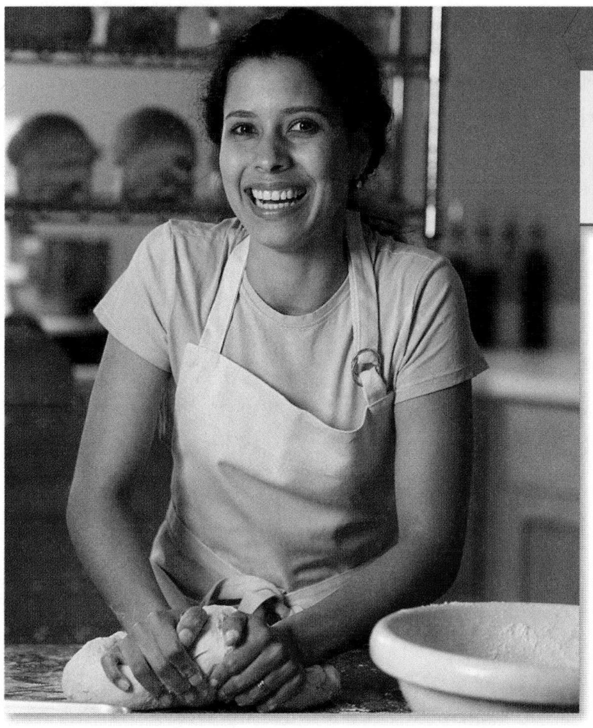

The Science of Cooking

In many ways, the kitchen is like a science lab. Learning how yeast reacts in dough, for example, can help you bake bread that rises just right. *How else does science help with cooking and eating?*

- **Food Processing** Improvements in processing methods help ensure a bountiful supply of nutritious food.
- **Food Safety** Scientists help to develop safe food handling methods and help to monitor the quality of the food supply.

✓ Reading Check **Explain** In what three areas does science help to ensure a healthy food supply?

The Joys of Food

Food offers more than nutrition. It also offers enjoyment. Food satisfies the senses and makes you feel good. Cooking and eating good food are two of the delights of living.

People who enjoy their food may absorb more nutrients from it. Why? When you see or smell appealing food, your brain reacts. It instructs your mouth and stomach to make chemicals that will help digest the food. When you see or smell unappealing food, the brain may not send these signals to the body. As a result, you may absorb fewer nutrients.

Many countries recognize the importance of enjoying food and making mealtimes pleasant. Some have issued dietary guidelines that encourage people to enjoy food. See **Figure 1.1** on page 8.

Family and Social Ties

The kitchen is one of the busiest and most enjoyable places in the house. Family members and guests gather there to enjoy snacks and conversation while food is prepared.

For many families, the kitchen is the social center of the home. Family members fix and share meals together and talk about the day's events. They join in the cleanup. As they work and eat together, family bonds strengthen.

Food helps strengthen social ties, too. Food is an important part of many social events, such as weddings, birthday parties, and holiday celebrations. Certain foods are linked to holidays, sporting events, and other special occasions.

Science in Action — Safety Through Science

Science helped develop refrigeration technology. A refrigerator keeps food cold and allows it to be stored for days or weeks. But does the temperature in a refrigerator stay the same?

Procedure Place a thermometer in a refrigerator and check the temperature. Record the temperature. In a pot, heat four cups of water. When the water is hot, but not boiling, turn off the heat and use potholders to put it in the refrigerator. Close the door, wait five minutes, and record the temperature again. Check the temperature a third time after 10 more minutes.

Analysis Write a paragraph detailing your results. How much did the temperature change due to the heat of the pot of water? Did the refrigerator return to its previous temperature? What does this tell you about refrigeration?

NSES G Develop an understanding of science as a human endeavor.

Figure 1.1 Enjoying Food Around the World

Wellness People from different parts of the world believe that when you take time to enjoy your food, you promote wellness. ***Even though food styles vary widely among cultures, what is one function that food fills for all people regardless of culture?***

Japan

In Japan, people strive to make all activities related to food enjoyable ones. They sit down to eat together and talk, and enjoy cooking at home.

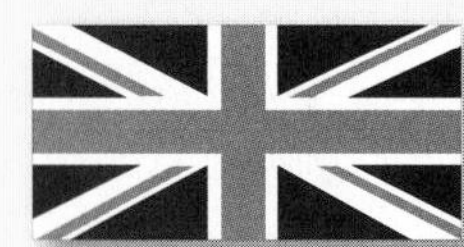

Great Britain

Residents of Great Britain take great pride in afternoon tea and scones. Sunday roast is also a centuries old tradition.

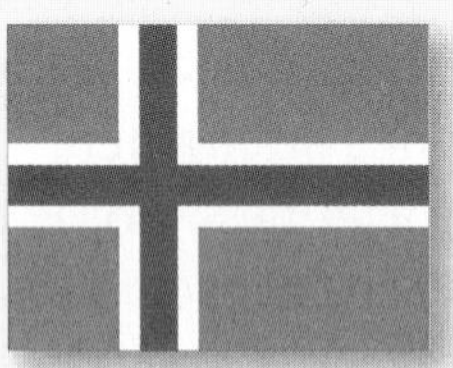

Norway

Norwegians believe that food plus joy equals health.

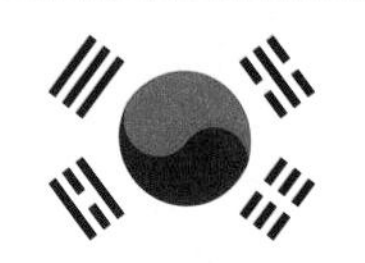

Korea

Koreans know it is important to enjoy meals, and keep harmony between diet and daily life.

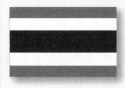

Thailand

Thailanders believe families are happy when they eat together and enjoy treasured family tastes and good home cooking.

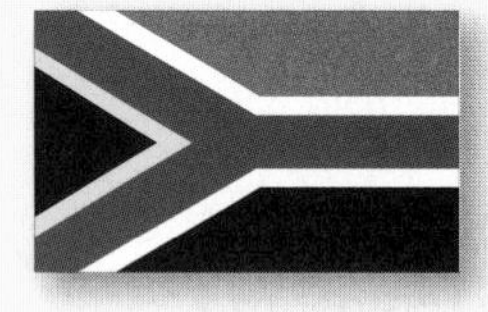

South Africa

South Africans take pride in Boerekos, or farmer's food. The traditional foods include lamb, vegetables, and potato dishes.

In fact, most social occasions include food. Food makes people feel welcome and at ease. Food can be a focus of conversation and activity. It can create a warm feeling of hospitality, making it easier for people to connect. **Hospitality** is kindness in welcoming guests or strangers.

Comfort

When people are stressed, troubled, bored, or unhappy, they often turn to food for comfort. **Comfort foods** are familiar foods that make people feel good.

Everyone has their own idea of what a comfort food is depending on their own tastes and experiences. Common comfort foods are ice cream, chocolate, macaroni and cheese, mashed or fried potatoes, bread with butter, pizza, and fried chicken. Comfort foods are often high in fat and calories.

Comfort foods often remind people of childhood. Comfort foods may also slow the release of **stress hormones**, making people feel better. Do any foods comfort you when you are unhappy or stressed?

Entertainment

Food entertains us in many ways. Eating at a restaurant is one form of entertainment. It is a way to explore new foods and spend time with family and friends. Cooking for guests is a way to show you care for them.

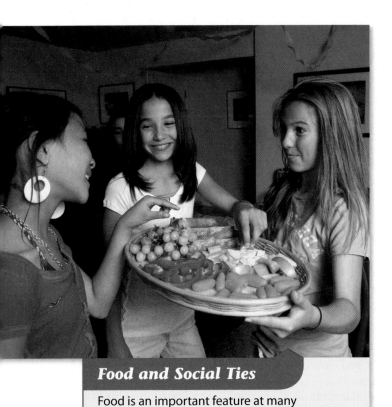

Food and Social Ties

Food is an important feature at many gatherings, such as parties, sporting events, and meetings. *How does food help strengthen family and social ties?*

TECHNOLOGY FOR TOMORROW

Global Awareness

Technology, international travel, and immigration are changing Americans' perspectives on food. As immigrants move from one country to another, they bring along their food customs. Modern transportation also makes it possible to import foods from around the globe. What is the result? Ethnic foods are changing the way many Americans cook. Foods that were once considered exotic are now sold side by side with traditional favorites. People are also more aware of the inequality in the global food supply. People in some nations have more food than they need, while people in other nations are starving. The challenge facing humanity is to ensure an adequate food supply for every person on the planet, so that no one goes hungry.

Investigate How can technology play a role in helping to provide food for every person on the planet?

NCSS VIII B Science, Technology, and Society Make judgements about how science and technology can transform the physical world and human society.

On television and on the Internet you can watch chefs at work, explore foods of the world, and go behind the scenes at farms and restaurants. Many people enjoy reading cooking blogs, magazines, and collecting cookbooks. Cookbooks cover an unlimited range of food topics, from general food preparation to specific foods such as bread or poultry. Many cookbooks cover regional and ethnic cooking.

In many areas of the country, annual food festivals draw big crowds. Some festivals celebrate specific foods such as strawberries, peaches, corn, lobster, or crawfish. Other festivals focus on ethnic foods, offering an opportunity to try new dishes.

Adventure

Do you enjoy adventure? Food can bring you new and different experiences. Try foods you have never tasted before. Look for unusual fruits and vegetables in the produce department of a supermarket. Experiment with recipes and cooking techniques. Browse ethnic markets to find different foods and seasonings. In ethnic restaurants, sample unfamiliar items on the menu. Ask friends with different cultural backgrounds to share their food customs with you. All of these ideas can bring the adventure of food into your life.

Creative Possibilities

Food can be an art, too. It provides constant opportunities to be creative. Even home cooks can turn ordinary recipes into dishes that are as appealing to the eye as they are to the palate. **Palate** is a person's ability to taste and judge the different flavors of food. Presenting and serving food attractively is as important as preparing it correctly.

Careers in Food

Joanne Larsen, MS RD LD
Dietitian

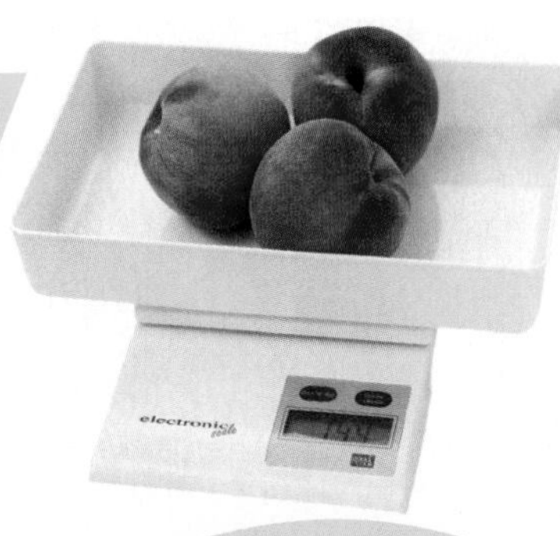

Q: What do dietitians do?

A: Dietitians working in health care or private practice use nutrition as a therapy to treat disease. We diagnose patients based on their dietary habits as well as their physical traits and prescribe nutrition intervention where certain foods are either encouraged or eliminated to change weight, blood values, or other symptoms.

Q: Do you work at a specific hospital or other facility, or do you run your own business?

A: I own a consulting company that develops nutrition software and content for Web sites. I have worked in hospitals, a nursing home, and out-patient clinics. I have also taught at a university and at community colleges.

Q: How do you become a dietition?

A: In order to call yourself a dietitian or registered dietitian, you must complete a 4-year American Dietetics Association program in college, complete an internship or planned experience program, and pass a national registration exam.

"I am passionate about helping people make healthier food choices."
—Joanne Larsen, *MS RD LD Registered Dietitian—State of Illinois*

Education and Training
The ADA requires a bachelor's degree to be eligible to take the national registration exam. Dietetic Technicians have a 2-year Associate of Arts degree and work under the supervision of dietitians.

Qualities and Skills
The ability to communicate with people through speaking and writing is important. An understanding of biology, chemistry, math, and health is important.

Related Career Opportunities
The knowledge a dietitian has is valuable in many other jobs. Related occupations include food service managers, health educators, diatetic technicians, and registered nurses.

Preparing and serving food lets you express your creativity. Turning ingredients into a delicious dish is satisfying. Sharing the dish with others makes the enjoyment even greater. Once you learn the principles of safe food preparation, you can experiment with your own creative food combinations.

Career Possibilities

There are thousands of careers in food. A **career** is a long-term job a person pursues. Would you like to manage a restaurant or make delicious dishes as a chef? Maybe you would enjoy decorating wedding cakes or coaching people about healthy food choices. These are just a few of the many careers related to food.

Exploration is the first step in choosing a satisfying career. If you like science, explore careers in food science. If you are interested in art, you might find out about jobs in food photography or cookbook design. If you like the outdoors, you might look into careers in agriculture. Talk to people in food careers, do research on the Internet, and learn about education and training options. As you learn about food, learn about related careers too. You just might find your life's work.

✓ **Reading Check** **Explain** How can food bring a sense of adventure to your life?

Skills You Will Build While Learning About Food

Your adventure in food is about to begin. As you work with food during this course, you will build skills and qualities that are useful in all areas of your life.

Self-Esteem

Self-esteem is the feeling that you are a worthwhile, capable person. Building food preparation skills and sharing your efforts with others can help raise your self-esteem. Working well in a team can also help you feel good about yourself.

Critical Thinking

Critical thinking means analyzing and evaluating what you hear and read. Critical thinking helps you understand and interpret information. For example, you can recognize when a health claim for a food product sounds too good to be true. You can notice and resist negative influences on your food choices.

Communication

As you work in the foods lab, you will work with others and practice your skills at verbal and nonverbal communication.

Verbal communication is the use of words to send and receive information, thoughts, and feelings. It includes speaking, listening, writing, and reading. A good communicator listens carefully, speaks clearly, and reads and writes well.

Nonverbal communication is sending and receiving information, thoughts, and feelings without words. Facial expressions are one form of body language. They offer clues to what you are thinking and feeling. Even if you say nothing, your feelings often show in your expression. Learning to notice other people's facial expressions, gestures, and body language can help you work well together.

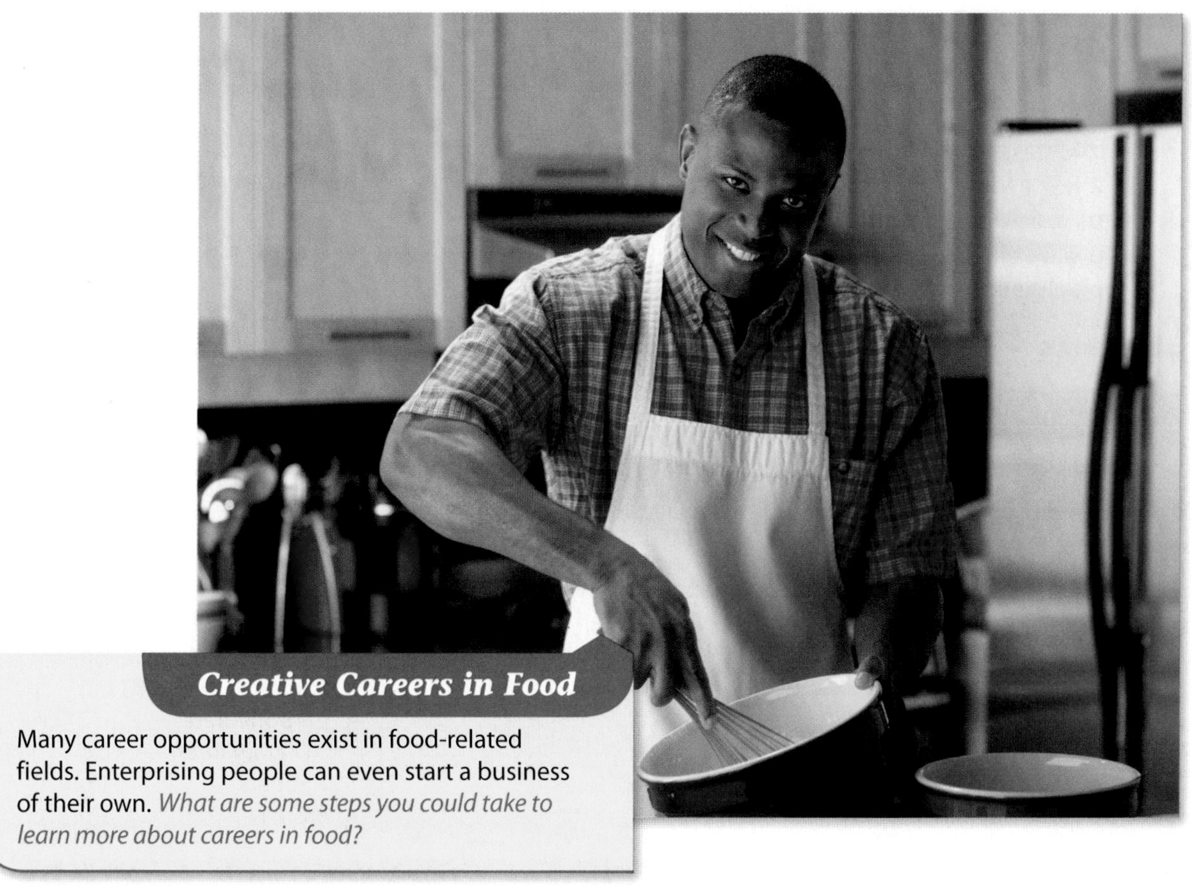

Creative Careers in Food

Many career opportunities exist in food-related fields. Enterprising people can even start a business of their own. *What are some steps you could take to learn more about careers in food?*

Leadership

Leadership is the ability to guide or direct people. You could practice your leadership skills as the captain of a team in the foods lab. As you learn more about nutrition, you could show leadership by helping others choose healthful foods.

Management

Handling resources wisely to reach goals is called **management**. Time, effort, money, and information are important resources. In your foods class, you will learn to manage time so that several dishes are ready to eat at a meal. You will learn about managing a food budget and sticking to it. You will learn to keep a food record and to plan meals. You will learn to evaluate your management skills and improve them.

Organization

Good organization is also part of management. **Organization** is an ordered manner of doing things. You practice your skill at organization when you arrange food and equipment in an orderly and logical way for quick and efficient meal preparation. You place kitchen items you need most often in places where they can be reached easily. Organization improves even simple tasks, like cleaning a kitchen or washing dishes.

What better place to learn skills for life than by exploring the world of food? So get ready for exploration. The amazing world of food awaits you.

✓ **Reading Check** **Describe** How is critical thinking useful in the world of food?

Light and Healthy Recipe

Caprese Salad

Ingredients

- **8 oz** Mozzarella, cut in circular slices
- **2** Roma tomatoes, cut in circular slices
- **1 cup** Fresh, whole basil leaves
- **½ cup** Olive oil
- **¼ cup** Balsamic vinegar

Directions

1. Arrange the slices of cheese and tomato in an alternating, circular pattern on a serving dish.
2. Sprinkle the basil leaves on top of the tomatoes and cheese.
3. In a small bowl, combine the olive oil and vinegar. Whisk together to make vinaigrette.
4. Cover and chill in a refrigerator until it is time to serve. Just before serving, drizzle the salad with the vinaigrette.

This dish uses the colors of the flag of Italy, where it comes from. It is a simple, healthy, and attractive salad.

Yield 6 servings

Nutrition Analysis per Serving

■ Calories	161
■ Total fat	13 g
Saturated fat	5 g
Cholesterol	15 mg
■ Sodium	192 mg
■ Carbohydrate	2
Dietary fiber	0 g
Sugars	1 g
■ Protein	7 g

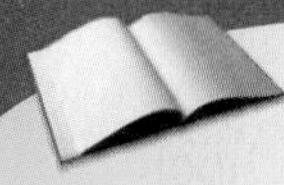

After You Read

Chapter Summary

Food has the power to keep you alive and healthy, and to affect the quality of your life. Food provides nutrients that promote wellness. Through science, we can understand more about food, including agriculture, food processing, and food safety. Food is recognized as a great source of pleasure around the world. It unifies friends and families, and provides comfort, entertainment, adventure, creativity, and career possibilities. Learning about food can build such personal skills as self-esteem, critical thinking, communication, leadership, and management. Food can influence virtually all areas of life.

Content and Academic Vocabulary Review

1. Write a sentence using two or more of these content and academic vocabulary words.

Content Vocabulary

- nutrient (p. 6)
- nutrition (p. 6)
- wellness (p. 6)
- hospitality (p. 8)
- comfort foods (p. 8)
- stress hormones (p. 8)
- palate (p. 9)
- self-esteem (p. 11)
- critical thinking (p. 11)
- verbal communication (p. 11)
- nonverbal communication (p. 11)
- leadership (p. 12)
- management (p. 12)

Academic Vocabulary

- career (p. 10)
- organization (p. 12)

Review Key Concepts

2. **Explain** what makes food powerful.
3. **Describe** the role of science in food.
4. **Summarize** the ways that food provides pleasure.
5. **Describe** the skills and qualities you can build as you learn about food.

Critical Thinking

6. **Explain** how food connects to many aspects of life, including wellness.
7. **Explain** how science can help people make smart choices when it comes to choosing a safe and healthy weight-loss plan.
8. **Analyze** how all cultures appreciate food and the pleasure it provides. Why do you think every culture has its own style of cuisine?
9. **Brainstorm** the potential dangers of routinely turning to food for comfort when you feel stressed, troubled, bored, or unhappy. What are two alternative ways to deal with these feelings?
10. **Examine** how food can be a form of communication. What specific messages can you send to others by making, serving, or sharing food?

Foods Lab

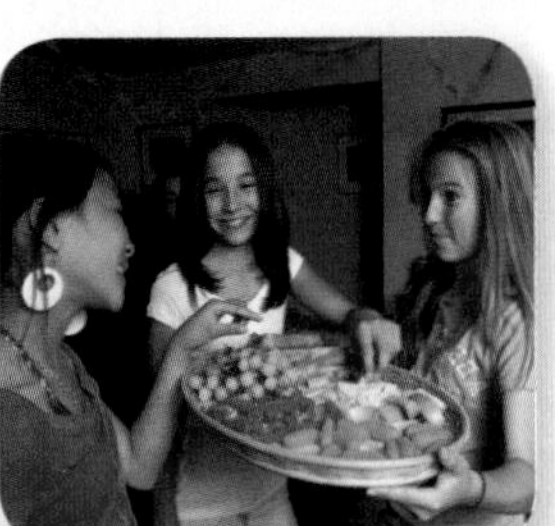

11. Foods and Emotions Think about comfort foods, then identify their common qualities. Identify the relationship between foods and emotions.

Procedure With your classmates, brainstorm a list of different comfort foods.

Analysis What qualities, such as those related to taste and texture, do the comfort foods have in common? How would you rate the overall healthfulness of the comfort foods on the list? What might this suggest about food and emotions? Write two paragraphs expressing your answers to these questions.

HEALTHFUL CHOICES

12. Increase Nutrients You return home from a long and difficult day at school ready to reach for your favorite comfort food. Using the knowledge you already have about nutrition and healthy eating, brainstorm one way to increase the nutritional value or healthfulness of your food choice. Make a list of ideas, including possible substitutions, and alternate ways of preparing the food.

TECH Connection

13. Research Food Festivals Food festivals are an entertaining way to explore and enjoy food. Look through food magazines or, under your teacher's supervision, use the Internet to research a food festival. Where and when does it take place? What type of food or foods does it focus on? What activities can festival participants enjoy? Share your findings with the class.

Real-World Skills

Problem-Solving Skills

14. Alleviate Food Boredom The Albani family eats the same seven dinners every week. They have become bored with their food, and less interested in eating dinner. What can the Albanis do to add excitement and interest to their meals?

Interpersonal and Collaborative Skills

15. Show Creativity Follow your teacher's instructions to form groups. Imagine you will prepare breakfast, lunch, or dinner for the famous artist of your group's choice. Work together to brainstorm ways to show creativity in preparing and serving the meal. As a group, discuss your ideas, write them down, and use art supplies to illustrate your plans for the meal's presentation.

Financial Literacy Skills

16. The Cost of Eating at Restaurants Petra visits her favorite Thai restaurant three times a month. She spends a total of $19 each visit. A local Thai market sells all the ingredients needed to make Petra's usual Thai meal. The total cost of ingredients needed to make the meal one time is $6. How much can Petra save if she prepares the dish at home twice a month and goes to the restaurant only once a month?

Academic Skills

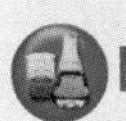

Food Science

17. Appearance and Preferences Can the appearance of a glass of juice influence a person's expectations of how it will taste?

Procedure Pour equal amounts of four different types of juice—into four clear glasses. Tint three glasses with one drop of food dye to create four different colored samples.

Ask a classmate to rate them in order of preference, based on appearance. Record the responses. Have your classmate taste each sample while blindfolded and rank them again. Compare the responses.

Analysis Write a paragraph to explain how the visual test compared to the taste test.

NSES A Develop abilities necessary to do scientific inquiry.

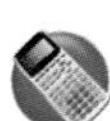

Mathematics

18. Find a Percent During a stressful week, Marge eats comfort food—whole-grain vegetarian pizza—for dinner on Monday, Tuesday, Thursday, and Friday. On Saturday, Marge has a comforting fried chicken meal for dinner. She eats soup and salad on the remaining two nights of the week. What percent of her dinners consisted of comfort food? What percent consisted of healthier meals?

Math Concept **Percentages as Ratios** Percent indicates the ratio of a number to 100. To find what percent a number is of another number, divide the first number by the second number, multiply by 100, and add the % symbol.

Starting Hint Count the number of nights Marge eats comfort food. Then divide by seven.

NCTM Number and Operations Compute fluently and make reasonable estimates.

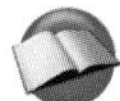

English Language Arts

19. Food Memories Food is often part of memorable holidays and celebrations. Write a paragraph about a special event in your life in which food played a role. Describe the event and the food. Your recollection might be humorous (a dish that did not turn out right), sentimental (a beautiful cake at a family wedding), or loving (a special dish prepared by a special friend or relative).

NCTE 4 Use written language to communicate effectively.

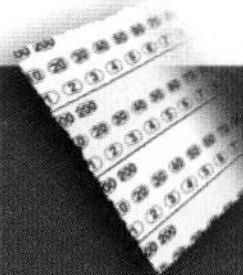

STANDARDIZED TEST PRACTICE

MULTIPLE CHOICE

Read the multiple choice question and choose the answer that best completes the sentence.

20. Why does science have an impact on the world of food?

a. Nutritious foods help scientists' brains function better.

b. Scientists are responsible for people's food choices.

c. Science leads to improvements in agriculture, food processing, and food safety.

d. The world of food is one mystery science cannot solve.

Test-Taking Tip Multiple choice questions may prompt you to select the best answer. They may present you with answers that seem partially true. The best answer is the one that is completely true, and can be supported by information you have read in the text.

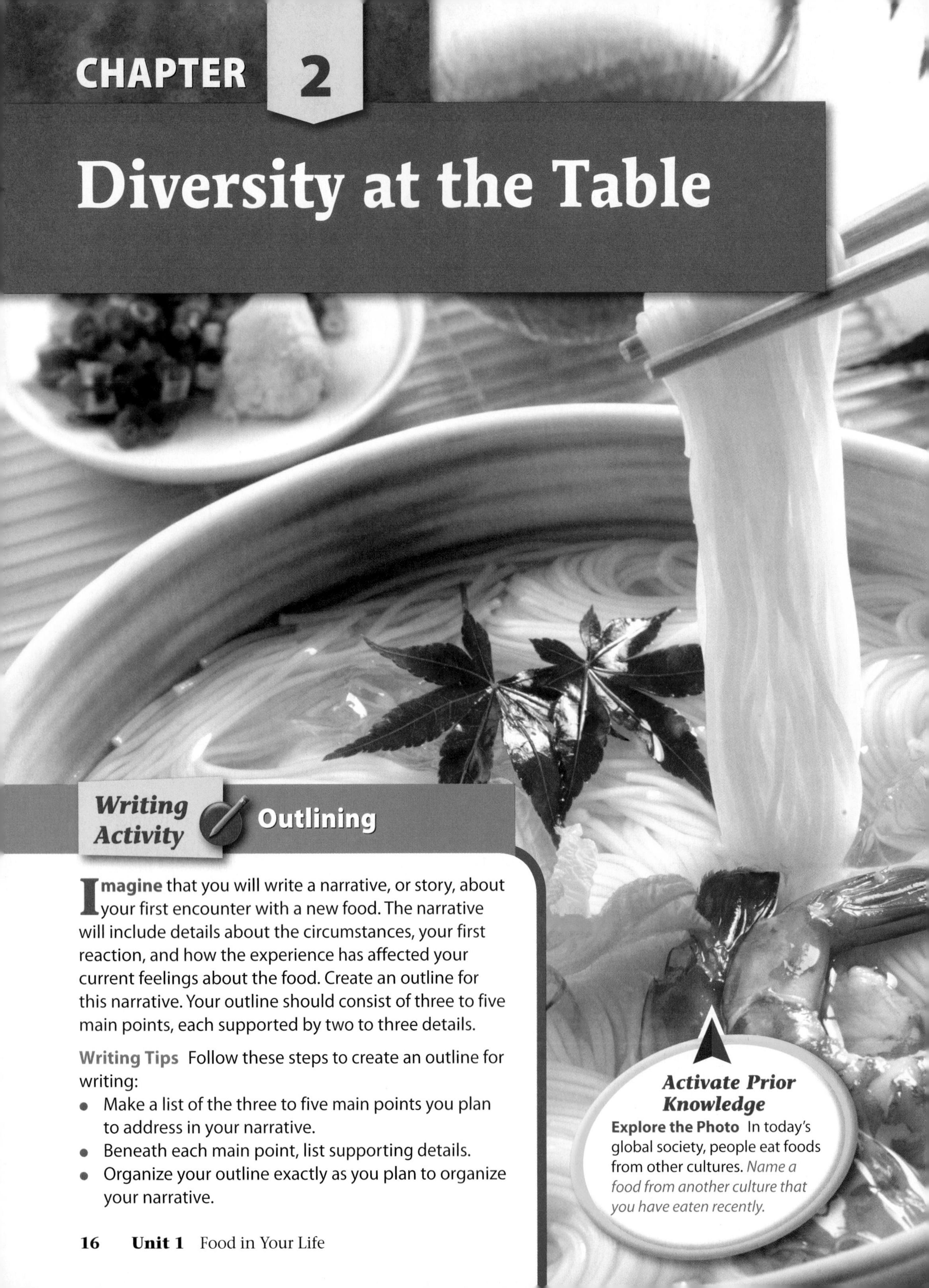

CHAPTER 2

Diversity at the Table

Writing Activity — Outlining

Imagine that you will write a narrative, or story, about your first encounter with a new food. The narrative will include details about the circumstances, your first reaction, and how the experience has affected your current feelings about the food. Create an outline for this narrative. Your outline should consist of three to five main points, each supported by two to three details.

Writing Tips Follow these steps to create an outline for writing:

- Make a list of the three to five main points you plan to address in your narrative.
- Beneath each main point, list supporting details.
- Organize your outline exactly as you plan to organize your narrative.

Activate Prior Knowledge

Explore the Photo In today's global society, people eat foods from other cultures. *Name a food from another culture that you have eaten recently.*

Reading Guide

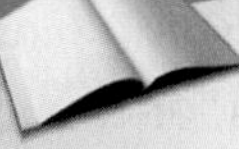

Before You Read

Preview Skim the photos, figures, and contents of this chapter, and start a list of the different cultures that you see mentioned.

Read to Learn

Key Concepts

- **Explain** culture and its relationship to food.
- **Summarize** influences on cuisines and customs.
- **Identify** similarities in global cuisines.
- **Explain** food customs today.
- **Describe** food customs in the United States.

Main Idea

People from all over the world maintain their traditional food customs and share them with other cultures, creating great diversity at the table.

Content Vocabulary

You will find definitions for these words in the glossary at the back of the book.

- ☐ culture
- ☐ ethnic
- ☐ cuisine
- ☐ custom
- ☐ staple food
- ☐ fasting
- ☐ fusion cuisine

Academic Vocabulary

You will find these words in your reading and on your tests. Use the glossary at the back of this book.

- provide
- impact

Graphic Organizer

Use a graphic organizer like the one below to note food preparation methods that are common to different cultures and the cultures that share them.

PREPARATION METHOD	CULTURES
Pasta/Noodles	
Raised Breads	
Flatbreads	
Dumplings with Filling	
Cured Meats	

Graphic Organizer Go to this book's Online Learning Center at **glencoe.com** to print out this graphic organizer.

Academic Standards

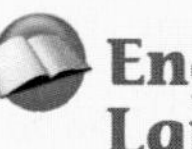

English Language Arts

NCTE 4 Use written language to communicate effectively.

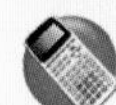

Mathematics

NCTM Measurement Understand measurable attributes of objects and the units, systems, and processes of measurement.

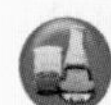

Science

NSES B Develop an understanding of motions and forces.

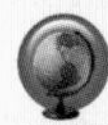

Social Studies

NCSS VIII B Science, Technology, and Society Make judgments about how science and technology have transformed the physical world and human society.

NCTE *National Council of Teachers of English*
NCTM *National Council of Teachers of Mathematics*
NSES *National Science Education Standards*
NCSS *National Council for the Social Studies*

What Is Culture?

Culture is a set of customs, traditions, and beliefs shared by a large group of people. Food, language, religion, history, style of dress, and form of government are all aspects of culture.

When people move around the world, they carry their culture with them. Immigrants from Germany, Japan, Italy, Mexico, and many other countries have brought their cultural traditions to North America. Many immigrants adopt some of the customs of the new culture while still preserving the culture of their former home. In a strong society, people value these cultural differences.

Food and Culture

Thanks to the many cultures in North American society, we can enjoy a range of ethnic foods. **Ethnic** means relating to a specific culture. The entire last unit of this book will take you around the globe to learn about foods of the world.

Different cultures have more than individual ingredients and dishes—they have entire cuisines. A **cuisine** (kwi-ˈzēn) is a culture's foods and styles of cooking. A cuisine may be particular to a country or a region, or it may be a blend from different areas. Tex-Mex cuisine combines foods from Texas and Mexico to create such specialties as tacos, burritos, and nachos. Most nations have different regional cuisines in their different geographic areas. Each regional cuisine is unique in its own way.

Different cultures also have different food customs. A **custom** is a group's specific way of doing things. Food customs include how and when foods are eaten. In some cultures, food is eaten with chopsticks, while in other cultures food is eaten with the fingers. In some cultures, the main meal is served at midday, while in other cultures the main meal is served in the evening. Different cultures also have different table manners.

✓ **Reading Check** **Define** What is culture?

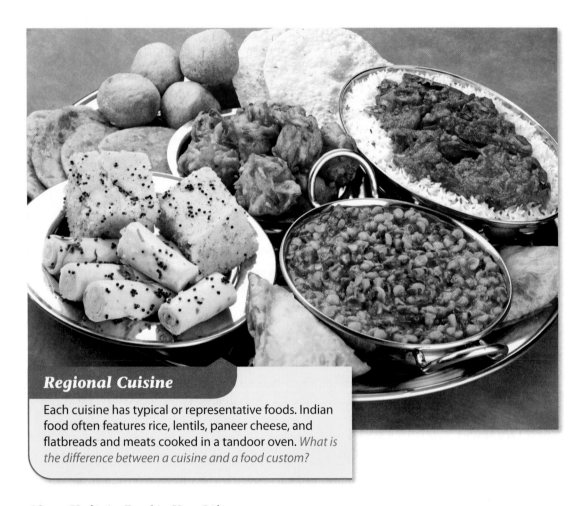

Regional Cuisine

Each cuisine has typical or representative foods. Indian food often features rice, lentils, paneer cheese, and flatbreads and meats cooked in a tandoor oven. *What is the difference between a cuisine and a food custom?*

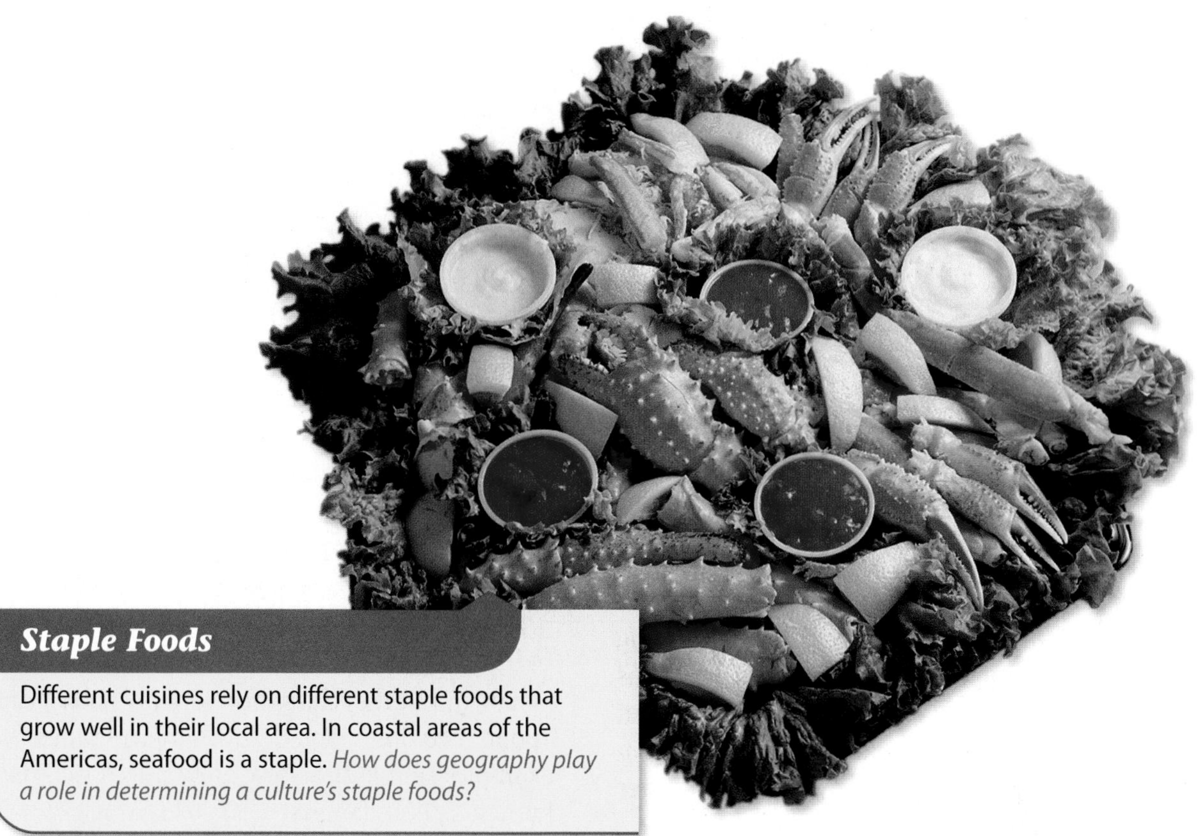

Staple Foods

Different cuisines rely on different staple foods that grow well in their local area. In coastal areas of the Americas, seafood is a staple. *How does geography play a role in determining a culture's staple foods?*

Influences on Cuisines and Customs

Why do different cultures have such different cuisines and food customs? A culture's history, its geographic origin, its contact with other cultures, and even its beliefs **provide**, or give, the answer.

Geography

For much of history, geography determined people's diet. Geography includes the climate, type of soil, elevation, temperature, and amount of sunlight. Different plants and animals thrive in different geographic regions. These local plants and animals became a culture's staple foods. A **staple food** is the most widely produced and eaten food in an area.

Geography and Staple Grains

Almost all cultures have a staple grain. Different grains grow well in different geographic areas. The primary grain in southeastern Asia is rice, which is ideally suited to the hot, humid conditions in much of that area.

Sorghum grows well in the hot, dry regions of Africa, India, and China. Wheat, rye, barley, and oats are the main grains in the cooler parts of Europe, Asia, and Africa. Corn, or maize, is the staple grain of most of the Americas.

Geography and Animal Foods

Geography also influences how people hunt or raise animals. In regions near oceans and rivers, people depend on fish for food. Salmon, cod, and other cold-water fish are staples in Finland and Norway. In the islands of the Pacific Ocean, such as Japan, meals may include squid, octopus, sea urchins, shark, and seaweed.

Historically, the woods and meadows of North America have been populated by large and small game, from squirrel to larger animals, like boar, deer, and elk. Inhabitants of the African plain hunted zebra and antelope for food. Where grazing land was good, people raised cattle. Where pasture was scarce or the land was hilly, as in the eastern Mediterranean, people rasied sheep and goats. Camels, yaks, or llamas are suited to harsher climates.

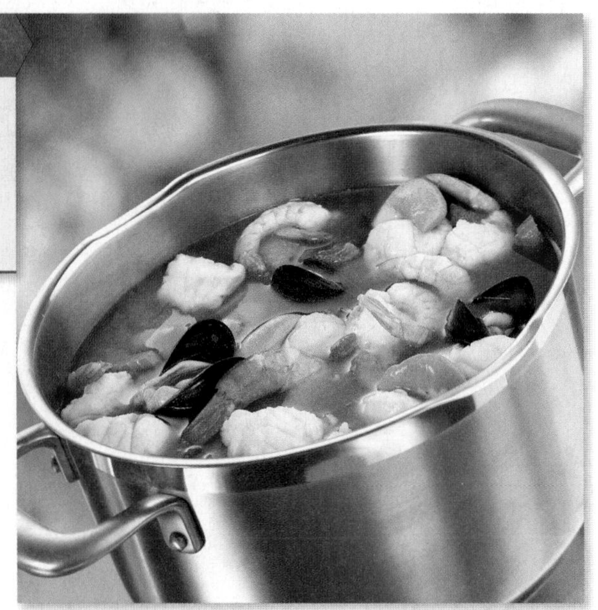

Humble Origins

Bouillabaisse is a highly seasoned stew made with at least two kinds of seafood. This celebrated and festive dish from France has its origins in an economical peasant stew. *Why did the rich and the poor develop different cuisines in many countries?*

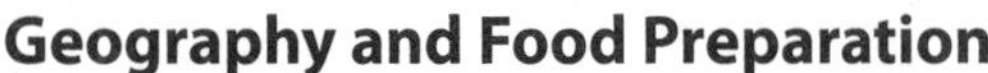

Geography and Food Preparation

Geography also affected the food-preparation methods of different cultures. Cooking required fire. If fuel was easy to come by, as in the forested areas of Europe, foods could cook slowly. Meals might feature long-simmering stews, for example. Where cooking fuel was scarce, as in some parts of Asia, food was cut into small pieces that cooked quickly. Frying in small amounts of fat and steaming were faster than roasting and baking.

Economics

Until relatively recent times, most societies had two classes, the wealthy and the poor. They ate differently and developed different cuisines.

The wealthy had more access to meat, poultry, and fresh fruits and vegetables. They could also afford to refine grain into white flour.

The poor had fewer food choices. They often relied on porridges and dark breads made from whole or coarsely ground grains. Soups and stews were based on whatever a family could hunt, catch, or raise. Wild berries and dried fruit satisfied the sweet tooth. Some people grew food, but had to sell most of the harvest.

Cooks grew resourceful in adding variety to meals. Edible odds and ends, from pigs' feet to oxtails, were cooked into zesty stews along with starchy, filling root vegetables. Meat from animals' feet, head, and organs was ground and stuffed into casings made from hog intestines—the recipe for sausage.

Cooks were equally creative with grains. Oats, corn, and barley could be baked into breads, steamed into puddings, cooked with milk, and sweetened with raisins.

As a middle class developed, "rich" and "poor" cooking merged. In southern France, for example, simple fish stew grew into a rich dish known as bouillabaisse (ˌbü-yə-ˈbās), which features costly shellfish, a tomato-based broth, and herbs.

Be a *Smart Consumer*

More for Your Money

Recipes created out of economic necessity are still very popular today. Some of today's favorite comfort foods started as "peasant" foods, including meatloaf, chicken noodle soup, rice pudding, and mashed potatoes. While they may not be peasants, most people today have to budget the amount of money they spend on food. Myra's budget for her upcoming dinner party is $50. She is deciding between two lamb recipes to prepare for the main course: roasted rack of lamb and lamb stew. The cost of rack of lamb to feed her 12 guests is $35. The cost of lamb stew meat, which can be combined with other ingredients such as vegetables to make a stew for 12, is $15.

Challenge Considering her budget, which recipe would you suggest Myra prepare and why? Write a paragraph explaining your reasoning.

Foreign Contacts

Cultures absorb new foods through immigration, through travel, and through trade with other peoples. Tea, for example, came to Europe from China in the seventeenth century. Before long, it was the national beverage in both England and Russia.

European explorers who reached the Americas brought back beans, corn, peanuts, vanilla, tomatoes, potatoes, sweet potatoes, peppers, and chocolate. European colonists introduced Native Americans to wheat, barley, chickpeas, and cattle.

Many foods that are part of our daily lives are actually recent imports. Bagels, cheesecake, and corned beef came to the United States with Jewish immigrants around 1900. Italian immigrants brought pizza to the United States around the same time.

War and conquest can have a big **impact**, or effect, on a culture's cuisine. From the twelfth to the seventeenth century, the Ottoman Turks swept through the Mediterranean and southeastern Europe. From the Persians they learned the art of making delicate, tissue-thin leaves of dough. The Turks layered this dough with spiced, ground nuts and steeped it in honey to make baklava (ˈbä-klə-ˌvä). As the Ottoman Empire spread into Hungary around 1535, the Hungarians adapted the technique to make a fruit-filled pastry roll called strudel.

Religious Beliefs

Many religions teach about the use of food, and these teachings affect a culture's food practices. Hindus do not eat beef because they consider cattle sacred. Most Jews and Muslims do not eat pork. Buddhists urge mindfulness about one's eating plan, which leads some followers to vegetarianism. Seventh Day Adventists often choose vegetarianism to express the value of simplicity and respect for the body.

Fasting, or abstaining from some or all foods for a period of time, is a practice in many religions. Most Catholics fast or refrain from eating meat on some holy days. During the month of Ramadan, Muslims do not eat or drink during daylight hours. Most Jews fast on Yom Kippur, the Day of Atonement.

Technology

In every age, advances in technology have changed the way people eat and cook. The stove was a great advance over open fire because it allowed cooks to control the strength of the heat. Refrigerators and freezers made it possible to store leftovers and other perishable foods such as fresh eggs and cream. Today, cooking can be as simple as using a microwave oven.

✓ Reading Check **Explain** How does geography influence a culture's cuisine?

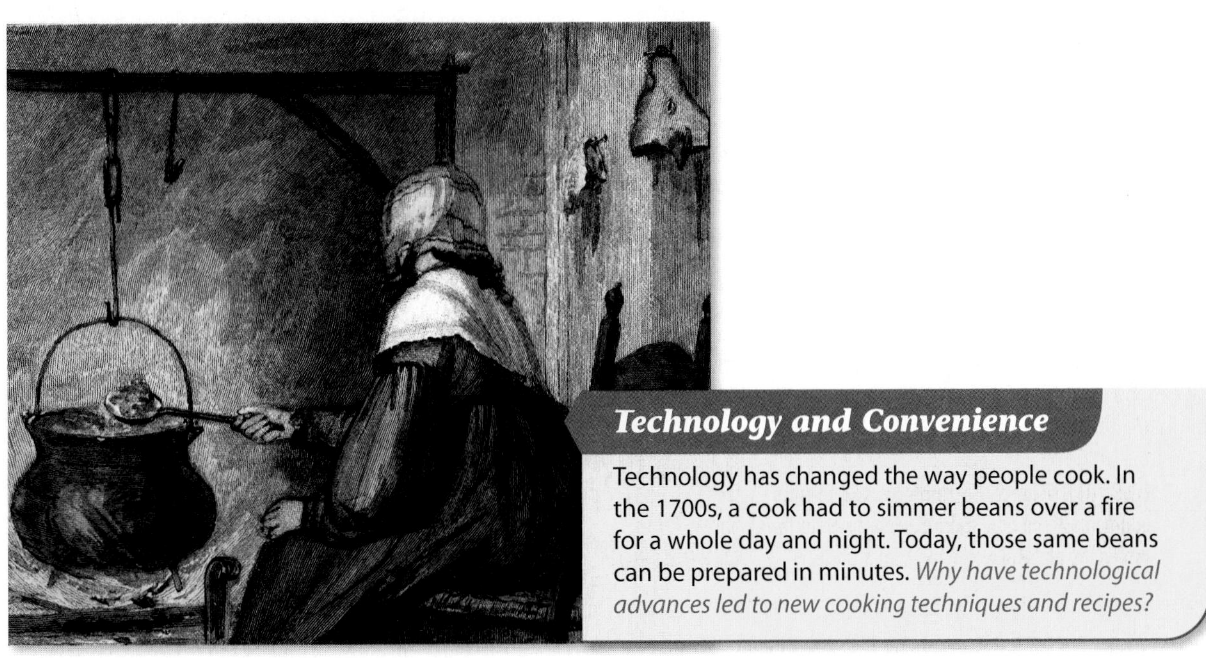

Technology and Convenience

Technology has changed the way people cook. In the 1700s, a cook had to simmer beans over a fire for a whole day and night. Today, those same beans can be prepared in minutes. *Why have technological advances led to new cooking techniques and recipes?*

Similarities in Global Cuisines

Different cuisines and food customs often have remarkable similarities. Chinese rice noodles are similar to Italian spaghetti. Greek feta cheese is not so different from Mexican queso fresco. In fact, the same principles of preparing food apply in every culture.

Preparation Methods

Many cuisines share similar food-preparation methods. For example, all cultures learned to grind grains into flour. Cooks mixed the flour with water to make dough, which they shaped into breads, rolls, and noodles. Raised, or leavened, breads were popular throughout Europe and parts of Asia. Flatbreads, which are rolled or patted into a circle and cooked on a griddle, were found in southwest Asia, North Africa, and Central and South America. Noodles, which are made from a dough that is rolled out and sliced to form different widths and lengths, are widely consumed in Europe, Asia, and North America.

Filled dumplings also appeared in cuisines worldwide. Thin sheets of noodle dough were made into pockets stuffed with cooked chopped meat, seafood, or vegetables. They were sealed and then steamed, boiled, or baked. Italians called them ravioli (ˌra-vē-ˈō-lē), the Chinese called them wontons (ˌwän-ˈtäns), and Jews named them kreplach (ˈkrep-lək).

Many cuisines preserved meats by drying and smoking. This is how the Italians made pepperoni and the Chinese produced *lop chong* (lahp chung). A Spanish version is chorizo (chə-ˈrē-(ˌ)zō), and a Polish variety is kielbasa (kēl-ˈbä-sə).

Unless forbidden by religion, thrifty cooks in many cultures saved the blood of butchered animals as a food ingredient. In parts of Europe, highly seasoned blood sausages combined animal blood with barley, oats, or rice. The English called their version blood pudding. In Poland, a nutritious soup, *czernina* (chär-ˈnē-nä), was made with duck blood and dried fruits. All of these foods are still eaten today.

TECHNOLOGY FOR TOMORROW

Futuristic Food

Technological advances have increased food choices and helped move cooking methods beyond the basics. Improved technology has also given people more leisure time, which has allowed them to develop new cooking techniques and recipes. Previously, preparing food was mostly a necessity. Now, thanks to technology, it can be a means of creative expression. Technology has also created a demand for specific types of foods that did not exist in the past. For example, the development of space exploration has created a demand for convenient foods that are easy to store and prepare in a space shuttle.

Investigate What do astronauts eat when they are in space? Investigate the foods as well as the storage and preparation methods used by astronauts.

NCSS VIII B Science, Technology, and Society Make judgments about how science and technology have transformed the physical world and human society.

Social Meanings

Food has symbolic meanings around the world. Food is a universal sign of hospitality. Sharing food is a way to show friendship and acceptance. In some cultures, hosts have a duty to offer food to their guests, and guests have a duty to accept the offer.

Food is an important part of religious, family, and cultural events around the world. In some countries, for example, Easter is celebrated with a feast of lamb and spring vegetables. The Scottish harvest festival of Lammas features breads made with flour from the first cutting of wheat. In the Czech Republic, people celebrate the fall harvest with sauerkraut and a cheese-filled pastry called kolacke (kō-ˈlä-chē).

✓ Reading Check **Identify** What is one social meaning that food can have?

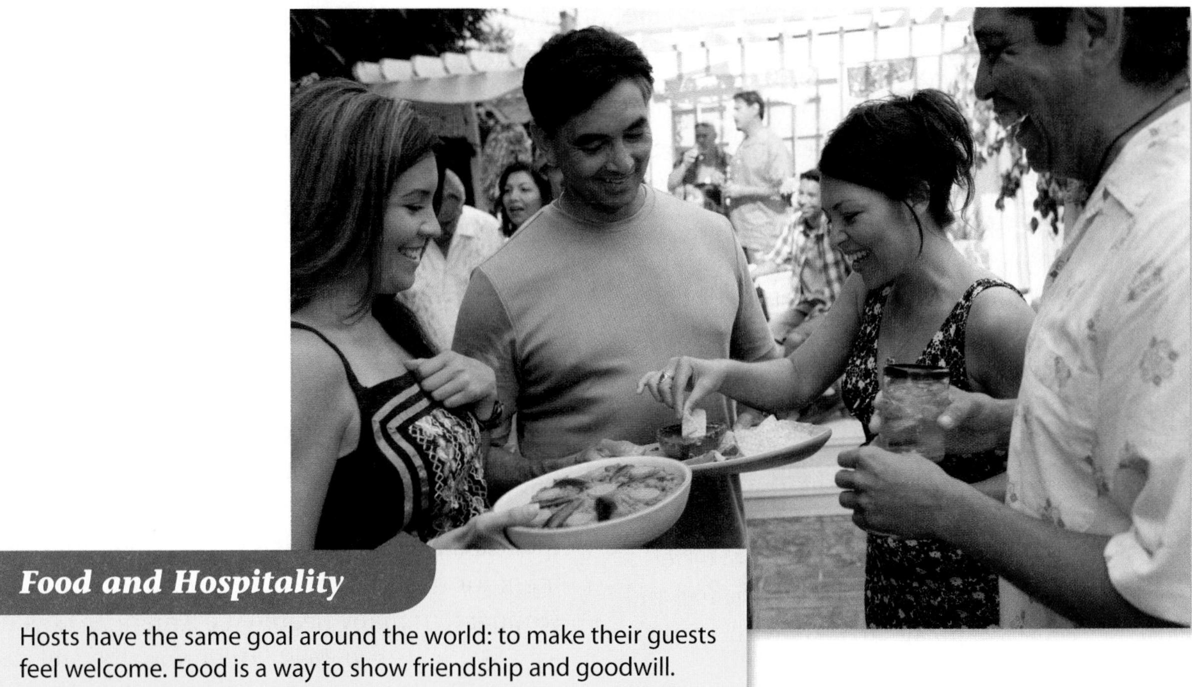

Food and Hospitality

Hosts have the same goal around the world: to make their guests feel welcome. Food is a way to show friendship and goodwill. *Why do you think sharing food shows hospitality and acceptance?*

Food Customs Today

Food customs change slowly. Tradition, cultural pride, and enjoyment keep our food customs stable from generation to generation.

Maintaining Food Customs

Many food traditions continue because people enjoy them. Chocolate remains a staple in Mexican cuisine, as it has been since the time of the Aztecs. People enjoy it over fried bananas, in hot chocolate, and in mole ('mō-lā), a spicy sauce for meat or eggs.

Some food customs are handed down as a matter of cultural pride. The custom is part of a people's tradition and identity.

In the Central American tradition, for example, tamales are made by spreading dough onto corn husks and then folding the husks over the filling. Today, you can also fold tamales using aluminum foil and coffee filters. Taking the time to learn and teach the original skill shows pride and respect for cultural heritage.

Keeping food customs can also provide a sense of security. Food traditions help people feel that they belong to something larger than themselves.

Changing Food Customs

Technology is changing what and how people eat. New methods for processing, transporting, and storing foods allow us to sample tastes from around the globe. We are no longer limited to foods that are grown locally or only in a particular season. Florida oranges are sold fresh in Norwegian groceries and Norwegian cod is served in restaurants in New York City. Unfortunately, transporting food over such long distances contributes to global warming. The cost of fuel also affects the price of food.

The trend of experimenting with foreign cuisines has given rise to a new school of cooking called fusion cuisine. **Fusion cuisine** is the practice of creating new recipes by mixing the influences and preparation techniques of different food traditions. For example, you might find French crepes filled with Caribbean-style shrimp in a coconut-lime sauce. Tex-Mex cuisine fuses ingredients available in Texas with cooking techniques from Mexico. Fusion sushi includes ingredients not typical in Japanese food.

✓ **Reading Check** **Explain** What is one reason people choose to maintain their food traditions?

Food Customs in the United States

The United States is home to people of countless ethnic backgrounds. The cuisines of each group add to the variety of American cooking. Some recipes retain their cultural identity. Hummus is still considered a Middle Eastern dish, for example. Others have become as American as apple pie. Pretzels, doughnuts, and coleslaw, for example, were contributed by the Dutch.

Many dishes blend ingredients and techniques from different cuisines. Pizza was originally an Italian dish. Now you can order a Tex-Mex pizza topped with refried beans and salsa, or a Creole pizza covered with shrimp, eggplant, and hot pepper sauce.

You might even enjoy foods from different cuisines at the same meal. At a food court, you could sample food from two continents by ordering a mango lassi and a bowl of gumbo. If you eat curried chicken and rice followed by a slice of Black Forest cake, you've sampled foods from India, China, and Germany.

Holiday foods from different cultures also have an influence on American food customs. Today, people may eat tamales at Christmas, rice dumplings around the Chinese New Year, or corned beef and cabbage on St. Patrick's Day.

Many respected American cookbooks have been written by chefs originally from other countries. There are many cookbooks that apply cooking techniques from foreign countries to foods found in abundance in America. Those authors found an opportunity to fuse their cooking knowledge with the wide assortment of foods available in America. It's no wonder that many people see American cuisine as a work in progress, a continually updated cookbook that blends the best of all cultures.

✓ **Reading Check** **Summarize** Why is American cuisine a work in progress?

Light and Healthy Recipe

Navy Beans Slow-Baked in Syrup

The navy beans in this recipe are high in protein and fiber.

Ingredients

- **3 cups** Navy beans
- **1 Tbsp.** Corn oil
- **1** Chopped small onion
- **½ cup** Tomato sauce
- **¼ cup** Corn syrup
- **¼ cup** Brown sugar
- **⅛ tsp.** Salt
- **⅛ tsp.** Pepper

Directions

1. Cover the beans with water and soak overnight. Drain and rinse the beans.
2. Preheat oven to 275 degrees.
3. Pour corn oil into a pan and add onions. Cook onions until tender and add to the pot with the beans.
4. Add remaining ingredients to the pot with the beans and cook, covered, for 5 hours.
5. Check beans frequently, adding water when necessary to keep mixture from drying out.

Yield 6 servings

Nutrition Analysis per Serving

Calories	292
Total fat	3 g
Saturated fat	1 g
Cholesterol	0 mg
Sodium	270 mg
Carbohydrate	54
Dietary fiber	18 g
Sugars	9 g
Protein	14 g

CHAPTER 2 Review & Applications

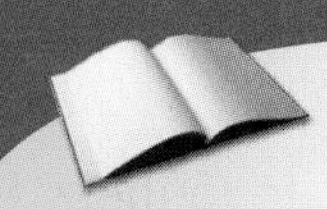

After You Read

Chapter Summary

Food is as diverse as the people who produce, prepare, and eat it. Cultures have their own distinct cuisines and food customs. These are influenced by geography, economics, foreign contacts, religious beliefs, and technology. Many cultures share similarities in their food preparation methods and in their beliefs about the social meanings of food. Today, people work hard to maintain their food customs. They also change their food customs and merge them with those of other cultures. In fusion cuisine, different food traditions are combined. The United States is an example of a place where many diverse food customs coexist and merge. The world of food is truly multicultural.

Content and Academic Vocabulary Review

1. Use these content and academic vocabulary words to create a crossword puzzle on graph paper. Use the definitions as clues.

Content Vocabulary

- ☐ culture (p. 18)
- ☐ ethnic (p. 18)
- ☐ cuisine (p. 18)
- ☐ custom (p. 18)
- ☐ staple food (p. 19)
- ☐ fasting (p. 21)
- ☐ fusion cuisine (p. 23)

Academic Vocabulary

- provide (p. 19)
- impact (p. 21)

Review Key Concepts

2. **Explain** culture and its relationship to food.
3. **Summarize** influences on cuisines and customs.
4. **Identify** similarities in global cuisines.
5. **Explain** food customs today.
6. **Describe** food customs in the U.S.

Critical Thinking

7. **Explain** how studying food can help you to understand how different groups of people have migrated around the world throughout history.
8. **Design** two different meals that are resourceful and inventive, using the same ingredients. You have tortillas, sliced turkey, cheese, a tomato, and a can of sliced black olives.
9. **Describe** a situation in which food can be an introduction to another culture or region.
10. **Explain** the challenge created by the need to balance the availability of food items from all over the world with the cost of transporting foods long distances. Consider the cost of damage to the environment.

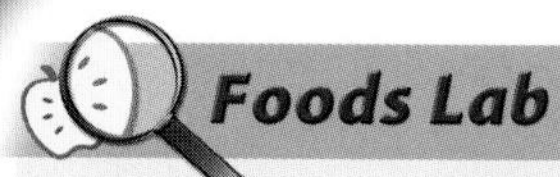

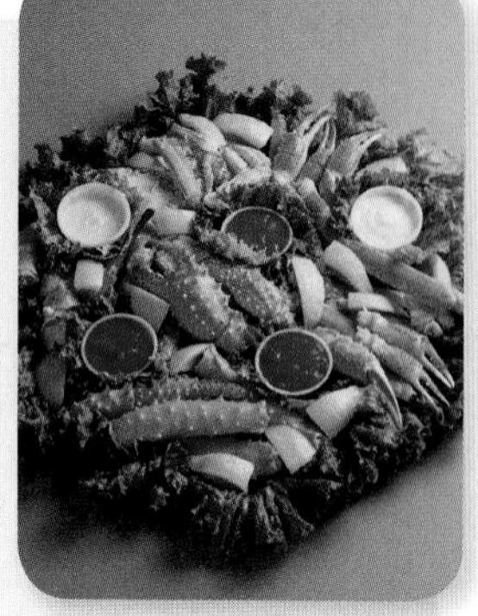

11. Regional Foods Regional foods are those that are grown or produced in a particular geographical area. There are many advantages to using foods from the region in which you live, including low cost, fresh taste, and less harm caused to the environment.

Procedure Identify the foods that are grown in or near your geographical region. Then choose a recipe that features one or more foods for which your region is known.

Analysis Evaluate the recipe. Give it between 1 and 5 stars in each of the following categories: visual appeal; taste; ease of preparation. Share your recipe with your classmates.

HEALTHFUL CHOICES

12. Maintain Healthy Traditions Since Miyako recently moved from Japan to the United States, her diet has changed. She eats more typical American food and less traditional Japanese food. Miyako's traditional Japanese diet is low in fat and offers many health benefits. Miyako spends her time socializing and eating with her friends after school and rarely prepares Japanese cuisine. Devise strategies Miyako can use to integrate more of her culture's food in her new environment.

TECH Connection

13. Native Origins Under your teacher's supervision use the library and Internet to research foods that are native to the Americas. Who first used and ate these foods? How were they first prepared? How are they used today? Use presentation software to create a presentation about your findings. Share your presentation with the class.

Real-World Skills

Problem-Solving Skills

14. Dinner Invitation Victor has been invited to a friend's home for dinner. The friend's cultural background is different from Victor's, which means the food might be quite different from what is familiar to Victor. He is concerned. How would you advise him?

Interpersonal and Collaborative Skills

15. Discuss Follow your teacher's instructions to form small groups. With your group, have a discussion about these questions: What will cuisines be like in 100 years? Will the cuisine be more distinct or less so? Why? How will this affect the relationship between food and culture?

Financial Literacy Skills

16. The Cost of Technology Technology, in the form of transportation, makes it possible to import and export food. To pay for the labor and fuel involved in transportation, this food may cost more. Visit your local supermarket's produce department and use labels to identify ten items in the produce department that come from distant places. Then figure out how far each item had to travel in miles to reach your local supermarket.

Academic Skills

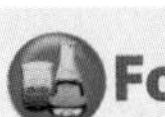

Food Science

17. Fat in Milk Milk is sold with varying amounts of fat. A type of milk used in Thai cuisine is coconut milk. Compare the fats in three kinds of milk.

Procedure Take three small paper plates and pour a different type of milk on each one so that the milk spreads to cover the bottom. Use coconut milk on one, heavy cream on another, and skim milk on the third. Add a drop of green food coloring in the middle of each plate.

Analysis Measure and record the diameter of each dot after 5, 15, 30, and 60 minutes. Write a paragraph explaining the changes in each dot and why you think they occurred.

NSES B Develop an understanding of motions and forces.

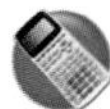

Mathematics

18. Comparing Temperatures Many cultures around the world use traditional cooking methods that involve very high temperatures. Such temperatures are typically obtained by burning wood in a special oven. For example, the tandoor is a clay oven used in India and elsewhere in Central Asia and the Middle East that can reach temperatures as high as 480°C. In Naples, Italy, traditional pizza preparation requires baking the pizza in a stone oven at 905°F. Which oven is hotter?

Math Concept **Converting Celsius to Fahrenheit** When comparing two temperatures, make sure the temperatures are in the same scale. Celsius temperatures (C) can be converted to the Fahrenheit (F) scale using the following formula: $F = (9/5 \times C) + 32$.

Starting Hint Convert 480°C into °F by multiplying 480 by 9/5 and adding 32 to the result. Compare that number to the temperature of the pizza oven.

NCTM Measurement Understand measurable attributes of objects and the units, systems, and processes of measurement.

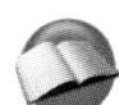

English Language Arts

19. Write a Narrative Use the outline you created at the beginning of the chapter to organize and write a one-page narrative, or story, about your first encounter with a new food. Include details about the circumstances, your first reaction, and your feelings about the food today.

NCTE 4 Use written language to communicate effectively.

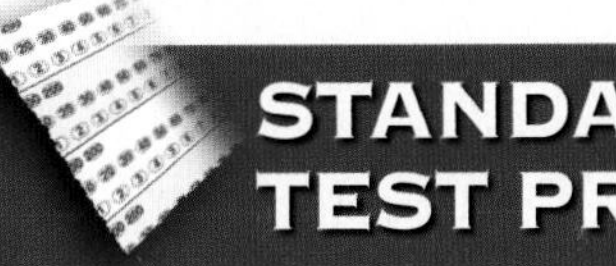

STANDARDIZED TEST PRACTICE

FILL IN THE BLANK

Read the sentence and choose the best word to fill in the blank.

20. A culture's _______ is defined as its foods and styles of cooking.
   a. ethnic
   b. custom
   c. staple food
   d. cuisine

Test-Taking Tip When answering a fill-in-the-blank question, silently read the sentence with each of the possible answers in the blank space. This will help you eliminate wrong answers. The best word results in a sentence that is both factual and grammatically correct.

CHAPTER 3

The Food Supply

Writing Activity — Freewriting

The Food Supply Think about the origin of all of the items in your most recent meal. Where did each item come from? How many hands did it pass through from the source to your plate? Spontaneously write anything that you know about the topic.

Writing Tips Follow these steps to freewrite:

- Try to write for ten minutes without stopping.
- Let your thoughts flow freely. Do not worry about organization, grammar, or spelling.
- Instead of planning, let each word or idea lead to another.

Activate Prior Knowledge

Explore the Photo Our food supply is the result of many elements working together. *Have you ever grown your own food?*

Reading Guide

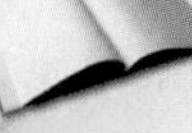

Before You Read

Preview On a sheet of paper, rewrite each of the main subject headings in this chapter in the form of questions.

Read to Learn

Key Concepts

- **Explain** ecosystems and their relationship to food.
- **Describe** the main sources of the U.S. food supply and the steps food takes from farm to consumption.
- **Identify** global food problems and explain their causes.
- **Explain** global water problems.
- **Describe** solutions to global food problems.

Main Idea

The world's food supply varies from place to place, and is influenced by many factors.

Content Vocabulary

You will find definitions for these words in the glossary at the back of this book.

- ☐ ecosystem
- ☐ food chain
- ☐ herbivore
- ☐ carnivore
- ☐ omnivore
- ☐ biodiversity
- ☐ shelf-stable
- ☐ shelf life
- ☐ food additive
- ☐ industrialized nation
- ☐ developing nation
- ☐ famine
- ☐ subsistence farming
- ☐ groundwater
- ☐ organic farming
- ☐ agroforestry
- ☐ hydroponics
- ☐ aquaculture
- ☐ sustainable living

Academic Vocabulary

You will find these words in your reading and on your tests. Use the glossary to look up their definitions, if necessary.

- domestic
- periodic

Graphic Organizer

Use a graphic organizer like the one below to take notes about the four main components of the food chain.

THE FOOD CHAIN

SUN	PRODUCERS
COMPOSERS	**DECOMPOSERS**

Graphic Organizer Go to this book's Online Learning Center at **glencoe.com** to print out this graphic organizer.

Academic Standards

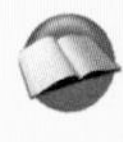

English Language Arts

NCTE 12 Use language to accomplish individual purposes.

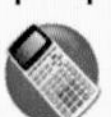

Mathematics

NCTM Data Analysis and Probability Formulate questions that can be addressed with data and collect, organize, and display relevant data to answer them.

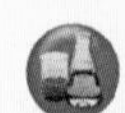

Science

NSES D Develop an understanding of energy in the earth system.

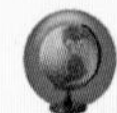

Social Studies

NCSS VIII Science, Technology, and Society Study relationships among science, technology and society.

NCTE *National Council of Teachers of English*
NCTM *National Council of Teachers of Mathematics*
NSES *National Science Education Standards*
NCSS *National Council for the Social Studies*

Ecosystems

The story of food begins with biology. All organisms, including humans, live as communities in environments. An environment can be as small as a pond or as large as a forest or ocean. An environment and its community of organisms, which all depend upon each other for survival, is called an **ecosystem**. The food we eat depends on the health of the world's ecosystems.

The Food Chain

In an ecosystem, organisms get food from other organisms and from the environment. The **food chain** is the flow of food energy from simpler to more complex organisms. The food chain is one part of a complex web of life. This web has four main components.

Sun The sun supplies the original energy for the planet in the form of light. This energy is needed to make food.

Producers Some organisms make, or produce, food. Green plants are important producers. Plants use the sun's energy to produce food for themselves.

Consumers Consumers are organisms that must eat other organisms to survive. In the ecosystem that includes humans, consumers come in three types. An **herbivore** (ˈ(h)ər-bə-ˌvor) is an organism that eats only plants. Cows and sheep are herbivores. While vegetarians are sometimes considered herbivores, the word is better used for animals whose stomachs cannot tolerate anything but plant food. A **carnivore** (ˈkär-nə-ˌvor) is an organism that feeds almost entirely on other animals. Cats, wolves, and hawks are carnivores. An **omnivore** (ˈäm-ni-ˌvor) is an organism that eats both plants and animals. Pigs, chickens, and most humans are omnivores.

Decomposers Decomposers are organisms such as bacteria and fungi that break down dead matter and return the nutrients to the environment. Decomposers are sometimes called recyclers, because they provide producers with the raw materials needed to start the cycle again.

Biodiversity

In a healthy ecosystem, all elements work together. Living organisms have a continuous set of relationships with every element within their ecosystem. If any part of an ecosystem disappears, food supplies are threatened.

To function properly, every ecosystem needs **biodiversity**, a wide variety of species. Biodiversity lessens the risk of a break in the chain, because each role is filled by more than one organism. For example, butterflies carry pollen from plant to plant so they can produce fruit. Recently, an unusually harsh winter killed many monarch butterflies in North America. With biodiversity, other butterfly species, as well as bees, could carry on the role of pollinating plants.

Natural Resources

Every ecosystem is supported by natural resources. Essential resources include land, water, and climate.

Land Nutrient-rich soil is needed for plant life, even underwater. Growing crops takes nutrients from the soil. Fertilizers can replenish nutrients, but they can also create pollution. Too much pollution can affect plants' ability to synthesize sunlight.

Water Clean water is crucial to all ecosystems, even deserts. Marine life needs clean fresh or salt water. On land, plants and animals get water from rainfall and snowmelt, which feeds lakes and rivers. Most farms and ranches are irrigated with water taken from lakes, rivers, or streams.

Climate Different plants and animals grow best in different climates. Mushrooms thrive in cool, moist surroundings. Citrus prefers heat. Brahman cattle are well adapted for the heat and humidity of their native India, while sheep prefer the cooler, wetter climates of Ireland and New Zealand. If global warming changes the climate, food production suffers.

✓ Reading Check **Identify** Which type of organism eats both plants and animals? Name an example.

The Food Supply in the United States

The earth provides resources in abundance, but these resources are not evenly distributed. The United States is fortunate to have abundant resources for raising food. Along with a temperate climate and a plentiful water supply, the U.S. has a wide expanse of good farmland and pastureland.

Food Producers

Farms, ranches, and fisheries produce much of the food you eat. Some foods may travel thousands of miles over land or sea to get to your table.

Farmers in the United States produce enough food not only for **domestic** use but also for export. A century ago, rural America was dotted with many small family farms. Today, many family farms have been absorbed into large operations.

Large farms often specialize in a single crop. Growing a single crop over a huge area is efficient, but harms biodiversity. Large operations may also apply more fertilizer and pesticides than small farms. Food shipped great distances may have reduced quality and flavor. Transportation of food also contributes to global warming.

The growth of industrial farms has contributed to a renewed interest in locally grown food. Many people are turning to farmers' markets, Community Supported Agriculture (CSA) projects, urban gardens, and other programs that make it possible to "eat local."

Food Processors

Once harvested, most food is shipped to processors to be cut, cooked, canned, dried, or frozen. When corn is shipped to a processor, for example, the kernels may be dried and ground to make cornmeal or soaked, pulverized, and treated with acids to release corn oil. When animals are processed for food, they are slaughtered and then processed into different forms of meat. Fruits and vegetables can be harvested at their peak of ripeness and frozen at that level of quality.

One important role of processing is to keep perishable foods from spoiling. Processing makes food **shelf-stable**, able to be stored at room temperature for weeks or months in the original, unopened containers. Such foods also have a longer **shelf life**, the length of time food holds its flavor and quality.

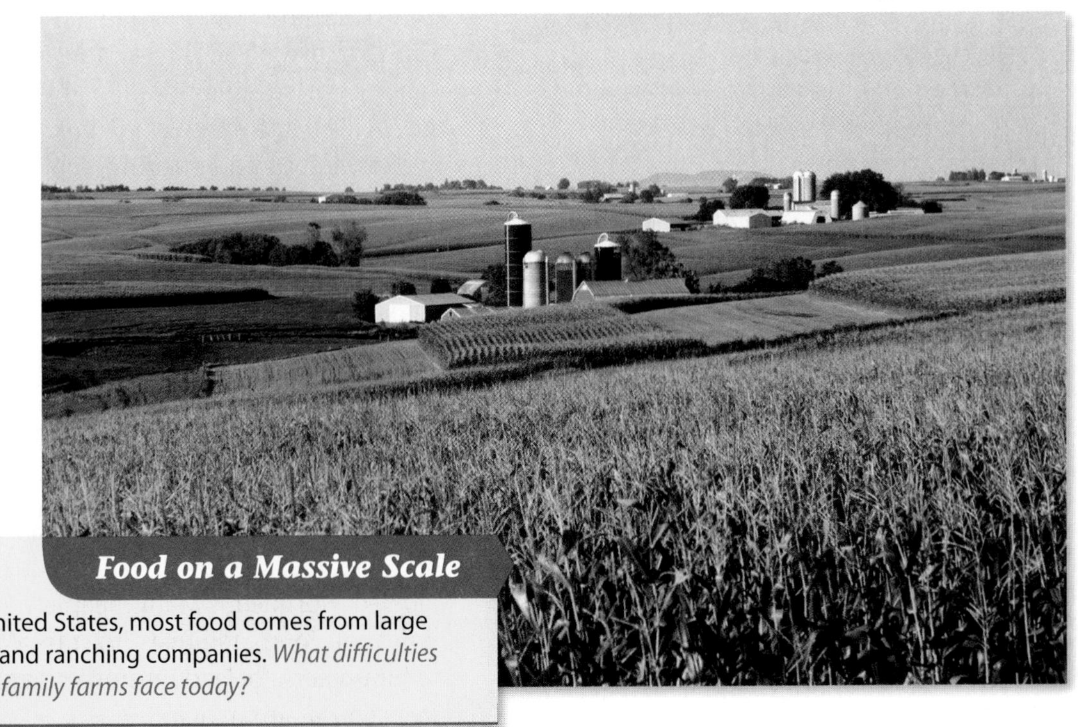

Food on a Massive Scale

In the United States, most food comes from large farming and ranching companies. *What difficulties do small family farms face today?*

Five common preservation processes are:

Canning Canning seals food in airtight metal or glass containers, which are then heated to destroy microorganisms that could cause spoilage or illness. Fruits, vegetables, legumes, meat, poultry, fish, and juices are examples of foods that are canned.

Freezing Foods are frozen quickly to slow the growth of any harmful organisms. Fruits and vegetables are often frozen shortly after picking. Meat, poultry, and fish are frozen to preserve their freshness until they are ready to be prepared. Many convenience foods come in frozen form.

Curing Salt, spices, sugar, and sodium nitrite are added when foods are cured. Nitrites prevent meat from turning grey. Curing is used to create products such as salami, pickles, sauerkraut, and kimchi. Many cured foods are high in sodium.

Drying Drying removes moisture from food, inhibiting the growth of harmful organisms. Grains, beans, milk, and fruit are often dried. Many dried foods require the addition of water during their preparation.

Freeze-Drying Freeze-drying first freezes and then dries food. This process retains more flavor, texture, and nutrients than drying alone. Freeze-drying is used to make instant coffee and dried soup mixes.

Controlled Atmosphere Storage This technique extends shelf life by holding foods in a cold area with specific amounts of nitrogen, oxygen, and carbon dioxide. Humidity and temperature are carefully regulated, inhibiting the growth of harmful organisms. It is especially useful for fruits.

TECHNOLOGY FOR TOMORROW

New Ways with Waste

Just as you throw out banana peels and egg shells, food makers also deal with inedible food parts. This waste poses an economic cost to food makers and an environmental cost to the planet. Researchers are refining a technology that includes nanofiltration and crystallization. The process purifies waste products to recover higher quality components. For example, to make cheese, the liquid part of milk is drained off. Some is powdered and sold for gravy and hot cocoa mixes, but it's often cheaper to throw it out. The new technology extracts a finer-grade powder that has medicinal value. The same technology is already used to recover wastewater left from food manufacturing. It may also save costly natural colors, flavors, and nutrients usually lost in processing sugars, fruits, and vegetables.

Investigate Now, natural grape flavoring is expensive and hard to come by. If this technology becomes widespread, what might the impact on grape growers be? On consumers?

NCSS VIII Science, Technology, and Society
Study relationships among science, technology, and society.

Food Additives

Have you ever wondered how jellybeans get their brilliant colors? Food additives are the answer. A **food additive** is a substance added to food for a specific reason during processing. Some additives have natural sources. Others are chemicals created in laboratories. The U.S. Food and Drug Administration monitors the safe use of additives. You can find information on specific additives by checking the FDA's Web site at www.fda.gov.

Besides adding coloring, food additives are frequently used for these five reasons:

Adding Flavoring Natural and artificial flavors, including sweeteners, enhance food's taste. Many packaged foods and beverages contain some sort of added flavoring. Try reading the labels of the foods you have on hand at home to see how many contain added flavors.

Improving Nutrition Vitamins and minerals are added to many foods, such as milk, juice, and breakfast cereal. These foods are often labeled "fortified." Many people rely on these types of food additives to meet their daily requirements for certain nutrients like vitamin D, calcium, and niacin.

Increasing Shelf Life Some additives delay spoilage. These are also known as preservatives. Sulfur dioxide, for example, is a preservative that keeps dried fruit from turning brown. Foods without preservatives must be consumed more quickly than those with them.

Maintaining Texture Additives are used to make the texture of processed food more appealing. Substances such as emulsifiers, stabilizers and thickeners are all added to make foods smooth, creamy, or spreadable. A chemical is even added to some pickles to keep them crisp after canning.

Helping Foods Age Many foods, including cheese, meats, and flour, are aged before they are sold. Additives can speed the aging process. Foods that are aged can be desirable because aging lends them a distinct flavor or texture.

Food additives are not new. Salts and spices have been used to cure meats for thousands of years. The use of artificial additives, however, has increased. Some people believe that added chemicals are unnecessary and possibly harmful. As a result, some food processors make products that are free of chemical additives.

Figure 3.1 Food Distribution Cycle

Apples on a Journey Foods pass through several stages before reaching a location where you can buy products and take them home for your table. ***What are some factors that can affect the price of applesauce?***

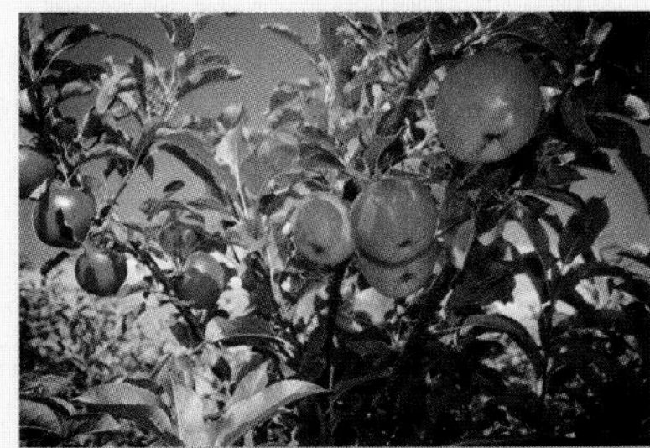

Ripe for the Picking
Apple growers try to wait until fruits are near or at their peak of ripeness before picking them. This ensures that the apple trees will bear as much fruit as possible. Once picked, apples are transported to a factory.

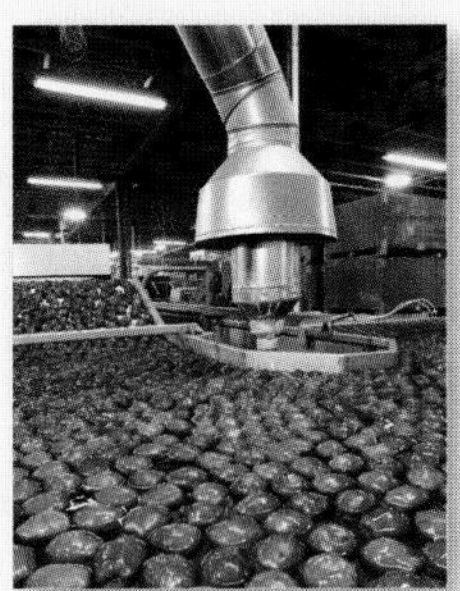

Processed and Packaged
At the factory, apples are cleaned. They may also be packaged, canned or crushed for applesauce. Additives may be added to increase the shelf life of packaged apple products. From there, apples and apple products are transported to grocery stores and supermarkets.

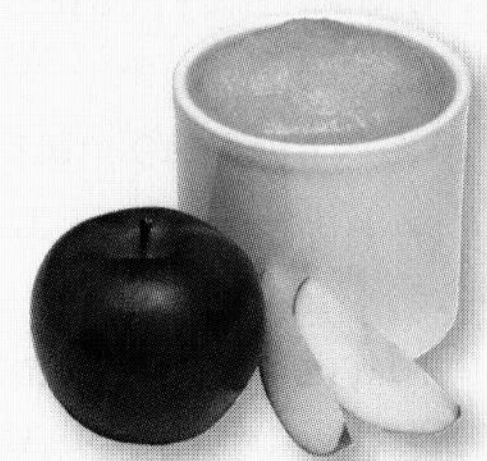

Time to Eat!
Once at the store, apple products may remain on shelves for months before being purchased and brought home where they may be consumed. Fresh apples kept in a refrigerator can last for weeks. Packaged apple products can last for months.

Packaging

Packaging, or putting food in containers, is the final step in processing. Containers help preserve the quality, shape, and appearance of food. They also make it easy to ship large quantities of a product. Familiar packaging materials include paper, plastic, glass, aluminum, and lightweight steel. Packaging methods are continually updated, allowing food manufacturers and processors to offer new products. Some containers allow a product to remain on a shelf for long periods of time.

Food Distributors

Food is shipped by truck, train, and plane to distribution centers throughout the world. Distribution centers are huge warehouses with controlled temperatures. **Figure 3.1** on page 33 shows a food distribution cycle. From here, food takes the last leg of its journey, to the store where you buy it.

Some distributors work regionally, while others work nationally or internationally. Some specialize in baked goods, meats, frozen foods, or gourmet items. Some distribution centers are owned by supermarket companies. Others are separate businesses that contract out space to different food sellers.

Food Retailers

Distributors ship food to retailers, which sell food directly to you. Supermarkets are the most popular food retailers in the United States. Specialty shops, neighborhood markets, farmer's markets and produce stands are smaller food retailers.

Food processors and manufacturers constantly develop new products in an effort to win consumers. Some stores review as many as 100 new products a week. Because shelf space is limited, however, only the most promising items are accepted. New foods that do not sell well are pulled from the shelves.

✓ Reading Check **List** Name five functions of food additives.

Global Food Problems

Some nations enjoy an abundant food supply, but other nations do not. In an **industrialized nation**, a country with a developed economy and a high standard of living, a sophisticated food industry provides people with a varied and nutritious diet. Industrialized nations that cannot produce enough food, such as Japan, Kuwait, and Switzerland, can afford to import it.

In developing nations, the situation is different. **Developing nations** are countries that are not yet industrialized or that are just beginning that process. People in these countries face many obstacles to feeding themselves and their families.

Imagine that one out of every seven people you know has only one meager meal on a good day and eats nothing for days at a time. That is the reality for about 15 percent of the world's population, some 800 million people. The most severe form of a food shortage is **famine**, which can last for months or years and cause thousands of deaths. Unfortunately, some people in industrialized countries face hunger and poverty too.

Global hunger has many complex causes, including economics, poor use of resources, rapid population growth, and political conflicts.

Economics

In developing countries, many people are too poor to buy food. Many families raise their own food on a small plot of land, a practice known as **subsistence farming**. Families live on what they can produce. They usually have a limited food supply with little variety and poor nutrition.

Some farmers accumulate enough land to grow cash crops—crops they can sell. However, since food prices change frequently, many cash-crop farmers cannot depend on a steady income.

In many countries, governments and utility companies cannot provide the services needed for a reliable food supply. Imagine trying to run a food processing plant in a city where the electricity shuts down for a few hours every day.

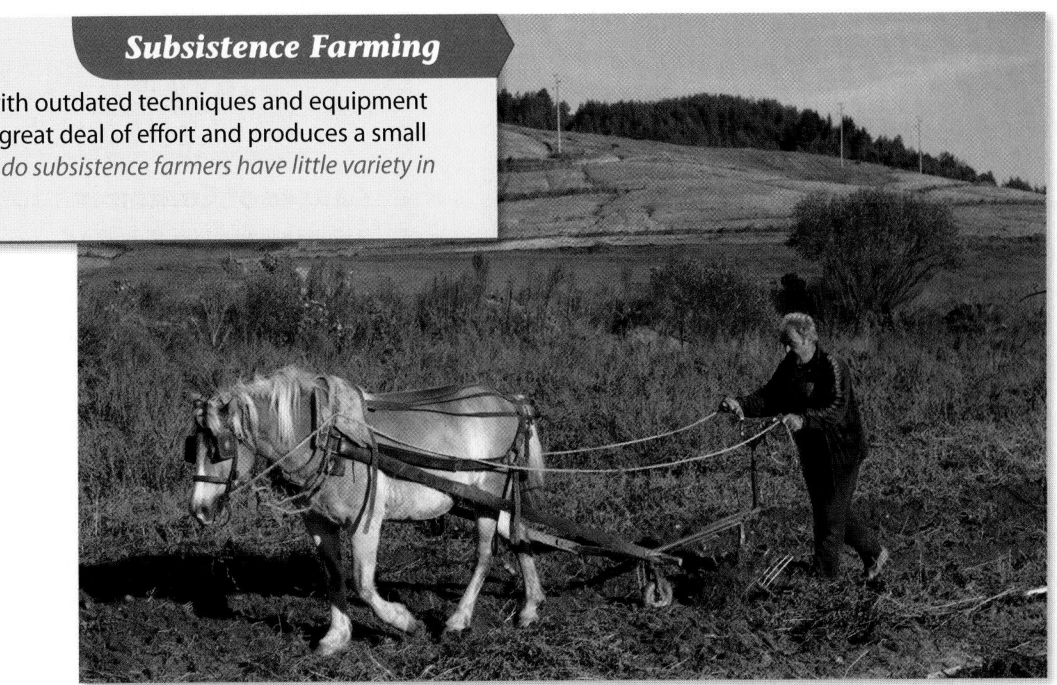

Subsistence Farming

Farming with outdated techniques and equipment requires a great deal of effort and produces a small yield. *Why do subsistence farmers have little variety in their diet?*

Inefficient Methods

Subsistence farming makes use of ancient methods. Animals supply power. Farm tools are simple. Food production is low. Modern equipment and methods are costly, however, and not always suited to the crops and conditions.

Developing countries also lack modern food storage facilities. Food is stored unprotected, where it can be damaged by animals, insects, and mildew. Refrigeration may be unavailable, so dairy foods, fresh produce, and meat spoil quickly.

Good roads are rare in developing nations, especially in the countryside. Bicycles and donkey carts are more common than trucks. City dwellers may have enough to eat, while villagers a few miles away are struggling. In times of famine, poor distribution keeps food aid from reaching starving people.

Natural Disasters

A natural disaster can cripple a region's food supply for years. A drought, an unusually long period without rain, kills crops and animals. Floods and hurricanes wash away soil and roads. In areas with poor food production and distribution systems, a natural disaster can bring about famine and starvation.

Rapid Population Growth

The world population is growing steadily and will reach nine billion by 2050. The most rapid population growth is in developing countries. As populations grow, so does the demand for food. Yet more land is taken for housing, leaving less land for farming. The population in many developing nations is too large for the food supply.

Fuel Shortages

Most food must be cooked to be eaten, so cooking fuel is essential. In developing countries, wood is the main fuel source. In many areas, the wood supply is dwindling as forests are cut for farming or construction. Gathering enough wood for a day's meal can mean walking for half a day. Without trees and shrubs for fuel, people use dung, dried animal manure. Dung produces a lot of smoke but little heat.

Conflict and Politics

Armed conflict can devastate food supplies. Animals are killed and crops are destroyed. Farmers are driven from their land, and fighting disrupts food distribution.

Fighting can disrupt planting and harvesting seasons. Seed for the following season may be destroyed. Workers who help with harvest may be driven away.

To escape the danger, many people flee to nearby regions. Thousands of refugees stream into an area, where the local food supply cannot support the surge in population. Everyone suffers.

Food is also used as a political weapon, to punish opponents or reward supporters. A ruling party may limit food distribution only to urban areas. This forces people to leave rural homes, which are then given to political allies. Efforts by relief agencies like the Red Cross, may be thwarted by ruling governments or warlords. Food aid may be stolen and sold on the black market, never reaching those in need. In recent decades, such tactics have left millions starving in Uganda, Rwanda, Zimbabwe, and Congo in Africa and Bosnia in southeastern Europe.

✓ **Reading Check** **Contrast** What is the difference between industrialized nations and developing nations?

Causes of Contamination

Pollution is a serious threat to the world's water supply. Even in industrialized countries with sanitation systems and water treatment plants, pollution is a problem. Rainwater carries oil, gasoline, and garden chemicals from streets and lawns into storm sewers. Animal waste from farms washes into streams. Factories release chemicals into rivers and the air, causing acid rain. In developing countries, more than two billion people have no sanitary system. Toxic chemicals and wastewater are dumped into rivers and lakes, which feed wells and streams where people draw water. Every year, contaminated water kills 1.4 million children under age five.

What Would You Do? You are helping your family with household chores. You mop the floor using a bucket full of strong cleaner. When you are done mopping, what should you do with the cleaner remaining in the bucket? Should you pour it down a sink drain, outside on the grass, into the gutter, or elsewhere?

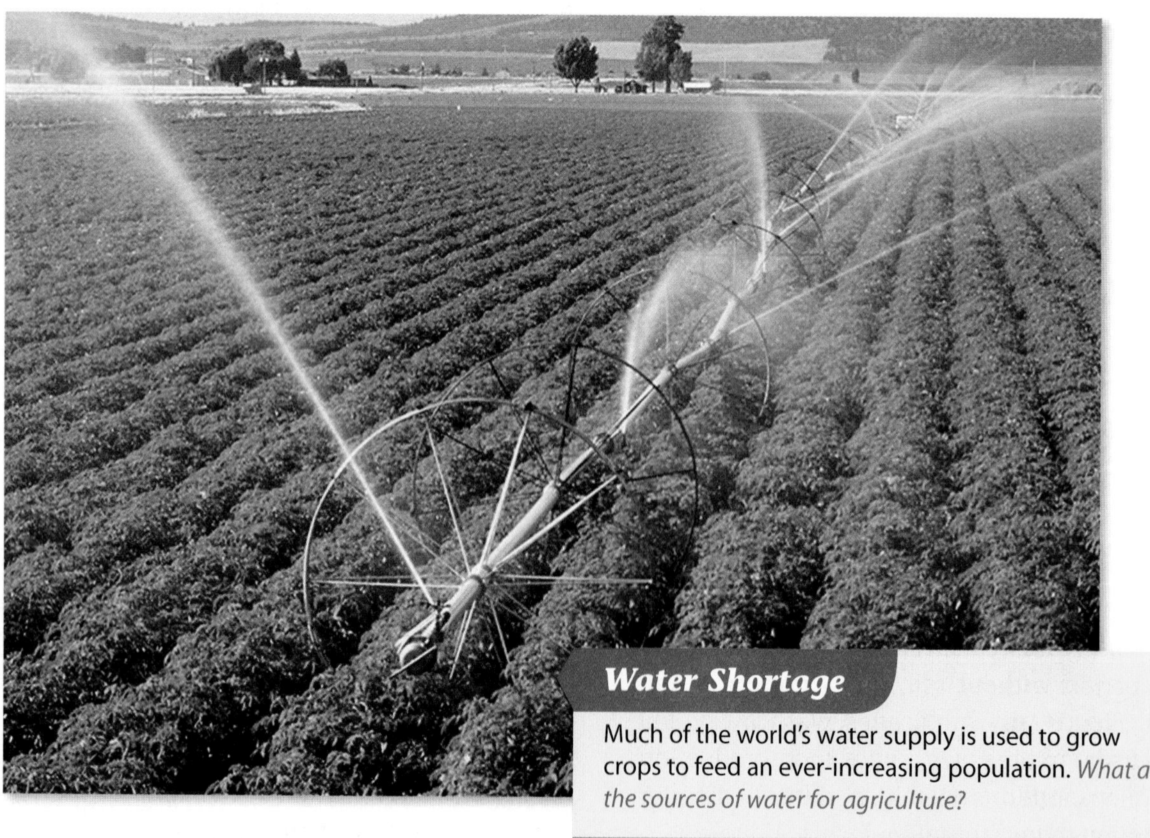

Water Shortage

Much of the world's water supply is used to grow crops to feed an ever-increasing population. *What are the sources of water for agriculture?*

Global Water Problems

Water covers three-fourths of the earth's surface. Ninety-eight percent of it is salt water, which is unusable for humans, crops, and farm animals. Seventy-five percent of the earth's fresh water is frozen in the polar regions. Of the total water on this planet, less than one percent is available for human needs.

Fresh water flows in lakes, rivers, and streams. **Groundwater** is water beneath the earth's surface, in the cracks and spaces between rocks and sediment. Groundwater is brought to the surface by digging wells.

Some areas of the earth have ample water, such as the land along the Amazon River in South America and around the Great Lakes in North America. Many other areas experience **periodic** or even permanent drought.

The earth's growing population is straining its water supply. Today, one billion people around the world lack access to clean water. About 70 percent of the world's fresh water is now used for agriculture. As populations grow, however, urban demands for water are expected to exceed rural ones.

✓ **Reading Check** **Identify** What percentage of the planet's water supply is available for human use?

Solutions to Global Food Problems

Oxfam International, the Food and Agriculture Organization of the United Nations and other organizations work in villages around the world to improve farming methods and provide access to clean water. Many organizations now offer microloans to farmers and other entrepreneurs to buy equipment and start businesses. People who once depended on food aid are starting bakeries, organizing fishing cooperatives, and growing cash crops. Farmers across the world are also creating seed banks of crops native to their region to preserve biodiversity.

Increase Food Supplies

To feed the world, we must create more food with the resources we have. Science can provide some solutions. For example, researchers are developing plant varieties that can resist disease and pests and tolerate drought and poor soil. Engineers have designed an irrigation system that uses a foot-powered pump to water a family garden—more efficient than hauling water in buckets. Organic and alternative farming methods can also help by keeping the earth healthy and fertile for future generations.

Organic Food Production

Organic farming is a way of farming that protects the environment and does not use pesticides or artificial fertilizers. Soil is fertilized with compost and animal manure rather than chemicals. Organically raised animals are treated more humanely and fed healthful feed that is free of chemicals and drugs. Farmers use an ecological approach to pest management and avoid pesticides.

Alternative Farming Methods The goal of alternative farming is to produce more food on less land and with less harm to the environment.

Agroforestry is an ancient practice of raising shade-loving crops, such as mushrooms and cocoa, under the shelter of trees. The trees control erosion, improve the soil, and preserve forest habitats. Some trees also provide lumber, oils, and extracts for medicine. Shade-grown coffee is one popular product of agroforestry.

Hydroponics (ˈhi-drə-ˈpä-niks) is growing plants without soil. Plants are grown in water or a lightweight medium such as coir or rockwool. They are fed with nutrient-enriched water. Hydroponic crops are usually grown in glass greenhouses.

Aquaculture is a method of raising seafood in enclosed areas of water. Fish farms may be ponds or enclosed areas of ocean. Aquaculture creates a large amount of food in a small area. It can also help to protect wild fish populations from overfishing. Unfortunately, aquaculture also generates a great deal of animal waste, which pollutes rivers and oceans.

Develop Alternative Fuel Sources

Most of the world's energy comes from fossil fuels such as oil, coal, and gas, which are nonrenewable. Alternative energy—from wind, water, and sun—offers the best hope for the future.

Solar Energy Solar power is renewable, non-polluting, and practical. Solar panels can be installed on almost any surface. Solar energy has countless uses. Solar water heaters, lights, and water purifiers are used around the world. Solar cookers, made from cardboard and aluminum, are inexpensive, versatile, and good for the environment.

Wind Power Wind is another source of power. Giant windmills and turbines turn with the wind and convert this motion into electricity. U.S. farmers and other landowners who install turbines are paid by their utility company for any excess electricity they produce.

Practice Sustainable Living

Solving global food and water problems will require a basic change in the way we live. If everyone lived like the average American, we would need six planets to have enough resources to go around! The alternative is **sustainable living**, making life choices to meet your own needs while still protecting the environment. When you live sustainably, you act with concern for the needs and quality of life of all people.

Simple steps can help you live sustainably. For example, you could buy locally grown foods, which require fewer preservatives to stay fresh and less fuel to transport. You could repair appliances and clothes rather than buying new ones. You can bike to school rather than taking a car, using less gas and creating no pollution. You could install low-flow aerators in all the sinks in your home to reduce water waste. Everyday choices like these can help to ensure that future generations can count on the same resources we enjoy today.

Light and Healthy Recipe

Chef's Salad

With protein and fiber, this salad makes a filling, nutritious lunch.

Ingredients

2 heads	Iceberg or romaine lettuce
2	Tomatoes, cut into quarters
½ cup	Shredded carrots
1	Cucumber, sliced
4 Tbsp.	Red wine vinegar
8 Tbsp.	Olive oil
1 Tbsp.	Chopped fresh parsley
2	Hard-boiled eggs, cut into quarters
½ pound	Sliced or cubed low-sodium turkey breast
4 oz	Sliced or cubed lowfat cheddar cheese

Directions

1. Chop the lettuce into bite-size squares and put into a large bowl with the tomatoes, carrots and cucumber slices.
2. In a separate mixing bowl, combine the vinegar, olive oil, and parsley. Pour the dressing over the salad and toss gently.
3. Divide the salad equally into four bowls. Top each with the quartered eggs, turkey and cheese.

Yield 4 servings

Nutrition Analysis per Serving

■ Calories	351
■ Total fat	22 g
Saturated fat	5 g
Cholesterol	141 mg
■ Sodium	607 mg
■ Carbohydrate	15 g
Dietary fiber	5 g
Sugars	9 g
■ Protein	24 g

CHAPTER 3 Review & Applications

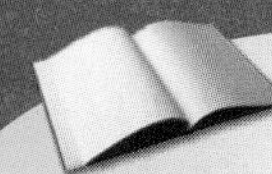

After You Read

Chapter Summary

Our food supply depends on the health of the world's ecosystems. Different components of the food chain work in harmony with natural resources to comprise a healthy ecosystem. In the United States, food is abundant. Food problems caused by economics, insufficient farming methods, natural disasters, population growth, fuel shortages, and political conflicts affect many people worldwide. Water contamination is also a global issue. To feed the world, we must create more food with the resources we have.

Content and Academic Vocabulary Review

1. Arrange the content and academic vocabulary words into groups of related words. Explain why you grouped the words together.

Content Vocabulary

- ecosystem (p. 30)
- food chain (p. 30)
- herbivore (p. 30)
- carnivore (p. 30)
- omnivore (p. 30)
- biodiversity (p. 30)
- shelf-stable (p. 31)
- shelf life (p. 31)
- food additive (p. 32)
- industrialized nation (p. 34)
- developing nation (p. 34)
- famine (p. 34)
- subsistence farming (p. 34)
- groundwater (p. 37)
- organic farming (p. 37)
- agroforestry (p. 37)
- hydroponics (p. 37)
- aquaculture (p. 37)
- sustainable living (p. 38)

Academic Vocabulary

- domestic (p. 31)
- periodic (p. 37)

Review Key Concepts

2. **Explain** ecosystems and their relationship to food.
3. **Describe** the main sources of the U.S. food supply and the steps food takes from farm to consumption.
4. **Identify** global food problems and explain their causes.
5. **Explain** global water problems.
6. **Describe** solutions to global food problems.

Critical Thinking

7. **Predict** what would happen to the food supply if several plant species within an ecosystem became extinct.
8. **Evaluate** this situation. Your garden produces an abundant supply of strawberries, and you cannot use the entire harvest right away. What would you do to prevent waste and ensure you could enjoy them later?
9. **Explain** the consequences to the food supply if a war in a developing nation sends refugees into a nearby country.
10. **Explain** why fuel is a necessary resource for the food supply.

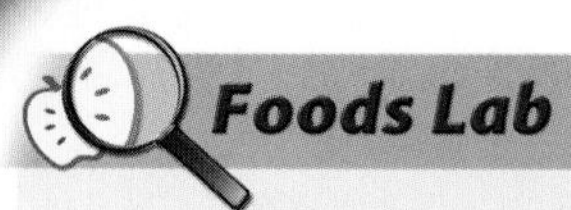

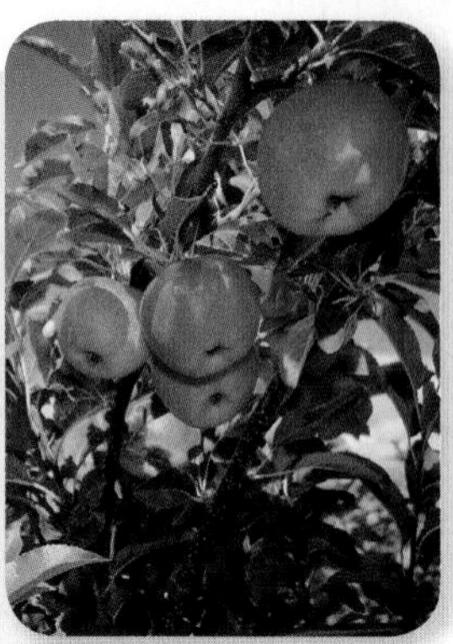

11. Comparing Food Forms The U.S. food supply is so abundant that we can often choose to buy a food in either its fresh or its processed form.

Procedure Compare a fresh fruit or vegetable with one of its processed forms. Prepare each food as needed for serving. Evaluate appearance, taste, texture, and amount of preparation required.

Analysis Write a persuasive paragraph in which you convince your reader that one form is better than the other. Support your opinion with specific reasons relating to taste, texture, preparation, and usefulness.

HEALTHFUL CHOICES

12. Health on the Go Anna likes to take prepackaged energy bars along when she goes on day hikes. At the grocery store, Anna can buy three of her favorite energy bars for $2.50. However, a three-pound bag of apples is on sale for $2. What is the better choice for Anna? What factors other than cost would be important to Anna? What would be your own preference? Write a paragraph explaining your answers.

TECH Connection

13. Spread the Message Research more about ways to practice sustainable living. Using word processing software, write a list of five specific suggestions for sustainable living. Include at least one thing you personally could do. Explain your suggestions and the possible challenges to putting them into practice. Give your list a title and a brief introduction. If possible, e-mail the information to your teacher.

Real-World Skills

Problem-Solving Skills

14. Develop Strategies for Sustainable Living Wanda recently learned about sustainable living and got excited about the idea. Wanda's mother insists on continuing to do all her shopping at the local supermarket where she has shopped for years because it is close and convenient. What can Wanda do?

Interpersonal and Collaborative Skills

15. Research Relief Follow your teacher's instructions to form groups. Work together to research one food relief organization that supplies food to people in need. Give a presentation about the organization to your classmates.

Financial Literacy

16. Evaluate Costs Josie is planning to make a peach pie. She can use fresh, canned, or frozen peaches. Fresh peaches are $3.50 a pound. A 15-ounce can of peaches costs $2.49. Frozen peaches are $2.99 per 16-ounce package. Which is the best value?

Academic Skills

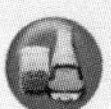

Food Science

17. Solar Energy Because solar energy uses no fuel, it is a form of sustainable living. Create sun tea to see solar energy in action.

Procedure Fill a 1-gallon glass jar with fresh cold water. Add 6–8 tea bags, and close the lid tightly. Place the jar outside in the direct sunlight for at least 4 hours. Remove the tea bags, and sweeten with sugar or honey. Serve over ice, or refrigerate for the next day.

Analysis What caused the water to change color? How is tea usually made? How was this method different? Write your answers in a paragraph.

NSES D Develop an understanding of energy in the earth system.

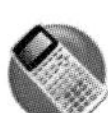

Mathematics

18. Graph and Analyze Population Trends Total world population was estimated to reach 5 billion in 1985 and 6 billion in 2000. Experts predict that global population levels will continue to grow, hitting 7 billion in 2015, 8 billion in 2030, and 9 billion in 2050. Draw a line graph showing these past and future population figures.

Math Concept **Line Graphs** A line graph can be used to display changes in data over time by showing a series of data points connected by lines.

Starting Hint Label the horizontal axis with years (use a five-year scale from 1985 to 2050) and the vertical axis with population in billions. Draw a point for each year for which you have data, and connect those points with a line.

NCTM Data Analysis and Probability Formulate questions that can be addressed with data and collect, organize, and display relevant data to answer them.

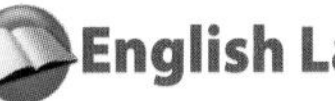

English Language Arts

19. Write a Song Write an educational song about the four main components of the food chain: the sun, producers, consumers, and decomposers. Write four verses, one each about the four different components: the sun, producers, consumers, and decomposers. Write one chorus about the food chain, which will be repeated between the verses. You can set your song to a melody you already know, or create a new one.

NCTE 12 Use language to accomplish individual purposes.

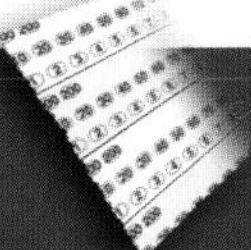

STANDARDIZED TEST PRACTICE

ANALOGY

Read the pairs of terms. Then choose the best word to pair with the term *food*.

20. sun : plants
soil : crops
snowmelt : lakes
food : ________

a. organic
b. people
c. biodiversity
d. water

Test-Taking Tip Analogies establish relationships between terms. When you look at the three pairs of terms listed here, identify the relationship that is common to all of them. Then try matching each possible answer with the term *food*. The one that establishes the same type of relationship as the other terms is correct.

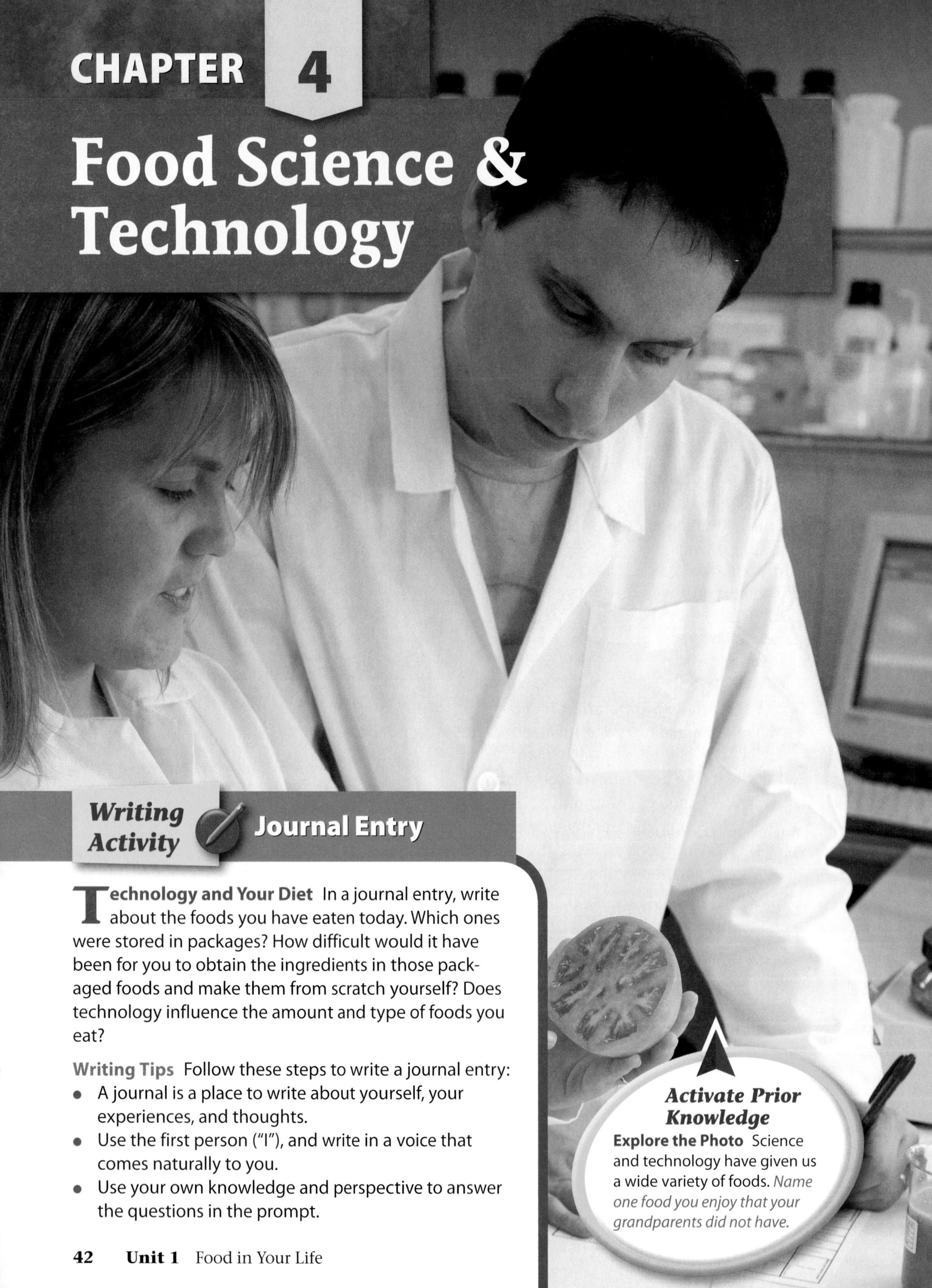

CHAPTER 4

Food Science & Technology

Writing Activity: Journal Entry

Technology and Your Diet In a journal entry, write about the foods you have eaten today. Which ones were stored in packages? How difficult would it have been for you to obtain the ingredients in those packaged foods and make them from scratch yourself? Does technology influence the amount and type of foods you eat?

Writing Tips Follow these steps to write a journal entry:

- A journal is a place to write about yourself, your experiences, and thoughts.
- Use the first person ("I"), and write in a voice that comes naturally to you.
- Use your own knowledge and perspective to answer the questions in the prompt.

Activate Prior Knowledge

Explore the Photo Science and technology have given us a wide variety of foods. *Name one food you enjoy that your grandparents did not have.*

Reading Guide

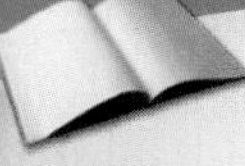

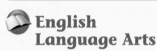

Before You Read

Preview Make a list of all the foods you consume on an average day. Circle all of those that you believe are influenced by science or technology. As you read through the chapter, verify whether you were correct.

Read to Learn

Key Concepts

- **Explain** the relationship between science and technology.
- **Explain** five ways technology affects food.
- **Identify** three ways science improves health.
- **Name** three ways cooks use technology in meal production.

Main Idea

Science and technology influence the types of foods we eat, increase the health benefits we obtain from our food, and make meal preparation easier.

Content Vocabulary

You will find definitions for these words in the glossary at the back of this book.

- ☐ science
- ☐ technology
- ☐ food science
- ☐ manufactured food
- ☐ analogs
- ☐ formed products
- ☐ MAP packaging
- ☐ aseptic packages
- ☐ retort pouches
- ☐ genetic engineering
- ☐ clone
- ☐ enrichment
- ☐ fortification
- ☐ functional foods
- ☐ ergonomics

Academic Vocabulary

You will find these words in your reading and on your tests. Use the glossary to look up their definitions if necessary.

- accelerate
- trait

Graphic Organizer

Use a graphic organizer like the one below to take notes about the three categories of functional foods.

Natural Foods	Enhanced Foods	Foods Created by Science

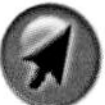

Graphic Organizer Go to this book's Online Learning Center at **glencoe.com** to print out this graphic organizer.

Academic Standards

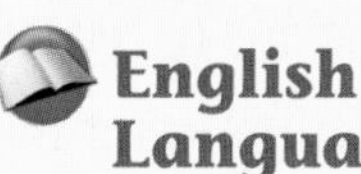

English Language Arts

NCTE 12 Use language for individual purposes.

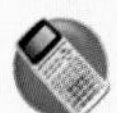

Mathematics

NCTM Data Analysis and Probability Select and use appropriate statistical methods to analyze data.

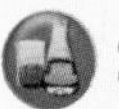

Science

NSES F Develop understanding of science and technology in local, national and global challenges.

NSES G Develop understanding of science as human endeavor.

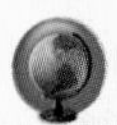

Social Studies

NCSS VIII A Identify and describe both current and historical examples of the interaction and interdependence of science, technology, and society in a variety of cultural settings.

NCTE *National Council of Teachers of English*
NCTM *National Council of Teachers of Mathematics*
NSES *National Science Education Standards*
NCSS *National Council for the Social Studies*

The Role of Science and Technology

Science and technology play an important role in every aspect of food, from farming through cooking. **Science** is the study of the physical world. **Technology** is the practical application of scientific knowledge. It is science in action. The microwave oven, for example, is a technology based on discoveries in the science of physics.

What Is Food Science?

Food is so important that there is an entire science devoted to it—food science. **Food science** is the study of all aspects of food, including processing, storage, and preparation. Food science is an applied science. An applied science uses the natural sciences, such as biology, chemistry, and physics, to solve practical problems. Food scientists help develop new products and keep the food supply safe.

Be a *Smart Consumer*

Food from a Distance

Many of the foods you find on supermarket shelves have traveled hundreds, if not thousands, of miles to get there. Once food growers and manufacturers finish processing foods, they must be distributed to retail stores where consumers can buy them. Ships, planes, trains, and trucks—all of which rely on polluting fuels—help with this task. In contrast, most of the foods you find at a community farmers market have been grown and processed nearby. Because local growers spend little in distribution costs, their crops may be more affordable than those that come from far away. Buying locally grown foods places less strain on both the environment and the pocketbook.

Challenge List the foods in your last meal. Visit the supermarket and find out where each food came from. How many total miles did your meal travel to get to your plate? Write one paragraph explaining your findings.

What Is Food Technology?

From food science comes food technology—tools and techniques that help with food production, processing, storage, and preparation. For example, food scientists study why food spoils and then develop technologies such as freeze-drying and controlled atmosphere storage to keep food fresh.

✓ **Reading Check** **Define** What is the difference between science and technology?

Technology Advances in Food History

Technology is not new. Technological advances have occurred throughout human history. Half a million years ago, people discovered that certain foods were more edible when held over a fire for a while—in other words, when they were cooked. Cooking over fire was the very first food technology.

Early Farming Advances

Throughout history, most farmers relied on simple tools and techniques such as animal power, human labor, and handmade tools. Advances in technology slowly began to make farming more efficient. In the eighteenth century, for example, the cotton gin made it easier to separate cotton fibers from the seeds. In the nineteenth century, the mechanical reaper made grain harvesting much faster.

Modern Advances

The pace of discovery in science and technology sped up dramatically in the twentieth century. Today, a single piece of machinery does the planting or harvesting work of hundreds of farmhands. On a wheat field in the spring, a machine called a planter drops hundreds of pounds of seed in rows at the precise depth and spacing. At harvest time, a huge combine (ˈkäm-ˌbīn) rolls up and down the field picking, threshing, and cleaning the grain. A grain elevator system measures the yield from each acre.

The pace of technological progress continues to **accelerate**, or speed up. New techniques are constantly being developed. Technology affects the way food is produced, processed, distributed, packaged, and transported.

Production

Modern advances are helping to make food production more efficient. For example, climatologists are better able to predict weather patterns, which help farmers manage their fields better. Veterinarians use new vaccines and antibiotics to protect livestock from diseases that once wiped out entire herds.

Processing and Distribution

A typical supermarket carries more than 50,000 different items. Food scientists are helping food manufacturers create new foods that meet the demand for variety. Scientists are also helping to improve existing foods by making them more nutritious or more shelf-stable.

Chances are good that you ate something today that did not even exist when your grandparents were your age. Fat-free, low-calorie, and flavored foods are relatively new products of technology. Perhaps you ate a **manufactured food**, a product developed as a substitute for another food. Manufactured foods increase choices for people on restricted diets or restricted incomes. Analogs, formed products, and egg substitutes are popular manufactured foods.

Analogs **Analogs** (ˈa-nə-ˌlȯgs) are foods made to imitate other foods. Some meat and dairy analogs are made from a vegetable protein, processed to replace animal-derived products. They may contain textured soy protein (TSP), tofu, vegetables, or grains. They can be made into meatless patties, bacon-flavored breakfast links, and imitation cheese.

Nutrition Check

Special Foods for Special Diets

Many people are on restricted diets for health reasons, such as to control their cholesterol or sodium levels. Others may be following a doctor's orders to decrease the amount of animal fats they consume. Still others may be allergic to dairy products. Some people are on restricted diets by choice. For example, vegetarians and vegans may choose to eliminate some or all animal products from their diets for ethical reasons. Manufactured foods may be valuable for all of these people.

Think About It Since his heart attack, Joseph has stuck to a low-cholesterol, meat-free diet. How might it be possible for Joseph to enjoy a breakfast of eggs and sausage links?

Formed Products Foods made from an inexpensive source and processed to imitate a more expensive food are called **formed products**. Surimi (su̇-ˈrē-mē), for example, is white fish flavored and shaped to resemble lobster or crab.

Egg Substitutes These are made from egg white and other ingredients. Because they have no yolks, they have little or no fat or cholesterol. People who cannot eat whole eggs for health reasons may buy egg substitutes.

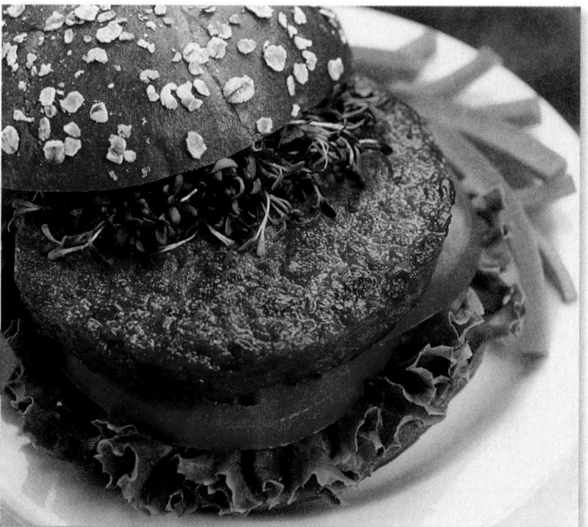

Creative Imitations

When is a food not what it appears to be? When the food is an analog. *Why might people choose analogs instead of the foods they imitate?*

Packaging

Packaging preserves quality and safety and adds convenience. Three examples of packaging methods in use today are shown in **Figure 4.1**.

Modified Atmosphere Packaging (MAP) **MAP packaging** uses carbon dioxide, oxygen, and nitrogen to slow bacterial growth. The ratio of gases depends on the product. Food retains quality without being subjected to damaging heat, as with canning. With MAP, cooked meats and fresh pasta keep in a refrigerator for weeks.

Aseptic Packages Also called "juice boxes," **aseptic packages** ((ˌ)ā-ˈsep-tik) consist of layers of plastic, paperboard, and aluminum foil. The food and package are sterilized separately and rapidly. The food is then packaged under sterile conditions. Aseptic packaging is used for many products, including liquids, cereals, grains, and other dry goods.

Retort Pouches **Retort pouches** are flexible packages made of aluminum foil and plastic film. Food is placed in the pouch and both are heat-processed. Retort pouches can store foods after opening. Some are adapted for use in the microwave.

Shrink-Wrap Packaging and Quick-Freezing Many kinds of plastic are used to package foods such as cheese, meat, and produce. Cheese and meat often come in shrink-wrapped plastic packages. Food is placed in the package and then the plastic is shrunk around the product to remove the surrounding air. Many fresh vegetables and prepared foods now come in plastic trays that can go directly in the microwave or conventional oven.

Quick-freezing, or flash freezing, preserves food by exposing it to temperatures below –238 °F (–150 °C). This process keeps foods fresher than standard freezing.

Transportation

Transportation and packaging technology combine to bring you foods from around the world. Foods can travel 1,000 miles or more from farm to store. Resources and labor are required to transport food. Planes, trains, trucks and other vehicles rely on fuel. Workers are needed to operate the different modes of transportation, and to load and unload product. Due to the combination of technology, resources, and labor, people now have access to a variety of foods that were once out of reach.

Figure 4.1 **Packaging Technology**

Packaging Methods The right kind of packaging can help foods retain their freshness, flavor, and nutrients. ***Which of these packaging methods is often used for cereals and grains?***

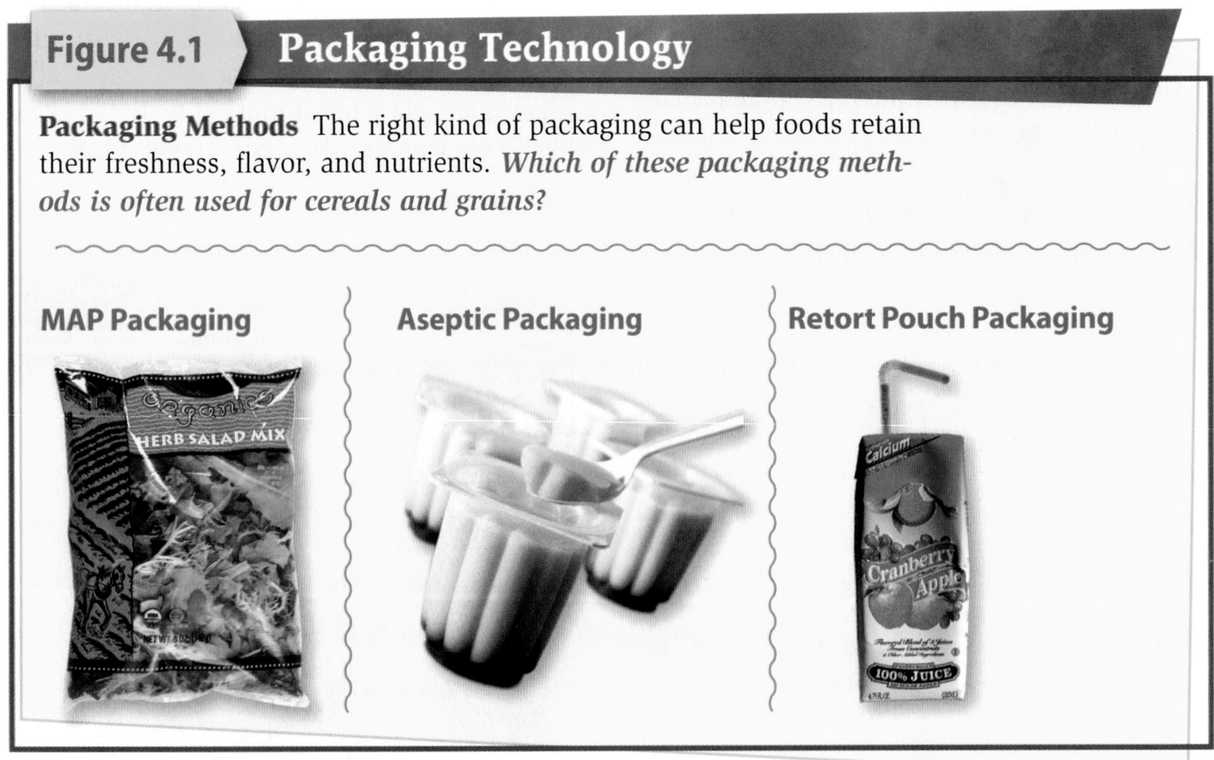

Genetic Engineering

Through **genetic engineering**, genes are removed from one organism, such as a plant, animal, or microorganism, and transferred to another organism. Plants and animals that are genetically engineered are known as genetically modified organisms (GMOs).

Genetic engineering can give plants and animals a **trait**, or characteristic, that they do not normally have. For example, corn, soybeans, and cotton have been modified to make them resistant to insects and weed killers. Tomatoes have been genetically modified to ripen without becoming mushy.

Advantages of Genetic Engineering

- Genetically modified foods may increase the food supply by helping crops survive pest and weed damage.
- Genetic engineering can improve the nutrition and taste of some foods and remove substances that cause allergic reactions.
- Farmers may need to use fewer pesticides on plants with built-in pest resistance.
- Modified foods may have greater resistance to spoilage.
- Science can engineer new and better varieties of food.

Disadvantages of Genetic Engineering

- Genetically modified foods may cause health problems, such as allergic reactions. For example, genes from Brazil nuts have been used in other foods. People allergic to nuts might become seriously ill by eating these new foods.
- Modified foods may threaten the environment and food supply. Pollen drifts on the wind and spreads to standard crops, harming biodiversity.
- Plants that have built-in pesticides may kill beneficial insects, such as bees and butterflies.
- Modified cotton, corn, and soybeans help create "superweeds" that resist herbicides. Such weeds result when herbicide-resistant plants pollinate weeds. Harmful insects feeding on pesticide-resistant plants could become immune to the pesticide.

TECHNOLOGY FOR TOMORROW

Transportation Technology

Today, people in Minnesota can enjoy fresh Florida oranges in December and residents of Rhode Island can eat recently harvested California artichokes. This was not always so easy. Advances in transportation technology have made moving foods from one place to another easier. Special storage units keep perishable foods at top quality during shipping. Railroad cars and trucks have separate, computer-controlled compartments for frozen, chilled, and dry foods. Containers made with vacuum insulation panels (VIP), an extremely thin plastic or Styrofoam™ layer coated with a metallic film, can keep ice cream frozen for a week. Thanks to technology, foods from distant locales can remain remarkably fresh.

Investigate Conduct research to find out when the first refrigerated train car was built. How did it work? Has transportation technology evolved much since then? Write your findings in one or two paragraphs.

NCSS VIII A Science, Technology, and Society
Identify and describe both current and historical examples of the interaction and interdependence of science, technology, and society in a variety of cultural settings.

- Genetically modified organisms are patented by large corporations.

Cloning

Cloning is another form of genetic engineering. A **clone** is a genetic copy of an organism. Scientists have cloned cattle, pigs, dogs, and other animals. Cloning allows scientists to create exact copies of animals with desirable traits.

Advocates believe that cloning will help to expand the food supply. Critics fear that it could destroy biodiversity. Many people oppose cloning because it produces animal suffering. Some cloned animals have painful health defects such as inflamed brains and spinal cords.

✓ Reading Check **Explain** What is genetic engineering?

Science in Action

A Controversial Development

Many scientists think that genetically modified foods are safe. However, many people worry that GMOs have not been tested enough. No one knows their long-term effects on the environment or human health. Consumer groups want GMOs to be identified on food labels. They also want better testing. Some food processors refuse to use GMOs in their products.

Procedure Conduct research to find answers to these questions: Where are GMOs currently grown? Which nations refuse to sell GMOs?

Analysis Write your findings in one paragraph. Explain your personal opinion about GMOs.

NSES G Develop understanding of science as a human endeavor.

Improving Health

In the last century, scientists have discovered an enormous amount about the relationship between diet and health. Science continues to reveal new facts and spur the development of new technologies. Science can be used to improve human health by improving food through enrichment and fortification and by providing information about nutrition research and ergonomics.

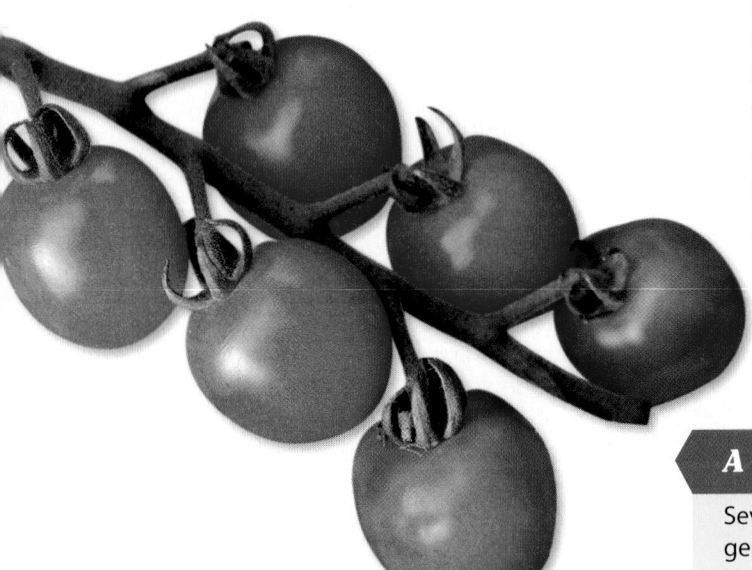

Better Nutrition in Foods

Technologies such as enrichment and fortification improve the nutrition in food. **Enrichment** is restoring nutrients that were lost in processing. For example, the iron and B vitamins found in whole grains are added back into breakfast cereals, white bread, and other foods made with refined grains. **Fortification** is adding a nutrient that is not normally found in a food. For example, milk is fortified with vitamin D.

Functional Foods

Functional foods are foods with ingredients that offer specific health benefits. They are one of the fastest growing types of food in North America. Currently, there are no special regulations governing them. Functional foods fit into three categories: natural whole foods, enhanced foods, and foods created by science.

Natural Whole Foods Blueberries, broccoli, salmon, garlic, and oats are "superfoods" with healthy natural chemicals. Blueberries, for example, have anti-oxidants that help prevent disease. Whole foods, or foods that have not been processed, fit well into a healthful diet.

Enhanced Foods Some foods have nutrients and other substances added. Cereals, for example, often have added fiber for digestive health. Some orange juice has added calcium for bone health.

Foods Created by Science Food scientists create new foods with specific health benefits. Some margarines, for example, are engineered to lower cholesterol. So-called designer foods or nutraceuticals (ˌnü-trə-ˈsü-ti-kəls) need long-term study. Do not rely too heavily on modified foods at the expense of naturally nutritious foods.

A Better Tomato?

Several companies are competing to develop genetically modified tomatoes with advantages such as intense flavor and resistance to rotting. *Would you buy genetically modified produce? Why or why not?*

Nutrition Research

Researchers have discovered about 40 nutrients and hundreds of chemical compounds that are essential to good health. No one knows how many others await discovery. Scientists spend years determining the role each nutrient plays in human health. How does the body use the nutrient? How much is needed? Which foods are the best sources? How is the nutrient affected by processing, storage, heat, and light? Scientists can use the information gathered through nutrition research to educate the public and reduce the risk of nutrition-related disorders in the population.

Nutrition research affects food production, too. For example, scientists try to improve soil and animal feed so that cattle produce leaner beef. Researchers look for ways to extend shelf life and fortify foods. Scientists experiment to find ways to grow wheat that yields more grain in limited space. New analogs are tested and developed.

Ergonomics

Ergonomics is another science that advances human health. **Ergonomics** (ˌər-gə-ˈnä-miks) is the study of ways to make space and equipment easier and more comfortable to use.

Ergonomics is essential in designing kitchens, appliances, and cookware that minimize strain on muscles, bones, and joints. For example, ergonomically designed countertops can be adjusted to different heights. Handles on tools are shaped to fit comfortably in the hand. Some are covered in soft plastic to cushion the grip.

Ergonomics researchers also study the movements people make as they work. This helps them figure out how people can work more efficiently. For example, moving a kitchen prep surface nearer to the stove could reduce extra repetitive steps and save time and energy.

✓ Reading Check **Identify** What is an example of an enhanced food?

Careers in Food

Professor Paul Dawson
Food Scientist

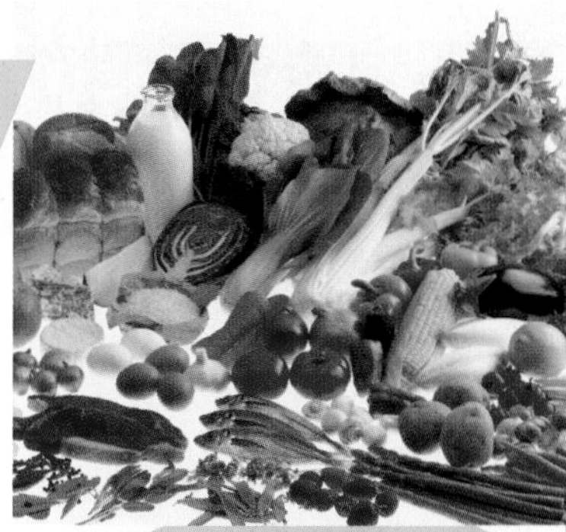

Q: What does a food scientist do?

A: A food scientist can study nutrition, microbiology, chemistry, even the texture of food. One of those is typically specialized in, and the scientist acquires basic understanding of the others. Research in these areas can lead to new food products, new ways to store or preserve food, and healthier ways to process food.

Q: You are a food microbiologist. Explain what that means.

A: I conduct research on microorganisms as they pertain to food and food products, both positively and negatively. A negative would be the bacteria, salmonella, for instance. A positive would be the lactose in milk, which helps us produce dairy products, cottage cheese and so forth. Most fermented products use some sort of bacteria in their production.

"Studying something as diverse and vital as food is attractive and fun."
— Paul Dawson, PhD
Professor, Food Science and Nutrition Department - Clemson University, SC

Education and Training

A PhD is required to be a professor. For non-academic food science positions a master's degree is necessary. Experience is needed, but education is the primary background needed.

Qualities and Skills

Obvious traits such as attention to detail and perseverance are important for research. A basic understanding of the steps of how to conduct research is essential.

Related Career Opportunities

Many scientists work for the U.S. Food and Drug Administration or state health departments. If they work for companies, they are often involved in product development.

Improving Meal Preparation

All cooks, whether they realize it or not, use food science and technology. Consider these contributions of science and technology to everyday life.

Cooking Techniques Foods are chemicals, and a recipe is a chemical formula. Even a slight change in one ingredient or condition can create a different product. Science explains how different foods react chemically and physically when they are heated, chilled, chopped, or mixed. Foods react differently to various cooking techniques. Understanding the science of food helps you cook skillfully.

Appliances Kitchen appliances make meal preparation easier and more successful. Chopping and washing tasks that were once done by hand can now be done using food processors and dishwashers. Refrigeration allows perishable foods to stay edible longer. Appliances are continually improved to make them easier to use and more reliable and energy efficient. Because there are so many appliances to choose from today, it is important to be a smart shopper. New products are constantly being developed and shoppers must make good decisions about how useful an appliance will be.

Computers Computers and the Internet are changing the way cooks shop, plan, and prepare meals. You can use computers to store recipes, create menus, research nutritional information, organize shopping lists, and shop for hard-to-find ingredients.

New technology brings new decisions. As you explore the world of food, use your critical thinking and decision-making skills to evaluate new technologies and make informed decisions.

Light and Healthy Recipe

Imitation Crab Salad

Imitation crab is made from ground whitefish. It is a good alternative for people who are allergic to shellfish.

Ingredients

12 oz Diced imitation crab
1 large Carrot, diced
1 stalk Celery, diced
2 Green onions, sliced thin
2 Tbsp. Mayonnaise
1 Tbsp. Mustard

Directions

1. In a large mixing bowl, combine the crab with the carrots, celery, and onions.
2. Mix the mayonnaise and mustard and add that to the crab mixture. Mix well.
3. Divide the salad equally into four bowls.

Yield 4 servings

Nutrition Analysis per Serving

■ Calories	121
■ Total fat	11 g
Saturated fat	1 g
Cholesterol	0 mg
■ Sodium	377 mg
■ Carbohydrate	7 g
Dietary fiber	2 g
Sugars	2 g
■ Protein	1 g

CHAPTER 4 Review & Applications

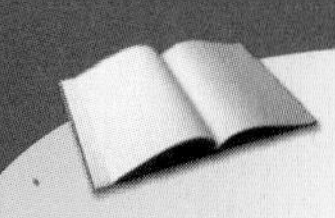

After You Read

Chapter Summary

Science and technology influence every aspect of food, from farming to cooking. Scientists develop new products and help keep the food supply safe. Food technology consists of the helpful tools and techniques that result from scientists' discoveries. Technology is not new. It has shaped the way we farm, cook, produce, process, and distribute food throughout history. Technology has also shaped the way we package and transport food, and has led to controversial developments like genetic engineering. Science and technology have worked in tandem to improve the health of our foods as well as the way we prepare them. Because of science and technology, the world of food is constantly evolving.

Content and Academic Vocabulary Review

1. Think about an example of each of these content and academic vocabulary terms in everyday life.

Content Vocabulary

- ☐ science (p. 44)
- ☐ technology (p. 44)
- ☐ food science (p. 44)
- ☐ manufactured food (p. 45)
- ☐ analogs (p. 45)
- ☐ formed products (p. 45)
- ☐ MAP packaging (p. 46)
- ☐ aseptic packages (p. 46)
- ☐ retort pouches (p. 46)
- ☐ genetic engineering (p. 47)
- ☐ clone (p. 47)
- ☐ enrichment (p. 48)
- ☐ fortification (p. 48)
- ☐ functional foods (p. 48)
- ☐ ergonomics (p. 49)

Academic Vocabulary

- accelerate (p. 45)
- trait (p. 47)

Review Key Concepts

2. **Explain** the relationship between science and technology.
3. **Explain** five ways technology affects food.
4. **Identify** three ways science improves health.
5. **Name** three ways cooks use technology in meal production.

Critical Thinking

6. **Explain** how science and technology might have worked together to lead to the invention of the refrigerator.
7. **Analyze** this scenario. Imagine that there is no such thing as food packaging, and you are limited to eating only foods that do not come in packages. How might this affect your health? Explain your reasoning.
8. **Evaluate** the pros and cons of genetic engineering.
9. **Explain** how scientists' discoveries about the relationship between diet and health may have contributed to a longer average human life span.
10. **Analyze** this situation. Just after you buy a new kitchen appliance, an improved version becomes available. What would you do? How does this relate to the concept of sustainable living from Chapter 3?

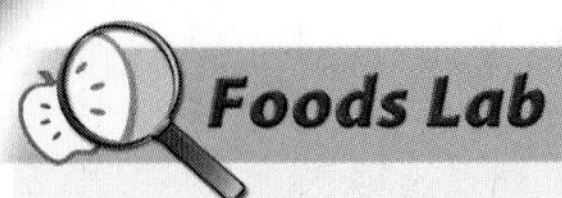

Foods Lab

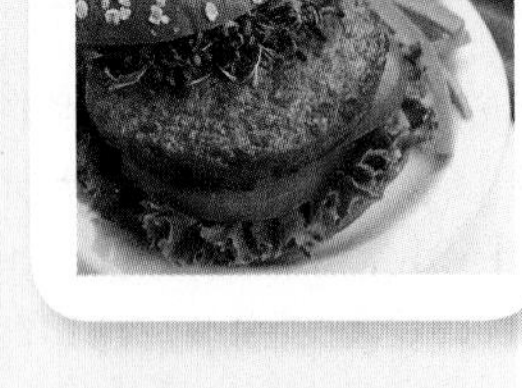

11. Evaluate Manufactured Food Do you prefer analogs, formed products, and egg substitutes, or the foods they are meant to replace?

Procedure Prepare a food and its manufactured food replacement. Compare the cost, ingredient lists, nutritional value, taste, texture, and appearance of both samples.

Analysis Create a chart that shows your assessment of both food samples. Use the chart to compare the food and its manufactured version in each of the six categories listed above. Write a paragraph summarizing your assessment. Explain under what circumstances you would choose the one you enjoy less.

HEALTHFUL CHOICES

12. Choosing Substitutes You are planning to make a breakfast of cheese omelets for several friends. One of your friends tells you he has high cholesterol and is allergic to dairy foods. How can you serve your friend the same dish as everyone else using ingredients that won't harm him? Can you incorporate some of your changes into what you are serving everyone else?

TECH Connection

13. Looking Back Under your teacher's supervision, use the Internet to research one of these topics: food preparation methods of the 19th century; food storage methods in the 19th century; baking methods in the 19th century; or traditional food preparation methods of indigenous cultures. Use presentation software to create a presentation outlining the results of your research. Include photos and art to illustrate your presentation. Share the presentation with the class.

Real-World Skills

Problem-Solving	**14. Create Comfort** Alma is 80 years old and she loves to cook. Complex kitchen appliances aggravate her arthritic joints. What can be done to help her?
Interpersonal and Collaborative Skills	**15. Innovate** Follow your teacher's instructions to form groups. Work together to identify a food-related need. Then brainstorm and describe a new food or technology that you would create to fulfill that need. Share your idea with the class.
Financial Literacy	**16. The Cost of Appliances** Visit a local home appliance retailer. Compare the costs and features of several types of ranges available for sale. How much are the least and most expensive models? What features do the more expensive models have that the less expensive ones lack? Do you think the extra technology is worth the additional cost?

Academic Skills

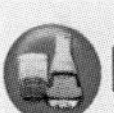

Food Science

17. Packaging Food Cryovac packaging is one of the latest methods developed to help keep food fresh.

Procedure Select a food you wish to keep fresh for several days. Put half the food in a sealable plastic bag. Squeeze as much of the air out of the bag as possible and seal the bag. Wrap the other half of the food in aluminum foil. Fold the ends of the foil and seal the food as tightly as possible. Store both packages in the same place for three days, then examine them.

Analysis Write a paragraph about your findings. Which package preserved the food better? What do you think are the advantages of cryovac packaging?

NSES F Develop understanding of science and technology in local, national and global challenges.

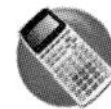

Mathematics

18. Calculate an Average One package of strawberries has traveled 475 miles to get to this store, while a second package originated 1,100 miles away, and a third comes from a farm 51 miles away. What is the average distance that these three packages traveled?

Math Concept **Finding the Mean** The mean, or average, is a statistical measure of data that is calculated by adding up all of the data amounts and dividing that total by the number of amounts.

Starting Hint Start by adding up the 3 mileage amounts, and then divide by 3.

NCTM Data Analysis and Probability Select and use appropriate statistical methods to analyze data.

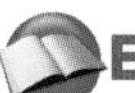

English Language Arts

19. Write an Advertisement Recall the new food or technology that you brainstormed with your group during the Interpersonal and Collaborative skills exercise on the previous page. Now, write a radio advertisement for the new product. Use language to compose an ad that not only describes the product, but draws attention, arouses interest, creates desire, and causes action. Make sure your ad is catchy and memorable.

NCTE 12 Use language to accomplish individual purposes.

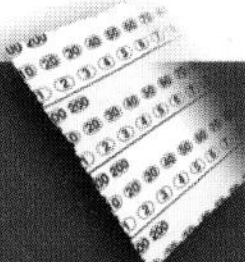

STANDARDIZED TEST PRACTICE

READING COMPREHENSION

Re-read the paragraph about Modified Atmosphere Packaging on page 46. Then select the best answer to the question.

20. How does modified atmosphere packaging work?

a. It subjects foods to long periods of heat to ensure their purification.
b. It speeds bacterial growth.
c. It refrigerates foods for several weeks.
d. It uses a mixture of carbon dioxide, oxygen, and nitrogen to slow bacterial growth.

Test-Taking Tip Before you answer reading comprehension questions remember that while some answers may seem identical, they contain subtle differences. Pay attention to every word.

UNIT 1

Thematic Project

Discover Local Foods

Foods come in diverse varieties from cultures and countries all around the world. Foods are also produced locally. In this project, you will explore local farms or farmers' markets to discover what foods are produced in your area. You will also learn about sustainable agriculture. You will use what you learn to create a poster about locally grown foods.

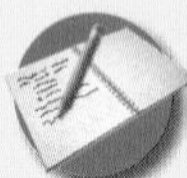

My Journal

If you completed the journal entry from page 3, refer to it to see if your thoughts have changed after reading the unit and completing this project.

Project Assignment

- Research and write a brief report about an issue related to sustainable agriculture.
- Visit a local farm or farmers' market.
- Talk with a farmer or vendors at the farmers' market about the goods they produce.
- Use what you learn from talking with the farmer or vendors to create a poster showing foods that are locally grown and available in your area.

Academic Skills You Will Use

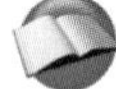

English Language Arts

NCTE 8 Use information resources to gather information and create and communicate knowledge.

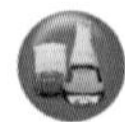

Science

NSES F Develop understanding of personal and community health; population growth; natural resources; environmental quality; natural and human-induced hazards; science and technology in local, national, and global challenges.

STEP 1 Choose a Topic

The topics below are examples of issues related to sustainable agriculture. Choose one of the topics to research.

- What is sustainable agriculture?
- How are nutrients in soil replenished?
- Monoculture (growing just one crop) versus polyculture (growing a mixture of crops)

Research Skills

- Use reputable Web sites such as government (.gov) or educational institutions (.edu).
- Use online dictionaries and encyclopedias.
- Cite the sources you use.

STEP 2 Research Your Topic and Write a Report

Conduct research on your topic, then create an outline for your report. Arrange your ideas in an order that makes sense. Then write a report on the topic you selected. As you write, be sure to use transition words and phrases; use repeated words, parallel structures, or synonyms to link sentences and paragraphs; and use pronouns to avoid unnecessary repetition.

STEP 3 Connect to Your Community

Arrange to visit a local farm or attend a farmers' market in your area. Find out what kinds of foods are grown in your local area. Take photographs of local foods, if possible. Talk with the farmer or vendors about sustainable agriculture. Use information gained from your research to pose questions about the vendor's thoughts on sustainable agriculture. Ask if the vendor uses sustainable methods and efficient practices for energy, water, waste, chemicals, and transportation.

Interview Skills

- Take notes during the interview.
- Use standard English to communicate.
- Listen attentively.
- When you transcribe your notes, write in complete sentences and use correct spelling and grammar.

STEP 4 Create a Poster

Use the Unit Thematic Project Checklist to plan and complete your project and create a poster showing local foods.

STEP 5 Evaluate Your Presentation

Your project will be evaluated based on:

- Content and organization of your information.
- Proper use of standard English.
- Mechanics—presentation and neatness.
- Speaking and listening skills.

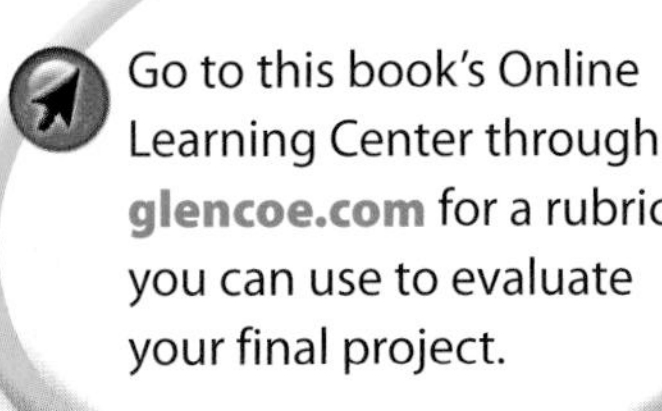

Go to this book's Online Learning Center through **glencoe.com** for a rubric you can use to evaluate your final project.

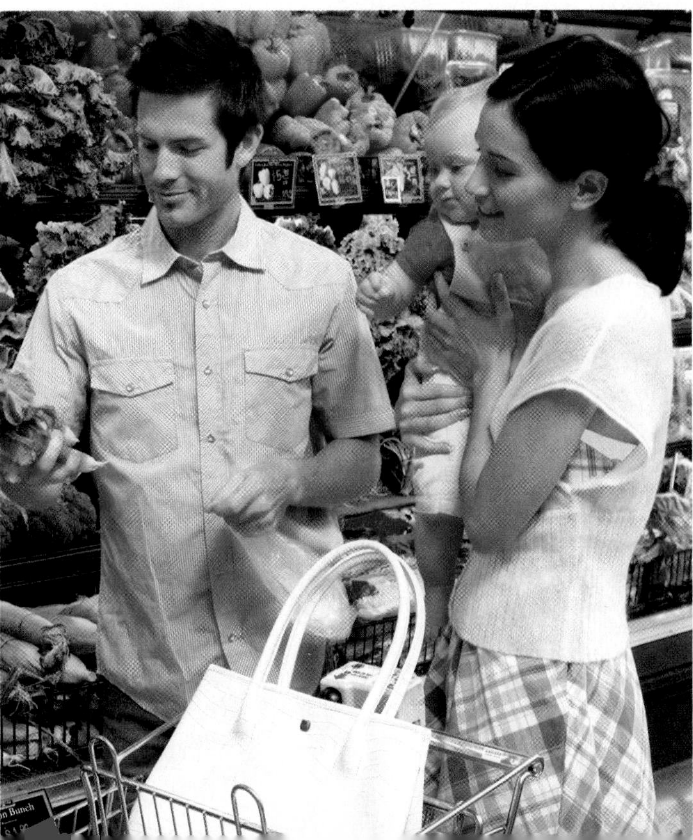

Unit Thematic Project Checklist

Category	Objectives
Plan	☑ Conduct research about an issue related to sustainable agriculture.
	☑ Write a report.
	☑ Visit a farm or farmer's market and interview farmers or vendors about local foods and sustainable agricultural practices.
	☑ Make a poster that illustrates the locally grown foods available in your area.
Present	☑ Make a presentation to your class to share your poster and discuss what you learned about local foods and sustainable agricultural practices.
	☑ Invite the students in your class to ask you any questions they may have. Answer three questions.
	☑ When students ask you questions, demonstrate in your answers that you respect their perspectives.
	☑ Turn in your report, the notes from your interview, and your poster to your teacher.
Academic Skills	☑ Be sensitive to the needs of different audiences.
	☑ Adapt and modify language to suit different purposes.
	☑ Thoughtfully express your ideas.

UNIT 2

Nutrition Basics

Activate Prior Knowledge

Explore the Photo Eating a variety of foods will supply your body with the nutrients it needs. *What kinds of foods do you typically eat?*

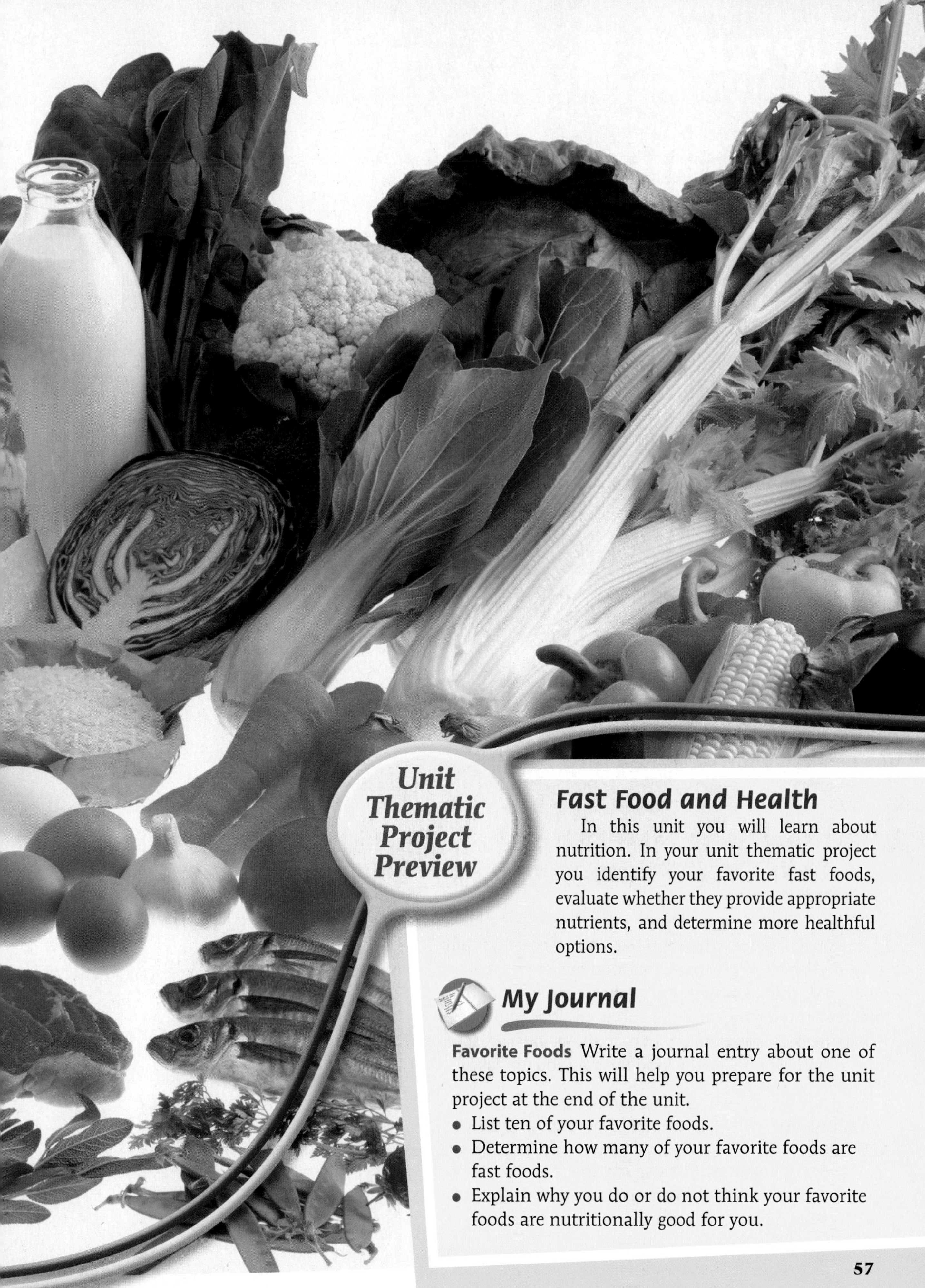

Unit Thematic Project Preview

Fast Food and Health

In this unit you will learn about nutrition. In your unit thematic project you identify your favorite fast foods, evaluate whether they provide appropriate nutrients, and determine more healthful options.

My Journal

Favorite Foods Write a journal entry about one of these topics. This will help you prepare for the unit project at the end of the unit.

- List ten of your favorite foods.
- Determine how many of your favorite foods are fast foods.
- Explain why you do or do not think your favorite foods are nutritionally good for you.

CHAPTER 5

Nutrients at Work

Writing Activity — Write Using Details

Foods That Help and Heal What kind of food makes you feel better when you are mentally or physically drained? Why do you think this food makes you feel better? Is the food special to you for reasons other than taste? For ten minutes, write about this food and its effect on you, using details that help the reader see, smell, taste, and experience the food the way you do. Take time to be specific.

Writing Tips Follow these steps to write using details:

- Avoid generalities. Be clear and specific.
- Use adjectives to help bring details to life.
- Include details that are relevant to the topic.

Activate Prior Knowledge

Explore the Photo The foods we eat have a big impact on how we look, feel, and function in life. *What foods make you feel strong and healthy?*

Reading Guide

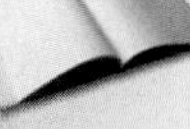

Before You Read

Preview List the things you know about how the body uses nutrients. Update your list after you read as needed.

Read to Learn

Key Concepts

- **Identify** the nutrients in foods and their main functions.
- **Describe** the digestive process and its stages.
- **Summarize** the body's absorption of nutrients.
- **Describe** how the body uses nutrients both now and later.
- **Explain** Basal Metabolic Rate and how it relates to calories.

Main Idea

The nutrients in foods affect on how we feel and function, and our bodies utilize many processes to use and absorb them.

Content Vocabulary

You will find definitions for these words in the glossary at the back of this book.

- □ malnutrition
- □ anemia
- □ Dietary Reference Intake (DRI)
- □ Recommended Dietary Allowance (RDA)
- □ Adequate Intake (AI)
- □ digestion
- □ enzyme
- □ esophagus
- □ peristalsis
- □ chyme
- □ pancreas
- □ absorption
- □ villi
- □ glucose
- □ glycogen
- □ metabolism
- □ oxidation
- □ calorie
- □ basal metabolism

Academic Vocabulary

You will find these words in your reading and on your tests. Use the glossary to look up their definitions if necessary.

- maintain
- vital

Graphic Organizer

Use a graphic organizer like the one below to take notes about what happens during and after nutrient absorption.

DURING NUTRIENT ABSORPTION	AFTER NUTRIENT ABSORPTION

Graphic Organizer Go to this book's Online Learning Center at **glencoe.com** to print out this graphic organizer.

Academic Standards

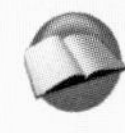

English Language Arts

NCTE 12 Use language to accomplish individual purposes.

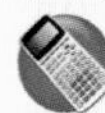

Mathematics

NCTM Number and Operations Compute fluently and make reasonable estimates.

NCTM Problem Solving Apply and adapt a variety of appropriate strategies to solve problems.

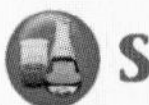

Science

NSES B Develop an understanding of chemical reactions.

NCTE *National Council of Teachers of English*
NCTM *National Council of Teachers of Mathematics*
NSES *National Science Education Standards*

The Nutrients in Foods

The nutrients in food keep your body healthy. Water is the most common nutrient in food. In fact, food can be up to 90 percent water. Carbohydrates (ˌkär-bō-ˈhī-ˌdrāts), fats, and proteins, make up the rest, along with a very small amount of vitamins, minerals, and phytochemicals (ˌfī-tō-ˈke-mi-kəls), which help keep your body free of disease.

- **Carbohydrates** provide the body's main source of energy.
- **Fats** provide a source of stored energy, as well as insulation for the body.
- **Proteins** help build, repair, and **maintain**, or preserve, body tissues.
- **Vitamins** help cells, tissues, and organs stay healthy.
- **Minerals** help the body work properly.
- **Water** helps with chemical reactions in the body and helps transport materials to and from cells.

Nutrients and Health

Different foods have different nutrients. Strawberries, for example, are rich in vitamin C but have almost no protein. The best way to get the nutrients you need is to choose a wide variety of healthful foods.

Unhealthy food choices or a lack of food can lead to **malnutrition**, poor nourishment resulting from a lack of nutrients. Shortages of specific vitamins and minerals can cause serious problems, too. People who do not eat enough iron, for example, may develop anemia. **Anemia** (ə-ˈnē-mē-ə), is a blood disorder that causes lack of energy, weakness, shortness of breath, and cold hands and feet.

Another form of malnutrition is caused by overeating. Eating sugary, fatty food instead of fruits, vegetables, and lean protein can lead to overweight.

Your health is influenced by your heredity, lifestyle, and food choices. Changing your lifestyle and your food choices can make a huge difference in your health. When you choose healthy habits and a nutritious diet, you can enjoy benefits such as:

- **Appearance** Good nutrition helps give you shiny hair, bright eyes, healthy nails and teeth, and smooth, clear skin.
- **Fitness** Good nutrition helps you stay energetic and alert throughout the day.
- **Weight** A healthy diet helps you reach and maintain a healthy weight.
- **Protection from Illness** Good nutrition helps your body defend against disease.
- **Healing** Nutrients help the body build new cells, repair breaks and sprains, and heal after illness or surgery.
- **Emotional Strength** Good nutrition helps your body and mind deal with stress.
- **Future health** Serious health problems, such as heart disease and some cancers, can result from poor eating habits. Good nutrition today can help you stay healthy as you grow older.

Nutrient Teamwork

Nutrients work together in your body. For example, proteins and minerals are both important for bone structure. Vitamin D helps your body absorb calcium. Nutrient teamwork means your body must have an adequate supply of all nutrients.

Nutrition Check

Not Enough Nutrients

When the body is not given sufficient nutrients, it suffers. Malnutrition is a term used to describe any of the health problems that may occur as a result of poor nutrition. Many different physical, mental, and emotional health problems can be a result of malnutrition. Malnourished people often do not have enough calories in their diet. This is why malnutrition is a serious problem in developing countries with inadequate food supplies. Anyone, however, can fail to consume a good variety of nutrients.

Think About It Conduct research about one specific form of malnutrition. What vitamin or mineral do sufferers of this form of malnutriton lack? What foods can they eat more of to improve their nutrition?

Nutrient Requirements

Everyone needs the same nutrients. However, different people need these nutrients in different amounts. For example, women and teenage boys need more iron than men. Nutrients are measured in the metric units of grams (g), milligrams (mg), and micrograms (µg).

To find out how much of each nutrient you need, consult a table of Dietary Reference Intakes. A **Dietary Reference Intake (DRI)** is the recommended daily amount of nutrients for people of a certain age and gender group.

The DRIs in **Figure 5.1** on page 62 show both Recommended Dietary Allowances and Adequate Intakes. A **Recommended Dietary Allowance (RDA)** is the amount of a nutrient needed by 98 percent of the people in a given age and gender group. An **Adequate Intake (AI)** is a nutrient standard that is used when a lack of scientific information makes it impossible to establish the RDA for a particular nutrient. DRIs include RDAs and AIs and are updated periodically.

Dietitians, nutritionists, and other health professionals use DRIs to shape nutrition policy and develop educational programs. The food industry also uses DRIs for product development.

Daily Values

The U.S. Food and Drug Administration (FDA) uses DRIs as the basis for Daily Values. Daily Values (DVs) are the nutrition standards used on nutrition labels. They are based on averages for all adults. **Figure 5.2** on page 63 shows the Daily Values in use today.

✓ **Reading Check** **Identify** What resource can you consult to determine how much of each nutrient you need daily?

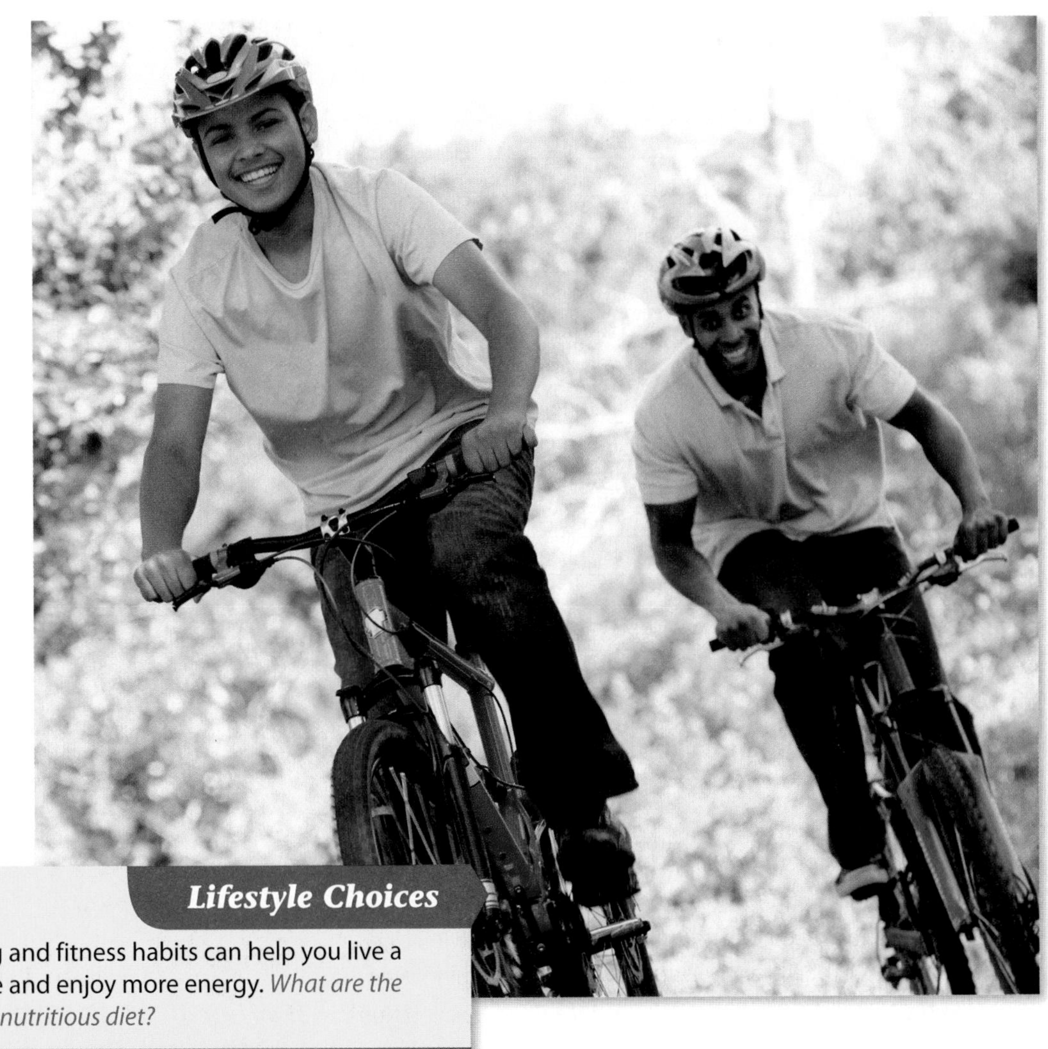

Lifestyle Choices

Good eating and fitness habits can help you live a healthier life and enjoy more energy. *What are the benefits of a nutritious diet?*

Figure 5.1 Dietary Reference Intakes for Teens (RDA or AI)

Necessary Nutrients Making sure your daily meals include choices that meet all the amounts listed below will help you as you grow. ***Why do you need more nutrients as you move from ages 9–13 to ages 14–18?***

Nutrient	Males 9–13	Males 14–18	Females 9–13	Females 14–18
Protein	34 g	52 g	34 g	46 g
Carbohydrate (total)	130 g	130 g	130 g	130 g
Dietary fiber	31 g	38 g	26 g	26 g
Fat (total)	*	*	*	*
Saturated fat	*	*	*	*
Cholesterol	*	*	*	*
Linoleic Acid	12 g	16 g	10 g	12 g
α-Linoleic Acid	1.2 g	1.6 g	1.0 g	1.1 g
Vitamin A	600 μg RAE	900 μg RAE	600 μg RAE	700 μg RAE
Thiamin	0.9 mg	1.2 mg	0.9 mg	1.0 mg
Riboflavin	0.9 mg	1.3 mg	0.9 mg	1.0 mg
Niacin	12 mg NE	16 mg NE	12 mg NE	14 mg NE
Vitamin B_6	1.0 mg	1.3 mg	1.0 mg	1.2 mg
Vitamin B_{12}	1.8 μg	2.4 μg	1.8 μg	2.4 μg
Folate	300 μg DFE	400 μg DFE	300 μg DFE	400 μg DFE
Biotin	20 μg	25 μg	20 μg	25 μg
Pantothenic acid	4 mg	5 mg	4 mg	5 mg
Vitamin C	45 mg	75 mg	45 mg	65 mg
Vitamin D	5 μg	5 μg	5 μg	5 μg
Vitamin E	11 mg α-TE	15 mg α-TE	11 mg α-TE	15 mg α-TE
Vitamin K	60 μg	75 μg	60 μg	75 μg
Calcium	1,300 mg	1,300 mg	1,300 mg	1,300 mg
Copper	700 μg	890 μg	700 μg	890 μg
Iodine	120 μg	150 μg	120 μg	150 μg
Iron	8 mg	11 mg	8 mg	15 mg
Magnesium	240 mg	410 mg	240 mg	360 mg
Phosphorus	1,250 mg	1,250 mg	1,250 mg	1,250 mg
Potassium	4.5 g	4.7 g	4.5 g	4.7 g
Selenium	40 μg	55 μg	40 μg	55 μg
Sodium	1.5 g	1.5 g	1.5 g	1.5 g
Zinc	8 mg	11 mg	8 mg	9 mg

*No value established

Key To Nutrient Measures

g gram
mg milligram (1,000 mg = 1 g)
μg microgram (1,000 μg = 1 mg; 1,000,000 μg = 1 g)
RAE retinol activity equivalents (a measure of vitamin A activity)
NE niacin equivalents (a measure of niacin activity)
DFE dietary folate equivalents (a measure of folate activity)
α-TE alpha-tocopherol equivalents (a measure of vitamin E activity)

Source: The National Academies, Institute of Medicine, Board of Nutrition

Figure 5.2 Daily Values

One Size Does Not Fit All The values used for nutrition labels are based on the nutrients necessary for adults. ***What does this mean for teenagers?***

Nutrient	Daily Value
Protein	50 g*
Carbohydrate (total)	300 g*
Dietary fiber	25 g
Fat (total)	65 g*
Saturated fat	20 g*
Cholesterol	300 mg
Vitamin A	5,000 IU (875 µg RAE)
Thiamin	1.5 mg
Riboflavin	1.7 mg
Niacin	20 mg NE
Vitamin B_6	2 mg
Vitamin B_{12}	6 µg
Folate	400 µg
Biotin	300 µg
Pantothenic acid	10 mg
Vitamin C	60 mg
Vitamin D	400 IU (6.5 µg)
Vitamin E	30 IU (9 mg α-TE)
Vitamin K	80 µg
Calcium	1,000 mg
Copper	2 mg
Iodine	150 µg
Iron	18 mg
Magnesium	400 mg
Phosphorus	1,000 mg
Potassium	3,500 mg
Selenium	70 µg
Sodium	2,400 mg
Zinc	15 mg

*Based on a diet of 2,000 calories per day

Key To Nutrient Measures

g gram
mg milligram (1,000 mg = 1 g)
µg microgram (1,000 µg = 1 mg; 1,000,000 µg = 1 g)
IU International Unit (an old measure of vitamin activity)
RAE retinol activity equivalents (a measure of Vitamin A activity)
NE niacin equivalents (a measure of niacin activity)
α-TE alpha-tocopherol equivalents (a measure of Vitamin E activity)

Source: U.S. Food and Drug Administration

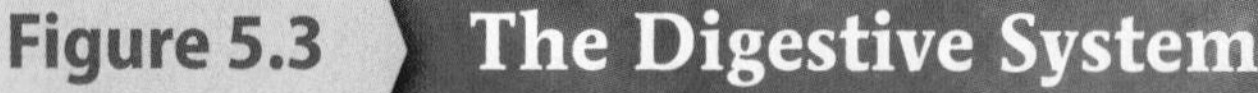

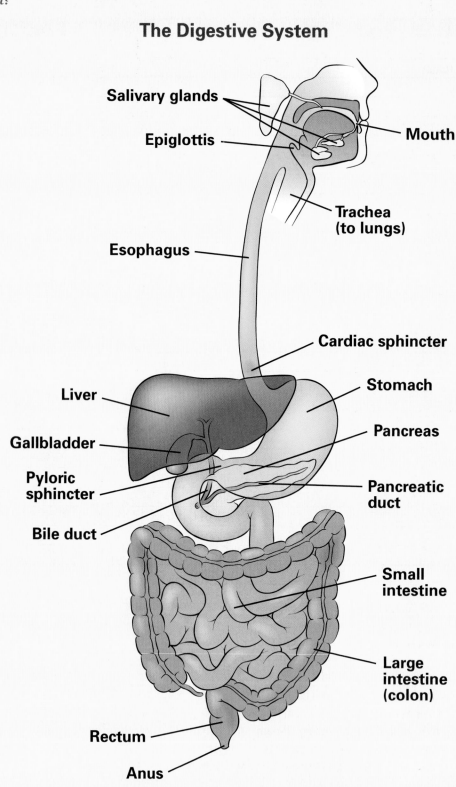

Figure 5.3 The Digestive System

Unlocking Nutrients Many organs are involved in the complex process of digestion. *What happens to food as it passes through each stage in digestion?*

The Digestive Process

Before your body can turn food into energy, it has to digest the food. **Digestion** is the mechanical and chemical process of breaking down food and changing nutrients into forms your body can use. Digestion takes place in the digestive tract, a flexible tube about 26 feet long. Your digestive tract extends from your mouth to your rectum ('rek-təm). **Figure 5.3** shows the major parts of the digestive system.

The Eyes

You eat with your eyes first. How? The sight and aroma of food starts saliva flowing in your mouth—your mouth "waters." Saliva is an important ingredient in digestion. This is why experienced cooks try to make the food they serve look as attractive as possible.

The Mouth

Digestion begins in the mouth. As you chew, your teeth grind food into smaller pieces that are easier to swallow and digest. This is the mechanical part of digestion. Chewing also increases the surface area of food, creating more space for chemical reactions to occur.

Try to chew solid food to the size and texture of applesauce. Your stomach cannot digest larger pieces of food completely, and you may miss out on nutrients.

The chemical part of digestion begins when saliva is released in the mouth. Saliva contains the enzyme ptyalin ('tī-ə-lən), which helps to break food down. An **enzyme** is a special protein that helps a chemical reaction take place. The ptyalin in saliva helps change carbohydrates into sugars.

Saliva also helps you taste food. Taste buds on the tongue can identify four general flavors: salty, bitter, sour, and sweet. Some researchers also list a savory fifth flavor, called umami (ü-'mä-mē). The taste buds need saliva to work well. The smell of food also helps your sense of taste. That is why food seems to have less flavor when you have a stuffy nose.

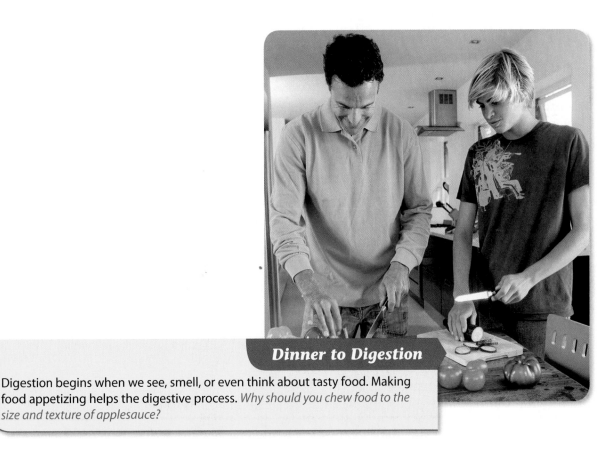

Dinner to Digestion

Digestion begins when we see, smell, or even think about tasty food. Making food appetizing helps the digestive process. *Why should you chew food to the size and texture of applesauce?*

The Esophagus

Once you swallow food, it passes into the **esophagus** (i-ˈsä-fə-gəs), the part of the digestive tract that connects the mouth and the stomach. Food moves through the esophagus by **peristalsis** (ˌper-əh-ˈstȯl-səs), rhythmic movements of muscles. The muscles of the esophagus contract and relax, forcing food into the stomach, as shown in **Figure 5.4.** A valve at the end of the esophagus closes to prevent food from moving back to the mouth.

The Stomach

The stomach is a muscular pouch just below the rib cage. It can hold up to six cups of food. The stomach produces gastric juices—acids and enzymes that help food break down chemically. It is lined with mucus, which protects it from damage by acids. Carbohydrates begin to break down in the mouth, but proteins and fats begin to break down in the stomach.

The stomach also breaks food down mechanically through peristalsis. The churned food turns into a thick liquid called **chyme** (ˈkīm).

Different foods take different amounts of time to break down and leave the stomach. Carbohydrates usually take one to two hours. Proteins take about three to five hours. Fats take up to 12 hours to break down and leave the stomach.

The Small Intestine

From the stomach, food moves a little at a time into the small intestine. The small intestine is a narrow, winding tube that connects the stomach with the large intestine. Three types of digestive juices help to break down carbohydrates, proteins, and fats in the small intestine.

- **Bile** Bile helps the body digest and absorb fats. Bile is produced in the liver and stored in the gall bladder until needed.
- **Pancreatic juice** Pancreatic (ˌpaŋ-krē-ˈa-tik) juice is a mixture of enzymes made by the **pancreas** (ˈpaŋ-krē-əs), a gland connected to the small intestine.
- **Intestinal juice** This works with other juices to break down food. Intestinal juice is produced in the small intestine itself.

✓ Reading Check **Describe** What is saliva's role in the digestion process?

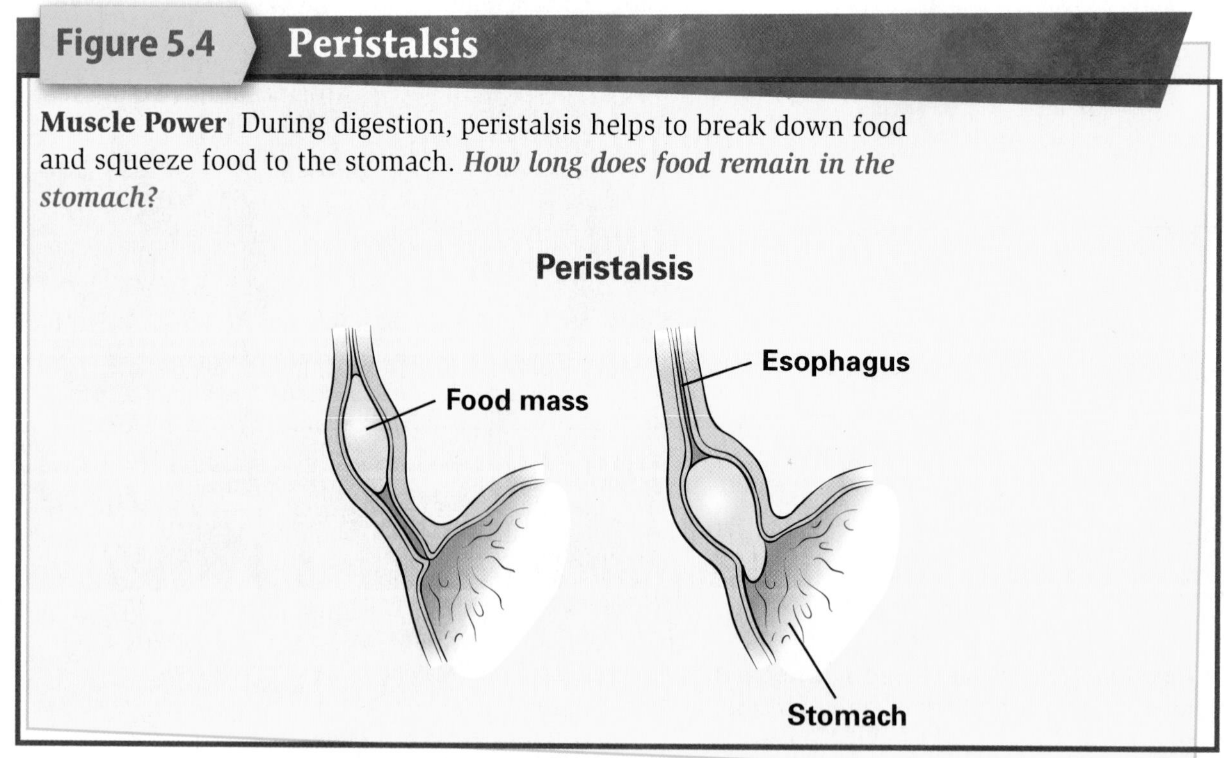

Figure 5.4 **Peristalsis**

Muscle Power During digestion, peristalsis helps to break down food and squeeze food to the stomach. ***How long does food remain in the stomach?***

Absorption of Nutrients

Once food is broken down, the body needs to absorb it. **Absorption** is the process by which nutrients move into the bloodstream. Most absorption takes place in the small intestine.

The inner wall of the small intestine has folds covered with billions of tiny, fingerlike projections called **villi** (ˈvi-ˌlī). The villi increase the surface area of the intestine so that it can absorb more nutrients. Although the small intestine is only about 20 feet long, its surface area is as big as a tennis court (see **Figure 5.5**).

After absorption, waste material, including dietary fiber, is left in the small intestine. Fiber helps with digestion and absorption but cannot be digested. Waste moves into the large intestine, also called the colon. The colon removes water, potassium, and sodium from the waste. The remainder is stored in the rectum, the lower part of the large intestine, until elimination.

Figure 5.5

Absorption in Action

Intestinal Fortitude Most nutrient absorption takes place in the small intestine. ***What digestive juices help the small intestine break down food?***

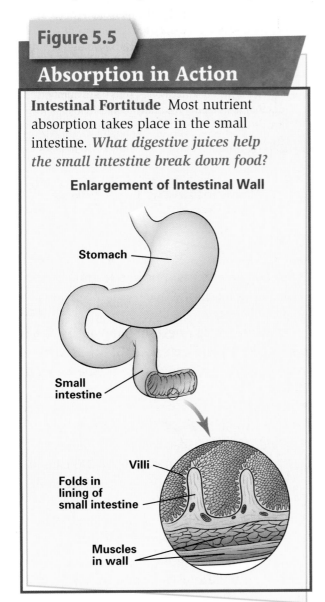

Enlargement of Intestinal Wall

✓ **Reading Check** **List** What three useful nutrients does the colon remove from waste?

Nutrient Transportation and Storage

After nutrients are absorbed by the villi of the small intestine, they are carried to the liver through a blood vessel called the portal vein. One of the liver's many jobs is to turn nutrients into forms the body can use.

When carbohydrates are fully broken down, they become a simple sugar called glucose. **Glucose** (ˈglü-ˌkōs), or blood sugar, is the body's basic fuel. Fats are changed into fatty acids. Proteins are broken down into amino acids. Vitamins, minerals, water, and phytochemicals, however, do not break down. Your body can use them without changing their form.

The bloodstream carries nutrients to individual cells, where they are put to work.

Some nutrients can be stored for future use. For example, the liver converts extra glucose into **glycogen** (ˈglī-kə-jən), a storage form of glucose. If your body has more glucose than it can store as glycogen, it converts the excess glucose to body fat. Your body also converts excess fatty acids and amino acids into body fat. Fats are your body's energy reserve.

Your body also stores minerals and vitamins. For example, iron is stored in the liver and in bone marrow. Some vitamins, such as vitamins A and E, are stored in the liver and in body fat. Other vitamins, such as vitamin C and the B vitamins, cannot be stored. If these vitamins are not needed right away, they leave the body in the urine.

✓ **Reading Check** **Identify** What parts of your body can store nutrients for later use?

Metabolism

Nutrients are **vital**, or necessary, for metabolism. **Metabolism** (mə-ˈta-bə-ˌli-zəm) is the use of nutrients to provide energy.

During metabolism, glucose in the cells combines with oxygen to produce energy and heat. A chemical reaction like this, in which molecules combine with oxygen, is called **oxidation** (ˌäk-sə-ˈdā-shən). When wood burns, it oxidizes and produces light and heat.

Energy is measured in units called kilocalories (ˈkē-lə-ˌka-lə-rēz), better known as calories. A **calorie** is the amount of energy needed to raise the temperature of 1 kilogram of water (a little more than 4 cups) by 1 degree Celsius. In the metric system, energy is measured in kilojoules (KJ). Calories measure the energy in food and the energy used by the body for activities.

Basal Metabolism

Your body uses energy for automatic processes as well as for physical activities. Automatic processes include breathing, digesting food, and building and repairing tissue. Because these processes go on 24 hours a day, your body uses small amounts of energy even when you are sleeping. The energy you need to maintain automatic processes is called **basal metabolism** (ˈbā-səl mə-ˈta-bə-ˌli-zəm).

The amount of energy your body uses for basal metabolism is called basal metabolic rate, or BMR. BMR varies greatly from person to person. Your body uses about two-thirds of the calories you consume for basal metabolism.

Energy Requirements

Different foods have different amounts of calories, depending on the amount of carbohydrates, protein and fat in each. Most foods have a combination of all three.

- There are four calories in one gram of pure carbohydrates. Carbohydrates are the body's first source of energy.
- There are four calories in one gram of protein. The body uses protein to build and maintain bones and muscles.

Kitchen Math

Calculate Calories

For lunch, Maria is making a ground turkey burger as a low-fat alternative to a beef burger. The ground turkey has 15 grams of protein, 7 grams of fat, and no carbohydrates. The burger bun has 4 grams of protein, 2 grams of fat and 21 grams of carbohydrates. The mayonnaise and mustard have 2 grams of fat and no protein or carbohydrates. Maria prepares baked sweet potato fries, which have 2 grams of protein, 4 grams of fat, and 23 grams of carbohydrates. How many calories does Maria's lunch contain?

Math Concept **Multi-Step Problems** This is a multi-step problem since you have to make more than one computation. Think through each step before beginning.

Starting Hint Remember that one gram of carbohydrates, protein, or fat does not equal one calorie. One gram of protein or carbohydrates has four calories. One gram of fat has nine calories. Use multiplication to convert the grams of protein, fat, and carbohydrate into calories. Add these numbers together to find out how many total calories are in this meal.

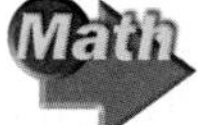

Math Appendix For math help, go to the Math Appendix at the back of this book.

NCTM Number and Operations Compute fluently and make reasonable estimates.

- There are nine calories in one gram of fat. Fat is stored in the body as a means of stored energy.

How many calories should you eat each day? That depends on your BMR, as well as your age, weight, gender and activity level. Here are some guidelines:

- Teen males, many active men, and some very active women need 2,800 calories per day.
- Older children, teen females, active women, and most men need 2,200 calories per day. Women who are pregnant or breast-feeding may need more.
- Younger children, women and most older adults need 1,600 calories per day.

If you are still growing, you need more calories to build muscles and bones. You also need more calories if you are physically active.

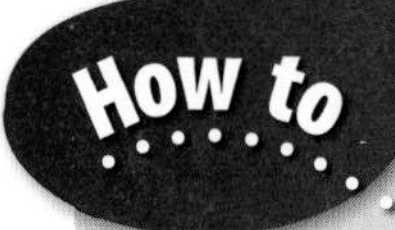

Calculate Your BMR

Use this formula to calculate your basal metabolic rate, the amount of energy your body uses for automatic metabolic processes.

Reference

Female	Male
BMR = 655 + (4.35 × weight in pounds) + (4.7 × height in inches) − (4.7 × age in years)	BMR = 66 + (6.23 × weight in pounds) + (12.7 × height in inches) −(6.8 × age in years)

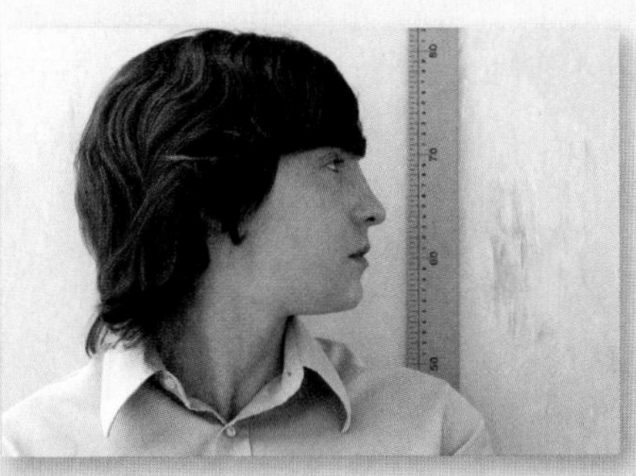

1. Have a partner use measuring tape to determine your height.

2. Use a scale to determine your weight. Remove heavy shoes and jackets to get an accurate measurement.

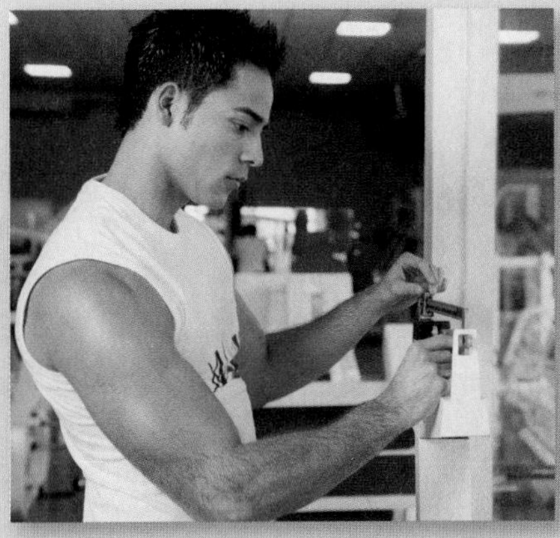

3. Complete the first part of the equation.
   Female: 655 + (4.35 × weight in pounds) + (4.7 × height in inches)
   Male: 65 + (6.23 × weight in pounds) + (12.7 × height in inches)

4. Complete the second part of the equation.
   Female: (4.7 × age in years)
   Male: (6.8 × age in years)

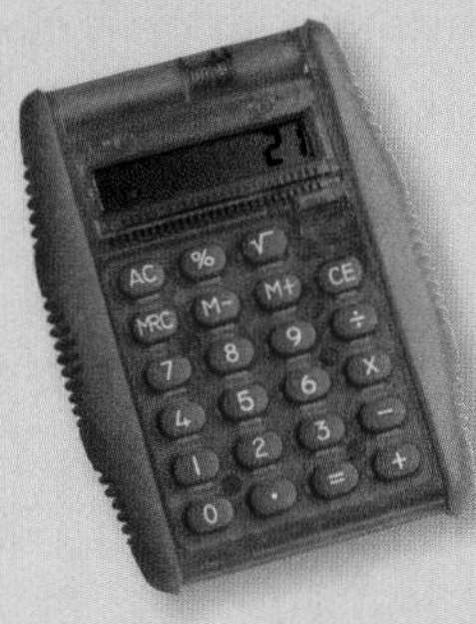

5. Subtract the number you calculated in Step 4 from the number you calculated in Step 3. This is your BMR.

The U.S. Department of Agriculture recommends daily calorie amounts. Increased muscle mass means an increased BMR, so weight-bearing muscle building exercise along with aerobic exercise raises your BMR. Some Olympic-level athletes need as many as 12,000 calories per day.

Recommended Sources of Calories

Most of your calories should come from carbohydrates. Limit fat to about a third of your daily calories. As little as 10 percent can come from protein. Adults need slightly more protein and less fat than teens.

- Teens need 45–65% of their calories from carbohydrates, 10–30% from protein and 25–35% from fats.
- Adults need 45–65% of their calories from carbohydrates, 10–35% from protein and 20–35% from fats.

Suppose a teen needs 2,200 calories a day. If she limits fat to 30 percent of her day's calories, that allows her 660 calories from fat (2,200 × .30 = 660). How many grams of fat will supply 660 calories? Since there are 9 calories in 1 gram of fat, divide 660 by 9. The answer is 73 grams. She can use information on food labels to make sure her fat intake is 73 grams or less.

Giving Your Body What It Needs

Your body has an amazing ability to use the nutrients in food. Help your body stay healthy by choosing a balanced diet that meets all your nutritional needs. Learning about the nutrients in different foods will help you make smart food choices. Learning what foods are high in protein, fat, and carbohydrates will help you make balanced meals even when time is short.

Light and Healthy Recipe

Trail Mix

Ingredients

1 cup Any whole grain cereal
¾ cup Raisins
½ cup Roasted peanuts
¼ cup Sunflower seeds
¼ cup Dried cranberries
¼ cup Chocolate chips

Yield: 4 servings, 3/4 cup each

Directions

1. Combine all ingredients and mix in a large bowl.
2. Store in an airtight container.

Yield 4 servings

Trail mix is a great lightweight snack food often used for long hikes. Its ingredients provide both short- and long-term energy.

Nutrition Analysis per Serving

■ Calories	357
■ Total fat	18 g
Saturated fat	4 g
Cholesterol	0 mg
■ Sodium	57 mg
■ Carbohydrate	49 g
Dietary fiber	5 g
Sugars	31 g
■ Protein	9 g

CHAPTER 5 Review & Applications

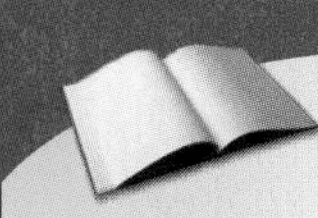

After You Read

Chapter Summary

Food contains nutrients that benefit the body in many ways. Some nutrients work together. While everyone needs the same nutrients, different people require different amounts. The body must digest food before it can use nutrients. Digestion involves the eyes, mouth, esophagus, stomach, and small intestine. Both the small and large intestine are involved in nutrient absorption. The body uses some nutrients right away, and stores others. The body metabolizes nutrients to provide energy. It is important to obtain calories from good sources and eat a balanced diet that meets nutritional needs.

Content and Academic Vocabulary Review

1. Use each of these content and academic vocabulary words in a sentence.

Content Vocabulary

- malnutrition (p. 60)
- anemia (p. 60)
- Dietary Reference Intake (DRI) (p. 61)
- Recommended Dietary Allowance (RDA) (p. 61)
- Adequate Intake (AI) (p. 61)
- digestion (p. 65)
- enzyme (p. 65)
- esophagus (p. 66)
- peristalsis (p. 66)
- chyme (p. 66)
- pancreas (p. 66)
- absorption (p. 67)
- villi (p. 67)
- glucose (p. 67)
- glycogen (p. 67)
- metabolism (p. 68)
- oxidation (p. 68)
- calorie (p. 68)
- basal metabolism (p. 68)

Academic Vocabulary

- maintain (p. 60)
- vital (p. 68)

Review Key Concepts

2. Identify the nutrients in foods and their main functions.
3. Describe the digestive process and its stages.
4. Summarize the body's absorption of nutrients.
5. Describe how the body uses nutrients both now and later.
6. Explain Basal Metabolic Rate and how it relates to calories.

Critical Thinking

7. Explain how eating the same healthful foods every day could harm your health.
8. Predict what will happen. Brian's mom serves an unappetizing dinner. The food is a strange color and gives off a foul odor.
9. Solve Lorenzo's dilemma. Lorenzo is overweight and unable to lose weight even though he has been eating less. What might Lorenzo be missing?
10. Explain why Rose feels hungry all the time. Rose, who is sixteen, eats breakfast, lunch, and dinner with her mom. Rose and her mom are the same height and weight. They eat the same portions.

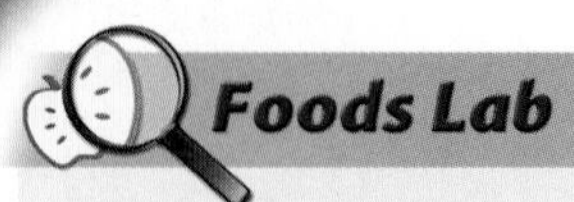

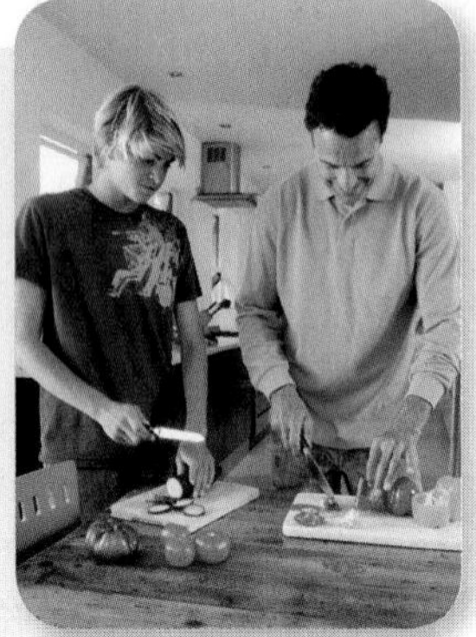

11. Meeting Nutrient Needs Many different foods supply the same nutrient. Taste, practicality, versatility, and cost can all determine which foods you prefer to use as sources of a certain nutrient.

Procedure Choose one nutrient. As a group, locate several foods that provide at least 15 percent of the daily requirement per serving of the same nutrient. Give a presentation about how they might be used in meals.

Analysis How do the different foods compare in terms of appeal, practicality, versatility, and cost? Do you think it is easy to meet nutrient needs from readily available foods? Why or why not?

HEALTHFUL CHOICES

12. How to Heal Beatrix has a broken leg. Her usual diet is heavy on pizza, milkshakes, and sweets. What changes should Beatrix make to her diet if she wants her leg to heal quickly? Why? Given that exercise will be more difficult with a broken leg, why should Beatrix be particularly concerned about diet? Write a paragraph explaining your suggestions.

TECH Connection

13. Digestive Aids Many herbs, teas, and supplements are considered to be digestive aids—that is, they help the body to digest foods more easily. With your teacher's permission, use the Internet to research one digestive aid. What is it? How does it work? Is it affordable? Is it safe? Are there natural ways of consuming it? Write one paragraph about your findings and share it with your class.

Real-World Skills

Problem-Solving

14. A Smart Start Each day, breakfast is the body's first chance to absorb a variety of useful nutrients, yet many people skip it. Brainstorm and write a menu for a week's worth of quick and convenient breakfasts, each one providing a different combination of nutrients. Note some of the nutrients that are provided by each breakfast.

Interpersonal and Collaborative Skills

15. An In-Depth Look Follow your teacher's instructions to get into groups. Select one nutrient to focus on. Work together to research the sources and benefits of the nutrient, as well as signs of its deficiency. Collaboratively create a poster board display that will educate others about the nutrient.

Financial Literacy

16. Compare Vitamin Costs Brenda wishes to supplement her regular diet with multivitamin pills, and is deciding between two competing products. Product A comes in a 120-pill bottle and directs that three pills be taken per day. Product B, which requires only one pill per day, comes in a 45-pill bottle. If both products cost $9.00 and provide the same amount of vitamins when taken according to directions, which is the better buy?

Academic Skills

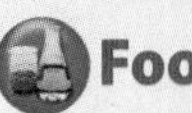

Food Science

17. Enzymes Aid Digestion Enzymes break down foods into smaller nutrients for absorption. As an example of enzyme action, observe how the enzyme in fresh pineapple (bromelin) breaks down the protein gelatin.

Procedure Prepare 2 small boxes of gelatin dessert, following the directions on the package. Add canned pineapple chunks to the first batch, and fresh pineapple chunks to the second batch. Chill overnight.

Analysis Describe the two gelatins. Explain your results, addressing the difference between the fresh versus canned pineapple.

NSES B Students should develop an understanding of chemical reactions.

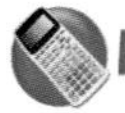

Mathematics

18. Translate Calories into Grams Dylan, a healthy and active teen male, has determined that he needs 2,800 calories each day. His goal is to limit his daily fat intake to 30 percent of his daily calories, while consuming 55 percent of his calories as carbohydrates and 15 percent as protein. How many grams of fat, carbohydrates, and protein does Dylan need each day?

Math Concept **Find the Percent of a Number** To find a percent of a given number, change the percent to a decimal by removing the percent sign and moving the decimal point two places to the left. Multiply this decimal by the number.

Starting Hint Determine the total calories for each nutrient by performing the percent calculations. Divide each total by the number of calories per gram.

NCTM Problem Solving Apply and adapt a variety of appropriate strategies to solve problems.

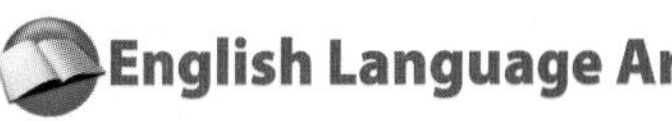

English Language Arts

19. Write a Letter Imagine you have a relative who is so concerned about her weight that she has changed her diet and refuses to eat anything but popcorn, crackers, and fruit. Write a letter to her that explains why she must change her diet, and offers specific suggestions for how she can. Offer her better ideas on how to control her weight while still getting proper nutrition. Explain to your relative that she needs carbohydrates, proteins, and fats. Tell her how many calories she needs to eat per day and explain how her body uses a minimum number of calories to carry out basic functions.

NCTE 12 Use language to accomplish individual purposes

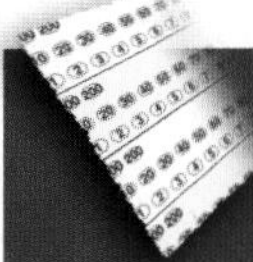

STANDARDIZED TEST PRACTICE

TRUE OR FALSE

Re-read the paragraph about the esophagus on page 66. Determine whether the following statement is true or false.

20. The muscles of the esophagus force food into the intestine by contracting and relaxing.

a. true

b. false

Test-Taking Tip Before deciding whether a statement is true or false, carefully read the text to which it relates. Then slowly review both the statement and the text again. Pay close attention to words. One word can make the difference between a true statement and a false one.

CHAPTER 6

Carbohydrates

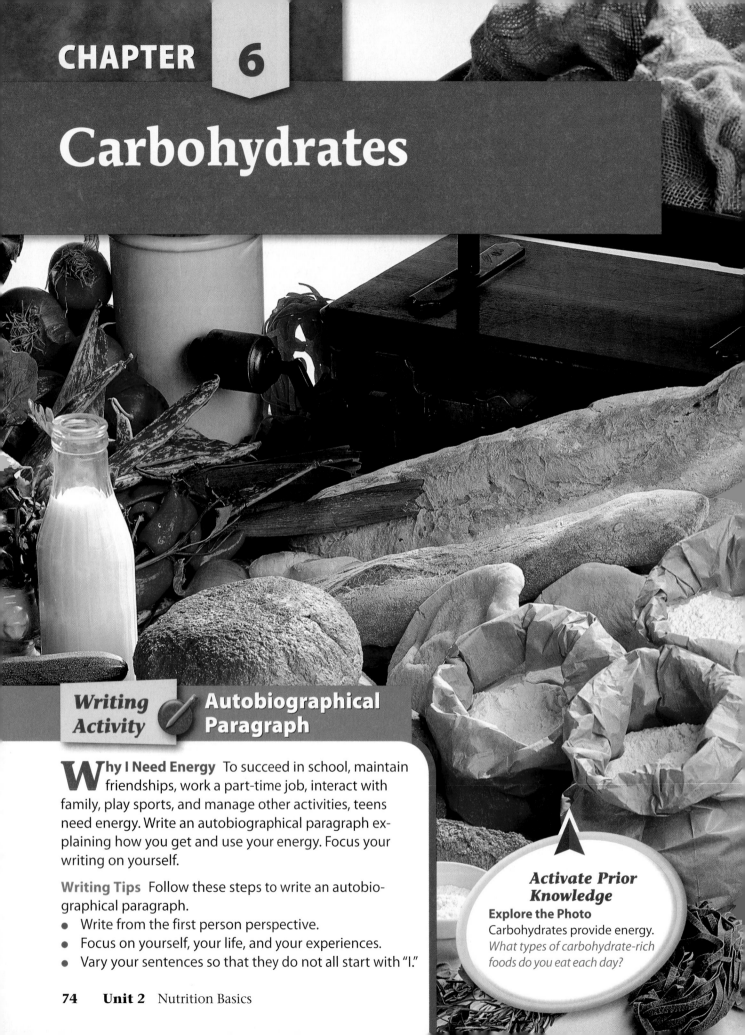

Writing Activity: Autobiographical Paragraph

Why I Need Energy To succeed in school, maintain friendships, work a part-time job, interact with family, play sports, and manage other activities, teens need energy. Write an autobiographical paragraph explaining how you get and use your energy. Focus your writing on yourself.

Writing Tips Follow these steps to write an autobiographical paragraph.

- Write from the first person perspective.
- Focus on yourself, your life, and your experiences.
- Vary your sentences so that they do not all start with "I."

Activate Prior Knowledge

Explore the Photo
Carbohydrates provide energy. *What types of carbohydrate-rich foods do you eat each day?*

Reading Guide

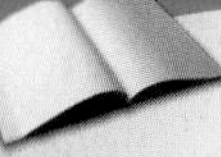

Before You Read

Preview Look at the photos and figures and read their captions. Think about the role that carbohydrates play in your daily diet.

Read to Learn

Key Concepts

- **Identify** the three types of carbohydrates.
- **Explain** how plants create carbohydrates.
- **Identify** and describe the forms that carbohydrates take in food.
- **Explain** how to meet the need for carbohydrates in a healthful diet.

Main Idea

Carbohydrates form the largest part of a healthy diet, are the body's main source of energy, and come in three different types.

Content Vocabulary

You will find definitions for these words in the glossary at the back of this book.

- ☐ carbohydrates
- ☐ photosynthesis
- ☐ chlorophyll
- ☐ sugar
- ☐ simple carbohydrate
- ☐ monosaccharide
- ☐ disaccharide
- ☐ starch
- ☐ polysaccharide
- ☐ complex carbohydrate
- ☐ dietary fiber
- ☐ added sugar
- ☐ sugar substitute

Academic Vocabulary

You will find these words in your reading and on your tests. Use the glossary to look up their definitions if necessary.

- observe
- adequate

Graphic Organizer

Use a graphic organizer like the one below to take notes about carbohydrates in the form of sugars and starches.

SUGARS	STARCHES

Graphic Organizer Go to this book's Online Learning Center at **glencoe.com** to print this graphic organizer.

Academic Standards

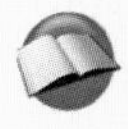

English Language Arts

NCTE 4 Use written language to communicate effectively.

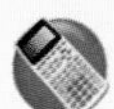

Mathematics

NCTM Number and Operations Compute fluently and make reasonable estimates.

NCTM Data Analysis and Probability Select and use appropriate statistical methods to analyze data.

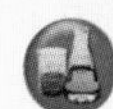

Science

NSES A Develop understanding about scientific inquiry.

NSES 1 Develop an understanding of science unifying concepts such as order and organization.

NCTE *National Council of Teachers of English*
NCTM *National Council of Teachers of Mathematics*
NSES *National Science Education Standards*
NCSS *National Council for the Social Studies*

What are Carbohydrates?

Carbohydrates are the largest part of a healthy diet. **Carbohydrates** (ˌkär-bō-ˈhī-ˌdrāts) are the body's main source of energy. Carbohydrates come mostly from plant foods such as fruits, vegetables, grain products, dry beans, nuts, and seeds.

There are three types of carbohydrates: sugars, starches, and fiber. Sugars, starches, and fiber all play an important role in a healthy diet.

✓ Reading Check **Identify** What are the three types of carbohydrates?

Figure 6.1

Photosynthesis

How Plants Make Food Carbohydrates are a product of photosynthesis in plants. ***What raw materials do plants need to make glucose?***

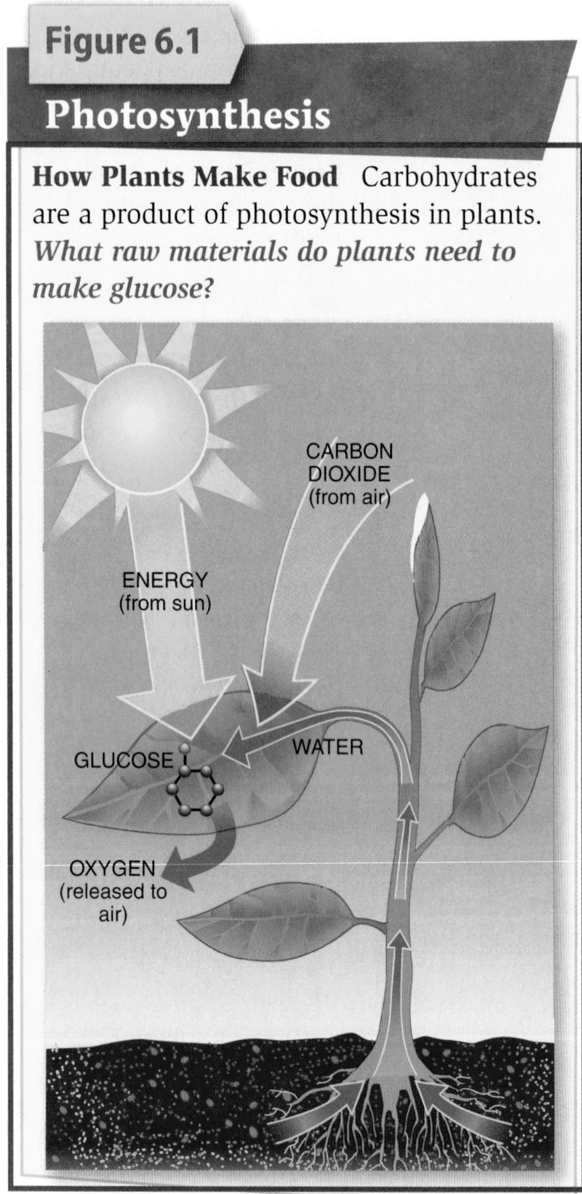

How Plants Create Carbohydrates

Plants create carbohydrates through photosynthesis. **Photosynthesis** (ˈfō-tō-ˈsin(t)-thə-səs) is the process by which plants use the sun's energy to convert carbon dioxide and water into oxygen and glucose. **Chlorophyll** (ˈklȯr-ə-ˌfil), the green pigment in plants, is necessary for photosynthesis. **Figure 6.1** shows the process of photosynthesis.

Plants use glucose to build leaves, flowers, fruits, and seeds. They also use it to help form the fiber that strengthens and supports their cell walls. Plants store extra glucose as starch in roots, stems, and leaves.

Sugars: Simple Carbohydrates

To make glucose, plants absorb water (H_2O) through their roots and carbon dioxide (CO_2) from the air. These sources provide carbon (C), hydrogen (H), and oxygen (O), the chemical elements needed to build sugars. A **sugar** is the form of carbohydrate that supplies energy to the body. Sugars end with the suffix *-ose*. **Figure 6.2** shows six different kinds of sugars.

Figure 6.2

Sugars: Simple Carbohydrates

Simple Sugars The six sugars shown here are important in nutrition. ***How are glucose and disaccharides linked?***

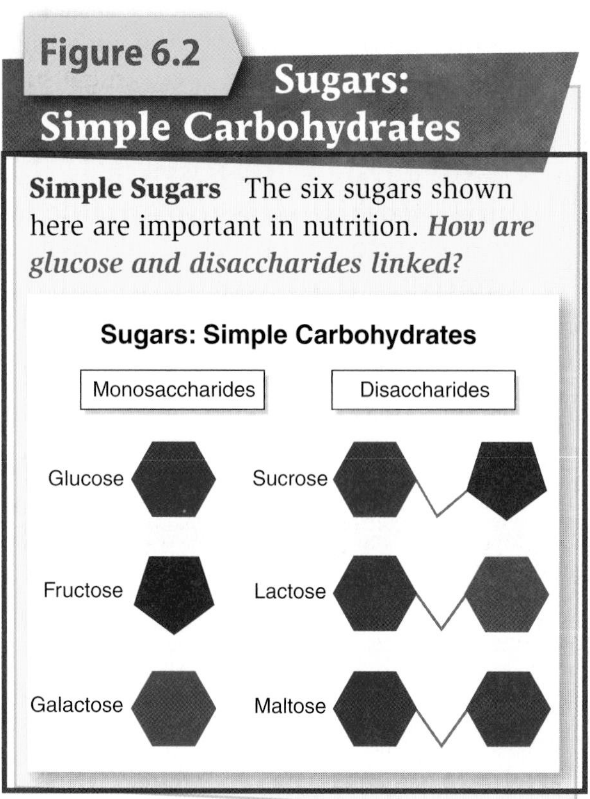

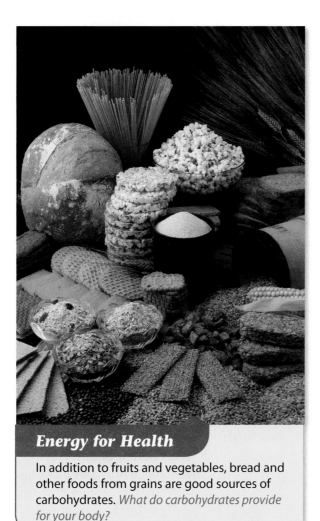

Energy for Health

In addition to fruits and vegetables, bread and other foods from grains are good sources of carbohydrates. *What do carbohydrates provide for your body?*

Science in Action **So Many Sugars**

Sugars, or simple carbohydrates, are present in a variety of foods, including those you do not typically think of as sweet, such as vegetables and milk. In addition to supplying energy to the body, many foods that contain simple carbohydrates offer other benefits, such as fiber, vitamins, minerals, and phytochemicals.

Procedure Consider this scenario: At a party, you are served a platter containing an assortment of sliced fresh fruits, vegetables, and cheese, along with a dip made from sour cream.

Analysis In list form, identify all of the simple carbohydrates that may be found in each of the foods served at the party.

NSES 1 Develop an understanding of science unifying concepts such as order and organization.

In nutrition, sugars are known as simple carbohydrates. A **simple carbohydrate** is a carbohydrate with a simple chemical structure.

Monosaccharides

A **monosaccharide** (ˌmä-nə-ˈsa-kə-ˌrīd) is a sugar with a single chemical unit. *Mono* means "one" and *saccharide* means "sugar." These are the monosaccharides most often found in food:

- **Glucose** This mildly sweet sugar is found in fruits, vegetables, honey, and corn syrup. Glucose is also known as dextrose.
- **Fructose** Fruits, many vegetables, and honey contain fructose, a highly sweet sugar.
- **Galactose** This sugar is in a few foods, including milk. Galactose helps create milk sugar (lactose). Galactose is not very sweet.

Disaccharides

A **disaccharide** ((ˌ)dī-ˈsa-kə-ˌrīd) is a sugar made of two monosaccharides. *Di* means "two." Disaccharides are combinations of glucose and another sugar. These are the disaccharides most often found in food:

- **Sucrose** (glucose + fructose) is found in fruits, sugar cane, and sugar beets.
- **Lactose** (glucose + galactose) is found only in milk and milk products.
- **Maltose** (glucose + glucose) forms when starch is digested.

Starches: Complex Carbohydrates

A **starch** is a carbohydrate with a more complex chemical structure than a sugar. The word *starch* is derived from the Middle English *sterchen*, meaning to stiffen. This is appropriate because starch can be used as a thickening agent when dissolved in water and heated.

Starches are polysaccharides. A **polysaccharide** (ˈpä-lē-ˈsa-kə-ˌrīd) is a sugar made of several monosaccharides. *Poly* means "many."

In nutrition, starches are known as complex carbohydrates. A **complex carbohydrate** is a carbohydrate that requires more work for the body to digest (see **Figure 6.3**).

Dietary Fiber

The third type of carbohydrate is fiber. **Dietary fiber** is plant material that cannot be digested. Fiber is not a nutrient, but it is essential for good health.

Digesting Carbohydrates

During digestion, your body converts carbohydrates to glucose. Glucose is a single-unit sugar that fuels body processes.

Digestive enzymes help break down disaccharides and polysaccharides into single units. For example, the enzyme lactase breaks down the disaccharide lactose, found in dairy products. People who do not produce enough lactase may feel discomfort after they eat milk products. Dietary fiber is not digested. It is important because it helps you feel full and creates weight that helps the body eliminate waste. It leaves the body in waste.

✓ Reading Check **Contrast** What is the difference between simple and complex carbohydrates?

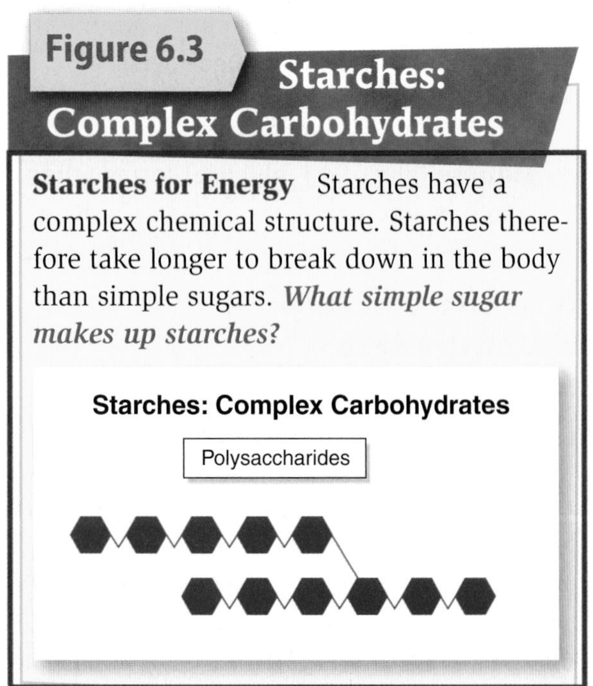

Figure 6.3 Starches: Complex Carbohydrates

Starches for Energy Starches have a complex chemical structure. Starches therefore take longer to break down in the body than simple sugars. ***What simple sugar makes up starches?***

Carbohydrates in Food

When you eat foods from plants, you get carbohydrates in all forms—sugar, starch, and fiber.

Sugars in Food

An apple tastes sweet because it has sugar. Strawberries, oranges, carrots, beets, and many other fruits and vegetables have a sweet taste that comes from natural sugars called sucrose, fructose and galactose. Another natural sugar, lactose, is found in milk.

Early people probably chewed on sweet plants such as sugarcane to satisfy their "sweet tooth." Sugarcane is a tall, thick grass that grows in tropical areas. People later discovered how to extract sucrose from sugarcane, as well as sugar beets. Sucrose from plants is made into brown, white, and powdered sugar.

A sugar that is extracted from plants and used to sweeten foods is an **added sugar**. Sucrose, corn syrup, honey, maple syrup, and molasses are added sugars. Added sugars give pastries, candies, and soft drinks their sweet taste.

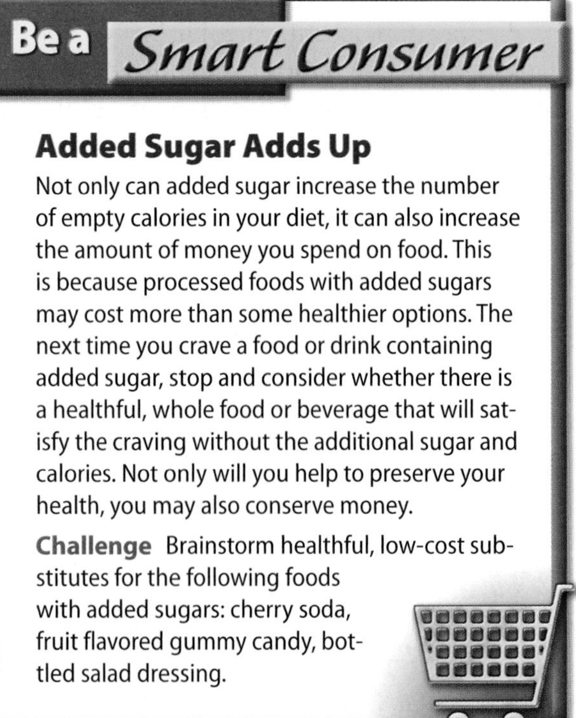

Be a Smart Consumer

Added Sugar Adds Up

Not only can added sugar increase the number of empty calories in your diet, it can also increase the amount of money you spend on food. This is because processed foods with added sugars may cost more than some healthier options. The next time you crave a food or drink containing added sugar, stop and consider whether there is a healthful, whole food or beverage that will satisfy the craving without the additional sugar and calories. Not only will you help to preserve your health, you may also conserve money.

Challenge Brainstorm healthful, low-cost substitutes for the following foods with added sugars: cherry soda, fruit flavored gummy candy, bottled salad dressing.

Starches in Food

In plants, glucose is stored as starch. Grains, or grass seeds, are rich in starch. Peas, corn, beans, winter squash, and potatoes also contain starch.

You may have heard someone say, "I like corn best early in the season when it's nice and sweet." Why is early-season corn sweeter than late-season corn? As a young plant grows, it makes glucose. As the plant matures, it converts glucose to starch. Glucose is sweeter than starch. That is why ears of corn from a young plant taste sweeter than ears of corn from an older plant.

Starches are made of sugars, but they do not taste sweet. Why? Starch molecules are too large to fit your taste buds' receptors. As starches break down in your mouth, however, they taste sweeter. Try chewing a cracker slowly to **observe** this change.

✓ Reading Check **Identify** What are the three forms of carbohydrates from plants?

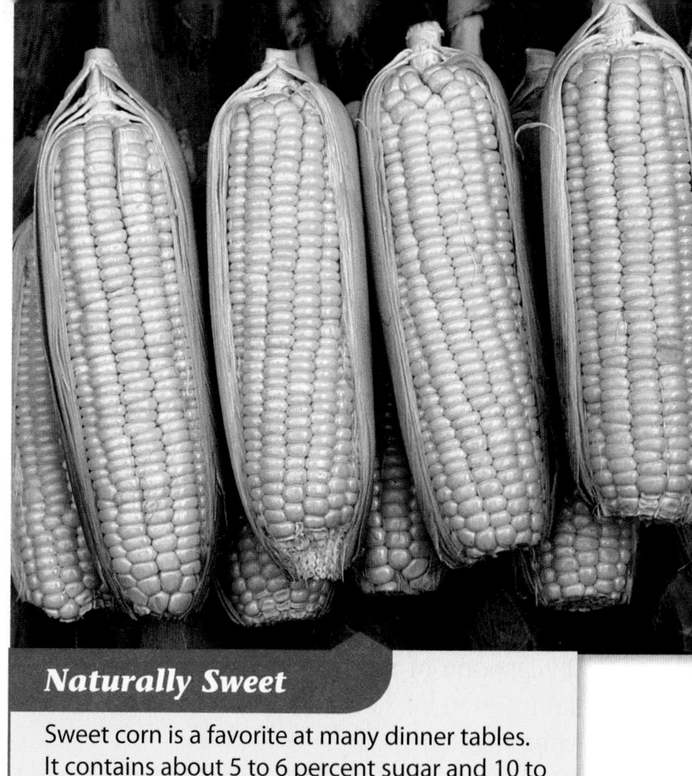

Naturally Sweet

Sweet corn is a favorite at many dinner tables. It contains about 5 to 6 percent sugar and 10 to 11 percent starch. *Why does early-season corn taste sweeter than late-season corn?*

The Need for Carbohydrates

If you do not eat enough foods with carbohydrates, your body will not have an **adequate** supply of glucose. Glucose powers all your activities — breathing, walking, running, thinking. Your brain runs on glucose. Although the brain is only a small part of the human body, it consumes around 20 percent of the body's energy. Fewer carbohydrates in your diet means less glucose for your body. Less glucose means less energy. The body stores glucose as glycogen in the muscles and liver. When your body needs energy, it converts glycogen back into glucose.

Carbohydrates in the Diet

Teens and adults should get 45 to 65 percent of their daily calories from carbohydrates. Choose mostly complex carbohydrates, which have more vitamins, minerals, and fiber than simple carbohydrates. Choose foods with natural sugars, not added sugars.

Carbohydrates cause bacteria in the mouth. The bacteria produce acids that stick to the teeth. This acid can cause tooth decay. This is one reason why it is very important to brush your teeth regularly for healthy teeth and gums.

No-Carb, Low-Carb Diets

What happens if you do not eat enough carbohydrates? Your body uses fat and protein for energy, which takes protein away from tissues. A low-carb diet may also rob your bones of minerals, raise your blood cholesterol, and increase your risk of developing kidney stones. Diets that rely on low-carbohydrates or no-carbohydrates may even cause problems in the nervous system.

Added Sugar in the Diet

Small amounts of foods with added sugar, such as cookies and fruit drinks, can be part of a healthy eating plan. Most people, however, eat far too much added sugar. Added sugars show up in soda, fruit drinks, and pies. Added sugars can lead to overweight and other health problems, such as diabetes and heart disease.

How Much Added Sugar Should You Eat?

The U.S. Department of Agriculture suggests a limit of 10 teaspoons of added sugars per day on a 2,000-calorie diet, and 18 teaspoons of added sugars on a 2,800-calorie diet. Very active people with high energy needs can eat a little more sugar.

How many calories do you get from sugar? Probably more than you realize. Sugar is used in many processed foods, such as ketchup, salad dressings, and convenience foods.

You can estimate the amount of sugar in food. Use the nutrition label to find the grams of sugar in a serving. Four grams of sugar equal 1 teaspoon of sugar, which has 15 calories. A tablespoon of ketchup contains about 2 teaspoons of sugar.

Read the ingredient list on the food label. Look for the terms in **Figure 6.4**. All of these are added sugars. Make a habit of examining food labels for these sugars so you can keep track of how much sugar you are consuming.

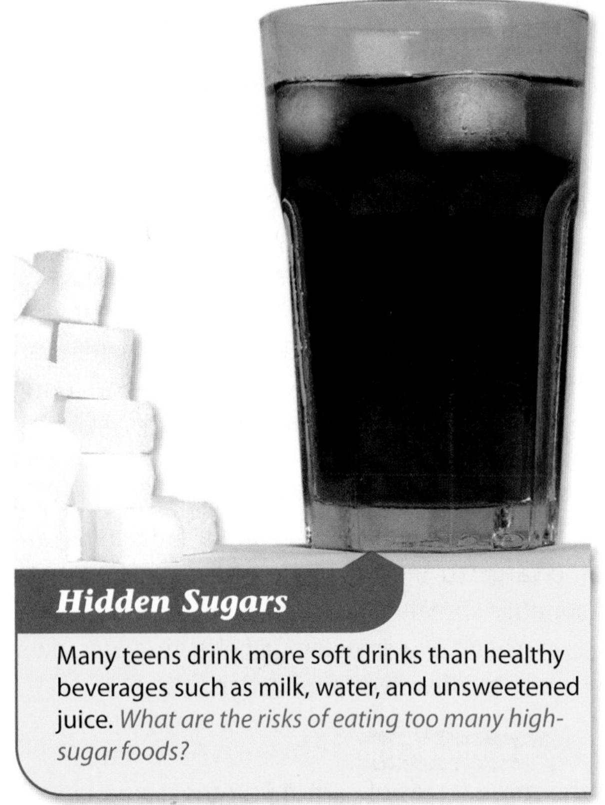

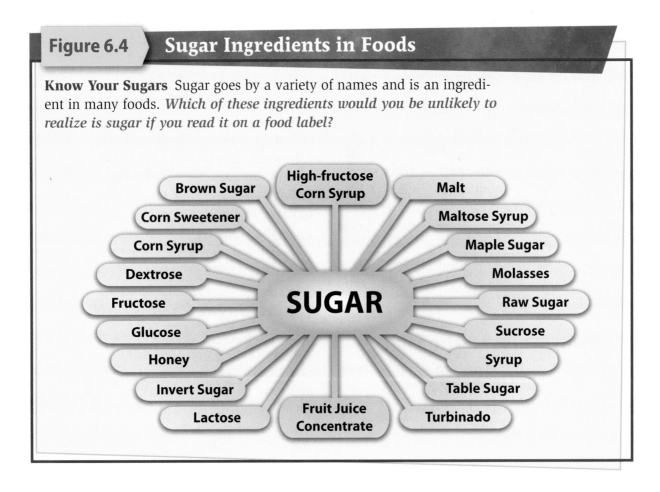

Hidden Sugars

Many teens drink more soft drinks than healthy beverages such as milk, water, and unsweetened juice. *What are the risks of eating too many high-sugar foods?*

Figure 6.4 **Sugar Ingredients in Foods**

Know Your Sugars Sugar goes by a variety of names and is an ingredient in many foods. ***Which of these ingredients would you be unlikely to realize is sugar if you read it on a food label?***

SUGAR

- High-fructose Corn Syrup
- Malt
- Maltose Syrup
- Maple Sugar
- Molasses
- Raw Sugar
- Sucrose
- Syrup
- Table Sugar
- Turbinado
- Fruit Juice Concentrate
- Lactose
- Invert Sugar
- Honey
- Glucose
- Fructose
- Dextrose
- Corn Syrup
- Corn Sweetener
- Brown Sugar

Sugar Substitutes

A **sugar substitute** is a substance that tastes sweet but has few or no calories. Foods sweetened with sugar substitutes can still be high in calories and fat, however. Artificial sweeteners and sugar alcohols are the most common types of sugar substitutes.

Artificial Sweeteners Artificial sweeteners have no calories. You can buy four kinds of artificial sweeteners: aspartame (ˈas-pər-ˌtām), ace-sulfame-K (ˈā-sē-ˌsəl-ˌfām-ˈkā), saccharin (ˈsa-k(ə)-rən), and sucralose (ˈsü-krə-ˌlōs). Food safety advocates question the safety of some artificial sweeteners.

Sugar Alcohols Despite their name, sugar alcohols do not contain sugar or alcohol. They are manufactured from carbohydrates and provide about one-half to one-third fewer calories than sugar. Common sugar alcohols include sorbitol (ˈsȯr-bə-ˌtȯl), mannitol (ˈma-nə-ˌtȯl), and isomalt (ˈī-sə-ˌmȯlt). Sugar alcohols are used in sugar-free candies, cookies, ice cream, and chewing gum. Eating too much sugar alcohol can cause diarrhea.

Starch in the Diet

To stay healthy, eat more complex carbohydrates than simple carbohydrates. Starchy foods not only provide glucose to keep your body running, but also supply protein, vitamins, minerals, phytochemicals, and fiber.

Some people believe that starchy foods like bread, potatoes, and pasta cause weight gain. These foods are not high in calories, but high-fat sauces, spreads, and gravies are. In fact, complex carbohydrates are filling and low in fat and can help people manage weight. A healthy meal is full of complex carbohydrates.

Fiber in the Diet

Dietary fiber is only found in foods from plant sources, such as fruits, vegetables, whole-grain products, nuts, seeds, and dry beans, peas, and lentils. Dietary fiber is sometimes called bulk, cellulose, or roughage. **Figure 6.5** shows the amount of fiber in several common foods.

Figure 6.5 Dietary Fiber in Selected Foods

Fiber in Focus Many foods provide the fiber that is vital for digestion. ***Which foods might you use to incorporate fiber into your lunch?***

Food	Approximate Measure	Grams of Dietary Fiber
Apple or pear	1	4
Orange	1	3
Strawberries	1 cup	4
Orange juice	¾ cup	0–1
Baked potato with skin	1 medium	4
Corn, cooked	½ cup	3
Broccoli or spinach, cooked	½ cup	2
Peanut butter	2 Tbsp.	2
Mixed nuts	¼ cup	2
Black-eyed peas, cooked	½ cup	8
Baked beans	½ cup	7

Food	Approximate Measure	Grams of Dietary Fiber
Refried beans	½ cup	6
Split pea soup	10 oz.	4
Raisin bran	1 cup	8
Cooked oatmeal	1 cup	4
Bran muffin	1	4
Whole wheat bread	2 slices	4
White bread or bagel	2 slices 1 bagel	1
Brown rice, cooked	1 cup	3
White rice, cooked	1 cup	1
Spaghetti, cooked	1 cup	2
Air-popped popcorn	3 cups	4

Dietary fiber is eliminated as waste, so why do you need it? Fiber does not provide energy, but it is vital to digestion. Fiber absorbs water, much like a sponge. It creates mass that helps food move through the large intestine. This promotes regular bowel movements and helps prevent constipation. Fiber may also help reduce blood cholesterol by absorbing it and helping remove it from the body.

Teens need between 26 and 38 grams of dietary fiber a day, depending on their age and gender. Adults need 19 to 38 grams.

How can you get more fiber in your diet? Choose whole-grain breads, cereals, and crackers instead of white bread or refined cereals and crackers. Try brown rice instead of white rice. Add wheat germ, barley, or bulgur to soups, stews, and casseroles. Eat more vegetables, fruits, and dry beans, peas, and lentils. These foods are rich in fiber as well as vitamins, minerals, and phytonutrients.

If you plan to increase the amount of fiber in your diet, do so gradually. This allows your body to adjust. Drink more water as you increase the amount of fiber you eat.

Kitchen Math

Menu Planning

One of your classmates is concerned about getting enough fiber in her diet, and has asked you for advice in choosing what to eat. Using Figure 6.5 as a guide, devise a full-day menu for your classmate consisting of three meals that, combined, will provide the necessary amount of fiber. Note that your classmate is allergic to nuts.

Math Concept **Problem Solving** When presented with a problem requiring calculations, read it carefully, and identify all facts. Make sure you understand what it is asking you to do.

Starting Hint First, determine how many grams of dietary fiber are necessary for your classmate. Select foods for your menu, being careful to avoid items that would trigger allergies. Add up the grams of fiber in your menu. If you do not have the recommended amount, adjust your menu.

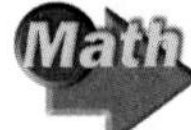

Math Appendix For math help, go to the Math Appendix at the back of the book.

NCTM Number and Operations Compute fluently and make reasonable estimates.

Light and Healthy Recipe

Polenta with Rosemary

Ingredients

- **1 cup** Lowfat milk
- **1 cup** Chicken stock
- **1 cup** Corn meal
- **2 tsp.** Fresh rosemary
- **1 Tbsp.** Butter

Yield 4 servings, ¾ cup each

Directions

1. Combine the milk and chicken stock in a pot and bring to a simmer.
2. Slowly pour in the cornmeal and begin stirring at once to avoid clumping. Keep heat at medium.
3. Stir occasionally until polenta begins to thicken. Add the rosemary and continue cooking and stirring occasionally.
4. Add butter and stir it in until melted just before serving.

The corn meal used in polenta makes it a good source of complex carbohydrates.

Yield 4 servings

Nutrition Analysis per Serving

■ Calories	205
■ Total fat	5 g
Saturated fat	3 g
Cholesterol	14 mg
■ Sodium	114 mg
■ Carbohydrate	32 g
Dietary fiber	1 g
Sugars	18 g
■ Protein	6 g

CHAPTER 6 Review & Applications

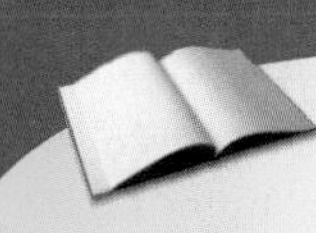

After You Read

Chapter Summary

Carbohydrates form the largest part of a healthy diet. Plants create carbohydrates through photosynthesis. Sugars are simple carbohydrates. Starches are complex carbohydrates. Fiber is plant material that cannot be digested, but is necessary for good health. During digestion, carbohydrates are converted to glucose. Carbohydrates create both sweet and starchy goods. They are an essential part of a healthful diet because they provide energy for all activities. No- or low-carb diets can be dangerous, as can too much added sugar. Some sugar in the diet is healthy. Sugar substitutes can replace added sugars. Starch and fiber are essential components to a healthful diet.

Content and Academic Vocabulary Review

1. Use each of these content and academic vocabulary words in a sentence.

Content Vocabulary

- ☐ carbohydrates (p. 76)
- ☐ photosynthesis (p. 76)
- ☐ chlorophyll (p. 76)
- ☐ sugar (p. 76)
- ☐ simple carbohydrate (p. 77)
- ☐ monosaccharide (p. 77)
- ☐ disaccharide (p. 77)
- ☐ starch (p. 77)
- ☐ polysaccharide (p. 77)
- ☐ complex carbohydrate (p. 78)
- ☐ dietary fiber (p. 78)
- ☐ added sugar (p. 78)
- ☐ sugar substitute (p. 81)

Academic Vocabulary

- observe (p. 79)
- adequate (p. 79)

Review Key Concepts

2. Identify the three types of carbohydrates.
3. Explain how plants create carbohydrates.
4. Identify and describe the forms that carbohydrates take in food.
5. Explain how to meet the need for carbohydrates in a healthful diet.

Critical Thinking

6. Describe how a severe drought might affect the body's access to energy.
7. Plan a meal that contains three different types of simple sugars. What foods would your meal include? Where would the simple sugars be found?
8. Describe a good choice of food for an athlete who has a long bike race coming up tomorrow. Explain your choice.
9. Explain why it is important to limit added sugars.
10. Design a menu that provides 26 grams of fiber for Mary. Mary is allergic to nuts and gluten, a type of protein found in wheat, rye, and barley. Bread, muffins, pasta, and cereals contain gluten.

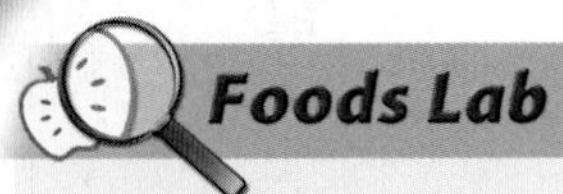

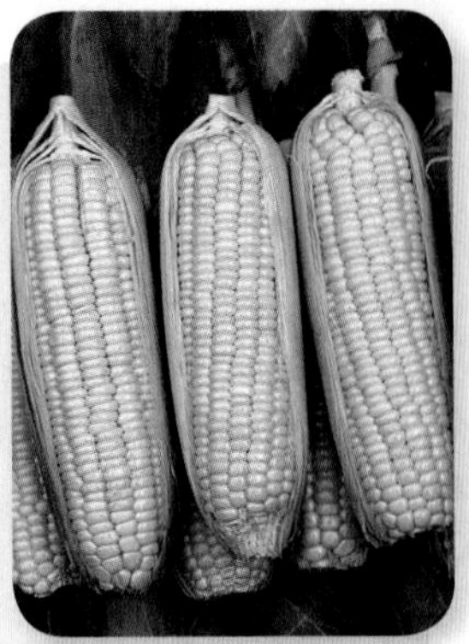

11. Carbohydrate Recipes How can you sustain your body's energy throughout the day, and enjoy tasty food? With the range of good foods that contain complex carbohydrates, it is easy to include them in every meal.

Procedure Create a simple recipe that uses at least two sources of complex carbohydrates, such as a salad, sandwich, main dish, or dessert. Prepare and evaluate your recipe.

Analysis Verbalize your responses to the following questions. What foods did you choose as carbohydrate sources? How did they increase your recipe's appeal? What are other advantages of choosing carbohydrate-rich foods?

HEALTHFUL CHOICES

12. Selecting Snacks You need a snack to eat before your big math test and you have two choices: a chocolate chip muffin sprinkled with sugar, or a whole grain bagel spread with peanut butter. Which should you choose and why?

TECH Connection

13. Simple or Complex How do you know whether a food is a simple or a complex carbohydrate? Conduct research to identify 10 foods that contain simple carbohydrates, and 10 foods that contain complex carbohydrates. Use word processing software to create a table that lists simple carbohydrate choices on one side and complex ones on the other. Include foods you eat often as well as foods you eat occasionally or have never tried. Rank the foods in order of the amount of carbohydrates in each food. Put the item with the most carbohydrates per ounce at the top and work down.

Real-World Skills

Problem-Solving

14. Naturally Sweet Most desserts, such as cakes, cookies, and ice cream, contain added sugars. Brainstorm three naturally sweet foods that you would serve for dessert at a party. What are they? How would you present them in an appealing way?

Interpersonal and Collaborative Skills

15. Conduct a Survey Follow your teacher's instructions to form into groups. Take a survey of each group member's five favorite snack foods. Categorize the results into simple and complex carbohydrates. What do the results show about your group's overall eating habits and health? Share your findings with the class.

Financial Literacy

16. Compare Cereal Costs Visit a local supermarket. Identify five types of fiber-rich cereals, and research their costs. Calculate their costs per ounce. Compare the amount of fiber per serving in each. If you are looking for maximum fiber, which is the best value? Why?

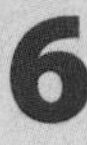

Academic Skills

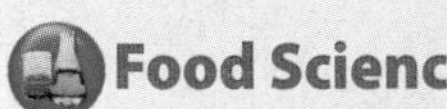

Food Science

17. Starch Indicator An easy way to detect the presence of starch in a food is with iodine. Chemically, the iodine slips into the starch coil, and changes color from brown to deep blue-black. If no starch is present, then the iodine stays brownish orange.

Procedure On a sheet of wax paper, place a cracker, pieces of bread, potato, meat, celery, and apple. Add a drop of iodine onto each. Record the color of each food.

Analysis Consider the color of each food. Record whether or not starch is present.

NSES A Develop understanding about scientific inquiry.

Mathematics

18. Comparing Carbohydrates A bottle of cranberry juice cocktail has 34 grams of carbohydrates per serving, while orange juice has 25 carbohydrate grams per serving. Per serving, a bottle of cola has 27 carbohydrate grams, a bottle of natural soda has 17, and milk has 12. Out of the figures observed, what is the minimum value of carbohydrate grams per serving? What is the maximum value? What is the range?

Math Concept **Range** Range is a statistical measure used with a set of numbers. It is calculated by subtracting the lowest value in the set from the highest value.

Starting Hint Find the largest (maximum) value of carbohydrate grams per serving, then find the minimum value given. Subtract to determine the range.

NCTM Data Analysis and Probability Select and use appropriate statistical methods to analyze data.

English Language Arts

19. Write a Paragraph Carbohydrate-rich foods are often the favorite part of a person's diet. Write a paragraph describing your favorite carbohydrate-rich food. In the paragraph, describe why you enjoy the food, how it looks, how it is made and what it tastes like. Identify whether it is rich in sugars, starches, or fiber. Exchange paragraphs with a classmate. Read each other's paragraph and suggest changes to make the paragraph better. Make your suggestions in writing. Rewrite your paragraph using at least one of the suggestions from your classmate.

NCTE 4 Use written language to communicate effectively.

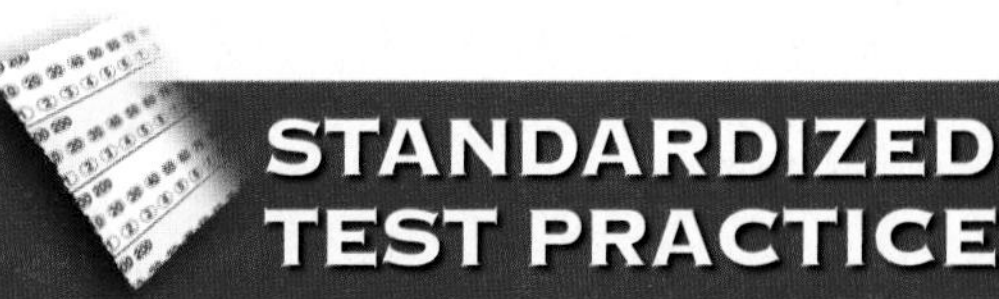

STANDARDIZED TEST PRACTICE

FILL IN THE BLANK

Read the statement and select the best word to fill in the blank.

20. Starches, carbohydrates with more complex chemical structures than sugar, are ____________.

a. disaccharides
b. bisacchardies
c. polysaccharides
d. monosaccharides

Test-Taking Tip When answering a fill-in-the-blank question, silently read the sentence with each of the possible answers in the blank space. This will help you eliminate wrong answers. The best word results in a sentence that is both factual and grammatically correct.

CHAPTER 7

Proteins & Fats

Writing Activity 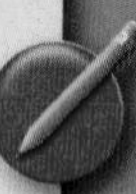 Autobiographical Paragraph

Your Growth As a teen, you have watched your own body change and grow. Write an autobiographical paragraph about your physical growth over the last five years. How has your growth affected the amounts and types of foods you eat? Was there a time in the last five years when you have felt hungry more often?

Writing Tips Follow these steps to write an autobiographical paragraph:

- Write from the first person perspective.
- Focus on yourself, your life, and your experiences.
- Vary your sentences so they do not all start with "I."

Activate Prior Knowledge

Explore the Photo While many people think fat is bad, the right amount and types of fats are essential. *Which foods have healthy fat?*

Reading Guide

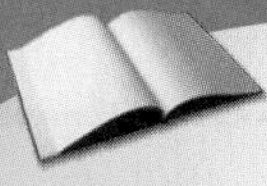

Before You Read

Preview Write one question about the role of proteins in a healthful diet and one question about the role of fats in a healthful diet. As you read, see if you can discover the answers to your questions.

Read to Learn

Key Concepts

- **Explain** protein, its structure, and its types.
- **Identify** the role of protein in a healthful diet.
- **Explain** lipids, their structure and their types.
- **Summarize** the role of cholesterol in a healthful diet.

Main Idea

Proteins help the body grow and repair itself, lipids are essential to nutrition, and both are necessary parts of a healthful diet.

Content Vocabulary

You will find the definitions for these words in the glossary at the back of this book.

- ☐ amino acid
- ☐ hemoglobin
- ☐ essential amino acid
- ☐ complete protein
- ☐ incomplete protein
- ☐ triglyceride
- ☐ fatty acid
- ☐ saturated fatty acid
- ☐ lipoprotein
- ☐ cholesterol
- ☐ hydrogenation
- ☐ trans fats

Academic Vocabulary

You will find definitions for these words in your reading and on your tests. Use the glossary to look up their definitions if necessary.

- continuous
- component

Graphic Organizer

Use a graphic organizer like the one below to take notes about the five most important roles of protein in the body.

5 ROLES OF PROTEIN				

Graphic Organizer Go to this book's Online Learning Center at **glencoe.com** to print out this graphic organizer.

Academic Standards

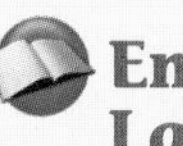

English Language Arts

NCTE 7 Conduct research and gather, evaluate and synthesize data to communicate discoveries

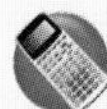

Mathematics

NCTM Measurement Understand measurable attributes of objects and the units, systems, and processes of measurement.

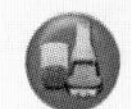

Science

NSES A Develop abilities necessary to do scientific inquiry.

NSES B Develop an understanding of the interactions of energy and matter.

NCTE *National Council of Teachers of English*
NCTM *National Council of Teachers of Mathematics*
NSES *National Science Education Standards*
NCSS *National Council for the Social Studies.*

Protein

Protein helps your body grow and repair itself. Proteins are found in animal products, including meat, poultry, fish, eggs, and dairy products. Proteins are also found in plant foods, especially dry beans and peas, nuts, vegetables, and grain products.

The Structure of Proteins

Proteins are part of every cell in your body. In fact, proteins make up one-fifth of your body weight.

Proteins are made of amino (uh-ˈmē-(ˌ)nō) acids. An **amino acid** is a molecule that combines with other amino acid molecules to make proteins. Twenty different amino acids are found in protein foods. Amino acids chain together to form thousands of different proteins.

Different proteins perform specialized tasks. Some amino acids wind together into long, rope-like spirals. These proteins are found in tendons and ligaments. Other amino acids combine into ball-shaped proteins, such as hemoglobin. **Hemoglobin** (ˈhē-mə-ˌglō-bən) is a protein that transports oxygen in the blood to all the cells in your body.

Nutrition Check

Complete Proteins

The nine essential amino acids that comprise a complete protein are phenylalanine, valine, threonine, tryptophan, isoleucine, methionine, histidine, leucine, and lysine. People who eat a diet that includes both animal and plant foods consume complete proteins with relative ease. People who follow a vegan diet, however, must make an effort. Vegans do not eat any animal foods, including milk and eggs. Since their diets are plant-based, they must combine different plant foods in order to consume complete proteins. For example, burritos containing beans, rice, and a wheat or corn tortilla contain complete protein. Pasta with broccoli is another combination that makes complete protein. Whole wheat bread with peanut butter is yet another.

Think About It Conduct research to find another example of a vegan recipe with ingredients that combine to form complete protein. Which ingredients are used? Can you discover which amino acids are present in each ingredient? Answer these questions in a paragraph.

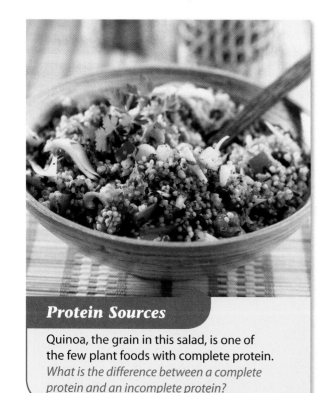

Protein Sources

Quinoa, the grain in this salad, is one of the few plant foods with complete protein. *What is the difference between a complete protein and an incomplete protein?*

Protein Digestion

How does protein in food become protein in your body? When you eat a protein food, your body breaks the protein down into amino acids. Then the amino acids combine into the proteins your body needs.

Protein digestion starts in the stomach. Acid changes the shape of the proteins, and enzymes break the proteins down. In the small intestine, the proteins break down into amino acids. The amino acids are then absorbed into the bloodstream and sent to the cells to make new proteins.

Complete and Incomplete Proteins

Your body makes some, but not all, amino acids for itself. An amino acid that your body needs but cannot make is called an **essential amino acid**. You must get essential amino acids from food.

A food that contains all nine essential amino acids is called a **complete protein**. Meat, poultry, fish, eggs, milk, and soy are complete proteins.

A food that lacks one or more essential amino acids is called an **incomplete protein**. Most plant foods are incomplete proteins. However, combining plant foods can provide complete protein. For example, legumes plus rice, corn, or nuts makes a complete protein. You can eat these combinations at different meals and still get the benefits of complete protein.

The Need for Protein

Proteins have countless roles in the body. Here are five of the most important.

Growth and Maintenance In a healthy body, proteins are constantly broken down and replaced. For example, the cells in your intestinal tract are replaced every few days. The body needs a **continuous**, or uninterrupted, supply of protein to grow and to repair itself.

Enzymes Chemical reactions take place in every cell in your body. Special proteins called enzymes make these reactions possible.

Hormones Hormones are chemical messengers that help regulate the body. Some hormones are made from amino acids. Two examples are insulin, which helps maintain the level of glucose (sugar) in your blood, and the thyroid hormone that regulates metabolism.

Antibodies Proteins play a role in the immune system in the form of antibodies. Antibodies are proteins that fight disease. If you get the flu, your body makes antibodies to fight it.

Fluid Balance Proteins inside cells and in the bloodstream help cells to maintain the right amount of fluid.

How Much Protein Do You Need?

Teens should get 10 to 30 percent of their calories from proteins. Adults should get 10 to 35 percent of their calories from protein.

Suppose a teen's daily calorie requirement is 2,800 calories. How many grams of protein should he eat? First, calculate how many calories should come from protein. Ten percent of 2,800 calories is 280 calories ($2800 \times .10 = 280$). Thirty percent of 2,800 calories is 840 calories ($2800 \times .30 = 840$). Protein has four calories per gram, so divide these numbers by four to determine the number of grams needed. The appropriate daily protein range for the

Figure 7.1 **Approximate Protein in Selected Foods**

Where to Get Protein Protein is found in many foods, including the ones on the following chart. ***How much protein is there in a roast beef sandwich with cheese?***

Food	Approximate Measure	Protein (Grams)
Beans, baked	½ cup	7
Beans, white, dried, cooked	1 cup	19
Beef, ground	3 oz.	22
Beef, roast	3 oz.	22
Bread	1 slice	2–5
Cheese, cheddar	1 oz.	7
Chicken, roasted	3 oz.	27
Egg	1	6

Food	Approximate Measure	Protein (Grams)
Green beans	½ cup	1
Halibut	3 oz	23
Milk	1 cup	8
Nuts, mixed	1 oz.	5–6
Peanut butter	2 Tbsp.	7–9
Peas	½ cup	2–4
Pasta	1 cup	7
Tofu	3 oz.	6–8
Yogurt, plain	8 oz.	7–13

for the teen is 70 to 210 grams. The chart in **Figure 7.1** on page 89 shows what foods the teen might eat in a day to get the right amount of protein.

People need more protein at certain times. For instance, pregnant women and nursing mothers need extra protein. Infants, children, and teens need more protein than adults, because they are still growing.

Excess Protein

Protein is essential for the body, but eating too much protein can be harmful. Excess protein is also hard on the digestive system. Excess protein is broken down and stored by the body as fat, which can lead to weight gain.

Most healthy people do not need supplements with protein or amino acids. Most people get plenty of protein by choosing a variety of healthy foods.

Inadequate Protein

Protein-energy malnutrition (PEM) occurs when a person does not get enough calories and protein. PEM is one of the most common forms of malnutrition in the world. Children with PEM do not grow properly. Some die of starvation. PEM can affect people who have eating disorders or drug addictions.

Protein Food Choices

Most Americans get most of their protein from animal sources. However, most health experts recommend eating more protein from plant sources. Plant foods have less fat and more fiber than animal foods—and they usually cost less.

Meatless dishes with complete proteins include rice and beans, a peanut butter sandwich, and hummus on pita bread. Soybeans, quinoa, and buckwheat offer complete protein, too. You could use tofu, tempeh (ˈtem-ˌpā), and soy milk in preparing main dishes. Nuts, lentils, and black beans also are good sources of protein.

Plant foods can also be mixed with a little animal protein to create dishes with complete protein. Macaroni and cheese, tuna-noodle casserole, and vegetable and chicken stir-fry all provide complete protein. Whole wheat pasta adds protein to meals.

Careers in Food

Corinne Trang
Food Author

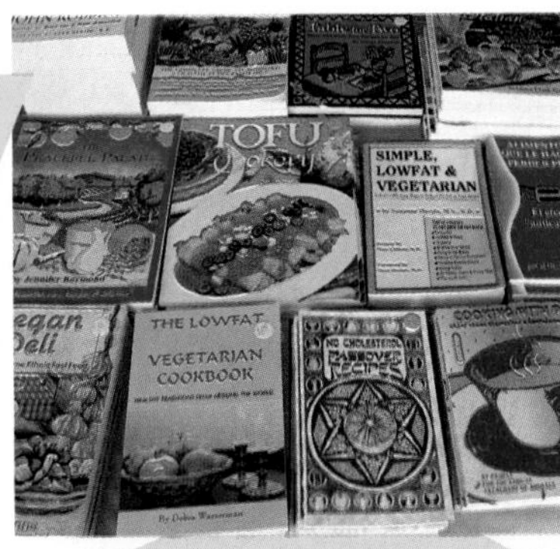

Q: What is your approach to writing a cookbook?

A: Cookbooks have recipes and are how-to's by definition. As an author, I instruct the reader on how to cook food through the recipes in my book and in published articles in other publications.

Q: What was your inspiration for becoming a cookbook author?

A: I took a fellow cookbook author to Chinatown in New York City and introduced her to my favorite noodle vendor. She went on to write about how to use Italian pasta to re-create Asian noodle recipes. In 1998, I left *Saveur* magazine to write my first cookbook, *Authentic Vietnamese Cooking: Food from a Family Table.*

Q: What do you like about your job?

A: Cooking and sharing meals while talking about food is my favorite thing to do.

"Have passion for what you do, otherwise you are just going through the motions."
— Corinne Trang
Food Author - New York, NY

Education and Training
On-the-job training at a food magazine. Degrees in English, journalism, or culinary arts also help.

Qualities and Skills
Creativity and a love of cooking is important. It also helps to be comfortable with change.

Related Career Opportunities
Journalist, chef/food stylist, consultant/spokesperson, public relations, hospitality management.

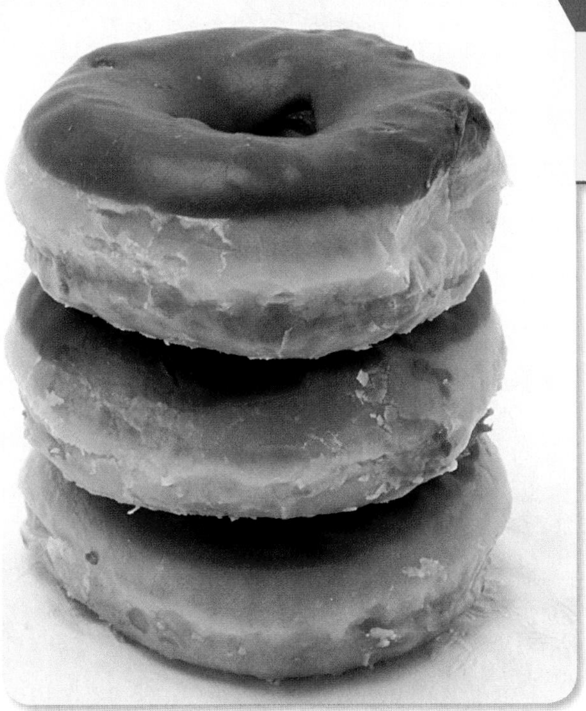

Finding the Fat

Fat is easy to see in some foods, like butter. Fat is not so easy to see in other foods, such as doughnuts. *How can you tell if a salad dressing or baked good is high in fat?*

✓ Reading Check **Explain** How does protein in your food become useful to your body?

The Lipid Family

Lipids are a family of chemical compounds found in every cell, both in foods and in the human body.

Two types of lipids are especially important in nutrition: triglycerides ((ˌ)trī-ˈgli-sə-ˌrīds) and sterols. A **triglyceride** is a basic fat molecule. Triglycerides are the main **component** of fatty tissue. Sterols are lipids found in cell membranes. Cholesterol (kə-ˈles-tə-ˌrōl) is one important type of sterol. You will read more about cholesterol on pages 93 and 94.

Fats

Fats are greasy substances, either solid or liquid, that will not dissolve in water. Liquid fats are called oils.

High-fat foods are usually high in calories. High-fat foods include butter, margarine, oils, cream, fried foods, ice cream, nuts and seeds, egg yolks, and whole milk. Many cheeses, salad dressings, baked goods, gravies, and processed meats (such as hot dogs) are also high in fat.

Some fats are easy to spot. The white portions of meats are fat. Butter, margarine, and oil are also easy to see. Fats you can see are called visible fats.

Many foods contain fats that cannot be seen. These invisible fats are part of the food's chemical composition. Egg yolks, nuts, whole milk, and avocados do not look greasy or oily, yet they are high in fat. This means that you cannot judge the amount of fat in a food just by how it looks.

When you eat fat in food, your body places it in adipose cells throughout the body. Adipose cells are cells in the body that store fat. The cells in adipose tissue grow larger as they store more fat.

Why Fats Are Needed

Are fats bad for you? No. In fact, fats have many important functions in the body.

- Fat helps the body absorb vitamins A, D, E, and K.
- Body fat serves as an energy reserve.
- Body fat cushions and protects the heart and other vital organs. It protects bones from injury.
- A layer of body fat under the skin provides insulation for warmth.
- Fat is a component of cell membranes.
- Because fats move slowly through the digestive system, they help you feel full longer after eating.

Know Your Fats

Saturated fats are solid at room temperature, and unsaturated fats are liquid at room temperature. *Chemically, what is the difference between saturated and unsaturated fats?*

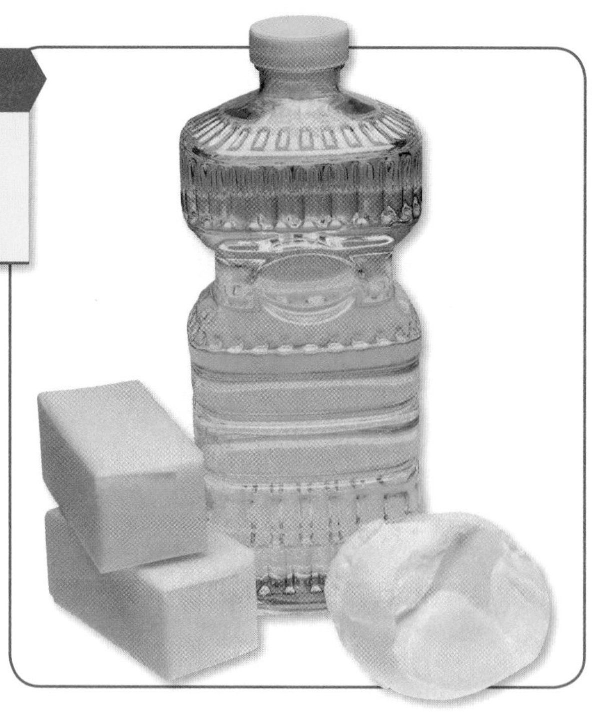

Fat also enhances the flavor and texture of many foods. Fats add moisture and tenderness to some foods and crispiness to others. The key is to eat fats in small, healthy amounts.

Structure of Fats

Fats are made from chemical structures known as fatty acids. A **fatty acid** is the basic building block of fats. It takes three fatty acids plus glycerol to make a triglyceride. Tri means three.

Different fatty acids have different chemical structures. Hydrogen is part of every fatty acid. A fatty acid that contains all the hydrogen it can chemically hold is called a **saturated** (ˈsa-chə-ˌrā-ted) **fatty acid**.

Unsaturated fatty acids are missing hydrogen units. A fatty acid with one hydrogen unit missing is a monounsaturated fatty acid (ˌmä-nō-ən-ˈsa-chə-ˌrā-ted). Mono means one. A fatty acid with two or more hydrogen units missing is a polyunsaturated (ˌpä-lē-ən-ˈsa-chə-ˌrā-ted) fatty acid. Poly means many.

Fats that are solid at room temperature, such as butter and the fat on meat, are made mostly of saturated fatty acids. Fats that are liquid at room temperature, such as corn oil and olive oil, are made mostly of unsaturated fatty acids. Melting does not change fat from one type to another. Melted butter, for example, is still a saturated fat.

Essential Fatty Acids

Your body makes some, but not all, fats for itself. A fatty acid that your body needs but cannot make is called an essential fatty acid. You must get essential fatty acids from food.

One important fatty acid is linolenic acid (ˌli-nə-ˈlē-nik), a type of omega-3 (ō-ˈmā-gə) fatty acid. An omega-3 fatty acid is a polyunsaturated essential fatty acid that may lower the risk of heart disease. It is found in fish oils, especially in fatty fish such as salmon, sardines, mackerel, trout, and herring. Plant sources include flax seeds, kiwifruit, walnuts, pumpkin seeds, sunflower seeds and leafy vegetables.

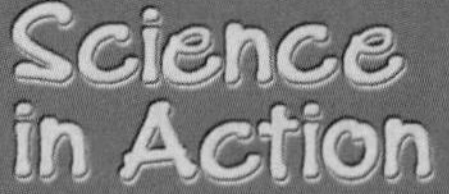

Butter or Margarine?

Before hydrogenation, animal products such as butter were used to add flavor and texture to foods. These animal products contain fat, cholesterol, and very small amounts of naturally occurring trans fats. The process of hydrogenation has introduced foods such as margarine, a low-fat, low-cholesterol food that is frequently substituted for butter. The process of hydrogenation creates trans fat.

Procedure Under your teacher's direction, use the library or the Internet to conduct research. Interview a chef or home cook about his or her preferences. Compare butter and hydrogenated margarine, noting the differences in their nutritional contents.

Analysis Write a one-page report noting the differences in the nutritional contents of butter and margarine. Make an argument for using one or the other based on taste and the amount of trans fat in each. Use specific examples from your research to back up your argument.

NSES A Develop abilities necessary to do scientific inquiry.

Fat Digestion

When you eat foods with fats, the digestive process breaks the fats down through a complex series of steps. Fats are mainly digested in the small intestine. The gallbladder releases bile, which is made by the liver, into the small intestine. The liver can make about 1 liter of bile a day. Bile helps to break down the fats into fatty acids.

Fatty acids are absorbed into the bloodstream, where they travel to the liver and to tissues that need them. Some form into triglycerides and join with protein in chemical packages that travel together through the bloodstream. A fat-protein unit is called a **lipoprotein** (lī-pō-ˈprō-ˌtēn).

Cholesterol

Cholesterol is a fatlike substance in cells that is needed for many body processes. Cholesterol helps digest fat, build cells, and make vitamin D and some hormones. Too much cholesterol, however, is linked to heart disease.

Your body makes all the cholesterol you need. You also get cholesterol, however, from eating animal foods. Fatty meat and poultry, egg yolks, liver and other organ meats, shrimp, and squid, are particularly high in cholesterol. Foods from plant sources have no cholesterol. **Figure 7.2** shows the amount of cholesterol in a variety of foods.

LDL and HDL

Cholesterol circulates in the blood as part of two lipoproteins—LDL and HDL.

LDL Low-density lipoprotein, or LDL, takes cholesterol from the liver to wherever it is needed in the body. Excess LDL can build up in the artery walls and increase the risk of heart disease and stroke. LDL cholesterol is often called "bad" cholesterol.

HDL High-density lipoprotein, or HDL, picks up excess cholesterol and takes it back to the liver for excretion. HDL cholesterol is known as "good" cholesterol. (To remember that HDL is the "good" one, you might associate the letter *H* with a positive word like "healthy" or "happy.") On a blood test, you would want your level of HDL to be high but your level of LDL to be low.

Figure 7.2 Approximate Cholesterol in Selected Foods

Keep Track of Cholesterol Since your body makes all the cholesterol it needs, it is wise to be aware of the amount of cholesterol in the foods you eat. ***How much cholesterol would you consume if you ate two eggs per day for a week?***

Food	Measure	Cholesterol (Milligrams)
Beef, ground, lean, broiled well done	3 oz.	77
Butter	1 Tbsp.	31
Candy bar	1	5
Chicken, roasted breast, without skin	3.4 oz.	77
Doughnut	1	18
Egg yolk	1	205

Food	Measure	Cholesterol (Milligrams)
Liver, pan-fried beef	3 oz.	324
Mayonnaise	1 Tbsp.	5
Milk, whole	1 cup	24
Milk, nonfat	1 cup	5
Shrimp, fresh cooked	3 oz.	166

Diet Affects Cholesterol

Eating foods with cholesterol raises the level of cholesterol in your bloodstream. But eating foods with fat raises it even more, because the liver uses the fat to make cholesterol.

Different types of fat have different effects on cholesterol levels.

Saturated Fat Foods with saturated fat appear to raise the level of LDL cholesterol in the bloodstream. Foods high in saturated fat include fatty meat, poultry skin, whole-milk products, and the tropical oils—coconut oil, palm oil, and palm kernel oil.

Polyunsaturated Fat Foods with polyunsaturated fat may help lower cholesterol levels if they are used instead of saturated fats. Many vegetable oils, such as corn oil, soybean oil, and safflower oil, are high in polyunsaturated fat. Fats in seafood are mostly polyunsaturated.

Monounsaturated Fat Foods with monounsaturated fat appear to lower LDL cholesterol levels and raise HDL cholesterol levels. These include olives, olive oil, avocados, nuts, peanut oil, and canola oil.

Kitchen Math

Determine Fat Intake

Maria needs 2,200 calories a day. Right now, Maria is consuming about 98 grams of fat per day. What percent of her total calories comes from fat? If she wishes to reduce her fat intake to 30% of daily calories, how many grams of fat should she have per day?

Math Concept **Calculating Percents** To find what percent a number is of another number, divide the first number by the second number, multiply by 100, and add the % symbol.

Starting Hint Remember, there are 9 calories in one gram of fat. Thus, Maria's total fat calories equal 98 x 9. Divide that total by 2,200 and multiply by 100 to find her current fat percentage. Reverse the process using the 30% amount to determine her optimal fat intake in grams.

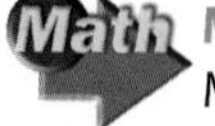

Math Appendix For math help, go to the Math Appendix at the back of the book.

NCTM Measurement Understand measurable attributes of objects and the units, systems, and process of measurement.

Trans Fats

When is a vegetable oil not an oil? When it is hydrogenated. The chemical process of **hydrogenation** (hī-ˌdrä-jə-ˈnā-shən) turns vegetable oils into solids. The missing hydrogen is added to the unsaturated fat, which increases saturation. Shortening and most margarines are hydrogenated vegetable oils.

Food producers often use hydrogenated fats to give products a longer shelf life and extra flavor. Many restaurants also use them when frying foods. Unfortunately, hydrogenation forms trans fatty acids, also called trans fats. **Trans fats** increase LDL cholesterol levels and lower HDL cholesterol levels.

Trans fats are common in margarine, salad dressings, crackers, snack foods, baked goods, fast foods, and convenience foods. Food producers are now required to list trans fats on nutrition labels. Some producers are changing their recipes to reduce trans fats. New York City, Philadelphia and California have recently adopted laws restricting or outlawing the use of trans fat in restaurants. Further research is being done to find ways to limit trans fats.

How Many Calories from Fat Do You Need?

Most Americans eat too much fat, especially too much saturated fat. Saturated fat increases the risk of heart disease and cancer. Eating too much fat can contribute to overweight and other health problems.

You need fat in your diet—in moderation. Some vitamins travel through the body in fat. Fat plays a key role in brain activity. Teens need about 25 to 35 percent of their calories from fat. Adults need about 20 to 35 percent. A teen who eats 2,400 calories each day should eat 67 to 93 grams of fat. **Figure 7.3** shows the amount of fat in a variety of common foods.

Keep track of your intake of saturated fat, trans fat, and cholesterol. Trans fats and saturated fats together should be less than 10 percent of your total calories. For a 2,000-calorie diet, that means under 22 grams a day. Limit the cholesterol you eat to under 300 milligrams per day.

Controlling Fat

Foods with fat taste good to most people. Eating fat in moderation allows you to enjoy the taste of fat and protect your health at the same time.

If you cut the amount of fat in your diet, you can actually eat more food without increasing calories. Try substituting carbohydrates and proteins for some fat. Per gram, these foods have about half the calories of fat and have needed nutrients.

Some people have actually gained weight when trying to cut fat from their diet. They thought they could eat larger quantities of fat-free and low-fat foods, not realizing that such foods often have a lot of calories. Use food labels to make decisions about what to eat.

Figure 7.3 Approximate Fat in Selected Foods

Finding the Fat in Foods Use nutritional labels to learn about the fat content of different foods. ***Do you get enough of your daily calories from fat?***

Food	Approximate Measure	Fat (Grams)	Saturated Fat (Grams)
Almonds, dry roasted	1 oz.	15	1
Apple, fresh	1 cup	Trace	Trace
Bagel, plain	1 (3½ in.)	1	Trace
Banana, fresh	1	1	0
Beef, ground, extra lean	3 oz.	14	5
Bread	1 slice	1	Trace
Brownie, plain	1 (0.8 oz.)	7	2
Butter	1 Tbsp.	11	7
Cake, angel food	1 piece	Trace	Trace
Cheesecake	1 piece	18	9
Chocolate, plain, milk	1 oz.	9	5.2
Chocolate cake, no frosting	1 piece	14	5
Cheese, cheddar	1 oz.	9	6
Cheese, mozzarella	1 oz.	6	4
Chicken breast, roasted with skin	½ breast	8	2
Chicken breast, with skin, batter dipped, fried	½ breast	18	5

Food	Approximate Measure	Fat (Grams)	Saturated Fat (Grams)
Cookies, chocolate chip with butter	1	5	2
Cookies, oatmeal	1	3	1
Doughnut, cake	1	11	2
Egg	1	5	2
French fried potatoes	Medium	27	7
Green beans, fresh	½ cup	Trace	Trace
Ice cream, chocolate	½ cup	7	4
Margarine, stick	1 Tbsp.	11	2
Margarine, tub	1 Tbsp.	7	1
Mayonnaise	1 Tbsp.	11	1.5
Milk, 1%	1 cup	3	2
Milk, whole	1 cup	8	5
Olive oil	1 Tbsp.	14	2
Potato chips	Small bag	11	2
Salad dressing, french homemade	1 Tbsp.	10	2
Shortening	1 Tbsp.	13	3.6

These suggestions can help you control the amount of fat you eat:

- Eat plenty of fruits, vegetables, and whole-grain foods. Consider these as snack options instead of fried or sweetened items.
- Choose fat-free or low-fat milk, yogurt, and cheese.
- Remove the skin from chicken and turkey before eating. Most of the fat is located just under the skin.
- Choose lean cuts of meat. Trim off and drain off fat.
- Choose lean ground beef or ground turkey.
- Watch portion sizes. A giant steak or hamburger includes much more fat than one with just a few ounces of meat. The recommended serving size for steak or hamburger is three ounces.
- Choose fish, lean poultry, or tofu instead of red meat.
- Limit fried foods. Choose chips that are baked over fried chips. If you are eating chips that are fried, look at the type of oil being used.
- Use smaller amounts of butter, margarine, oily salad dressings, sour cream, gravy, and rich sauces.
- Eat high-fat desserts only occasionally. Make servings small.
- Watch for new products that offer lower fat, but conduct research to learn about health concerns.
- Avoid trans fats and foods made with trans fat.
- Limit the amount of cheese in your diet.

✓ **Reading Check** **Identify** Which type of fat raises HDL cholesterol?

Light and Healthy Recipe

3-Bean Salad

Ingredients

1(15-ounce) can	Black beans
1(15-ounce) can	Kidney beans
1(15-ounce) can	Green beans
¼ cup	Rice vinegar
¼ cup	Olive oil
1 tsp.	Sugar
¼ tsp.	Dill weed
½ tsp.	Oregano
½ tsp.	Minced garlic

Yield: 8 servings

Directions

1. Open the cans of beans and drain off any liquid. Combine all three kinds of beans in a large serving bowl.
2. In a separate bowl, combine the vinegar, oil, sugar, dill, oregano and garlic. Mix well.
3. Pour over the beans and mix gently so that the beans are not smashed. Chill in the refrigerator for at least one hour before serving.

Beans are a great source of protein and fiber. One serving of this recipe contains 28% of the RDA of protein.

Yield 8 servings

Nutrition Analysis per Serving

■ Calories	162
■ Total fat	7 g
Saturated fat	1 g
Cholesterol	10 mg
■ Sodium	440 mg
■ Carbohydrate	18 g
Dietary fiber	7 g
Sugars	1 g
■ Protein	6 g

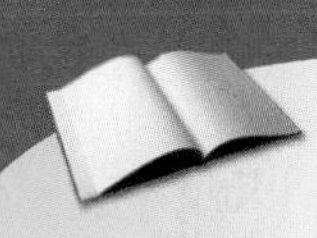

After You Read

Chapter Summary

Proteins are found in both animal and plant foods. They help the body to grow and repair itself. They are made of amino acids, which are sent into the cells during digestion. Proteins may be complete or incomplete. A teen's daily calories should contain 10 to 30 percent proteins. Lipids are a family of chemical compounds found in every cell. Both fats and cholesterol are lipids, and both are needed for the body to function properly. Controlling fat consumption can help manage cholesterol levels. The body needs both proteins and lipids to be healthy.

Content and Academic Vocabulary Review

1. Use at least six of these content and academic vocabulary terms in a short essay about wellness.

Content Vocabulary

- amino acid (p. 88)
- hemoglobin (p. 88)
- essential amino acid (p. 89)
- complete protein (p. 89)
- incomplete protein (p. 89)
- triglyceride (p. 91)
- fatty acid (p. 92)
- saturated fatty acid (p. 92)
- lipoprotein (p. 93)
- cholesterol (p. 93)
- hydrogenation (p. 94)
- trans fats (p. 94)

Academic Vocabulary

- continuous (p. 89)
- component (p. 91)

Review Key Concepts

2. **Explain** protein, its structure, and its types.
3. **Identify** the role of protein in a healthful diet.
4. **Explain** lipids, their structure and their types.
5. **Summarize** the role of cholesterol in a healthful diet.

Critical Thinking

6. **Construct** a day of meals to meet, but not go over, your protein requirement using only food from animal sources.
7. **Consider** that as an active teen, Ruben needs 2,800 calories per day. Construct two days of meal plans to meet Ruben's protein need between 280 and 840 calories, or 70 and 210 grams.
8. **Examine** the two menus you designed for Ruben. Which is easier and why? What are the differences in fat and cholesterol content between the two days?
9. **Compare and contrast** saturated and unsaturated fat.
10. **Compare** the effect of trans fats on LDL and HDL.

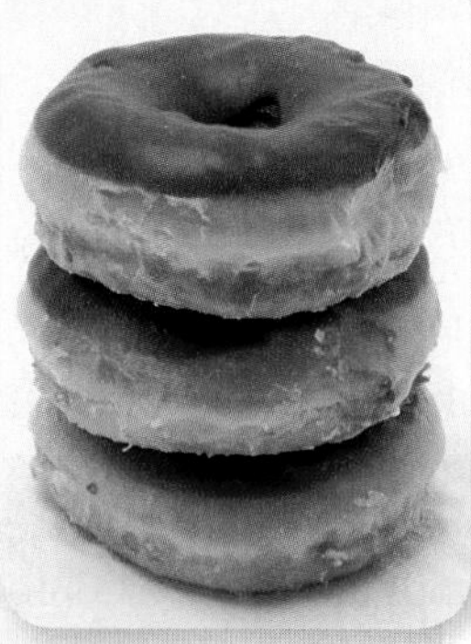

11. Reduced-Fat Recipes As consumers become more concerned with controlling consumption of fatty foods, food manufacturers have created many reduced-fat and fat-free versions. How do they measure up?

Procedure Evaluate a regular dairy product and its reduced-fat variety, comparing the foods on taste, texture, and appearance. Prepare two versions of a simple recipe using one of the foods in each version.

Analysis Write a paragraph comparing and contrasting the similarities and the differences between the regular and reduced-fat varieties. Describe noticeable differences between the two recipes.

HEALTHFUL CHOICES

12. Protein with Fat Margaret is deciding what to order from a restaurant menu. She wants her dinner to include protein. She also wants to consume the most nutritious foods for her body. She is torn between steak and salmon. Which should she choose and why?

TECH Connection

13. International Fare Select a country outside of North America. Under your teacher's supervision use the Internet to research traditional cuisine in that country. Focus on one dish that contains both a source of protein and a source of fat. Describe the other ingredients in the dish and any special equipment used to make it. Prepare an outline of your findings and use it to share what you learned with your class in a five-minute oral report. Study the topic well enough to be able to answer the questions about it.

Real-World Skills

Problem-Solving Skills

14. Revising Recipes Dominic runs a bakery. Many of his recipes call for ingredients such as butter, cheese, and milk. Some of his customers are requesting reduced-fat desserts. How can Dominic provide them without finding all new recipes?

Interpersonal and Collaborative Skills

15. Create a Pamphlet Some teens are so concerned with weight that they try to eliminate all fat and extra calories from their diets. Work with your group to create a pamphlet that targets teens. Explain why fat is essential, how much is needed, and which fats are beneficial. Make copies of the pamphlet and give them to the school health center.

Financial Literacy Skills

16. The Price of Protein When combined, beans and rice make a complete protein. Visit your local supermarket to find the cost per pound of both dry beans and rice. Then research the cost per pound of chicken breasts. Which is the more affordable source of complete protein?

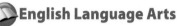

Academic Skills

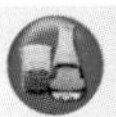

Food Science

17. Protein Coagulation Proteins consist of tight coils of amino acids. With heat, these coils unwind, and the protein becomes denatured. These denatured strands form new bonds to make a solid network.

Procedure Using low heat, pan-fry an egg in a small amount of butter. When the egg is mostly solid, but still jiggles in the middle, carefully flip it over with a spatula, taking care not to break the yolk. After a minute or so, turn it over onto a plate.

Analysis Write a paragraph to explain what you observed as the egg cooked.

NSES B Develop an understanding of the interactions of energy and matter.

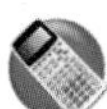

Mathematics

18. Measure Weight and Volume A dry ounce is a measure of weight. A fluid ounce is measure of volume. Fill an eight-ounce measuring cup with flour and weigh it. Now empty the cup, fill it with water, and weigh it. How much does the water weigh, and how much does the flour weigh? As a percentage, how much heavier is the water than the flour?

Math Concept **Turn Fractions into Decimals** Fractions and decimals both represent parts of a whole. Use long division to divide the numerator by the denominator.

Starting Hint Divide the weight of the water by the weight of the flour. Then transform the result from a decimal into a percentage.

NCTM Measurement Understand measurable attributes of objects and the units, systems, and processes of measurement.

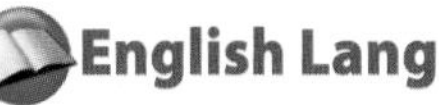

English Language Arts

19. Analyze Messages About Fat Spend one day paying attention to the media's attitude toward dietary fat. What messages do television advertisements, magazine articles, and other media sources send about dietary fat? Are the messages positive, negative, or mixed? Do you think they are helpful to people who want to eat a nutritious diet? Write a one-page analysis of your observations. Include specific examples of media messages.

NCTE 7 Conduct research and evaluate data to communicate discoveries.

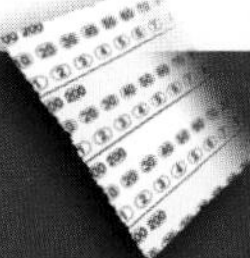

STANDARDIZED TEST PRACTICE

MULTIPLE CHOICE

Read the question and select the best answer.

20. Why are some proteins incomplete?

a. They come from animal sources.
b. They do not contain all nine essential amino acids.
c. They do not contain the necessary essential fatty acids.
d. They lack the fat and fiber that make proteins complete.

Test-Taking Tip Multiple-choice questions may prompt you to select the best answer. They may present you with answers that seem partially true. The best answer is the one that is completely true, and can be supported by information you have read in the text.

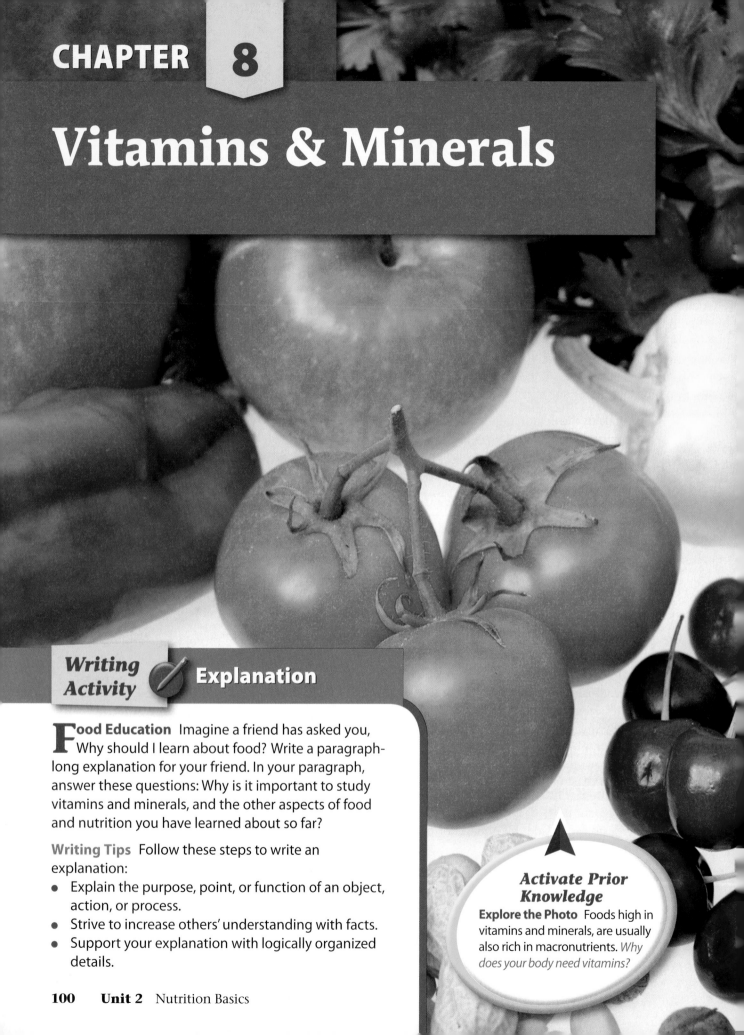

CHAPTER 8

Vitamins & Minerals

Writing Activity — Explanation

Food Education Imagine a friend has asked you, Why should I learn about food? Write a paragraph-long explanation for your friend. In your paragraph, answer these questions: Why is it important to study vitamins and minerals, and the other aspects of food and nutrition you have learned about so far?

Writing Tips Follow these steps to write an explanation:

- Explain the purpose, point, or function of an object, action, or process.
- Strive to increase others' understanding with facts.
- Support your explanation with logically organized details.

Activate Prior Knowledge

Explore the Photo Foods high in vitamins and minerals, are usually also rich in macronutrients. *Why does your body need vitamins?*

Reading Guide

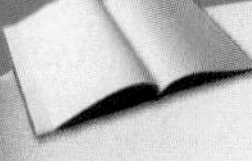

Before You Read

Preview Look at each of the photos in the chapter without reading their captions. Then write your own captions for the photos.

Read to Learn

Key Concepts

- **Explain** how vitamins work.
- **List** the two types of vitamins and their functions.
- **Explain** minerals and describe their functions and types.

Main Idea

Vitamins and minerals are valuable micronutrients that the body needs to be strong and healthy.

Content Vocabulary

You will find definitions for these words in the glossary at the back of the book.

- ☐ antioxidant
- ☐ free radical
- ☐ water-soluble vitamin
- ☐ fat-soluble vitamin
- ☐ toxicity
- ☐ major mineral
- ☐ electrolyte mineral
- ☐ hypertension
- ☐ trace mineral
- ☐ iron-deficiency anemia
- ☐ pica

Academic Vocabulary

You will find these words in your reading and on your tests. Use the glossary to look up their definitions if necessary.

- stabilize
- regulate

Graphic Organizer

Use a graphic organizer like the one below to list, define, and give examples of major minerals and trace minerals.

MAJOR MINERALS	TRACE MINERALS

Graphic Organizer Go to this book's Online Learning Center at **glencoe.com** to print out this graphic organizer.

Academic Standards

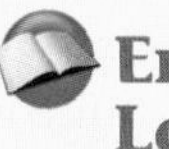

English Language Arts

NCTE 8 Use information resources to gather information and create and communicate knowledge.

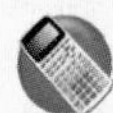

Mathematics

NCTM Number and Operations Understand numbers, ways of representing numbers, relationships among numbers, and number systems.

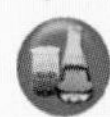

Science

NSES G Develop an understanding of science as a human endeavor.

NSES C Develop an understanding of the cell.

NCSS II F Time, Continuity, and Change Apply ideas, theories and modes of historical inquiry to analyze multiple historical developments.

NCTE *National Council of Teachers of English*
NCTM *National Council of Teachers of Mathematics*
NSES *National Science Education Standards*
NCSS *National Council for the Social Studies*

What are Vitamins?

Vitamins are important to health, but they do not supply energy or become part of the body's structure in the form of body tissue. Instead, vitamins work with enzymes, the special proteins that help chemical reactions take place in body cells, to keep cells healthy and active. Your body cannot produce energy without vitamins.

Vitamins and minerals are needed in much smaller amounts than other nutrients such as carbohydrates, protein, and water. That is why they are called micronutrients. Micro means very small.

When vitamins were first discovered, they were assigned letters of the alphabet, such as A, B, and C. When scientists learned that vitamins are chemicals, they gave them chemical names to replace the letters. For example, vitamin C is also called ascorbic acid.

Some vitamins, such as vitamin C, are found in a wide range of foods. Others, such as vitamin B_{12}, come from just a few foods. A healthy diet full of vegetables, fruits, and grains provides all the vitamins and minerals your body needs. Many vitamins your body needs have to be supplied daily so loading up on a particular vitamin does not help. Maintaining healthy eating habits is important.

Figure 8.1 Free Radicals and Antioxidants

Powerful Protection Antioxidants protect the body by creating a barrier between cells and free radicals. ***How do antioxidants protect the body?***

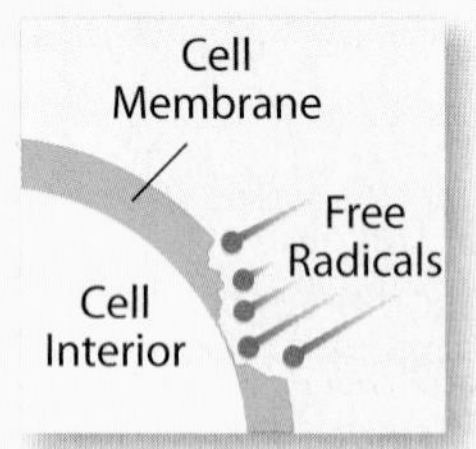

Disease

Free radicals are linked to over 200 diseases. When free radicals are linked to damaged body cells and DNA, they cause the body to age more rapidly, and increase the risk of disease.

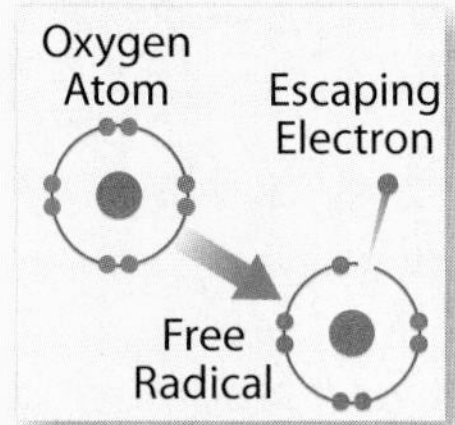

Production

Where do free radicals come from? They are produced by oxidation, a chemical reaction in which a material combines with oxygen and loses some of its electrons.

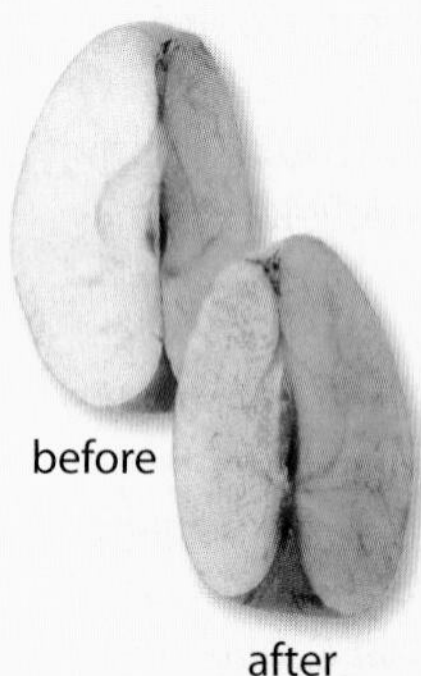

Oxidation

If you leave a sliced apple exposed to the air, it will begin to turn brown. Oxidation is occurring, and free radicals are attacking the apple. The aging and damage that oxidation causes to the human body can be slowed or prevented.

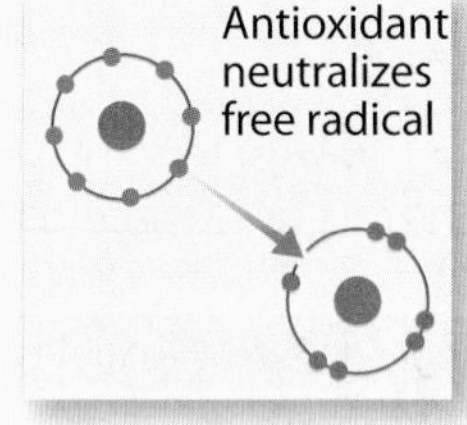

Antioxidants

Antioxidants work to defend the body's cells against free radicals. They give their own electrons to the material that has lost electrons through oxidation. Because they are stable molecules, they do not become free radicals themselves.

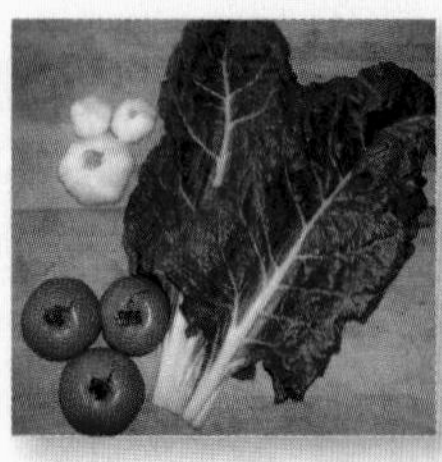

Diet

The best way to obtain antioxidants is through diet. Plants contain natural stores of antioxidants. When you eat plant foods that are rich in antioxidants, you increase your body's defenses against oxidation and free radicals.

Figure 8.2 Food Sources of Water-Soluble Vitamins

Water Soluble There are many opportunities to obtain water-soluble vitamins through the foods you eat. ***Which foods would you include if you wanted a breakfast that is rich in riboflavin?***

Vitamin	Sources
Vitamin C (ascorbic acid)	Citrus fruits, including oranges, grapefruit, and tangerines; other fruits, including cantaloupe, guava, kiwi, mango, papaya, and strawberries; vegetables, including bell peppers, broccoli, cabbage, kale, plantains, potatoes, and tomatoes.
Thiamin (vitamin B_1)	Enriched and whole-grain breads and cereals; dry beans and peas; lean pork and liver.
Riboflavin (vitamin B_2)	Enriched breads and cereals; milk and other dairy products; green leafy vegetables; eggs; meat; poultry; fish.
Niacin (vitamin B_3)	Meat; poultry; fish; enriched and whole-grain breads and cereals; dry beans and peas; peanuts.
Vitamin B_6 (pyridoxine)	Poultry; fish; pork; dry beans and peas; nuts; whole grains; some fruits and vegetables; liver and kidneys.
Folate (folacin, folic acid, vitamin B_9)	Green leafy vegetables; dry beans and peas; fruits; enriched and whole-grain breads.
Vitamin B_{12} (cobalamin)	Meat; poultry; fish; shellfish; eggs; dairy products; some fortified foods; some nutritional yeasts.
Pantothenic acid (vitamin B_5)	Meat; poultry; fish; eggs; dry beans and peas; whole-grain breads and cereals; milk; some fruits and vegetables.
Biotin (vitamin H)	Green leafy vegetables; whole-grain breads and cereals; liver; egg yolks

Antioxidants

Some vitamins and minerals, including vitamins C and E and the mineral selenium, are also antioxidants (ˌan-tē-ˈäk-sə-dənts) **Antioxidants** are substances that protect cells and the immune system from damage by harmful chemicals. Antioxidants may help prevent heart disease, cancer, and other ailments by protecting and repairing cells.

Why does your body need antioxidants? When cells burn oxygen to produce energy, free radicals are made. A **free radical** is an unstable substance that can damage body cells. Antioxidants change free radicals to make them less damaging. Antioxidants also repair damaged cells (see **Figure 8.1**).

Water-Soluble Vitamins

Vitamins fall into two groups: water-soluble and fat-soluble. The difference is how the vitamin is absorbed and transported in the bloodstream.

A **water-soluble vitamin** dissolves in water and passes easily into the bloodstream during digestion.

Water-soluble vitamins remain in your body for a short time. If they are not used right away, they are passed out of the body in urine. That is why you need to drink ample amounts of water and eat foods with water-soluble vitamins each day (see **Figure 8.2**). It is also why consuming large doses of one vitamin is a poor strategy.

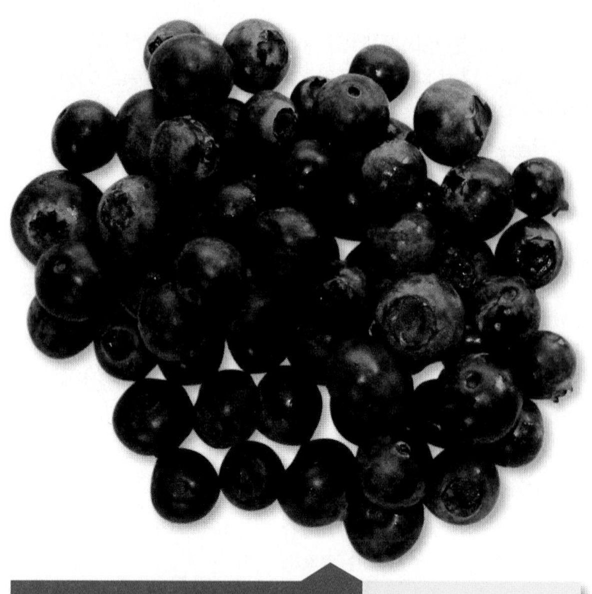

Stabilizing Force

Foods high in antioxidants work to protect cells from damage and aging. *What are some antioxidant-rich foods?*

TECHNOLOGY FOR TOMORROW

Diagnosing Deficiencies

Throughout history, many scientific discoveries pertaining to nutrition were made by accident. For example, thanks to some chickens. Thiamin deficiency was recognized as the cause of the disease beriberi, a nervous system ailment. Before 1900, prisoners in East Asia were stiff and weak from beriberi. A physician observed that chickens at the prison displayed similar symptoms. When the chickens ate the discarded bran removed from the prisoners' rice, their symptoms disappeared. When the prisoners also ate the discarded bran, they improved, too. This observation led to the identification of something valuable in the bran of whole grains—thiamin. Modern scientists rely on technology to identify deficiencies of both vitamins and minerals.

Investigate Conduct research to find out how modern scientists use technology to test for vitamin and mineral deficiencies in humans. Write two or more paragraphs to explain your findings.

NCSS II F Time, Continuity, and Change Apply ideas, theories and modes of historical inquiry to anlyze historical developments.

Vitamin C (Ascorbic Acid)

Vitamin C helps maintain healthy capillaries, bones, skin, and teeth. Vitamin C is necessary for the enzyme that forms and takes care of the protein called collagen. Collagen gives structure to bones, cartilage, and muscle. Vitamin C helps your body heal wounds and resist infections. It also aids in the absorption of iron and works as an antioxidant.

Lack of vitamin C can cause poor appetite, weakness, bruising, and soreness in the joints. A severe lack of vitamin C causes a disease called scurvy. Scurvy used to be common among sailors at sea, who did not have access to fresh fruits and vegetables. Large doses of Vitamin C, on the other hand, may cause nausea, cramps, and diarrhea. Vitamin C is found in citrus fruits, other fruits such as cantaloupe and berries, and some vegetables, including tomatoes, green peppers, potatoes, broccoli, and cabbage.

Thiamin (Vitamin B_1)

Thiamin helps turn carbohydrates into energy. Your body needs thiamin for muscle coordination and a healthy nervous system.

Nausea, apathy, and loss of appetite are early symptoms of a thiamin deficiency. Today most people get the thiamin they need by eating a variety of nutritious foods, including enriched and whole-grain breads and cereals, brown rice, asparagus, kale, oranges, ham, and eggs.

Riboflavin (Vitamin B_2)

Riboflavin helps the body release energy from carbohydrates, proteins, and fats. It contributes to body growth and red blood cell production.

Riboflavin deficiency is rare. Signs include light sensitivity, gritty eyes, sore tongue, mouth and lip sores, and dry, flaky skin.

Most people get riboflavin from whole grains and milk products. Riboflavin is easily destroyed by light, so milk containers are made to prevent light from entering.

Niacin (Vitamin B_3)

Niacin helps your body release energy from carbohydrates, proteins, and fats. You also need niacin for a healthy nervous system and mucous membranes.

Lack of niacin can cause pellagra (pə-ˈla-grə), a disease that produces skin lesions and mental and digestive problems. In the early 1900s, this disease was widespread in parts of the U.S. where people ate a diet based mainly on cornmeal. Cornmeal is low in the essential amino acid tryptophan (ˈtrip-ˌtə-fan), which the body uses to make niacin. Tryptophan is found in most other protein foods, however. Niacin can be found in meat, chicken, fish, milk, broccoli, tomatoes, carrots, nuts, and mushrooms.

Vitamin B_6 (Pyridoxine)

Vitamin B_6 helps the body release energy from carbohydrates, proteins, and fats. Vitamin B_6 also promotes a healthy nervous system and helps to make nonessential amino acids. B_6 helps the body convert tryptophan to niacin.

Deficiency in vitamin B_6 is rare because it is found in many meats, whole grains, vegetables and nuts. Symptoms include skin disorders, confusion, irritability, and insomnia. Serious deficiencies can produce convulsions. Taking in too much vitamin B_6 through supplements may cause nerve problems, such as difficulty walking.

Folate (B_9)

Folate, also called folic acid and folacin, teams with vitamin B_{12} to help build red blood cells and form genetic material (DNA). Folate also helps the body use proteins.

The word folate is related to the word foliage, meaning leaves. Leafy green vegetables, like spinach, are good sources of folate.

Too little folate can cause anemia, which alters red blood cells so they carry less oxygen. People with anemia feel tired and weak, and may develop diarrhea and lose weight.

Folate helps prevent birth defects in the brain and spinal cord. Folate is so important that it is now added to grain products. A health professional may prescribe additional folate during pregnancy and lactation (milk production).

Vitamin B_{12}

Like many other B vitamins, vitamin B_{12} helps the body process carbohydrates, proteins, and fats. It also helps maintain healthy nerve cells and red blood cells and is used in making genetic material. Vitamin B_{12} and folate work together.

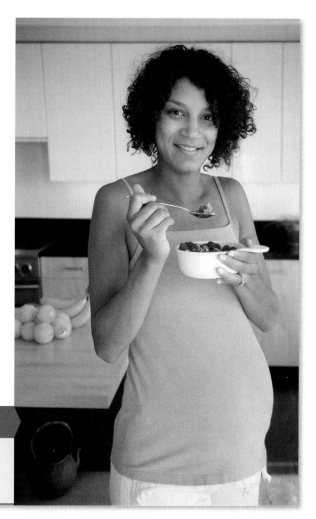

The Power of Vitamins

Folate is very important for women who may become pregnant. *Why do pregnant women need folate?*

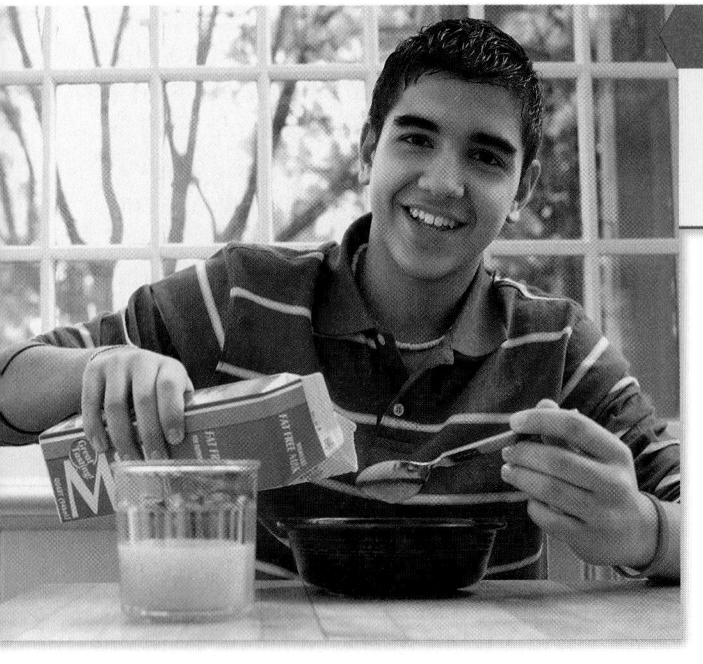

Vitamin Chemistry

Proper packaging protects vitamins in food. Milk, for example, is often sold in opaque, not clear, containers to protect riboflavin. *How does the opaque container protect riboflavin?*

Vitamin B_{12} is found in meat and milk products, but not in plant foods. Vegetarians can get B_{12} in fortified grain products.

Signs of B_{12} deficiency include fatigue, weakness, nausea, a sore mouth or tongue, loss of appetite, weight loss, and numbness or tingling in the hands and feet. Some older adults take B_{12} supplements because they have trouble absorbing the vitamin. People who cannot absorb B_{12} may develop a chronic condition called pernicious anemia.

Pantothenic Acid (Vitamin B_5)

Pantothenic acid helps the body release energy from carbohydrates, proteins, and fats. It helps the body produce cholesterol and promotes normal growth and development. Pantothenic acid is also needed for a healthy nervous system.

Deficiencies of pantothenic acid are rare. This vitamin is abundant in food and can also be manufactured by bacteria in the intestine.

Biotin

Biotin helps your body use carbohydrates, proteins, and fats. Biotin also helps **stabilize** the level of sugar (glucose) in the blood.

Deficiency of biotin is rare because it is abundant in many foods, including grains, eggs, and milk.

Fat-Soluble Vitamins

A **fat-soluble vitamin** is a vitamin that is absorbed and transported by fat. The most important fat-soluble vitamins are A, D, E, and K. See **Figure 8.3** on page 107.

Excess fat-soluble vitamins are stored in the liver. Your body draws on the stored vitamins when needed. The liver stores enough of the fat-soluble vitamins to satisfy the body's needs for several months if they are absent from the diet. Large amounts of fat-soluble vitamins can harm the body, so use caution with vitamin supplements.

Vitamin A

Three forms of vitamin A are active in the body: retinol, retinal, and retinoic acid. They promote good vision and help maintain tissues and skin. Vitamin A also supports reproduction and growth.

Orange and green vegetables such as carrots and chard are a good source of beta-carotene, an antioxidant that the body converts to vitamin A. Too much beta-carotene may turn the skin yellow, but this is harmless.

Vitamin A deficiency can cause rough, scaly skin and infections in the respiratory tract and other areas of the body. Deficiency is a serious problem in developing countries. Lack of vitamin A causes night blindness and even total blindness in many children.

Too much vitamin A, on the other hand, can build up in the body and lead to toxicity. **Toxicity** is poisoning from too much of a substance. Taking too many vitamin A supplements can cause headaches, vomiting, double vision, abnormal bones, and liver damage.

Figure 8.3 Food Sources of Fat-Soluble Vitamins

Fat-Soluble Your liver will store excess fat-soluble vitamins for future use. ***If you eat green leafy vegetables each day, which vitamins might your body store for later use?***

Vitamin	Sources
Vitamin A	Dairy products; liver; egg yolks; foods high in beta-carotene, such as carrots, sweet potatoes, broccoli, and dark green, leafy vegetables.
Vitamin E	Nuts; seeds; green leafy vegetables; wheat germ; vegetable oils and products made from them; soybean oil.
Vitamin D	Fortified dairy products; egg yolks; fatty fish, such as herring, salmon, and mackerel; fortified breakfast cereals.
Vitamin K	Green leafy vegetables; other vegetables; some fruits.

Vitamin D

Vitamin D works with calcium and phosphorus to ensure that bones grow properly.

Your body makes vitamin D when sunlight touches your skin. Ten to 15 minutes of sun on the hands, face, and arms three times a week is enough for most people. More sunlight will not cause your body to make too much vitamin D, but it may lead to sunburn and even skin cancer. Make sure to wear sunscreen and eye protection.

Fortified milk is a good source of vitamin D. Other sources of vitamin D include egg yolks and fatty fish.

In children, vitamin D deficiency causes a disease called rickets. Rickets was a serious problem in the United States until the 1930s, when vitamin D was added to milk. In adults, vitamin D deficiency causes osteomalacia (ˌäs-tē-ō-mə-ˈlā-sh(ē)ə), a disease that weakens the bones. Osteomalacia and rickets cause weak and sometimes deformed bones. Children with rickets may have bowed legs.

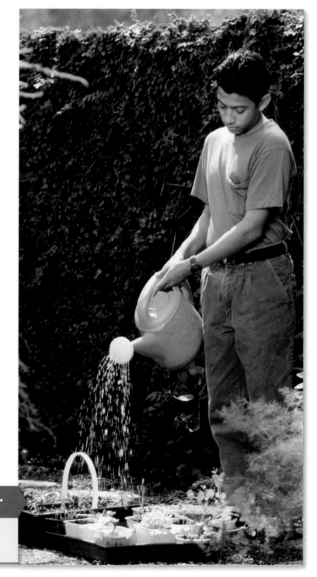

Herbs Add Flavor

Try using herbs and spices instead of salt. *How else can you limit your sodium intake?*

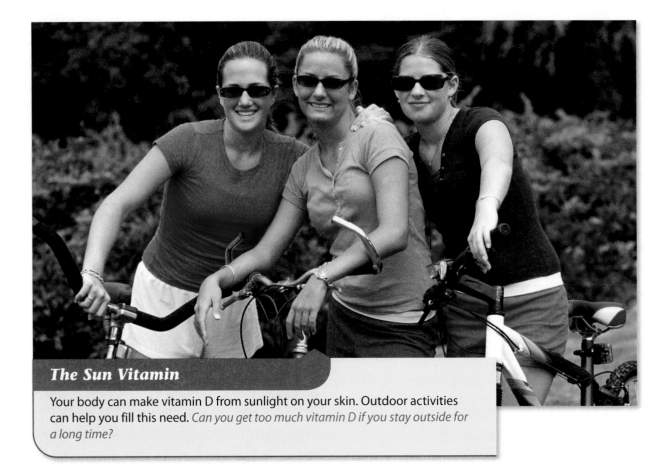

The Sun Vitamin

Your body can make vitamin D from sunlight on your skin. Outdoor activities can help you fill this need. *Can you get too much vitamin D if you stay outside for a long time?*

Too much vitamin D from supplements can cause nausea, vomiting, and hardening of body tissues.

Vitamin E

Vitamin E is a powerful antioxidant. It protects cells from oxidation damage, particularly in the lungs. Vitamin E may reduce the risk of heart disease and some cancers.

Vitamin E is found in many foods, and deficiency is rare. Toxicity from excess amounts is also rare.

Vitamin K

Vitamin K helps blood clot so that wounds stop bleeding. It also helps with bone health.

Vitamin K deficiency and toxicity are rare in people who eat a healthy diet. Vitamin K is found in green leafy vegetables and is made in the intestine.

✓ **Reading Check** **Explain** Why is it important to eat foods with water-soluble vitamins each day?

What Are Minerals?

Minerals are just as important to good health as vitamins. Minerals are part of your body, especially in your teeth and bones. In fact, minerals make up four to five percent of your body weight.

Minerals often team with vitamins in chemical reactions. For example, vitamin C boosts iron absorption.

Major Minerals

Every mineral is either a "major mineral" or a "trace mineral." A **major mineral** is a mineral that you need in the amount of 100 mg or more a day. See **Figure 8.4** on page 109.

Calcium

Calcium helps regulate blood clotting, nerve activity, and other body processes. It is needed for the contraction of muscles, including the heart. Calcium also helps keep teeth and gums healthy.

Calcium's most important role is keeping your bones strong. If you do not get enough calcium, you may develop osteoporosis (ˌäs-tē-ō-pə-ˈrō-səs). Osteoporosis is a condition in which bones become porous, and therefore weak and fragile. People with osteoporosis may develop a stooped posture and suffer bone breaks. About 10 million Americans, both men and women, have osteoporosis. Another 34 million are at risk for developing it.

Bone mass builds up during childhood, the teen years, and young adulthood. To build strong, healthy bones and avoid osteoporosis:

- Eat plenty of calcium-rich foods, including dry beans and peas, dark green, leafy vegetables, and dairy products.
- Eat a healthy diet. Since nutrients work in teams, you need vitamin D and other nutrients to build healthy bones.
- Include vitamin D and calcium in each meal, if possible because children can only absorb so much at a time.
- Exercise or play sports. Weight-bearing exercises, such as walking, jogging, and weight training, help strengthen bones.
- Avoid caffeine, which is found in coffee, tea, and some soft drinks. Do not use tobacco products or alcohol.

Science in Action

Manufacturing and Microminerals

Both salt and water are manufactured to contain microminerals. This ensures that consumers will reap the benefits provided by the trace minerals and avoid dangerous deficiencies. Iodine is added to table salt in the form of potassium iodide, either as a dry or liquid solution when the salt is manufactured.

Procedure Conduct research to learn why scientists chose to add iodine to salt rather than a different food product.

Analysis Write a paragraph explaining why this was done. Cite your research. Why do you think scientists chose to add iodine to salt?

NSES G Develop an understanding of science as a human endeavor.

Phosphorus

Phosphorus works with calcium to build strong bones and teeth. It helps release energy from carbohydrates, proteins, and fats. It also helps to build cells and tissues. Protein foods are rich in phosphorus, so deficiencies are rare.

Figure 8.4 **Food Sources of Major Minerals**

Major Minerals These six minerals play an important role in keeping your body healthy. ***Which two minerals are obtained through table salt?***

Mineral	Sources
Calcium	Dairy products; canned fish with edible bones; dry beans, peas, and lentils; dark green, leafy vegetables, such as broccoli, spinach, and turnip greens; tofu made with calcium sulfate; calcium-fortified orange juice and soy milk.
Phosphorus	Meat; poultry; fish; eggs; nuts; dry beans and peas; dairy products; grain products.
Magnesium	Whole-grain products; green vegetables; dry beans and peas; nuts and seeds.
Sodium (Electrolyte)	Table salt; processed foods.
Chloride (Electrolyte)	Table salt.
Potassium (Electrolyte)	Fruits, including bananas and oranges; vegetables; meat; poultry; fish; dry beans and peas; dairy products.

Magnesium

Magnesium helps build bones and make proteins. It helps nerves and muscles work normally and helps regulate body temperature. Magnesium also contributes to proper heart function. Deficiency is uncommon because magnesium can be found in many foods including nuts, yogurt, beans, dairy products, bananas, and raisins.

Sodium, Chloride, and Potassium

In your body, fluids flow in and out of cells through cell walls. Fluids on the inside and outside of cells must be in balance, or the cells will burst or collapse. Sodium, chloride, and potassium help with this balance.

Sodium, chloride, and potassium are important electrolyte (i-ˈlek-trə-ˌlīt) minerals. An **electrolyte mineral** is a mineral that helps form particles called electrolytes, which help cells function. Electrolytes pull fluid with them. Cells move electrolytes back and forth through cell walls to help fluids stay in balance. If an illness, such as vomiting or diarrhea, causes excessive fluid loss, electrolytes will be lost and must be replaced.

Sodium, chloride, and potassium also have other functions. Sodium helps muscles and nerves work and helps **regulate** blood pressure. Chloride helps nerves send signals. In the stomach, chloride helps maintain the acidity needed to digest food. Potassium, found in bananas, cantaloupe, milk, oranges, and squash, helps maintain a steady heartbeat and helps with muscle and nerve action. Potassium also helps maintain normal blood pressure. Sodium, chloride, and potassium deficiencies are uncommon.

Table salt contains sodium and chloride, so you get both of these minerals when you eat salt. Some foods naturally contain sodium. Sodium is added to many foods during processing.

Eating too much potassium is not a problem, but eating too much sodium is. **Hypertension**, or high blood pressure, is linked to high salt intake. Hypertension can lead to heart disease and stroke. Eating too much sodium can also cause your bones to lose calcium and can increase the risk of kidney stones.

Limit sodium to 2,300 mg or less each day. This is one rounded teaspoon of table salt.

Figure 8.5 Food Sources of Trace Minerals

Trace Minerals While the body only requires small quantities of trace minerals, their effects on health are significant. ***Which trace mineral can find its way into vegetables through the soil in which they grow?***

Mineral	Sources
Iron	Meat; fish; shellfish; egg yolks; dark green, leafy vegetables; dry beans and peas; enriched and whole-grain products; dried fruits.
Zinc	Meat; liver; poultry; fish; shellfish; dairy products; dry beans and peas; peanuts; whole-grain breads and cereals; eggs; miso (fermented soybean paste).
Copper	Whole-grain products; seafood; variety meats; dry beans and peas; nuts; seeds.
Iodine	Saltwater fish; iodized salt.
Selenium	Whole-grain breads and cereals; vegetables (amount varies with content in soil); meat; variety meats; fish; shellfish.
Fluoride	Water supplies in many communities (added to help improve dental health); also in some bottled waters.

Fluoride

Fluoride helps strengthen bones and teeth. It is sometimes added to drinking water. *Why do some people oppose adding fluoride to drinking water?*

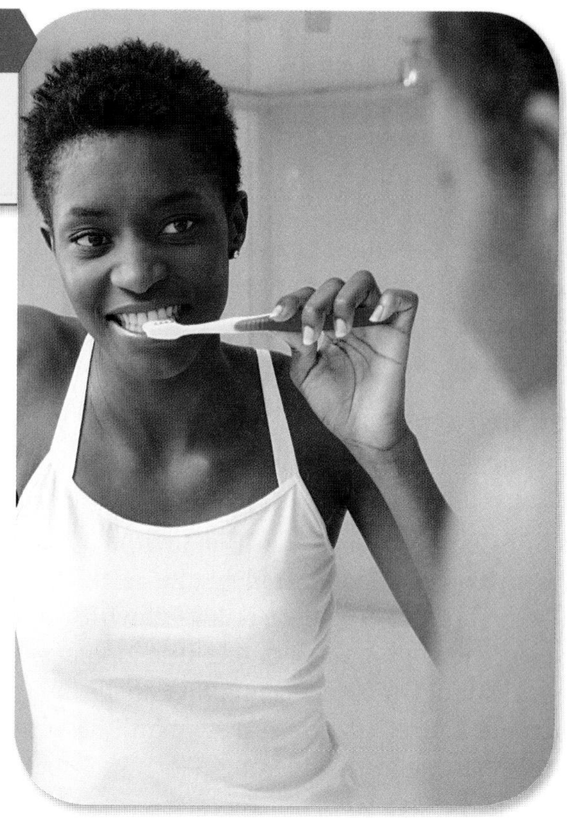

To limit your sodium intake, try these suggestions:

- Choose foods that are naturally low in sodium, including fresh fruits and vegetables, fresh meats and poultry, and grains such as brown rice and bulgur.
- Limit the amount of processed foods you eat, and choose processed foods with the lowest sodium.
- Limit high-salt condiments such as soy sauce, ketchup, mustard, pickles, and olives.
- Limit salty snacks, such as chips, crackers, pretzels, and nuts. Choose unsalted snacks where possible.
- Use herbs and spices instead of salt to flavor food. Many spice and herb mixes are available to use as substitutes.
- Add little or no salt to food when cooking and eating.

Nutrition Check

Sneaky Salt

Did you know that salt can sneak into your diet without your knowledge? Most people take in more than 4,000 milligrams of sodium each day—1,700 milligrams above the recommended amount. Much of the salt we consume is considered "hidden sodium." This hidden sodium is found in many everyday foods we don't typically think of as salty. For example, two slices of bread may contain 900 milligrams of sodium.

Think About It Where does sodium hide? Uncover five foods that are common sources of hidden sodium. Explain how people can become more aware of hidden sodium in their diets.

Trace Minerals

A **trace mineral** is a mineral that you need in the amount of less than 100 mg a day. Trace minerals are sometimes called microminerals. Even though you only need small amounts of trace minerals, they serve vital functions.

You can get all the trace minerals you need from food. Excess amounts can be harmful, so only take mineral supplements if a health professional recommends it. See **Figure 8.5** on page 110.

Scientists continue to study trace minerals. It is believed that other minerals perform functions in the body, but those are not yet determined.

Iron

Iron is essential for making hemoglobin, the substance in red blood cells that carries oxygen to all body cells.

Without enough iron, your blood cannot carry enough oxygen to your cells. Too little iron can lead to **iron-deficiency anemia**, having too few red blood cells. People with anemia are often tired, weak, short of breath, and pale. They may feel cold.

Sources of iron include red meat, fish, poultry, lentils, beans, leafy vegetables, and chickpeas.

Anemia is common around the world. Women who are menstruating should be sure to get enough iron. Vitamin C helps your body absorb iron, so it is good to combine foods rich in vitamin C with foods rich in iron.

Some people who are iron deficient have an unusual appetite for ice, clay, or other nonfood items. A craving for things that are not normally eaten is called **pica**. Pica usually goes away when the iron deficiency is fixed.

Other Trace Minerals

Other important trace minerals include iodine, zinc, selenium, copper, and fluoride.

Iodine Iodine is stored in the thyroid gland. The thyroid gland, located in the neck, produces substances needed for growth and development. Too much or too little iodine can cause thyroid problems. Infants can be born with mental retardation if a woman does not get enough iodine during pregnancy.

Zinc Zinc helps enzymes do their work. It also aids the immune system, helps wounds heal, and helps children grow. Zinc deficiency can cause growth retardation, poor appetite, loss of taste, dry skin, and depression.

Selenium Selenium (sə-ˈlē-nē-əm) is an antioxidant. It maintains muscles, red blood cells, hair, and nails. It may also protect against certain cancers.

Copper Copper helps several enzymes do their work. Copper also helps form hemoglobin and collagen. Deficiencies are rare.

Fluoride Fluoride helps prevent tooth decay and strengthen bones. Foods contain little fluoride, so some communities add it to drinking water. Some toothpastes have added fluoride. Some health advocates are against adding fluoride to water because of possible health risks and because fluoride does not need to be swallowed to strengthen teeth.

Light and Healthy Recipe

Jicama Slaw

Ingredients

- **1 cup** Cabbage, sliced thin
- **½ cup** Jicama, peeled and diced
- **1 large** Apple, cut into matchstick-sized strips
- **¼ cup** Diced red onion
- **2 Tbsp.** Pine nuts
- **1** Lime
- **1 Tbsp.** Olive oil
- **1 tsp.** Chopped mint

Yield 4 servings

Directions

1. Combine the cabbage, jicama, apple, onion and pine nuts in a serving bowl and mix.
2. In a separate bowl, squeeze the juice out of the lime and whisk it with the olive oil and mint to make a dressing.
3. Cover both bowls and chill for at least an hour. Pour the dressing over the slaw and mix just before serving.

Jicama is a root vegetable that is high in fiber and provides a mildly sweet crunch.

Yield 4 servings

Nutrition Analysis per Serving

■ Calories	115
■ Total fat	7 g
Saturated fat	1 g
Cholesterol	0 mg
■ Sodium	22 mg
■ Carbohydrate	14 g
Dietary fiber	5 g
Sugars	14 g
■ Protein	2 g

CHAPTER 8 Review & Applications

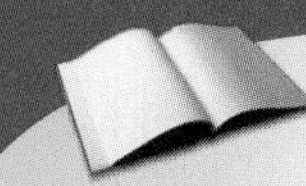

After You Read

Chapter Summary

Vitamins and minerals are micronutrients that help to keep the body healthy. Vitamins work with enzymes to keep cells healthy and active. Antioxidants are special vitamins and minerals that protect against free radicals. Water-soluble vitamins dissolve in water and pass easily through the bloodstream during digestion. Fat-soluble vitamins are stored in the liver for the body to use when needed. Minerals often team with vitamins in chemical reactions. Major minerals are those that the body requires 100 mg or more of each day. The body needs less than 100 daily mg of trace minerals. The best way to obtain vitamins and minerals is through a healthful and varied diet.

Content and Academic Vocabulary Review

1. Use each of these content and academic vocabulary words in a sentence.

Content Vocabulary

- antioxidants (p. 103)
- free radical (p. 103)
- water-soluble vitamin (p. 103)
- fat-soluble vitamin (p. 106)
- toxicity (p. 106)
- major mineral (p. 108)
- electrolyte mineral (p. 110)
- hypertension (p. 110)
- trace mineral (p. 111)
- iron-deficiency anemia (p. 111)
- pica (p. 112)

Academic Vocabulary

- stabilize (p. 106)
- regulate (p. 110)

Review Key Concepts

2. **Explain** how vitamins and antioxidants work.
3. **List** two types of vitamins and their functions.
4. **Explain** minerals and describe their functions and types.

Critical Thinking

5. **Explain** to Trey the specific substances he should eat in order to slow the aging of his body's cells.
6. **Explain** which foods a pregnant woman should eat to prevent birth defects in her baby.
7. **Predict** which vitamin deficiency Mike is at risk for. He lives in Seattle, Washington, where sunny days are rare. He also works indoors.
8. **Detail** what steps you can take to avoid osteoporosis.
9. **Explain** why salt, a major mineral, should be consumed in moderation to protect heart health.
10. **Detect** what might be missing from Amy's diet. She never eats fruit or fruit juice. Despite an iron-rich diet, Amy has been diagnosed with an iron deficiency.

Foods Lab

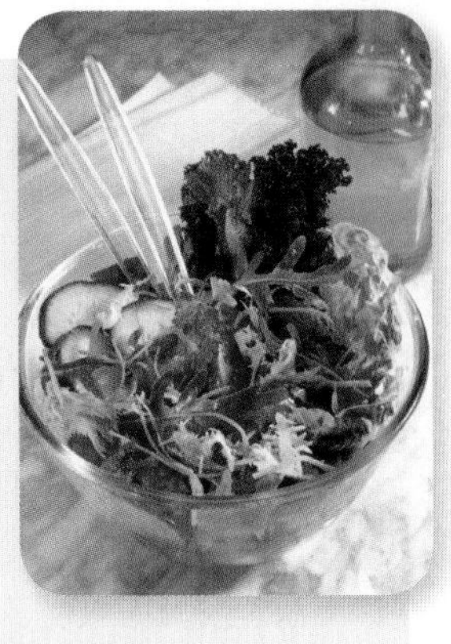

11. Vitamin Salad A fresh and colorful salad is one of the easiest ways to include a wide variety of vitamins and minerals in a single delicious dish.

Procedure Follow your teacher's directions to form teams. Work with your team to create a recipe for a vitamin- or mineral-rich salad. Plan a dish that is visually appealing and nutritious. Prepare your salad.

Analysis Present an oral evaluation of your salad. What foods did you choose? What vitamins, minerals, and other nutrients did each ingredient provide? How did your salad promote appearance, taste, and texture?

HEALTHFUL CHOICES

12. Evaluate Supplements Examine the label of a multivitamin and mineral supplement. What percentage of the daily recommended amount of various vitamins and minerals does it provide? What might be the consequences of overusing supplements? Write a paragraph to explain your answers. Include an explanation of reasons why someone might need the supplement.

TECH Connection

13. Antioxidant Slideshow Research twenty foods that contain powerful antioxidants. Use slideshow software to create a presentation for your classmates. Each food should have its own slide containing a description, main ingredients, image, and idea for use in a recipe. Prepare a narration to give while you present your slideshow.

Real-World Skills

Problem-Solving Skills

14. Saving Sight You are a doctor on an aid mission in a developing nation with a poor food supply. You notice that many of the children are suffering from vision problems and blindness. What might be your first course of action and why?

Interpersonal and Collaborative Skills

15. Diagnose Deficiencies Write and perform a skit in which one group member portrays a patient with specific symptoms. The other group members portray a panel of doctors who ask the patient questions. Perform your skit for the class without giving away what is wrong with the patient. Have the class determine which vitamin or mineral deficiency the patient suffers from.

Financial Literacy

16. Dollars and Sense Monday through Friday, Daniel spends $7.50 on a fast food lunch. He orders a burger, fries, soda, and ice cream. Visit a supermarket and research how much five days worth of vitamin- and mineral-rich salad ingredients would cost. What would be the daily cost of the salad? Which lunch makes more financial sense? Which makes more health sense?

Academic Skills

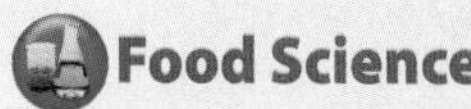

17. **Effects of Salt** Salt dissolves in water. A membrane is a very thin layer of tissue that covers a surface. When the concentration of salt is higher on one side of a membrane than the other, water will pass through the membrane to equalize both sides.

Procedure Get 2 small bowls and fill each halfway with water. To the first bowl, add 2–3 tablespoons of salt, and mix until the salt is dissolved. Label the bowl "S." Add a thin slice of raw potato to each bowl. Wait 30 minutes, and examine each potato slice.

Analysis What is the difference between the potato slices? Write a paragraph to explain what happened. How do you think salt intake affects fluids in the body?

NSES C Develop an understanding of the cell.

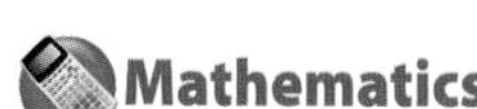

18. **Tracking Salt Intake** Lydia's breakfast had 450 mg of sodium, her lunch had 1,200 mg of sodium, her dinner had 1,500 mg, and her dessert added 300 mg. What fraction of her recommended maximum daily intake did Lydia consume?

Math Concept **Changing Fractions to Mixed Numbers** Convert fractions greater than 1 to a mixed number by dividing the numerator by the denominator. Write the whole-number portion of the quotient, and remainder over the original denominator.

Starting Hint Find the daily recommended salt intake and make it the denominator with Lydia's total intake as the numerator.

NCTM Number and Operations Understand numbers, ways of representing numbers, relationships among numbers, and number systems.

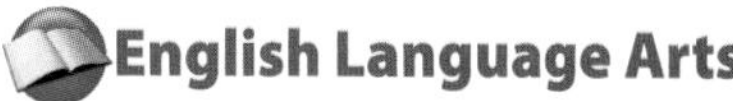

19. **Read and Report** Read a recent article about vitamins or minerals. You may find one in a magazine, newspaper, or online. The article can be about a single vitamin or mineral or vitamins and minerals in general. Pay close attention to new research on vitamins and minerals. Summarize the article in one page, using your own words. Share your summary with the class. Cite the article you are using. Include your opinion about the main points the article makes. Do you agree with the main points? Do you disagree? Explain why.

NCTE 8 Use information resources to gather information and create and communicate knowledge.

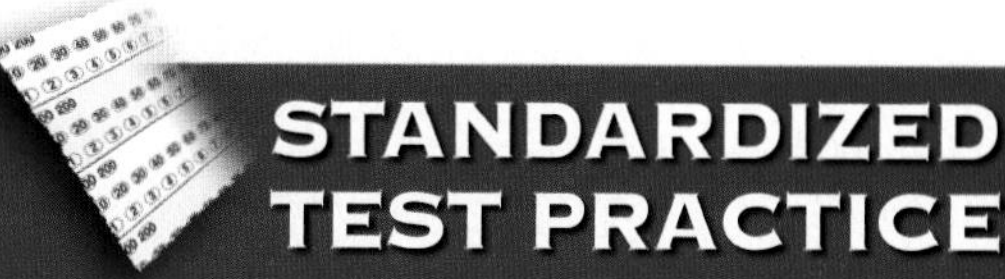

TRUE OR FALSE

Re-read the section on iron on pages 111 to 112. Then determine whether this statement is true or false.

20. Iron-deficiency anemia is a condition in which a person has too many red blood cells.
    a. True
    b. False

Test-Taking Tip Before deciding whether a statement is true or false, carefully read the text to which it relates. Then slowly review both the statement and the text again. Pay close attention to words. One word can make the difference between a true statement and a false one.

CHAPTER 9

Water & Phytochemicals

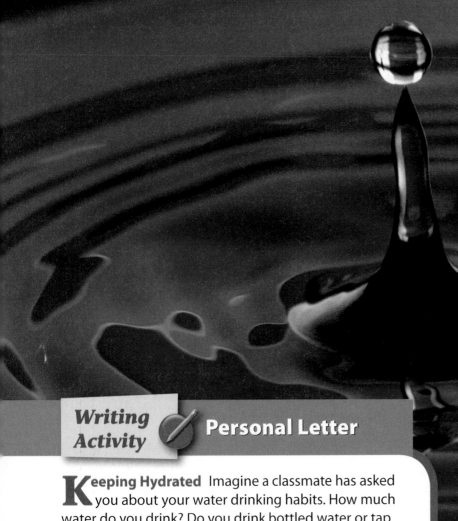

Writing Activity — Personal Letter

Keeping Hydrated Imagine a classmate has asked you about your water drinking habits. How much water do you drink? Do you drink bottled water or tap water? Do you like it room temperature or on ice? Where and when do you drink it? How do you make sure you are drinking enough water? Write a personal letter to your classmate in which you respond to these questions.

Writing Tips To write a personal letter:

- Include a date, salutation, body, closing, and signature.
- Divide the letter into paragraphs just as you would an essay.
- Share your information, thoughts, and experiences.

Activate Prior Knowledge

Explore the Photo Water is essential to the body's survival. *What is one way that water helps your body to function?*

Reading Guide

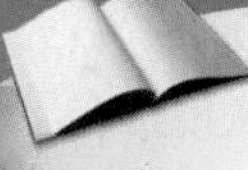

Before You Read

Preview List two things you know about water and two questions you have about phytochemicals. As you read, confirm your knowledge and find answers to your questions.

Read to Learn

Key Concepts

- **List** seven ways water is crucial to your body's health.
- **Describe** phytochemicals and five benefits they provide.

Main Idea

Water is a nutrient that is needed to sustain life, phytochemicals offer many benefits, and both play important roles in keeping the body healthy.

Content Vocabulary

You will find the definitions for these words in the glossary in the back of the book.

- ☐ hydration
- ☐ dehydration
- ☐ phytochemical
- ☐ beta-carotene
- ☐ cruciferous vegetable

Academic Vocabulary

You will find these words in your reading and on your tests. Use the glossary to look up their definitions if necessary.

- essential
- resistance

Graphic Organizer

Use a graphic organizer like the one below to take notes about the colors, sources, and benefits of three types of carotenoids.

BETA-CAROTENE	LYCOPENE	LUTEIN

Graphic Organizer Go to this book's Online Learning Center at **glencoe.com** to print out this graphic organizer.

Academic Standards

English Language Arts

NCTE 5 Use different writing processes to communicate effectively.

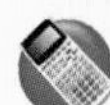

Mathematics

NCTM Number and Operations Understand meanings of operations and how they relate to one another.

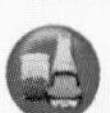

Science

NSES A Develop understandings about scientific inquiry.

NCTE *National Council of Teachers of English*
NCTM *National Council of Teachers of Mathematics*
NSES *National Science Education Standards*
NCSS *National Council for the Social Studies*

The Nutrient Water

Water is one of the six types of nutrients needed to sustain life. Water makes up about 55 to 75 percent of the human body. People can live for about six weeks without food but only a few days without water.

The Need for Water

Water is part of every cell, tissue, and organ in your body. Without water in the right balance, body cells would die. Water is in blood, saliva, digestive juices, urine, and all other body fluids. What does water do?

Chemical Reactions Water participates in chemical reactions in cells. For example, water helps break food down into nutrients before passing them through the intestinal wall and into the bloodstream.

Transportation Minerals, vitamins, glucose, and other substances dissolve in water and can then be absorbed by the body. Blood, which is mostly water, carries oxygen and nutrients to the cells.

Cushioning and Moisturizing Water cushions joints, tissues, and organs to protect them from shock. This is particularly important for the spinal cord. Water keeps your eyes, mouth, nose and skin from drying out.

Waste Removal Water helps filter out pollutants and toxins and get rid of waste. Waste washes out of the body in urine. Water also keeps solid wastes moist to prevent constipation.

Temperature Regulation When you exercise, your body heats up. Your body cools itself by releasing heat in the form of perspiration or sweat. This keeps your body at its normal tem-

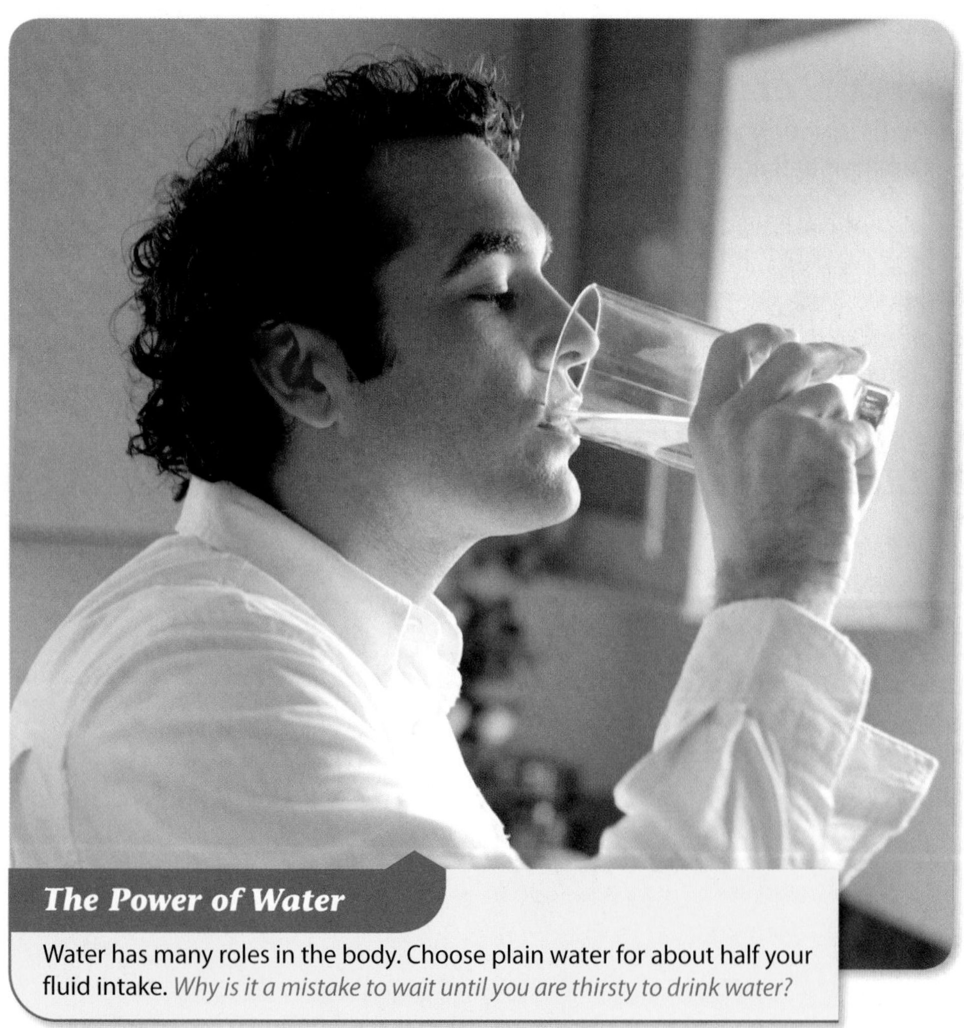

The Power of Water

Water has many roles in the body. Choose plain water for about half your fluid intake. *Why is it a mistake to wait until you are thirsty to drink water?*

perature of 98.6°. As perspiration evaporates from the skin, the body cools.

Breathing When you inhale, your body adds moisture to the air so the lungs can process it. As you exhale, water leaves the lungs. On a cold day, you can see this water as a small cloud in the air.

Overall Well-Being You feel better and have more energy when you have enough water.

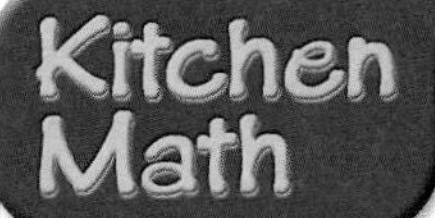

Calculate Your Water Consumption

Use the formula described on this page to calculate the number of ounces you should consume in one day. If you use an 8-ounce water glass, how many glasses of water a day should you drink? What if you use a 10.5-ounce water glass?

Math Concept **Dividing Decimals** To divide decimals, convert the divisor to a whole number by multiplying by a power of 10. Multiply the dividend by the same power of 10.

Starting Hint You can calculate half of your weight by multiplying your weight by 0.5, or dividing your weight by 2. Divide that total by 8 to find the number of 8-ounce glasses. To find the number of 10.5-ounce glasses, multiply the total ounces needed by 10, and divide by 105.

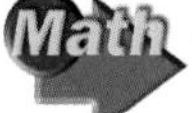

Math Appendix For math help, go to the Math Appendix at the back of the book.

NCTM Number and Operations Understand meanings of operations and how they relate to one another.

How Much Water Do You Need?

You get water from food and drink. The body also makes some water during metabolism. Water exits the body in four ways: through sweat, breathing, urine, and feces.

You lose about two to three quarts of water each day. That is why hydration is important. **Hydration** (hī-ˈdrā-shən) means getting enough water to meet all the body's needs. When you consume enough water, you are hydrated.

Teens and adults should drink 8 to 12 cups of water or other beverages every day. To see how much you need, divide your weight in pounds by half. The result is the number of ounces of water you need. For example, someone who weighs 130 pounds needs at least 65 ounces of water (130 ÷ 2 = 65). This is about 8 cups (65 ounces ÷ 8 ounces per cup = 8.1). This formula works for anyone who is 100 pounds or more.

Check your favorite water glass or bottle to see how much it holds. You can also estimate the amount of water you drink by counting gulps, which are hearty swallows. One gulp equals about one ounce of water.

You will need more water than usual if you work strenuously, have an illness with fever or diarrhea, or take certain medications. Extremely hot or cold weather, pregnancy, breast-feeding a baby, and eating high-fiber foods can also increase water needs. A healthy body does not store water. If you drink more than you need, your body will get rid of it in urine.

Dehydration

People who do not drink enough water every day become dehydrated. **Dehydration** is a condition in which the body has too little water. Signs of dehydration include dark urine, dry lips and skin, and constipation. Dehydration can also cause headaches, dizziness, nausea, light-headedness, and muscle fatigue. Extreme dehydration can produce seizures, brain damage, and even death.

Thirst is one of the warning signs of dehydration. By the time you feel thirsty, however, you have already lost water. Prevent dehydration by drinking water regularly throughout the day, even before you get thirsty.

Other Fluids

At least half of the fluids you drink should be plain water. The rest can come from milk, juice, and other beverages. Limit beverages that contain caffeine, which can have negative effects in large amounts. Coffee, tea, and many soft drinks have caffeine. Be careful in choosing flavored waters and sports drinks, which may have a lot of added sugar.

Figure 9.1 Approximate Water Content of Food

Water Everywhere Almost everything you eat is at least partly made of water. *Does this mean you don't need to drink water?*

Food	Percentage of Water
Fruits and vegetables	80–90%
Milk	90%
Cooked cereals	85%
Eggs	75%
Pasta	65%
Seafood	60–85%
Meats	45–65%
Cheeses	35%
Breads	35–40%
Nuts	2–5%
Oils	0%

Most solid foods contain some water. You cannot rely on food alone to meet your water needs, however. Fruits and vegetables have a higher percentage of water than other foods, as shown in **Figure 9.1**.

Drinking More Water

These simple habits can help you increase your water intake.

- Drink at least eight ounces of water when you get up in the morning, when you go to bed, and before meals. A good habit is to drink a glass of water after brushing your teeth.
- Carry a sports bottle filled with water. Reach for the bottle instead of a soft drink.
- Drink water before, during, and after physical activities.
- Each time you pass a water fountain, take a drink.

✓ **Reading Check** **List** What are three signs of dehydration?

Phytochemicals

Plant-based foods have phytochemicals that have many health benefits. A **phytochemical** is a chemical compound that occurs naturally in plants. *Phyto* means plant.

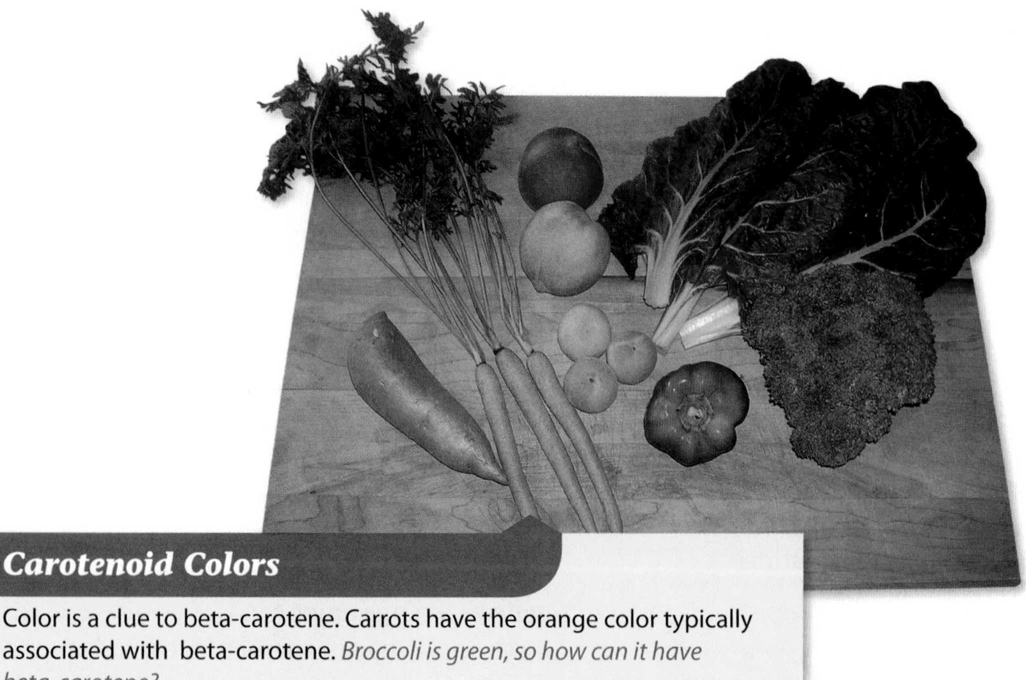

Carotenoid Colors

Color is a clue to beta-carotene. Carrots have the orange color typically associated with beta-carotene. *Broccoli is green, so how can it have beta-carotene?*

The Colors of Health

Phytochemicals have several health benefits. *Which of these foods contain phytochemicals? Explain.*

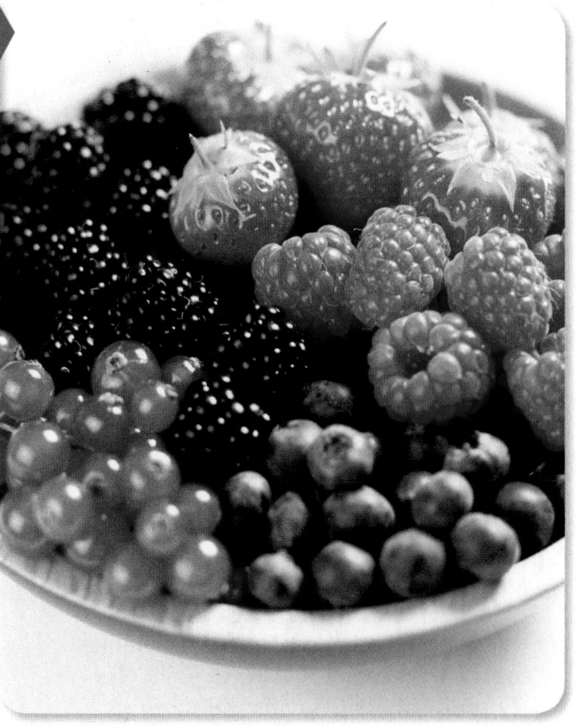

Plants produce phytochemicals for protection from insects, viruses, fungi, and the sun. Some phytochemicals give plants their color, flavor, and aroma.

Scientists have identified thousands of phytochemicals in plant foods. Every plant contains at least 200 different phytochemicals.

Phytochemicals are not considered **essential**, or necessary, for life, so they are not classified as nutrients. As research uncovers more about the role of phytochemicals in the body, they may one day be called nutrients too.

Benefits of Phytochemicals

Scientists have recently begun to discover the roles that phytochemicals play in the human body. These are some of the tasks that phytochemicals perform:

- Act as antioxidants.
- Boost **resistance**, or immunity, to disease.
- Keep cancer cells from forming and multiplying.
- Influence the production of cholesterol.
- Protect the body against diseases such as cancer, diabetes, heart disease, high blood pressure, and blindness caused by aging.

How do specific phytochemicals act in the body? How much of each phytochemical do you need? Do phytochemicals work alone or together? Scientists are trying to answer these questions through research.

Examples of Phytochemicals

Scientists categorize phytochemicals by structure and function. Here are important categories of phytochemicals.

Carotenoids

A carotenoid (kə-ˈrä-tə-ˌnȯid) is a yellow, orange or red phytochemical that gives color to fruits and vegetables such as carrots and red peppers. You may recognize these well-known carotenoids:

Nutrition Check

Healing with Phytochemicals

Because of the healing powers of phytochemicals, plants have been used medicinally for centuries. In 400 BCE, Hippocrates prescribed willow tree leaves to relieve fever. Today, research shows that phytochemicals in tomatoes and broccoli may prevent prostate cancer. Diindolylmethane, a phytochemical found in kale, is currently used in clinical trials to treat several types of cancer. The world's most widely-used cancer drug, Taxol, is based on a phytochemical from the Pacific Yew Tree.

Think About It Health experts emphasize the importance of prevention—stopping diseases before they start. A person with a history of cancer in her family eats a diet comprised mostly of animal products. What changes would you suggest for her and why?

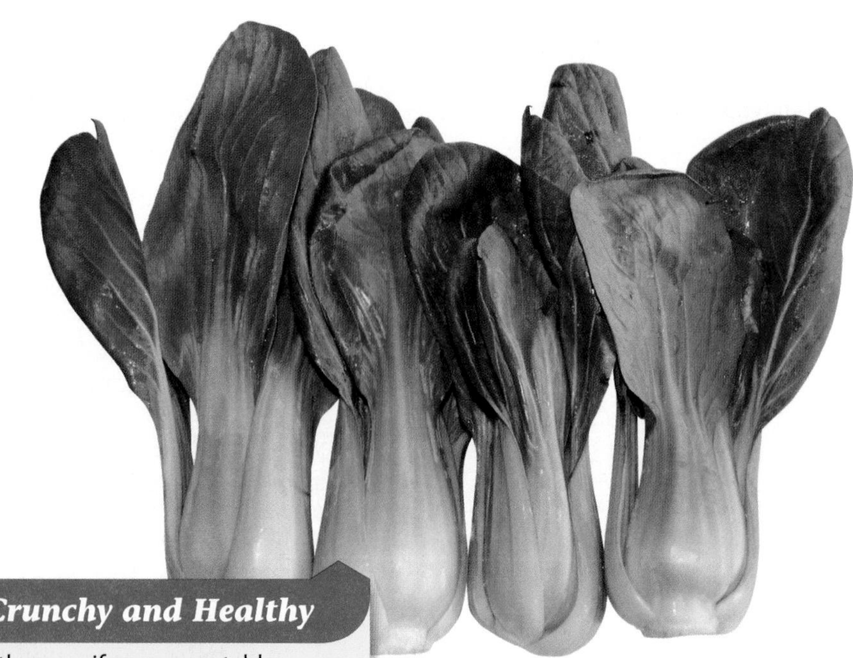

Crunchy and Healthy

Bok choy and other cruciferous vegetables supply phytochemicals known as indoles. Try adding these to salads and stir-fries. *Besides vegetables, what plant foods are good sources of phytochemicals?*

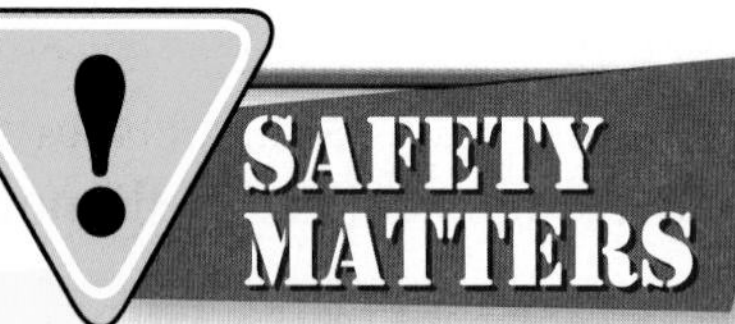

SAFETY MATTERS

Safe Sports

Dehydration can cause serious complications—even death—for athletes. On a hot day, a runner loses about two *pounds* of water an hour. You should drink 8 ounces of fluid for every 20 minutes of athletic activity, more if heat is extreme. But do not wait until you are done exercising before you guzzle fluids. Hydrate your body before and after physical exercise. Do not wait for thirst to drink. By the time you notice being thirsty, you are already in need of water. Athletes need 2 ounces of water for every three pounds they weigh each day. If you plan to exercise for an hour, calculate how much water you will need, and drink half before you begin. And remember that you still need fluids in cool weather, when dehydration may not be noticeable, but is still a risk.

What Would You Do? Throughout August, your friends play basketball every afternoon for about two hours. You want to join them. How much water will you plan on drinking, and when will you drink it?

Beta-carotene **Beta-carotene** (ˈbā-tə-ˈkar-ə-ˌtēn) is an orange or red phytochemical found in dark green and orange vegetables and fruits, such as carrots. The body uses beta-carotene to make vitamin A. Beta-carotene also acts as an antioxidant and may help prevent cancer.

Good sources of beta-carotene are yellow and orange fruits and vegetables, such as apricots, cantaloupes, papayas, peaches, carrots, pumpkins, sweet potatoes, and winter squash. Chlorophyll in green plants can mask beta-carotene's orange color. Spinach, mustard greens, green peppers, broccoli, green peas, and kale are rich in beta-carotene.

Lycopene Red fruits and vegetables contain a carotenoid called lycopene (ˈlī-kə-ˌpēn). Tomatoes and tomato products are good sources. Others are pink grapefruit, guava, and watermelon. Lycopene may reduce the risk of cancer and heart disease.

Lutein Another well-known carotenoid is lutein (ˈlü-tē-ən), which is found in kale, spinach, collard greens, romaine lettuce, broccoli, and brussels sprouts. Lutein may help protect against blindness.

Flavonoids

Flavonoids (ˈflā-və-ˌnȯids) are another important group of phytochemicals. Many fruits and vegetables are rich in a flavonoids. Flavonoids include the following:

Anthocyanins Anthocyanins (ˌan(t)-thə-ˈsī-ə-nəns) are found in blackberries, blueberries, cherries, cranberries, kiwifruit, strawberries, eggplant skin, plums, red cabbage, and red or purple grapes. They are antioxidants and may lower cancer risk.

Isoflavones Soybeans and soy-based foods contain isoflavones (ˌī-sō-ˈflā-ˌvōns). They may prevent cancer, lower cholesterol, and help reduce symptoms of menopause. Menopause is the point in life when a woman's menstrual cycle slows and stops.

Quercetin Quercetin (ˈkwər-ˌsi-tən) is found in onions, tea, and many vegetables. It acts as an antioxidant and may slow the growth of cancer cells.

Resveratrol Red grapes and juice have resveratrol (rez-ˈvir-ə-ˌtrȯl). Resveratrol is an antioxidant and may contribute to heart health and reduce cancer risk.

Other Phytochemical Categories

Besides carotenoids and flavonoids, a few other notable phytochemical categories are:

Allyl Sulfides Allyl sulfides (ˈa-ləl ˈsəl-ˌfīds) are found in garlic, onions, chives, leeks, and shallots. They may prevent cancer and lower blood pressure and cholesterol. Allyl sulfides also are thought to aid in preventing or helping the body cope with colds, blood circulation, high blood pressure, diabetes and insomnia.

Indoles Indoles (ˈin-ˌdōls) are found in cruciferous (krü-ˈsi-f(ə-)-rəs) vegetables. A **cruciferous vegetable** is a vegetable from the cabbage family, such as cabbage, broccoli, brussels sprouts, cauliflower, kale, Swiss chard, and bok choy. Indoles are antioxidants and may reduce cancer risk. Indoles also assist in detoxifying human tissues and promote hormone balance.

Careers in Food

Michael Kristof
Menu Designer

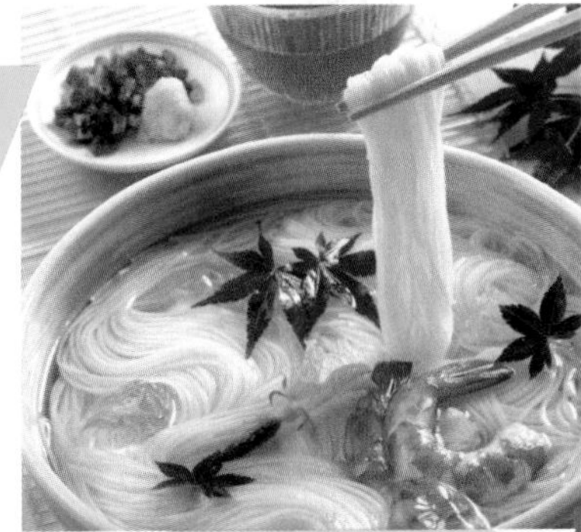

Q: What does a menu designer do?

A: Menu designers create visually appealing displays of a restaurant's food items in a way that makes people want to purchase them.

Q: How does a person typically get into that line of work?

A: It comes from a love of design in general. Menu designers are interested in the client, and the message they want to convey. They become interested in the psychology—the reason things are put into a menu in a certain order.

Q: Are the opportunities for menu designers on the rise?

A: Yes. If you want to be a menu designer, you could get a job every single day if you know what you're doing. Restaurants understand the need and benefit of having their menus professionally designed.

"You have to really love what you do. If you don't, you will not produce quality work."
— Michael Kristof
Owner/Designer,
Kristof Creative
– Mount Juliet, TN

Education and Training

Most menu designers go to school and take graphic arts courses at a junior college, a university, or a private design school.

Qualities and Skills

The ability to visualize quality designs. Patience is important because education is involved in every project. The ability to learn the goals of the project and understand how the goals were formulated.

Related Career Opportunities

Advertising, public relations, and, graphic arts.

Phytosterols Phytosterols (fī-ˈtäs-tə-ˌrōls) are found in vegetable oils. They may have a positive effect on cholesterol levels. Phytosterols also aid the immune system, helping to guard against viral infections, allergies, and cancer.

Saponins Whole-grain products, soy products, and dry beans, asparagus, beets, olives, quinoa, spinach, peas, and lentils contain saponins (ˈsa-pə-nəns). Saponins aid the immune system and have been shown to lower cholesterol and prevent cancer.

How Much Do You Need?

You can get all the phytochemicals in the right combinations by eating plant foods. Manufacturers are creating supplements, called neutraceuticals, that supply phytochemicals. Health experts do not recommend these supplements, because no one knows exactly how much of each phytochemical you need and how much is safe to take.

Getting Phytochemicals

Color counts when choosing fruits and vegetables: the brighter the color, the greater the supply of phytochemicals. Aim for at least five to nine servings of fruits and vegetables each day in different colors. Choose a variety of cruciferous vegetables.

Whole-grain products have phytochemicals too. Try whole-grain breads, cereals, pasta, and crackers, as well as brown rice, kasha, bulgur, and millet. Dry beans, peas, garlic, flax seeds, broccoli, and lentils are good sources of phytochemicals. Herbs, spices, and herbal tea have phytochemicals as well. Garlic and leeks are also good sources of phytochemicals. Eat a variety of plant foods to get the benefits of phytochemicals. These foods are a delicious way to protect your health. If you are having trouble consuming five to nine servings of vegetables per day, consider juicing vegetables and fruits.

Light and Healthy Recipe

Carotenoid-rich Fruit Salad

Ingredients

- **2 cups** Watermelon, cut into cubes
- **2 cups** Cantaloupe, cut into cubes
- **1 cup** Strawberries, quartered
- **1 cup** Red grapes, halved lengthwise
- 2 Kiwi fruits, sliced in circles

Directions

1. Combine the fruit pieces in a large serving bowl and gently mix them.
2. Chill for at least an hour before serving.

This recipe is packed with carotenoids, including lycopene, anthocyanin, beta-carotene, lutein, and resveratrol.

Yield 4 servings

Nutrition Analysis per Serving

■ Calories	111
■ Total fat	1 g
Saturated fat	1 g
Cholesterol	0 mg
■ Sodium	16 mg
■ Carbohydrate	28 g
Dietary fiber	3 g
Sugars	22 g
■ Protein	2 g

CHAPTER 9 Review & Applications

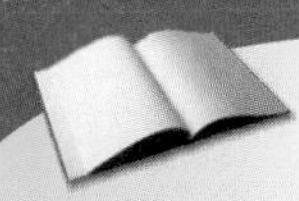

After You Read

Chapter Summary

Water is a nutrient that is necessary to sustain life. It assists with many body functions and with overall well-being. To be adequately hydrated, teens and adults need 8 to 12 cups of fluids daily. Dehydration poses serious risks. Half of a person's daily fluids should be plain water. To drink more water, gradually increase the amount consumed. Phytochemicals are chemical compounds in plants that offer many health benefits, including protection against diseases. There are carotenoids, flavonoids, and other categories of phytochemicals. Five to nine daily servings of colorful plant foods will provide adequate amounts of phytochemicals.

Content and Academic Vocabulary Review

1. Use each of these content and academic vocabulary words in a sentence.

Content Vocabulary

- hydration (p. 119)
- dehydration (p. 119)
- phytochemical (p. 120)
- beta-carotene (p. 122)
- cruciferous vegetable (p. 123)

Academic Vocabulary

- essential (p. 121)
- resistance (p. 121)

Review Key Concepts

2. List seven ways water is crucial to your body's health.

3. Describe phytochemicals and five benefits they provide.

Critical Thinking

4. Describe three problems, symptoms, or sensations a person might have if he or she lacked water. Review the seven functions of water for help.

5. Advise Jeremiah about water intake. Jeremiah weighs 160 pounds, lives in a hot, arid region, and plays soccer every day.

6. Evaluate whether Marisol's fluid intake is ideal. Marisol weighs 130 pounds. Most days, she drinks 50 ounces of juice, milk, soda, and coffee. She drinks 10 ounces of water.

7. Decide who has the better plan. Frances, 15, plans to consume many phytochemicals now in order to reap their benefits in the future. Katya, also 15, plans to wait until later in life before eating phytochemicals regularly.

8. Examine what many restaurants call a "green salad." What is right and/or wrong with this offering?

9. Explain why tofu is often recommended as a dietary addition for women who experience uncomfortable menopause symptoms.

10. Describe how the following statement is specifically relevant to phytochemicals: "Eat a variety of foods to stay healthy."

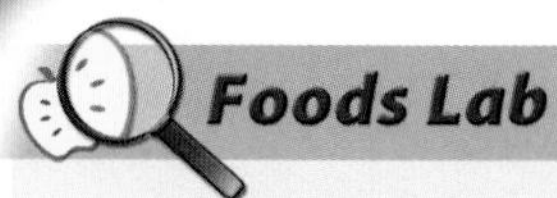

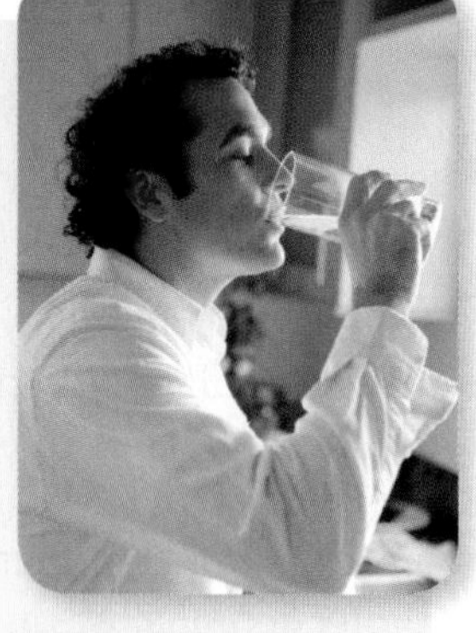

11. Water Taste Test It is easier to stay hydrated when your water tastes great. Using members of your lab team as tasters, conduct a blind taste test of different water samples.

Procedure Assemble samples of bottled, softened, and regular tap water. Include tap water from different parts of your community, if possible. Serve all samples to tasters at the same temperature.

Analysis Have your tasters evaluate and rank the samples in order of preference. Create a chart in which you note the characteristics of each water sample, as well as the most preferred and least preferred samples.

HEALTHFUL CHOICES

12. Determine Quantity Without a labeled water bottle, you may not know how many ounces of water you are drinking. Pour exactly 8 ounces of water into a glass. Count the number of gulps you take to empty the glass. How many gulps equal a cup for you? Calculate the number of gulps needed for you to drink four ounces.

TECH Connection

13. Packed with Phytochemicals Under your teacher's supervision, conduct research on the Internet to find a recipe for a dish that includes at least four different types of phytochemicals. Then use presentation software to create a presentation that describes the recipe. In your presentation, identify the foods in the recipe that provide phytochemicals, and explain the type of phytochemicals they contain. Also use the presentation software to explain how the recipe is prepared.

Real-World Skills

Problem-Solving Skills

14. An Early Start Yolanda's toddler is a slightly picky eater. He will not eat many fruits or vegetables, but he is open to most other foods. What else can Yolanda feed him to make sure he consumes phytochemicals?

Interpersonal and Collaborative

15. The Rainbow Connection Work with your group to create a paper or cardboard mobile that will hang in your classroom. Mobiles should include the following: a rainbow; one fruit or vegetable matching each color of the rainbow; the names of phytochemicals contained in each fruit and vegetable.

Financial Literacy

16. Compare Water Prices Suppose you need 70 oz. of water a day. Determine the cost per ounce of your favorite bottled water brand. How much would it cost to meet all of your water requirements for a week? If tap water costs $0.00002 per ounce, how much would you save in one week drinking tap water instead?

Academic Skills

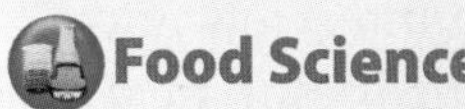

Food Science

17. Ubiquitous Water Water is the most common food molecule, composing most of the weight of many foods. By evaporating water, we can concentrate the flavor in sauces, which is known as reduction.

Procedure Pour a third of a can of beef broth into a bowl. Put the remaining broth into a small pot. Simmer the broth until half of it evaporates. Pour the reduced broth into another small bowl. Compare.

Analysis Write a paragraph describing the differences between the 2 bowls.

NSES A Develop understandings about scientific inquiry.

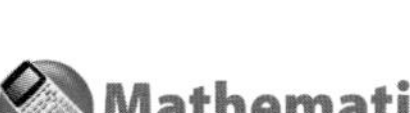

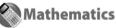

Mathematics

18. Compare Water Content A fig is 4/5 water, while blackberries are 17/20 water. A grapefruit is typically 9/10 water, an orange is 87% water, and an apple is 21/25 water. Which of these fruits has the highest percentage of water? Which has the lowest?

Math Concept **Comparing Fractions** When comparing fractions, convert all fractions to equivalent fractions which have common denominators. Then, compare the numerators. If you are comparing fractions and percents, change all numbers to the same format: percents, decimals, or fractions with common denominators.

Starting Hint Since a percent is involved, convert each amount to a fraction with 100 as the denominator.

NCTM Number and Operations Understand meanings of operations and how they relate to one another.

English Language Arts

19. Phytochemical Pamphlet Create and write a 250-word supermarket pamphlet that will inform shoppers about phytochemicals and the foods that contain them. Your pamphlet may also include illustrations or images. Make it clear, educational, and factual. Include a chart listing the amounts and types of phytochemicals needed.

NCTE 5 Use different writing processes to communicate effectively.

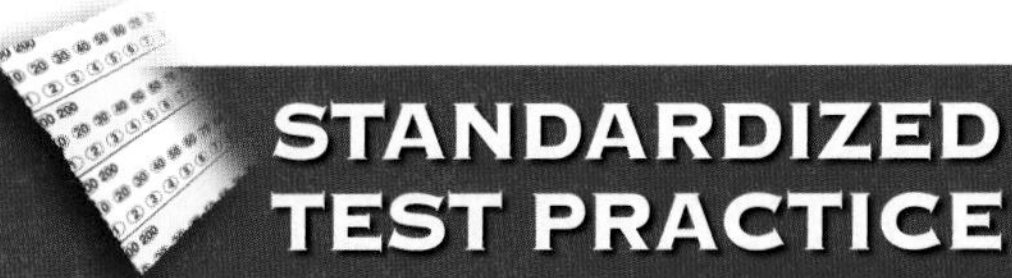

STANDARDIZED TEST PRACTICE

Analogy Read the pairs of terms. Then choose the best word to match with the term *phytochemical.*

20. chicken breast : protein
olive oil: fat
pasta: carbohydrate
_____ : phytochemical

a. cell
b. plant
c. fruit
d. blueberry

Test-Taking Tip Analogies establish relationships between terms. When you look at the three pairs of terms listed here, identify the relationship that is common to all of them. Then try matching each possible answer with the term *phytochemical*. The one that establishes the same type of relationship as the other terms is correct.

UNIT 2

Thematic Project

Fast Food and Health

Foods contain nutrients that are essential for good health. Carbohydrates, proteins and fats, vitamins and minerals, and water and phytochemicals are a necessary part of a healthy diet. In this project you will analyze the nutrients in your favorite fast foods. You will use what you learned to interview the manager of a fast food restaurant and to develop a healthful meal plan.

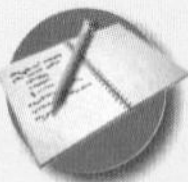

My Journal

If you completed the journal entry from page 57, refer to it to see if your thoughts have changed after reading the unit.

Project Assignment

- Describe your favorite fast food meal.
- Search the fast food restaurant's Web site for the nutritional value of specific foods.
- Visit a fast food restaurant and interview the manager about recommendations for healthful food choices.
- Arrange, take notes, and type the interview with the manager.
- Use what you learn in the interview and your research to create a healthful meal plan. The meal plan should show total calories and calories from fat for each food.

Academic Skills You Will Use

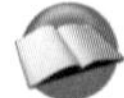

English Language Arts

NCTE 12 Use language to accomplish individual purposes.

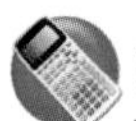

Mathematics

NCTM Numbers and Operations Compute fluently and make reasonable estimates.

STEP 1 Choose Your Favorite Fast Food Meal

Fast food has become ingrained in American culture. Most Americans eat fast food often. What is your favorite fast food restaurant? What do you like to order when you visit this restaurant? Choose a fast food restaurant that you like to eat at, and write down what you typically order when you eat there.

STEP 2 Evaluate a Fast Food Meal

Go to the Web site of the fast food restaurant you chose. Find the nutritional values of each item in the meal you wrote down in Step 1. Make a table listing the following information for each food item you selected: Total calories, total calories from fat, fat, saturated fat, trans fat, cholesterol, sodium, carbohydrates, dietary fiber, sugars, and protein. Then calculate the total calories and total calories from fat for the entire meal. Use these research skills as you compile the information.

Research Skills

- Identify appropriate resources.
- Synthesize and organize information.

STEP 3 Connect to Your Community

Arrange to talk with the manager of a local fast food restaurant, preferably the one that serves your favorite fast food meal. Plan your meeting well in advance and be on time. Take the information you compiled in Step 2. Show the manager the nutritional information you compiled about your favorite fast food meal. Ask for advice about making more healthful choices at fast food restaurants. Ask the manager for advice on developing an alternate meal plan that is low in calories and fat and that provides valuable nutrients. Take notes during the interview and type the notes of your interview.

Interpersonal Skills

- Be polite; do not interrupt the manager while he or she is talking.
- Listen attentively.
- Ask additional questions to better understand the manager's answers.

STEP 4 Create a Healthy Meal Plan

Use the Unit Thematic Project Checklist to plan and complete your project and give your presentation to the class.

STEP 5 Evaluate Your Presentation

Your project will be evaluated based on:

- Content and organization of your presentation.
- Speaking and audience interaction skills.
- Mechanics—presentation and neatness.

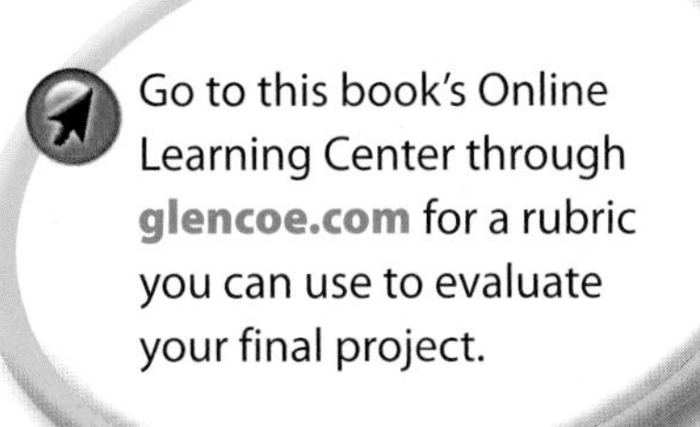

Go to this book's Online Learning Center through **glencoe.com** for a rubric you can use to evaluate your final project.

Unit Thematic Project Checklist

Category	Objectives
Plan	☑ Research the nutritional values of your favorite fast foods.
	☑ Talk with the manager of a fast food restaurant about strategies for choosing healthful fast foods.
	☑ Develop an alternate meal plan for a fast food meal that is low in calories and fat and that provides valuable nutrients.
Present	☑ Make a presentation to your class to share your original meal plan and your revised meal plan and discuss what you learned.
	☑ Invite the students in your class to ask you any questions they may have. Answer three questions.
	☑ When students ask you questions, demonstrate in your answers that you respect their perspectives.
	☑ Turn in the nutritional information you compiled about your favorite fast food meal, your notes from your interview, and your revised healthier meal plan to your teacher.
Academic Skills	☑ Organize your presentation so the audience can follow along easily.
	☑ Be sensitive to the needs of different audiences.

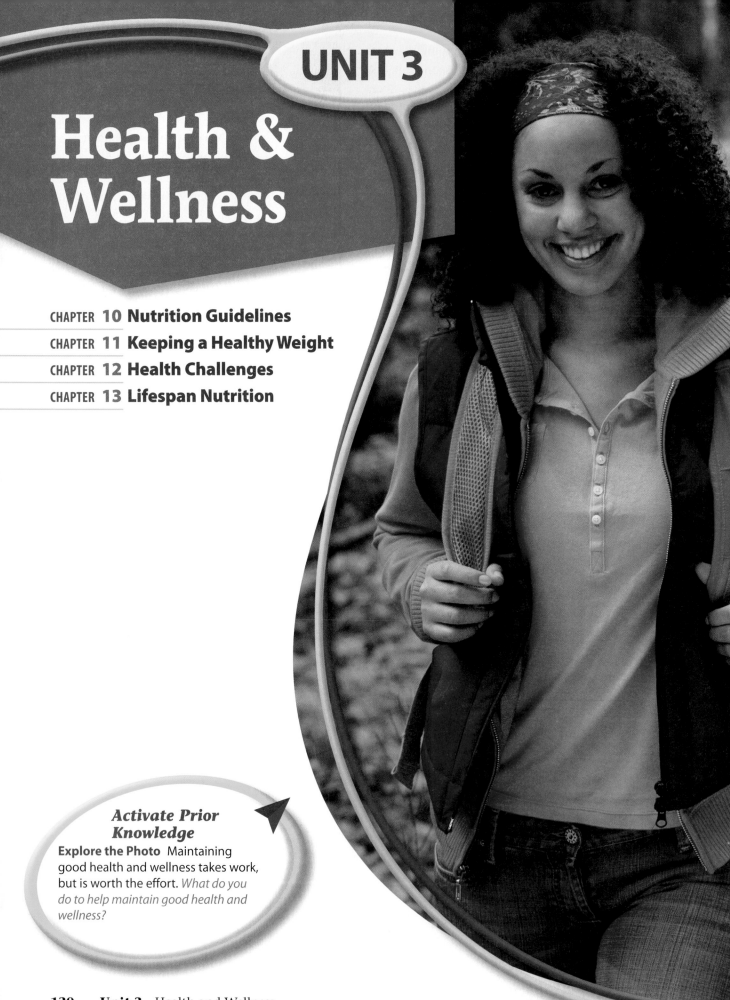

UNIT 3

Health & Wellness

Activate Prior Knowledge

Explore the Photo Maintaining good health and wellness takes work, but is worth the effort. *What do you do to help maintain good health and wellness?*

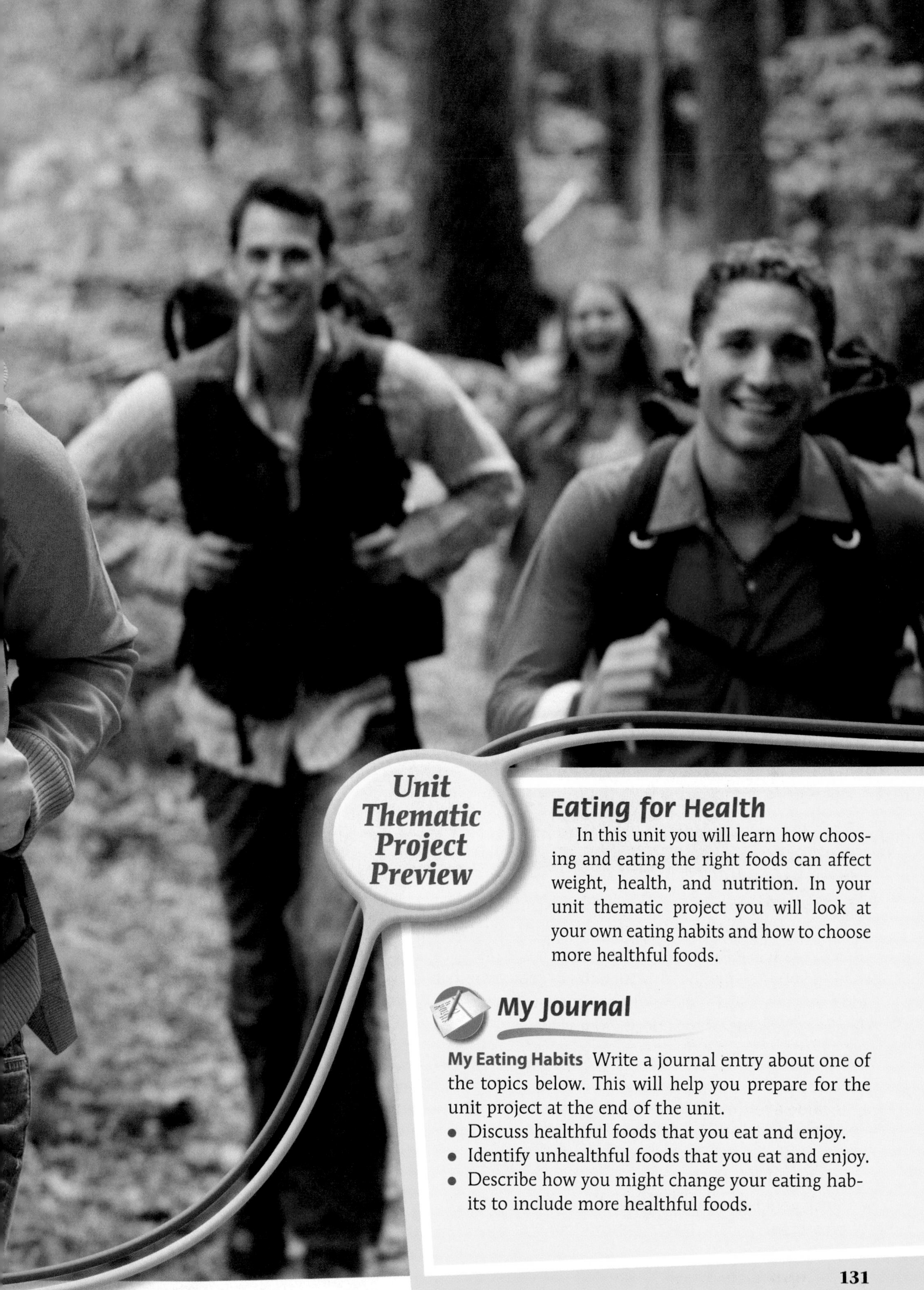

Unit Thematic Project Preview

Eating for Health

In this unit you will learn how choosing and eating the right foods can affect weight, health, and nutrition. In your unit thematic project you will look at your own eating habits and how to choose more healthful foods.

My Journal

My Eating Habits Write a journal entry about one of the topics below. This will help you prepare for the unit project at the end of the unit.

- Discuss healthful foods that you eat and enjoy.
- Identify unhealthful foods that you eat and enjoy.
- Describe how you might change your eating habits to include more healthful foods.

CHAPTER 10

Nutrition Guidelines

Writing Activity — Letter to the Editor

A Teen's Perspective A magazine has published an article suggesting that teens make poor dietary choices. Write a letter to the editor of the magazine sharing your perspective. In your letter, explain whether you think this statement is right or wrong, using specific details and examples to support your view.

Writing Tips Follow these steps to write a letter to the editor:

- Include a return-address heading, date, inside address, salutation, closing, and signature.
- Respond to, correct, or elaborate on a previously published statement.
- Since your letter may be published, make it error-free.

Activate Prior Knowledge

Explore the Photo Nutrition experts have categorized foods to help people make nutritious dietary choices. *Can you name the five food groups?*

Reading Guide

Before You Read

Preview Examine this chapter's photos and figures. With a partner, list three facts you can infer about nutrition. Verify your inferences as you read.

Read to Learn

Key Concepts

- **Explain** the Dietary Guidelines for Americans.
- **Describe** MyPyramid and its recommendations.
- **Describe** a Nutrition Facts panel, its contents, and how to use it.
- **Explain** dietary supplements, their different forms, and their pros and cons.
- **Discuss** the importance of separating nutrition facts from fiction.

Main Idea

Nutrition guidelines are sources of information that help people to make smart dietary choices, stay healthy, and separate fact from fiction.

Content Vocabulary

You will find the definitions to these words in the glossary in the back of the book.

- ☐ nutrient density
- ☐ Nutrition Facts panel
- ☐ Daily Value
- ☐ dietary supplement
- ☐ herbal
- ☐ fraud

Academic Vocabulary

You will find these words in your reading and on your tests. Use the glossary at the back of the book.

- reliable
- moderate

Graphic Organizer

Use a graphic organizer like the one below to take notes about the types, forms, pros, and cons of dietary supplements.

DIETARY SUPPLEMENTS			
TYPES	FORMS	PROS	CONS

Graphic Organizer Go to this book's Online Learning Center at **glencoe.com** to print out this graphic organizer.

Academic Standards

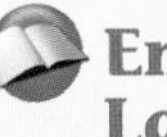

English Language Arts

NCTE 12 Use language to accomplish individual purposes.

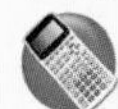

Mathematics

NCTM Data Analysis and Probability Develop and evaluate inferences and predictions that are based on data.

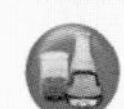

Science

NSES A Develop understanding about scientific inquiry.

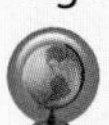

Social Studies

NCSS VIII B Science Technology, and Society Make judgments about how science and technology have transformed the physical world and human society.

NCTE *National Council of Teachers of English*
NCTM *National Council of Teachers of Mathematics*
NSES *National Science Education Standards*
NCSS *National Council for the Social Studies*

Dietary Guidelines for Americans

With so much information in the media about health and nutrition, how can you know what is really true? Use sources of information you can trust. Three of the best **reliable**, or trustworthy, sources of information are the Dietary Guidelines for Americans, MyPyramid, and Nutrition Facts panels. These sources come from the U.S. Department of Agriculture (USDA).

The Dietary Guidelines for Americans is a source of science-based advice on nutrition and fitness. **Figure 10.1** summarizes key topics in the guidelines.

Following the Dietary Guidelines for Americans can help you stay healthy and avoid chronic disease. The guidelines are updated every five years and are the basis for federal nutrition programs.

✓ Reading Check **Respond** When are the Dietary Guidelines for Americans updated?

MyPyramid

MyPyramid is an easy-to-use food guidance system that can help you make smart choices from every food group and find a balance between food and physical activity. MyPyramid is shown in **Figure 10.2**.

MyPyramid is divided into bands of different colors. Each band except the yellow band represents a food group. The yellow band represents oils. You need to eat more from the food groups with wide bands and less from the food groups with thin bands.

The MyPyramid Web site offers free food and exercise recommendations. These recommendations are based on your individual needs, such as age, gender, and activity level.

The MyPyramid Web site can give you individualized evaluations of your calorie needs based on your age, gender, and physical activity level. You can use the Web site, **www.MyPyramid.gov**, to create and track menus and exercise plans.

Figure 10.1 Dietary Guidelines for Americans

Dietary Do's and Don'ts These guidelines help people know just what to do, and what to avoid, in order to remain healthy. ***How much physical activity do teens need daily?***

Factor	Guidelines
Nutrients and Calories	• Choose a variety of nutrient-dense foods and beverages. • Choose foods low in saturated and trans fats, cholesterol, added sugars, and salt.
Weight Management	• Balance calories consumed with calories used to maintain a healthy weight. • Reduce calorie intake and increase activity to prevent weight gain.
Physical Activity	• Engage in at least 60 minutes of moderate-intensity physical activity, above usual activity, on most days of the week. • Increase exercise while not exceeding calorie intake requirements to lose weight and be healthier.

Factor	Guidelines
Food Choices	• Choose a variety of foods from the different food groups.
Fats	• Choose lean, low-fat, and fat-free foods. • Limit intake of fats and oils high in saturated and trans fat. • Consume less than 10 percent of calories from saturated fat. • Teens: Limit fat to 25 to 35 percent of calories.
Carbohydrates	• Choose fiber-rich fruits, vegetables, and whole grains often. • Limit foods and beverages with added sugars.
Sodium and Potassium	• Consume less than 2,300 mg (about 1 teaspoon) of sodium per day. • Choose potassium-rich foods, such as fruits and vegetables.

Figure 10.2 MyPyramid

A Visual Tool MyPyramid provides a visual tool that uses shape, color, and words to help people understand the food groups and make smart dietary choices. ***Why does MyPyramid show a figure walking up stairs?***

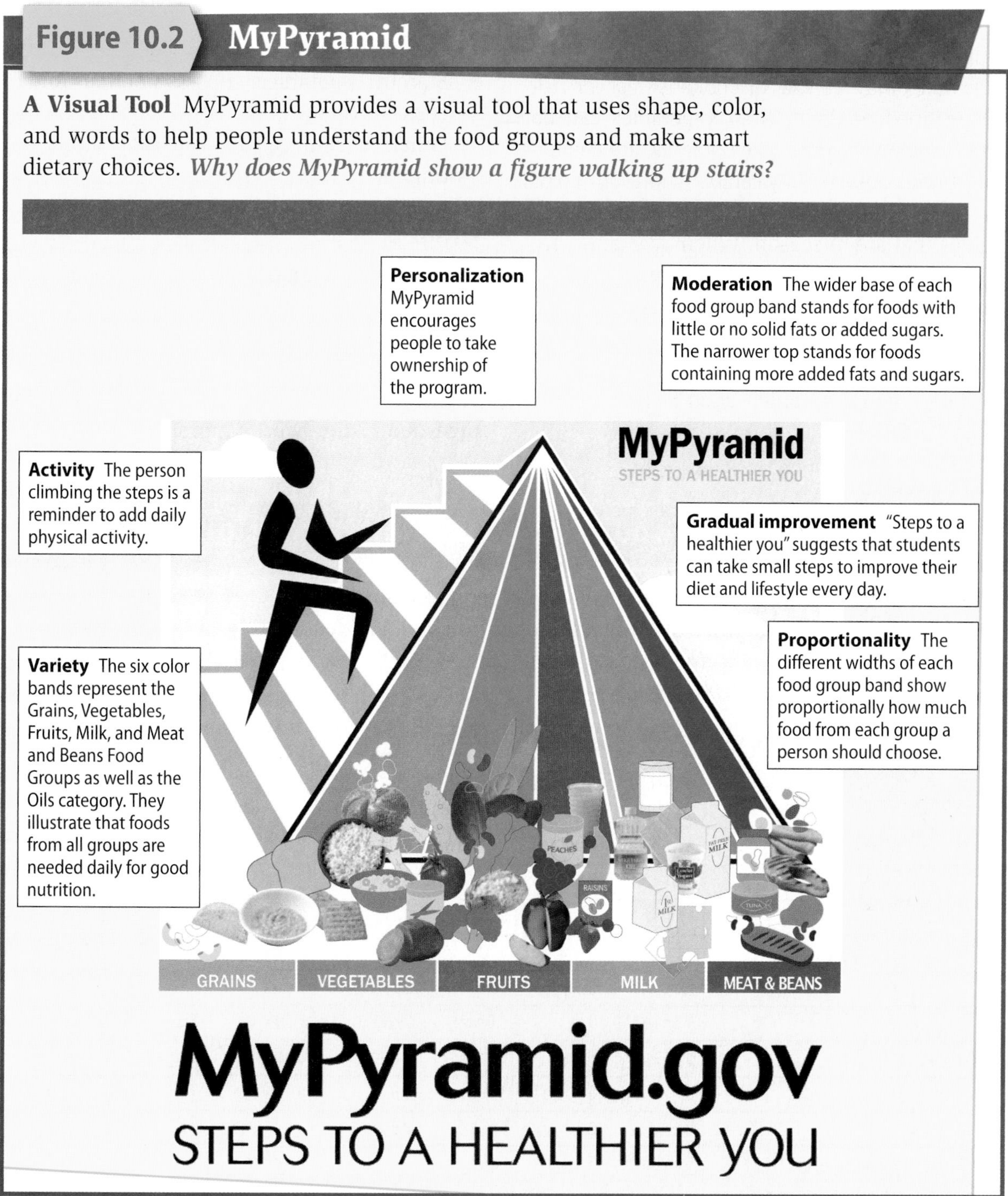

Personalization MyPyramid encourages people to take ownership of the program.
Moderation The wider base of each food group band stands for foods with little or no solid fats or added sugars. The narrower top stands for foods containing more added fats and sugars.
Activity The person climbing the steps is a reminder to add daily physical activity.
MyPyramid
STEPS TO A HEALTHIER YOU
Gradual improvement "Steps to a healthier you" suggests that students can take small steps to improve their diet and lifestyle every day.
Proportionality The different widths of each food group band show proportionally how much food from each group a person should choose.
Variety The six color bands represent the Grains, Vegetables, Fruits, Milk, and Meat and Beans Food Groups as well as the Oils category. They illustrate that foods from all groups are needed daily for good nutrition.
PEACHES
RAISINS
MILK
TUNA
GRAINS
VEGETABLES
FRUITS
MILK
MEAT & BEANS
MyPyramid.gov
STEPS TO A HEALTHIER YOU

Food Groups

There are six color bands in the MyPyramid chart, representing five food groups and a sixth category, oils. Each band is a different color and some bands are thicker than others, to point out that you need to eat more from some food groups than from others. Oils are a category rather than a group because they should be consumed in small amounts.

Fruit Group

Any fruit or 100 percent fruit juice is part of the Fruit Group. Common fruits include apples, bananas, strawberries, and oranges. Because fruit juices are high in calories and do not contain fiber, whole fruits are a better choice. Fruits have many of the same benefits as vegetables, including maintaining a healthy heart and blood vessels and helping to control body weight.

Vegetable Group

Any vegetable or 100% vegetable juice counts as a member of the Vegetable Group. Vegetables may be raw or cooked, fresh or frozen, canned or dried. Most vegetables can be eaten raw, while some, like potatoes, are usually only eaten cooked. They can be whole, cut up or mashed. Whenever possible, choose fresh vegetables that are in season. When vegetables are in season, they cost less and taste better because they are likely to be at their peak flavor.

Vegetables are divided into these categories based on the nutrients they contain:

- Dark green vegetables, such as broccoli and spinach
- Orange vegetables, such as carrots and pumpkin
- Dry beans and peas
- Starchy vegetables, such as potatoes and corn
- Other vegetables, such as celery and onions

Grain Group

The Grain Group includes any food made from wheat, rice, cornmeal, barley, or other grains. Examples include bread, pasta, oatmeal, and tortillas. The nutrients in grain reduce the risk of heart disease and keep the digestive system working properly.

Figure 10.3 Daily Food Group Amounts by Calorie Level

Determine Quantities Your total daily calorie requirement can help you determine the quantities of individual foods you should consume. ***How many ounces of protein foods are recommended for a person who requires 2,200 total calories per day?***

Food Groups	Calorie Levels						
	1,600	1,800	2,000	2,200	2,400	2,600	2,800
Fruits	1 c (3 srv)	1 c (3 srv)	1.5 c (4 srv)	1.5 c (4 srv)	1.5c (4 srv)	2c (4 srv)	2c (4 srv)
Vegetables	1.5 c (4 srv)	2 c (4 srv)	2 c (4 srv)	2c (4 srv)	2.5c (4 srv)	3c (4 srv)	3c (4 srv)
Dark Green	2 c/wk	3 c/wk	3 c/wk	3 c/wk	3 c/wk	3 c/wk	3 c/wk
Orange	1.5 c/wk	2 c/wk	2 c/wk	2 c/wk	2 c/wk	2.5 c/wk	2.5 c/wk
Dry beans/peas	2.5 c/wk	3 c/wk	3 c/wk	3 c/wk	3 c/wk	3.5 c/wk	3.5 c/wk
Starchy	2.5 c/wk	3 c/wk	3 c/wk	6 c/wk	7 c/wk	7 c/wk	7 c/wk
Other	5.5 c/wk	3	6.5 c/wk	7 c/wk	7 c/wk	8.5 c/wk	8.5 c/wk
Grains	5 oz-eq	6 oz-eq	6 oz-eq	7 oz-eq	8 oz-eq	9 oz-eq	10 oz-eq
Whole	3	3	3	3.5	4	4.5	5
Other	2	3	3	3.5	4	4.5	5
Meat, poultry, fish, dry beans, eggs, nuts, and seeds	5 oz-eq	5 oz-eq	5.5 oz-eq	6 oz-eq	6.5 oz-eq	6.5 oz-eq	7 oz-eq
Milk, yogurt, and cheese	3 c	3 c	3 c	3 c	3 c	3 c	3 c
Oils	20 g	22 g	24 g	26 g	27 g	30 g	34 g
Discretionary calorie allowance*	132	195	267	290	362	410	426

Note: Food group amounts are shown in cups (c), cups per week (c/wk), and ounce-equivalents (oz-eq). Where it applies, the number of servings (srv) is in parentheses. Oils are shown in grams (g).

* This number shows calories that can be eaten in addition to the amounts of nutrient-dense foods in each group. Solid fats and added sugars are counted here.

Grains are divided into whole grains and refined grains. Whole grains, such as whole-wheat flour and oatmeal, contain the entire grain kernel. Refined grains have been milled, causing parts of the grain to be removed. This gives them a finer texture and slows down the rate at which they spoil. However, refining also removes fiber, iron, and some vitamins. Examples of refined grain products include white bread and white rice. Most refined grains are enriched. This means that some vitamins and iron have been added back into them. However, they are still missing the fiber and some of the vitamins of whole grains. Because whole grains are more nutritious than refined grains, it is recommended that at least half of the grains eaten be whole grains.

Meat and Bean Group

All foods made from meat, poultry, fish, dry beans or peas, eggs, nuts and seeds are considered part of the Meat and Bean Group. Include more fish, nuts and seeds, which contain healthy oils, than meat and poultry. Dry beans and peas are part of the Meat and Bean Group as well as the Vegetable Group. When you choose meat and poultry, choose lean or low-fat cuts.

Milk Group

The Milk Group is made up of all liquid milk products and many of the foods made from milk. Foods made from milk that retain little or no calcium, like cream cheese, cream, and butter, are not part of the group. Foods that retain their calcium, like yogurt and many hard cheeses, are part of the group. Yogurt is particularly good because it contains healthful bacteria in addition to the benefits of milk. Most of your choices from the milk group should be fat-free or lowfat.

Oils Category

Oils are fats that are liquid at room temperature. MyPyramid recommends choosing oils over solid fats. Solid fats are not recommended because they are higher in saturated fat and may be by hydrogenated. Oils that come from plants are preferred because they are low in saturated fats. Also, because they come from plant sources, they have no cholesterol.

Nutrient Density

MyPyramid recommends foods that are nutrient dense. **Nutrient density** is the relationship between nutrients and calories in a food. Foods with low nutrient density are low in nutrients, but high in calories from fat and added sugars. For example, a candy bar has over 200 calories from fat and sugar but hardly any vitamins, minerals, or phytochemicals.

Foods with high nutrient density offer more nutrients for fewer calories. Nutrient-dense foods are also low in fat and added sugars. For example, a slice of whole-grain bread has only about 100 calories but is rich in complex carbohydrates, B vitamins, and fiber.

Adding fat or sugar to nutrient-dense foods makes them less nutrient dense. For example, spreading a tablespoon of butter on that slice of whole-grain bread doubles its calories.

How Many Calories Do You Need?

People have different needs for calories and nutrients depending on their age, gender, body size, and activity level. In general, the more active you are, the more you can eat. Women who are pregnant and breast-feeding may also need more calories. If you want to gain or lose weight, you have to adjust your calories, too.

Active You are active if you do **moderate** or heavy physical activity for at least 60 minutes each day. A very active teen male may need 3,000 calories or more each day. An active teen female may need around 2,500 or more calories a day.

Moderately Active You are moderately active if you do moderate or heavy physical activity for 30 to 60 minutes each day. A moderately active teen male may need around 2,700 calories a day. A moderately active teen female may need around 2,000 calories a day.

Sedentary You are sedentary if you do less than 30 minutes of moderate or heavy physical activity each day. A sedentary teen male may need around 2,400 calories a day. A sedentary teen female may need around 1,800 calories per day.

Figure 10.4 How Much Is a Cup? How Much Is an Ounce?

Do the Math Thinking of foods in terms of ounces and cups can help you to make smart food choices. *How many nuts equal three ounces?*

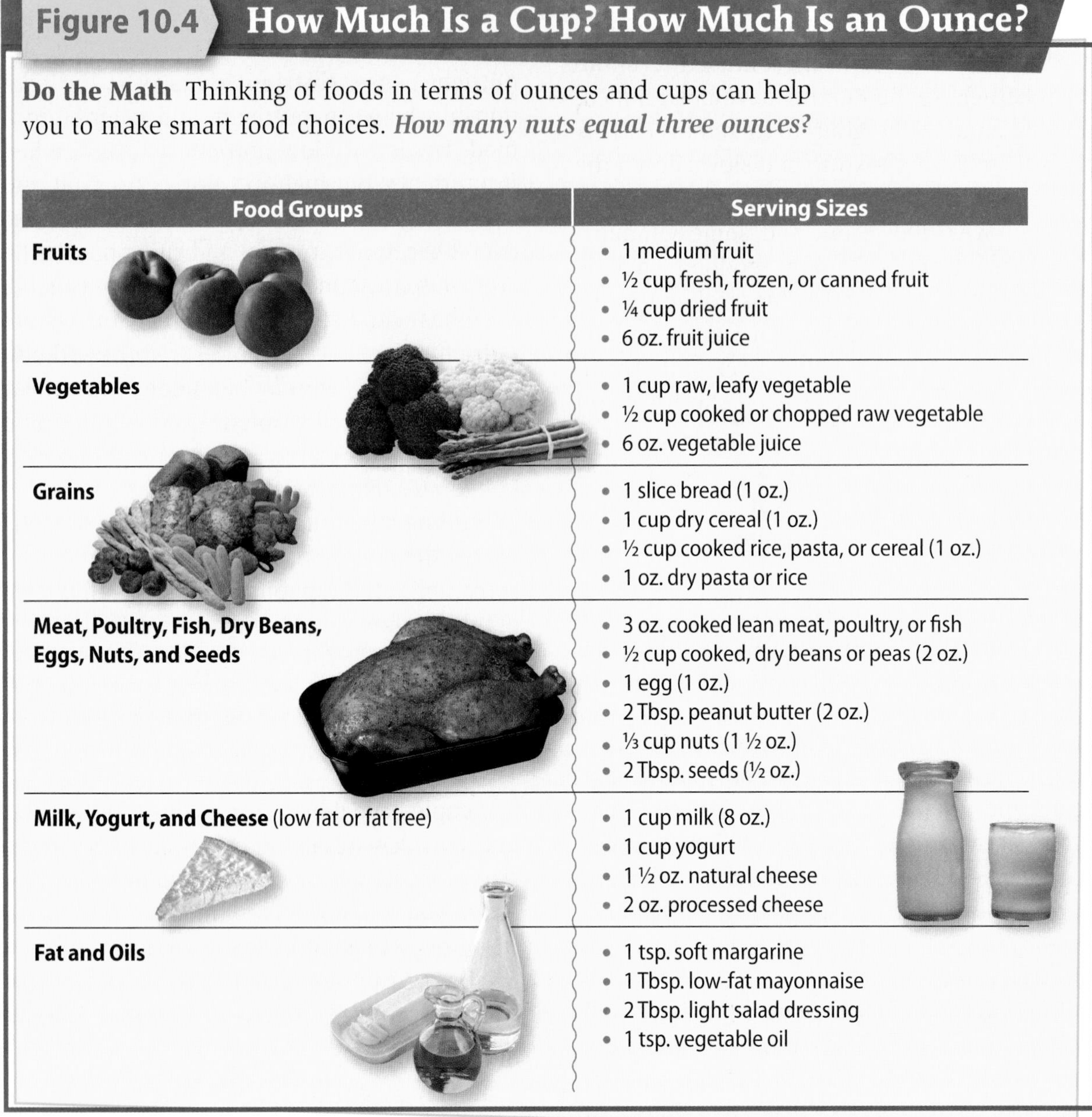

Food Groups	Serving Sizes
Fruits	• 1 medium fruit • ½ cup fresh, frozen, or canned fruit • ¼ cup dried fruit • 6 oz. fruit juice
Vegetables	• 1 cup raw, leafy vegetable • ½ cup cooked or chopped raw vegetable • 6 oz. vegetable juice
Grains	• 1 slice bread (1 oz.) • 1 cup dry cereal (1 oz.) • ½ cup cooked rice, pasta, or cereal (1 oz.) • 1 oz. dry pasta or rice
Meat, Poultry, Fish, Dry Beans, Eggs, Nuts, and Seeds	• 3 oz. cooked lean meat, poultry, or fish • ½ cup cooked, dry beans or peas (2 oz.) • 1 egg (1 oz.) • 2 Tbsp. peanut butter (2 oz.) • ⅓ cup nuts (1 ½ oz.) • 2 Tbsp. seeds (½ oz.)
Milk, Yogurt, and Cheese (low fat or fat free)	• 1 cup milk (8 oz.) • 1 cup yogurt • 1 ½ oz. natural cheese • 2 oz. processed cheese
Fat and Oils	• 1 tsp. soft margarine • 1 Tbsp. low-fat mayonnaise • 2 Tbsp. light salad dressing • 1 tsp. vegetable oil

Recommended Serving Sizes

Visit the MyPyramid Web site at **www.MyPyramid.gov** to calculate how many calories you need on most days. Once you know how many calories you need each day, you can plan your food choices. Use **Figure 10.3** on page 136 to figure your daily food intake. Find the column with your calorie level. That column shows how much you should eat from each food group. For example, if you need to eat 2,200 calories a day, you should choose 2 cups of fruit and 7 ounces of grains.

MyPyramid lists daily amounts of grains, meat, and beans in ounces, and it lists daily amounts of fruits, vegetables, and milk in cups. **Figure 10.4** and **Figure 10.5** show how much food counts as an ounce or a cup. For example, a large orange equals one cup of fruit, and a slice of toast equals one ounce of grains.

Mixed foods include foods from two or more groups. For example, tacos have food from the grains group (taco shell), meat & beans group (meat or bean filling), milk group (cheese), and vegetable group (lettuce and tomatoes).

Figure 10.5 How Much Do You Eat?

Know Your Portions These common objects can help you get to know the size of common measures, such as ½ cup, one cup, or one ounce. The column on the right shows the amount of food needed for a 2,000 calorie diet. ***How do these common objects compare to your usual portion sizes?***

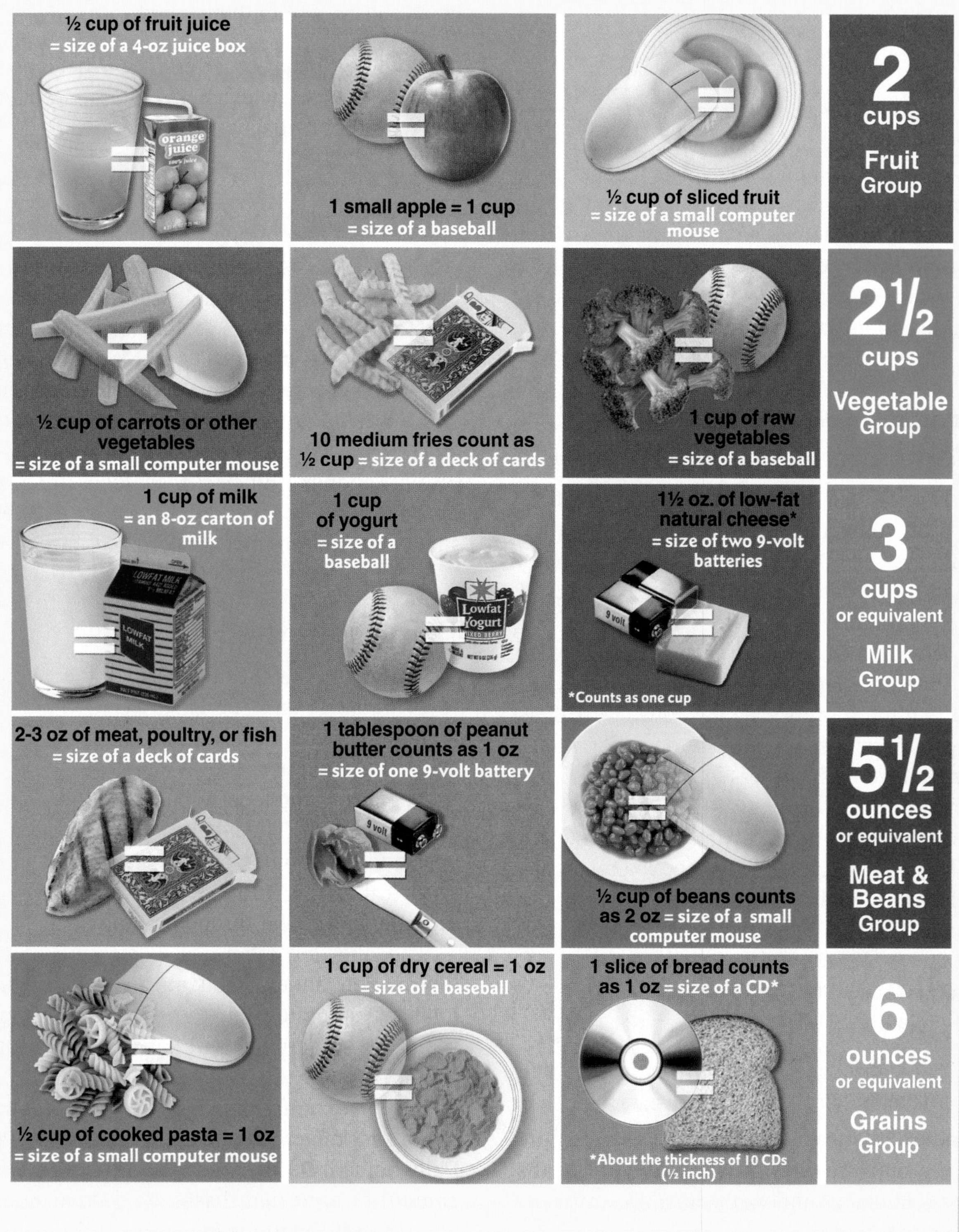

Portion Sizes

Portion sizes have increased dramatically in recent years. Today's bananas and apples are much more than one cup. A bagel can contain as many calories as five slices of bread. A half-pound burger is nearly three standard portions.

It is easy to eat too much and gain weight. An extra 100 calories a day without added exercise can increase your weight by 10 pounds in a year.

At home, measure a recommended serving size of food and put it on a plate. Make a mental note of how much of the plate it covers. You can also compare the size of the food to the size of a familiar object, such as your palm, your fingertip, or a deck of cards. **Figure 10.5** on page 139 shows some common objects you can use to measure portions.

Tracking What You Eat and How Much You Eat

Do you eat the right amount? Keep track of what you eat from each food group for several days. Add up the totals. Then compare the totals to the amounts shown in Figure 10.3. Are you on target?

If you need to make changes, be specific and realistic. For example, you might say, "I'll eat two more fruits each day, one at breakfast and one for a snack." Make one change at a time. Move from success to success.

According to a recent study, keeping a log of what you eat makes you twice as likely to adhere to a diet. Keeping a food log might also help you to make better food choices.

Building Healthy Eating Habits

Three principles of healthy eating can help you develop healthy food habits.

Aim for Balance Choose foods from all of the food groups. Each group has nutrient strengths. If you miss a group on one day, you can make it up on the next.

Choose Variety Even within a food group, different foods have different nutrients. Eat many different foods in each group. Eat small amounts of many different foods rather than large amounts of a few favorites.

Eat in Moderation Include all types of foods, but in reasonable amounts. There are no "good" and "bad" foods. You can eat foods with fat and added sugars, but in moderation.

✓ **Reading Check** **Identify** What is an example of a food with a high nutrient density and why does it qualify as nutrient dense?

Nutrition Facts Panel

The Dietary Guidelines for Americans and MyPyramid are two reliable nutrition sources. A third reliable source is the Nutrition Facts panel. A **Nutrition Facts panel** is a label with easy-to-read information about the calories and nutrients of foods sold in containers. The federal Nutrition Labeling and Education Act of 1990 requires all packaged foods to have Nutrition Facts panels. Nutrition Facts panels show information in a standardized format.

What's on the Panel?

The top of the Nutrition Facts panel shows "Serving Size" and "Servings Per Container." A container with 3 servings of ½ cup each has 1½ in the container.

The rest of the label is based on the single-serving amount. The label shows total calories per serving, number of calories from fat per serving. Use this information to keep track of the calories you eat throughout the day.

The nutrition label also gives per-serving information about some nutrients. Look for total fat, saturated fat, trans fat, cholesterol, sodium, total carbohydrates, dietary fiber, sugars, and protein.

For most nutrients and for certain vitamins and minerals, the label also lists "% Daily Value." **Daily Value** (DV) is the needed amount of a nutrient based on current nutrition recommendations for a 2,000-calorie diet.

Nutrition Facts

Serving Size 3/4 cup (50g)
Servings Per Container 30

Amount Per Serving	
Calories 200	Calories from Fat **35**
	% Daily Value*
Total Fat 3.5g	**6%**
Saturated Fat 0.5g	**3%**
Trans Fat 0g	
Polyunsaturated Fat 2g	
Monounsaturated Fat 1g	
Cholesterol 0mg	**0%**
Sodium 65mg	**13%**
Total Carbohydrate 37g	**12%**
Dietary Fiber 6g	**22%**
Soluble Fiber less than 1g	
Insoluble Fiber 2g	
Sugars 9g	
Protein 6g	**12%**

Vitamin A	0%	• Vitamin C	60%
Calcium	4%	• Iron	15%
Thiamin	20%	• Riboflavin	15%
Niacin	20%	• Vitamin B6	20%
Folate	20%	• Vitamin B12	15%

* Percent Daily Values are based on a 2,000 calorie diet. Your daily values may be higher or lower depending on your calorie needs:

	Calories	2,000	2,500
Total Fat	Less than	65g	80g
Sat Fat	Less than	20g	25g
Cholesterol	Less than	300mg	300mg
Sodium	Less than	2,400mg	2,400mg
Total Carbohydrate		300g	375g
Dietary Fiber		25g	30g
Protein		50g	65g

Just the Facts

Nutrition Facts panels show what nutrients are in a food and how much of each nutrient the food contains. *How much of the Daily Value for protein does this food contain? How much for fiber?*

Using the Panel

The Nutrition Facts panel and other resources can help you evaluate your nutrient intake.

When you eat from packages that have more than one serving, adjust the informaton on the label to the amount you really eat. Suppose the label on a jar of vegetable juice lists 50 calories and 1 gram of protein per 8-ounce serving. If you drink 12 ounces (1½ servings) you are taking in 75 calories and 1.5 grams of protein.

The serving size on a label may differ from the recommended portion in MyPyramid. A label on a six-ounce juice can may say that it has one serving, even though MyPyramid says that 8 ounces is a typical portion.

✓ **Reading Check** **Define** What is Daily Value?

Dietary Supplements

Dietary supplements such as vitamin tablets are not good replacements for real food. A **dietary supplement** is a nutrient substance taken to supplement, or add to, nutrients in the food you eat. Common dietary supplements include vitamins, minerals, amino acids, and herbals. They are available as tablets, capsules, liquids, and powders.

Dietary supplements may be useful for some people. They are sometimes helpful for people taking certain types of medication, for pregnant and nursing women, for people recovering from illness, and for infants, the elderly, and people with special nutrition needs.

Most people do not need supplements, because they can get all the nutrients they need through a balanced diet. Supplements lack the great variety of compounds in foods. No one should eat a poor diet and then rely on supplements to fix the problem.

Nutrient Megadoses

Some people take megadoses (ˈme-gə-ˌdōs-əs) of dietary supplements. A megadose is a very large amount of a supplement. Such supplements are sometimes called high-potency.

Use caution with vitamin supplements. Excess amounts of some nutrients can accumulate in the body and cause harm. The water-soluble vitamins that are not stored simply pass out of the body unused. Fat-soluble vitamins are stored in your body, so they can build up to dangerous levels. If a health professional advises you to take supplements, avoid megadoses. They could be harmful to your health.

Herbals

A plant used for medicinal purposes is called an **herbal**. Many herbals have been used for centuries. Aloe is used for lotions to keep skin moist. Many modern medicines are made from plants. One is digitalis (ˌdi-jə-ˈta-ləs), which is used to treat heart failure.

Some herbal products are safe and effective. Other herbals may be poisonous or may interfere with medications. Still other herbals are ineffective. Few long-term studies have been done to determine the safety of herbals.

TECHNOLOGY FOR TOMORROW

Nutrition Analysis Software

What if your computer could tell you whether all the food you ate yesterday fulfilled your daily need for vitamin C? What if it could tell you whether you are eating enough calories? To make nutrition analysis easier, computer software developers have put nutrient data into programs that do the work for you. You enter information about your physical condition, including age, height, weight, gender, and activity level. Then, the program creates your nutrition needs profile. When you enter a type of food and serving size, the program computes the major nutrients and calories provided, both as a figure and a percentage of your daily needs.

Investigate Could you use nutrition analysis software to determine the percentage of your recommended DV (Daily Value) for protein that your breakfast provided? How?

NCSS VIII B Science, Technology, and Society Make judgments about how science and technology have transformed the physical world and human society.

Buying Dietary Supplements

Check with a reliable health professional before taking any supplement, If you need to buy supplements, read the "Supplement Facts" label on the container. It shows the serving size, number of servings, and the amount of each ingredient. Look for the expiration date as well.

Health experts recommend that people avoid supplements with more than 100 percent of the DV. Never take a supplement that has ingredients you do not understand.

✓ **Reading Check** **True or False**
Herbals are always safe to use because they are natural.

Separating Fact from Fiction

Information about nutrition is everywhere—television, radio, magazines, books, the Internet. Advertisements promote supplements. Web sites offer health advice. Television news reports findings of nutrition studies. How do you know what to believe? To separate fact from fiction, learn about different types of food information and how to evaluate them.

Food Myths

A food myth is a mistaken belief about food. For example, some people say that brown eggs are more nutritious than white eggs. In fact, the color of the shell depends on the breed of hen. Shell color has no effect on nutrition. Another common myth claims that sea salt is more nutritious than regular salt. In truth, both have the same amount of sodium chloride, but table salt comes from salt mines and sea salt comes from evaporated seawater. Sea salt has a few minerals found in the ocean, but not enough to make a difference.

Advertising

The purpose of advertising is to sell. Food ads usually emphasize the pleasure of eating. The nutrition information in ads is often missing or misleading.

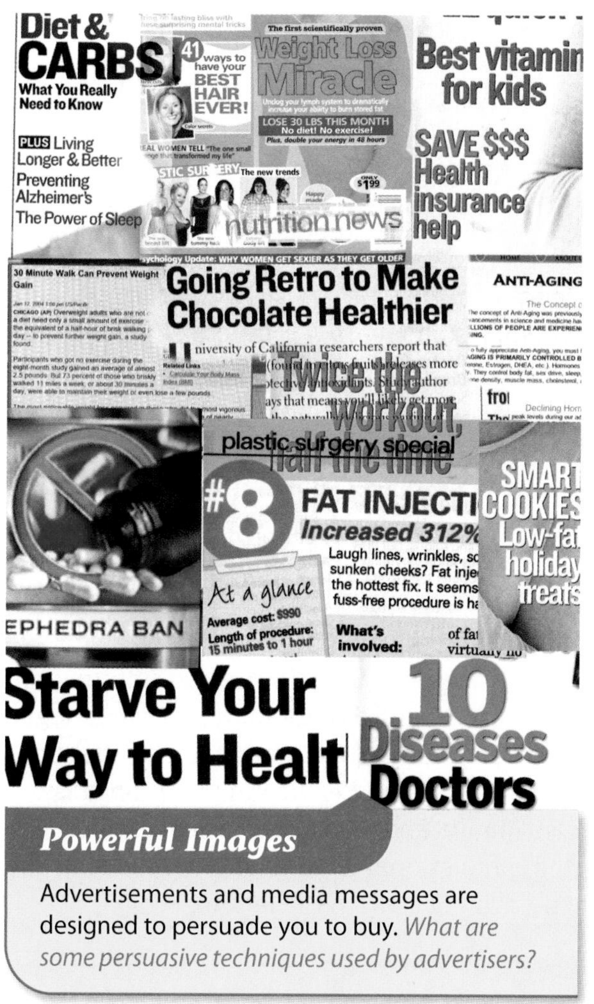

Powerful Images

Advertisements and media messages are designed to persuade you to buy. *What are some persuasive techniques used by advertisers?*

Companies use many techniques to promote products. Food companies pay to have their products shown in movies. Coupons and store displays encourage you to buy. Even product packages are a form of advertising.

Advertisers try to convince you to buy through strategies like these:

Limited Information Advertisements give only the facts that encourage you to buy. A snack food is praised for its flavor and crispiness, but nothing is said about the high amount of fat.

Positive Images Some advertisers use positive images, such as attractiveness and social status, to convince you that their product will make you feel or look better. You associate positive images and feelings with the product, which makes you more likely to buy it.

Celebrity Endorsement Some ads show popular performers or athletes promoting a product. The endorsement may not mean that the product is worth buying.

Scare Tactics Advertisers sometimes play on people's fears of aging or disease. They claim or imply that their products can prevent or relieve problems.

Studies Advertisers sometimes use findings from nutrition studies to support product claims. Such ads rarely tell you who funded the study. Studies are often biased in favor of the organization funding the study.

Infomercials These ads look like regular consumer programs on television or ordinary stories in a magazine or newspaper. These ads can trick you into believing that you are getting unbiased information. However, these are just commercials paid for by advertisers.

False Claims Be alert for statements that sound unrealistic. "Fast results guaranteed!" "Eat all the desserts you want and still lose weight!" Look out for claims that sound too good to be true.

The Internet

The Internet is a great information source. However, some Web sites have incorrect, even deceptive, information. Check who runs a Web site before you believe what you read. Is it a reliable organization, such as the Mayo Clinic or the National Institutes of Health? Or is it a company that is trying to sell something?

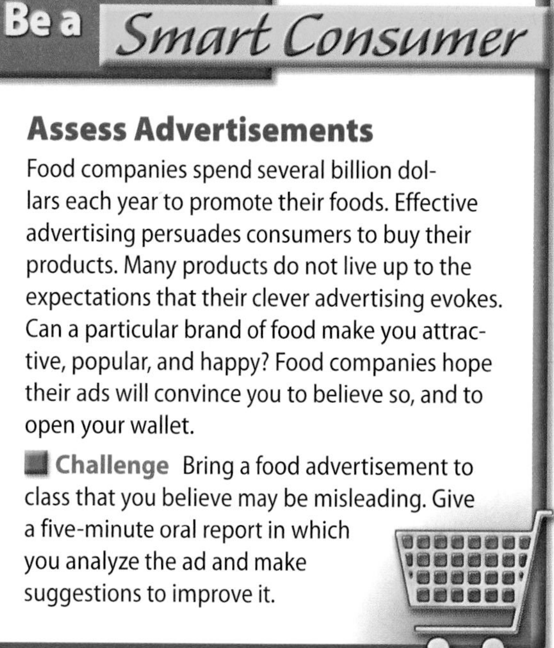

Be a Smart Consumer

Assess Advertisements

Food companies spend several billion dollars each year to promote their foods. Effective advertising persuades consumers to buy their products. Many products do not live up to the expectations that their clever advertising evokes. Can a particular brand of food make you attractive, popular, and happy? Food companies hope their ads will convince you to believe so, and to open your wallet.

Challenge Bring a food advertisement to class that you believe may be misleading. Give a five-minute oral report in which you analyze the ad and make suggestions to improve it.

Nutrition Fraud

Fraud occurs when people gain something of value, often money, by deceiving others.

Fraudulent nutrition and health claims often appear in advertising and on the Internet. For example, people may promote a useless supplement or an ineffective cure. To stop fraud, you can file a complaint with the Food and Drug Administration (FDA) or the Federal Trade Commission (FTC).

Evaluating Information

Evaluating information is a skill that you can learn with practice. This skill can save you time and money and help you avoid harm. Use these steps to evaluate information:

Look for the source. When you hear or read a health claim, find the source of the information. Is the source trustworthy? Most food producers have a toll-free number for their consumer service department, or you can contact them on their Web site.

Identify Web sites. Beware of nutrition information on Web sites operated by companies. Be skeptical if a claim seems too good to be true. Conduct your own research to verify or disprove it. Look for sites operated by governments, universities, and hospitals and other health organizations.

Read carefully. As you read, ask yourself whether statements are opinions or are facts backed by science and research. Check dates to find current information. Read more than one reliable source of information.

Identify funding. Companies and industries fund many scientific research studies. Some studies omit findings that do not support the funder's objectives. Sometimes this funding influences the results.

Choose experts. When you need information, go to an expert. Expert sources include registered dietitians (RDs) and licensed dietitians (LDs), nutritionists, health care professionals, family and consumer sciences teachers, and professional organizations, such as the American Dietetic Association.

Light and Healthy Recipe

Fruit and Nut Oatmeal

Ingredients

- **3 cups** Water
- **1½ cups** Quick rolled oats
- **1 cup** Raisins
- **¼ cup** Chopped walnuts
- **2 Tbsp.** Brown sugar

Directions

1. Pour the water into a pot and begin heating it.
2. While you wait for the water to boil, blend the oats, raisins, walnuts and sugar in a mixing bowl.
3. When the water boils, carefully add the mixture to the pot. Cook the oatmeal, stirring constantly, for one minute.
4. Turn off the heat and let the mixture sit 1–3 minutes.
5. Serve in bowls.

Oats and raisins are nutrient-dense foods. Raisins are high in fiber, folate and calcium.

Yield 4 servings

Nutrition Analysis per Serving

■ Calories	322
■ Total fat	7 g
Saturated fat	1 g
Cholesterol	0 mg
■ Sodium	12 mg
■ Carbohydrate	62 g
Dietary fiber	5 g
Sugars	32
■ Protein	7 g

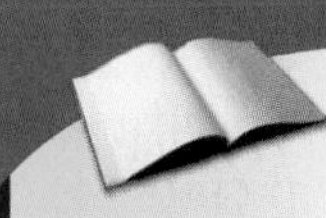

After You Read

Chapter Summary

People need reliable sources of information to make smart dietary choices. Dietary Guidelines for Americans is a source of science-based advice on nutrition and fitness. MyPyramid is a guidance system that categorizes foods into groups. Nutrition Facts panels are labels with information about the calories and nutrients and Daily Values of foods sold in containers. Dietary supplements can be useful additions to a healthful diet for some people. It is important to separate fact from fiction when making choices about diet and nutrition.

Content and Academic Vocabulary Review

1. Write each of the content and academic vocabulary terms on an index card. Write the definition for each term on another index card. Then work with a partner to match each term to its definition.

Content Vocabulary

- nutrient density (p. 137)
- Nutrition Facts panel (p. 140)
- Daily Value (p. 140)
- dietary supplement (p. 141)
- herbal (p. 142)
- fraud (p. 144)

Academic Vocabulary

- reliable (p. 134)
- moderate (p. 137)

Review Key Concepts

2. **Explain** the Dietary Guidelines for Americans.
3. **Describe** MyPyramid and its recommendations.
4. **Describe** a Nutrition Facts panel, its contents, and how to use it.
5. **Explain** dietary supplements, their different forms, their pros and cons.
6. **Discuss** the importance of separating nutrition facts from fiction.

Critical Thinking

7. **Compare and contrast** various ways to determine appropriate portion sizes.
8. **Determine** what Annie is forgetting about the Nutrition Facts label on the large package of her favorite snack. She eats the whole package of crackers, saying, "Only 100 calories—great!"
9. **Evaluate** this scenario. Lena's doctor has prescribed a medication for a minor health problem. In addition, Lena plans to use an herbal remedy. She says, "It will not do any harm because it is all-natural." Do you agree? Why or why not?
10. **Evaluate** this television ad: A famous and fit athlete says that a certain supplement improves her strength and endurance. What criticisms, if any, would you have of such an ad?

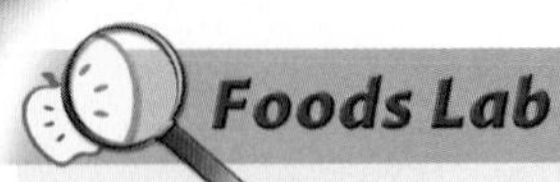

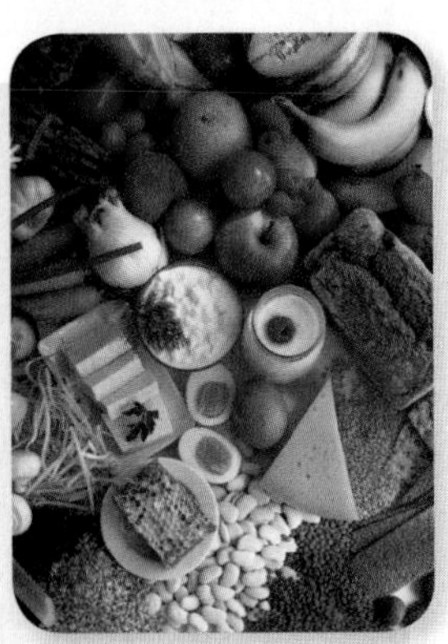

11. Food Group Combo MyPyramid encourages a daily diet that combines foods from all the groups and limits fats and sugars. Can you follow this recommendation in just one meal?

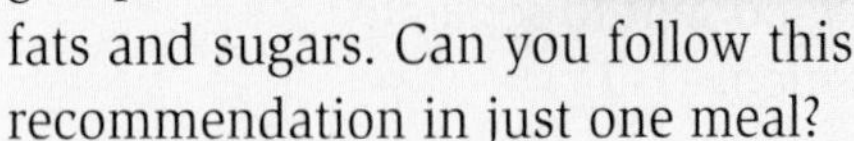

Procedure Create a dish, such as a sandwich or salad, that combines foods from all the MyPyramid groups. Use two grain servings as a base, adding other foods from each group. Consider appeal and nutrition.

Analysis Write a one-page report summarizing the specific nutrients in each food you chose, how you limited fats and sugars in choosing foods, and how you would improve this recipe.

HEALTHFUL CHOICES

12. Smart Sweetening Jackson is preparing an oatmeal cookie recipe. The recipe provides two options for sweetening the cookie batter: fruit juice or brown sugar. If Jackson wants to follow the recommendations of MyPyramid, which sweetening option should he choose and why? What are the consequences of choosing not to follow the MyPyramid recommendations?

TECH Connection

13. Web Assessment Under your teacher's supervision, use the Internet to find a Web site that is devoted to a particular dietary supplement. Use the suggestions for evaluating information that are presented in this chapter. Look for the techniques listed in the chapter and note their use on the site you are evaluating. Write a one-page report analyzing the reliability of the information and your opinion on whether the site can be trusted.

Real-World Skills

Problem-Solving Skills

14. A MyPyramid-Friendly Menu Using the MyPyramid dietary recommendations, analyze a restaurant menu. Would the food choices on the menu allow people to follow MyPyramid's recommendations? Why or why not? How could you alter the food items to better follow the recommendations?

Interpersonal and Collaborative Skills

15. Advertising Analysis Work together to find seven advertisements. Each should illustrate one of the seven tactics used in food and nutrition advertising. Label and write a one-paragraph analysis of each advertisement. Compile the advertisements and your analyses of them in a booklet to educate consumers about misleading advertising.

Financial Literacy Skills

16. Actual Serving Size Find the amount of servings in a box of cereal to calculate the cost per serving. Then pour the amount you typically eat into a bowl. Measure and record the amount. Then pour the recommended serving size. Measure and record that amount. Compare the two amounts. What is the actual serving size and cost per serving for you?

Academic Skills

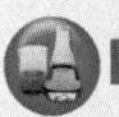

Food Science

17. Comparing Nutrition Different kinds of a certain product can have different levels of nutrition. A bowl of one kind of cereal might have more protein and fiber than another.

Procedure Obtain Nutrition Facts labels from two similar, but different foods. You might use two different types of breakfast cereal or two different kinds of canned tomato soup. Make a chart listing the amounts of calories, fat, cholesterol, sodium, dietary fiber, sugars and protein in each of the two foods.

Analysis When you have completed your chart, write a paragraph explaining which of the two foods is the more nutritious choice and why you believe this is the case. Use the data you have collected to support your analysis.

NSES A Develop understandings about scientific inquiry.

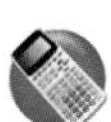

Mathematics

18. Evaluate Survey Data Infomercials are long commercials that look like informational shows on television. Of 191 infomercials broadcast during one month, 73 sold a weight-loss or health care product. What percent of infomercials does this represent?

Math Concept **Percents** A fraction can be expressed as a percent by first converting the fraction to a decimal and then converting the decimal to a percent by moving the decimal point two places to the right.

Starting Hint Set up a ratio, with the number of health care infomercials as the numerator and the total number of infomercials as the denominator.

NCTM Number and Operations Understand numbers, ways of representing numbers, relationships among numbers, and number systems.

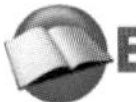

English Language Arts

19. Role Play Imagine you are an advertising copywriter in charge of promoting vegetables. Write an advertisement that encourages teens to buy and eat vegetables in season. Be sure to make all the relevant points about the savings consumers can get by buying what is in season.

NCTE 12 Use language to accomplish individual purposes.

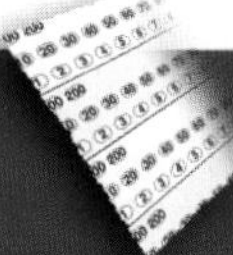

STANDARDIZED TEST PRACTICE

READING COMPREHENSION

Re-read the section about portion sizes on page 140. Then read the question and select the best answer:

20. Why do increased portion sizes contribute to weight gain?

a. An extra 10 calories a day without added exercise can increase your weight by 100 pounds in a year.

b. One of today's large slices of bread can contain as many calories as a bagel.

c. An extra 100 calories a day without added exercise can increase your weight by 10 pounds in a year.

d. An average burger today is twice as large as an average burger 20 years ago.

Test-Taking Tip Closely read the text to which the question refers. Then read the question and each of the answer choices. Re-read the text to confirm which answer is correct. Some answers may seem identical, but they contain subtle differences. Pay attention to every word.

CHAPTER 11

Keeping a Healthy Weight

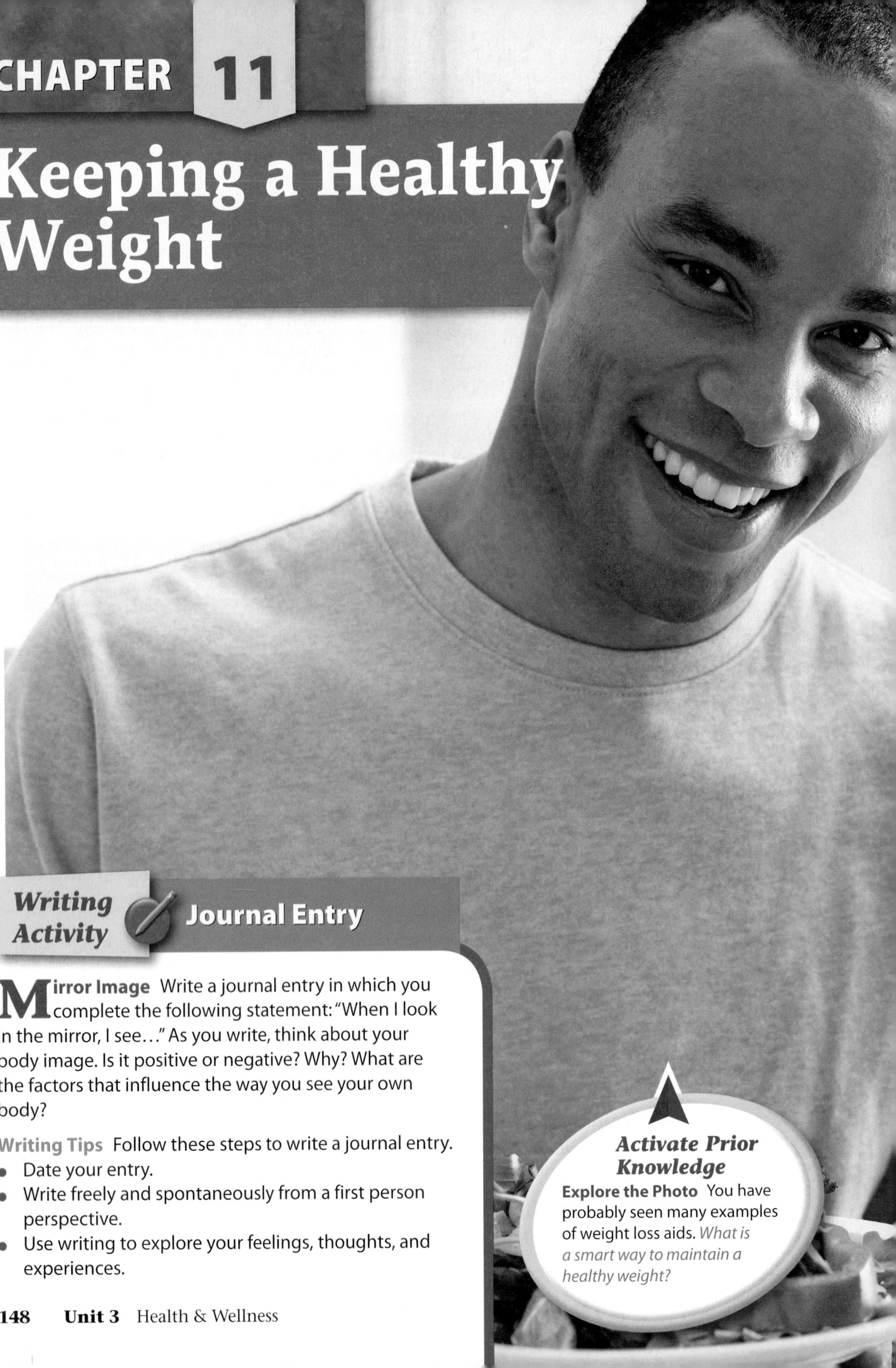

Writing Activity — Journal Entry

Mirror Image Write a journal entry in which you complete the following statement: "When I look in the mirror, I see…" As you write, think about your body image. Is it positive or negative? Why? What are the factors that influence the way you see your own body?

Writing Tips Follow these steps to write a journal entry.

- Date your entry.
- Write freely and spontaneously from a first person perspective.
- Use writing to explore your feelings, thoughts, and experiences.

Activate Prior Knowledge

Explore the Photo You have probably seen many examples of weight loss aids. *What is a smart way to maintain a healthy weight?*

Reading Guide

Before You Read

Preview Before you read, write down what you think an ideal body is for a person of your gender. As you read, make notes about why ideal body myths are problematic.

Read to Learn

Key Concepts

- **Explain** why the ideal body myth is problematic.
- **Discuss** reasons for and consequences of the overweight epidemic.
- **Explain** how to determine what a healthy weight is for you.
- **Describe** how to manage weight in a healthy way.

Main Idea

To keep a healthy weight, you must determine the weight that is right for you, and make smart choices to maintain it.

Content Vocabulary

You will find the definitions for these words in the glossary at the back of the book.

- ☐ Body Mass Index (BMI)
- ☐ overweight
- ☐ obese
- ☐ body fat percentage
- ☐ behavior modification
- ☐ emotional eating
- ☐ aerobic exercise
- ☐ anaerobic exercise
- ☐ fad diet

Academic Vocabulary

You will find these words in your reading and on your tests. Use the glossary to look up their definitions if necessary.

- minimize
- chronic

Graphic Organizer

Use a graphic organizer like the one below to compare aerobic and anaerobic exercise.

AEROBIC EXERCISE	ANAEROBIC EXERCISE

Graphic Organizer Go to this book's Online Learning Center at **glencoe.com** to print out this graphic organizer.

Academic Standards

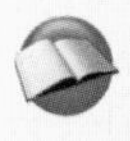

English Language Arts

NCTE 7 Conduct research and gather, evaluate, and synthesize data to communicate discoveries.

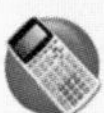

Mathematics

NCTM Algebra Represent and analyze mathematical situations and structures using algebraic symbols.

NCTM Number and Operations Compute fluently and make reasonable estimates.

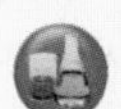

Science

NSES A Develop abilities necessary to do scientific inquiry.

NCTE *National Council of Teachers of English*
NCTM *National Council of Teachers of Mathematics*
NSES *National Science Education Standards*
NCSS *National Council for the Social Studies*

The Ideal Body Myth

Images of "ideal" bodies are everywhere in advertising and the media. In our society, the ideal female body is tall and ultra-thin, and the ideal male body is tall, slender, and muscular.

This ideal does not reflect how most people actually look. For example, most female fashion models are several inches taller than the average American woman and weigh 25 percent less. Most male models are taller and more muscular than the average American man.

Many teens and adults try to lose weight or build muscle to look more like celebrities and models. Diet cannot change a person's height or body shape. Height and overall shape are determined by genes. Genes also influence how easily a person gains or loses weight.

Ultra-thin models and celebrities often follow strict diets and workout plans. Plus, even models have flaws. Photos are altered to make these flaws invisible.

Be a Smart Consumer

Money for Muscle

While some people try to lose weight in order to look more like the "ideal," others try to build muscle. They may stick to high-protein eating plans, or spend money on protein shakes, bars, and powders. These foods and supplements do not help build muscle, and they may harm the body. Muscle size is determined by genes and exercise, not by how much protein you eat. In fact, eating extra protein can lead to increased fat, not muscle. Excess protein also stresses the kidneys and can dehydrate the body.

Challenge Name one naturally protein-rich food you could include in a well-rounded diet. What is the difference in cost between that food and a container of protein powder?

Health Risks

Many people risk their health to try to get the kind of body that they see in the media. Some people diet until they are underweight, depleting the body of muscle and fat. Muscle loss can lead to fatigue and injury to bones and joints. Without fat, the body cannot store fat-soluble nutrients. Calcium is lost. The immune system weakens. Hormones that regulate growth in teens and brain chemicals that stabilize mood may go out of balance.

✓ **Reading Check** **Identify** What factor determines height and overall shape?

The Overweight Epidemic

In industrialized nations such as the United States and Canada, overweight and obesity are serious problems. Thirty years ago, one in 20 teens was overweight. Today, one in five teens is overweight. Two-thirds of adults are overweight.

Carrying excess weight has serious consequences. It strains bones, muscles, and organs. Walking and even breathing take extra effort. Heat and humidity increase the stress, because fat traps body heat. Overweight contributes to high blood pressure, heart disease, stroke, diabetes, and certain kinds of cancer.

Why Weights Are Increasing

Why are people getting fatter? Portions are growing and access to food is becoming easier. In most places, junk food and fast food are cheaper and easier to find than healthful food. Supermarkets are packed with high-calorie, highly processed foods in giant portions. People also eat out more than in the past, and restaurant meals tend to be higher in calories, fat, and salt than home-cooked meals.

People eat more calories, but they are less active. Labor-saving devices, television, and computers encourage a sedentary lifestyle.

Some people also have a genetic tendency to gain weight easily. Maintaining a healthy weight is a challenge.

✓ **Reading Check** **List** What are three consequences of carrying excess weight?

Figure 11.4 Computing Calories

Calories In, Calories Out Weight depends on the relationship between calories taken in and calories burned. ***If energy intake and energy expenditure are out of balance, what can happen?***

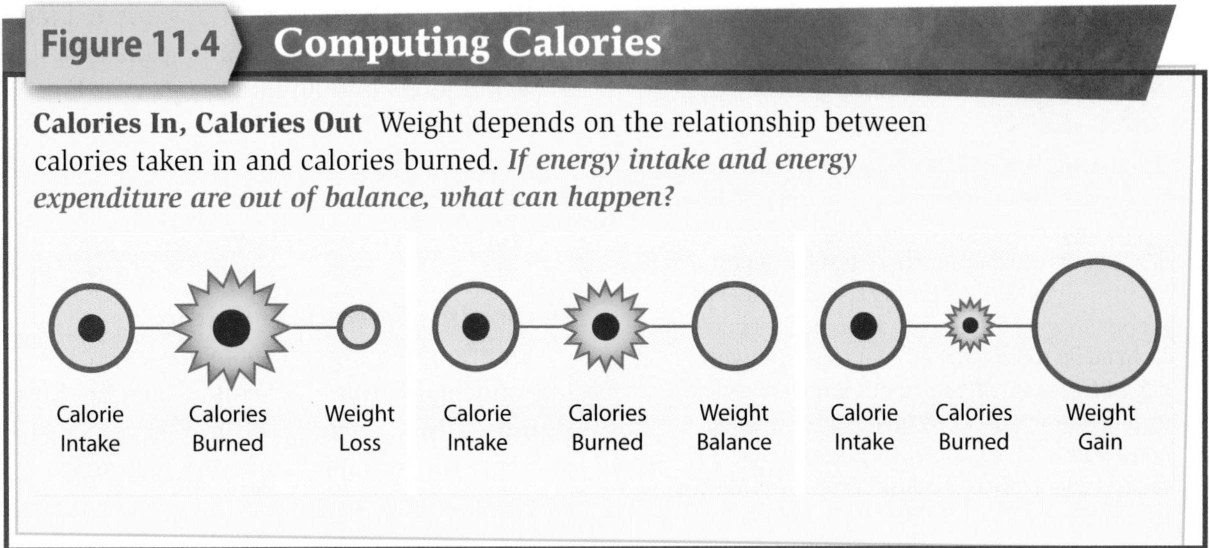

A Healthy Weight for You

Many teens grow at an uneven rate. For example, a teen may be overweight just before a growth spurt. The increase in height balances out the weight. It is normal for teen females to develop some fat stores. In this case, gaining fat does not mean getting fat.

Different parts of the body can grow at different rates. Legs may grow and gain muscle before arms do.

If you're concerned about your weight, talk to a dietitian, a nutritionist, or your health care provider. Do not compare yourself to friends or pictures in a magazine.

✓ Reading Check **Identify** What is the absolute minimum percentage of body fat a woman needs to be healthy?

Managing Weight

Achieving a healthy weight takes effort and discipline. To manage your weight, you use a budget—a calorie budget. Calories measure the energy supplied by food for life processes and physical activities. If you take in more calories than you burn, you gain weight. If you take in fewer calories than you burn, you lose weight. And if you take in the same number of calories as you burn, your weight stays the same (see **Figure 11.4**).

A Healthy Weight-Loss Plan

If you eat fewer calories than you need, your body uses its energy reserves—fat—to make up the difference. One pound of body fat equals 3,500 calories. If you eat 500 fewer calories than you need every day, you will lose one pound per week ($500 \times 7 = 3{,}500$).

The most successful way to achieve and maintain weight loss is through **behavior modification**, making gradual, permanent changes in eating and activity habits. Limiting calories and increasing activity are the two keys to lasting weight control.

See a doctor before changing your eating or exercise habits, to make sure that losing weight is necessary and safe. A physician may make a referral to a dietitian or nutritionist, who can help you find healthy ways to cut calories without neglecting nutrition.

Setting Reasonable Goals

A successful weight-loss plan has realistic goals. First, set a healthy goal weight. A health professional can help you identify a healthy weight based on your age, height, gender, and body shape.

Aim to lose weight gradually. This helps the body adjust more easily to its lower weight. Gradual weight loss also makes it likely to come from body fat and not muscle. Losing one or two pounds a week is a reasonable weight-loss goal for many people.

Kitchen Math

Counting Calories

On Tuesday, Marcus eats a 500-calorie breakfast, 750-calorie lunch, 300-calorie snack, and 1000-calorie dinner. During the day, he spends a total of 2 ½ hours walking. At school, he plays tennis for 30 minutes during P.E. After school, he spends ½ hour mowing the lawn, and another half hour cleaning his room. After an hour playing basketball with friends (which requires ½ hour of cycling to get there and back), he spends 2 hours doing homework at his computer. He burns another 350 calories doing miscellaneous activities. Will Marcus gain or lose weight that day?

Math Concept **Multi-Step Problems** When solving problems with more than one step, think through the steps before you start.

Starting Hint Add the calories Marcus consumed during meals. Use the table in Figure 11.5 to determine the calories burned by Marcus during each activity. (Note that those figures are for 30 minutes, so you will need to adjust them for longer activities.)

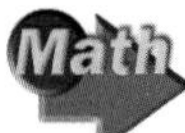

Math Appendix For math help, go to the Math Appendix at the back of the book.

NCTM Number and Operations Compute fluently and make reasonable estimates.

Changing Eating Habits

A healthy weight-loss plan focuses on developing positive eating habits that contribute to long-term health. These positive habits can help you reach and maintain a healthy weight:

- Enjoy a variety of flavors. Try many types of foods and herbs and spices.
- Focus on vegetables, fruits, whole-grain products, and dry beans. These foods are rich in nutrients and in fiber, which helps you feel full with fewer calories.
- Drink enough liquid. Drinking a glass of water before you eat decreases your appetite.
- Do not skip meals. Skipping meals can lead to overeating.
- Watch your portion sizes.
- Control emotional eating. Look for healthy alternatives such as gardening, playing sports, bicycling, or going for a walk.
- Eat moderate amounts of unsaturated fats. Minimize saturated fats and trans fats.
- Avoid foods high in fat or sugar, such as soft drinks, chips, cookies, and candy. Avoid adding sugar to foods.
- Check Nutrition Facts labels. Compare products before you buy.

Managing Emotional Eating

Emotional eating can get in the way of reaching and maintaining a healthy weight. **Emotional eating** is using food to relieve negative feelings. For example, someone may reach for chips or a chocolate bar to deal with feelings of stress, anger, loneliness, and boredom. Fatty, sugary food can provide a sense of security and comfort. However, the comfort soon fades, and the person may reach for food again.

Managing emotional eating requires identifying your triggers—the situations or feelings that lead to overeating. Find healthy ways to deal with your triggers. For example, take a short walk or call a friend.

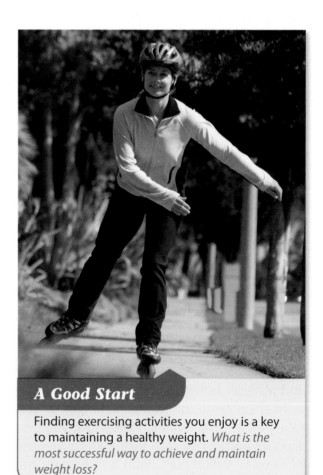

A Good Start

Finding exercising activities you enjoy is a key to maintaining a healthy weight. *What is the most successful way to achieve and maintain weight loss?*

Increasing Physical Activity

Physical activity is just as important for weight loss as cutting calories. Exercise burns calories and speeds metabolism. It also builds muscles, which burn calories than fat. Imagine that you adding activities that use 100 calories a day. This will help you shed 10 pounds in a year (100 calories × 365 days a year = 36,500 calories ÷ 3,500 = 10.4). **Figure 11.5** shows how many calories you can burn through exercise and everyday activities.

Staying active has other benefits as well. It boosts energy and builds endurance. It supports healthy bones, muscles, and joints. Regular exercise lowers cholesterol, strengthens the heart, and lowers the risk of heart disease, high blood pressure, diabetes, and some cancers.

Physical exercise also eases stress and anxiety. Active people often have a brighter outlook on life.

Types of Exercise

Any activity that uses muscles is exercise. Even active chores, such as cleaning, cooking, and washing the car, are mild exercise.

There are two basic types of exercise: aerobic exercise and anaerobic exericse. Both are necessary to health.

Aerobic exercise (ˌer-ˈō-bik) is activity that increases the heart and breathing rate for at least 20 minutes. Aerobic means "using oxygen." During aerobic exercise, the heart and lungs send more oxygen to the blood, allowing the muscles to work harder. The oxygen also helps the body metabolize fat.

Teens should aim for 60 minutes of aerobic exercise each day. Try walking, jogging, climbing stairs, bicycling, aerobic dancing, or swimming.

Anaerobic exercise (ˌa-nə-ˈrō-bik) involves short, intense bursts of activity. Anaerobic means "without oxygen." During anaerobic exercise, the muscles work hard and quickly.

Figure 11.5 Calories Used in Common Activities

Staying Active Even the most common, everyday activities can help you to burn calories and maintain a healthy weight. The calories listed here are average numbers for someone weighing 150 pounds. Heavier people burn more calories than people who weigh less. ***How many calories would you burn if you shopped for groceries for one hour?***

Activity	Calories Used in 30 Minutes
Standing in line	50
Working at a computer	50
Cooking	90
Mowing lawn with power mower	100
Auto repair	100
Playing table tennis	100
Recreational swimming	110
Walking 3 miles an hour	120
House cleaning	120

Activity	Calories Used in 30 Minutes
Food shopping with a cart	125
Cycling at 5 miles per hour	125
Vigorous dancing	150
Raking leaves	150
Rollerblading	160
Playing tennis	180
Heavy physical labor	180
Playing basketball	180
Shoveling snow	200

They burn glycogen, the form of glucose stored in the cells. Anaerobic exercise builds muscle and raises the metabolic rate.

Running a 100-meter dash is an anaerobic activity. So is resistance training, which increases muscle strength and endurance. Resistance training conditions muscles by requiring them to resist force. The greater the resistance, the stronger the muscles become. Resistance can be provided by weights, machines, or your own body weight, as in push-ups. Teens should do resistance training at least twice a week.

Enjoying the Activity Habit

If you want to become more active, start slowly. Prevent injury by learning proper technique. Even healthy people should get a medical checkup before starting an exercise plan.

Choose an activity that holds your interest and fits your lifestyle, schedule, budget, and personality. Games and sports, from bowling to rollerblading, offer chances to meet people and have fun with friends. Many people enjoy dancing, working out to music, or doing yoga or pilates. Setting achievable goals adds challenge and motivation to an exercise routine.

Short periods of exercise can be as effective as a single longer workout. Look for ways to add activity throughout the day. Take the stairs instead of the elevator. Walk places where you can. As you get more fit, you can explore new sports and ways to exercise, too.

Commercial Weight-Loss Plans

Weight loss has become big business. Weight-loss diets, weight-loss centers, and weight-loss shakes, meals, and pills make claims about quick, easy weight loss.

Many commercial weight-loss plans are fad diets. A **fad diet** is a popular weight-loss

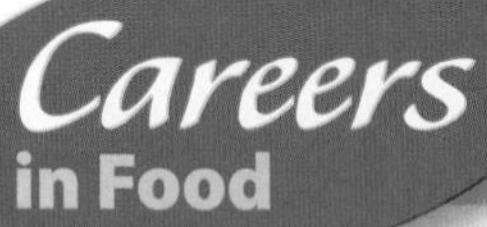

Denise Tryner
Fitness Consultant

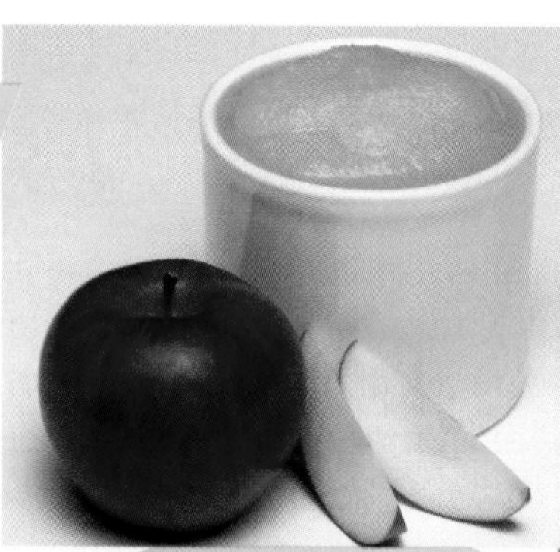

Q: What is the difference between a fitness consultant and a fitness instructor?

A: I started off as an instructor, teaching classes at a health club. A consultant covers the whole ball instead of just part of it – physical fitness, nutrition, healthy habits. So now I teach classes, do personal training one-on-one – actually groups of four or five people at a time – and nutrition counseling and coaching.

Q: What is your personal philosophy on diet and nutrition?

A: Everything in moderation. You don't have to deprive yourself in order to reach your end goal. Eat healthy, exercise every day, and anything is possible.

Q: Do you go to clients or do they come to you?

A: Both. I go to clients' offices and homes, or sometimes meet at a park. And I also have the basement of my home so they can come to me in my studio.

"Motivating someone to push his or her body to its limit is exhilarating."
— Denise Tryner
Professional Fitness
Consultant – Denver, *CO*

Education and Training

Certification in personal training and group fitness training is available through the American Council on Exercise.

Qualities and Skills

Patience, understanding, and a passion to motivate and inspire people to reach their personal goals.

Related Career Opportunities

Physical therapists also help people figure out what's going on with their bodies and help them make changes to reach their goals.

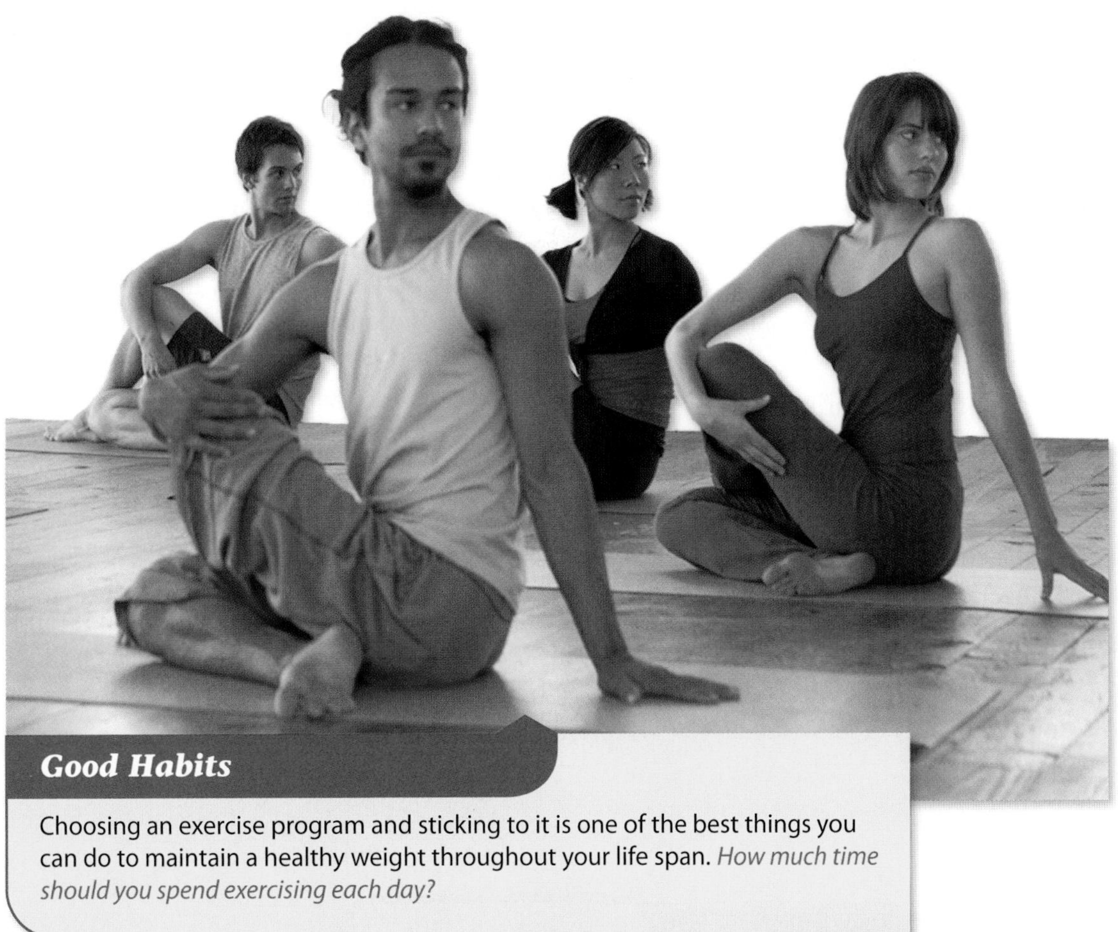

Good Habits

Choosing an exercise program and sticking to it is one of the best things you can do to maintain a healthy weight throughout your life span. *How much time should you spend exercising each day?*

method that is not based on sound nutrition principles. Fad diets often promise dramatic results—lose 10 pounds a week while you sleep, for example. Some require fasting or cutting out entire food groups. For example, some popular fad diets require you to avoid carbohydrates and eat high-fat protein foods instead.

Fad diets may lead to weight loss for a while, but they create unhealthy habits. People quickly regain the weight as dieters return to their old ways. Some people become **chronic** dieters, losing and regaining weight again and again. This is sometimes called yo-yo dieting.

Evaluating Weight-Loss Plans

How can you spot a plan that is based on sound nutrition? Test it with these questions:

- Is the program developed by a qualified health professional, such as a dietitian or nutritionist?
- Does it include nutritional counseling and an individualized eating plan?
- Does it offer a variety of appealing foods from all food groups?
- Does it supply enough nutrients?
- Does it align with the recommendations of the Dietary Guidelines for Americans and MyPyramid?
- Does it make reasonable claims?
- Does it teach healthful eating habits?

Gaining Needed Weight

Gaining weight can be just as challenging as losing weight. People who are concerned about being too thin should talk to a health professional. They may have a naturally high metabolic rate, or a medical issue.

Here are some ways for underweight people to gain weight:

- Eat three meals a day and frequent snacks. Eat snacks two to three hours before meals so you are hungry at mealtime.
- Eat the higher number of recommended servings from each of the food groups.

- Add extra calories to the food you eat. For example, add nonfat dry milk or wheat germ to puddings, pancakes, mashed potatoes, soups, stews, casseroles, vegetables, and cooked cereals. Add nuts and lowfat cheese to vegetables and salads.
- Drink fluids only between meals or at the end of the meal. Do not drink fluids just before or with a meal because they can make you feel full.
- Choose nutritious high-calorie beverages such as juice, milk, milk shakes, and smoothies.
- Stay active. Exercise can increase the appetite. Exercise also assures that the weight gained is muscle, not fat.
- Use nutrition facts labels to find nutrient dense foods with more calories.
- Avoid skipping meals.

Maintaining a Healthy Weight

Maintaining a healthy weight requires balancing energy eaten in food with energy used in physical activity. Healthy eating and exercise habits are as important for maintaining a healthy weight as they are for losing weight.

Changes in body size change your metabolism and your calorie needs. Do not be alarmed if you suddenly seem to be gaining weight. It probably means you are growing. As you grow, you will need more calories. After you lose weight, you will need fewer calories than you did before. Understanding the basics of weight maintenance is one of the keys to supplying your body with a lifetime of good nutrition. Work on developing good exercise habits. Habits you form now will help you throughout your life.

Light and Healthy Recipe

Fruit Smoothie

Ingredients

1 cup Ice cubes
1 Banana, frozen
1½ cups Strawberries (fresh or frozen)
1 cup Lowfat milk
1 cup Orange juice

Yield 4 servings

Directions

1. Put the ice cubes into a carefully cleaned blender. Add the banana and strawberries. Pour in half the milk.
2. Turn the blender on. Stop to add the rest of the milk and the orange juice in parts. Adding the liquid slowly and in stages will aid the blender if it has difficulty with the ice.
3. Serve in chilled glasses.

A lowfat smoothie can be a great dessert choice for someone trying to gain weight.

Yield 4 servings

Nutrition Analysis per Serving

■ Calories	120
■ Total fat	2 g
Saturated fat	1 g
Cholesterol	5 mg
■ Sodium	27 mg
■ Carbohydrate	25 mg
Dietary fiber	2 g
Sugars	12 g
■ Protein	3 g

CHAPTER 11 Review & Applications

After You Read

Chapter Summary

The ideal body myth does not reflect how most people look. Many people risk their health to attain the kind of body they see in the media, rather than embrace their natural overall shape and height, which are shaped by genetics. The overweight epidemic is a serious problem with many consequences and causes. To maintain a healthy weight, you should determine the weight that is right for you. Setting reasonable goals, managing emotions, and evaluating weight-loss plans are part of achieving a healthy weight. It is possible to lose, gain, and maintain weight through effort, discipline, and healthful eating and activities.

Content and Academic Vocabulary Review

1. Use each of these content and academic vocabulary words in a sentence.

Content Vocabulary

- body mass index (BMI) (p. 151)
- overweight (p. 151)
- obese (p. 151)
- body fat percentage (p. 152)
- behavior modification (p. 153)
- emotional eating (p. 154)
- aerobic exercise (p. 155)
- anaerobic exercise (p. 155)
- fad diet (p. 156)

Academic Vocabulary

- minimize (p. 151)
- chronic (p. 157)

Review Key Concepts

2. Explain why the ideal body myth is problematic.
3. Discuss reasons for and consequences of the overweight epidemic.
4. Explain how you can determine what a healthy weight is for you.
5. Describe how to manage weight in a healthy way.

Critical Thinking

6. Evaluate Lindsay's plan. Lindsay covers her bedroom walls with pages from magazines featuring tall, thin models. She says the images will motivate her to exercise. Do you think this is a good idea?

7. Determine three instant changes to culture or technology in the United States that you would make if you could to help and solve the overwieght epidemic. What would you do and why?

8. Examine Janet's complaint. Janet complains she is overweight. She is twenty-six, 5 feet 8 inches, and 152 pounds. Is she overweight? Explain.

9. Evaluate Renee's behavior. She comes home from school stressed and eats comfort foods. What are the consequences and alternatives to her behavior?

10. Examine Johnny's plans. Concerned that he is too thin, Johnny plans to increase his calorie intake by eating more healthful foods, and to decrease his activity level by ceasing to exercise.

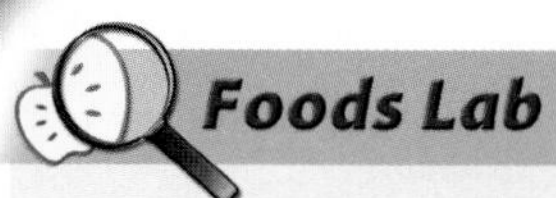

Foods Lab

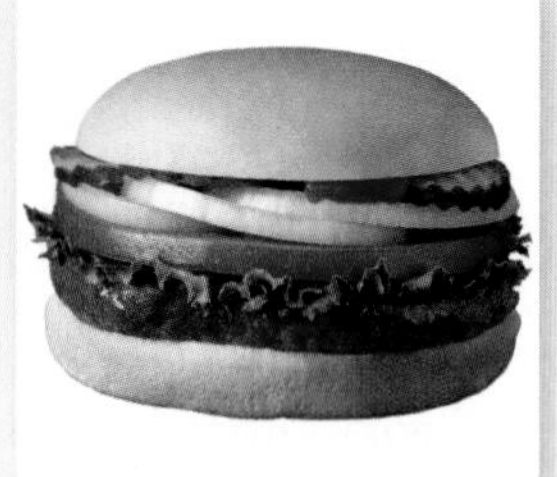

11. Weight-Friendly Snacks Snacks can be a smart way to obtain nutrients, calories, and energy between meals. Some snacks are healthier than others, especially for people who want to manage their weight.

Procedure With your team, list ten snacks for people managing their weight. The snacks should be convenient, low in fat and calories, nutritious, and tasty. Choose two snacks to prepare and sample.

Analysis Write complete responses to these questions: If someone wants to lose weight, how might snacks cause problems? How might they help? How would you rate your two snacks on fat and calorie content, nutrition, and taste?

HEALTHFUL CHOICES

12. Diet Decision Zoe wants to lose five pounds. After a few minutes searching on the Internet, she finds a diet endorsed by a celebrity who says it worked for her. The diet plan suggests eating only citrus fruits for five days. The plan is supposed to be safe and healthy, because citrus fruits are rich in vitamins and minerals. Should Zoe use this diet? Explain.

TECH Connection

13. Exercise Chart How much aerobic and anaerobic exercise should teens get in a week? Use spreadsheet or word processing software to create a one-week calendar with specific suggestions for exercise on each day. Make sure to indicate how much time should be spent on each exercise. Write a paragraph explaining why you think your plan is a good one. Also, explain what types of foods and beverages you might eat before and after exercising.

Real-World Skills

Problem-Solving Skills

14. A Solution for Stress Dean is feeling stressed and anxious. School and work are very demanding. In his free time, he tries to unwind with video games, but still feels tense and tired. What should Dean do?

Interpersonal and Collaborative Skills

15. Critique Commercial Diet Plans Work with a partner to evaluate two commercial weight-loss plans, using the criteria in this chapter. How do the plans rate? Would you recommend one, both, or neither? Suggest changes to the plans where needed that would help dieters be more successful.

Financial Literacy Skills

16. Save on Snacks Every afternoon, Hector spends $5 on a snack from his favorite fast food restaurant. He orders fries and a milkshake. Brainstorm healthier, more nutritious snacks that Hector could eat for less than $5.

Academic Skills

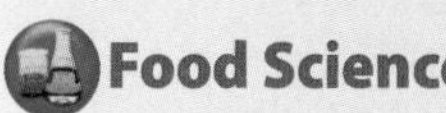

Food Science

17. Spotting Fat Fats will leave a stain on absorbent paper, while water will evaporate. Using this concept, show the fat content in different foods.

Procedure Label 6 paper lunch bags with foods to be tested: apple slice, raisins, bread, pretzels, french fries, and donut. Next rub the food item vigorously onto the paper bag, and leave it for about 10 minutes. Record your results.

Analysis Observe the stains to rank the fat content from 1-6. Use these findings to help you make choices about your diet.

NSES A Develop abilities necessary to do scientific inquiry.

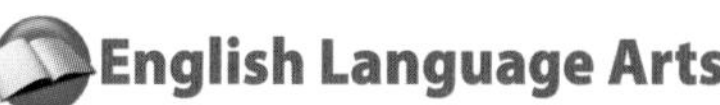

English Language Arts

19. Interview Identify a person who has been overweight and lost weight and kept the weight off. List ten questions relating to the person's diet and exercise habits, their struggles, and their secrets for success. Then interview the person, and write down their responses. In your interview, be sure to ask about particular diet plans the person used to lose weight and how those eating plans changed once the person achieved his or her desired weight. Ask the person what challenges they had to overcome to achieve their weight loss. Use your notes to write a one-page profile.

NCTE 7 Conduct research and gather, evaluate, and synthesize data to communicate discoveries.

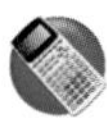

Mathematics

18. BMI Calculations Robert is a 15-year-old boy who is 62 inches tall. If Robert's BMI is 21.9, approximately how much does he weigh? Mia is a 14-year-old girl who weighs 105 pounds. If Mia's BMI is 22.7, approximately how tall is Mia in inches?

Math Concept **Solving Algebraic Equations** Use a variable to represent an unknown quantity. Rearrange the equation step by step so that the variable is on one side of the equals sign, and all other numbers are on the other.

Starting Hint For each calculation, use the formula: $(703 \times \text{weight}) \div (\text{height in inches})^2 = \text{BMI}$. Put in the two values (BMI, height, or weight) that you know, and use x to represent the third. Solve for x.

NCTM Algebra Represent and analyze mathematical situations and structures using algebraic symbols.

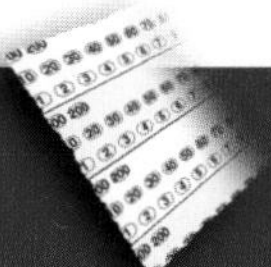

STANDARDIZED TEST PRACTICE

TRUE OR FALSE

Re-read the paragraphs about anaerobic exercise on pages 155–156. Then determine whether the statement is true or false.

20. During anaerobic exercise, muscles burn glycogen.

a. True

b. False

Test-Taking Tip Before deciding whether a statement is true or false, carefully read the text to which it relates. Then slowly review both the statement and the text again. Pay close attention to every word. One word can make the difference between a true statement and a false one.

CHAPTER 12

Health Challenges

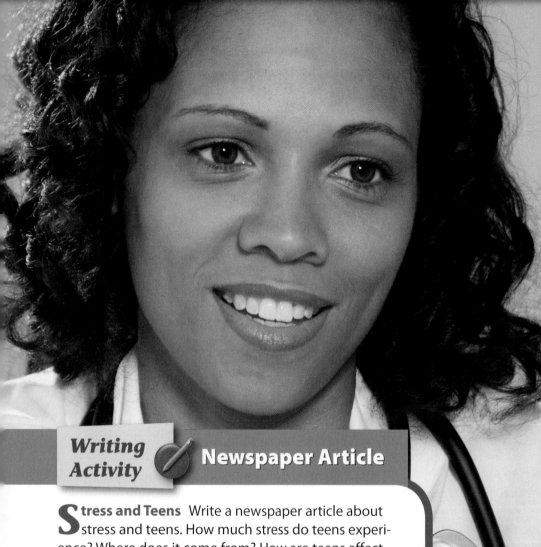

Writing Activity — Newspaper Article

Stress and Teens Write a newspaper article about stress and teens. How much stress do teens experience? Where does it come from? How are teens affected? How do they cope? Newspaper articles should inform readers of the following: who, what, where, when, why, and how. Address those questions, and proofread to eliminate grammar, spelling, and punctuation errors.

Writing Tips Follow these steps to write a newspaper article:

- Keep sentences clear, simple, and to the point.
- Focus on informing your reader.
- Explain who, what, where, when, why, and how.

Activate Prior Knowledge

Explore the Photo Many health problems can be improved by changing eating habits. *What is one health problem dietary changes can improve?*

Reading Guide

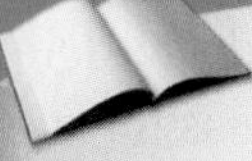

Before You Read

Preview Before you read, list three causes of stress in your life. As you read, note three smart ways that you can cope with each stressor.

Read to Learn

Key Concepts

- **Explain** stress and its relationship to nutrition.
- **Describe** the role food plays in illness and recovery.
- **Examine** how food can help to resolve or manage chronic health problems.
- **Identify** eating disorders and explain their causes and solutions.

Main Idea

Diet plays an important role in dealing with many health challenges, including stress, temporary illness, chronic problems, and eating disorders.

Content Vocabulary

You will find definitions for these words in the glossary at the back of this book.

- ☐ stress
- ☐ chronic
- ☐ diabetes
- ☐ HIV/AIDS
- ☐ food allergy
- ☐ food intolerance
- ☐ eating disorder
- ☐ anorexia nervosa
- ☐ binge eating disorder
- ☐ bulimia nervosa

Academic Vocabulary

You will find these words in your reading and on your tests. Use the glossary to look up their definitions if necessary.

- defuse
- stabilize

Graphic Organizer

Use a graphic organizer like the one below to take notes about four common chronic disorders and dietary changes that can improve them.

CHRONIC DISORDERS	DIETARY CHANGES

Graphic Organizer Go to this book's Online Learning Center at **glencoe.com** to print out this graphic organizer.

Academic Standards

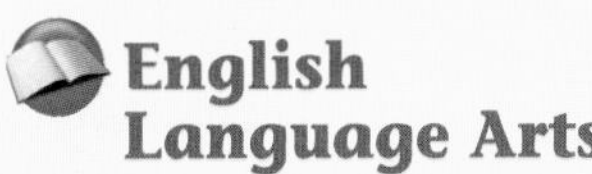

English Language Arts

NCTE 8 Use information to gather information and create and communicate knowledge.

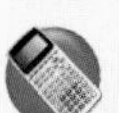

Mathematics

NCTM Data Analysis and Probability Select and use appropriate statistical methods to analyze data.

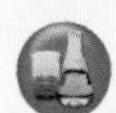

Science

NSES C Develop an understanding of organization in living systems and behavior of organisms.

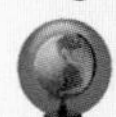

Social Studies

NCSS VIII A Science, Technology, and Society Identify and describe both current and historical examples of the interaction and interdependence of science, technology, and society in a variety of cultural settings.

NCTE *National Council of Teachers of English*
NCTM *National Council of Teachers of Mathematics*
NSES *National Science Education Standards*
NCSS *National Council for the Social Studies*

Stress

Everyone has to cope with stress. **Stress** is physical or mental tension caused by a person's reaction to a situation. Situations do not cause stress by themselves. Instead, stress comes from how you react to events in your life. Different events trigger stress for different people. Going on a date, for example, may be fun for one person and stressful for another. Major changes, such as graduating, getting married, or moving to a new home, are stressful for most people.

Stress upsets the body and the mind. Stress can lead to headaches, backaches, insomnia, and irritability. Prolonged stress can weaken the immune system, your body's defense against disease. Unmanaged stress is a risk factor for hypertension.

Stress and Nutrition

Stress can have two effects on eating. Moderate stress can cause people to engage in emotional eating. Severe stress can shut down the appetite. Stress makes demands on the muscles and organs, so healthy eating is more important than ever during stressful times.

Follow good nutrition when you are under stress. If stress dulls your appetite, schedule time for nourishing meals. Avoid filling up on fluids before or during meals.

If you overeat when you are stressed, choose fruit, yogurt, and other healthful choices. Avoid comfort foods such as ice cream, chips, and cookies. Heavy foods like these can lead to digestive upset, which is already more likely in times of stress.

Avoid caffeinated beverages. Caffeine is a stimulant that can worsen stress.

Coping Skills

Exercise and relaxation techniques are two good ways to deal with stress and anxiety. *How can physical fitness help you deal with stress?*

Coping with Stress

Despite its negative effects, stress serves a valuable purpose. It readies you to take action in difficult situations. Taking action is a good way to **defuse** stress, or make it less harmful. Are you worried about a major school assignment? Make a schedule and begin work. Is a friendship in trouble? Reach out to heal the relationship.

What should you do if stress is draining and not helpful? Learn positive coping skills, or ways of dealing with challenging situations. Try these coping strategies:

- Distinguish between what you can change and what you cannot change. Often, you cannot change situations or people, but you *can* change the way you react to them. Learning to recognize what you can change and what you can not can help you manage stress.
- Develop a sense of humor. Laughter relieves tension.
- Take one step at a time. Break big tasks into small parts and handle them one by one.
- Reach out. Talk over problems with a close friend, relative, health professional, or counselor. Talking about problems often makes them seem more manageable. Talking with someone about a problem often helps you understand it better.
- Keep physically fit. A fit body copes with life's situations more easily. Physical activity, like yoga, can work off tension.
- Take time for rest and recreation. Get enough sleep each day and make time for leisure activities such as hobbies, music, reading, and time with friends.
- Criticize less and praise more. Instead of finding fault, look for something positive in people and situations. Focus on solutions.
- Do not use drugs to relieve stress, and do not use medications unless your physician recommends it. Alcohol, tranquilizers, pep pills, and antacids do not solve the underlying problem, and they may even lead to more serious problems.

✓ Reading Check **Explain** How can laughter affect your body?

TECHNOLOGY FOR TOMORROW

Safe Substitutes

People with food allergies must be very careful to avoid even the tiniest amount of problem foods. Fortunately, science and technology have made it possible for food makers to create safe substitutes for some allergenic foods. For example, people with lactose intolerance can substitute lactose-reduced or lactose-free products. Lactose-free milk is made by adding lactase to the milk. Lactase is an enzyme that breaks down lactose into glucose and galactose, digestable sugars. This process removes 70-100 percent of the lactose. In all other aspects, the lactose-free milk is nutritionally the same as regular milk..

Investigate Research a safe substitute for a food that can cause allergies or intolerance in people. Discover how the substitute is produced, which food or foods it can replace, and its nutritional benefits.

NCSS VIII A Science, Technology, and Society
Identify and describe both current and historical examples of the interaction and interdependence of science, technology, and society in a variety of cultural settings.

Illness and Recovery

A well-nourished body is better equipped to handle any ailment—fever, cold, or broken ankle. A person who is ill or recovering from illness should pay special attention to the foods they choose.

Food-Drug Interactions

Foods and supplements can change the effect of drugs on the body. Some drugs can change the effect of food and supplements on the body. For example, your body uses some medicines better when taken with a meal. Some antibiotics should not be taken with dairy foods, because calcium binds to them and prevents the body from absorbing either one. A physician or pharmacist can give detailed instructions for when and how to take medication.

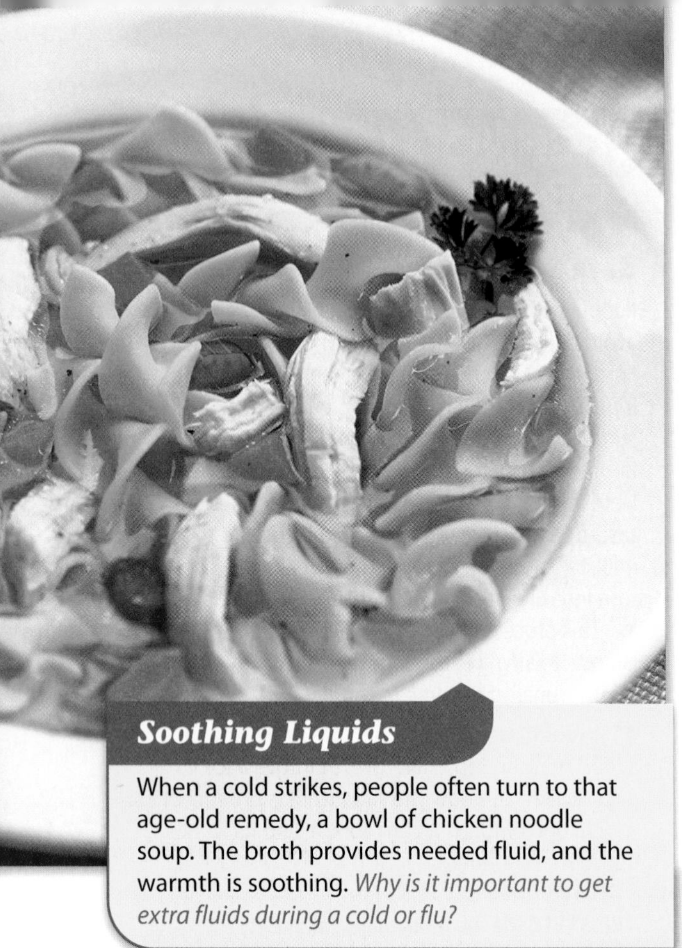

Soothing Liquids

When a cold strikes, people often turn to that age-old remedy, a bowl of chicken noodle soup. The broth provides needed fluid, and the warmth is soothing. *Why is it important to get extra fluids during a cold or flu?*

Be a Smart Consumer

Caffeine Consumption

Have you ever felt shaky, anxious, irritable, or jittery after drinking certain beverages? Chances are that the drinks were high in caffeine. Many people consume excess amounts of caffeine without even knowing it. They may not know just how much caffeine is in the beverages they regularly drink. Coffee contains between 80–175 milligrams of caffeine. Energy drinks contain about 80 milligrams. Sodas contain about 35 to 55 milligrams. Tea contains between 15 and 60 milligrams. Even decaffeinated tea and coffee retain small amounts of caffeine. Keeping your kitchen stocked with caffeine-free beverages will help you decrease your caffeine consumption, and your stress.

Challenge What are good drink options if you want to avoid caffeine? Write a shopping list for a person on a caffeine-free diet that includes at least five caffeine-free beverages.

Fluids

Fluids are particularly important during illness, especially a cold or flu. Drink fluids to replace water lost to vomiting or fever. Cool liquids also help a high temperature. Fluids help moisten nasal and sinus tissues to prevent irritation. Liquid foods like the chicken soup in the Light and Healthy Recipe in this chapter are soothing to sore throats. Because they are mostly made of water, soups are easily digested and provide nutrients your body needs to get better.

Calories

Your nutrient needs remain the same during mild illnesses and injuries, but your calorie needs may drop if you are inactive for a long period. Choose nutrient-dense foods to prevent weight gain.

✓ **Reading Check** **Describe** What can happen if antibiotics are taken with dairy foods?

Chronic Health Problems

Chronic means recurring or taking place over a long period of time. Chronic health problems can occur over years or even decades, such as diabetes and HIV/AIDS.

Common Chronic Disorders

Many chronic health problems require special eating plans or medical nutrition therapy. A dietitian or nutritionist will make specific recommendations. Here are general guidelines for some major chronic health disorders:

High Cholesterol

High cholesterol increases the risk of heart disease and stroke. Medical nutrition therapy for this condition includes cutting back on foods high in cholesterol and saturated fat and adding foods high in fiber. Soy proteins may also help control cholesterol.

High Blood Pressure

High blood pressure is a risk factor for heart disease and other medical problems. People who need to reduce blood pressure often follow a diet low in sodium and saturated fat and rich in calcium, potassium, and magnesium.

Diabetes

Diabetes is a condition in which the body cannot control blood sugar levels. Untreated diabetes can do serious damage to the kidneys, eyes, and heart. People with diabetes can **stabilize**, or regulate, blood sugar levels by rationing their carbohydrate intake through regular meals and careful food choices. High-fiber foods may slow carbohydrate digestion and absorption and help to stabilize blood sugar.

HIV/AIDS

Human Immunodeficiency Virus/Acquired Immune Deficiency Syndrome (HIV/AIDS) is a disorder that weakens the immune system. People who are HIV positive can experience a variety of nutrition-related problems, including poor appetite, nausea, diarrhea, weight loss, and changes in body composition. Proper nutrition and exercise can help with these problems. People with HIV/AIDS are sensitive to foodborne illness, so safe food handling is also essential.

Food Sensitivities

Some chronic conditions are actually caused by certain foods. A **food allergy** is an abnormal response to certain foods by the body's immune system. Even a trace amount of the food can trigger symptoms such as a rash, stomach cramps and nausea, or even trouble breathing. In rare cases, food allergy can cause death. Fish, shellfish, eggs, nuts, and peanuts are the most common allergens (allergy-causing substances) for adults. Children are more often allergic to cow's milk, eggs, peanuts, wheat, and soy.

A **food intolerance** is a negative physical reaction to food that does not involve the immune system. Food intolerance usually causes digestive problems. For example, people who cannot digest lactose, the sugar in cow's milk, experience an upset stomach after they eat dairy foods. People with food allergies or a food intolerance need to avoid problem foods.

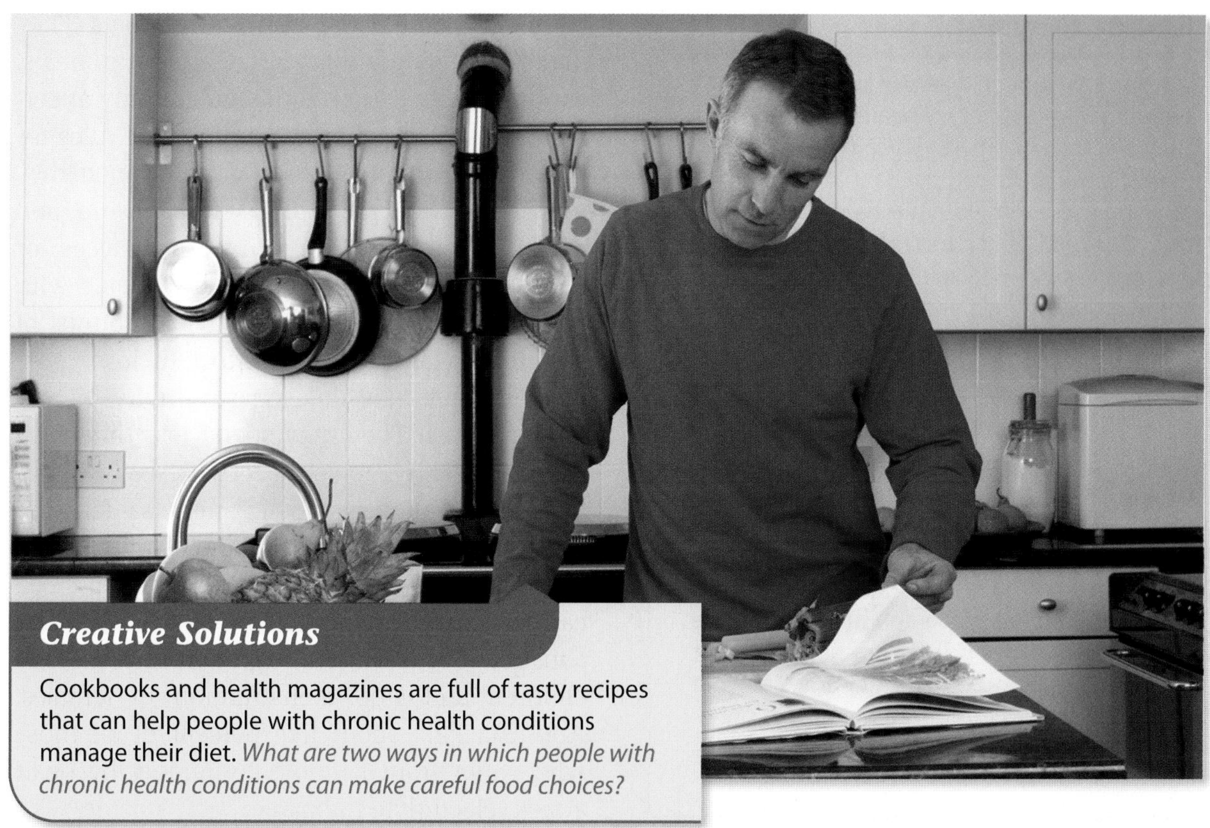

Creative Solutions

Cookbooks and health magazines are full of tasty recipes that can help people with chronic health conditions manage their diet. *What are two ways in which people with chronic health conditions can make careful food choices?*

Eating Plan Strategies

People with chronic health conditions who follow a special eating plan need to pay close attention to their food choices. For example, they must carefully check food labels for ingredients they need to limit or increase. They must ask restaurant staff about how foods are prepared and request special orders if menu items contain potentially harmful ingredients.

A special eating plan does not have to be boring. It can be an opportunity to explore new foods and learn new cooking skills. For instance, a fresh tomato sauce with blended herbs and spices fits a low-fat, low-sodium diet.

Many medical centers offer cooking classes for different nutritional needs. Family and friends can help try new recipes and share healthful habits, making the experience even more positive.

✓ Reading Check **Explain** Why are high-fiber foods recommended for people with diabetes?

Nutrition Check

Recipe Revision

Low-fat, low-sodium diets can benefit people suffering from a variety of health conditions. Such diets can be smart for healthy people, too. Avoiding too much saturated fat and sodium can help to prevent potential health challenges down the road. Eating healthfully, however, does not mean you must eliminate your favorite flavorful recipes from your diet. Instead, you can use your knowledge and creativity to revise recipes and make them healthier.

Think About It Find an appealing recipe in a book or online. Write a revised version of the recipe that lowers its fat and sodium content. You might eliminate ingredients, substitute ingredients, or alter quantities. Consider alternate preparation methods for the recipe. Along with your recipe, write a paragraph summarizing the changes you made and your reasoning. Present the old recipe along with the new one and your paragraph to your class. Read the recipes presented by your classmates and discuss changes you made.

Eating Disorders

An **eating disorder** is a condition marked by extreme emotions, attitudes, and behaviors related to food, eating, and weight.

Eating disorders can damage health and even threaten life. They occur most often among teens and young adults, especially girls and women. People of all ages can develop eating disorders, however, even children. Up to ten percent of all teens and young adults may develop an eating disorder at some point. People with eating disorders work hard to hide them from others. Knowing the signs of these disorders can help you protect yourself and your friends and family.

Anorexia Nervosa

Anorexia nervosa (ˌa-nəh-ˈrek-sē-ə (ˌ)nər-ˈvō-sə) is an intense fear of gaining weight that leads to unhealthy eating and dangerous weight loss. People with anorexia nervosa become extremely underweight, but they still see themselves as fat.

Food, eating, and dieting become obsessions for people with anorexia nervosa. People with anorexia nervosa develop unusual, and often very rigid, eating habits and rituals. They may deny being hungry or avoid group meals, eat only a few certain foods, or eat only at certain times. They may set complicated rules for themselves about when and how much they may eat. They may precisely measure and arrange their food, cut it into tiny pieces, or chew it more than normal. Many people with anorexia nervosa get excessive amounts of strenuous exercise in an effort to lose more weight. They may develop sensitivity to cold temperatures. They may spend less time with friends and give up some activities.

The starvation of anorexia nervosa damages the body, lowering the heart and breathing rate, blood pressure, and body temperature. Anorexia can lead to heart problems, osteoporosis, and constipation. It can stunt growth in teens and children and stop menstruation in females. Anorexia kills about five percent of all those who suffer from it, most commonly by heart attack, electrolyte imbalance, and suicide.

Binge Eating Disorder

A **binge eating disorder** is an eating disorder that causes people to binge, or eat enormous amounts of food in a short time. It is the most common eating disorder. When people binge, they cannot control what or how much they eat. They may eat up to 5,000 calories in one sitting.

An eating binge usually occurs when the person is alone. After the binge, the person may feel guilty, disgusted, or depressed.

Binge eating disorder leads to excessive weight gain, with related problems of high blood pressure, high cholesterol, heart disease, and diabetes.

Bulimia Nervosa

Bulimia nervosa (bü-ˈlē-mē-ə) is an eating disorder that combines bingeing with purging, or ridding the body of the food to prevent weight gain. Purging methods include self-induced vomiting, fasting, excessive exercise, and abuse of laxatives, diet pills, and diuretics (water-removal pills). People with bulimia may binge and purge twice a week.

People with bulimia fear getting fat, but they usually stay within 10 to 15 pounds of a healthy weight. Signs include missing food, empty food containers, the presence of laxatives or diuretics, and long periods spent in the bathroom after meals.

Bulimia creates many serious health problems. Vomiting damages the teeth, gums, and stomach and can rupture the esophagus. Loss of fluid causes electrolyte imbalance, which can lead to an irregular heartbeat and even heart failure.

Causes of Eating Disorders

Eating disorders have complex causes. Emotional problems are usually the underlying cause. Genetics and chemical imbalances in the brain may also play a role.

People who have eating disorders struggle with issues of identity and control. They may use food to cope with stress, low self-esteem, and fears about the future. Family troubles, loneliness, anger, depression, and being teased about their weight add to the problem. Often, people with eating disorders hate the way they look. They have unrealistic ideas about body shape and weight.

Stopping the Cycle

The earlier an eating disorder is recognized and treated, the better the chance for recovery. Few people can stop these self-destructive behaviors without professional help. Resistance is common, however. People may not see that their behavior is unhealthy, or they may be ashamed to admit the problem.

Family and friends may have to step in and persuade a person with an eating disorder to accept help. A person with an eating disorder can seek advice from a trusted adult, such as a family member or a school nurse or counselor. Then, a mental health counselor can provide expert help.

People with eating disorders need physical and emotional treatment. Physicians and nurses deal with the disorder's physical complications. Psychotherapists try to uncover and heal the emotional causes. Behavior therapists and dietitians help the person learn healthy eating habits. Self-help groups offer support from others who have the disorder. Recovery can be a long process, and support from family and friends is very important.

Finding an open door to communication is difficult for many. Choosing a private place to talk can help. Some people write down their concerns and specific history to make opening up a little easier. Realizing that health now, and in the future, is more important than moments of embarrassment gets many people started on the road to recovery.

Preventing Eating Disorders

Eating disorders are serious and complex problems. Education and counseling can help prevent eating disorders by showing people positive ways to cope with life's challenges.

It is important to identify problem eating behaviors early, because these behaviors can lead to eating disorders. People with eating disorders often may not recognize or be able to admit that they have a problem.

Embarrassment can also get in the way. For this reason it is very important that family members and friends can recognize the symptoms and help the person find treatment. For example, someone who goes on extreme diets may be at risk for developing an eating disorder. Speak up early—do not wait until the problem grows. Express your concerns clearly in a caring manner. Encourage the person to seek trained professional help.

Another way to prevent eating disorders is to find healthy models of beauty. The human body comes in diverse shapes and sizes. Reject the ultra-thin standard of beauty and encourage your family and friends to do the same. Discourage the idea that obtaining a particular weight or body size will lead to happiness. When you value people for who they are and praise their positive accomplishments, you show that you base personal worth on much more than appearance.

Light and Healthy Recipe

Chicken Noodle Soup

A favorite comfort food, this Chicken Noodle Soup is low in fat and full of lean meat and vegetables.

Ingredients

- **1 Tbsp.** Vegetable oil
- **¼ cup** Chopped carrots
- **¼ cup** Chopped celery
- **½ cup** Chopped onion
- **1 tsp.** Minced garlic
- **1** Diced tomato
- **10 oz.** Cubed grilled chicken breast
- **4 cups** Low-sodium vegetable broth
- **1 cup** Dry pasta, any shape that will fit on a spoon
- **1 tsp.** Chopped parsley
- **1 tsp.** Chopped oregano
- **¼ tsp.** Pepper

Directions

1. Pour the vegetable oil into a pot and warm it under medium heat.
2. Add the carrots, celery, onions, and garlic and cook them under medium heat until all the vegetables are tender enough to be pierced easily by a fork. Stir the vegetables often to avoid browning.
3. Add the vegetable broth and the chicken and bring to a simmer.
4. Allow the soup to simmer for 20 minutes. Then add the pasta and allow it to cook through as the soup continues to simmer.
5. As the pasta cooks, it will absorb some of the water. If the soup looks too thick, adjust it by adding water.
6. Add the diced tomato and let the soup cook 10 more minutes.
7. Add the parsley, oregano, and pepper and let the soup cook five more minutes.
8. Serve piping hot in bowls. Garnish with a parsley leaf.

Yield 6 servings

Nutrition Analysis per Serving

■ Calories	186
■ Total fat	2 g
Saturated fat	0 g
Cholesterol	25 mg
■ Sodium	329 mg
■ Carbohydrate	26
Dietary fiber	1 g
Sugars	3 g
■ Protein	15g

CHAPTER 12 Review & Applications

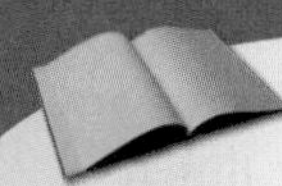

After You Read

Chapter Summary

Food plays a role in many health challenges. Stress can contribute to numerous ailments. People may eat more or less during stress. Good nutrition and coping skills can minimize its effects. A well-nourished body can recover more quickly from illness. It is important to eat foods that do not interact with medicines, and to consume enough fluids and nutrient-dense calories. Many chronic health problems can be improved or managed by making dietary changes. Eating disorders are health challenges marked by extreme emotions and behaviors related to food. They can be prevented through education and counseling.

Content and Academic Vocabulary Review

1. Use each of these content and academic vocabulary words in a sentence.

Content Vocabulary

- stress (p. 164)
- chronic (p. 166)
- diabetes (p. 167)
- Human Immunodeficiency Virus/Acquired Immune Deficiency Syndrome (HIV/AIDS) (p. 167)
- food allergy (p. 167)
- food intolerance (p. 167)
- eating disorder (p. 168)
- anorexia nervosa (p. 168)
- binge eating disorder (p. 169)
- bulimia nervosa (p. 169)

Academic Vocabulary

- defuse (p. 165)
- stabilize (p. 167)

Review Key Concepts

2. **Explain** stress and its relationship to nutrition.
3. **Describe** the role food plays in illness and recovery.
4. **Examine** how food can help to resolve or manage chronic health problems.
5. **Identify** eating disorders and explain their causes and solutions.

Critical Thinking

6. **Evaluate** Angela's actions. Angela is stressed about an upcoming test. Instead of her usual run, she goes out for ice cream with a friend.
7. **Explain** why you should drink more fluids when you have a fever.
8. **Explain** what Jessica should do and why. Jessica knows that drinking cow's milk upsets her stomach.
9. **Analyze** this situation and provide advice. Your friend Jane's parents are getting a divorce. Jane is stressed, and the situation is affecting her sleeping and eating patterns.
10. **Compare and contrast** anorexia nervosa and bulimia nervosa.

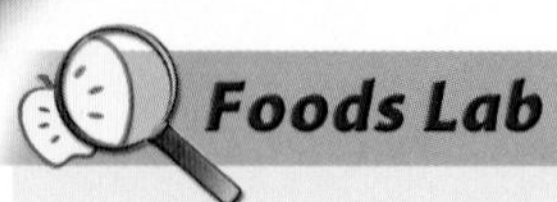

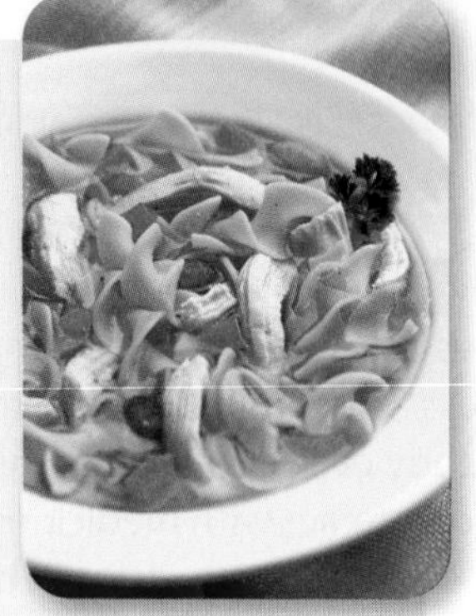

11. Modified-Diet Recipes A person with a health challenge may stick to a modified diet in which they avoid certain foods, such as salt, or make an effort to eat others, such as fiber.

Procedure Find a suitable recipe for someone on a modified diet due to a specific health challenge. The recipe should have accessible ingredients. Prepare and evaluate the recipe.

Analysis Give an oral presentation explaining how the recipe fit the modified diet, how you would rate it for convenience and ease, and whether it has appeal for people who are not following a modified diet.

HEALTHFUL CHOICES

12. Presentation Jitters Marie has to give an oral presentation to her class after lunch. She is feeling stressed and anxious about standing in front of her classmates and speaking. At lunch, her beverage options are: iced tea; water; cranberry juice; and iced coffee. What should Marie choose and why? Which of the options would be the worst choice? Besides making wise choices at lunch, what else can Marie do to ease her anxiety?

TECH Connection

13. E-mail Reminder People under stress can benefit from laughter, physical activity, and taking a break. Compose an e-mail message that will be sent to your classmates to encourage them to do one of those three things. Explain why it is important to defuse stress and how the activity you have chosen will help. Send the e-mail to two of your classmates and copy your teacher.

Real-World Skills

Problem-Solving Skills

14. Recovering from Injury After Kyle spent his summer recovering from a broken leg, he has been gaining weight. What changes should he make to his diet and why?

Interpersonal and Collaborative Skills

15. Interview Follow your teacher's instructions to pair up with a classmate. Take turns interviewing each other about: common causes of stress in your lives, the effects stress has on you, and how you cope with stress. Write down your partner's responses to the interview questions. Then participate in a class discussion about teens and stress.

Financial Literacy Skills

16. Milk Money Visit a local supermarket. Research the cost per gallon of regular cow's milk, lactose-free cow's milk, soy milk, and rice milk. Which is the least expensive and which is the most expensive? Which of the latter three varieties would be the best value for a lactose-intolerant person?

Academic Skills

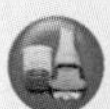

Food Science

17. Taste Is Mainly Smell Our taste buds can recognize only a few flavors: sweet, sour, salty, bitter, and savory, or umami. In contrast, we can smell thousands of different odors, greatly enhancing our ability to taste food.

Procedure You will need 3 jars of baby food: a fruit, a vegetable, and a meat. Have your partner close his eyes (or use a blindfold) while you feed him a small bite of each food. Before each bite, have your partner hold his nose while trying to taste the food. Ask your partner what the food is after each bite. Repeat the experiment with an open nose.

Analysis How does smell affect our ability to taste food? What happens to this ability when we have a cold?

NSES C Develop an understanding of organization in living systems and behavior of organisms.

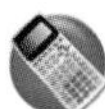

Mathematics

18. Compare Caffeine Content Many beverages contain caffeine in large or small amounts. The typical cola contains 35 mg of caffeine, although some diet colas contain 46 mg. Other sodas have 55 mg of caffeine, while "energy" drinks contain 80 mg. A cup of green tea has 15 mg, the typical iced tea has 47 mg, and coffee can reach 175 mg. Even a cup of hot chocolate contains caffeine (14 mg). What is the median caffeine amount for all of these beverages?

Math Concept **Find the Median** Median is a statistical measure that indicates the middle number in an ordered set of values. If you have an even number of values, the median is the average (mean) of the two middle numbers.

Starting Hint Arrange the caffeine values in order from lowest to highest. Locate the two values in the middle, add them together, and divide by two.

NCTM Data Analysis and Probability Select and use appropriate statistical methods to analyze data.

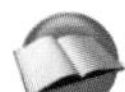

English Language Arts

19. Research and Report Use three sources to research one of the eating disorders discussed in this chapter. Write a one-page report about your findings. Include information that is not discussed in this chapter, such as statistics and quotes from experts. Also include a list of your sources.

NCTE 8 Use information resources to gather information and create and communicate knowledge.

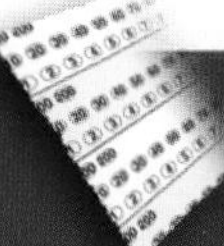

STANDARDIZED TEST PRACTICE

FILL IN THE BLANK

Read the sentence and choose the best word to fill in the blank.

20. People with high cholesterol should cut back on foods high in cholesterol and saturated fat and add foods high in ______.

a. salt **c.** fiber
b. vitamin C **d.** lactose

Test-Taking Tip When answering a fill-in-the-blank question, silently read the sentence with each of the possible answers in the blank space. This will help you eliminate wrong answers. The best answer results in a sentence that is both factual and grammatically correct.

CHAPTER 13

Lifespan Nutrition

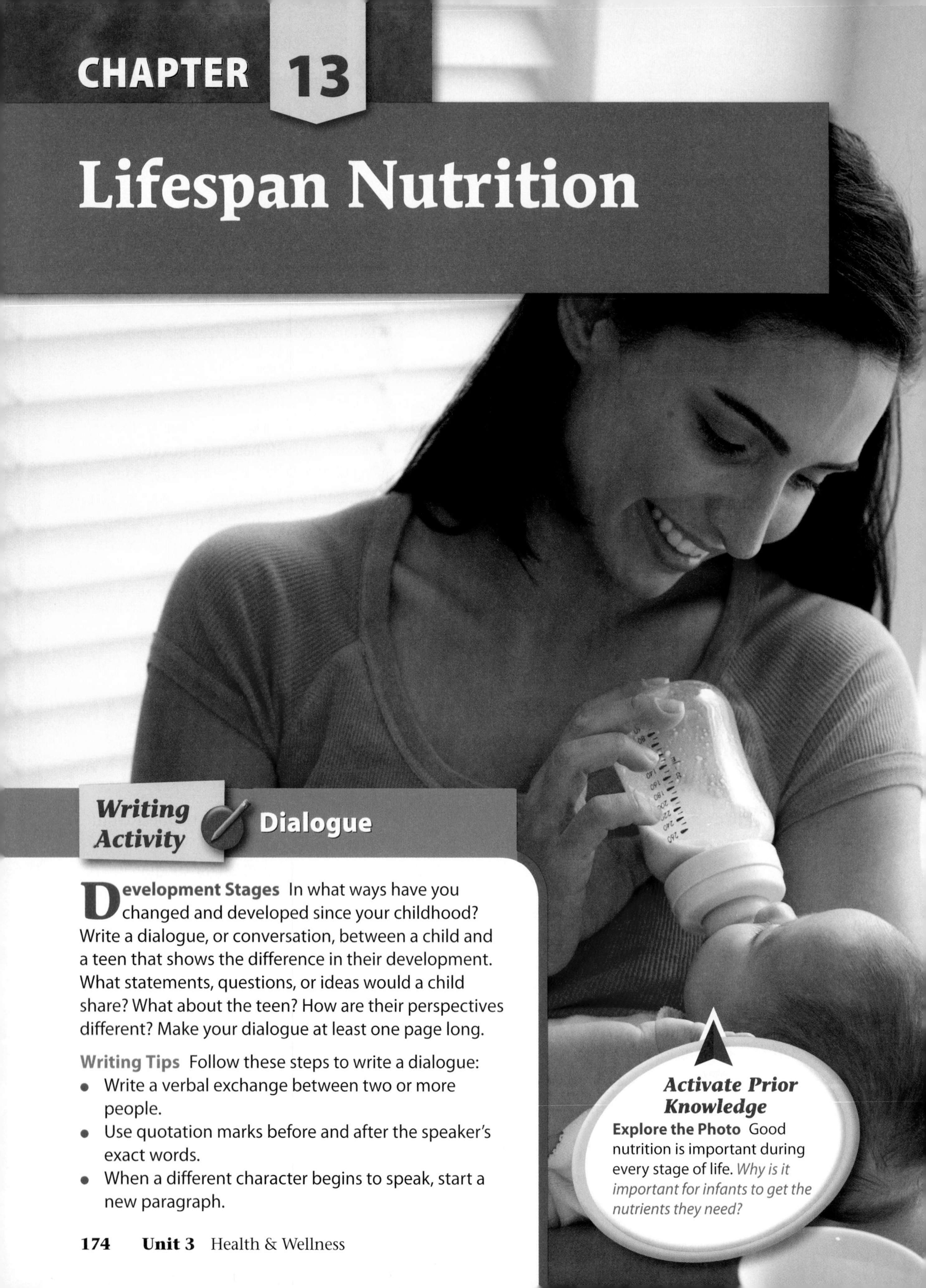

Writing Activity — Dialogue

Development Stages In what ways have you changed and developed since your childhood? Write a dialogue, or conversation, between a child and a teen that shows the difference in their development. What statements, questions, or ideas would a child share? What about the teen? How are their perspectives different? Make your dialogue at least one page long.

Writing Tips Follow these steps to write a dialogue:

- Write a verbal exchange between two or more people.
- Use quotation marks before and after the speaker's exact words.
- When a different character begins to speak, start a new paragraph.

Activate Prior Knowledge

Explore the Photo Good nutrition is important during every stage of life. *Why is it important for infants to get the nutrients they need?*

Reading Guide

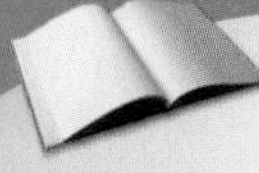

Before You Read

Preview Examine the figures and photos in this chapter. Think about how your nutrient needs have changed from the time you were born until now.

Read to Learn

Key Concepts

- **List** the five stages of the life span.
- **Evaluate** why good nutrition is important to a fetus and the mother
- **Compare and contrast** breast feeding and bottle feeding.
- **Explain** why snacks are important to a child's diet.
- **Explain** why nutrient needs increase during your teens.
- **Explain** why calorie needs drop in older adulthood but nutrition needs often rise.

Main Idea

Nutritional needs change throughout the five stages of the life span, and meeting them promotes good development and health for life.

Content Vocabulary

You will find the definitions for these words in the glossary at the back of this book.

- ☐ life span
- ☐ fetus
- ☐ obstetrician
- ☐ osteoporosis
- ☐ colostrum
- ☐ lactation
- ☐ pediatrician
- ☐ peer pressure

Academic Vocabulary

You will find these words in your reading and on your tests. Use the glossary to look up their definitions if necessary.

- replenish
- dilemma

Graphic Organizer

Label a graphic organizer like the one below to write notes about eight guidelines to help children develop good eating habits.

ENCOURAGING GOOD EATING HABITS

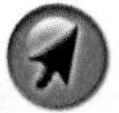

Graphic Organizer Go to this book's Online Learning Center at **glencoe.com** to print out this graphic organizer.

Academic Standards

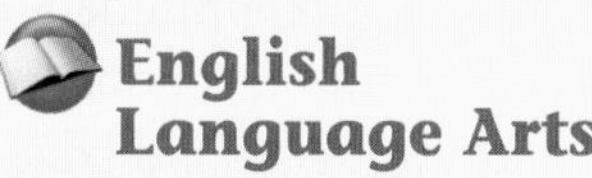

English Language Arts

NCTE 12 Use language to accomplish individual purposes.

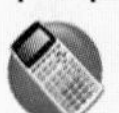

Mathematics

NCTM Measurement Understand measurable attributes of objects and the units, systems, and processes of measurement.

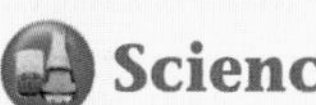

Science

NSES B Develop an understanding of the structure and properties of matter.

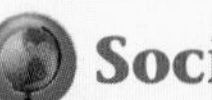

Social Studies

NCSS IA Culture Analyze and explain the ways groups, societies, and cultures address human needs and concerns.

NCTE *National Council of Teachers of English*
NCTM *National Council of Teachers of Mathematics*
NSES *National Science Education Standards*
NCSS *National Council for the Social Studies*

Nutrition for a Lifetime

Your nutritonal needs change throughout your life span. A **life span** is all the stages of growth and development throughout life, from before birth to old age. The human life span includes five stages: the prenatal period, infancy, childhood, adolescence, and adulthood.

Each life stage brings its own growth and nutrition needs and challenges. Meeting these demands promotes good health at each time of life and builds a solid base for the future.

✓ Reading Check **List** What are the five stages of the human life span?

Prenatal Period

Good food choices are especially important for pregnant women. Good nutrition is the single most important requirement during pregnancy. During nine months in the womb, a single cell multiplies into an embryo and then into a fetus. A **fetus** (ˈfē-təs) is an unborn baby from the age of eight weeks to birth. The baby's growth and development, including crucial brain development, depend on nutrients from the mother.

A woman often does not learn that she is pregnant until a month or more into the pregnancy. A woman who has been enjoying healthful foods from the beginning of the pregnancy is more likely to have a healthy baby. Poor eating habits by the mother place the baby at risk for serious problems throughout life.

Poor nutrition can damage the mother's health as well. If the fetus does not get enough nutrients from the mother's diet, it draws them from her body tissue. This creates a deficiency.

Teen pregnancies are particularly risky because teens need added nutrients for their own growth and development. Poor nutrition increases the chance that the baby will have a low birth weight (under 5½ pounds) as well as physical and learning problems later in life. Most teens are physically immature, so they are also more likely to have difficult pregnancies.

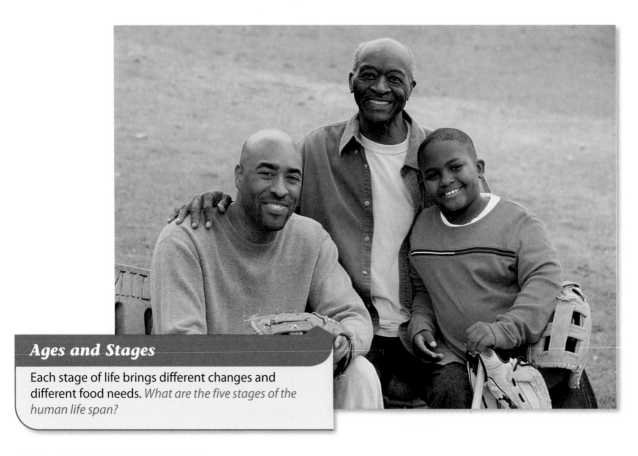

Ages and Stages

Each stage of life brings different changes and different food needs. *What are the five stages of the human life span?*

Mother's Nutrition

MyPyramid for Moms divides foods into five basic groups, plus oils. *How can pregnant women meet most of their nutrients?*

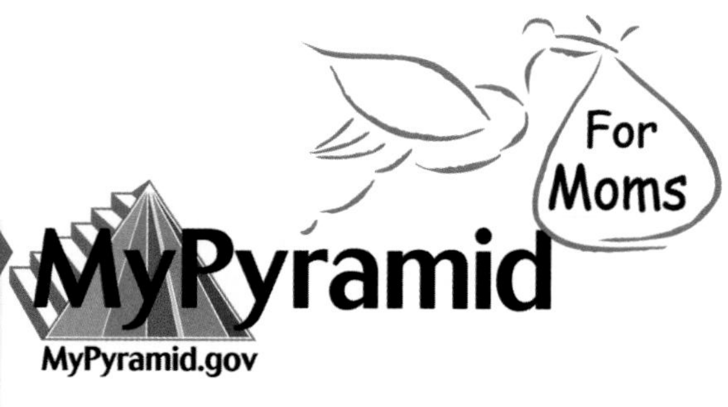

MyPyramid for Moms

As soon as a woman learns that she is pregnant, she should see an **obstetrician** (ˌäb-stə-ˈtri-shən), a physician who specializes in the care of women during pregnancy and childbirth. An obstetrician will recommend specific kinds and amounts of food and possibly supplements.

The United States Department of Agriculture has developed nutritional guildelines for pregnant women. These guidelines are known as MyPyramid for Moms. MyPyramid for Moms gives recommendations for pregnant and breast-feeding women. Pregnant women can meet most of their nutrient needs by choosing low-fat, nutrient-dense foods.

You learned about the five good groups and oils category in Chapter 10. Expecting mothers need a variety of nutrients to keep themselves and their developing babies healthy. The following information about the five food groups and oils category is specific to pregnant women.

Grains

Eating grains is essential to any well-balanced diet. They contain carbohydrates, which provide our body with energy. Grains fortified with folic acid can help prevent defects to the baby's nervous system.

Vegetables

Eating vegetables keeps the mother's heart healthy. They also can reduce the chances of her getting diabetes, high blood pressure, and some kinds of cancer. They are rich in potassium and dietary fiber. Many are rich in folic acids and vitamins A, C, and E. Most are low in fat and calories, and therefore can help to control the mother's weight.

Fruits

Pregnant women should try to eat seven or more servings of fruits and vegetables combined every day. Fruits and vegetables are rich sources of fiber, vitamins and minerals. Fruits with vitamin C help mother and baby have healthy gums and other tissues. Vitamin C also helps the body to heal wounds and to absorb iron.

Milk Products

Nutrients in milk products include calcium, potassium, vitamin D, and protein. Calcium is vital for building healthy bones and teeth. It is important that pregnant women get adequate calcium to prevent osteoporosis. **Osteoporosis** is a condition in which bones become fragile and break easily. Choosing milk products that are low fat or fat-free is also important.

Meat and Beans

Meat, poultry, fish, dried beans, nuts, and eggs belong to this group. Choose meat and poultry cuts that are low-fat. They provide protein, which is vital to the baby's growth and development of bones and teeth. Protein also helps keep the mother's body healthy. Expectant mothers need more protein than they did before they were pregnant.

Oils

Oils are fats that are liquid at room temperature. Solid fats, such as margarine and shortening, contain hydrogenated oils that are higher in saturated fats and trans fats than oils. While some fat is needed for brain development, pregnant women, like everyone else, should try to limit their intake of saturated and trans fat.

Vitamins and Minerals

A variety of vitamins and minerals are vital to both the fetus and the mother. Whenever possible, it is best to get these from a healthy diet, rather than by taking supplements. Pregnant women should take vitamins, minerals, or other supplements only with their doctor's approval.

Vitamins

Vitamins help to maintain a healthy pregnancy. Research has determined some birth defects, such as spina bifida, are linked to vitamin deficiency.

Women usually need more vitamins during pregnancy. Some important ones are listed below.

- Vitamin A ensures proper eye development and helps keep skin healthy.
- The B vitamins assist in general fetal development.
- Vitamin C helps build healthy teeth and gums. It also helps form the connective tissue of skin, bone, and organs.
- Vitamin D aids in the creation of bones and teeth.
- Folic acid is necessary for normal spinal development in the fetus. Lack of folic acid can lead to spina bifida. Pregnant women need twice the normal amount. Even women who are considering becoming pregnant should increase their intake of folic acid.

Minerals

Pregnant women need iron, a mineral that helps prevent anemia and assists in developing the baby's own blood supply. Extra iron is stored in the baby's liver and is used in the months

Figure 13.1 MyPyramid for Moms

Sample Nutrition Plan This nutrition plan is for a 30-year-old woman who weighs 140 pounds. ***Amounts in which groups increase over the course of the pregnancy?***

	1st Trimester	2nd Trimester	3rd Trimester	
	Jan - Mar	Apr - Jun	Jul - Oct	
▶ Grains	7 ounces	9 ounces	9 ounces	tips
▶ Vegetables	3 cups	3½ cups	3½ cups	tips
▶ Fruits	2 cups	2 cups	2 cups	tips
▶ Milk	3 cups	3 cups	3 cups	tips
▶ Meat & Beans	6 ounces	6½ ounces	6½ ounces	tips

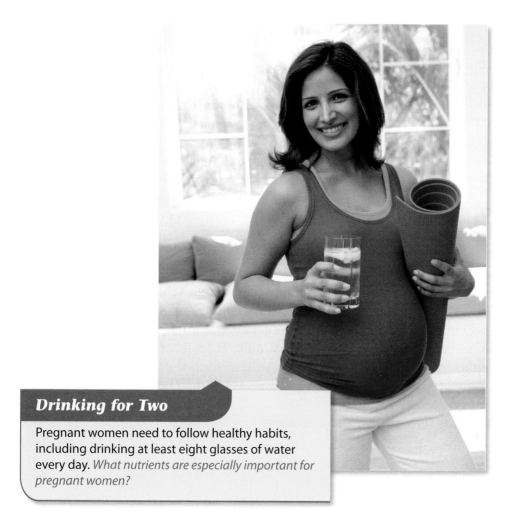

Drinking for Two

Pregnant women need to follow healthy habits, including drinking at least eight glasses of water every day. *What nutrients are especially important for pregnant women?*

right after birth. During this period, a baby who lives on breast milk lacks iron in the diet. The mother can get iron from dried beans, raisins, dates, meat, and leafy green vegetables.

Calcium and phosphorous are also important minerals during pregnancy. These nutrients work together to produce strong bones and teeth and ensure regular elimination of waste from the body. Milk and other dairy products are key sources of calcium and phosphorous.

Food Quantities

All pregnant women should eat a wide variety of healthy foods. However, the exact quantities vary depending on the mother's age, weight, and activity level, as well as the stage of pregnancy. When you visit the MyPyramid for Moms Web site you can create a specific plan based on these factors. **Figure 13.1** shows a sample nutrition plan made using this Web site.

Pregnancy and Weight Gain

Most women gain 25 to 35 pounds during pregnancy. Overweight women should gain less, and underweight women should gain more. Women carrying twins should also gain more—as much as 45 pounds.

Pregnant women gain weight from the growth of the baby and from physical changes of pregnancy. Healthy women need only about 300 calories per day more than usual. These extra calories should come from nutrient-rich foods.

Pregnancy is not a good time for a weight-loss diet, even for women who are overweight. Limiting food deprives the fetus of vital nutrients. Women can lose weight after delivery by eating healthfully.

✓ Reading Check **Explain** Why can poor nutrition damage a mother's health as well as the health of her fetus?

Infancy

Good nutrition is the single most important requirement during pregnancy. The baby's growth and development, including crucial brain development, depend on nutrients from the mother. By eating a nutritious, balanced diet, a pregnant woman promotes her baby's development and maintains her own health.

Feeding Newborns

Parents have two choices for feeding a newborn—breast-feeding and bottle-feeding.

Breast milk has exactly the right balance of fat, carbohydrates, and protein for a baby. The protein in breast milk is better digested and absorbed than the protein in formula.

Breast-feeding also helps protect infants from infection. The mother passes her immunity to disease to the baby through colostrum. **Colostrum** (kə-ˈläs-trəm) is a thick, yellowish fluid that a mother produces for about three days after birth and that is rich in nutrients and antibodies (proteins that protect against infection). Antibodies form in response to the environment, so each mother's colostrum is tailored to her infant's needs.

A breast-feeding woman should eat well and drink plenty of liquids to ensure that she produces enough milk. **Lactation**, or breast milk production, burns added calories that make a weight-loss diet unnecessary and unwise. A breast-feeding woman may need to adjust her food choices if the infant is sensitive to certain foods.

Infant formula also provides good nutrition. A mother may choose to feed formula if she cannot produce milk or if she takes medications that could be passed to her infant in breast milk. Formula allows a mother to have a more flexible schedule and can be stored longer. However, formula can be expensive and it does not give the baby natural immunities to disease.

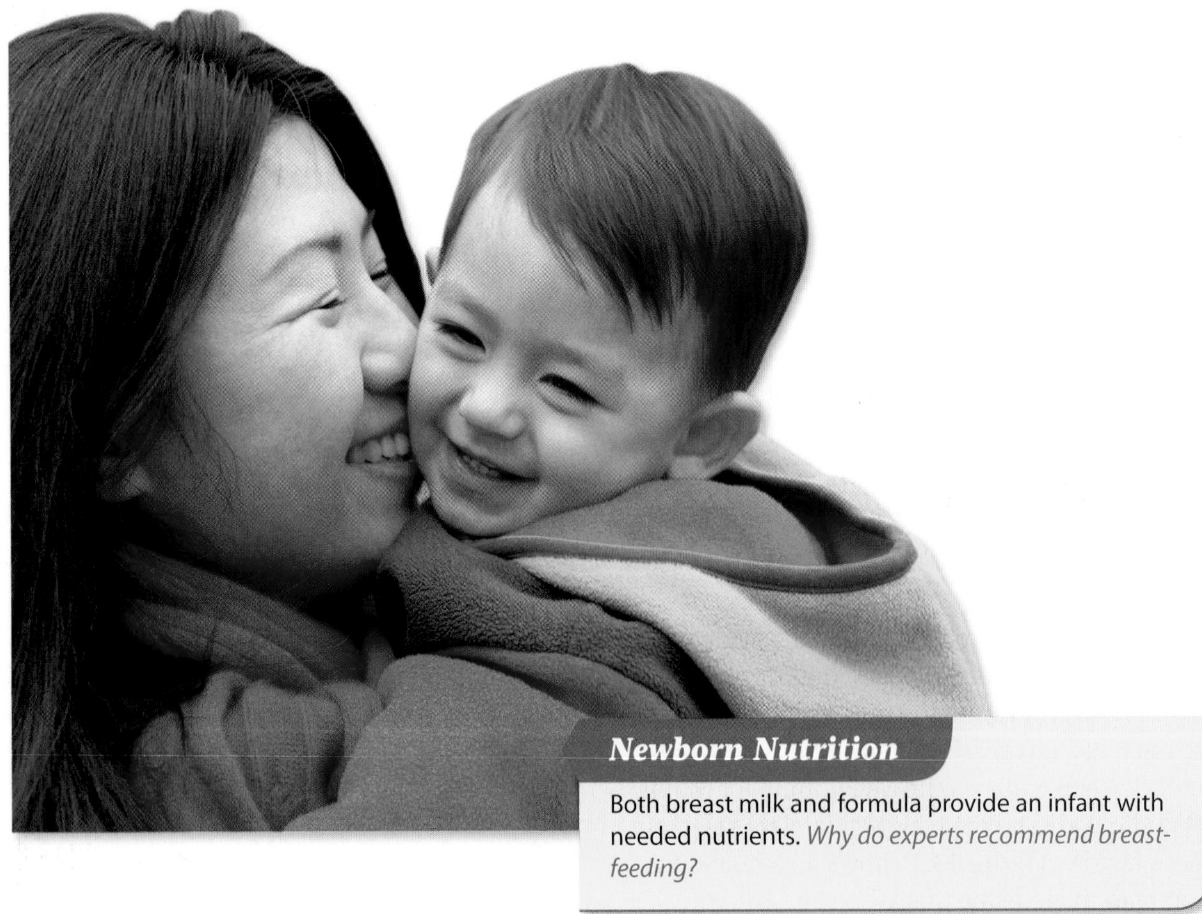

Newborn Nutrition

Both breast milk and formula provide an infant with needed nutrients. *Why do experts recommend breast-feeding?*

Science in Action: Easing Digestion

Some babies who do not drink breast milk have problems digesting formula. Predigested baby formula, called protein hydrolysate formula, is often recommended by doctors. It is easier to digest and less likely to cause allergic reactions than other formulas.

Procedure Use the Internet to research protein hydrolysate. Hydrolysate formula is made by breaking down the protein in cow's milk into smaller units. The smaller proteins are easier to digest than whole proteins, and enter into the baby's bloodstream faster.

Analysis Write one or more paragraphs to answer these questions: Who else besides infants consumes this broken-down, easily absorbed form of protein? Why?

NSES F Develop an understanding of personal and community health.

TECHNOLOGY FOR TOMORROW

Big Steps in Baby Foods

Baby food makers use technology to make their products more appealing. New processing methods reduce cooking time, so baby foods retain more nutrients, taste, and color. Whole-grain and multi-grain cereals are more available. So are organic baby foods, which are free of pesticides and additives. To make feeding babies easier, food makers apply the same technology used in adult foods. Instant rice cereals come in single-serving packets to eliminate the need for measuring. Combination meals for infants on the go come in portable, microwave-safe bowls. To keep up with toddlers' developing motor skills, baby food makers are creating finger foods, allowing them to feed themselves with nutritious bite-sized foods.

Investigate Some parents prefer to make their babies' food at home. What forms of technology, either new or old, can help them with this task?

NCSS IA Culture Analyze and explain ways groups, societies cultures and address human needs and concerns.

Adding Solid Food

Between four and six months of age, a baby is ready to start the transition to solid food. For easier swallowing and digestion, solids are strained to resemble a mash or paste. Iron-fortified rice cereal mixed with breast milk or formula is a good first solid food. There is no rush to start, however. Once babies have started to eat cereal, other new foods can be introduced. Vegetables and fruits come next.

It is not unusual for a baby to have an allergic reaction to a new food. Some foods may cause a skin rash or digestive trouble. By keeping track of what the baby has eaten and by introducing new foods one at a time and four days apart, you can know which food the baby is reacting to.

At about eight months, a baby is ready for protein foods. Introduce new choices one at a time. That makes it easier to tell whether a food is causing a negative reaction. The child's **pediatrician**, a physician who cares for infants and children, should be notified if a problem persists. The baby may have a food allergy or sensitivity.

At around nine months, infants' eating skills improve. They are able to sit up steadily in a high chair. They start to self-feed, picking up and chewing soft finger foods. Cutting food into small pieces makes it easier to handle and guards against choking. Healthful finger foods include pieces of peeled fruit, cooked vegetables, and cheese. Small pieces of a bagel or hard roll can help relieve gum irritation when a baby is teething. Being able to self-feed is an important step for an infant because it allows increased independence.

A one-year-old child can usually eat the same foods as the rest of the family if they are cut into small pieces. Children under two have high energy needs, so caregivers should not limit fat in their diet.

✓ **Reading Check** **Describe** How can a mother pass antibodies to her infant?

Childhood

Young children are active and growing. They need to eat a wide selection of nutritious foods. Children have small stomachs and short attention spans, so small servings and regular snacks are better than heavy meals. A rule of thumb for portions is 1 tablespoon of food for each year of the child's life. For example, 3 tablespoons of vegetables are a good portion for a three-year-old. A child who is still hungry can have a second helping. Milk, juice, yogurt, pieces of fruit or vegetables, unsweetened cereal, whole-grain crackers, and cooked meat, poultry, and fish all make healthful snacks. Avoid foods high in fat or sugar.

A child's appetite can vary from day to day. During growth spurts, children often eat more than usual. Children sometimes go on food jags, insisting on a certain food at every meal. Humor these phases until they pass.

Encouraging Good Eating Habits

Eating habits and attitudes that are learned in childhood can last a lifetime. Follow these guidelines to help children develop a healthy approach to food and nutrition.

- Serve foods that vary in color and texture. Cut foods into imaginative shapes. This adds interest and encourages children to appreciate food's sensory appeal.
- Share meals with children and make mealtime enjoyable. Model good manners and eating habits.
- Do not use food as a reward or punishment. This practice gives the wrong impression about the purpose of food.
- Allow children to leave food on their plates if they are not hungry. Insisting that they finish all their food can lead to overeating.
- When possible, let children choose meals and snacks from several nutritious options. Keep plenty of nutritious snacks on hand.
- Teach children how to prepare a few simple, healthful foods by themselves, with your supervision. Depending on their age, they might tear lettuce or make sandwiches. As children grow older, allow them to help in preparing meals.
- Make shopping trips with children fun and educational. Help them identify fruits and vegetables. Point out flavorful foods of different cuisines.
- Encourage children to drink water when thirsty rather than sugary drinks.

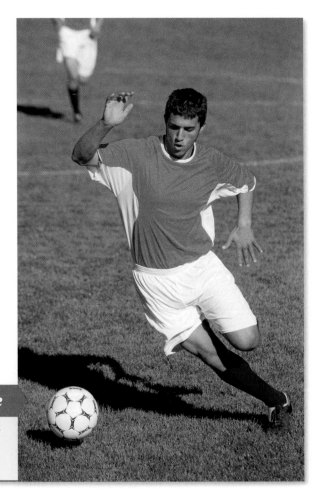

Eat to Compete

Successful physical and mental performance requires good nutrition. *Why do teen athletes need to make sure to get enough carbohydrates and water?*

Nutrition and Special Needs

Children with special physical, emotional, or cognitive needs may need extra help with eating and nutrition. A child with limited mobility, for example, may need family support to follow a low-calorie eating plan. A child with a physical disability may need extra time to learn self-feeding skills.

Some physical disorders can cause nutritional challenges. For example, metabolic disorders can prevent the body from absorbing nutrients.

Caregivers, family members, physicians, and dietitians need to work together to help children with special needs cope with daily challenges. Caregivers may need to learn special skills, such as how to use a feeding tube or how to respond to disruptive behavior at mealtime.

✓ **Reading Check** **Explain** Why are small servings of food and regular snacks appropriate for children?

Adolescence

Adolescence is the second most rapid growth period of life. Dramatic physical changes increase a teen's need for almost all nutrients. Iron and calcium are especially important for building muscle and bone, which continues even after growth stops.

During growth spurts, teens' calorie and nutrient needs increase. Every teen's growth rate is different, and your needs are different from your friends' needs. Base your food choices on your own body cues, such as hunger and height gain. You may need to resist **peer pressure**, the influence of people in your age group, to eat more or less than you need.

Nutrition for Teen Athletes

Conditioning and nutrition are the keys to top athletic performance. Daily food choices can make the difference between a good performance and a poor one. Without proper nutrition, an athlete will not be able to achieve his or her maximum athletic potential.

Be a Smart Consumer

Sports Drinks vs. Water

Sports drinks contain several ingredients that distinguish them from plain water. These include electrolytes, which are salts that conduct electricity and are found naturally in the body, carbohydrates, which are the main source of energy in the human body, and vitamins. In addition, most sports drinks contain artificial colors, flavors, and sugar. The most useful ingredients in sports drinks are carbohydrates, which feed muscles and delay fatigue during a workout. To reap the benefits of a sports drink, consume 8 ounces twenty minutes before exercise and 4-6 ounces every 15 minutes during exercise.

Challenge List three situations when a sports drink would be an appropriate choice, and three situations when water would be better.

Most athletes can meet their nutrition needs by following the Dietary Guidelines for Americans. Athletes who eat a varied, nutritious diet do not need sports bars or dietary supplements. Extra protein from foods or supplements does no good and can be harmful. All athletes should make sure to get enough carbohydrates and water.

Carbohydrate Needs

Carbohydrates are the body's source of glucose, which is used for energy. Extra carbohydrates are stored in the liver and muscles as glycogen. Glycogen fuels the body during vigorous, extended periods of training and competition, when an athlete may use two or three times as much energy as the average person. When glycogen runs out, so does energy.

Athletes need to eat plenty of carbohydrates to build their glycogen stores. Teen athletes should get 55 to 60 percent of their daily calories from carbohydrates, 20 to 25 percent from fat, and 15 to 20 percent from protein.

Water Needs

During a strenuous workout, you can lose up to 5 quarts of water through perspiration.

To avoid dehydration, athletes should drink water before and after an event, even if they do not feel thirsty. Athletes should also drink water about every 15 minutes during an event. Do not wait for thirst, which signals that dehydration has already begun.

How much water do you need to drink? An athlete should drink two ounces of water for every three pounds he or she weighs. So, an athlete who weighs 100 pounds should drink 66 ounces of water per day.

Sugary beverages can cause stomach cramps, diarrhea, and nausea. Dilute them with water or drink plain water instead. Sports drinks that contain carbohydrates and electrolytes are valuable for activities lasting longer than 90 minutes. Salt, potassium, and other minerals lost in shorter events are easily replaced through meals and snacks.

Even well-hydrated athletes should never exercise in extreme heat and humidity. The result can be heat exhaustion or heat stroke.

Pre-Event Meals

If you eat just before a competition, the digestive process competes with your muscles for energy. Eat three to four hours before an event to allow time for proper digestion.

A good pre-event meal features foods high in complex carbohydrates. Fats and proteins take longer to digest than carbohydrates. Sugary foods can cause a sudden rise and fall in blood sugar levels, leaving energy stores empty. Eat familiar foods that you enjoy and drink at least two cups of fluids.

Soon after a hard workout, refuel the body with nutritious foods and fluids. Popular choices include juice and a bagel, a bowl of cereal with fruit and milk, or fruit and yogurt. Your body will convert the carbohydrates to glycogen to **replenish** your energy supply.

✓ **Reading Check** **Identify** Why don't all teens have the same calorie and nutrient needs?

Careers in Food

Cheryl Lesiak
Food Technologist/Test Kitchen Professional

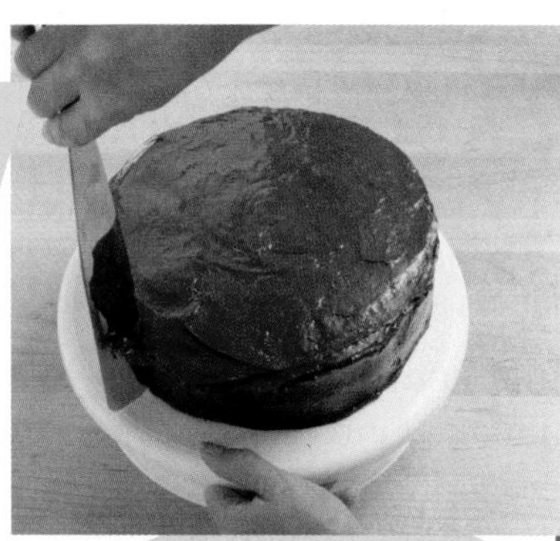

Q: What does a food technologist do?

A: Food technologists create new food products. We look at restaurants, at recipes, at what is happening in the world with food. We take ideas and turn them into products—starting from scratch in the kitchen all the way to manufacturing.

Q: What are some of your responsibilities?

A: I test ingredients and new food products in the lab, checking for cook times, ease of use, taste, and nutritional value. I also work with suppliers of various ingredients to find information I can use in the lab.

Q: What do you love about your job?

A: I love to cook. I love to bake, and I love to experiment. I have taken two things I like very much, cooking and science, and put them together as a career.

"I get to bake cakes for a living!"
— Cheryl Lesiak
Senior Food Technologist
Duncan Hines–Cherry Hill, NJ

Education and Training

A degree in food sciences and nutrition is required for many positions. Culinary school background and other experience with food is useful.

Qualities and Skills

Food scientists need the ability to apply statistical techniques and use computers to analyze data.

Related Career Opportunities

Related careers include research chef, product developer, research technician, and laboratory technician.

Nutrition for Older Adults

Calorie needs drop in older adulthood, but nutrition needs rise. *Why should older adults choose nutrient-dense foods?*

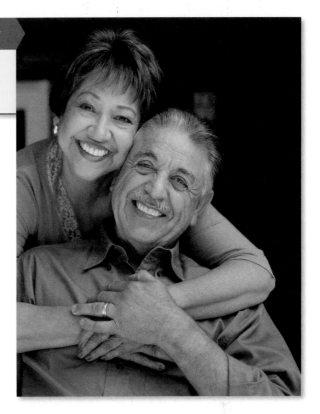

Adulthood

Many adults face a nutrition **dilemma**, or problem. They need the same amount of nutrients as they get older, but they need fewer calories. The demands of work and family leave less time for exercise and balanced meals. Adults may find their weight rising, along with their risk of heart disease, various types of cancer, and other assorted health problems.

It is easier and healthier to maintain a healthy weight than to gain weight and then try to lose it. Adults need to choose a variety of healthful, low-calorie foods and make regular physical activity a priority. Your study of foods and nutrition today can help you keep those commitments as an adult.

Nutrition Check

Educate to Encourage

In the United States, the incidence of childhood obesity has grown dramatically. Too many children eat high-calorie foods that are low in nutrients. Good eating habits begin in early childhood and can last a lifetime, and parents and other caregivers have the most influence over how well a child eats. Education may be the key to improving children's eating habits. When parents have the information they need to encourage good eating habits in their children, they are more likely to promote positive changes.

Think About It Using one or more tips for encouraging good eating habits in children, design a colorful, educational poster. Imagine your poster will be displayed in a supermarket to help caregivers teach their children to develop good eating habits.

Older Adults

Good nutrition plays a major role in wellness and disease prevention in older age. Healthy food helps older adults and seniors stay healthy, active, and energetic. Calorie needs drop in older adulthood, but nutrition needs often rise. Aging and disease cause the body to use some nutrients, notably calcium and vitamins D and B_{12}, less efficiently. Older adults must therefore take in more of these nutrients than younger adults. Low-fat milk and yogurt are good sources of these nutrients, and are easy to eat for people who have trouble chewing. To make every calorie count, older people should choose nutrient-dense foods.

Thirst signals also decline with age, although fluid needs remain the same. Older people need to make a point of drinking eight cups of water, milk, or juice each day. Moist foods, such as soups and cooked cereals, add fluids and ease chewing problems. Milk-based beverages and homemade smoothies boost nutrition without many calories. As the sense of taste and smell weaken, older adults can keep meals appealing with flavorful foods and seasonings.

Nutrition Challenges

Older adults face challenges that can get in the way of healthy eating. Seniors who live alone or on fixed incomes may not have the desire or the means to prepare nourishing meals. It may take longer to prepare meals.

Lifestyle changes also affect food choices. Older adults may have health problems that require a special diet and limit the foods they can eat. Disabilities can make kitchen tasks painful. The death of loved ones can depress the appetite as well as the spirit.

Most older adults want to stay independent for as long as possible. To do this, they can use the same strategies used by busy families, such as buying convenience foods, cooking ahead and freezing meals. Health care aides can teach new cooking skills to people with physical limitations.

Social service programs in many communities address all of these needs. At churches and community centers, older people can share good meals and the company of others for a modest price. Community services may provide shopping and meal assistance. Volunteer groups and public agencies put together food baskets and deliver meals. Through nutrition education and screening, they help older adults make good food choices for their individual health needs.

Families and neighbors can take an active role as well. Go grocery shopping for an older relative or invite an elderly neighbor for a meal. This kindness satisfies more than a nutrition need—it nourishes the whole person.

Light and Healthy Recipe

Pre-Game Pasta

Pasta with pear slices, walnuts, and a light dressing provides long-term and short-term energy.

Ingredients

- **2 cups** Bowtie pasta
- **2** Diced pears
- **2 Tbsp.** Walnuts
- **2 Tbsp.** Balsamic vinegar
- **1 Tbsp.** Olive oil
- **1 Tbsp.** Lime juice
- **½ tsp.** Finely chopped mint

Directions

1. Bring a large pot of water to a boil and add the pasta. Stir to make sure the pasta does not stick to itself.
2. While the water is heating and the pasta is cooking, dice the pears and crush the walnuts.
3. In a separate bowl, mix the vinegar, olive oil, lime juice and mint.
4. Test the pasta to see if it is done. When it is finished cooking, drain the pasta in a colander and rinse it with cold water.
5. In a large serving bowl, mix the pasta with the pears and walnuts. Mix gently so that the pasta does not break. Pour on the vinaigrette and mix again.
6. Serve cold in bowls.

Yield 4 servings

Nutrition Analysis per Serving

■ Calories	374
■ Total fat	7 g
Saturated fat	1 g
Cholesterol	0 mg
■ Sodium	6 mg
■ Carbohydrate	70
Dietary fiber	5 g
Sugars	13 g
■ Protein	11 g

CHAPTER 13 Review & Applications

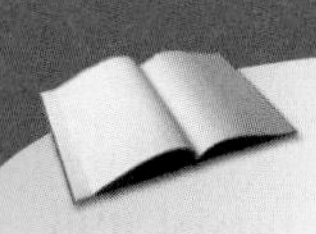

After You Read

Chapter Summary

There are five stages to the human life span, and each brings its own growth and nutrition needs. Pregnant women should use MyPyramid for Moms to promote good nutrition during the prenatal period. To provide nutrition during infancy, caregivers can breastfeed or bottle-feed infants before transitioning to solid foods. There are several ways to encourage good eating habits in children, to provide a large selection of nutritious foods, and to meet their special needs. Adolescents have an increased need for almost all nutrients. Good nutrition helps teen athletes perform optimally. It also promotes wellness and disease prevention in adulthood.

Content and Academic Vocabulary Review

1. Write your own definition for each of these content and academic vocabulary words.

Content Vocabulary

- ☐ life span (p. 176)
- ☐ fetus (p. 176)
- ☐ obstetrician (p. 177)
- ☐ osteoporosis (p. 177)
- ☐ colostrum (p. 180)
- ☐ lactation (p. 180)
- ☐ pediatrician (p. 181)
- ☐ peer pressure (p. 183)

Academic Vocabulary

- replenish (p. 184)
- delemma (p. 185)

Review Key Concepts

2. **List** the five stages of the life span.
3. **Evaluate** why good nutrition is important to a fetus and the mother.
4. **Compare and contrast** breast feeding and bottle feeding.
5. **Explain** why snacks are important to a child's diet.
6. **Explain** why nutrient needs increase during your teens.
7. **Explain** why calorie needs drop in older adulthood but nutrition needs often rise.

Critical Thinking

8. **Explain** why a woman pregnant with twins should not start a weight-loss diet because she is five pounds over the 35-pound weight-gain limit in her eighth month.
9. **Describe** a parent's reasons for offering a young son "trees" of broccoli. The parent also puts raisins on sliced celery smeared with peanut butter and calls it "ants on a log."
10. **Identify** why elderly people need more of certain nutrients than young people.

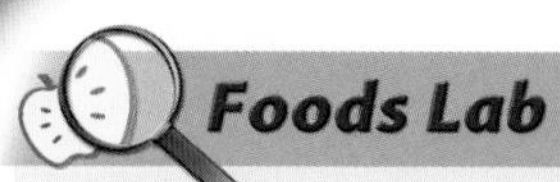

Foods Lab

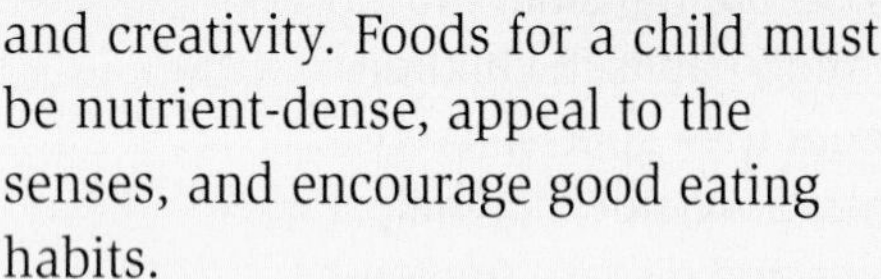

11. Recipes for Children Preparing food for children requires thoughtfulness and creativity. Foods for a child must be nutrient-dense, appeal to the senses, and encourage good eating habits.

Procedure Create and prepare a recipe for a healthful snack for a five-year-old. Consider nutrition, appeal, self-feeding skills, and taste preferences of children at that age. Give your recipe a name.

Analysis Write answers to each of the following questions: What colors, tastes, textures, or other techniques did you use to make the recipe appealing? What nutrients does it supply? How could a child help prepare the recipe?

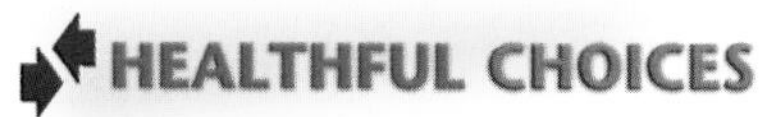

HEALTHFUL CHOICES

12. Newborn Nutrition Cleo is the new mother of a healthy baby. Cleo produces breast milk and takes no medications. Her mother-in-law tells her to breast-feed her baby. Her mother tells her to feed the baby formula. What other factors should Cleo consider? Which choice would be most healthful and why? How can Cleo's mother-in-law and mother help Cleo with her choice?

TECH Connection

13. Eating Plan for Pregnancy Develop a one-week eating plan that meets nutrition guidelines for a pregnant woman in the third trimester of her pregnancy. Use My-Pyramid for Moms to construct the eating plan. Consider that the pregnant woman works full time and is moderately active. Use computer software to create a chart that shows your meal recommendations for each day of the week. Include a list of nutrient amounts recommended and the amounts found in your eating plan.

Real-World Skills

Problem-Solving Skills

14. Infant Digestion James, a one-month-old infant, has a hard time digesting cow's milk. His mother cannot breastfeed because she takes medication that would be harmful to James. How can James get the nutrients he needs?

Interpersonal and Collaborative Skills

15. Pre-Event Meal Follow your teacher's instructions to form groups. Collaborate with your group to plan a pre-event meal for one of your school's sports teams. Select recipes that fulfill nutrition requirements. If possible, use the food lab to prepare the meal for the team.

Financial Literacy Skills

16. Provide Nutrition Advice Since retiring, Mary's fixed income means she buys less food. How can she still obtain adequate nutrients?

Academic Skills

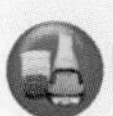

Food Science

17. Practice Pureeing Purees are made by crushing food tissue, breaking apart cells and cell walls. Purees are fluid versions of the original tissue. Most purees are cooked first to soften cell walls.

Procedure Peel, core, and cut up three apples into chunks and put them in a pan. Cover with cold water. Cover and cook until fork tender, then drain most of the water. Mash the apples with a fork. Adjust the consistency by cooking over low heat.

Analysis Write a paragraph describing the experience. How long did it take for the apples to get tender? How would you make this into a smoother consistency?

NSES B Develop an understanding of the structure and properties of matter.

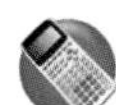

Mathematics

18. Measure Weight and Volume A dry ounce is a measure of weight. A fluid ounce is measure of volume. Fill an eight-ounce measuring cup with flour and weigh it. Empty the cup, fill it with water, and weigh it. How much does the water weigh. How much does the flour weigh? As a percentage, how much heavier is the water than the flour?

Math Concept **Transform Fractions into Decimals** Fractions and decimals are parts of a whole. Use long division to divide the numerator by the denominator to transform a fraction into a decimal.

Starting Hint Divide the weight of the water by the weight of the flour. Then transform the result from a decimal into a percentage.

NCTM Measurement Understand measurable attributes of objects and the units, systems, and processes of measurement.

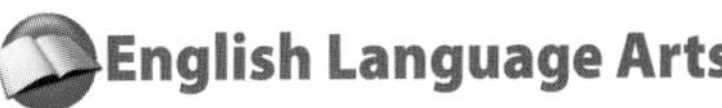

English Language Arts

19. Create an Invitation Use computer software or art supplies to design and write an invitation for a children's potluck party. Your invitation should explain the party's theme, date, time, and place. The theme should be about healthful eating for children. It should also include a descriptive list of 6 healthful snacks that reflect the theme of the party.

NCTE 12 Use language to accomplish individual purposes.

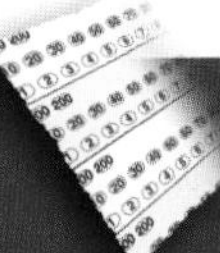

STANDARDIZED TEST PRACTICE

READING COMPREHENSION

Re-read the section on older adults on page 185. Then select the best answer to the question.

20. Aging and disease cause the body to ________________________.

  a. use some nutrients less efficiently.
  b. lose some nutrients through illness.
  c. absorb greater quantities of nutrients, leading to weight gain.
  d. need fewer fluids due to less activity.

Test-Taking Tip Before you answer a reading comprehension question, closely read the text to which the question refers. Then read through the question and each of the answer choices. Next, take a second look at the text to confirm which answer is correct. Some answers may seem identical, but they contain subtle differences. Pay attention to every word.

UNIT 3

Thematic Project

Eating for Health

In this unit you have learned that each stage in the human life span brings its own growth and nutrition needs. You also learned that adolescents have an increased need for all nutrients. In this project, you will create a food rubric and talk with a professional. You will also develop a personal food plan that will include healthier options.

My Journal

If you completed the journal entry from page 131, refer to it to see if your thoughts have changed after reading the unit and completing this project.

Project Assignment

- Create a rubric of foods from each food group that you enjoy.
- Arrange to talk with someone qualified to discuss food, nutrition, and healthful food choices for adolescents.
- Use what you learn in the interview to develop a one-week personal eating plan that includes healthful options.

Academic Skills You Will Use

English Language Arts

NCTE 4 Use written language to communicate effectively.

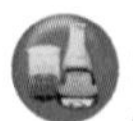

Science

NSES F Develop understanding of personal and community health; population growth; natural resources; environmental quality; natural and human-induced hazards; science and technology in local, national, and global challenges.

STEP 1 Create a Food Rubric

To help you make the best and most healthful food choices throughout your life, it is useful to make a food list. First, write down all the names of the healthful foods that you already enjoy. Then add to the list some of the healthful foods that you would like to try. You can add new foods whenever you find one that you enjoy, and use the rubric to plan future meals.

Create a spreadsheet with six columns. Label each column at the top with the name of one of the five food groups: grains, vegetables, fruits, milk, and meat and beans. The sixth column is for the oils category. In the rows under each heading, list foods from each food group that you enjoy and that will help you make healthful food choices. This rubric can serve as your menu-planning guide. Keep it in a handy place in your kitchen for easy reference.

STEP 2 Choose Someone to Interview

Choose someone qualified to interview about food and nutrition. Before the interview, think about the questions you would like to ask him or her. Write them down for easy reference during the interview. Focus the interview on the ways in which food choices affect aspects of a person's health and well-being. If your conversation takes place in person, bring the rubric that you have created to the interview. If your interview is taking place over the telephone, mail, e-mail or fax the rubric to your interviewee in advance of your interview time. Discuss the items that are in your rubric and ask for advice about other nutritious food choices to add to create a well-rounded menu plan. Examples of people to interview include:

- Registered dietitian
- Medical doctor
- Nurse

Writing Skills

- Use complete sentences.
- Use proper spelling and grammar.
- Organize your interview questions in the order you want to ask them.

STEP 3 Connect to Your Community

Interview a member of the community who is qualified to discuss food and nutrition. Use the interview questions you wrote in step 2. Ask the professional to help you evaluate your food rubric and to make suggestions for your menu plan.

Interviewing Skills

- Include in your notes any additional thoughts and ideas that occur to you during the interview, such as other sources to check and more questions to ask.
- Listen attentively.
- Record responses and take notes.
- When you transcribe your notes, write in complete sentences and use correct spelling and grammar.

STEP 4 Create Your Menu Plan

Use the Unit Thematic Project Checklist to plan and complete your project and evaluate your work.

STEP 5 Evaluate Project

Your project will be evaluated based on:

- Thoroughness in creating your food rubric.
- Thought devoted to developing your menu plan.
- Content of your visual representation.
- Mechanics — presentation and neatness.

Unit Thematic Project Checklist

Category	Objectives
Plan	☑ Create a rubric complete with healthful food choices you can use to create a realistic menu plan for your daily life.
	☑ Interview someone qualified to discuss food and nutrition, and take notes during the interview.
Create	☑ Use your rubric to create a menu plan for one week that includes breakfast, lunch, dinner, and snacks.
	☑ Include a variety of food group foods in the proper portion sizes in each meal.
	☑ Turn in your food rubric, interview notes, and menu plan to your teacher.
Academic Skills	☑ Be creative when writing your menu plan.
	☑ Adapt and modify language to suit different purposes.

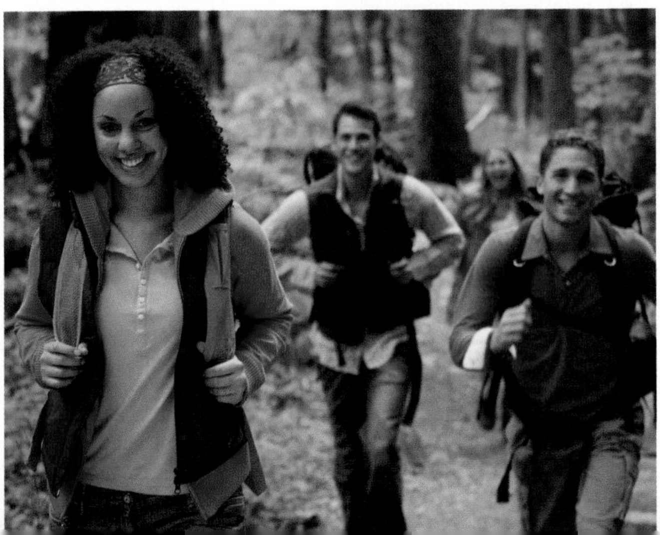

Go to this book's Online Learning Center through **glencoe.com** for a rubric you can use to evaluate your final project.

UNIT 4

Food Decisions

Activate Prior Knowledge

Explore the Photo Shopping for good, healthful foods takes skill. *How do you plan for a grocery shopping trip?*

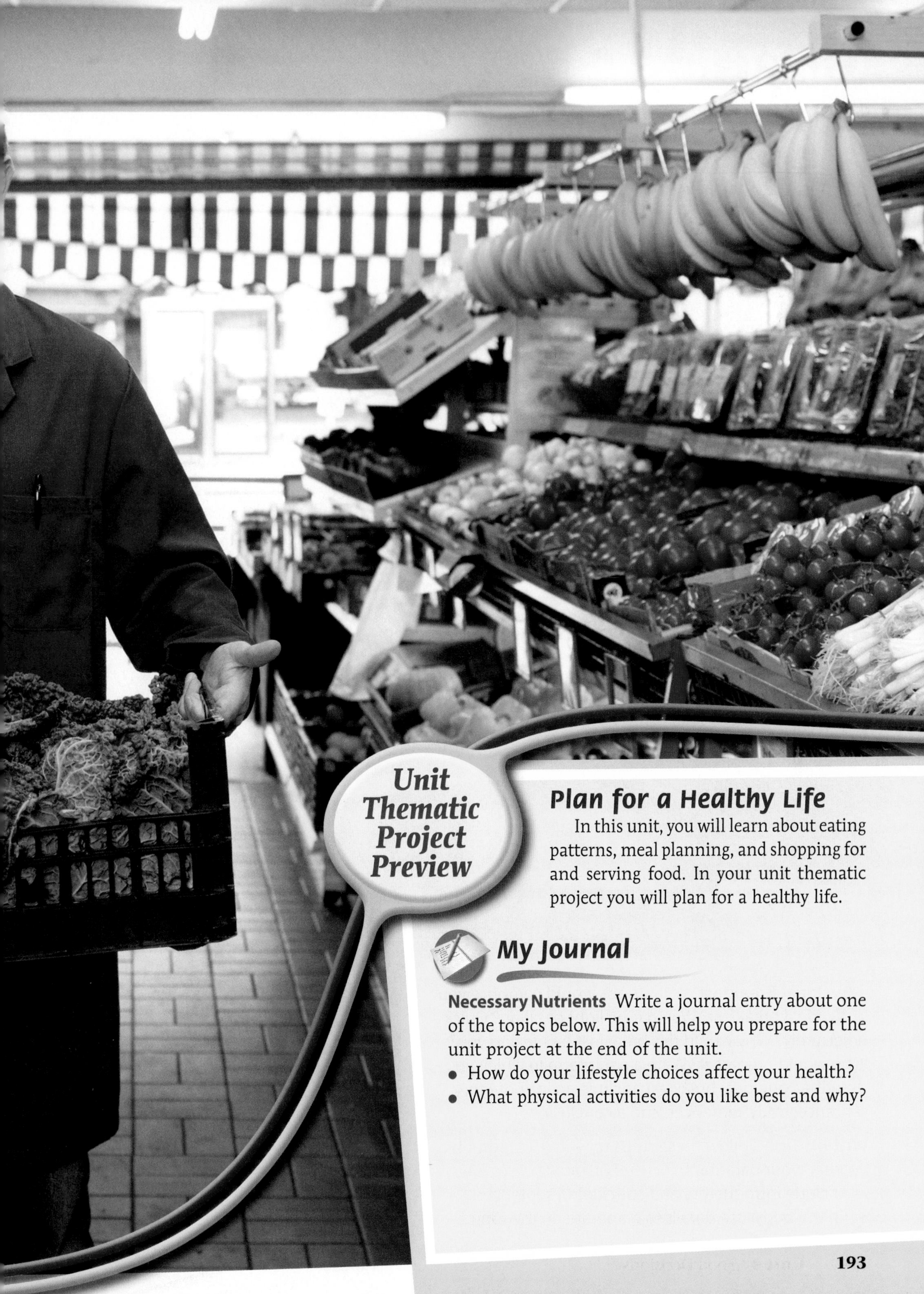

Unit Thematic Project Preview

Plan for a Healthy Life

In this unit, you will learn about eating patterns, meal planning, and shopping for and serving food. In your unit thematic project you will plan for a healthy life.

My Journal

Necessary Nutrients Write a journal entry about one of the topics below. This will help you prepare for the unit project at the end of the unit.

- How do your lifestyle choices affect your health?
- What physical activities do you like best and why?

CHAPTER 14

Eating Patterns

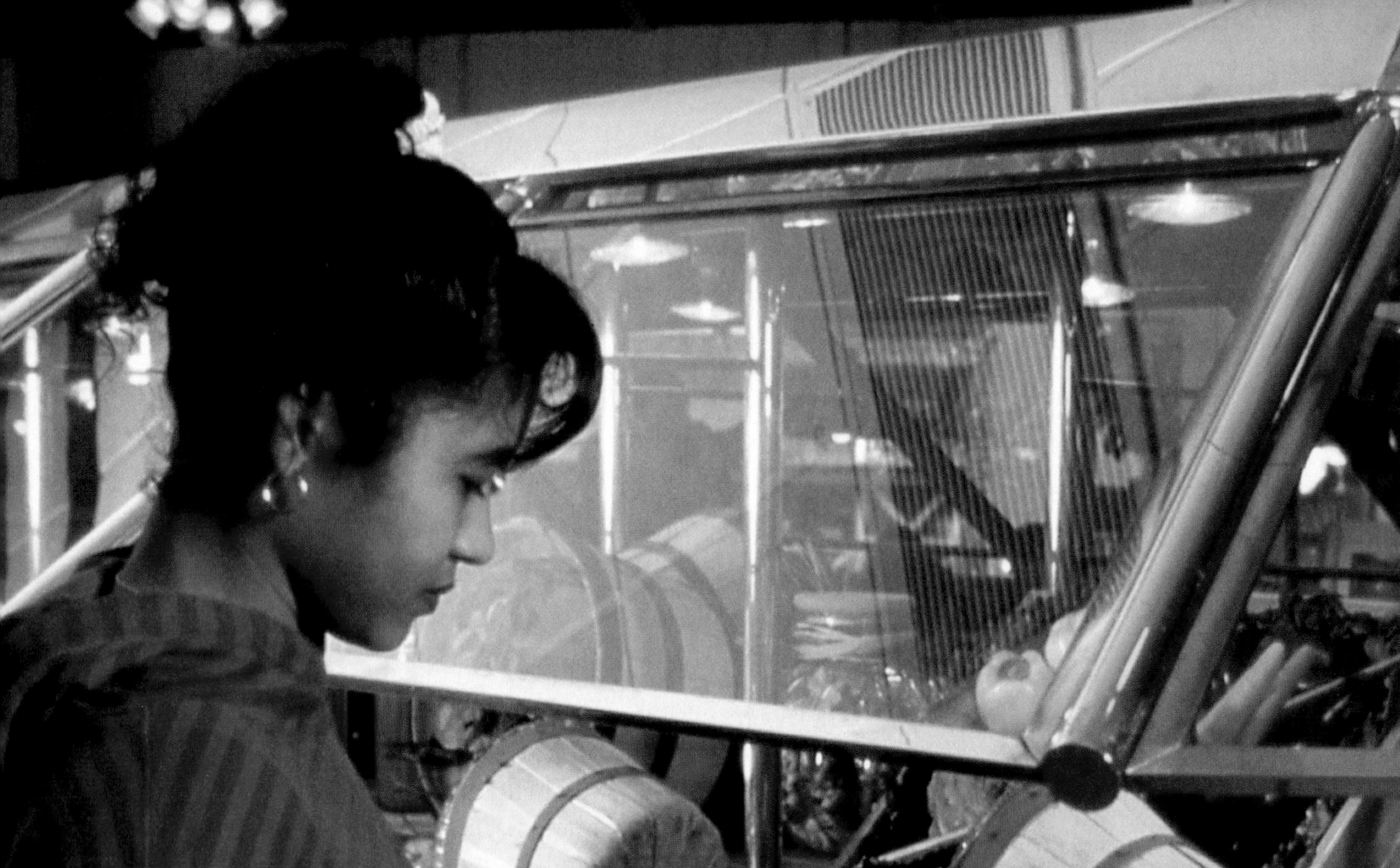

Writing Activity — Paragraph

An Ideal Breakfast What foods would comprise your ideal breakfast? Would it be light or filling? Quick or leisurely? Why would this breakfast be ideal to you? Who would prepare it? Write a paragraph in which you describe your ideal breakfast. Include an introductory sentence, body sentences, and a conclusion.

Writing Tips Follow these steps to write a paragraph:

- Keep your paragraph focused on one topic or idea.
- Include introductory and concluding sentences.
- In the body, use details to elaborate on the topic.

Activate Prior Knowledge

Explore the Photo It is possible to make healthful food choices in all kinds of circumstances. *How can you eat healthfully while dining out?*

Reading Guide

Before You Read

Preview Look through the chapter and examine the photos and their captions. Based on what you see, write one sentence in your own words about eating patterns.

Read to Learn

Key Concepts

- **Identify** different influences on food choices.
- **Explain** historical and current eating patterns.
- **Discuss** choices for dining out and how to do so healthfully.
- **Explain** why and how people should evaluate their food choices.
- **Explain** how to make good decisions about food.

Main Idea

Eating patterns are shaped by many factors, and it is possible to make healthful food choices in a variety of circumstances.

Content Vocabulary

You will find definitions for these words in the glossary at the back of this book.

- ☐ resources
- ☐ values
- ☐ perishable
- ☐ eating patterns
- ☐ grazing
- ☐ entree

Academic Vocabulary

You will find these words in your reading and on your tests. Use the glossary to look up their definitions if necessary.

- significant
- reinforce

Graphic Organizer

Use a graphic organizer like the one below to take notes about choices for dining out and what each choice offers.

FULL-SERVICE RESTAURANTS	SELF-SERVE RESTAURANTS	FAST-FOOD RESTAURANTS

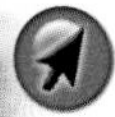

Graphic Organizer Go to this book's Online Learning Center at **glencoe.com** to print out this graphic organizer.

Academic Standards

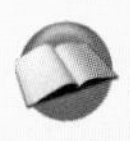

English Language Arts

NCTE 12 Use language to accomplish individual purposes.

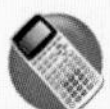

Mathematics

NCTM Number and Operations Understand numbers, ways of representing numbers, relationships among numbers, and number systems.

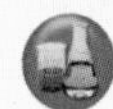

Science

NSES B Develop an understanding of chemical reactions.

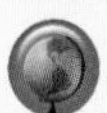

Social Studies

NCSS V F Individuals, Groups, and Institutions Evaluate the role of institutions in furthering both continuity and change.

NCTE *National Council of Teachers of English*
NCTM *National Council of Teachers of Mathematics*
NSES *National Science Education Standards*
NCSS *National Council for the Social Studies*

What Influences Your Food Choices?

You can learn a lot about yourself by investigating your food habits and choices. Important influences on your food choices include the resources available to you, local customs, messages from the media, and your individual preferences and habits.

Resources

Resources are people, things, and qualities that can help you reach a goal. This textbook is a resource that helps you learn about food and nutrition. Time is a resource.

Your food choices depend on the resources available to you. For example, the greater your food budget is, the wider your eating options are. If you have cooking skills, you can try more recipes and new foods.

You can often substitute one resource for another that is in short supply. If you have more time and skills than money, you can make delicious dishes with less costly foods. Businesses often use information on resource use to plan menus and set prices.

Family Food Customs

For most people, family is the most powerful influence on food choices. Children learn food preferences and habits from the example of older family members. For example, you may have learned to like—or dislike—certain foods because they were served at home. Parents foster eating habits their children will carry throughout their lives.

Families often enjoy special food customs handed down through generations. Such customs can create memories and family bonds. In one family, every young adult learns to make the "secret recipe" at Thanksgiving.

Food customs can unite families with a sense of pride and identity in their cultural heritage. Jewish families, for example, eat matzo (unleavened bread), hard-boiled egg, and other symbolic foods at the Passover Seder.

Friends

Food and friendship go together. In fact, the word companion comes from the Latin for "with bread." Sharing tastes in food fosters a sense of belonging and identity, especially during the teen years.

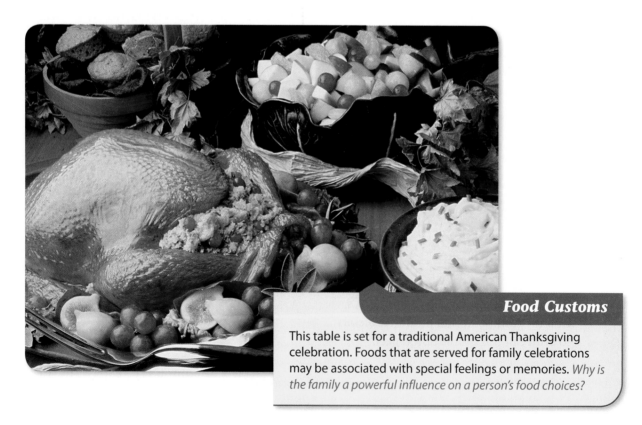

Food Customs

This table is set for a traditional American Thanksgiving celebration. Foods that are served for family celebrations may be associated with special feelings or memories. *Why is the family a powerful influence on a person's food choices?*

Many teens feel pressure to make food choices that please their friends. In the school cafeteria, you might plan on the baked fish and fruit salad—until friends ask for pizza and french fries. Friends can have a positive influence, too. Friends of different cultural backgrounds can share new food choices, and friends can offer each other support for healthy eating habits.

The Media

Advertisements and news reports can alert you to food trends, new products, and the latest nutrition advice. They can also persuade you to choose certain foods and avoid others.

Advertising is a powerful influence. People often respond to ads without even realizing it. People may buy a snack because the package makes it seem fun, or try a cereal because a television commercial promises health benefits.

Use the principles covered in Chapter 10 about evaluating information. Become aware of the media's influence on you. Measure products and claims using logic rather than emotion.

Personal Influences

Your food choices do not depend entirely on external forces. They also depend on your lifestyle and your choices.

Daily Routine

Your daily routine affects your food choices. If you are rushed in the morning, for example, you might grab a cereal bar instead of preparing a full breakfast. If you have lots of school activities, you might find yourself too busy for a regular lunch or dinner. If you have an after-school job, you may choose different foods on days you work than on days when you eat at home.

It is important to follow healthy food habits even if you have a busy schedule. As teens gain independence, they have more choices about what, when, and where to eat. One part of independence is taking good care of yourself by planning healthful meals and snacks.

Be a Smart Consumer

Assess Advertisements

Have you ever been influenced by advertising to make unhealthful food choices? How can you avoid this in the future? Try to assess advertisements with a critical eye and ear. Determine what message an advertisement is trying to send, and decide whether it is logical. Then identify the specific claims advertisements make. For example, will drinking a certain brand of sports drink make you a better athlete? Why or why not? Can eating one type of cereal make you lose weight? Use the knowledge you already have and conduct research to assess the truthfulness of claims in advertising.

Challenge Identify the claims of a print or television ad for a food product. Write a paragraph explaining whether the claims are based on actual nutrition facts.

Values

Values are beliefs and concepts that a person holds as important. People make choices based on their personal values. Someone who believes that eating local is important might shop at a farmers' market, for example.

As a teen, you are developing the critical thinking skills to determine your own values. You also have more chances to act on your values. Learning about foods and nutrition can help you make food choices that support your values.

Emotions

Your emotional state can strongly influence your food choices. For example, you may reach for comfort foods when you feel stressed or unhappy.

Food carries strong associations, both pleasant and unpleasant. For one person, corn on the cob may bring back happy memories of summer grill parties. For another, it may be a reminder of working long hours every summer in a vegetable processing plant.

✓ **Reading Check** **Identify** For most people, what is the most powerful influence on food choices?

Eating Patterns

Eating patterns are a mix of food customs and habits that include when, what, and how much people eat. Eating patterns vary over time and among different cultures. For example, a breakfast of rice, dried sardines, and pickled vegetables would not be a typical breakfast in many American homes, but it would be a typical breakfast in a Korean home.

Family Eating Patterns and History

Eating patterns have changed over the centuries along with changes in society. Until the Industrial Revolution that began in the mid-1800s, extended families often lived, worked, and ate together. Families worked together to produce food through hunting, fishing, or raising crops. Preparing food took most of the day for women and older girls.

As families moved to the city in the 1800s and 1900s, they adopted new food habits. Mealtimes depended on job schedules. More foods were available, and waves of immigrants introduced a wide range of cuisines. Diners sprang up, as men arrived from rural areas in search of work and in need of places to eat.

The 1930s and 1940s

Families of the 1930s struggled through the Depression, when necessities such as bread were very costly. Scraps and leftovers were saved for casseroles, hashes, and other thrifty, filling recipes.

Food shortages continued in the 1940s, during World War II. Massive food shipments to troops overseas required rationing, or food allowances, at home. Each family member received a ration book with coupons that listed what food could be bought. Having the coupons, however, was no guarantee of finding the food. Many staples, especially butter, sugar, meat, and canned goods, were scarce or unavailable. Eggs, cheese, and fish, which were too perishable to ship to troops, became popular protein foods. A **perishable** food is one that can spoil quickly. Growing and canning vegetables from home gardens, nicknamed victory gardens, kept millions of families from going hungry.

World War II had other **significant**, or important, impacts on eating habits. Women became a major part of the labor force, working long shifts in factories and shipyards. They relied more on convenience foods, such as boxed dessert mixes and boxed macaroni and cheese dinners. Military technology led to the invention of instant rice and microwave ovens.

Some troops fighting in the war developed health problems from poor nutrition. This spurred the federal government to develop food guides based on nutrition research. In 1943, the Food and Nutrition Board of the National Research Council developed the first recommended daily allowances (RDAs). They specified levels of nutrients needed for almost all healthy people in the United States. Food and nutrition guides play a large role in people's food choices.

The 1950s

With relative peace and prosperity in the 1950s, many women gave up their jobs outside the home. New appliances and new technologies saved time in the kitchen and encouraged home cooks to prepare interesting, nutritious family meals. More diverse restaurants became more common throughout the country.

Nutrition Check

Smart Choices at School

Just as at a restaurant, students face decisions about food while at school. In the past, some schools have included outlets of national fast-food franchises. This earned income for the schools, and students liked the fast food. Parents and educators, however, worried that this encouraged unhealthful eating. In response, some school districts have created their own low-fat recipes for popular fast foods. Others are working with students to find appealing, healthful options.

Think About It What food options do you think schools should provide for students? How healthful are the options that your school provides? Ask your school principal how decisions are made about your school's food offerings.

A Healthy Start

After a full night's sleep, your body and brain need to "break" the "fast" with breakfast. Everyone can incorporate at least a small breakfast into their routine. *What is wrong with eating a donut for breakfast?*

Recent Decades

Changes continue to affect how and what we eat. Shifting social and family roles, new nutrition discoveries, and evolving food technology have all strongly influenced our food habits. Today, for example, Americans spend about half their food budget on eating away from home. More men are helping to cook for the family. Consumers are also demanding more healthful and organic menu options, which is changing the way many restaurants do business.

Stages of Family Life

Like individuals, families go through different stages. Family eating patterns change as circumstances change.

While young children are at home, families tend to eat meals together. If parents are employed, take-out meals may be common. As children become teens with hearty appetites, food costs go up. Teens can also eat out on their own, giving them more food choices.

When children have grown and left the family home, spending on food and other child-related costs may go down. Family members may have the time and money to eat out more frequently or try new foods. Older adults often become less active and eat lighter meals. Health concerns may play a greater role in food choices.

Daily Meal Patterns

Regular daily meals—breakfast, midday, and evening—give you nutrition and energy. In most cultures, meals are also a relaxing, enjoyable time. Many people use mealtime to give thanks for a secure food supply.

Breakfast

When you get up in the morning, you may have been fasting for 10 or 12 hours. Breakfast gives you much-needed energy. That is why breakfast is often called the most important meal of the day.

Breakfast also helps you feel alert throughout the morning. Research reveals that students who eat breakfast do better in school than those who go without it.

Not all breakfasts are equal, however. A nutritious combination of carbohydrates, proteins, and a little fat—a bowl of cereal and fruit, for example—gives long-lasting energy. A high-sugar, high-fat breakfast, such as a doughnut and soda or coffee, provides a spurt of energy that quickly fades.

Midday and Evening Meals

The midday and evening meals go by different names, depending on their size and on the area of the country. Most Americans eat a light midday meal, or lunch. The largest meal of the day, traditionally called dinner, is served in the evening, often at a time when family members can eat together. In some cultures, people eat the largest meal at midday and a lighter meal, sometimes called supper, in the evening.

Some individuals and families change their usual pattern on weekends or special occasions. On Sunday, for instance, they may eat dinner as their midday meal, and have a light supper in the evening. Another choice is brunch, a late morning meal that combines breakfast and lunch.

All of these meal patterns can be healthful. Some nutritionists recommend that you get most of your calories by mid-afternoon and use the evening meal to fill in any nutrition gaps in the day's food choices. Some people find they sleep better if their evening meal is light. As long as the midday meal supplies the energy and nutrients to carry you through the rest of the day, you can follow the pattern that fits your personal preference and schedule.

Grazing

Many people prefer an eating pattern called grazing. **Grazing** is eating five or more small meals throughout the day instead of three large ones. Someone might have a vegetable salad during a work break, for example, and a sandwich later at home.

Grazing can be as healthful as more conventional meal patterns, and it can work well for people with busy schedules. Grazing may also help control appetite and calorie intake. Grazing is not healthy, however, if it turns into continuous snacking. Overeating and poor nutrition can result if people lose track of their food choices. Healthful grazing takes the same planning as eating three larger meals. By day's end, you should still have taken in the needed nutrients from a variety of wholesome foods.

Snacks

A snack is a small amount of food eaten between meals. Snacking can help meet teens' increased nutrient and calorie needs. Choose snack foods carefully—many are high in fat and added sugar.

Pay attention to serving size when choosing snacks. A cup of tortilla chips is a snack, but when covered with refried beans and cheese, it has the calories of a meal. Watch timing too.

If you snack too close to mealtime, you may miss out on nutrients because you are too full to eat. Limit snacks while watching television. It is easy to overeat when you are not paying attention.

Many people like crunchy snacks, so they reach for chips and cookies, which are high in fat and added sugars. More nutritious choices are apples, carrots, whole-grain cereal or breadsticks.

Any healthful food that you enjoy at a meal can make a good snack if it fits your eating plan for the day. A bowl of soup, a slice of pizza, or leftover pasta salad may be just what you need when hunger strikes.

✓ Reading Check **Explain** Why should students always make sure to eat breakfast?

Choices for Dining Out

Americans buy about 70 billion meals and snacks from restaurants, caterers, food carts, and vendors each year. In fact, Americans spend about $300 billion on restaurant food alone—almost half the money spent on food.

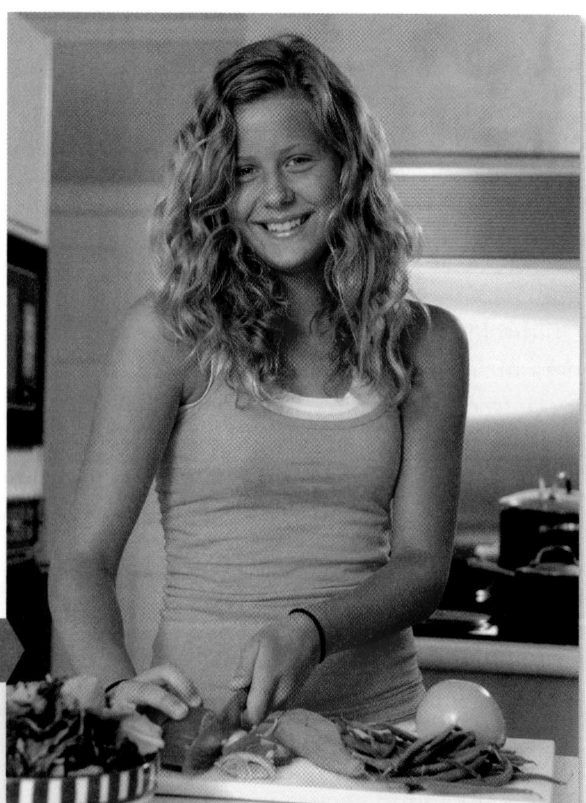

Energy for the Afternoon

By midday, energy from breakfast is used up and you need to recharge your body with healthful foods. *Should a midday meal be large or small?*

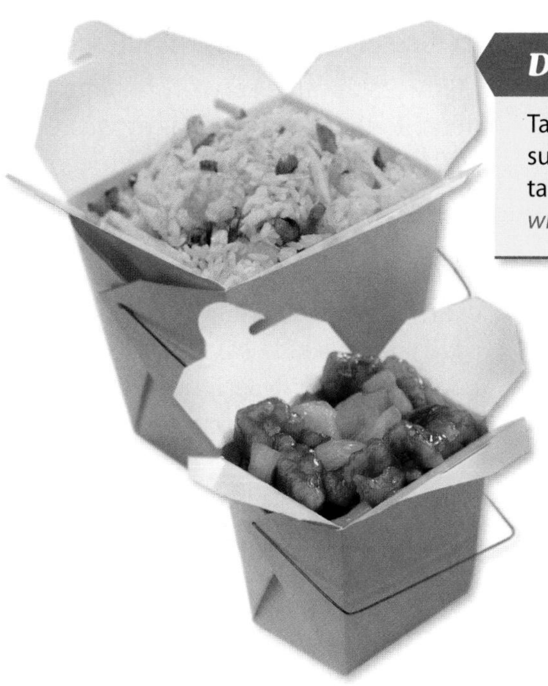

Dinner on the Go

Takeout food is more popular than ever. Many supermarkets have ready-to-eat meals that can be taken home for a quick dinner. *What should you look for when choosing foods from a take-out center?*

Restaurants

Three main types of restaurants claim most of the business. These establishments vary in selection and healthfulness of food choices.

Full-Service Restaurants

Full-service restaurants offer table service. Guests are seated and a server takes their order. Some restaurants offer a wide range of choices. Others specialize in seafood, steak, vegetarian or vegan food, or ethnic cuisine.

Self-Serve Restaurant

At self-serve restaurants, you order at a counter or help yourself from a buffet, then pay and take your food to a table. Cafeterias, buffets or food bars, and food courts in malls are self-service restaurants. Some self-serve restaurants invite diners to return for second and third helpings, which is an invitation to overeat.

Fast-Food Restaurants

Fast-food restaurants offer quick service from a limited menu, often in large portions. Fast food is not typically made with concern for healthfulness. It is often fried and high in calories and fat. Most fast-food restaurants are self-serve restaurants. Some fast-food chains are adding more healthful choices, such as grilled and roasted foods, salads, low-fat milk, and fruit juice.

Takeout Meals

Takeouts, or carryout meals, are ready-to-eat meals purchased at a restaurant, deli, or market and taken elsewhere. Takeout meals often cost more than home-cooked meals, but they appeal to people who have little time to cook.

In the food service industry, takeouts are known as home meal replacements. Many delicatessens, fast-food chains, and restaurants have take-out menus for delivery or customer pick-up. More supermarkets are adding take-out centers. They feature a variety of items, including chilled foods such as salads and hot food such as cooked meats and vegetables.

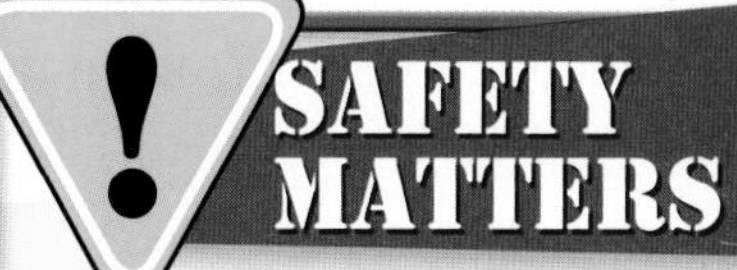

Handling Takeout Food

Protect yourself from foodborne illness when eating takeout food. To prevent bacterial growth, hot food should be served hot and cold food should be served cold. If you are concerned about the safety of takeout food or a self-service food bar, talk to an employee. Restaurant delivery vehicles are equipped to keep food at the right temperature until it reaches your door. Time your order so it is delivered when you plan to eat. Takeout food that is not eaten within an hour should be refrigerated and then reheated. Always eat it within a day of purchase.

What Would You Do? At a salad bar, you notice that one of the salad dressing containers has been left out of ice. When you touch the container, it feels warm. What would you do?

TECHNOLOGY FOR TOMORROW

Snacking for Health

Technology can help to create healthier snacks. That's good news, because studies show that about 75 percent of Americans eat at least one snack each day, accounting for about 25 percent of their daily calories. While fruits and nuts are favored for their healthfulness, consumers want nutrition in their processed snacks as well. In response, food manufacturers are using technology to develop processing methods that increase healthfulness. Health concerns are not behind every trend, however.

Investigate Identify a processed snack with enhanced nutrition or healthfulness. Research how technology plays a role in making the snack more healthful. Write your findings in a paragraph.

NCSS V F Individuals, Groups, and Institutions Evalute the role of institutions in furthering both continuity and change.

Food is priced by weight or by the size of the container. Look for foods that are nutrient dense, without a lot of fat, added sugar, or salt.

Dining Out Healthfully

If you eat in restaurants only on special occasions, you can indulge in a high-calorie meal without worry. If you often eat at restaurants, plan your menu choices carefully.

Most restaurant meals are higher in fat, sodium, and calories than home-cooked meals. Many restaurants now offer nutrition information for items on their menu. Ask a server if you do not see the information posted. You can also find information on some restaurant Web sites. You can also spot healthful choices by learning foreign words and phrases that are clues to how the food is prepared. Which of the preparation methods defined in **Figure 14.1** are healthy choices?

To dine out healthfully, try these strategies:

- Many restaurants serve very large portions. Rather than overeat or waste food, ask for a container to take leftovers home for another meal.
- Build your meal around several appetizers or side dishes instead of one large main dish, or **entrée** (ˈän-ˌtrā). For example, order soup, a side salad, and fruit.
- Look for menu descriptions like broiled, poached, steamed, roasted, or au jus. These are fat-free cooking methods.
- Avoid items described as batter-dipped, fried, creamy, rich, scalloped, or crispy. All are high in fat.
- Choose salads with care. Chicken, tuna, shrimp, potato, and macaroni salads are often made with creamy dressings, which average around 100 calories per tablespoon.
- Choose salads with fresh vegetables or topped with grilled or baked meat. Ask that dressings be served on the side, or use seasoned vinegar instead of dressing.
- Choose pasta dishes served with tomato sauces rather than cream sauces. Ask if sauces can be served separately.
- Ask that fish and vegetables be prepared without added fat.

✓ **Reading Check** **Identify** Which terms would you look for if you wanted your dish to use fat-free cooking methods?

Evaluating Your Food Choices

How healthy are your food choices? To answer this question, you need to take an honest look at your food habits. Then you can work to replace poor habits and **reinforce**, or strengthen, good ones.

Keeping a Food Record

The best way to become more aware of your eating habits is keeping a food record. A food record is a list of everything you eat and drink for a period of time. A food record is a way to gather information.

For three days, including a weekend day, record each meal and snack you eat. List specific foods and fluids (water too), the approximate amounts, and the time of day. Add a brief description of the eating situation: the setting, your mood, what you were doing, who you were with, and any other details that could help you understand your food habits. Studies have found that keeping a food record helps you maintain a healthy weight.

Using Your Food Record

When your record is completed, look it over. Do you notice any patterns in your food choices? Are some of your choices linked to certain situations or emotions?

Once you have noted your habits, look for explanations. For example, did you overeat during stressful times? Did you make some choices just from force of habit, without even thinking?

Figure 14.1 Food Terms to Know

In Writing Many of the foodservice industry words in the chart below originated with French chef Marie Antoine Careme in the 1800s. These terms are still used, mostly because Careme was the first to write them down. ***If you were allergic to dairy foods, which terms would you avoid?***

Term	Pronunciation	Definition
à la carte	(ˌä lə-ˈcärt)	Listed and priced individually on the menu. Compare with table d'hôte.
flambé	(fläm-ˈbā)	Dish is set on fire while cooking.
à la king	(ˌä lə-ˈkiŋ)ˈ	Served in a cream sauce with mushrooms, pimientos, and green peppers.
Florentine	(ˈflȯr-ən-ˌtēn)	With spinach and Mornay sauce.
à la mode	(ˌä lə-ˈmōd)	With ice cream.
fricassee	(ˈfri-kə-ˌsē)	Poultry stewed with vegetables.
amandine	(ˌäm-ˌmän-ˈdēn)	Garnished with almonds.
hors d'oeuvre	(ȯr-ˈdərv)	Any food served as an appetizer.
au gratin	(ō-ˈgrä-tən)	Topped with buttered crumbs or grated cheese, then browned.
jardinière	(ˌjär-də-ˈnir)	Garnished with mixed vegetables.
au jus	(ō-ˈzhü(s))	Served with its natural juices, such as "beef au jus."
julienne	(ˌjü-lē-ˈen)	Cut in two-inch-long thin strips.
au lait	(ō_ˈlā)	Served with milk. "Café au lait" is equal parts hot milk and coffee.
Lyonnaise	(ˌlī-ə-ˈnāz)	Served with cooked onion.
béarnaise	(ˈbā-är-ˌnāz)	Rich sauce made with egg yolks, butter, vinegar, wine, and herbs.
meunière	((ˌ)mə(r)n-ˈyer)	Floured, then sautéed in butter.
béchamel	(ˌbä-shə-ˈmel)	Thick, white cream sauce.
Mornay	(mȯr-ˈnā)	Cream sauce with cheese.
du jour	(dü-ˈzhər)	"Of the day," or today's specialty.
mousse	(ˈmüs)	Molded, chilled dessert made with sweetened, flavored whipped cream or egg whites and gelatin.
en brochette	(ˌän brō-ˈshet)	Broiled and served on a skewer.
pâté	(pä-tā)	Finely ground mixture of seasoned meat or poultry.
en coquille	(ˌän kō-ˈkēl)	Served in a shell.
table d'hôte	(ˈtä-bəl-ˈdōt)	Complete meal offered at a fixed price.
en croûte	(ˌän ˈkrüt)	Prepared with a flaky pastry crust.
vinaigrette	(ˌvi-ni-ˈgret)	Dressing of vinegar, oil, and seasonings.

Next, decide on specific and realistic actions to correct any problems. For instance, if you skip lunch, you might decide to get up ten minutes earlier to pack a lunch. Gradual changes are more likely to be permanent.

✓ **Reading Check** **Explain** Why is a food record helpful?

Decision Making

Making good choices is easier when you follow a sound decision-making process.

1. **Identify the decision to be made by setting your goals**. Knowing what you want to accomplish makes the decision clearer. Suppose you want to make a snack for a party. Your goals might include finding a recipe that other guests will like, that you can make ahead of time, and that will not cost a lot of money.
2. **Consider your resources.** Your choice should reflect available resources. If time is short, you might rule out complicated recipes.
3. **Identify your options.** Look at all the possibilities. Be realistic, but also creative.
4. **Consider each option.** Imagine the results of each possible choice. If necessary, gather more information. List advantages and disadvantages of each option. Compare pros and cons.
5. **Choose the best option.** After weighing pros and cons, choose the option that seems best. If none of them is acceptable, go back to Step 3 to see whether you missed one.
6. **Carry out your decision.** Make a plan based on your choice.
7. **Evaluate the results.** If your decision worked out well, take pride in your success. If it did not work out well, take pride in having done your best. Either way, try to learn something new from the experience.

Light and Healthy Recipe

Marinated Julienned Vegetables

Ingredients

- **1 cup** Red bell pepper, julienned
- **1 cup** Carrots, Julienned
- **½ cup** Red onion, julienned
- **1 cup** Cabbage, julienned
- **1 Tbsp.** Rice vinegar
- **2 tsp.** Low-sodium soy sauce
- **2 tsp.** Peanut oil
- **1 tsp.** Chopped garlic

Yield: 4 servings, 3/4 cup each

Directions

1. Mix the julienned vegetables and put them in a sealable plastic bag.
2. Mix the vinegar, soy sauce, peanut oil and garlic and add it to the bag.
3. Seal the bag and store the vegetables in a refrigerator overnight. If possible, turn the bag over every few hours. Serve cold.

The vinegar in the marinade contains an acid that breaks' down the fibers in the vegetables. This softens the vegetables without cooking.

Yield 4 servings

Nutrition Analysis per Serving

■ Calories	58
■ Total fat	3 g
Saturated fat	0 g
Cholesterol	0 mg
■ Sodium	136 mg
■ Carbohydrate	8 g
Dietary fiber	2 g
Sugars	16 g
■ Protein	1 g

CHAPTER 14 Review & Applications

After You Read

Chapter Summary

Many factors affect why, when, what, and how much people eat. A person's food choices are influenced by a variety of elements, such as family and emotions. Eating patterns have changed over time, but many people eat breakfast, midday, and evening meals, as well as snacks. There are different options for dining out, and strategies for eating healthfully while doing so. To make improvements to your diet, you can evaluate your food choices by keeping a food record. Understanding and applying the steps of good decision making will help you to make smart food choices.

Content and Academic Vocabulary Review

1. Write your own definition for each content and academic vocabulary term.

Content Vocabulary

- ☐ resources (p. 196)
- ☐ values (p. 197)
- ☐ eating patterns (p. 198)
- ☐ perishable (p. 198)
- ☐ grazing (p. 200)
- ☐ entrée (p. 202)

Academic Vocabulary

- significant (p. 198)
- reinforce (p. 202)

Review Key Concepts

2. **Identify** and explain different influences on food choices.
3. **Explain** historical and current daily eating patterns.
4. **Discuss** choices for dining out and how to do so healthfully.
5. **Explain** how and why people should evaluate their food choices.
6. **Explain** how to make good decisions about food.

Critical Thinking

7. **Explain** how your values might affect your food choices.
8. **Assess** how your eating patterns have changed over the last decade. Explain what has caused the changes and whether the changes have been beneficial or harmful to your health.
9. **Categorize** the restaurants in your neighborhood according to the three main types named in this chapter. Which ones offer the most healthful meal selections? Explain your answer.
10. **Compare and contrast** snacking and grazing.

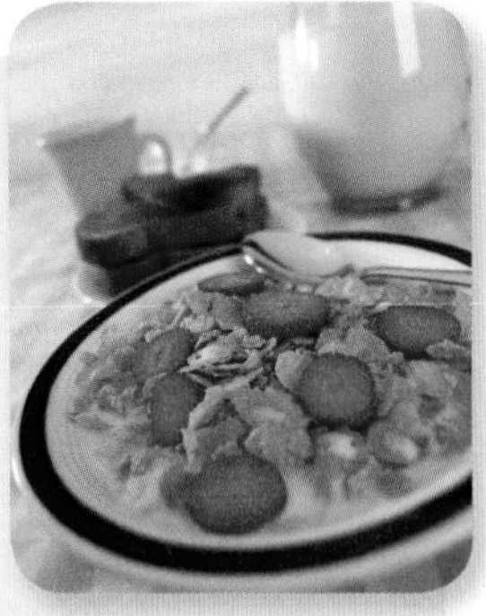

11. Quick Breakfasts Today, many people lack the time to prepare and eat an elaborate breakfast. Some rely on convenience foods to "break the fast" they experienced while sleeping. Which convenience foods make a nutritious and tasty breakfast?

Procedure Prepare and evaluate one kind of store-bought, convenience breakfast food, such as frozen waffles, toaster pastries, instant oatmeal, or cereal bars.

Analysis Write a product review of the food that will help others determine if it is right for them. Describe the food's appeal, cost, nutritional value, and method of preparation. Read your review aloud for the class.

HEALTHFUL CHOICES

12. Translate Terms To keep her heart healthy, Marie follows a low-fat diet plan. She visits a restaurant where the daily specials are trout amandine, chicken en brochette, chicken Mornay, chicken béarnaise, and steak meunière. Which special is the healthiest choice? Which options should she avoid and why?

TECH Connection

13. Historical Comparison Conduct research into the life of a typical teen in colonial America (1600–1775). Compare the influences on a teen's food choices in colonial America with the influences on a teen's food choices today. Did colonial American teens have healthful choices? What did they take to school for lunch? How did teens typically help with preparing meals? Give an oral presentation to the class explaining the similarities and differences. Explain how technology affects food choices.

Real-World Skills

Problem-Solving Skills	**14. What to Order?** Sal joins his friends for dinner at a restaurant. His friends are all hungry and order big, filling entrees. Sal is not that hungry, but still wants to eat with his friends. What can he do?
Interpersonal and Collaborative Skills	**15. Decision Making** Follow your teacher's directions to form groups. Imagine your group is in charge of deciding what beverage will be served at an upcoming class party. Together, use the steps of the decision-making process to determine which beverage you will serve. Explain your decision to the class.
Financial Literacy Skills	**16. Takeout or Homemade?** Think of a takeout meal that you like, such as pizza or Chinese food. Identify the ingredients used in that meal, and visit a local supermarket to determine their prices. Then compare the money and time spent on the take-out meal to that spent on a similar version prepared at home. Which option is the better value?

Academic Skills

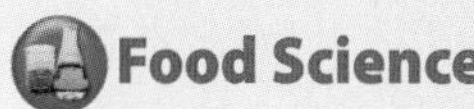

Food Science

17. Starch as Thickener Gelatinization is caused by starches absorbing water. The starches form a network of molecules that entrap water. Roux (Rü) is an equal mixture of flour (starch) and fat, and acts as a base for many sauces.

Procedure Make a roux with a tablespoon of melted butter and a tablespoon of flour, stirring together for several minutes over medium heat. Slowly add 1 cup of milk, stirring constantly. Stir until it reaches a simmer.

Analysis What happened to the sauce as it cooked? What did the sauce taste like after five minutes and after 10 minutes?

NSES B Develop an understanding of chemical reactions.

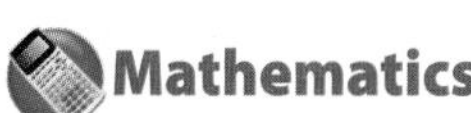

Mathematics

18. Comparing Trends A study forecasts that average annual spending on supermarket "ready-to-eat" meals will increase from $160 per person to $360 per person in five years. The study also predicts that average annual spending on other types of take-out meals will increase from $1,600 per person to $2,400 in five years. Which of the two forecasts shows a higher percentage increase in spending?

Math Concept **Percentage Increase** To find the percent of increase, determine the total increase by subtracting the original amount from the new amount.

Starting Hint Calculate each total increase. Divide the total increase by the original amount, and convert to a percent.

NCTM Number and Operations Understand numbers, ways of representing numbers, relationships among numbers, and number systems.

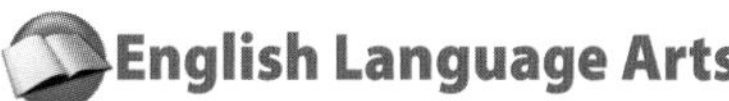

English Language Arts

19. Food Record Keep a food record for three days, following the procedure described in the chapter. Review your food record and look for patterns. What do you notice about your food choices? What changes do you want to make? Write a letter to your teacher describing what you can conclude about your own eating habits and patterns and what actions, if any, you need to take.

NCTE 12 Use language to accomplish individual purposes.

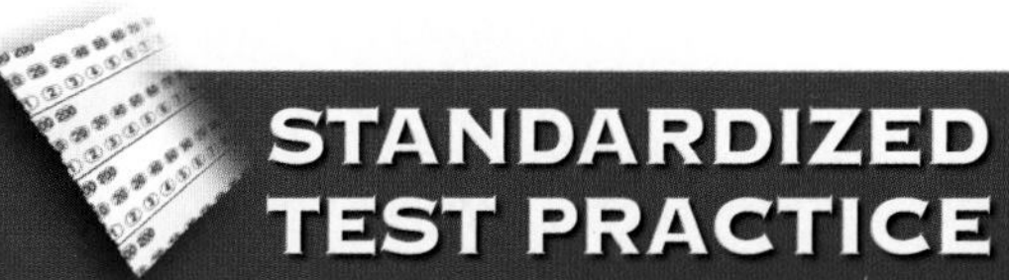

MULTIPLE CHOICE

Read the question and select the best answer.

20. Why were there food shortages during World War II?

a. Food shipments to the United States were intercepted by Germany.

b. Food shipments to troops overseas required rationing at home.

c. Women cooked less because they joined the labor force.

d. Women in the labor force could not maintain the victory gardens.

Test-Taking Tip Multiple-choice questions may prompt you to select the best answer. They may present you with answers that seem partially true. The best answer is the one that is completely true, and can be supported by information you have read in the text.

CHAPTER 15

Vegetarian Food Choices

Writing Activity — Dialogue

Conversation Imagine a conversation between two teens about food. One teen does not eat meat. The other teen does. What questions would they ask each other? What views might they express? What reasons might they give for their views? Write a script of their conversation.

Writing Tips Follow these steps to write a script:

- Precede every statement by the speaker's name.
- Do not use quotation marks.
- Make your script sound realistic and conversational.

Activate Prior Knowledge

Explore the Photo There are thousands of recipes for meat-free dishes. *What is one dish usually served with meat that might taste good without it?*

Reading Guide

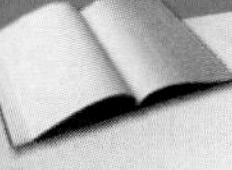

Before You Read

Preview Before you read, make a list of what you believe are the pros and cons of being a vegetarian. As you read, make changes to your list as you see fit.

Read to Learn

Key Concepts

- **Describe** different types of vegetarian diets.
- **Identify** and explain reasons why people choose a vegetarian diet.
- **Explain** the challenges of vegetarian nutrition.
- **Describe** daily food choices for vegetarians.
- **Discuss** ways to explore vegetarian foods.

Main Idea

People who choose a vegetarian diet can obtain needed nutrients and eat a wide variety of tasty and healthful foods.

Content Vocabulary

You will find definitions for these words in the glossary at the back of this book.

- ☐ vegetarian
- ☐ vegan
- ☐ raw vegan
- ☐ macrobiotics
- ☐ lacto-vegetarian
- ☐ ovo-vegetarian
- ☐ lacto-ovo vegetarian
- ☐ fruitarian
- ☐ pescatarian
- ☐ semi-vegetarian
- ☐ tempeh
- ☐ seitan
- ☐ quorn

Academic Vocabulary

You will find these words in your reading and on your tests. Use the glossary to look up their definitions if necessary.

- advocate
- abundant

Graphic Organizer

Use a graphic organizer like the one below to note important nutrients for vegans and which vegan foods provide them.

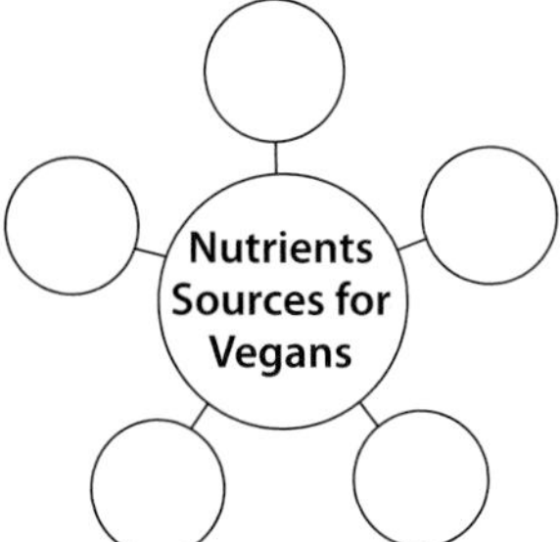

Graphic Organizer Go to this book's Online Learning Center at **glencoe.com** to print out this graphic organizer.

Academic Standards

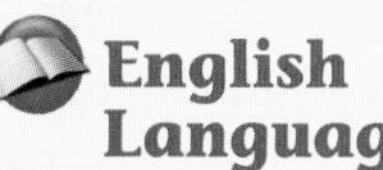

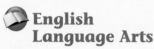

English Language Arts

NCTE 7 Conduct research and gather, evaluate, and synthesize data to communicate discoveries.

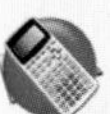

Mathematics

NCTM Data Analysis and Probability Formulate questions that can be addressed with data and collect, organize, and display relevant data to answer them.

NCTM Algebra Represent and analyze mathematical situations and structures using algebraic symbols.

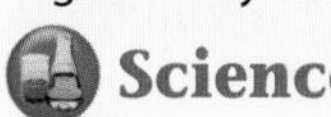

Science

NSES C Develop an understanding of matter, energy and organization in living systems.

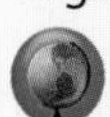

Social Studies

NCSS VIII A Identify and describe both current and historical examples of the interaction and inter dependence of science, technology, and society in a variety of cultural settings.

NCTE *National Council of Teachers of English*
NCTM *National Council of Teachers of Mathematics*
NSES *National Science Education Standards*
NCSS *National Council for the Social Studies*

Types of Vegetarians

What does it mean to be a vegetarian? A **vegetarian** is a person who does not eat meat, poultry, or fish. Vegetarians eat a plant-based diet that is rich in whole grains, fruits, vegetables, legumes, nuts, and seeds. These form the foundation for thousands of delicious dishes.

A large percentage of the world's population practices vegetarianism. However, vegetarians differ in their food choices:

A **vegan** (ˈvē-gən) eats only foods from plant sources. Many vegans choose not to use or wear anything made from, or containing, animal by-products. A **raw vegan** eats only unprocessed vegan foods that have not been heated above 115 degrees Fahrenheit. Also called raw foodists, raw vegans believe that cooked food is harmful to the body because cooking destroys valuable enzymes in foods and causes nutrient loss.

Macrobiotics is a diet that includes unprocessed foods, mostly whole grains, beans, and organically grown fruits and vegetables, particularly Asian vegetables, such as daikon, sea vegetables, and seaweed. Not all macrobiotics are vegan, as some allow the occasional consumption of small amounts of fish. Sugar and refined oils are avoided. People who follow a macrobiotic diet chew their food thoroughly before swallowing, and they make an effort not to overeat.

A **lacto-vegetarian** eats foods from plant sources, plus dairy products.

An **ovo-vegetarian** eats foods from plant sources, plus eggs.

A **lacto-ovo-vegetarian** eats foods from plant sources, plus dairy products and eggs.

A **fruitarian** eats only the ripe fruits of plants and trees, such as grains, nuts, fruits, and some vegetables. Fruitarians try to choose foods that can be harvested without killing the plant. For example, a fruitarian would eat squash but not carrots.

A **pescatarian** eats fish and shellfish and foods from plant sources. A pescatarian may or may not eat dairy products.

Many people incorporate some, but not all, elements of a vegetarian diet. A **semi-vegetarian**, for example, avoids certain kinds of meat, poultry, or fish. Many semi-vegetarians eat fish or poultry but not red meat.

Some people eat a vegetarian diet part of the time and have meat only occasionally. Others eat a semi-vegetarian diet as a first step toward becoming a vegetarian.

Reading Check **Contrast** What is the difference between a vegan and a fruitarian?

The Vegetarian Decision

A growing number of Americans are exploring meals without meat. A vegetarian diet is full of flavor and can benefit human health, the environment, and animal welfare.

Kitchen Math

Track Your Meals

Even non-vegetarians eat vegetarian-style meals on occasion. Think back to each of the meals you consumed over the past five days. Count the total number of meals where you ate red meat. Count the total meals where you ate fish or poultry. Then count the total meals that you ate in each of the categories of vegetarianism. Display your results in a bar graph.

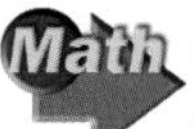

Math Concept **Bar Graphs** A bar graph uses vertical bars to display data. Typically, the vertical axis indicates quantity, while the horizontal axis can show categories or time periods.

Starting Hint Place evenly spaced labels for each of the meal categories across the horizontal axis of your graph. Label the vertical axis with quantity units (with zero at the bottom and 15 at the top). Draw a vertical bar above each category label representing the number of meals of that type you consumed.

Math Appendix For math help, go to the Math Appendix at the back of the book.

NCTM Data Analysis and Probability Formulate questions that can be addressed with data and collect, organize, and display relevant data to answer them.

Health Benefits

Health benefits are one attraction of a vegetarian diet. Plant foods such as vegetables, fruits, nuts, and seeds are usually high in fiber and low in saturated fat and cholesterol. Vegetarians live about seven years longer than non-vegetarians, according to medical studies. Vegetarians have a lower risk of heart disease, high blood pressure, obesity, and some forms of cancer than meat eaters. In addition, they are less likely to have digestive disorders, diabetes, strokes, and gallstones.

Animal Rights

Many people choose vegetarianism out of concern for animal welfare. Many vegetarians are concerned about the conditions under which animals are raised and slaughtered. Some people oppose the killing of animals entirely. Certain religions, including Hindu and Buddhist sects, **advocate**, or support, vegetarianism as part of an ethic of non-violence and respect for living things.

Ecology

A vegetarian diet also benefits the earth. Livestock and poultry must eat about 7 to 8 pounds of grains or soybeans to produce 1 pound of meat. Growing crops used to feed livestock requires nearly half of the U.S. water supply and 80 percent of the country's agricultural land. As the global population increases and farmland dwindles, land is better used to grow grains and vegetables for people than for livestock feed. Raising animals for food also creates an enormous amount of pollution in the form of animal waste and gas.

Cost

Vegetarian foods usually cost less than animal foods, so going meat-free can save money. For example, a pound of ground meat can cost three to five times as much as a pound of dry beans. When cooked, the meat gives about four 3-ounce servings, while the beans provide five or six 1-cup servings.

✓ **Reading Check** **Identify** Name one way a vegetarian diet benefits the earth.

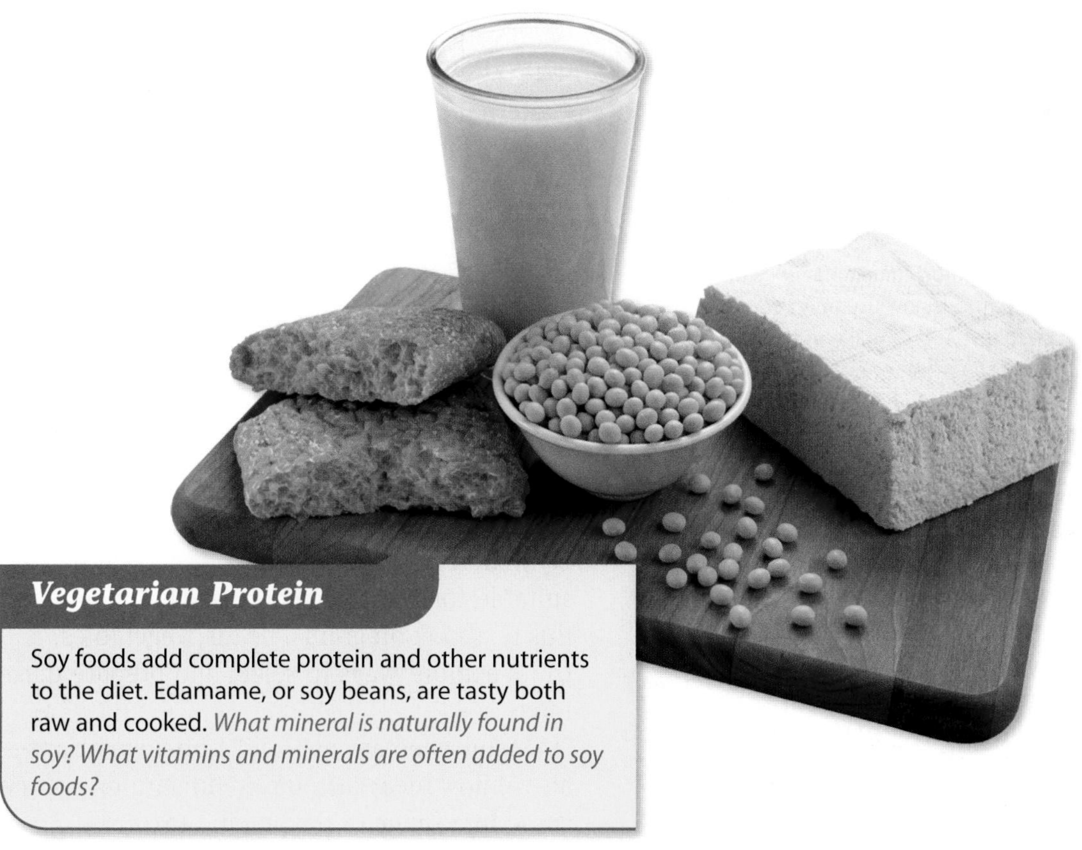

Vegetarian Protein

Soy foods add complete protein and other nutrients to the diet. Edamame, or soy beans, are tasty both raw and cooked. *What mineral is naturally found in soy? What vitamins and minerals are often added to soy foods?*

Vegetarian Nutrition

Vegetarians need to choose a healthy, nutritionally sound eating plan. Vegetarianism does not guarantee good nutrition. After all, plenty of high-calorie, low-nutrient foods, such as potato chips, candy, soda, and ice cream, are meatless. Eating too many high-fat foods is bad for your health, whether the fat comes from meats, dairy products, or fat-laden desserts. Healthful choices make a difference.

Vegetarians have many healthful food choices in the Grain, Vegetable, Fruit, Milk, and Beans & Meat Group. In the Beans & Meat Group, soy foods, dry beans and peas, peanut butter, and eggs are good options. Vegetarians who do not eat dairy products can substitute calcium-fortified soy milk or soy yogurt.

Even children can fulfill nutrient needs through vegetarian eating. Food choices, however, should be evaluated by a nutritionist.

Maintaining a healthy weight can be just as challenging for vegetarians as for meat eaters. Maintain a healthy weight by balancing calories consumed with calories burned.

Be a Smart Consumer

Avoiding Animal-Derived Ingredients

In response to consumer demands and health concerns, some restaurant chains are shifting away from animal-derived products when possible. Major fast-food chains that once used beef tallow to fry foods now use only vegetable oils. Some pizza restaurants make pizza and pasta sauces without meat or beef flavoring. Consequently, it is getting easier for vegetarians to split a pizza or plate of onion rings with nonvegetarian friends. However, animal-derived ingredients are not always listed on restaurant menus and can still hide in seemingly meatless dishes. Vegetarians who dine out might pay for foods they would prefer to avoid.

Challenge As a vegetarian, how would you make sure that you did not inadvertently pay for and eat animal-derived products while dining out? Write your ideas in one paragraph.

Important Nutrients for Vegans

Some nutrients that are **abundant**, or plentiful, in meat and dairy foods are less common in plants. Vegetarians, especially vegans, must make sure to choose foods that provide the nutrients below. They may also benefit from a vitamin-mineral supplement.

Zinc Zinc is largely supplied by meat, poultry, and fish, but it also comes in whole-grain breads and cereals, dry beans and peas, nuts, and soy foods.

Calcium Vegans can get calcium from dry beans and peas, nuts, dark green vegetables, fortified grain products, and fortified soy milk products. Calcium is vital for bone development, so ovo-vegetarians and vegans need to make sure to get enough.

Iron Many foods that contain zinc and calcium are also good sources of iron. Eating foods that are high in vitamin C boosts absorption of iron from plants.

Vitamins B_{12} and D Vegans may find it difficult to get vitamins B_{12} and D, which are found in meat, eggs, and dairy products but not in plant foods. Some cereals and soy foods, especially soy milk, are fortified with both vitamins.

Protein Plant foods that contain complete protein include soy, quinoa, buckwheat, and amaranth. Vegans can also get complete protein from combining plant foods, such as rice and beans or wheat and nuts.

✓ **Reading Check** **Respond** Do any plant foods contain complete protein?

Daily Food Choices

Meatless eating plans can be full of variety. There is vast selection of foods that are suitable for most vegetarians. The chapters in this textbook on grains, beans, vegetables, and fruits explore ways to select and prepare these foods.

Many vegetarians—and non-vegetarians—also enjoy meat and dairy substitutes, which come in a range of flavors and textures.

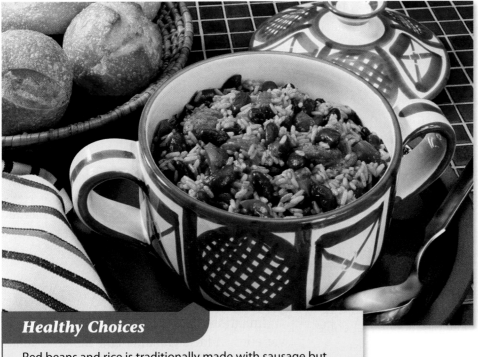

Healthy Choices

Red beans and rice is traditionally made with sausage but can be a vegetarian dish if made with meatless sausage or without sausage at all. *What are meat substitutes made from?*

Meat Substitutes

Meat substitutes, or analogs, are made from blends of plant proteins. They provide quality protein with little or no cholesterol and saturated fat. Spices and flavorings are added to create tastes ranging from smoked salmon to Italian sausage. You can find meat substitutes in prepared meals, such as deli slices, in recipe crumbles that substitute for ground meat, and in patties.

Firm Tofu

Firm tofu, or soya bean curd made from coagulated soy milk, is amazingly versatile. It is high in protein, low in fat, and a good source of calcium and vitamins B_1, B_2, and B_3. A half-cup serving provides nearly 20% of your daily protein, has less than 100 calories, and provides more calcium than a cup of milk. Like many soy products, it absorbs flavors from other foods easily, especially if frozen and thawed. It is widely used instead of meat in dishes such as stir-fries. It can be cubed for grilling, mashed into patties, or crumbled into chili.

Tempeh

Tempeh (ˈtem-ˌpā) is a pressed cake of fermented, cooked soybeans mixed with a grain, usually rice. Tempeh is a popular source of protein in Indonesian cooking. Fermentation gives tempeh a chewy consistency and a nutty, yeasty flavor. You can use tempeh cubed or shredded. You can also marinate and grill tempeh or add it to soups, casseroles, and stir-fries.

Nutrition Check

Obtaining Omegas

Omega-3 fatty acids, which are found in fish, have been recognized for their heart, brain, joint, and digestive health benefits. Vegetarians who do not eat fish may wonder whether they are denying themselves an important nutrient. They can add foods that contain linolenic acid to their diet. Linolenic acid is converted to an omega-3 acid in the body.

Think About It Walnuts, canola and soybean oils, flax seed, and soy nuts are all good, vegetarian sources of linolenic acid. How might walnuts and flax seeds be incorporated into an eating plan?

Seitan

Wheat gluten with seasonings is called **seitan** (ˈsā-tän). Seitan is made by simmering flour in a broth flavored with ginger, garlic, soy sauce, and seaweed. Sometimes called "wheat meat," seitan has a firm, chewy texture and brown color, and can be used like firm tofu in recipes. Seitan is popular in Asian cooking.

Quorn

Quorn (ˈkwórn) is a meat substitute made of protein from a type of edible fungus. The protein is fermented and mixed with egg whites and vegetable oils to make a product with a meaty texture. Quorn was developed in Great Britain in the 1970s and is popular in Europe. It was introduced in the United States with FDA approval in 2002. A small percentage of people have reported allergic reactions to Quorn.

Dairy Substitutes

Dairy substitutes have the taste and texture of dairy foods and can be used instead of dairy in recipes. Like meat substitutes, many dairy substitutes are based on soy.

Silken Tofu

Silken tofu is similar to firm tofu, but it has a smooth, custard-like texture. It can replace eggs in homemade mayonnaise and cream in whipped toppings. Soft tofu is used in baking and in smoothies, soups, and sauces.

Beverages

Soy, rice, almond, oats, and other grains are used to make nondairy milks. These milks are usually made by grinding the grain and soaking it in water. Enzymes are sometimes added to break down complex carbohydrates for a sweeter, less starchy taste. The liquid is drained, often fortified, and sometimes flavored.

Imitation Cheeses

Imitation cheeses come in both soft and firm varieties. Added vitamins and minerals make some cheese substitutes nutritionally comparable to milk-based cheeses. Yeast extract or vinegar is added to a soy and starch base to create the cheese flavor. Nondairy cheese is also made from rice. Most imitation cheeses are not vegan because they contain casein, which is derived from milk.

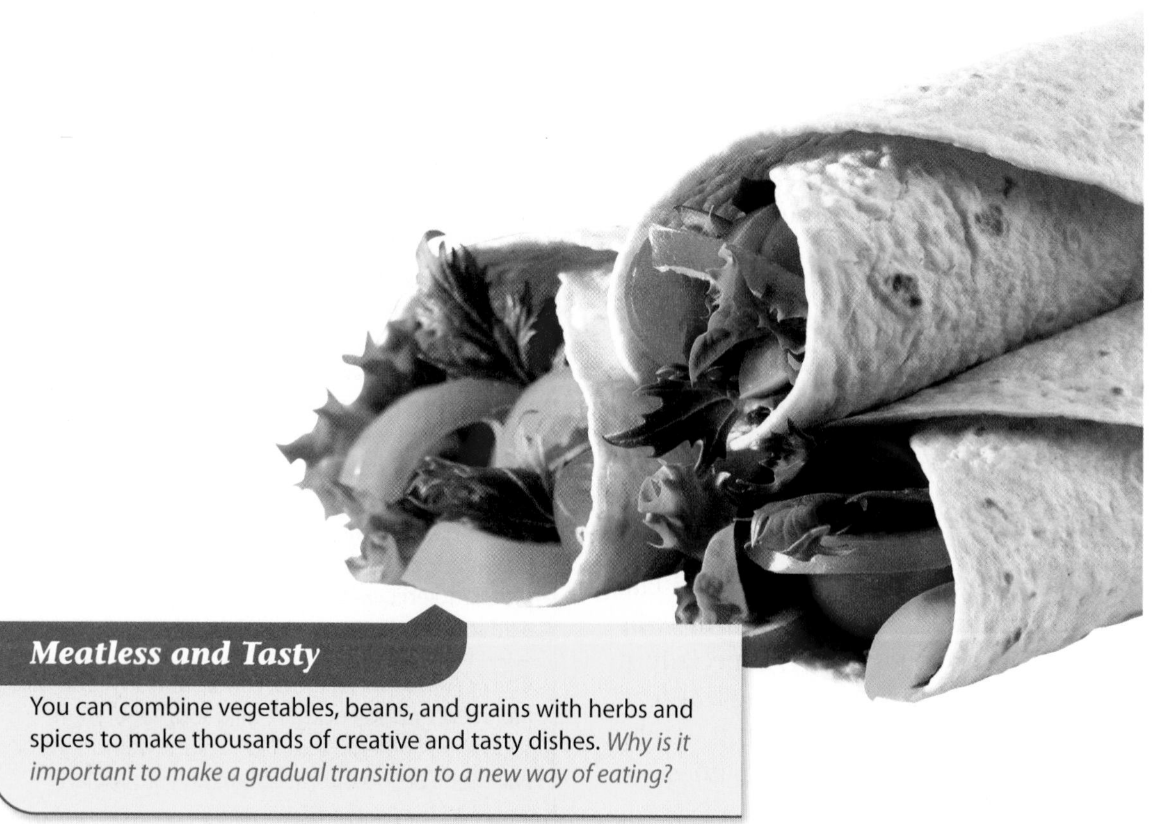

Meatless and Tasty

You can combine vegetables, beans, and grains with herbs and spices to make thousands of creative and tasty dishes. *Why is it important to make a gradual transition to a new way of eating?*

Spreads

Nondairy spreads are sold as powders and prepared mixes in a range of flavors, from butter to cheese to ranch dressing. Most nondairy spreads are soy protein combined with gums, starches, sugars, and seasonings. Margarine is a common nondairy spread made from vegetable oil and salt.

Frozen Desserts

Frozen nondairy desserts taste very similar to frozen dairy desserts. Soy or rice milk and vegetable oils imitate the richness of cream. Chocolate flavor comes from cocoa powder, not milk chocolate.

Vegetarian Recipes

A wide selection of vegetarian cookbooks is available, including cookbooks focusing on vegetarian dishes from different cuisines. Many vegetarians also learn to modify recipes with meat by substituting different ingredients. For example, chunks of sautéed eggplant can add texture in a pasta sauce instead of meat. Liquid smoke, rather than bacon, can give a smoky flavor to baked beans.

Many ethnic cuisines are rich in vegetarian foods. Indian, Thai, Italian, and Mexican cooking, for example, have many delicious meatless dishes.

Dining Out

More and more restaurants offer meatless choices. Lacto-vegetarians and lacto-ovo-vegetarians have the widest range of choices when eating out. However, foods may be prepared with animal products that are not mentioned on the menu. Lard is often used in pastry crusts, for example, and many soups have chicken or beef stock. Check with the server to be sure.

For vegans, eating out can be frustrating. Many restaurants have few or no satisfying vegan choices. Vegans and vegetarians can often make a meal of appetizers, salads, and side dishes, which are more likely to be meatless than main dishes. Some ethnic restaurants offer a wide choice of vegetarian meals.

If you do not see any meatless options on the menu, it is acceptable to ask whether a vegetarian option is available. Some restaurants will be willing to make a special vegetable or pasta plate upon request. Many restaurants will also honor a request for special preparation of items on the menu. Typically sauces are made with milk or chicken or beef stock but some sauces, like marinara, are made without meat products. Ask your server how a sauce is made if you are unsure.

Vegetarians who eat away from home often might suggest some simple additions to make restaurant menus more vegetarian friendly. A vegetable soup in a tomato base or a zucchini lasagne would satisfy vegans and vegetarians as well as diners who want lighter, healthful meals.

✓ **Reading Check** **List** What are four types of meat substitutes?

TECHNOLOGY FOR TOMORROW

Fast and Fresh Soymilk

Just as farmers can drink milk fresh from their own cows, people today can enjoy fresh, homemade soymilk at the push of a button. Vegetarians who use soy products to fill some of their protein needs can purchase a small appliance that turns dried soybeans and water into soymilk. The machine sells for about $100 and is available at many department stores. The appliance is similar to a coffeemaker, but contains a motor that is fueled by electricity. The motor grinds presoaked soybeans, and electricity boils the water. Then the steaming water is filtered through the beans, becoming suffused with their taste and nutrients. The process takes about 15 minutes. The appliance can also be used to turn soybeans into tofu.

Investigate What other foods can be turned into milk at home with a soymilk maker? How can soymilk makers help the supply of milk?

NCSS VIII A Identify and describe both current and historical examples of the interaction and interdependence of science, technology and society in a variety of cultural settings.

Exploring Vegetarian Foods

Are you interested in trying a vegetarian eating plan? Make a gradual transition. Start by planning a single day of vegetarian meals. As you become comfortable, add more days. Plan how you will get the nutrients that you may be getting now from meat. You may also discuss your options with a dietitian.

The following ideas are valuable for vegetarians and meat eaters alike:

- Identify vegetarian foods that you enjoy now and explore new recipes using these foods. For example, try new ways to prepare dried beans, make a new pasta sauce, or experiment with new ways of preparing your favorite vegetables in a sandwich or wrap.
- Get creative with substitutions. What can your favorite chili seasoning mix do for chunks of carrots, turnips, and other root vegetables?
- Try new products from your supermarket. Does your local store carry soy milk? Bok choy? Hummus? Explore each department. You might be surprised at the variety.
- Explore new places to shop. Farmers' markets, ethnic groceries, health-food shops, and online retailers offer unusual and tasty products. Some products might inspire recipe ideas of your own.
- Keep up with new research on vegetarianism and vegetarian foods. Read recipes for vegetarian foods.
- Explore cookbooks and cooking magazines. Recipes that use meats might still provide ideas for combining vegetables with different spices.
- Examine all the ingredients listed on food labels. Some products that might seem like vegetarian foods are actually made with meat products. Some jams, for example, use gelatin for thickening. Gelatin is made from the bones, hooves, and dried skin of horses, cows, and pigs.

Light and Healthy Recipe

Hummus

Ingredients

- **1 cup** Canned garbanzo beans (chick peas)
- **¼ cup** Tahini (sesame seed paste)
- **2 Tbsp.** Lemon juice
- **1 clove** Garlic, minced
- **Dash** Salt
- **1 Tbsp.** Minced fresh parsley

Yield 4 servings

Directions

1. Drain and rinse the beans, then puree them in a blender.
2. Add tahini, lemon juice, garlic and salt. Blend until smooth.
3. Place mixture in a serving bowl. Garnish with minced parsley.
4. Serve as a spread or a dip for toasted pita chips or raw vegetables.

When combined with bread, hummus provides complete protein.

Yield 4 servings

Nutrition Analysis per Serving

■ Calories	93
■ Total fat	5 g
Saturated fat	1 g
Cholesterol	0 mg
■ Sodium	161 mg
■ Carbohydrate	8 g
Dietary fiber	2 g
Sugars	1g
■ Protein	4 g

CHAPTER 15 Review & Applications

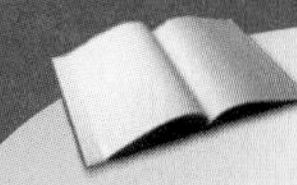

After You Read

Chapter Summary

There are different types of vegetarians who make different food choices. People choose a vegetarian diet because of health benefits, concern for animal rights, concern for ecology, and financial reasons. Vegetarians must choose a healthful eating plan. Vegans must make an effort to obtain certain nutrients. There are many tasty, meatless, and dairy-free foods that vegetarians can incorporate into their diets. Recipes allow cooks to prepare diverse vegetarian dishes. Many vegetarians can dine out and make choices that fit into their eating plans. It is best to make a gradual transition to a vegetarian diet.

Content and Academic Vocabulary Review

1. Write a journal entry using at least four of these content and academic vocabulary terms.

Content Vocabulary

- vegetarian (p. 210)
- vegan (p. 210)
- raw vegan (p. 210)
- macrobiotics (p. 210)
- lacto-vegetarian (p. 210)
- ovo-vegetarian (p. 210)
- lacto-ovo vegetarian (p. 210)
- fruitarian (p. 210)
- pescatarian (p. 210)
- semi-vegetarian (p. 210)
- tempeh (p. 213)
- seitan (p. 214)
- quorn (p. 214)

Academic Vocabulary

- advocate (p. 211)
- abundant (p. 212)

Review Key Concepts

2. **Describe** different types of vegetarian diets.
3. **Identify** the reasons why people choose a vegetarian diet.
4. **Explain** the challenges of vegetarian nutrition.
5. **Describe** daily food choices for vegetarians.
6. **Discuss** ways to explore vegetarian foods.

Critical Thinking

7. **Explain** to your friend why his decision to become a vegetarian starting today might need careful thought and planning.
8. **Infer** why many vegans, raw vegans, and macrobiotics choose not to consume refined oils.
9. **Evaluate** this scenario. John's parents are opposed to his vegetarian diet and say it will inhibit his body's growth and development. Are they right or wrong?
10. **Conclude** whether Meredith can make good recipe substitutions. Meredith has recently become a vegan. Can she prepare lasagna similar in taste and texture to the beef-and-cheese lasagna she used to eat?

CHAPTER 15 Review & Applications

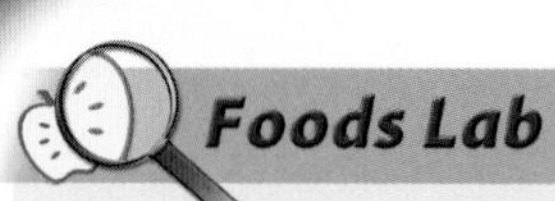

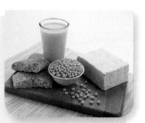

11. Using Soy Foods Soy products are a staple in many vegetarian diets. They provide complete protein, are often enriched with other nutrients such as calcium, and can replace milk, meat, cheese, eggs, and other foods.

Procedure Find and prepare a recipe that uses a soy-based meat or cheese substitute, such as meatless tacos or tofu vegetable dip. Offer samples to five classmates for tasting.

Analysis Survey the five people who tasted your dish. Ask them how its texture, taste, and appearance compare to those of a similar, nonvegetarian dish. Write a paragraph summarzing the tasters' feedback.

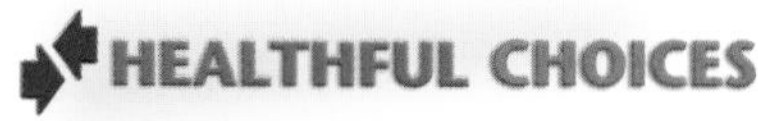

12. A Smart Snack Kirsten, a vegan, usually opts for a bag of potato chips, candy, or pretzels for an after-school snack. She likes her snacks to be both vegan and crunchy. What are some healthier, more nutrient-dense snack options you would suggest to Kirsten? How easy are these snack options to prepare?

TECH Connection

13. Three-Day Plan Use computer software to create a table with three columns and five rows. Use the table to create a three-day eating plan for a lacto-ovo vegetarian. Each day should include three meals and two snacks. Write a paragraph summarizing your choices and your reasoning for the choices. Explain how your meal plan meets the nutrient needs for a lacto-ovo vegetarian. Make sure calories come from carbohydrates, proteins, and fats in the proper proportions.

Real-World Skills

Problem-Solving Skills

14. Stuck in a Rut Janie is a vegetarian who eats no meat, eggs, or dairy. For years, she has eaten a peanut butter and jelly sandwich for her lunch every day. She is so bored with her lunch routine that now she has begun skipping lunch. What should Janie do?

Interpersonal and Collaborative Skills

15. Problem Solving Follow your teacher's instructions to form pairs. With your partner, imagine you are roommates. One of you is a vegetarian and the other is not. Plan a week of dinners that will be convenient and satisfy you both.

Financial Literacy Skills

16. Compare Costs Visit your local supermarket to determine the cost of ingredients for a non-vegetarian dish, such as beef lasagna, and the cost of ingredients for a vegetarian version of the dish. Which is less expensive and why?

Academic Skills

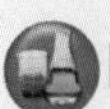

Food Science

17. Seed Germination There are variables that affect the process of seed germination.

Procedure Soak several beans overnight. Line two glasses with moist paper towels. Place soaked beans between the glass and paper towel. Place one glass in the refrigerator, and keep the other at room temperature. Record your results over the next several days, making sure the towel is kept moist.

Analysis Judging from the root and shoot growth, what conclusions can you draw about temperature's effect on germination?

NSES C Develop an understanding of matter, energy and organization in living systems.

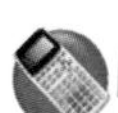

Mathematics

18. Nutrients from Vegetable Products Boneless, skinless chicken breast typically has 8.8 grams of protein per ounce. Vegetarian stir-fry strips made from seitan have 7.3 grams of protein per ounce. How much seitan is needed to duplicate the protein content of a 3-ounce chicken breast?

Math Concept **Solving Algebraic Equations** Use a variable to represent an unknown quantity. Rearrange the equation so that the variable is on one side of the equals sign, and all other numbers are on the other.

Starting Hint The chicken's protein content equals 8.8. $\times$ 3. In an equation, let this total equal the protein content in the seitan ($7.3x$), where x represents the ounces of seitan. Solve for x.

NCTM Algebra Represent and analyze mathematical situations and structures using algebraic symbols.

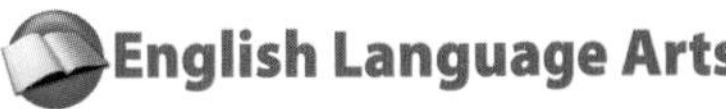

English Language Arts

19. Write a Profile Research a famous person, living or dead, who was or is a vegetarian. Write a one-page profile of the person, describing their biography, their accomplishments, and their reasons for choosing vegetarianism. Include quotes from the person if possible. Include with your profile a list of sources you read for your research.

NCTE 7 Conduct research and gather, evaluate, and synthesize data to communicate discoveries.

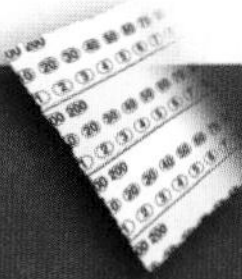

STANDARDIZED TEST PRACTICE

ANALOGY

Read the pairs of terms. Then choose the best word to match with the term *vegan*.

20. politician: governor

flower: daisy

book: novel

______: vegan

a. vegetarian

b. plant

c. fruit

d. meat

Test-Taking Tip Analogies establish relationships between terms. When you look at the three pairs of terms listed here, identify the relationship that is common to all of them. Then try matching each possible answer with the term *vegan*. The one that establishes the same type of relationship as the other terms is correct.

CHAPTER 16

Meal Planning

Writing Activity: Criticism

Restaurant Review Identify a restaurant you have visited. Rate the restaurant on a scale of one to five stars, with five stars being the best. Then write a review of the restaurant that explains your rating. Consider the restaurant's atmosphere, service, menu, quality of food, and cost. Use descriptive language to help the reader experience the restaurant in their imagination.

Writing Tips Follow these steps to write a restaurant review:

- Highlight strengths, weaknesses, or both.
- Use specific, descriptive language.
- Support all judgments with details and examples.

Activate Prior Knowledge

Explore the Photo Planning ahead for meals can ensure good nutrition and save money. *How does your family decide what to eat?*

Reading Guide

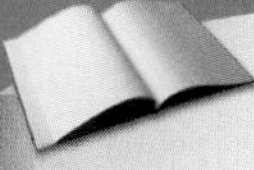

Before You Read

Preview Make a list of three factors that you think influence the meals a family eats. As you read, see if your factors are addressed in the chapter and, if so, note how.

Read to Learn

Key Concepts

- **Explain** the benefits of meal planning.
- **Explain** how to create and meet a food budget.
- **Describe** convenience foods and how they can be used to save time while cooking.
- **Describe** ways to make a meal appealing to the senses.
- **Explain** how to develop a meal plan for a week.

Main Idea

Meal planning can save money, ensure good nutrition, and make meals appealing and enjoyable.

Content Vocabulary

You will find the definitions for these words in the glossary at the back of the book.

- ☐ role
- ☐ budget
- ☐ staples
- ☐ commodity
- ☐ scratch cooking
- ☐ convenience foods
- ☐ bulk foods
- ☐ speed-scratch cooking

Academic Vocabulary

You will find these words in your reading and on your tests. Use the glossary to look up their definitions, if necessary.

- consecutive
- complement

Graphic Organizer

Use a graphic organizer like the one below to take notes about six types of food assistance programs and who they help.

FOOD ASSISTANCE PROGRAMS	WHO IS HELPED?

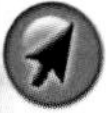

Graphic Organizer Go to this book's Online Learning Center at **glencoe.com** to print out this graphic organizer.

Academic Standards

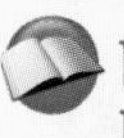

English Language Arts

NCTE 4 Use written language to communicate effectively

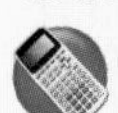

Mathematics

NCTM Number and Operations Understand numbers, ways of representing numbers, relationships among numbers, and number systems.

NCTM Algebra Represent and analyze mathematical situations and structures using algebraic symbols.

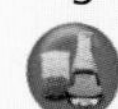

Science

NSES B Develop an understanding of chemical reactions.

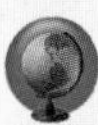

Social Studies

NCSS II B Time, Continuity, and Change Apply key concepts such as time, chronology, causality, change, conflict, and complexity to explain, analyze, and show connections among patterns of historical change and continuity.

NCTE *National Council of Teachers of English*
NCTM *National Council of Teachers of Mathematics*
NSES *National Science Education Standards*
NCSS *National Council for the Social Studies*

Resources for Meal Planning

There are many benefits to meal planning. Meal planning lets you enjoy nutritious, flavorful meals even when time or money are tight. Meal planning helps ensure good nutrition. A smart meal plan can save money, too.

Like any good plan, a plan for meals starts with identifying available resources. Resources include time and energy, skills and equipment, and available food, as well as money.

Time and Energy

Your time and energy are limited, and are affected by your multiple roles. A **role** is a set of responsibilities based on your different relationships to others. You have many different responsibilities in your roles as student, family member, and friend. You may also have responsibilities as a sibling, worker, teammate, or volunteer. Roles make demands on your time and energy. With so many responsibilities, planning what to eat can be challenging.

Planning healthful meals ahead of time can help you get good nutrition and stay energized for your busy life. Meal planning is also a skill you need for independence. Families can work as a team by pooling their time and energy. Meal planning and preparation tasks can be assigned based on who can do them most conveniently.

TECHNOLOGY FOR TOMORROW

High-Tech Kitchens

Just as it does in many other areas of life, technology saves time and labor in the kitchen. The high-tech products found in today's average kitchen would have made a significant difference in the lives of families who lived a hundred years ago. Then, most families prepared foods from scratch using basic equipment. Now, microwaves, food processors, juicers, food dehydrators, and bread making machines are just some of the tools that families can use to help them prepare foods with the push of a button. Thanks to technology, families can plan a wide variety of meals, knowing that they can complete many preparation steps in mere moments.

Investigate Plan two meals: one that can be prepared in 15 minutes using modern kitchen technology; and one that could be prepared in 15 minutes a century ago.

NCSS II B Time, Continuity, and Change Apply key concepts such as time, chronology, causality, change, conflict, and complexity to explain, analyze, and show connections among patterns of historical change and continuity.

Skills and Equipment

Successful meal planning takes advantage of each family member's cooking skills. Less experienced cooks can do simpler tasks at first and can learn more complicated techniques from more skilled family members. Less experienced cooks should also learn important rules for kitchen safety and cleanliness.

Kitchen equipment can help you use time and energy efficiently. A sharp knife, for example, makes slicing and chopping faster and safer. Often there is more than one right tool for the job. For example, you can make a stir-fry in a skillet instead of a wok. You can use two small pans instead of one large pan to bake a cake.

Available Food

Some foods are more plentiful at certain times of the year or in certain areas. For example, tomatoes are abundant in late summer and citrus fruits are abundant in winter. Foods are usually a good buy when they are in season. Use grocery store ads to determine what foods are in season as you plan your meals. Building meals around seasonal foods can help you ensure a high-quality, nutritious diet. You can preserve foods by canning or freezing to get even more value.

✓ Reading Check **Explain** What is a role and how does it relate to meal planning?

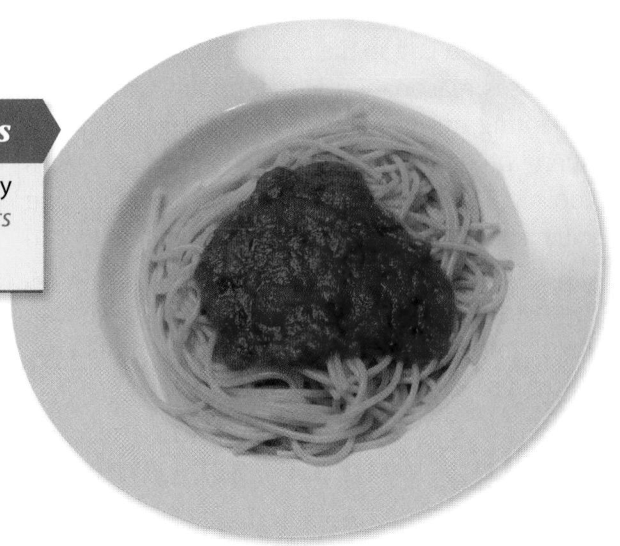

Home-Cooked Savings

Many people discover that they can save a lot of money by cooking meals at home. *What are some other benefits of home-cooked meals?*

The Food Budget

One of the most important resources you need for healthy eating is money. A budget helps you get the most from your money. A **budget** is a plan for managing money. When you budget, you decide how much money to spend for food, housing, clothing, transportation, health care, savings, entertainment, and any other expenses.

Americans spend about 10 percent of their disposable income (after taxes) on food each year. This includes food eaten at home and food eaten away from home. The percentage of income that Americans spend on food has decreased since the 1960s, but the percentage that they spend eating out has increased greatly.

Influences on Food Spending

One major influence on food spending is income. High-income families spend more dollars on food than low-income families, but their food spending represents a smaller percentage of their income. The challenge for any family is to provide wholesome, enjoyable meals without spending more than the budget allows. Good planning can help families create tasty, nutritious meals without spending a lot of money.

Besides income, several other factors influence how much money a family spends on food:

- The number of family members. It takes more money to feed a larger family than a smaller one, but a large family can also save money per serving by buying in bulk.
- The age of family members. It costs more to feed growing teens than elderly adults, for example.
- Time and skills available for food preparation. Buying takeout and prepared foods costs more than cooking from scratch.
- How often family members eat out.
- The amount of food wasted. Food may be wasted if it is not stored or prepared properly. If servings are larger than people can eat, leftovers may be thrown away.

Setting Up a Food Budget

Follow these steps to set up a family food budget:

1. Find out how much you spend on food. Record all food purchases for at least two **consecutive** weeks. Consecutive means sequential. Keep separate records for foods bought at the store and for foods eaten out, including restaurant meals, school lunches, takeouts, and vending machine snacks. Keep receipts or enter the amounts in a small notebook.
2. Determine the amount you spent on food each week. After two weeks, add up all the money you spent on groceries and all the money spent on food eaten out. Then add both amounts together. Divide that total by two to find the average amount you spent on food per week.
3. Find the percentage of food expenses used for eating at home and eating at restaurants. First divide the amount spent on food eaten out by the total food expense. Then multiply the result by 100.
4. Now find the percentage of income spent on food. Divide the average amount spent on food by the family's weekly income. Then multiply that figure by 100. Is it more or less than the average of 10 percent?

Now you can make decisions. Are your food expenses reasonable? Is the amount you spend on eating out in balance with the amount you spend on groceries? If your food expenses seem too high, you will need to create a budget that cuts spending. Try a 10 percent reduction to start. If you spend a lot on eating in restaurants, try cutting expenses there first. Your budget can be a simple dollar amount that represents how much you want to spend on food each week.

Meeting Your Budget Goals

Developing a workable budget often takes time and fine-tuning. Families need to continue tracking their food expenses to stay within their budget. In some weeks, you may spend more to stock up on sale items. In other weeks, you may buy only staples. **Staples** are basic items that are used on a regular basis, such as milk, cereal, eggs, and bread. You can use any money left over for unexpected needs, special occasions, or savings.

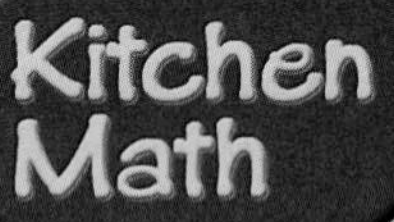

Buying In Bulk

Emiko can buy a quart (32 oz.) of milk for $3.50 at her local convenience store. Or she can go to the supermarket and buy a half gallon (64 oz.) for $4.00, or a gallon (128 oz.) for $5.00. She can also drive to the warehouse store and buy 2 gallons for $6.00, but it will take $5 worth of gas to get there and back. Which milk is the best buy, assuming that Emiko can consume all the milk before it expires?

Math Concept **Calculate Unit Price** The unit price of an item indicates the cost for every 1 unit of measurement. Calculate unit price by dividing the price of an item by the quantity.

Starting Hint Calculate the unit price of each size milk container by dividing its price by the number of ounces in the container. This calculation will give you the price per ounce. Find the item with the lowest price per ounce.

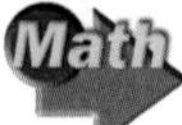

Appendix For math help, go to the Math Appendix at the back of the book.

NCTM Number and Operations Understand numbers, ways of representing numbers, relationships among numbers, and number systems.

What if a family spends more on food than budgeted, week after week? If they made only basic purchases and did not eat out, they probably need to allow more money in their budget for food. They may be able to cut back on other expenses to increase food spending.

Families can trim food costs by planning meals with the budget in mind. Cost-cutting strategies include:

Prepare simple meals at home more often. Homemade meals, such as casseroles, hearty soups, stews, and stir-fries, can cost less and taste better than convenience meals and food eaten out. By sharing kitchen tasks, family members can cut preparation time and have fun together.

Choose economical main dishes. Meat is usually the most expensive item in a food budget. Stretching or replacing animal proteins with high-protein plant foods, such as dry beans and peas and whole grains, can save money.

Look for store advertisements. Newspaper ads and flyers can point out good prices on many nutritious foods.

Reduce food waste. Avoid waste by preparing food properly. Reduce recipes for smaller families or appetites. Save money and avoid overeating by serving smaller portions. Use safe storage to protect leftovers for future meals.

Food Assistance Programs

Healthy citizens contribute productively to the economy, to their families, and to their communities. When people cannot afford healthy food due to old age, illness, or job loss, society suffers.

Many private organizations and religious groups run food banks and soup kitchens. Volunteering for these programs can be a rewarding experience.

Governments also support good nutrition by supplying service agencies with funds and commodities. A **commodity** is a product of agriculture, often surplus food purchased from farmers. Many food programs are funded by the federal government and carried out by state and local authorities. Here are six of the most important government food programs.

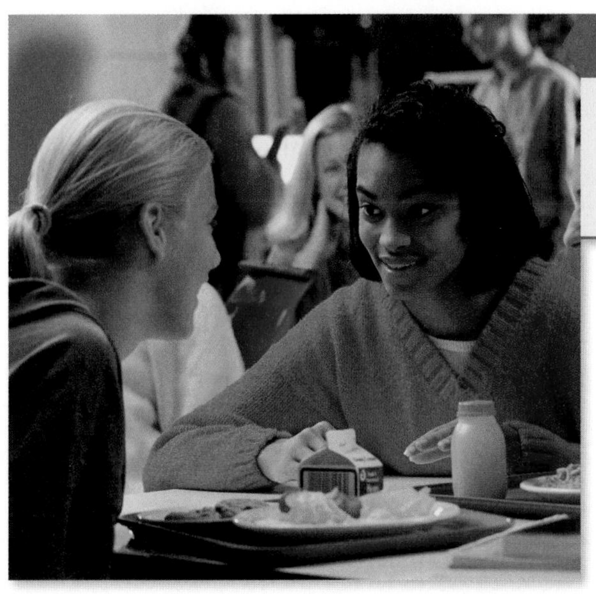

School Lunch

The National School Lunch Program helps children get the nutrition they need to grow and develop properly and to do well in school. *What government programs help older adults get the food they need?*

National School Lunch Program

This program began with the National School Lunch Act of 1946, which recognized that many low-income students lacked nutritious, balanced meals. The National School Lunch Program supplies cash and commodities to nonprofit food services in grade schools, high schools, and residential child care centers to serve free or reduced-price meals to children in need. The Summer Food Service Program offers breakfast and lunch during summer vacation in some communities.

Food Stamp Program

The Food Stamp Program was created by the Food Stamp Act of 1964. The goal of this program is to improve nutrition among low-income households. Families of a certain size and income can receive food help in the form of food stamps or an Electronic Benefits Transfer (EBT) card. Families can only use these funds for essential food purchases. Food stamps do not pay for nonfood items, tobacco, alcohol, pet food, or restaurant meals.

School Breakfast Program

Created by the Child Nutrition Act of 1966, the School Breakfast Program ensures that all children have access to a healthy breakfast at school. Eligible students can receive nutritionally balanced breakfasts at little or no cost.

Child and Adult Care Food Program

The Child and Adult Care Food Program began in 1968. Like the National School Lunch Program, it is funded by the National School Lunch Act of 1946. This program provides healthful meals and snacks to children in day care. The Child and Adult Care Food Program was expanded in the 1980s and 1990s to include older adults in adult care centers and families in homeless shelters.

Women, Infants, and Children Program (WIC)

First implemented in the early 1970s, the Women, Infants, and Children Program (WIC) is now funded by the Healthy Meals for Healthy Americans Act of 1994. The goal of the WIC program is to improve nutrition and health of low-income pregnant women, breast-feeding women, and children up to five years of age. Participants in WIC receive vouchers to use at retail food stores for wholesome foods. WIC also provides **supplemental** foods, nutrition education, and health services.

Elderly Nutrition Program (ENP)

The Elderly Nutrition Program began in 1972 and is funded by the Older Americans Act of 1965. The program provides grant money and commodities for meals served to aging citizens. Meals are delivered to community centers, to elder care facilities, and to older people in their homes.

✓ Reading Check **List** List four strategies for cutting food costs.

Nutrition Check

Skimp Now, Pay Later

When setting a food budget, remember the phrase, "An ounce of prevention is worth a pound of cure." Some people skimp on healthful foods in order to allow room in their budget for processed foods and snacks. This habit, however, can end up costing more money over time. A poor diet can also lead to health problems that can require expensive treatment or even prevent people from earning an income.

Think About It A college student tells you, "I'm really short on money, so I live on popcorn and candy bars." What health problems might the student face now and in the future? What advice would you offer?

Planning for Convenience

Home cooking, or **scratch cooking**, means preparing a dish from basic ingredients. Chicken soup from scratch, for example, is made from whole chicken, water, onions, carrots, seasonings, and rice or noodles. At its best, scratch cooking produces flavorful, economical meals. It uses fresh, quality ingredients, prepared the way you like them. People who cook from scratch often enjoy maintaining an herb or vegetable garden that provides healthy, home-grown produce.

Meals made from scratch can take a lot of time and energy. Even an experienced cook could easily spend half a day on one recipe. Many people do not have time for scratch cooking very often. Instead, they turn to time- and energy-saving products and techniques.

Convenience Foods

Convenience foods are foods that have been processed to make them easier and faster to use. You can find single-serving, microwavable containers of foods, ranging from Chinese-style noodles to oatmeal with chopped peaches. Retort packages can be boiled in water for a hot pasta entrée or broccoli in cheese sauce. Chunks of cleaned, peeled fruits are sold in plastic containers, ready for snacks or salads. In the refrigerator case are fresh potatoes, shredded or diced for home recipes.

Convenience foods can help with meal planning, but consider their pros and cons before you buy.

Cost Every additional step in processing adds to the price of the food. A ready-to-cook meatloaf purchased at the supermarket may cost twice as much as an equal amount of ground beef. Cut-up chicken pieces usually cost more per serving than a whole chicken.

Nutrition Processing removes some nutrients. Heat destroys vitamin C. Grains lose much of their fiber and nutrients during milling. Some convenience foods are high in fat, sodium, and added sugar, so it is important to read the Nutrition Facts panel.

Meal Appeal Processing affects food's flavor, color, and texture. As a result, convenience foods may lack the appeal of foods prepared at home.

Be a Smart Consumer

Hectic Lives Versus Healthful Meals

In one study, consumers cited a lack of time and information as the two biggest obstacles in planning healthful meals. Most believed that meals made from scratch, including children's lunches, were more nutritious than those bought away from home. But not all consumers are knowledgeable about what a good diet includes, and many said that busy schedules make it hard to learn about healthful options and prepare them at home. It is possible that a person could take the time to make a lunch from scratch that is less nutritious than a convenient pre-packaged lunch from a supermarket.

Challenge At a supermarket, assess the nutritional value of a pre-packaged lunch product. Compare this to a typical school lunch that you would prepare at home. Which is the better option?

Additives Some processed foods contain preservatives, artificial colors, or other additives. Check the ingredients list.

Packaging The more convenient a convenience food is, the more packaging it may need. Each ingredient in a casserole kit, for instance, may be sealed in a separate container inside the box. Both producing and disposing of packaging materials, even those that are recyclable, take a toll on the environment. In contrast, you can buy **bulk foods**, shelf-stable foods sold loose in covered bins or barrels, in just a single bag or reusable container.

Using Convenience Foods

Like restaurant meals, convenience foods can be part of a healthful, balanced diet. Look for directions and recipe suggestions on the label. Canned foods may need only heating. Boxed mixes require more preparation and often other ingredients. Be sure to read labels to find out what other ingredients you will need to prepare boxed mixes. Read the Nutrition Facts panel to see whether the information listed includes everything added to the mix or just what is in the mix.

Speed-Scratch Cooking

More and more cooks are enjoying a satisfying way to blend convenience with scratch cooking known as speed-scratch cooking. **Speed-scratch cooking** is an approach to cooking that uses a few convenience foods along with basic ingredients for easier meal preparation. With the shortcuts of speed-scratch cooking, recipes that took hours to prepare can be made in 30 minutes or less. As a result, many families are eating at home more often.

Speed-scratch cooking can also help you add variety and creativity to your food choices without spending a lot of money. For example, you could add taco seasoning to whipped cream cheese to make a Tex-Mex dip for tortilla chips, or use bottled Chinese dipping sauce as a topping for a baked potato. You could sauté fresh bell peppers with precooked chicken to make fajitas. Or you could add cooked beans and chopped tomatoes to boxed macaroni and cheese for a heartier meal with more vitamins, minerals, and fiber.

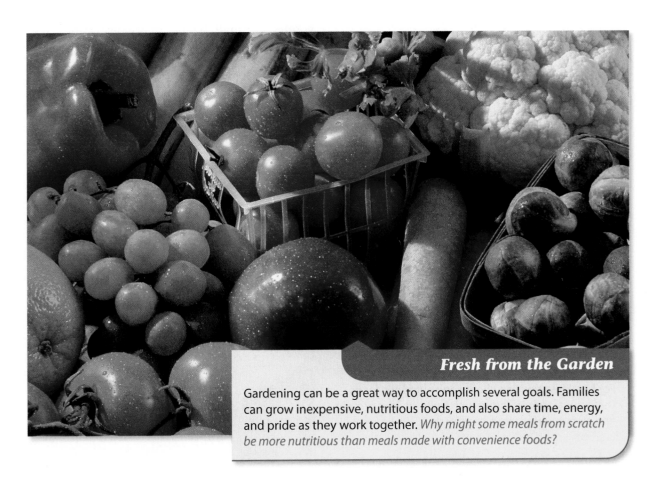

Fresh from the Garden

Gardening can be a great way to accomplish several goals. Families can grow inexpensive, nutritious foods, and also share time, energy, and pride as they work together. *Why might some meals from scratch be more nutritious than meals made with convenience foods?*

Always make sure to check the nutrition facts labels when using speed-scratch items. When food is processed, chemicals are sometimes added. Check to make sure fats and sugars are not added.

Time-Saving Techniques

In addition to using convenience foods, you can enjoy home-cooked meals more often with these time-saving strategies:

- Cut large pieces of meat or whole poultry into smaller portions. Small pieces cook more quickly and can be easier to serve.
- Prepare quick-cooking, one-dish meals. Choose casseroles, hearty salads, and stir-fries that combine vegetables, grain products, and protein foods.
- Try fish, a natural convenience food that is easily prepared and quickly cooked.
- Use a microwave oven to cook food from scratch, to defrost foods, and to heat leftovers.
- Work as a family team to plan and prepare meals. Teens can handle grocery shopping and many cooking tasks. Younger children can set the table. Everyone can help clean up.
- Set aside a weekend day to make and freeze lunches or dinners for the week ahead. Package dishes in single servings and include any needed instructions.
- Look for recipes that can be used in different ways. A lightly seasoned meat-and-bean mixture can be a base for chili, burritos, and taco salad. Prepare a large amount and freeze it in the quantity needed for each variation.
- If schedules keep family members from eating together at home, find another place to meet for a shared meal.

Saving Time at Breakfast

Breakfast is the nutritional foundation for the day. Nevertheless, many people do not have much time or appetite in the morning—at least, not for traditional breakfast foods, which can be heavy.

Plan ahead for healthy breakfasts that fit your schedule and appetite. Keep a supply of quick foods on hand, like instant hot cereal packets or fresh fruit and yogurt. Include breakfast foods when you cook for the freezer. Prepare a whole recipe of pancakes, freeze them individually, and reheat a few in the microwave for a quick pancake breakfast. You could even organize a "breakfast bar." Store cereals, bowls, spoons, and glasses near the refrigerator. Keep milk, juice, and fresh fruit in easy reach on one refrigerator shelf.

What if your appetite does not wake up until mid-morning? Try eating a small amount of food that you can grab without a lot of preparation. Any healthful combination of carbohydrates and protein will work: a handful of raisins and nuts and a glass of milk or a slice of cold pizza and a glass of pineapple juice. Later in the morning, another snack such as yogurt, a small bagel, or cheese cubes will keep you going until lunch.

✓ **Reading Check** **Identify** At its best, what benefits does traditional scratch cooking offer?

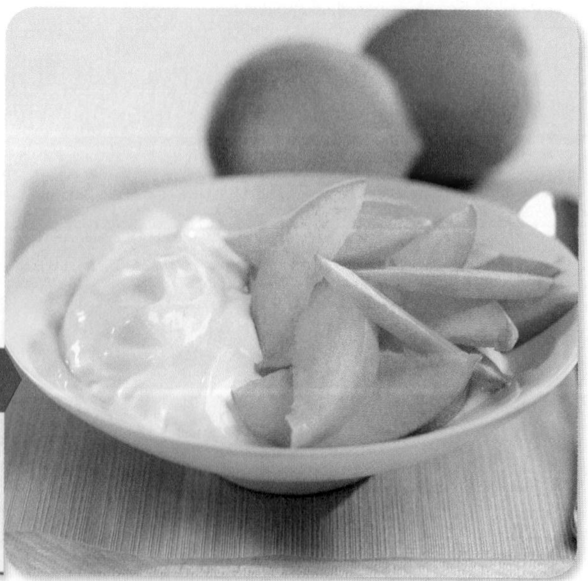

A Tasty Start

For breakfast, you can choose any nutritious foods that appeal to you. Yogurt with fruit provides protein and carbohydrates for a healthy start. *How can you fit breakfast into a busy schedule?*

Planning for Appeal

Apppealing meals have an interesting combination of flavors, colors, and textures. Like the musicians in your favorite band, foods in an appetizing meal are not only good but also good together. Some foods **complement** each other, or go together, better than others.

You can make a meal appealing by paying attention to these factors:

Flavor Food flavors should harmonize. Foods in a meal should keep the taste buds interested, but not overwhelmed. Avoid using foods with similar flavors in the same meal. If you serve a fruit salad with the main course, for example, choose a dessert without fruit.

Color Select foods in a variety of colors. Imagine a dinner of roast chicken, mashed potatoes, and jicama salad. The meal is tasty, but because all three foods have a similar off-white color, the plate may not look as appealing as a plate with more color variety. Colorful fruits and vegetables brighten a meal. Garnishes can also add color.

Texture Texture refers to the way food feels when you chew it. Different foods have different textures. Brown rice is firmer than white rice, for example. You also can change the texture of foods through how you prepare them. Raw carrots are crunchier than cooked carrots, for example. Aim for a variety of textures in meals, and think of ways to add an appealing crunch. For example, toast Italian bread slices to serve with soup.

Shape and Size It is easy to add variety by changing food's shape and size. You can create different effects with a single food. You can slice a tomato vertically into wedges or horizontally into a wagon wheel pattern, or serve corn on the cob or as kernels.

Careers in Food

Lucy Zaunbrecher
Television Chef

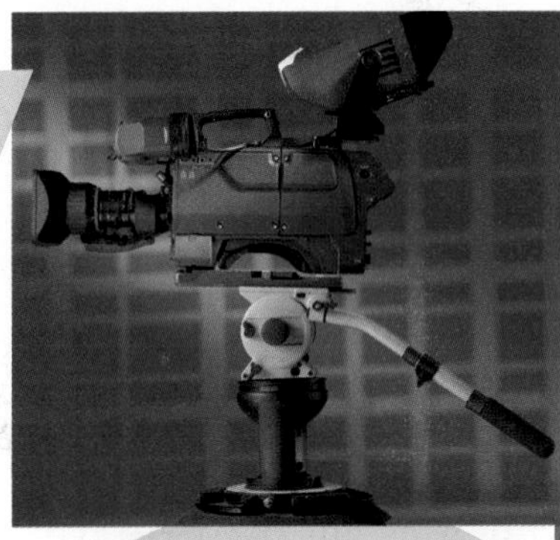

Q: How did you become a TV chef?

A: I am a 69-year-old homemaker who pursued a career at the age of 55. First, I wrote a cookbook and promoted it on morning cooking shows. I would get a five- or ten-minute segment and demonstrate one cooking technique.

Q: What advice can you give a young cook or chef who wants to have a TV show like yours?

A: You have to love cooking and be prepared for hard work, because doing what I do is not as easy as it looks. You have to practice cooking at home, and figure out how to demonstrate cooking techniques on television.

Q: What are your favorite aspects of cooking on TV?

A: When I do what I do, and I do it well, it makes me happy. I get a warm and fuzzy feeling!

"Follow your heart because life is too precious to waste."
— Lucy Zaunbrecher
Host, Ms. Lucy's Classic Cajun Culture & Cooking Show
– Baton Rouge, LA

Education and Training

A culinary school background is important, but so is experience working with an established chef or cook. Formal training in broadcasting is valuable.

Qualities and Skills

In addition to cooking skills, you need to have a pleasant personality and be able to engage people. Being able to put people at ease is important.

Related Career Opportunities

Television chefs must entertain their audiences, so their work is similar to other entertainment-related occupations.

Temperature A food's temperature affects its taste and texture, as well as its safety. To help keep hot and cold foods at their most appealing temperature, serve them on separate, preheated or chilled plates. Use potholders when pulling a plate from the oven. Remember that the outside temperature affects what foods people enjoy. Hot cider, for example, is more appealing on a winter day than in the middle of summer.

✓ Reading Check **List** What are five things to think about when planning how to make meals more appealing?

Weekly Meal Planning

Planning meals in advance can help keep meals interesting. It is also easier to think about variety and meal appeal ahead of time, when you are alert and not hungry.

Planning meals by the week can save time and money and help you follow a healthful eating plan. **Figure 16.1** shows a sample meal plan. For good nutrition, the plan includes servings of foods from all the food groups, sometimes called exchanges.

Figure 16.1 Sample Meal Plan

Plan for a Week A meal plan like this takes time but pays off since all items can be purchased with one trip to the grocery store. ***What are some items from the grocery store that will be used in multiple meals throughout the week?***

Meal	Monday	Tuesday	Wednesday
Breakfast	• Bran cereal • Sliced bananas • Rye toast • Milk/tea	• Fruit smoothie • Bran muffin • Coffee	• Orange juice • Bagel with low-fat cream cheese • Milk/coffee
Lunch	(Packed) • Turkey sandwich on whole-wheat bread • Red, yellow, and green pepper sticks • Apple • Fortified almond milk or yogurt	(Packed) • Peanut butter sandwich on whole-wheat bread • Carrots • Pear • Milk or yogurt	• Adults-eat lunch out • Jake and Crystal-school lunch
Dinner	• Baked fish • Coleslaw • Broccoli • Whole-wheat rolls • Milk/tea	• Spaghetti with meatballs • Tossed salad • Italian bread • Milk/coffee	• Baked chicken • Mashed potatoes • Spinach • Sliced tomato salad • Whole-wheat rolls • Milk/coffee
Snacks	• Fresh fruits or vegetables • Trail mix	• Fresh fruits or vegetables • Popcorn	• Fresh fruits or vegetables • Pretzels
Notes	Crystal not home for dinner—swim team banquet.	Everyone home for dinner.	Dad has dinner meeting.

Another benefit of meal planning is that it makes grocery shopping much easier and quicker. Before planning, check the refrigerator, freezer, and fruit bowl for leftovers and fresh produce that need to be used up. Then make your plan and decide what you need to buy. Arrange your grocery list by supermarket aisle to save time. Remember that time is a resource. Label your grocery list by store section so you do not spend time going back and forth in the store. Once in the store, keep your eyes open for unadvertised specials that fit into your meal plan. If your plan called for baked potatoes, but sweet potatoes are on special, you might substitute one for the other.

Some families set aside a regular time and place for meal planning. This helps with organization and lets family members discuss scheduling issues that may affect the week's menus and recipes. Family members can also agree on how to share the shopping, cooking, and clean-up tasks.

It is also wise to develop a few meal plans based on nutritious convenience foods that you can keep on hand. If time is short, you can fall back on these quick meals.

For example, if the whole family will be attending a school play on one night, a meal prepared in a slow cooker might help get dinner on the table on time.

Thursday	Friday	Saturday	Sunday	Meal
• Orange juice • Oatmeal • Whole-wheat toast • Milk/tea	• Toaster waffles • Strawberries • Milk/coffee	• Grapefruit • Omelet • Whole-wheat toast • Milk/coffee	• French toast with syrup • Sliced oranges • Milk/coffee	**Breakfast**
(Packed) • Leftover chicken sandwich on whole-wheat bread • Carrot and celery sticks • Banana • Milk or fortified almond milk	(Packed) • Leftover chili • Cucumber sticks • Tortilla chips • Mixed fruit cup • Milk or yogurt	• Hearty vegetable soup • Swiss chard • Corn muffin • Milk/coffee	• Sandwiches on assorted breads • Tomato-cucumber salad • Milk/coffee	**Lunch**
• Spicy chili with beans • Butternut squash • Tossed salad • Cornbread • Milk/coffee	• Chinese takeout • Milk/coffee	• Chicken stir-fry with vegetables • Brown rice • Whole-wheat roll • Milk/coffee • Frozen yogurt with chocolate syrup	• Pot roast with vegetables • Fruit salad • Whole-wheat rolls • Milk/tea • Angel food cake	**Dinner**
• Fresh fruits or vegetables • Popcorn	• Fresh fruits and vegetables with yogurt	• Popcorn • Flavored yogurt • Mixed fruit juice	• Fresh fruits or vegetables • Rice cakes	**Snacks**
Jake's basketball game—eat early. Plan next week's meals.	Mom working late shift. Dad will pick up Chinese takeout on way home from work.	Shop for food. Rob and Cindy coming for dinner.	Aunt Clara coming for dinner.	**Notes**

Meal Planning for One

Meal planning is just as essential for single people as for families. Planning menus, shopping for food, and cooking may not seem worth the effort for just one person. Without definite plans, single adults may slip into poor eating habits, relying on frozen convenience meals or takeout foods, or substituting snacks for regular meals.

Meal planning for one poses a few challenges. Foods are often packaged to serve a group, and some packages of food need to be used quickly after opening. Smaller size packages often cost more per serving than larger packages with more servings.

Singles can share large food packages with a friend or freeze them into single-serving packages. Single people can also buy bulk foods in the exact amount they need. Buying prepared foods from a supermarket deli can sometimes save money by reducing food waste.

Many recipes can be creatively adapted for people eating alone. For example, stuffing can be used with a chicken breast or a tofu cutlet rather than a whole bird. Larger recipes can serve as multiple meals. A meatloaf eaten with rice and roasted vegetables for dinner on Monday can be the filling for a sandwich for lunch on Tuesday. Cooking for the freezer also comes in handy. By choosing recipes that freeze well, a single person can prepare enough individual servings for several more meals. Those frozen meals can be especially useful when cooking for one seems like too much of an effort.

Like grocery items, larger recipes can also be shared. Singles who enjoy eating with others can meet regularly and take turns cooking for each other. Some clubs have a weekly or monthly potluck, with each member bringing a dish.

Meals alone can be enjoyable, too. Enjoying flavorful, healthful foods, accompanied by your favorite music, can be a soothing end to a busy day.

Light and Healthy Recipe

Versatile Chicken Salad

Chicken salad can be served as a sandwich for lunch, with crackers for a snack, or on a bed of lettuce for a nutritious dinner.

Ingredients

- **1 cup** Lowfat plain yogurt
- **2 tsp.** Lemon juice
- **¼ tsp.** Paprika
- **1 pound** Diced grilled chicken
- **¼ cup** Diced carrots
- **¼ cup** Diced celery
- **¼ cup** Raisins
- **2 Tbsp.** Diced almonds

Directions

1. Mix the yogurt, lemon juice, and paprika in a small bowl.
2. In a larger mixing bowl, combine the chicken, carrots, celery, raisins, and almonds.
3. Fold the yogurt mixture into the chicken mixture.
4. Chill the chicken salad in the refrigerator for at least one hour.

Yield 4 servings

Nutrition Analysis per Serving

■ Calories	224 g
■ Total fat	5 g
Saturated fat	1 g
Cholesterol	65 mg
■ Sodium	601 mg
■ Carbohydrate	16
Dietary fiber	1 g
Sugars	11 g
■ Protein	31 g

CHAPTER 16 Review & Applications

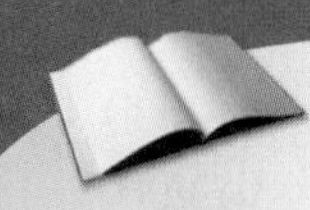

After You Read

Chapter Summary

Meal planning can save money and help to ensure good nutrition. It requires time and energy, and utilizes family members' skills as well as available equipment and foods. A food budget helps with meal planning. There are many strategies for setting up and meeting a budget. Food assistance programs help people have access to nutritious foods. When planning meals, people may look to convenience foods to help them save time. To plan appealing meals, pay attention to factors such as flavor, color, and texture. It is possible to plan a week's worth of meals, and to plan meals for just one person.

Content and Academic Vocabulary Review

1. Use each of these content and academic vocabulary words in a sentence.

Content Vocabulary

- role (p. 222)
- budget (p. 223)
- staples (p. 224)
- commodity (p. 224)
- scratch cooking (p. 226)
- convenience foods (p. 226)
- bulk foods (p. 227)
- speed-scratch cooking (p. 227)

Academic Vocabulary

- consecutive (p. 223)
- supplemental (p. 225)
- complement (p. 229)

Review Key Concepts

2. **Explain** the benefits of meal planning.
3. **Explain** how to create and meet a food budget.
4. **Describe** convenience foods and how they can be used to save time while cooking.
5. **Describe** ways to make a meal appealing to the senses.
6. **Explain** how to develop a meal plan for a week.

Critical Thinking

7. **Describe** what might happen to Lisa's holiday dinner in December. She plans on serving a salad of fresh, locally grown tomatoes bought from the farmers market.
8. **Contrast** the Bova and the Schmitt families. Both families are well-fed. The Bova family has five members. The Schmitt family has three. Both families spend the same amount of money on food. Why do you think this might be?
9. **Conclude** what changes the Browns can make. The Browns eat frozen, microwavable dinners every night. They notice that they are spending too much of their income on food. What changes can they make to save money and eat more healthfully?
10. **Explain** how you would change a meal that consists of broiled halibut, white rice, steamed cauliflower, and applesauce to save time and energy.

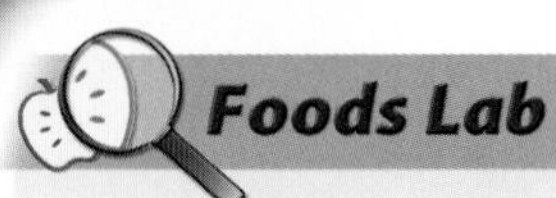

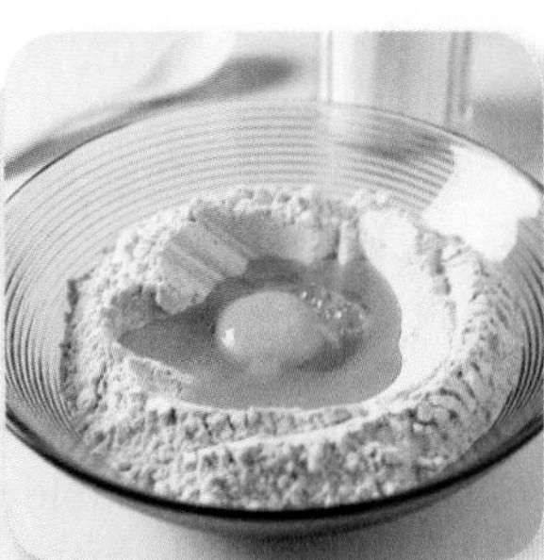

11. Using Dry Mixes Dry mixes, such as those used to season tacos, make dressings and gravies, or bake cakes, are a common convenience food. Creative cooks can use them to add fast flavor to a variety of foods.

Procedure Create a recipe that uses a dry mix in a creative way. Look through cookbooks for ideas on ingredients and proportions, if needed. Prepare the recipe.

Analysis In an oral presentation, explain how the mix added flavor, color, and texture to the recipe, shortened preparation time, and affected the dish's nutritional value.

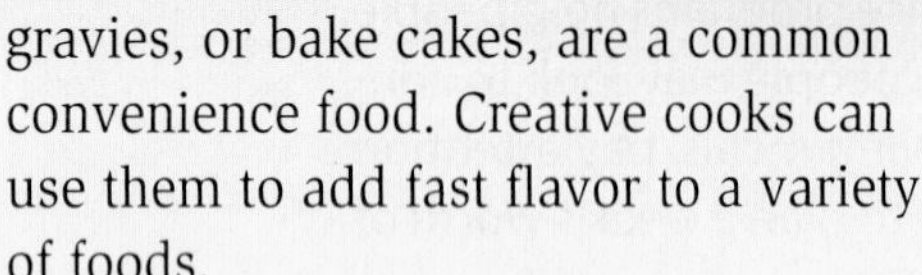

HEALTHFUL CHOICES

12. Speedy Breakfast Walter's refrigerator is short on supplies. He is in a hurry to get to work one morning, and his stomach is growling. In his pantry, Walter has a can of soda, a bag of mixed nuts, a package of cookies, and a box of crackers. What should Walter eat for breakfast? Why are some of the items in Walter's pantry a poor choice for breakfast?

TECH Connection

13. Finding Food Assistance Imagine you are in need of food assistance. Conduct research to identify a local or federal food assistance program in your area. How does the program work? Where is it located? Who is eligible to participate? What assistance is provided? Is the program in need of volunteers? Create a multimedia presentation to show your findings to your classmates.

Real-World Skills

Problem-Solving Skills

14. Evaluate Meal Preparation Observe someone making a meal. Write notes about how the meal was prepared. Then write an evaluation identifying what was efficient about the process and what steps could be improved to be more efficient.

Interpersonal and Collaborative Skills

15. Meal Plan Meeting Follow your teacher's instructions to form groups. You are a family holding a weekly meal-planning meeting. Each person should list 5 foods they want to eat. Work together to create a meal plan for the next week. Plans must be cost- and time-efficient and include at least three of each person's preferences.

Financial Literacy Skills

16. Food Spending Suppose two families of four each spend $360 on food every month. Family A has a net monthly income of $3,000 and Family B, $1,900. What percentage of income does each family spend on food? Compare how the overall budgets for the two families may be affected.

Academic Skills

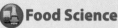

Food Science

17. Vegetables and Acids Green vegetables contain chlorophyll, while red-purple vegetables contain anthocyanins. These pigments are affected by the acidity level of the liquid they are cooked in. To demonstrate this, acid will be added to the cooking water for two different vegetables.

Procedure Add 1 cup of water to two small pots. Add five green beans to each pot. Add ½ cup of vinegar to one of the pots. Wait 15 minutes then take notes about any changes in the color of the vegetables. Put both pots on a stove and bring them to a boil. Boil for three minutes and note any other changes. Repeat the process with five slices of red onion in two pots.

Analysis What conclusions can you draw about the affects of acid on the two different pigments, chlorophyll and anthocyanins? Write a paragraph detailing your conclusions.

NSES B Develop an understanding of chemical reactions.

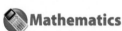

Mathematics

18. Food Spending Joey is trying to work out his budget and is trying to figure out how much he wants to spend on food. If Joey makes $875 per week and wants to limit his total food budget to 10% of his income, how much money can he spend each week on food?

Math Concept **Percentages** To work out the dollar amount from a percentage, multiply the total by the percentage you are trying to find.

Starting Hint Multiply Joey's salary of $875 by 10% to find his food budget.

NCTM Algebra Represent and analyze mathematical situations and structures using algebraic symbols.

English Language Arts

19. Persuade to Plan Write a persuasive letter directed toward a family that fails to plan its meals. Your letters should clearly state the advantages of meal planning, what it entails, and what families miss if they do not plan meals.

NCTE 4 Use written language to communicate effectively.

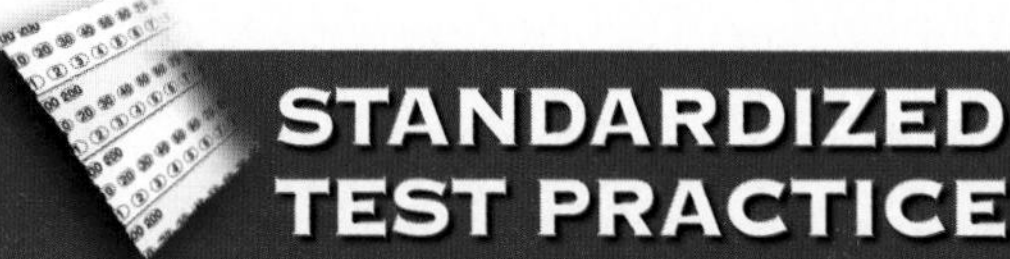

STANDARDIZED TEST PRACTICE

READING COMPREHENSION

Re-read the paragraph about the National School Lunch Program on page 225. Then select the best answer to the question.

20. The National School Lunch Program supplies cash and commodities to ______________________.

a. nonprofit food services in preschools, grade schools, high schools, and residential child care centers.

b. children under 16 in need throughout America.

c. children in need all summer.

d. nonprofit food services in grade schools, high schools, and residential child care centers.

Test-Taking Tip Before you answer a reading comprehension question, carefully read the text to which the question refers. Then read through the question and each of the answer choices. Next, take a second look at the text to confirm which answer is correct. Some answers may seem identical, but they contain subtle differences. Pay attention to every word.

CHAPTER 17

Shopping for Food

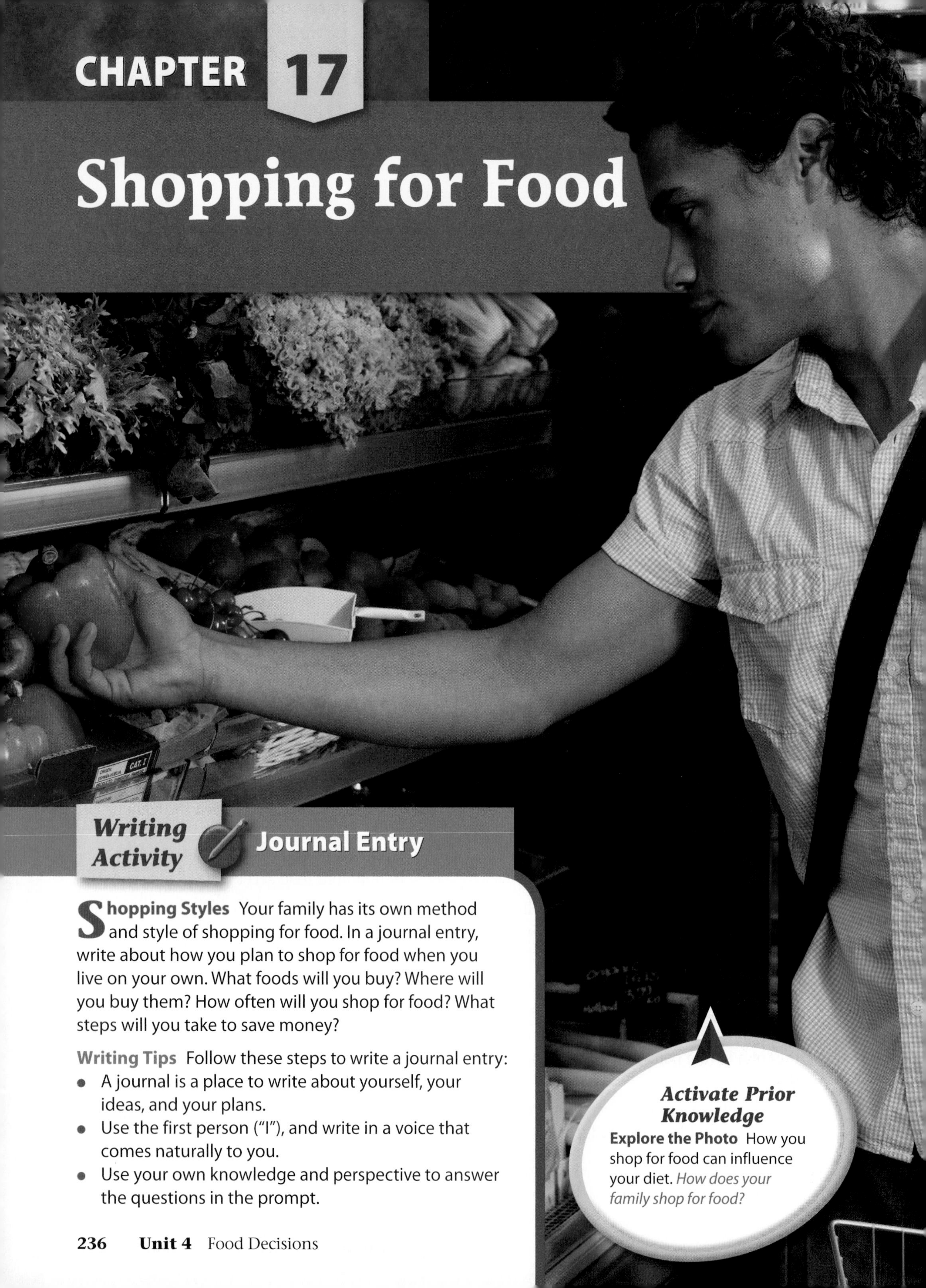

Writing Activity — Journal Entry

Shopping Styles Your family has its own method and style of shopping for food. In a journal entry, write about how you plan to shop for food when you live on your own. What foods will you buy? Where will you buy them? How often will you shop for food? What steps will you take to save money?

Writing Tips Follow these steps to write a journal entry:

- A journal is a place to write about yourself, your ideas, and your plans.
- Use the first person ("I"), and write in a voice that comes naturally to you.
- Use your own knowledge and perspective to answer the questions in the prompt.

Activate Prior Knowledge

Explore the Photo How you shop for food can influence your diet. *How does your family shop for food?*

Reading Guide

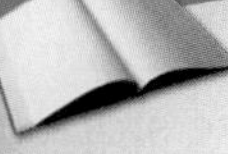

Before You Read

Preview Examine the photos, figures, and captions in this chapter. Then brainstorm three ways that smart shopping can affect your overall quality of life.

Read to Learn

Key Concepts

- **Identify** places to shop for food and explain how to choose a store.
- **Explain** how to plan your shopping to be effective and easy.
- **Describe** how to use food labels to understand the foods you eat.
- **Summarize** how to shop smart to get quality foods and save money.

Main Idea

Shopping for food is a skill that can help you to conserve time, select quality products, and save money.

Content Vocabulary

You will find definitions for these words in the glossary at the back of this book.

- ☐ natural food
- ☐ organic food
- ☐ food cooperative
- ☐ perishable food
- ☐ impulse buying
- ☐ code dating
- ☐ open dating
- ☐ sell-by date
- ☐ use-by date
- ☐ universal product code (UPC)
- ☐ comparison shopping
- ☐ unit price
- ☐ rebate
- ☐ store brand

Academic Vocabulary

You will find these words in your reading and on your tests. Use the glossary to look up their definitions, if necessary.

- representative
- customize

Graphic Organizer

Use a graphic organizer like the one below to note the differences between foods that are labeled Organic, Made with Organic Ingredients, and Natural.

Organic	Made with Organic Ingredients	Natural

Graphic Organizer Go to this book's Online Learning Center at **glencoe.com** to print out this graphic organizer.

Academic Standards

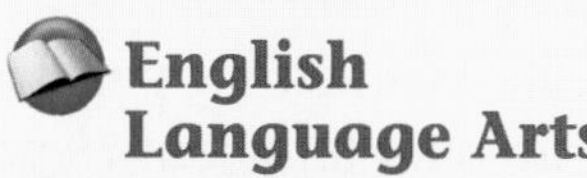

English Language Arts

NCTE 8 Use information resources to gather information and create and communicate knowledge.

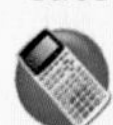

Mathematics

NCTM Problem Solving Apply and adapt a variety of appropriate strategies to solve problems.

NCTM Algebra Represent and analyze mathematical situations and structures using algebraic symbols.

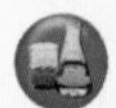

Science

NSES B Develop an understanding of chemical reactions.

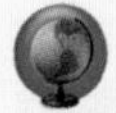

Social Studies

NCSS III I People, Places, and Environments Describe and assess ways that historical events have been influenced by, and have influenced, physical and human geographic factors in local, regional, national, and global settings.

NCTE *National Council of Teachers of English*
NCTM *National Council of Teachers of Mathematics*
NSES *National Science Education Standards*
NCSS *National Council for the Social Studies*

Where to Shop

Just like preparing food, shopping for food is a skill. Practicing this skill helps you to save time, choose the best quality food, and get the best value for your money. You have many choices in buying food. Food stores go by many names, but they fall into two basic types: supermarkets and specialty stores such as food cooperatives and farmers' markets.

Supermarkets

Supermarkets are popular, all-purpose stores that account for about 75 percent of all grocery sales. Most supermarkets are part of a regional or nationwide chain, which gives them the buying power to offer competitive prices. Large supermarkets may stock 50,000 items—all kinds of food and drinks, as well as paper products, cleaning supplies, pet items, and health and beauty aids. Many supermarkets have their own bakeries, butcher shops, and take-out food departments. Local banks may operate a small banking center inside. Supermarkets have different variations that emphasize low prices or convenience.

Supercenters Supercenters are huge stores that combine a supermarket with other types of shops in one building. They may include a full-service pharmacy, a hair salon, a vision center, or a department store.

Warehouse Stores Warehouse stores are large stores with low prices. Warehouse stores usually offer limited customer service. They sell basic food items, like canned goods and bread, in bulk. Shoppers bag or box their own groceries when checking out, using their own bags or spare store boxes. Larger "super warehouse" stores have separate food departments.

Warehouse Clubs Warehouse clubs, or wholesale clubs, are large stores that require an annual membership fee. Members can buy a large variety of food items at low prices, but usually in extra-large quantities only—four-pound bags of tortilla chips and one-gallon jugs of salsa, for example. Some stores carry gourmet items, along with clothing, housewares, and small appliances.

Health Food Supermarkets Health food supermarkets carry only natural foods. A **natural food** is a food that has been minimally processed and has few additives such as dyes and added sugars. Health food supermarkets are sometimes called natural food stores. Health food supermarkets offer many vegetarian foods, including various grains, beans, and

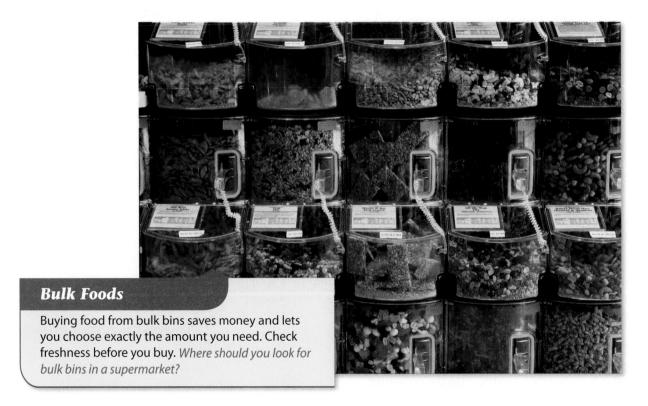

Bulk Foods

Buying food from bulk bins saves money and lets you choose exactly the amount you need. Check freshness before you buy. *Where should you look for bulk bins in a supermarket?*

other healthful foods. Most health food supermarkets have a wide array of organic foods. An **organic food** is a food produced without the use of pesticides, artificial fertilizers, growth hormones, or antibiotics, and without genetic modification or irradiation. Some health food supermarkets sponsor cooking classes and lectures on health and nutrition.

Specialty Stores

Specialty stores focus on specific foods or offer special services.

Independent Grocers Independent grocers are markets that are not part of a chain. Independent grocers may charge higher prices than big supermarkets, but they have more freedom to choose the local foods and specialty foods that their customers prefer.

Specialty Stores Specialty stores are small, independent stores that sell one specific type of food, such as fish, cheese, wine, or baked goods. Specialty stores are good places to find high-quality, fresh food and gourmet items. Ethnic grocers offer grains, produce, and spices of different cultures. Prices at specialty stores are generally higher than prices at supermarkets.

Food Cooperatives A **food cooperative**, or co-op, is a food distribution business owned and operated by its members. The cooperative keeps food costs down by buying food in quantity and having members do much of the work. Members receive a discount for the hours they work. This hands-on approach gives members more control over the food in their store. Many cooperatives emphasize fresh or natural foods. Some co-ops sell to nonmembers also.

Convenience Stores Convenience stores include service station food marts and drugstores. Like convenience foods, they're quick and easy to use. Some stores never close. Their line of groceries is limited and based on staples and snacks. Shoppers pay for the convenience: food prices are generally higher than in most other types of stores.

Farmers' Markets Farmers' markets are groups of stalls where farmers sell their produce during the growing season. Farmers' markets are growing more and more popular in cities. The produce at farmers' markets is often fresher and lower in cost than produce at supermarkets.

Online Food Retailers Many food sellers operate partly or entirely on the Web. You can find nearly any specialty item online, from gourmet chocolates to exotic spices. Some supermarket chains also allow shoppers to order groceries online. The stores prepare orders for pick-up or deliver them for a fee.

Be a Smart Consumer

Farmers' Markets

Farmers' markets are a vital resource, even in urban areas. Produce growers are usually experts on the foods they sell. Some provide nutritional facts and recipes. Most farmers' markets in the United States participate in the federal government's Farmers' Market Nutrition Program, which provides coupons for fresh foods to low-income families and older adults. Some contribute produce to food banks and other social service agencies. Farmers' markets make shopping a social activity, and strengthen communities. In discussing food, farming, and the news of the day, growers and consumers gain a better appreciation for each other.

Challenge By shopping at farmers' markets, consumers support them. List three specific ways that your choice to support a farmers' market can benefit others in your community.

Choosing a Store

Most stores claim to offer friendly service, low prices, convenient locations, and a wide selection. To evaluate whether these claims are true, ask yourself the following questions:

- How do the store's regular prices and sale prices compare with the prices at other stores?
- Are prices clearly marked?
- Are the employees courteous, knowledgeable, and helpful? Is there an information center to answer your questions?

TECHNOLOGY FOR TOMORROW

Cyber Shopping

Virtually anything can be ordered with the click of a computer mouse, including groceries. To buy food online, shoppers create an account at a supermarket's Web site. There, they can compare prices and select the foods they want, even specifying forms, such as husked corn on the cob. As early as one day after ordering, groceries are delivered to shoppers' homes in vehicles equipped with refrigeration and freezer units. Online grocery shoppers pay service and delivery fees. For some, these costs are comparable to what they would spend on transportation to and from the supermarket, and are worth the time they save by shopping from home.

Investigate Compare the costs of online shopping with those of shopping in person. Which method would provide the best value for your family and why?

NCSS III I People, Places, and Environments Describe and assess ways that historical events have been influenced by, and have influenced, physical and human geographic factors in local, regional, national, and global settings.

- If the store is large, is it easy to find your way around?
- Are all parts of the store, including shelves and bulk bins, clean and neat? Are food packages in good condition? Does the store smell clean?
- Are shelves and cases well stocked with a variety of brands and sizes?
- Does the produce department feel cool? Do fresh fruits and vegetables look fresh? Are greens kept moist and berries dry?
- Are the meat and dairy cases cold enough to keep the foods at a safe temperature?
- Does the store have a fair return policy?

If you answer "no" to any of these questions, you may want to choose another store. It may be worth your time and effort to go further from home to get better quality food.

✓ Reading Check **Describe** Describe five places where you can shop for food.

Plan Your Shopping

The typical American shopper goes to the supermarket once every three days. Some of these trips result from forgetting to buy items on the previous trip. A well-planned shopping trip helps you avoid these extra trips, spend less time in the store, and manage your spending.

Getting to Know a Store

Some stores are so big that you need a map to find your way around. Look for a map or directory at the entrance showing **representative** items, or samples of products, found in each aisle.

Most supermarkets have the same general layout. In the middle of the store are numbered aisles of shelves stocked with packaged, shelf-stable foods, as well as household goods and health and beauty aids. Products are arranged by type. For example, breakfast cereals and bars are grouped together on one aisle, and pet items are grouped together on another aisle.

Around the edges of the store are coolers and cases for perishable foods. A **perishable food** is a food that spoils quickly without proper storage. Many perishable foods must be refrigerated or frozen. Most stores have these sections for perishable foods:

- A produce department for fresh fruits and vegetables.
- A refrigerated meat, poultry, and fish department.
- Refrigerated sections for dairy products, eggs, cured luncheon meats and sausages, and fresh pasta.
- A freezer section for all frozen foods, including many convenience foods.

Look for bulk foods in their own department or with other foods of the same type. For example, bins of nuts are often found in the produce department, and barrels of flour are kept with the baking supplies. To buy bulk foods, you fill a container, usually a bag, with the desired amount of food. You then write the food's identification number on a tag or sticker so that the checkout clerk can identify the contents.

Timing Your Trip

To save time and stress, avoid the store's busiest hours. Most supermarkets are crowded between 4:30 p.m. and 6:30 p.m. Weekends are also busy. If you can shop during less congested hours, you may feel less rushed and make better choices.

Writing a Shopping List

A shopping list helps you remember what you need to buy and get through your shopping trip quickly. A list can also help prevent **impulse buying**, buying items you did not plan to purchase and do not really need. Impulse buying can ruin your food budget. Start writing your shopping list during your weekly meal planning. Do you need to buy anything for the menus and recipes you have planned? List these items in the amounts you need, increasing the quantities if you plan to cook additional meals to freeze. Check your supply of food, paper products, and cleaning supplies to see what you already have on hand. Also check local store ads for sale items that you might want to use in meals.

Group items on your shopping list in the order they are arranged in the store. For example, group items that are in the same department. Take a pen or pencil with you to the store and cross off items as you add them to your cart so you will not overlook anything.

Many families keep a shopping reminder list in the kitchen and jot down items that are running low. Some people use the computer to keep a shopping list with all the things they usually buy. Each week, they **customize**, or tailor, and print the list. Many people use online grocery lists.

✓ Reading Check **Identify** When do supermarkets tend to be the most crowded?

Organized and Ready

A well-organized shopping list makes it easier to find needed items once you get to the store. *Why is it a good idea to list frozen foods at the end of the list?*

Using Food Labels

Wrappers on food packages are full of details about the food inside. Food labels are part advertising and part information. Understanding labels and distinguishing facts from claims is an important shopping skill.

Basic Information

The Nutrition Facts panel on a food package lists the calories, nutrients, number of servings, and portion size of a food. Food labels must also tell you other information.

Kind of Food Labels identify the kind of food, such as chicken pot pie or peaches in light syrup. Analogs are not called by the name of the food they imitate. For example, soy-based sausages may be labeled "breakfast links." Food labels also identify the form of the food, if more than one form is commonly available. For example, a food label on canned tomatoes should say whether the tomatoes are whole, diced, or crushed.

Amount of Food Labels give the amount of food in the package in both customary and metric measurements. The amount may be written as a volume, such as 2 liters, or as a net weight, such as 12 ounces. Net weight is the weight of the food and any added liquid without the packaging. Labels also give nutrition information per serving. Make sure to note the number of servings in a package before consuming it.

List of Ingredients Labels on foods with more than one ingredient must list all the ingredients. Ingredients are listed in order from the largest to the smallest amount by weight. Ingredients must be identified by their common name. For example, a label would list baking soda, not sodium bicarbonate. The purpose of any additives must be explained, such as "to inhibit mold growth."

Name and Address of the Manufacturer, Packer, or Distributor An e-mail address, Web site, or toll-free phone number may be included in addition to a physical address.

Instructions for Safe Storage Labels also list storage methods that are recommended to maintain quality or safety, such as "Refrigerate after opening."

Some products have special labeling requirements. For example, the USDA requires that safe handling instructions be printed on packages of raw meat, poultry, and eggs. Beverages that contain fruit juice must have the percentage of juice listed on their labels.

Most labels include a picture of the product and directions for use. If the product is not shown exactly as it is found in the package, the photo must be labeled "serving suggestion."

Figure 17.1 Decoding Food Labels

What's in It? Understanding the content of labels can help you to choose quality, nutritious foods. ***If your breakfast cereal box says "High in Fiber," and the recommended Daily Value for fiber is 25 grams, at least how much fiber does it contain?***

Term	What It Means
High	Provides at least 20 percent of the Daily Value for the nutrient per serving.
Good source	Contains 10 to 19 percent of the Daily Value for the nutrient per serving.
More	Contains at least 10 percent more of the Daily Value for the nutrient than a comparable food per serving.
Free	Contains no significant amount of the ingredient. This term is used for fat, saturated fat, cholesterol, sodium, sugar, and calories. "Free" may be written with a percentage, such as "97 percent fat-free." "Nonfat" is sometimes used instead of "fat-free" for dairy foods.
Low	Can be eaten frequently without exceeding recommended amount of fat, saturated fat, cholesterol, sodium, and calories.
Reduced	Contains at least 25 percent less of the ingredient or 25 percent fewer calories than the regular version.
Lean	Contains less than 10 g total fat, 4.5 g or less saturated fat, and less than 95 mg cholesterol per serving. Used on meat and poultry products.
Extra lean	Contains less than 5 g fat, less than 2 g saturated fat, and less than 95 mg cholesterol per serving. Used on meat and poultry products.
Healthy	Low in fat and saturated fat and contains limited amounts of sodium and cholesterol. Single-item foods marked "healthy" provide at least 10 percent of the Daily Value of vitamins A or C, iron, calcium, protein, or fiber.
Fresh	Raw and free of preservatives, and has not been heated or frozen.
Fresh frozen	Frozen while still fresh.

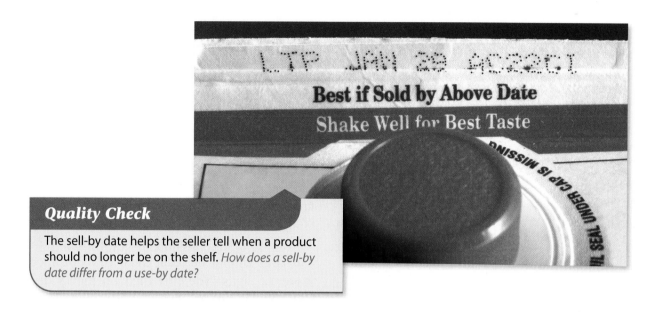

Quality Check

The sell-by date helps the seller tell when a product should no longer be on the shelf. *How does a sell-by date differ from a use-by date?*

Claims on Labels

Food makers also use labels to promote the product and make claims about its nutritional advantages. The FDA has precise definitions for many terms used on labels. Manufacturers must follow these definitions.

The FDA also allows manufacturers to make claims about the health benefits of foods. However, manufacturers have to follow strict rules:

- The claim must be supported by science and research.
- The food must meet specific nutrient levels that are set by the government.
- The label must be carefully worded to explain the relationship between the food or nutrient and a particular disease or health condition.
- The label must state that eating the food is only part of managing the condition. For example, the label on a box of oat bran might carry this claim: "Studies show that a diet high in fiber helps reduce the risk of heart disease."

The Organic Seal

The word "organic" on a food label means that the food is not genetically modified, that it was produced without pesticides, artificial fertilizers, growth hormones, or antibiotics, and that it was not irradiated. The USDA uses state and private agencies to inspect farms and meat producers to certify that their products are organic. Certified products are labeled as "Certified organic by" plus the name of the agency that did the inspection. Foods that contain only certified organic ingredients can also be marked "100 percent organic." Foods that have 95 percent or more certified organic ingredients can be called "organic." Look for the USDA organic seal on these foods.

Processed products that contain at least 70 percent organic ingredients cannot carry the USDA organic seal, but their label may say "Made with organic ingredients." If the product has less than 70 percent organic ingredients, the word "organic" can appear only on individual items in the ingredients list.

There is controversy over the term "natural." On meat and poultry labels, "natural" means that the product is minimally processed and contains no artificial ingredients, colorings, or chemical preservatives. However, a product labeled "natural" is not necessarily healthy, nutritious, or environmentally friendly.

Product Dating

Some packages are stamped with a date that indicates how fresh a product is and how long you can use it before it expires. Different states have different laws regarding dating of foods. Nationally, dating is required only on infant formula and some baby foods. There are two types of dating: code dating and open dating.

Code Dating

Code dating is the use of a series of numbers or letters that indicate where and when the product was packaged. Processors use date codes to identify shelf-stable products. If a recall is necessary, the products can be tracked quickly and removed from the shelves. Federal law requires code dating on most canned food.

Open Dating

Open dating is the use of a day, month, and sometimes a year to indicate a product's freshness. It is called "open" dating because it uses an easy-to-read calendar date, rather than a date code. Open dating is found mainly on perishable foods, such as meat and dairy products.

Open dating comes in two basic formats.

Sell-by Date The **sell-by date** is the last day the product should remain on the store shelf. The package may state "Sell by" or "Best if purchased by." The sell-by date allows for a reasonable amount of time for home storage and use after the date. Although intended for the retailer, the sell-by date is useful to consumers.

Use-by Date The **use-by date** is the last day on which the product will still have high quality. Sometimes the use-by date is called a quality assurance date. If a date appears without wording on baked goods, it is usually a use-by date. "Best if used by" shows the last day that the product will have high quality or best flavor.

Open dating does not guarantee quality, but it helps you pick the freshest food on the shelf. Foods are still safe to eat after the date, although nutrition and flavor have passed their peak. Stores should remove products from their shelves that have passed their use-by dates.

Buyer Beware

Examine food items for quality as you take them from the supermarket shelf. *What signs tell you that these foods may be unsafe?*

Universal Product Code

A small rectangle of black bars on almost every food package is the **universal product code (UPC)**. The UPC is a bar code that can be read by a scanner, which makes checkout faster and more accurate. An electronic scanner identifies the product, enters the correct price on a screen for the customer to see, and adds it to the receipt. The store computer automatically deducts the item from inventory.

Below the black bars on the UPC is a series of numbers. These numbers are a backup if the bar code cannot be read. Most UPCs on food have 12 digits. The first digit on the far left identifies the code. The next five digits identify the manufacturer. The following five digits identify the product. The last digit checks whether the number scanned correctly.

Countries outside the United States use a slightly different code called the European Article Number (EAN). Scanning equipment in the U.S. will eventually recognize these codes as well.

✓ Reading Check **Organize** Are ingredients on food labels listed from the smallest to largest amount or largest to smallest?

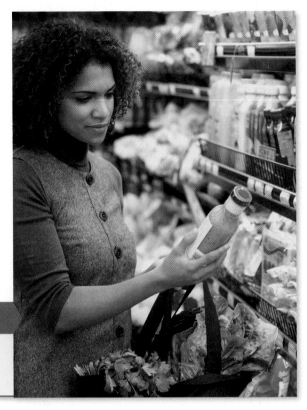

Shopping Smarts

A smart shopper knows how to select the best quality food and get good value for the money. This section describes strategies to accomplish both these goals.

Getting Quality

Getting the best value for your money means balancing food price with food quality. Quality foods are fresh and nutritious. Poor quality food is no bargain, no matter how low the price. It may even be unsafe to eat.

Practice these strategies for checking quality in food you buy:

- Check product dates for freshness.
- Plan your shopping trip so that you pick up perishable foods last. Bring the food directly home and store it properly.
- Check products for signs of spoilage. Avoid packages that are dirty, rusty, leaking, or damaged. They may have harmful bacteria.
- Put meat, poultry, and fish packages in plastic bags so they do not drip onto other foods in your cart or shopping bag.
- Choose frozen foods that are frozen solid and that are not frosted with ice. Packages with frost may have started to thaw and then been refrozen, which can damage food.
- Place fragile items on top of heavier ones when adding food to a cart or bag.

Getting Your Money's Worth

You should pay a fair price for high-quality food. You cannot control what stores charge for food, but you can look carefully for food that gives you a good value for your money.

What Affects Food Prices?

Why do some foods seem to cost so much, and others so little? Why do food prices go up and down during the year? Many complex factors affect food prices.

Processing, Transportation, and Marketing Costs As food travels from farm to processor to store, its cost goes up. Processing and packaging food costs money. Transporting food to the store costs money. Food workers' wages cost money. Food advertisements cost money. These costs also depend on many other factors. A rise in oil prices, for example, can add to the cost of operating farm machinery, processing plants, and delivery trucks.

Supply and Demand The principle of supply and demand also affects food prices. Supply is how much of something is available. Demand is how much of something people want. Prices go up as demand goes up and supply goes down. Prices go down as demand goes down and supply goes up. Given the rising cost of gas, biofuels have increased in popularity. The use of corn as a biofuel has increased its demand and the price has risen. Stores often change their prices based on changes in supply and demand. If a late freeze destroys part of the peach crop, for example, the supply of peaches is less than the demand for peaches,

Kitchen Math

Find the Best Buy

Laura needs 4 cups (32 ounces) of chicken broth for a recipe. She can buy one 32-ounce container of Brand A at $2.79. Or she can buy two 16-ounce containers of Brand B, normally $1.89 each but now on sale at 10% off. Or she can buy four 8-ounce containers of Brand C, which is normally $0.99 per can but is on sale at 35% off. Which brand should Laura buy?

Math Concept **Discounts and Sale Prices** When an item is on sale for a certain percent, calculate the discount amount by multiplying the percent by the original price. The sale price equals the original price minus the discount.

Starting Hint Calculate the sale prices of Brand B and Brand C by multiplying the discount percentage by the regular price and subtracting that amount from the regular price. Find the unit price of each brand by dividing the cost per can by ounces per can. Find the lowest unit price.

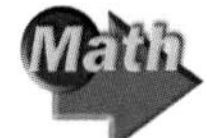

Appendix For math help, go to the Math Appendix at the back of the book.

NCTM Problem Solving Apply and adapt a variety of appropriate strategies to solve problems.

and stores can charge more. If there is a huge peach harvest, the supply of peaches is greater than the demand for peaches, and stores must charge less to get people to buy.

Consumer Carelessness Careless consumers sometimes damage food when they shop. Stores throw out most of this damaged food and sell some of it at a discount. Shoplifting and grocery cart theft cost stores money, too. Stores have to raise prices to make up for their losses.

Government Policies Governments buy crops or foods for their commodities programs or pay growers subsidies, or bonuses, to grow certain foods. These practices are meant to stabilize food prices and help farmers stay in business. Government price supports for corn keep the prices of foods made with corn syrup artificially low. International trade deals can also affect the price of both domestic and imported foods.

Comparison Shopping

With so many different products, brands, and sizes from which to choose, how can you find the best buy? The best way to choose the best product is through comparison shopping. **Comparison shopping** means matching prices and characteristics of similar items to determine which offers the best value.

Personal preference plays a role in comparison shopping, too. You might buy your favorite cereal even if it costs more than another cereal because you know you will eat it all—and enjoy it.

Two pieces of information can help you with comparison shopping: unit price and cost per serving.

Unit Price The **unit price** is the cost per ounce, quart, pound, or other unit of an item. Most stores show the unit price on the shelf tab below the item, next to the total price. For example, if a 12-ounce jar of spaghetti sauce costs $1.32, its unit price is 11 cents per ounce. If a 16-ounce jar of spaghetti sauce costs $1.52, its unit price is 9.5 cents per ounce. You can use the unit price to tell if a safe item is really a better buy.

If no unit price is given, you can calculate it yourself by dividing the item's total price by the number of units.

Larger packages of food often have a lower unit price than smaller packages—but not always. Check to make sure. Also check the unit price of items that you buy often. Manufacturers often reduce the size of the package instead of raising a food's price. Do not buy a bigger container than you need just because the unit price is lower. If a food loses quality before you finish it, you lose money and food.

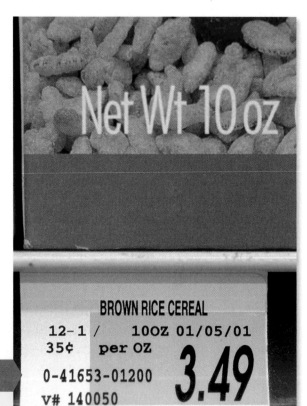

Unit Pricing

Unit pricing helps you compare different sizes of the same or similar product to see which is the best value. *How can you calculate the unit price if it is not listed?*

Figure 17.2 Servings per Pound of Meat, Poultry, and Fish

Serve It Up Though a serving of meat is 3 ounces, some meats contain fewer servings per pound than others due to the presence of more bones and fat. ***If you want to have as many servings per pound as possible, should you buy ground lamb or lamb chops?***

Food	Characteristics	Servings Per Pound
Meat	• Lean, boneless or ground	3 to 4
	• Some bone or fat	2 to 3
	• Large amount of bone or fat	1 to 2
Poultry	• Boneless or ground	4
	• With bones	2
Fish	• Fillets or steaks	4

Cost Per Serving Unit price does not always tell you a product's real value. For example, boneless chicken costs more per unit than bone-in chicken, but it may be a better value because it has more edible meat. Cost per serving is a good way to compare foods like these.

To find the cost per serving, determine how many servings are in a certain food. Divide the price by the number of servings. The result is cost per serving. You can also use this math to find the cost per serving of prepared foods by dividing the item's price by the number of servings shown on the label.

To estimate the cost per serving of a homemade recipe, add the cost of the ingredients. Divide the sum by the number of servings the recipe makes. Remember that meat, poultry and fish are heavier before cooking than after. The proper portion size for meat of any kind is three ounces after cooking. This is why a pound, or 16 ounces, of boneless chicken makes four three-ounce servings after cooking.

Suppose fish fillets are on sale at $1.80 per pound, and a whole broiling chicken is $1.06 per pound. At first, the chicken might seem to be a better buy. The chicken includes bones and fat, however, so there is less meat. A pound of fish makes four servings, while a pound of chicken — with bones — makes only two. The cost per serving for a pound of the filets is 45 cents ($1.80 ÷ 4 servings). The cost per serving for a pound of chicken is 53 cents ($1.06 ÷ 2 servings). **Figure 17.2** shows the typical number of servings per pound of meat, poultry, and fish.

Using Coupons

Coupons offer savings on specific products. You can find coupons in newspapers, magazines, product packages, mailed advertisements, in-store displays, and on the Internet. In some stores, the checkout computer prints coupons for you based on what you buy.

Coupons come in two basic types. A cents-off coupon offers a reduced price on a certain item. When you check out, the coupon's face value is subtracted from your bill.

The second type of coupon is a **rebate**, a partial refund from the maker of an item. You pay the full price at the store. Later you fill out the rebate coupon and mail it, with a proof of purchase, to the address given. The maker sends you a check for the rebate.

Some people save a lot with coupons, especially if their supermarket doubles the discount. Other people save just as much money through careful shopping.

If you collect coupons, be selective. Focus on items you usually buy or want to try. Avoid the temptation to buy an item just because you have a coupon. Read coupons closely. Some are good only on one size of a product or at a certain store. Most coupons have an expiration date. Stores cannot accept coupons after they expire.

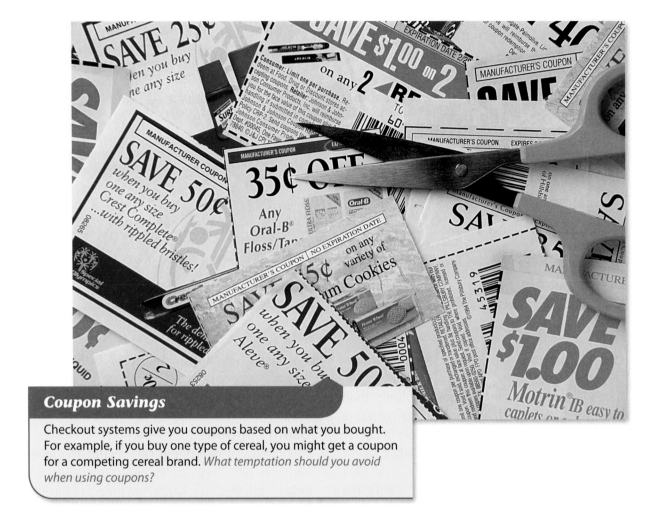

Coupon Savings

Checkout systems give you coupons based on what you bought. For example, if you buy one type of cereal, you might get a coupon for a competing cereal brand. *What temptation should you avoid when using coupons?*

Other Money-Saving Strategies

Savvy consumers avoid shopping when they are hungry. People spend up to 15 percent more on food when they are hungry, because they give in to impulse buys. Eat before you shop.

Other ideas to help control supermarket spending include:

- Take only enough money to cover planned purchases, plus a little extra. Take a small calculator to keep track of your spending.
- Resist impulse spending traps. Stores may offer free samples, product promotions, and discount bins. Candy, magazines, and other small, high-profit items are placed at checkout lanes to tempt you. Foods that are often served together may be displayed side by side. Seeing packages of shortcake next to the strawberries might entice you to buy them both.
- Use your shopping list, but be flexible. Be alert for unadvertised specials and sale items that you can substitute for the ones on your list.
- Consider store brands. A **store brand** is a line of food produced and packaged for a specific store chain. Store brands are sometimes manufactured by the makers of name-brand goods. Store brands cost less than name brands but are usually just as good. Store brands are sometimes called private labels.
- If a package of meat, poultry, or produce has more than you can safely store or use, ask if a clerk can repackage it for you.
- Buy a membership at a wholesale discount club to get reduced prices on certain items.
- Some stores offer large, packaged quantities of food staples at a reduced per-unit cost. Consider these but buy them only if you have room to store them and plan on using all of the product before its use-by date.

- Some grocery store chains offer customer loyalty cards that provide discounts or other store benefits based on what you purchase. Make use of these cards when they benefit you.

Checking Out

Your final stop in shopping is the checkout lane. Have ready any coupons or store discount cards you plan to use. You may be able to use an express lane if you have a limited number of items or if you are paying cash. Some stores offer a self-checkout counter where customers can check out their purchases themselves to save time.

Be aware of the store's policy regarding forms of payment. To pay by check, you may need a store check-cashing card. Most supermarkets accept credit cards and automated banking cards, but do not let the ease of using credit tempt you to go over your food budget.

Most checkout counters are stocked with point-of-sale items like chewing gum, chocolate, and magazines. Be aware that these counters are designed to encourage impulse buying.

Watch the checkout screen as items are listed to make sure the prices are correct. Sometimes items are priced incorrectly. Sometimes clerks enter incorrect codes, so pay attention. Review the register tape before leaving the store to make sure that discounts and coupons registered correctly. If a charge seems incorrect, ask the cashier to check it for you.

Take your purchases home right away and store them properly. Store frozen foods immediately, quickly followed by refrigerated foods, and finally shelf-stable ones. Repackage bulk foods in airtight, durable containers.

Responsible Shopping

Courtesy makes a shopping trip more pleasant. Apply the rules of the road to grocery store aisles. Push your cart at a safe speed, keeping to the right-hand side. If you bump another shopper or want to pass someone, excuse yourself. Avoid blocking aisles or other busy areas when you "park" to look for specific items.

Handling food carefully helps maintain its quality for other shoppers. Return a product to its proper place if you choose not to buy it. If you find food that is past its expiration date, notify a store clerk. Use the scoop or tongs provided for bulk foods rather than your hands, and close the bin when you are done. Never open a package to sample the contents. The costs of damage and theft are passed along to all consumers.

If you take a shopping cart to the car for unloading, return the cart to the proper area to keep it out of traffic lanes.

Resolving Purchasing Problems

What should you do if a food is spoiled or of poor quality? Return it to the store with your receipt as soon as possible. The manager should replace the product or refund your money, according to the store policy.

If you find foreign particles such as stones or insects in packaged foods, report the problem to the consumer complaint coordinator at your regional FDA office. For a meat or poultry problem, call the USDA.

Nutrition Check

FDA Approved

Additives are substances added to processed foods to improve their flavor, taste, and appearance. In the United States, all food additives must be approved by the Food and Drug Administration (FDA) before use. The FDA determines the safety of each additive, and issues specific instructions for its use and appearance on food labels. Additives are assigned specific names and numbers. Despite the FDA's efforts to establish their safety, many food additives have been controversially linked to a variety of health complaints. Visit the FDA's Web site to learn about specific additives.

Think About It Your neighbor, a chemist, has created his own preservative and used it to prolong the shelf life of his homemade strawberry jam. He is selling the jam in unlabeled jars at a farmers' market. Is it safe to eat?

You may also want to comment or complain to a food processor. You can write to the address on the label, send an e-mail, or call a toll-free consumer service number. If no number is given, try calling toll-free directory assistance. If you write or e-mail, follow these guidelines:

- Be brief but include all relevant facts. Give the product name, size, and the product code from the package. Mention the date of purchase and the store name and address. If you talked to anyone at the store where you purchased the product, include that information.
- Express your problem or comments clearly. Explain what action, if any, you want the company to take.
- Include your name, address, phone number and e-mail address so that the company can let you know how it is addressing your concerns.

You have rights as a consumer. You have the right:

- to buy safe products.
- to be truthfully informed.
- to choose from a variety of reasonably priced goods and services.
- to have your opinions about legislation and decisions heard.
- to have problems corrected.
- to have helpful consumer facts presented in writing.

The law protects these rights. If you have questions about your rights as a consumer, contact the Federal Trade Commission or consult its Web site. There are organizations that can offer additional help. There are local consumer protection offices. Each state has a Better Business Bureau. When you stand up for these rights by alerting a store or company to a problem with a product, you protect yourself and the safety of the food supply.

Light and Healthy Recipe

Potato Salad

Ingredients

2 cups Diced potatoes
2 each Diced pickles
¼ cup Diced celery
2 each Diced green onions
¼ tsp. Pepper
½ cup Low-fat, low-sodium mayonnaise
¼ cup Prepared mustard

A serving of potatoes contains 45 percent of the recommended daily amount of vitamin C.

Directions

1. Boil the potatoes in water until they are tender enough to be easily pierced with a fork. Remove the potatoes from the water and cool them with running cold water.
2. Put the potatoes in a large mixing bowl and add the pickles, celery and green onions.
3. In a separate bowl, mix the mayonnaise, mustard and pepper until combined. Fold the mixture into the potato salad until well blended.
4. Chill in the refrigerator for at least one hour and serve cold.

Yield 4 servings

Nutrition Analysis per Serving

■ Calories	141
■ Total fat	6 g
Saturated fat	1 g
Cholesterol	7 mg
■ Sodium	217 mg
■ Carbohydrate	20 g
Dietary fiber	3 g
Sugars	2 g
■ Protein	3 g

CHAPTER 17 Review & Applications

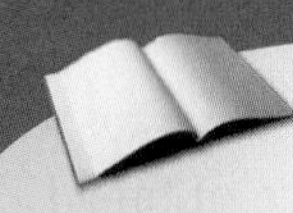

After You Read

Chapter Summary

Shopping for food is a skill. Places to shop for food include supermarkets and specialty stores. Use several criteria to choose a suitable store. Planning shopping can save time and money. It is helpful to get to know a store's layout and to make shopping lists. Understanding food labels is important. Labels contain basic information, make claims, indicate whether a food is organic, contain sell-by or use-by dates, and feature a universal product code. There are many strategies for smart shopping, including assessing food quality before buying, getting a good value, using coupons, and resolving purchase problems.

Content and Academic Vocabulary Review

1. Write each of these content and academic vocabulary words on an index card, and the definitions on separate index cards. Work in pairs or small groups to match each term to its definition.

Content Vocabulary

- natural food (p. 238)
- organic food (p. 239)
- food cooperative (p. 239)
- perishable food (p. 240)
- impulse buying (p. 241)
- code dating (p. 244)
- open dating (p. 244)
- sell-by date (p. 244)
- use-by date (p. 244)
- universal product code (UPC) (p. 244)
- comparison shopping (p. 246)
- unit price (p. 246)
- rebate (p. 247)
- store brand (p. 248)

Academic Vocabulary

- representative (p. 240)
- customize (p. 241)

Review Key Concepts

2. **Identify** places to shop for food and explain how to choose a store.
3. **Explain** how to plan your shopping to be effective and easy.
4. **Describe** how to use food labels to understand the foods you eat.
5. **Summarize** how to shop smart to get quality foods and save money.

Critical Thinking

6. **Explain** why food prices are generally higher in convenience stores than in most other types of stores.
7. **Describe** steps consumers can take to avoid buying foods they do not need.
8. **Evaluate** the ingredient list on two bottles of juice. One bottle says "orange juice." Another bottle of the same size lists "water, orange juice from concentrate, and sugar" as ingredients.
9. **Evaluate** the 100 percent organic Thanksgiving dinner Jason plans to cook for his friends. Does a turkey labeled "All Natural" fit into his plans?
10. **Explain** how weather can influence the price of certain foods.

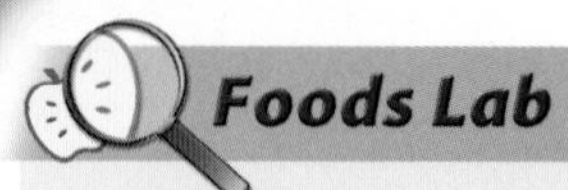

Foods Lab

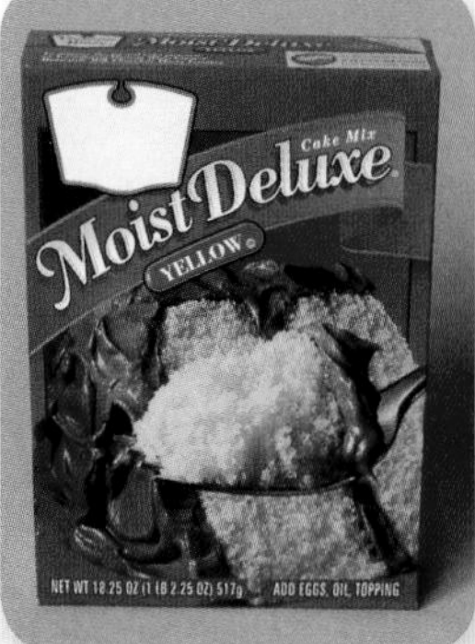

11. Using Package Directions Many food labels include directions for how to prepare the food. This is especially true of convenience foods, such as frozen entrees, canned soups, or boxed rice and pasta dishes.

Procedure Prepare a convenience food that offers two preparation methods, such as heating on the stove and in the microwave. Use the preparation method assigned by your teacher, following the directions exactly.

Analysis In an informal oral presentation, address the following: Were the directions clear and complete? What would you add or change? What other information or instructions on the package were helpful? Overall, were you satisfied with the outcome?

HEALTHFUL CHOICES

12. Deciphering Stamps At the supermarket on May 7th, Alicia found a package of bread stamped with the words "Sell by: May 8." Another package was stamped "Quality Assurance Date: May 8." What do these stamps mean and which package should Alicia choose?

TECH Connection

13. Cost Comparison Identify a food that you can buy prepared, semi-prepared, or make at home. Research the difference in cost among the three forms. Calculate the amount of time it would take you to prepare each version of the food. Then use computer software to create a chart showing the cost difference between a prepared, semi-prepared, and homemade food. Write a paragraph explaining when and under what circumstances you might choose each of the three versions of the food. Explain how your choice is affected by both the cost of the food and how long it takes to prepare.

Real-World Skills

Problem-Solving Skills

14. Homebound and Hungry The Villenos, a married couple, are both sick with the flu. They are staying home to try to recover. Neither feels strong enough to go shopping, but their supply on food is running low. What can they do?

Interpersonal and Collaborative Skills

15. Map and Plan Pair up with a classmate who is familiar with the same supermarket, warehouse store, specialty store, or food cooperative as you. Using your shared knowledge of the store, work together to draw a map of it, noting where different types of merchandise are placed. Then prepare a well-organized shopping list to use in the store.

Financial Literacy Skills

16. Convenient Cookies Calculate the cost per serving of a batch of homemade chocolate chip cookies. Then compare it to cost per serving of similar cookies that can be conveniently purchased in a bakery. Which is more expensive? When and why might you use the more expensive cookies?

Academic Skills

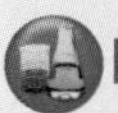

Food Science

17. Cabbage as pH Indicator Red cabbage contains a pigment called anthocyanin. Anthocyanin shows different colors depending on the pH level where it is found. Anthocyanin appears red in acids, violet in neutral solutions, and green in basic solutions. Because the color changes with the pH, it can serve as a pH indicator.

Procedure Grate half a head of red cabbage. Place the cabbage in a pot, and cover in water. Boil for 30 minutes. Strain the fluid, noting the color. Add a few drops of the fluid to the following: distilled water, white vinegar, lemon juice, and baking soda in water. Record your results, noting the color changes.

Analysis Write a list labeling each sample as acidic, basic, or neutral. Research other tools used to measure pH, like litmus paper. Write a paragraph explaining your conclusions.

NSES B Develop an understanding of chemical reactions.

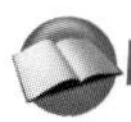

Mathematics

18. Bulk Weight Emily needs 4 cups of uncooked brown rice to prepare for dinner. To save money, she would like to purchase the ingredients from her local grocery store's bulk food bins. She brings a measuring cup with her to the store, and takes exactly 4 cups from the bin. If the bulk rice is selling for $1.44 per pound (16 ounces), and Emily is charged $2.52 for her 4 cups, how much does a cup of rice weigh?

Math Concept **Solving Problems with Proportions** You can set up two equal ratios (known as a proportion) to relate a quantity you already know to another you are solving for. Use x to represent the unknown amount in the second ratio.

Starting Hint Write one ratio as $1.44 over 16 oz., and set it equal to a second ratio of $2.52 over x ounces. Solve for x, which represents the weight (in oz.) in 4 cups of rice. Divide by 4.

NCTM Algebra Represent and analyze mathematical situations and structures using algebraic symbols.

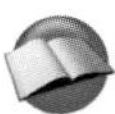

English Language Arts

19. Analyze and Predict Conduct research about statistics related to organic farming. Analyze your findings in a one-page report in which you predict the future of organic farming and the potential changes organic farming may cause in people's diets.

NCTE 8 Use information resources to gather information and create and communicate knowledge.

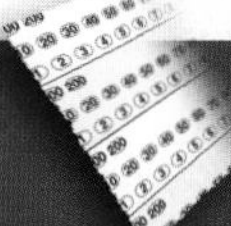

STANDARDIZED TEST PRACTICE

FILL IN THE BLANK

Read the sentence and choose the best word to fill in the blank.

20. The ________ is the cost per ounce, quart, pound, or other unit of an item.
    a. cost per serving
    b. unit price
    c. serving unit cost
    d. base cost

Test-Taking Tip When answering a fill-in-the-blank question, silently read the sentence with each of the possible answers in the blank space. This will help you eliminate wrong answers. The best word results in a sentence that is both factual and grammatically correct.

CHAPTER 18

Serving Food

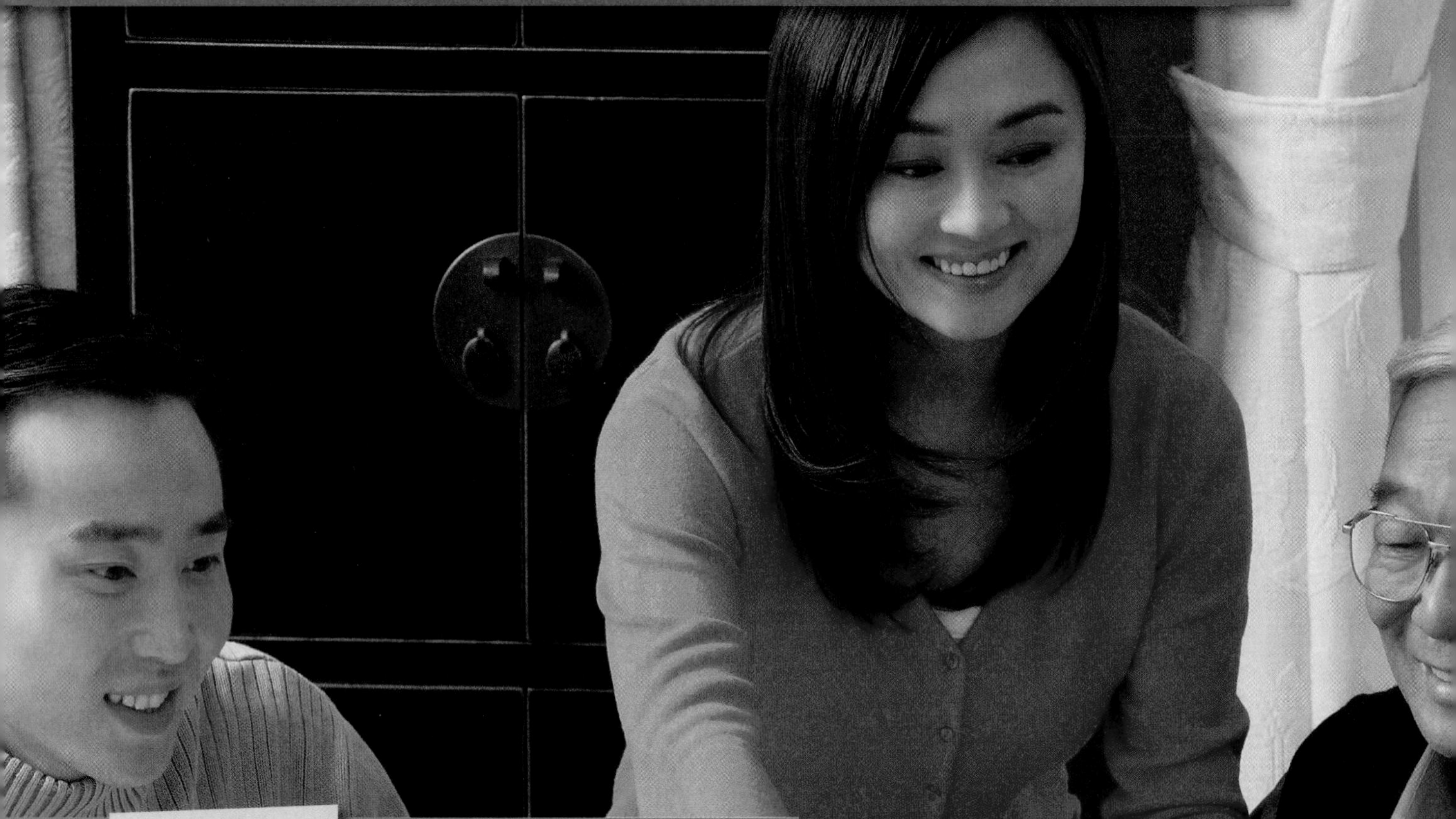

Writing Activity — Step-By-Step Guide

Etiquette Imagine your younger sister is about to dine at a restaurant for the first time. What would you tell your sister about showing good manners while eating out? Write a step-by-step guide that explains how to demonstrate etiquette while eating out, from the time you enter the restaurant until you leave it.

Writing Tips Follow these steps to write a step-by-step guide:

- Include a minimum of five specific steps, and number them.
- List steps chronologically in the order in which they should be completed.
- Briefly explain the purpose of or reason for each step.

Activate Prior Knowledge

Explore the Photo Food is served in different styles. *How would you adjust your behavior if you sat down to eat at a table like this?*

Reading Guide

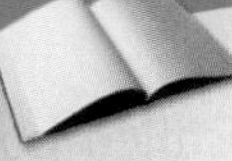

Before You Read

Preview Think about three times you or your family has served food to others. Consider what made these times memorable, and connect them to the text as you read.

Read to Learn

Key Concepts

- **List** four types of tableware and describe their uses.
- **Describe** how to arrange flatware on a cover.
- **List** and describe four ways of serving meals at home.
- **List** the things that should be included on an invitation.
- **Describe** how knowing proper table etiquette can help you.
- **Explain** how to calculate a standard tip.

Main Idea

Eating is more enjoyable when you know how to serve food and how to show good etiquette when it is served to you.

Content Vocabulary

You will find definitions for these words in the glossary at the back of this book.

- tableware
- place setting
- flatware
- crystal
- cover
- family service
- plate service
- modified English service
- buffet
- hors d'oeuvre
- canapé
- formal service
- service plate
- appetizer
- etiquette
- reservation
- à la carte
- gratuity

Academic Vocabulary

You will find these words in your reading and on your tests. Use the glossary to look up their definitions if necessary.

- complement
- principle

Graphic Organizer

Use a graphic organizer like the one below to note ways to pack chilled food, hot food, and nonperishable food for a picnic.

Packing Chilled Food	
Packing Hot Food	
Packing Nonperishable Food	

Graphic Organizer Go to this book's Online Learning Center at **glencoe.com** to print out this graphic organizer.

Academic Standards

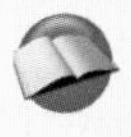

English Language Arts

NCTE 12 Use language to accomplish individual purposes.

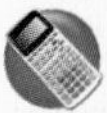

Mathematics

NCTM Problem Solving Solve problems that arise in mathematics and in other contexts.

NCTM Geometry Use visualization, spatial reasoning, and geometric modeling to solve problems.

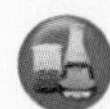

Science

NSES B Develop an understanding of interactions of energy and matter.

NCTE *National Council of Teachers of English*
NCTM *National Council of Teachers of Mathematics*
NSES *National Science Education Standards*
NCSS *National Council for the Social Studies*

Tableware

Meals are more satisfying when the food, serving style, and table setting suit the occasion. A table setting is the arrangement of tableware on the table and at each person's place setting. **Tableware** is any item used to serve or eat food. A **place setting** is the tableware needed by one person to eat a meal. A basic place setting includes a plate, a glass, and a knife, fork, and spoon.

Tableware has three basic components: dinnerware, flatware, and glassware, plus a special type of serving container called holloware.

Dinnerware Dinnerware includes the largest pieces in a place setting—the dinner plate, salad plate, cup, and saucer—as well as the serving dishes and trays. Dinnerware is made from a range of materials, from plastic to bamboo. Most dishes are fine china, earthenware, ironstone, or stoneware, which are made by baking clay at a high temperature and coating it with a liquid glass glaze.

Flatware **Flatware** is eating and serving utensils, such as knives, forks, spoons, ladles, and cake servers. Most flatware is made from stainless steel. Finer flatware is crafted from sterling silver or silver plate. By law, sterling silver must contain 92.5 percent silver. Copper is added for strength. Silver plate has a thin coat of silver over a base metal, making it much less expensive than sterling. Both types of silver tarnish unless polished regularly. Stainless steel resembles silver but is more durable and needs no polishing.

Glassware Glassware is containers for serving and drinking beverages. Drinking glasses come in two main types, stemware and tumblers. Stemware, such as wine glasses, has a thin stem between the bowl and the base. Tumblers, such as juice glasses, have a flat bottom with no stem. **Crystal** is a type of glassware that contains lead, which gives clarity and sparkle. Glassware is traditionally made of glass, but stemware and tumblers also come in plastic.

Holloware Serving containers made of silver, silver plate, or stainless steel are called holloware. A silver cake tray is considered holloware, for example, but a glass cake tray is not.

Buying Tableware

Tableware is typically sold by the place setting or as boxed sets with an even number of place settings. Some brands of tableware are also available as open stock, in individual pieces sold separately. Open stock tableware usually costs more, but it is convenient if you need to replace a single piece. Flatware and serving utensils are also sold in sets and individually.

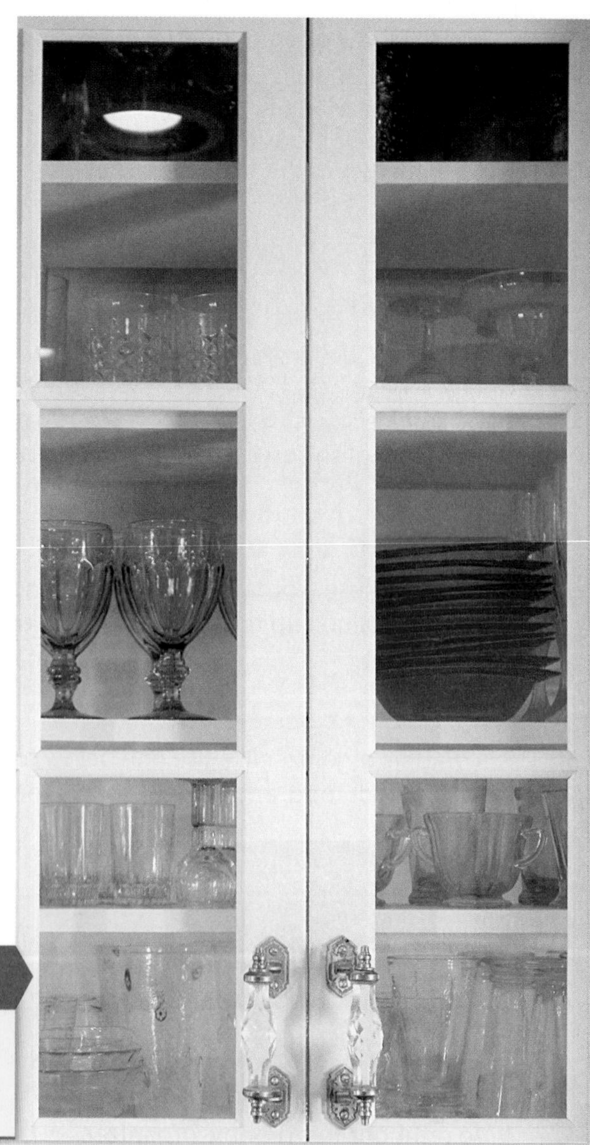

Glassware

Some types of glassware have stems, while other types of glassware have no stem and a flat base. *What three materials are most often used for glassware?*

Tableware is available in many different patterns, and even in different shapes. You can buy a complete set of one pattern or combine patterns that **complement**, or enhance, each other.

Tableware can be very expensive, very inexpensive, or anywhere in between. Price depends on the material, the quality, and the brand name. The most expensive choices are fine china, sterling silver flatware, and crystal glassware. These require more care when handling and washing. People who have expensive tableware tend to save it for special occasions.

Tableware that is safe for the microwave and dishwasher is practical for everyday use. Some dinnerware is also oven-safe and can be used for both cooking and serving. Pieces that stack easily are convenient to store.

Table Linens

Table linens protect the dining table and the diner during a meal and add beauty and interest.

Tablecloths Tablecloths are coverings for the entire table. They can be formal or informal. Tablecloths look most attractive if they hang at least 6 inches below the tabletop on all sides.

Runners Runners are long, narrow cloths that run down the center of the table. They create a decorative effect.

Place Mats Place mats cover the area of a single place setting. They can be made of fabric, straw, or plastic.

Napkins Napkins come in different sizes and materials. They should be large enough to be useful for diners but small enough to handle comfortably.

Stain-resistant table linens with a permanent-press finish are practical choices, because they are easy to wash and do not need ironing. Linens made with lace or delicate fabrics may require special care, such as dry cleaning.

Place mats and napkins are sometimes sold in sets. You can also mix and match designs to add contrasts of color and texture.

✓ Reading Check **Explain** What is open stock tableware?

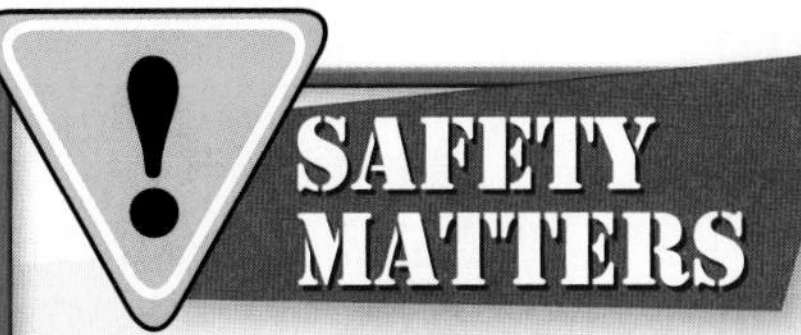

Lead Precautions

Lead is a toxic metal that has long been recognized as a health hazard. When absorbed into the body, it can cause problems with blood pressure, fertility, and brain function. While lead is no longer used in paints, small amounts of it can still be found in lead crystal glassware and in cookware made from improperly glazed ceramic pottery. Lead can travel from a container to foods, especially acidic foods. In most cases, the risk is small. For safety, however, avoid storing beverages in lead crystal for more than a few hours, especially fruit juices. Limiting the use of lead crystal is another precaution.

What Would You Do? At a special dinner honoring your grandparents' 50th wedding anniversary, you want to use their antique lead crystal. How can you use it at the dinner in a way that poses few or no health risks?

Table-Setting Basics

A table should be set before people sit down to eat. Even a simple table setting can make a meal feel special.

Start with a clean, uncluttered table. Place the linens, such as the tablecloth and place mats. You may want to add a simple decoration, such as a single flower in a vase or one or more unscented candles, as a focal point.

Now place the tableware. The area containing each person's tableware is called a **cover**. The arrangement of a cover is based on tradition and function. You will want people to fit comfortably around the table, so each cover should be at least 20 inches wide to have enough room for the guest and the tableware. Set the cover in this order:

1. Dinner Plates Center the plate on the cover, with its edge about 1 inch from the edge of the table. If diners will not be filling their own plates at the table, leave a space for the plate to be served.

2. Flatware Arrange flatware in the order in which it will be used, starting at the outside and working toward the plate. For example,

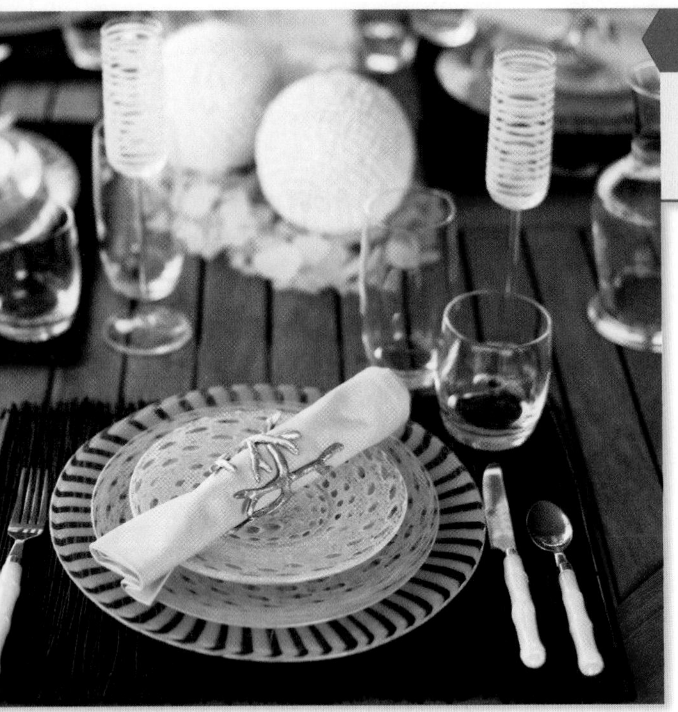

Everyday Elegance

Even simple table settings can make a meal feel relaxing and special. *What other factors can make a meal special?*

the salad fork should sit further from the plate than the entrée fork. Place knives to the right of the plate, with the blades facing the plates. Place spoons to the right of the knives. If you have both a soupspoon and a teaspoon, put the soupspoon to the right of the teaspoon. Place forks to the left of the plate, tines up. If dessert forks are needed, bring them to the table later, when dessert is served.

3. Glassware Place the beverage glass just above the tip of the dinner knife. If each cover also has a water glass, put the water glass above the tip of the dinner knife and put the beverage glass to its right. A cup and saucer for coffee or tea can go to the right of the spoon or be brought to the table after the meal.

4. Bread and Salad Plates If you are using a plate for bread and butter, place it above the forks. Place the salad plate or bowl either to the left of the forks or above them, depending on the space available.

5. Napkin As a final step, place a folded napkin to the left of the forks. You can also arrange it on the dinner plate or tuck it into a glass.

✓ Reading Check **Describe** When setting a table, how should you position the entrée forks and salad forks?

Serving Meals

Meals can be served in many different ways depending on the setting, the occasion, and the number of people. Meals may be served at a dinner or banquet table, set up on a buffet, or eaten outdoors or on the go.

Serving Meals at Home

Most families set up their daily meals for speed and convenience. For parties and special occasions, a buffet or a formal type of table service is common. Sometimes combining styles gives the best results.

Family Service

Family service is a way of serving meals in which food is placed in serving dishes and passed around the table. Food is usually passed to the right to avoid confusion. People have a dinner plate at their place, and they help themselves to as much or as little as they want.

Family service is popular for everyday meals at home, and some restaurants use it as well. The main advantage of family service is that diners can serve themselves.

Family service also has drawbacks. Hot food in serving dishes may quickly cool to room temperature, allowing harmful bacteria to grow. Easy access to second helpings may tempt some people to overeat. Uneaten food left on plates must usually be thrown away, which wastes food.

Plate Service

Plate service is a way of serving meals in which food is portioned out on individual plates in the kitchen and brought to the table. Space is left at each place for the plate when the table is set.

Plate service has several advantages. Food can be kept hot on the range or in the oven. Portion control is easier. Cleaning up takes less time and effort because no serving dishes are used.

Modified English Service

Modified English service is a more formal way of serving a meal for a small group. Foods for the main course are brought to the table in serving dishes. They are placed in front of the host, along with a stack of dinner plates. The host carves the meat, if necessary, and then places meat and vegetables on each dinner plate. The first plate is passed to the right, down to the person at the end of the table. When all the people on the right have received their plate, those on the left are served.

The salad may be served in the same way, or placed on individual plates in the kitchen and set on each cover before guests are seated. Rolls, butter, salad dressings, and other accompaniments are usually passed at the table so people can serve themselves. Dessert is served after the table has been cleared.

Buffet

What if there are more people than can fit at a dining table? A practical solution is a **buffet**, a method of serving food in which people help themselves to food set out on a table. A buffet can be as informal as a sit-down meal.

To set up a buffet, place prepared foods in serving dishes and arrange them on a kitchen counter, a large table, or furniture draped in tablecloths. Put the buffet in a place that is easy for several guests to reach at once. If you need extra serving space, try creating tiers. Set clean, cloth-covered boxes or overturned bowls and flowerpots on the table and place serving dishes on top. Guests can sit at small tables or hold plates of food on their laps.

When you set up the buffet, stack plates where you want the guests to start serving themselves. Then set the appetizer and main dish, followed by side dishes and condiments such as vegetables, salad, rolls, and butter. Place flatware last. Napkins can go at the end of the buffet or at the start. Rolling flatware into a napkin makes a bundle that is easy to pick up.

Foods in a buffet should be easy to serve and to eat. Foods that do not require cutting are good choices, such as casseroles, stir-fries, sandwiches, and salads. You may want to serve beverages after guests are seated.

It is important to keep buffet foods at safe temperatures. Use an electric skillet, slow cooker, chafing dish, or electric warming tray for hot foods. Keep cold food on ice or in insulated containers.

Service for Large Groups

Serving many guests at once requires skill and style. Large gatherings take two basic forms: receptions and sit-down banquets.

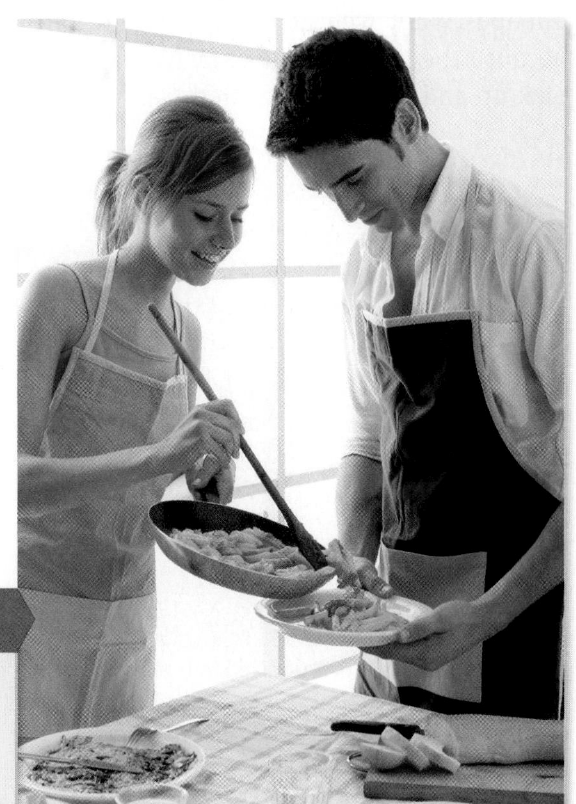

Dishing It Up

Plate service is an easy, practical way to serve family dinners. It helps with portion control and makes clean-up a snap. *What is the difference between plate service and family service?*

Receptions

A reception is a social gathering with food to honor a person or to celebrate an event. Receptions often follow weddings, graduations, and other ceremonies.

Receptions are meant as much for meeting as for eating. Buffet service helps to encourage mingling. The same foods are often served along both sides of the buffet table, allowing people to move in two lines instead of one. Coffee is poured at one end of the table and tea at the other.

At receptions, the menu is usually light, varied, and imaginative. Smaller events may offer nuts, candies, small sandwiches, fruit, and cheese. Formal receptions usually feature hors d'oeuvres (ȯr-ˈdərvs). An **hors d'oeuvre** is a small serving of hot or cold food served as an appetizer. Stuffed mushroom caps and dates wrapped in prosciutto are two popular hors d'oeuvres.

Canapés are a popular are receptions as well. A **canapé** (ˈka-nə-pā) is an hors d'oeuvre consisting of a small piece of bread in an interesting shape with flavorful toppings. For example, toasted bread triangles might be topped with melted cheese and olive slices. Crackers or pastry are sometimes used instead of bread. Canapés work well at receptions and parties because they are attractive, tasty, and easy to pick up and eat with one hand.

Formal Service

Formal service is the most elaborate style of serving food. Banquets in restaurants and hotels often use formal service. Banquets often offer two or more choices, called a selective menu.

For formal service, the cover is set with glassware and flatware. Formal service often has several courses, and every course requires its own fork, spoon, and possibly knife. Instead of a dinner plate, the cover includes a service plate. A **service plate** is a large, often beautifully decorated plate that holds other plates. An **appetizer** is a small portion of food served at the beginning of a meal to whet the appetite. The appetizer is served on a separate plate, which is placed on the service plate. After the first course, the service plate is removed. Each course that follows—and there are several—arrives on its own plate.

Enjoyable Family Meals

A family meal is a chance to enjoy food and catch up on family news. A relaxing family meal is free of television and other distractions, and conversation is pleasant.

Simple table settings are common for family meals. Most meals need only a dinner plate, fork, knife, teaspoon, and beverage glass. A more formal place setting would include

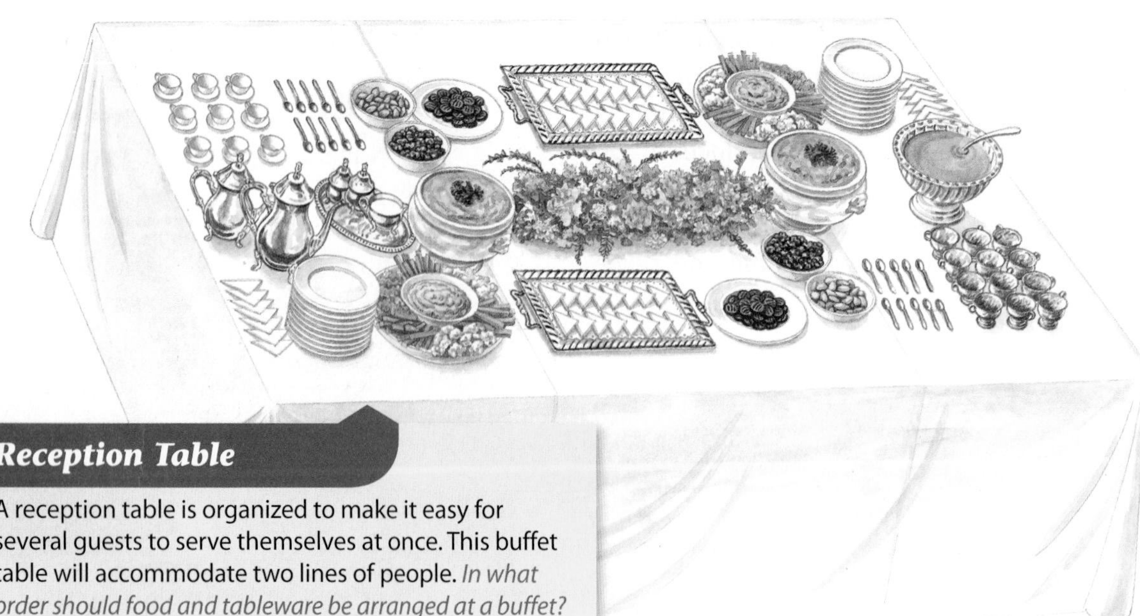

Reception Table

A reception table is organized to make it easy for several guests to serve themselves at once. This buffet table will accommodate two lines of people. *In what order should food and tableware be arranged at a buffet?*

Organized and Fresh

A container with compartments, like this Japanese bento box, creates a unique presentation and helps ensure that foods remain undamaged. *When packing food, how can you ensure that hot foods stay hot and cold foods stay cold?*

separate forks for the salad and main dish. Add a cup and saucer or a mug for a hot beverage, if needed, and a soup or salad bowl if either food is on the menu.

It can be hard to find time to eat meals as a family, but it is worth the effort. Eating together promotes positive relationships and good nutrition. Meals are good opportunities for teens and parents to communicate and spend time together.

Creating Atmosphere

Many restaurants are as popular for the atmosphere as the food. A lunch counter might have an upbeat, fun atmosphere, while a fancy restaurant might have an elegant and sophisticated atmosphere.

You can create atmosphere when serving meals at home, too. Use your creativity to make the dinner table interesting and special. Here are a few ideas:

- Add a cheerful touch of nature by filling a small basket with flowers, fresh fruit, colorful gourds, or clean leaves and nuts.
- For an elegant air, tuck a fresh or silk flower into every napkin. Arrange a centerpiece using candles. Place tall candles in candleholders or float small candles in glass dishes of colored water. Play soft music.
- Add humor with cartoon character glasses, souvenir salt and pepper shakers, and other offbeat tableware that expresses your sense of fun.

Packing a Lunch

Packing a nutritious, delicious lunch saves money and ensures that you have a healthful meal ready to keep you going during the middle of the day.

Lunch-Packing Pointers

Packing lunch requires some organization. Set aside a section in the freezer, refrigerator, and cabinet for lunch foods and packing supplies. Plastic wraps and bags, aluminum foil, and wax paper all work well as wrapping materials. Family members might take turns packing lunches for everyone, or two people might work together.

To save money and avoid waste, save an assortment of clean, empty margarine tubs, cottage cheese cartons, and other reusable containers. Make sure caps and covers seal securely to help keep liquids from leaking out and moisture from getting in. Tuck a wet washcloth in a plastic bag for cleaning hands and wiping up spills, rather than packing paper napkins or pre-moistened wipes.

When possible, start packing the night before. For example, if pasta from dinner will be someone's lunch, set aside a lunch portion before putting the rest of the leftovers away. In the morning, work assembly-line style—for example, make all the sandwiches, then wrap all the sandwiches, and finally add all the utensils.

Flavor and Fun

Grilling is fun and gives food a delicious, smoky flavor. *What safety rules should you follow when grilling food?*

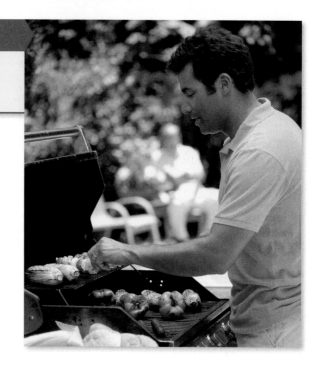

Keeping Lunch Foods Safe

Food must stay at the right temperature. For hot dishes such as soup, stew, chili, and stir-fries, use a wide-mouth vacuum bottle. A vacuum bottle is a container made of plastic or metal with a glass lining, and a vacuum between the outside of the container and the inner lining. Preheat the bottle before filling it with hot food. Fill it with hot tap water and let it stand a minute or two. Empty the water, fill the bottle with the piping hot food, and close tightly. If the food is still steaming at lunchtime, you know the bottle is doing its job.

A vacuum bottle also works well for cold food, such as milk and pudding. Chill the bottle first by filling it with cold water. You can also pack a reusable frozen gel pack with lunch to keep food cold. You can even make edible freezer packs by freezing sandwiches and juice boxes. They will thaw by lunchtime. Keep the food in the refrigerator or freezer as long as possible. Pack hot and cold foods separately or in different compartments of an insulated lunch bag.

Create a cheerful lunch by packing reusable utensils and brightly colored plastic plates. Add an upbeat note, cartoon, or inspiring thought from a page-a-day calendar.

Food Choices

Any nutritious food can make a tasty lunch. Choose foods that travel well and that will not fall apart or be messy to eat. A sturdy lunch container can help keep your food from getting squashed or soggy.

Some foods taste best if you assemble them just before eating. Lettuce leaves stay crisper if packed separately and added to a sandwich at lunchtime. For a salad, keep the dressing and croutons in individual containers and toss with the greens when you sit down to eat.

Serving Meals Outdoors

Many people enjoy eating outdoors to enjoy the fresh air and change of scene. There are many options for outdoor cooking.

Outdoor Grilling

Grilling is cooking food outdoors over an open flame. Grilling does not require expensive equipment or a lot of outdoor space. Tabletop grills are available for grilling in small spaces. Many parks provide picnic areas with grills. You can also achieve the effect of grilling with a grill pan that you use on the stovetop.

A few basic tools can make cooking outdoors safer and more convenient. Large trays are useful for carrying foods and utensils in and out. Long-handled tongs, spatulas, and heavy mitts protect your hands as you turn food on the grill and serve it onto plates.

Many foods can be prepared on the grill. Make vegetable kebabs by stringing whole mushrooms and cherry tomatoes and chunks of green pepper and onion onto wooden or metal skewers. Grill fish in a long-handled basket. You can also place large pieces of food directly on the grill, such as meat, poultry, and some shellfish; corn on the cob, still in the husk; and sliced bread or eggplant. Even homemade pizza can be cooked on the grill.

Grilling is less controllable than range-top or oven cooking, so cooking times are less predictable. Start early enough to have food ready on time. Set the grill a safe distance from trees and buildings that could catch fire, but with easy access to the kitchen. If you plan to eat outdoors, burn citronella candles to keep bugs away. Do not bring food outside until you are ready to cook it. Nest bowls of chilled foods in bowls of ice.

Picnics

Picnics are outings to enjoy eating food outdoors, often in a scenic spot such as a park. Good planning makes a successful picnic. Make a list of everything you want to take, including all the foods, utensils, and blankets or tablecloths. You may also need tools, such as a bottle opener, a cutting board, a paring knife, and cleanup supplies such as washcloths, trash bags, and smaller plastic bags for dirty utensils. As you pack each item, check it off your list.

Picnic Safety Follow the same safety rules when packing a picnic as when packing a lunch:

Chilled Food Use an insulated cooler lined with frozen gel packs to keep perishable food chilled. If possible, use a separate cooler for cold beverages to avoid frequently opening the cooler that holds the perishables. Keep frozen foods in the freezer until you are ready to leave for the picnic. If possible, arrange frozen foods around the outer edges so they can help keep other chilled foods cold.

Hot Food Take hot foods on a picnic only if you will be able to eat them within two hours. Pack them in a separate insulated container. If you are taking raw meat or poultry to cook at the picnic site, pack it in its own cooler to prevent juices from contaminating other foods. Keep the meat cold and covered until you are ready to cook it. Do not partially cook foods at home and then finish cooking them at the picnic. Harmful bacteria may grow in the half-cooked food.

Careers in Food

Bob Waggoner
Executive Chef

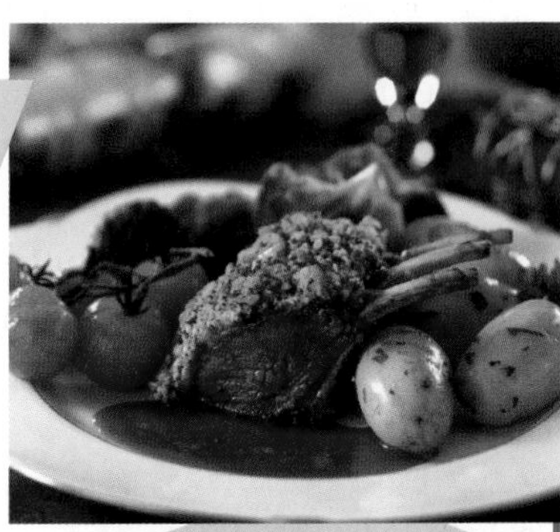

Q: What is the difference between a chef and an executive chef?

A: The executive chef is in charge of the entire menu and the staff in the kitchen and the dining room. An executive chef is also responsible for interacting with the county Health Department.

Q: How many chefs/cooks in a fine restaurant have been to culinary school?

A: We have 12 or 13 chefs, plus three who do pastries. About half are classically trained, and the other half are not.

Q: Why do you love your job?

A: There is nothing better than being a chef. I am treated like an owner, and I am respected and honored in this city.

"You have to be passionate about the work, and not just trying to become famous."
— Bob Waggoner
Executive Chef, The Charleston Grill – Charleston, SC

Education and Training

Culinary school is valuable but not the only way to get into the business. Your experience is just as important. Some chefs get their knowledge from working as an apprentice to a chef.

Qualities and Skills

A positive attitude is extremely important. People skills are very important. Being able to listen and learn is important and so is being able to speak and teach. Patience is also necessary.

Related Career Opportunities

Teaching at a culinary school is one job alternative. Other related jobs include food and beverage manager at a hotel, restaurant manager, butcher, and baker.

Party Decorations

A festive table adds to the pleasure of a party. Choosing a party theme can inspire decorating ideas. *What is the benefit of choosing foods that can be prepared ahead of time?*

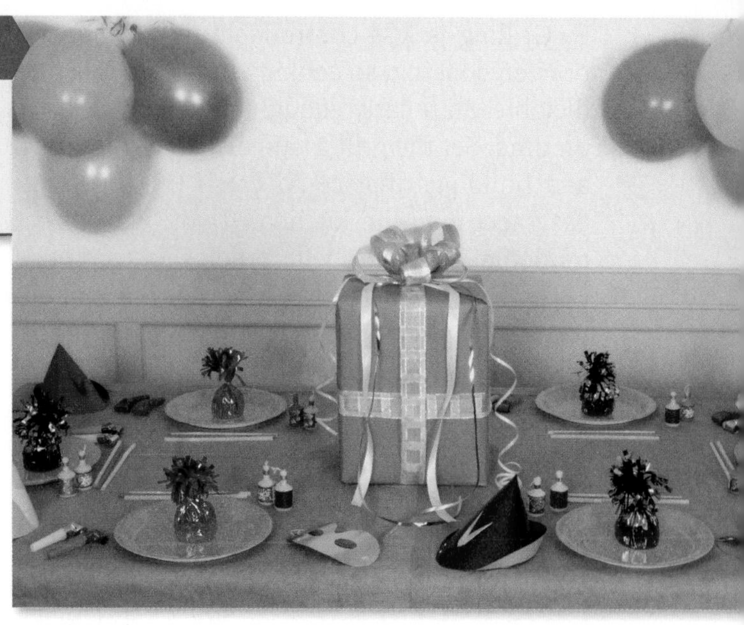

Nonperishable Food Pack nonperishable items, such as crackers and cookies, in a basket or other container.

When packing a cooler, place the items you will need last on the bottom, so the ones you need first will be on top. You will not need to look through the cooler every time you want something. Put fragile foods in crush-resistant plastic containers.

When you are traveling, keep the cooler in the air-conditioned interior of the car, not in a hot trunk. Keep it closed at all times. At the picnic site, keep the cooler in a cool, shady spot. Even an insulated cooler does not stay cool in the sun, in a hot car, or a car trunk.

Bring only as much food as you think you will need—leftovers may not be safe to eat after the trip home.

Before you leave the picnic, clean up the picnic site. If there are no trash containers, take the trash with you and dispose of it at home. Leave the site in good, usable condition for the next group of people to enjoy.

✓ **Reading Check** **Describe** What is one way you can create atmosphere when serving meals at home?

Entertaining

Food is an important part of most gatherings of friends and family. With preparation and organization, entertaining can be as much fun for the host as it is for the guests. Before planning a party, check with the adults in your home. Make sure the time and type of event fit with their schedule. Next, check your budget. How much money do you have for food and decorations? Now choose the type of party you want to give. Think about your entertaining skills. A buffet is easier to manage than a sit-down meal.

For inspiration in planning a party, consider a theme, or a unifying idea that is reflected in the menu, decorations, and activities. Holidays, birthdays, and graduations provide ready-made themes. You might also choose an interest you and your guests share, such as sports or old movies. Surprise friends with the unexpected. Invite them to an indoor beach party in the middle of winter, for example.

Invitations

Once you have planned the budget and theme, it is time to make a guest list and send invitations. For an impromptu gathering, you can ask friends in person or by phone. If you are planning a party for a larger group, written or e-mailed invitations help guests remember the date and time.

Send invitations at least ten days before the party. Be sure to include the date, location, start and end time of the event, and your name. Mention the theme or occasion, if there is one.

Formal invitations usually include the letters R.S.V.P. This is an abbreviation for the French phrase "Répondez, s'il vous plaît" (rā-pōn-dā-sē-vü-ple), or "Please reply." It is followed by your phone number or e-mail address and a date by which guests are to reply. Asking for a reply helps you determine the number of guests and plan how much food to buy.

Food for Entertaining

Before planning your menu, learn whether any guests have special food needs or preferences. Look for recipes that can be prepared ahead of time. Think of creative ways to connect foods to your theme, such as by color or ingredient. For a simple dessert for an Italian theme party, represent the colors of the Italian flag with red and green apple wedges and a white cream cheese dip. Aim for variety to ensure that every guest finds foods to enjoy.

Prepare enough food so guests do not feel self-conscious about how much they take. Consider how popular a food is likely to be and how many other foods there are to choose from. Pay attention to presentation, too. An attractive table can help make your party a hit.

Making a Schedule

A schedule helps to keep party plans on track. Start by listing everything that needs to be done. Include food shopping and preparation, decorating, setting the table, and cleanup. Use this master list to make two separate lists. On one list, write tasks you need to do before the day of the party. On the other list, write tasks you need to do on the day of the party. Next to each task, write the time it must be done. List the tasks in the order you need to do them. Check the lists often to make sure you are on schedule. As you complete each task, cross it off the list.

A big advantage of planning is that it helps you get everything done on time so that you can relax and enjoy the party. Of course, things do not always go according to plan. Keep a positive attitude and focus on enjoying your guests' company. A welcoming, upbeat attitude makes an event a success.

✓ Reading Check **Identify** What should you learn about your guests before planning a menu for a party?

Table Etiquette

Whether at a banquet, a picnic, or a simple family meal, table etiquette is an important part of serving and enjoying food. **Etiquette** is the courtesy you show to others by using good manners when eating. Learning the rules of etiquette can also help you feel at ease in social situations by helping you know how to act.

Knowing table etiquette can also be an asset in the working world. Some job interviews and business meetings take place during a restaurant meal. Workers who order with confidence, eat politely, and treat servers with consideration inspire trust.

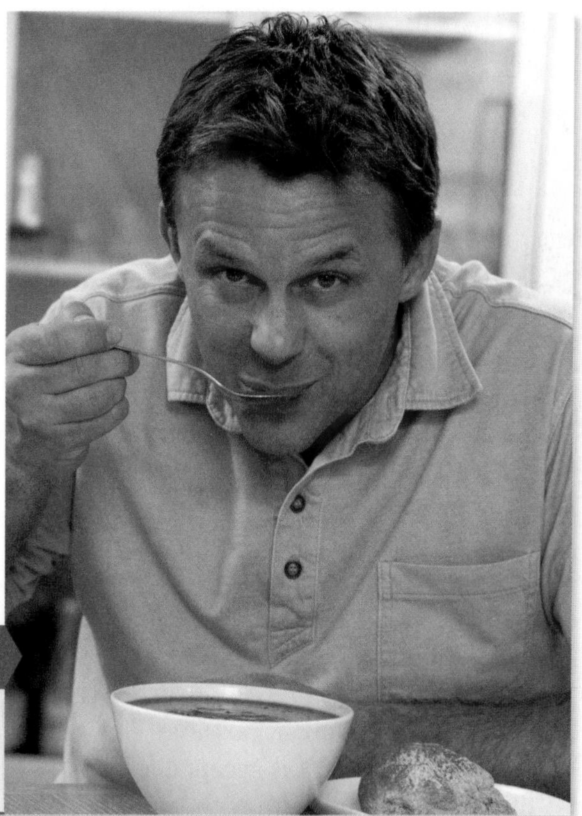

Table Manners

Knowing the basics of table etiquette can help you feel more at ease in social situations. *What should you do after you finish eating?*

International Customs

Sipping soup from the side of a bowl is appropriate in some cultures. *What is the basic rule of table etiquette in all cultures?*

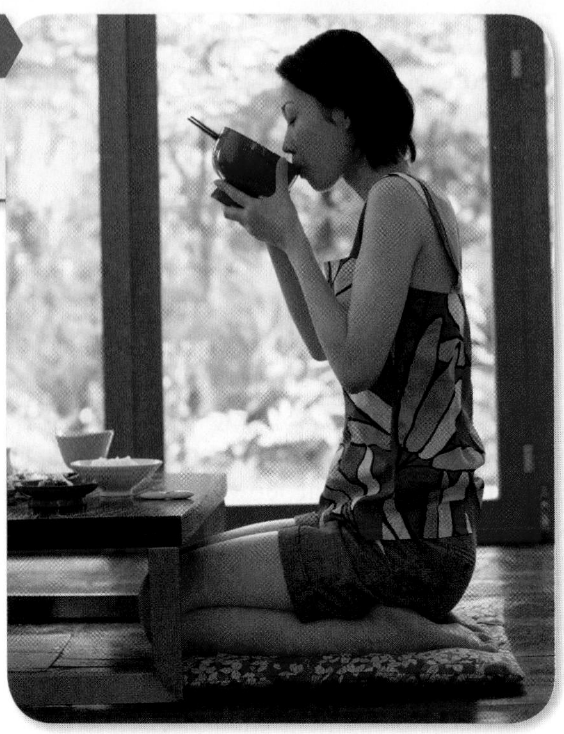

Courteous Behavior at the Table

A few basic etiquette skills cover most dining situations:

- Unfold your napkin on your lap before you start eating. Do not tuck your napkin into your belt or shirt collar.
- Sit up straight when you eat. Bring the food to your mouth rather than bending toward the food. You may lean slightly forward so any food that drops will land on the plate. Avoid resting your elbows on the table.
- Cut each food into manageable pieces as you eat it, rather than all at once.
- If you have trouble getting peas or other food onto your fork, push it on with a piece of bread or the tip of your dinner knife.
- Chew with your mouth closed and swallow food before speaking.
- When eating soup, dip the soup spoon away from you in the soup bowl. Sip soup from the side of the spoon without making a slurping sound.
- If you feel a cough or sneeze coming on, cover your mouth and nose with a handkerchief or a napkin and turn away from the table. If the coughing continues, excuse yourself and leave the table.
- If you cannot reach the food easily, politely ask the person nearest the food to pass it to you.
- After stirring a beverage with a spoon, place the spoon on the saucer. A spoon sticking out of a cup may be hit accidentally, knocking over the cup.
- Remove inedible parts of food from your mouth as discreetly as possible. Fish bones are very small, so it is acceptable to remove them from your mouth with your fingers.
- When you have finished eating, place your fork and knife across your plate, side by side, pointing toward the center. Fold your napkin and place it to the left of the plate.
- Do not use a toothpick in front of others.
- Never comb your hair or apply makeup at the table.
- Wait for others to finish before leaving the table. Excuse yourself if you must leave.

Respecting Cultural Differences

Table etiquette varies among cultures. In traditional Japanese etiquette, slurping noodles shows appreciation for the meal. In Thailand, the practice is thought rude. Americans apologize for burping. In Indonesia, a loud burp at the end of the meal is a compliment to the cook. In the United States, soup is sipped from the side of the spoon. In many cultures in Asia it is drunk directly from the bowl.

Rules for eating and serving food grow out of each culture's customs, cuisine, and history. However, all cultures place value on showing respect and consideration for others and making the meal experience pleasant. When you are eating a meal with people from a different culture, take your cue from their behavior.

STEP 3 Connect to Your Community

Some volunteer activities may count toward your daily physical activity requirements. Identify someone in your community qualified to discuss community volunteer opportunities. Here are some suggestions:

Listening Skills

- A school counselor
- A community official
- Someone who works for an organization that needs the help of volunteers, like a soup kitchen, a homeless shelter, or a food pantry. Arrange to interview the person. Take notes during the interview, and transcribe your notes in complete sentences after the interview. Use these listening skills while you conduct the interview.

STEP 4 Develop Your Eating Plan

Use the Unit Thematic Project Checklist to plan and complete your plan for healthful living and evaluate your work.

STEP 5 Evaluate Presentation

Your project will be evaluated based on:

- Creativity used in creating your plan.
- Understanding and application of research.
- Mechanics, presentation, and neatness.

Unit Thematic Project Checklist

Category	Objectives
Plan	☑ Choose an eating plan that appeals to you.
	☑ Identify physical activities you enjoy.
	☑ Interview a member of your community.
Create	☑ Make a chart, spreadsheet, calendar or other visual that illustrates a realistic and healthful eating and physical activity plan for one week.
	☑ Include 60-minutes of physical activity each day in your plan.
	☑ Include ways to incorporate volunteer activities into your plans for physical activity.
	☑ Turn in your research summary, interview notes, and your weeklong eating and physical activity plan to your teacher.
Academic Skills	☑ Conduct research to gather information.
	☑ State your findings clearly.
	☑ Cite your sources.

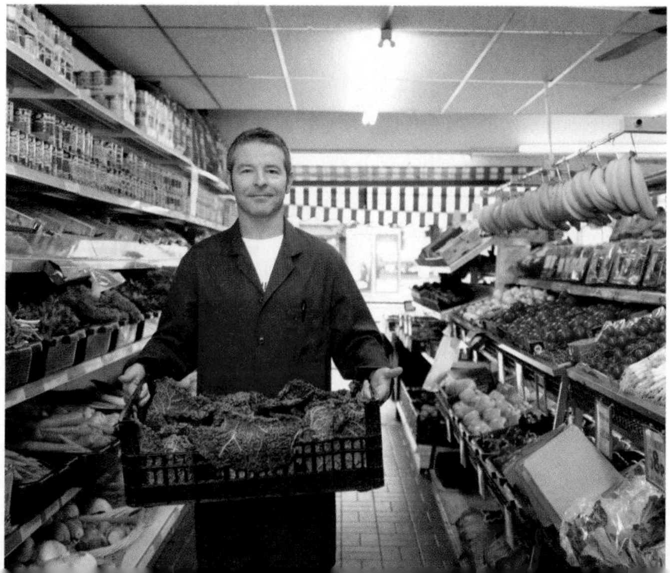

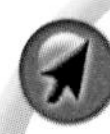
Go to this book's Online Learning Center through **glencoe.com** for a rubric you can use to evaluate your final project.

UNIT 5

Kitchen Basics

Activate Prior Knowledge

Explore the Photo Proper food storage is important in helping to prevent foodborne illnesses. *Have you ever contracted a foodborne illness?*

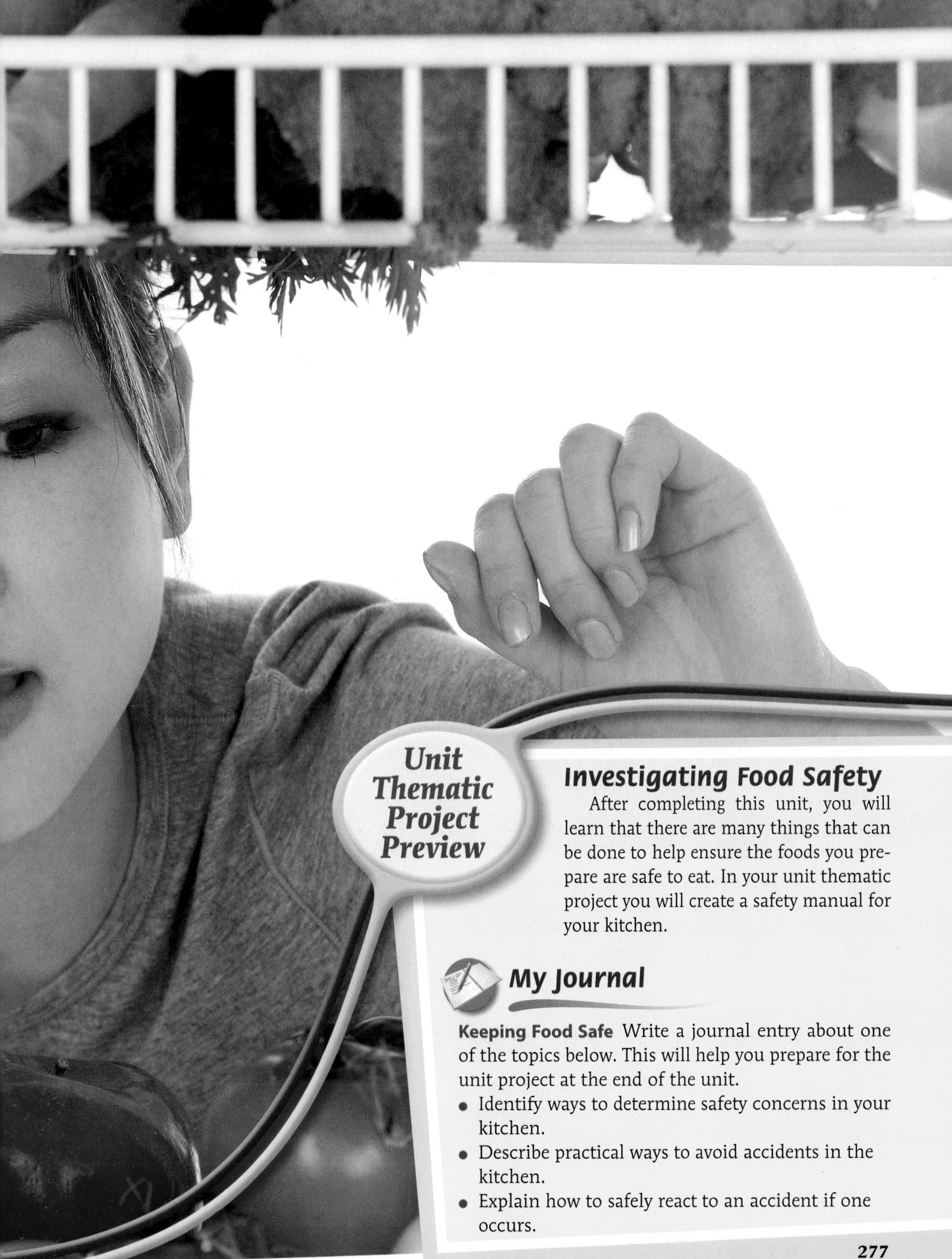

Unit Thematic Project Preview

Investigating Food Safety

After completing this unit, you will learn that there are many things that can be done to help ensure the foods you prepare are safe to eat. In your unit thematic project you will create a safety manual for your kitchen.

My Journal

Keeping Food Safe Write a journal entry about one of the topics below. This will help you prepare for the unit project at the end of the unit.

- Identify ways to determine safety concerns in your kitchen.
- Describe practical ways to avoid accidents in the kitchen.
- Explain how to safely react to an accident if one occurs.

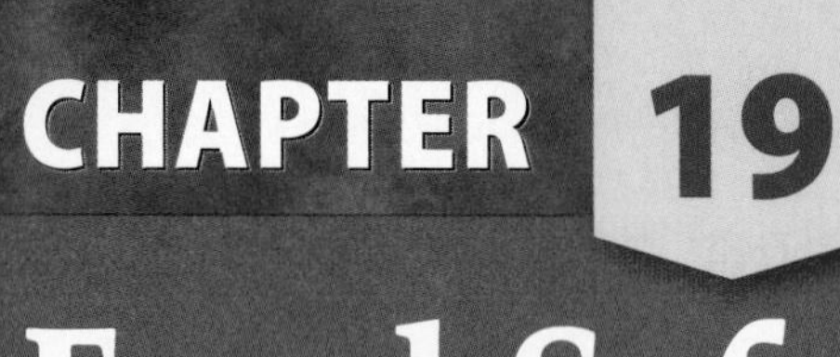

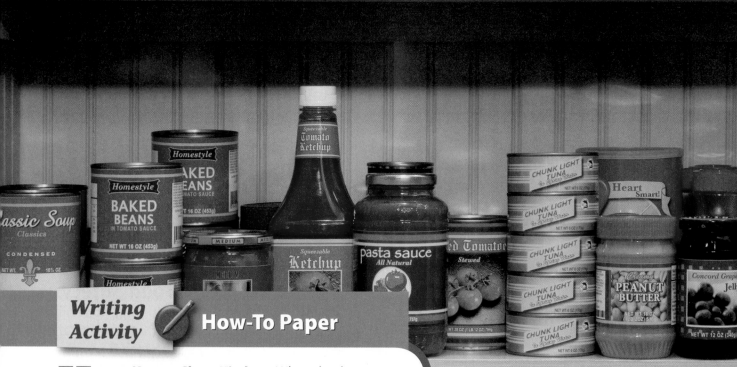

CHAPTER 19

Food Safety & Storage

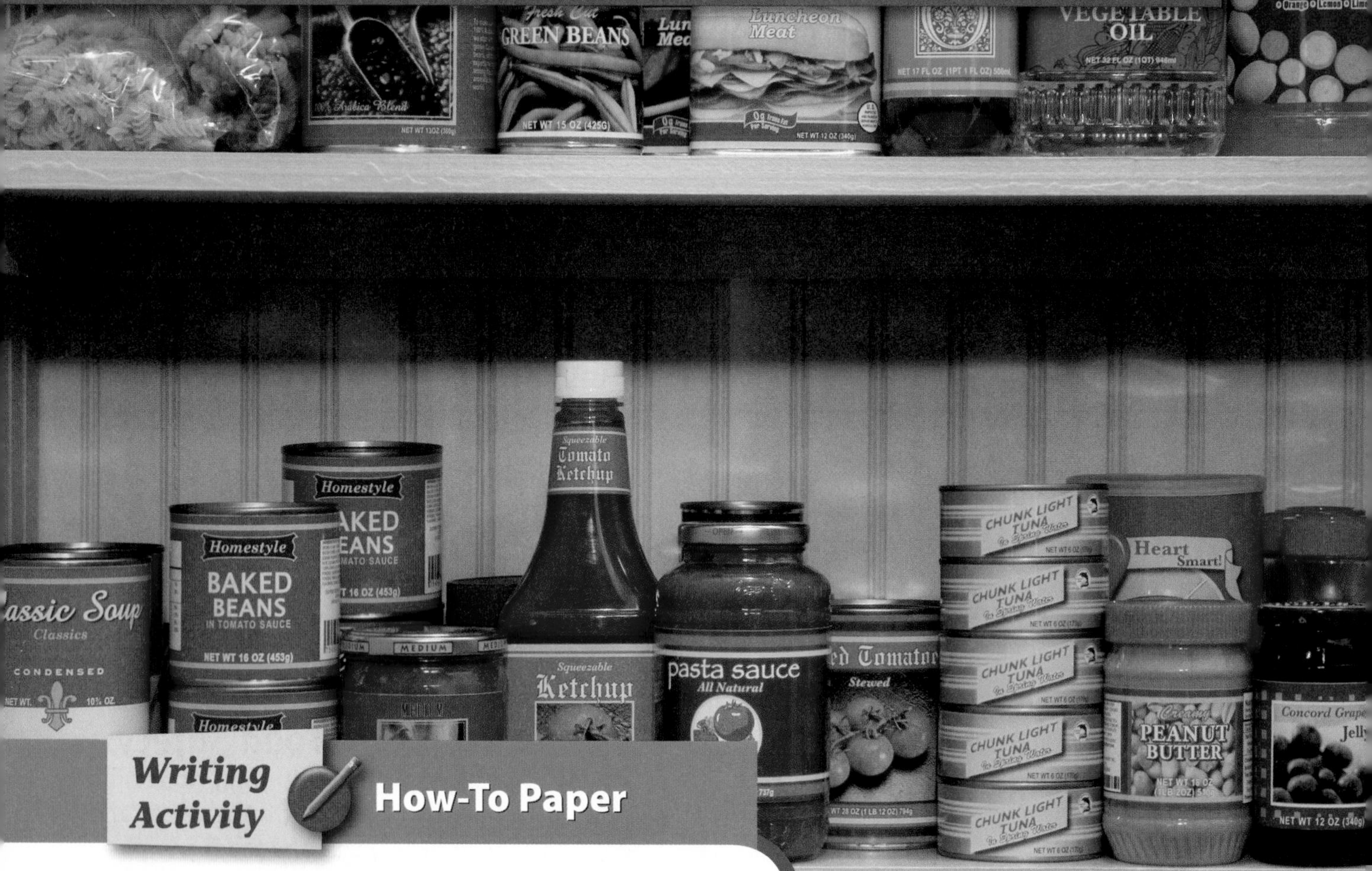

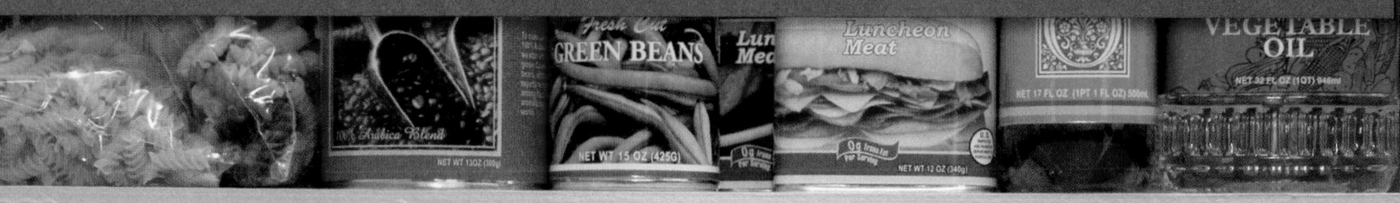

Writing Activity — How-To Paper

How to Keep a Clean Kitchen Why is kitchen cleanliness important? What steps should a person take to keep their kitchen clean? What supplies will they need in order to complete the steps? Write a How-To paper for a person who is moving into his or her own apartment.

Writing Tips Follow these steps to write a How-To Paper:

- Discuss the steps required to complete the task.
- Identify the supplies you will need to complete the task.
- Include an introduction and conclusion.

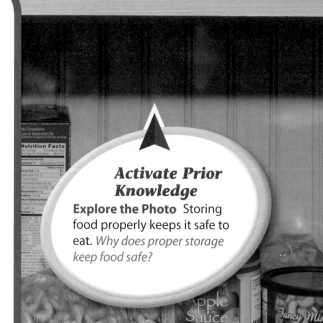

Activate Prior Knowledge

Explore the Photo Storing food properly keeps it safe to eat. *Why does proper storage keep food safe?*

Reading Guide

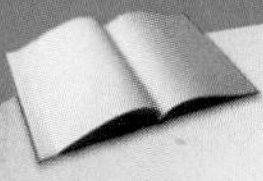

Before You Read

Preview Look at the photos in the chapter and write your own caption relating to food safety and storage for each photo.

Read to Learn

Key Concepts

- **Identify** the causes of foodborne illness.
- **Explain** the importance of cleanliness in the kitchen.
- **Summarize** ways to cook, thaw, and serve food safely.
- **Describe** safe food storage practices.
- **Summarize** methods for safely preserving food at home.
- **Describe** the roles of government agencies in protecting the food supply.

Main Idea

Prepare, store, and preserve foods safely to maximize nutrition and enjoyment and prevent foodborne illness.

Content Vocabulary

- ☐ contaminant
- ☐ foodborne illness
- ☐ microorganism
- ☐ toxin
- ☐ spore
- ☐ food safety
- ☐ sanitation
- ☐ personal hygiene
- ☐ 20-second scrub
- ☐ cross-contamination
- ☐ internal temperature
- ☐ rancidity
- ☐ freezer burn
- ☐ preserve
- ☐ sugar-pack method
- ☐ syrup-pack method
- ☐ tray-pack method
- ☐ dry-pack method
- ☐ blanching
- ☐ headspace
- ☐ raw-pack method
- ☐ hot-pack method
- ☐ boiling-water bath
- ☐ pressure canning
- ☐ rehydrate
- ☐ GRAS list
- ☐ irradiation
- ☐ recall
- ☐ tolerance

Academic Vocabulary

- tolerate
- reserve

Graphic Organizer

Use a graphic organizer like the one below to take notes about the four methods of freezing fruit.

Sugar-Pack	Syrup-Pack	Tray-Pack	Dry-Pack

Graphic Organizer Go to this book's Online Learning Center at **glencoe.com** to print out this graphic organizer.

Academic Standards

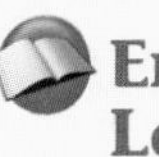

English Language Arts

NCTE 12 Use language to accomplish individual purposes.

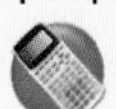

Mathematics

NCTM Geometry Use visualization, spatial reasoning, and geometric modeling to solve problems.

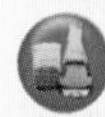

Science

NSES B Develop an understanding of the structures and properties of matter.

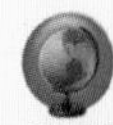

Social Studies

NCSS VIII A Science, Technology and Society Identify and describe both current and historical examples of the interaction and interdependence of science, technology, and society in a variety of cultural settings.

NCTE *National Council of Teachers of English*
NCTM *National Council of Teachers of Mathematics*
NSES *National Science Education Standards*
NCSS *National Council for the Social Studies*

Foodborne Illness

Contaminants in food cause over 76 million illnesses and 5,000 deaths in the United States each year. A **contaminant** is a substance, such as a chemical or organism, that makes food unsafe to eat.

Sickness caused by eating food that contains a contaminant is known as **foodborne illness**. Fever, headache, and digestive troubles are symptoms of foodborne illness. Children, pregnant women, older adults, and chronically ill people are most at risk.

Roots of Foodborne Illness

Most foodborne illness is caused by microorganisms. A **microorganism** is a living thing so small that it can only be seen through a microscope. Bacteria are single-celled microorganisms that cause most cases of foodborne illness. Thousands of species of bacteria are present in the human body. Many bacteria are harmless. Some bacteria, like those that aid in food digestion, are essential for health.

A few bacteria are dangerous to human health. These bacteria produce a **toxin**, or poison, that can cause illness. Some bacteria also produce spores. A **spore** is a protected cell that develops into a bacterium when it has the right conditions of food, warmth, and moisture. **Figure 19.1** lists some of the bacteria that cause foodborne illness and where they might be found.

Bacteria cannot travel far by themselves. They are carried on people, animals, insects, and objects. Harmful bacteria are sometimes already in food when you buy it. More often, bacteria multiply through careless handling. In just a few hours, one bacterium can multiply into thousands—yet the food may look, taste, and smell completely safe to eat. A healthy human body can **tolerate**, or allow, small amounts of harmful bacteria. Large amounts of harmful bacteria are a health hazard.

You can help prevent foodborne illness through **food safety**, keeping food safe to eat by following proper food handling and cooking practices. The basic food safety rules are:

- Keep yourself and your kitchen clean.
- Do not cross-contaminate. Store and handle uncooked meat, poultry, seafood, and eggs separately from other foods.
- Cook food thoroughly.
- Refrigerate food promptly.

✓ Reading Check **Identify** What are the symptoms of food borne illness?

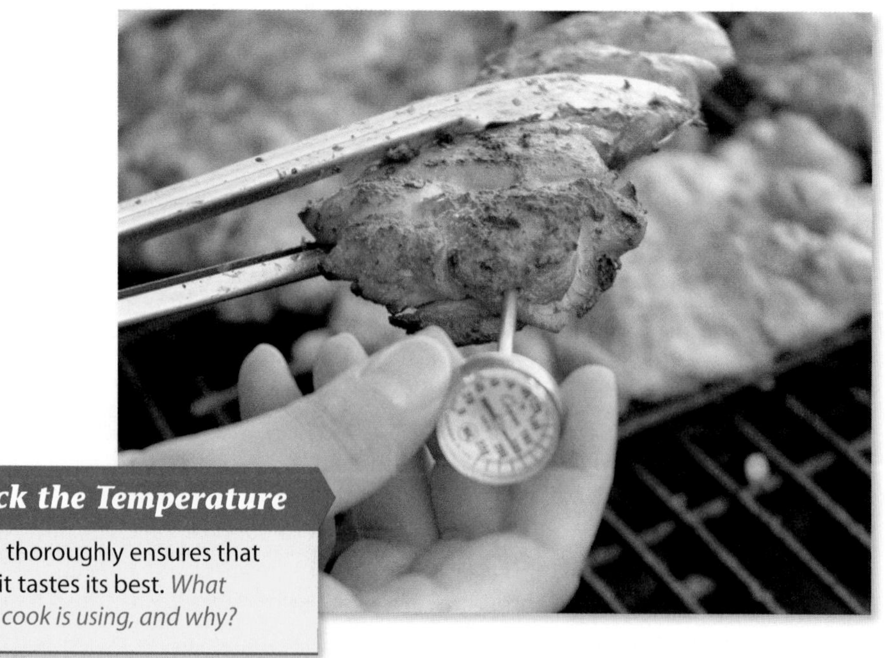

Check the Temperature

Cooking food correctly and thoroughly ensures that food is safe to eat and that it tastes its best. *What instrument do you think this cook is using, and why?*

Figure 19.1 Selected Bacteria that Cause Foodborne Illness

Completely Cooked Harmful bacteria are the most common cause of foodborne illness. Different species of bacteria are found in different foods, as shown below. ***What harmful bacteria are sometimes found in raw or undercooked meat, poultry, and seafood?***

Bacteria and Disease	Common Sources
Campylobacter jejuni (disease: campylobacteriosis)	Contaminated water; unpasteurized milk; undercooked meat, poultry, and seafood.
Clostridium botulinum (disease: botulism, which can be fatal)	Improperly processed, home-canned and commercially canned foods; garlic in oils; vacuum-packed or tightly wrapped food.
Clostridium perfringens (disease: perfringens food poisoning)	Environments where there is little or no oxygen. Sometimes called the "cafeteria germ" because it is often found in food served in quantity and left for long periods on a steam table or at room temperature.
Escherichia coli (disease: hemorrhagic colitis)	Unchlorinated water; raw or rare ground beef; raw alfalfa sprouts; unwashed produce; unpasteurized milk or apple cider.
Listeria monocytogenes (disease: listeriosis)	Raw or undercooked meat, poultry, or fish; unwashed produce; soft cheeses; unpasteurized milk; ready-to-eat foods, such as hot dogs, cold cuts, dry sausages, and deli-style meats and poultry.
Salmonella (disease: salmonellosis)	Raw or undercooked poultry, eggs, meat, and seafood; unpasteurized milk.
Staphylococcus aureus (disease: staphylococcal food poisoning)	Prepared foods left too long at room temperature. Typical sources are meat, poultry, egg products, and such mixtures as tuna, chicken, potato, and egg salad; cream-filled pastries.

Cleanliness in the Kitchen

A clean kitchen plays an important role in **sanitation**, the prevention of illness through cleanliness. Habits of cleanliness help to ensure food safety and make your kitchen a more pleasant place to work.

Personal Hygiene

Bacteria on your body can contaminate work surfaces, utensils, and food. By practicing **personal hygiene**, thoroughly washing your body, face, and hands, you help to avoid transferring harmful bacteria when handling food.

Your hands come in frequent contact with food, so keeping them clean is the single most effective way to prevent the transfer of bacteria. Make a habit of the **20-second scrub**, using soap and warm water to scrub your hands for 20 seconds. Use a brush to clean underneath your fingernails. Keep your nails trimmed.

Do a 20-second scrub before working in the kitchen. Scrub your hands right after handling raw meat, poultry, fish, shellfish, and eggs. Scrub your hands immediately after you use the toilet, blow your nose, handle pets, or touch your face, hair, or any other part of your body.

Bacteria get into food by other routes as well, such as sneezing or coughing. Bacteria can even grow in spots and stains, so wear clean clothes covered with a clean apron. Remove dangling jewelry and roll up long sleeves. Tie back your hair if it is long. Cover any wounds on your hands with rubber or plastic gloves, and wash gloved hands as often as bare ones.

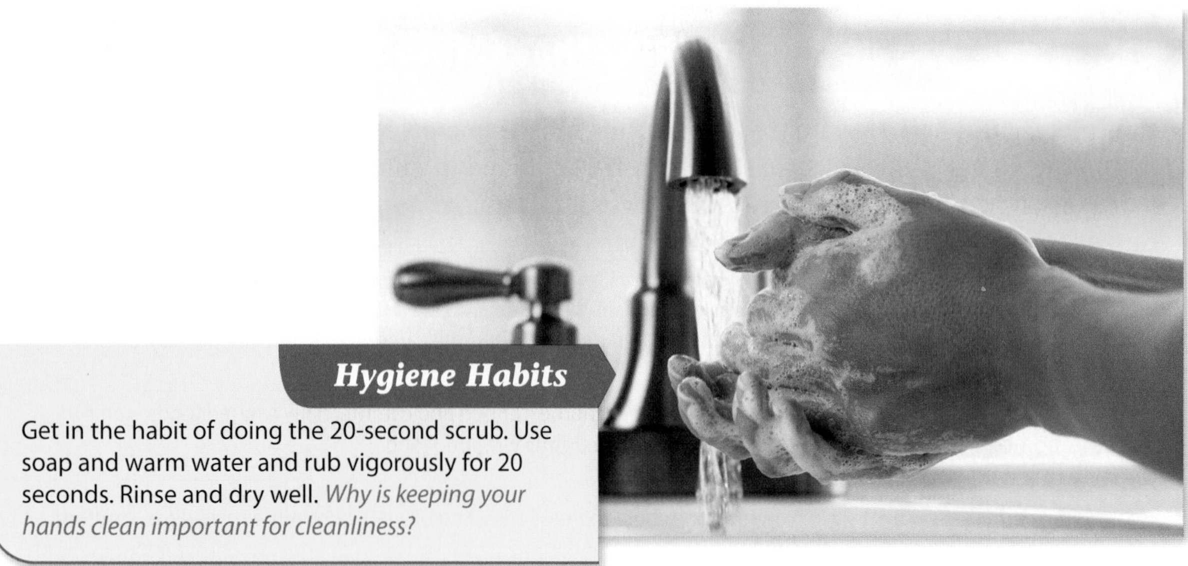

Hygiene Habits

Get in the habit of doing the 20-second scrub. Use soap and warm water and rub vigorously for 20 seconds. Rinse and dry well. *Why is keeping your hands clean important for cleanliness?*

A Clean Kitchen

A clean kitchen also helps to limit the growth of bacteria. Practice these kitchen routines until they become habits:

- Wash work surfaces and utensils in hot, sudsy water before you prepare food.
- Wash the tops of cans before opening them.
- Use a clean spoon to taste food during cooking.
- Change dishtowels often. Use separate towels for wiping hands, wiping dishes, and any other purposes.
- At the end of the day, put the dishcloth in the laundry and replace it with a clean one. Wash sponges by hand or in a dishwasher and let them air-dry overnight.
- Keep pets out of the kitchen. Pet hairs carry bacteria.

Pest Control

Insects can bring harmful bacteria into the kitchen. Clean up crumbs and food spills from floors, counters, and tables that might attract insects. Take garbage to an outside, covered can at least once a day. Wash garbage cans regularly.

Chemical insecticides can be hazardous to people and the environment. Try prevention first. Repair holes in walls and screens where pests get in. Caulk cracks and crevices. Sprinkle chili powder, paprika, or dried peppermint across ant trails. If you must use a commercial insecticide, follow the label directions carefully, and do not let the spray get onto dishes, countertops, or food.

Clean-up

Thorough clean-up is essential for food safety. Wash all the work areas and tools you have used, and wipe down all appliances. As you work, rinse your dishcloth or sponge often in hot, sudsy water.

Mop up any spills on the floor. Wash the sink to remove grease and bits of food. If the sink has a disposal, run it. Put any garbage in a plastic bag and close tightly.

Washing Dishes

If your kitchen has a dishwasher, use it according to the owner's manual. You can also wash dishes thoroughly by hand by following these steps:

- Scrape and rinse soiled dishes and place them to one side of the sink.
- Group dishes. Put glasses closest to the sink, then flatware, plates and bowls, kitchen tools, serving pieces and containers, and cookware. Keep sharp knives separate.
- Presoak any cookware that has food stuck to it. Pour in a little detergent, add hot water, and let it stand while you wash the other dishes.

- Fill a dishpan or sink with sudsy water that is hot enough to remove grease but not so hot that it burns your hands.
- Use a sponge or dishcloth to wash dishes in order, from glasses first to greasy cookware last. Refill the sink or dishpan with clean, hot, soapy water as needed.
- Rinse dishes thoroughly in hot water. Make sure to thoroughly rinse the insides of containers.
- Let dishes air-dry in a rack or dry them with a clean, dry towel.
- Wash knives after the other dishes. Handle them with care and towel them dry.

Avoid Cross-Contamination

Cross-contamination is the spread of harmful bacteria from one food to another. Cross-contamination can occur with any food, raw or cooked, but it is most common with raw meat, poultry, seafood, and eggs. Keep these foods separate in your shopping cart and grocery bags. Store them in the refrigerator in sealed containers or plastic bags.

When you prepare raw meat, poultry, or seafood, wash every surface the food touched with hot, soapy water. Wash plates, tools, and utensils, as well as your hands. Always put cooked food on a clean plate, not a plate that held the raw food.

Wash the dining table before and after eating. Always handle cooked foods with clean utensils, never by hand. Place a serving utensil in every serving dish so that people are not tempted to use their own utensils. Do not refill a used serving dish. Instead, get a clean dish.

Hold cups and flatware by their handles and glassware by the lower third, away from the lip. When you carry more than one plate of food, do not let the plates touch.

Cutting Boards

Cutting boards are a common source of cross-contamination. Keep two cutting boards and always use the same one for meat, poultry, and seafood. **Reserve**, or set aside, the other cutting board for foods other than meat.

Keep cutting boards clean by washing them in hot, sudsy water after each use. Rinse and air-dry the boards, or dry them with a clean towel. Some plastic boards can be washed in a dishwasher. Discard boards with hard-to-clean cuts and grooves. Many studies have been done about the safety of cutting board materials. Microorganisms are easier to wash from plastic than from wood, so consider choosing plastic cutting boards.

✓ Reading Check **Explain** Why is it smart to have at least two cutting boards in your kitchen?

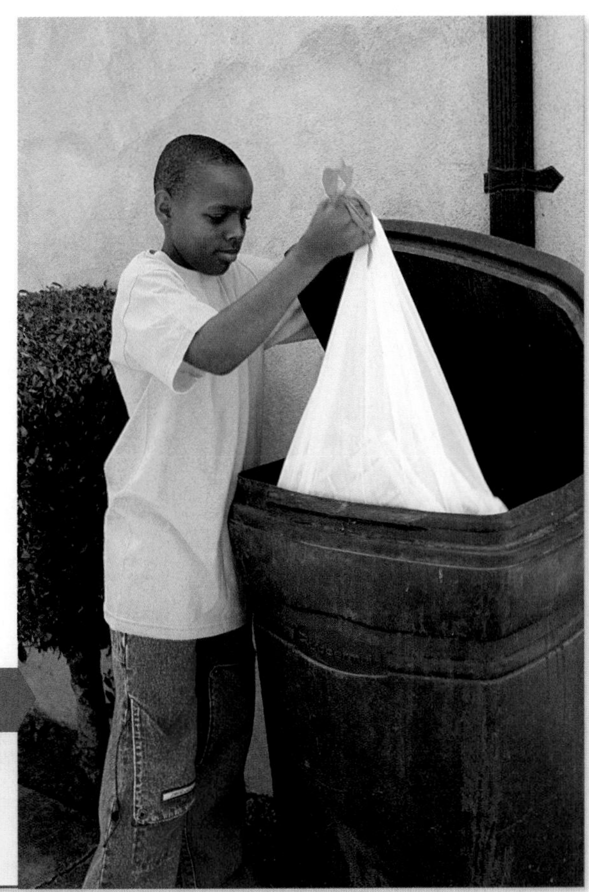

Conscientious Clean-Up

Remove kitchen garbage to an outside garbage can at least once a day to prevent pest infestations and reduce germs and odors. *What are the drawbacks of using insecticides to manage pests?*

Cooking Food Safely

Food temperature affects how quickly bacteria grow. The danger zone given by the USDA for home use is the temperature range in which bacteria grow fastest: 40°F to 140°F (4°C to 60°C). See **Figure 19.2**. (Foodservice businesses use a slightly different set of temperatures from a system called Hazard Analysis Critical Control Point.) The less time food spends at room temperature, the more slowly bacteria will multiply.

High temperatures during cooking kill most bacteria, but spores and some toxins can survive. Bacteria grow more slowly when food is in the refrigerator and freezer, but some bacteria can survive freezing. When food warms up, the bacteria start to grow again. No amount of heating or chilling, however, will make food safe to eat if it has been improperly stored.

How do you know when meat and poultry have been cooked thoroughly enough to kill bacteria? You cannot tell by appearance alone whether the meat has reached the proper temperature. Use a food thermometer to check the **internal temperature**, the temperature deep inside the thickest part of the food. The internal temperature must reach at least 160°F for most foods, and must be held at that temperature for a short time. Upcoming chapters give safe internal temperatures for meat, poultry, and other specific foods. To help prevent the growth of harmful bacteria, follow these guidelines when you cook:

- Taste foods containing ingredients from animal sources only after they are fully cooked.
- Never partially cook food and then wait to finish the cooking later. Cook the food completely all at once.

Figure 19.2 Temperature Danger Zone

Danger Zone Bacteria die when foods are thoroughly cooked at high temperatures. *Do bacteria die when food is frozen?*

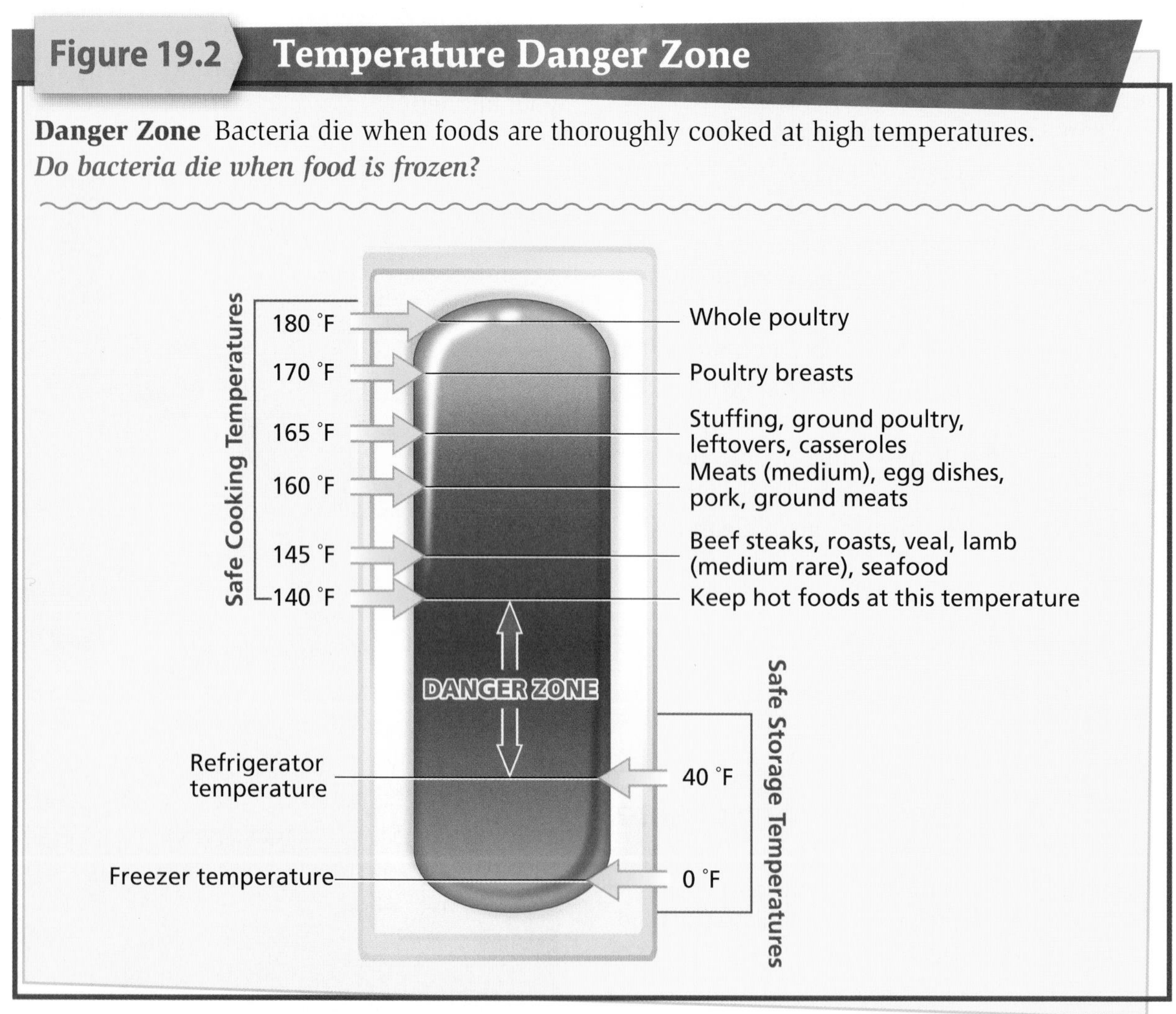

- When microwaving, cover the food and stir or rotate it. Some foods cook unevenly in a microwave oven, and cool spots may remain where bacteria can survive.
- When reheating food that has been refrigerated, bring it to an internal temperature of 165°F or higher.

Thawing Food

Bacteria can multiply when food is thawing, so you should never defrost frozen food at room temperature. By the time the inside is thawed, millions of bacteria will have grown on the outside. Instead, put the food into a container in the refrigerator. The container prevents the frozen food from leaking onto other foods as it thaws. The cold temperature slows bacterial growth.

For faster thawing, you can put the food into a watertight plastic bag and submerge it in a bowl or sink filled with cold water. Change the water every 30 minutes to keep it cold. You can also defrost food in the microwave according to the manufacturer's directions. Defrosting in the microwave starts the cooking process, so do this only if you plan to cook the food right away.

You can also skip the thawing step altogether. Just cook the food longer and make sure it reaches the proper internal temperature.

Serving Food

When serving food, remember these three rules:

1. Keep hot foods hot. Keep hot foods at a temperature higher than 140°F. Keep extra quantities of food hot on the range, on a warming tray, or in an electrical serving dish.

2. Keep cold foods cold. Refrigerate cold foods until serving time.

3. Follow the two-hour rule. Perishable foods that contain meat, poultry, fish, eggs, or dairy products should not sit at room temperature longer than two hours. If the air temperature is higher than 90°F, the limit is one hour.

✓ **Reading Check** **Explain** Is it safe to defrost food at room temperature?

Storing Food Safely

Food that is stored improperly or for too long loses quality and nutrients, and eventually spoils. Some types of spoilage cause foodborne illness. Protect your health by using proper storage techniques.

Identifying Spoiled Food

Why does food spoil? Dirt, heat, and moisture promote the growth of harmful bacteria, yeasts, and molds. Dry air wilts some fresh foods and causes staleness in others. Air and light can destroy nutrients. Heat speeds the action of enzymes in food, which trigger chemical changes that lessen food quality.

Food spoilage is often obvious. Fresh produce may look wilted, wrinkled, bruised, or brown. Meats may become slimy. Spots of mold and a foul taste or smell are also sure signs that food has gone bad.

Food packages can also warn of spoiled contents. Damaged packaging makes the food inside more likely to spoil. Bulging cans, liquids that spurt when you open a container, and cloudy fluids that should be clear all indicate bacterial action.

What should you do if you think food is spoiled? Throw it away—do not taste it first. If the food is moldy, prevent the spread of spores by gently wrapping the food in a bag before discarding it. Examine other foods that may have been in contact with the moldy item. If you suspect that mold is spreading to other foods, wash out the refrigerator.

Food-Storage Guidelines

Proper storage prevents spoilage and preserves food's nutrients, flavor, texture, and appearance. Follow these guidelines to protect quality in stored food:

- Follow package directions for storing food.
- Follow the principle of "first in, first out." Store newly purchased food behind older food of the same kind so that you use the older items first.
- If containers have no sell-by or use-by dates, write the purchase date on them before storing. Use canned food within a year.

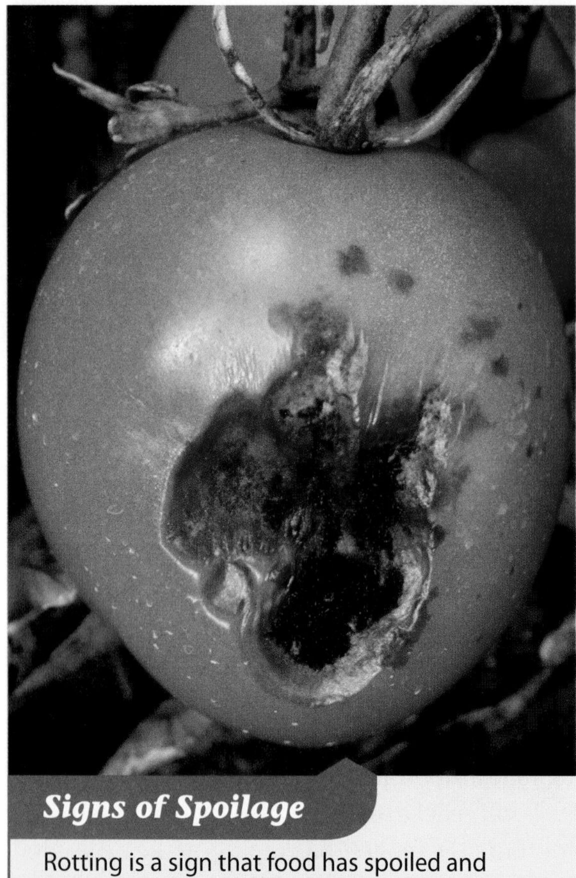

Signs of Spoilage

Rotting is a sign that food has spoiled and is no longer safe to eat. *What should you do with spoiled food?*

- Clean storage areas regularly. Wipe up spills right away.
- Buy only as much food as you need before your next shopping trip. Restaurants call this barstock. Extra food is likely to go bad.

Room Temperature Storage

Shelf-stable foods can be stored at normal room temperatures, generally below 85°F and above freezing, 32°F. Shelf-stable foods include unopened canned foods, dry beans and peas, oils and shortening, and many grain products except whole grains, which should be refrigerated. Most fruits and vegetables should not be stored at room remperature.

Storage cabinets should be clean and dry, with doors to keep out light, dirt, and pests. They should not be near heat sources, such as a range, radiator, toaster, or refrigerator coils. Do not store food in damp areas such as under the sink.

Keep stored food away from household chemicals, such as cleaners. Keep chemicals in their original packages, never in empty food packages or other food storage containers. Someone might mistake a poisonous chemical for food.

After you open canned goods, store the leftovers in a glass or plastic container in the refrigerator. Dry goods and bulk foods such as dry beans and cereal can stay in the cabinet at room temperature. Reseal the package as much as possible to keep out dirt and insects, or move the food to a storage container with a tight-fitting cover.

Nutrition Check

Killing Bacteria...and Nutrients

When handled properly, the process of canning destroys many harmful bacteria. Unfortunately, it can also destroy valuable nutrients. When foods are subjected to high temperatures and immersed in water, they lose between 60 and 80 percent of their valuable vitamins, enzymes, and other nutrients. Nutrients are also lost when the excess liquid is poured off of simmered and canned foods. Instead of discarding this liquid, try using it in soups, stews, or sauces.

Think About It Nora says, "One raw apricot contain 15 percent of the daily value for vitamin A. I eat a jar of 7 canned apricots every day, so I know I'm meeting 100% of my daily needs for vitamin A." Is she correct? Explain.

Refrigerator Storage

Bacteria thrive at room temperature, so it is important to refrigerate food promptly. Put away any perishable food you are not using in the refrigerator or freezer.

Keep the temperature inside your refrigerator under 40°F but above 32°F to avoid freezing liquids. If you see frost or ice forming, the temperature is too low. Read the owner's manual to learn how to set the temperature control on your refrigerator. It is a good idea to keep a thermometer in the refrigerator to monitor the temperature.

Help air circulate to all parts of the refrigerator by not overloading the fridge. Be sure that foods are tightly covered, too. This keeps them from drying out or picking up odors from other foods. Storage areas in the door are exposed to warm air every time you open the fridge, so save that space for soft drinks and other less perishable items.

These foods need refrigeration:

- Foods that are refrigerated in the store, including dairy products, eggs, and deli items.
- Most fresh fruits and vegetables. Exceptions are onions, garlic, potatoes, and sweet potatoes, which should be kept in a cool, dry place. Wash produce before storing it only if you need to remove dirt. Dry fruits and vegetables before storing.
- Whole-grain products, seeds, and nuts. Their high oil content makes them prone to **rancidity** (ran-ˈsi-də-tē), or spoilage due to the breakdown of fats. Rancid foods have a stale, bitter flavor.
- Baked products with fruit or cream fillings.
- Any food with a label that says "refrigerate after opening."

Refrigerating Cooked Food

Refrigerate or freeze leftovers immediately. Do not wait for them to cool to room temperature first. To ensure quick chilling, put leftovers in tightly closed, shallow containers. Cut large chunks of food into smaller pieces. Label containers with the date you stored them. Eat leftovers within three or four days, or freeze them for longer storage. You may want to keep all leftovers on the same refrigerator shelf so it is easy to see them all at a glance. Throw away perishable food that has been left at room temperature for too long.

Freezer Storage

Frozen food keeps longer than refrigerated food. At temperatures of 0°F or below, foods keep from one month to a year, depending on the type of food and its packaging. **Figures 19.3** and **19.4** on pages 288–289 give a general timetable for storing perishable foods in the refrigerator freezer.

A full refrigerator works poorly, but a fairly full freezer functions best. Frozen items act like ice blocks, keeping each other cold.

When you buy frozen food, put it in the freezer right away. You can also freeze other foods to lengthen their shelf life. You can freeze tofu, meat, poultry, and seafood; baked products; and home-prepared meals and leftovers.

Foods with high water content, such as salad greens and celery, do not freeze well. As the water freezes, it expands and explodes the food's cells, making it soft and soggy when thawed.

Thickened sauces, gravies, fillings, yogurt, and sour cream tend to separate in the freezer. Custards and cream fillings, meat and poultry stuffing, and raw or cooked whole eggs also do not freeze well.

Packaging Foods for Freezing

Foods that are sold frozen are specially packaged to preserve quality. Foods that you freeze at home need special protection to avoid freezer burn. **Freezer burn** is moisture loss caused by improper packaging or overly long storage in the freezer. Cold air gets into the package, damaging the food's quality. Food with freezer burn may have tough, grayish-brown spots and a stale taste and aroma.

Containers for freezing food should be airtight and should resist vapor and moisture.

Science in Action

From Firm to Floppy

Not all foods look or taste as good after freezing as they do before it. Foods with high water content, such as spinach and celery, do not freeze well. Because water molecules expand when they freeze, they stretch and explode foods' cells. Consequently, frozen foods that contain a lot of water become soft and soggy when thawed. Textural changes due to freezing are not as apparent in products that are cooled before freezing because cooking softens the cell walls.

Procedure Imagine this scenario: A busy restaurant prepares its cucumber salad side dishes in advance and stores them in the freezer.

Analysis What might customers complain about? What will be the cause of their complaints?

NSES B Develop an understanding of the structures and properties of matter.

Figure 19.3 Cold Storage of Meats, Poultry, and Fish

Clean, Cold, Covered Both cooked and uncooked meats keep for only a few days in the refrigerator. Cured meats keep longer. ***Which kind of meat keeps the longest in the refrigerator? The shortest?***

Food	Refrigerator Storage 40°F	Freezer Storage 0°F
Uncooked		
Beef, lamb, pork, or veal chops; steaks; roast	3–5 days	4–12 mos.
Chicken or turkey, whole	1–2 days	1 yr.
Chicken or turkey, pieces	1–2 days	9 mos.
Ground meats or poultry	1–2 days	3–4 mos.
Lean fish (cod)	1–2 days	6 mos.
Fatty fish (salmon)	1–2 days	2–3 mos.
Shellfish (shrimp)	1–2 days	3–6 mos.
Cooked/Leftover		
Cooked meats; meat dishes	3–4 days	2–3 mos.
Fried chicken	3–4 days	4 mos.
Poultry, in broth	3–4 days	6 mos.
Fish stews, soups (not creamed)	3–4 days	4–6 mos.
Cured Meats		
Hot dogs, opened	1 wk.	1–2 mos.
Lunch meats, opened	3–5 days	1–2 mos.
Hot dogs, lunch meats, unopened	2 wks.	1–2 mos.
Bacon	7 days	1 mo.
Smoked sausage (beef, pork, turkey)	7 days	1–2 mos.
Hard sausage (pepperoni)	2–3 wks.	1–2 mos.
Ham, canned, unopened	2–3 wks.	*
Ham, fully cooked, whole	7 days	1–2 mos.
Ham, fully cooked, half or slices	3–5 days	1–2 mos.

**Food should not be stored here.*

Good choices include plastic containers with tight-fitting lids, heavy-duty plastic freezer bags, and heavy-duty foil and freezer wrap. Regular refrigerator storage bags and plastic margarine or yogurt tubs do not give enough protection. The lightweight store wrap on fresh meat, poultry, and seafood also needs added layers for freezing.

To freeze meat, wrap it tightly and seal the package with freezer tape. When filling a container, leave enough space for food to expand as it freezes, about 1 inch of space per quart. Then seal the container tightly. Label all items with the contents, amount or number of servings, the date frozen, and any special instructions.

For best quality, freeze food quickly. Spread packages out in one layer so they touch the cooling coils or sides of the freezer. Leave enough space between packages for air to circulate. Give the food at least 24 hours to freeze, then stack similar items together. Keep an inventory of the food in the freezer. List the food, date frozen, and quantity. Update the inventory as you use food so that you know how much is left.

When the Power Goes Off

If the power goes off or the refrigerator-freezer breaks down, chilled food can spoil. Carry the frozen foods to another refrigerator or freezer in coolers or heavily wrapped in paper or plastic. If you cannot move the food, keep the freezer or refrigerator door closed to help keep the temperature down.

After losing power, a full freezer should keep food frozen for about two days. A half-full freezer may keep food frozen for only one day. If the freezer is not full, quickly stack packages closely together so they will stay cold. Separate frozen raw meat, poultry, and seafood from other foods to avoid any cross-contamination if they start to thaw.

If the power will be off longer than two days, you can nest foods in the freezer in bags of ice cubes from the store. Place a blanket or several layers of newspaper on the outside of the freezer to insulate it. You can also use dry ice (frozen carbon dioxide), but be very careful. Never touch dry ice with your bare hands or breathe its vapors in an enclosed area. Carbon dioxide gas in high concentration is poisonous.

Figure 19.4 Cold Storage of Dairy Products and Other Foods

Stay Cool Some cultured dairy products, such as butter and sour cream, keep longer than fresh milk or cream. ***Can you store any egg products in the freezer? If so, which ones?***

Food	Refrigerator Storage 40°F	Freezer Storage 0°F
Dairy Products		
Fresh milk, cream	7 days	3 mos.
Butter, margarine	1–3 mos.	6–9 mos.
Buttermilk	2 wks.	3 mos.
Sour cream	1–3 wks.	*
Yogurt, plain or flavored	1–2 wks.	1–12 mos.
Cottage cheese	1 wk.	*
Hard cheese, opened (cheddar)	3–4 wks.	6 mos.
Hard cheese, unopened	6 mos.	6 mos.
Ice cream, sherbet	*	2–4 mos.
Miscellaneous Foods		
Bread	7–14 days	3 mos.
Cakes; pies (not cream-filled)	7 days	2–3 mos.
Cream pies	1–2 days	*
Fresh eggs, in shell	3 wks.	*
Raw yolks, whites	2–4 days	1 yr.
Hard-cooked eggs	1 wk.	*
Egg substitutes, opened	3 days	*
Egg substitutes, unopened	10 days	*
Mayonnaise, opened	2 mos.	*
Salad dressing, opened	3 mos.	*
Salsa, opened	3 mos.	*
Cookies	2 mos.	8–12 mos.

**Food should not be stored here.*

Once the freezer is back in service, use the coldest setting to quickly refreeze any salvageable items. A food is safe to refreeze if ice crystals are visible, though it may have lost quality. Use these foods as soon as possible. Food that has thawed but is still cold can be refrigerated and used as soon as possible. Raw meat, poultry, and seafood can be refrozen after cooking. Throw out any food that has a strange odor.

Food will usually keep in a nonworking refrigerator for four to six hours, depending on the temperature of the room and how often you open the door. If the power will be out for a long time, try to keep foods cold by placing a large bag of ice cubes in the refrigerator.

When the power returns, check all foods for signs of spoilage, especially butter, margarine, and fresh produce. Clean up any food spills and wipe surfaces dry. If odors remain, wash surfaces with a solution of 2 tablespoons of baking soda dissolved in 1 quart of warm water. Put an open box of baking soda in the refrigerator to absorb odors.

✓ Reading Check **Respond** How soon should you eat leftovers after refrigerating them?

Careers in Food

Tom Nerney
Food Safety Inspector

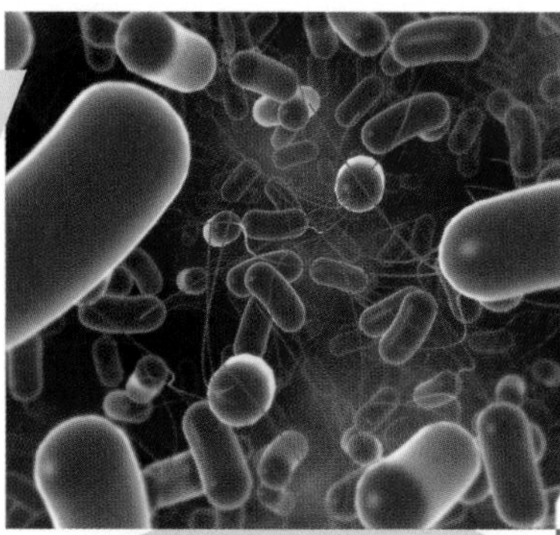

Q: What does a food safety inspector do?

A: Food safety inspectors identify hazards in food establishments and verify that those hazards are eliminated. They also assist in investigations of foodborne illnesses, collect food samples for laboratory analysis, and investigate consumer complaints. In addition, they often provide 24-hour response to disasters or accidents involving food products.

Q: What are some of the business and government entities that might hire a food safety inspector?

A: Local and state health departments, the U.S. Food and Drug Administration, The Centers For Disease Control, and the U.S. Department of Agriculture all need health inspectors. In the private sector, there are food consulting firms, food safety certification organizations, and chain food service establishments and markets.

Q: If an inspector deems something unsafe or hazardous, what typically happens next?

A: The person in charge of the facility is asked to dispose of the food product voluntarily. However, these people do not always cooperate. Most local and state regulations grant inspectors the power to embargo food that is deemed unsafe, meaning to initiate a legal process to have it removed or eliminated. In some cases, the product may be able to be re-processed rather than destroyed.

"Food safety inspectors are dedicated to protecting all consumers."
— Tom Nerney Compliance Officer, *Rhode Island Department of Health*

Education and Training

Most agencies require a bachelor's degree with an emphasis on the sciences. There are also certification classes for food safety inspectors.

Qualities and Skills

Communication skills and organization skills are very important, as is computer competency.

Related Career Opportunities

The most closely related is a manager of quality assurance or quality control for a food manufacturer or retailer.

Preserving Food Safely

Canning, freezing, and drying have long been used as safe methods for food preservation. To **preserve** is to prepare food in a way that allows it to be safely stored for later use. Many people still preserve food, especially vegetables and fruits, by canning, freezing, or drying. Preserving saves money and can be satisfying.

Some people preserve foods they raise themselves. They enjoy the seasonal fruits, vegetables, and herbs they grew themselves all year long. Use correct techniques to ensure the quality and the safety of the food.

Preserving food can be a fun family activity and a way to preserve traditions. A recipe for an unusual family favorite like red pepper jam might be handed down for generations. A store of preserved jam jars is good to have on hand.

Preserving food at home can also give you more control over what you eat. You can choose high-quality food and decide whether it will contain salt, sugar, or other additives. You can create your own delicious recipes and give them as gifts to friends and family. To avoid foodborne illness, it is important to follow safety rules when preserving food.

Preparing to Preserve

Get off to a good start by doing some planning first.

- Decide what foods to preserve, how much, and by what method. Buy only as much as you can prepare in the time available.
- Select foods to preserve based on what is in season. Selecting foods that are in season also allows you to get great value for your money.
- Be sure that all supplies are in usable condition.
- Always use high-quality food: ripe, firm fruit and young, tender vegetables.
- Follow recipes exactly. Do not take shortcuts or experiment.
- Wash food carefully and prepare it according to recipe directions.
- Have all equipment and supplies ready before you begin to work with the food.
- Follow all food-safety rules.

Freezing Fruits and Vegetables

Freezing preserves food at a temperature of 0°F or below. Freezing is the most convenient way to preserve produce, except for fruits and vegetables with a high water content, such as salad greens and celery. Frozen tomatoes and citrus fruits are fine for juice or sauce but not appealing raw.

Freeze foods quickly. Slow freezing allows large ice crystals to form, damaging food texture. To promote quick and even chilling, freeze foods in small containers and small batches.

Freezing Fruits

Prepare fruit the way you plan to use it—sliced or peeled, for example. Some fruits need to be treated with ascorbic acid (vitamin C) to disable their enzymes. Follow the directions on the package. Certain fruits, like apples, apricots, peaches, and nectarines, particularly need this treatment.

TECHNOLOGY FOR TOMORROW

Unsafe Preservation Methods

The open kettle method was once a standard way to preserve foods. Foods were simply cooked and then sealed in jars with no further treatment. This technique is now recognized as unsafe because the food never gets hot enough to kill all microorganisms. In more recent years, some people have misused technology by processing canned foods by heating them in a conventional or microwave oven. This method is also unsafe, because the foods cannot reach temperatures higher than the boiling point of water, and the jars could explode. Today's pressure canners are an example of how smart technology can be appropriately used to increase food safety.

Investigate Find out what a modern pressure canner looks like, how it operates, and how much it costs.

NCSS VIII A Science, Technology, and Society Identify and describe both current and historical examples of the interaction and interdependence of science, technology, and society in a variety of cultural settings.

Freeze the fruit with one of these methods:

Sugar-Pack Method The **sugar-pack method** is the technique of freezing fruit coated in sugar. Toss the fruit in sugar until it is well coated, then pack it into freezer-safe containers. The sugar helps retain the fruit's color and texture and combines with the juice to form a syrup when defrosted.

Syrup-Pack Method The **syrup-pack method** is the technique of freezing fruit in sugar water. Make a syrup by dissolving sugar in water. Pack fruit in freezer-safe containers and cover it with the chilled syrup. Keep the fruit under the syrup with a small piece of crumpled wax paper on top of the fruit.

Tray-Pack Method The **tray-pack method** is the technique of freezing fruit whole on a tray. This method works well with blackberries, blueberries, cranberries, and other small fruits. Place the fruit on a tray or baking sheet, leaving space between pieces. Cover tightly with aluminum foil and freeze just until frozen. Then pack the pieces into freezer-safe containers.

Dry-pack method The **dry-pack method** is the technique of freezing fruit directly in freezer continers. This method works best for small whole fruits.

Freezing Vegetables

All vegetables except tomatoes require **blanching**, or brief cooking in boiling water, before freezing. Blanching neutralizes enzymes. To blanch vegetables, use 1 gallon of boiling water in a large pot for 1 pound of vegetables. Place the prepared vegetables in a large strainer and immerse them in the water. A blanching chart shows how long to blanch different vegetables. Another clue that vegetables are done is their color. Look for an intensified color change.

When the time is up, remove the vegetables and plunge them into a large pot of ice water until cool. Add ice cubes as needed to keep the water ice-cold. Drain the vegetables on clean, dry towels. Pat them dry to prevent ice crystals from forming as they freeze. Pack them into freezer-safe containers.

Do not use a microwave oven for blanching. Microwaves do not cook evenly, so they do not blanch evenly.

Packing and Freezing

When you pack foods in containers to freeze, leave 1 inch of headspace between the food and the lid of the container. **Headspace** is room left in a container for food to expand. If you are freezing food in plastic bags, squeeze out as much air as possible before sealing. Wipe containers clean and label them with the date, contents, and amount.

Freeze foods as soon as they are packed. Arrange containers in a single layer with plenty of space between them. This promotes air circulation and rapid, even freezing. Do not place food in the freezer door, because the door is warmer than the rest of the compartment.

Canning Fruits and Vegetables

Canning is the process of cooking and preserving food in glass jars. You need to follow specific instructions and use special equipment to can food safely. The time, effort, and expense are worth the result.

Jars and Lids

Canning jars are strong, reusable glass jars with a flat rim and a threaded neck that creates an airtight seal with the lid. The airtight seal prevents harmful microorganisms from getting into the jar. Jars from mayonnaise, peanut butter, and other commercial products do not work for canning, because they lack these features. Only use canning jars in perfect condition. Inspect the jar's rim for chips or nicks. Discard any jars with tiny cracks that could fracture when heated.

Canning lids have two metal pieces, a top and a screw band. The flat top is rimmed with a rubber compound that molds to the jar. The screw band holds the top in place. **Figure 19.5** shows what these parts look like. Bands can be reused as long as they remain in good condition, but tops are used only once. Do not use older, porcelain-lined lids or one-piece lids with separate rubber rings.

Just before canning, wash the jars and lids in hot, sudsy water or in the dishwasher. Rinse the jars well. Keep them immersed in clean, hot water until you are ready to use them.

Packing Methods

Pack food into jars with either the raw-pack method or the hot-pack method.

Raw-Pack Method The **raw-pack method** is the technique of canning raw foods. Put the prepared raw food into the jars. Pour in a hot liquid, such as syrup, water, or juice. Raw packing helps delicate foods retain their shape and texture.

Hot-Pack Method The **hot-pack method** is the technique of canning simmered foods. Simmer the food briefly, then place it and some of the liquid into the jars. Light cooking "preshrinks" foods. They fit together more closely, leaving less air in the jar. This increases the vacuum effect.

When you pack jars, leave about ½ to 1 inch of headspace for the food to expand. Run a spatula between the food and the jar to remove any air bubbles. Wipe the jar top clean. Apply the lid and screw on the band until just tight. A lid that's too tight might not allow air to escape during processing.

Some microorganisms may survive the heat of blanching and packing. It is very important to boil the jars after canning, as described in the next section.

Processing Methods

For home canning, foods are divided into two classes—high acid and low acid. Each type is processed differently.

Boiling-Water Bath High-acid foods, including most fruits, can be processed in a boiling-water bath. A **boiling-water bath** is a large, deep kettle with a tight-fitting lid. The jars are covered with boiling water and processed for a specified length of time. A removable, divided rack separates and holds the jars off the bottom of the kettle, allowing water to circulate around all sides of the jars.

Pressure Canning Low-acid foods, including tomatoes and other vegetables, need pressure canning. **Pressure canning** is canning using a pressure canner, which is like a large pressure cooker. Jars of food are processed in steam under pressure. Pressure canning raises the temperature above the boiling point of water to kill the deadly botulinum bacteria, which can survive the heat of boiling.

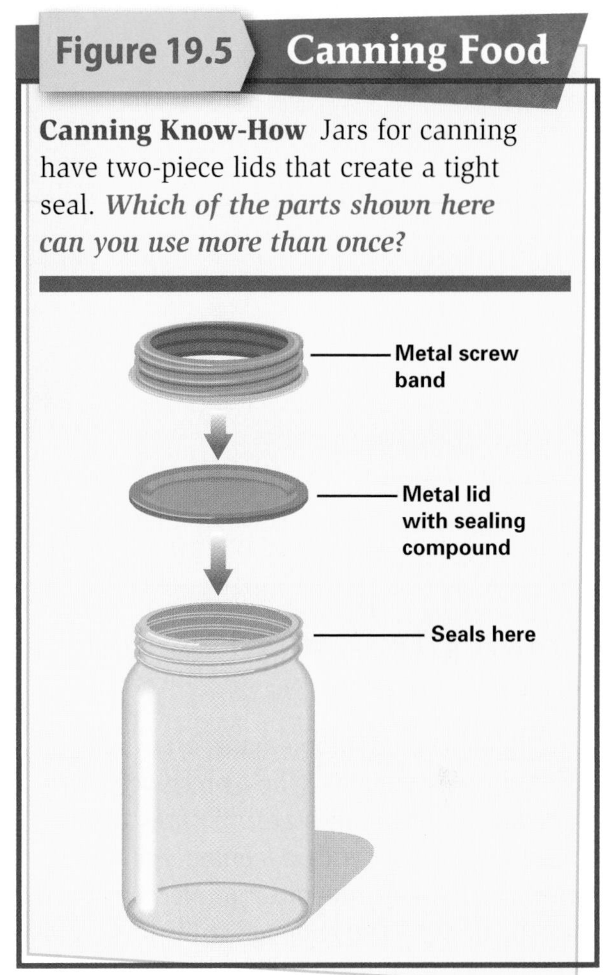

Canning Know-How Jars for canning have two-piece lids that create a tight seal. ***Which of the parts shown here can you use more than once?***

Read the manufacturer's directions carefully before using a canner. Have the gauge on the pressure canner checked every year to make sure it is accurate.

After processing, place the jars on a rack or clean dish towel away from drafts until completely cool, usually 12 hours or longer. During this time, the lids should "pop." This sound indicates that the jar and lid have formed the perfect seal needed to prevent spoilage. To make sure, press down on the center of the lid. It should stay down when released because of the vacuum inside.

Jars that do not seal properly in the pressure canner can be reprocessed within 24 hours using a new lid. Food quality will suffer, however. You may want to remove the food from the can and refrigerate or freeze it.

To allow flavors to develop, you should store home-canned foods in a clean, cool, dry area for at least two weeks before using. Remove or loosen the screw bands to prevent them from rusting. A rusted band can cause a faulty seal.

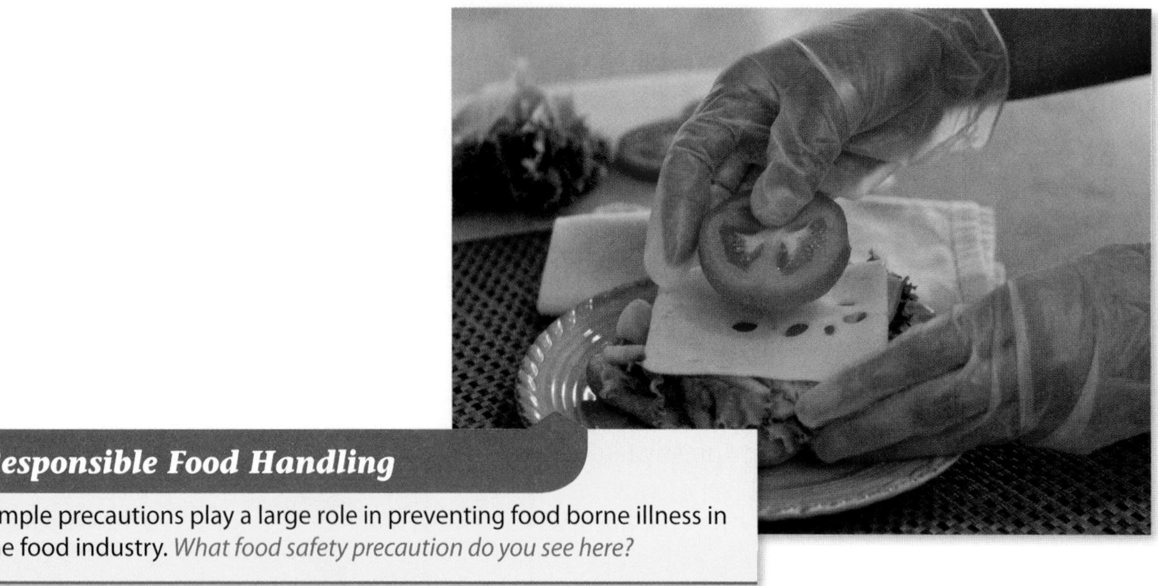

Responsible Food Handling

Simple precautions play a large role in preventing food borne illness in the food industry. *What food safety precaution do you see here?*

Canning Fruit and Vegetable Spreads

You can also can homemade fruit and vegetable spreads, such as jellies, preserves, jams, and fruit butters. Jellies are mixtures of juice and sugar, firmed with a gelling agent. Preserves are whole fruits or large pieces cooked with sugar. Jams use chopped fruits or vegetables. Butters are puréed fruit pulp cooked with sugar and spices until smooth and creamy.

Cook jellies, preserves, jams, and fruit butters in a large, wide pot with a flat bottom so the mixture has room to boil and foam without bubbling over. Prepare small batches so the food cooks quickly. Process the mixture in a boiling-water bath.

There are thousands of recipes for tasty fruit and vegetable spreads, including many that are low in added sugar.

Pickling Food

Pickling means packing food in a mixture of pickling salt, vinegar, water, and spices. Pickling turns cabbage into sauerkraut or kimchi and cucumbers into pickles. You can also pickle mixed vegetables and beans and sweetened combinations of chopped fruits, vegetables, or both. Hard-cooked pickled eggs are a regional favorite. Pickled fruits are simmered in a spicy, sweet-sour syrup that complements naturally tart foods, including crabapples and watermelon rind.

The vinegar in pickling liquid is high in acid, so all pickled recipes can be processed in a boiling-water bath.

Drying Food

Drying, or dehydration, preserves food by depriving microorganisms of the moisture they need for survival. This method is the oldest type of preservation, yet it requires special equipment. Food must dry slowly and evenly, retaining enough water to be edible but not enough water to breed microorganisms.

The most convenient, reliable way to dry food is to use a food dehydrator. A food dehydrator dries foods safely through a balance of moderate temperatures, low humidity, and good air circulation. Most dehydrators have a 24-hour timer and an adjustable thermostat to dry each food in the proper time and at the proper temperature.

Food can also be dried in an oven set to 140°. A convection oven works better, since the temperature can be kept even and air can circulate, drying the food. If the temperature gets over 140°, the food will cook, rather than dry. Another concern is the cost of running the oven for the eight hours it takes to dry most foods.

Almost any kind of food can be dried. Apples, berries, peaches, and pears are delicious dried. Peppers, peas, corn, onions, and green beans also dry well. Treat fruits with ascorbic acid before drying, and blanch vegetables before drying them.

The owner's manual for your dehydrator should give recommendations for drying different foods.

Store home-dried produce just as you would store dried store-bought produce: in glass jars or sturdy plastic containers or bags. Choose containers that close securely to keep out moisture.

Using Home-Preserved Foods

Dried foods make nutritious snacks and are great for dipping. You can add dried foods to soups or soften them in warm water. The warm water causes dried foods to **rehydrate**, or absorb water and become soft again. For example, you can soften dried blueberries by soaking them in warm water before adding them to muffin or pancake batter.

Properly frozen fruits and vegetables keep their quality for 12 to 18 months. Thawed frozen fruits and vegetables tend to have a softer, mushier texture than fresh fruits and vegetables. This is less noticeable if you cook frozen foods in recipes. Try serving frozen fruits when they are still slightly frozen. Except for corn on the cob, which should be partially thawed, vegetables can be cooked frozen without thawing.

Before using canned foods, examine jars carefully. Bulging lids and liquids trickling from under the lid are signs of spoilage. Examine jars when you open them, too. Check for mold, unusually soft food, or cloudy, bubbling, or spurting liquid. Discard the food without tasting it.

Never taste canned low-acid foods cold. Canned foods containing botulinum bacteria often look and smell normal, but even a teaspoon can be fatal. Boil low-acid foods for 10 to 15 minutes before tasting them. Use a conventional cooktop only. A microwave oven heats too unevenly to kill all the microorganisms.

✓ **Reading Check** **Identify** What is the oldest method of food preservation?

Safeguarding the Food Supply

Just as you work to keep your own food supply safe, the government works to keep the nation's food supply safe. Several government agencies work to help ensure that foods are handled properly from farm to marketplace. Each agency has responsibilities, such as examining ingredients, testing new processing technologies, and preventing contamination.

Food and Drug Administration

The Food and Drug Administration (FDA) is the division of the Department of Health and Human Services that oversees the overall safety of the food supply. The FDA has an impact on every food and beverage you buy.

Food Additives

The FDA examines food additives such as preservatives and dyes to see whether they are safe. After conducting public hearings and reviewing test results, the FDA determines how the additive may be used and in what amount. It also decides how the ingredient should be listed on the food label, like the one shown in **Figure 19.6.**

Figure 19.6 **Extra Ingredients**

Know Your Additives Some food additives improve quality and lengthen shelf life. ***What ingredient in this bread is likely to be an additive?***

INGREDIENTS: ENRICHED FLOUR (NIACIN, REDUCED IRON, THIAMINE MONONITRATE, RIBOFLAVIN), WATER, HIGH FRUCTOSE CORN SYRUP. CONTAINS 2% OR LESS OF WHEY, SOYBEAN OIL, YEAST, SALT, CULTURED WHEY, SOY FLOUR, DOUGH CONDITIONERS (SODIUM STEAROYL LACTYLATE, AMMONIUM SULFATE, CALCIUM SULFATE, CALCIUM PEROXIDE, AND/OR ASCORBIC ACID, PROTEASE), MONOCALCIUM PHOSPHATE.

Be a *Smart Consumer*

Protecting the Food Supply

All companies that process, package, or sell food in the United States are required to register with the FDA. This helps health officials track sources of tainted food in case of an outbreak of foodborne illness. The rule applies to makers and distributors of fresh and processed items, even chewing gum and animal foods, whether they are located in the United States or overseas. A few types of businesses, including farms, restaurants, and supermarkets, are excluded. Meat, egg, and poultry producers, which are regulated by the USDA, are also exempt.

Challenge With your teacher's permission, use the FDA's Web site to learn about food-related recalls, market withdrawals, and safety alerts for the last 60 days. What foods are mentioned? Why? Where did they come from?

The FDA classifies additives with a long history of safe use as "Generally Recognized as Safe" (GRAS). Items on the **GRAS list**, or safe list, range from sugar to seaweed and can be used by food processors for specific uses without further testing.

No additive is approved permanently. If new evidence shows that an additive might be unsafe, the FDA may require retesting and may tell manufacturers to stop using it.

Fat Replacers

The FDA also oversees the use of "fat replacers" found in many fat-free and reduced-fat processed foods. Fat replacers mimic the smoothness and creaminess of fat, without the calories. They are made from carbohydrates, proteins, fats, or a combination of these.

Carbohydrate-based fat replacers include modified food starch, cellulose, dextrin, and guar gum, which thicken foods. These ingredients are common in fat-free salad dressings.

Fat replacers based on carbohydrates cannot survive much heat, so they do not work well in fried foods.

Protein-based fat replacers are made from egg whites and fat-free milk. They are often used in frozen and refrigerated products. Low-fat cheese, ice cream, baked products, and cream soups contain protein-based fat replacers. Fat replacers based on protein cannot survive much heat, so they also do not work well in fried foods.

Fat-based fat replacers are made from chemically altered fats. They are stable in heat and very versatile, making them suitable for baked foods, cake mixes, frostings, dairy foods, and some fried foods. Olestra (ō-ˈles-trə) is a fat-based replacer that passes through the body without being absorbed. Foods made with olestra are fortified with vitamins A, D, E, and K to boost the absorption of fat-soluble vitamins. Olestra causes mild digestive problems for some people. Salatrim is another fat-based replacer found in baked goods, dairy products, and sweet products.

Most fat replacers have fewer calories per gram than fat, but some fat-free and low-fat foods are still high in calories. Check the Nutrition Facts panel for the fat, sugar, and calories per serving.

Hazard Analysis and Critical Control Point

Some outbreaks of foodborne illness have been traced to contamination during processing. To avoid contamination, the FDA requires some processors to use a system called Hazard Analysis and Critical Control Point (HACCP, pronounced "hassip"). HACCP is an individualized plan or set of procedures that predicts and prevents threats to food safety during food processing and service. For example, meat can become contaminated while it is being handled to make packaged sandwiches. A delicatessen that makes sandwiches might have a HACCP plan that requires specific safety procedures to prevent contamination. Workers might be required to wear sanitary gloves and change them whenever they need to handle money. A set of procedures might be followed each time sandwich meat is moved from the refrigerator to the counter. Still another set of rules might be set each time food is received at the delicatessen.

International food agencies and manufacturers around the world follow HACCP. Manufacturers that use HACCP keep records to show whether the program is working. Public health agencies usually evaluate food service and business compliance with HACCP procedures.

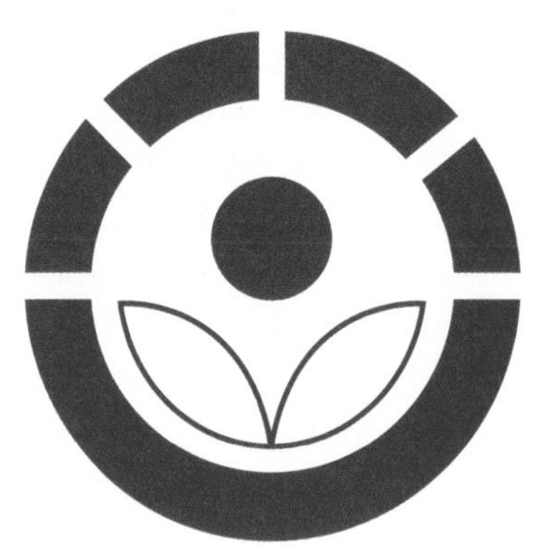

Radura Symbol

The radura symbol is used around the world to show that a food has been irradiated. *What kinds of foods may be irradiated?*

Irradiation

The FDA also judges the safety of food processing methods, including new and sometimes controversial methods such as irradiation. **Irradiation** is the process of exposing food to high-intensity energy waves to increase shelf life and kill harmful microorganisms. Irradiation does not make foods radioactive. Like other processing methods, irradiation can slightly affect flavor, texture, and vitamin levels.

The FDA first approved the use of irradiation for spices and wheat flour in 1963. The process proved successful, with no known negative health effects. The FDA gradually extended approval for irradiation to produce, poultry, pork, beef, and seafood. Irradiated foods must be identified with the radura symbol.

Some people support irradiation because it can reduce cases of foodborne illness and control pests without poisons. Other people oppose irradiation because they worry that the radioactive elements used in irradiation plants may create harmful byproducts.

Recalls

What happens if a manufacturer or the FDA learns that a food is unsafe? Usually, a food maker issues a **recall**, the immediate removal of a product from store shelves. The brand name and package code numbers are publicized in the media. Consumers who have purchased the food are urged to return it to the store for a refund. If the company does not voluntarily recall an item, the FDA may take legal action.

Environmental Protection Agency

The Environmental Protection Agency (EPA) is an agency of the federal government that helps to protect the environment. It helps to monitor the impact of food production on land, air, and water.

The EPA also regulates the use of pesticides. Just as the FDA regulates which additives can be used in foods, the EPA also decides when, how, and in what amounts pesticides can be used in growing food.

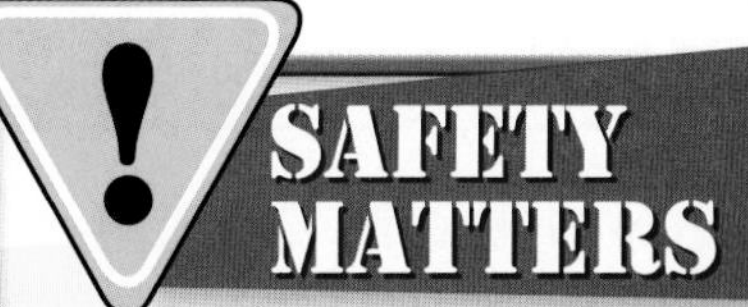

Predict, Prevent, Protect

There are seven principles of HACCP. These seven principles require food manufacturers to predict what may go wrong during food processing. They encourage food manufacturers to identify ways to prevent potentially dangerous errors. And they ask food manufacturers to think of specific ways to protect the food from hazards in the event that something does go wrong. Each of the seven principles of HACCP promotes prediction, prevention, and protection in a different way. For example, the fifth principle asks food manufacturers to establish "corrective actions"—or brainstorm steps to take in order to correct a mistake or accident that occurs during food processing.

What Would You Do? What corrective actions would you take if you broke a dish or glass while working in the foods lab? How would you prevent this from happening in the future? Develop your own specific HACCP plan of procedures.

The EPA and other government agencies regularly test levels of chemical residues on food. Residues are substances left in food as byproducts of processing or agriculture. For example, the EPA monitors the amount of pesticides in grains, produce, and animal feed. Pesticides in animal feed can build up in animals' tissues, harming them and the people who eat them.

A build-up of pesticides and other chemical residues can lead to serious health problems in people and other inhabitants of an ecosystem. For every pesticide, the EPA establishes a **tolerance**, or a maximum safe level in food. If a pesticide is found above tolerance levels, it may be banned or restricted.

Food Safety and Inspection Service The Food Safety and Inspection Service (FSIS) is the branch of the United States Department of Agriculture (USDA) responsible for the wholesomeness of meat, poultry, and eggs. FSIS inspectors check the sanitation of packing plants and storage facilities. They test food products for residues of hormones, antibiotics, and other drugs used in raising animals. They keep diseased animals out of the food supply. FSIS officials work with foreign governments to ensure that imported animal products meet U.S. safety standards. Like the FDA, the FSIS can request a recall if it believes that a meat, poultry, or egg product poses a health risk.

Centers for Disease Control and Prevention The Centers for Disease Control and Prevention (CDC) is the lead federal agency for protecting the health and safety of people. Foodborne and waterborne diseases are one concern of the CDC's National Center for Infectious Diseases (NCID). The NCID works with governmental and nongovernmental organizations at the federal, state, and local level to monitor foodborne and waterborne diseases, to train people to identify them, to research causes of these diseases, and to promote prevention and control.

Light and Healthy Recipe

No-Bake Oatmeal Raisin Cookies

Ingredients

- **1 cup** Sugar
- **4 oz.** Butter
- **½ cups** Low-fat milk
- **1 cup** Oats
- **½ cups** Raisins
- **½ cups** Chocolate chips

Yield 12 servings (two cookies per serving)

These cookies provide enough fiber and protein to make a good snack without driving your calorie count up.

Directions

1. Put the sugar, butter and milk in a pot and bring to a boil, stirring constantly. Allow the mixture to cook for five minutes.
2. Turn off the heat and add the oats and raisins and mix them in.
3. Add the chocolate chips and mix again.
4. Drop tablespoonfuls of the mixture onto wax paper. They will stiffen as they cool. Refrigerate uneaten cookies.

Nutrition Analysis per Serving

■ Calories	186
■ Total fat	7 g
Saturated fat	4 g
Cholesterol	11 mg
■ Sodium	5 mg
■ Carbohydrate	31g
Dietary fiber	1 g
Sugars	25 g
■ Protein	2 g

CHAPTER 19 Review & Applications

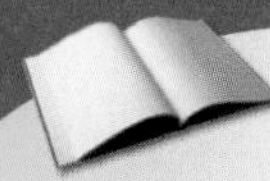

After You Read

Chapter Summary

Proper food safety and storage prevents foodborne illness. Practicing personal hygiene, maintaining kitchen cleanliness routines, cleaning up properly, and avoiding cross-contamination are all ways to keep a clean kitchen and ensure food safety. Cook, thaw, and serve food properly and at the right temperature. Store food correctly and prevent spoilage. Preserve food safely by freezing, canning, pickling, or drying. Government organizations inspect food, prevent diseases, and safeguard the food production process.

Content and Academic Vocabulary Review

1. Create multiple-choice test questions for each of these content and academic vocabulary terms.

Content Vocabulary

- contaminant (p. 280)
- foodborne illness (p. 280)
- microorganism (p. 280)
- toxin (p. 280)
- spore (p. 280)
- food safety (p. 280)
- sanitation (p. 281)
- personal hygiene (p. 281)
- 20-second scrub (p. 281)
- cross-contamination (p. 283)
- internal temperature (p. 284)
- rancidity (p. 287)
- freezer burn (p. 287)
- preserve (p. 291)
- sugar-pack method (p. 292)
- syrup-pack method (p. 292)
- tray-pack method (p. 292)
- dry-pack method (p. 292)
- blanching (p. 292)
- headspace (p. 292)
- raw-pack method (p. 293)
- hot-pack method (p. 293)
- boiling-water bath (p. 293)
- pressure canning (p. 293)
- rehydrate (p. 295)
- GRAS list (p. 296)
- irradiation (p. 297)
- recall (p. 297)
- tolerance (p. 298)

Academic Vocabulary

- tolerate (p. 280)
- reserve (p. 283)

Review Key Concepts

2. **Identify** the causes of foodborne illness.
3. **Explain** the importance of cleanliness in the kitchen.
4. **Summarize** ways to cook food safely.
5. **Describe** safe food storage practices.
6. **Summarize** methods for safely preserving food at home.

Critical Thinking

7. **Explain** the pros and cons of irradiation.
8. **Conclude** whether a sandwich maker is practicing food safety if he touches cooked chicken, his face, and cutting boards with gloved hands.
9. **Explain** whether Mona should throw away all of the food in her full freezer and refrigerator. Upon returning from a trip, she learns her power was out for 46 hours.
10. **Describe** how income, time, and the size of a family might affect which methods are used to preserve foods.

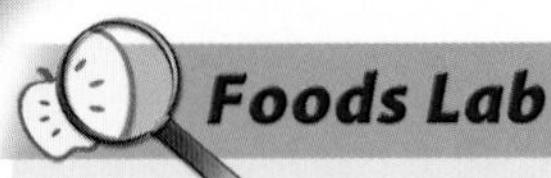

Foods Lab

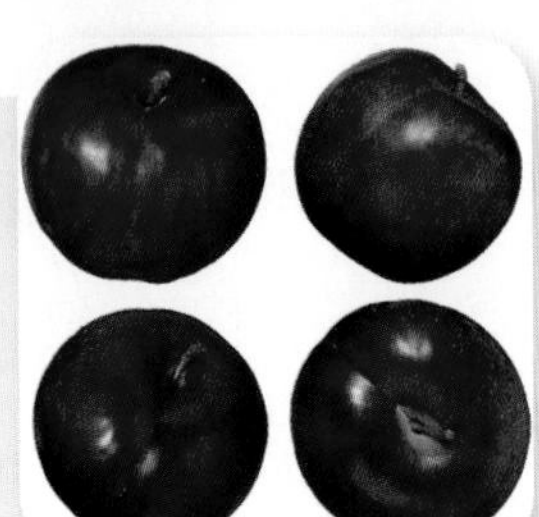

11. Dehydrating Foods Drying is the oldest method of food preservation. Food dehydrators balance temperature, humidity, and air to dry foods safely. Different foods, however, are dehydrated in different ways.

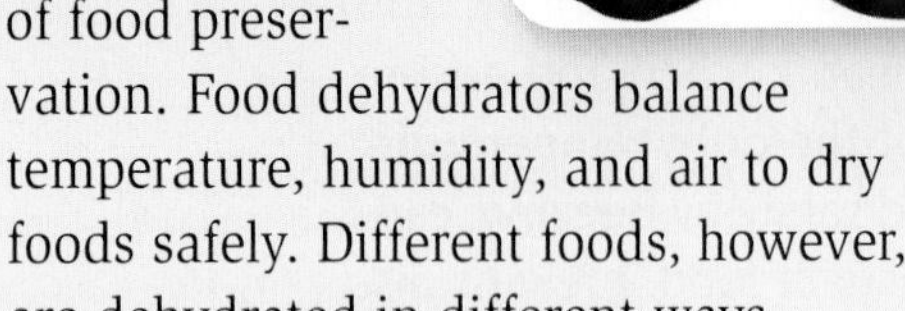

Procedure Use a dehydrator to dry two different fruits. Consult the dehydrator manual for recommendations for drying different fruits. Contrast the methods and evaluate the results.

Analysis Write answers to these questions: How did you prepare the two fruits for dehydration? Why was each preparation needed? Which of the foods gave better results?

HEALTHFUL CHOICES

12. Thawing Methods To prepare for tomorrow's barbecue, Mike wants to defrost several frozen steaks. He wants to defrost them on the kitchen counter to ensure they will be ready for grilling. His wife wants to defrost them in the refrigerator. Who is correct? Why is it important they begin defrosting the steaks tonight?

TECH Connection

13. Preserving History Under your teacher's supervision, use the Internet to research the history of either canning or freezing foods. How did these methods begin? What challenges did the pioneers of these processes encounter? What improvements has technology brought to this process? Use comptuer software to create a slide show that depicts your findings, and share it with the class.

Real-World Skills

Problem-Solving Skills	**14. Mystery Foods** The Ling family has a freezer stocked with carefully wrapped food. Unfortunately, they have forgotten which foods most of the packages contain. What can they do to prevent this in the future?
Interpersonal and Collaborative Skills	**15. Demonstrations** Follow your teacher's instructions to form a small group. In the food lab, work with your group to demonstrate one of these topics: cross-contamination prevention; personal hygiene when handling food; proper dishwashing procedure; serving food safely; defrosting techniques; action during a power failure. Enact your demonstration in front of the class, and have the class identify which topic you are demonstrating.
Financial Literacy Skills	**16. Calculate Savings** The Swansons have peach trees in their yard. They consume 30 jars of jam a year. A jar of peach jam costs $4 at the market. A pressure canner costs $75. Empty canning jars cost $1 each. Is it cheaper for the Swansons to can their own peach jam or to buy 30 jars of it from the market each year?

Academic Skills

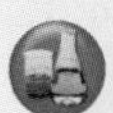

Food Science

17. Food Contaminants Mold spores are everywhere, and given the right conditions, can grow into fungal colonies.

Procedure Cut two bread slices in half. Label four plastic sandwich bags: dry, water, lemon juice, and simple syrup (equal parts sugar and water). Put one of the bread pieces into the "dry" bag. Put 8–9 drops of water on the next bread piece, and repeat with the lemon juice and the syrup. Seal up all 4 bags, and put in a dark warm place. Check the bread daily over the next 12 days. Record the results.

Analysis Create a bar graph with percentages of mold on bread on the y axis, and the labels from the bags as the x axis. Which showed the most growth and which the least?

NSES B Develop an understanding of the structures and properties of matter.

Mathematics

18. Choosing Containers Ramona knows that she will be very busy at work next week and won't have time to do a lot of cooking. She would like to make a big pot of soup this week and freeze it to eat next week. Ramona has several cylindrical, resealable, freezer-proof containers that measure 6 inches wide and 4.1 inches tall. If she makes 6 quarts (346.5 cubic inches) of soup, how many containers will she need?

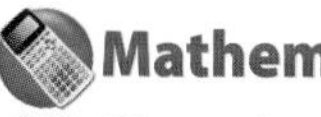

Cylindrical Volume A cylinder is a solid with circular parallel bases. Calculate the volume (V) of a cylinder as $V = \pi r^2 h$, where r is the radius of the circular base, and h is the cylinder's height.

Starting Hint The container's radius is half of its diameter (width). Remember to subtract 1 in. from the height to allow for a proper headspace. Use 3.14 for π.

NCTM Geometry Use visualization, spatial reasoning, and geometric modeling to solve problems.

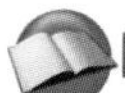

English Language Arts

19. Public Service Announcement Develop, write, and record a 30-second public service announcement about food safety. Your announcement should capture listeners' attention and inform them about one important aspect of food safety. Air it on the school's public address system.

NCTE 12 Use language to accomplish individual purposes.

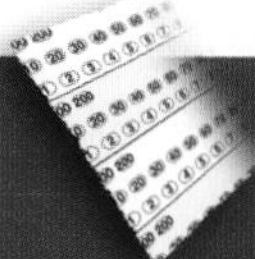

STANDARDIZED TEST PRACTICE

MULTIPLE CHOICE

Read the question and select the best answer.

20. Which government organization oversees the overall safety of the food supply?

a. The senate
b. The FDA
c. The HACCP
d. The USFA

Test-Taking Tip Multiple-choice questions may prompt you to select the "best" answer. They may present you with answers that seem partially true. The best answer is the one that is completely true, and can be supported by information you have read in the text.

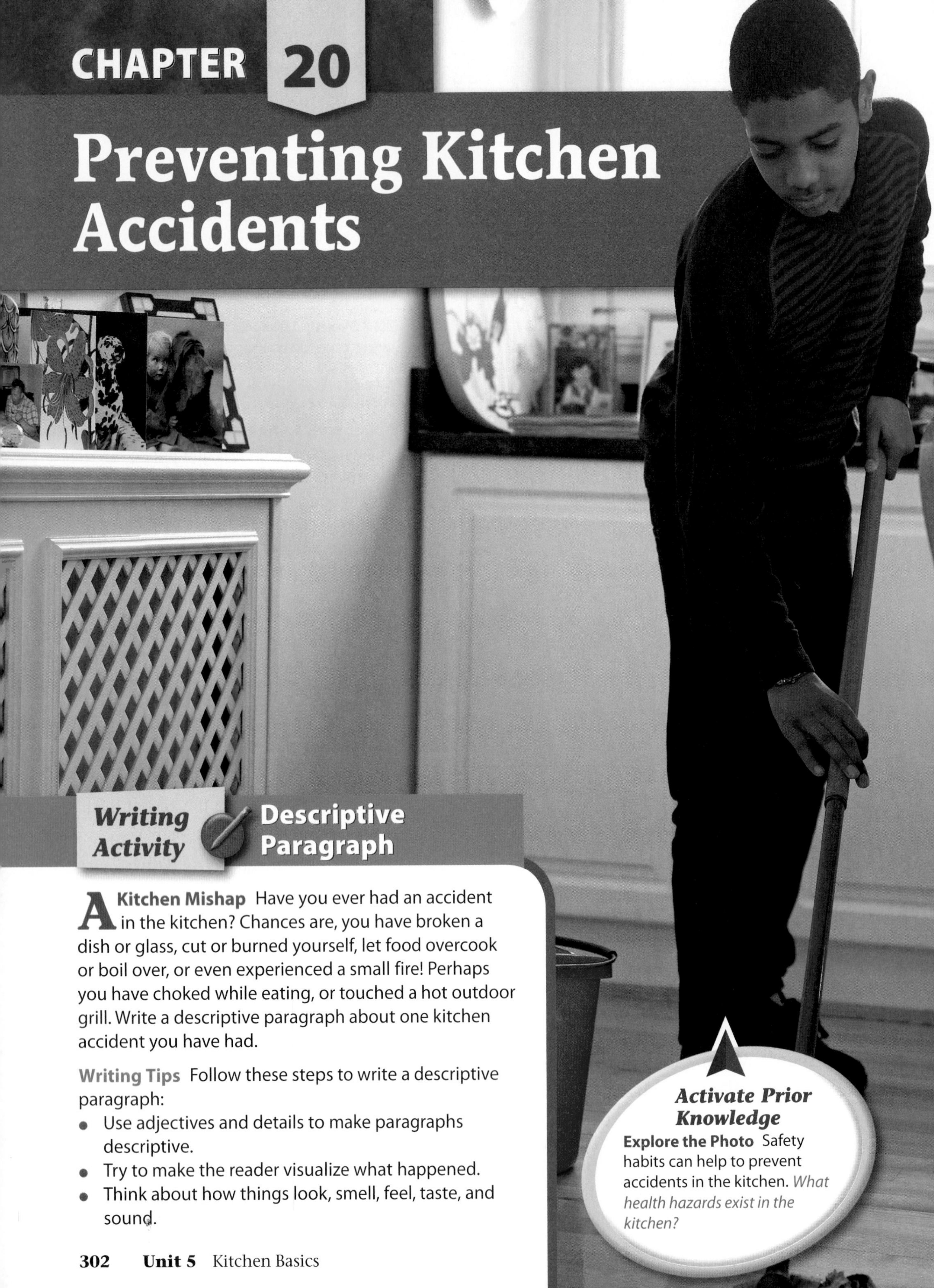

CHAPTER 20
Preventing Kitchen Accidents

Writing Activity: Descriptive Paragraph

A Kitchen Mishap Have you ever had an accident in the kitchen? Chances are, you have broken a dish or glass, cut or burned yourself, let food overcook or boil over, or even experienced a small fire! Perhaps you have choked while eating, or touched a hot outdoor grill. Write a descriptive paragraph about one kitchen accident you have had.

Writing Tips Follow these steps to write a descriptive paragraph:

- Use adjectives and details to make paragraphs descriptive.
- Try to make the reader visualize what happened.
- Think about how things look, smell, feel, taste, and sound.

Activate Prior Knowledge

Explore the Photo Safety habits can help to prevent accidents in the kitchen. *What health hazards exist in the kitchen?*

Reading Guide

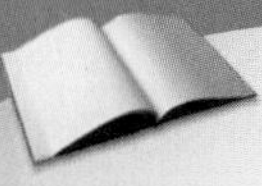

Before You Read

Preview Make a list of three kitchen safety hazards. Write a way to prevent each hazard. As you read, see if your suggestions for prevention are correct.

Read to Learn

Key Concepts

- **List** six ways to prevent accidents in the kitchen.
- **Explain** why keeping a kitchen clean can prevent a kitchen fire.
- **List** five things to remember when using household chemicals.
- **Explain** why it is important to follow safety guidelines when cooking outdoors.
- **Summarize** five precautions to make kitchens safe for children.
- **Describe** two first aid procedures you should know to prepare you to respond to kitchen emergencies.

Main Idea

Good safety habits can prevent accidents and protect you against a variety of hazards in the kitchen.

Content Vocabulary

You will find definitions for these words in the glossary at the back of this book.

- polarized plug
- carbon monoxide
- Heimlich maneuver
- cardiopulmonary resuscitation (CPR)

Academic Vocabulary

You will find these words in your reading and on your tests. Use the glossary to look up their definitions if necessary.

- inspect
- vulnerable

Graphic Organizer

Use a graphic organizer like the one below to note six ways to prevent accidents in the kitchen.

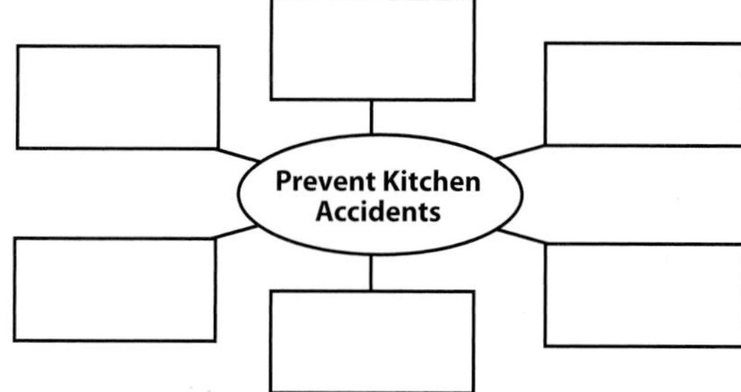

Graphic Organizer Go to this book's Online Learning Center at **glencoe.com** to print out this graphic organizer.

Academic Standards

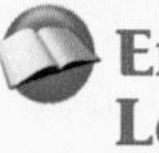

English Language Arts

NCTE 5 Use different writing process elements to communicate effectively.

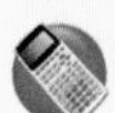

Mathematics

NCTM Data Analysis and Probability Formulate questions that can be addressed with data and collect, organize, and display relevant data to answer them.

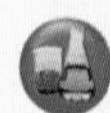

Science

NSES B Develop an understanding of interactions of energy and matter.

NSES C Develop an understanding of chemical reactions.

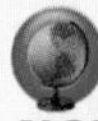

Social Studies

NCSS VIII A Make judgments about how science and technology have transformed the physical world and human society.

NCTE *National Council of Teachers of English*
NCTM *National Council of Teachers of Mathematics*
NSES *National Science Education Standards*
NCSS *National Council for the Social Studies*

Kitchen Safety Basics

Kitchens are full of hazards that can cause accidents: slippery surfaces, sharp edges, electrical appliances, heat and flame, and household chemicals, to name a few. These six safety habits can help protect you against these hazards.

- Focus on what you are doing, especially when cutting, cooking, or using appliances.
- Dress for safety. Wear short or snug sleeves and tie back long hair and apron strings. This prevents loose items from tangling in appliances or catching fire.
- Use all tools and equipment safely and use the right tool for the job. For example, use a can opener to open a can—never pry it open with a knife.
- Close drawers and doors completely to avoid bumps, bruises, and cuts.
- Store large pots and other heavy or bulky items that could fall on low shelves, within easy reach.
- Control clutter. Put items back where they belong as soon as you finish using them.

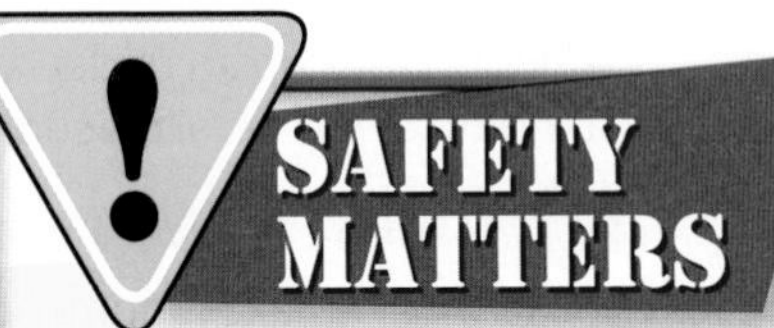

Dull, But Dangerous

Imagine you are teaching a group of young students how to safely cut vegetables. To keep them from cutting themselves, would you provide them with dull knives? Actually, a dull knife is more dangerous than a sharp knife. Why? You have to use more force to cut with a dull knife, which makes it more likely to slip. A dull knife applied to the skin with great force can do harm. A sharp blade, in contrast, cuts with less effort, and is less likely to slip. Keep knives sharp by using a sharpening stone or by having them professionally sharpened. A sharpening steel keeps a blade straight.

What Would You Do? In your foods lab, you notice one of your peers trying to forcefully cut a tomato with a dull knife. "Gee," she says, "this knife works slowly, but at least I won't cut myself." What would you do?

Preventing Falls

Falls are a common cause of household injuries. Prevent falls by removing hazards that could cause slips and trips. Wear snug shoes without trailing shoelaces, and choose pants or skirts that are not so long as to cause tripping.

Keep the floor clear of clutter. Wipe up spills and spatters right away. If you spray oil on baking pans, hold the pan over the sink. Otherwise, oil can create slick spots on the floor or the stovetop. Secure slippery throw rugs with tacking or tape or replace them with non-skid mats. Repair damaged or worn flooring. Use a sturdy stepstool to reach higher shelves rather than a chair, box, or stool, which may tip over.

Handling Sharp Edges

Sharp edges in the kitchen can cause serious cuts. Handle and wash knives, graters, and other sharp-edged tools carefully.

Knife Safety

Knives can cause serious cuts, so manage them with care. Store knives in a divided drawer, knife block, or knife rack so that you can pick them up by the handle, not the blade. Learn when and how to use different types of knives, so that you use the right knife for the task. Always use a cutting board when cutting.

Take extra care when cleaning knives, as well as other tools with sharp edges. Do not soak them in a sink or dishpan, where suds or other dishes can hide them from view. Dry knives by wiping them carefully, with the blade pointed away from you.

Sharp Edges

Graters, peelers, chopping tools, mixers, and can lids also have sharp edges and require caution. Keep fingers away from rough surfaces, slicing edges, and rotating beaters. Keep tools away from mixers and blenders when they are switched on. If a cake recipe says "Scrape the bowl while beating," for example, stop the mixer before using the scraper. If a sharp-edged tool starts to fall, resist the impulse to catch it. Step back and pick it up when it comes to a complete rest.

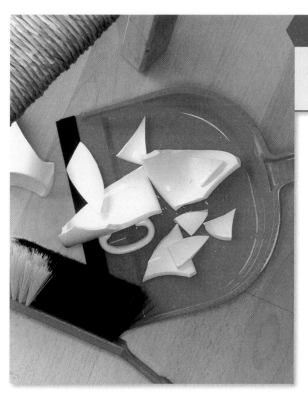

Sharp Edges

If you break a glass, carefully sweep up all the pieces using a broom, never your bare hands. *What is a safe way to pick up fine particles of broken glass?*

Broken glasses and dishes also have dangerously sharp edges. Sweep up broken items right away with a broom or a whisk broom and dustpan. If you need to pick up very small pieces by hand, use a wet paper towel instead of your bare fingers. Seal broken bits or pieces in a bag and place it in the waste-basket. Take out the trash as soon as possible.

✓ **Reading Check** **Identify** Where, besides knives, can you encounter sharp edges in the kitchen?

Preventing Fires and Burns

There are many sources of heat and flame in a kitchen, including the stovetop, range, microwave, and toaster. Help prevent fires and burns by keeping the kitchen clean. Regular, thorough cleaning prevents grease and bits of food from building up in burners, ovens, range hoods, and toasters, where they can catch fire.

Use cookware that is in good condition. A glass baking dish with a hairline crack can fracture. **Inspect**, or carefully examine, pots, pans, and dishes before each use to make sure they are safe.

Cooktop Safety

On a cooktop, pots and pans can get hotter than the food inside. Handle cookware with dry potholders or oven mitts. Wet potholders are not effective, because water carries heat. When cooking, turn the handles of pans toward the back or center of the range top so that they are less likely to be jostled and knocked over. To remove a lid from a pot or the top from a microwave container, lift the far edge first so the steam rises away from you. Steam can deliver a worse burn than hot metal or boiling water. Make sure that burners are turned off before you reach over them.

Keep flammable items such as curtains, kitchen linens, paper goods, aerosol cans, and potholders away from heat and flame. Use only heatproof utensils when cooking. Regular plastics are flammable and give off poisonous fumes when they burn.

Oven Safety

How hot is a hot oven? Water as hot as 130°F can burn your skin, yet oven temperatures of 325°F and above are common. Several strategies can help you avoid contact with the high temperatures of an oven:

- Arrange oven racks as you want them before you turn on the oven, not when the oven is already hot.
- Stand to one side when you open a hot oven. This protects you from the heat that rushes out.
- Use a sturdy potholder or oven mitt to remove a pan from a hot oven. Pull the oven rack forward a little first, then grab and lift the pan.
- Turn the oven and broiler off right after using them.
- Clean up spills and crumbs inside the oven after the oven has cooled.

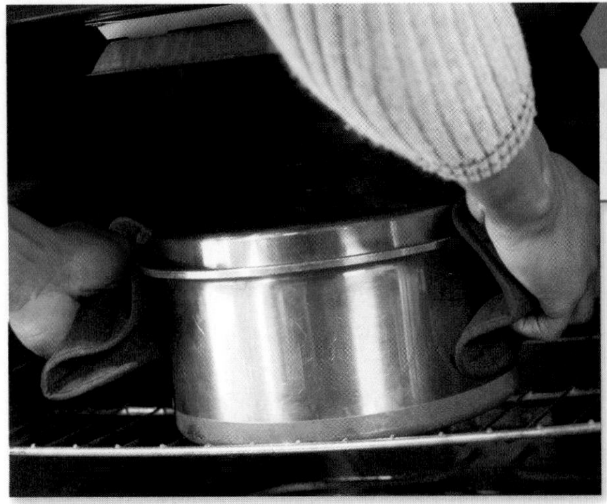

Protect Yourself

Oven mitts protect your hands and lower arms from burns when you reach into a hot oven. *What is the correct way to remove a pan from the oven?*

Gas Safety

Gas ranges carry risks from the gas as well as the heat and flame. If you smell gas, check to see whether any pilot lights have gone out. If so, light a match first; then turn on the burner and light it. If you turn on the burner first, gas will accumulate and could explode when you strike the match.

If all the pilot lights are on, turn off all range controls and open the windows for ventilation. Do not try to find the source of the gas leak yourself. Alert others and go outside immediately. Call the gas company from another location.

Science in Action **Fighting Flames**

To start and survive, a fire requires three elements: fuel, heat, and an oxidizing agent—usually oxygen. Removing any one of these elements can extinguish a fire.

Procedure Conduct research about extinguishing fires. Firefighters remove the fuel that would start wildfires through controlled burning. They remove the heat from some types of fires with water. They can remove oxygen using the aqueous foam found in fire extinguishers.

Analysis In a kitchen fire, you can smother flames with a lid, pan, salt, or baking soda. Why is this method effective?

NSES C Develop an understanding of chemical reactions.

If a Fire Starts

Catching a fire early saves lives and property. Install smoke detectors. Test them every six months and check inside for cobwebs. Learn how to use a fire extinguisher and read its label. Keep the extinguisher handy in the kitchen.

Quick action can also keep a fire from getting out of hand. If a fire starts in the kitchen:

- Do turn off the burner if the fire is on the cooktop.
- Do unplug the cord if the fire is in an electric skillet, a toaster, or another electrical appliance.
- Do turn off the heat if the fire is in the oven. Keep the oven door closed until the fire dies out.
- Do smother the fire with a lid, with another pan, or with salt or baking soda.
- Do smother flames on clothes: stop, drop, and roll.
- Do use a fire extinguisher, if you know how to do so.
- Do not use baking powder or flour on a fire, because they can explode.
- Do not use water on a kitchen fire. Water makes grease spatter, which spreads the flames and can inflict a severe burn.
- Do not carry a burning pan to the sink or outside, because you could hurt yourself and start a bigger fire when air fans the flames.

If you cannot put a fire out quickly, alert others and leave the building at once. Call the fire department from another location.

✓ **Reading Check** **Explain** Can steam burn worse than hot metal or boiling water?

Handling Electricity and Chemicals

Electrical appliances and household chemicals are big helpers in the kitchen, but they can cause burns, shocks, and other injuries. Handling cords, appliances, and chemicals carefully can prevent injuries.

Cord Safety

Check cords for damage before each use. An exposed wire could catch fire or shock you. Keep cords away from hot surfaces. Keep cords tidy so that they do not get snagged and pull an appliance down. Do not staple or nail cords in place. To disconnect an appliance, grasp the plug at the electrical outlet rather than tugging on the cord.

Limit the number of cords in an electrical outlet. An overloaded circuit can start a fire. If you need an extension cord, choose a heavy-duty cord or surge protector designed for appliances.

Newer appliances have polarized plugs. A **polarized plug** is a plug that has one blade wider than the other. Polarized plugs reduce the risk of shock if used with a polarized outlet. Do not try to fit a polarized plug into a non-polarized outlet. Buy an adapter at a hardware store or supermarket.

Appliance Safety

Read the owner's manual carefully before using any electrical appliance. Turn off small appliances as soon as you are finished with them. Never put your fingers or a kitchen tool inside an appliance that is plugged in. You may get a painful shock, and you can seriously hurt yourself if you accidentally turn on the appliance. Unplug a mixer before removing the beaters, for example.

Unplug an appliance immediately if it starts to overheat or gives a shock. Have it repaired before using it again.

Water conducts electricity, so appliances and water can be a deadly mix. Never use an electric appliance with wet hands or while standing on a wet floor. Do not run a cord around the sink. If an electric appliance falls into water or gets wet, unplug it immediately before touching it. Check the owner's manual to see how to clean an appliance. If an owner's manual recommends cleaning the appliance with a wet cloth, unplug the appliance first.

Household Chemical Safety

Many household chemicals are hazardous to your health. Cleaners, lighter fluid, drain cleaners, and pesticides can harm eyes, lungs, and skin.

Less toxic substitutes are often just as effective. Baking soda and boiling water dissolve some sink clogs. Borax sprinkled outside the door discourages ants. Diluted vinegar cleans glass.

Here are five things to remember when using household chemicals:

1. Read the label before buying. Read the instructions carefully. Material Safety Data Sheets will list all potential hazards.

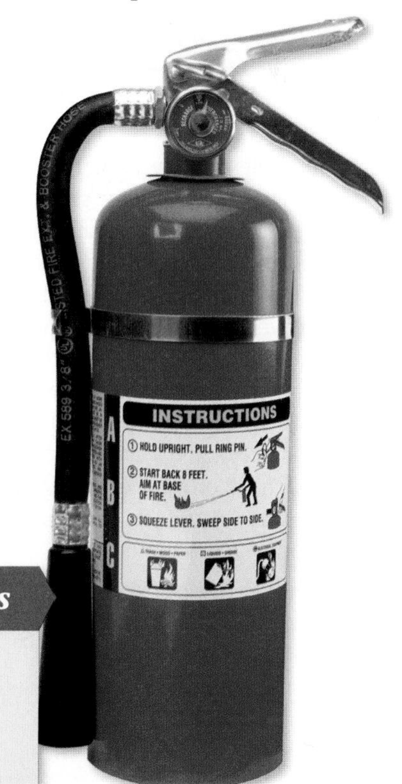

Fire Extinguishers

Letters and drawings on fire extinguishers show how to use them. This extinguisher works on ordinary combustibles like wood and paper (A), flammable liquids like grease (B), and electrical fires (C). *Why should you not use water to put out a grease fire?*

2. Keep hazardous products in their original containers so you can refer to the directions each time you use them.
3. Follow all directions for proper ventilation and protection for people and pets. Consult the label for first aid steps if someone accidentally swallows or inhales a chemical.
4. Never mix household chemicals, such as bleaches, chlorine, ammonia, toilet bowl cleaners, or rust removers. Chemicals in the mixtures may interact and release poisonous gases.
5. Make sure the nozzle is pointed away from people and pets when using a spray bottle.

Store hazardous chemicals away from food. Store flammable products, including kerosene, lighter fluid, and aerosol sprays, away from all sources of heat. In households with children, all hazardous household chemicals belong in a locked cabinet.

Never throw unused chemicals in the trash or pour them down the drain. Take them to a nearby household hazardous waste collection center.

✓ **Reading Check** **Explain** Why don't water and appliances mix?

Be a Smart Consumer

A Childproof Kitchen

Watchful adults can buy a variety of protective gadgets to help keep children safe in the kitchen. A clear plastic stove guard attaches to the edge of the cooktop, angling up and outward, to block burners from a child's reach. Rounded plastic covers fit over knobs to make them harder for small hands to grip. A two-piece freezer lock can secure refrigerators and freezers. Magnetic locks seal cabinet doors from inside and can be opened by holding a magnetic "key" to the outside of the door. None of these products, however, is a substitute for adult supervision when children are in the kitchen.

Challenge Use the Internet to find a device that prevents children from tampering with dishwashers, which may be full of sharp utensils. Write a summary of the options and costs.

Cooking Outdoors Safely

Burning coals can generate temperatures up to 1,000°F. Burning charcoal also gives off large amounts of **carbon monoxide**, an odorless, highly poisonous gas. Follow these safety guidelines to help you grill food safely:

- Start with a clean grill. Baked-on food and grease can cause flames to flare up when you light the charcoal. Clean the grill with a hard-bristle brush after each use. Wipe and wash the grate in hot, soapy water.
- Set the grill on a level, paved surface where it will not tip over. Keep the grill away from buildings, shrubs, trash containers, and anything else that could catch fire.
- Keep a fire extinguisher handy.
- Never use a charcoal grill or hibachi inside the home or garage. Carbon monoxide can build up in an enclosed area, causing drowsiness, headaches, nausea, and even death.
- If you use starter fluid or fuel, apply enough before striking the match. Adding fluid to lighted coals could trigger an explosion.
- Use fireproof gloves and heavy-duty grilling tools with long handles that let you reach food while staying a safe distance from the heat.
- Extinguish a flare-up by raising the grate off the grill, covering the grill, or spreading the coals with a long-handled tool. You can also use a pump-spray bottle filled with water to mist the flare-up. Do not pour water directly on burning charcoal, because this creates a dangerous cloud of steam.
- Let the coals burn down to ashes when you are finished grilling. Douse the ashes with water and put them in a metal trash can. Do not dump hot coals or ashes on the ground. They can burn grass and people and may even start a fire.

✓ **Reading Check** **List** List the tools and supplies you need to safely grill outdoors.

Protecting Family Members

Kitchen safety protects the entire household. However, more **vulnerable** members of the family, such as children and people with physical impairments, need extra protection. Vulnerable means susceptible to harm.

Five Precautions to Protect Children

Children can enjoy and learn from their time in the kitchen when you take a few simple precautions:

- Never leave young children alone in the kitchen, even for a few seconds.
- Protect toddlers by using safety latches on drawers and cabinet doors.
- Teach children to stay away from heat sources such as the oven, range, and toaster.
- If children want to help you work, set up a child-size table or a safe stepstool. Provide small utensils that children can handle for simple tasks, such as mixing and mashing. Do not let young children use knives or work near heat sources. Supervise them at all times.
- Model safe work habits. Teach by example.

People with Physical Challenges

Simple changes in tools and workspaces can make it easier for people with physical challenges such as limited eyesight or arthritis to use the kitchen safely. These steps can help everyone in the family stay safe in the kitchen:

- Add more or better lighting.
- Use unbreakable dishes and glassware and heatproof utensils.
- Store frequently used tools and foods in easy-to-reach places.
- Keep a magnifying glass in the kitchen for reading small print. Re-label items in larger letters with stick-on labels and a marking pen.

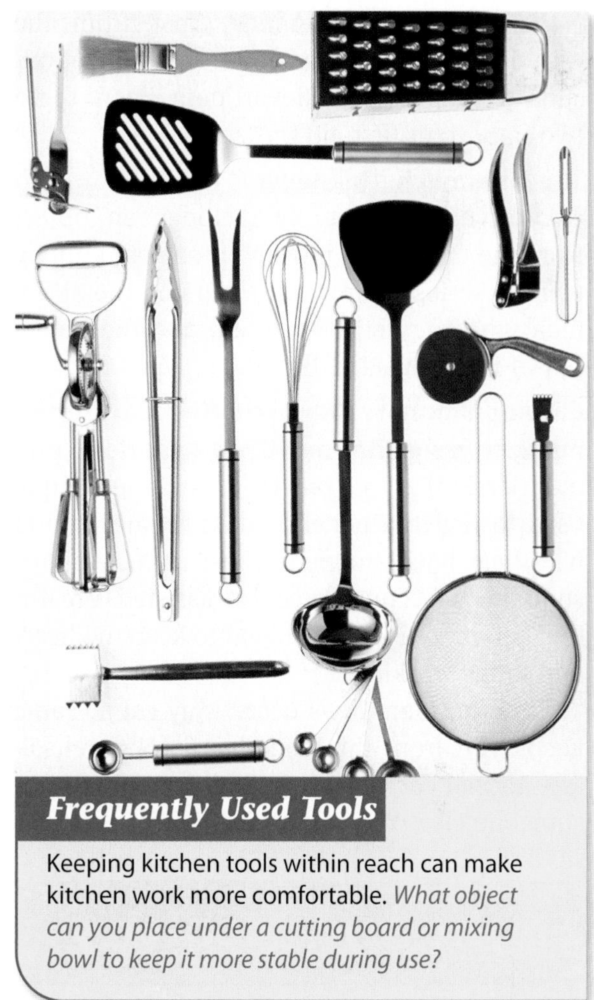

Frequently Used Tools

Keeping kitchen tools within reach can make kitchen work more comfortable. *What object can you place under a cutting board or mixing bowl to keep it more stable during use?*

- Buy round rubber jar openers for gripping appliance knobs.
- Put mixing bowls on a damp dishcloth or on a round, rubber jar opener to keep them on the countertop during mixing.

✓ **Reading Check** **Explain** Why might a magnifying glass be useful in a kitchen?

Handling Emergencies

You cannot prevent every kitchen accident—but you can be prepared. Keep emergency numbers next to the phone. Keep a well-stocked first-aid kit in a handy location. Learn to use a fire extinguisher and keep one ready in the kitchen. Have the fire extinguisher tested each year and recharged when necessary.

Take a first-aid training class from the American Red Cross or another organization, such as your local fire department. Learn these two important first-aid measures:

The Heimlich Maneuver The **Heimlich maneuver** is a way to dislodge an object from the throat of a person who is choking by using a series of upward thrusts on the abdomen with the fist to force air, and the object out of the lungs and throat.

Cardiopulmonary Resuscitation **Cardiopulmonary resuscitation (CPR)** (ˌkär-dē-ō-ˈpu̇l-mə-ˌner-ē ri-ˌsə-sə-ˈtā-shən) is a technique used to revive a person whose breathing and heartbeat have stopped. Chest compressions, sometimes accompanied by assisted breathing, get oxygen into the blood to keep the heart and lungs working.

If an accident does occur, stay calm. Panic keeps you from thinking clearly. Never hesitate to call for help, whether for yourself or someone else. You could save a life.

TECHNOLOGY FOR TOMORROW

A Silent Alarm

Your home's smoke detector can awaken you with loud beeps. But what if you're hearing impaired? Inventors in Japan have created a new smoke detector that uses food, not sound, to alert the deaf during a fire. Wasabi is a Japanese horseradish that has a strong odor and taste. When the Wasabi Smoke Detector senses smoke, it sprays potent wasabi extract into a room to alert deaf people to a fire. In tests, this silent alarm woke up 13 out of 14 people.

Investigate What other types of alarms can alert the hearing impaired to a kitchen fire?

NCSS VIII B Science, Technology and society. Make judgments about how science and technology have transformed the physical world and human society.

Light and Healthy Recipe

Grilled Vegetable Sandwich

Ingredients

- **1 Tbsp.** Olive oil
- **1 tsp.** Balsamic vinegar
- **¼ tsp.** Salt
- **⅛ tsp.** Cayenne pepper
- **1** Red bell pepper
- **1** Red onion
- **1** Zucchini
- **2** Portabella mushrooms
- **4** Rolls (kaiser, sesame or other)

Directions

1. Mix the olive oil, vinegar, salt and cayenne pepper in a small bowl.
2. Cut the bell pepper lengthwise to make four wide, flat slices. Cut the onion into four thick circles. Slice the zucchini lengthwise into four long strips, then cut the strips in half. Remove the stems from the mushrooms and slice them in half so that you have two circular pieces.
3. Place the vegetables on a tray and brush them with the marinade. Grill the vegetables on a grill or bake them on a wire rack in an oven set to 375°. Watch the vegetables closely and remove them from the heat when they are done.
4. Stack the vegetables on the bread to make the sandwich. Slice the sandwich in half and serve.

This mixture of grilled vegetables creates a hearty sandwich without added fat and cholesterol.

Yield 4 servings

Nutrition Analysis per Serving

Calories	232
Total fat	6 g
Saturated fat	1 g
Cholesterol	0 mg
Sodium	315 mg
Carbohydrate	37
Dietary fiber	3 g
Sugars	4 g
Protein	7 g

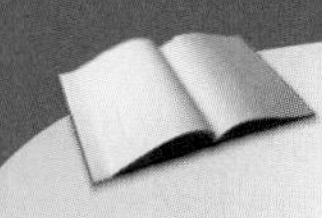

After You Read

Chapter Summary

Good safety habits protect against many kitchen hazards. Make six safety habits part of your kitchen routine. In addition, prevent falls by removing hazards, and handle sharp edges with care. Prevent fires and burns by practicing cooktop, oven, and gas safety, and take the correct steps to respond if a fire starts. Handle cords, appliances, and household chemicals properly to prevent injuries. When cooking outdoors, follow safety guidelines. Protect family members, including children and people with physical challenges, by taking precautions and providing safe and useful tools. Be prepared to handle emergencies by keeping important tools handy and learning safety measures.

Content and Academic Vocabulary Review

1. Create a fill-in-the-blank sentence for each of these content and academic vocabulary words.

Content Vocabulary

- polarized plug (p. 307)
- carbon monoxide (p. 308)
- abdominal thrusts (p. 310)
- cardiopulmonary resuscitation (CPR) (p. 310)

Academic Vocabulary

- inspect (p. 305)
- vulnerable (p. 309)

Review Key Concepts

2. **List** six ways to prevent accidents in the kitchen.
3. **Explain** why keeping a kitchen clean can prevent a kitchen fire.
4. **List** five things to remember when using household chemicals.
5. **Explain** why it is important to follow safety guidelines when cooking outdoors.
6. **Summarize** five precautions to make kitchens safe for children.
7. **Describe** two first aid procedures you should know to prepare you to respond to kitchen emergencies.

Critical Thinking

8. **Evaluate** this situation. After breaking a glass in the foods lab, Jarred quickly swept up the pieces and put them directly into the wastebasket.
9. **Explain** what the cook might have done wrong. After a severe kitchen fire, firefighters learned that it started small, but the cook's attempts to put out the fire made it worse.
10. **Examine** the safety issues illustrated by this scenario. A child stands on a chair at the kitchen counter. She uses a dull knife to cut a sandwich while her parent answers a phone call.

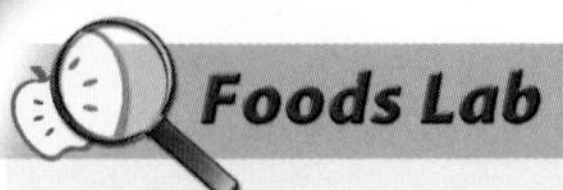

Foods Lab

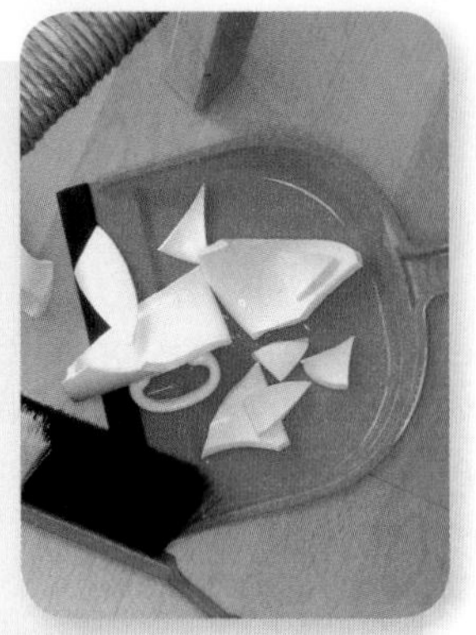

11. Safety Demonstration One way to develop good kitchen safety habits is to practice. By giving a lab demonstration of how to safely complete a kitchen task, you will be prepared to practice safety in your own kitchen.

Procedure With your lab team, demonstrate a simple kitchen task, such as chopping vegetables or heating soup, verbally pointing out the necessary safety precautions.

Analysis Analyze another team's demonstration. Take notes about the following: the correctness of their actions; the clarity of their verbal narration; their demonstration's ability to inform and educate others. Also write one question you have about the task. Share your analysis and question with the team.

HEALTHFUL CHOICES

12. Stirring Safely Eladio is sautéing an assortment of vegetables in a hot pan. He has a variety of utensils to choose from with which he can stir the vegetables. Should he choose a wooden spoon or a regular plastic spoon? Explain your reasoning. What might happen if Eladio uses the wrong utensil?

TECH Connection

13. First Aid Education Under your teacher's supervision, use the Internet to find out where people in your community or state can take a class to learn either the Heimlich maneuver or CPR. Your local Red Cross usually offers first aid classes. Then use basic word processing software to create an informative and visually interesting flyer telling where and when people can learn these safety measures. Explain in the flyer why it is valuable to know how to use these two important first aid procedures.

Real-World Skills

Problem-Solving Skills

14. Curious Child The Tamakos have a curious toddler who is constantly opening the lower cabinet doors in their kitchen. Yesterday, he pulled out a heavy pan, and his mother tripped on it. Today, he smashed his finger in a cabinet door. What can the Tamakos do?

Interpersonal and Collaborative Skills

15. Assess Safety Follow your teacher's instructions to form small groups. Work together to evaluate the safety of one aspect of your school's foods lab, such as tools, equipment, cords, accessibility to first aid, or handiness of fire extinguishers. What changes would be helpful?

Financial Literacy Skills

16. The Cost of Carelessness Research the average cost of a doctor's visit in the United States. Then research the cost of a basic knife sharpener. How much money could a person save by buying a sharpener to prevent a dangerous cut and avoid a visit to the doctor?

Academic Skills

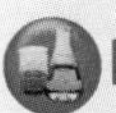

Food Science

17. Carbon Dioxide Fire Extinguishers A carbon dioxide fire extinguisher works by eliminating oxygen and replacing it with carbon dioxide. Combining baking soda (a base) with vinegar (an acid) creates carbon dioxide to put out a flame.

Procedure Under your teacher's supervision, place a small candle in a flameproof safe container. In a large glass, place a tablespoon of baking soda, then add about 2 tablespoons of white vinegar, mixing. Watch the foam until it dies down. Light the candle, and pour the contents of the glass (carbon dioxide gas) over the flame. (Don't pour out the liquid.)

Analysis Why did the flame go out? How did the carbon dioxide stay in the glass? Write a paragraph to summarize the results of the experiment.

NSES B Develop an understanding of interactions of energy and matter.

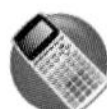

Mathematics

18. Kitchen Hazards You have read the results of a survey comparing the various types of kitchen accidents. According to this survey, 50% of all kitchen accidents are cuts; 25% are burns; 15% are falls; 7% are due to electric shock; and 3% are poisoning. Create a circle graph to show this data.

Math Concept **Circle Graphs** A circle graph (or pie chart) can be used to indicate parts of a whole, which are shown as sections (wedges) of the circle.

Starting Hint Multiply each percent by 360° to find the angles of each section.

NCTM Data Analysis and Probability Formulate questions that can be addressed with data and collect, organize, and display relevant data to answer them.

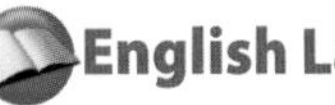

English Language Arts

19. A–Z Safety Lists Write an A–Z list of safety tips for the kitchen in which each tip corresponds to one letter from the alphabet. For example, the first tip might be "Appliances should be unplugged when not in use." The second could be "Bake safely by using oven mitts to handle hot items." Each tip should be a complete sentence, and be written in your own words.

NCTE 5 Use different writing process elements to communicate effectively.

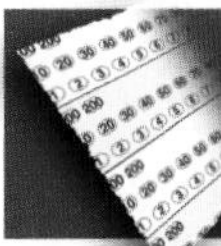

STANDARDIZED TEST PRACTICE

READING COMPREHENSION

Re-read the section about cord safety on page 307. Then select the best answer to the question.

20. What can you do to prevent accidents caused by cords in the kitchen?

a. Keep cords tidy and away from water by stapling or nailing them in place.

b. Keep cords organized by putting as many as possible in one electrical outlet.

c. Do not try to fit a polarized plug into a non-polarized outlet.

d. Avoid electrocution by unplugging cords by pulling on the cord, not the plug.

Test-Taking Tip Before you answer a reading comprehension question, closely read the answers. Some answers may seem correct, but they contain subtle errors. Pay attention to every word.

CHAPTER 21

Equipping the Kitchen

Writing Activity Cause-and-Effect Paragraph

A Disorganized Kitchen What makes a kitchen organized? What are the consequences if a kitchen is disorganized? Write a cause-and-effect paragraph in which you explore kitchen disorganization and its consequences. The disorganization will be the cause, and the consequences will be the effect.

Writing Tips Follow these steps to write a cause-and-effect paragraph:

- Describe a cause and explain its result, or effect.
- Use detailed, specific language.
- Explain why the effect results from the cause.

Activate Prior Knowledge

Explore the Photo A well-equipped kitchen has plenty of work and storage space. *How can you make the most of your space?*

Reading Guide

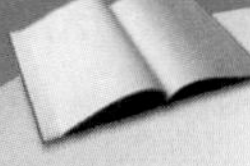

Before You Read

Preview Skim through the chapter. As you skim, think about how your home kitchen is equipped. What makes it easy or difficult to use?

Read to Learn

Key Concepts

- **Explain** the items that make up a work triangle.
- **Describe** factors to consider when selecting kitchen components.
- **Contrast** a warranty and a service contract.
- **List** three large kitchen appliances and nine small kitchen appliances.
- **Describe** seven common types of cookware.

Main Idea

In a well-designed and equipped kitchen, you can store, prepare, and serve foods with ease.

Content Vocabulary

- work flow
- work center
- work triangle
- peninsula
- island
- universal design
- grounding
- task lighting
- EnergyGuide label
- warranty
- service contract
- credit
- down payment
- principal
- interest
- annual percentage rate (APR)
- finance charge
- heating unit
- convection oven
- cookware
- bakeware

Academic Vocabulary

- assess
- versatile

Graphic Organizer

Use a graphic organizer like the one below to compare and contrast glass and enamel cookware.

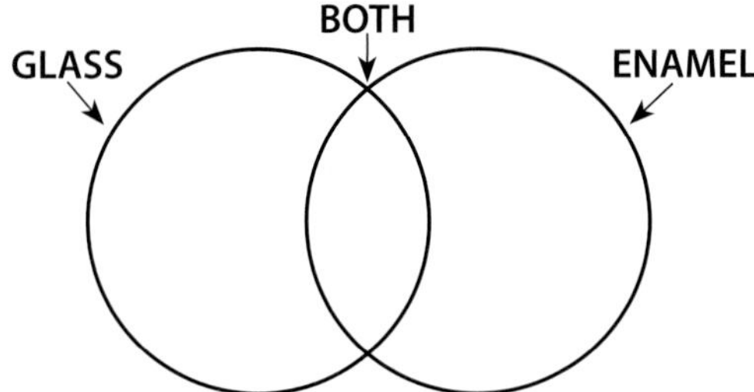

Graphic Organizer Go to this book's Online Learning Center at **glencoe.com** to print out this graphic organizer.

Academic Standards

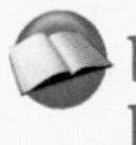

English Language Arts

NCTE 4 Use written language to communicate effectively.

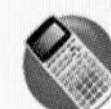

Mathematics

NCTM Number and Operations Compute fluently and make reasonable estimates.

NCTM Measurement Apply appropriate techniques, tools, and formulas to determine measurements.

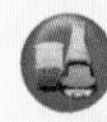

Science

NSES B Develop an understanding of interactions of energy and matter.

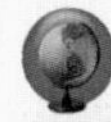

Social Studies

NCSS VIII A Science, Technology, and Society Identify and describe both current and historical examples of the interaction and interdependence of science, technology, and society in a variety of cultural settings.

NCTE *National Council of Teachers of English*
NCTM *National Council of Teachers of Mathematics*
NSES *National Science Education Standards*
NCSS *National Council for the Social Studies*

Kitchen Design Basics

A well-designed kitchen is organized for efficiency so that you get the most from your time and effort. An efficient kitchen starts with a floor plan that promotes the work flow. In a kitchen, **work flow** is all the steps involved in removing food from storage, preparing it, and serving it.

Work Centers

Kitchens are organized around work centers. A **work center** is an area designed for performing specific kitchen tasks, such as chopping vegetables or washing dishes. A well-designed work center has the equipment you need to do a task, plus convenient and adequate storage and work space.

A typical kitchen has three major work centers:

Cold-Storage Center The focus of the cold-storage center is the refrigerator-freezer. Plastic storage bags, food wraps, and containers for leftovers might also be stored here.

Sink Center The sink center is the place to do tasks that require running water, including cleaning fresh fruits and vegetables, draining foods, and washing dishes. Dishpans and other cleanup supplies should be stored in this area. The garbage disposal and dishwasher are also part of the sink center.

Cooking Center The cooking center includes the range, small cooking appliances, and related tools. Pots and pans, cooking tools, and possibly canned and packaged foods are also stored in the cooking center.

Larger kitchens may have additional work centers. A mixing center, for example, is a place to mix and prepare foods. Here you would find measuring cups, mixing spoons, and appliances such as a food processor, along with baking ingredients such as flour and spices. Even small kitchens often have a shelf for baking tools and ingredients.

Large kitchens might have a laundry center with a washer and dryer. Some kitchens even have a computer desk or a play or study area for children.

The Work Triangle

The arrangement of the three main work centers in a kitchen forms the **work triangle**. Each work center is one point in the triangle. For an efficient work flow, the distance between any two centers should be between 12 and 26 feet. The work triangle should be away from through-traffic, the path of people walking from one room to another.

When one person works in the kitchen alone, the work triangle can be compact. If people share kitchen tasks, additional work space is useful. For example, a second sink lets one person scrub vegetables while another washes dishes. This arrangement might create adjacent or overlapping work triangles.

Kitchen Plans

A kitchen's floor plan determines its work triangle. The four most common floor plans are shown in **Figure 21.1** and described here:

One-Wall Small kitchens often have a one-wall plan, with all three work centers on one wall. Kitchens with a one-wall plan often have limited storage and counter space.

L-Shaped Kitchens with an L-shaped plan have work centers on two connecting walls. This layout keeps through-traffic away from the work flow.

Corridor Kitchens with a corridor plan have work centers on facing walls. This design is convenient for a single cook. If doorways are located at opposite ends of the kitchen, however, through-traffic can be disruptive.

U-Shaped Kitchens with a U-shaped plan have work centers on three connecting walls, forming a U shape.

Peninsulas and Islands

Many kitchen plans also include a peninsula or an island. A **peninsula** is a countertop extension that is open on two sides and on one end. An **island** is a freestanding counter that is open on all sides and is often placed in the center of the kitchen. Peninsulas and islands often have storage space below the countertop. They sometimes have a sink, a cooktop, or a countertop that doubles as an eating area.

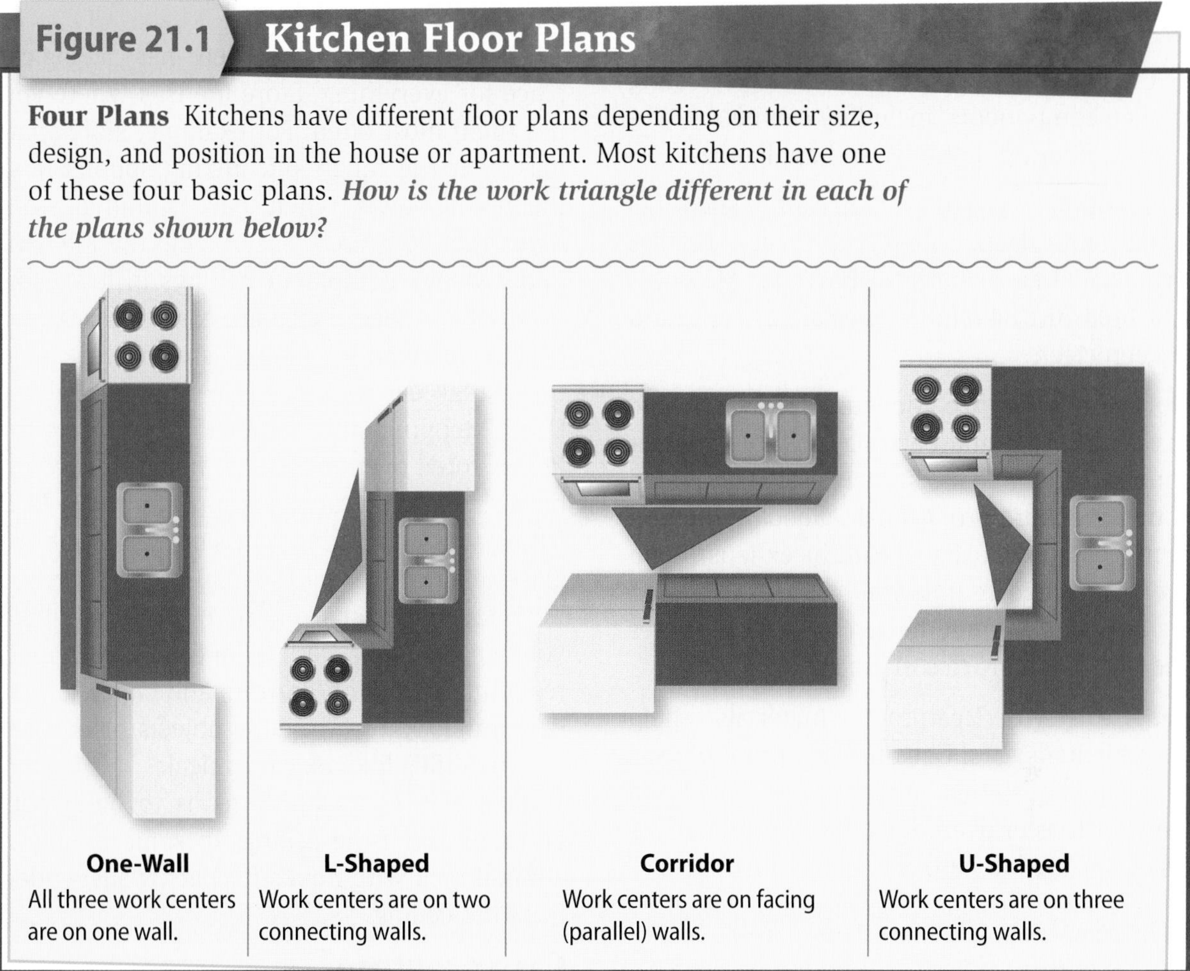

One-Wall
All three work centers are on one wall.
L-Shaped
Work centers are on two connecting walls.
Corridor
Work centers are on facing (parallel) walls.
U-Shaped
Work centers are on three connecting walls.

Figure 21.1 Kitchen Floor Plans

Four Plans Kitchens have different floor plans depending on their size, design, and position in the house or apartment. Most kitchens have one of these four basic plans. ***How is the work triangle different in each of the plans shown below?***

Universal Design

To make kitchens easier and more pleasant to use, designers and appliance makers use universal design, also called lifespan design. **Universal design** is a way of making objects and spaces easy to use by everyone, regardless of age or physical ability. Kitchens created using universal design often have wider doorways and work areas to accommodate wheelchairs and walkers. They have adjustable countertops and work surfaces at various heights so that tasks may be completed while sitting or standing. They may also have open shelves and drawer spaces, which are more accessible than closed cabinets.

Small changes can make kitchens better suited to individual needs. For example:

- Replacing cabinet knobs with large handles can help people who have trouble grasping small objects.
- Kitchen sinks can be made 6½-inches deep.
- Sinks can be fitted with handles rather than knobs.
- Push-button or touchpad controls make operating microwaves, stovetops, and other appliances easier.
- Adding Braille labels to appliance controls can help people with limited vision.
- Carts with wheels can be used to move food and equipment.
- Tongs or grippers can be used to grab items.
- Stools or tall chairs can make working at counters more comfortable.
- Fire extinguishers can be located in an easy-to-reach place.

✓ **Reading Check** **Contrast** In a kitchen, what is the difference between a peninsula and an island?

Kitchen Components

Consider these three factors when selecting kitchen components, including cabinets, countertops, flooring, lighting, and appliances.

Washability Washable materials, such as metal and plastic, help you keep surfaces clean and free of harmful bacteria. Materials that hold dirt or require special care are hard to keep clean.

Moisture Resistance Moisture promotes the growth of mold and bacteria, so kitchen components should be moisture resistant or treated with a moisture-proof finish. Good ventilation from a window, exhaust fan, or exhaust hood over the range is important. An exhaust fan system can also limit the spread of mold spores and airborne particles of grease.

Heat Resistance Heatproof materials help keep kitchens safe. Use only heatproof objects near appliances that produce heat, such as a range or toaster oven. Keep flammable materials out of the kitchen.

Cabinets

Kitchen cabinets that rest on the floor under a countertop are called base cabinets. Standard cabinet size is 24 inches deep and 36 inches high. Wall cabinets attach to the wall above the countertop. Tall, floor-to-ceiling cabinets are called pantries. Pantries may include a shelf for a microwave oven.

Cabinets can be made of solid wood or stainless steel, but laminates are the most popular option. A laminate is made of several layers of paper that are compressed and bonded with liquid plastic. Laminates resemble more costly materials but need less care. The sides of laminate cabinets are often made from compressed wood that is chemically treated to resist water.

Special features make cabinets handy for storing various foods and tools. Some cabinets have roll-out shelves, pop-up shelves, or vertical dividers for organizing baking sheets and trays. Pull-out ventilated baskets provide cool, dry storage for produce. Storage helpers such as door racks and shelves, stackable bins, and turntables make items easy to reach. Shelf lining makes cabinet shelves easy to keep clean.

Storage Strategies

A well-organized kitchen has a logical place for everything. Store utensils where you use them most often. For example, store spatulas near the range and mixing spoons near the mixing bowls. When space is limited, store items that you rarely use outside the kitchen. Large, heavy equipment belongs in low cabinets, where bulky items are easy to reach and lift. Try to avoid stacking glass items, because they break easily. Be careful of high shelves. Use a stepping stool rather than reaching for items stored over your head. Items stacked on high shelves can fall on you. If you have limited space, stack lighter glass on top of heavier glass, and do not stack too many items together. Keep tools with sharp parts in drawers where you can see and access them easily. Use child-restraint devices on drawers and cabinets that contain sharp or breakable objects or hazardous materials like toxic chemicals.

One way to avoid clutter is to hang pots and pans from the ceiling. In some kitchens, a metal rack with hooks for pots is suspended from the ceiling.

Countertops

Countertops come in many different materials, including wood, concrete, metal, tile, stone, and laminates. Some kitchens have more than one kind of countertop. For example, counters near sinks might be made of moisture-resistant glazed tile, and counters near the range might be made of heat-resistant granite.

Laminates are usually the most affordable countertop material. Wood and stone are usually the most costly. Some countertop materials need special care, which costs time and money. For example, wood countertops need to be oiled on a regular basis.

Countertops are valuable work space, and many cooks wish they had more counter space. A cart, a table, or a portable base cabinet can add more work space. Flip-down shelves, pull-out breadboards, and adjustable cutting boards that fit over the sink also increase work space. Keeping the work space you have clear of clutter is one of the best ways to increase work space. Store small appliances that you do not use often in a pantry or in cabinets.

Floors and Walls

Kitchen flooring should be durable and comfortable. To be easy on the feet, floors should be resilient, which means that they spring back under pressure. Vinyl and linoleum are resilient and do not need waxing or polishing, but they can be nicked by sharp objects. Stone floors are hard to damage but can be uncomfortable to stand on for long periods. Mats or throw rugs can make hard floors easier on the feet and joints. Mats and non-slip shoes also prevent kitchen falls. Hardwood floors are attractive in the kitchen, but are easily damaged by water.

Easy cleaning is the most important quality in kitchen wall coverings, especially near the sink and range. Wallpaper and paint are both practical. Vinyl-coated wallpaper can be wiped clean with a sponge. Paint with a semigloss finish helps to repel dirt. Ceramic tile is also a good choice, but cleaning the grout can be time-consuming.

The Electrical System

A kitchen electrical system should be safe and sufficient for the number of appliances you use. Make sure you have enough power coming into the kitchen, as well as sufficient outlets and a grounded electrical system. **Grounding** is the process of providing a path for electrical current to travel back through the electrical system, rather than through your body. Grounding helps to prevent shocks.

The National Electric Code requires grounded wires in new homes. In some states, homes without grounded wiring need to have it installed before the home can be sold. Outlets with three holes usually have grounded wiring. Check with an electrician to be certain, however. Grounded outlets accept three-pronged plugs from grounded appliances.

Keep electrical cords away from heat sources and blades. If a cord becomes frayed, have it repaired or replace it immediately.

If appliances work slowly or poorly or lights dim or go out when you use an appliance, the wiring does not provide enough power to meet your needs. Have a qualified electrician **assess**, or evaluate, the electrical system.

Lighting

Good lighting is essential for comfort and safety. Injuries can happen if you cannot see what you are doing. A ceiling light or lighted panels can provide good general lighting. Close work takes **task lighting**, bright, shadow-free light over specific work areas. Light fixtures mounted beneath overhead cabinets provide good task lighting for countertops. Recessed spotlights or track lights on the ceiling can be arranged to shine on specific spots in the kitchen. A dimmer switch lets you make the lighting as bright or as dim as you need. Indirect lighting from windows also brightens a kitchen.

✓ Reading Check **Explain** Why should kitchen components be moisture-proof?

Kitchen Math

Equipment Budget

Mandy is moving into her first apartment. The apartment comes with all the kitchen appliances she will need (refrigerator, stove, oven, and microwave). Mandy does not own any other kitchen supplies or tools, and she will need to purchase them. She cannot afford to buy everything, so you are going to help her to determine which equipment she will need the most, and develop a budget for those supplies.

Math Concept **Working with Tables** When using tables to track information and calculations, label the columns and be sure that the type of information within each column is consistent.

Starting Hint Decide on at least 10 items Mandy will need. Use the Internet or advertisements to find out the prices of the items you select. Create a table in a spreadsheet program or on a piece of paper with a proposed budget. One column should list each item needed. The next column should list the price of each item. The third column should list the quantity of each item needed. The fourth column should list the total cost (price multiplied by quantity) of the item. Add all of the total costs together.

Math Appendix For math help, go to the Math Appendix at the back of the book.

NCTM Number and Operations Compute fluently and make reasonable estimates..

Buying for the Kitchen

There are tens of thousands of items available for your kitchen. With some thoughtful planning, you can select the right tools and avoid wasting money on items that you do not really need.

Before You Buy

Be a smart shopper. First, consider whether you really need the item. Second, prioritize features. Third, do research to make an informed decision.

1. Consider your needs. Before you decide to buy, consider whether you really need the item. Ask yourself these questions:

- Does the usefulness of this item justify the cost?
- Can tools I already own perform the same tasks?
- Do I have room to store the new item?
- Do I have time and energy to use, clean, and maintain the new item?
- How much can I afford to spend?
- How will I pay?

2. Prioritize features. Identify the most important features of the item based on your needs and wants. Know the measurements of the space where an appliance must fit. Items in your price range might not have all the features you want, so rank your wants from most to least important.

3. Conduct research. The third step is to gather information about products that fit your needs. Some consumer magazines such as Consumer Reports conduct unbiased tests to compare brands of similar items. Most appliance manufacturers have Web sites with up-to-date information on products, including features, dimensions, and warranty information.

When you make a large purchase, choose a reliable dealer or retailer. If you shop by catalog or on the Internet, make sure the seller is reputable. Check with the Better Business Bureau to see if customers have made complaints about a company and whether the complaints have been settled. Use only secure sites when ordering online.

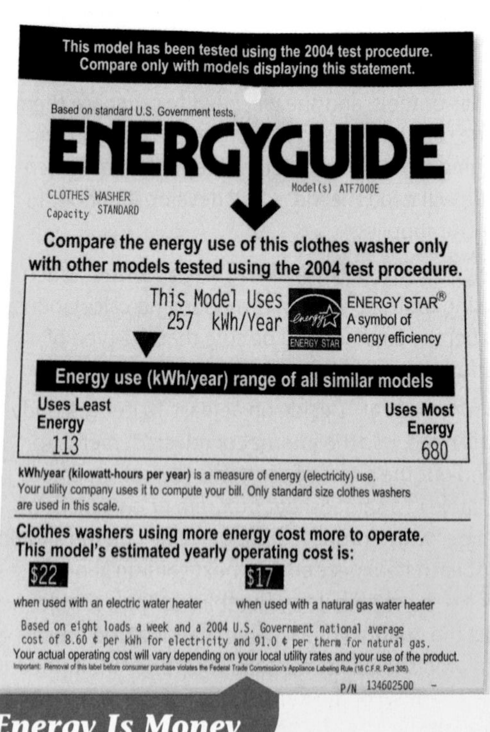

Energy Is Money

The EnergyGuide label helps you compare energy efficiency of different appliance models. *What does it cost to run this appliance for a year? How does this appliance's energy use compare to that of other models?*

Consumer Safeguards

Government agencies, manufacturers, and dealers help ensure that consumers are treated fairly. Look for these consumer safeguards as you shop.

EnergyGuide Label

The **EnergyGuide label** is a yellow label on large appliances that shows the average cost per year of using the appliance. EnergyGuide labels are required on refrigerators, freezers, dishwashers, and other major appliances. Use the EnergyGuide label to compare operating costs of different brands and models. You can also estimate energy expenses based on the cost of gas or electricity in your area.

EnergyGuide labels usually say whether an appliance has earned the Energy Star. The Energy Star symbol shows that an appliance meets strict energy efficiency guidelines set by the Environmental Protection Agency and U.S. Department of Energy.

Seals of Approval

Testing agencies give seals of approval to show that a product meets certain safety and performance standards. One widely recognized group is Underwriters Laboratories (UL). On electric appliances, the UL mark certifies that the appliance design is reasonably free from risk of fire, electric shock, and other hazards. The American Gas Association (AGA) seal attests to the design, performance, and reliability of gas appliances.

If you see a seal of approval from an organization that you do not recognize, do some research. A seal is only as reliable as the group that issues it.

Warranties

A **warranty** is a manufacturer's guarantee that a product will perform as advertised. If you have problems with the product, the manufacturer promises to replace or repair it. Warranties have time limits, and coverage is usually conditional. For example, most warranties only cover damage that occurs when you are following the rules in the owner's manual.

Service Contracts

A **service contract** is insurance that covers repair and maintenance of a product for a specific length of time. Service contracts are usually offered by dealers who sell appliances. Service contracts are often expensive, and they often do not cover the total cost of repairs and parts. Before signing up for a service contract, check the free warranty to see if you are already well covered.

Be a Critical Shopper

Comparison shopping helps you get the best value for your money. These strategies can help you make a smart buying decision, especially when shopping for an expensive item:

- Keep written notes as you shop. List your likes and dislikes for each product.
- Check items carefully for potential hazards and for features that guard against injuries, such as heatproof handles.
- Pick up tools, cookware, and appliances. Do they seem well made and a good fit?
- Look at the owner's manual. Will the item be easy to use and care for? What does the warranty cover?
- Compare prices. High-quality items with lots of features usually cost more, but may be worth the money. An item from a well-known brand may not be better than an item from an unfamiliar brand—do research to find out.
- Ask the dealer about additional costs, such as delivery and installation charges.

Be a Smart Consumer

Be Careful with Credit Cards

Credit cards can be helpful tools for making purchases. They can also create enormous debt. If you do not pay off your credit card each month, interest can accumulate. High interest rates and compounding interest can cause you to pay much more for an item than it originally cost. Compounding interest means that any unpaid interest becomes part of your principal debt, which continues to have interest added to it each month. To avoid drowning in debt, pay off your monthly credit card balance. Choose a card with a low- or no-interest plan.

Challenge Research the cost of an item you want to purchase. If you buy it on credit with a 3% compounding monthly interest rate, how much will you owe after three months?

Paying for Your Purchase

Most major purchases are bought with credit. **Credit** is a financial arrangement that delays payment for an item. Using credit is more expensive than paying with cash, but you can use the product while you pay for it.

When you buy on credit, there may be a **down payment**, a portion of the purchase price that you must pay before you take the item home. The purchase price minus the down payment is the **principal**, the amount to be financed. You borrow the principal from a lender, such as a credit card company, a bank, or a finance company. The lender charges interest.

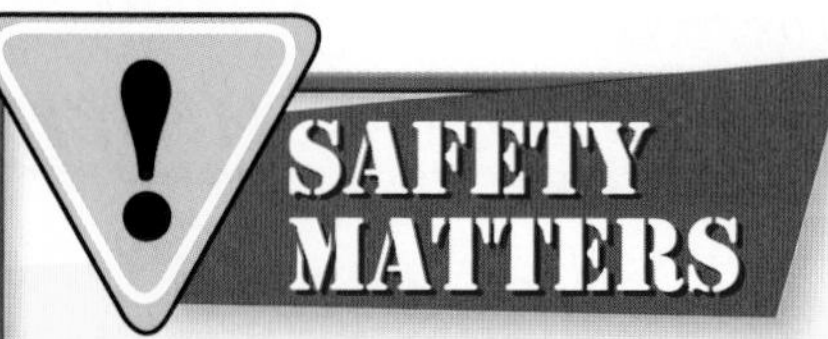

Prevent Carbon Monoxide Poisoning

The natural gas that fuels gas ranges requires oxygen to burn completely. Incomplete burning creates carbon monoxide, a colorless, odorless gas that is a common cause of fatal poisoning. Signs of incomplete burning include a pilot light that burns yellow instead of blue, and a buildup of soot near the range. To ensure a good air supply to a gas range, keep air vents open. Do not line the burner bowls with foil. If a burner lights only partially, try clearing the holes with a metal wire or paper clip. Do not use toothpicks, which can break and plug the holes.

What Would You Do? For the summer, your family has rented a cabin with an old gas range. What steps would you take to make sure your family will be safe from carbon monoxide poisoning?

Interest is a fee for the loan expressed as a percentage of the amount borrowed.

When you buy something on credit, you also agree to pay the fee that a creditor adds to the purchase price. For example, if you do not pay your credit card bill in full every month, you will be charged interest on the amount you have not paid.

Interest rates can vary greatly. By law, lenders must state the **annual percentage rate (APR)**, or the yearly rate of interest that you must pay on the principal. Annual percentage rates can be very high, up to 30 percent a year. Interest can add up quickly, making the total price of an item much higher than you originally planned.

Lenders may also charge fees, such as a service charge or insurance premiums. Fees plus interest make up the **finance charge**, the total amount you pay for borrowing. The finance charge is written as a dollar figure, not a percentage. Monthly payments usually equal the total cost (principal plus finance charges) divided by the number of months that you have to pay off the account.

Shop for credit carefully. Compare APRs and other fees to find the lowest cost of borrowing. Do not use credit to spend more than you can afford. If you do not make payments on time, you may lose the item and have trouble getting credit in the future.

Protecting Your Purchase

Keep the warranty, owner's manual, and sales receipt for every appliance and kitchen tool you buy. File these documents together in a safe place where you can easily find them. If you have to use the warranty, you will need the receipt to show the date of purchase. Fill out and send in the warranty registration card, if there is one. This validates the warranty if you lose the receipt. Sending the card also enables the manufacturer to notify you if the product has a danger or defect.

Read the owner's manual before using the item. Then test it to make sure it works. If it does not work, return the item to the store or call the dealer.

✓ Reading Check **Describe** What resources can you use to conduct research about products for the kitchen?

Kitchen Appliances

Appliances are devices powered by gas or electricity that help you prepare food and clean up afterwards. A kitchen typically has three major, or large, appliances: a range, a refrigerator-freezer, and a dishwasher. Most kitchens also have several small appliances including a blender, food processor, electric mixer, toaster, toaster oven, electric skillet, slow cooker, broiler/grill, and rice cooker.

Ranges

The conventional range is a single, freestanding unit consisting of a cooktop, an oven, and a broiler. Cooking heat is generated by heating units. A **heating unit** is an energy source in the range. Most ranges have either gas or electric heating units. Dual-fuel ranges use electricity for the oven and gas for the cooktop.

You control the heat on a cooktop with dials, buttons, or touchpads marked with settings from low to high. You control the heat in an oven with a dial, button, or touchpad marked with temperatures. Settings range from warm, which is below 200°, to broil, which is about 500°. The broiler cooks and browns foods using direct heat.

Ovens are available with many different features. Some ovens have a self-cleaning cycle that uses intense heat to burn off spatters and spills. Some ovens have digital displays instead of dials, and some are built with racks to hold oversize pans. Some have pull-out warming drawers that create a slightly humid environment that helps to raise yeast breads or to hold cooked foods safely without drying them out.

Gas Ranges

The heating units in a gas range are called burners. Burners heat with a visible flame that is easy to turn up or down. Newer ranges use an electronic spark that ignites the gas when you turn the burner on. Older ranges use pilot lights, small flames that burn continuously. When you turn the burner on, the pilot light ignites the gas.

Some gas ranges have sealed burners that are easy to clean. Others have one continuous grate so that cookware can slide from one burner to another. The oven and broiler in a gas range are in separate compartments. The broiler is usually below the oven.

Electric Ranges

The heating units in an electric range are called elements. Elements stay hot longer than gas burners, so many electric ranges have a warning light that stays on until the cooktop has cooled.

Electric ranges come in two basic styles. One style has exposed metal coils that turn red when the heating unit is on. The other style has a glass-ceramic smoothtop covering ribbon heating elements. Some smoothtops have a bridge that connects several heating elements, which works well for oblong pots and pans. Some smoothtops also have a low-heat, warming zone to keep food hot without burning. All smoothtops are easy to clean. Unlike gas ranges, electric ranges do not have separate broiler compartments. A heating element at the bottom of the oven bakes food. An element on the ceiling of the oven comes on for broiling.

Convection Ovens

Ovens use convection currents, which are created by the natural tendency of hot air to rise. A **convection oven** also has a fan that circulates heated air to equalize temperatures throughout the oven. The result is faster and more even cooking and browning.

Some ranges combine convection and microwave cooking. These powerful models are similar to those used in professional kitchens. Food cooks twice as fast, which helps it retain moisture and flavor.

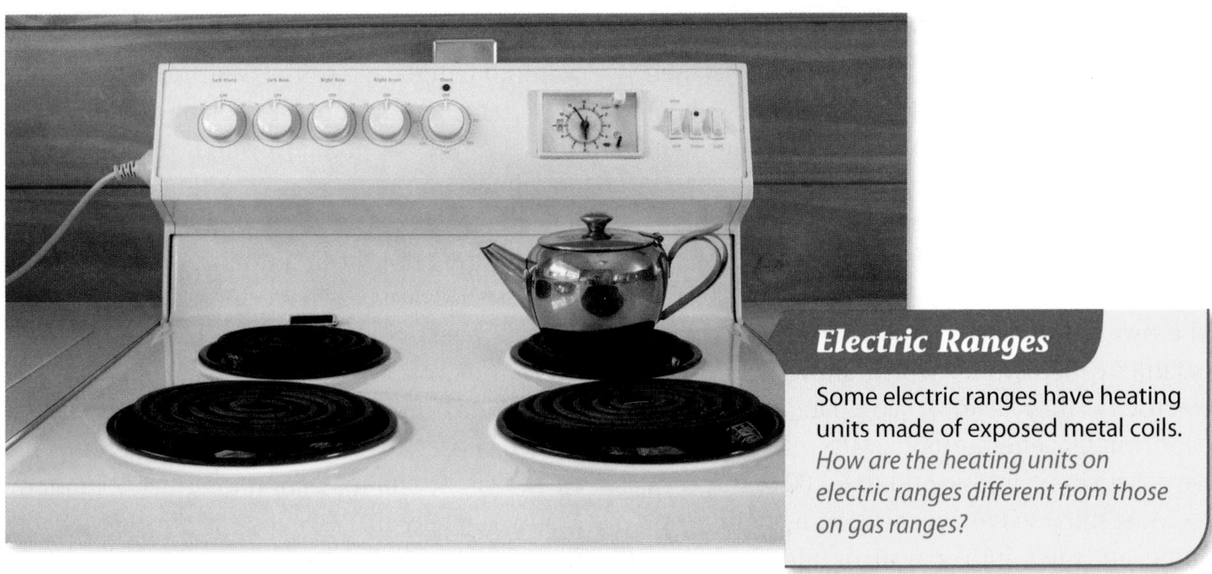

Electric Ranges

Some electric ranges have heating units made of exposed metal coils. *How are the heating units on electric ranges different from those on gas ranges?*

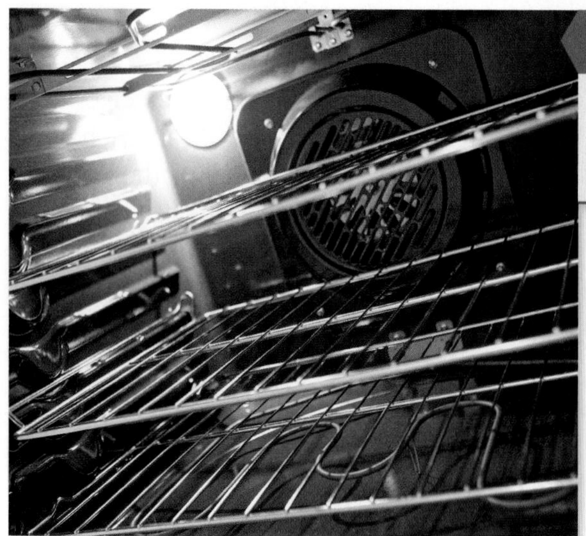

Fast and Even

A convection oven has a fan that forces air to circulate around food. *What are the benefits of a convection oven?*

Built-In Range and Oven Units

Some kitchens have separate cooktop and oven units. Ovens are built into walls, with added insulation to protect adjacent areas. Cooktops are set in cabinets. Some built-in units also have modules for grills and griddles. A downdraft exhaust system draws heated air into a duct below the cooktop.

Microwave Ovens

A microwave oven has a magnetron (ˈmag-nə-ˌträn) tube that converts electricity into microwaves, a form of energy that travels through space like radio waves. A fanlike device called a stirrer blade distributes the microwaves through the oven, where they bounce off the walls and floor. Microwaves pass through paper, glass, and plastic. The molecules in food, however, absorb the microwaves and vibrate against each other, which produces friction. This friction produces heat that cooks the food up to four times faster than in a conventional oven.

Microwave ovens vary in size from about ½ cubic foot to 2 cubic feet. Large models produce more microwaves and cook food faster. Microwave ovens have power ratings measured in units called watts, which show how much electricity they use. A compact microwave oven might generate 600 watts of electricity. Large versions produce up to 1,100 watts.

Most microwave ovens sit on a countertop. Some are built into a wall or mounted over a range. Most newer microwaves have turntables that rotate food for more even cooking. Some have racks that increase oven capacity. Many microwave ovens have presets that can cook food automatically by weight or type. Some have sensors that adjust cooking conditions based on the amount of moisture left in a food.

Refrigerator-Freezers

Refrigerator-freezers create cold storage using a chemical blend called refrigerant. The refrigerant expands into a gas as it circulates in the refrigerator walls. The gas absorbs heat, which escapes through coils on the outside of the refrigerator.

Full-size refrigerator-freezers range in size from 10 to 30 cubic feet. Most have two doors, one for the refrigerator and one for the freezer. The freezer may be on the top, the bottom, or the side. The freezer maintains a temperature of 0°. It can freeze fresh foods and store foods that are already frozen.

Dishwashers

Dishwashers save time and tend to use less water than hand-washing. Built-in dishwashers fit under a countertop and attach to a hot water line, drain, and standard outlet. Dishwashers on wheels connect to the sink faucet and drain into the sink. You can also buy small, in-sink dishwashers that fit in a double sink.

Most dishwashers have several wash cycles, from a basic rinse to a sanitizing cycle that heats the water to above 140°. Popular dishwasher features include adjustable racks, a food disposer to keep food from resettling on clean dishes, and insulation for quiet operation. Dishwashers with a delayed-start feature let you program the washer to start at a later time.

Figure 21.2 Small Appliances

Little Luxuries Small appliances can cook, chop, mix, and more. *If you were equipping your first kitchen, which small appliances would you buy first?*

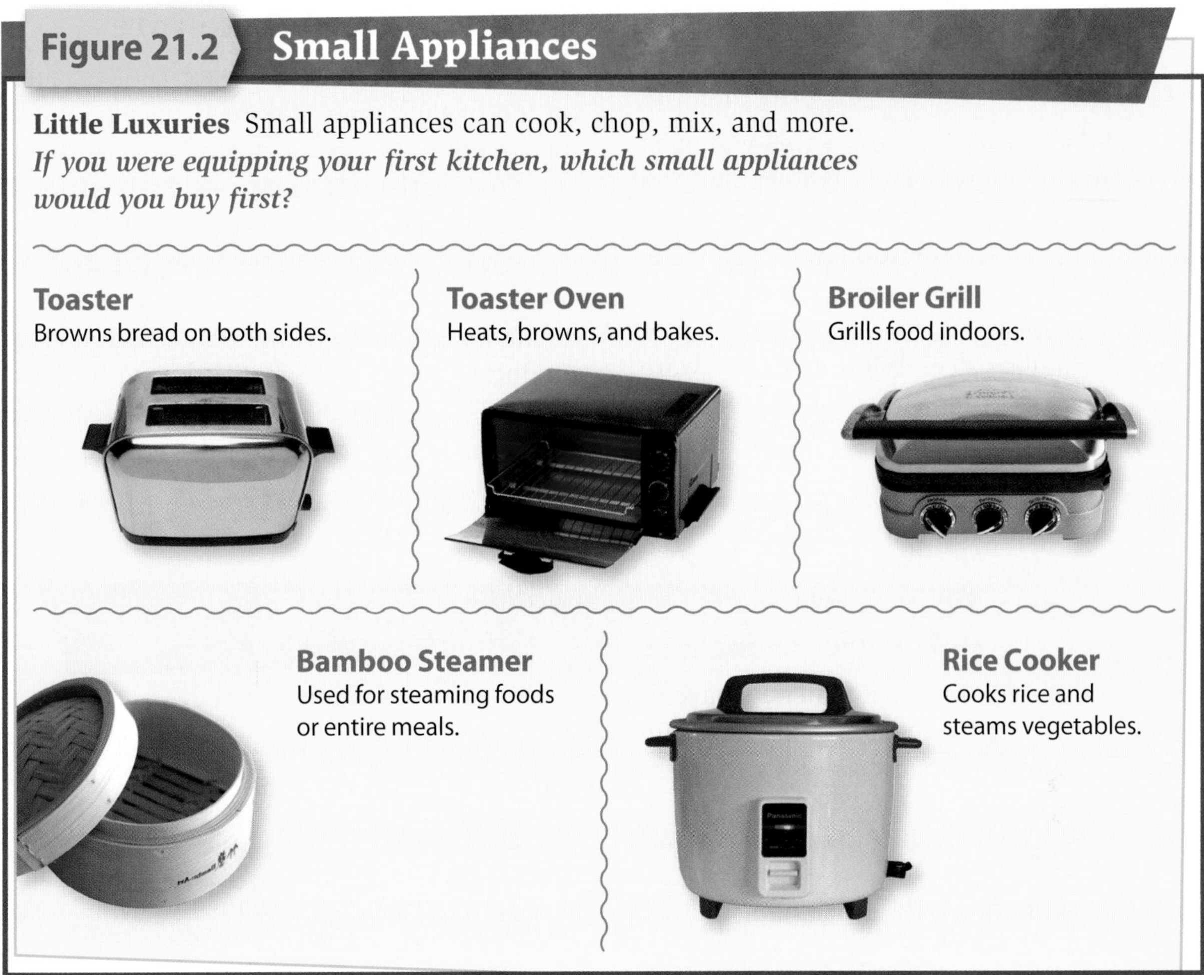

Toaster
Browns bread on both sides.

Toaster Oven
Heats, browns, and bakes.

Broiler Grill
Grills food indoors.

Bamboo Steamer
Used for steaming foods or entire meals.

Rice Cooker
Cooks rice and steams vegetables.

Small Appliances

Small appliances are electrical devices that perform a simple task, such as toasting or blending. Small appliances can save time and are cheaper and use less energy than major appliances. **Figure 21.2** shows some small appliances.

Small appliances exist for almost every kitchen task, from dicing onions to blending ice cream. Accumulating appliances can create clutter, however. Before buying an appliance, think about how often you will really use it.

Useful small appliances include:

Blender A blender chops, blends, and liquefies foods. Blenders have several speeds for different food preparation tasks.

Food Processor A food processor is more **versatile**, or capable of many uses, than a blender. Food processors have blades and discs for specialized jobs, such as juicing fruit.

Electric Mixer An electric mixer blends, beats, and whips ingredients.

Toaster A toaster browns slices of bread and small flat pastries on both sides at the same time.

Toaster Oven A toaster oven heats, browns, or bakes small amounts of food. Some toaster ovens can broil.

Electric Skillet An electric skillet fries, roasts, steams, and bakes. Electric skillets have thermostatic temperature control.

Slow Cooker A slow cooker is a deep pot with a heating element in the base that cooks food slowly for hours. Slow cookers are convenient for one-dish meals.

Broiler/Grill A broiler/grill is used to grill food indoors.

Rice Cooker/Steamer A rice cooker cooks rice perfectly and can also be used to steam vegetables.

✓ **Reading Check** **List** What are the three major appliances in a typical kitchen?

Food Preparation Tools and Equipment

In addition to appliances, a well-equipped kitchen has a variety of tools and cooking and serving equipment such as cookware, bakeware, and handheld tools. Cookware and bakeware can be made from many different types of materials, including aluminum, copper, cast iron, and stainless steel. While most cookware and bakeware is cylindrical, the size and shape of a cooking vessel is determined by how it will be used.

Cookware and Bakeware

Cookware is equipment for cooking food on top of the range. **Bakeware** is equipment for cooking food in an oven. Both are available in a variety of materials. Each material has advantages, disadvantages, and rules for use and care as you can see in **Figure 21.3**.

Cookware and bakeware are major investments that should last for years. High-quality products have durable materials and finishes, heat-resistant handles, heavy and seamless construction, smooth edges, flat bottoms, and secure lids.

Figure 21.3 Cookware and Bakeware Materials

Kitchen Basics Different materials have different pros and cons. Some pots and pans combine materials, for example with a stainless steel layer over an aluminum base. ***What materials work well for both cooking and serving?***

Material	Advantages	Disadvantages	Use and Care
Aluminum	• Conducts heat quickly and evenly if heavy. • Lightweight and durable. • Comes in a variety of finishes. • Comparatively inexpensive. • May be clad (covered) with stainless steel for benefits of both materials.	• Warps, dents, and scratches easily. • Darkens and stains, especially in dishwasher. • Pits if used with salty or acidic foods.	• Wash by hand, not in dishwasher. • Cool before washing to prevent warping. • Avoid sharp tools like knives and beaters. • Do not use to store salty or acidic foods.
Anodized Aluminum (coated with a hard protective finish)	• Maintains even, consistent cooking temperature. • Durable. • Will never peel, chip, or crack. • Less reactive to salty or acid foods than non-anodized aluminum. • Anodizing makes aluminum easier to clean. • Resists sticking and scratching.	• Heavy. • Can be expensive.	• Wash by hand, not in dishwasher. • Use nonabrasive cleaners and nylon scrubbers.
Stainless Steel	• Durable, tough, hard. • Lightweight. • Will not dent easily. • Can withstand use of metal utensils. • Attractive; keeps bright shine. • Moderately priced.	• Conducts heat unevenly; thick aluminum or copper core bottom helps. • Stains when overheated or from use with starchy foods. • Can develop hot spots. • Pits if salty or acidic foods used.	• Use nonabrasive cleaners and nylon scrubbers. • Use stainless steel cleaner to remove stains. • Do not use to store salty or acidic foods.

Figure 21.3 Cookware and Bakeware Materials (continued)

Material	Advantages	Disadvantages	Use and Care
Copper	• Excellent heat conductor. • Heats quickly and evenly and cools quickly. • Attractive.	• Discolors easily. • Discolors food and may create toxic compounds, so must be lined with tin, silver, or stainless steel.	• Dry after washing. • Do not scour inside—the thin lining can be worn away. • Expensive. • Polish with copper cleaner or mixture of flour and vinegar.
Cast Iron	• Distributes heat evenly. • Retains heat well. • Good for browning, frying, and slow cooking.	• Heavy. • Heats and cools slowly. • Rusts if not wiped dry after washing.	• Store in dry place. • Store lid separately—pan may rust if stored covered.
Glass	• Attractive. • Can be used for cooking and serving. • Easy to clean.	• Breaks easily, especially if exposed to extreme temperature changes. • May need a wire grid if used on an electric cooktop. • Holds heat, but does not conduct heat well.	• Some can be used only on the cooktop, others only in the oven. • Use nonabrasive cleaners and nylon scrubbers. • Do not plunge hot pan into cold water or put into the refrigerator.
Glass-Ceramic	• Goes from freezer to oven or cooktop. • Durable, attractive, heat-resistant. • Dishwasher-safe. • Holds heat well—reduce oven temperatures by 25° for baked goods.	• May break if dropped. • May heat unevenly. • May develop hot spots.	• Used for roasting, broiling, and baking in conventional or microwave ovens. • Use nonabrasive cleaners and nylon scrubbers. • Use manufacturer's care instructions.
Stoneware	• Attractive. • Dishwasher-safe. • Can be used for cooking and serving. • Retains heat.	• Breaks easily.	• Use nonabrasive cleaners and nylon scrubbers.
Enamel (glass fused to a base metal)	• Attractive. • Dishwasher-safe. • Can be used to cook and serve.	• Chips easily.	• Use nonabrasive cleaners and nylon scrubbers.
Microwave-Safe Plastic	• Durable. • Dishwasher-safe. • Stain-resistant. • Easy to clean.	• Can be scratched by sharp kitchen tools. • Some cannot be used in conventional ovens.	• Use nonabrasive cleaners and nylon scrubbers.
Nonstick Finishes	• Keeps food from sticking—fat may not be necessary for browning, sautéing, or frying. • Easy to clean.	• Easily scratched by metal kitchen tools or abrasive cleaners. • High heat may stain finish or warp pan.	• Follow manufacturer's directions. Some cannot be washed in dishwasher. • Use nonmetal tools to prevent scratching.

Types of Cookware

Cookware comes in two basic types: pots and pans. Pots are deep containers that usually come with a lid. Pans are broad, shallow containers that often come without a lid. Pots and pans come in different shapes and sizes for different uses, as shown in **Figure 21.4**.

Skillet A skillet, also called a frying pan, is a shallow pan for browning and frying foods. Skillets come in many sizes and often have matching lids. A griddle is a skillet without sides.

Saucepan A saucepan is a deep pan with one long handle. Large saucepans may have a small handle on the opposite side as well. Saucepans are usually made of metal or heatproof glass, and they come in sizes ranging from ½ quart to 4 quarts. Many saucepans come with a lid. They are used for simmering or boiling.

Pot A pot is larger and heavier than a saucepan. Pots range in size from 3 to 20 quarts. They have two small handles, one on each side, for lifting. Most pots come with lids.

Double Boiler A double boiler is a small saucepan with a lid that fits into a larger saucepan. You simmer water in the lower pan to gently heat food in the upper pan. Double boilers are useful for heating foods that scorch easily, such as chocolate, sauces, and cereals, and for keeping food warm over a long period of time.

Figure 21.4 Types of Cookware

Kitchen Basics You can buy cookware in matching sets or as individual pieces. A set of quality cookware is a good investment for a beginning cook. ***Which cookware would you use for making soup? Which would you use for scrambling eggs?***

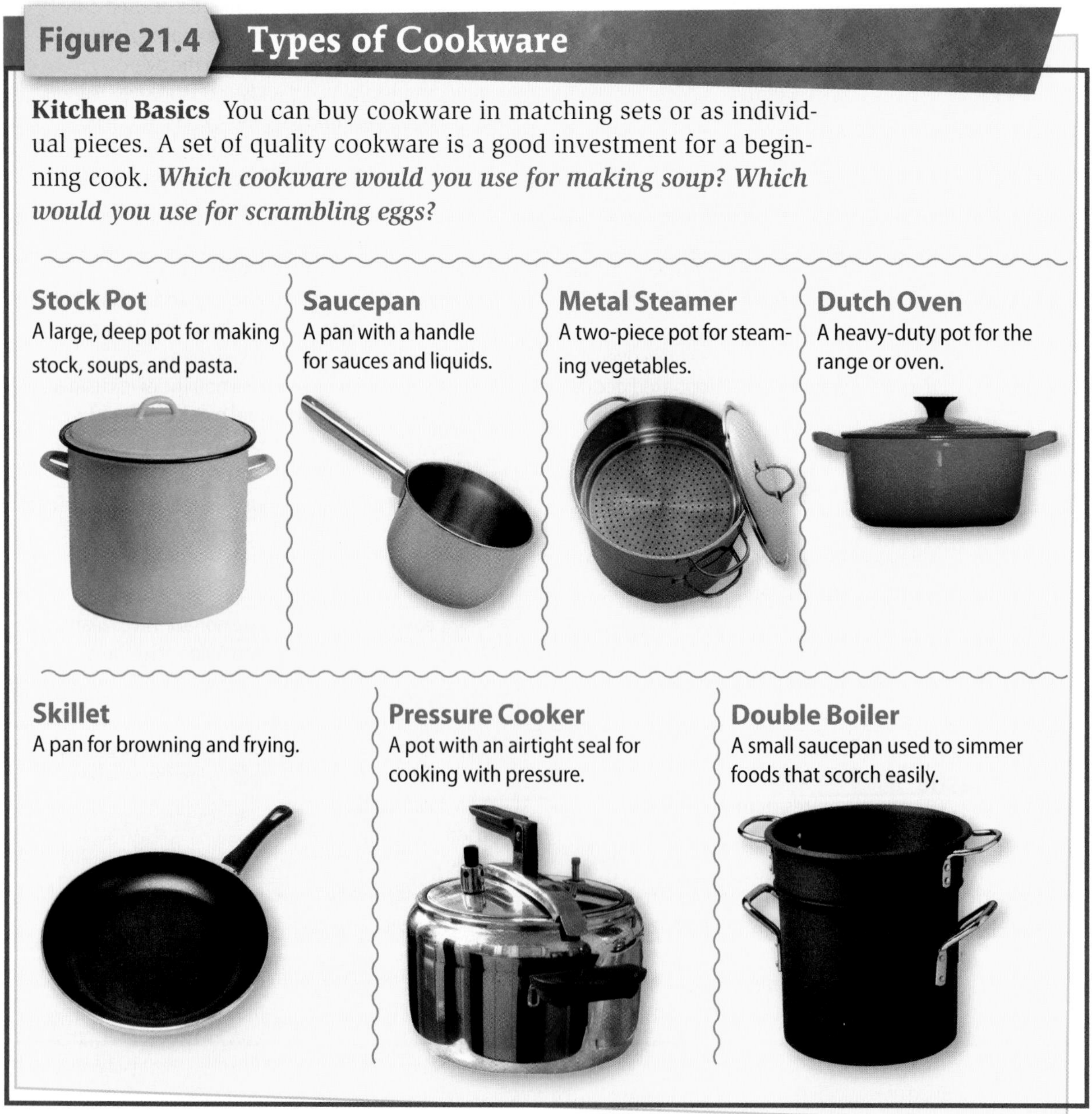

Stock Pot
A large, deep pot for making stock, soups, and pasta.
Saucepan
A pan with a handle for sauces and liquids.
Metal Steamer
A two-piece pot for steaming vegetables.
Dutch Oven
A heavy-duty pot for the range or oven.
Skillet
A pan for browning and frying.
Pressure Cooker
A pot with an airtight seal for cooking with pressure.
Double Boiler
A small saucepan used to simmer foods that scorch easily.

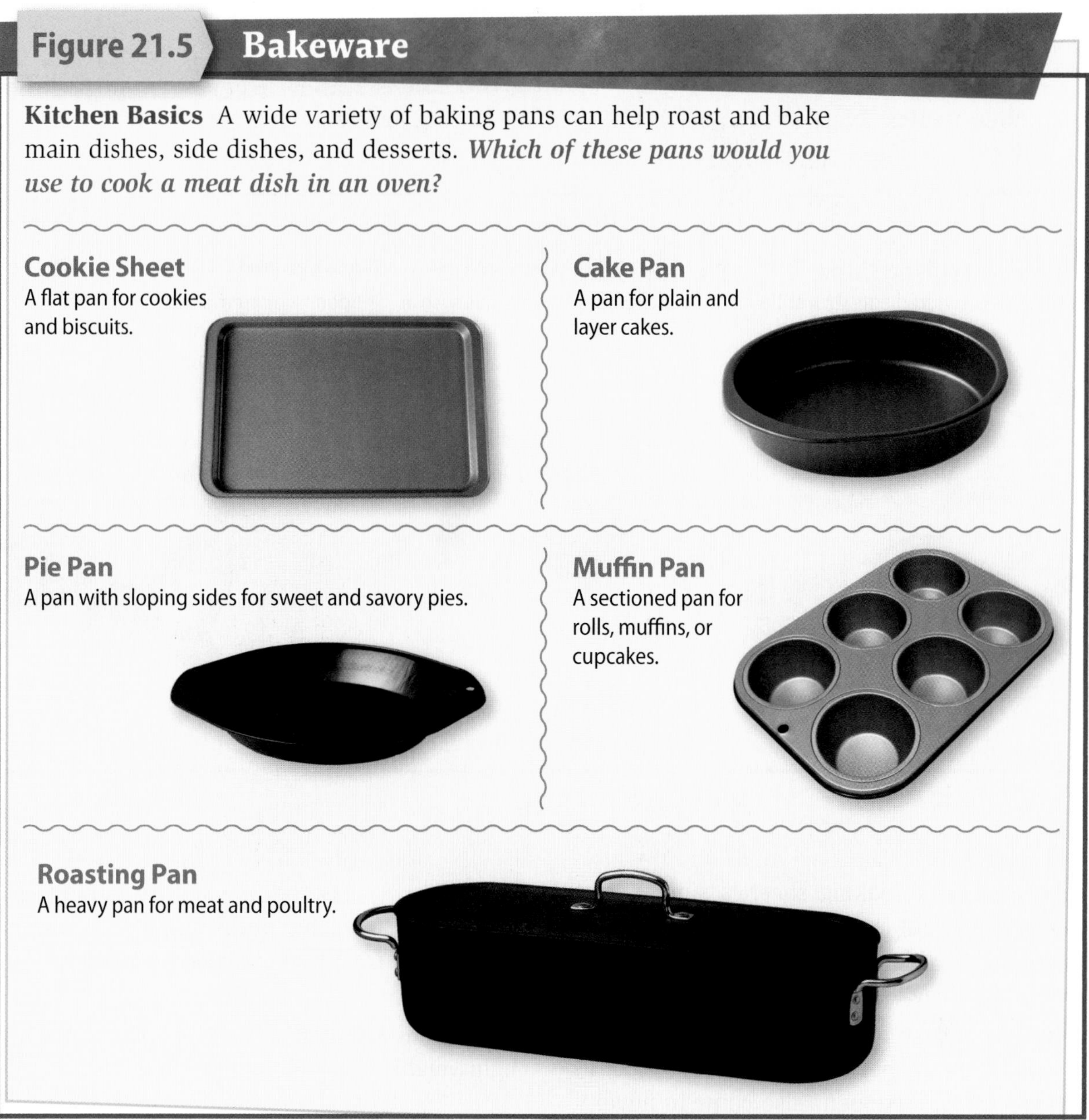

Figure 21.5 Bakeware
Kitchen Basics A wide variety of baking pans can help roast and bake main dishes, side dishes, and desserts. Which of these pans would you use to cook a meat dish in an oven?
Cookie Sheet
A flat pan for cookies and biscuits.
Cake Pan
A pan for plain and layer cakes.
Pie Pan
A pan with sloping sides for sweet and savory pies.
Muffin Pan
A sectioned pan for rolls, muffins, or cupcakes.
Roasting Pan
A heavy pan for meat and poultry.

Dutch Oven A Dutch oven is a heavy pot with a close-fitting lid that can be used on the range or in the oven. Some Dutch ovens have a rack to keep meat and poultry from sticking to the bottom.

Steamer A steamer is a covered saucepan with an insert that holds food over a small amount of boiling water. Holes in the insert allow steam to pass through and cook the food. Steamer inserts are made of metal or bamboo.

Pressure Cooker A pressure cooker is a heavy pot with a locked-on lid and a steam gauge. Steam builds inside the pot, creating very high temperatures that cook food quickly.

Types of Bakeware

Baking pans come in a wide variety of shapes, sizes, and materials, as shown in **Figure 21.5**. The type and quality of the bakeware you choose affects the texture and appearance of the finished product. You may need to adjust baking times and temperatures to fit to the pan you use. Basic bakeware includes:

Loaf Pan A loaf pan is a deep, narrow, rectangular pan that is used for baking loaves of bread or meat.

Cookie Sheet A cookie sheet is a flat, rectangular pan with two or three open sides that is used to bake cookies and biscuits.

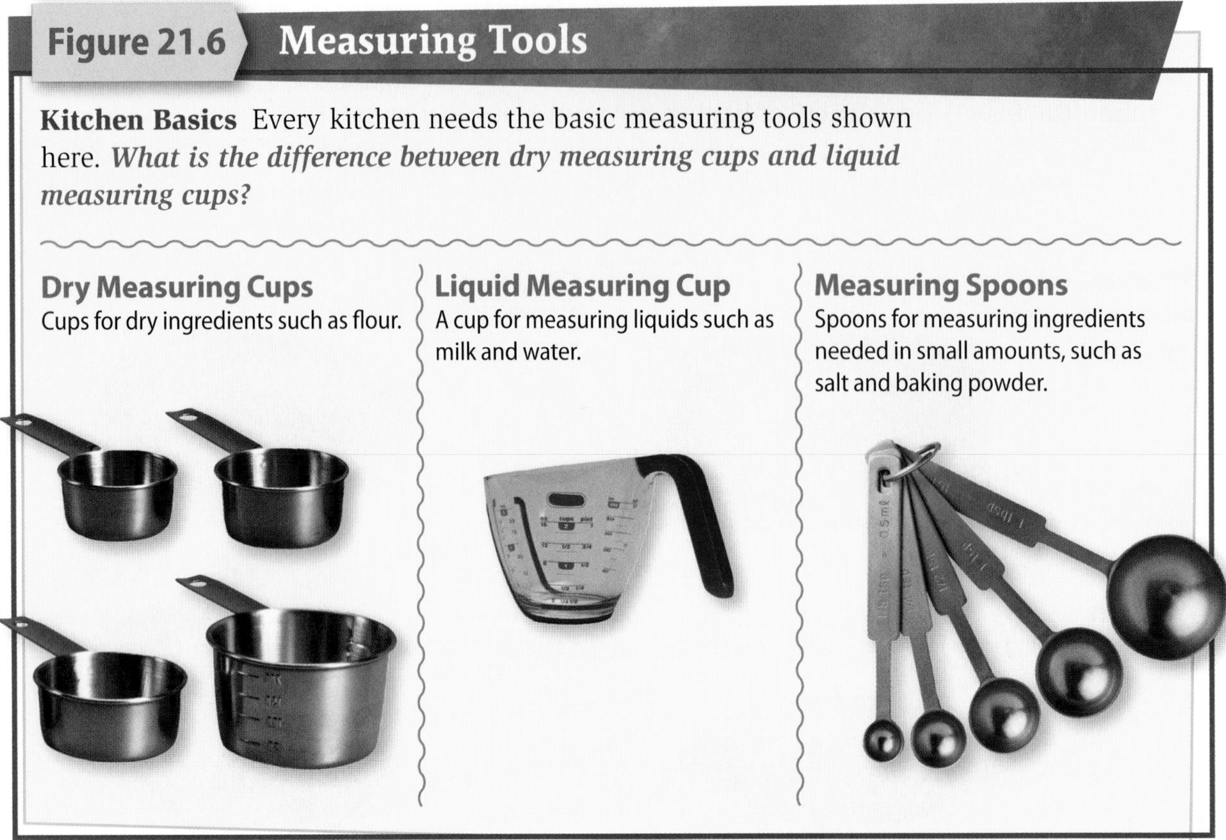

Dry Measuring Cups
Cups for dry ingredients such as flour.
Liquid Measuring Cup
A cup for measuring liquids such as milk and water.
Measuring Spoons
Spoons for measuring ingredients needed in small amounts, such as salt and baking powder.

Figure 21.6 Measuring Tools

Kitchen Basics Every kitchen needs the basic measuring tools shown here. ***What is the difference between dry measuring cups and liquid measuring cups?***

Baking Sheet A baking sheet is similar to a cookie sheet, but is about 1 inch deep. Baking sheets are used for sheet cakes, pizza, chicken pieces, and fish.

Cake Pan A cake pan is a round or square pan that is a few inches deep and about 8 to 10 inches across. Cake pans also come in novelty shapes.

Tube Pan A tube pan is a deep, one- or two-piece cake pan with a center tube. Tube pans are used for angel food cakes and sponge cakes.

Springform Pan A springform pan is a round pan with a removable bottom. The side is latched, which allows you to open it gently to remove cheesecake or another delicate dessert.

Pie Pan A pie pan is a round pan with slanted sides. Tart pans are similar in shape, but are smaller.

Muffin Pan A muffin pan, also called a muffin tin, holds 6 to 12 muffins, rolls, or cupcakes.

Roasting Pan A roasting pan is a large, heavy oval or rectangular pan. Roasting pans are used for roasting meats and whole poultry.

Casserole A casserole is used for baking and serving main dishes and desserts. Casseroles come in many different sizes, with or without lids.

Aluminum Foil Pan Aluminum foil pans are lightweight recyclable pans.

Handheld Tools

Handheld implements help you measure, cut, mix, and cook food. (See **Figure 21.6**.) Handheld tools are made from a variety of materials including wood, plastic, glass, metal, and heat-resistant silicone.

Measuring Tools

Measuring tools help you follow recipes exactly. The basic measuring tools include:

Dry Measuring Cups Dry measuring cups come in a set of several sizes, usually ¼ cup, ⅓ cup, ½ cup, and 1 cup. A metric set includes 50 mL, 125 mL, and 250 mL measures.

Liquid Measuring Cups Liquid measuring cups are transparent glass or plastic cups with measurements marked on the side. They are typically marked in fluid ounces, in fractions of a cup, and in milliliters. Liquid measuring cups have a headspace of about ¼ inch, which helps prevent spills when you move a filled cup. A spout helps with pouring. Common sizes are 1 and 2 cups.

Measuring Spoons Measuring spoons usually come in sets of four or five. Standard sets include four sizes: ¼ teaspoon, ½ teaspoon, 1 teaspoon, and 1 tablespoon. Metric sets include five measures: 1 mL, 2 mL, 5 mL, 15 mL, and 25 mL.

Kitchen Scales Kitchen scales measure food by weight rather than volume. Both spring scales and digital, plug-in scales are available.

Cutting Tools

Knives are the basic cutting tools in the kitchen. A quality knife has a sturdy handle firmly attached to the blade by at least two rivets, or bolts with heads. Peelers, shears, and choppers also help with cutting tasks in the kitchen. It is important to choose the right cutting tool for the job.

TECHNOLOGY FOR TOMORROW

Nonstick Technology

The nonstick finish that coats some bakeware and cookware is the most slippery substance known. If it is so slippery, how do manufacturers make it stick to the pan? The process involves both mechanics and chemistry. Cookware is coated with a film of microscopic grains of ceramic, and sometimes titanium. This mix is liquified and sprayed on with force, creating a textured surface. An adhesive layer is applied next, which also helps hold the top, nonstick surface coat. The cookware is baked at 800° for about five minutes, melding the layers.

Investigate Nonstick technology makes cooking easier. Conduct research to learn how cooks prevented food from sticking before nonstick technology was invented.

NCSS VIII A Science, Technology, and Society Identify and describe both current and historical examples of the interaction and interdependence of science, technology, and society in a variety of cultural settings.

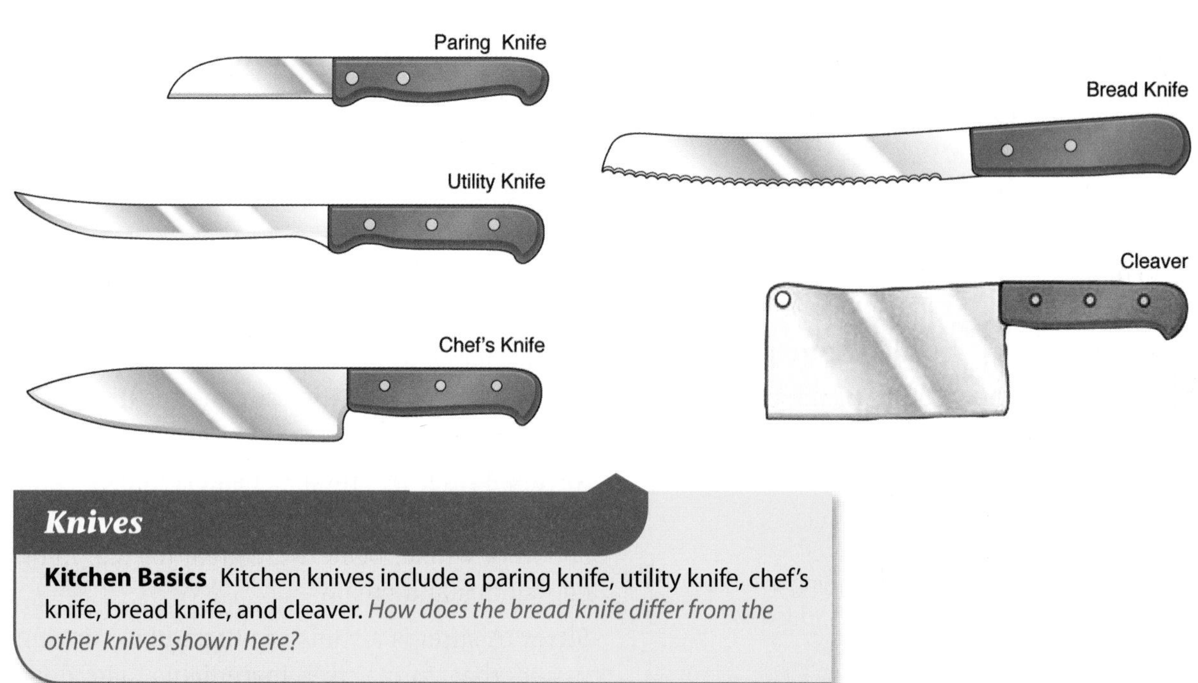

Knives

Kitchen Basics Kitchen knives include a paring knife, utility knife, chef's knife, bread knife, and cleaver. *How does the bread knife differ from the other knives shown here?*

Here are some common cutting tools:

Bread Knife A bread knife has a serrated or saw-tooth blade for slicing bread.

Slicing Knife A slicing knife is a large knife used for meat and poultry.

Chef's Knife Also called a French knife, a chef's knife has a large, triangular blade for slicing, chopping, and dicing.

Utility Knife A utility knife is a small slicing knife that is good for cutting small foods such as tomatoes and apples.

Boning Knife A boning knife has a thin, angled blade suited for removing bones.

Paring Knife A paring knife is a small knife for removing the peel from fruits and vegetables.

Vegetable Peeler A peeler has a swivel blade for quickly paring fruits and vegetables.

Kitchen Shears Shears are powerful scissors used for snipping, trimming, and cutting.

Food Chopper A food chopper is a small food processor. Choppers come in various sizes, from small handheld nut choppers to large electric models with several blades.

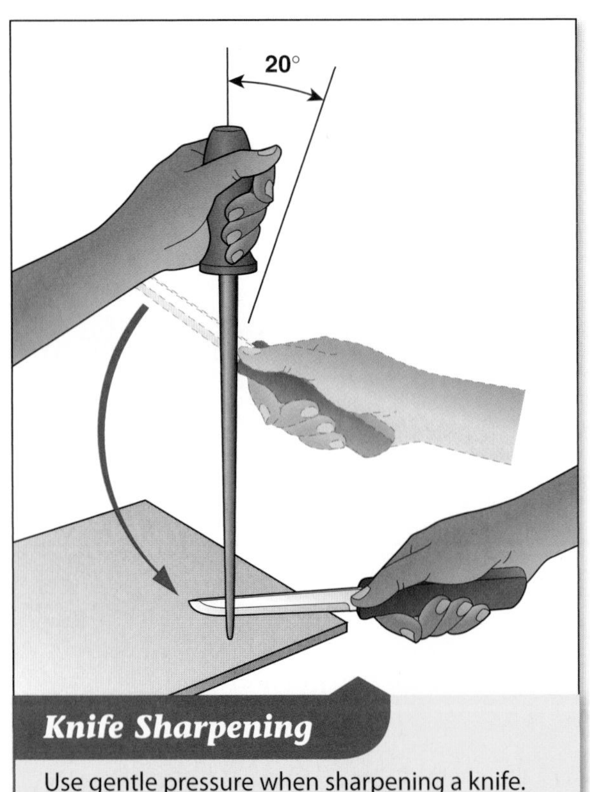

Knife Sharpening

Use gentle pressure when sharpening a knife. Follow the technique shown here, which is described in the text on this page.

Food Grinder A food grinder grinds meat, poultry, nuts, and other foods. Grinders can also be used for grating and shredding.

Pizza Wheel A pizza wheel is a round revolving blade on a handle for slicing pizza and cutting rolled-out dough.

Cutting Board A cutting board protects the countertop and the knife. Plastic cutting boards resist bacteria better than wood boards.

Keeping Knives Sharp

Knives need regular sharpening on a sharpening stone. You can also keep most conventional knives sharp longer with a sharpening steel, a long, steel rod with a handle. Use the steel regularly, following these directions:

1. Hold the handle of the steel in your left hand (or in your right hand if you are left-handed). Place the point straight down, very firmly, on a secure cutting board. Hold the knife by the handle, blade down, with your right hand (or your left hand, if you are left-handed).
2. Hold the knife blade at a 20-degree angle against the side of the steel. The knife blade and steel should touch near the handles.
3. Draw the blade down the steel and toward you, keeping a 20-degree angle to the steel. Use gentle pressure.
4. When the tip of the knife reaches the tip of the steel, repeat the process, holding the knife against the steel. Draw the blade down along the steel four or five times, alternating right and left sides.

Mixing Tools

Spoons, bowls, whisks, and other small tools like the ones shown in **Figure 21.7,** make quick work of mixing ingredients.

Wire Whisk A whisk is an instrument made of wire loops that are held together by a handle. Whisks are used for stirring, beating, and whipping.

Rotary Beater A rotary beater mixes and whips food more quickly and easily than a spoon or whisk. Beaters are great for whipping egg whites and cream.

Sifter A sifter is a canister with a blade or ring inside that forces dry ingredients like flour

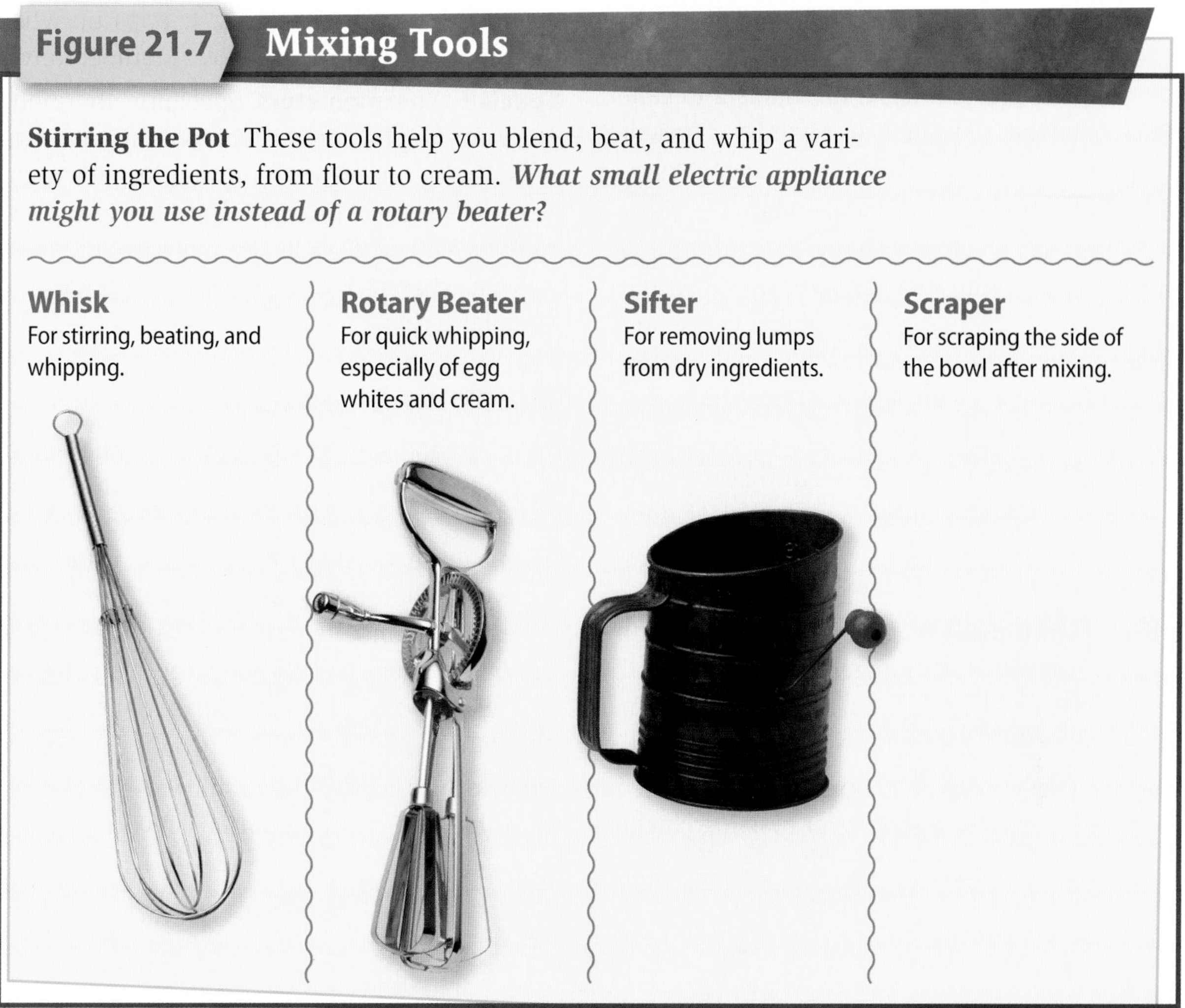

through a wire screen at the bottom to make finer particles.

Figure 21.7 Mixing Tools

Stirring the Pot These tools help you blend, beat, and whip a variety of ingredients, from flour to cream. ***What small electric appliance might you use instead of a rotary beater?***

Whisk
For stirring, beating, and whipping.
Rotary Beater
For quick whipping, especially of egg whites and cream.
Sifter
For removing lumps from dry ingredients.
Scraper
For scraping the side of the bowl after mixing.

Scraper A scraper quickly scrapes food from bowls, pans, and other containers. Scrapers can also be used for light mixing.

Cooking and Baking Tools

A variety of hand tools, as shown in **Figure 21.8**, help with a variety of cooking and baking tasks.

Turner A turner, or spatula, lets you lift and turn flat foods, such as pancakes on a griddle or cookies on a cookie sheet.

Tongs Tongs are like giant tweezers for gripping and lifting foods.

Baster A baster is a long tube with a bulb on the end that is used to suction up meat juices or other sauces for basting food that is cooking.

Ladle A ladle is a large, angled spoon with a long handle. It is used for dipping hot liquids from a pan.

Pastry Brush A pastry brush lets you brush a sauce on foods or glazes on pastry.

Rolling Pin A rolling pin helps you roll out dough for biscuits, cookies, and pies.

Wire Cooling Rack A wire cooling rack holds baked goods safely until they cool.

Potholder/Oven Mitt Potholders and mitts are thick cloth pads that protect your hands while you handle hot containers.

Food Thermometers

Food thermometers measure a food's exact temperature, which helps with safe and successful cooking. Some thermometers measure internal temperature, which reveals whether meats, poultry, egg dishes, and leftovers are safely cooked. Choose a thermometer that is easy to read and that has a mechanism to calibrate, or adjust, the gauge for accuracy. Types of thermometers are described on the next page.

Oven-Safe Thermometer An oven-safe thermometer has a large dial or indicator on a probe, which you stick into roasts or whole poultry and leave in during cooking. Oven-safe thermometers do not work with small pieces of food. Some oven-safe thermometers are designed for microwave ovens.

Instant-Read Thermometer An instant-read thermometer has a probe with a dial or digital display. You stick the thermometer into the food and get an instant temperature reading.

Disposable Indicator A disposable indicator is a heat sensor that changes color when food reaches the proper internal temperature. You use it once, then throw it away.

Pop-Up Thermometer A pop-up thermometer is sometimes used in turkeys or roasting chickens sold by food processors. It pops up when food reaches the proper internal temperature.

Specialty Thermometers Specialty thermometers are helpful for certain cooking methods. A candy thermometer, for example, clips to the side of a pan to measure the temperature of candy syrup as it cooks. A frying thermometer is used to record the temperature of oil in a deep-fat fryer.

Cleanup Supplies

Keep food safe by cleaning tools and equipment after every use. Disease-causing bacteria can grow even in tiny bits of food. Most tools can be washed in hot, soapy water. Use a towel to thoroughly wipe off tools and appliances that cannot be immersed in water. Check the owner's manual for cleaning instructions. You will need these cleanup supplies in the kitchen:

Dishcloths Use dishcloths for washing dishes and cleaning work surfaces. Have at least a

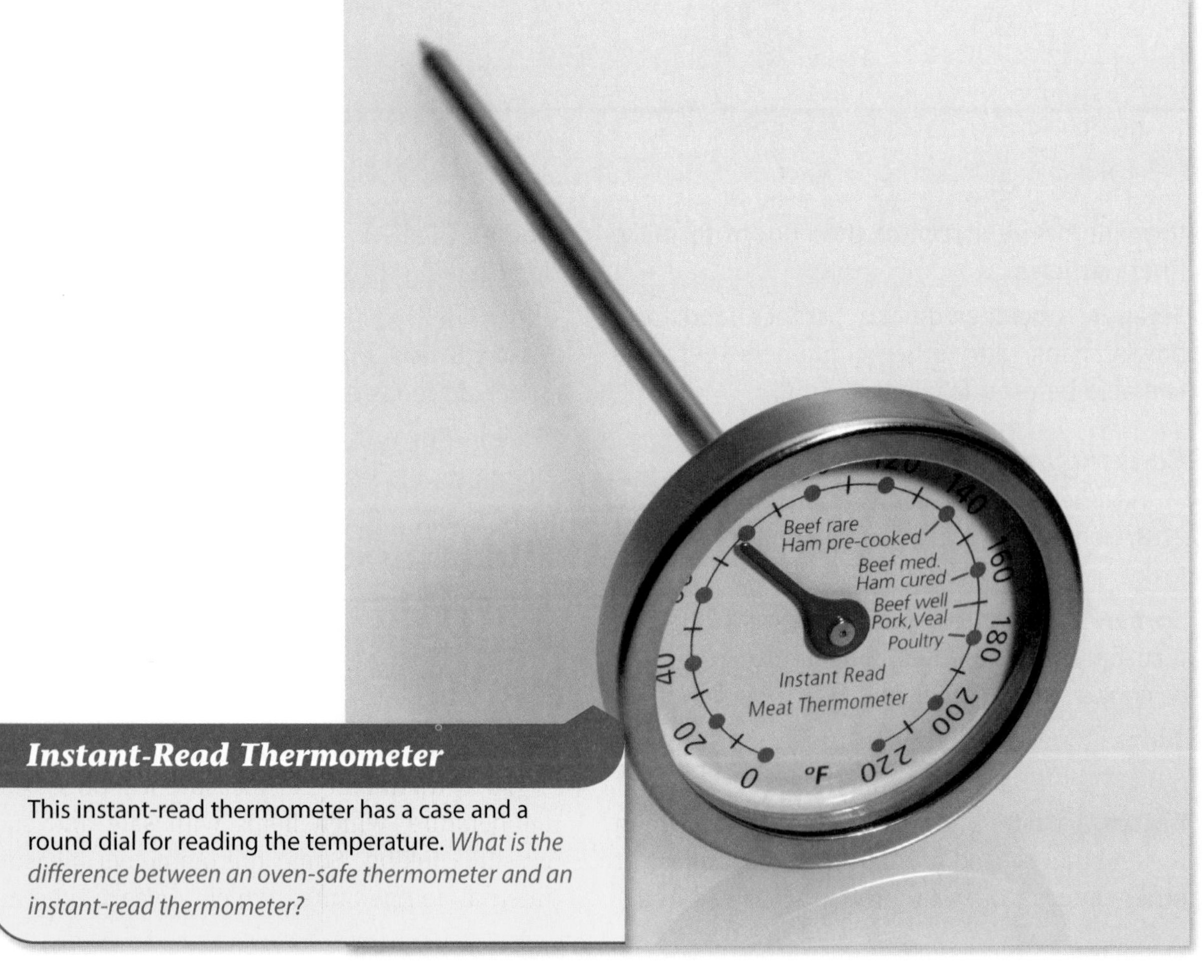

Instant-Read Thermometer

This instant-read thermometer has a case and a round dial for reading the temperature. *What is the difference between an oven-safe thermometer and an instant-read thermometer?*

Figure 21.8 Baking and Cooking Tools

Kitchen Basics These tools can cook food, serve food, or remove it from the range or oven. ***How would you use each one?***

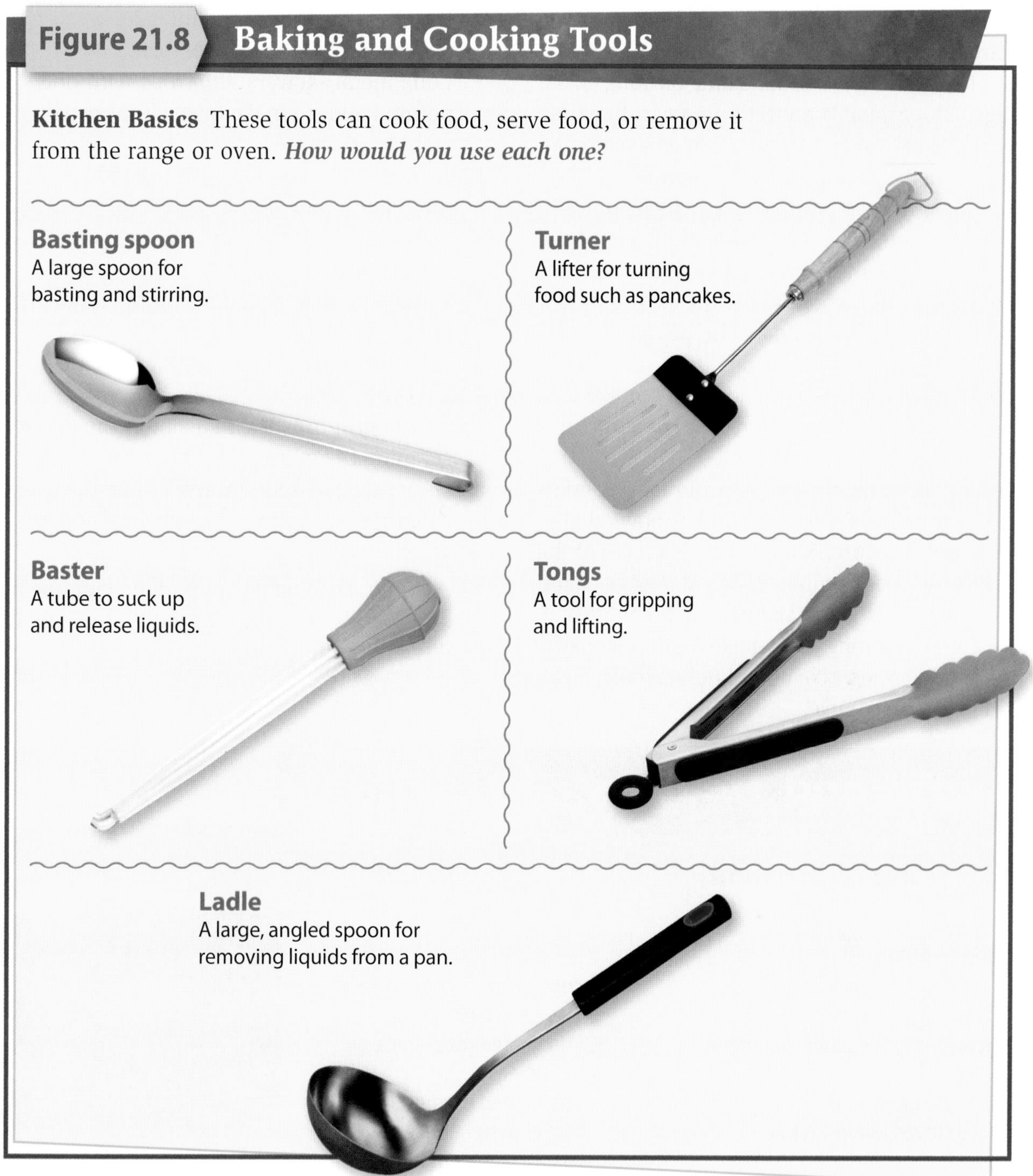

dozen dishcloths so that you can use a fresh one every day.

Basting spoon
A large spoon for basting and stirring.
Turner
A lifter for turning food such as pancakes.
Baster
A tube to suck up and release liquids.
Tongs
A tool for gripping and lifting.
Ladle
A large, angled spoon for removing liquids from a pan.

Dishtowels Use dishtowels, which are larger than dishcloths, to dry dishes and equipment. Have plenty on hand and keep them clean.

Scouring Pads Use scouring pads to scrub hard-to-clean spots on pots and pans. Steel wool pads work for cooked-on food, but will scratch some surfaces. Nylon pads are needed for some metals and finishes.

Bottle Brush Use a bottle brush to clean the inside of jars, bottles, and similar containers.

Dish Drainer Use a dish drainer to let dishes air-dry.

Grills and Grilling Tools

Most outdoor grills have a fire bowl, which is a box- or bowl-shaped metal container that holds the burning charcoal. A metal grate fits over the fire bowl to hold food over hot coals.

Grills with a fire bowl and grate come in many variations, from a portable hibachi to a 6-foot stretch grill. Kettle grills stand on long metal legs. Other models are set into a cart-like base with a work table attached. Some have domed lids to help maintain even temperatures.

Gas grills use propane gas, which comes in a heavy tank that attaches to the base of the grill. Gas grills are more expensive than charcoal grills. Some cooks prefer the taste imparted by grilling with charcoal. The advantage of a gas grill is that you do not have to wait for coals to warm before cooking. A smoker is a covered grill that burns aromatic wood chips, flavoring food as it cooks.

A good grill is stable and durable. A grill's legs should be level, and the fire bowl should be evenly balanced on the legs. All parts of the grill should be securely attached. Heavy, stainless steel grills withstand rust, wear, and tear.

Quality grilling tools make outdoor cooking safer and easier. Like other kitchen tools, clean them after each use.

Handy items for grilling include:

- A basket for grilling vegetables.
- Long metal skewers, thin rods with one pointed end, to make meat, fruit, or vegetable kebabs.
- A work table near the grill to hold tools, food, and other supplies.
- Long tongs for gripping, placing and turning food on the grill.
- A long metal spatula for flipping food such as hamburgers.
- A baster or spray bottle to put out flare-ups.
- Fireproof mitts.
- A wire grill brush with a slot in the end for scraping the grate.
- Heavy-duty aluminum foil to line the grill, catch grease, and hold small foods on the grate.

As with all kitchen tools and equipment, the best grills and grilling tools are high in quality and built to last.

Light and Healthy Recipe

Slow-Cooked Lasagna

This recipe allows you to make a healthy meal ahead of time.

Ingredients

- **1 pound** Italian sausage
- **1 cup** Diced onion
- **1 jar (15 oz.)** Prepared spaghetti sauce
- **2 cups** Water
- **3 cloves** Minced garlic
- **½ cup** Fat-free ricotta cheese
- **1 tsp.** Chopped oregano
- **½ cup** Grated mozzarella cheese
- **½ cup** Grated parmesan cheese
- **8 oz.** Lasagna noodles

Directions

1. Chop and cook the sausage and onions in a pan.
2. In a large bowl, combine the sausage and onions with the sauce, water, garlic, ricotta cheese, and oregano. Combine and mix the mozzarella and parmesan cheeses.
3. Spread ⅓ of the sauce across the bottom of the slow cooker crock.
4. Top the mixture with ⅓ of the cheese. Lay lasagna noodles over the sauce and cheese, breaking the noodles as needed.
5. Repeat steps 3 and 4 twice.
6. Turn the slow cooker on low for five to six hours. Serve hot.

Yield 10 servings

Nutrition Analysis per Serving

■ Calories	236
■ Total fat	6 g
Saturated fat	3 g
Cholesterol	19 mg
■ Sodium	391 mg
■ Carbohydrate	28 g
Dietary fiber	2 g
Sugars	7 g
■ Protein	15 g

CHAPTER 21 Review & Applications

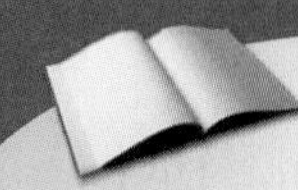

After You Read

Chapter Summary

A well-designed kitchen is organized for efficiency and promotes good work flow. Work centers and universal design make kitchens easy to use. Kitchen components must withstand heat, moisture, and food. Ample cabinets and countertops, durable floors and walls, safe electrical systems, and good lighting are important. Before buying items for the kitchen, consider needs, prioritize features, and conduct research. Shop critically, pay carefully, and protect your purchase. Appliances, including ranges, refrigerators, and dishwashers, help you prepare food and clean up. Preparation tools and equipment, including cookware, bakeware, and utensils, help with cooking and serving.

Content and Academic Vocabulary Review

1. Use at least eight of these key terms and academic vocabulary words in a descriptive paragraph about your dream kitchen.

Content Vocabulary

- work flow (p. 316)
- work center (p. 316)
- work triangle (p. 316)
- peninsula (p. 316)
- island (p. 316)
- universal design (p. 317)
- grounding (p. 319)
- task lighting (p. 319)
- EnergyGuide label (p. 320)
- warranty (p. 321)
- service contract (p. 321)
- credit (p. 321)
- down payment (p. 321)
- principal (p. 321)
- interest (p. 322)
- annual percentage rate (APR) (p. 322)
- finance charge (p. 322)
- heating unit (p. 322)
- convection oven (p. 323)
- cookware (p. 326)
- bakeware (p. 326)

Academic Vocabulary

- assess (p. 319)
- versatile (p. 325)

Review Key Concepts

2. **Explain** the items that make up a work triangle.
3. **Describe** three factors to consider when selecting kitchen components.
4. **Explain** the difference between a warranty and a service contract.
5. **List** three large kitchen appliances and nine small kitchen appliances.
6. **Describe** seven common types of cookware.

Critical Thinking

7. **Explain** how Henry can have more counter space to his kitchen without doing any construction.
8. **Describe** a good approach to buying a new dishwasher.
9. **Decide** the best course of action for washing dishes during a drought period. Explain your answer.
10. **Explain** why using dry measuring cups to measure both liquid and dry ingredients might cause a cake to fall.

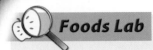

Foods Lab

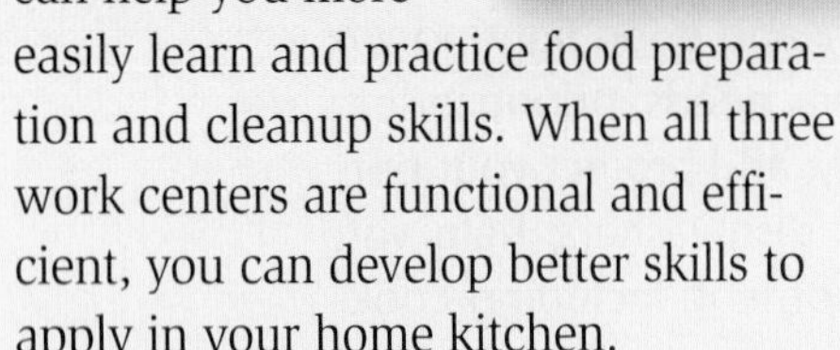

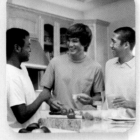

11. Work Centers in the Foods Lab Having a well-designed foods lab can help you more easily learn and practice food preparation and cleanup skills. When all three work centers are functional and efficient, you can develop better skills to apply in your home kitchen.

Procedure Prepare a simple recipe that requires the use of all three basic work centers in the foods lab. Pay attention to how well the lab layout and design of each station accommodates more than one person at a time.

Analysis In a class discussion, provide feedback to these questions: Is the lab convenient for more than one person to use? Are items arranged conveniently in each work center? Are the lab, cookware, and supplies accessible to people of varying abilities? Why or why not? How might any problems be corrected?

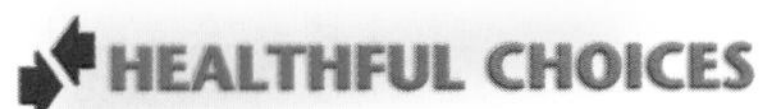

HEALTHFUL CHOICES

12. Low-Fat Cookware Harold is on a low-fat diet recommended by his doctor. He is shopping for a frying pan that will allow him to sauté vegetables without adding too much fat. Should he choose stainless steel or nonstick? Why?

TECH Connection

13. Appliance Comparison Under your teacher's supervision, use the Internet to comparison shop for one of these appliances: refrigerator-freezer, gas or electric range, convection or microwave oven, or dishwasher. Examine several models of the appliance you choose. Learn what features are available and decide on the make and model you want. Set a dollar amount you are willing to spend before you begin shopping. What features does each model have? What is covered by the warranty? Which product would you recommend buying and why? Prepare a summary of the product you chose to present to your class. Include an explanation of the product, your reasons for choosing that particular model, and the best price you could find.

Real-World Skills

Problem-Solving Skills	**14. Tight Spaces** Gwen noticed a milk residue inside a narrow drinking glass that had already been through the dishwasher. What type of cleanup supply can she use to get the glass clean where her hand cannot reach?
Interpersonal and Collaborative Skills	**15. Kitchen Floor Plans** Follow your teacher's instructions to form pairs. Using images from magazines, work together to create a photo display of a kitchen floor plan. Label work centers, peninsulas and islands, indicate work triangles, and evaluate your plan for efficency.
Financial Literacy Skills	**16. Cash or Credit?** You can buy a new $1,500 dollar range on credit, and spend three years paying it off at a 12% APR. How much would you save if you paid for it entirely in cash?

Academic Skills

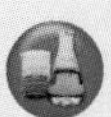

Food Science

17. The Right Cookware Non-stick pans have advantages and disadvantages. Sometimes we do not want food to stick, but other times we like caramelization, browning of surface sugars, to occur. Determine how this is affected by nonstick surfaces.

Procedure Get a non-stick skillet and a regular skillet, filming the bottoms with a small amount of cooking oil. Dip two thin pork chops in flour seasoned with salt and pepper. Heat the skillets first, carefully adding the chops. Cook on the first side until nicely browned, then repeat on the opposite side. Remove. Create a table to contrast both effects, including color, appearance, taste.

Analysis Is caramelization affected by the non-stick surface? Which skillet would work best for pancakes or fried eggs? Make a list of advantages and disadvantages for non-stick equipment for various cooking tasks.

NSES B Develop an understanding of interactions of energy and matter.

Mathematics

18. Calculate Counter Space Sam has decided to remodel his kitchen. According to the plans, the counter to the left of the sink measures 2 feet by 4 feet, while another to the right of the sink measures 2 feet by 5 feet. On the other wall, counters on both sides of the stovetop will each measure 2 feet by 3 feet. The kitchen will also have a 7 feet by 4 feet island. How much total counter space will Sam's new kitchen have?

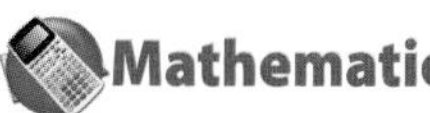

Math Concept **Area of a Rectangle** The area of a rectangle is equal to its length times its width: $A = lw$. If necessary, convert the length and the width to the same units before multiplying.

Starting Hint Multiply the length and width of each of the counters to find each counter's surface area in square feet. Then, add the areas together.

NCTM Measurement Apply appropriate techniques, tools, and formulas to determine measurements.

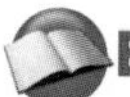

English Language Arts

19. Equipping a Kitchen You write an advice column. A reader, Mary, has sent you a letter asking what appliances and supplies she will need to equip the kitchen in her new home. Write her a response explaining what she will need immediately and what she can buy in the future.

NCTE 4 Use written language to communicate effectively.

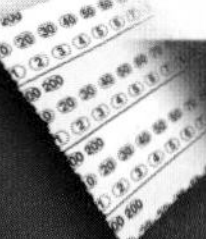

STANDARDIZED TEST PRACTICE

ANALOGY

Read the pairs of terms. Then choose the best word to match.

20. dishwasher : large appliance
measuring cup: handheld tool
blender: small appliance
____________ : cookware

a. knife
b. saucepan
c. food processor
d. range

Test-Taking Tip When you look at the three pairs of terms listed here, identify the relationship that is common to all of them. The answer that establishes the same type of relationship as the other terms is correct.

CHAPTER 22

Conserving Resources

Writing Activity — Advertisement

Earth-Friendly Appliances Kitchen appliances that conserve energy and water are better for the environment. Write an original magazine advertisement for an earth-friendly kitchen appliance. Your advertisement may be for a product that you imagine, or one that already exists. Your advertisement should contain about 100 words.

Writing Tips Follow these steps to write an advertisement:

- Capture readers' attention with a catchy phrase.
- Educate readers about your product using details and descriptions.
- Persuade readers to buy your product using relevant facts.

Activate Prior Knowledge

Explore the Photo Preparing food uses resources like food, water, and energy. *What are some ways to conserve energy and water?*

Reading Guide

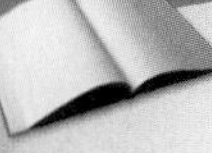

Before You Read

Preview Skim the chapter, noting photos, figures, captions, and headings. Then list three habits you have that may use up valuable environmental resources.

Read to Learn

Key Concepts

- **Explain** how conservation benefits people and the environment.
- **Describe** how to use large kitchen appliances efficiently.
- **List** eight ways to conserve water in the kitchen.
- **Summarize** two guidelines for reducing trash.
- **Explain** how population growth is affecting the world's resources.

Main Idea

Conserving resources saves money, improves efficiency in the kitchen, and helps future generations to enjoy a healthy environment.

Content Vocabulary

You will find definitions for these words in the glossary at the back of this book.

- ☐ conservation
- ☐ nonrenewable resource
- ☐ greenhouse gas
- ☐ renewable resource
- ☐ biodegradable
- ☐ sanitary landfill
- ☐ food waste
- ☐ recycle

Academic Vocabulary

You will find these words in your reading and on your tests. Use the glossary to look up their definitions if necessary.

- consumption
- synthetic

Graphic Organizer

Use a graphic organizer like the one below to list eight ways you can conserve water while preparing and serving a meal.

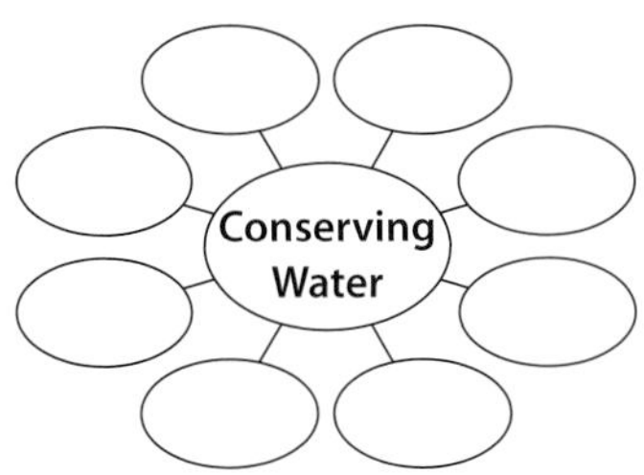

Graphic Organizer Go to this book's Online Learning Center at **glencoe.com** to print out this graphic organizer.

Academic Standards

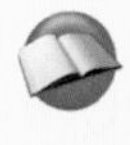

English Language Arts

NCTE 7 Conduct research and gather, evaluate, and synthesize data to communicate discoveries.

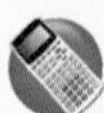

Mathematics

NCTM Number and Operations Understand numbers, ways of representing numbers, relationships among numbers, and number systems.

NCTM Problem Solving Solve problems that arise in mathematics and in other contexts.

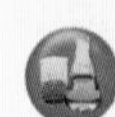

Science

NSES C Develop an understanding of the structure and properties of matter.

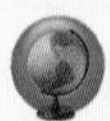

Social Studies

NCSS I A Analyze and explain the ways groups, societies, and cultures address human needs and concerns.

NCTE *National Council of Teachers of English*
NCTM *National Council of Teachers of Mathematics*
NSES *National Science Education Standards*
NCSS *National Council for the Social Studies*

Why Conserve?

Conservation is the protection of the environment to preserve it for the future. When you conserve, you use only as much food, water, energy, and other resources as you need so that future generations can enjoy a healthy environment. Conserving also helps you save money and work more efficiently in the kitchen.

Renewable and Nonrenewable Resources

Most of the electricity we use in our homes is generated by power plants that burn fossil fuels. A fossil fuel is an energy source such as coal, oil, or natural gas that is formed in the earth by the remains of plants and animals.

Fossil fuels are a **nonrenewable resource**. Nonrenewable resources are produced so slowly that they cannot be replaced as quickly as they are used. Coal, for example, takes hundreds of millions of years to form.

The burning of fossil fuels releases pollutants and greenhouse gases into the environment. A **greenhouse gas** is a gas that traps heat in the earth's atmosphere and contributes to global warming. Conserving nonrenewable resources helps reduce global warming and ensure that we leave resources for future generations.

Conservation is equally important for renewable resources, such as water, timber, and solar energy. A **renewable resource** is a resource that can be replaced once it is used. Some renewable resources, such as sun and wind, are plentiful. Other renewable resources, such as clean water, topsoil, and wood from trees, are being used faster than they can be replaced. Food is a renewable resource, but producing food requires the use of nonrenewable resources, such as fuel for farm equipment and transportation. Meat is processed using fossil fuels, as well. Your food choices have a large impact on the environment.

✓ **Reading Check** **Define** What is a fossil fuel?

Using Energy Efficiently

Small steps can help you reduce your use of gas and electricity and save money on your energy bill. For example, you can save up to 75 percent on lighting by replacing incandescent bulbs with compact fluorescent bulbs. Major appliances use most of the energy in the kitchen, so it is important to use them efficiently.

Refrigerator

Refrigerators use about 15 percent of all the energy in a typical home, so it is important to take steps to keep your refrigerator efficient:

- Help the condenser coils release heat by vacuuming them at least twice a year.
- Keep the refrigerator and freezer doors closed as much as possible. Decide what you want before opening the door. Keep the refrigerator and freezer well organized so you can find food quickly.

Kitchen Math

Avoid Wasting Water

Oscar's kitchen faucet has been dripping for four days at a steady rate of one drip every 3 seconds (or 20 drips per minute). If it takes 8,000 drips to fill up a 2-liter soda bottle, how many 2-liter soda bottles could Oscar fill with all of the water that dripped in four full days?

Math Concept **Solving Problems with Proportions** Write two equal ratios (known as a proportion) to relate a quantity you already know to another you are solving for. Use *x* to represent the unknown amount in the second ratio.

Starting Hint Determine the total minutes in four days by multiplying $4 \times 24 \times 60$. Use a proportion and solve for *x* to find the number of drips during that period: 20 drips / 1 minute = *x* drips / (total minutes in 4 days). Divide by 8,000 to find the number of 2-liter bottles.

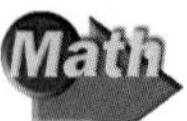

Appendix For math help, go to the Math Appendix at the back of the book.

NCTM Number and Operations Understand numbers, ways of representing numbers, relationships among numbers, and number systems.

- Check that the doors on your refrigerator have a tight seal. Hold a dollar bill against the frame and close the door on it. If the door does not hold the dollar securely, it is not holding cold air in or keeping warm air out. Repair or replace the rubber gasket around the door to create a tighter seal.
- When choosing a refrigerator-freezer, consider models with a top-mount freezer, which use less energy than side-by-side models.

Oven

Save energy by using your oven wisely:

- Open the oven only when needed. Each time you open the door, heat escapes. When the oven temperature drops, more energy is needed to raise it again. Use the oven light to check on foods instead of opening the door.
- Plan meals that allow you to cook several foods at the same time.
- Use glass cookware if possible. Glass absorbs heat better than metal, so oven temperatures in recipes can be lowered by 25°F.
- Only preheat the oven if you are making baked goods. Most recipes do not require a preheated oven.
- Consider whether you can use a smaller appliance, such as an electric skillet, slow cooker, or microwave oven instead of a conventional oven. Microwave ovens use about half the energy of conventional ovens.

Cooktop

When you use a cooktop, you can save energy with these simple habits:

- Cover pots that have cooking liquid inside them. Liquid in a covered pot boils more quickly than liquid in an uncovered one. The cover holds the heat inside, allowing the temperature to rise faster. Lower the heat after liquids come to a boil, using just enough heat to keep them bubbling.
- On an electric cooktop, match the size of the pan to the size of the heating element. Using a small pan on a large heating element wastes energy.

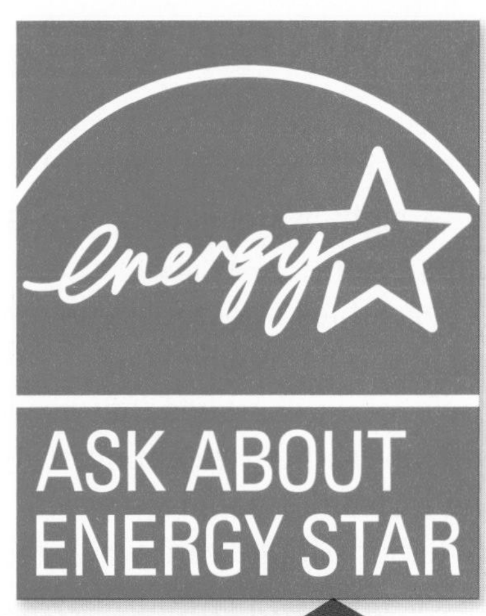

Good Buy

Appliances and light fixtures with the ENERGY STAR label help conserve resources and cost less money to operate. *What is the difference between the EnergyGuide label and the ENERGY STAR label?*

- Turn off the heat a few minutes before the food is done. Enough heat will remain in the food to finish the job.
- Make more than one serving of food, such as pasta or soup, at a time.

Shopping for Energy Efficiency

When it is time to replace an appliance, compare EnergyGuide labels, which list energy efficiency and average annual cost to operate, to find the most efficient model. Also look for the ENERGY STAR® label. This mark is found on refrigerators, dishwashers, lighting fixtures, and other appliances and indicates that the item meets strict government standards for energy efficiency. All appliances with the ENERGY STAR label also have an EnergyGuide label.

✓ **Reading Check** **Explain** When shopping for an appliance, how can you find the most energy-efficient model?

Using Water Wisely

Many people take water for granted, but clean water is a precious natural resource. Make these eight water-saving habits part of your kitchen routine:

- Wash vegetables under just enough running water to get them clean.
- Choose cooking methods that use less water—for example, steaming or microwaving instead of boiling.
- Ask whether people want water to drink with their meal before pouring.
- Wash dishes in a filled sink or basin instead of under constantly running water. Then rinse them as quickly as possible.
- If you use a dishwasher, scrape dishes instead of rinsing them before loading. Run the appliance with full loads only.
- Do not dump hazardous household chemicals into the water system. Call your local sanitation department to learn how to dispose of them safely.
- Make sure your kitchen faucet does not drip. Water dripping at the rate of one drop per second can waste about 700 gallons, or 11,200 cups, a year.
- Install a low-flow aerator on your faucet. An aerator is a simple attachment that mixes air with water to maintain water pressure but reduce water flow. It can save about 3 gallons of water a day.

Reading Check **Describe** Describe a way to conserve water while cooking.

SAFETY MATTERS

Hazardous Chemicals

Have you ever wondered what happens to the hazardous chemical waste people produce? When leftover household chemicals like cleaners, paints, and pesticides are disposed of down the drain or in rain gutters, they may be out of sight and out of mind, but their effects on land, oceans, and drinking water can be devastating. Community sanitation departments have strict regulations for hazardous chemical disposal, and many will pick up chemicals from your home. At treatment facilities, chemicals like drain cleaner and poisons are neutralized or incinerated. Some chemicals are placed in hazardous waste landfills, which must be strictly managed to protect the health of the people, animals, land, and water around them.

What Would You Do? You have decided to "go green" and keep a chemical-free household. You still have several chemical cleaners under your kitchen sink. What will you do?

Reducing Trash and Waste

The average American produces about 4.5 pounds of trash each day. It is easy to reduce the amount of trash you create by reusing materials and recycling wherever possible. It is also important to reduce your **consumption**, or the amount of resources you use.

Trash contains both biodegradable and non-biodegradable materials. **Biodegradable** materials can be broken down by microorganisms. Yard trimmings and kitchen waste are biodegradable. A banana peel, for example, will break down in about two weeks.

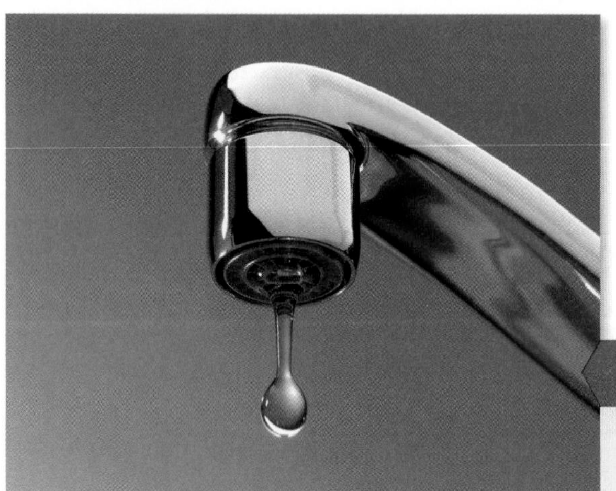

Easy Savings

Make sure your water faucets do not drip. *How can you save water when washing dishes?*

Figure 22.1 What's in the Trash?

Headed for the Landfill A large amount of trash in the United States consists of materials that could be recycled or composted. ***Which of these components of trash could be recycled? Which could be composted?***

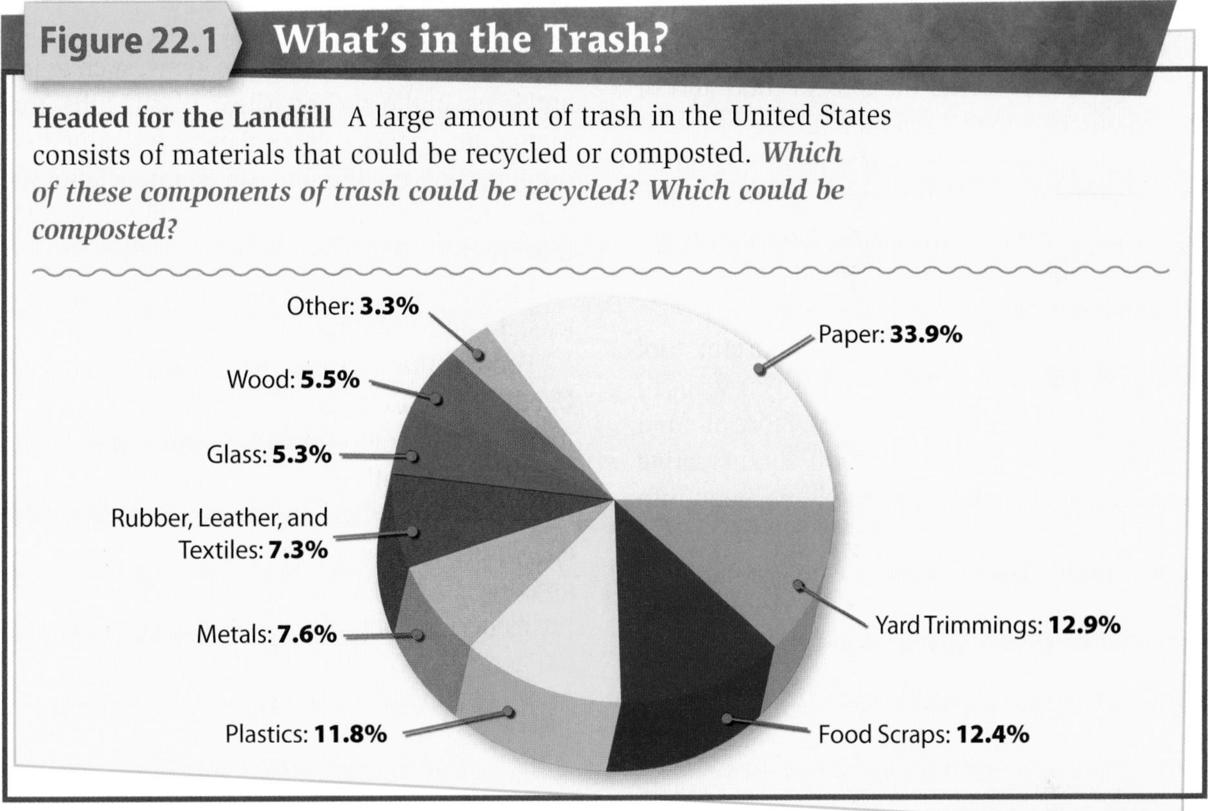

Non-biodegradable materials include plastic and styrofoam. Some materials biodegrade, but very slowly. A cigarette filter may take 12 years to break down. A disposable diaper may survive for 500 years. Some plastics and **synthetic**, or man-made, textiles may last forever.

Where does trash go? Some trash is burned, which reduces its volume but adds to air pollution. Most of our trash ends up in dumps, where it attracts pests, breeds harmful bacteria, and pollutes the land and water.

About half of our trash is buried in sanitary landfills, as shown in **Figure 22.1**. A **sanitary landfill** is a landfill insulated with clay and plastic liner. Trash is thinly spread, compacted, and covered with a layer of soil. The process is repeated until the area is full. Covering and compacting trash interferes with elements necessary for decay, such as oxygen and bacteria. Biodegradable items break down more slowly in sanitary landfills, and some materials may not break down at all.

Landfills are not a long-term solution to our waste problems. Despite precautions, landfills can leak or overflow and pollute soil and water. Landfills fill up quickly. They also can release greenhouse gases, such as methane.

Reduce

Reducing the quantity of materials you consume is the most important way to reduce the amount of trash you create. Reducing is sometimes called source reduction or precycling. Reducing helps the environment and can also save money. Follow these two guidelines to reduce the amount of trash you create.

- Choose minimally packaged fresh foods and bulk items over heavily packaged processed foods. Packaging is a major source of trash and accounts for 10 cents of every dollar you spend on food. Buy large containers of juice and pour them into reusable bottles rather than buying single-serving juice boxes.
- Limit your use of paper goods, which make up over a third of all trash. Use paper cups, plates, and napkins only if washing reusable tableware is impossible. Instead of paper towels, use a mop for spills on floors and a dishcloth for spills on countertops. Reducing, even in small ways, can make a big difference. By carrying your groceries in your own canvas bags or used paper bags, you can save a tree.

Food Waste

Food waste is edible food that is discarded. Food waste represents the loss of food and of the resources used to produce it.

People in the United States are accustomed to abundance and waste large amounts of food. Up to 20 percent of all edible food is thrown out. This adds up to half a pound of garbage per person each day.

Good meal planning is an important tool to reduce food waste. Know what you want to serve, and buy the right amounts. Store all food properly so that it does not spoil. Find creative ways to use leftovers. Cut dried-out bread into cubes for croutons, for example, or grate it for breadcrumbs. Use leftover mashed potatoes to top meat pies, thicken soups, and make yeast rolls. Get creative with casseroles, salads, soups, stews, meat pies, stir-fries, and omelets.

Reuse

Find ways to reuse inedible items, such as jars and bags, in the kitchen. Clean plastic tubs from margarine, yogurt, cottage cheese, and other food products and use them for refrigerating leftovers. Keep glass jars and bottles with tight-fitting lids to store rice, pasta, and dry beans. Wash the jars and lids carefully. Let open containers dry for at least 24 hours to remove odors.

Food containers can hold more than food. Used egg cartons can be used to store small items such as nuts and bolts or golf balls. Empty cereal boxes, with one corner and side cut diagonally, can be used to organize manila folders. Cut lengthwise, they make trays for letters, greeting cards, or school papers. Convert smaller boxes into coupon organizers. Boxes of all sizes are good for wrapping gifts or storing things.

Careers in Food

Dr. Edward Zimney
Consumer Advocate

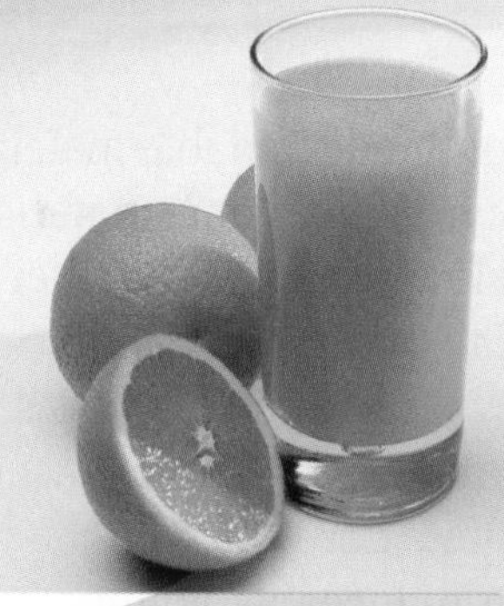

Q: How does someone become a consumer advocate?

A: To be a qualified consumer advocate, you need an understanding of science, medicine, and nutrition. Once you have that, all you need is the Internet for research, the willingness to write about it consistently and compellingly, and the honesty and courage to tell the truth.

Q: What specific things interest you?

A: I look for obvious fraud, scams, cons, and other examples of medical quackery that are advertised or promoted in the media. Unfortunately for consumers, such rip-offs are common.

Q: In your opinion, what is the single most vital food-related danger facing Americans today?

A: Obesity, no question. Over-eating of inexpensive, sugary, and fat-filled food products has led to an epidemic of health problems ranging from diabetes to heart disease, and even cancer.

"I try to expose fraud and provide information understandable by the average person."
— Dr. Ed Zimney
Medical Director, *HealthTalk.com – Seattle, WA*

Education and Training

A medical degree is useful, and a bachelor's degree in science is valuable. Experience as a physician or a specialist in any industry that affects consumers can provide a deeper context for understanding certain issues.

Qualities and Skills

You need to know how to get accurate information quickly. Technology skills and communication skills are essential. You have to be able to write and edit what you write.

Related Career Opportunities

Careers in the medical and food industries are closely related. Journalism careers also are related.

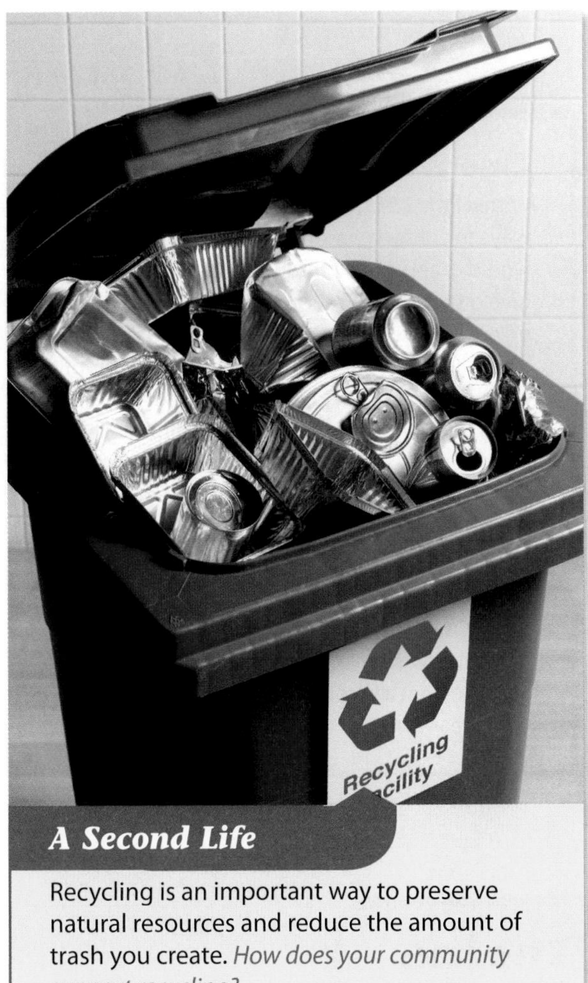

A Second Life

Recycling is an important way to preserve natural resources and reduce the amount of trash you create. *How does your community support recycling?*

TECHNOLOGY FOR TOMORROW

Bioplastics

Conventional petroleum-based plastic is not biodegradable. Recent technology has led to the creation of bioplastics—plastic products made from natural substances such as corn starch, pea starch, or vegetable oil. Bioplastics dissolve when exposed to heat and water, can be composted, and are biodegradable. These plastics are more earth-friendly because they are made from renewable resources rather than petroleum, a fossil fuel. Petroleum is still used as a source of energy during the manufacturing of bioplastics, because it is needed to power farm machinery, irrigate and transport crops, and more. Consequently, there is still room for improvement in this evolving technology.

Investigate Under your teacher's supervision, use the Internet to research how and where bioplastics are currently being used. Write a brief report on the results of your research.

NCSS I A Analyze and explain the ways groups, societies, and cultures address human needs and concerns.

Recycle

To **recycle** is to reprocess discarded products so they can be used again. Products are collected and sent to processing plants, where the raw materials are recovered to make something new.

Recycling cuts down on trash and pollution. It conserves energy and other resources. For example, it takes 90 percent less energy to manufacture a product from recycled aluminum than from the raw material. Recycling also reduces the need to mine for metal, cut down trees, and drill for oil.

Many kitchen items can be recycled. Learn which materials are recyclable in your area and how they should be sorted or prepared. Some communities have curbside pickup for recycled materials. In others, residents bring items to collection centers. In most communities, you can recycle clean newspapers, steel ("tin") cans, aluminum cans and foil, glass bottles, and some plastics. Many supermarkets accept clean plastic shopping bags.

When you shop, look for paper goods and plastics made from recycled materials. Look for the phrase "post-consumer" on cardboard and plastic containers. This supports the recycling industry and lets manufacturers know that protecting the environment matters to you.

✓ **Reading Check** **List** List three reasons that landfills are not a long-term solution to waste problems.

A World of Perspective on Conservation

As the world's population grows, so does the strain on the world's resources. A few years ago, the World Wildlife Fund, a conservation group, figured that the earth has about 28 billion acres of natural resources. With a global population of over 6.5 billion, that comes to 4.3 acres for each person.

The problem is that humans use about 5.6 acres per person—and some use far more. Each European uses about 12.4 acres per person, and Americans average 23.7 acres per person.

People around the world are practicing conservation and looking for solutions. Even simple actions such as carpooling, composting food scraps, and using refillable containers and bags can make a difference.

Be a Smart Consumer

Creative Conservation

With a little creativity, you can devise clever ways to conserve resources and reuse items that would otherwise be thrown away. For example, give grocery bags a second career as trash bags or wastebasket liners. Reuse paper bags to hold lawn clippings. Cut small holes into the sides of plastic milk cartons, fill them with birdseed, and hang them outside as birdfeeders. Empty glass jars can make great candle holders. Use egg cartons as planters for germinating seeds, and then transfer the plants to empty coffee cans.

Challenge Brainstorm a creative way to reuse a kitchen- or food-related item that may otherwise be thrown away. In one paragraph, write clear instructions for how to give the item a second life. Share your idea with your classmates.

Light and Healthy Recipe

Croutons

Croutons make a big impact on a salad by providing crunch and seasoning. Cooks often use stale bread to make croutons, reducing waste.

Ingredients

- **1 loaf** Bread
- **2 Tbsp.** Olive Oil
- **1 tsp.** Oregano
- **¼ tsp.** Paprika
- **¼ tsp.** Pepper

Directions

1. Preheat oven to 350°.
2. Cut the bread into ½-inch cubes and put into a large bowl. Drizzle the olive oil over the bread. Sprinkle the bread with the oregano, paprika, and pepper.
3. Toss the bread lightly in the oil and spices. Spread the bread out on a sheet tray and put the tray into the oven. Bake the croutons 15 minutes, or until crispy and browned.
4. Store in an airtight container until use.

Yield 24 servings

Nutrition Analysis per Serving

Calories	58
Total fat	1 g
Saturated fat	0 g
Cholesterol	0 mg
Sodium	123 mg
Carbohydrate	11 g
Dietary fiber	1 g
Sugars	1 g
Protein	2 g

CHAPTER 22 Review & Applications

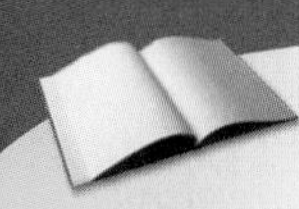

After You Read

Chapter Summary

Conservation protects the environment for future generations, saves money, and increases efficiency in the kitchen. Conservation is equally important for both nonrenewable and renewable resources. To conserve energy, it is important to use major appliances efficiently. Water can be conserved by using eight water-saving habits. Decrease trash and waste by reducing consumption, reusing materials, and recycling wherever possible. As the world's population increases, there are fewer resources available for each person, and people often use more than they need. By looking for solutions and taking simple actions, we can conserve valuable resources.

Content and Academic Vocabulary Review

1. Arrange the content and academic vocabulary words into groups of related words. Explain why you put the words together.

Content Vocabulary

- conservation (p. 342)
- nonrenewable resource (p. 342)
- greenhouse gas (p. 342)
- renewable resource (p. 342)
- biodegradable (p. 344)
- sanitary landfill (p. 345)
- food waste (p. 346)
- recycle (p. 347)

Academic Vocabulary

- consumption (p. 344)
- synthetic (p. 345)

Review Key Concepts

2. **Explain** how conservation benefits people and the environment.
3. **Describe** how to use large kitchen appliances efficiently.
4. **List** eight ways to conserve water in the kitchen.
5. **Summarize** two guidelines for reducing trash.
6. **Explain** how population growth is affecting the world's resources.

Critical Thinking

7. **Explain** how buying several small appliances can actually help conserve energy.
8. **Analyze** the policy at Smith's Diner. The restaurant's policy has always been to provide a glass of water for every diner and keep it filled at all times. What can the restaurant do to become more resource friendly?
9. **Explain** how one person can make a difference when it comes to saving our planet's resources.
10. **Conclude** which areas of resource conservation you think are the most critical. Explain why.

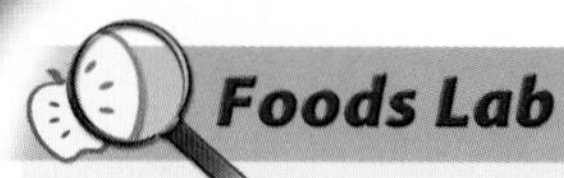

Foods Lab

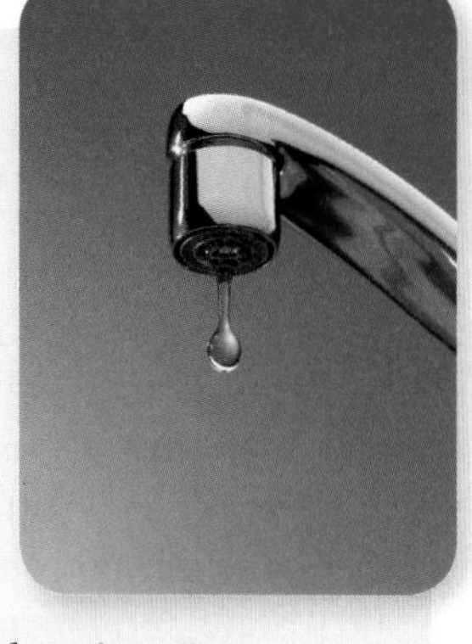

11. Recipes and Resources Conservation can begin before you even turn on a light, oven, or faucet. How? It can start with a good recipe. Some recipes require the use of many resources. Others do not.

Procedure Prepare a recipe you think is resource-friendly. Determine what resources were used to process, package, and store the ingredients. How much water and energy is needed for preparation?

Analysis With your lab team, list factors that make the recipe resource-friendly. Then brainstorm and list ways you might modify the recipe to use even fewer resources.

HEALTHFUL CHOICES

12. Energy-Efficient Cooking Dominic is a chef who wants to use his oven's energy efficiently. Should he stock his kitchen with glass cookware or use only metal cookware? Explain your answer in one or more paragraphs. Name at least three other things Dominic could do to conserve energy in his kitchen.

TECH Connection

13. Chemical-Free Cleaning Many of the household cleaners used to keep a kitchen clean contain hazardous chemicals. Under your teacher's supervision, use the Internet to research chemical-free alternatives to common household cleaners that you can make yourself. Write a recipe for one cleaner and note its uses. Note any precautions for anyone using the cleaner, as well as precautions necessary for storage. Write a paragraph to summarize your findings. Under your teacher's supervision, try making and using the cleaner.

Real-World Skills

Problem-Solving Skills

14. Eating without Waste After a large dinner including mashed potatoes, rolls, roast beef, gravy, and assorted vegetables, the Abbey family has a lot of leftover food. In one or more paragraphs, describe how you would advise the Abbeys to conserve their resources.

Interpersonal and Collaborative Skills

15. Post a Reminder Follow your teacher's instructions to form pairs. Work together to design and create a colorful poster to be hung in your school's food lab. The poster should relate to reducing, reusing, or recycling. It should include specific tips related to using the food lab.

Financial Literacy Skills

16. Saving Money and Resources The Ruiz family spends $90 each month on the electricity required to light their home. If they replace their incandescent bulbs with compact fluorescent bulbs, they can save up to 75 percent on lighting costs. How would this change their monthly lighting expenses?

Academic Skills

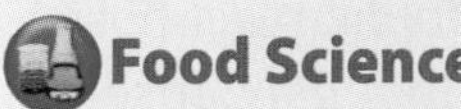

Food Science

17. Water Expansion For most substances, the solid phase is denser than the liquid phase. However, solid water has more space between molecules than its liquid phase due to the need for even distribution of hydrogen bonds. This causes water to expand when freezing.

Procedure Get a small plastic bottle with a screw cap and fill it completely with water. Put the bottle in the freezer and leave it there overnight.

Analysis Write a paragraph to explain what happened to the bottle of water.

NSES C Develop an understanding of the structure and properties of matter.

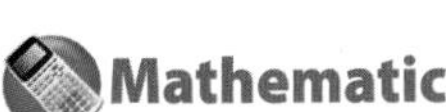

Mathematics

18. Save Energy and Money An incandescent light bulb costs $0.49 and burns for 1,000 hours. It also uses $0.01 of electricity for each hour it burns. A compact fluorescent light bulb costs $3.44, burns for 10,000 hours, and uses $0.0026 of electricity per hour. What will Chris' total savings be after 10,000 hours with the new bulbs?

Math Concept **Multiplying Decimals** Multiply decimals as you would whole numbers, but count the number of decimal places in all of the factors. The final product will have that total number of decimal places.

Starting Hint Figure out the total bulb cost and total electricity cost for 10,000 hours using eight incandescent bulbs. Then figure out the same costs for eight CFL bulbs.

NCTM Problem Solving Solve problems that arise in mathematics and in other contexts.

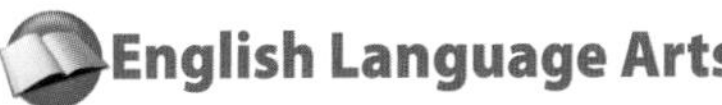

English Language Arts

19. Read and Report Find a magazine, book, or Web site about conservation. Read an article, chapter, or Web page from your source and consider how it relates to what you learned in this chapter. Write a one-page report summarizing what you read. Connect the article to conservation during food preparation and consumption. Include in your report your evaluation of the article. Is it relevent to what you see in your home kitchen? Also include the three most important details you learned about conservation.

NCTE 7 Conduct research and gather, evaluate, and synthesize data to communicate discoveries.

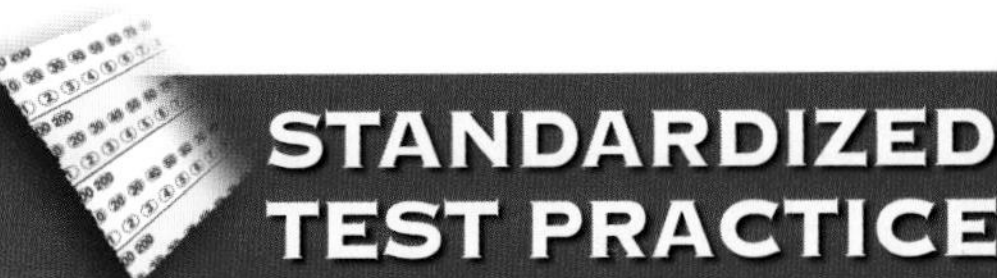

STANDARDIZED TEST PRACTICE

FILL IN THE BLANK

Read the sentence and choose the best word to fill in the blank.

20. In the United States, up to __________ of all edible food is thrown out.
    - **a.** 20 percent
    - **b.** 30 percent
    - **c.** 10 percent
    - **d.** 40 percent

Test-Taking Tip When answering a fill-in-the-blank question, silently read the sentence with each of the possible answers in the blank space. This will help you eliminate wrong answers. The best answer results in a sentence that is both factual and grammatically correct.

UNIT 5

Thematic Project

Investigating Food Safety

In this unit you have learned that there are many things that can be done to help ensure the safety of those working in the kitchen and the safety of foods prepared in the kitchen. In this project, you will create a safety manual to use in your kitchen as a reference.

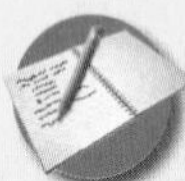

My Journal

If you completed the journal entry from page 277, refer to it to see if your thoughts have changed after reading the unit.

Project Assignment

- Research home kitchen safety and sanitation regulations.
- Compile the results of your research in an organized and easily understood way.
- Create a resource list of community experts or agencies that raise awareness of safety issues or help the public react positively to safety situations that may arise in your kitchen.
- Create a graphic that includes call-outs that explain the parts of the kitchen and how they promote food and kitchen safety.
- Create a reference guide that explains food and safety concerns, how to prevent them, and how to solve problems when they occur.

Academic Skills You Will Use

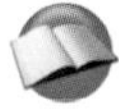

English Language Arts

NCTE 8 Use information resources to gather information and create and communicate knowledge.

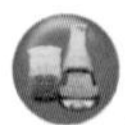

Science

NSES F Develop understanding of personal and community health; population growth; natural resources; environmental quality; natural and human-induced hazards; science and technology in local, national, and global challenges.

STEP 1 Choose a Food Safety Topic

There are several issues that can affect food and kitchen safety, including food and equipment storage, safe use of appliances, fire prevention, and protection against electrical shock. Research safety and sanitation regulations set by your local health department. Write a summary of your research. In your summary:

- Identify safety and sanitation regulations.
- Explain how to prevent illness and injury.
- Describe practical ways to react to safety issues.

STEP 2 Plan Your Talk

Arrange to interview someone in your community whose job involves food safety and/or kitchen safety. Write a list of interview questions to ask this person. Keep these writing skills in mind when you develop your questions.

Writing Skills

- Use complete sentences.
- Be descriptive.
- Use correct spelling and grammar.
- Write your questions in the order you want to ask them.

STEP 3 Connect to Your Community

Talk with a member of your community whose job involves food and/or kitchen safety. Possible choices include: grocery store produce or dairy manager or restaurant chef or manager.

Ask them to describe policies and procedures they use to ensure the safety of food and safety in the kitchen.

STEP 4 Create and Illustrate Your Brochure

Use the Unit Thematic Project Checklist to plan and complete your project and evaluate your work. As you conduct research for your food and kitchen safety manual, keep these research skills in mind.

Internet Research Skills

- Look for sources with .gov or .edu as the three-letter extension at the end of the domain name.
- Check your information at more than one Web site to make sure the advice is consistent.

STEP 5 Evaluate Your Presentation

Your project will be evaluated based on:

- Accuracy of the information presented.
- Content of the brochure.
- Layout and design of the brochure.
- Mechanics—presentation and neatness.

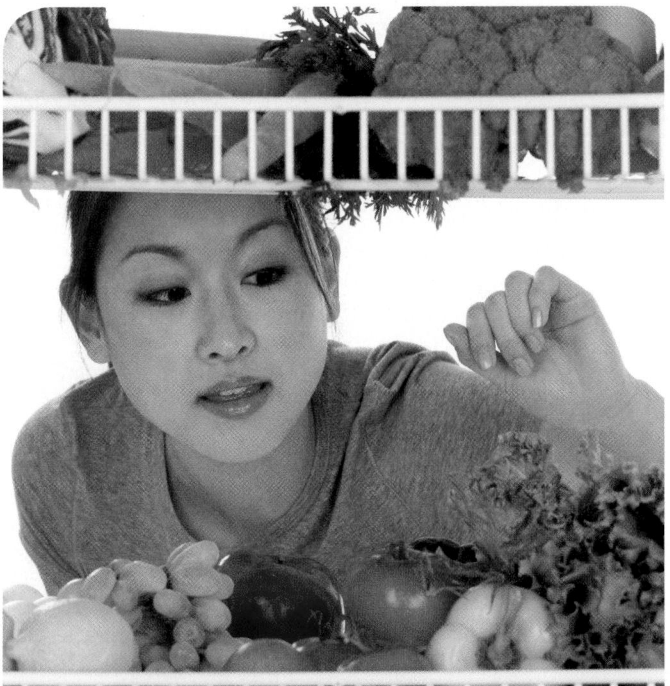

Unit Thematic Project Checklist

Category	Objectives
Plan	☑ Research home kitchen safety and sanitation regulations.
	☑ Summarize the results of your research in an organized and easily understood way.
	☑ Create a safety manual that explains food and kitchen safety concerns, how to prevent them, and how to solve problems when they occur.
	☑ Use graphics to illustrate your manual.
Present	☑ Make a presentation to your class about what you learned during this project.
	☑ invite students to ask any questions they may have. Answer these questions.
	☑ Turn over your research summary, the notes from your interview, and your food and kitchen safety manual to your teacher.
Academic Skills	☑ Conduct research to gather information.
	☑ Communicate effectively.
	☑ Organize your food and kitchen safety manual so subjects are easily found.

Go to this book's Online Learning Center through **glencoe.com** for a rubric you can use to evaluate your final project.

UNIT 6

The Art of Cooking

Activate Prior Knowledge

Explore the Photo There are many different ways to prepare foods. *With what cooking methods are you familiar?*

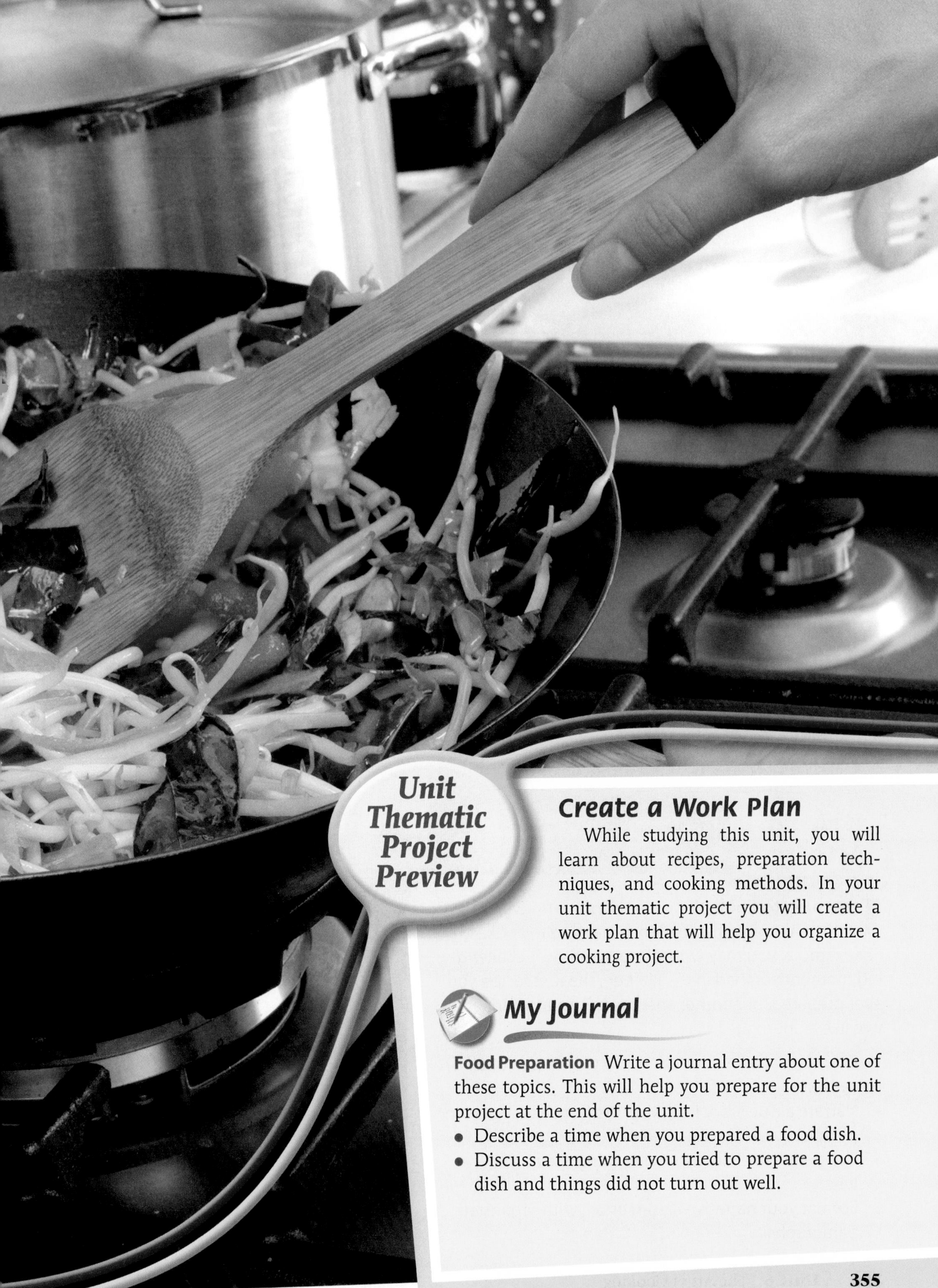

Unit Thematic Project Preview

Create a Work Plan

While studying this unit, you will learn about recipes, preparation techniques, and cooking methods. In your unit thematic project you will create a work plan that will help you organize a cooking project.

My Journal

Food Preparation Write a journal entry about one of these topics. This will help you prepare for the unit project at the end of the unit.

- Describe a time when you prepared a food dish.
- Discuss a time when you tried to prepare a food dish and things did not turn out well.

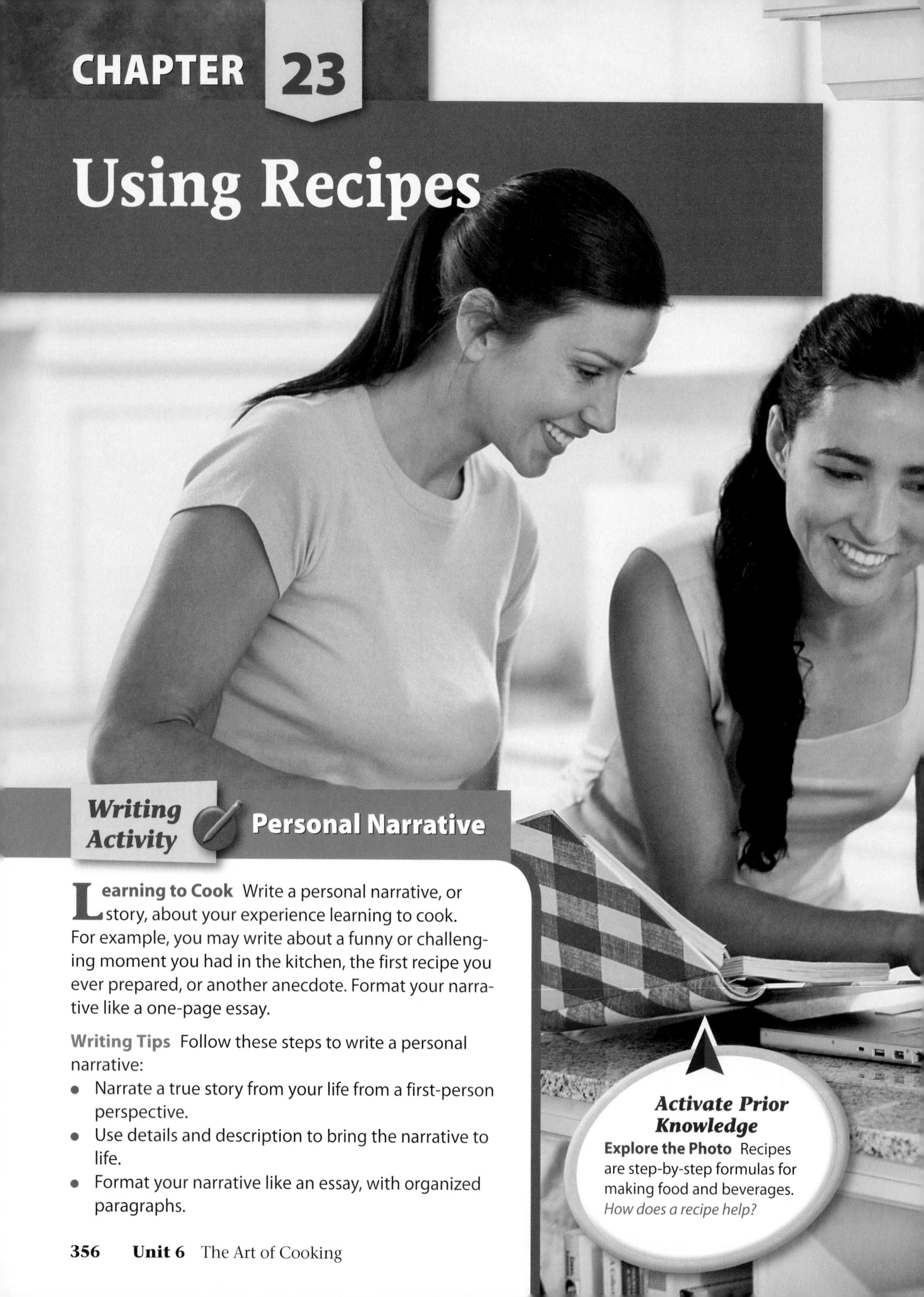

CHAPTER 23

Using Recipes

Writing Activity — Personal Narrative

Learning to Cook Write a personal narrative, or story, about your experience learning to cook. For example, you may write about a funny or challenging moment you had in the kitchen, the first recipe you ever prepared, or another anecdote. Format your narrative like a one-page essay.

Writing Tips Follow these steps to write a personal narrative:

- Narrate a true story from your life from a first-person perspective.
- Use details and description to bring the narrative to life.
- Format your narrative like an essay, with organized paragraphs.

Activate Prior Knowledge

Explore the Photo Recipes are step-by-step formulas for making food and beverages. *How does a recipe help?*

Reading Guide

Before You Read

Preview Before you read, locate a recipe online or in a cookbook. As you read, refer to the recipe to see real-life examples of the topics discussed in this chapter.

Read to Learn

Key Concepts

- **List** the six types of information a recipe provides.
- **Define** the different units and systems of measurement used in recipes.
- **Explain** how and why a recipe might be modified.
- **Describe** ways to find and organize recipes.

Main Idea

Recipes are directions for preparing foods and beverages that are useful to cooks and offer helpful information.

Content Vocabulary

You will find definitions for these words in the glossary at the end of this book.

- ☐ recipe
- ☐ yield
- ☐ customary system
- ☐ metric system
- ☐ volume
- ☐ weight
- ☐ equivalent
- ☐ high-altitude cooking

Academic Vocabulary

You will find these words in your reading and in your tests. Use the glossary to look up their definitions, if necessary.

- omit
- compensate

Graphic Organizer

Use a graphic organizer like the one below to list and explain four steps for decreasing the yield of a recipe.

DECREASING RECIPE YIELD

1.
2.
3.
4.

Graphic Organizer Go to this book's Online Learning Center at **glencoe.com** to print out this graphic organizer.

Academic Standards

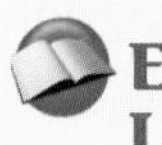

English Language Arts

NCTE 12 Use language to accomplish individual purposes.

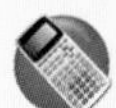

Mathematics

NCTM Measurement Understand measurable attributes of objects and the units, systems, and processes of measurement.

NCTM Number and Operations Compute fluently and make reasonable estimates.

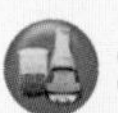

Science

NSES A Develop understandings about scientific inquiry.

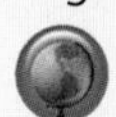

Social Studies

NCSS VIII B Science, Technology, and Society Make judgments about how science and technology have transformed the physical world and human society.

NCTE *National Council of Teachers of English*
NCTM *National Council of Teachers of Mathematics*
NSES *National Science Education Standards*
NCSS *National Council for the Social Studies*

What Is a Recipe?

A **recipe** is a set of directions for making a food or beverage. Recipes are useful for all cooks, from beginner to expert. A well-written recipe offers six types of information.

List of Ingredients Ingredients are given in exact amounts and they are listed in the order that they are used.

Yield The **yield** is the amount or the number of servings that the recipe makes.

Cooking Method, Temperature, and Time Recipes tell you how long to cook or chill food and at what temperature. The temperature describes the control settings for cooking equipment used during preparation. Some recipes give temperatures and times for both conventional and microwave ovens. Recipes may remind you to preheat the oven. Temperature and time may also be written with instructions such as "fry until golden" or "chill until set."

Container Size and Type Containers are described in as much detail as needed. A brownie recipe may specify "a large bowl" for mixing or "an 8-inch square pan" for baking.

Step-by-Step Directions Good recipes have clear, easy-to-follow directions that describe all of the steps in a logical order. Some recipes number the steps to help you keep your place.

Nutrition Analysis Choose recipes that provide the calories and nutrients you need. Information on the nutrient and calorie content in a recipe can help you choose recipes that fit your eating plan. Many recipes list the number of calories and grams of fat, sodium, and fiber per serving. Some recipes include information on carbohydrates, protein, cholesterol, vitamins, and minerals.

✓ **Reading Check** **Explain** Why do some recipes provide information on nutrient and calorie content?

Step by Step

Recipes tell you how much of each ingredient to use and give instructions for preparing and cooking. *What are the six types of information in a good recipe?*

Be a *Smart Consumer*

Recipe Trends

Today's fast-paced world has led to a trend for 30-minute meals—recipes that take just thirty minutes or less to prepare. Another recipe trend is one-dish meals—meals such as casseroles that combine an assortment of ingredients and nutrients in one container. Other trends have centered around low-fat recipes. Sometimes trends can introduce consumers to styles of cooking, such as ethnic recipes, that they would not have otherwise tried. Trends in cooking, like in fashion, tend to come and go, but certain qualities—good nutrition, flavor, ease of preparation—are always valued.

Challenge Visit a bookstore or library that contains recently published cookbooks and cooking magazines. What recipe trends do you perceive? Share your findings with the class.

Figure 23.1 **Units of Measurement**

Customary and Metric Customary and metric measurements describe tools, ingredients, and cooking methods by volume, weight, dimensions, and temperature. ***What is the difference between volume and weight?***

Type of Measurement	Customary Units of Measurement	Metric Units of Measurement
Volume	teaspoon (tsp.) tablespoon (Tbsp.) cup (c.) pint (pt.) quart (qt.) gallon (gal.) fluid ounce (fl. oz.)	milliliter (mL) liter (L)
Weight	ounce (oz.) pound (lb.)	milligram (mg) gram (g); kilogram (kg)
Dimensions	inches (in.)	centimeter (cm)
Temperature	degrees Fahrenheit (°F)	degrees Celsius (°C)

Weights and Measures

Recipes usually turn out best when you use each ingredient in exactly the right amount. Ingredient amounts are written in different ways, depending on whether the recipe uses customary or metric measurements. The **customary system**, also called U.S. standard or English, is a system of measurement used in the United States. Cups, tablespoons, and teaspoons are customary measures. Most other countries use the **metric system**, a system of measurement based on multiples of ten. For instance, just as one dollar contains 100 pennies, one meter contains 100 centimeters. Grams and liters are metric measures.

The United States is gradually converting to metric. Metric measurements are easy to find. Scientists work in metric. Food service operations often measure in metric. Beverages are sold by the liter, and food labels indicate weight in grams.

You can use recipes written in either system. You just need measuring tools that are sized or marked for the particular system, and a kitchen scale to weigh ingredients.

Units of Measure

The customary and the metric systems use different units of measurement for volume, weight, dimensions, and temperature.

Volume **Volume** is the amount of space an ingredient takes up. For example, a salad recipe might list "½ cup chopped celery" or "250 mL milk." A bread recipe might ask for 1½ tsp. of yeast.

Weight **Weight** measures the heaviness of an ingredient, as in "1 lb. ground beef" or "50 g chopped walnuts." A can of tomatoes may be labeled "Net wt. 24 oz."

Dimensions Dimensions are used to describe bakeware lengths and widths. A baking pan might be described as "8.5 in. round" or "20 × 4 cm." Some recipes even ask for the height of a pan, "20 × 4 × 2."

Temperature Temperatures in the customary system are given in degrees Fahrenheit (°F). Temperatures in the metric system are given in degrees Celsius (°C).

Figure 23.1 compares several basic customary and metric units of measurement and shows common abbreviations.

Using Dry and Fluid Ounces

In the customary system, an ounce (or dry ounce) is a measure of weight, and a fluid ounce is a measure of volume. What is the difference? Suppose you measure a cup of popcorn and a cup of brown rice. Both ingredients have the same volume, or number of fluid ounces. However, the popcorn is much lighter in weight than rice—it weighs fewer ounces. You can use a kitchen scale to find out how many ounces each ingredient weighs.

Calculating Equivalents

Your math skills can help you succeed with recipes. What if you want to make a fruit salad recipe that calls for 1½ cups of blueberries, but the store only sells them by the pint? How many pints should you buy? Use equivalents to get the answer. An **equivalent** is a different way of measuring. For example, one cup is the equivalent of 16 tablespoons, and one pint is the equivalent of two cups. **Figure 23.2** shows common volume and weight equivalents.

Figure 23.2 Volume and Weight Equivalents

Conversions You can convert measurements between customary and metric by using this chart. ***How many teaspoons are in 30 mL?***

	Customary Measurements		Metric Measurements*
	Measurements	fl. oz.	Millileters
Volume	¼ tsp.		1 mL
	½ tsp.		2 mL
	1 tsp.		5 mL
	1 Tbsp. (3 tsp.)	½ fl. oz.	15 mL
	⅛ c. (2 Tbsp.)	1 fl. oz.	30 mL
	¼ c. (4 Tbsp.)	2 fl. oz.	50 mL
	⅓ c. (5 Tbsp.)	3 fl. oz.	75 mL
	½ c. (8 Tbsp.)	4 fl. oz.	125 mL
	⅔ c. (11 Tbsp.)	5 fl. oz.	150 mL
	¾ c. (12 Tbsp.)	6 fl. oz.	175 mL
	1 c. (16 Tbsp.)	8 fl. oz.	250 mL
	1 pt. (2 cups)	16 fl. oz.	500 mL
	1 qt. (2 pints or 4 cups)	32 fl. oz.	1 L
	1 gal. (4 quarts or 8 pints or 16 cups)	128 fl. oz.	4 L

	Customary Measurements		Metric Measurements*
	Pounds	Ounces	Grams/Kilo
Weights		1 oz.	28 g
	1 lb.	16 oz.	448 g
	2.2 lb.	35 oz.	1000 g or 1 kg

*Volumes have been rounded to correspond to metric measuring tools.

Legend of Abbreviations

Customary measurements

tsp. . .teaspoon
Tbsp. . .Tablespoon
c. . .cup
qt. . .quart
pt. . .pint
gal. . .gallon
oz. . .ounce
fl. oz. . .fluid ounce
lb. . .pound

Metric measurements

mL . .milliliter
L . .liter
g . .gram
kg . .kilogram

Figure 23.3 Conversion Chart

Convert International Recipes Learning the most common weights and measures in the customary and metric systems helps you to use and convert international recipes. ***Which is a greater volume, a quart or a liter?***

	To Convert From	Multiply By	To Get
Volume	fl. oz.	30	mL
	mL	0.03	fl. oz.
	c.	0.2368	L
	L	4.22675	c.
	pt.	0.47	L
	L	2.1	pt.
	qt.	0.95	L
	L	1.06	qt.
	gal.	3.8	L
	L	0.26	gal.

	To Convert From	Multiply By	To Get
Weights	oz.	28.35	g
	g.	0.03527	oz.
	lb.	0.45	kg
	kg	2.2	lb.

Converting Between Customary and Metric

Knowing how to convert from one measuring system to the other helps you to use international recipes. Converted measurements are close, but not exact. For example, 8 fluid ounces equals 236.5 mL, or 240 mL rounded. Metric markings on a liquid measuring cup do not list this measurement, so you would measure almost to the 250-mL mark. Inexact conversions are fine for most recipes. Converting precisely is more critical for baked goods than for most other recipes.

To convert measurements, you will use multiplication. Conversion charts and formulas help with converting recipes. It also helps to have a calculator handy for conversions in the kitchen. **Figure 23.3** shows formulas for converting amounts.

Converting Temperatures

You may also need to convert temperatures between Fahrenheit and Celsius. Here is how to convert quickly.

Celsius to Fahrenheit Multiply the Celsius temperature by 9. Then divide by 5 and add 32. For example, to convert 175°C, multiply 175 by 9 to get 1,575. Divide 1,575 by 5, which yields 315. Now add 32 to get 347°F, or about 350°F.

Fahrenheit to Celsius Subtract 32 from the Fahrenheit temperature. Then multiply by 5 and divide by 9. For example, to convert 350°F, subtract 32 from 350 to get 318. Multiply 318 by 5, which yields 1,590. Divide 1,590 by 9, which yields 176.66°C, or about 175°C.

✓ **Reading Check** **Contrast** In the customary system, what is the difference between a dry ounce and a fluid ounce?

Changing Recipes

You can personalize recipes for many reasons. You may need to increase or decrease the yield. You may want to substitute an ingredient for health reasons or because you want a certain flavor. You might want to be creative and try something new.

Some recipes handle change better than others. Substitutions usually work fine in recipes where the ingredients act more or less independently of each other—fruits in a salad, for example, or vegetables in a stir-fry. You can experiment with different flavors and textures.

Other recipes, including most recipes for baked goods, require exact ingredients and precise measurements. Recipes for baked items are like chemical formulas. Ingredients blend together to create a certain effect. If you change one amount or **omit** (leave out) one ingredient, the food may be ruined.

Kitchen Math

Metric Conversions

A popular restaurant chain sells a quarter-pound hamburger in the United States. However, in Europe and elsewhere around the world, the hamburger goes by a different name, since those countries use the metric system and are unfamiliar with pounds. How much does a quarter-pound (4 oz.) hamburger patty weigh in grams? If the weight of the beef after cooking is 85.05 g, how much is that to the nearest ounce?

Math Concept **Converting Weights** To convert ounces into grams, multiply ounces by 28.35. To convert grams into ounces, divide grams by 28.35.

Starting Hint To find the weight of a 4-ounce hamburger patty in grams, multiply 4 by 28.35, and round to the nearest gram. To convert 85.05 grams into ounces, divide 85.05 by 28.35. Round to the nearest ounce.

Math Appendix For math help, go to the Math Appendix at the back of the book.

NCTM Measurement Understand measurable attributes of objects and the units, systems, and processes of measurement.

Changing the Yield

Most recipes, including those for baked goods, can be doubled. Multiply the amount of each ingredient by two and follow the same steps. You may need to cook the food for a longer time, because there is more of it. You will also need larger bowls and cookware for mixing and cooking. For a double recipe of a baked product, use two baking pans of the original size rather than one large pan.

Recipes for casseroles, stews, and other mixtures can usually be decreased as well. Do not decrease the yield of baked goods unless a recipe for a baked product can be cut in half exactly. What should you do if decreasing a recipe is not workable? Prepare the original amount and freeze the leftovers for another meal or share them with friends.

Here are four steps to follow to decrease the yield of a recipe.

1. Divide. Divide the desired yield by the recipe's yield. Suppose a lasagne recipe yields 12 servings and you want only 6. Divide 6 by 12, which gives 0.5, or ½.

2. Multiply. Multiply each ingredient amount by the fraction or decimal you got in Step 1. This keeps the ingredients in the same proportion as in the original recipe. Suppose the lasagne recipe calls for 16 ounces of tomato sauce. Multiply 16 ounces by 0.5 to get 8 ounces.

3. Convert. Convert the measurements into logical, manageable amounts. You may need to use equivalents. Suppose the lasagne recipe calls for ¼ cup of parsley. Half of ¼ cup is ⅛ cup. Since ⅛ cup equals 2 tablespoons, you can measure the parsley easily by using a tablespoon.

4. Adjust. Make any needed adjustments in equipment, temperature, and time. Try to use a pan that maintains the depth and shape of the original recipe. If a 13 × 9 inch baking dish holds the larger lasagne, a 10 × 6 inch dish will hold your 6-serving version proportionally. Because the amount is smaller, however, you may still need to decrease the oven temperature or cooking time. If this is a recipe you plan to cut in half again, pencil in your calculations so that you do not have to figure them again.

Figure 23.4 Ingredient Substitutions

Trade Offs The ingredient substitutions listed here give good results in most recipes. ***Based on the information in this chart, which would you predict to give a stronger flavor: one tablespoon of fresh herbs or one tablespoon of dried herbs?***

When You Don't Have...	Substitute ...
Baking chocolate, unsweetened, 1 oz.	3 Tbsp. cocoa + 1 Tbsp. butter, margarine, or vegetable oil
Bread crumbs, fine, dry	Equal amount cracker or cornflake crumbs
Buttermilk, 1 cup	1 Tbsp. lemon juice or vinegar + enough fat-free milk to equal 1 cup, or use 1 cup plain, nonfat yogurt
Cake flour, 1 cup	⅞ cup (¾ cup + 2 Tbsp.) sifted all-purpose flour
Corn syrup, 1 cup	1 cup granulated sugar + ¼ cup water
Cornstarch (for thickening), 1 Tbsp.	2 Tbsp. flour
Garlic, 1 clove	⅛ tsp. garlic powder
Herbs, 1 Tbsp. fresh, chopped	1 tsp. dried, crushed herbs
Lemon juice	Equal amount vinegar
Milk, fat-free, 1 cup	⅓ cup nonfat dry milk powder + ⅞ cup water
Mustard, dry, 1 tsp.	1 Tbsp. prepared mustard
Onion, 1 small	1 Tbsp. dried, minced onion or 1 tsp. onion powder
Tomato sauce, 1 cup	6 Tbsp. tomato paste + ½ cup water
Worcestershire sauce, 1 Tbsp.	1 Tbsp. soy sauce + dash red pepper sauce

Substituting Ingredients

Substituting, or changing, ingredients is another way of working with recipes. You might substitute ingredients if you do not eat a certain food, if you do not have a certain ingredient on hand, if you are trying to use up an ingredient you have on hand, or if you want to achieve a different flavor. For example, you may use strawberries instead of blueberries in pancakes or soy crumbles instead of ground beef in marinara sauce. You might also change a recipe to use an ingredient that is more healthful than one in the recipe. **Figure 23.4** shows a list of reliable substitutions.

Recipes for baked goods are sensitive to substitutions. Changing nonessential ingredients—exchanging walnuts for raisins in cookie dough, for instance—has little effect on the final product. Changing basic ingredients—whole-wheat flour for cake flour, for example—will change the recipe's appearance, taste, and texture. Experienced cooks often make these changes intentionally.

Nutrition Check

A New Nutritional Value

Substituting ingredients does not only change a recipe's flavor, texture, or appearance. It also changes its nutritional value. Incorporating ingredients different from those specified in a recipe can increase or decrease its calories, alter its fat, carbohydrate, sodium, protein, and sugar content, and change the types of vitamins and minerals it contains. It can also change the way a recipe tastes. For example, topping a salad with chopped walnuts rather than croutons will give the recipe a new nutritional value that is higher in protein and healthy omega-3 fatty acids.

Think About It A cake recipe with 10 grams of fat calls for ½ cup of buttermilk. Buttermilk contains 2.2 grams of fat per cup. How would the fat content of the recipe change if you substituted lemon juice and fat-free milk for the buttermilk?

Converting International Ingredients

International recipes often use ingredients that differ from those used in the United States. For example, crème fraîche (ˈkrem ˈfresh), which is used in European cuisine, has a texture like sour cream but is less tart. Thai eggplant tastes similar to other eggplants but has a different shape and texture.

Using substitutions, or other similar ingredients, will affect the flavor of a recipe. Many recipes written for North American cooks specify what substitutes work well, and how they will affect the flavor or texture.

High-Altitude Cooking

Altitude, or elevation, makes a difference in cooking. A cook in Denver, which has an elevation of 5,280 feet, needs to cook differently than a cook in New Orleans, which is below sea level. Most recipes are developed for altitudes of 3,000 feet or below. Many recipes include directions to adjust for cooking at higher altitudes.

As the altitude gets higher, air pressure gets lower. This has two effects. First, water boils at a lower temperature. Liquids come to a boil sooner, but foods simmered in them take longer to cook. For example, you may need to simmer soup for 40 minutes instead of 30, and you may also need to add liquid to replace evaporated water. You may need to do this more than once and may have to adjust seasonings as you go.

Second, gas bubbles in liquids escape from mixtures more readily at high altitudes. Baked products may rise before the batter is set, causing them to collapse in the center. Cooks at high altitudes usually need to use less baking powder and sugar, increase the oven temperature, and add a little extra liquid to **compensate** for (make up for) the drier air.

Adjusting for higher elevations is called **high-altitude cooking**. Many packaged foods include directions for high elevations.

✓ Reading Check **Describe** Describe two ways that high-altitude cooking affects food preparation.

Careers in Food

Natasha Miller
Caterer

Q: What does a caterer do?

A: A caterer cooks and delivers food to any event that requires food being served, whether it is buffet style or plated meals.

Q: What are the differences between a caterer and a chef?

A: A traditional restaurant has a fixed menu. Caterers have more flexibility. We do what we need to do to fit the clients' needs. Each event is unique in its own way, and so is the food we prepare for that event.

Q: Does catering require specialized culinary skills?

A: Caterers are responsible for preparation, transportation, and presentation. Some venues have kitchens, where I can heat certain dishes before serving, and some venues do not have kitchens. That is when I have to make sure food that needs to be hot is hot, and food that needs to be cold is cold.

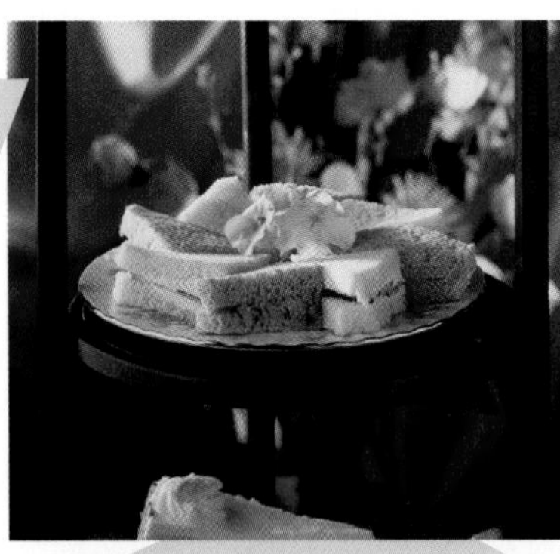

"Elegance is only the beginning. You want to exceed expectations."
— Natasha Miller
Executive Chef, Simply Soul Catering – Indianapolis, IN

Education and Training

A culinary degree is valuable but it is also important to learn about entrepreneurship.

Qualities and Skills

Being able to make and follow a budget, make menu decisions, and cook good food.

Related Career Opportunities

Restaurant manager, restaurant owner, food and beverage manager, personal chef.

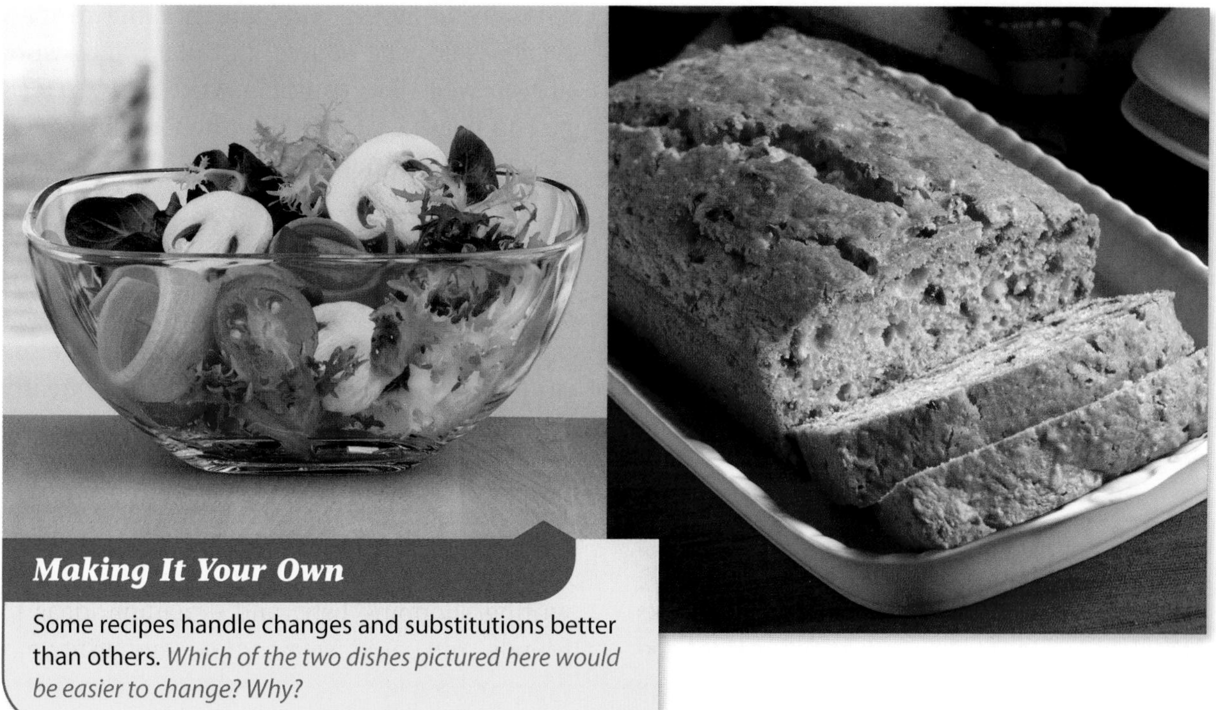

Making It Your Own

Some recipes handle changes and substitutions better than others. *Which of the two dishes pictured here would be easier to change? Why?*

Collecting Recipes

Now is a good time to start a recipe collection. What you learn in this course will help you choose recipes that you can prepare successfully, as well as troubleshoot problems that might arise. As you develop your skills, you can tackle more and more challenging recipes.

Sources of Recipes

You can find recipes in many places. Cookbooks are reliable sources. Basic cookbooks give a broad range of foods and help you to develop cooking skills. Your classroom or school library probably has at least a few cookbooks. The public library is another source. If you do not find a cookbook you like, ask your teacher for recommendations. You can also ask family and friends, look in magazines and newspapers, and browse package labels. Most newspapers devote space to cooking and recipes at least once a week. Millions of recipes are available for free on the Web, along with comments, tips, and ratings. Cooking magazines often have Web sites with searchable databases that contain thousands of recipes.

TECHNOLOGY FOR TOMORROW

Clicking Before Cooking

With a quick click of a computer mouse, cooks can quickly access thousands of recipes and plenty of valuable information using recipe software programs. Using the software, cooks can search recipes by cuisine, food group, or occasion, and avoid recipes that use certain ingredients. They can save a photo with a recipe, convert between metric and customary measuring systems, and change a recipe's yield. The software also estimates the cost of ingredients for a recipe, does nutrition analysis, and suggests recipes based on ingredients the user enters. Cooks can also use the software to broaden their horizons and access online databases to swap recipes with people all over the world.

Investigate Use the Internet to find one type of recipe software that is available, its cost, and its features.

NCSS VIII B Science, Technology, and Society Make judgments about how science and technology have transformed the physical world and human society.

Before you decide to try a recipe, study it carefully. Does it suit your cooking skills and budget? Does it give all the needed information? Are directions clear? If ingredients are given without directions, or if directions refer to an ingredient that is not listed, look for another recipe.

If you plan to use a new recipe for a special occasion, try it ahead of time. Practice helps you work out any problems. You can make sure the recipe turns out as expected and decide whether to add it to your collection.

Organizing Recipes

An organized recipe collection makes cooking easier and more enjoyable. Many cooks write or paste recipes on index cards and store them in a card file box. Recipe cards are specially designed with lines for the recipe's name, yield, and source, but plain ones work just as well. You can also write or type recipes on pages of a divided notebook or binder. Label each tab with a category based on food types or your interests, such as vegetarian, low-fat, or dessert recipes. An expanding file with tabbed, accordion-like pouches also holds clipped recipes. Expanding wallets fit smaller papers and cards. Photo albums not only store recipes but also display them conveniently under easy-to-clean plastic film. Many people use recipe software or store their recipes online using bookmarks or recipe Web sites. You can then sort and search your recipes easily. Electronic recipes are handy for planning meals, writing shopping lists, and e-mailing ideas to friends. You could even compile and print your own cookbook.

Light and Healthy Recipe

Granola

Ingredients

- **2 cups** Old fashioned oats
- **½ cup** Wheat germ
- **¼ cup** Brown sugar
- **½ tsp.** Cinnamon
- **⅛ tsp.** Salt
- **¼ cup** Maple syrup
- **1 Tbsp.** Water
- **1 Tbsp.** Canola oil

Directions

1. Preheat oven to 275°.
2. Lay parchment paper over a sheet tray.
3. In a large bowl, combine oats, wheat germ, brown sugar, cinnamon, and salt. Mix well.
4. Combine syrup, water, and oil and bring to a simmer. Carefully pour the mixture over the oat mixture and mix well.
5. When the mixture cools enough to handle, use your hands to make small clumps and drop them onto the tray. Bake for 45 minutes, stopping once to turn the clumps over.
6. Store in an airtight container.

Granola makes a great low-sugar addition to a cereal but can be expensive when purchased at a grocery store. Making it yourself is much less expensive.

Yield 6 servings

Nutrition Analysis per Serving

■ Calories	219
■ Total fat	5 g
Saturated fat	0 g
Cholesterol	0 mg
■ Sodium	52 mg
■ Carbohydrate	36 g
Dietary fiber	5 g
Sugars	15 g
■ Protein	7 g

CHAPTER 23 Review & Applications

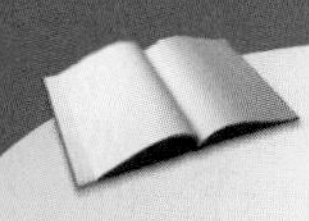

After You Read

Chapter Summary

Recipes are directions for making foods and beverages that are useful for cooks. Recipes offer six types of information. Ingredient amounts in recipes are written differently depending on whether the recipe uses customary or metric measurements, which use different units of measurement. It is possible to convert between the two systems. Recipes can be changed for several purposes. Cooks can change the yield, substitute ingredients, or adjust a recipe for high-altitude cooking. Now is a good time to start collecting recipes. Recipes can be found in many places, and organized in different ways.

Content and Academic Vocabulary Review

1. Use each of these key terms and academic vocabulary words in a sentence.

Content Vocabulary

- ▫ recipe (p. 358)
- ▫ yield (p. 358)
- ▫ customary system (p. 359)
- ▫ metric system (p. 359)
- ▫ volume (p. 359)
- ▫ weight (p. 359)
- ▫ equivalent (p. 360)
- ▫ high-altitude cooking (p. 364)

Academic Vocabulary

- omit (p. 362)
- compensate (p. 364)

Review Key Concepts

2. **List** the six types of information a recipe provides.
3. **Define** the different units and systems of measurement used in recipes.
4. **Explain** how and why a recipe might be modified.
5. **Describe** ways to find and organize recipes.

Critical Thinking

6. **Describe** the problems with Jen's apple pie recipe. Jen wrote the list of ingredients along with their exact amounts. What is missing?
7. **List** the challenges Anna might have when she travels to France. Anna is visiting her uncle and will bring her favorite cookbook of American recipes. What will Anna have to do when shopping for ingredients in France?
8. **Explain** whether it is better to decrease the yield for baked goods by exactly half or to make no changes to the yield.
9. **Describe** how you can create a great recipe collection without buying cookbooks and software.
10. **Explain** whether you think using recipe software takes the creativity from cooking.

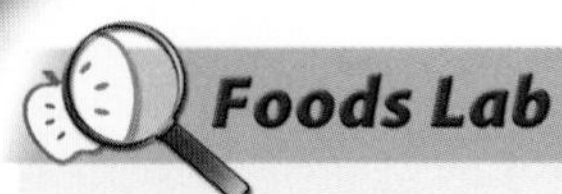

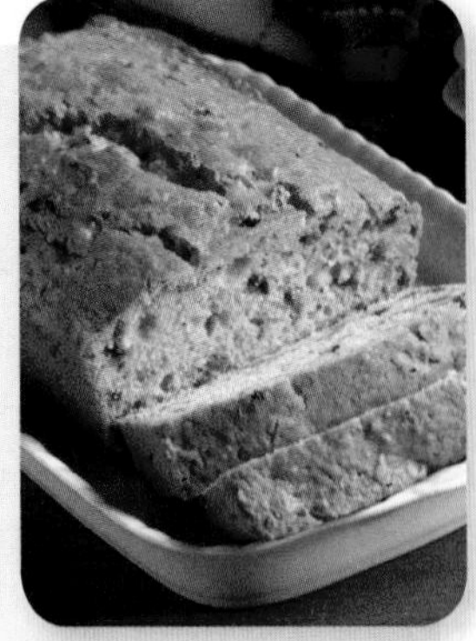

11. Altering Recipes By altering recipes, cooks can change their nutritional value. Care must be taken, however, to maintain the recipe's appeal, taste, and texture when changes are made.

Procedure Choose a recipe and change it in some way to improve its nutritional value. Depending on the recipe, you might reduce or replace some ingredients or increase others. Prepare and evaluate your modified recipe.

Analysis Write the original recipe and your modified version. In a paragraph, explain how you improved the recipe nutritionally. Was this recipe a good choice for the change you made? Why or why not?

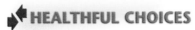

HEALTHFUL CHOICES

12. Recipe Resource Kate is on a low-fat, low-sodium diet to maintain her heart's health. While shopping for cookbooks, she finds one that provides a nutritional analysis with each recipe, and one that does not but is titled "Healthy Recipes." Which should she choose and why? Conduct research to find a "healthy recipe" and examine it to see if it really is healthy. Write a paragraph outlining your conclusion.

TECH Connection

13. Online Options Millions of recipes are available online at no cost. Identify two ingredients that you have a craving for. Conduct an online search for a recipe that contains both ingredients. How many recipes came up on your search? How many recipes come up when you search for both ingredients separately? Which recipe would you be most likely to try and make? Share your findings with the class.

Real-World Skills

Problem-Solving Skills

14. Cake in the Mountains The Sanders family is celebrating a birthday party at their mountain cabin, which is at an elevation of 3,600 feet. They plan to bake a cake from scratch, but do not want the elevation to ruin it. What can they do?

Interpersonal and Collaborative Skills

15. Collaborative Conversion Follow your teacher's instructions to form pairs. Work with your partner to find a recipe that contains a minimum of 12 ingredients. Then work together to convert each ingredient from the customary measurement system to the metric measuring system, or vice versa. Write out your converted recipe, and check it for accuracy.

Financial Literacy Skills

16. Bake Sale Leah baked brownies for her school's bake sale. The recipe yielded 24 brownies measuring 3 inches square. She sold them for $1.50 each. How much more money would she earn if the recipe had yielded 36 brownies of the same size?

Academic Skills

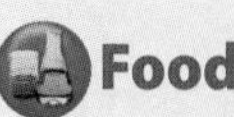

Food Science

17. Measurements The old adage, "a pint is a pound the world round," is true only for water and other liquids like it. For most ingredients, it is far more accurate to weigh rather than use volumetric measurements.

Procedure Weigh 8 ounces of flour, 8 ounces of sugar, and 8 ounces of water, each put in its own labeled container. Then measure 1 cup of each ingredient. Check your classmates' results by exchanging the measured ingredients.

Analysis Which measurements were in agreement, and which were not? Explain why 8 ounces might mean two different things.

NSES A Develop understandings about scientific inquiry.

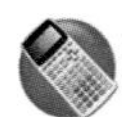

Mathematics

18. Changing Recipe Yield A recipe for home-made granola calls for 4 cups of rolled oats, 1 cup of wheat germ, ½ cup of almonds, ½ cup of coconut, ½ cup of raisins, ½ cup of sesame seeds, 1 cup of honey, and ¼ cup of oil. The recipe makes 8 cups of granola. Rewrite the recipe so that it yields 6 cups instead.

Math Concept **Multiplying Fractions** Convert any mixed or whole numbers to improper fractions. Then multiply all numerators to get the new numerator, and multiply the denominators to get the new denominator. Reduce to lowest terms.

Starting Hint The new recipe yields 6/8, or ¾, of the original recipe. To reduce each ingredient by the same proportion, multiply each ingredient amount by ¾.

NCTM Number and Operations Compute fluently and make reasonable estimates.

English Language Arts

19. Writing Recipes Right Choose a snack that you usually prepare without a recipe, such as a fruit smoothie, sliced apples and peanut butter, or cheese and crackers. Write a recipe for the snack in correct form. Include the six types of information that a well-written recipe features. Make sure your directions are clear and easily understandable. Use computer software to organize all the information on one-half page.

NCTE 12 Use language to accomplish individual purposes.

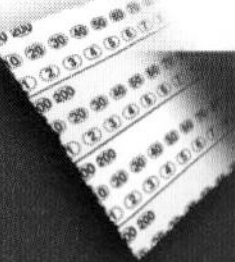

STANDARDIZED TEST PRACTICE

MULTIPLE CHOICE

Read the question and select the best answer.

20. What is an equivalent?

a. a substitute used to replace a recipe ingredient

b. an identical way of measuring a volume or a weight

c. a different way of measuring a volume or a weight

d. a metric volume that matches a customary weight

Test-Taking Tip Multiple-choice questions may prompt you to select the "best" answer. They may present you with answers that seem partially true. The best answer is the one that is completely true, and can be supported by information you have read in the text.

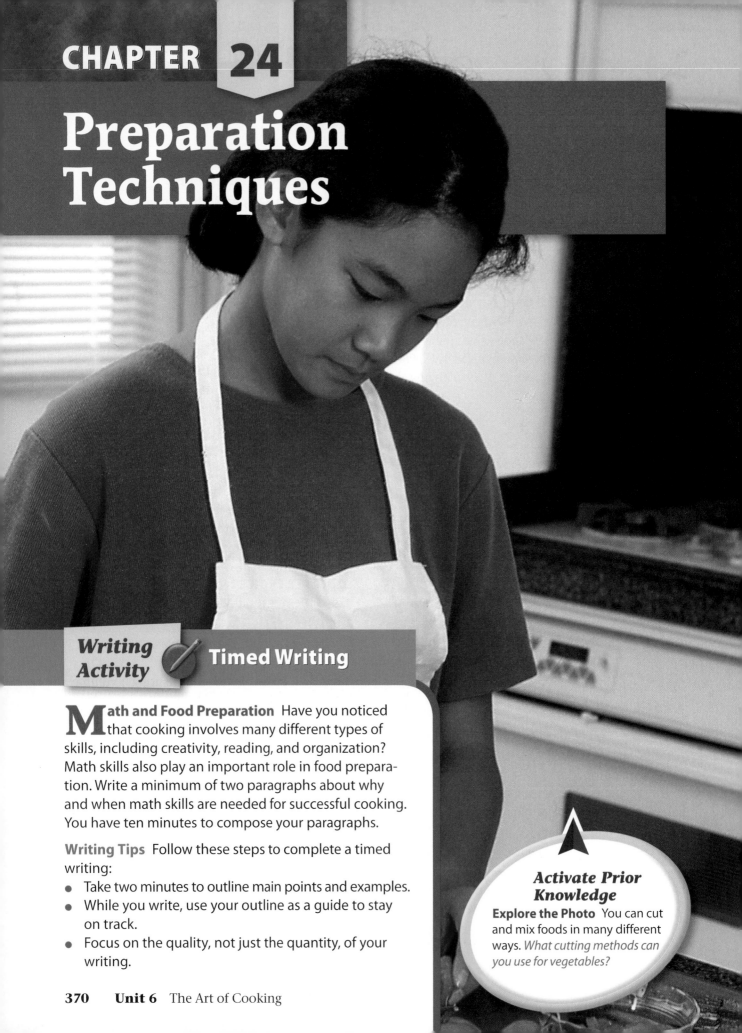

CHAPTER 24

Preparation Techniques

Writing Activity — Timed Writing

Math and Food Preparation Have you noticed that cooking involves many different types of skills, including creativity, reading, and organization? Math skills also play an important role in food preparation. Write a minimum of two paragraphs about why and when math skills are needed for successful cooking. You have ten minutes to compose your paragraphs.

Writing Tips Follow these steps to complete a timed writing:

- Take two minutes to outline main points and examples.
- While you write, use your outline as a guide to stay on track.
- Focus on the quality, not just the quantity, of your writing.

Activate Prior Knowledge

Explore the Photo You can cut and mix foods in many different ways. *What cutting methods can you use for vegetables?*

Reading Guide

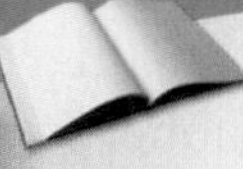

Before You Read

Preview Find a recipe, and underline each of the preparation techniques mentioned, such as "dice," "baste," or "marinate." As you read this chapter, note the definition of each preparation technique mentioned in the recipe.

Read to Learn

Key Concepts

- **List** three different types of ingredients and the tools you need to measure them.
- **Explain** guidelines for proper knife safety.
- **List** eight different ways to mix ingredients.
- **Describe** coating and why it is a useful cooking technique.
- **Explain** the benefits of learning specialized cooking techniques.

Main Idea

Different food preparation techniques have varied effects on foods, and mastering them is essential for success in the kitchen.

Content Vocabulary

- ☐ taring
- ☐ cutting
- ☐ mixing
- ☐ coating

Academic Vocabulary

- affect
- effect

Graphic Organizer

Use a graphic organizer like the one below to note how to stir, toss, and whip foods.

STIR	TOSS	WHIP

Graphic Organizer Go to this book's Online Learning Center at **glencoe.com** to print out this graphic organizer.

Academic Standards

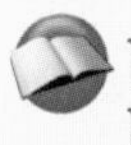

English Language Arts

NCTE 12 Use language to accomplish individual purposes.

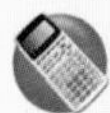

Mathematics

NCTM Number and Operations Understand meanings of operations and how they relate to one another.

NCTM Measurement Understand measurable attributes of objects and the units, systems, and processes of measurement.

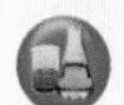

Science

NSES C Develop an understanding of matter, energy and organization in living systems.

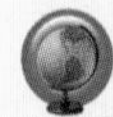

Social Studies

NCSS VIII B Science, Technology, and Society Make judgements about how science and technology have transformed the physical world and human society.

NCTE *National Council of Teachers of English*
NCTM *National Council of Teachers of Mathematics*
NSES *National Science Education Standards*
NCSS *National Council for the Social Studies*

Measuring Ingredients

Mastering food-preparation techniques is essential for success in the kitchen. Most recipes give amounts measured in standard units, such as cups, teaspoons, and tablespoons. That is why you need standard measuring cups and spoons to follow recipes correctly. Coffee mugs, soup spoons, and juice glasses do not work well as measuring tools, because they come in all different sizes.

Liquids, dry ingredients, and fats each take slightly different measuring methods.

Measuring Liquids

Liquid measuring cups are used for larger amounts of flowing ingredients, including oils and syrups. To measure liquids, follow these steps:

1. Set the cup on a level surface. If you hold the cup in your hand, it may tip over or sit at an angle, resulting in an inaccurate reading.
2. Pour the liquid into the measuring cup.
3. Bend down to check the measurement at eye level. Looking down at an angle can distort the reading.
4. Add more liquid or pour some out, if needed, until the top of the liquid is at the desired mark.
5. Pour the ingredient into the mixing container. You may want to use a rubber scraper to empty the cup completely.

Do not measure ingredients over a mixing bowl. Anything you spill will land in the bowl.

Using Measuring Spoons for Liquids

For amounts of liquids smaller than ¼ cup, use measuring spoons instead of cups. Most sets of measuring spoons have a ¼-teaspoon measure as their smallest size. To measure ⅛ teaspoon, dribble the liquid into the ¼-teaspoon measure until it looks half full.

Measuring Dry Ingredients

Dry measuring cups are used for larger amounts of dry ingredients. They are also used for moist but not flowing ingredients, such as jam, yogurt, and peanut butter.

Before measuring dry ingredients, check whether you need to sift first. Flour, granulated sugar, and confectioners' sugar are often sifted to add air and remove small lumps. Whole-grain flours are too coarse to go through the sifter. Stir them with a spoon before measuring.

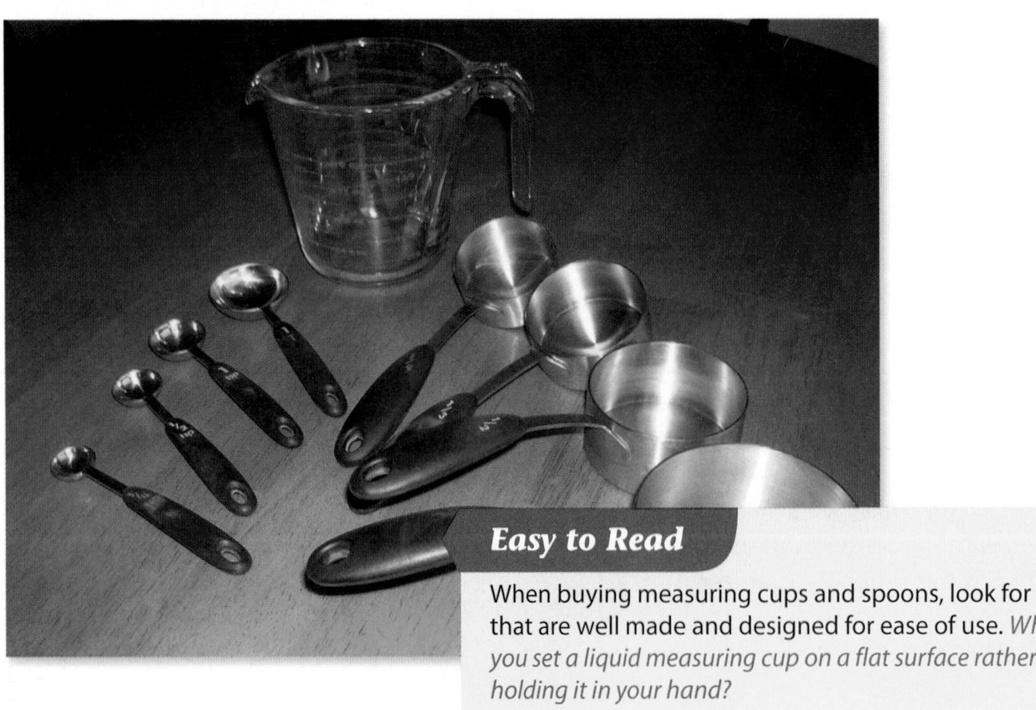

Easy to Read

When buying measuring cups and spoons, look for products that are well made and designed for ease of use. *Why should you set a liquid measuring cup on a flat surface rather than holding it in your hand?*

To measure dry ingredients, follow these steps:

1. Lay out a piece of wax paper.
2. Set out the proper size measuring cup. If you need ¾ cup, use the ½-cup and ¼-cup measures. For ⅔ cup, measure ⅓ cup twice.
3. Fill the cup with the ingredient. Do not pack down flour, granulated sugar, or confectioners' sugar. Do pack down brown sugar, which tends to be fluffy. Use the back of a spoon to pack it firmly into the cup.
4. Level off the top of the cup using the straight edge of a spatula unless the recipe calls for a "heaping," or rounded, measure. Let the excess fall on the wax paper and return it to its original container.
5. Pour the ingredient into the mixing container. Moist foods can be spooned or scraped into and out of the cup. You may want to use a rubber scraper to empty the cup completely.

Do not measure ingredients over the bowl in which you are mixing. Anything you spill will land in the bowl.

Using Measuring Spoons for Dry Ingredients

To measure dry ingredients in amounts smaller than ¼ cup, you need measuring spoons instead of cups. Level dry ingredients in spoons unless the recipe calls for a "heaping," or rounded, measure. A heaping teaspoon is almost twice as much as a leveled teaspoon. If you need ⅛ teaspoon of a dry ingredient, fill the ¼-teaspoon measure and level it off. Then remove half the ingredient with the tip of a straightedge spatula or table knife. Add smaller measurements if you do not have a measuring spoon in the size you need.

Dashes and Pinches Some recipes ask for a dash or a pinch of an ingredient, typically an herb, spice, or other seasoning. This is an even smaller quantity, measured as the amount that can be held between the thumb and finger.

Measuring Solid Fats

Solid fats such as butter and margarine can be measured in several ways, depending on their type.

Be a *Smart Consumer*

Consider Costs

When it comes to supplying their kitchens with measuring tools, consumers can choose from a variety of materials and a range of costs. A set of plastic measuring cups can be purchased for a few dollars, while a set of ceramic measuring cups costs five times as much. A basic electronic scale shows the weight of food in a digital display. A version that also displays the food's nutritional values costs twice as much. When shopping for tools to measure volume and weight, consumers can save money by paying only for the features they need.

Challenge Use the Internet to shop for liquid and dry measuring cups, measuring spoons, and a kitchen scale. Can you buy the necessary tools to measure volume and weight with a budget of 100 dollars? Share your findings verbally.

Stick Method

The stick method works for fat that comes in ¼-pound sticks, such as butter and margarine. The wrapper is marked in tablespoons and in fractions of a cup. You simply cut off the amount you need, cutting through the paper with a serrated knife.

Dry-Measure Method

The dry-measure method works well for measuring shortening. Pack the fat into a spoon or dry measuring cup, pressing firmly to eliminate pockets of air. Level off the top. Use a rubber scraper to remove as much of the fat as possible from the spoon or cup.

Water-Displacement Method

The water-displacement measuring technique works for any kind of fat. First, subtract the amount of fat you want to measure from one cup. Pour that amount of cold water into a 1-cup liquid measuring cup. If you need ¼ cup of shortening, for example, use ¾ cup of cold water. Cold water keeps the fat from melting. Now add fat until the water reaches the 1-cup mark. Hold the fat down to keep it completely

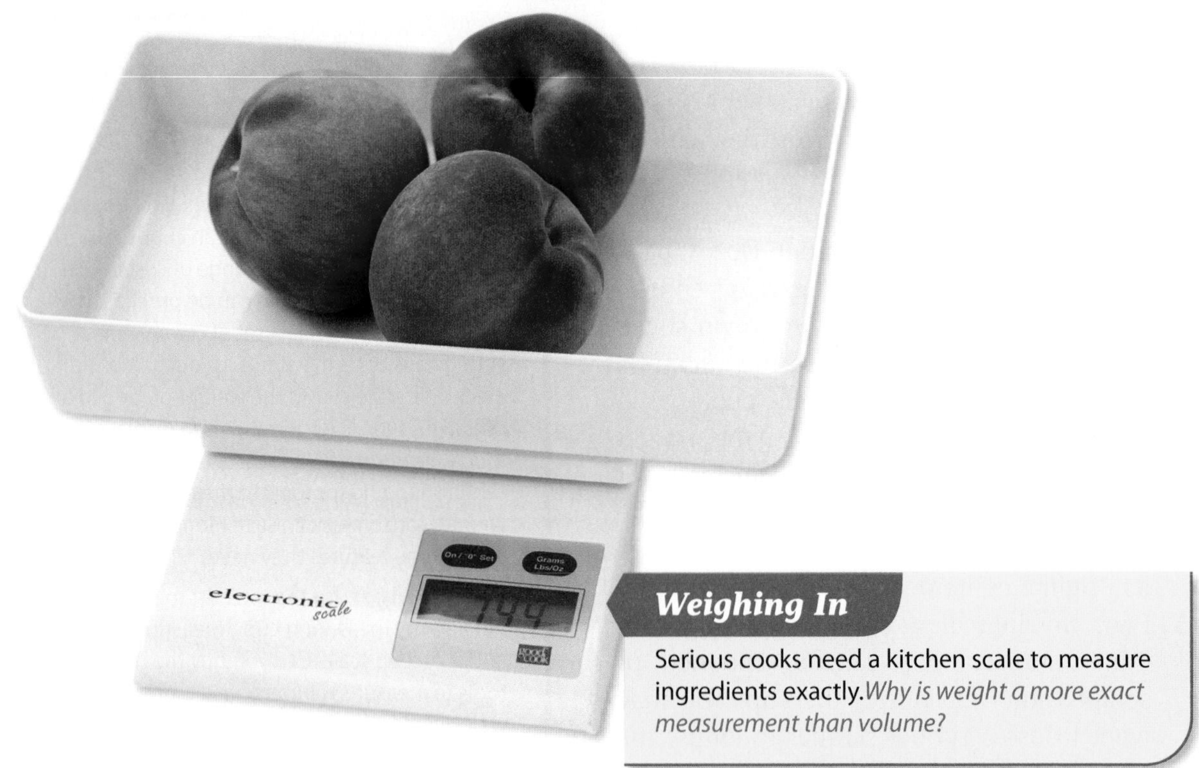

Weighing In

Serious cooks need a kitchen scale to measure ingredients exactly. *Why is weight a more exact measurement than volume?*

below the surface of the water. Do not push the utensil under the water, however, or it could **affect**, or change, the measured amount. Finally, lift the fat from the water with a slotted spoon.

Measuring by Weight

Many recipes list ingredients by weight. Some recipes call for a certain package weight, such as a 10-ounce bag of frozen peas or a 28-ounce can of peeled tomatoes. Others call for specific weights, such as 1 pound of chicken breasts.

Weight is a more exact measurement than volume. For example, four ounces of shredded cheese may fill between 1 and 1½ cups, depending on how firmly it packs. Professional chefs typically weigh ingredients to get accurate results.

You need a kitchen scale to weigh ingredients. A spring scale is used differently from an electronic scale, so follow the manufacturer's directions for the type of scale you use. To weigh small pieces of food, such as rice or chopped vegetables, you need to put them in a container. Remember to adjust the scale by **taring**, or subtracting the weight of the container from the total weight in order to find the weight of the food. First place the empty container on the scale. Press the tare button to set the scale back to zero. Then add the ingredient. The scale will register that weight only.

Measuring Unusual Amounts

You can use your math skills and your knowledge of equivalents to measure nearly any unusual amount.

To measure amounts that are not marked on your measuring cups, use a combination of standard-size measures that add up to what you need. For example, suppose you halve a recipe and need ⅝ cup of flour. Measure out ½ (4/8) cup, then add ⅛ cup more. You can measure ⅛ cup using measuring spoons. ⅛ cup equals 2 tablespoons. So ⅝ cup equals ½ cup plus 2 tablespoons.

You can also measure some amounts by subtracting a smaller quantity from a larger quantity. To get ⅞ cup of milk, for instance, you can pour one cup and then remove 2 tablespoons.

✓ **Reading Check** **List** What are three methods of measuring solid fats?

Cutting Foods

Cutting means dividing a food into smaller parts by using a tool with a sharp blade. The most common cutting tool is a knife.

Think safety first. Use a sharpened knife to help prevent accidents and make the work easier. Use a cutting board to protect the countertop and your hands. Place a wet paper towel or dishcloth under the board to prevent it from slipping.

Hold the food firmly on the board *with* your hand but not *in* your hand. Curl your fingertips away from the blade. Grasp the knife securely by its handle with the other hand, avoiding the sharp edge of the blade. Face the blade away from your body. For rounded foods such as potatoes and onions, cut a thin slice from the bottom first so that the food sits flat on the board.

Knife Cutting Techniques

You can use a knife to cut food into different sizes and shapes. Here are the cutting terms most often found in recipes. **Figure 24.1** shows several of these techniques.

Chop, Mince To chop is to cut food into small, irregular pieces. To mince is to chop finely. Use a chef's knife for both tasks. Hold the knife handle with one hand, pressing the tip against the cutting board. Guide the blade by resting the other hand lightly on the back of the blade near the tip. Rock or pump the knife handle up and down carefully, keeping the tip of the blade on the board as the blade chops the food.

Cube, Dice To cube is to cut food into square pieces about ½ inch on a side. To dice is to cut food into square pieces about ⅛ to ¼ inch on a side.

Pare To pare is to cut off a very thin layer of peel with a paring knife or peeler.

Score To score is to make straight, shallow cuts with a slicing knife in the surface of a food. Scoring helps to tenderize meat and let sauces sink in.

Slice To slice is to cut a food into large, thin pieces with a slicing knife. Use a sawing motion while pressing the knife down gently.

Sliver To sliver is to cut a food, such as almonds, into very thin strips.

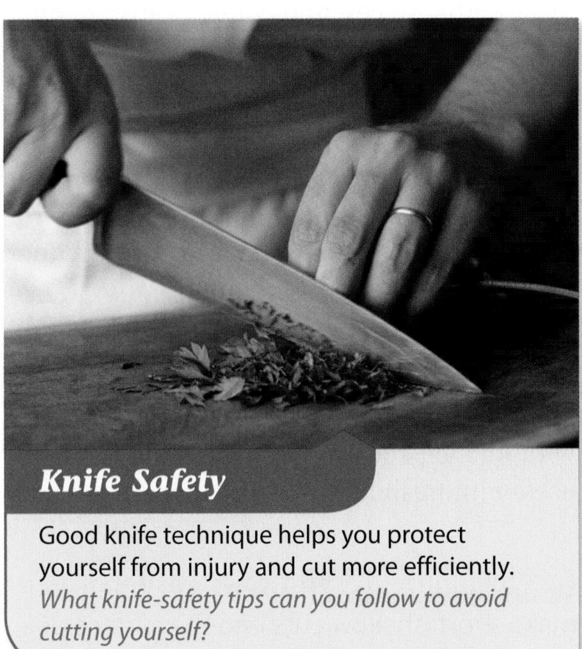

Knife Safety

Good knife technique helps you protect yourself from injury and cut more efficiently. *What knife-safety tips can you follow to avoid cutting yourself?*

TECHNOLOGY FOR TOMORROW

Cutting-Edge Technology

The first knives were made of rock, wood, and bone. Since then, technology has evolved to bring modern cooks lightweight and efficient cutting tools—made with cutting-edge materials. Today, tough substances like titanium, carbon fiber, alloy tool steel, and ceramic give knives strength and durability. Ceramic blades are so hard that they stay sharp for years with no sharpening! Technology also influences knife-making processes. Instead of the old-fashioned method of forging, or shaping red-hot metal with a hammer, many knives are drop forged. This means hot metal is poured into a pre-shaped mold. In other cases, lasers are used to cut knife blades out of sheets of metal. Lasers are also used to make blade edges sharp and precise.

Investigate Some modern kitchen knives are labeled "self-sharpening." Can these knives really sharpen themselves? If so, how? Share your findings in a paragraph.

NCSS VIII B Science, Technology, and Society Make judgements about how science and technology have transformed the physical world and human society.

Figure 24.1 Cutting Techniques

Slice and Dice Different cutting tools and techniques let you shape food into different shapes and sizes. ***Why are foods cut into small pieces?***

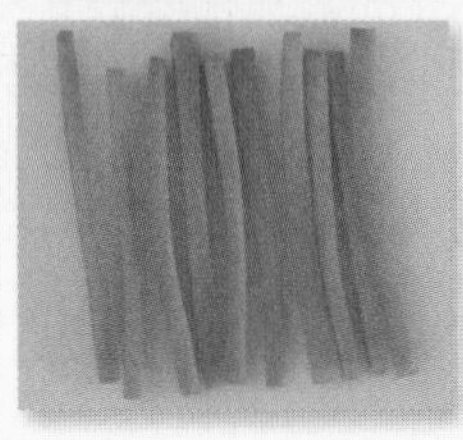

Julienne

Cutting food into ⅛- × ⅛- × 2-inch strips

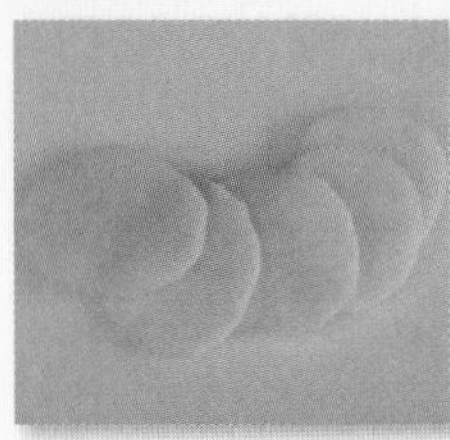

Chip

Cutting food into small, ⅛-inch thick slices

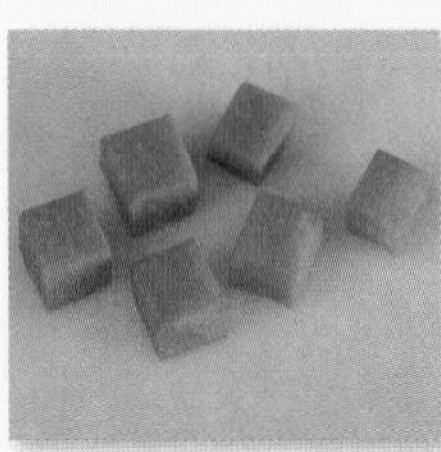

Dice

Cutting food into small, square pieces

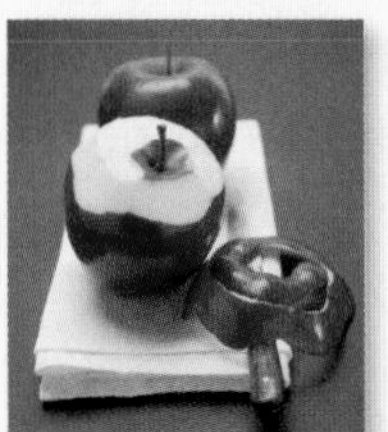

Pare

Cutting off a very thin layer of peel

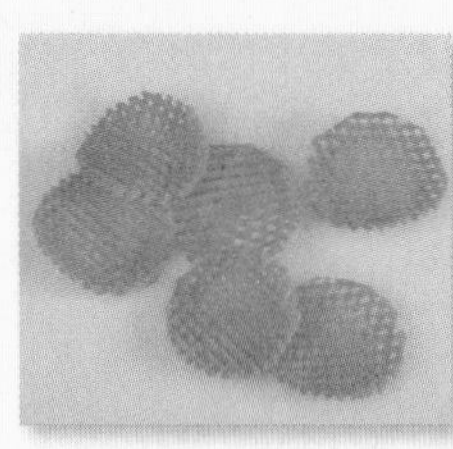

Waffle

Cutting food into ⅛-inch thick perforated slices

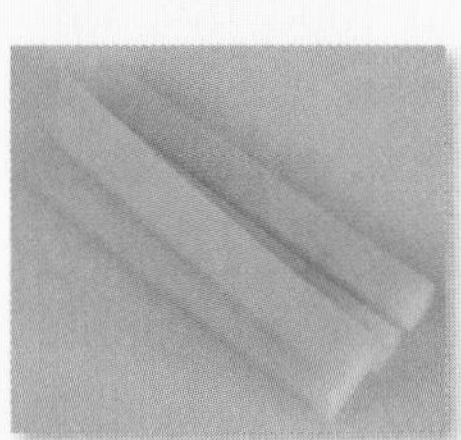

French Fry

Cutting very long lengthwise pieces

Other Cutting Techniques

You can use a variety of kitchen tools besides a knife to produce a different **effect**, or result.

Crush To crush is to pulverize food into crumbs, powder, or paste with a rolling pin, blender, or food processor.

Flake To flake is to break or tear off small layers of food with a fork. Flaking is often used for fish.

Grate, Shred To grate or shred is to cut food, such as cheese or carrots, into smaller pieces or shreds by rubbing the food against the rough surface of a grater or microplane. You can also shred cooked meat by pulling it apart with a fork.

Grind To grind is to use a grinder to break food into coarse, medium, or fine particles. Meat herbs, spices, and coffee beans are often ground.

Mash To mash is to crush food into a smooth mixture with a masher or beater.

Purée To purée is to grind or mash cooked fruits or vegetables until they are smooth. You can use a blender, a food processor, a food mill, or a sieve to purée food.

Quarter To quarter is to divide a food, usually by cutting it with a knife into four equal pieces.

Snip To snip is to cut food into small pieces with kitchen shears. This technique is usually used with fresh herbs or dried fruit.

✓ **Reading Check** **Identify** When you make short, shallow cuts into the surface of a food, what do you do?

Mixing Ingredients

Most recipes require some form of **mixing**, combining two or more ingredients thoroughly so they blend. Spoons and forks work well for basic mixing. Appliances such as blenders and food processors help with bigger mixing jobs. The terms *mix*, *combine*, and *blend* all refer to basic mixing. More specific techniques are shown in **Figure 24.2** and include the following:

Beat To beat is to mix thoroughly and add air to foods. Use a spoon and a vigorous over-and-over motion, or a mixer or food processor.

Cream To cream is to beat ingredients, such as shortening and sugar, until they are soft and creamy.

Cut in To cut in is to combine solid fats with dry ingredients such as flour to make small coarse pieces. Cutting in is used for many baked goods such as scones, biscuits, and pie crust. This is done by using a knife or fork to mash the fat into the flour.

Fold To fold is to gently mix a light, fluffy mixture into a heavier one. Egg whites are often folded into a cake batter. Place the light mixture on top of the heavier one in a bowl. With a rubber scraper or spoon, cut down through the mixture and move the tool across the bottom of the bowl to the side. Bring it back up to the surface, along with some of the mixture from the bottom. Do not lift the tool out of the mixture. Give the bowl a quarter-turn and repeat until well blended. Do this as gently and with as few passes of the scraper as possible.

Stir To stir is to mix with a spoon or a wire whisk in a circular motion. Stirring is often used for food that is cooking. It distributes heat and keeps foods from sticking to a pan.

Toss To toss is to mix ingredients, such as salad greens and dressing, by tumbling them with tongs or a large spoon and fork.

Whip To whip is to beat quickly and vigorously to incorporate air into a mixture, making it light and fluffy.

Knead To knead is to work a dough to blend the ingredients and make it smooth and springy. You can knead dough by hand or with a mixer.

✓ **Reading Check** **List** What three recipe terms all refer to basic mixing?

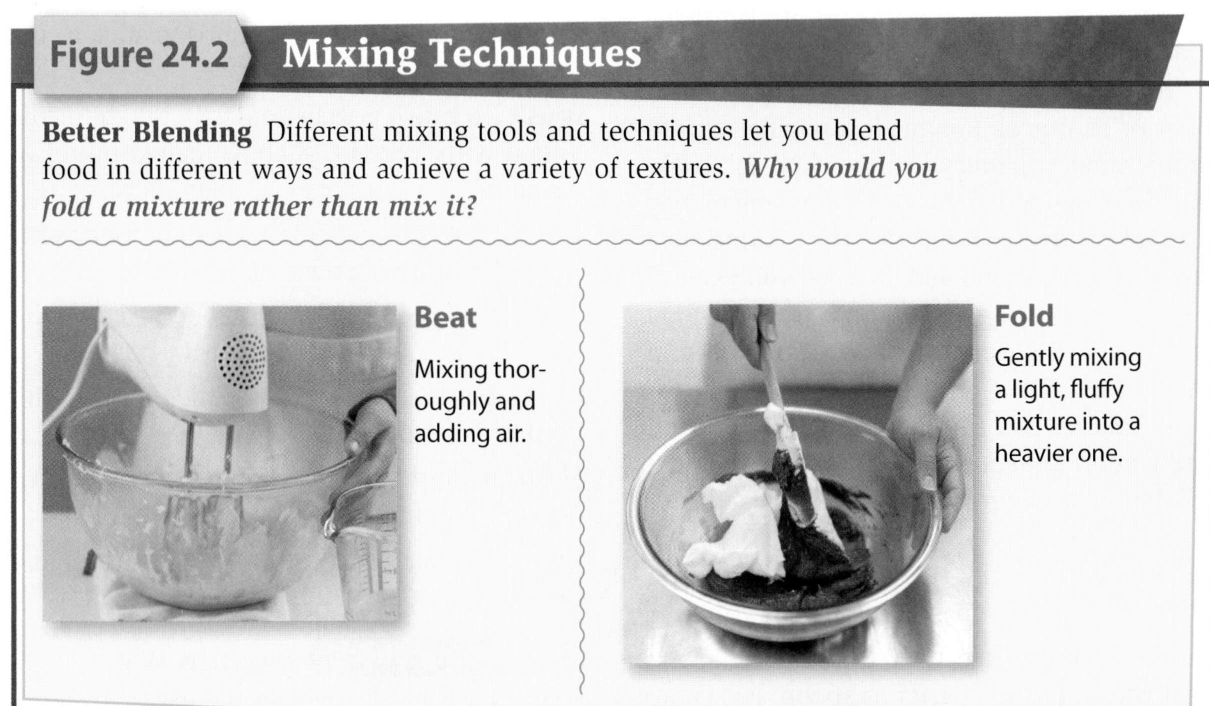

Figure 24.2 Mixing Techniques

Better Blending Different mixing tools and techniques let you blend food in different ways and achieve a variety of textures. ***Why would you fold a mixture rather than mix it?***

Beat

Mixing thoroughly and adding air.

Fold

Gently mixing a light, fluffy mixture into a heavier one.

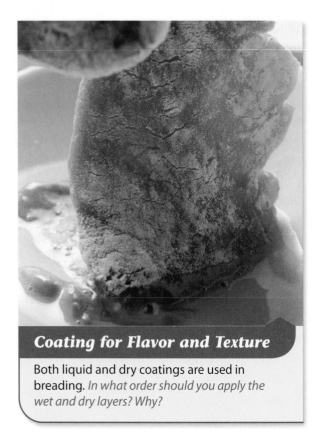

Coating for Flavor and Texture

Both liquid and dry coatings are used in breading. *In what order should you apply the wet and dry layers? Why?*

Coating Techniques

Another common preparation technique is coating. **Coating** means adding a thin layer of food on top of another food. Coating also refers to the food you use for the thin layer. Coating adds flavor and texture. It also helps food brown better and retain moisture.

A coating can be a dry ingredient, such as flour or cornmeal. Coating is a popular way to prepare meat, poultry, and seafood for cooking. Shaking food in a bag is a convenient way to apply a dry coating. Put the coating in a large plastic bag and add the food you want to coat. Close the bag and shake it until the food is completely covered. Remove the food from the bag and shake off the excess coating.

A coating can also be a liquid ingredient. You can brush foods with a sauce or dip them in a batter. A batter is a dry coating mixed with liquid.

Different coating techniques help you achieve a variety of tasty results:

Baste To baste is to pour liquid over a food as it cooks, using a baster or spoon. Foods are often basted in sauces or pan juices.

Kitchen Math

Dicing Potatoes

Miranda is preparing a recipe for home fries, which calls for diced potatoes. After peeling a potato, she squares off the sides, leaving a rectangular block. She slices this block into 20 long sticks, each measuring $5/8$ inch by $5/8$ inch by $6\frac{1}{4}$ inches. How many $5/8$ inch cubes can she get out of the potato?

Math Concept **Dividing Fractions** To divide fractions, convert any mixed or whole numbers to improper fractions. Multiply the first fraction by the reciprocal of the second fraction. Reduce to lowest terms.

Starting Hint To find the number of cubes in each stick, divide $6\frac{1}{4}$ by $5/8$. Do this by changing $6\frac{1}{4}$ into an improper fraction, and then multiplying it by $8/5$ (which is the reciprocal of $5/8$). Multiply the answer by 20 (since there are 20 sticks).

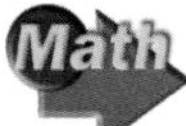

Math Appendix For math help, go to the Math Appendix at the back of the book.

NCTM Number and Operations Understand meanings of operations and how they relate to one another.

Bread To bread is to coat a food with three different layers: first flour, second a liquid such as milk or beaten egg, and third seasoned crumbs or cornmeal, which provide a crunchy surface. The flour helps the liquid to stick to the food, and the liquid helps the crumbs to stick to the food.

Brush To brush is to use a pastry brush to coat a food with a liquid, such as melted butter or a sauce.

Dot To dot is to put small pieces of food, such as butter, on the surface of another food.

Dredge To dredge is to coat food heavily with flour, breadcrumbs, or cornmeal.

Dust To dust is to lightly sprinkle a food with flour or confectioners' sugar.

Flour To flour is to coat a food, such as chicken or fish, with flour.

Glaze To glaze is to coat a food with a liquid that forms a glossy finish.

✓ **Reading Check** **Explain** Which coating technique involves the use of a handheld utensil and why?

Specialty Food-Preparation Techniques

Some food-preparation techniques are useful for specific situations, such as canning vegetables, grilling, or preparing fruit salad.

Blanch To blanch is to dip a food briefly into boiling water, then into cold water to stop the cooking process. Blanching is used in canning and freezing fruits and vegetables. Blanching foods with a thin coating or peel, such as peppers and almonds, makes them easier to peel. Blanching is useful when you want to partially cook food ahead of time so that you can finish it and serve it with other items in a complete meal.

Candy To candy is to cook a food in a sugar syrup. Some root vegetables, fruits, and fruit peels are prepared this way.

Caramelize To caramelize is to heat sugars on the surface of foods until they liquefy and darken in color. Other foods, such as onions, are sometimes caramelized to release their sugar content.

Clarify To clarify is to make a liquid clear by removing solid particles. These particles are usually mostly fat. Broth is clarified by cooking it with vegetables and egg whites that absorb the fat and remove it from the broth. Clarify butter by melting it and skimming off milk solids. The remaining butterfat is useful for frying.

Core To core is to remove the center of a fruit or vegetable, such as an apple, tomato, or pineapple.

Deglaze To deglaze is to loosen the flavorful food particles in a pan after food has been browned. Pour off the excess fat and push the food to the outside edges of the pan. Then add a small amount of liquid, and scrape the particles from the pan with a wooden spoon. The liquid will cook off but the flavor will be absorbed into the food.

Drain To drain is to separate water from solid food, such as vegetables or cooked pasta, by putting the food in a colander or strainer and letting the water run off.

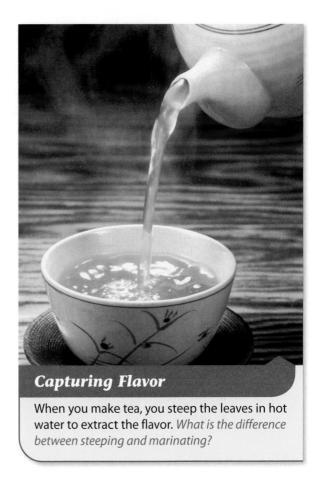

Capturing Flavor

When you make tea, you steep the leaves in hot water to extract the flavor. *What is the difference between steeping and marinating?*

Glaze To glaze is to finish cooking blanched foods, usually vegetables, in a syrup of water, sugar and butter.

Marinate To marinate is to add flavor to a food by soaking it in a cold, seasoned liquid. The liquid is usually discarded but sometimes can be used as a base for a sauce. In addition to adding flavor, marinades can be used to break down tough pieces of meat. The acid in a marinade loosens muscle fibers.

Mold To mold is to shape a food by hand or by placing it in a decorative mold.

Pit To pit is to remove a stone or seed from fruit using a sharp knife.

Reduce To reduce is to simmer a mixture in order to evaporate the liquid and intensify the flavor. When reducing, be careful not to bring mixtures to a boil as this can burn the liquid and give it a bitter flavor. Reducing is also called cooking down.

Scald To scald is to heat liquid to just below the boiling point. Many baking recipes call for scalded milk. A liquid is scalded when very small bubbles begin to form.

Score To score is to cut shallow lines into the bottom of a piece of meat that is going to be pan fried. This prevents the meat from puffing up in the middle and curling at the edges as it is heated during cooking.

Season To season is to add flavorings such as salt, pepper, herbs, and spices to a food before or during cooking.

Shell To shell is to remove the tough outer coating of a food, such as eggs, nuts, and shellfish.

Steep To steep is to soak dry ingredients, such as tea or herbs, in hot liquid to extract the flavor or soften the texture. You then strain the mixture and discard the solids. The longer the ingredients steep, the stronger the mixture will be.

Strain To strain is to separate solid particles from a liquid, such as broth, by pouring the mixture through a strainer or sieve. Sometimes it is necessary to strain a liquid more than once.

Vent To vent is to leave an opening, usually a small slit, in a container so steam can escape during cooking.

Practice these preparation techniques to expand your kitchen skills and try new flavors. Mastering a wide range of food-preparation techniques will help you to add new recipes to your list of favorites. Knowing a wide range of techniques and understanding how they can be applied to different foods allows you to create your own recipes. It allows you to base your cooking decisions on ingredients you have available. By knowing a wide range of cooking techniques you can find uses for whatever ingredients you have on hand and avoid waste.

Light and Healthy Recipe

Pico de Gallo

Ingredients

3 Roma tomatoes, diced
1 White onion, diced
2 tsp. Cilantro, chopped fine
2 tsp. Lime juice

Directions

1. Put the diced tomatoes, onions, and cilantro in a bowl and fold together.
2. Squeeze or pour the lime juice onto the mixture and fold again.
3. Serve with chips or as a condiment to a dinner of tacos or burritos.

Pico de Gallo gets its attractive look not just from the colors of red, white and green, but also from the precise cuts of tomato and onions.

Yield 4 servings

Nutrition Analysis per Serving

■ Calories	22
■ Total fat	0 g
Saturated fat	0 g
Cholesterol	0 mg
■ Sodium	4 mg
■ Carbohydrate	5
Dietary fiber	1 g
Sugars	3 g
■ Protein	1 g

CHAPTER 24 Review & Applications

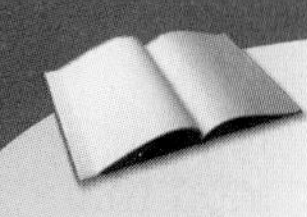

After You Read

Chapter Summary

Food preparation techniques are essential for success in the kitchen. Liquid and dry ingredients, as well as solid fats, require specific measuring tools. Foods may be measured by either volume or weight. Cutting foods requires care to ensure safety. Different cutting techniques each have varied effects on food. Most recipes require some form of mixing. There are eight mixing techniques, each having a different result. Coating techniques add a thin layer of food on top of another food. There are eight ways to coat foods. Specialty food preparation techniques are useful for specific situations, and help cooks expand their kitchen skills.

Content and Academic Vocabulary Review

1. Use each of these content and academic vocabulary words in a sentence.

Content Vocabulary

- ☐ taring (p. 374)
- ☐ cutting (p. 375)
- ☐ mixing (p. 377)
- ☐ coating (p. 378)

Academic Vocabulary

- affect (p. 374)
- effect (p. 376)

Review Key Concepts

2. **List** three different types of ingredients and the tools you need to measure them.
3. **Explain** guidelines for proper knife safety.
4. **List** eight different ways to mix ingredients.
5. **Describe** coating and why it is a useful cooking technique.
6. **Explain** the benefits of learning specialized cooking techniques.

Critical Thinking

7. **Explain** which tools you will use to measure each ingredient, and whether you will measure weight or volume. The recipe calls for 2 cups of milk, 1 cup of brown sugar, 1 teaspoon of baking soda, and 1½ pounds of chocolate chips.
8. **Describe** a meal that uses six knife cutting techniques on six different ingredients.
9. **Identify** the technique to make egg whites light, fluffy, and full of air so that they may be folded into heavier mixtures.
10. **Explain** why breaded foods are typically higher in fat than dredged foods.

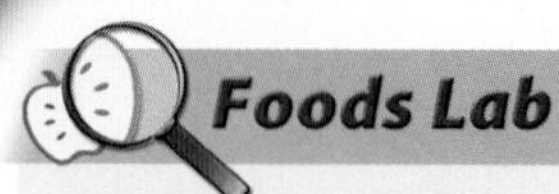

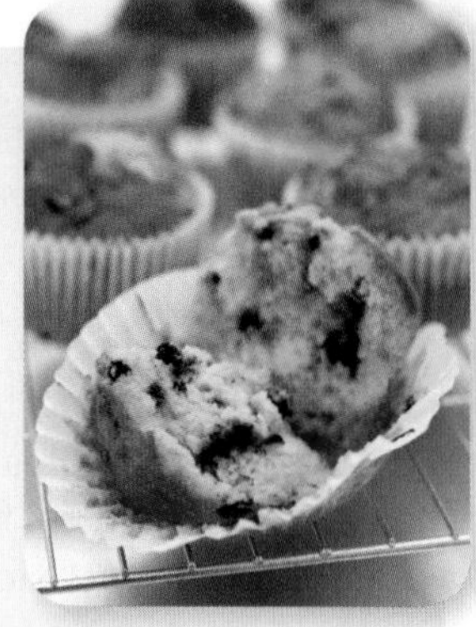

11. Making a Streusel Streusel is a topping for baked goods that is supposed to be crumbly. Different techniques for making streusel can produce very different results.

Procedure Prepare two recipes for streusel, using different techniques. For both recipes, use 2 Tbsp. flour, 2 Tbsp. sugar, and 2 Tbsp. margarine. For the first recipe, sift together the flour and sugar; then cut in the margarine. For the second recipe, cream the margarine and the sugar; then cut in the flour.

Analysis In a paragraph, compare your results and explain which technique produced the more crumbly mixture and why.

HEALTHFUL CHOICES

12. Measuring Fats Laura is careful not to include more saturated fats in her food than her recipes require. She uses butter in a tub, not stick butter. What can she do to ensure that she measures her butter accurately when her recipes call for it? What is the best way for Laura to measure accurately? What other ways can she measure?

TECH Connection

13. Terms and Techniques Under your teacher's supervision, conduct research on the Internet to find a recipe that involves one of the four following food preparation terms: purée; glaze; caramelize; marinate. Share your recipe in a brief oral report to the class. Include a picture of the completed dish and display it while you give your report. Explain how to use the food preparation technique that the recipe requires.

Real-World Skills

Problem-Solving Skills	**14. A Cutting Conflict** Ron, a cook at a restaurant, scored a piece of beef. Then his boss noticed and said, "I asked you to cube that, not to score it." What can Ron do?
Interpersonal and Collaborative Skills	**15. Techniques Quiz** Follow your teacher's instructions to form pairs. Each person should find a recipe that uses at least four preparation techniques from the chapter, then write a four-question quiz that asks for explanations of each technique. Exchange recipes and quizzes with your partner. Grade your partner's completed quiz.
Financial Literacy Skills	**16. Measuring and Money** The owner of a restaurant is upset. When she buys a week's worth of ingredients for recipes, they only last three days. She is spending extra money on ingredients, serving the usual amount of food. Explain why her kitchen staff's measuring techniques could be causing the problem.

Academic Skills

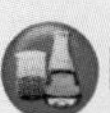

Food Science

17. Surface Tension Water molecules cling together to act as an elastic sheet at the surface, causing surface tension. Molecules not only cling to themselves, but have an attraction to the glass as well. Notice the curve at the top called the meniscus. It is higher at the edges than in the middle, or concave.

Procedure Fill a glass to the brim with water, and place in a bowl on a level surface. Drop paper clips into the water, one at a time. Record how many you can add before any water spills.

Analysis How many paper clips did it take to overflow? Did the meniscus change shape? Explain how this is possible.

NSES C Develop an understanding of matter, energy and organization in living systems.

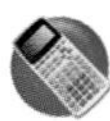

Mathematics

18. Measuring Volume
Brendan has a two-cup container of frying oil that is ¾ full. Whenever he has friends over for dinner he likes to prepare his famous wok-fried shrimp, which requires 2 tablespoons of oil each time. How many dinners can Brendan prepare with the oil he has on hand?

Math Concept **Equivalent Measurements** There are 2 tablespoons in one ounce and 8 ounces in a cup. To convert ounces to cups, multiply by 8.

Starting Hint Compute the number of tablespoons that fit in the two-cup container and divide by ¾.

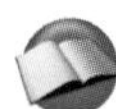

English Language Arts

19. Methods Demonstration Write and perform an oral presentation for your class in which you demonstrate and explain one of the following food preparation methods: cutting safely with knives; measuring solid fats; coating techniques; measuring by weight in a bowl. Use your own words when you write and present your demonstration. As a handout for your presentation, create a list of tips to remember what goes along with your chosen topic. Pass the tip sheet out to your classmates before you begin your presentation.

NCTE 12 Use language to accomplish individual purposes.

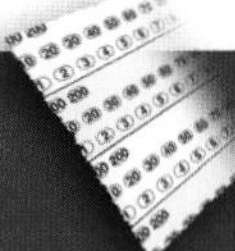

STANDARDIZED TEST PRACTICE

TRUE OR FALSE.
Read the statement and determine if it is true or false.

20. It is possible to sliver almonds after grinding them.
a. True
b. False

Test-Taking Tip Before deciding whether a statement is true or false, read it carefully, and recall what you have learned from reading the text. Does the statement reflect what you know? Pay close attention to individual words. One word can make the difference between a true statement and a false one.

CHAPTER 25

Cooking Methods

Writing Activity: Persuasive Paragraph

The Value of Cooking Today, restaurants and prepared foods make it possible to eat well without cooking. Do you think knowing how to cook is still a valuable skill? Why or why not? Write a persuasive paragraph in which you convince your reader of cooking's value, or lack thereof. Support your stance with specific examples, details, and facts.

Writing Tips Follow these steps to write a persuasive paragraph:

- Take a definite stance on an issue.
- Use specific examples, details, and facts to support your stance.
- Be persuasive by appealing to readers' logic and emotions.

Activate Prior Knowledge

Explore the Photo Different cooking methods create different flavors, and textures. *What cooking method is the cook using here?*

Reading Guide

Before You Read

Preview Skim through the chapter, noting each of the cooking methods mentioned. Think about whether you have personally used each method.

Read to Learn

Key Concepts

- **Describe** three main ways to transfer heat to food.
- **Identify** three factors that affect the rate at which food cooks.
- **Describe** seven techniques for moist-heat cooking.
- **Explain** five techniques for cooking in fat.
- **Describe** three techniques for dry-heat cooking.
- **Describe** the best method for preserving nutrients in vegetables.

Main Idea

Different cooking methods change the texture and flavor of foods, and add nutrition and appeal to meals.

Content Vocabulary

You will find definitions for these words in the glossary at the back of this book.

- conduction
- convection
- radiation
- Maillard reaction
- moist-heat cooking
- smoking point
- sear
- wok
- dry-heat cooking
- microwave cooking
- cooking power
- arcing
- microwave time
- standing time

Academic Vocabulary

You will find these words in your reading and on your tests. Use the glossary to look up their definitions if necessary.

- uniform
- withstand

Graphic Organizer

Use a graphic organizer like the one below to categorize the 15 methods of cooking described in this chapter.

MOIST-HEAT COOKING	DRY-HEAT COOKING	COOKING IN FAT

Graphic Organizer Go to this book's Online Learning Center at **glencoe.com** to print out this graphic organizer.

Academic Standards

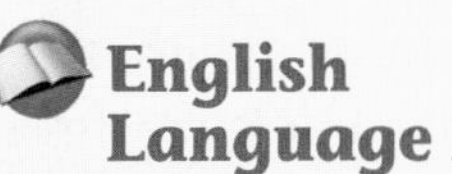

English Language Arts

NCTE 4 Use written language to communicate effectively.

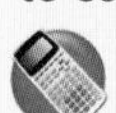

Mathematics

NCTM Problem Solving Apply and adapt a variety of appropriate strategies to solve problems.

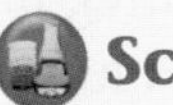

Science

NSES G Develop an understanding of science as a human endeavor.

NSES A Develop understandings about scientific inquiry.

NCTE *National Council of Teachers of English*
NCTM *National Council of Teachers of Mathematics*
NSES *National Science Education Standards*
NCSS *National Council for the Social Studies*

How Food Cooks

Why are foods cooked in so many different ways? What happens to food as it cooks? Knowing the answers to these questions can help you choose cooking methods that add nutrition and appeal to meals.

All cooking methods have one thing in common: heat. You heat food by putting it in contact with a heat source, such as a cooktop or a campfire. If you add enough heat to a substance, the molecules vibrate. The greater the heat, the more intense the vibration. Vibration is invisible, but it creates results that you can see, feel, and taste. You can transfer heat to food using conduction, convection, and radiation.

Conduction

Conduction is a method of transferring heat by direct contact. Heated molecules pass their vibration to neighboring molecules, spreading heat, as you see in **Figure 25.1**.

As an example, think of a pancake cooking in a skillet. Heat in the heating unit is conducted to the skillet. Heat in the skillet is conducted to the bottom of the pancake. Heat in the bottom of the pancake is conducted to the rest of the pancake. To cook the pancake evenly, you flip it over so that both sides come in contact with the hot pan.

Convection

Convection is a method of transferring heat through the movement of molecules in air or liquid. Warm air is less dense than cool air because the molecules vibrate more quickly, driving them farther apart. Warm air rises. As it rises, it pushes cool air out of the way, driving the cool air down until it warms and rises back up. The movement of warm air up and cool air down forms a convection current. The convection current continues until the air is evenly heated.

Convection also occurs in liquids. Suppose you heat a pan of water. As the water at the bottom of the pan warms, it rises toward the surface. The rising warm water forces the cool water downward. Now the cool water absorbs heat and rises back toward the surface again until the water boils.

Figure 25.2 shows the process of convection at work in an oven and on a stovetop.

Radiation

Radiation is a method of transferring heat as waves of energy. Unlike convection, which relies on rising heat, radiant heat flows evenly from the source in every direction. This is how the sun warms the earth and how flames from a broiler cook food on the pan below it. **Figure 25.3** shows radiation in action.

Figure 25.1 Conduction

Heavy Heat In conduction, heat moves from one object to another through direct physical contact. Here, the heating element heats the pan, which in turn heats the food. ***How does a heated molecule pass heat to an unheated molecule?***

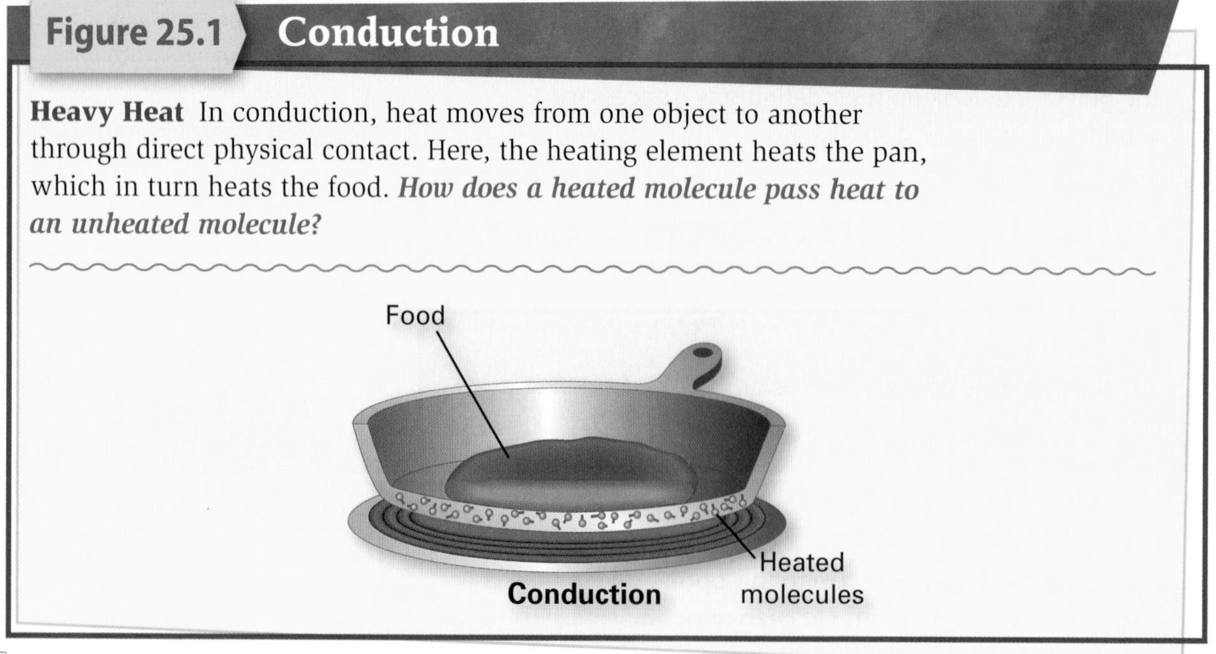

Figure 25.2 Convection

Currents for Cooking In convection, heat transfer occurs as molecules move through air or water, creating currents. ***What keeps convection currents moving?***

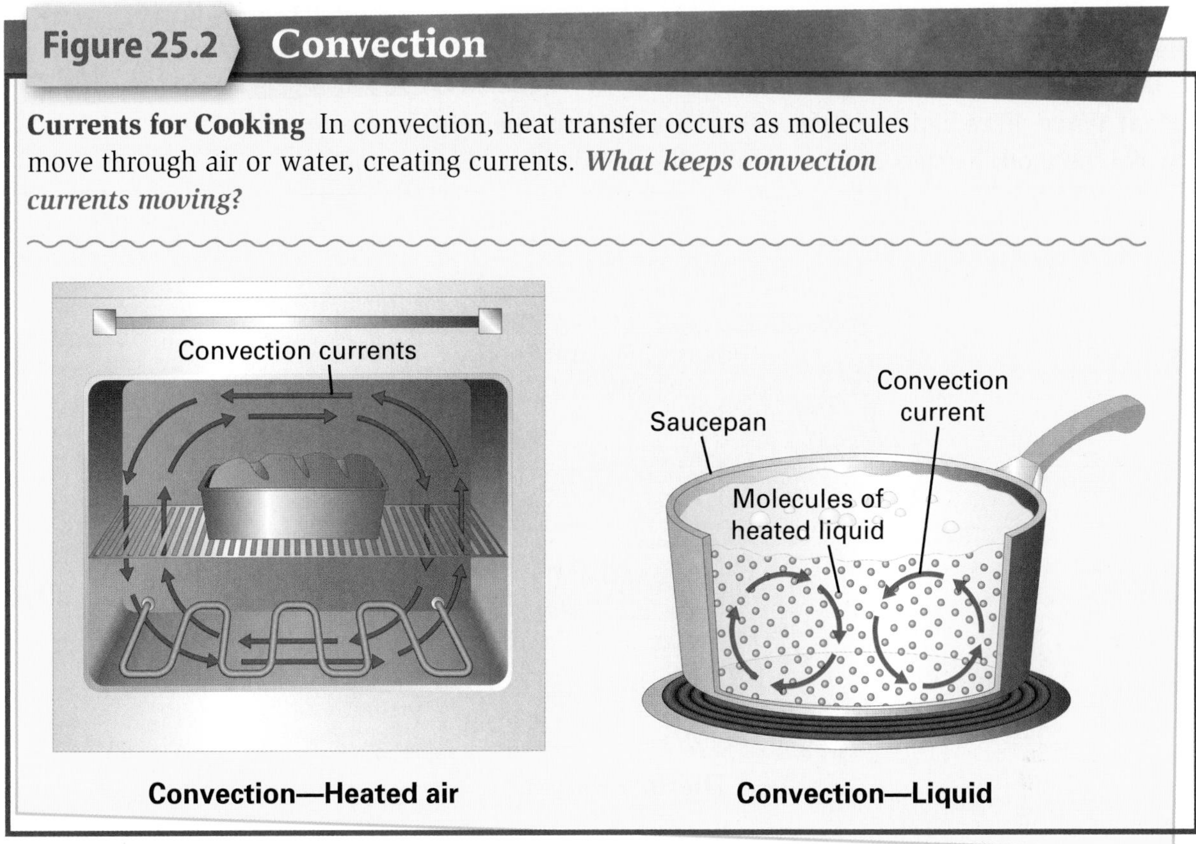

Combining Cooking Processes

Most cooking methods use a combination of heat-transfer processes. In baking, for example, the surface of a food is heated by convection. The heat then travels through the food by conduction.

All ovens use convection as well as radiation to cook foods; however, a convection oven has a fan to circulate the heated air. The moving air delivers more heat energy, which promotes browning and crispness. Depending on the food, you can reduce oven temperatures in recipes by 25°F to 50°F when using a convection oven.

Effects on Food and Nutrients

When you apply heat properly, you create delicious changes in food's sensory qualities. Heat releases flavor and aroma. Sometimes heat changes food's texture and color. Cookie dough becomes crisp and meat becomes tender. Some vegetables grow brighter and some become duller.

Heat has positive and negative effects on nutrients. Cooking breaks down some forms of fiber, making them easier to digest and more useful to the body. However, heat destroys some nutrients, especially vitamin C and the B vitamins. Heat usually has little effect on minerals. Heat does not damage protein, although animal proteins are sensitive to high temperatures. When cooked too long, eggs become rubbery and meat becomes chewy and tough.

The browning that you see on roasted, fried, or baked foods adds flavor and color. Browning occurs when heat provokes a series of chemical reactions between certain sugars and proteins in the food. This is known as the **Maillard reaction**, named for the person who discovered it, Dr. L.C. Maillard.

How heat is applied—that is, the cooking method you choose—also affects food's color, texture, taste, and nutritional value. Food can be cooked in several ways, including in moist heat, in fat, and by microwave.

✓ **Reading Check** **Describe** What happens to the molecules of a substance when it is heated?

Figure 25.3 Radiation

Heat Wave In radiation, waves of heat energy from the heat source strike the food. Broilers and toasters both use radiation. ***What is the difference between radiation and convection?***

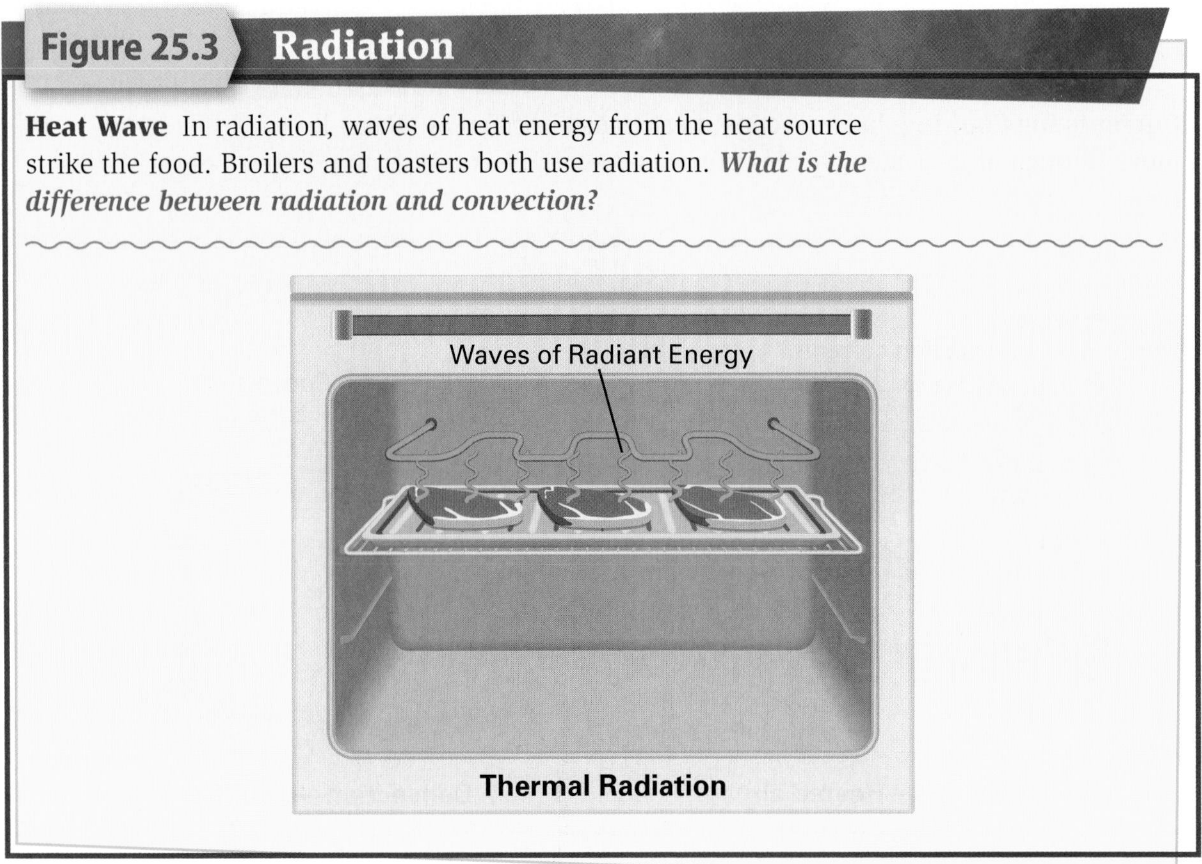

Cooking Rates

Different cooking processes transfer heat at different rates. This affects the time foods need to cook. The speed at which food cooks is also influenced by these three factors:

Density Density is a food's weight divided by its volume. A 3-inch cube of meat weighs more than a 3-inch cube of potato, so it is more dense. Foods that are denser cook more slowly than foods that are less dense.

Shape and Size The more surface area a food has, the greater its exposure to heat. Two thin carrot slices cook more quickly than one thicker carrot slice, for example. Cutting foods to a **uniform**, or same, size also helps them cook at the same rate. Suppose you put a whole carrot in a pot of soup. Which end will finish cooking first, the narrow end or the thick end?

Amount The more food you put in the pot, pan, or other cooking area, the longer it takes heat to reach each item. Foods closer to the heat source cook more quickly as well. The impact varies with food size, shape, density, and other factors. A small potato still takes less time to cook than a large potato, but four potatoes do not necessarily take four times longer to cook than one.

✓ Reading Check **Explain** What is density and how does it influence cooking rates?

Moist-Heat Cooking

Food can be cooked in several ways, including in moist heat, in dry heat, in fat, and by microwave. **Moist-heat cooking** is a method of cooking food in hot liquid, steam, or both. Moisture allows heat transfer by both conduction and convection. Moist-heat cooking helps tenderize food and blend flavors. Moist-heat cooking is the only way to prepare rice, dry beans, and other foods that must absorb liquid to be edible.

You can cook with moist heat in a slow cooker, in a microwave oven, or in a pot or pan, either with or without a tight-fitting lid.

A lid prevents liquid from evaporating so that foods do not dry out or burn. Sometimes you may want water to evaporate, however, to concentrate flavors or thicken sauces.

Match the moist-heat cooking method to the food to get the best results.

Boiling

Boiling is cooking food in a liquid that has reached the highest temperature possible under normal conditions. The temperature varies depending on the liquid. Water boils at 212°F. In boiling, air bubbles continuously rise, break the surface, and escape as steam. This vigorous, rolling action propels pieces of food against each other. These tiny collisions can break up foods and break down texture, color, and flavor.

Boiling works well for the few foods that need this high degree of energy, such as corn on the cob and pasta. Boiling toughens animal proteins and results in the greatest loss of nutrients of all cooking methods, particularly if food is overcooked. Water-soluble vitamins dissolve in boiling liquid.

When you boil foods, use a pot or saucepan large enough to hold the liquid and the food, plus some space for bubbling. Bring the liquid to a boil and add the food. Be sure the liquid continues to boil as the food cooks. To save any water-soluble vitamins, save the liquid to make a sauce or to cook rice.

Simmering

Simmering is cooking food in a liquid at temperatures just below boiling. Water simmers at about 185°F to 210°F. When a liquid simmers, air bubbles rise slowly and just barely break the surface. Simmering is gentler on foods than boiling and is less destructive to shape, flavor, color, and texture. Simmering does remove water-soluble vitamins, however, so save the liquid for another recipe.

Simmering is useful for cooking many types of foods, including fish, rice, firm or dried fruits, and less tender cuts of poultry. Some foods, such as meat and dry beans, can be simmered in a slow cooker.

Poaching

Poaching is cooking food in a small amount of liquid at temperatures just below simmering. You can use a covered or an uncovered pan. Poaching is a gentle cooking method that helps retain the shape and tenderness of delicate foods such as fish, fruit, and eggs without the shell. You can add flavor by seasoning or sweetening the liquid.

Steaming

Steaming is cooking food over, but not in, boiling water. You place the food in a perforated steamer basket that fits inside a pan, and fill the pan with water to just below the level of the basket. Cover the pan with a tight-fitting lid to trap the steam created as the water boils.

It takes longer to steam foods than to boil or simmer them, but they retain their appearance, flavor, and nutrients better. You may need to add water to keep the pan from boiling dry. An electric steamer does not boil dry.

Most types of food can be steamed, including vegetables, seafood, poultry, and meat. Steamed breads and puddings are holiday traditions in some cuisines.

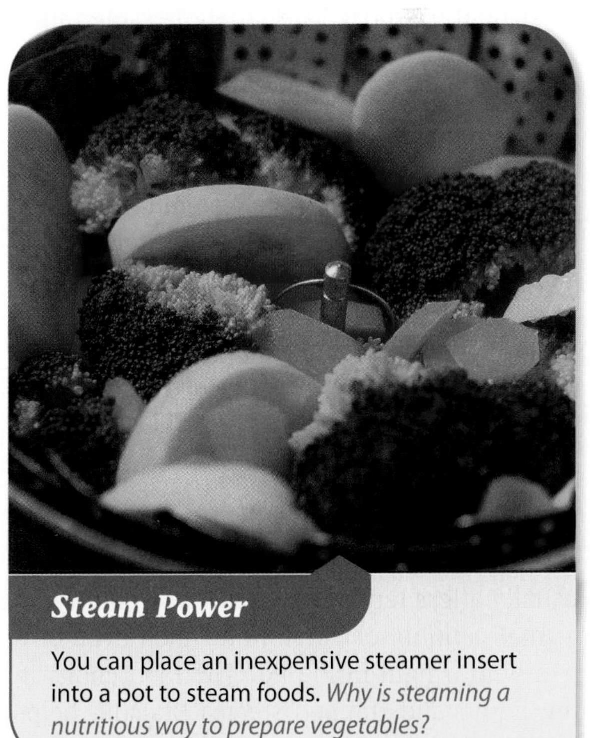

Steam Power

You can place an inexpensive steamer insert into a pot to steam foods. *Why is steaming a nutritious way to prepare vegetables?*

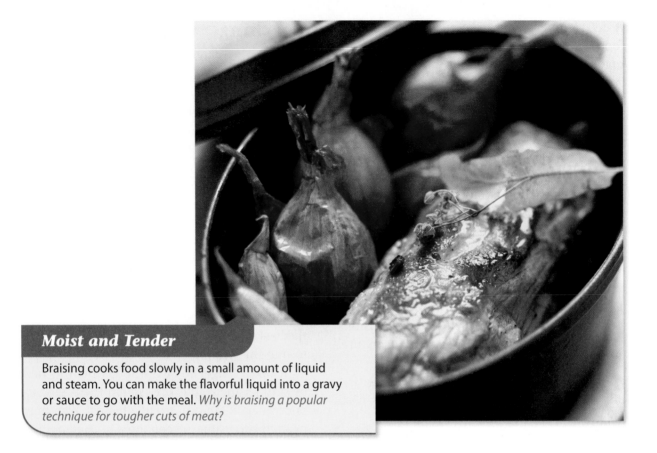

Moist and Tender

Braising cooks food slowly in a small amount of liquid and steam. You can make the flavorful liquid into a gravy or sauce to go with the meal. *Why is braising a popular technique for tougher cuts of meat?*

Pressure-Cooking

Pressure-cooking is cooking food in a pressure cooker, a special lidded pot that creates a high-pressure atmosphere by trapping steam in an airtight chamber. The added pressure raises the boiling point. Water can reach temperatures of around 250°F in a pressure cooker, so foods cook in less time. Shorter cooking times mean that fewer nutrients are lost.

Pressure-cooking is convenient for foods that normally have long cooking times, such as potatoes, dry beans, and less tender cuts of meat. Foods that cook quickly, however, soon turn to mush. Follow the manufacturer's directions carefully when using a pressure cooker.

Braising

Braising is cooking food in simmering liquid and steam. You place a large piece of food, usually a less tender cut of meat or poultry, in a small amount of liquid in a Dutch oven or a pan with a tight-fitting lid. The food cooks in the liquid and trapped steam. Braising helps tough meats break down and become tender.

Meats are usually browned before braising. You can add carrots and other vegetables near the end of the braising time. You can flavor tender foods, such as fish or pork chops, by using a seasoned sauce as the braising liquid.

You can braise food on a cooktop, in the oven, in a slow cooker, or in a pressure cooker. On a cooktop, let the liquid simmer just enough to create steam. In the oven, use a low temperature around 325°F. Check the pan occasionally. Add a little hot liquid if more is needed. Cold liquid slows the cooking process.

Stewing

Stewing is cooking small pieces of food by covering them completely with a liquid and simmering them slowly in a covered pan. Stewing is often used for less tender cuts of meat and for poultry, fish, and fruit.

✓ **Reading Check** **Identify** In which moist-heat cooking method does the food not touch the water?

Cooking in Fat

Cooking food in oil or melted fat applies heat through convection and conduction. Fats can be heated to much higher temperatures than liquids. Fried foods turn brown, develop a crisp crust, and acquire a characteristic fried flavor.

Every type of fat has a **smoking point**, the temperature at which a fat begins to break down and burn. Fats heated above their smoking point give off smoke, discolor, develop an unpleasant odor and flavor and may set off smoke alarms.

Animal fats have low smoking points. Butter starts to break down at around 300°F, lard at 375°F. Vegetable oils have relatively high smoking points—450°F for corn oil, 495°F for soybean oil. You can add a little oil to butter to raise its smoking point, which makes it useful for more frying tasks.

An oil's smoking point drops about 10°F each time you re-use it, because exposure to food, heat, and air lowers its quality. Therefore, fresh oil gives the best results.

Moisture in food can make fats spatter, burning anyone in range. Water falling into oil can cause burns as the oil bubbles violently. Fats ignite easily at temperatures over 600°F. To fry safely, use only dry food and keep a fire extinguisher nearby.

There are many different ways to cook foods in fat, including frying, sautéing, pan-broiling, deep-fat frying, and stir-frying. Surprisingly, some methods add little fat to food.

Frying and Sautéing

Frying and sautéing are methods of cooking food in a small amount of hot fat in a skillet over moderate heat.

Frying uses more fat than sautéing and is designed for larger pieces of food, including seafood, eggs, and tender cuts of meat and poultry. Allow the food to cook undisturbed as long as possible so that it can brown. However, you may need to turn the food a few times to cook it completely and evenly. If the pieces are thick, you can cover the pan to retain heat. Frying is also called pan-frying.

Sauté comes from the French word for jump. You shake the pan from time to time as you sauté food, which makes the food "jump." This technique lets food cook quickly in small amounts of fat without burning. Sautéing is often used to precook vegetables for use in a recipe, such as chopped onions and celery for a poultry stuffing. You can also sauté small pieces of fish and tender meats.

Pan-Broiling

Pan-broiling is cooking food in an uncovered skillet in its own natural fat, with no fat added. Pan-broiling is most often used for thin cuts of tender meat that cook quickly, including hamburgers, steak, and some cuts of pork. The fat liquefies as it cooks, and you drain it away before serving. Pan-broiled food therefore retains a minimal amount of fat. Pan-broiling is often used to **sear** meat, or brown it quickly over high heat, before the meat is cooked in moist heat. The high heat and a hot skillet give an attractive, flavorful brown crust that moist-heat cooking does not provide. You can also use a broiler to sear meat.

Be a Smart Consumer

Cooking Classes

Community-sponsored cooking classes are popular with consumers who want to develop their culinary skills and have fun. The classes vary to meet almost every interest. A registered dietitian may give a one-day demonstration on preparing nutritious meals on a budget. A professional chef might lead a six-week course that includes practicing sophisticated techniques, growing fresh herbs, and touring a farmers market. Candy and cookie making classes are popular around the holidays. Some classes even travel to foreign countries such as Italy or France to learn regional cooking techniques.

Challenge Besides classes, what are other resources for consumers who want to learn more about cooking? Write a paragraph describing your findings or ideas.

Deep-Fat Frying

Deep-fat frying is cooking food by immersing it in hot fat, without making contact with the cooking vessel. Seafood and vegetables are breaded or coated with a batter first. Sweet doughs are deep-fat fried to produce a variety of breads and pastries, such as doughnuts. Deep-fat frying is often called "French frying."

To deep-fat fry, fill a deep kettle no more than half full of oil. Bring the oil to the temperature specified in the recipe, usually around 350°F. Monitor the temperature with a deep-fat frying thermometer. If the temperature is too low, the food soaks up the fat. If the temperature is too high, the food burns on the outside but remains undercooked on the inside.

Add food carefully to the hot oil. Place small pieces of solid food in a wire frying basket, which can be gently lowered and easily removed. Do not poke or prod food while it is frying. This can cause breading or batter to fall off. Turn large pieces of food with tongs or a slotted spoon, not a fork. A fork will pierce the food, releasing its juices. This lowers the temperature of the fat and allows fat to enter the food. The juices may also cause the fat to bubble over or ignite. Overcrowding the kettle also lowers the oil's temperature.

Nutrition Check

Taking the Fat Out of Frying

Many people limit deep-fat fried food for health reasons. One way to add the flavor and crunch of deep-fat frying to food while limiting the amount of fat is to first steam or bake food until almost done, then deep-fat fry it for one minute. Another alternative cooking method is oven-frying. Oven-fried food is coated in a textured mixture—such as bread crumbs, shredded cheese, and melted butter—and then baked in the oven.

Think About It How do you think these alternative cooking techniques cut down on the fat that is present in traditional deep-fat fried foods? Describe your thoughts in a paragraph.

After the food is fully cooked, carefully remove it from the kettle and drain it on a baking sheet lined with paper towels. Some people use a cooling rack so that food does not sit in its own fat. Let the fat return to the proper temperature before adding another batch of food. When you are done cooking, allow the oil to cool and then discard it.

Stir-Frying

Stir-frying is stirring small pieces of food over high heat in a small amount of oil until just tender. Use thin, uniformly sliced pieces of food to ensure fast, even cooking. Begin with the foods that will take the longest to cook and add others as you work. For example, begin with chicken strips and stir in sliced green pepper a few minutes later. Add firm vegetables like onions and carrots before softer ones like celery and squash. Vegetables in a stir-fry remain crisp.

When you are almost done stir-frying, add a small amount of seasoned liquid. The liquid thickens as it cooks, glazing the ingredients and helping their flavors blend. Some stir-fry recipes call for covering the pan toward the end.

A special bowl-shaped pan called a **wok** is the traditional cookware for stir-frying. A skillet with a tight-fitting lid makes a fine substitute.

✓ Reading Check **Identify** Which cooking method is often used for thin cuts of tender meat that cook quickly?

Dry-Heat Cooking

Dry-heat cooking is cooking food uncovered without added liquid or fat. Despite its name, this method produces soft, chewy brownies in the oven and juicy hamburgers on the grill. Dry, radiant heat gives food a crisp brown crust with a distinctive flavor, while the inside remains moist and tender. Dry-heat cooking also helps retain water-soluble vitamins.

Dry-heat methods include roasting, baking, broiling, and grilling. The main difference among these methods is the position of the heat source.

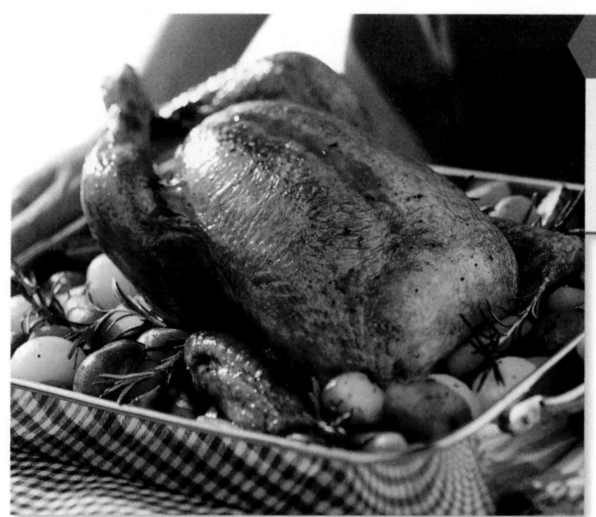

Roasted Foods

Roasted and baked foods cook in dry heat, without liquid or fat. Vegetables can cook alongside meat or poultry in the roasting pan. *Why is moisture lost as food bakes?*

Roasting and Baking

Roasting and baking refer to cooking foods surrounded by heat in an oven. The word *roasting* is used for meat and poultry. The word *baking* is more often used for vegetables, fruits, casseroles, fish, and baked goods such as cakes.

To roast meat or poultry, place a large, tender cut in a shallow roasting pan without a cover. You can place the food on a rack inside the pan to allow fat to drain away.

When you bake vegetables, fruits, casseroles, fish, and baked goods, moisture is lost from the food as it cooks. Moisture loss is sometimes desirable in baking, however. A baked potato, for example, gets fluffy inside as steam escapes from it.

Broiling

Broiling is cooking food under direct heat. Place food on a pan below the heating unit, which may be in a special compartment or in the oven. The heat radiates down from the heating unit and cooks the food rapidly. Turn large pieces of food so they can brown on both sides.

Tender cuts of meat and poultry broil well. So do seafood, fruits, and some vegetables. A broiler pan is used for broiling meat. It has two pieces: a slotted grid that holds the food and a shallow pan below that catches the fat drippings. The lower pan is usually called the drip pan.

Most ranges have only one broil setting, which turns on the broiling unit. You control the cooking by adjusting the distance of the pan from the heat. For example, you might place tomato slices 4 inches below the heat source and chicken pieces 6 inches below the heat source.

Be sure food is dry before broiling it. Moisture can keep food from browning and getting crisp. Salt foods after broiling, not before. Salt draws moisture to the surface, which interferes with browning and dries the food.

Help keep foods from sticking by starting with a cold broiler pan. Remove the pan before preheating the broiler. Make sure the pan is clean in case you want to use the drippings to make gravy or sauce. Do not line the broiler grid with foil to keep it clean. Liquid that drips from the food will turn to steam, which defeats the purpose of broiling. Fat that drips onto the foil may also start to smoke, spoiling the food's taste or even catching fire.

Broiling requires careful attention. Food near an open flame can go from nearly done to completely burned in only seconds.

Science in Action

Browning

The brown exterior on cooked roasts and baked and fried foods adds flavor as well as color. Browning of foods is known in food science as the Maillard reaction, a chemical reaction between amino acids and sugars when food is exposed to heat.

Procedure Julienne a small onion and add it to a pan with a little hot oil. Sauté the onion until it is browned. Taste the onion.

Analysis Write a paragraph detailing your evaluation of the onion. Does it taste sweet? What else do you notice about the taste of the caramelized onion compared to the way a raw onion tastes? Knowing what you know now, why do you think onions often are used in recipes?

NSES G Develop understanding of science as a human endeavor.

Grilling

Grilling is cooking food on a grate over an open flame. Grilling is like broiling, but with the flame below the food rather than above it. As with broiling, the cooking time depends on the type of food, the thickness of the food, and the food's distance from the heat.

You can grill countless foods, including vegetables, kebabs, meat, poultry, and fish. Corn on the cob and potatoes grill well when placed in a skillet on top of the grill or wrapped in heavy-duty aluminum foil. You can also use a skillet or foil to warm breads and rolls.

Some people worry that rapidly cooking meat over high heat creates chemicals that can cause cancer. Fat that drips onto hot coals may also create unsafe chemicals. Take these precautions for grilling safety:

- Marinate food before grilling. Marinating can reduce cancer-causing agents.
- Raise the grate a few inches to cook food farther from the flame.
- Precook meat and poultry in the microwave oven to limit grilling time. Finish cooking immediately to stop bacterial growth.
- Cut food into small pieces to speed cooking.
- Turn food frequently while grilling so that it does not char.
- Be attentive to everything cooking on your grill. Watch items you are grilling closely so that you can remove them from the grill as soon as they are done.
- Be aware of hot spots. Different areas of your grill will be hotter than others. Use these spots to your advantage by rotating foods over them. Avoid letting any item stay in a hot spot for too long.

✓ Reading Check **List** What types of food are suitable for grilling?

Microwave Cooking

Microwave cooking is cooking food with energy in the form of electrical waves. Microwave ovens cook food quickly with little or no added water. Microwaving retains more nutrients, especially water-soluble vitamins, than most other cooking methods.

How Microwaves Cook

Microwaves are a form of radiant energy, but they are not a form of heat energy. Microwaves flow in an electric current that causes food molecules to vibrate. Vibration creates friction, which produces the heat that cooks the food. Microwaves cook fast, but they are relatively weak. They penetrate food to a depth of 1½ inches at most. Conduction is a slower process than microwaving, but it moves the heat deeper into thick foods.

Microwaves penetrate foods unevenly. They affect water molecules most, so foods with high water content cook more quickly. Fat, sugar, and salt also absorb microwaves. Concentrations of these ingredients can become "hot spots." If you microwave a jelly doughnut, you might burn your mouth on scorching jelly, while the doughnut itself feels only warm.

Use caution when microwaving foods with a peel or skin such as potatoes and squash. Steam can build up inside, causing the food to split open and even explode.

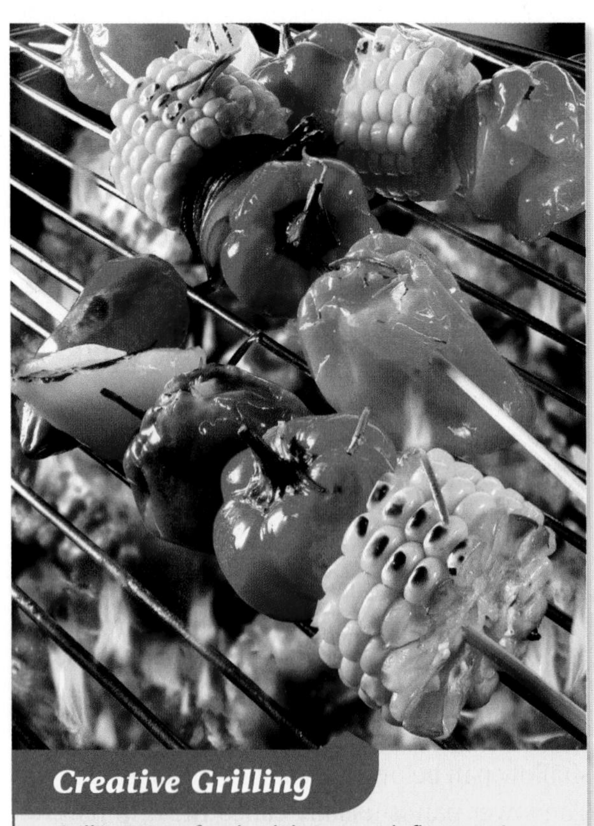

Creative Grilling

Grilling gives food a delicious, rich flavor. *What other foods besides meats and poultry can be grilled?*

Power Settings

Microwaves generate power but not heat, so oven controls are not marked with temperature settings. Instead of a temperature, you choose a **cooking power**, the amount of energy the microwave oven uses to generate microwaves. The energy is measured as watts of electricity rather than as degrees Fahrenheit. The higher the cooking power is, the more quickly foods cook.

On some microwave ovens, the power setting is expressed as a percentage, such as 50 percent or 100 percent power. On others, it is a description, such as "low" or "medium." **Figure 25.4** compares the two kinds of settings.

Microwave ovens have different power levels. The larger the number of watts, the more powerful the microwave. A 900-watt oven at 30 percent power cooks with more energy than a 700-watt oven at 30 percent power. To avoid overcooking or undercooking, check the owner's manual for information on power settings.

When a microwave is set at less than full power, it cycles on and off during cooking. At 50 percent power, for example, microwaves are created only during half the cooking time. By working with your microwave you can learn which foods taste better if cooked slower.

Microwave Cookware

You can buy special cookware for microwave ovens or use tableware and conventional cookware that you already have. You can use containers made of glass, china, pottery, or paper. Microwaves pass through these materials to heat only the food. Avoid products containing recycled paper, which may contain metal fragments or chemicals that could catch fire. Use containers that can **withstand**, or resist, the heat transferred from the food.

You can use plastic containers, but only if they are marked as microwave-safe. Plastic and Styrofoam™ containers from store-bought or take-out foods may blister, warp, or melt. Chemicals from the plastic may contaminate the food. Do not reuse containers from microwavable foods, such as cups from shelf-stable soups.

Figure 25.4 Microwave Power Levels

Know the Wattage Microwaves have power settings instead of temperature settings to let you control how a food is cooked. ***A 500-watt microwave set on high cooks as quickly as a 1000-watt microwave set at what level?***

Description	Percentage of Power
High	100
Medium-High	70
Medium	50
Medium-Low	30
Low	10

Metal is a microwaving hazard. Metals reflect microwaves, which can cause **arcing**, the production of electrical sparks that can damage the oven or start a fire. Never leave a metal tool or utensil in any food while microwaving. Even small bits of metal, such as the trim on a bowl, can cause a fire.

Use aluminum foil only as the owner's manual or recipe specifies. Small pieces of foil are sometimes used to shield the bony end of chicken legs, for instance.

How can you tell if a container is microwave-safe? Use this simple test. Put a cup of cold water in a glass measuring cup and place it in the microwave oven next to the empty container you want to test. Heat them for 2 minutes on high (100 percent power). If the water has heated and the empty container is still cool, the container is microwave-safe. If the container is warm or hot, it is not safe. It has trapped heat rather than letting it pass through, the way a microwave-safe container should.

The size and shape of microwave cookware also affect the way food cooks and the cooking time. Pans should be shallow, with straight sides. Round pans promote even cooking. Food in square or rectangular pans may overcook in the corners.

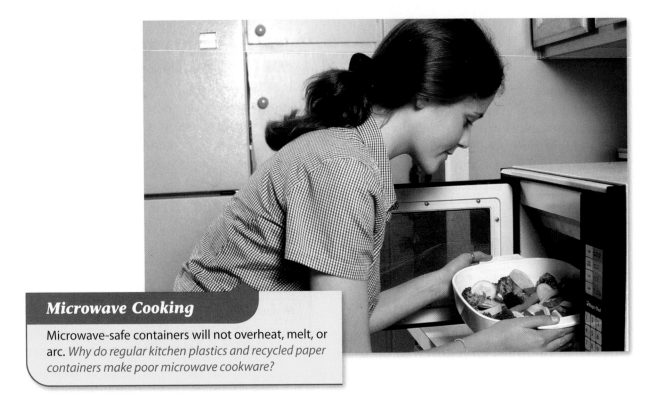

Microwave Cooking

Microwave-safe containers will not overheat, melt, or arc. *Why do regular kitchen plastics and recycled paper containers make poor microwave cookware?*

Techniques for Microwave Cooking

Microwaves heat water, fat, sugar, and salt more quickly than other parts of food. You can ensure thorough, even cooking by following a few basic microwaving techniques. Microwave recipes and cookbooks also give specific instructions on how to prepare particular foods.

Proper Food Placement

Food should be arranged to let microwaves enter from as many sides as possible. A ring is the most effective shape for microwave cooking. You can mold meatloaf into a ring, for example, or make a circle of potatoes. Leave space between them to allow microwaves to get in from all sides.

Food in the center of a microwave oven cooks more slowly than food toward the edges. Arrange food like the spokes of a wheel, with the thickest or toughest parts toward the outside and the thinnest or most tender parts toward the center. For example, place asparagus spears in a dish with stalks pointing outward. Some recipes call for rearranging the food partway through cooking.

Covering Food

Covering helps foods retain moisture as well as cook more evenly in the microwave oven. Covering also keeps food from spattering in the oven. The kind of cover you use depends on the results you want.

Heat and steam can build up under any type of cover. Remove a cover with a potholder or an oven mitt, tilting the cover away from you to shield against escaping steam.

Paper Towels Paper towels absorb excess moisture. When you heat breads and sandwiches, keep them from getting soggy by wrapping them in paper towels. Choose paper towels labeled "microwave-safe." Other towels may contain synthetic fibers that could melt.

Wax Paper and Cooking Parchment Wax paper and silicone-coated parchment paper retain heat while allowing some moisture to escape. They are sometimes used for microwaving frozen entrées.

Plastic Wrap Plastic wrap works well for holding in moisture. It is used for foods that may dry out, such as casseroles, or to keep liquids from evaporating. Use only microwave-safe plastic wrap, never plastic storage bags or other wrappers. Cover the container loosely or slit the wrap so steam can escape. Keep the plastic from touching the food to prevent chemical contamination. Some plastic wrap calls for at least 1 inch of space between food and plastic.

Lids You can cover food with an upside-down plate or a loose-fitting glass or plastic lid. Avoid tight-fitting lids, which may cause the contents to erupt.

Stirring, Rotating, and Turning

Microwaves are not distributed evenly in a microwave oven. That is why microwaved foods can have hot spots. Stirring or turning foods halfway through cooking is helpful, even if you are using an oven with a turntable that rotates food as it cooks. Stir food to bring the less cooked food in the center of the container toward the edges. Foods such as pasta and rice, which need to absorb liquid as they cook, take the same amount of time in a microwave oven as on a cooktop. Turn dense foods over with tongs. To rotate a pan by hand, grasp it with a potholder and turn it half way.

Cooking Times

Most microwave recipes give two kinds of time: microwave time and standing time. **Microwave time** is the time the food needs to cook with microwave energy. Most recipes give a range of time, such as 2 to 2½ minutes. Check the food after the shorter time. Continue microwaving only if some of the food is still cool. Food overcooks quickly in a microwave oven, which can cause it to become hard or tough. You can test whether food is done or not with an instant-read thermometer.

Food may be slightly undercooked even after the maximum time. Cooking should finish during standing time. **Standing time** is the time after microwave time during which foods continue to cook on their own. During standing time, heat becomes more evenly distributed throughout the food. Cover food and let it stand on a potholder or a solid surface such as a countertop. The food molecules will continue to vibrate until they lose energy and the food starts to cool.

Careers in Food

Rocky Durham
Chef Instructor

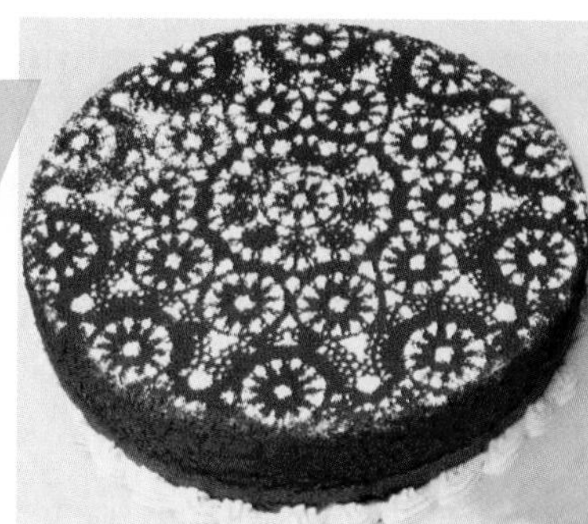

Q: What do you have to do to be a chef instructor?

A: There is no specific degree required. There are two types of instructors, those who teach the public how to cook and those who teach aspiring professional chefs. A thorough knowledge of your chosen specialty is essential.

Q: What kind of schedule is typical for a chef instructor?

A: The biggest difference between being an instructor and a traditional chef is that the hours are much more kind. The day may start earlier because you have some prep work to do, but a long day would be eight hours. You teach one or two classes per day, and the classes are two to two-and-a-half hours long.

"Few things that are worthwhile are easy."
— Rocky Durham, *Instructor, Santa Fe School of Cooking – Santa Fe, NM*

Education and Training

Chefs can get training from independent cooking schools, professional culinary institutes, or 2- or 4-year college degree. Chef instructors require many years of training and experience. Many have advanced degrees.

Qualities and Skills

Chef instructors must be comfortable with public speaking. Manual dexterity is required for teaching students knife skills. Chef instructors need creativity and a keen sense of taste and smell.

Related Career Opportunities

Executive chefs are in charge of all food service operations. A chef de cuisine is responsible for the daily operations of a single kitchen. A sous chef runs the kitchen in the absence of the chef.

To be sure that meat, poultry, fish, and casseroles are thoroughly cooked, use an instant-read food thermometer after the standing time. Insert the thermometer in several different areas to check for cold spots.

Getting the Most from a Microwave Oven

Keep your microwave in safe working condition with some simple, regular maintenance.

Clean the interior. Clean the microwave oven regularly, wiping the inside with a clean, wet dishcloth and drying it thoroughly. Use a mild detergent if needed, but not an abrasive (scratchy) cleanser. Built-up dried food is unsanitary and can absorb energy, reducing cooking power.

Clean the door seal. Keep the door seal clean so that the door shuts tightly.

Clean the exterior. The touch pad controls, door hardware, and other exterior trim pieces will last longer if they are clean.

Never run the oven empty. Never turn on an empty oven, because the microwaves could build up and cause damage.

Avoid magnets. Do not attach kitchen magnets to a microwave. They can affect the oven's electronic controls.

Review the owner's manual. Check the owner's manual for care directions. Keep the manual handy and review it from time to time.

Know what to do in case of leakage. Microwaves rarely leak if properly used and cared for. If you suspect a leak, however, the manufacturer or the state health department can explain how to have the oven tested by a qualified service. You can buy a leakage meter to use at home, but they are not very reliable.

Explore recipes. A good microwave cookbook can help you get the most from your microwave. It describes basic cooking techniques and helps you get the best results. As you grow familiar with microwave recipes, you can try adapting some conventional ones, making your oven and your recipe files more useful.

Light and Healthy Recipe

Roasted Asparagus

Ingredients

- **12 oz** Whole asparagus spears
- **1 Tbsp.** Olive oil
- **¼ tsp.** Pepper
- **⅛ tsp.** Paprika
- **1 tsp.** Balsamic vinegar

Directions

1. Preheat oven to 350°.
2. Wash and trim the bottoms of the asparagus spears. Toss with olive oil and place them in a single layer in a roasting pan.
3. Sprinkle with the pepper and paprika. Place in the oven and roast for 30 minutes.
4. Remove the asparagus from the oven and place in a serving dish. Drizzle the asparagus with the vinegar just before serving.

The balsamic vinegar and light caramelization from roasting gives the asparagus a sweet taste. Asparagus is high in vitamin A.

Yield 4 servings

Nutrition Analysis per Serving

■ Calories	50
■ Total fat	4 g
Saturated fat	1 g
Cholesterol	0 mg
■ Sodium	2 mg
■ Carbohydrate	4
Dietary fiber	2 g
Sugars	2 g
■ Protein	2 g

CHAPTER 25 Review & Applications

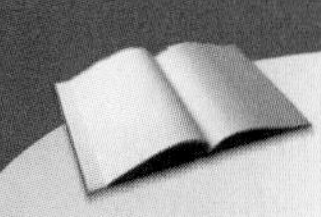

After You Read

Chapter Summary

All cooking methods transfer heat to foods through conduction, convection, or radiation. Cooking affects the appearance, flavor and nutrients of foods. Different factors influence the rate at which foods cook. Moist-heat cooking uses hot liquid, steam, or both. Cooking food in fat or oil applies heat through convection and conduction. Dry heat cooking is cooking food uncovered without added liquid or fat. Microwave cooking uses energy in the form of electrical waves. It requires careful timing and proper cookware.

Content and Academic Vocabulary Review

1. Think of a visual example of each of these content and academic vocabulary words.

Content Vocabulary

- ☐ conduction (p. 386)
- ☐ convection (p. 386)
- ☐ radiation (p. 386)
- ☐ Maillard reaction (p. 387)
- ☐ moist-heat cooking (p. 388)
- ☐ smoking point (p. 391)
- ☐ sear (p. 391)
- ☐ wok (p. 392)
- ☐ dry-heat cooking (p. 392)
- ☐ microwave cooking (p. 394)
- ☐ cooking power (p. 395)
- ☐ arcing (p. 395)
- ☐ microwave time (p. 397)
- ☐ standing time (p. 397)

Academic Vocabulary

- uniform (p. 388)
- withstand (p. 395)

Review Key Concepts

2. Describe three main ways to transfer heat to food.
3. Identify three factors that affect the rate at which food cooks.
4. Describe seven techniques for moist-heat cooking.
5. Explain five techniques for cooking in fat.
6. Describe three techniques for dry-heat cooking.
7. Describe the best method for preserving nutrients in vegetables.

Critical Thinking

8. Explain how a person's nutrient intake can be influenced by their cooking methods. Josie is deficient in several nutrients found in vegetables. "But I eat plenty of vegetables," she says.

9. Determine who is right. Jack and Billie are planning a party. They want to serve meat, fruit, vegetables, rolls, and fish. Jack says, "We will have to use several different cooking methods." Billie says, "We can cook everything using one method."

10. Explain what went wrong. Jude cooked several turkey drumsticks in the microwave. He was disappointed to find that the narrow parts were overcooked, and the larger meaty parts were undercooked.

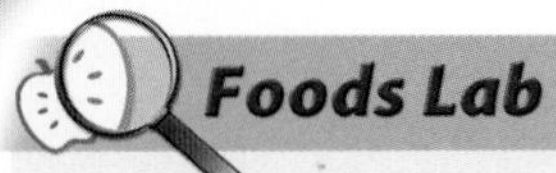

Foods Lab

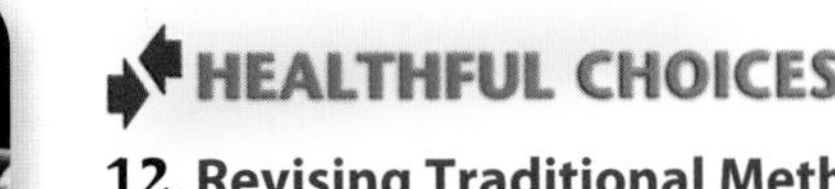

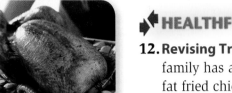

11. Effects on Color Exposing food to heat can change its texture and color. Some vegetables grow brighter, and some lose their vibrant hues. Which cooking method is best for preserving the color of vegetables?

Procedure Conduct a cooking experiment with fresh broccoli to test color change, using three different cooking methods of your choosing. Cook the broccoli for the same amount of time using each method.

Analysis Create a chart that shows the results of your experiment. Which cooking method preserved color best? Worst? Share your chart and explain your findings to the class.

HEALTHFUL CHOICES

12. Revising Traditional Methods The Greer family has a traditional recipe for deep-fat fried chicken that they prepare every Sunday. Many family members, however, struggle with heart problems and obesity. How can they prepare their traditional recipe in a more healthful way?

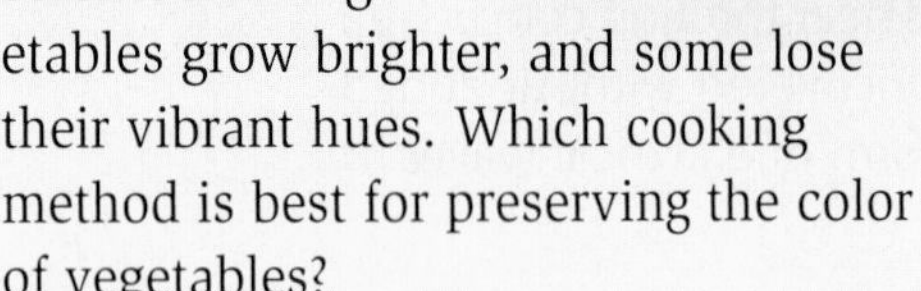

TECH Connection

13. Cooking Methods Under your teacher's supervision, use the Internet to find four recipes that use different cooking methods for the same food. Then create a slide show that explains four different cooking methods and gives recipes that utilize each method. If possible, include photos that show the results of each method. Include an explanation of how each cooking method affects the healthfulness of the recipe. Conduct research to learn how many calories the food has with each preparation method. Include this information in your presentation.

Real-World Skills

Problem-Solving Skills

14. Making Microwave-Friendly Recipes Imagine you live in a small studio apartment that has a microwave oven, but no cooktop or oven. Find a recipe that calls for a cooking method other than microwaving. Modify it so it can be prepared in a microwave oven. What steps will you take to make sure food is properly and safely cooked?

Interpersonal and Collaborative Skills

15. Heat Transfer Graphic Follow your teacher's instructions to form pairs or small groups. Using art supplies provided by your teacher, work togethether to create one graphic for each of the three methods of heat transfer. Show your graphics to the class, and explain how the methods differ.

Financial Literacy Skills

16. Wasting Money Elsa roasted a small, whole chicken in the oven at the proper temperature. The chicken cost 8 dollars. When she thought the chicken would be cooked to perfection, she opened the oven to find that it was badly overcooked, and her 8 dollars had gone to waste. What did she fail to consider during cooking?

Academic Skills

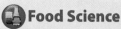

Food Science

17. Popcorn Thermodynamics Popcorn pops because the outer covering of the kernel, the pericarp, is strong. Like a pressure cooker, it keeps the steam inside until the whole thing blasts apart. Popcorn can be made on the stovetop, in the microwave, or with an air popper.

Procedure Count out 4 samples of 50 kernels. Freeze the first sample in a plastic bag. Spread out the second onto a baking sheet to leave in a 200° oven for 1 hour. Place the third into a bowl of water. Leave the last as is in a plastic bag. The next day, pop all 4 samples using one of the methods listed above.

Analysis Which sample left the most unpopped kernels? Were all the kernels the same size? Explain your results.

NSES B Develop an understanding of the interactions of energy and matter.

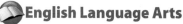

Mathematics

18. Measuring Volume For tonight's dinner, Doris would like to prepare breaded, pan-fried turkey cutlets according to a recipe that she has found, but she is not sure if she has enough of the required ingredients. The recipe calls for the cutlets to be fried in olive oil poured into a frying pan so that it is one-half inch deep. If Doris's frying pan is 11 inches wide, how many fluid ounces of olive oil will she need?

Math Concept **Volume of Liquids** Calculate the volume (V) of a cylinder as $V = \pi r^2 h$, where r is the radius of the circular base, and h is the cylinder's height. Use 3.14 for π. Multiply cubic inches by 0.554 to convert into fluid ounces.

Starting Hint Find the oil's volume in cubic inches using the formula above, with r equal to ½ the pan's width, and h equal to the depth of the olive oil. Convert to fluid ounces.

NCTM Problem Solving Apply and adapt a variety of appropriate strategies to solve problems.

English Language Arts

19. Cultural Cuisine Choose a culture with which you are not familiar. Research that culture's traditional cuisine. What cooking methods are used to prepare food in that culture? What affects do the cooking methods have on the foods? Write a letter to your teacher describing your findings.

NCTE 4 Use writing to communicate effectively.

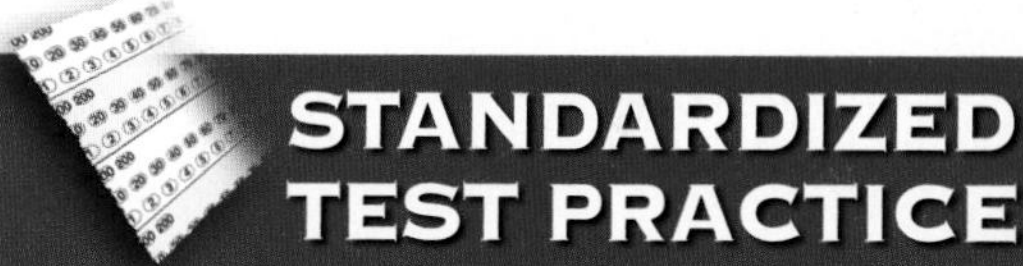

STANDARDIZED TEST PRACTICE

TRUE OR FALSE

Read the statement and determine if it is true or false.

20. In convection, heat is transferred through the movement of molecules in air or liquid.
    a. True
    b. False

Test-Taking Tip Before deciding whether a statement is true or false, read it carefully, and recall what you have learned from reading the text. Does the statement reflect what you know? Pay close attention to individual words. One word can make the difference between a true statement and a false one.

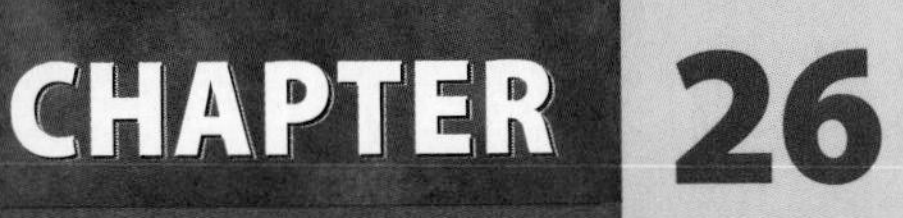

Develop a Work Plan

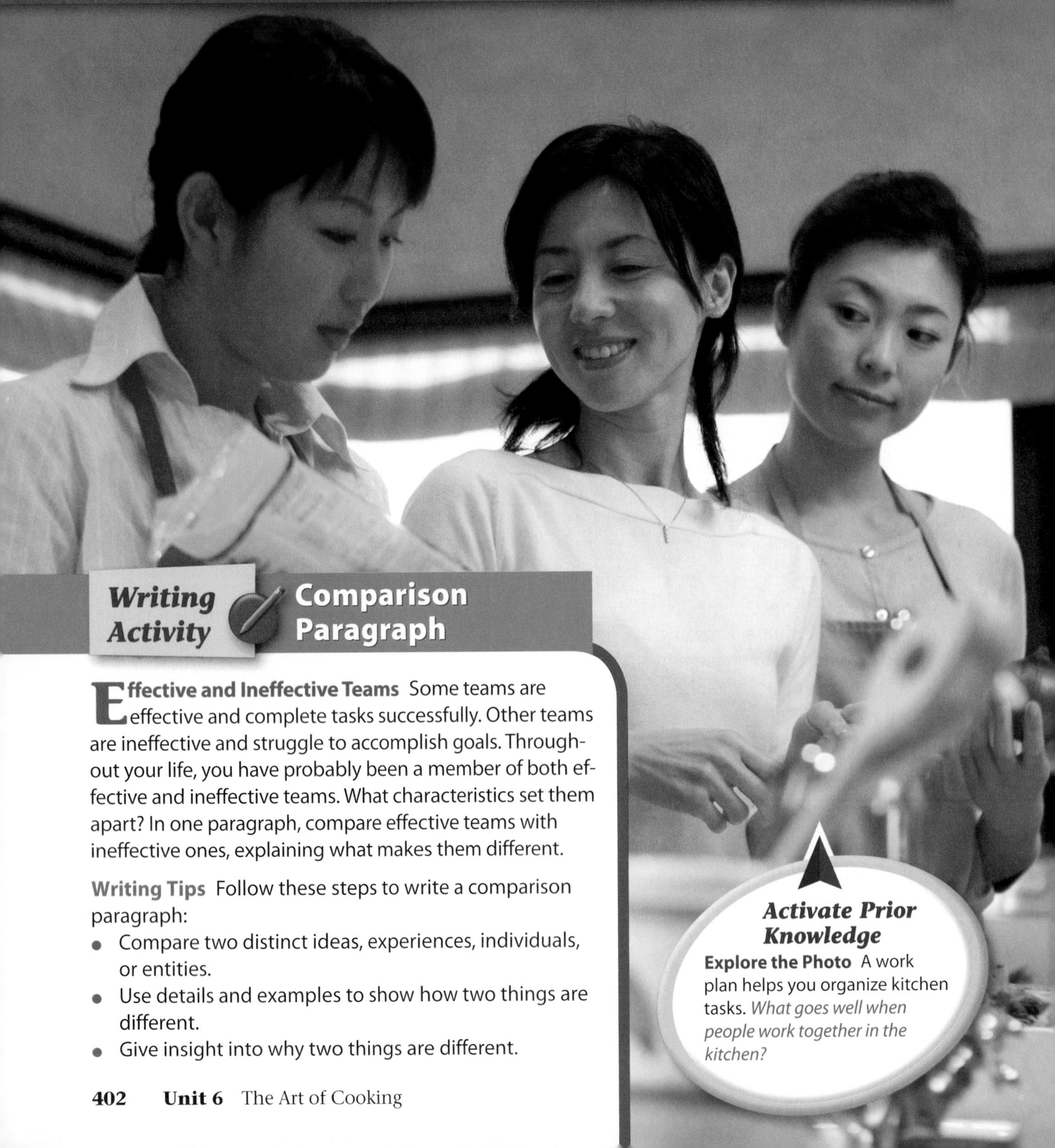

Writing Activity — Comparison Paragraph

Effective and Ineffective Teams Some teams are effective and complete tasks successfully. Other teams are ineffective and struggle to accomplish goals. Throughout your life, you have probably been a member of both effective and ineffective teams. What characteristics set them apart? In one paragraph, compare effective teams with ineffective ones, explaining what makes them different.

Writing Tips Follow these steps to write a comparison paragraph:

- Compare two distinct ideas, experiences, individuals, or entities.
- Use details and examples to show how two things are different.
- Give insight into why two things are different.

Activate Prior Knowledge

Explore the Photo A work plan helps you organize kitchen tasks. *What goes well when people work together in the kitchen?*

Reading Guide

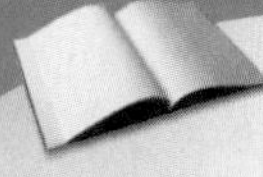

Before You Read

Preview Look at the chapter's headings, photos, figures, and captions. List three other tasks in life besides cooking that require a work plan and good teamwork.

Read to Learn

Key Concepts

- **Explain** how to create and evaluate a work plan.
- **State** the value of teamwork in the foods lab.
- **Explain** the benefits of fostering teamwork at home.

Main Idea

A work plan helps you manage time and tasks in order to prepare meals successfully. Teamwork makes meal preparation fun and efficient.

Content Vocabulary

You will find definitions for these words in the glossary at the back of this book.

- ☐ work plan
- ☐ pre-preparation
- ☐ dovetail
- ☐ timetable
- ☐ teamwork

Academic Vocabulary

You will find these words in your reading and on your tests. Use the glossary to look up their definitions, if necessary.

- chronological
- stagger

Graphic Organizer

Use a graphic organizer like the one below to take notes about the five steps of a work plan.

The Work Plan

1.
2.
3.
4.
5.

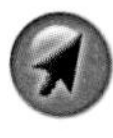

Graphic Organizer Go to this book's Online Learning Center at **glencoe.com** to print out this graphic organizer.

Academic Standards

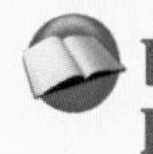

English Language Arts

NCTE 12 Use language to accomplish individual purposes.

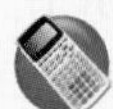

Mathematics

NCTM Number and Operations Compute fluently and make reasonable estimates.

NCTM Problem Solving Solve problems that arise in mathematics and in other contexts.

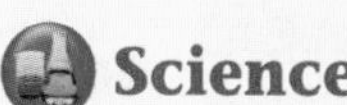

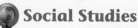

Science

NSES B Develop an understanding of interactions of energy and matter.

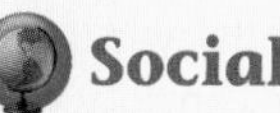

Social Studies

NCSS I A Analyze and explain the ways groups, societies, and cultures address human needs and concerns.

NCTE *National Council of Teachers of English*
NCTM *National Council of Teachers of Mathematics*
NSES *National Science Education Standards*
NCSS *National Council for the Social Studies*

The Work Plan

How can you make sure that all the foods in a meal are ready to eat at the right time? By using a work plan. A **work plan** is a list of all the tasks you need to do in order to prepare a meal. A work plan lists tasks in **chronological** order based on their starting time. Chronological means organized according to time.

A work plan is one part of the meal planning process, which also includes reading recipes beforehand, listing the tasks for each recipe, developing a timetable, making and carrying out the work plan, and evaluating your success.

Read Recipes Beforehand

Read the recipes you plan to use ahead of time. Also read the instructions on any packaged food you plan to use. Make note of the following:

- The food and equipment you need. Do you have everything you need?
- The oven temperature and whether preheating is required.
- The cooking time for each food.
- The food preparation techniques to use. Consider your skill at each one.

> **Kitchen Math** **Adjusting a Work Plan**
>
> At 9:30 a.m., you receive a call from one of your invited Sunday brunch guests, who informs you that she will be delayed until 11:45 a.m. Although she attempts to convince you to start brunch without her, you insist on waiting until she arrives to serve the food. Rewrite the work plan in Figure 26.2 on page 406 to account for the new brunch start time of 11:45.
>
> **Math Concept** **Adding Time** When adding two times together, add the hours and minutes separately. If the sum of the minutes exceeds 60, subtract 60 from the minutes and add 1 to the hours.
>
> **Starting Hint** First, determine the length of the delay by subtracting the old start time from the new start time. Then add that same amount of time to each time in the work plan, going through each item one by one.
>
> 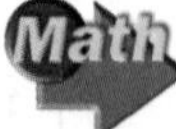
>
> **Math Appendix** For math help, go to the Math Appendix at the back of the book.
>
> **NCTM Number and Operations** Compute fluently and make reasonable estimates.

List the Tasks

Now list the tasks involved in preparing each recipe and in doing related jobs, such as setting the table and gathering food and equipment. As you identify each task, look for ways to speed and simplify the work. Ask yourself the following questions:

- Could any appliances or prepared foods save time or effort? Would a different cooking method be more efficient?
- Can any foods be prepared safely ahead of time? A dessert might be baked the day before, for example.
- Can any steps be done as pre-preparation? **Pre-preparation** includes tasks that can be done before you begin to put the recipes together. You might open packages, chop and measure ingredients, and grease baking pans. Having ingredients and equipment ready when you need them saves time. List all pre-preparation tasks.
- How many tasks can be dovetailed? To **dovetail** means to fit different tasks together to make good use of time. Not every preparation step needs your undivided attention. For example, clean-up tasks can often be dovetailed with others. Fill the sink or dishpan with hot, sudsy water before you start to work. Whenever you have a few free minutes, wash the equipment you have finished using. Keep a clean, wet dishcloth handy to wipe up spills as they happen. Put away leftover ingredients after using them.

Develop a Timetable

Now that you have listed all your tasks, you can make a timetable. A **timetable** shows the amount of time you will need to complete preparation tasks and lists when you should start each task. The timetable serves as the basis for your work plan.

To make a timetable, work backwards from the time you want to have everything ready to serve the meal. To serve brunch at 11:00 a.m., for example, you might want to have everything ready by 10:55 a.m. Work back from 10:55 a.m. Be sure to allow enough time for each task. You might also want to allow time in case you need to greet guests who arrive early. To prepare a timetable like the one in **Figure 26.1**, follow these steps:

1. Create a grid. Divide a sheet of paper into five columns with these headings: Task; Preparation Time; Cooking Time; Total Time; and Starting Time.

2. List tasks. List tasks in the first column. Group tasks that do not have to start at a specific time, such as setting the table.

3. Estimate times. Estimate preparation and cooking times for each dish or beverage and write these in the second and third columns. Allow extra time for dishes you have never prepared before. Double-check your entries and make sure you have left adequate time to complete your work.

4. Calculate time per dish. Add the preparation time to the cooking time to find the total time needed for each dish or beverage. Write these totals in the fourth column.

Figure 26.1 Sunday Brunch Timetable

Game Plan A timetable helps you plan how long it will take to make a meal so that you can make a work plan to have everything ready at the right time. ***Which of the tasks listed here could be dovetailed? How?***

Task	Preparation Time	Cooking Time	Total Time	Starting Time
Tasks with Optional Start Times				
Set table.	10 min.	—	10 min.	To be decided
Gather food and equipment.	10 min.	—	10 min.	To be decided
Pre-preparation: Open packages; measure ingredients; wrap muffins in paper towels and put in microwave; fill coffeemaker; arrange cleanup area.	20 min.	—	20 min.	To be decided
Food Preparation and Serving Tasks				
Broil ham steak: Put ham steak on broiler pan and into broiler; set timer to remind.	2 min.	13 min.	15 min.	10:40 a.m.
Prepare French toast: Mix batter; heat skillet; dip bread; fry.	5 min.	15 min.	20 min.	10:35 a.m.
Prepare orange juice: Mix frozen concentrate in pitcher; refrigerate.	5 min.	60 min. (to chill)	65 min.	9:50 a.m.
Prepare cherry sauce: Pour cherries into pan; mix cornstarch and water; stir in and cook.	2 min.	3 min.	5 min.	10:50 a.m.
Warm bran muffins: Start microwave.	—	2 min.	2 min.	10:50 a.m.
Prepare coffee: Turn on coffeemaker.	—	10 min.	10 min.	10:45 a.m.
Serve food on plates in kitchen; pour beverages.	5 min.	—	5 min.	10:55 a.m.

Figure 26.2 Work Plan for Sunday Brunch

Tight Schedule A work plan lists steps for preparing and cooking a meal in the order you need to start them. ***Why is mixing frozen juice the first step here?***

Time	Task
9:50 a.m.	Mix frozen juice in pitcher; refrigerate.
9:55 a.m.	Set table.
10:05 a.m.	Gather equipment and ingredients.
10:15 a.m.	Do pre-preparation: Open packages; measure ingredients; wrap muffins in paper towels; fill coffeemaker; get cleanup area ready.
10:35 a.m.	Start French toast: Mix batter; heat skillet; dip bread in batter; fry.
10:40 a.m.	Put ham in broiler; set timer.
10:45 a.m.	Start coffee.
10:50 a.m.	Prepare cherry sauce. Finish French toast.
10:50 a.m.	Warm bran muffins in microwave oven.
10:55 a.m.	Put food on plates in kitchen. Pour beverages.
11:00 a.m.	Start brunch.

5. Determine start times. Determine when you need to start preparing each food by deducting the time needed to prepare the food from the time the meal should be ready. Enter this starting time in the last column. For example, the ham steak for the brunch menu shown in Figure 26.1 takes 15 minutes. To be ready at 10:55, it should go on the broiler pan at 10:40 (10:55 − 15 = 10:40). Tasks that can be done ahead or dovetailed do not need a specific start time. You will pick times to do these later, when you make the work plan. For example, you might set the table while food bakes or coffee brews.

Make and Carry Out the Work Plan

A work plan organizes the information in the "Starting Time" column of your timetable into a start-to-finish road map for getting your meal to the table. **Figure 26.2** shows a work plan based on the timetable in Figure 26.1.

To make a work plan, list all the tasks in the order in which you need to start them. For tasks with optional start times, choose times that fit with other tasks. For example, you might set the table before you start cooking or during a lull in the activity. Dovetail tasks when you can.

What if you are making a meal with several courses? You will need to **stagger**, or arrange in order, the timing of different courses. For example, you might want a fresh-baked pie to be ready 30 minutes later than the main course. The more complicated the meal, the more important a work plan is.

Once you have your work plan, you are ready to start. First, get organized. Gather all the equipment, tools, and ingredients you will need. A tray or cart may be helpful for this. Arrange your work area so that everything is at hand. Then begin work. Check off each task as you complete it so that no step is left out.

Evaluate the Work Plan

After the meal is over, review your work plan. Ask yourself these questions:

- Did I complete the meal on time?
- Did I feel hurried or pressured at any point? If so, when?
- Was the work plan flexible enough to handle problems?

- Could I have worked more efficiently? How?
- What changes, if any, would I make in the work plan to prepare the same meal again?

Evaluating your work plan helps you improve your skills and become more efficient and confident.

✓ Reading Check **Explain** What simple formula can you use to determine when you should start preparing a food?

Teamwork in the School Foods Lab

Teamwork in the kitchen can be fun and can make food preparation easier and more efficient. **Teamwork** means combining individual efforts to reach a shared goal. A good team uses each team member's special skills and talents to achieve the best result.

TECHNOLOGY FOR TOMORROW

Advanced Kitchens

Many modern advancements in kitchen design and technology have made it easier for people with disabilities to prepare food. To accommodate people who use wheelchairs, sinks, cooktops, and cabinets can be raised or lowered at the push of a button. The button activates a motor that adjusts the appliance to a convenient height. Heat-resistant countertops can be installed beside the stove, allowing wheelchair users to slide hot pots and pans without the danger of trying to lift them. Motion detector faucets with anti-scald valves turn on automatically and keep water at a comfortable temperature. Mobile islands equipped with locking wheels make it easier to transport food and equipment from one area to another.

Investigate Brainstorm a list of five ways you could adapt or redesign a kitchen to accommodate the needs of people who are disabled.

NCSS I A Analyze and explain the ways groups, societies, and cultures address human needs and concerns.

A team is strong when its members cooperate and communicate well. Good teamwork includes the following skills:

Organizing Jobs In a foods lab, several people work on different tasks at the same time. Teams need a well-organized work plan to manage their efforts. Team members need to decide when each task should start and who will do it. They need to consider work space and equipment. It may be helpful to use a work plan marked with five-minute blocks of time down the left and each person's name across the top. This lets all team members know what everyone should be doing.

Cooperation Team members should help each other. Ask for help if you have a question or problem. In return, be willing to help someone who falls behind or makes a mistake. Keep a sense of humor. Show respect and use tact to promote a cooperative spirit.

Communication Share information as you work. Keep your team aware of your progress and of any problems. After the work is done, use your communication skills to evaluate the process and the result. Honest and thoughtful discussion helps you learn from experience.

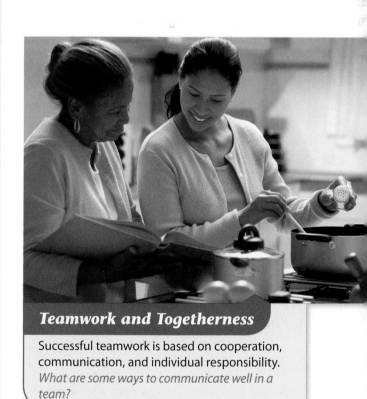

Teamwork and Togetherness

Successful teamwork is based on cooperation, communication, and individual responsibility. *What are some ways to communicate well in a team?*

If the team faced a problem, suggest creative ways to improve your performance. Avoid blaming others.

Taking Responsibility Teams are successful when each person does his or her part. Take responsibility by learning your job and doing your share of the work carefully, efficiently, and in a timely manner. Follow safety rules at all times. When you finish your assigned tasks, ask if you can help others. Leave the lab as you like to find it yourself. Be sure all equipment, appliances, and work surfaces are clean and dry. Return everything to its proper place. Dispose of waste properly. Cleaning as you go makes end-of-class cleanup easier and faster.

✓ **Reading Check** **List** What are at least three things you can do to be a cooperative team member?

Teamwork at Home

Teamwork skills help work run smoothly at home as well as in the lab. Teamwork can also foster a relaxed, enjoyable atmosphere at home. Teaching a younger brother or sister how to master a new skill can build your confidence and your cooking skills.

Trying out a new recipe with your family might be the start of a new family food tradition. Showing your family new techniques you have learned or sampling foods at home that you have made in class can be fun for your whole family. Enjoying meal times with your family builds family bonds and feelings of togetherness and love. Sharing provides a positive and supportive environment for everyone in the family. Perhaps a family member has an idea about a recipe that will improve it. Maybe you will learn new techniques for managing your workplan.

Light and Healthy Recipe

Hot Chicken Salad

Ingredients

- **12 oz** Chopped grilled chicken breast
- **1** Hard-boiled egg, diced
- **½ cup** Chopped celery
- **½ cup** Chopped onion
- **¼ cup** Chopped pickle
- **½ cup** Lowfat, low-sodium mayonnaise
- **¼ cup** Prepared mustard
- **1 cup** Corn flake cereal

Directions

1. Preheat oven to 375°.
2. In a large mixing bowl, combine chicken, hard-boiled egg, celery, onion, and pickle.
3. In a separate bowl, mix mayonnaise and mustard. Fold mixture into chicken mixture.
4. Place the mixture in a small baking pan and spread it out evenly. Place in oven and bake for 30 minutes.
5. While casserole is baking, pour the cereal into a plastic bag and crush it. After 30 minutes, remove casserole from the oven and sprinkle the cereal crumbs evenly over the top. Bake another 10 minutes and serve hot.

A casserole can be a big help to meal planning because it can be prepared ahead of time.

Yield 4 Servings

Nutrition Analysis per Serving

■ Calories	219
■ Total fat	9 g
■ Saturated fat	1 g
Cholesterol	106 mg
Sodium	682 mg
■ Carbohydrate	13 g
Dietary fiber	1 g
Sugars	3 g
■ Protein	21 g

CHAPTER 26 Review & Applications

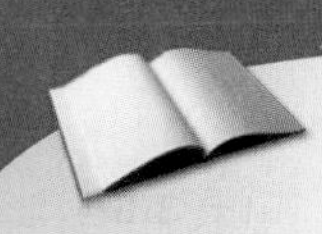

After You Read

Chapter Summary

The meal planning process results in a work plan that makes food preparation more efficient and fun. To plan a meal, follow these steps: read recipes beforehand; list the tasks; develop a timetable; make and carry out the work plan; evaluate the work plan. Teamwork also plays a role in successful food preparation. Good teamwork involves the organization of jobs, cooperation, communication, and taking responsibility. The same teamwork skills that are applied in the foods lab at school can also be applied at home.

Content and Academic Vocabulary Review

1. Use each of these content and academic vocabulary words in a sentence.

Content Vocabulary

- work plan (p. 404)
- pre-preparation (p. 404)
- dovetail (p. 404)
- timetable (p. 404)
- teamwork (p. 407)

Academic Vocabulary

- chronological (p. 404)
- stagger (p. 406)

Review Key Concepts

2. **Explain** how to create and evaluate a work plan.
3. **State** the value of teamwork in the foods lab.
4. **Describe** the benefits of fostering teamwork at home.

Critical Thinking

5. **Explain** whether you think setting the table needs a specific start time in a timetable for meal preparation.
6. **Explain** why serving temperature influences where tasks are listed on timetable, using specific examples from Figure 26.1.
7. **Detail** three possible consequences to this scenario: Brandon failed to create a work plan before preparing an elaborate meal with several courses.
8. **Describe** whether each foods lab team should have a team leader to encourage good teamwork. Why or why not?
9. **Identify** three specific ways that one team member's failure to take responsibility can adversely affect other team members.
10. **Describe** why Nora and David's attitudes changed. After they began helping their parents prepare meals at home, they had a new appreciation for them.

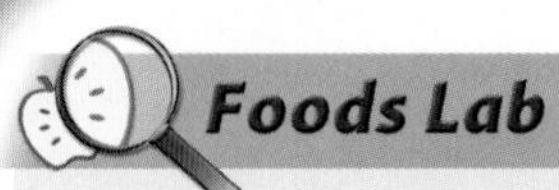

Foods Lab

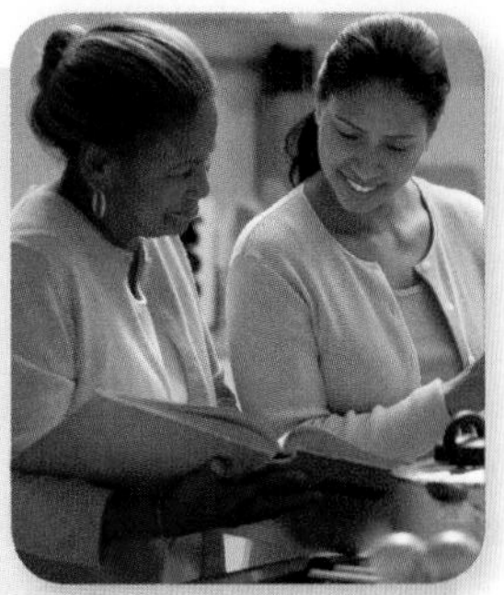

11. Implementing a Work Plan The steps to create and carry out a work plan may seem numerous and complicated. By practicing them with a team in the foods lab, you can more easily carry them out when preparing food on your own at home.

Procedure With your team, plan a lunch menu to prepare and eat together. Gather and read recipes. List tasks. Develop a timetable and create a work plan. Then prepare, serve, and eat the meal.

Analysis As a team, evaluate your work plan by discussing your responses to the evaluation questions listed on page 406–407, replacing the "I" in each question with "we." In writing, have one team member summarize your responses to each question. Then share them with the class.

HEALTHFUL CHOICES

12. An Overworked Cook Adrienne is a busy wife and mother who works full time and also prepares her family's dinner each night. Her busy lifestyle is affecting her health. She experiences fatigue, stress, and irritability. What can her family do to help Adrienne and why is it important to help her as soon as possible?

TECH Connection

13. Evaluation Form Using word processing or spreadsheet software, develop an evaluation form students can use after working in teams in the foods lab. Present at least four questions in a clear format that will encourage students to assess their teamwork skills. Try to phrase the questions so that answers can be given in a positive manner. For example, ask students to list things their team did well. Present an additional two questions that encourage students to assess their team's success. Exchange forms with another student and fill them out.

Real-World Skills

Problem-Solving Skills

14. Cold Stew Jose created a meal plan for a lunch he prepared for his friends. However, he was disappointed to find that when he served the stew it was already cold. What can he do to prevent this if he prepares the same meal in the future?

Interpersonal and Collaborative Skills

15. Pre-Preparation Tasks Follow your teacher's instructions to form pairs. Working with your partner, plan menus and locate recipes for the three meals in one day. Examine these, and list specific pre-preparation tasks for each meal and when the tasks could be done.

Financial Literacy Skills

16. Time is Money Caitlin runs a catering business. She hires cooks to prepare the food, and pays them by the hour. How can creating a work plan for each recipe save Caitlin money?

Academic Skills

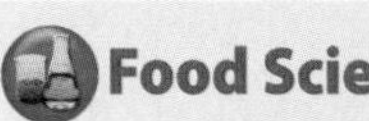

Food Science

17. Blanching Blanching is cooking a food partially in boiling water, then plunging it into ice water to stop the cooking. Fresh vegetables have air between cells, which clouds the color. With heat, the air expands and leaves a much brighter color.

Procedure Bring a pot of water to a boil. Drop in 10 broccoli florets, and cook for 3 minutes. Remove and plunge into a bowl of ice water. Repeat with 10 green beans, but cook for 1–2 minutes. Compare the color and texture before and after blanching.

Analysis Think about blanching and write a paragraph about how blanching can help in planning a timetable.

NSES B Develop an understanding of interactions of energy and matter.

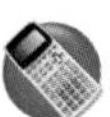

Mathematics

18. Timing a Meal For her dinner guests, Claudia wants to serve chocolate soufflés for dessert. Soufflés cannot be prepared in advance. Claudia wants to serve dessert at 7:30 p.m., and the soufflés require 10 minutes of preparation, 26 minutes to cook, and 2 minutes for plating. What time should Claudia begin preparing dessert?

Math Concept **Subtracting Time** When subtracting one time from another, subtract the hours and minutes separately. If the difference of the minutes is a negative number, add 60 to the minutes and subtract 1 from the hours.

Starting Hint Determine the start time by starting with 7:30 and subtracting the time needed for each step.

NCTM Problem Solving Solve problems that arise in mathematics and in other contexts.

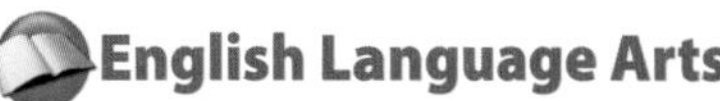

English Language Arts

19. Skit Performance Follow your teacher's instructions to form groups. Work together to write and perform a short skit that presents a problem within a kitchen team. Include a method to resolve or prevent the problem that corresponds to one of the four teamwork skills. Show how using the skill can help resolve conflict. Agree on who will play each part. Use appropriate props for your skit. Rehearse before performing. Ask your audience to assess which teamwork skill was used to solve or prevent the problem.

NCTE 12 Use language to meet individual purposes.

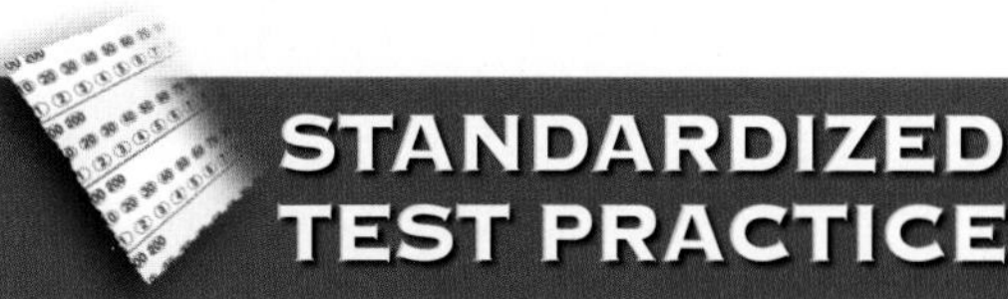

STANDARDIZED TEST PRACTICE

MULTIPLE CHOICE

Read the question and select the best answer.

20. What does it mean to dovetail tasks?

a. To delay until just before meal time.

b. To divide a task between two team members.

c. To assign two tasks to each team member.

d. To fit different tasks together to make good use of time.

Test-Taking Tip Multiple-choice questions may prompt you to select the best answer. They may present you with answers that seem partially true. The best answer is the one that is completely true, and can be supported by information you have read in the text.

CHAPTER 27

Creative Additions

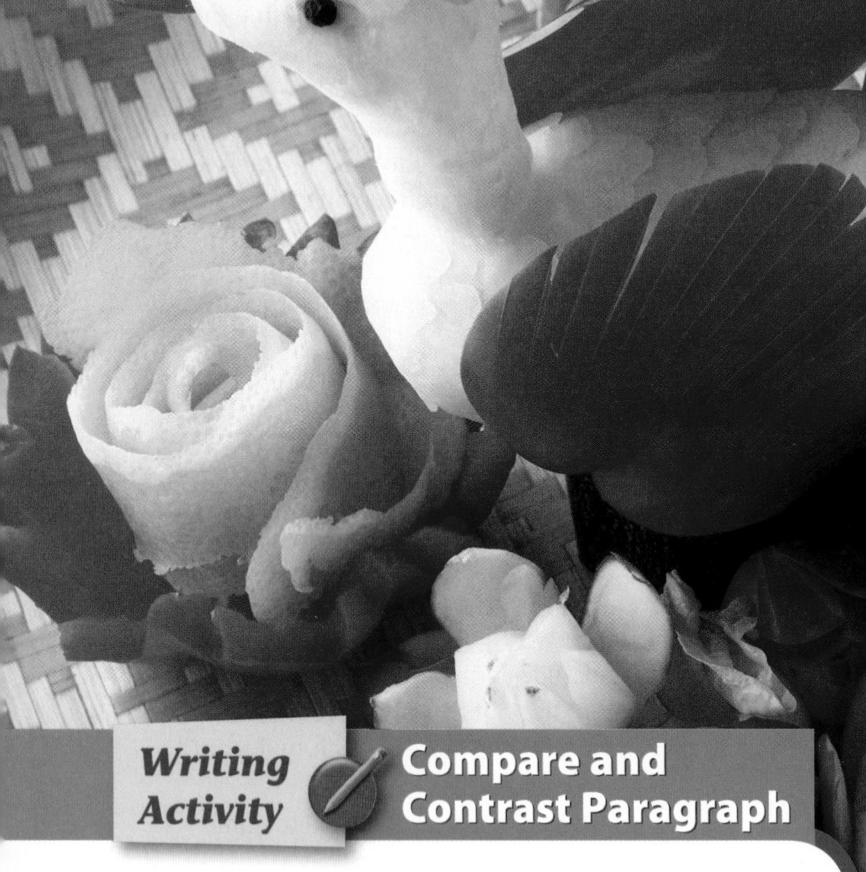

Writing Activity: Compare and Contrast Paragraph

Art and Cooking Many people have noted the similarities between art and cooking. Some may liken preparing a meal to painting a picture or building a sculpture. But there are also differences. In a compare and contrast paragraph, compare art and cooking by highlighting their similarities. Then contrast them by noting their differences.

Writing Tips Follow these steps to write a compare and contrast paragraph:

- Identify two objects, ideas, actions, or people.
- Compare two things by highlighting their similarities.
- Contrast two things by noting their differences.

Activate Prior Knowledge

Explore the Photo Garnishes add flavor, color, and texture to food. *What vegetables, herbs, and spices are familiar to you?*

Reading Guide

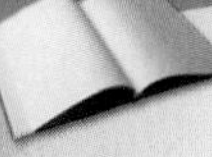

Before You Read

Preview Identify a food to which you make creative additions. What do you add to the food and how do your additions influence its appeal and taste?

Read to Learn

Key Concepts

- **Identify** common herbs and spices.
- **Describe** the role of garnishes.
- **Identify** techniques for varying the presentation of your favorite recipe.
- **Explain** how homemade food can be a meaningful gift.

Main Idea

Learning about different types of creative additions and how to use them can help you enhance food's appeal and texture.

Content Vocabulary

You will find definitions for these words in the glossary at the back of this book.

- herb
- spice
- bouquet garni
- seasoning blend
- condiment
- garnish

Academic Vocabulary

You will find these words in your reading and on your tests. Use the glossary to look up their definitions if necessary.

- opaque
- complement

Graphic Organizer

Use a Venn diagram like the one below to compare and contrast herbs and spices.

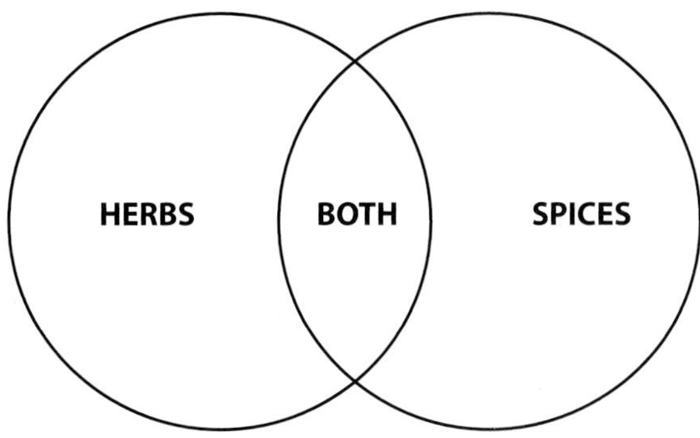

Graphic Organizer Go to this book's Online Learning Center at **glencoe.com** to print out this graphic organizer.

Academic Standards

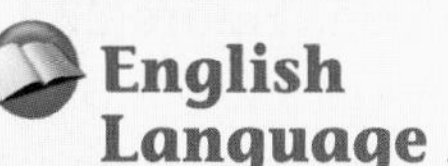

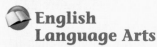

English Language Arts

NCTE 7 Conduct research and gather, evaluate, and synthesize data to communicate discoveries.

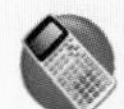

Mathematics

NCTM Problem Solving Build new mathematical knowledge through problem solving.

NCTM Algebra Represent and analyze mathematical situations and structures using algebraic symbols.

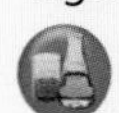

Science

NSES B Develop an understanding of the structure and properties of matter.

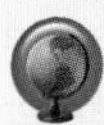

Social Studies

NCSS VIII A Science, Technology, and Society Identify and describe both current and historical examples of the interaction and interdependence of science, technology, and society in a variety of cultural settings.

NCTE *National Council of Teachers of English*
NCTM *National Council of Teachers of Mathematics*
NSES *National Science Education Standards*
NCSS *National Council for the Social Studies*

Seasonings

Creative additions, such as seasonings and garnishes, enhance food's flavor and visual appeal. Exploring seasonings is fun and helps you create rich flavor with minimal salt.

Herbs and Spices

An **herb** is the flavorful leaf or stem of a soft, succulent (fleshy and moisture-rich) plant that grows in a temperate climate. You can buy herbs fresh or dried. **Figure 27.1** and **Figure 27.2** on pages 415–417 show a wide variety of herbs and spices and describe their flavors and uses.

A **spice** is the dried form of various buds, bark, fruits, seeds, stems, or roots, typically from an aromatic plant or tree that grows in a tropical or subtropical region. You usually buy spices whole or ground. A few spices, such as ginger root, are also sold fresh.

TECHNOLOGY FOR TOMORROW

From the Source to the Supermarket

How does the bark of a tree become a finely ground topping for your oatmeal? From the moment they are harvested until they appear on supermarket shelves, spices take a journey. Technology is involved every step of the way. Many spices are grown on cultivated land that has been prepared with farming equipment. From there, they are transported via plane, boat, or vehicle to a processing plant. Factory machines dry, clean, grind, and package the spices. Most machines run on fossil fuels, but new technology is changing the way spices are processed. Solar spice drying technology utilizes the sun's renewable energy to operate equipment that dries mass quantities of spices in a short period of time.

Get Involved What is food irradiation, and how are spices irradiated? Use the Internet or library to research this technology.

NCSS VIII A Science, Technology, and Society
Identify and describe both current and historical examples of the interaction and interdependence of science, technology, and society in a variety of cultural settings.

Herb and Spice Blends

You can buy herbs and spices individually or in bundles or blends. A **bouquet garni**, for example, is a bundled or bagged collection of herbs that flavors foods while cooking and is later removed.

A **seasoning blend** is a pre-mixed combination of herbs and spices. Popular seasoning blends include the following:

Curry Powder Curry powder is a blend of up to 20 herbs and spices in different combinations. Cinnamon, ginger, and various peppers are part of most curry powders. Curry flavor is often used in Indian cooking.

Five-Spice Powder Five-spice powder contains equal parts of ground cinnamon, cloves, fennel seed, star anise, and Szechuan peppercorns. It is a staple in Chinese and Japanese cuisine.

Chili Powder Chili powder is a mix of ground, dried chiles, garlic, oregano, cumin, coriander, and cloves. It is the hallmark of Tex-Mex dishes and chili.

Creole Seasoning This blend has a lot of paprika along with onion powder, garlic powder, dried oregano, dried basil, dried thyme, pepper, and cayenne pepper. Cajun seasoning is similar but usually has a little more heat, provided by ancho chili powder. It also has ginger and oregano.

Taco Seasoning This blend is sold in individual packets so that you can easily brown and spice ground beef or poultry for use in tacos. It is a blend of cayenne, chili powder, cumin, garlic, and oregano.

Using Herbs and Spices

Certain herbs and spices are often used with specific foods, but no combination is right or wrong. Try different combinations to see which ones you enjoy.

Use these guidelines to get the best flavor from herbs and spices:

- Use dried herbs in recipes unless fresh herbs are specifically listed.
- Begin with a few of the basic herbs and spices. Learn how to use them, then add others.
- Add herbs and spices in small amounts, tasting as you go. Some herbs and spices are stronger than others. Start with ¼ teaspoon of spices or dried herbs for every four servings. Add more if desired.

Figure 27.1 Commonly Used Herbs

Flavor Enhancers Herbs are the flavorful leaves and stems of plants. The taste of herbs ranges from sweet to musky to bitter. ***Which of the herbs shown here is used in desserts? Which are used in breads?***

Basil

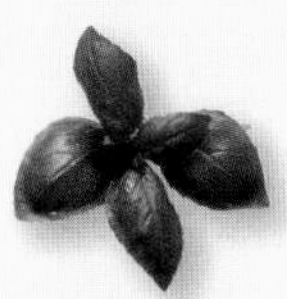

Whole or ground leaves. Sweet, with a hint of mint and cloves. Use in meat, poultry, dry beans, soups, strews, and tomato dishes.

Mint

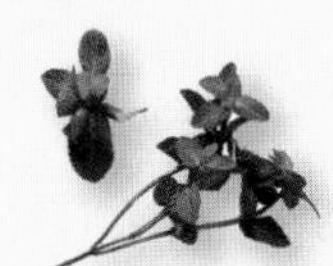

Whole or chopped leaves. Refreshing and strong. Use in poultry, lamb, pork, beverages, desserts, salads, jellies, and vegetables.

Bay Leaf

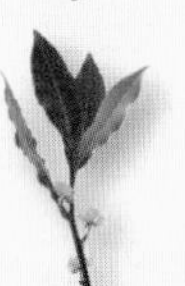

Whole leaves. Strong and pungent. Use in braised meats, soups, stews, and dry beans. Remove before serving.

Oregano

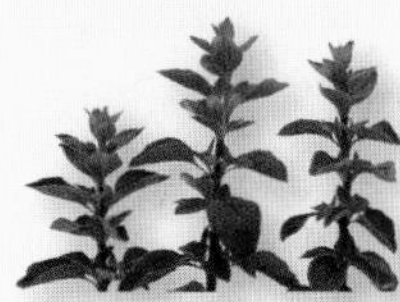

Whole or ground leaves. Strong, slightly bitter. Use in seafood, meat, soups, stews, and Italian and Mexican cuisine.

Chervil

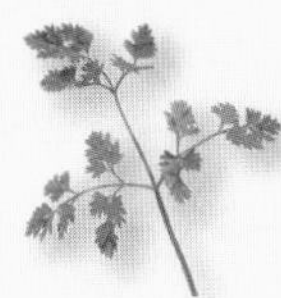

Whole or chopped leaves. Mildly peppery. Use in egg dishes, poultry, fish, cream soups, and spring vegetables.

Parsley

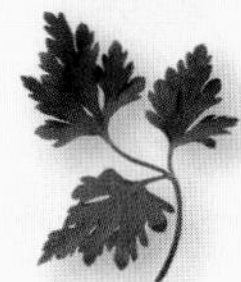

Whole or flaked leaves and stems. Refreshing and slightly sweet. Use in fish, stuffing, soups, and sauces.

Chives

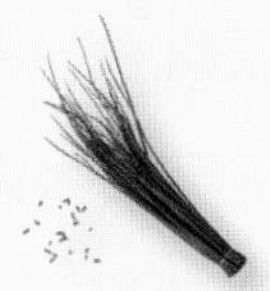

Chopped leaves. Mildly onion-like. Use in fish, potatoes, egg dishes, and herb cheeses.

Rosemary

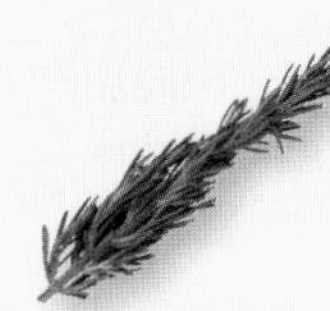

Whole leaves. Pungent, with hints of pine. Use in lamb, pork, chicken, soups, and salads.

Cilantro

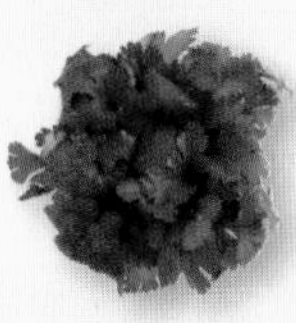

Whole or chopped leaves. Pungent and slightly citrusy. Use in stews, root vegetables, and Tex-Mex dishes.

Sage

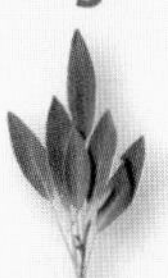

Whole or ground leaves. Strong and musky. Use in bread, stuffing, pork, poultry, and dry beans.

Dill

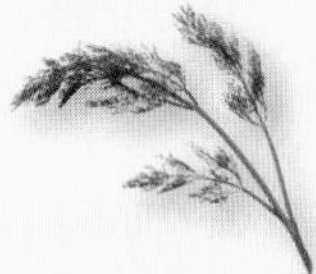

Whole leaves. Strong and sharp. Use in fish, bread, root vegetables, and sauces.

Tarragon

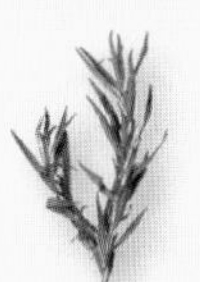

Whole or crushed leaves. Hints of licorice. Use in meats, poultry, vegetables, and egg dishes.

Marjoram

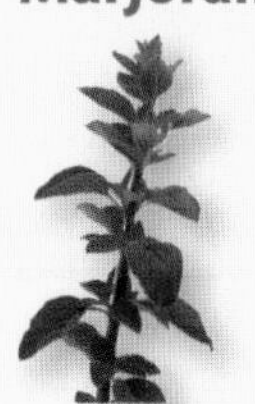

Crushed or ground leaves. Mild and sweet. Use in poultry, meat, soups, and tomato dishes.

Thyme

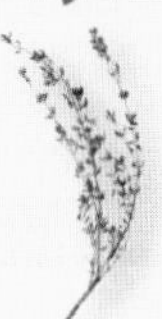

Crushed or ground leaves. Strong and clove-like. Use in meats, soups, seafood, and vegetables.

Figure 27.2 Commonly Used Spices

Flavor Enhancers Spices are the dried buds, bark, fruits, seeds, stems, or roots of plants or trees. They are usually used dried. ***Which of the spices shown here have a licorice-like flavor? Which are made from ground peppers?***

Allspice

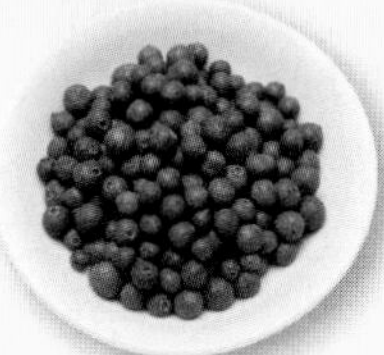

Whole or ground berries. Sweet and slightly peppery. Use in meats, baked goods, and Caribbean cuisine.

Celery Seed

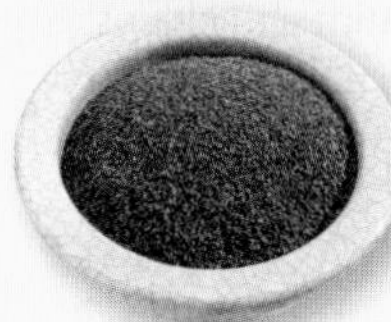

Whole or ground flower seed of the celery plant. Celery-like and slightly bitter. Use in fish, soups, and salads.

Anise

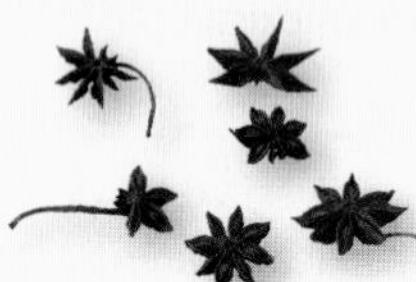

Whole or ground flower seed. Licorice-like flavor. Use in baked goods, fish, and Middle Eastern and Indian cuisines.

Chili Powder

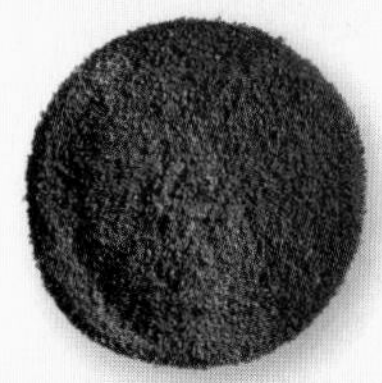

Ground pepper fruit. Hot and peppery. Use in meats, stews, and salsas.

Caraway Seed

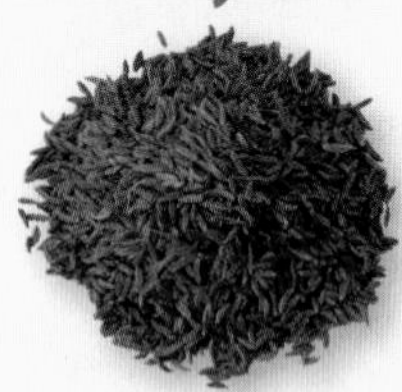

Whole or ground fruits. Slightly sweet and tangy, with a licorice-like flavor. Use in breads, soups, and German cuisine.

Chiles

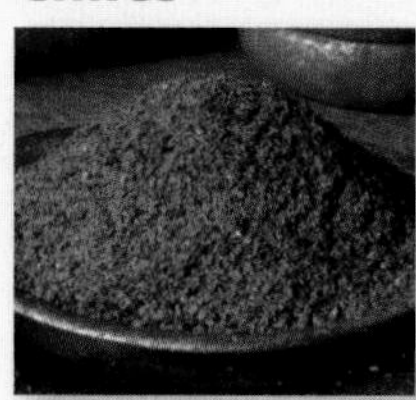

Whole or ground pepper fruit. Mildly to very hot. Use in meats, stews, and salsas.

Cardamom

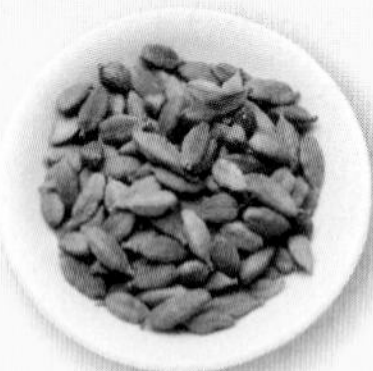

Whole or ground flower seed. Slightly sweet and lemony. Use in baked goods, cheese dishes, and Indian cuisine.

Cinnamon

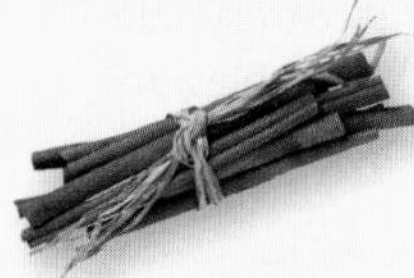

Whole or ground tree bark. Warm and sweet. Use in baked goods and beverages.

Cayenne

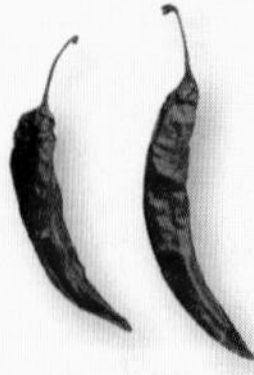

Ground pepper fruit. Pungent and very hot. Use in meats, poultry, and egg dishes and in Cajun cuisine.

Cloves

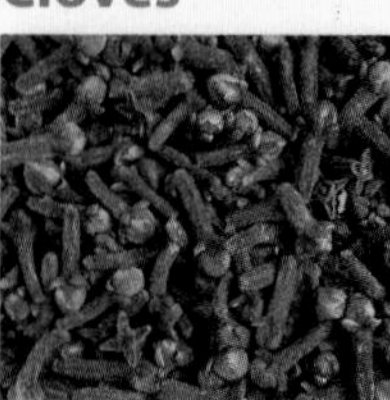

Whole or ground flower buds. Pungent and slightly hot. Use in pork, baked goods, and beverages.

Figure 27.2 Commonly Used Spices (continued)

Coriander Seed

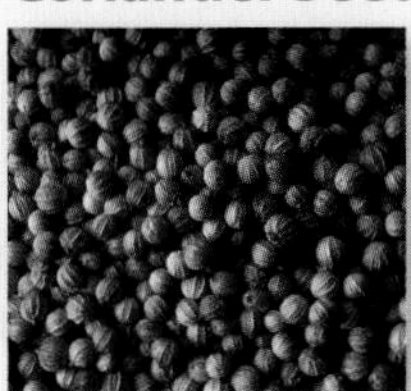

Whole or ground flower seed of the cilantro plant. Musky and slightly citrusy. Use in meats, baked goods, and Indian cuisine.

Mustard Seed

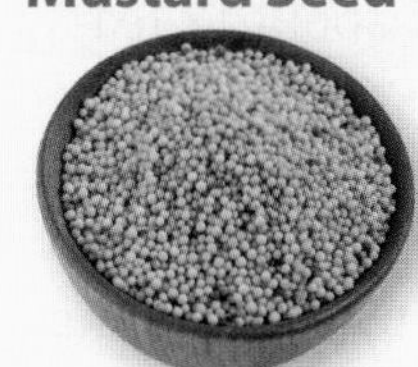

Whole or ground flower seed. Pungent and moderately to very hot. Use in egg dishes, salad dressings, and sauces.

Cumin

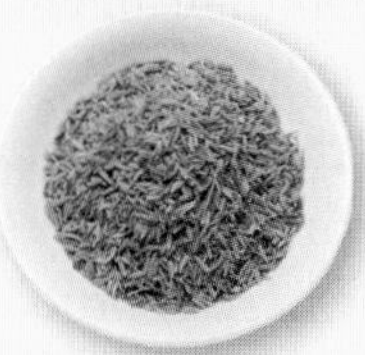

Whole or ground flower seed. Musky and slightly bitter. Use in legumes, soups, rice, vegetables, and in Middle Eastern, Asian, and Tex-Mex cuisines.

Nutmeg

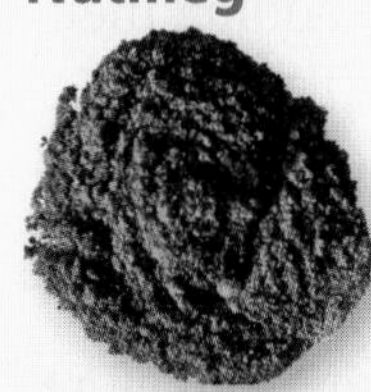

Whole or ground tree seed. Mellow, nutty, and sweet. Use in baked goods, milk-based soups and sauces, fruits, and vegetables.

Dill Seed

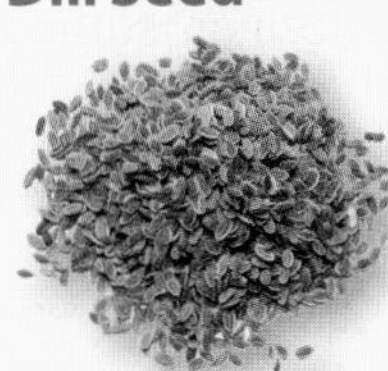

Whole flower seed of the dill plant. Sharp and slightly bitter. Use in seafood, breads, and salad and slaw dressings.

Paprika

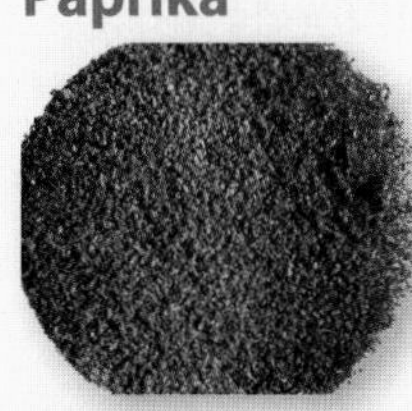

Ground, dried pepper fruit. Sharp, and from sweet to moderately hot. Use in fish, poultry, and egg and cheese dishes.

Fennel Seed

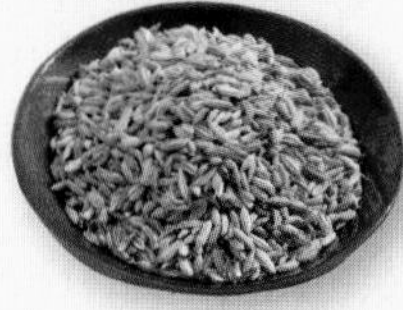

Whole, cracked, or ground seed of the fennel plant. Licorice-like flavor. Use in seafood, breads, and pasta sauces.

Pepper

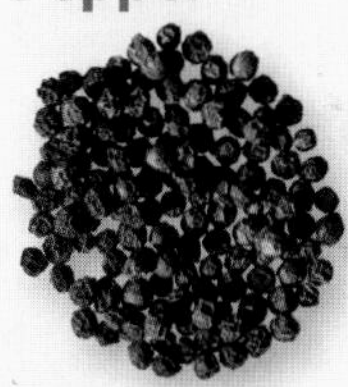

Whole, cracked, or ground dried fruits. Sharp; from moderately to very hot. Use with meat, poultry, fish, soups, and sauces.

Garlic

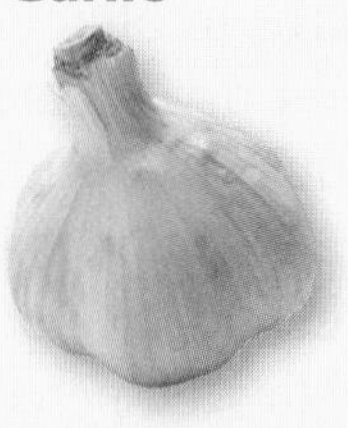

Whole, minced, ground or flaked cloves of a bulb. Sharp and pungent when raw, sweet and nutty when cooked. Use in meats, poultry, soup, tomato dishes, and in Italian and Mediterranean cuisines.

Poppy Seed

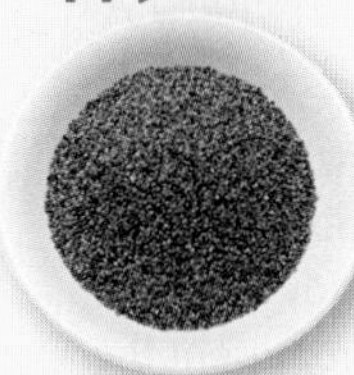

Whole flower seeds. Mild and nutty. Use in breads, pasta dishes, and salad dressings.

Ginger

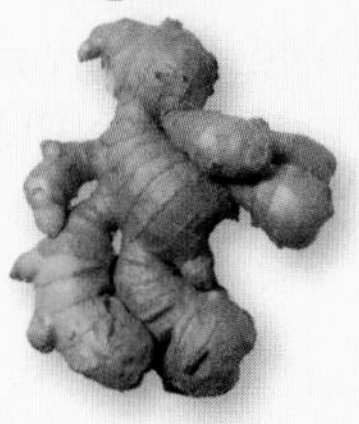

Whole, ground, or candied root. Sweet, hot, and pungent. Use in baked goods, vegetables, and Asian cuisines.

Sesame Seed

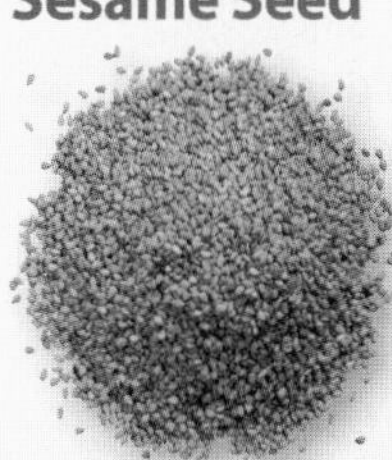

Whole flower seeds. Mild and nutty. Use in poultry, breads, pasta dishes, and stir-fries. Ground for tahini sauce.

- Use a smaller quantity of dried herbs than of fresh herbs, because dried herbs have a stronger flavor than fresh. One tablespoon of fresh herbs equals about 1 teaspoon of dried or crushed herbs, and about ¼ teaspoon of ground herbs.
- Wash fresh herbs before using them. Shake off the excess water. Snip them with scissors or chop them by hand. If the stems are tough, use only the leaves.
- Crush the leaves of dried herbs, such as oregano and rosemary, before adding them to foods. This helps to release flavors.
- Add herbs and spices to hot foods at least 10 minutes before the end of cooking time to let the heat activate their oils. However, add herbs no more than 30 minutes before serving. They lose flavor if overcooked.
- Add herbs and spices to cold foods 30 minutes to several hours before serving so that flavors can be released.

Kitchen Math

Using Fresh Herbs

While shopping at your local farmers' market, you are inspired to make a tomato sauce by the selection of fresh herbs on display. The tomato sauce recipe calls for one teaspoon of dried oregano, ¼ teaspoon of dried parsley, and ½ tablespoon of dried basil. What amount of fresh herbs should you use in place of the dried herbs?

Math Concept **Solving Problems with Proportions** Write two equal ratios (known as a proportion) to relate a quantity you already know to another you are solving for. Use *x* to represent the unknown amount in the second ratio.

Starting Hint One tablespoon of fresh herbs equals one teaspoon of dried herbs. Since 3 tsp. = 1 Tbsp., the ratio of fresh to dried herbs is $3/1$. The ratio of fresh basil to dried basil needed is $x/0.5$ Tbsp. Write a proportion with $3/1 = x/0.5$ and solve for *x*. Repeat for the other two herbs.

Math Appendix For math help, go to the Math Appendix at the back of the book.

NCTM Algebra Represent and analyze mathematical situations and structures using algebraic symbols.

Buying and Storing Dried Herbs and Spices

Dried herbs and spices are used in small amounts. Buy a small amount at a time so you always have a fresh supply.

Store dried herbs and spices in a cool, dark place in tightly closed, **opaque**, light-shielding, containers. A container is opaque if you cannot see through it. This protects them from light, air, and heat, which degrade the oils that carry their flavor. Mark containers with the purchase date. Dried, crushed herbs keep their flavor for about six months if properly stored. To test for freshness, rub a bit of the herb in the palm of your hand with your thumb for five to ten seconds. If the aroma is weak, the herb is probably too old to use. It might impart a bitter flavor.

Ground spices hold their flavor for about a year. Whole spices last much longer, some for several years.

Buying and Storing Fresh Herbs

Fresh herbs are often sold in bundles or packages. Look for bright color with no wilting, browning, or damage. Fresh herbs keep for about five days in the refrigerator, wrapped in a slightly damp paper towel and sealed in a plastic bag with the air pressed out. For longer storage of fresh herbs, dry or freeze them. If you buy fresh herbs that are damp, dry them with a paper towel before storing them in your refrigerator.

Drying Fresh Herbs Tie the herbs in bunches, label them, and hang them in a dry, shaded, well-ventilated area. They should dry within two weeks. To dry herbs in the microwave oven, place them between several layers of paper towels. Microwave on high (100 percent power) for 15 to 30 seconds at a time until they are crumbly.

Freezing Fresh Herbs Spread the herbs on a baking sheet in a single layer and freeze them overnight. You can store them in a freezer container for up to a year.

Growing Fresh Herbs Many herbs can be successfully grown in large containers on a deck or patio. Clay, wooden, or ceramic pots are good choices. Move planted herbs indoors when the weather turns cold enough for frost.

Be a *Smart Consumer*

Do-It-Yourself Dried Herbs

Drying your own herbs can be fun and cost-effective. Packages of fresh herbs can be expensive. Fresh herbs are less flavorful than dry herbs, so you need to use more of them. You may not use all of the fresh herbs in a package, however, and this leads to waste. Instead of throwing the unused stems away, hang and dry them. You can save even more money by growing your own herbs from seeds or plants. This way, you will always have fresh herbs available, and can dry what you don't use.

Challenge Create a poster that illustrates how to dry herbs and explains why drying herbs can save money.

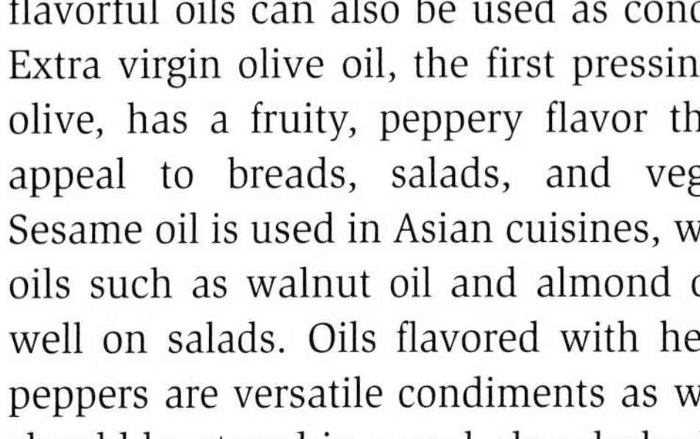

Condiments

Like herbs and spices, condiments are creative seasonings for food. A **condiment** is a liquid or semi-liquid accompaniment to food. Mayonnaise, barbecue sauce, and wasabi are just a few of the many condiments you can choose from.

You can use condiments in creative ways. Tomato ketchup, for example, can add spicy sweetness to soups or beans. Salsa can add mild spice or fiery heat. How would you use the following condiments to liven up a dish?

Mustards American mustard has a relatively mild flavor and a bright yellow color, which comes from the spice turmeric. It is a tangy spread made from ground or powdered mustard seeds with vinegar and seasonings. French, German, and Chinese mustards are darker in color and more intense in flavor. You can also buy specialty mustards that range from spicy hot to honey sweetened.

Vinegars Vinegar is a mildly acidic liquid made by souring or fermenting cider, wine, fruit, or grain. Vinegars come in many different colors and flavors. Distilled white vinegar, a product of grain or white grapes, has a sour, pungent taste. Rice vinegar, used in Asian cooking, adds a slight sweetness and a golden color to recipes. Balsamic (bȯl-ˈsa-mik) vinegar is a sweet, dark vinegar made from grapes. It is aged in wood barrels for years, giving it a pungent flavor and a dark color. Herb vinegars are flavored by soaking or blending various herbs in the vinegar.

Oils Oils are used for cooking, but certain flavorful oils can also be used as condiments. Extra virgin olive oil, the first pressing of the olive, has a fruity, peppery flavor that adds appeal to breads, salads, and vegetables. Sesame oil is used in Asian cuisines, while nut oils such as walnut oil and almond oil work well on salads. Oils flavored with herbs and peppers are versatile condiments as well. Oils should be stored in a cool, dry, dark place.

Sauces Sauces are zesty, sometimes intensely flavored, liquids. Hot pepper sauce is made from chili peppers and is so fiery that it is doled out in drops. Worcestershire (ˈwu̇s-ˌtə-shir) sauce combines vinegar, soy sauce, garlic, molasses, and a tropical fruit called tamarind. Soy and tamari (tə-ˈmär-ē) sauces are made from fermented soybeans. Soy sauce has a sharp, pungent flavor, and tamari is thicker and mellower. Barbecue sauce is a sweet sauce often served with grilled meats. What other sauces can you name?

✓ **Reading Check** **Explain** How should you store dried herbs?

Nutrition Check

Big Benefits in Small Packages

Many herbs and spices are rich in vitamins, minerals, flavonoids, and antioxidants. For example, paprika, cayenne, and red chili peppers all contain capsaicin, an antioxidant that may lower the risk of cancer. Rosemary may lower heart attack risk. Cinnamon can decrease cholesterol. Large quantities of herbs are not necessary to reap benefits. Just 100 grams of oregano contains 244 percent of the daily value for iron.

Think About It Oregano is also rich in calcium and vitamin C, and is the most antioxidant-rich herb. Use the Internet to find five recipes that contain this powerful herb.

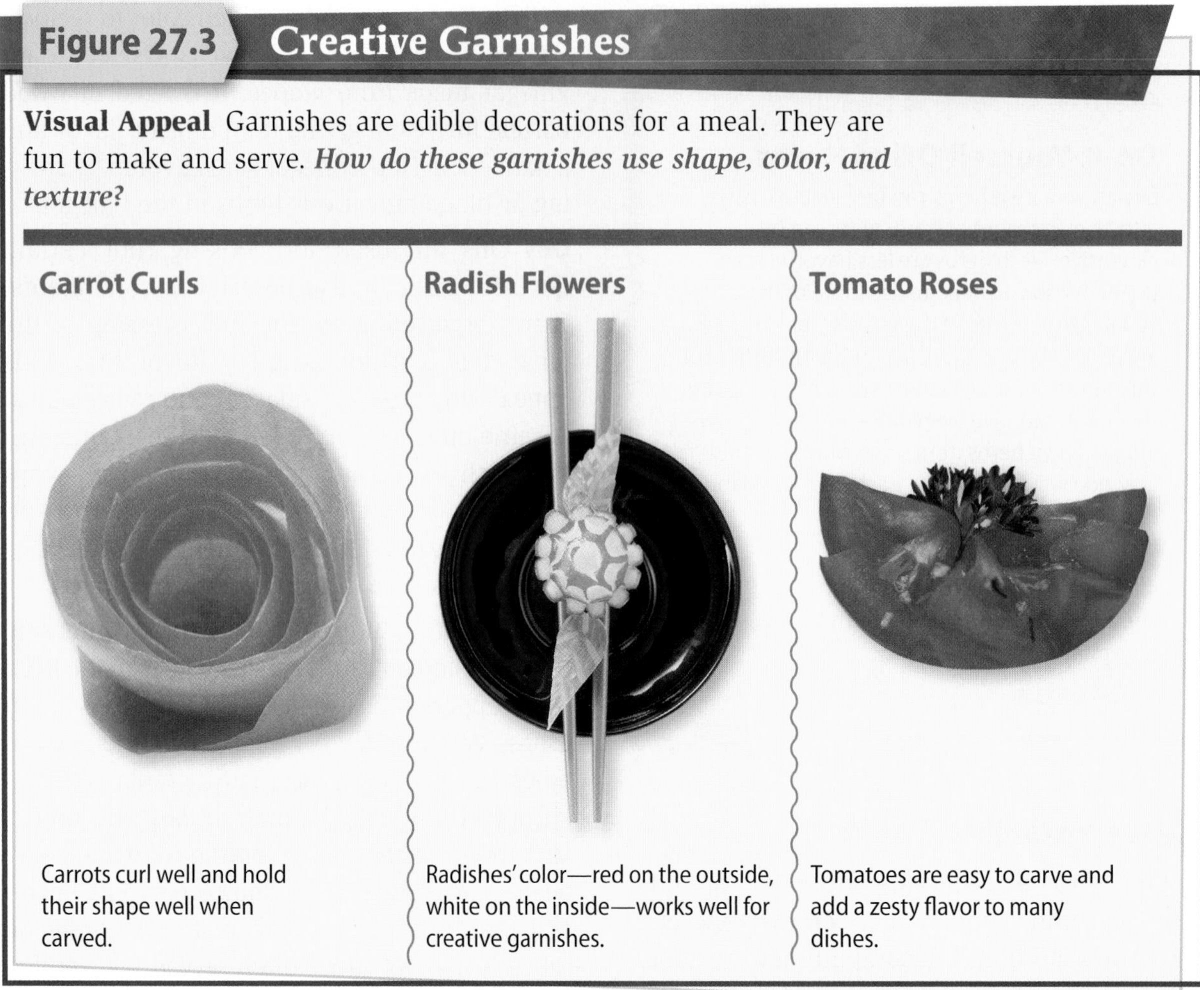

Figure 27.3 Creative Garnishes

Visual Appeal Garnishes are edible decorations for a meal. They are fun to make and serve. ***How do these garnishes use shape, color, and texture?***

Carrot Curls

Carrots curl well and hold their shape well when carved.

Radish Flowers

Radishes' color—red on the outside, white on the inside—works well for creative garnishes.

Tomato Roses

Tomatoes are easy to carve and add a zesty flavor to many dishes.

Garnishes

Garnishes give meals visual appeal. A **garnish** is a small, decorative piece of food used to enhance the appearance of a dish. Garnishes are edible as well as colorful. Garnishes are the finishing touch on a meal. They use color, shape, and texture in creative ways.

A garnish should **complement**, or add something to a meal, but not compete with the rest of the food. It should be small in comparison to the food and serving container. Food and garnish should be compatible in color and flavor.

Making Garnishes

Fruits and vegetables are the most common garnishes. Radishes, carrots, and tomatoes are popular for garnishes, as you can see in **Figure 27.3**. You can create fun, eye-catching effects with garnishes.

Carrot Curls Peel carrots, then use a vegetable peeler to cut them into long, paper-thin strips. Roll up the strips and fasten them with a wooden pick. Chill in ice water. Remove the picks right before serving. You can also use paper-thin carrot strips as an attractive ribbon around green beans or asparagus spears.

Radish Roses Remove the stems from several radishes and cut thin petal-shaped slices around the edges of each one. Chill them in ice water to open the petals and make them crisp.

Citrus Twists Slice unpeeled oranges or lemons across the middle. Cut each slice just to the center, then separate and twist.

Celery Curls Cut celery stalks into 3-inch lengths. Starting at one end, make several parallel cuts to about one third of the way down each stalk. Repeat on the other end. Do not cut through the center. Chill in ice water until the ends curl.

Use your creativity to create spur-of-the-moment garnishes. Add a sprig of fresh mint and a small crunchy cookie or bit of peanut brittle to a dish of vanilla ice cream. Hook a candy cane over the rim of a mug of hot cocoa or frame a sandwich on a bed of lettuce with cheese strips at the corners. Cut a sandwich into thirds and stack them on top of each other. Float croutons, chopped fresh herbs, a spoonful of yogurt, or a sprinkling of cheese in a bowl of soup. Any ingredient in a salad can also serve as a garnish: olives, grapes, chopped nuts, cherry tomatoes, croutons, tomato wedges, or rings of green bell pepper or red onion. Remember that contrasting colors surprise the eye in a pleasing way.

✓ **Reading Check** **Describe** How can you make sure a garnish complements, but does not compete with, a meal?

Freshening Up Favorites

When people get tired of how a room looks, they often rearrange the furniture. The same approach works when a favorite recipe starts to grow boring. Paying attention to which foods are available and in season can help you avoid growing bored with meals. If blackberries are in season try substituting them for the strawberries in strawberry shortcake. Vary the presentation or try new seasonings or condiments. Instead of serving a bowl of chili and a square of cornbread, spread the cornbread batter in muffin cups, top with the cooked chili, and bake. Garnish the chili with shredded cheese or green bell pepper. You could also try serving the chili with polenta, a soft bread made with corn meal, instead of corn bread. For dessert, cut a thin slice off the top of an angel food

Careers in Food

David Holloway
Food Editor

Q: What does a food editor do?

A: My job is to coordinate the entire scope of food coverage for the newspaper. That means coming up with story ideas, lining up art and photos for stories, editing articles and writing headlines. I manage freelance food writers who contribute stories.

Q: How much of your time is spent on restaurant related coverage as opposed to home cooking?

A: Eighty to 90 percent of our content is about home cooking. A separate restaurant review column runs in another section of the newspaper.

Q: What qualities benefit a food editor?

A: It helps to have a good appetite, a healthy curiosity about food, and a good sense of humor about what you do.

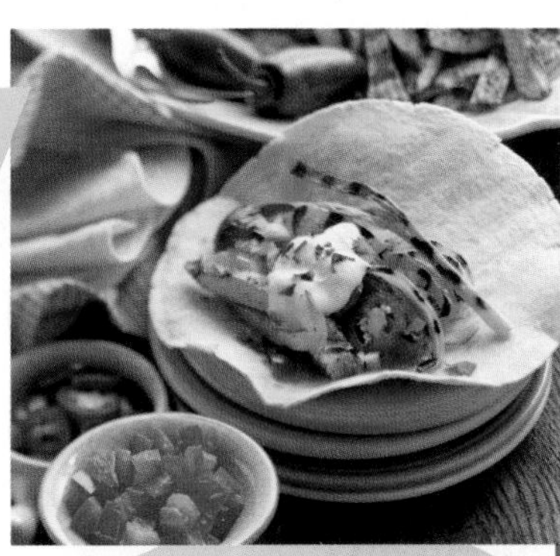

"The food section is the one section of the newspaper that everyone can relate to."
— David Holloway, *Food Editor, Press-Register, Mobile, AL*

Education and Training

A college degree in Journalism or English with a writing focus is a necessary, entry-level requirement. Since you will be writing about food, a culinary education is valuable. Nutrition knowledge also is useful.

Qualities and Skills

You need to have enough kitchen skill to understand what goes into preparing something you are reviewing. You need to be able to write well and under deadline pressure. You need to be accurate with lots of detailed information.

Related Career Opportunities

General assignment reporting and working in a newsroom as a copy editor, layout editor or features editor are all related opportunities. Essentially, they are the same types of positions except the emphasis is on something other than food or dining.

cake, dig out a channel in the center, and fill it with fresh fruit and chunks of cake.

Find new uses for kitchen tools such as a pastry bag, which is normally used to decorate cakes. Use the pastry bag to swirl mashed potatoes into a fluffy basket filled with colorful cooked broccoli. Ring a roast with a decorative border of mashed sweet potato. For snacks or appetizers, pipe a creamy tuna salad or seasoned cheese spread into celery sticks or onto crackers or bread rounds.

✓ **Reading Check** **Explain** Why is it helpful to vary the presentation of a meal?

Food as Gifts

Homemade food is a gift from the heart. Cakes, cookies, and pies are often given at holidays and birthdays. Homemade breads and jams provide thoughtful host or hostess gifts. Preparing a meal is a traditional way to show care for a person going through a period of illness or grief. Food takes time, skill, and attention to make, so giving food is a good way to show that you care.

Food gifts can also be beautiful when you take as much care with the wrapping as with the food. For example, tie ribbon around a jar of jam or wrap cookies in colorful plastic wrap. A special container can even be part of the present. Give bread baked in a clay flowerpot to a gardener or small cakes made in jelly jars to a home canner. There are thousands of recipes for spicing and pickling vegetables. With the skills you learned in Chapter 18 you will be able to can things like pickled vegetables to give as gifts. You can make dozens of jars of canned foods ahead of time to have on hand as gifts when you are invited to a barbecue or dinner party.

When choosing food for a gift, keep the person's dietary needs in mind. The extra effort of finding a diabetic or low-fat recipe makes the gift even more meaningful.

Light and Healthy Recipe

Spiced-Up Chili

Ingredients

- **1 Tbsp.** Olive oil
- **1 cup** Chopped onion
- **8 oz.** Ground turkey
- **2 cups** Prepared salsa
- **1 can (15 oz.)** Kidney beans
- **1 can (15 oz.)** Black beans
- **1 can (15 oz.)** Crushed tomatoes
- **1 can (6 oz.)** Tomato paste
- **1 tsp.** Chili powder
- **1 tsp.** Paprika
- **½ tsp.** Cumin
- **¼ tsp.** Pepper
- **⅛ tsp.** Cayenne pepper

Directions

1. In a large pot, add the olive oil and cook the onions on low heat until nearly tender.
2. Add the ground turkey to the pot and continue cooking until the meat is cooked through.
3. Add the salsa, beans, tomatoes and tomato paste and bring to a simmer, stirring often.
4. Let everything cook together for 30 minutes. Stir in the spices and let the chili cook for another 10 minutes.
5. Serve hot in bowls.

With ground turkey and beans, this chili recipe packs protein.

Yield 8 Servings

Nutrition Analysis per Serving

Calories	180
Total fat	3 g
Saturated fat	0 g
Cholesterol	11 mg
Sodium	606 mg
Carbohydrate	25 g
Dietary fiber	7 g
Sugars	4 g
Protein	14 g

CHAPTER 27 Review & Applications

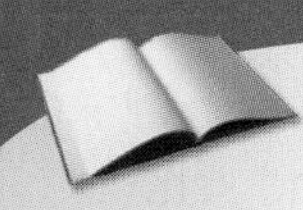

After You Read

Chapter Summary

Many different types of creative additions can be used to add appeal and flavor to meals. Seasonings are ingredients used in small amounts to flavor foods. They include herbs, spices, and condiments. Follow guidelines to use, buy, and store them properly. Garnishes are small, edible pieces of food that give meals visual appeal. They add color, flavor, and texture. Freshen up favorite foods by varying their presentation, adding garnishes, and finding new uses for kitchen tools. Giving homemade food as a gift takes time and skill, and shows thoughtfulness.

Content and Academic Vocabulary Review

1. Write a memo introducing yourself to the class. Use each of the following content and academic vocabulary terms in your memo.

Content Vocabulary

- ☐ herb (p. 414)
- ☐ spice (p. 414)
- ☐ bouquet garni (p. 414)
- ☐ seasoning blend (p. 414)
- ☐ condiment (p. 419)
- ☐ garnish (p. 420)

Academic Vocabulary

- opaque (p. 418)
- complement (p. 420)

Review Key Concepts

2. **Identify** common herbs and spices.
3. **Describe** the role of garnishes.
4. **Identify** techniques for varying the presentation of your favorite recipe.
5. **Explain** how homemade food can be a meaningful gift.

Critical Thinking

6. **Explain** whether Leah's statement is accurate: "I really enjoy curry powder. It is such a tasty herb."
7. **Describe** two solutions for the following problem: While preparing a recipe that calls for dried sage, Lin realizes he forgot to buy some, but he does have plenty of fresh sage.
8. **Identify** five of your favorite dishes and suggest how the foods might be garnished for added visual appeal.
9. **Describe** how the Campbell family can freshen up their favorite meal—broiled chicken, steamed wild rice, and sautéed broccoli—without eliminating ingredients.
10. **Describe** an idea for a specific edible gift that Janelle, who has extra time but not much extra money, can present to her friends and family during the holiday.

Foods Lab

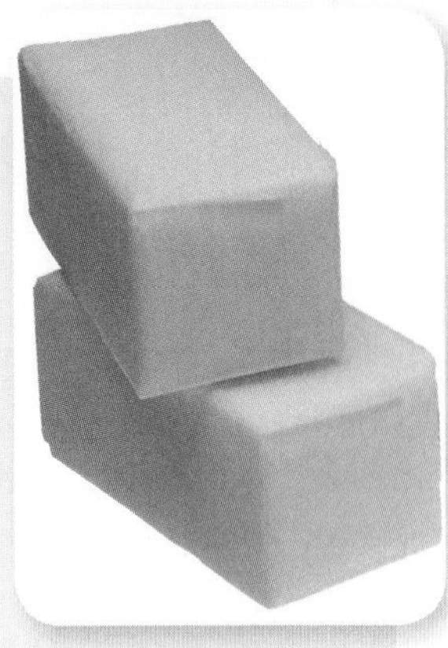

11. Herb Butters Mixing butter with herbs and spices makes a flavorful, appealing spread for bread, crackers, and other foods.

Procedure With your lab team, experiment with a variety of seasonings to develop a recipe for an herb butter. Keep track of amounts and proportions as you work. Make a batch to share with other lab teams.

Analysis Verbally answer the following questions in an oral presentation: How did your team agree on a final recipe? Was compromise needed? What improvements, if any, might still be needed? Which herbs do you think made the best herb butters? Why?

HEALTHFUL CHOICES

12. Health-Friendly Flavor Typically, Isaac flavors his noodles with butter and salt. Isaac's nutritionist has suggested he stick to a diet low in sodium and saturated fats. Suggest at least two specific changes Isaac can make to add flavor to his noodles in a more healthful way.

TECH Connection

13. Research Saffron Under your teacher's supervision, use the Internet to research the history and uses of saffron, a popular spice. Learn which countries export saffron. Examine saffron as a crop and how its production and sale impacts a particular country. Research the steps involved in growing and harvesting saffron and its price on the world market. Write a paragraph about saffron production. Then, use word processing software to create a chronology showing the history of this spice.

Real-World Skills

Problem-Solving Skills

14. Spontaneous Salad Dressing After serving an elaborate meal, including salad, to several friends, Dominic realizes he is out of salad dressing. He does have several seasonings and condiments on hand. Suggest specific ingredients he might use to make his own salad dressing.

Interpersonal and Collaborative Skills

15. Demonstration Area Follow your teacher's instructions to form groups. In the foods lab, work with your group to effectively use space, dishes, utensils, signs, and labels to set up a demonstration area where classmates can see, smell, and taste various seasonings.

Financial Literacy Skills

16. Fund-Raiser Plan a food gift that your class could make and sell as a fund-raiser. For example, you could make and package a Valentine cookie for students to buy and give to someone special. Determine the cost of making the item. How much would you need to charge for it to make a 50 percent profit?

Academic Skills

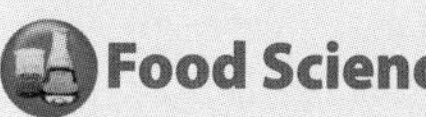

Food Science

17. Sugar Crystals If dissolved sugar molecules get too crowded for the water to keep them apart, as in a supersaturated solution, the sugar molecules bond to each other and form crystals. You will need a pot, two cups of water, five cups of sugar, a glass jar, Popsicle sticks or skewers and a plastic lid for this activity.

Procedure Bring the water to a boil. Stir in the sugar and bring the mixture back to a simmer. Remove from heat and let cool for 5 minutes. Carefully pour the syrup into the glass jar. Punch the skewers through a plastic lid and set the lid over the glass jar so the sticks hang down into the syrup, but don't touch the bottom of the jar. Set aside for 7–14 days.

Analysis Explain the science of crystal formation and supersaturated solutions in paragraph form.

NSES B Develop an understanding of the structure and properties of matter.

Mathematics

18. Growing Herbs Jordan frequently uses fresh herbs while cooking, but purchasing fresh herbs at the grocery store can be expensive. He decided to plant his own small herb garden. He started in June by planting an 11″–tall basil plant and a 1′–4″-tall mint plant. In July, the basil plant is now 1′–9″, and the mint has grown to 3′–1″. How much did each of Jordan's plants grow during the month?

Math Concept **Subtracting Lengths** When subtracting measurements given in feet and inches, subtract the feet and inch amounts separately. If you wind up with a negative number of inches, add 12 to the inch amount, and subtract one foot.

Starting Hint For the mint, subtract 1′ from 3′ to get the new foot amount, and 4″ from 1″ to get the inch amount. Rewrite the answer to eliminate the negative number of inches. Repeat for the basil.

NCTM Problem Solving Build new mathematical knowledge through problem solving.

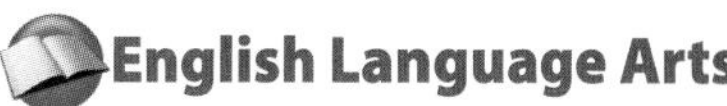

English Language Arts

19. Interview Write ten interview questions to ask an herb gardener in your family or community. Then conduct your interview. In a presentation to the class, share the information you gained in your interview. Then apply it to grow one or more herbs in your classroom.

NCTE 7 Conduct research and gather, evaluate, and synthesize data to communicate discoveries.

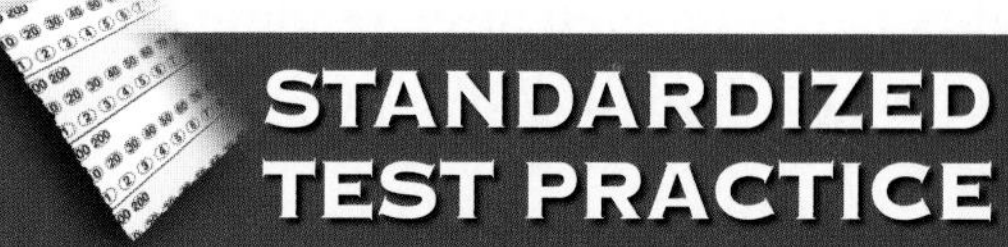

STANDARDIZED TEST PRACTICE

Fill in the Blank Read the sentence and choose the best word to fill in the blank.

20. Vinegar is a mildly acidic liquid made by fermenting ________________

a. cider, wine, fruit, or grain
b. spices, herbs, and fruits
c. herbs and flowers
d. wine, spices, fruit, and flowers

Test-Taking Tip When answering a fill-in-the-blank question, silently read the sentence with each of the possible answers in the blank space. This will help you eliminate wrong answers. The best word results in a sentence that is both factual and grammatically correct.

UNIT 6 Thematic Project

Create a Work Plan

In this unit you have learned that to be successful in the kitchen, you must use recipes, preparation techniques, and cooking methods appropriately. You have also learned that a work plan is an easy and useful way to accomplish your goals in the kitchen. Work plans also help minimize the stress you may feel when you are cooking a new or large meal. In this project, you will choose a recipe, discuss it with an adult in your community qualified to discuss it, and develop a work plan for preparing it.

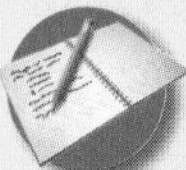

My Journal

If you completed the journal entry from page 355, refer to it to see if your thoughts have changed after reading the unit and completing this project.

Project Assignment

- Choose a recipe to discuss with a friend or family member.
- Write a list of discussion questions about tips and advice for preparing the recipe you have chosen.
- Discuss your recipe with a friend or family member. Ask questions you have prepared.
- Take notes during the discussion.
- Create a work plan for a recipe of your choice.
- Share your work plan with your class.

Academic Skills You Will Use

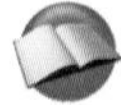

English Language Arts

NCTE 8 Use information resources to gather information and create and communicate knowledge.

NCTE 12 Use language to accomplish individual purposes.

STEP 1 Choose a Recipe

The list below includes examples of different types of recipes. Choose a recipe for which you will create a work plan.

- Ethnic foods
- Breads
- Cakes, pies, candies
- Meat, fish, poultry
- Salads
- Soups
- Comfort food
- Family recipe

STEP 2 Write Interview Questions

Make a list of questions to ask someone who is qualified to give you advice about developing a work plan. Use the time you spend in your interview to ask questions that will help you dovetail the preparation of your recipe. Write interview questions that elicit advice about these topics:

- How to best prepare the recipe you have chosen.
- How to collect all the ingredients required.
- The types or forms of ingredient, such as fresh versus dried herbs.
- Changes or substitutions to help give the recipe unique flair.
- Planning the timing of the preparation of the recipe.

Take careful notes during the interview.

STEP 3 Connect to Your Community

Choose an adult member of your community whom you consider to be a good cook. This may be a chef at a local restaurant, a family member, or a friend. Set up a time to discuss with them the recipe you chose. Ask for advice or tips for preparing the recipe. Also ask for any modifications they might make. Speak clearly and politely. Maintain eye contact, and encourage the person you interview to share his or her ideas.

Writing Skills

- During the discussion, record responses and take notes.
- Use standard English to communicate.
- Listen attentively.
- After the interview, transcribe your notes into complete sentences.

STEP 4 Create and Present Your Work Plan

Use the Unit Thematic Project Checklist to plan and complete your project and evaluate your work.

STEP 5 Evaluate Your Presentation

Your project will be evaluated based on:

- Thoroughness of your work plan.
- Notes from your interview.
- Mechanics—demonstration and neatness.

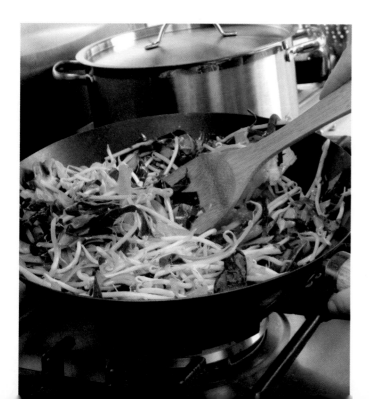

Unit Thematic Project Checklist

Category	Objectives
Plan	☑ Choose a recipe.
	☑ Interview someone about the recipe and strategies for creating a work plan for executing the recipe.
	☑ Create a work plan for the recipe you selected. Make sure all steps are in a logical order.
	☑ Plan a presentation in which you will explain your work plan.
Present	☑ Make a presentation to your class to share your work plan and discuss what you learned.
	☑ Invite the students in your class to ask you any questions they may have. Answer three questions.
	☑ When students ask you questions, demonstrate in your answers that you respect their perspectives.
	☑ Turn in your recipe, the notes from your interview, and your work plan to your teacher.
Academic Skills	☑ Be sensitive to the needs of different audiences.
	☑ Adapt and modify language to suit different purposes.
	☑ Speak clearly and concisely.

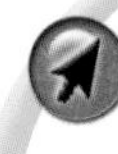

Go to this book's Online Learning Center through **glencoe.com** for a rubric you can use to evaluate your final project.

UNIT 7

Food Preparation

Activate Prior Knowledge

Explore the Photo Preparing healthy food can be fun, especially when you work together with family members or friends. *What are some ways to use teamwork in the kitchen?*

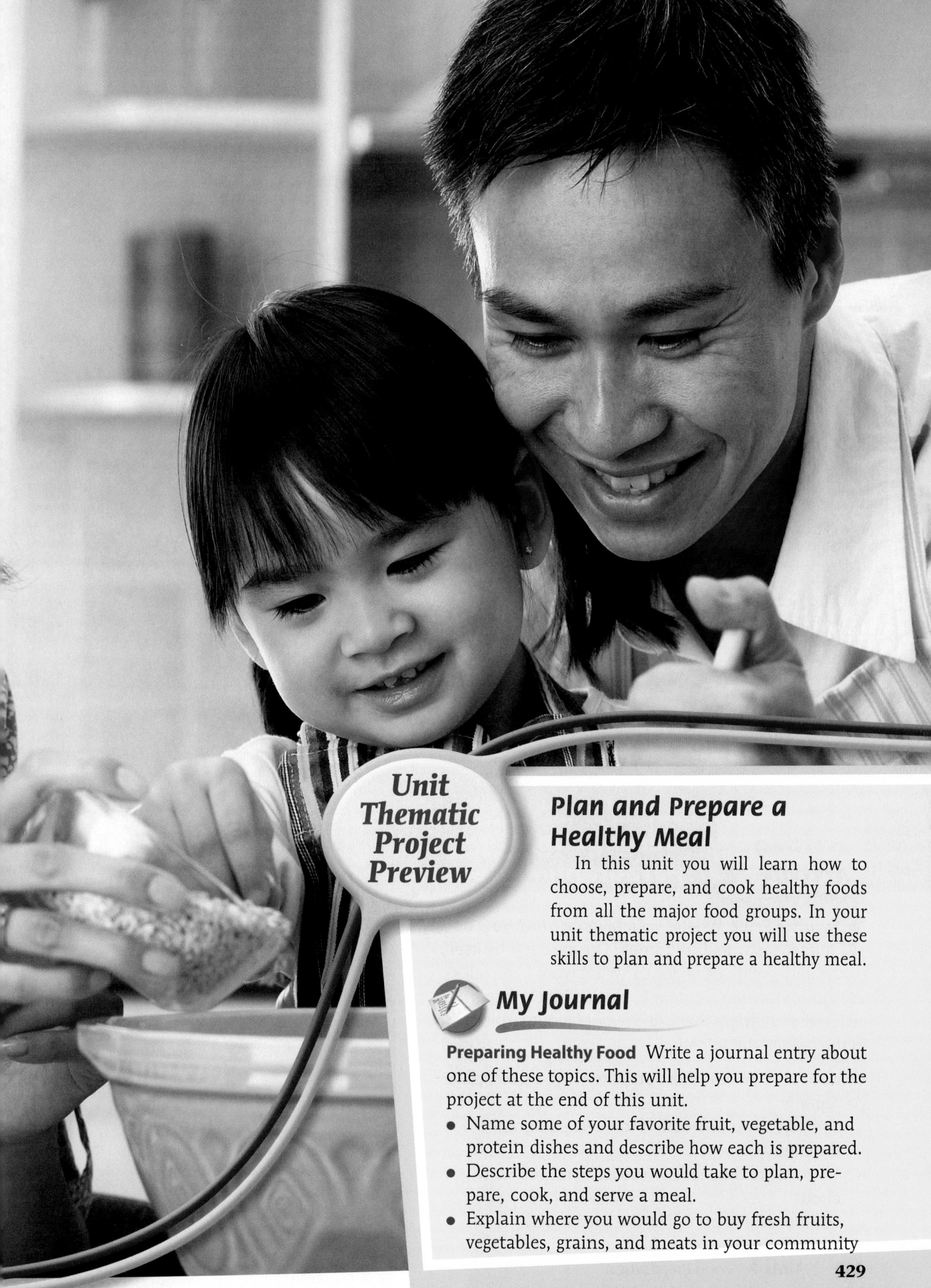

Unit Thematic Project Preview

Plan and Prepare a Healthy Meal

In this unit you will learn how to choose, prepare, and cook healthy foods from all the major food groups. In your unit thematic project you will use these skills to plan and prepare a healthy meal.

My Journal

Preparing Healthy Food Write a journal entry about one of these topics. This will help you prepare for the project at the end of this unit.

- Name some of your favorite fruit, vegetable, and protein dishes and describe how each is prepared.
- Describe the steps you would take to plan, prepare, cook, and serve a meal.
- Explain where you would go to buy fresh fruits, vegetables, grains, and meats in your community

CHAPTER 28

Fruits

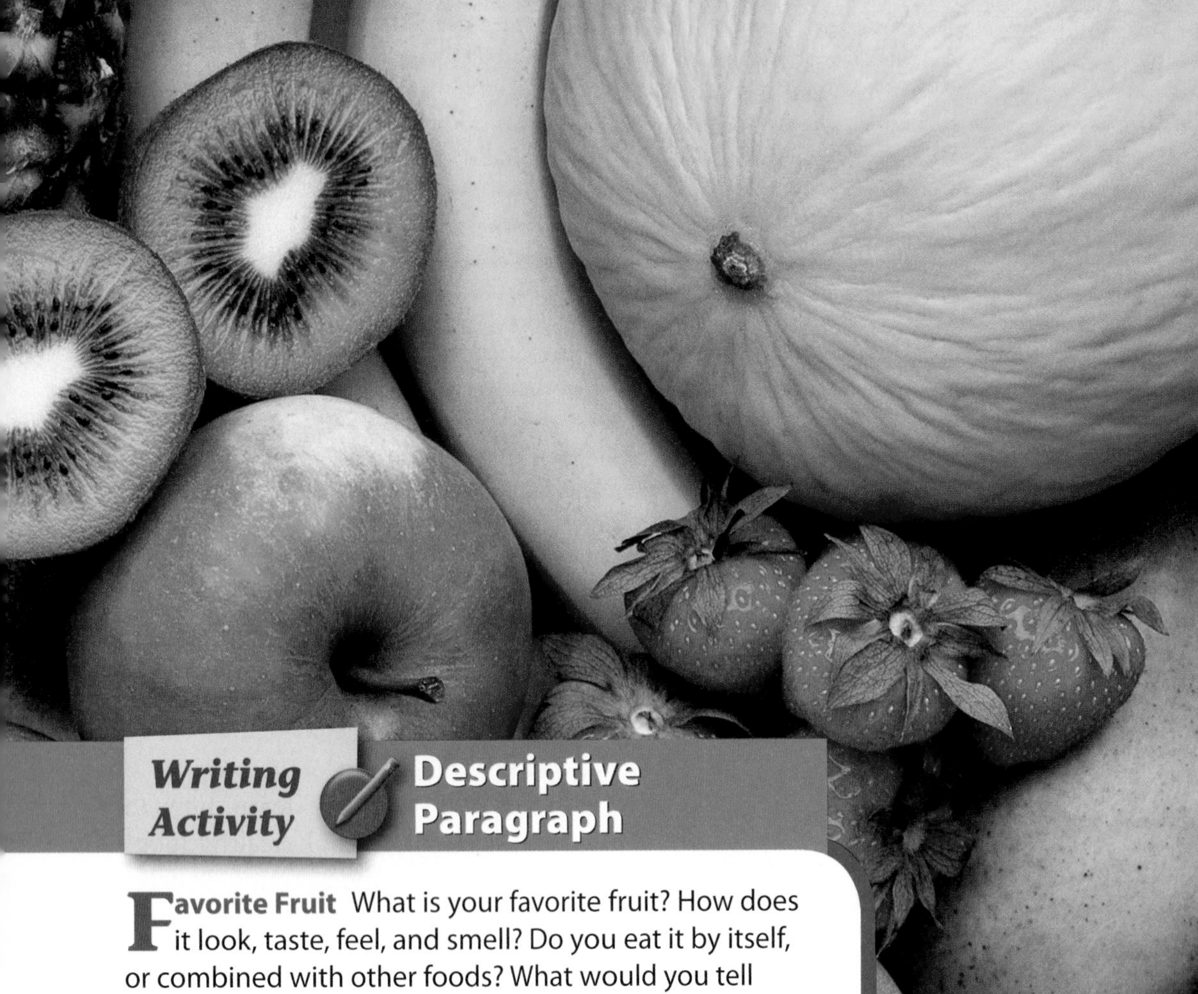

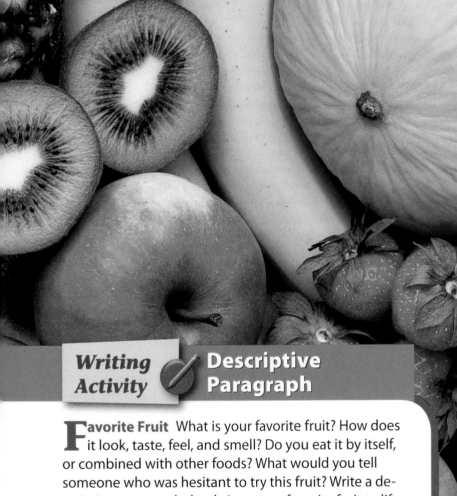

Writing Activity — Descriptive Paragraph

Favorite Fruit What is your favorite fruit? How does it look, taste, feel, and smell? Do you eat it by itself, or combined with other foods? What would you tell someone who was hesitant to try this fruit? Write a descriptive paragraph that brings your favorite fruit to life in the reader's imagination.

Writing Tips Follow these steps to write a descriptive paragraph:

- Use adjectives and details to make paragraphs descriptive.
- Try to make the reader visualize what you write about.
- Use words that appeal to the five senses.

Activate Prior Knowledge

Explore the Photo Fruit provides nutrients plus something important to your diet. *What else does fruit supply?*

Reading Guide

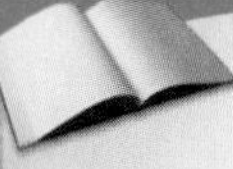

Before You Read

Preview Examine the photos in this chapter. How many of the fruits pictured have you tasted? Make a list.

Read to Learn

Key Concepts

- **Describe** the nutritional benefits of fruits.
- **Identify** the six major types of fruits.
- **Explain** how to store fresh fruits.
- **Describe** enzymatic browning and how to prevent it.
- **Identify** the types and uses of convenience forms of fruits.
- **Describe** methods for cooking fruits.

Main Idea

Fruits are nutrient-rich, come in a variety of forms, and are colorful, flavorful, and easy to prepare.

Content Vocabulary

You will find definitions for these words in the glossary at the back of this book.

- ☐ fruit
- ☐ drupe
- ☐ pome
- ☐ savory
- ☐ produce
- ☐ mature fruit
- ☐ ripe fruit
- ☐ immature fruit
- ☐ under ripe fruit
- ☐ regreening
- ☐ enzymatic browning
- ☐ enzyme
- ☐ trifle
- ☐ reconstitute
- ☐ fritter

Academic Vocabulary

You will find these words in your reading and on your tests. Use the glossary to look up their definitions if necessary.

- membrane
- characteristic

Graphic Organizer

Use a graphic organizer like the one below to note and briefly explain three steps you should take to make fruit ready for serving.

Washing	Paring and Preparing	Preventing from Darkening

Graphic Organizer Go to this book's Online Learning Center at **glencoe.com** to print out this graphic organizer.

Academic Standards

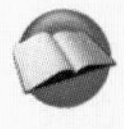

English Language Arts

NCTE 7 Conduct research and gather, evaluate, and synthesize data to communicate discoveries.

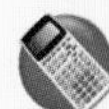

Mathematics

NCTM Algebra Represent and analyze mathematical situations and structures using algebraic symbols.

NCTM Measurement Apply appropriate techniques, tools, and formulas to determine measurements.

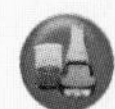

Science

NSES B Develop an understanding of chemical reactions.

NCTE *National Council of Teachers of English*
NCTM *National Council of Teachers of Mathematics*
NSES *National Science Education Standards*
NCSS *National Council for the Social Studies*

Nutrients in Fruits

A **fruit** is the part of a plant that holds the seeds. Fruits are colorful, flavorful, and easy to prepare, making them ideal for snacks as well as meals. Fruits also supply a wide variety of nutrients. Dietary fiber and carbohydrates are abundant in fruit. Fruits are also fat-free, low in calories, and low in sodium.

Fruits are an excellent source of vitamin C, potassium, and phytochemicals such as beta carotene. Some fruits are good sources of other nutrients as well. For example, oranges provide folic acid. Bananas are a source of magnesium. Raisins and other dried fruits provide iron.

✓ Reading Check **Explain** Why do fruits make ideal snacks?

Identifying Fruits

Fruits are sorted into six major types, based on their structure and origin.

Berries Berries are small, juicy fruits with a thin skin. Strawberries, cranberries, grapes, and blackberries are berries.

Melons Melons have a thick rind, or outer skin. They are juicy and usually have many seeds. Watermelons, cantaloupes, and casaba (kə-ˈsä-bə) are popular types of melon.

Nutrition Check

A Daily Dose of Fruit

Because fruit provides so many valuable nutrients, it is an important part of a healthful diet. A person on a 2,000 to 2,600 calorie diet should eat at least 2 cups of fruit each day. Simply eating two cups of apples, however, is not as beneficial as eating a variety of fruits. Different colors provide different phytochemicals and antioxidants. Instead of 2 cups of one type of fruit, try eating four ½ cup servings of different types of fruit.

Think About It Plan to eat four ½ cup servings of different types and colors of fruit today. Which fruits will you choose? Make a list.

Citrus Fruits Citrus fruits have a thick rind and a thin **membrane** separating inner flesh segments. A membrane is a thin layer of tissue. Oranges, tangerines, grapefruits, lemons, and limes are citrus fruits.

Drupes A **drupe** is a fruit with a single hard seed, also called a pit or stone, and soft inner flesh covered by a tender, edible skin. Cherries, apricots, peaches, nectarines, and plums are drupes.

Pomes A **pome** is a fruit with several small seeds and thick, firm flesh with a tender, edible skin. Apples and pears are pomes.

Tropical Fruits Tropical fruits are grown in tropical and subtropical climates. Bananas, guavas, papayas, and mangoes are popular tropical fruits.

Figure 28.1 shows many fruits and their uses in sweet and savory dishes. **Savory** means flavorful but not sweet.

Unusual Fruits

Identifying an apple and a banana is easy, but would you recognize a carambola or a cherimoya? Many less familiar fruits are gaining popularity in the United States as interest in international cooking grows.

Carambola (ˌka-rəm-ˈbō-lə) Also called star fruit, a carambola has an oval shape with four to six prominent ribs and edible skin. When sliced horizontally, it forms a star. Ripe carambolas are yellow-gold, with a slight browning on the ribs. Their flavor is similar to a combination of plums, apples, and citrus. The fruit does not darken when cut.

Cherimoya (ˌcher-ə-ˈmȯi-ə) Called a "custard apple," the cherimoya has a custard-like texture when chilled. It is heart-shaped, with green skin that is imprinted with petal shapes. A cherimoya tastes like a blend of strawberries, pineapples, and bananas. Eat the fruit by spooning the flesh from the shell.

Feijoa (fā-ˈyō-ə) This small, egg-shaped fruit has thin, bright green skin and fragrant, cream-colored flesh. It tastes like a combination of pineapple and mint. Peel the fruit before eating.

Figure 28.1 Fruits and Their Uses

Fruit Quiz A wide variety of fruit can be used in main dishes, side dishes, and desserts. ***Based on text descriptions, can you identify these fruits?***

Apples

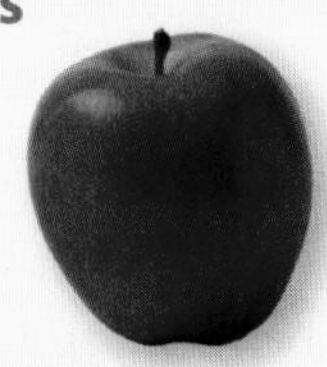

- Red, green, or yellow roundish fruits. Some varieties hold their shape well when cooked. Look for vibrant color and firm texture, with no bruises. Eat unpeeled.
- Use Braeburn apples raw or cooked. Eat Gala, Golden Delicious, McIntosh, and Red Delicious varieties raw. Eat Granny Smith and Rome varieties cooked.
- Use raw in salads or cooked in desserts, sauce, cider, and some savory dishes.

Apricots

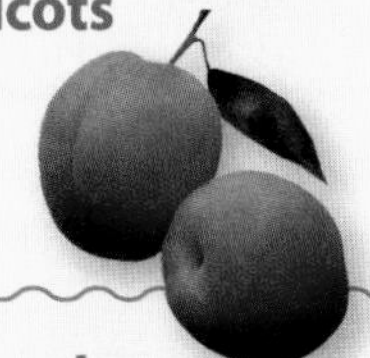

- Small oval fruit with even, golden color and slightly fuzzy skin. Smaller than peaches with drier, tarter flesh. Pit removes easily. Eat unpeeled. Flavor is sweet and slightly tart.
- Use raw, cooked in jams, or baked with other stone fruits in crisp or tart.

Avocados

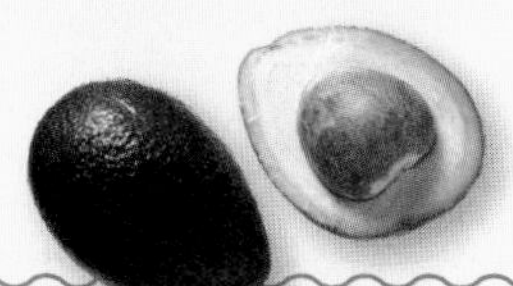

- Green to black oval-shaped fruit with a single large seed. Ripens after harvesting, turning dark. Gives to slight pressure when ripe, but should not be too soft or sunken. Light green flesh darkens with oxygen exposure. Peel before eating. High in monounsaturated fat.
- Use raw in guacamole dips and salads.

Bananas

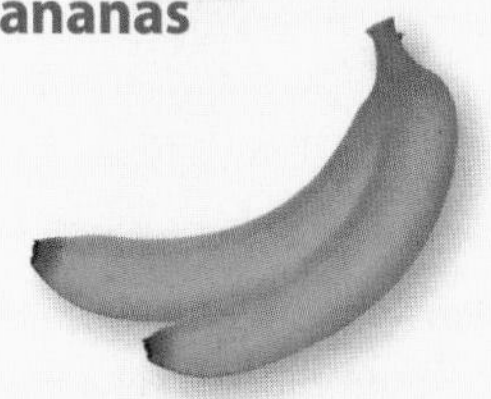

- Distinctive fruit comes in yellow, baby, and red varieties. Picked green. Ripe when fully yellow, with only a few black spots. Spots indicate starch is turning to sugar. Plantains are similar and look like overripe yellow bananas. Red are very sweet with a creamy texture. Peel before eating.
- Use raw in fruit salads and smoothies or cooked in pancakes, quick bread, and pies.

Blueberries

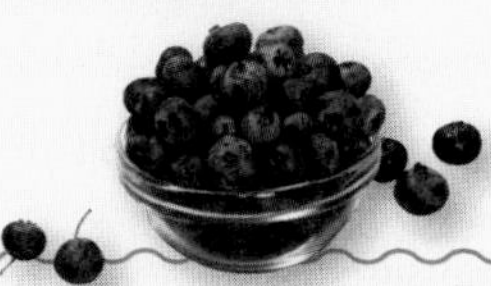

- Dark bluish purple berries, often with a silvery surface. No aroma. Choose plump and unwrinkled berries. Eat unpeeled.
- Use raw, dried as a cereal topping or snack, or cooked in syrup, sauce, jam, muffins, desserts, and pancakes.

Cherries

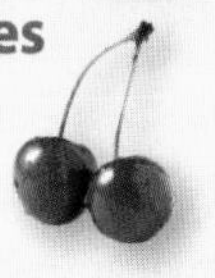

- Small pome with varieties including dark red Bing and light red Queen Anne. Bright, plump, and firm. Cherries do not ripen after harvesting. Eat unpeeled. Flavor is sweet to tart. Dark cherries are usually sweeter.
- Use raw, marinated, or cooked in pie or cobbler.

Clementines

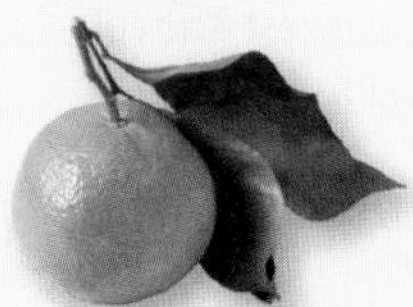

- Orange citrus fruits smaller than tangerines and oranges, with loose, easy-peel rind. Peel before eating. Very sweet and nearly seedless.
- Use raw or cooked in savory and sweet dishes, especially sauces. Substitutes for orange sections in recipes to save peeling time.

Figure 28.1 Fruits and Their Uses *(continued)*

Cranberries

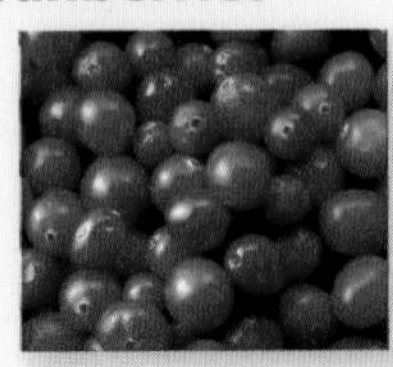

- Small, hard berries. Light to dark red. Should be shiny and plump, not shriveled. Eat unpeeled. Flavor is tart, dry, and sour.
- Use dried, raw in relish, as juice, or cooked in sauces, jellies, quick breads, and desserts and savory dishes.

Gooseberries

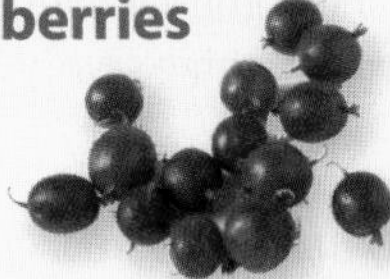

- Small berries with green, red, purple, golden, and milky-white varieties. Should be firm, not hard. Eat unpeeled. Flavor is tart, like green grapes.
- Use cooked with sugar added in jams, jellies, crisps, and pies.

Grapefruits

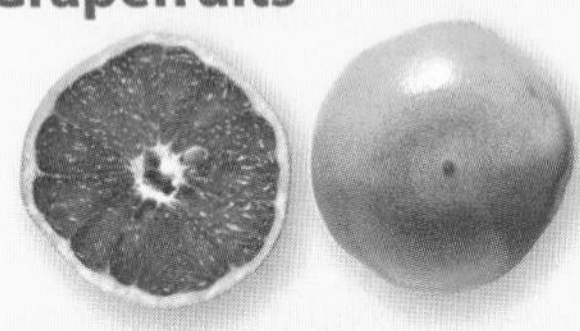

- Large citrus fruits with a yellow rind and a rosy blush. Flesh is white/yellow or pink. Pink flesh is sweeter. Peel before eating. Flavor is tart to sweet and juicy.
- Use raw in salads or as juice.

Grapes

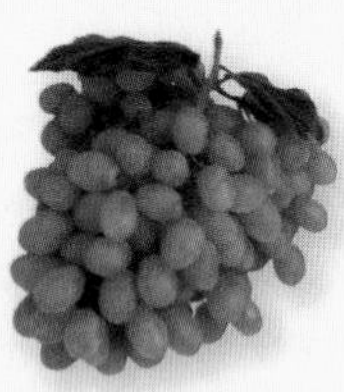

- Small berry with varieties including green seedless; deep purple, red, or white Concord; and red seedless. Plump, bright, and firm when ripe. Eat unpeeled. Dry into raisins.
- Use raw, dried, as juice, and in jams, jellies, and salads.

Kiwifruit

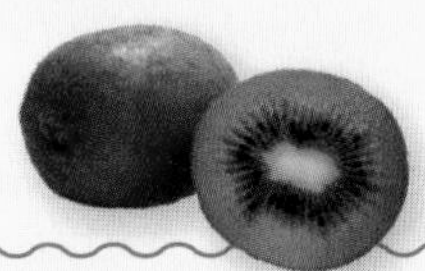

- Small and egg-shaped fruit with thin, fuzzy brown skin and soft green flesh. Tiny, black edible seeds. Slightly soft when ripe. Peel before eating. Flavor is sweet and slightly tart.
- Use raw in smoothies and fruit salad.

Kumquats

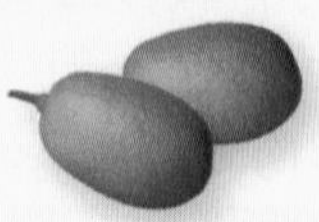

- (ˈkəm-ˌkwäts) Small, round or oval citrus fruits. Orange in color. Skin is sweet and flesh is tart and juicy, with sour-orange flavor. Eat unpeeled.
- Use raw in salads, cooked in jelly, marmalade, and desserts, or candied, pickled, or preserved.

Lemons and Limes

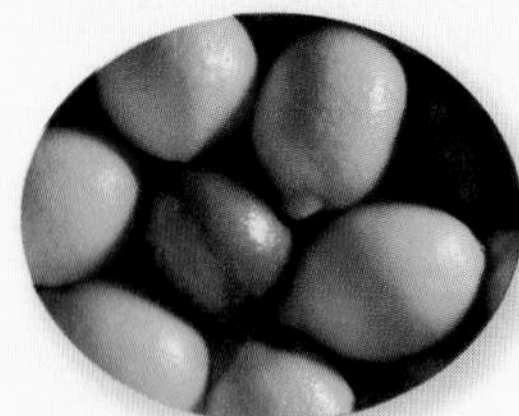

- Small citrus fruits. Lemons are yellow, limes are green. Both are plump, with glossy skin. Key limes are very small and light green. Fruits that are heavy for their size have more juice. Peel before eating. Flavor is very tart.
- Use juice or zest raw or cooked in soups, stews, rice and bean dishes, fish, vegetables, fruit and vegetable salads, and desserts. Get zest (the colorful outer layer of rind) by shaving small strips from the skin.

Figure 28.1 Fruits and Their Uses *(continued)*

Mangoes

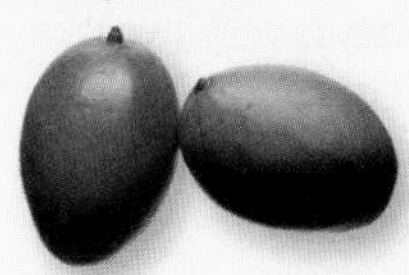

- Large, oval fruit with single large seed. Red, yellow, green, orange, or a combination. Usually tinged yellow when ripe. Flesh is golden orange, juicy, and sweet. Peel before eating. Fruity aroma from stem end.
- Use raw in fruit salads, chutneys, and marinades, or cooked in sauces and desserts.

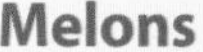

Melons

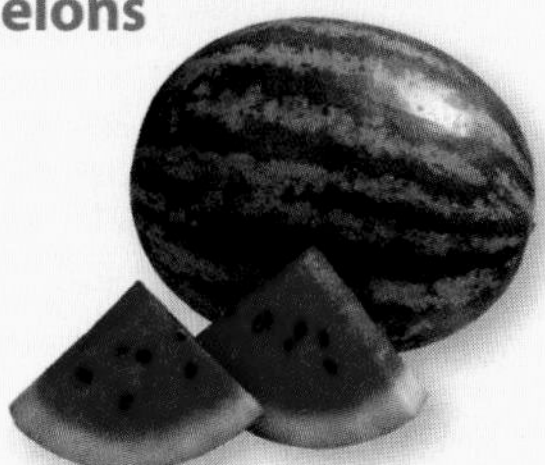

- Large round or oval fruits with many varieties including: cantaloupe with sweet, juicy, orange flesh and rough rind; honeydew with green juicy flesh; muskmelon with bright orange flesh; watermelon with sweet, juicy, red flesh. Watermelon may be seedless. Peel before eating.
- Use raw in fruit salads.

Oranges

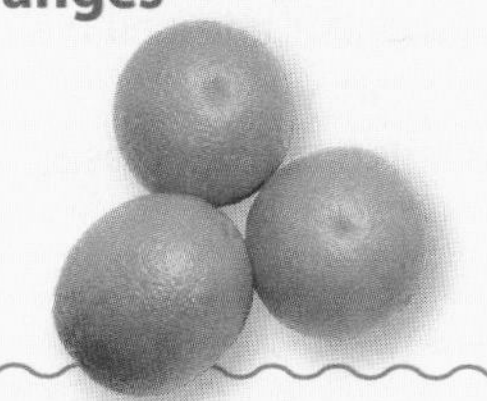

- Round citrus fruits with a thin or thick rind. Orange in color. Navel orange is large, seedless, and easy to peel. Blood orange is red inside. Peel before eating. Flavor is usually sweet.
- Use raw in salads, as juice, or cooked in marmalade.

Papayas

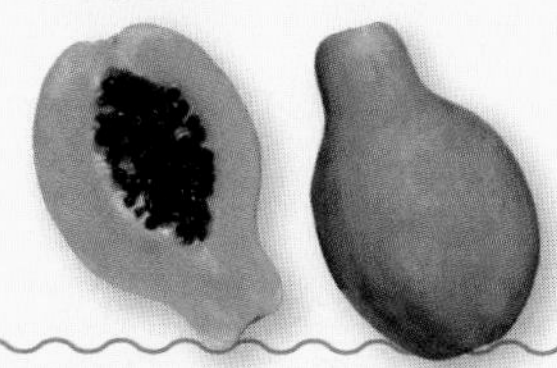

- Oval fruits with yellow skin when ripe. Small, black, edible seeds. Peel before eating. Flesh is sweet, seeds are bitter.
- Use raw in salads or cooked in main dishes. Papaya enzyme is used in meat tenderizers.

Peaches and Nectarines

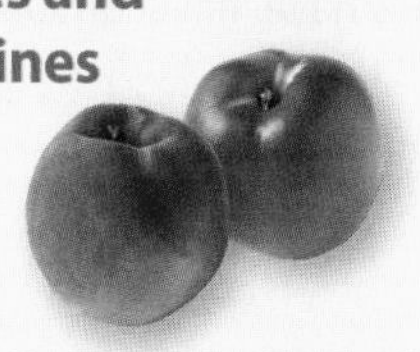

- Round fruits. Peaches are yellow with a reddish blush and have fuzzy skin. "Freestone" varieties have flesh that is not attached to the pit. Nectarines are similar to peaches, but with smooth skin. Both are juicy with a pleasing aroma. Eat unpeeled. Flavor is sweet.
- Use raw, dried, or cooked in pies, cobbler, and other desserts.

Pears

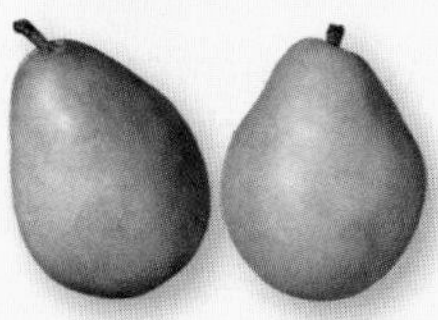

- Oval fruit with many varieties including: Bartlett, yellow or red; Bosc, brown with a long neck; D'Anjou, yellow. Pears soften but do not ripen after picking. Eat unpeeled. Flavor is sweet.
- Use raw, poached, or baked.

Persimmons

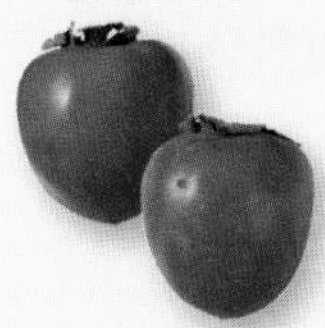

- Roundish fruits. Fuyu variety is shaped like a tomato and is firm when ripe, with a sweet-spicy flavor. Hachiya variety tastes sour until ripe and is soft when ripe. Eat unpeeled.
- Use raw or cooked in pudding and other desserts.

Figure 28.1 Fruits and Their Uses *(continued)*

Pineapples

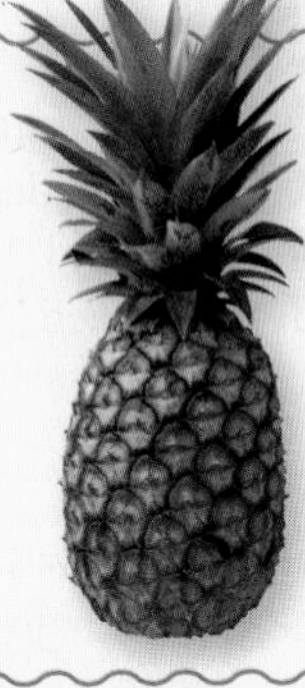

- Large oval fruit with a spiky leaf crown and tough, prickly skin. Golden cast indicates ripeness. Juicy flesh is white to yellow. Gold variety is very sweet, with deep yellow flesh. Pineapples do not ripen or sweeten after picking. Peel before eating. Fresh pineapple has an enzyme that prevents gelatin from setting.
- Use raw in salads, as juice, or cooked as a meat accompaniment and in desserts.

Plums

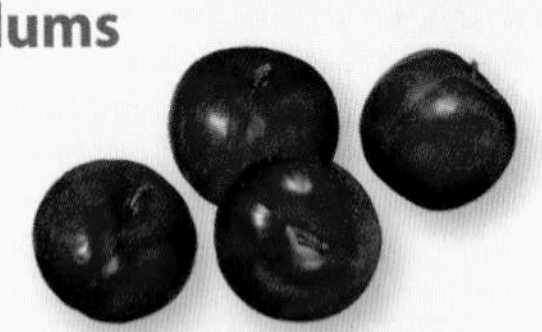

- Small roundish fruits with varieties in green, red, and purple shades and different sizes. Smooth skin. Slightly soft and very juicy when ripe.
- Use raw, dried (as prunes), or cooked in jam and cobbler.

Pomegranates

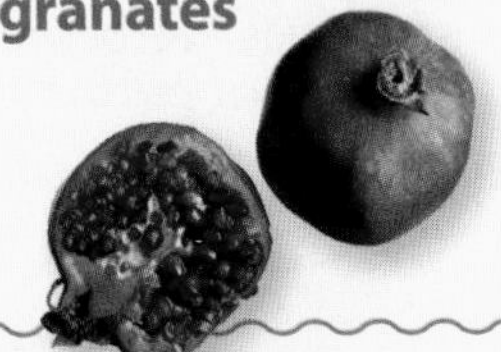

- Round red fruits with red flesh and many seeds. Remove peel and inedible membrane around flesh before eating. Flavor is sweet-tart.
- Use raw, as juice, or cooked in sauces. Sprinkle raw seeds on salads, roasts, ice cream, and pie.

Quinces

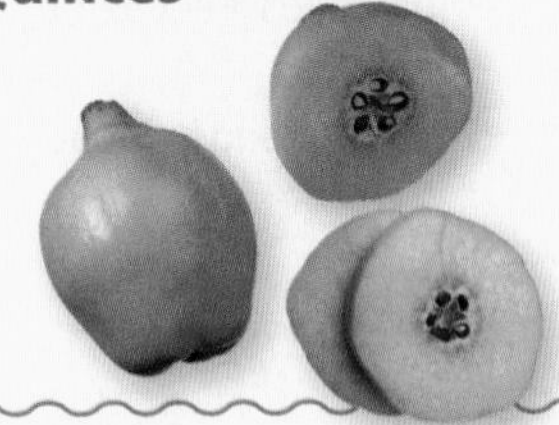

- Large, round to pear-shaped fruits. Yellow, fuzzy skin with dry, white flesh. Peel before cooking. Flavor is pineapple-like.
- Use poached, stewed, baked, or braised.

Raspberries

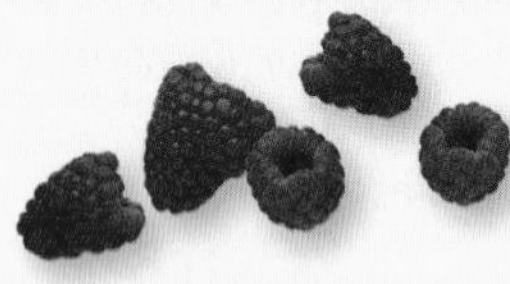

- Small cup-shaped red, black, or white berries. May have "hairs" on surface. Bright, plump, juicy, and firm. Flavor is sweet and tart.
- Use raw or cooked in syrup, jam, jellies, and desserts.

Strawberries

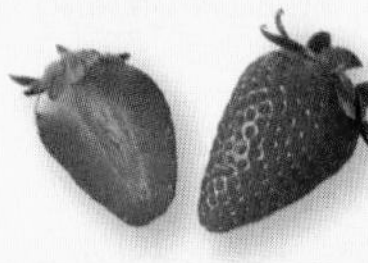

- Bright red berries with edible exterior seeds and green stem cap attached. Remove stem cap before eating. Flavor is sweet and slightly tart.
- Use raw or cooked in jam, jellies, shortcake, cobbler, pie, and other desserts.

Tangerines

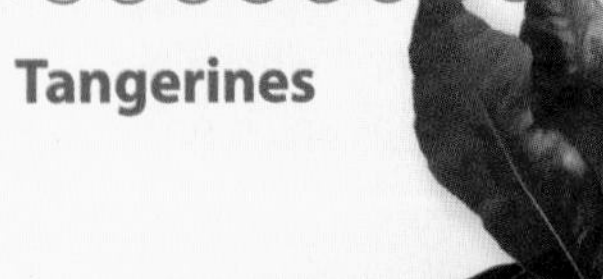

- Small citrus fruits with deep orange color. Skin is loosely attached. Juicy, usually with many seeds. Peel before eating. Flavor is sweet to tart.
- Use raw or as juice.

Lychee (ˈlē-(ˌ)chē) Lychees, or litchis, are small fruits with a rough leathery red shell and a single seed. The lychee is a tropical fruit tree native to Southern China. The flesh of the lychee fruit is creamy white, juicy, and sweet. Remove the shell and seed before eating. When lychees are dried, they are called "lychee nuts" because the shell turns dark brown and the flesh turns crisp and brown.

Prickly Pear Prickly pears are the delicious fruit of several varieties of cactus. They are also called cactus pears. Prickly pears are like pears in size and shape and range in color from yellow to red. Their flesh is soft and yellow, with a melon-like aroma and sweet flavor. They are often used to make candies and jelly. Prickly pears can also be used in salads. Peel, section, and remove the seeds and serve the fruits cold.

Sapote (sə-ˈpō-tē) Sapote fruits are medium-size and plum-shaped with thin, olive-green skin. Their creamy, custard-like flesh has a sweet flavor that resembles a combination of peach and vanilla. Peel and remove the seeds before eating.

Tamarillo (ˌta-mə-ˈri-(ˌ)lō) Tamarillos are small, egg-shaped fruit with a tough, bitter, skin of several colors and flavorful, tart, pink flesh. Peel, remove the seeds, and add sugar before eating. To more easily peel a tamarillo, blanch it for two minutes, then place it in cold water.

Ugli Fruit An ugli fruit is about the size of a grapefruit. It has a rough, thick, yellow-green skin and juicy, yellow-orange flesh that is divided into sections. You can eat ugli fruit like grapefruit.

✓ **Reading Check** **Describe** What does a sapote look like?

Selecting and Storing Fresh Fruits

Some fresh fruits are available all year. Other fresh fruits are seasonal. This means that they are only available during certain months. Fresh fruits and vegetables are agricultural products known as **produce**.

Maturity and Ripeness

For best quality, fruits should be picked when they are mature. A **mature fruit** is a fruit that has reached its full size and color. When a mature fruit reaches its peak of flavor and is ready to eat, it becomes a **ripe fruit**. Ripe fruits are tender and have a pleasant aroma.

Some fruits continue to ripen after they are picked. Others do not. Grapes, berries, cherries, citrus fruits, pineapples, and melons, for example, do not ripen after harvest. These fruits must be picked when fully ripe.

A fruit that is still growing and is not yet mature is an **immature fruit**. Immature fruits are usually small for their size and have a poor color and texture. If a fruit is picked while it is still immature, it may never ripen.

Most fruits are picked when they are mature but still under ripe. An **under ripe fruit** is a very firm mature fruit that lacks flavor and has not reached top eating quality. Fruits are picked when they are under ripe to prevent them from spoiling during shipping. They ripen during shipping and after you buy them.

Be a *Smart Consumer*

Fluctuating Fruit Costs

Many factors—including seasonality, weather, transportation, and even insects—can affect the cost of fruit. For example, peaches may be affordable in July during the peak of their season. This is because they are abundant, and there is enough supply to meet consumers' demand. If unexpected weather or pests destroy a large amount of the peach crop, there will not be enough supply to meet demand. Even the threat of bad weather can affect the cost of peaches, or other fruits. The price of peaches will increase because their scarcity will make them more valuable. If peaches come to your community from a great distance, their price will be higher to compensate for the cost of transporting them.

Challenge Visit a supermarket to find out which seasonal fruits are available in your community now. Are some more expensive than others? Why? Share your insights with the class.

Choosing Quality Fruit

Buy only good-quality fruits. Immature, overripe, and damaged fruits have fewer nutrients, have poor flavor and texture, and do not keep well. Most fruits are highly perishable and lose quality quickly, so buy only what you can use and store for about a week.

To find the best-quality fruit, look for the following:

Ripeness Buy fruits that are at the stage of ripeness you want. For example, choose ripe fruits if you want to use them right away and less ripe fruits if you plan to use them a few days later. For cooking, choose fruits that are ripe but firm so that they will hold their shape. Test fruits for ripeness by pressing very gently. Ripe fruit gives slightly under the pressure. Do not press so hard that you damage the fruit, however. Damaged fruit spoils quickly.

Condition Avoid fruits with bruised or damaged spots or decay. Some fruits, especially fruits with inedible peels, may have natural blemishes that do not affect their quality. Grapefruits and oranges may have harmless brownish spots, for example.

Denseness Fruit should be plump and firm. Avoid fruits that are dry, withered, very soft, or very hard.

Color Color should be typical for the type of fruit you are buying. Many fruits, such as apples, pears, and plums, come in different varieties with a range of colors. Get to know what to expect from these different varieties.

Some oranges may look greenish if they have experienced a process known as regreening. **Regreening** is the return of chlorophyll, the greening substance in plants, to the skin of ripe oranges during warm weather or under bright light. Green oranges are fully ripe and have the same sweet flavor as those with an orange color.

Aroma Ripe fruit usually has a pleasant, **characteristic** aroma. If it has been refrigerated and is still cold, however, it may not have an aroma. A few fruits, such as blueberries, have only a very mild aroma.

Size Fruit should be heavy for its size. Heaviness usually means the fruit is juicy. This is especially important if you want to use the fruit for juice.

Shape Each type of fruit has its own characteristic shape. Misshapen fruit probably has poor flavor and texture.

Kitchen Math

Planning to Serve Fruit

Nicola is planning to serve fruit skewers at an upcoming dinner party. She would like the ratio of banana to kiwi to mango on each skewer to be 3:2:1, and she would also like each skewer to have 12 total pieces of fruit. How many total pieces of each type of fruit will Nicola need if she serves six people one skewer each?

Math Concept **Like Terms** When an algebraic expression has like terms (terms containing the same variable), combine the like terms into one term. For example, $5y + 2y$ simplifies to $7y$.

Starting Hint Represent each skewer as the equation $3x + 2x + x = 12$, with x = mango pieces, $2x$ = kiwi pieces, and $3x$ = banana pieces. Solve for x, and use that number to determine the amount of each type of fruit on one skewer. Multiply each amount by 6 to find the totals for all skewers.

Math Appendix For math help, go to the Math Appendix at the back of the book.

NCTM Algebra Represent and analyze mathematical situations and structures using algebraic symbols.

Storing Fresh Fruit

How long fruits keep depends on how fresh they were when you bought them, how they were handled, and the storage temperature. Most fresh fruits should be used within a few days. Citrus fruits can last longer.

Different fruits require different storage methods. Use the right method for the fruit.

Under Ripe Fruits Keep under ripe fruits at room temperature to ripen. To speed ripening, put the fruit in a brown paper bag. You can add an apple, which gives off ethylene, a harmless gas that helps fruit to ripen. If you use a plastic bag for storage, make holes in the bag to allow moisture to evaporate.

Bananas Store bananas uncovered at room temperature. They can be refrigerated after ripening. Bananas' skin turns dark, but they keep their quality.

Berries, Cherries, and Grapes Sort these fruits to remove any that are damaged or decayed. Refrigerate in a perforated plastic bag or container, in a covered shallow container, or uncovered in the refrigerator crisper. Use the fruits as soon as possible.

Citrus Fruits Store citrus fruits at room temperature. Refrigerate them uncovered for longer storage.

All Other Ripe Fruits Refrigerate other fruits uncovered in the crisper or in a perforated plastic bag. To keep melon's aroma from flavoring other foods, store it in a closed container or plastic bag.

Cut Fruits Refrigerate cut fruits in an airtight container or plastic bag.

✓ **Reading Check** **List** What are seven factors to consider when choosing fruit?

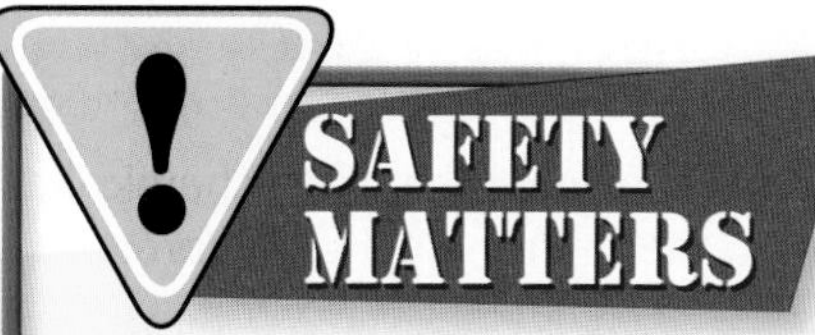

Washing Fruit

From growers to processors to transporters to sellers, fruit is handled by a variety of people in many different environments. By the time you buy it, it may be covered with a coat of dirt and invisible bacteria. This is why it is so important to thoroughly wash all fruit, whether raspberries or watermelons, before use. Even if you plan to pare a fruit or not eat the skin, washing prevents substances from transferring to the flesh of the fruit through paring or slicing. The mere slicing action on a watermelon, for example, can move harmful substances to the flesh.

What Would You Do? You visit a farmstand where fresh strawberries are sold. The seller says, "We just picked these today. Here, try a few." What should you do?

Preparing and Serving Fresh Fruits

Fresh fruits are easy to prepare. First, wash the fruit, then prepare it for serving. Wait until you are ready to use fruits before washing them. If you wash fruits before storing, moisture can encourage bacteria to grow. The fruit will spoil faster and get moldy.

When you are ready to prepare fruits, wash them under cool, running water, even if you are planning to peel them. The running water washes away dirt and microorganisms that can cause illness. You can use a clean brush to loosen dirt on thick-skinned fruits. Do not soak fruits in water, because this can cause flavor and nutrients to be lost.

Some fruits, such as apples and oranges, are waxed. The wax layer makes them look more attractive and prevents moisture loss so they last longer. Food waxes are on the FDA list of GRAS chemicals, meaning they are safe to eat. They are not water-soluble and therefore cannot be washed off.

Many fruits also have pesticide residues. To remove the wax and pesticides, pare a thin layer of skin from the fruit. Never use detergents to wash fruits. Detergents may react with pesticides and waxes to create harmful compounds.

Paring and Preparing Fresh Fruit

To prepare fruits, remove any stems or damaged spots. Then pare the fruit (remove the peel) if needed. Pare thinly in order to retain nutrients that are right under the skin. Many fruits, including apricots, apples, peaches, and pears, have a tender, edible skin. In many cases, the skin of the fruit is the most nutrient-dense portion. You can pare them or eat the skin, which has many nutrients. Some fruits, such as oranges and bananas, must be peeled before using. Melons must be cut open and their seeds removed. Fresh fruits are easier to eat when cut into pieces. To retain nutrients, keep the chunks fairly large and serve them as soon as possible. If you need to store cut fruit, cover it tightly with plastic wrap and squeeze out as much air as possible. Refrigerate until serving time.

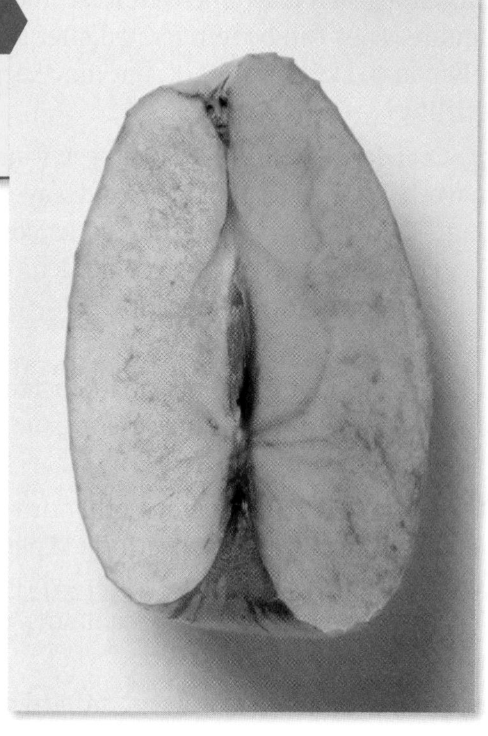

Enzymatic Browning

Some fruits have enzymes that react chemically with oxygen in the air, turning the fruit brown. *How can you prevent this reaction?*

Blanching Fresh Fruit

Blanching fresh fruits can make them easier to peel. Suppose you are freezing a large quantity of peaches and you want to remove the skin as quickly as possible. Lower the fruit gently into simmering water for about 15 seconds, then use a slotted spoon to move the fruit into a bowl of ice water. Let it sit for two minutes. The skin should slide off easily.

Preventing Fruits from Darkening

When you see the flesh of an apple, banana, or peach turn brown, you are seeing a scientific process known as enzymatic (ˌen-zəh-ˈma-tik) browning. **Enzymatic browning** is a chemical reaction in which oxygen in the air reacts with an **enzyme**, a special protein, in the fruit and turns it brown. Enzymatic browning involves oxygen, so it is a type of chemical reaction called oxidation. The longer a piece of cut fruit is exposed to the air, the more it will turn brown, or oxidize.

Ascorbic acid (vitamin C) destroys the enzyme that causes browning. The juice of lemons, limes, grapefruits, and oranges contains ascorbic acid, so you can dip the fruit into one of these juices to prevent browning. You can also buy ascorbic acid powder to mix with water and sprinkle on the cut fruit.

Serving Fresh Fruit

Fresh fruit is nutritious and delicious, making it the perfect meal accompaniment, snack, or party fare. Here are a few ideas for serving fresh fruit. What other ideas can you add?

- Experiment with shapes. Slice bananas and kiwifruit. Cut peaches into wedges. Section citrus fruits. Try cutting fruits into bite-size pieces and stringing them on a small skewer to make fruit kebabs, or serving bite-size pieces with wooden picks.
- Arrange different fruits in circles or wedges on a large platter. Use color contrasts to make a fun display. Cover the arrangement tightly with plastic wrap and refrigerate it until serving time.
- Use a melon baller or a small scoop to make balls of soft fruits. For an eye-catching centerpiece, place balls in a basket made from the rind.
- Serve fruit with dip. You can make flavorful dips with yogurt or caramel, for example.
- Make frozen fruit bites. Freeze whole berries or grapes on trays to make frozen candy-like snacks.
- Make a **trifle** (ˈtrī-fəl), a refrigerated dessert with layers that may include cake, jam or jelly, fruit, custard, and whipped cream. Try alternating layers of fruit, sponge cake, and sweetened whipped cream or yogurt. You can experiment with other layers, such as nuts or oatmeal.

✓ **Reading Check** **Explain** How and why do you blanch fresh fruit?

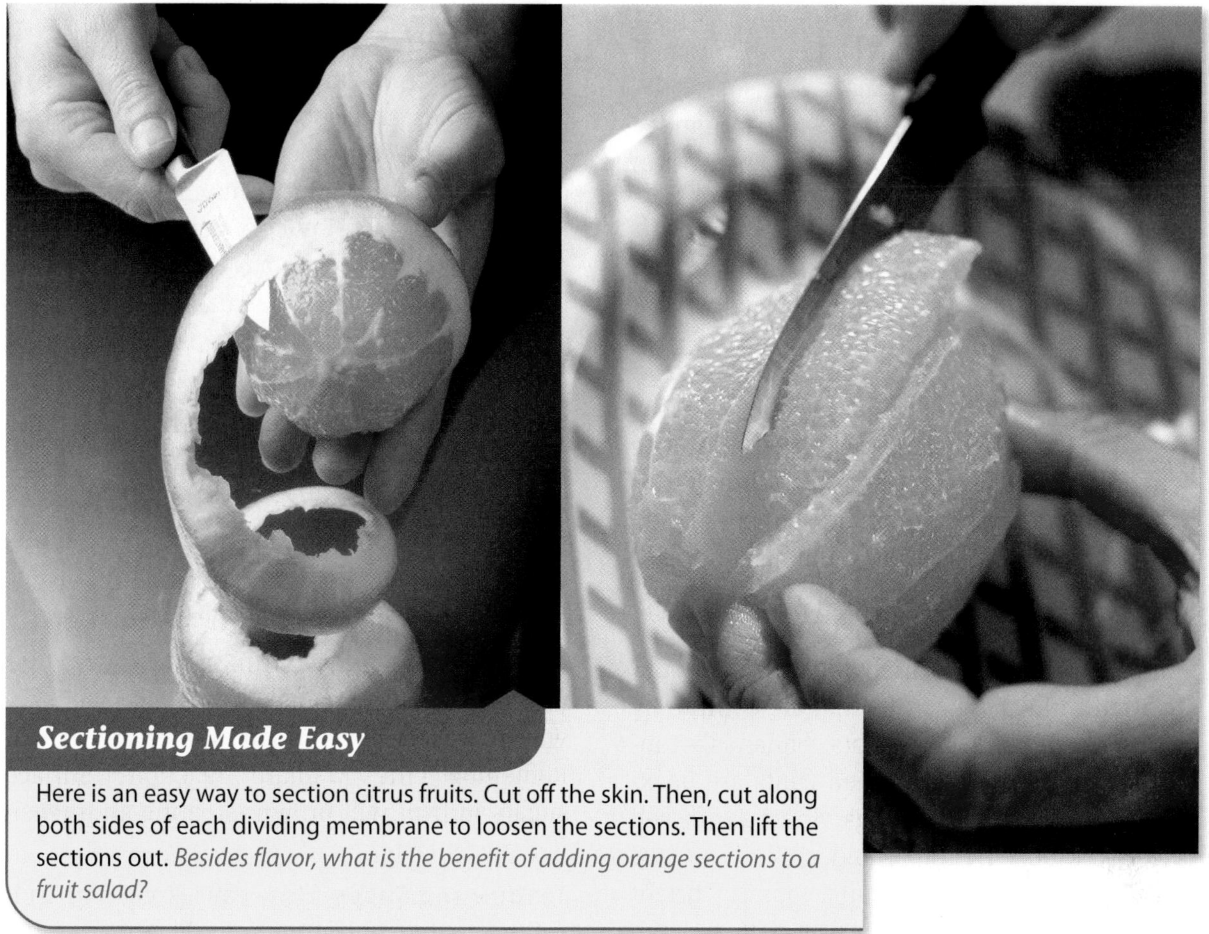

Sectioning Made Easy

Here is an easy way to section citrus fruits. Cut off the skin. Then, cut along both sides of each dividing membrane to loosen the sections. Then lift the sections out. *Besides flavor, what is the benefit of adding orange sections to a fruit salad?*

Using Convenience Forms of Fruits

Canned, frozen, and dried fruits have many uses in snacks and meals. Fresh and frozen fruits are usually more nutritious than canned and dried fruits. Canned and dried fruits, however, are convenient and easy to store.

Canned Fruits

Canned fruits come in many forms—whole, halved, sliced, and in pieces. Some fruits are packed in light or heavy syrup, which adds sugar. Heavy syrup is sweeter and higher in calories than light syrup or juice. Fruits packed in water or in their own juices are healthy choices. They have no added sugar and about the same number of calories as fresh fruit.

Canned fruits also come with various flavors. For example, you can find pears flavored with vanilla or apples flavored with cinnamon. Read the label carefully to be sure you get the kind you want. Buy the form best suited for your needs.

Canned fruits can often be served in place of fresh. Canned fruits are also good to have on hand for last-minute recipes. For a quick dessert, for example, you could purée canned fruits in a blender and serve them over angel food cake.

Frozen Fruits

Frozen fruits taste similar to fresh fruits, but have a softer texture when they are defrosted. Freezing damages the cell walls, allowing water to run out as fruits thaw. When serving frozen fruit plain, thaw it only partially so that ice crystals help keep the fruit firm.

Freezing also damages the attractiveness of fruit so frozen fruit is best used for baking or for making smoothies. Because fruits that are picked for freezing are usually at their peak of ripeness, they are a reliable, consistent product.

Frozen fruits are sold with and without added sugar, so check the label to be sure. If you have enough freezer space, consider buying frozen fruit in large bags. You can remove just the amount you need and leave the rest in the freezer.

To freeze your own fresh fruit, spread the fruit out in a single layer on a tray. Once the fruit is frozen you can put it in sealable bags.

Dried Fruits

Many fruits are delicious dried. Because dehydration results in water loss, dried fruit has a stronger flavor than fresh fruit. Dried fruit is rich in vitamins and minerals, although most of the vitamin C in the fruit is destroyed during the drying process. Raisins (dried grapes) and prunes (dried plums) are popular dried fruits. Other fruits that are commonly dried include apples, apricots, bananas, cranberries, and dates. Most dried fruits are packaged in boxes or plastic bags. Some stores sell dried fruit loose by the pound.

When you buy dried fruits, look for bright color. Choose fruit that is fairly soft and pliable. Hard fruits have become too dry. Store unopened packages in a cool, dry place. After opening, store dried fruits in an airtight container in the refrigerator.

Dried fruits are nutritious, although they have a high concentration of natural sugar. They make nutritious snacks, especially when combined with other foods such as nuts and seeds. Dried fruits are also useful for cooking and baking. Some recipes call for reconstituting dried fruit so it cooks faster. To **reconstitute** is to restore a dried food to a rehydrated condition by adding water. This will not restore the fruit to its pre-dried condition, but it will rehydrate it.

Many dried fruits are preserved with sulphur dioxide. It helps preserve the fruit and keep its bright color. Some people are sensitive to sulphur dioxide, however, and should only eat unsulphured fruit.

✓ Reading Check **Identify** Which form of convenience fruit comes with added flavors such as cinnamon or vanilla?

Cooking Fruits

Cooked fruits are part of many desserts, such as pies and cobblers. Fruit can also be part of a main course, or a sweet or savory side dish. Mango salsa adds a highlight to shrimp. Apple sauce is a sweet contrast to a spicy pork dish. Cooking is a good way to use overripe fruit, such as very soft bananas.

Several changes happen to fruit during cooking.

Nutrients Heat-sensitive nutrients, especially vitamin C and dietery fiber are lost during cooking. To prevent loss of nutrients, leave the skin on.

Color Colors change in many cooked fruits. Some become lighter or deeper in color.

Flavor Cooking gives fruit a mellower, less acidic flavor. Overcooked fruits lose their flavor and may develop an unpleasant flavor. Remember the Maillard reaction? Surface sugars in fruit will brown, creating an intensified sweet taste.

Texture and Shape Heat causes cells in fruit to lose water and grow soft. This causes the fruit to lose shape. Adding sugar to the cooking water helps cooked fruit keep its shape. Sugar draws some water back into fruit's cells, which strengthens them. Tougher fruits like apples and pears become softer and milder.

Cooking Fruits in Moist Heat

You can cook fruit in moist heat when you want it to hold its shape or when you want to make fruit sauce. Use a saucepan with a tight-fitting lid.

One of the more popular methods for cooking fruit is poaching. Poaching softens and tenderizes fruit. Poached fruits retain their shape. Use firm fruits, such as apples, peaches, plums, or pears. Leave them whole or cut them into fairly large pieces. Quarters and eighths work well. Place the fruits in a saucepan, then add sugar and enough water to cover them. The sugar helps keep the fruit from breaking down. Cover the pan and simmer gently just until tender. Do not boil, because boiling breaks the fruit apart.

To make a sauce, cut fruits into small pieces. Leave small berries whole. Add a small amount of water, just enough to cover the bottom of the pan. You want the fruit to break down, so do not add sugar yet. Simmer in a tightly covered pan, stirring occasionally to break the fruit apart. At the end of the cooking time, you can add sugar, honey, or another sweetener if you wish.

You can add extra flavor to poached fruit or fruit sauce with lemon juice, lemon or orange rind, vanilla, a cinnamon stick, or other spices.

Frying Fruits

Some fruits are fried, usually as a side dish. Fried apple slices, for instance, are often served with pancakes or roast pork. Pineapple slices and banana slices or halves also fry well.

Fruits for frying should be firm enough to hold their shape. If you use canned fruits, drain them well.

Sauté fruit in a small amount of butter or margarine until they are lightly browned. A tasty way to fry fruit is to make fritters. A **fritter** is cut-up fruit dipped in batter and fried until golden brown.

Baking Fruits

Fruits are used in many baked goods, including pies, cakes, cobblers, and muffins. Fruits can also be baked alone or as part of another dish. For example, you can bake pineapples or dried prunes with pork. You can bake fruits whole, peeled, or in pieces. Use apples, pears, bananas, or other firm fruits that hold their shape well.

Baked apples are easy to prepare and make a delicious ending to a meal. Before cooking, core the apples and cut a thin strip of skin from around the middle. This allows the apples to expand as they cook so they do not burst. You can fill the empty core with raisins, nuts, and a spicy sugar mixture. Place the apples in a baking dish and pour hot water around them to a depth of ¼ inch. Bake at 350°F until tender, about 45 to 60 minutes, depending on the size of the apples.

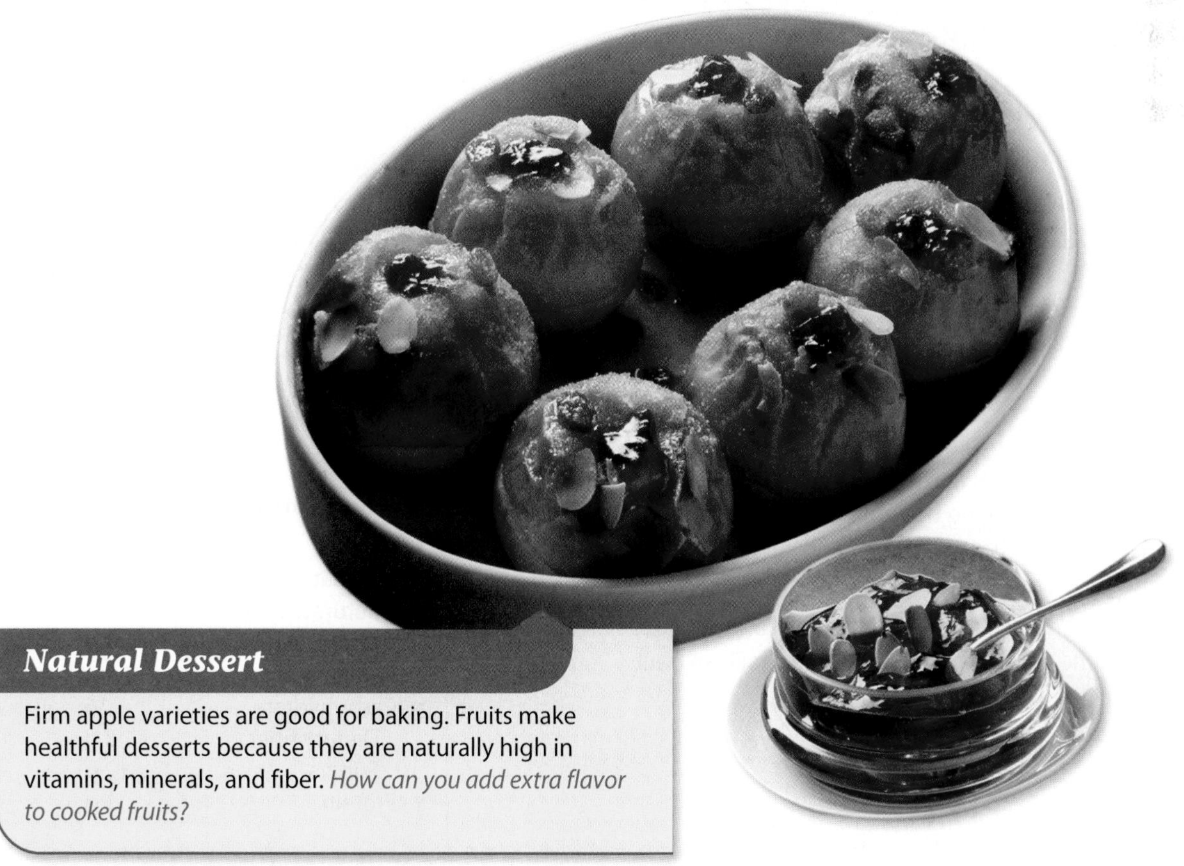

Natural Dessert

Firm apple varieties are good for baking. Fruits make healthful desserts because they are naturally high in vitamins, minerals, and fiber. *How can you add extra flavor to cooked fruits?*

Broiling Fruits

Broiling cooks fruits slightly and browns them. You can broil any tender fruit that holds its shape. For example, you might try bananas, peaches, grapefruit halves, or pineapple slices. You can also broil canned fruits.

Fruits have no fat, so you need to protect them from drying out during broiling. Brush the surface with melted butter or margarine or use a topping, such as brown sugar or seasoned crumbs.

Grilling Fruits

Grilling fruits gives them a delicious flavor and a caramelized color. Choose firm, ripe fruits. Fruits that are overripe fall apart too easily. Cantaloupes, apples, pears, or peaches can be cut into slices for grilling. Pineapples take on an intense sweetness when grilled. Banana halves also grill well. You can also cut the fruits into pieces and thread them on a small skewer.

Before grilling fruit, clean the grate well, then, brush a little oil on the grate. Place the fruits on the grate and grill them until grill marks form. Then turn them to cook the other side. Use a high heat and make sure the grate is hot before putting the fruit on. You want to cook the fruit quickly then get it away from the heat before it gets too soft. The fruit should soften but not be mushy.

Microwave Cooking

Fruits are easy to prepare in the microwave oven. They cook quickly, keep their flavor and shape, and retain most of their nutrients. Fruits can easily overcook in the microwave oven, however.

Cover fruits when you microwave them, but leave a small opening for steam to escape. If you are cooking whole fruits, such as plums, pierce them with a fork in several places to keep them from bursting. Refer to the owner's manual or a microwave cookbook for power levels and cooking times.

Light and Healthy Recipe

Citrus Fruit Salad

Ingredients

- **2** Grapefruits
- **2** Oranges
- **1** Lime
- **¼ tsp.** Vanilla extract

Directions

1. Carefully wash and pat dry the fruits. Carefully remove the peel and as much pith as possible without damaging the fruit. On a cutting board, lay the grapefruit on its side and cut round slices. Remove any seeds. Repeat with the oranges.
2. Place the fruit slices in a salad bowl and squeeze the lime juice over them. Add the vanilla extract and toss gently.
3. Chill for at least 30 minutes and serve.

One serving of this tangy fruit salad has 110% of your daily vitamin C needs.

Yield 6 servings (two cookies per serving)

Nutrition Analysis per Serving

■ Calories	65
■ Total fat	0 g
Saturated fat	0 g
Cholesterol	0 mg
■ Sodium	0 mg
■ Carbohydrate	16
Dietary fiber	3 g
Sugars	12 g
■ Protein	1 g

CHAPTER 28 Review & Applications

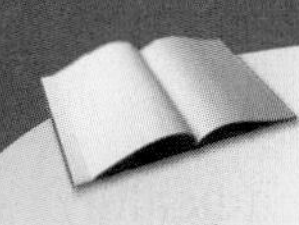

After You Read

Chapter Summary

Fruits are colorful, flavorful, and easy to prepare. They are rich in many nutrients. There are six major types of fruits. Unusual fruits are gaining in popularity. There are several factors to consider when selecting quality fresh fruit. Different fruits must be stored in different ways to keep them fresh. Fruits must be properly prepared before serving. They may be served in a variety of ways. Convenience forms of fruits have many uses in snacks and meals. It is also possible to cook fruits using several cooking methods.

Content and Academic Vocabulary Review

1. Find a visual example in the textbook of six of these content and academic vocabulary words.

Content Vocabulary

- ☐ fruit (p. 432)
- ☐ drupe (p. 432)
- ☐ pome (p. 432)
- ☐ savory (p. 432)
- ☐ produce (p. 437)
- ☐ mature fruit (p. 437)
- ☐ ripe fruit (p. 437)
- ☐ immature fruit (p. 437)
- ☐ under ripe fruit (p. 437)
- ☐ regreening (p. 438)
- ☐ enzymatic browning (p. 440)
- ☐ enzyme (p. 440)
- ☐ trifle (p. 440)
- ☐ reconstitute (p. 442)
- ☐ fritter (p. 443)

Academic Vocabulary

- membrane (p. 432)
- characteristic (p. 438)

Review Key Concepts

2. Describe the nutritional benefits of fruits.
3. Identify the six major types of fruits.
4. Explain how to store fresh fruits.
5. Describe enzymatic browning and how to prevent it.
6. Identify the types and uses of convenience forms of fruits.
7. Describe methods for cooking fruits.

Critical Thinking

8. Describe and give an example of how the increased availability of unusual fruits can actually educate consumers about other cultures.
9. Explain why you think the length of time that many fresh fruits are available in supermarkets has increased.
10. Conclude the consequence of harvesting fruit without carefully considering how mature it is.
11. Summarize how Jack can prepare a recipe using berries that will not be available in their fresh form for another six months.

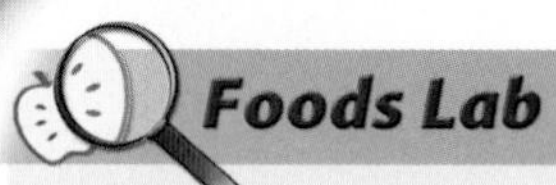

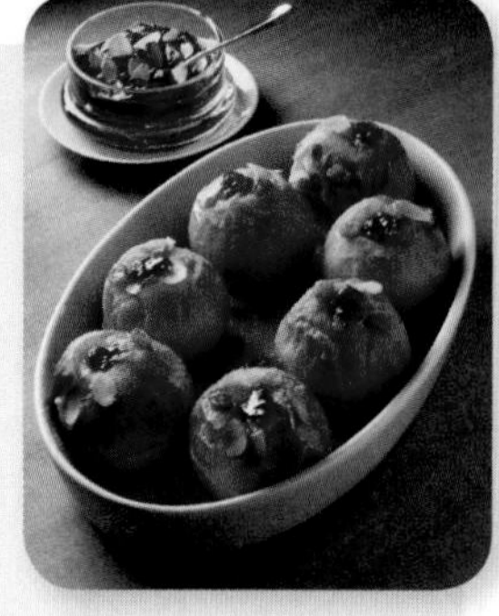

12. Baking Apples Baked apples are a versatile desert that can be prepared using a variety of seasonings, apple types, and fillings. What do you think would make a tasty combination?

Procedure With your lab team, create an original recipe for stuffing a baked apple. What kind of apple and ingredients will you use? Write your recipe, and then make it. Conduct a taste test of teams' recipes.

Analysis With your team, create a chart that displays your rating of other teams' baked apple recipes as well as your own. What criteria will you use to rate the recipes? Show and explain your chart to the class.

HEALTHFUL CHOICES

13. Canned Fruit and Calories Gia is on a low-calorie eating plan to achieve a healthy weight. She is shopping for canned fruit to keep on hand for healthful deserts, recipes, and snacks. What type of canned fruit should she avoid and why? What type should she choose? What should Gia look for on the labels of canned fruit she is thinking about purchasing?

TECH Connection

14. Origins of Unusual Fruits Under your teacher's supervision use the Internet to research one of the unusual fruits mentioned in this chapter. Find out where the fruit originated, which culture or cultures eat it, and how they prepare it. Explain how the fruit was carried from its original location and cultivated in other parts of the world. Use word processing software to write a paragraph about your findings.

Real-World Skills

Problem-Solving Skills	**15. Shapeless Berries** While preparing a warm berry sauce to put on top of a cheesecake, Paul was disappointed to see the berries lost their shape and turned mushy. What can he do next time to help prevent this from happening?
Interpersonal and Collaborative Skills	**16. Demonstration** Follow your teacher's instructions to form small groups. Work together to plan, write, and give a demonstration about cooking fruit. Choose a fruit and a method for preparing it. Demonstrate and explain the cooking method in the foods lab.
Financial Literacy Skills	**17. Cost Comparison** Visit a supermarket. Compare the cost per ounce of fresh, frozen, canned, and dried versions of three fruits. Then chart the results. What do you conclude? Share your chart and conclusion with the class.

Academic Skills

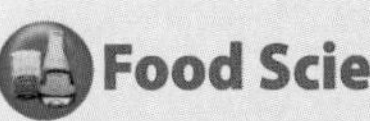

Food Science

18. Preserves Fruit preserves are a kind of gel forming a sponge-like network that traps water. The key to creating this gel is pectin, found in the plants' cell walls. Once the pectin is free of the cells, it traps the other ingredients.

Procedure Place 1 cup blackberries, 1 cup halved strawberries, ½ cup cranberries, and ½ cup blueberries into a 4 quart microwave safe bowl. (Rinse fruit first.) Mix in 2 cups sugar. Put the bowl in the microwave and cook the fruit uncovered on full power for 10 minutes. Stir, then cook another 5 minutes. Cool, cover, and refrigerate. Evaluate taste and texture.

Analysis Write a paragraph describing the fruit after you've tried it. Which of the fruits do you think contains the most pectin? Why do you think the sugar was added?

NSES B Develop an understanding of chemical reactions.

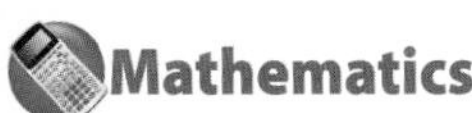

Mathematics

19. Measure Surface Area Two small limes each measure 1½ inches in diameter. One lemon measures 2 inches in diameter. Assume that each of the fruits is a perfect sphere. If you were to remove the peel from each of the fruits, would you have a larger total amount of lime peel, or a larger amount of lemon peel? (Assume that the amount of peel for each fruit is equal to its surface area.)

Math Concept **Surface Area of a Sphere** Calculate the surface area (A) of a sphere with the following formula: $A = 4\pi r^2$, where r = the radius of the sphere. Use 3.14 for π.

Starting Hint Since radius equals ½ of diameter, multiply each measurement by ½, and plug each result into the area formula as r.

NCTM Measurement Apply appropriate techniques, tools, and formulas to determine measurements.

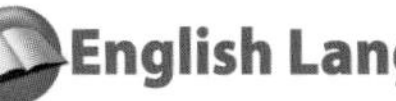

English Language Arts

20. Report Ripening Rates Conduct research about the ripening rates of four green bananas. Leave each one in a different location. Record changes twice a day until all are ripe. Write a one-page report explaining how different environments affect ripening.

NCTE 7 Conduct research and gather, evaluate, and synthesize data to communicate discoveries.

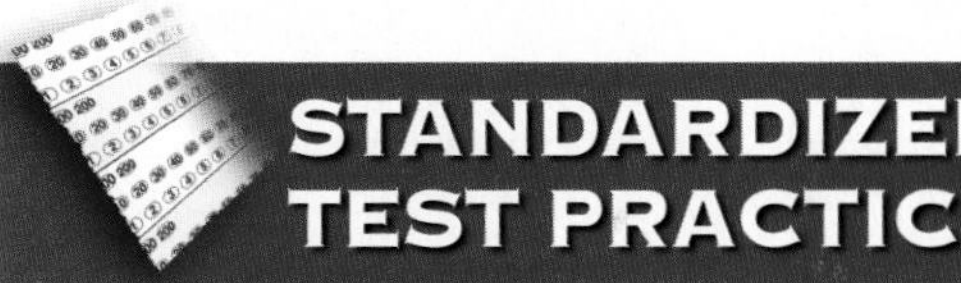

STANDARDIZED TEST PRACTICE

READING COMPREHENSION

Re-read the section about maturity and ripeness on page 437. Then read the question and select the best answer:

21. When are most fruits picked?
  - **a.** when they are mature and ripe
  - **b.** when they are fully ripe
  - **c.** when they are mature, but still under ripe
  - **d.** when they are juicy and soft to the touch

Test-Taking Tip Before you answer a reading comprehension question, closely read the text to which the question refers. Then read through the question and each of the answer choices. Some answers may seem correct, but they contain subtle errors. Pay attention to every word.

CHAPTER 29

Vegetables

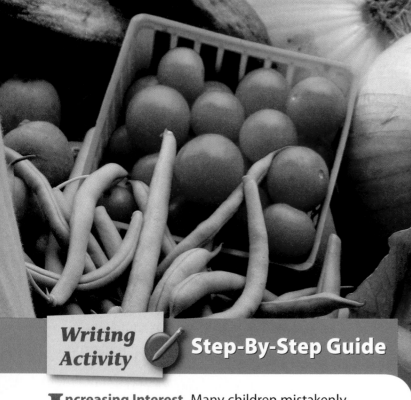

Writing Activity — Step-By-Step Guide

Increasing Interest Many children mistakenly believe that all vegetables taste bad. Imagine you have a young sibling who refuses to eat vegetables. What steps will you take to increase her interest in vegetables and motivate her to eat them? Write a step-by-step guide that explains your ideas.

Writing Tips Follow these steps to write a step-by-step guide:

- Consider what steps are necessary to achieve a desired outcome.
- Present steps in chronological order with an introduction and conclusion.
- Explain the purpose of each step.

Activate Prior Knowledge

Explore the Photo Vegetables are versatile as main dishes, sides, and snacks. *What is your favorite way to prepare vegetables?*

Reading Guide

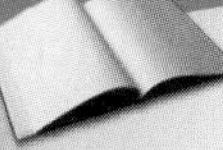

Before You Read

Preview Examine the photos in this chapter. How many of the vegetables pictured have you tried? Make a list.

Read to Learn

Key Concepts

- **List** the nutrients found in vegetables.
- **Identify** the eight types of vegetables.
- **Explain** how to store fresh vegetables.
- **Describe** how to prepare fresh vegetables.
- **Describe** methods for cooking vegetables.
- **Identify** the types and uses of convenience forms of vegetables.

Main Idea

Vegetables contribute to good health, can be prepared in many ways, and add flavor, color, and texture to meals.

Content Vocabulary

You will find definitions for these words in the glossary at the back of this book.

- tuber
- salad greens
- cooking greens
- sea vegetables
- solanine
- crudités
- aromatic vegetable

Academic Vocabulary

You will find these words in your reading and on your tests. Use the glossary to look up their definitions if necessary.

- dainty
- compound

Graphic Organizer

Use a graphic organizer like the one below to note signs of quality to look for when choosing vegetables.

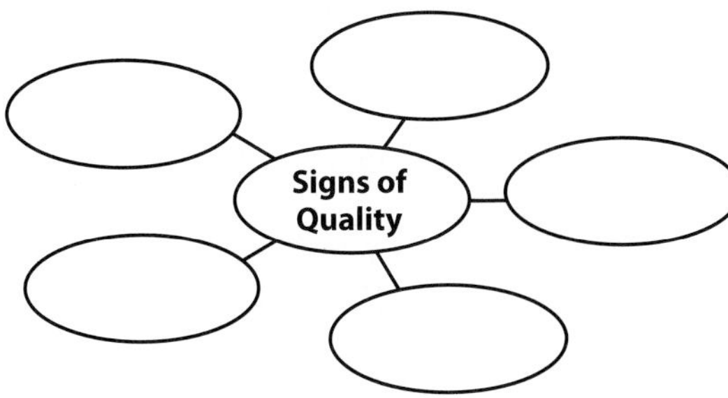

Graphic Organizer Go to this book's Online Learning Center at **glencoe.com** to print out this graphic organizer.

Academic Standards

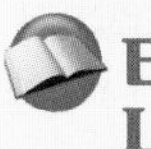

English Language Arts

NCTE 8 Use information resources to gather information and create and communicate knowledge.

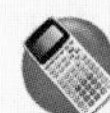

Mathematics

NCTM Data Analysis and Probability Formulate questions that can be addressed with data and collect, organize, and display relevant data to answer them.

NCTM Problem Solving Build new mathematical knowledge through problem solving.

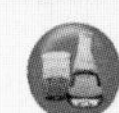

Science

NSES B Develop an understanding of the structure and properties of matter.

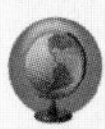

Social Studies

NCSS VIII A Science, Technology, and Society Identify and describe both current and historical examples of the interaction and interdependence of science, technology, and society in a variety of cultural settings.

NCTE *National Council of Teachers of English*
NCTM *National Council of Teachers of Mathematics*
NSES *National Science Education Standards*
NCSS *National Council for the Social Studies*

Nutrients In Vegetables

There are countless ways to prepare and serve vegetables as main dishes, side dishes, appetizers, and snacks. Vegetables add flavor, color, and texture to meals. They also contribute to your health.

Vegetables are rich in many vitamins and minerals, making them among the most nutritious foods. For example, bell peppers, tomatoes, and raw cabbage are good sources of vitamin C. Leafy green vegetables provide folic acid, vitamin K, calcium, and magnesium.

Vegetables are also an important source of fiber, carbohydrates, and phytochemicals. They contain no cholesterol, and most are low in calories, fat, and sodium. Many vegetables contain antioxidants, including vitamins A and C and lycopene, that may lower your risk of some cancers and heart disease.

✓ **Reading Check** **Identify** Which vegetables are good sources of vitamin C?

Types of Vegetables

Different vegetables come from different plant parts as shown in **Figure 29.1**. There are eight types of vegetables:

Flowers Broccoli and cauliflower are the flowers of a plant. They can be eaten raw or cooked.

Fruits Most vegetables from the fruit part of a plant, such as tomatoes, cucumbers, and peppers, can be eaten raw. Eggplant and squash are usually cooked.

Seeds High in nutrients and requiring minimal cooking, seeds are the plant part that grows new plants. Beans, corn, and peas are seeds.

Stems Edible stems are tender and need very little cooking. Some stems, such as celery, onions, and leeks can be eaten raw. Some vegetables, such as asparagus, have both the stem and the flower.

Leaves Leaf vegetables include cabbage, lettuce, Brussels sprouts, and spinach. Most leaves are tender and can be eaten raw or with just a little cooking.

Figure 29.1 Types of Vegetables

Many Choices Vegetables come from different parts of plants, from the roots to the flowers. ***What vegetables can you name that come from each of these parts?***

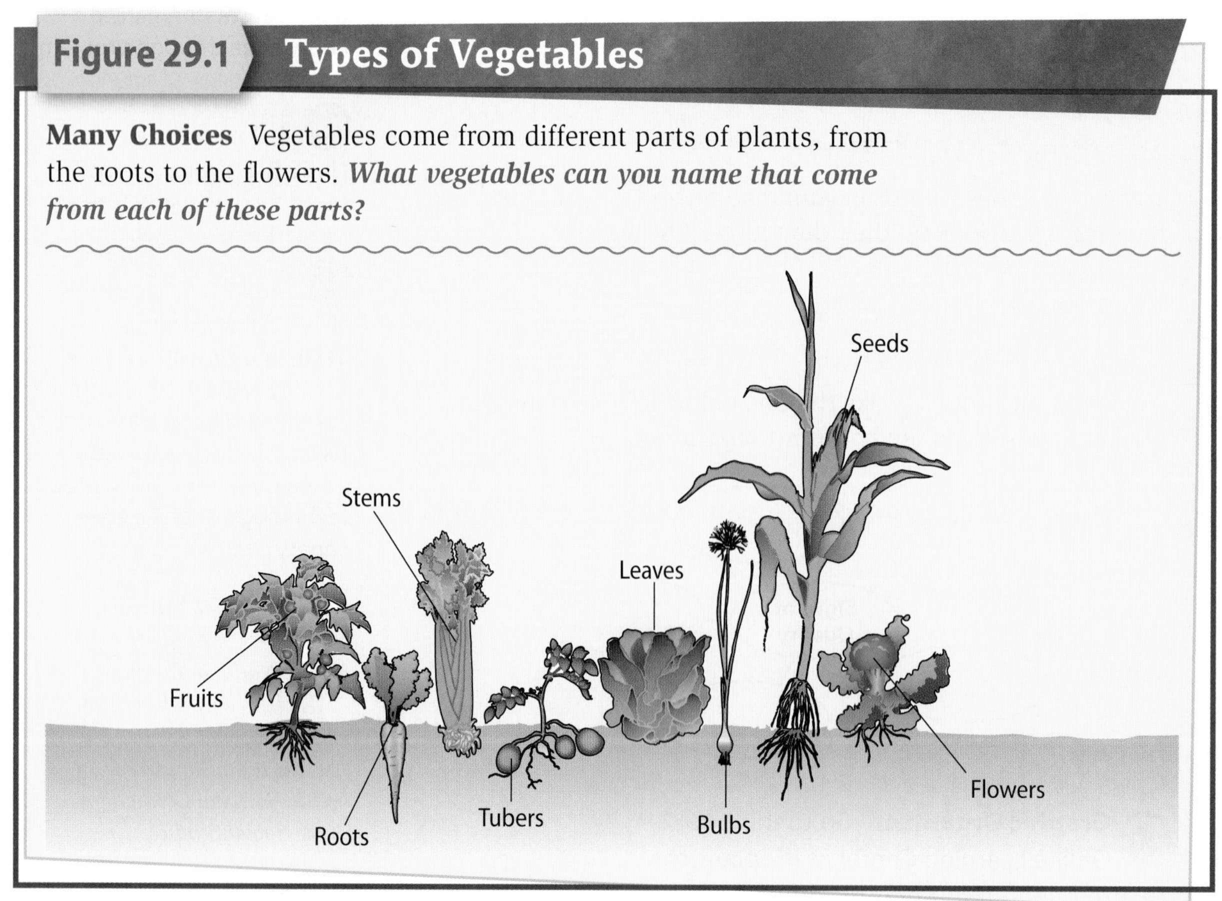

Roots A plant's food supply is stored in its roots. The purpose of a plant's roots are to absorb water and nutrients and anchor the plant to the ground. Many roots can be eaten raw, but others must be cooked. Carrots, beets, turnips, and radishes are roots.

Tubers A **tuber** is a large underground stem that stores nutrients. This part of the plant must be cooked. The potato is the most popular tuber. Other tubers include yams and jicama.

Bulbs Found in the underground part of the stem, bulbs are fleshy structures surrounded by layers of fleshy leaves. They can be eaten raw or cooked and used in many recipes. Onions and garlic are bulbs.

Identifying Vegetables

Vegetables come in an incredible array of shapes and sizes, from the **dainty**, or delicate, green pea to the hefty orange pumpkin. **Figure 29.2** describes nearly three dozen vegetables and their uses.

Vegetables that come from leaves are called leafy greens. Leafy greens that are eaten raw are called **salad greens**. Many lettuce varieties are salad greens. Leafy greens that are eaten cooked are called **cooking greens**. Cooking greens are usually tougher and thicker than salad greens. Cooking greens can be added to soups, sauces, and other recipes. Cooking greens include collards, dandelion greens, kale, mustard greens, chard, and spinach.

Figure 29.2 Vegetables and Their Uses

Plant Parts Vegetables come from many different plant parts, including leaves, stems, fruit, and seeds. ***Which vegetables shown here are types of cabbage? Which vegetable is a type of fungus?***

Artichokes

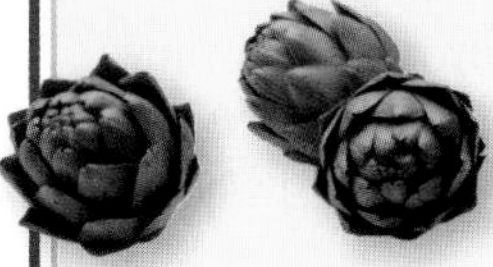

- Large, unopened flower bud of a plant in thistle family with thick, green, compact scales. Nutty flavor.
- Pull off outer leaves.
- Use raw with dip.
- Use cooked in appetizers, salads, and entrées.

Asparagus

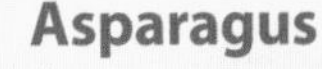

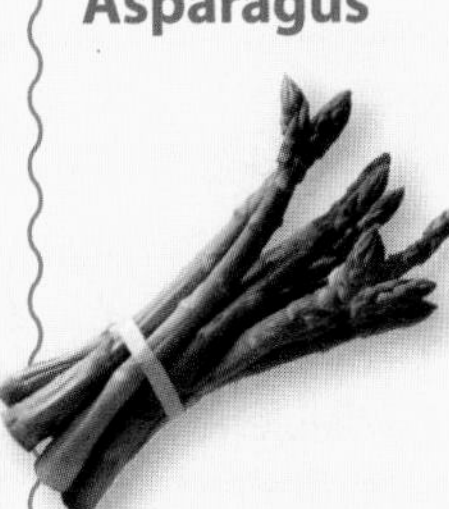

- Green stem vegetable. Tall stalks with closed, compact, rich green tips. Related to onions, garlic, and leeks.
- Comes in green, purple, and white varieties.
- Use raw with dip.
- Use cooked in salads, pasta dishes, and as a side dish.

Beans

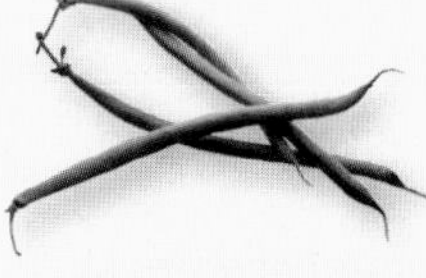

- Seed vegetable.
- Young and tender, with firm, crisp pods.
- Varieties include yellow wax beans and snap beans (also known as green beans or string beans).
- Beans are fresh if they make a snapping sound when bent.
- Choose unblemished beans with a bright appearance and good color. Avoid wilted, flabby, or tough pods.
- Use raw plain or with dip. Use cooked in salads, stir-fries, and as a side dish.

Beets

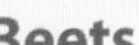

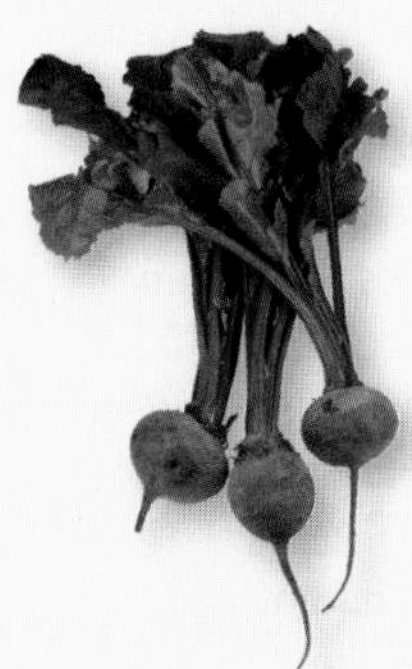

- Root vegetable.
- Firm, round, and smooth, with deep red color and a slender tap root.
- Crisp with sweet flavor. Color bleeds into other foods.
- Avoid elongated or wilted beets. Beet greens are the crisp, dark green leaves of beets, used as cooking greens.
- Use cooked in salads and as a side dish.

Figure 29.2 Vegetables and Their Uses *(continued)*

Bok Choi

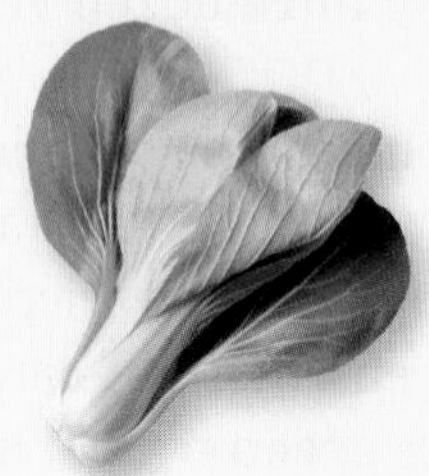

- Head of dark green leaves on thick, crisp, edible white stalks.
- Mild flavor like cabbage.
- Use raw in salads. Use cooked in stir-fries and as a side dish.

Broccoli

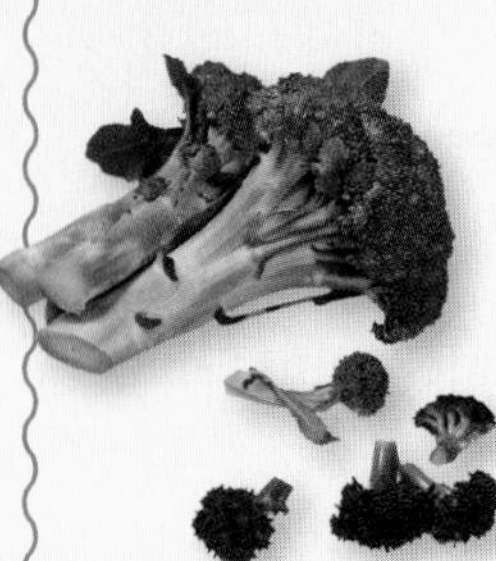

- Type of cabbage.
- Related to cauliflower.
- Firm, compact cluster of tiny buds on stout, edible stems. Deep emerald green, with possible purple tinge. Avoid yellowing or open buds, watery spots on cluster, and very thick stems.
- Use raw with dip or in salads. Use cooked as a side dish.

Brussels Sprouts

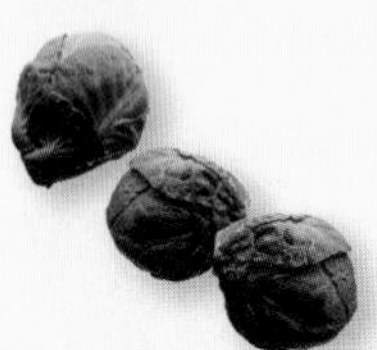

- Enlarged buds cut from tall stem.
- Look like small cabbages.
- Bright green color, compact leaves, and a firm body.
- Avoid wilted leaves or yellow or black spots.
- Use raw with dip. Use cooked in soups and stews and as a side dish.

Cabbage

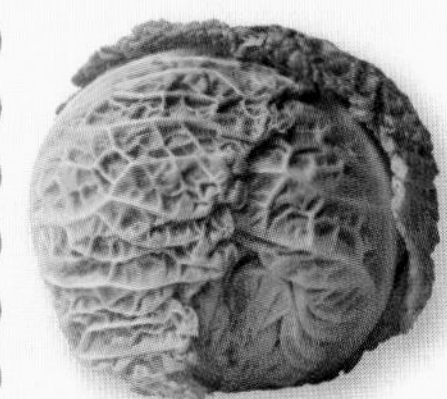

- Leaf vegetable with a short, broad stem and a compact, heavy head of leaves or flowers.
- Strong flavor.
- Varieties include green, red, savoy (milder flavor), kale.
- Napa cabbage has elongated head and thick-veined, cream-colored crinkly leaves with a mild flavor.
- Use raw, shredded, in salads or slaws. Use cooked in stir-fries and as a side dish. Use leaves to wrap meat fillings.

Carrots

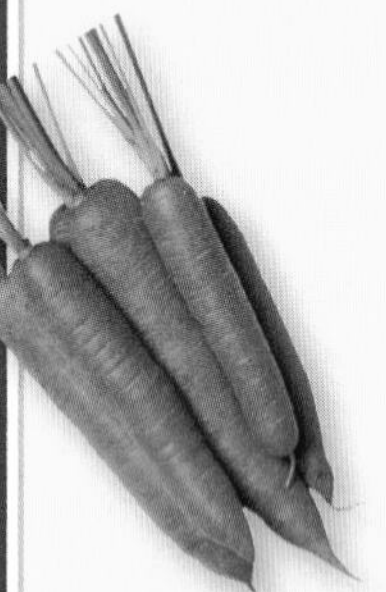

- Root vegetable.
- Lacy greens and long, slender, orange root.
- Crunchy.
- Avoid wilted, flabby carrots. Baby variety is available.
- Use raw as crudités or shredded or sliced in salads. Use cooked in breads, soups, stews, roasts, and as a side dish.

Cauliflower

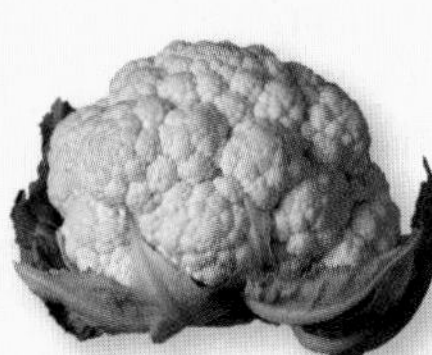

- Type of cabbage.
- Compact, tiny white or creamy white florets in clusters on stalks surrounded by green leaves.
- Avoid brown spots.
- Use raw with dip or in pasta salad. Use cooked in stir-fries and soups.

Celery

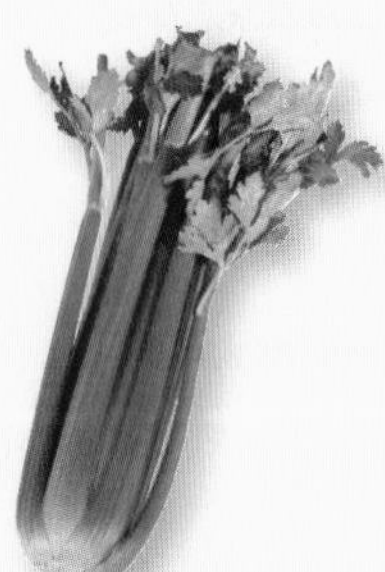

- Stem vegetable.
- Green stalk containing individual ribs with green leaflets.
- Crisp; bitter to slightly sweet flavor. "Hearts" are innermost tender ribs.
- High water content.
- Use raw with dip.
- Use cooked in soups, stews, stir-fries, and stuffing.

Collards

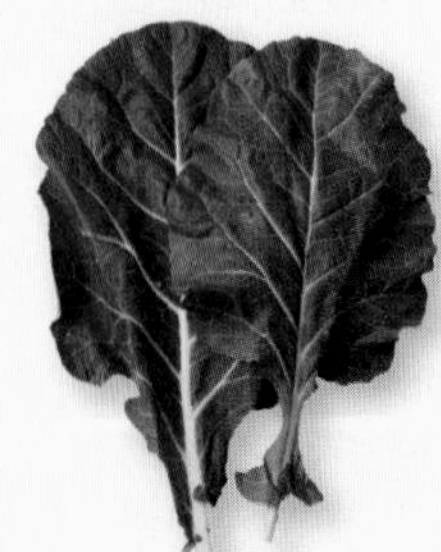

- Large, dark green leaves on tall stems.
- Flavor is a cross between cabbage and kale.
- Use raw, shredded, in salads or slaws.
- Use cooked in stir-fries and as a side dish.
- Use leaves to wrap meat fillings.

Figure 29.2 Vegetables and Their Uses *(continued)*

Corn

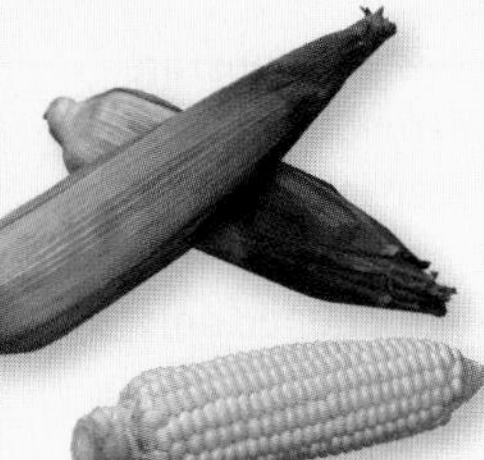

- Seed vegetable.
- Ears of plump kernels enclosed in green husks with moist, golden silk.
- Kernels may be yellow, white, or both.
- Sweet and juicy.
- Silk ends should not be decayed or have worm injury.
- Use cooked, on the cob or as loose kernels.

Cucumbers

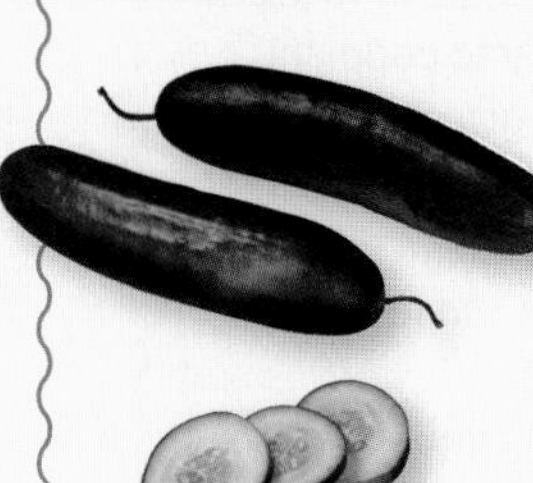

- Fruit vegetable related to pumpkins, watermelon, and squash.
- Deep green skin covering cool, moist, whitish flesh with edible seeds.
- Often waxed to keep in moisture.
- Avoid cucumbers with an overly large diameter or shriveled ends.
- Use raw, plain or with dip, or sliced or shredded in salads.

Eggplant

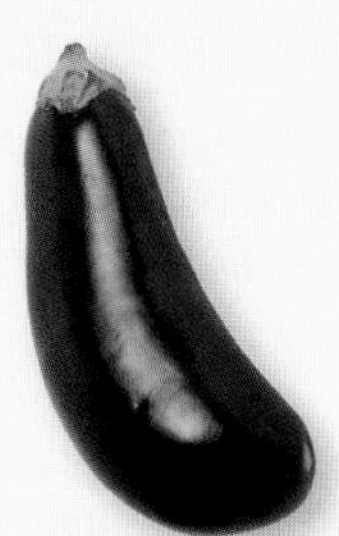

- Fruit vegetable related to tomatoes and potatoes.
- Many varieties.
- Most common is dark purple, elongated, and rounded horn-shaped. Firm, smooth, and glossy, with meaty flesh.
- Use cooked in stir-fries, stews, and baked dishes.
- Often stuffed.

Garlic

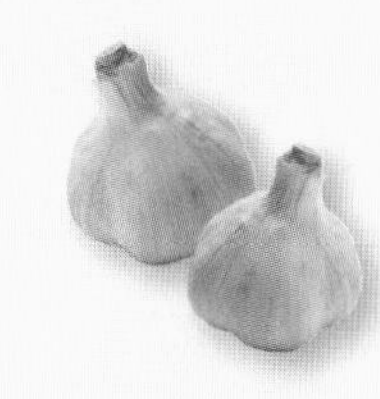

- Bulb vegetable related to onions and leeks.
- Plump white bulbs made of several small cloves encased in thin skin.
- Strong flavor mellows with cooking but becomes bitter when overcooked.
- Use raw in oils, dressings, and spreads.
- Use cooked in soups, stews, and roasts, or baked whole.

Jicama

- Tuber shaped like a turnip. Tough brown skin.
- White flesh.
- Slightly sweet flavor, crunchy texture, juicy.
- Peel before using.
- Use raw as a snack and in salads.
- Use cooked in stir-fries.

Kohlrabi

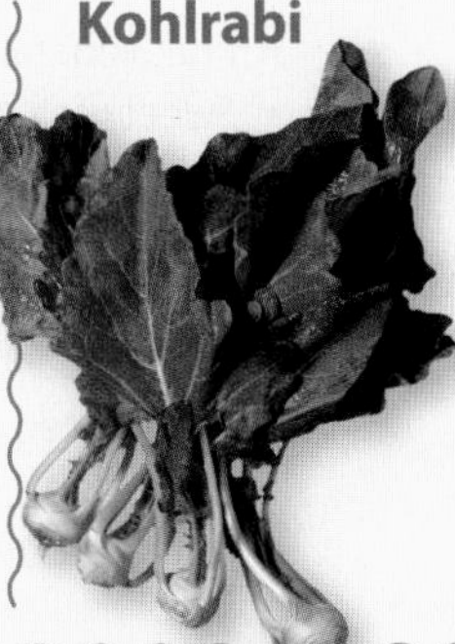

- Short, white stem shaped like a globe with green leaves.
- Tastes like a mild, sweet turnip.
- Use cooked in soups, stews, stir-fries, and as a side dish.

Leeks

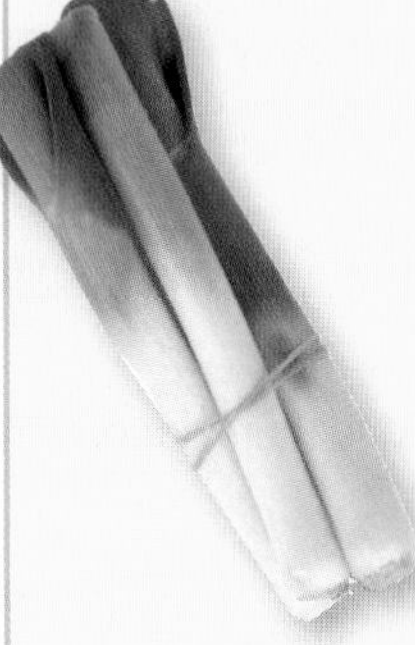

- Related to onion and garlic, with a milder, sweet flavor.
- Thick, short white stalks with crisp, blue-green leaves.
- Use raw in thin slices in salads.
- Use cooked in casseroles, soups, stews, and a side dish.

Mushrooms

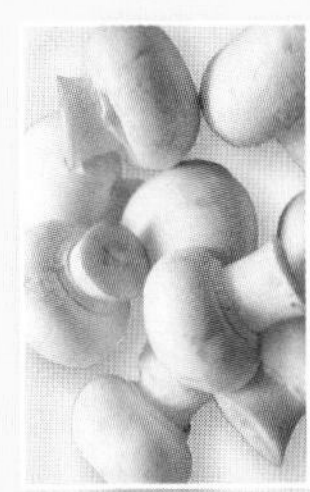

- Type of fungus.
- Many edible varieties, including white, portobello, and shiitake.
- Short stem with pink or light-tan gills and a white, creamy, or light brown cap.
- Moist with mild to bold flavor.
- Use raw as a snack, in salads, or stuffed.
- Use cooked in soups, stews, omelets, and stir-fries, or marinated.

Figure 29.2 Vegetables and Their Uses *(continued)*

Okra

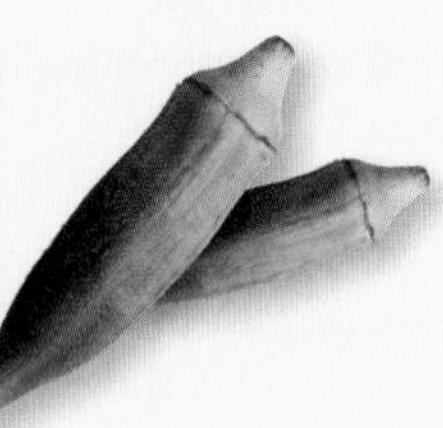

- Fruit vegetable. Tapered, oblong fuzzy pods with a taste similar to eggplant.
- When cut, gives off a sticky substance that thickens soups.
- Dark green and red varieties.
- Bends with slight pressure.
- Use raw, marinated, in salads.
- Use cooked in soups and stews, or breaded and fried.

Onions

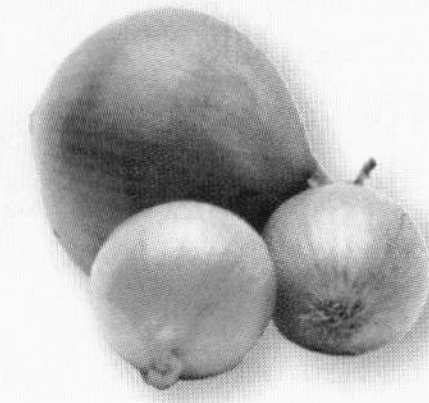

- Bulb vegetable.
- Green onions (scallions) are mild young onions with long, straight green leaves and a small white bulb.
- Yellow, white, and red onions are firm, round, and dry with small necks, juicy flesh surrounded by papery skin, and mild to strong flavor.
- Vidalia onions are crisp, juicy, and sweet.
- Use raw, chopped, in salads and as fillings.
- Use cooked in soups, stews, stir-fries and roasts.

Parsnips

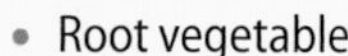

- Root vegetable.
- Whitish color, similar in shape to carrots.
- Firm with a sweet, nutty flavor.
- Use cooked, mashed, or added to stews.

Peas

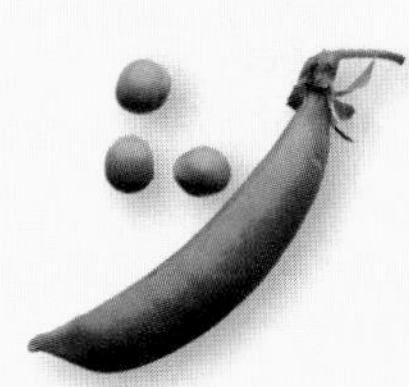

- Crisp, bright green pods filled with small, sweet peas.
- Snow pea pods are flat.
- Sugar snap pea pods are plump.
- Use raw as a snack or in salads.
- Use cooked in pasta dishes, baked dishes, soups, and as a side dish.

Peppers

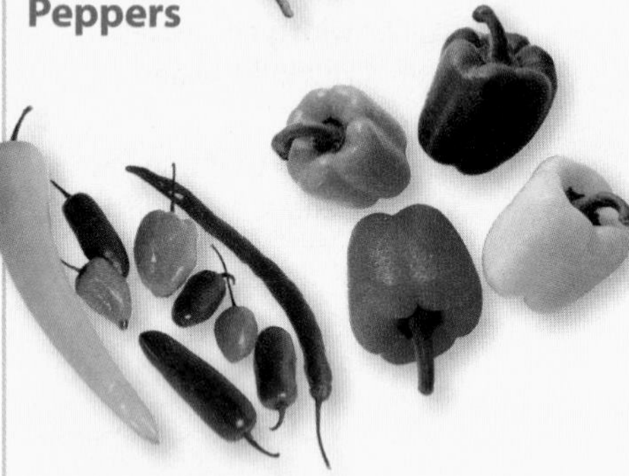

- Fruit vegetable.
- Sweet (bell, banana, pimiento) or hot (chile).
- Bell peppers are bright and glossy and may be green, red, yellow, orange, or purple.
- Bell-shaped, firm, and hollow, with a short, thick stem and three to four lobes.
- Green peppers are less sweet. Hot chile peppers include jalapeño, cayenne, and habanero.
- Use raw as a snack or sliced or chopped in salsa and salads.
- Use cooked in stir-fries, soups, stews, and chili.
- Often stuffed with cooked rice and meats.

Potatoes

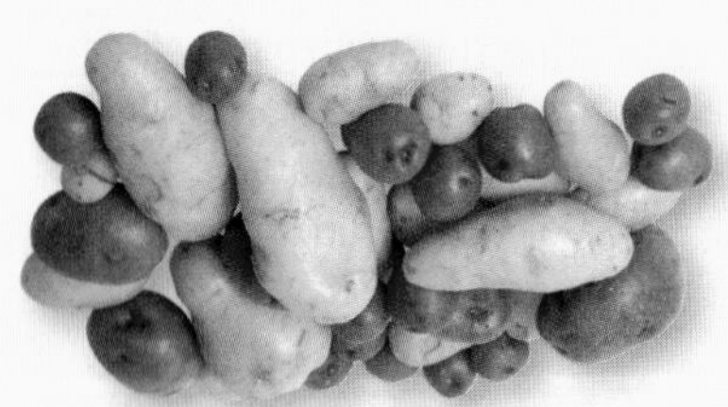

- Tubers.
- Varieties include: Idaho or russet (dark brown), new (freshly harvested), white, round red, and blue or purple.
- Firm, heavy, round to oval, with thin skin.
- White, starchy flesh.
- Purple has purple flesh.
- Texture varies with type.
- New, whites, and round reds keep their shape, making them good for boiling, frying, and salads.
- Russets loosen up easily and bake well.
- Use cooked in soups, stews, cold salads, and as a side dish.

Figure 29.2 Vegetables and Their Uses *(continued)*

Pumpkins

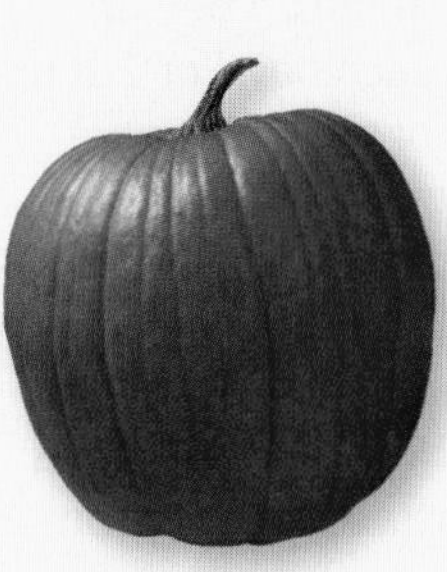

- Fruit vegetable.
- Large, round, orange gourd, related to squash.
- Sweet, mild flavor.
- Seeds can be husked and roasted.
- Nutty taste.
- Small pumpkins are best for cooking.
- Use cooked in soups, casseroles, and pies.

Radishes

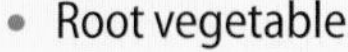

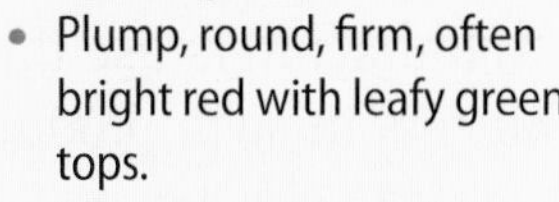

- Root vegetable.
- Plump, round, firm, often bright red with leafy green tops.
- Crunchy and flavorful.
- May be spongy if very large and not firm.
- Use raw as a snack or garnish and in salads and sandwiches.

Rutabagas

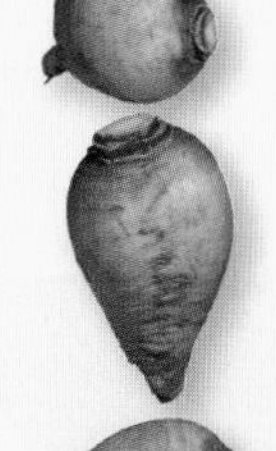

- Root vegetable related to turnips.
- Large, smooth, round or elongated; firm, dense.
- Sweet, yellow flesh.
- Strong flavor.
- Skin may be waxed to prevent the loss of moisture.
- Peel before cooking.
- Use cooked, mashed or puréed.

Spinach

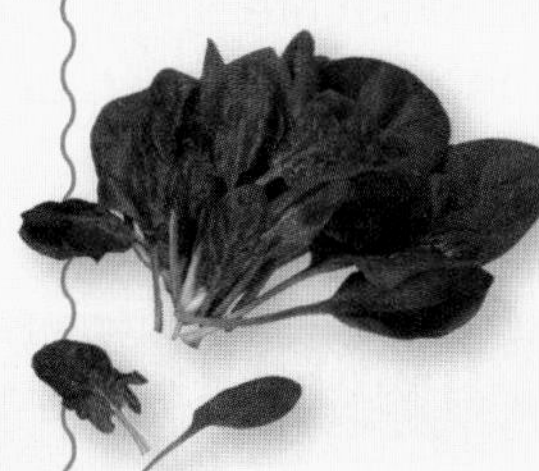

- Small, dark green, tender leaves with slightly bitter flavor.
- Cooks quickly.
- Baby spinach has very small leaves.
- Use raw in salads and sandwiches.
- Use cooked in casseroles and as a side dish.

Squash

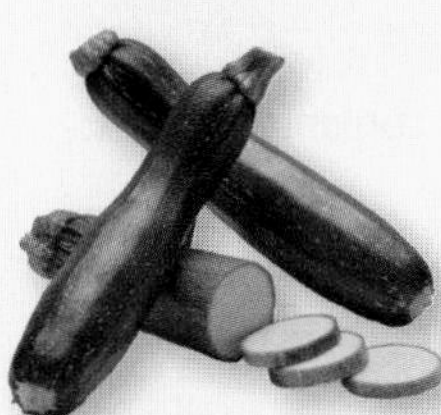

- Fruit vegetable.
- Varieties include winter, summer, and spaghetti.
- Use winter and summer squash cooked in casseroles and as a side dish.
- Use summer squash raw as a snack or shredded in slaws.
- Use spaghetti squash cooked in place of pasta.

Sweet Potatoes

- Root vegetable.
- Pale-skinned variety has light-colored, thin skin and pale yellow, dry flesh.
- Dark-skinned variety (called "yam" but not related to the true yam) has thicker, dark orange skin with sweet, moist orange flesh.
- Use cooked in soups, stews, and as a side dish.

Tomatoes

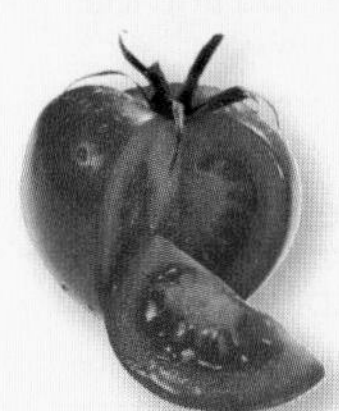

- Fruit vegetable. Juicy flesh with seeds.
- Varieties include vine, plum, cherry, and beefsteak.
- Fully ripe tomatoes are bright red and slightly soft.
- Use raw in salads, sandwiches, and salsa.
- Use cooked in sauces, casseroles, and for canning.

Turnips

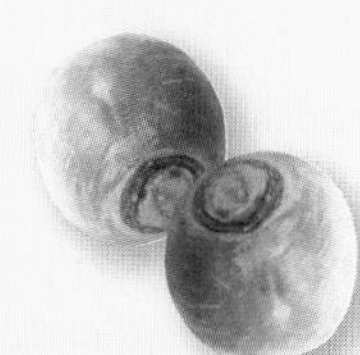

- Root vegetable.
- Smooth, fairly round, firm, and small to medium in size.
- White skin with purple tinge and white flesh.
- Turnip greens can be cooked.
- Use cooked, mashed or puréed.

Sea Vegetables

Sea vegetables are seaweeds used as vegetables. They have been used as food for centuries in coastal regions around the globe. Sea vegetables are more common than you might realize. Manufacturers use them as thickeners and stabilizers in such products as ice cream, pudding, salad dressing, and even toothpaste! Sea vegetables grow in water with filtered sunlight. Many are grown in Japan. Sea vegetables are actually algae, not plants. They are low in fat and a rich source of vitamins and minerals. However, they contain more sodium than other vegetables. **Figure 29.3** describes several varieties of sea vegetables.

✓ Reading Check **Contrast** What are the differences between a tuber and a bulb?

Nutrition Check

Colorful Vegetables

Vegetables play a key role in a healthful diet. In a diet of 1,800 to 2,000 daily calories, a person needs 2½ cups of vegetables each day. For 2,200 to 2,400 daily calories, 3 cups of vegetables are recommended. Eat 5 or 6½-cup servings of different colored vegetables each day. Remember that raw vegetables like carrots and celery make convenient snacks. Different colored vegetables provide different nutrients. Choosing vegetables in all colors of the rainbow ensures you will consume a wide variety of nutrients.

Think About It What are some easy ways to increase vegetable servings in an eating plan? Make a list of your ideas.

Figure 29.3 Common Sea Vegetables

Under the Sea Sea vegetables are rich in minerals and add an interesting flavor to soups, salads, and stir-fries. ***What flavor do the sea vegetables shown here have?***

Name	Description	Uses
Arame	Dark brown with a mild, slightly sweet flavor.	Used without cooking in salads; sautéed.
Kombu, or kelp	Dark brown or black with a delicate flavor. Sold in sheets or strips. White powder covering the surface adds flavor.	Used in soups, stews, stir-fries, and salads or cooked as a vegetable.
Carrageen	Mossy with color ranging from yellow-green, through red to purplish-brown.	It is used as a thickener in ice cream and other milk products.
Laver	Dark purple with a strong, tangy, slightly sweet flavor. Sold in sheets.	Used in soups or deep-fried as an appetizer.
Wakame	Deep green. Mild flavor. Treated as vegetable.	Adds richness to soups and salads.
Nori	Dark green, dark purple, or black with a sweet flavor. Comes in sheets.	Used to wrap seafood and rice rolls, sushi.
Dulse	Dark pink to brick red with a pungent, salty flavor.	Used in soups or as a condiment. Also eaten like beef jerky.
Hijiki	Black with a mild, salty, sea-like flavor. Highest mineral content of all sea vegetables.	Used as a vegetable in soups, stews, and stir-fries.
Agar	Tasteless. Sold in blocks, flakes, or powder.	Can be used as a substitute for gelatin. Will set at room temperature.

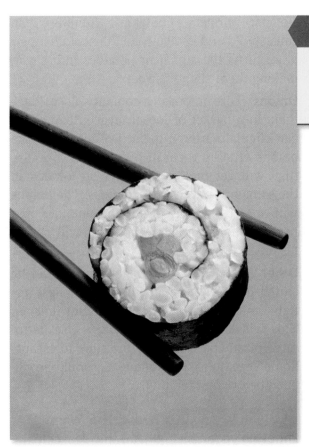

Ocean Food

Sea vegetables, sometimes called seaweeds, are often used in Asian dishes. Seaweeds are used both fresh and dried. *What moss is sometimes used in ice cream and other creamy foods? Why?*

Selecting and Storing Fresh Vegetables

Fresh vegetables taste good, look appealing, are full of nutrients, and can be used in countless ways. The quality of fresh vegetables generally peaks during the summer months, and prices are typically lower then, too. Exploring seasonal vegetables is a good way to try new flavors and get the benefits of fresh vegetables throughout the year.

Many people grow their own vegetables. Growing vegetables saves money and helps you enjoy the freshest produce. For information on starting a vegetable garden, visit a garden center, consult gardening books or Web sites, or visit the Web site of your local Cooperative Extension office.

Choosing Quality Vegetables

Depending on where you shop, fresh vegetables may be available loose, in a plastic-covered tray, or pre-packaged in a plastic bag. Some vegetables, such as broccoli and parsley, usually come in bunches held together with a rubber band or plastic tie. When you buy vegetables, look for these signs of quality:

Ripeness Vegetables are harvested when ripe, so buy only what you can use during the storage life of the vegetable. Most fresh vegetables should be used within two to five days, although root vegetables last from one to several weeks. Underripe vegetables have poor texture and flavor.

Color and Texture Vegetables should have a bright color and crisp texture. Avoid green potatoes. The green color, which is usually caused by exposure to light, may indicate the presence of a bitter, toxic **compound** called **solanine**. A compound is a combination of two or more substances. If green parts develop on potatoes during storage, cut them away before cooking.

Shape Each type of vegetable has its own characteristic shape. Misshapen vegetables usually have poor flavor and texture.

Size A vegetable should be heavy for its size. Avoid very large or very small vegetables. Extra-large vegetables may be overripe, tough, and have poor flavor. Extremely small vegetables may be immature and lack flavor.

Condition Choose crisp, fresh vegetables and avoid wilted, decayed, or damaged ones. Unless you plan to use the tops of root vegetables, such as carrots and beets, buy them without the tops. The tops draw moisture from root vegetables, making them wilt. Root vegetables, bulbs, and tubers should not have any sprouts (new growth in the form of offshoots). Sprouts indicate that the vegetables have been stored too long.

Storing Fresh Vegetables

Except for roots, tubers, and bulbs, most vegetables are highly perishable and should be refrigerated as soon as you bring them home. Only wash vegetables before refrigerating them if dirt is visible. Moisture can encourage bacteria to grow, and the vegetables may spoil faster or get moldy. If you do wash vegetables before storing them, dry them thoroughly.

To maintain the freshness of vegetables, store them according to their type:

Potatoes Store potatoes, including sweet potatoes, in a cool, dark, dry place. Storing potatoes in a dark place prevents them from turning green. If you do not have a dark storage area, put potatoes in a paper bag. If you must store potatoes at room temperature, buy only what you can use within a few days. Do not refrigerate potatoes. Humidity can cause mold and spoilage, and the cold temperature turns the starch in potatoes into sugar, making them slightly sweet.

Onions Store onions in a cool, dry place. Place them in a basket or loosely woven bag so air can circulate around them. Do not refrigerate onions or store them in plastic bags, because they will get moldy. Do not store onions in the same bag or bin with potatoes. The onions will absorb moisture from the potatoes and become moldy, and the potatoes will sprout faster.

Other Vegetables Most vegetables should be stored in the refrigerator in plastic bags, airtight containers, or the refrigerator crisper. This will keep them fresh longer. Use perforated plastic bags to allow moisture to escape. Some vegetables, like tomatoes, should be ripened before refrigerating.

Kitchen Math

Track Your Vegetable Consumption

Do you know which vegetables are part of your diet? For three days, write down every vegetable that you eat, making a tally mark next to the vegetable name for every serving of that vegetable that you have. Then, create a table that shows the names of the vegetables and the number of servings that you had of each one.

Math Concept **Create a Table** A common method of displaying data is a table. Each row and column in a table should be carefully labeled to explain what data is being displayed.

Starting Hint Label your first column "Vegetables" and the second column "Number of Servings," then list out your results below the headings, using one row for each vegetable. Order your table in a logical way, such as in alphabetical order by vegetable name, or ranked from most-consumed to least-consumed. At the bottom, provide a total of all vegetable servings eaten during the three days.

Math Appendix For math help, go to the Math Appendix at the back of the book.

NCTM Data Analysis and Probability Formulate questions that can be addressed with data and collect, organize, and display relevant data to answer them.

✓ **Reading Check** **Describe** When choosing vegetables, what is the ideal color and texture?

Preparing Fresh and Raw Vegetables

Most fresh vegetables are easy to prepare. First wash the vegetables, then prepare them for serving raw or cooking.

Washing Fresh Vegetables

Wash vegetables even if you are planning to peel or cook them. Most vegetables grow close to the ground, so they may carry dirt and harmful bacteria.

Wash tender vegetables under cool, running water. Scrub potatoes, root vegetables, and thick-skinned vegetables, such as winter squash, with a stiff brush to remove dirt. Wash salad greens by the leaf and pat them dry with a clean towel.

Do not soak vegetables in water, because soaking causes nutrient loss. Do not use detergents, because detergents may react with pesticides and waxes on the vegetables to create harmful compounds.

Paring and Peeling Fresh Vegetables

After washing, remove any inedible parts of the vegetable, including stems and soft spots. A few vegetables, such as peppers, have inedible seeds that should be removed. Some recipes call for peeling vegetables with a vegetable peeler. To retain more nutrients, eat edible skins instead of peeling them away. You do not have to peel cucumbers, potatoes, or carrots, for example.

Preparing Raw Vegetables

Many vegetables taste great and look appetizing without cooking because of their bright colors and crunchy texture. You can serve many vegetables raw, including celery, cucumbers, radishes, tomatoes, peppers, turnips, carrots, cabbage, cauliflower, and broccoli.

Raw vegetables can be served in salads, as a snack, or as crudités on a relish tray. **Crudités** are sliced or small whole vegetables served raw, often with dip, as an appetizer. Ranch dressing is a popular choice for a crudité dip. Flavored yogurt also makes a simple tasty dip for vegetables.

To prepare crudités, cut vegetables into small pieces that can be picked up easily. Experiment with a variety of shapes for extra appeal. On a serving plate, you might arrange rings, wedges, and sticks in a design that shows off colors and shapes. When you are deciding what to serve on a vegetable plate, consider including a variety of tastes. Sweet cherry tomatoes, for example, nicely complement the mild flavor of green beans and a more distinctive tasting asparagus.

To keep a supply of nutritious vegetable snacks on hand, simply cut up raw vegetables and refrigerate them in a covered container or sealed plastic bag. Add a few ice cubes or a tablespoon or two of cold water to the container to keep the vegetables crisp. You can restore crispness to a vegetable like celery by placing it in ice water for a few minutes.

✓ **Reading Check** **List** What are three ways to serve raw vegetables?

Be a Smart Consumer

Munchable Miniatures

Two-inch ears of corn and egg-size eggplants are not agricultural accidents. They are "baby" vegetables. Some baby vegetables are regular vegetables picked while immature, but most are full-grown miniatures. First introduced in restaurants, baby vegetables are now available in supermarkets, where consumers respond favorably to the "teardrop tomatoes," "turnip pearls," and other novelties. Baby vegetables are just as nutritious as regular varieties, but cook more quickly and must be used sooner. Given their small size, that is not difficult. You might eat half a dozen ears of baby corn, cob and all, in one serving.

Challenge Why do you think baby vegetables may be more appealing to consumers than regular-sized vegetables? Conduct research about baby vegetables. Research the production and consumption of the vegetables. What does the research show about the appeal of baby vegetables? Learn about at least two types. Write a paragraph expressing your critical thinking and insights.

Cooking Fresh Vegetables

Many vegetables, including most roots and tubers, must be cooked to make them edible and easy to digest. Fresh vegetables can be cooked several different ways. The method you choose and the length of cooking time depends on the vegetable, its tenderness, the size of the pieces, and your own taste preferences.

How Cooking Affects Vegetables

Cooking affects vegetables' nutrient content, texture, color, and flavor.

Nutrients Some nutrients dissolve in cooking water, are destroyed by heat, or both. Vitamin B is lost in water, for example, while vitamin C is lost in water and through heat.

Texture Heat softens the cellulose, or fiber, in cell walls of vegetables, making them tender. Cooked vegetables are most appealing and nutritious when they are still somewhat firm. Vegetables become mushy if overcooked. Cooking vegetables for a short time in a small amount of water usually gives the best results. The idea is to get the vegetables a bit more tender than when they are raw but still maintain some of the crispness.

Color Properly cooked vegetables are colorful. Green vegetables get their color from chlorophyll, the chemical compound that plants use to turn the sun's energy into food. Green vegetables can turn an unpleasant olive color if overcooked. Heat does not destroy the carotene that gives some vegetables their yellow or orange color.

Flavor Cooking releases flavors, making vegetables taste more mellow and delicious. Overcooked vegetables become bland or may even develop an unpleasant flavor.

Simmering Vegetables

Simmer vegetables by putting a small amount of water in a medium-size saucepan, covering it, and bringing it to a boil. Add the vegetables, recover the pan, and bring the water to a boil again. Then lower the heat until the water simmers. Cook covered until the vegetables are tender, yet somewhat firm. Keep the heat low enough to prevent scorching. Drain the vegetables before serving. Using a small amount of water helps keep nutrients from being lost.

To allow the true flavor of vegetables to come through, do not add salt during or after cooking. Instead, experiment with flavor by adding herbs or spices or use the cooking water to make a seasoned sauce. The cooking liquid contains nutrients. Serve it with the vegetables or save it to use in sauces, soups, or stews. Do not add water to cook greens such as spinach or chard. The water left from washing these leaves is enough to cook them.

Careers in Food

Alex Miller
Grocer/Produce Professional

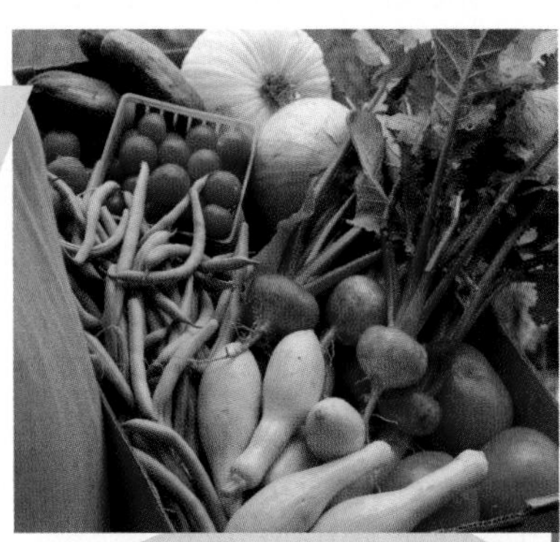

Q: What is the difference between a green grocer and a grocer?

A: Grocers work with food that can last two years before it is no longer usable. Green grocers work with fresh food that might not last two days.

Q: How are the two in common with each other?

A: Both involve stocking, and customer service—knowing what you have available to shoppers.

Q: How do you feel about working in a profession that helps provide people with a basic staple of life?

A: There is a lot more involved in this job than most people realize, and it is very important that it be done right and consistently to a very high standard.

"The joy I get from my job is opening a box of cauliflower and finding it fresh and alive."
— Alex Miller
Mustard Seed Market & Café - Akron, OH

Education and Training

Experience is important. You can get a degree in management, but not in grocery store management or produce management. You have to learn by working under someone who has learned from someone else.

Qualities and Skills

Customer service skills are important. Paying attention to detail is important. A grocer has to learn what fruits and vegetables are in season and about subtle differences in produce from different regions.

Related Career Opportunities

People who have worked in produce can go on to working in produce distribution, sales, or grocery store management.

In hard-water areas, minerals in cooking water can change the color of red vegetables, such as red cabbage, to purple or purplish-green. To prevent this undesirable color change, add a small amount of acid—vinegar or lemon juice—to the cooking water. Tomatoes retain their color when cooked because they have natural acid.

Simmering Root Vegetables

Potatoes and beets take longer to cook than many other vegetables. Cover them with water, put on the lid, and simmer until the vegetables are tender. To help retain nutrients, cook both potatoes and beets with skins on. If you prefer to eat them without the skins, peel them after the vegetables have been cooked.

Mashed is one favorite way to prepare potatoes. After the potatoes are cooked, drain the water, add seasonings, and mash with an electric mixer or by hand. A little butter adds rich flavor. Gradually adding a little milk as you beat produces a fluffy texture.

Steaming Vegetables

Steaming helps vegetables retain their water-soluble nutrients. Place a steamer basket in a saucepan with a tight-fitting lid. Fill the pan with water to just below the bottom of the basket. Cover the pan and bring the water to a boil. Then add the vegetables to the steamer basket and re-cover then pan. Steam the vegetables until they are tender. Green beans and other tender vegetables steam more quickly than such firm vegetables as potatoes and carrots. Thicker pieces of vegetables also take longer to steam.

Pressure-Cooking Vegetables

Pressure-cooking is a handy way to prepare vegetables that need a long cooking time, such as beets, turnips, whole carrots, and potatoes. These vegetables cook quickly under the high temperature in a pressure cooker. Like steaming, pressure-cooking preserves most of the nutrients in vegetables. Follow the manufacturer's directions carefully when using a pressure cooker.

TECHNOLOGY FOR TOMORROW

Talented 'Taters

You may have eaten potatoes today without even knowing it. Potatoes are a surprising ingredient in many processed foods. Technology aids in the processing of these potatoes. They are steam-peeled, machine-scrubbed, partially cooked, cooled, and then cooked again. The resulting mash is thinly spread onto a hot drum and dried. This sheet of pulverized potato is crumbled into fine flakes, which are used in breads, noodles, dry soup mixes, muffin mixes, meat and fish products, and many other foods. To make a variety of crunchy snacks, bits of processed potato are forced from a high-pressure machine called an extruder. As each piece shoots out, it rapidly expands. This process is called "explosion puffing."

Get Involved Examine the labels of ten different packaged foods. Which ones contain potatoes? In a paragraph, describe your findings and explain why you think the potatoes were included.

NCSS VIII A Science, Technology, and Society
Identify and describe both current and historical examples of the interaction and interdependence of science, technology, and society in a variety of cultural settings.

Braising Vegetables

Braising is similar to stewing but uses less liquid. Braising vegetables develops greater nuances of flavor. It also preserves more color in vegetables. Onions, carrots, parsnips, and potatoes are often added to braised dishes, such as pot roast. You can also braise vegetables by themselves for a side dish. Carrots, potatoes, and eggplant work well braised. Celery hearts lose much of their bitter flavor when braised. Cut the vegetables into large pieces and place them in a heavy pan with a small amount of water or other liquid. Season them as you like. Cover tightly and bake in the oven at 375°F until the vegetables are tender and browned and the liquid is reduced to a sauce. Braising times depend on the variety of vegetables used, their shape and size, and their maturity and tenderness.

Frying Vegetables

Vegetables can be sautéed, fried, stir-fried, or deep-fried. Aromatic vegetables are often sautéed to bring out their flavor. **Aromatic vegetables** are vegetables such as onion, garlic, celery, and carrots, that add flavor and aroma to dishes.

Frying cooked vegetables in a small amount of butter or margarine gives them a tasty crust. Hash browns are made this way from shredded cooked potatoes. You can also fry raw vegetables, although they take longer to cook. To speed cooking time for raw vegetables, add a small amount of water to the pan and then cover it so the vegetables also cook in moist heat. Add the water carefully to prevent spatters.

Potatoes are often deep-fried. Eggplant, onion rings, zucchini, and mushrooms can be dipped in batter and then deep-fried as well.

Baking Vegetables

Baking is a simple way to cook many vegetables, including onions, tomatoes, winter squash, potatoes, and eggplant. You can cut winter squash in half, remove the seeds, and place the halves on a baking sheet. Bake the squash at 350°F until tender.

Baking potatoes makes them fluffy inside and crispy outside. Poke holes in potatoes before you bake them, to allow steam to escape and keep them from exploding. Place the potatoes directly on the oven rack. If you like crispy skin, rub them with oil before placing in the oven. Potatoes can bake at any temperature between 300°F and 450°F, so you can bake them with other foods that require exact temperatures. For example, you can bake muffins at 375°F and bake potatoes at the same time. Baked potatoes are done when a fork easily pierces the potato.

Roasting Vegetables

Any vegetable can be roasted. Brussels sprouts, carrots, onions, turnips, and asparagus taste particularly good roasted. Cut the vegetables into pieces of similar size. Drizzle with oil, sprinkle with seasonings, and toss lightly to coat. Then place them on a baking sheet in a single layer. Roast at 425°F until browned, tender, and caramelized. To assure even roasting, turn the vegetables over about halfway through the cooking time.

Potatoes, onions, and carrots can be roasted in the same pan with meat. Pare the vegetables and place them in the pan around the roast. Cut large vegetable pieces into halves or quarters. Turn them occasionally to moisten them with the meat drippings. This method adds fat to vegetables, but it browns them and produces a tasty crust.

Grilling Vegetables

Follow these guidelines for the best results grilling vegetables:

- Brush the grate of the grill with oil to keep vegetables from sticking.
- To shorten grilling time, blanch less tender vegetables, such as carrots, before grilling.
- Marinate vegetables for added flavor.
- Keep vegetables from drying out by brushing them with an oil and herb mixture.
- When making skewers, group vegetables that have similar cooking times. For example, make one skewer for onions and another for mushrooms.
- Use the center of the grill, the hottest part, for vegetables that take time to cook.
- Wrap large pieces of potatoes, and other vegetables that take time to cook, in heavy-duty foil before placing them on the grate.
- Grill small pieces in a vegetable basket or on skewers.

Microwaving Vegetables

Microwave ovens cook vegetables quickly, using only a small amount of water. As a result, vegetables lose few nutrients and retain color, texture, and flavor.

Large vegetable pieces take longer to cook than small ones. Arrange the tender parts of the vegetable toward the center of the plate and the less tender parts toward the edge. For example, arrange broccoli spears so that the stems are pointing toward the edge.

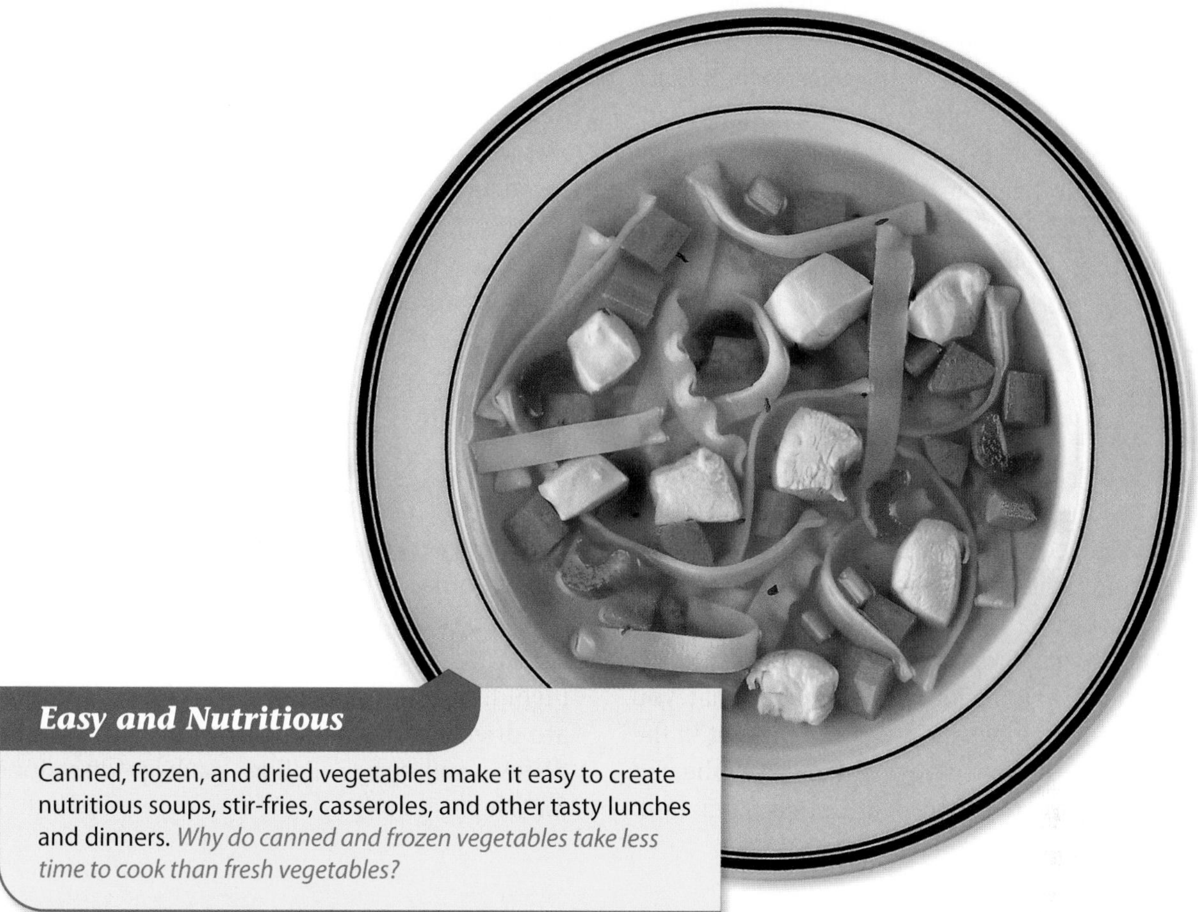

Easy and Nutritious

Canned, frozen, and dried vegetables make it easy to create nutritious soups, stir-fries, casseroles, and other tasty lunches and dinners. *Why do canned and frozen vegetables take less time to cook than fresh vegetables?*

Cover the container to retain moisture, and stir or turn the vegetables during cooking to allow heat to reach all the parts so that the vegetables cook evenly. When cooking potatoes, squash, and other whole vegetables that have a skin, first pierce the skin with a fork to keep the vegetables from bursting.

Follow the directions in the oven's owner's manual for cooking times, power settings, and any special instructions.

Using Leftover Vegetables

Leftover vegetables, both raw and cooked, have many uses in recipes. Marinate cold, cooked vegetables in a tangy salad dressing and serve them on a bed of lettuce. Add cooked vegetables to a stir-fry dish or mix them into a casserole. Add cooked vegetables to a soup, fold them into an omelet, or sauté them with garlic and onions for a side dish.

✓ **Reading Check** **Explain** How can you cook vegetables evenly in a microwave?

Using Convenience Forms of Vegetables

Vegetables come in many convenience forms, including canned, frozen, and dried. Convenience vegetables are handy and easy to use. They can be stored longer than fresh vegetables and can be prepared quickly. Convenience vegetables are available all year long, often at a lower cost than fresh vegetables.

Canned and frozen vegetables may have a different texture and taste than fresh vegetables, but they have about the same amount of vitamins and minerals as fresh vegetables.

Canned Vegetables

Vegetables are canned whole, sliced, or in pieces. Most canned vegetables are packed in water. Some, such as Harvard beets and creamed corn, are packed in sauces. Salt is generally added to canned vegetables as a preservative, but you can also find no-salt and low-salt vegetables.

Use canned vegetables the same way you use cooked fresh vegetables. Season them for a side dish, for example, or toss them in a salad. Canned vegetables are already cooked, so you only need to heat the vegetables in their liquid until they are heated through. Do not overcook cooked vegetables, because they will soften and lose nutrients and color.

Frozen Vegetables

Frozen vegetables are closest in nutrients, color, and flavor to fresh vegetables, although their texture may be different. Frozen vegetables are packaged whole or in pieces. You can also buy combinations of vegetables, such as peas and carrots, or vegetables packed in cheese or butter sauces. Frozen vegetables usually come in cartons or plastic bags. Remove what you need from the package and store the rest in the freezer. Some frozen vegetables can be heated in the microwave oven right in their container.

Frozen vegetables take less time to cook than fresh vegetables because they are preheated prior to freezing. To cook frozen vegetables, follow the directions on the package. In general, it is best to use as little water as possible when preparing frozen vegetables. It is not necessary to thaw frozen vegetables before cooking them. Frozen vegetables keep their flavor, color, and nutrients best if they are heated for the least amount of time necessary.

Dried Vegetables

Dried vegetables come in different forms. Mushrooms, tomatoes, and potatoes are available dried. You can add water to reconstitute them for use in recipes. Many vegetables, including onions, parsley, chives, and garlic, are dried for use as flavorings in entrées, side dishes, and soups. Follow package directions for use.

Light and Healthy Recipe

Vegetable Stir-Fry

Ingredients

- **1 cup** Julienned white onion
- **1 cup** Julienned carrots
- **1 cup** Julienned zucchini
- **1 cup** Julienned green bell pepper
- **1½ tsp.** Vegetable oil
- **1 cup** Bean sprouts
- **2 tsp.** Low-sodium soy sauce
- **¼ tsp.** Ground ginger

Directions

1. Heat a wok or large skillet over high heat. Add the oil, then the onion and carrots. Stir-fry for 3 minutes.
2. Add the zucchini and bell pepper. Continue stir-frying for 1 minute.
3. Add the bean sprouts. Stir-fry for 45 to 60 seconds or until sprouts are heated through.
4. Turn off the heat. Add the soy sauce and ginger and mix gently. Serve immediately.

If served over rice, this recipe provides complete protein.

Yield 4 Servings

Nutrition Analysis per Serving

■ Calories	74
■ Total fat	2 g
■ Saturated fat	0 g
Cholesterol	0 mg
Sodium	129 mg
■ Carbohydrate	12 g
Dietary fiber	3 g
Sugars	6 g
■ Protein	4 g

CHAPTER 29 Review & Applications

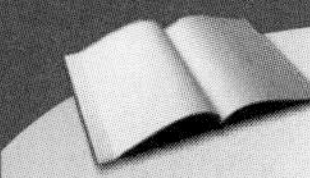

After You Read

Chapter Summary

Vegetables can be prepared and served in a variety of ways. They supply many nutrients. There are eight types of vegetables that come in an array of shapes and sizes. Select vegetables by looking for specific signs of quality. To maintain their freshness, store vegetables properly according to their type. Wash vegetables to ensure safety. Preparing vegetables may involve removing inedible parts, paring, or peeling. Vegetables may be eaten raw or cooked, which affects vegetables' nutrients, texture, color, and flavor. Vegetables may be cooked using several methods. Convenience forms of vegetables are handy and easy to use.

Content and Academic Vocabulary Review

1. Use these content and academic vocabulary words to create a crossword puzzle on graph paper. Use the definitions as clues.

Content Vocabulary

- tuber (p. 451)
- salad greens (p. 451)
- cooking greens (p. 451)
- sea vegetables (p. 456)
- solanine (p. 457)
- crudités (p. 459)
- aromatic vegetable (p. 462)

Academic Vocabulary

- dainty (p. 451)
- compound (p. 457)

Review Key Concepts

2. **Describe** the nutrients found in vegetables.
3. **Identify** the eight types of vegetables.
4. **Explain** how to store fresh vegetables.
5. **Describe** how to wash and prepare fresh vegetables.
6. **Describe** methods for cooking vegetables.
7. **Identify** the types and uses of convenience forms of vegetables.

Critical Thinking

8. **Explain** whether Denise's statement is accurate: "I have a very well-rounded diet. I get my daily recommended serving of vegetables by eating 3 cups of spinach every day."
9. **Compare and contrast** salad greens and cooking greens.
10. **Explain** whether Jude should buy potatoes that the seller says "are green because they are very fresh and still ripening."

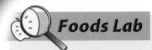

Foods Lab

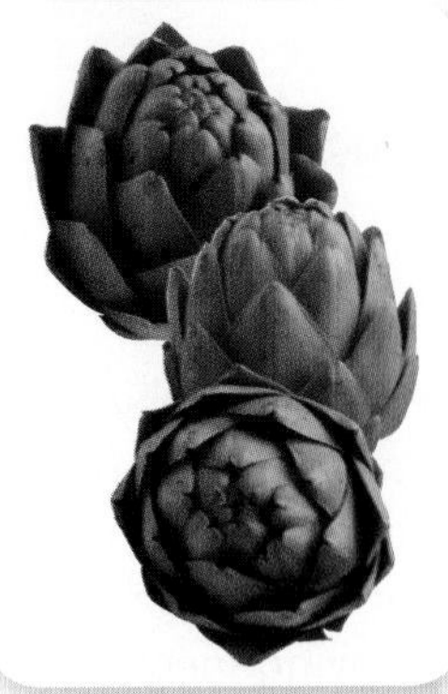

11. Vegetable Recipes There are thousands of vegetable recipes. You can let the plant part that you want to eat be your guide in choosing a recipe.

Procedure With your team, find a recipe that uses vegetables from the plant part assigned to you (for example, flower, stem, root, or bulb). Prepare the recipe.

Analysis Write answers to these questions: How did the plant part used in the recipe react to the cooking method? Did the other ingredients complement or compete with the vegetable? What changes might you make to this recipe? Do you think there is a better method for cooking this type of vegetable?

HEALTHFUL CHOICES

12. Snack Solution After school, Jackie usually reaches for unhealthy snacks, such as chips and cookies. "I would snack on vegetables," she says, "but it is never convenient to prepare them." What advice would you give Jackie to help her make healthier choices? How can Jackie prepare vegetables suitable for quick snacking?

TECH Connection

13. Nutrition Comparison Chart Using computer software, make a chart that compares the nutritional value of three of your favorite vegetables and three of your least favorite vegetables. Then evaluate the nutritional values of your favorite vegetables and determine what nutrients you are not getting from your favorite vegetables. Below the chart, summarize your conclusions in writing. Make suggestions for how you can add more variety to your eating plan to diversify your nutrient intake.

Real-World Skills

Problem-Solving Skills

14. A Suitable Substitute Dario is a vegetarian who avoids gelatin because it is an animal product. However, he wants to prepare an appealing recipe that calls for gelatin. What vegetable substitute can he use?

Interpersonal and Collaborative Skills

15. Puppet Play Follow your teacher's instructions to form groups. Work together to develop a puppet play for young children about the benefits of eating vegetables. Write the play and create the puppets. Perform the play for young children.

Financial Literacy Skills

16. Cost Comparison Visit a supermarket and conduct a cost comparison of fresh, canned, frozen, and dried forms of one type of vegetable. Which form is the least expensive? Why? Which form is the most expensive? Why? Report your findings and explain your insights in a paragraph.

Academic Skills

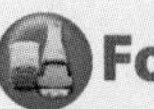

Food Science

17. Onions and Tears Cutting an onion can be a tearful experience because onions contain lacrimator, a chemical that causes the eyes to water.

Procedure Chill an onion for an hour in ice water. Then peel and dice it using a sharp knife. For comparison, peel and dice another onion without chilling. Was there a difference in the amount of irritation experienced?

Analysis How does chilling affect the onion's chemistry? Do you think the sharpness of the knife matters?

NSES B Develop an understanding of the structure and properties of matter.

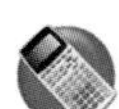

Mathematics

18. Using a Pressure Cooker Leslie does not eat artichokes as often as she would like because they take a long time to cook. As a solution, she purchased a pressure cooker that claims to cook vegetables 3½ times faster than regular cooking methods. If it typically takes Leslie about 40 minutes to cook an artichoke in boiling water, how long would it take in the pressure cooker?

Math Concept **Working with Time** To convert decimal minutes (such as 14.87) into minutes and seconds, keep the whole number portion (as minutes), and multiply the decimal portion by 60 (which represents the seconds).

Starting Hint Find the new cooking time by dividing 40 minutes by 3½. Convert the decimal portion into seconds by multiplying by 60. Round to the nearest second.

NCTM Problem Solving Build new mathematical knowledge through problem solving.

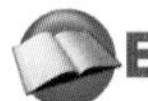

English Language Arts

19. Vegetable Exploration Use three different resources, including two books, to research one of the following topics: baby vegetables, starting a vegetable garden, or production and distribution of less familiar vegetables (for example, fiddlehead ferns, celeriac, broccoflower, fennel). Write an informative report based on your research. Remember to cite all the sources you use in your report. Include pictures or drawings in your report to illustrate your topic.

NCTE 8 Use information resources to gather information and create and communicate knowledge.

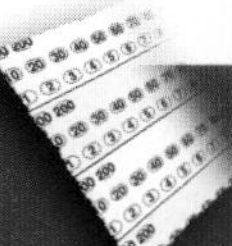

STANDARDIZED TEST PRACTICE

TRUE OR FALSE

Read the statement and determine if it is true or false.

20. Of the three convenience forms of vegetables, canned vegetables are closest in nutrients, color, and flavor to fresh vegetables.

a. True

b. False

Test-Taking Tip Before deciding whether a statement is true or false, read it carefully, and recall what you have learned from reading the text. Does the statement reflect what you know? Pay close attention to individual words. One word can make the difference between a true statement and a false one.

Grain Products

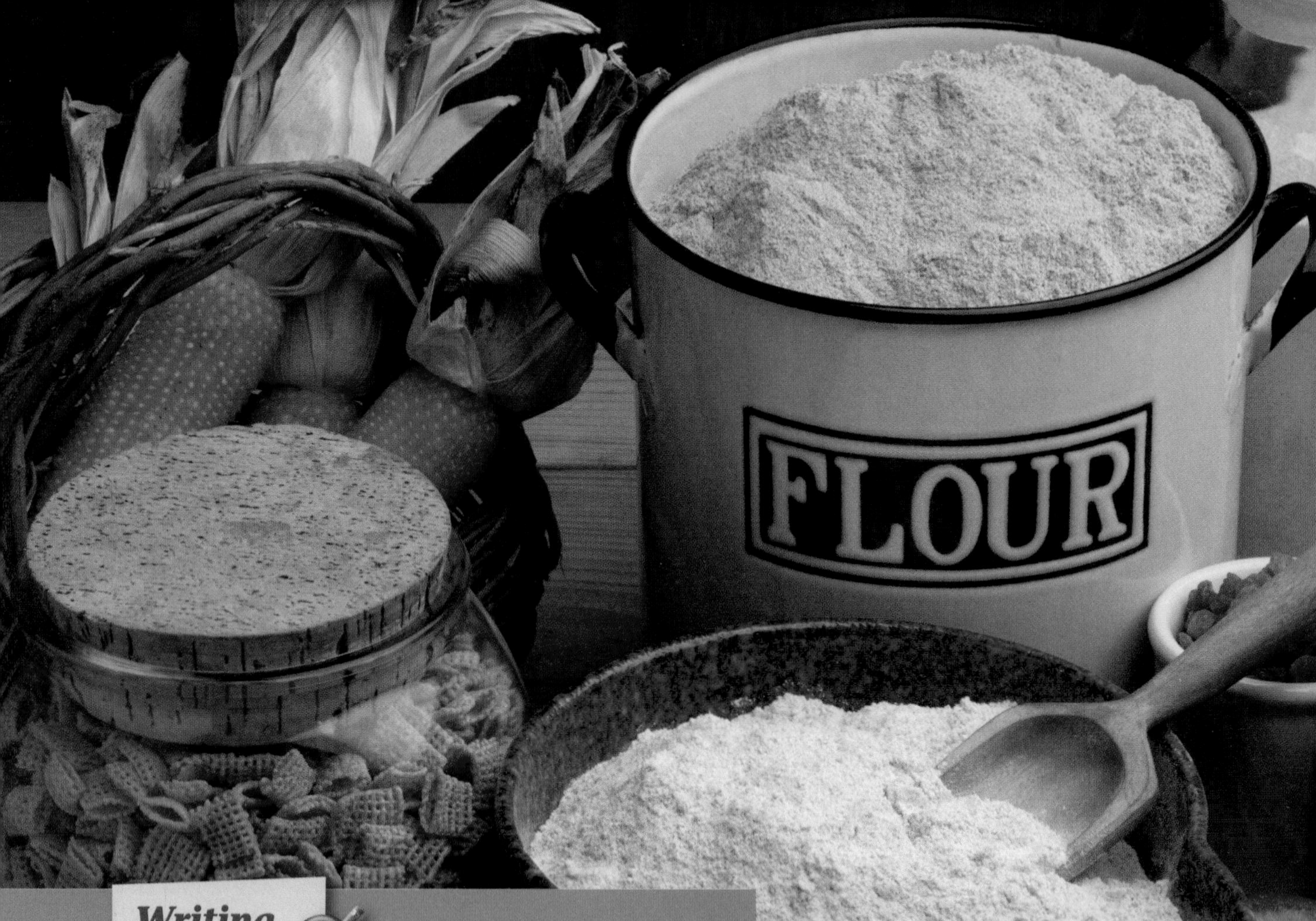

Writing Activity **Report**

Great Grains Chances are, grains play a significant role in your diet. What do you know about their flavors, forms, and uses? Choose a type of grain you like and write a report about it.

Writing Tips Follow these steps to write a report:

- Locate sources of information.
- Take notes on what you find.
- Organize the information into an introduction, a body, and a conclusion.

Activate Prior Knowledge

Popular Grains Pasta is just one of many grains. *What other grain foods can you name?*

Reading Guide

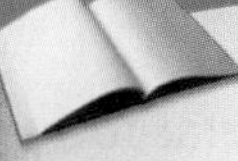

Before You Read

Preview Skim through the chapter, and examine the photos and figures. Think about how frequently you eat grains.

Read to Learn

Key Concepts

- **Describe** how food is made from grains.
- **Explain** how the processing of grains can affect their nutritional value.
- **Name** and describe six grains used around the world.
- **Explain** what to look for when buying grain products.
- **Describe** how to prepare grains for eating.

Main Idea

Grains are a versatile, nutritious, and flavorful addition to meals and an economical way to stretch a food budget.

Content Vocabulary

You will find definitions for these words in the glossary at the back of this book.

- ☐ grains
- ☐ kernels
- ☐ bran
- ☐ endosperm
- ☐ germ
- ☐ hull
- ☐ whole grain
- ☐ wheat
- ☐ rice
- ☐ pasta
- ☐ macaroni
- ☐ noodles
- ☐ leavened bread
- ☐ flatbread
- ☐ whole wheat
- ☐ al dente

Academic Vocabulary

You will find these words in your reading and on your tests. Use the glossary to look up their definitions if necessary.

- considerable
- translucent

Graphic Organizer

Use a graphic organizer like the one below to identify and briefly describe three common types of rice grains.

RICE GRAINS		

Graphic Organizer Go to this book's Online Learning Center at **glencoe.com** to print out this graphic organizer.

Academic Standards

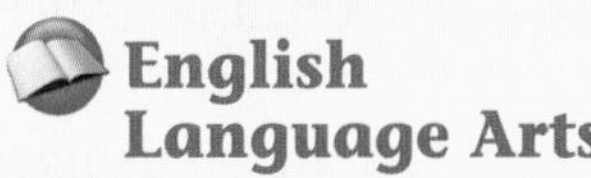

English Language Arts

NCTE 4 Use written language to communicate effectively.

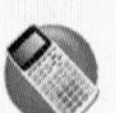

Mathematics

NCTM Algebra Represent and analyze mathematical situations and structures using algebraic symbols.

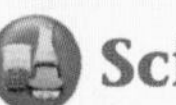

Science

NSES B Develop an understanding of the structure and properties of matter.

NCTE *National Council of Teachers of English*
NCTM *National Council of Teachers of Mathematics*
NSES *National Science Education Standards*
NCSS *National Council for the Social Studies*

Grain Sourcing and Harvesting

Few foods are as versatile as grains. Grains are a nutritious, flavorful addition to meals and an economical way to stretch a food budget.

Grains are plants in the grass family cultivated for their fruits or seeds. Common grains in North America include wheat, corn, rice, oats, rye, barley, buckwheat, and millet. Grains produce many small, separate dry fruits called **kernels**, which are harvested and processed for food. Because grain kernels are fruits, grains are sometimes called berries, as in wheat berries.

Every grain kernel has three main parts. The **bran** is the edible, outer layer of the kernel. The **endosperm** is the largest part of the kernel, which is made of proteins and starches that supply the plant with food. The **germ** is the seed that grows into a new plant. Some grains are covered with an inedible outer coat called the **hull**, which is removed after harvesting. **Figure 30.1** shows the parts of a grain kernel without a hull.

Grains are processed into several forms for different uses. For example, oats are rolled and flaked for use in hot cereals and cookies and ground into flour.

✓ **Reading Check** **Identify** What are the three main parts of a grain kernel?

Nutrients in Grains

Whole grains are rich in nutrients. The endosperm consists mostly of complex carbohydrates and proteins. The bran contains dietary fiber, B vitamins, and minerals. The germ provides protein, unsaturated fats, B vitamins, vitamin E, iron, and zinc, as well as other minerals and phytochemicals.

Figure 30.1 **Parts of a Grain Kernel**

Three Parts A grain kernel has three main parts. All three parts are used to make whole-grain products. The parts are separated and used individually to make other grain products. ***Which part of the kernel contains the plant's food supply?***

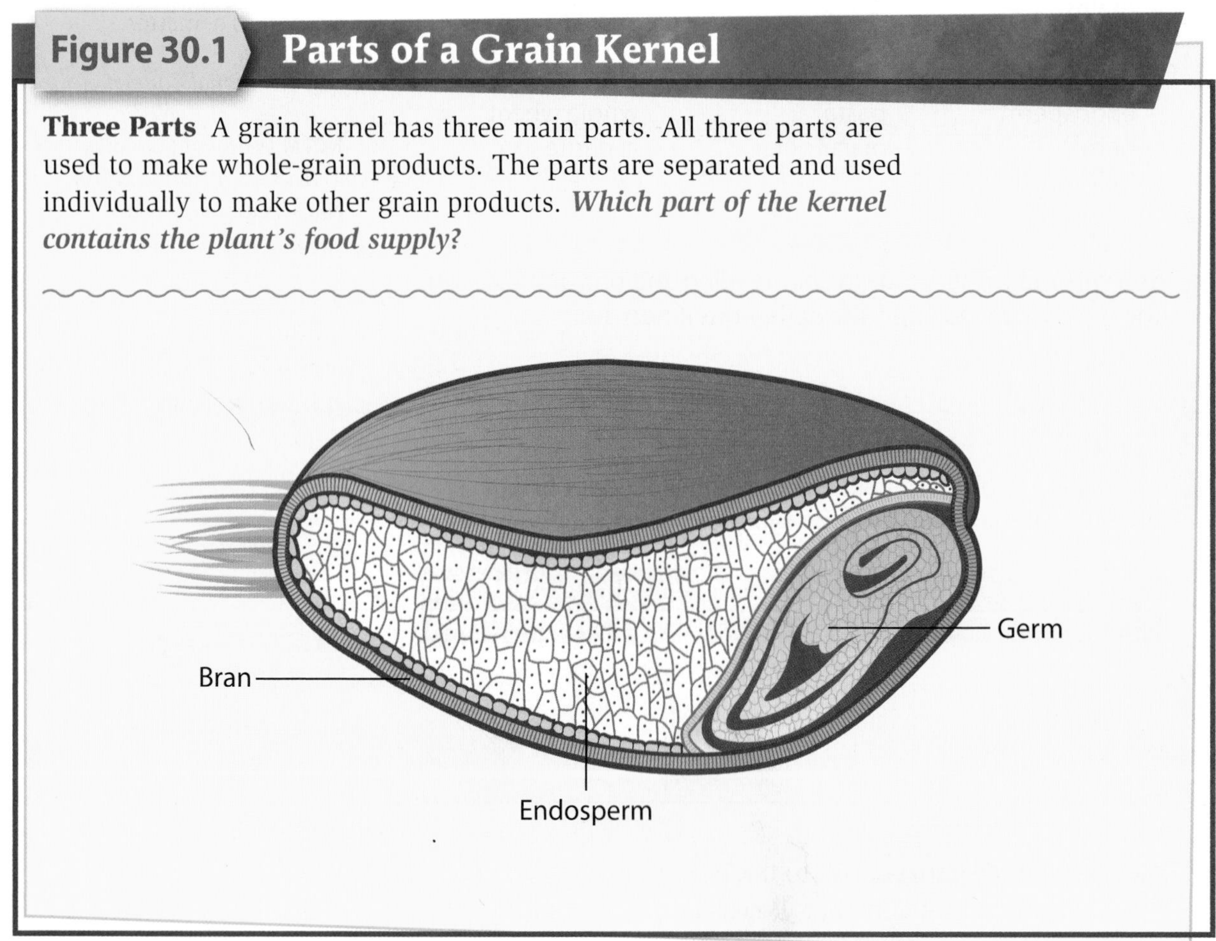

All grains must be processed before you eat them. The type of processing affects a grain's nutrient value. **Whole-grain** products, including whole-wheat flour and whole-grain breakfast cereals, are made of the entire kernel and so contain most of the original nutrients.

Grains' bran and germ are often removed during processing, leaving only the endosperm. White flour and many breakfast cereals are made this way. Removing the bran and germ removes most of the vitamins, minerals, phytochemicals, and dietary fiber. According to federal law, some of nutrients lost in processing must be replaced. Replacing nutrients lost through processing is called enrichment. Some grain products are also fortified with nutrients such as iron to make them more nutritious.

✓ **Reading Check** **Define** What is a whole-grain product?

Nutrition Check

Daily Grain Needs

The foundation of a healthy diet, grains make up the biggest portion of MyPyramid. On a 2,000-calorie diet, a person needs 6 ounces of grains each day. Half of these should be whole grains. The following servings equal one ounce: ½ cup of cooked rice, pasta, or cooked cereal, 1 ounce of dry pasta or rice, 1 slice of bread, 1 small muffin, or 1 cup of ready-to-eat cereal flakes.

Think About It What do you think is the reason behind MyPyramid's advice to make half of the grains you eat each day be whole grains?

Grains and Grain Products

Grains can be prepared in many different ways:

- Served plain or topped with vegetables, seasonings, and sauces.
- Used in side dishes, casseroles, soups, and baked goods.
- Added to soups and stews to thicken them.
- Cooked and eaten hot as breakfast cereals.
- Cooked into desserts by adding sweeteners or fruits.

Most meals include at least one grain. If you eat oatmeal for breakfast, a sandwich on wheat bread for lunch, and rice for dinner, you have eaten three different grains in three different ways.

Wheat

Wheat is one of the oldest cereal grains. Thousands of wheat varieties exist. Most bread and pasta is made with wheat. Other grain products made from wheat or other grains include:

Wheat Berries Wheat berries are the entire wheat kernel, including the bran and germ. Wheat berries are very chewy and can be cooked as a cereal or used in grain dishes.

Buckwheat Buckwheat is the seed of a non-grass plant that is used like a grain. It has a nutlike, earthy flavor and is high in protein and other nutrients. Buckwheat is often ground into flour or crushed and used as breakfast cereal. Buckwheat flour makes tasty pancakes.

Bulgur Bulgur is wheat kernels that have been steamed, dried, and crushed. Bulgur is tender and has a chewy texture. It is used in main dishes, in salads, and as a side dish. It is also used in baked goods and as stuffing. Bulgur is the main ingredient in tabbouleh, a Middle Eastern salad with chopped tomatoes, onions, parsley, mint, lemon juice, and olive oil.

Couscous (ˈküs-,küs) Couscous is the steamed, cracked endosperm of durum wheat. It is a staple in North African cuisines. Couscous has a flavor similar to pasta and is used as a cereal, in salads and main dishes, or sweetened for dessert. It is traditionally served under a meat or vegetable stew.

Cracked Wheat Cracked wheat is made from crushed wheat berries. Cracked wheat is debranned during processing. Cracked wheat has a tough, chewy texture and is often added to bread.

Kasha (ˈkä-shə) Kasha is hulled, roasted, and crushed buckwheat. It is used extensively in Eastern European, Middle Eastern, and Asian cuisines. Kasha has a pleasant, nutty flavor and is used in the United States as a breakfast cereal or a side dish.

Quinoa (ˈkēn-ˌwä) Quinoa is a small, ivory-colored, rice-like grain that has more protein than any other grain which makes it a popular staple with vegeterians. Quinoa is also gluten free, which makes it a popular grain with people allergic to gluten. It is popular in South American cuisines and was a staple of the Incas. Quinoa cooks quickly and has a unique, mild flavor. It is used as a side dish and in soups, puddings, and salads.

Spelt Spelt is a type of wheat that has been used for thousands of years in southern Europe. Spelt has a mellow, nutty flavor, and spelt flour can be substituted for wheat flour in baking. Spelt also is used in pasta. Spelt is sometimes tolerated by people who have wheat allergies.

Triticale (ˌtri-tə-ˈkā-lē) Triticale is a cross between wheat and rye, with more protein than wheat. It can be used in cereals and main dishes and combined with other cooked grains.

Rice

Rice is the starchy seed of plants grown in flooded fields in warm climates. Much of the world's rice grows in Asian paddies, or wetlands, but some is grown in parts of the United States.

Types of Rice Grains

Rice is often described by the length of its grain. Each type of rice has a different purpose.

Long-Grain Rice Long-grain rice is the most popular rice in the United States. When cooked, the grains are fluffy and stay separated. Long-grain rice hardens when it cools, so it does not work well for puddings and cold salads. It is often used as a side dish. Basmati (ˌbäz-ˈmä-tē) rice is a long-grain rice with a fine texture and a nutlike aroma and flavor.

Medium-Grain Rice Medium-grain rice is plump, tender, and moist. The grains of medium-grain rice stick together, but not as much as the grains of short-grain rice do. Medium-grain rice works well for puddings and cold salads.

Short-Grain Rice The grains of short-grain rice are almost round, and they have the highest starch content of the three types of rice. When cooked, the grains are moist and stick together. Short-grain rice is usually used for creamy dishes and molded rice rings. Asian cuisine uses short-grain rice because it is easy to pick up with chopsticks. Italian arborio (ˌär-ˈbȯr-ē-ō) rice is a short-grain rice used to make risotto (ri-ˈsȯ-(ˌ)tō), a creamy rice dish.

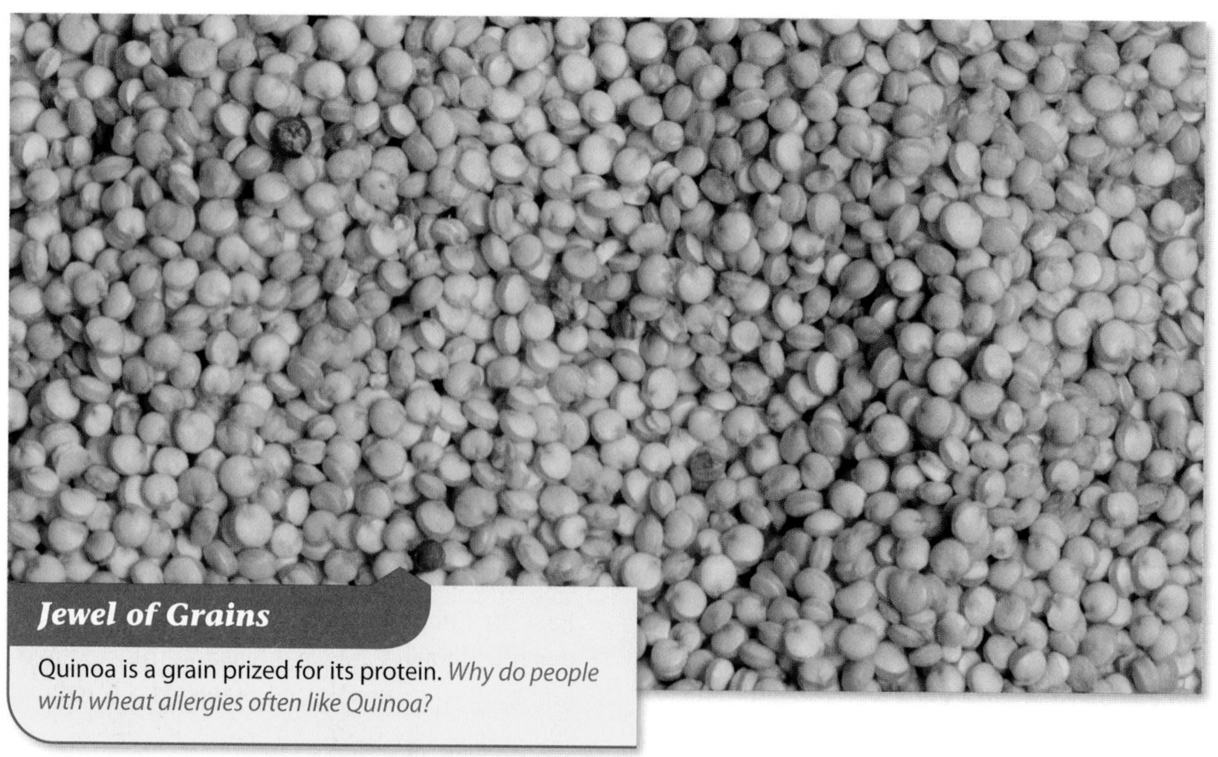

Jewel of Grains

Quinoa is a grain prized for its protein. *Why do people with wheat allergies often like Quinoa?*

Rice Processing

Rice is processed in several different ways, yielding products with different colors, textures, and nutritional values.

Enriched Rice Enriched, or white, rice has its bran and germ removed, leaving only the endosperm. White rice loses some of the nutrients, phytochemicals, and dietary fiber found in brown rice when it is processed.

Brown Rice Brown rice is the whole-grain form of rice. Only the hull has been removed. The bran, endosperm, and germ remain, along with all the nutrients and dietary fiber. Brown rice takes longer to cook than white rice and has a nutlike flavor and chewy texture. Brown rice and white rice have similar amounts of calories, carbohydrates, fat, and protein. Brown rice should not be stored for more than six months.

Converted Rice Converted rice is steamed under pressure to save nutrients before the hull is removed. It takes longer to cook than white rice but it has more nutrients than white rice because it is enriched.

Instant Rice Instant rice is precooked and dehydrated before packaging. It takes only a few minutes to prepare, but it is not as nutritious as rice that takes longer to cook.

Corn

Corn is the most popular food plant in the world and the most widely grown crop in the United States. As far back as 3500 BCE, people were raising corn in Central America. Today the corn plant is also used for many purposes other than food, including making plastics, dyes, and ethanol fuel.

Corn is popular as a vegetable, on the cob or as kernels. Hominy is the dried kernel with the hull and germ removed, leaving only the endosperm. When hominy is coarsely ground, it becomes grits, which can be served as a side dish or used in casseroles. Cornmeal, which is used to make cornbread, comes from ground, dried, corn kernels. Cornmeal is also used to make polenta. The endosperm of corn is also ground into a fine flour called cornstarch, which is used as a thickener in sauces and fillings.

Be a Smart Consumer

Adding Oats

Inexpensive and easy to find, oats have uses that go beyond breakfast cereal and granola. Grind rolled oats in a food processor to make oat flour. Use oat flour to replace up to one-quarter of the wheat flour in recipes for baked goods. Coat foods with oat flour or oatmeal before baking or pan-frying. Toast oats to give them a nutty taste and crunchy texture and make a fat-free alternative to nuts and seeds. Use oat groats, also called Scotch oats or Irish oatmeal, instead of rice or barley in stuffing, stews, or casseroles.

Challenge Find a recipe in which you can substitute oats for another grain. In a paragraph, explain how you think oats would change the flavor, texture, or appearance of the recipe.

Oats

Oats have a pleasant, slightly sweet flavor. Most of the oat grain produced in the world is used to feed livestock. In North America, oats are usually eaten as a hot breakfast cereal or used in baked goods. Oats contain **considerable**, or large, amounts of nutrients and dietary fiber. Quick-cooking oats and oatmeal are available.

Other Grains

Wheat, rice, corn, and oats are the most popular grains in North America. However, many other grains are used around the world.

Amaranth (ˈa-mə-ˌran(t)h) These tiny round seeds that get thick and sticky when cooked were the staple crop of the Aztecs. Amaranth has a sweet, nutty flavor, and it can be used as a hot cereal, as a side dish, or in puddings.

Barley Unlike other grains, the entire kernel of barley contains dietary fiber. Barley is one of the most ancient grains and a staple in Asia, the Middle East, and parts of Europe. Barley is mild-flavored and chewy and is usually used in soups and stews. Hulled barley lacks the outer hull but has the bran, so it has more dietary fiber than other types of barley. Pearl barley,

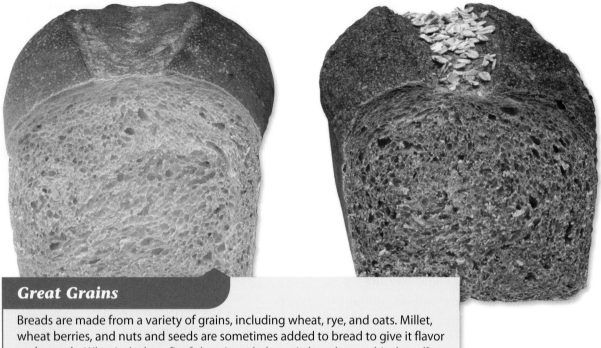

Great Grains

Breads are made from a variety of grains, including wheat, rye, and oats. Millet, wheat berries, and nuts and seeds are sometimes added to bread to give it flavor and crunch. *What is the benefit of choosing whole-grain bread over white bread?*

the most common form sold in supermarkets, lacks the outer hull and bran, but still contains half of the original fiber. Scotch (or pot) barley is less processed than pearl barley and is used in salads, soups, and casseroles.

Millet These small, round, yellow grains are a staple in Europe, Asia, and North Africa. Millet has a mild flavor and is used in breads and as a breakfast cereal or side dish. Millet porridge is a traditional Russian food.

Rye Often used in breads and crackers, rye is a dark grain with a hearty flavor. It is less nutritious than other grains but is high in minerals. Rye is popular in northern Europe.

Teff Available in brown and white varieties, teff is a tiny grain with a mild, nutty flavor. It is native to North Africa and has been a staple in Ethiopian cuisine for thousands of years. Teff is used in flatbread, as a cooked cereal, and in puddings.

Wild Rice Not a rice at all, wild rice is actually the seed of a water grass. Wild rice has a crisp texture and nutlike flavor, and it is high in protein and dietary fiber. The supply of wild rice is limited, which makes it very expensive. Wild rice is often sold combined with long-grain rice.

Pasta

Pasta is an Italian word meaning "paste" that refers to dough made from flour and water. Pasta includes **macaroni**, which is made from durum (ˈdu̇r-əm) wheat flour and water, and **noodles**, which have egg solids added for tenderness.

Durum wheat is grown especially for pasta. It is processed into semolina (ˌse-mə-ˈlē-nə) flour, which gives pasta its characteristic yellow color and nutlike flavor. Durum wheat products hold their shape and firm texture when cooked.

Pasta dough is rolled thin and then formed by machines into hundreds of different shapes. **Figure 30.2** shows some common pasta shapes. Certain sauces go best with specific shapes. For instance, smooth tomato sauces, cream sauces, and sauces with small pieces of food complement long, flat pasta. Large, hollow shapes are usually stuffed with a meat, vegetable, fish, or cheese mixture and baked in a sauce.

Pasta is sold in both dried and fresh forms. Dried pasta is the more common form. Packages of dried pasta are found with other shelf-stable foods. Fresh pasta is perishable and is found in the refrigerated section.

Figure 30.2 Common Types of Pasta

Shapes and Sizes Pasta shapes are both functional and decorative. Larger shapes work well for baking, while smaller shapes are versatile for sauces, soups, salads, and casseroles. ***Which of these pasta shapes work well in pasta salads? Why?***

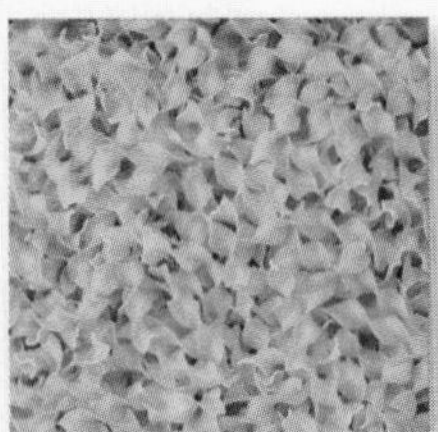

Egg Noodles
Egg noodles have egg solids added for tenderness.

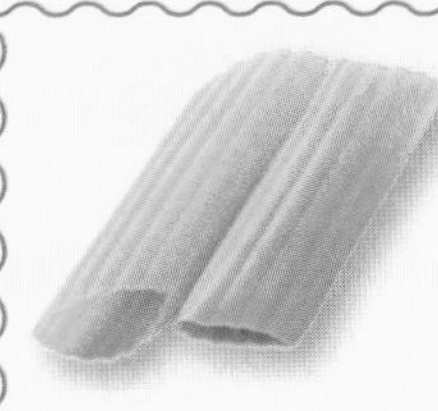

Manicotti
(ˌma-nə-ˈkä-tē) Large tube-shaped pasta, usually stuffed.

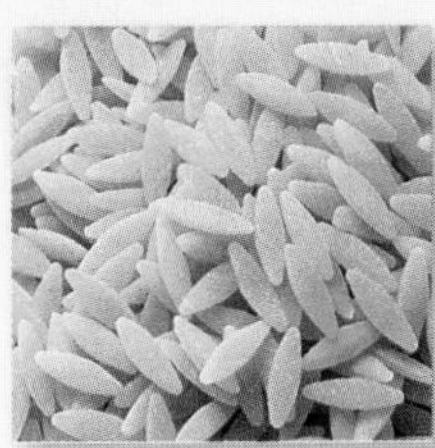

Orzo
(ˈȯrd-(ˌ)zō) Small, rice-shaped pasta, good for salads and soups.

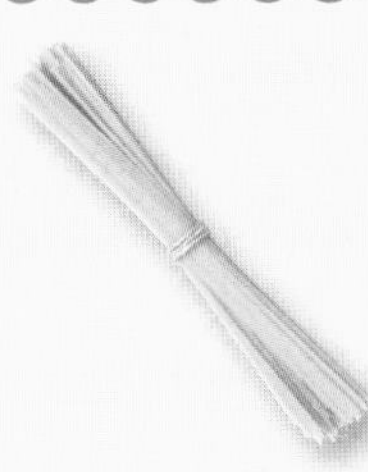

Linguine
(liŋ-ˈgwē-nē) Long, narrow, flat pasta. Holds sauces well.

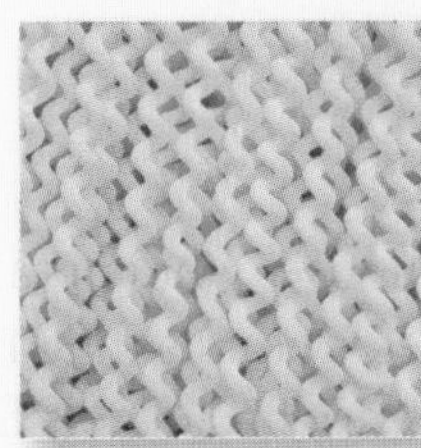

Fusilli
(fyü-ˈsi-lē) Corkscrew pasta. Holds smooth sauces well and works well in salads.

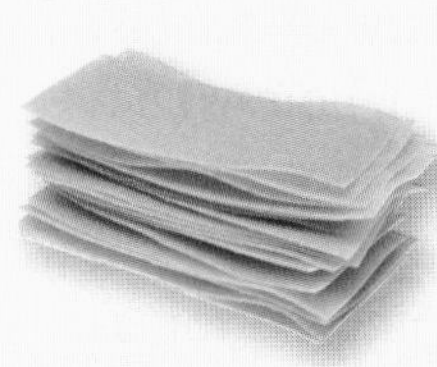

Lasagne
(lə-ˈzän-yə) Wide, flat noodles, usually baked with sauce.

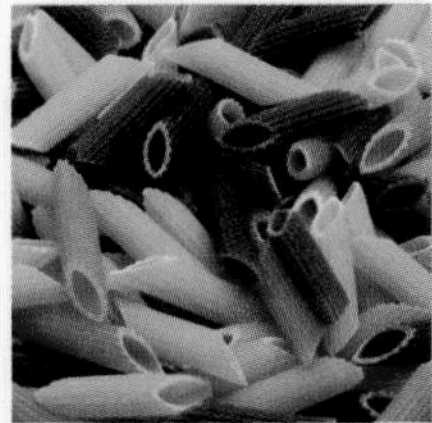

Penne
(ˈpe(n)-(ˌ)nā) Straight tube-shaped pasta cut diagonally on the ends. Works well with most sauces and in baked dishes.

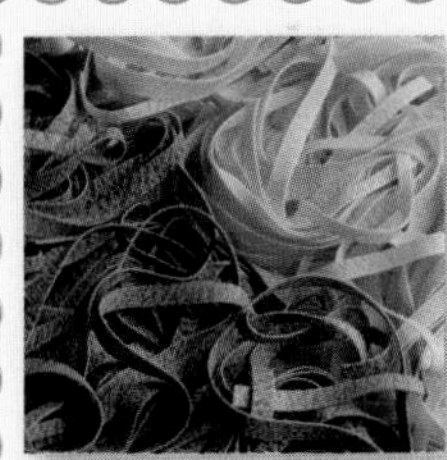

Fettuccine
(ˌfe-tə-ˈchē-nē) Long, flat pasta, wider than linguine. Holds sauces well.

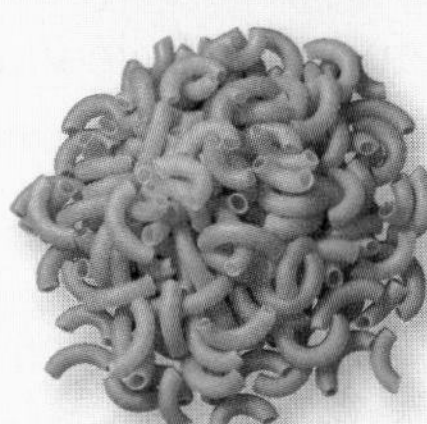

Elbow Macaroni
Small, curved tube-shaped pasta. Works well in soups, salads, and baked dishes.

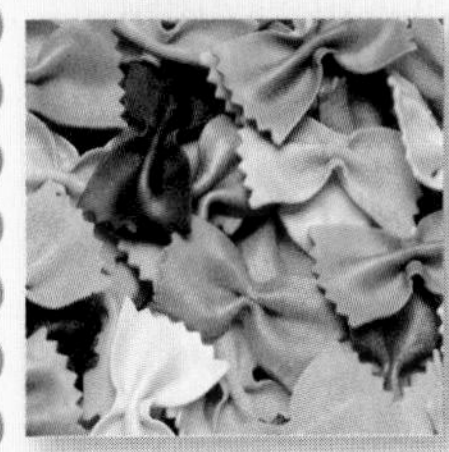

Farfalle
(fär-ˈfä-(ˌ)lā) Bowtie pasta. Works well with sauces and in pasta salads.

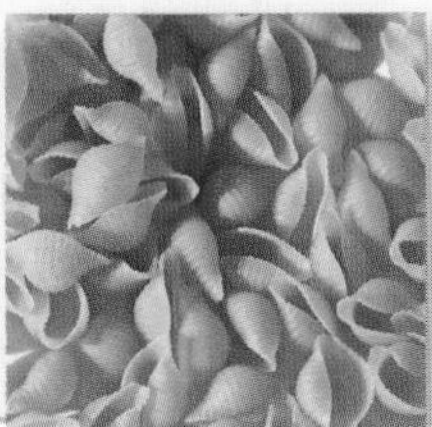

Conchiglie
(kon-ˈkēl-yā) Seashell pasta. Holds sauce well.

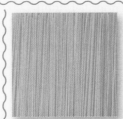

Spaghetti
Long, thin round pasta. Angel hair is thin spaghetti.

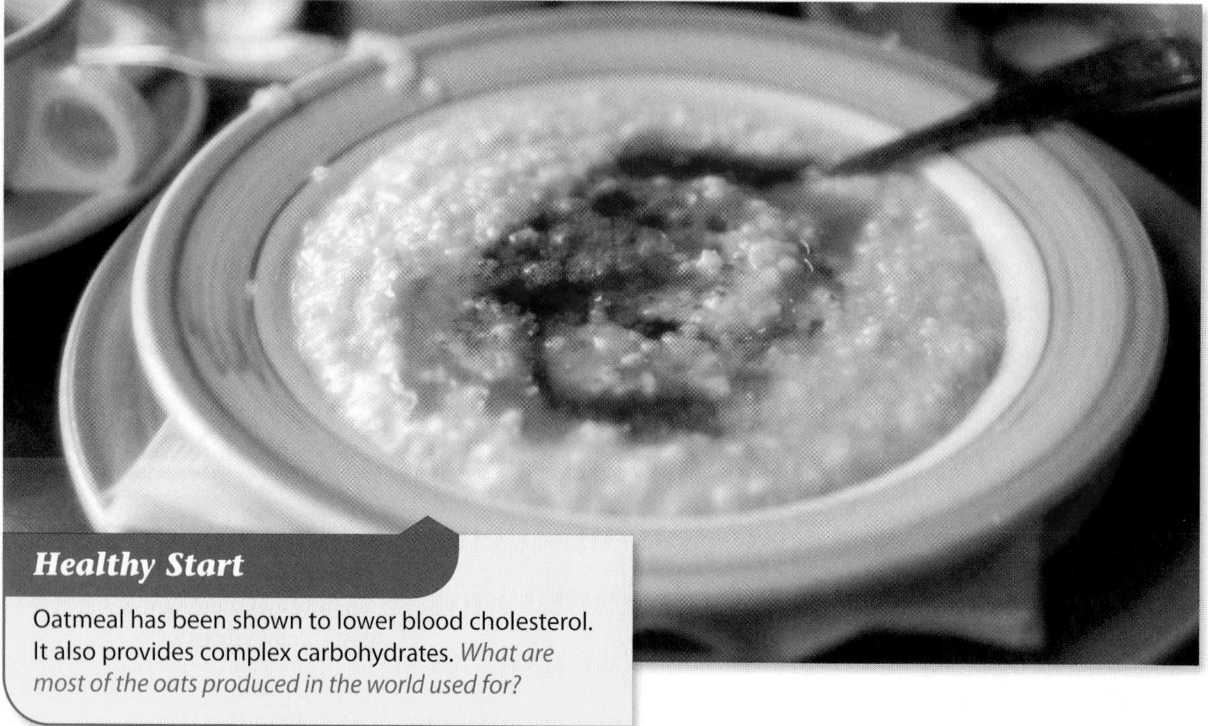

Healthy Start

Oatmeal has been shown to lower blood cholesterol. It also provides complex carbohydrates. *What are most of the oats produced in the world used for?*

You can choose from a variety of pastas, including enriched, flavored, and whole-wheat pastas. Whole-wheat pasta has more dietary fiber than enriched pasta. Some pastas are blended with herbs, carrots, spinach, tomatoes, and other foods for flavor and color.

Asian Noodles

Asian noodles are similar in texture to pasta but are made from different flours, such as rice, potato, cornstarch, bean, and soy. Most Asian noodles are made without eggs. Chinese cellophane noodles, for instance, are thin, **translucent** noodles made from mung-bean starch. Translucent means almost transparent. The Chinese are fond of wheat noodles, which they use in soups, and wheat and egg noodles, which they use in stir-fries and chow mein, their famous fried noodle dish. The Japanese like to serve noodles in soups and salads. Kishimen, udon, hiyamugi, ramen, chuka soba, and somen are all wheat noodles, while soba is made from buckwheat, shirataki from yams, and harusame from mung bean or other starches. Pad Thai, the national dish of Thailand, is made with stir fried rice noodles.

✓ Reading Check **Identify** Which type of rice contains the whole grain?

Buying and Storing Grains

When buying grains, choose whole-grain products as often as possible. Products that are not whole grain should be enriched. Look for products that are low in fat, sugar, and sodium, and try different grains for variety and nutrition. Read the label carefully to be sure you are getting the product you want.

Fresh Pasta and Whole Grains

When buying pasta and whole grains, inspect the product carefully. Whole-grain kernels should be plump and uniform in size and color, and pasta should not be cracked or broken.

Refrigerate fresh pasta, whole grains, and whole-grain products. Because whole-grain products contain oil, they can spoil at room temperature if not used quickly. Store other uncooked grains and grain products, such as white rice and dried pasta, in a cool, dry place in tightly covered containers. Refrigerate cooked grains if you plan to use them within a few days, or freeze them for longer storage.

Convenience Forms of Grains

Convenience forms of grain products, such as cereals and breads, make preparation of grain dishes quick and easy. Read the Nutrition Facts panels and compare products to make sure you are getting a good nutrition value.

Breakfast Cereals

Wheat, oats, and corn are made into many different breakfast cereals. Breakfast cereals may consist of whole grains, refined and enriched grains, or both. Dry breakfast cereals are ready to eat out of the container. Other cereals, such as oatmeal, need to be cooked first.

Ready-to-eat cereals come in puffed, rolled, flaked, granulated, and shredded types. Some are coated with sugar or other sweeteners, and they may have fruit, nuts, and other flavorings added. Breakfast cereals do not need to be refrigerated. Keep them in a cool, dry place.

Oats and other cereals that require cooking come in regular, quick-cooking, and instant forms. Some have sugar and other flavorings added. Instant cereal is usually precooked, so all you need to do is mix it with boiling water.

You do not need a cereal that provides 100 percent of the recommended daily requirement for fiber, vitamins, or minerals, because you will also get these nutrients from other foods you eat. Cereals that are highly fortified often cost more than other cereal as well.

Breads

Breads, rolls, and buns are made from enriched white flour, whole wheat, and mixed whole grains. **Leavened bread** (ˈle-vənd) is bread made with a leavening agent, such as yeast or baking powder, which makes the bread rise. **Flatbread** is any bread that is unleavened, or made without leavenings. Tortillas, naan, lavash, and pita bread are types of flatbread.

Read the label carefully when choosing bread. **Whole wheat** means that the product is made from the whole wheat grain. 'Wheat' on a bread package means that the product is made from white flour. Look for bread that has at least 2 to 3 grams per serving.

A bread's color is not always a clue to its nutritional value. Pumpernickel bread, for example, is made with white and rye flour and then colored with caramel or molasses. Words such as multigrain, cracked wheat, and 7-grain also do not tell you very much about a bread's nutritional value. Unless the label lists whole wheat or another whole grain first, the bread is made mostly of white flours.

Store bread in a cool, dry place. Refrigerating bread can cause it to turn stale more quickly. In humid weather, however, refrigerating bread keeps mold from growing. If you need to keep bread for more than a few days, freeze it in a freezer-safe container.

✓ Reading Check **Explain** Why should you refrigerate whole-grain products?

Figure 30.3 Dried Pasta Yields

Pasta Portions Pasta expands in size as it cooks because it absorbs water. One cup of cooked pasta is considered a typical portion. ***About how many ounces of small dry pasta shapes do you need to make one cup of cooked pasta?***

Type of Pasta	Dry Weight	Dry Volume	Cooked Yield (approximate)
Small pasta shapes: macaroni, shells, spirals, twists	4 ounces	1 cup	2½ cups
Long, slender pasta strands: spaghetti, angel hair, vermicelli	4 ounces	1-inch-diameter bunch	2 cups

Preparing Grains and Grain Products

Grains must be cooked in liquid. Grains are full of complex carbohydrates, also known as starches. Starch granules have many layers of tightly packed molecules. When you heat a grain in water, the molecules start moving, the chemical bonds break, and the tight layers loosen. This lets water enter the starch, causing it to become softer and swell.

Cooking methods and times vary depending on the type of grain product you are using. Always follow package or recipe directions.

Grains are one of the few foods that do not cook faster in the microwave. Grains need time to absorb liquid and soften, so microwaving does not usually save time.

Cooking Pasta

Pasta must be boiled. Boiling helps circulate the pasta for even cooking and prevents pieces from sticking together. Package directions tell how much water to use for a particular serving size of pasta. For example, dry spaghetti takes about 1 quart of water for every 4 ounces of spaghetti. Choose a pot large enough to keep the water from boiling over. **Figure 30.3** on page 477 shows the cooked yields of dried pasta.

To cook pasta, boil the water first. Then add the pasta slowly so that the water continues to boil. If boiling stops, the pasta will stick together. Stir the pasta occasionally as it cooks to keep it from sticking. Do not add oil to the cooking water. Oil forms a slippery surface layer that keeps sauce from clinging to pasta.

Dried pasta is generally cooked al dente. To cook **al dente** (äl-den-(ˌ)tā) is to cook so that the pasta is firm to the bite, rather than soft and mushy. The cooking time of pasta varies. Dried angel hair pasta, a very thin form of spaghetti, can cook in as little as one minute. Large, thick pasta shapes may take up to 20 minutes to cook. If you plan to add the pasta to a dish that will cook longer, such as lasagne, reduce the boiling time to keep the pasta slightly firmer. Fresh pasta cooks much more quickly than dried pasta. The best way to tell if pasta is done is to taste it.

After cooking, drain the pasta in a colander or strainer. Do not rinse cooked pasta, because rinsing removes nutrients. To keep cooked pasta hot, set the colander or strainer over a pan of hot water, and cover. For best results plan to have the pasta finished just as you are ready to serve it.

You can freeze leftover cooked pasta by itself, but it freezes best with a sauce. Freeze in serving-size portions.

Figure 30.4 Cooking Grains

Cooking Times and Yields Some grains need more liquid to cook than others. ***What should you do if liquid is still left in the pan near the end of the cooking time?***

Grain (1 cup dry)	Liquid	Cooking Time	Yield (approximate)
Barley, pearl	3 cups	40 minutes	3 cups
Bulgur	2 cups	30 minutes of standing time	2½ cups
Cornmeal	4 cups	25 minutes	3 cups
Grits (regular)	4 cups	25 minutes	3 cups
Kasha	2 cups	20 minutes	2½ cups
Millet	2½ to 3 cups	35 to 40 minutes	3½ cups
Rice, brown (long grain)	2½ cups	45 minutes	3 cups
Rice, white (long or medium grain)	2 cups	15 minutes	3 cups

Nutrient-Rich Rice

Brown rice takes longer to cook than white rice but has more nutrients, including fiber, vitamins, and minerals. *What is similar about enriched rice and converted rice? What is different?*

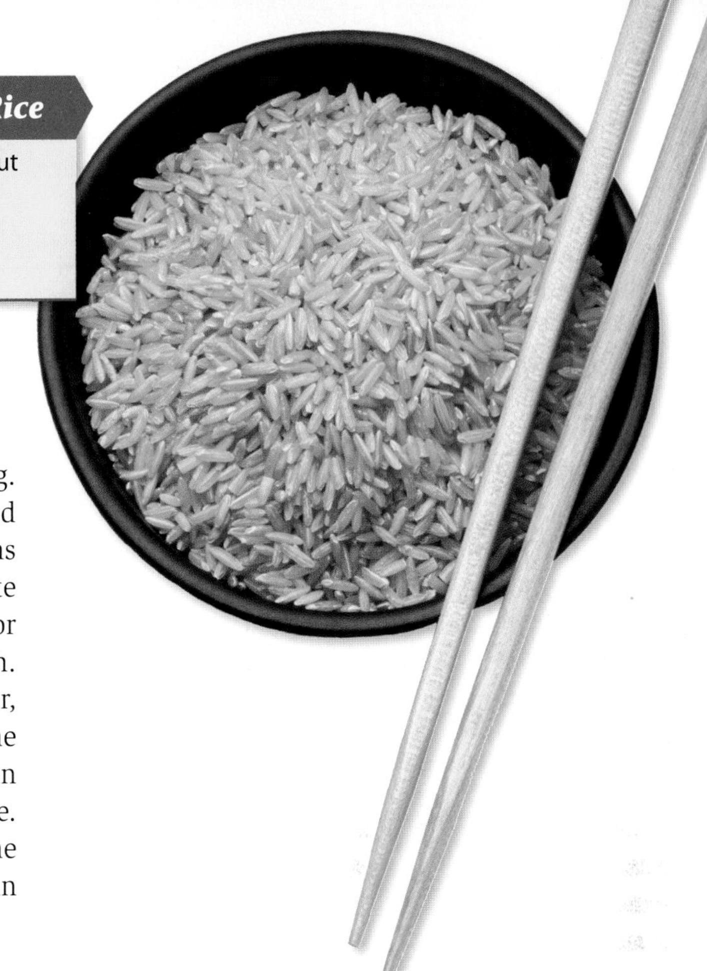

Cooking Rice

Rice is usually cooked by simmering. **Figure 30.4** shows how much liquid you need to cook 1 cup of different types of grain, as well as the cooking time and approximate yield. You can use water or add extra flavor to rice by cooking it in milk, juice, or broth. Bring the liquid to a boil. Add the rice, cover, and bring to a boil again. Then reduce the heat so the rice simmers gently. Keep the pan covered and stir the rice as little as possible. Stirring scrapes off the starch and makes the rice sticky. Brown rice needs more liquid than white rice, and takes longer to cook.

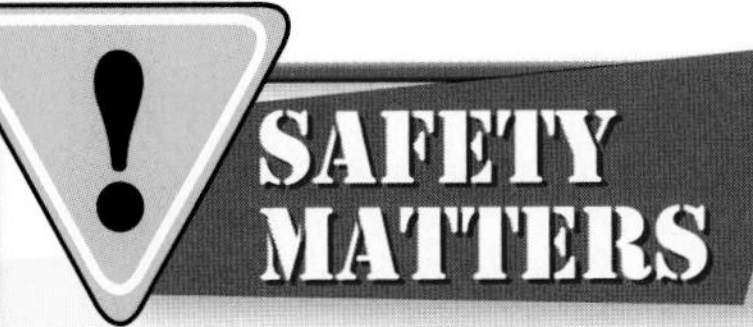

To Rinse or Not to Rinse

Some cookbooks direct you to rinse rice. Others state rice should not be rinsed. This is because rice grown in Asia has to travel a great distance to get to your store. When it is packed for transport, it sometimes is packed with talc, a fine powder that is not edible. Even if it is not packed with talc, it could pick up impurities on the way. Rice grown in the U.S. does not have the same problem. Rinsing clean rice removes some of the starch and other nutrients that make rice a good food choice. Rinse any rice you have not used before. When you add water to rinse the rice, look at the water. If it stays clear, the rice does not need to be rinsed.

What Would You Do? Bob eats a lot of rice. Because of the large discount he was able to get, Bob purchased a 50-pound bag of rice online. It arrived in a burlap bag. Should Bob rinse his rice before cooking?

Near the end of the cooking time, check the rice for doneness. It should be moist and tender but firm, with no liquid left in the pot. If any liquid remains, remove the lid and continue cooking until the liquid is absorbed or evaporates. Undercooked rice is hard and gritty. Overcooked rice is soft and sticky. To cook converted and instant rice, follow the directions on the package.

If you plan to use cooked rice in a recipe that needs further cooking, undercook the rice slightly. This prevents it from getting mushy.

Keep rice warm by placing it in a colander and setting the colander over a pan of simmering water. Cover the pan to allow the steam to warm the rice without making it sticky. You can also reheat rice using this method.

Refrigerate leftover rice immediately and use it within a few days. You can also freeze it for longer storage. To reheat rice, add 2 tablespoons of water for each cup of cooked rice, then microwave it or reheat it on top of the range.

Cooking Other Grains

Barley, grits, kasha, and many other grains are cooked in much the same way as rice: Boil the water, add the grain, cover, and bring to a boil again. Reduce the heat so the grain simmers gently. The cooking time varies from 20 to 45 minutes, depending on the grain.

Stir grains occasionally during cooking to keep them from sticking, lumping, or scorching. Do not over-stir, however, because they will turn gummy and pasty. Grains are usually chewy if not cooked long enough and sticky if overcooked. Most grains have a delicate flavor, so only a little seasoning is needed.

Bulgur requires a different preparation method: Pour boiling water on the dry grain and let it stand for 30 minutes.

Preparing Convenience Forms of Grains

Instant forms of grains take less time to cook than regular forms, and they can be served in the same ways. Instant forms may have more sodium than regular forms, so check labels carefully.

Both dry and hot breakfast cereals can be a tasty and nutritious way to start your day. Dry cereals are ready to eat. You can add milk, yogurt, soy, or rice milk. You can also add fresh or dried fruit for flavor and nutrition. Some dry cereals add more sugar than others so read nutrition facts labels carefully. To prepare instant hot breakfast cereals, follow the package directions. Usually, you just add boiling water and stir.

Light and Healthy Recipe

Wheat Germ Pancakes

Wheat germ adds folate, iron and zinc into these pancakes. It also gives them a smoky flavor.

Ingredients

- **2 cups** All-purpose flour
- **½ cup** Whole wheat flour
- **3 Tbsp.** Sugar
- **2 tsp.** Baking powder
- **1 tsp.** Baking soda
- **1** Egg
- **½ cup** Toasted wheat germ
- **2 cups** Lowfat buttermilk
- **1 Tbsp.** Canola oil
- **6 oz.** Maple syrup

Directions

1. Combine the flours, wheat germ, sugar, baking powder and baking soda in a large mixing bowl.
2. In another bowl, beat the egg and mix it with the buttermilk. Add the wet ingredients to the dry ingredients and combine.
3. Heat a little of the oil on medium heat in a skillet or large pan and pour the batter into the pan to make pancakes. Adjust the amount of batter to make the size of pancake you want.
4. When pancakes start to bubble on top, flip them over with a spatula.
5. Repeat until all batter is used.
6. Serve with maple syrup.

Yield 6 Servings

Nutrition Analysis per Serving

■ Calories	408
■ Total fat	6 g
Saturated fat	1 g
Cholesterol	43 mg
■ Sodium	476 mg
■ Carbohydrate	80 g
Dietary fiber	4 g
Sugars	33 g
■ Protein	12 g

CHAPTER 30 Review & Applications

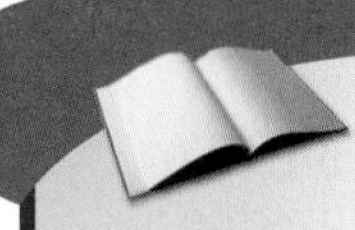

After You Read

Chapter Summary

Grains are a versatile, nutritious, flavorful addition to meals. They provide many nutrients. Wheat, rice, corn, and oats are popular grains in North America, but many other grains are used around the world. Buy whole-grain products as often as possible. Store grains properly to maintain their freshness. Convenience forms of grains make preparation of grain dishes easy. Grains must be cooked in liquid, but specific cooking methods and times vary. Pasta is boiled, rice is simmered, and other grains are cooked much like rice. Convenience forms of grains take less time to cook than regular forms.

Content and Academic Vocabulary Review

1. Think of an example of each of these content and academic vocabulary words in everyday life.

Content Vocabulary

- grains (p. 470)
- kernels (p. 470)
- bran (p. 470)
- endosperm (p. 470)
- germ (p. 470)
- hull (p. 470)
- whole grain (p. 471)
- wheat (p. 471)
- rice (p. 472)
- pasta (p. 474)
- macaroni (p. 474)
- noodles (p. 474)
- leavened bread (p. 477)
- flatbread (p. 477)
- whole wheat (p. 477)
- al dente (p. 478)

Academic Vocabulary

- considerable (p. 473)
- translucent (p. 476)

Review Key Concepts

2. Describe how food is made from grains.

3. Explain how the processing of grains can affect their nutritional value.

4. Name and describe six grains used around the world.

5. Explain what to look for when buying grain products.

6. Describe the ways in which grains can be prepared for eating.

Critical Thinking

7. Summarize why you think grains have been a food staple around the world for thousands of years.

8. Explain how it is possible for Casey to eat wheat at lunch when she does not have any bread products or pasta.

9. Describe three ways that grains can be combined with other foods to produce tasty dishes.

10. Infer the reason why Harry, who has only cooked dry pasta in the past, cooked fresh pasta and it came out too soft and mushy.

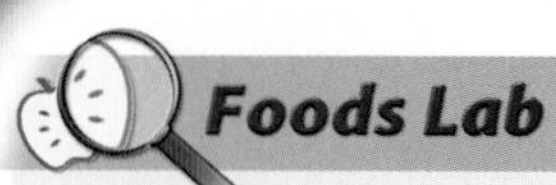

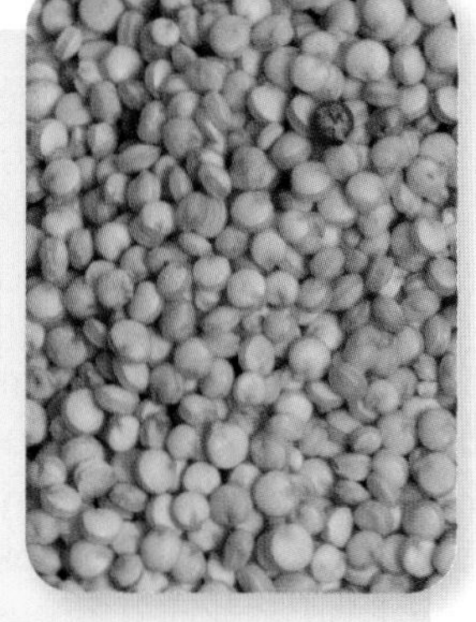

11. Evaluate Grain Dishes Grains vary widely in their taste, texture, appearance, and ease of preparation. By experimenting with different grains in your cooking, you can learn about your preferences.

Procedure Find three simple recipes that use rice, bulgur, and couscous. Follow package instructions to prepare the grains for the recipes. Prepare the three recipes. Compare the grains on appearance, taste, and texture.

Analysis Using a scale of 1 to 10, rate the grains on the following categories: appearance, taste, texture, and ease of preparation. Then create a chart that shows your ratings of each grain in each category.

HEALTHFUL CHOICES

12. Good Grains During his weekly grocery shopping trip, Jeremiah always buys the same grain products: enriched white flour, spaghetti and macaroni pasta made with enriched flour, enriched white bread, ready-to-eat corn flakes, white rice, and instant oatmeal. What changes would you suggest Jeremiah make to his shopping list to increase the healthfulness of his grains? How can Jeremiah continue to enjoy the same kinds of products by making minor changes?

TECH Connection

13. Grain Origins Under your teacher's supervision, use the Internet to research where three different grains originated. Then research where the same three grains are grown today. Next, search for and find a map of the world online, and print it out. Use the world map to locate where the three grains originated and are grown currently. Label the map to reflect your findings. Share your map with the class.

Real-World Skills

Problem-Solving Skills

14. Storing Grains Paul pulled a bag of whole-grain bread from the cupboard, and used two slices to prepare a sandwich. When he ate it, however, he noticed the bread had a rancid taste. Why, and what can he do to prevent this in the future?

Interpersonal and Collaborative Skills

15. Radio Advertisement Follow your teacher's instructions to form groups. Work together to write an attention-getting and informative radio advertisement for one type of grain. The ad should describe some of the grain's characteristics, uses, and nutritional benefits in one minute. Read your ad for the class.

Financial Literacy Skills

16. Homemade vs. Storebought Find instructions for making your own bread crumbs. As a homework assignment, make one cup of breadcrumbs. Bring your breadcrumbs to the foods lab and compare their quality and cost to prepared crumbs purchased from the supermarket. Express your analysis in a paragraph.

Academic Skills

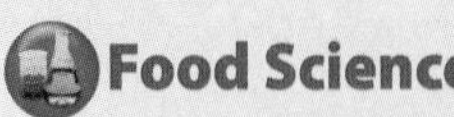

Food Science

17. Gluten in Dough Gluten, an important protein in bread making, is made from 2 proteins found in wheat, gliadin and glutenin. It is formed when water and kneading are added. The amount of kneading influences how much gluten is developed.

Procedure Add ½ cup water gradually to about 2 cups of flour, mixing as you go. Turn out onto a lightly floured surface and form into a dough ball. Separate the dough into 3 equal smaller balls. Leave the first alone. Knead the second for 1 minute. Knead the third for 5 minutes. Roll out each with a pin, noticing how easily it stretches or snaps back.

Analysis Which sample has the most gluten development? How might this experiment help you to make better bread?

NSES B Develop an understanding of the structure and properties of matter.

Mathematics

18. Preparing Pasta Nisha has invited a group of friends over for a spaghetti dinner. There will be eight people dining, and Nisha would like to prepare 1½ cups of cooked spaghetti per person. How many 16 oz. packages of dry spaghetti must Nisha use, and in how much water should she cook the pasta? Remember, it takes 4 oz. of dry spaghetti to produce 2 cups of cooked spaghetti, and each 4 oz. of dry spaghetti requires 1 quart of water.

Math Concept **Solving Problems with Proportions** Write two equal ratios (known as a proportion) to relate a quantity you already know to another you are solving for. Use x to represent the unknown amount in the second ratio.

Starting Hint Since the ratio of dry spaghetti to cooked spaghetti is 4 oz./2 cups, set $4/2 = x/(8 \times 1\frac{1}{2})$ and solve for x to find the total dry weight of spaghetti needed.

NCTM Algebra Represent and analyze mathematical situations and structures using algebraic symbols.

English Language Arts

19. The Need for Grains In recent years, several fad diets have suggested limiting grains for weight loss. Write a persuasive article that counters this view. Review the information in Chapter 11 on maintaining a healthy weight, and include specifics on the valuable role of grains in the diet.

NCTE 4 Use written language to communicate effectively.

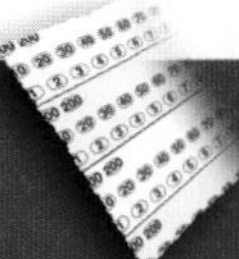

STANDARDIZED TEST PRACTICE

MULTIPLE CHOICE

Read the question and select the best answer.

20. What is leavened bread?

- **a.** Bread such as tortillas, naan, lavash, and pita.
- **b.** Bread made with a leavening agent.
- **c.** Bread made without bran.
- **d.** Bread made with bran.

Test-Taking Tip Multiple-choice questions may prompt you to select the best answer. They may present you with answers that seem partially true. The best answer is the one that is completely true, and can be supported by information you have read in the text.

CHAPTER 31

Legumes, Nuts, & Seeds

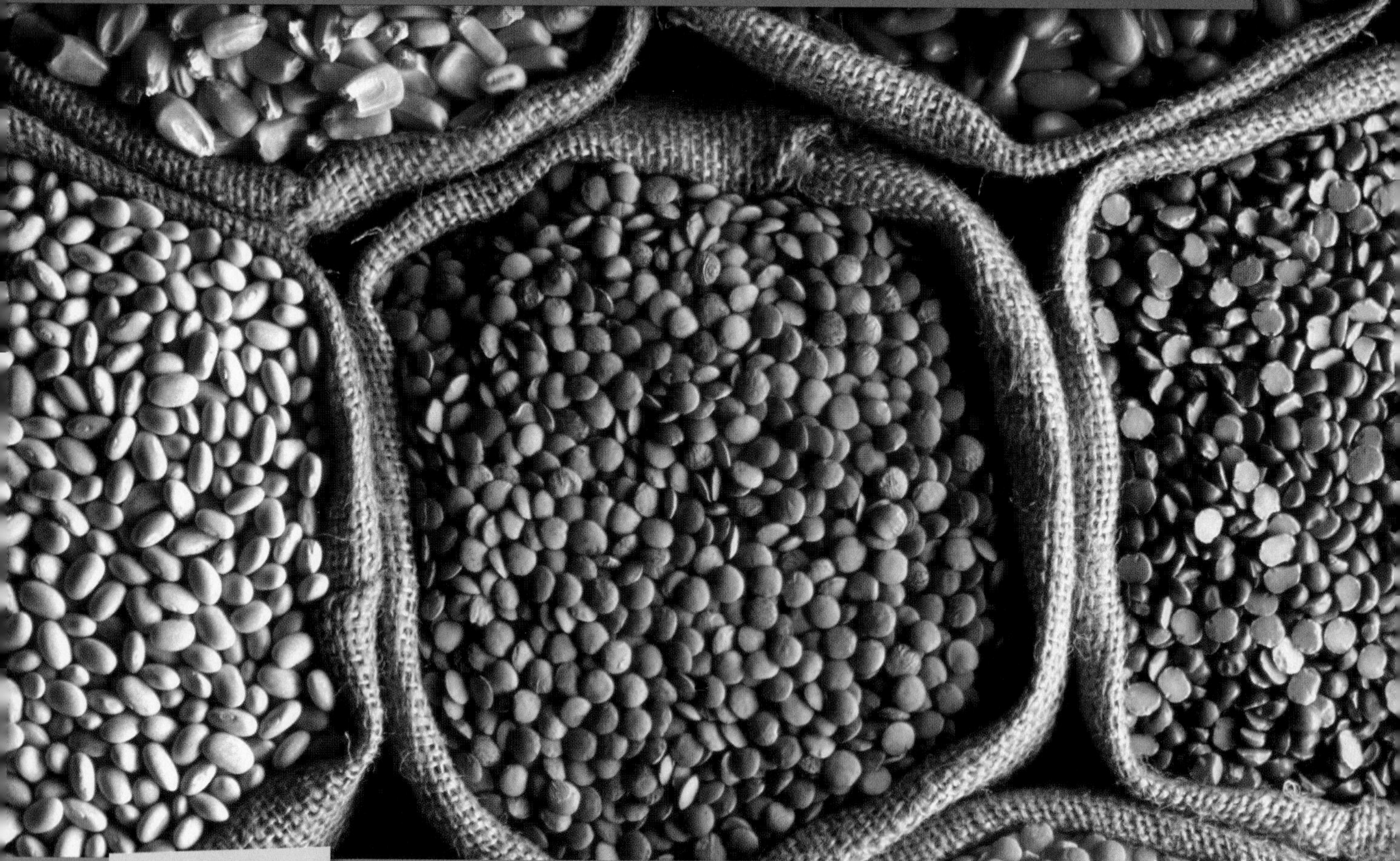

Writing Activity 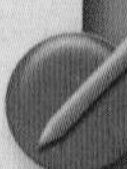 Creative Writing

Spilling the Beans "One night, over a dinner of bean soup, Jamie made an announcement." After reading the previous sentence, did you wonder what happened next? Using the sentence as your introduction, write a one-page short story called "Spilling the Beans." Use your imagination and your writing skills to create fictional characters and events.

Writing Tips Follow these steps for creative writing:

- Create characters, dialogue, and events.
- Let your imagination inspire you.
- Write vividly and descriptively.

Activate Prior Knowledge

Packed with Protein Legumes, nuts, and seeds are tasty and full of protein. *What is your favorite recipe with legumes, nuts, or seeds?*

Reading Guide

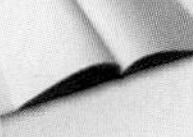

Before You Read

Preview Examine the photos of different legumes, nuts, and seeds. Then make a list of the ones you have tried.

Read to Learn

Key Concepts

- **Explain** the nutritional benefits of legumes.
- **Describe** how to prepare beans before cooking.
- **Identify** ten types of nuts.
- **Describe** three types of seeds and their uses.

Main Idea

Legumes, nuts, and seeds offer valuable nutrients and satisfying flavor, are easy to prepare, and have many uses.

Content Vocabulary

You will find definitions for these words in the glossary at the back of this book.

- legume
- fresh legume
- dry legume
- hilum
- tofu
- nut
- seed

Academic Vocabulary

You will find these words in your reading and on your tests. Use the glossary to look up their definitions if necessary.

- aseptic
- reconstitute

Graphic Organizer

Use a graphic organizer like the one below to note and briefly describe the five different forms of nuts.

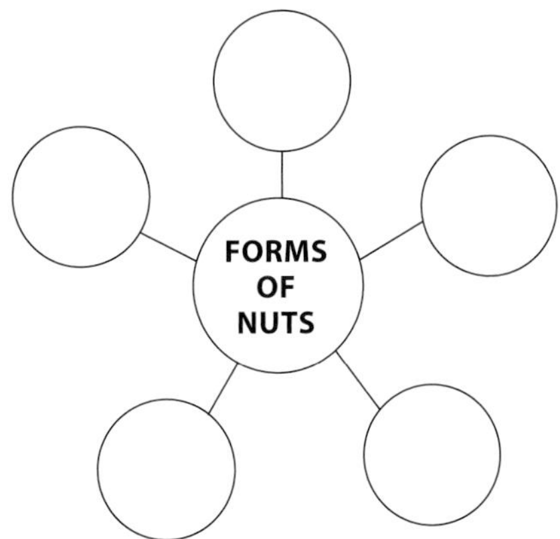

Graphic Organizer Go to this book's Online Learning Center at **glencoe.com** to print out this graphic organizer.

Academic Standards

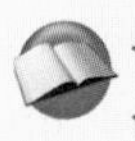

English Language Arts

NCTE 4 Use written language to communicate effectively.

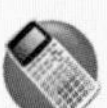

Mathematics

NCTM Data Analysis and Probability Understand and apply basic concepts of probability.

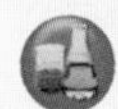

Science

NSES B Develop an understanding of the structure and properties of matter.

NCTE *National Council of Teachers of English*
NCTM *National Council of Teachers of Mathematics*
NSES *National Science Education Standards*
NCSS *National Council for the Social Studies*

Recognizing Legumes

Legumes, nuts, and seeds are packed with nutrients and flavor. A **legume** is a plant with seed pods that split along both sides when ripe. Beans, lentils, and peas are legumes.

A **fresh legume** is a seed or seed pod from a young plant sold as a vegetable. Green beans, green lima beans, and green peas are fresh legumes.

A **dry legume** is a seed or seed pod from a mature plant that has been left in the field to dry. Dry beans, peas, and lentils are dry legumes. Dry legumes are more nutritious than fresh legumes because they are allowed to mature before drying. In food preparation, the word legumes refers to the dry legumes, not fresh legumes.

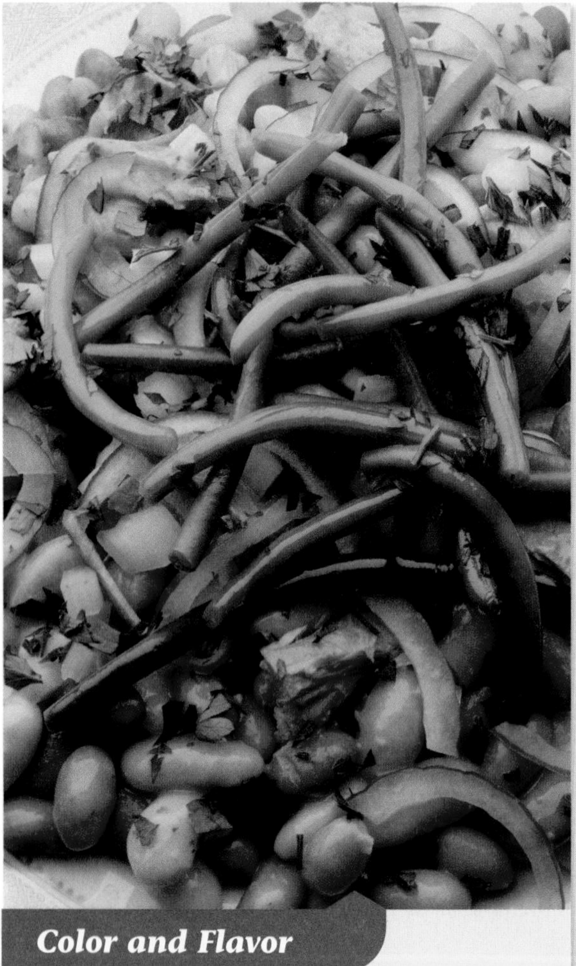

Color and Flavor

Legumes come from plants, which makes them like vegetables. Legumes also supply protein, which makes them like meats. *What is the difference between fresh legumes and dry legumes?*

Nutrients in Legumes

Because seeds contain the food supply for a new plant, dry legumes are rich in nutrients. They are an excellent source of protein and fiber. Mixing legumes with grains provides complete protein, because each has amino acids the other lacks. You can eat legumes and grains at the same meal or at different meals to get the benefits of complete protein. Combined grains and legumes make up about two-thirds of the proteins eaten by people throughout the world.

Legumes are also an inexpensive source of protein. One-half cup of cooked legumes contains the same amount of protein as one ounce of cooked meat, but costs less. Beans also double in volume when cooked, whereas meat, poultry, and other high-protein foods lose moisture and shrink during cooking. An ounce of dry beans, therefore, goes further than an ounce of meat.

Legumes are rich in complex carbohydrates and dietary fiber, as well as protein. They are also high in iron, calcium, potassium, and some trace minerals. Legumes are a healthful alternative to meats because they are low in fat, calories, and sodium and contain no cholesterol.

Types of Legumes

Beans, split peas, and lentils vary from small to large and come in white, pink, red, green, orange, and black varieties. **Figure 31.1** shows many types of legumes and their uses. Each variety has its own distinctive flavor and texture, although some are interchangeable in recipes. Look for interesting varieties of legumes in supermarkets and ethnic markets.

Some legumes are traditional in ethnic dishes. Pinto beans, for instance, are used in Tex-Mex cuisine, including burritos, enchiladas, nachos, and refried beans. Lentils are the main ingredient in dal, a traditional dish in India.

Academic Skills

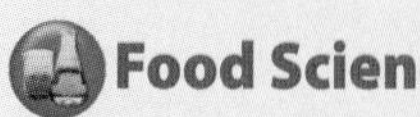

Food Science

17. Peanut Brittle Syrup is a solution of sugar and water. As it boils, the water evaporates, and the temperature of the syrup rises. Syrup cooked to a high temperature is harder when it cools.

Procedure Mix 1 cup sugar, ½ cup light corn syrup, 1 cup peanuts, and ⅛ tsp salt in a 2 quart microwave bowl. Microwave on high 8 minutes, stirring after 4 minutes. Add 1 tablespoon butter, and microwave for 2 minutes. Stir in 1 teaspoon vanilla and 1 teaspoon baking soda until light and foamy. Spread thinly on buttered baking sheet. Cool. Break into pieces.

Analysis Research how brittles differ from other hard candies. What effect does the baking soda have? The corn syrup?

NSES B Develop an understanding of the structure and properties of matter.

Mathematics

18. Mixed Nuts The description on a bag of mixed nuts indicates that it contains 20 peanuts, 14 almonds, 10 Brazil nuts, 7 cashews, and 4 walnuts. If you randomly pull out one nut, what is the probability that you will select a Brazil nut? What is the probability that you will select a peanut?

Math Concept **Calculate Probability** The probability that an event will occur is a fraction comparing the number of favorable outcomes (as the numerator) to the number of all possible outcomes (the denominator).

Starting Hint The number of possible outcomes will be the total number of nuts.

NCTM Data Analysis and Probability Understand and apply basic concepts of probability.

English Language Arts

19. Food Review Imagine you are a food writer for a popular magazine. Prepare one type of bean using dry beans. Compare this with the canned version of the same bean. Rate the appearance, taste, and texture of each. Write a descriptive, 150-word food review in which you inform your readers which form is best and why. Cut out pictures or use photo-editing software to design a magazine-style page layout for your article.

NCTE 4 Use written language to communicate effectively.

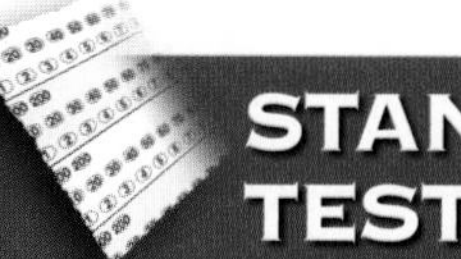

STANDARDIZED TEST PRACTICE

20. Analogy Read the pairs of terms. Then choose the best word to match with the term legumes.

vegetables : frozen peas
grains: ready-to-serve cereal
fruits: dried apricots
legumes: __________

a. peas
b. canned beans
c. pinto beans
d. dry peas

Test-Taking Tip Analogies establish relationships between terms. When you look at the three pairs of terms listed here, identify the relationship that is common to all of them. Then try matching each possible answer with the term legumes. The one that establishes the same type of relationship shared by the other terms is correct.

CHAPTER 32

Dairy

Writing Activity 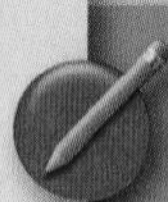 Descriptive Paragraph

Brochure Text Imagine you are writing the text for a food store's brochure. The brochure is from a gourmet food store called Dairy Delights. Write a descriptive paragraph about one of these items: fruit-flavored ice cream, chocolate milk, or extra-sharp cheddar cheese.

Writing Tips Follow these steps to write a descriptive paragraph:

- Use details and adjectives to bring your subject to life.
- Think about the five senses as you write.
- Be specific in your word choices and avoid generalities.

Activate Prior Knowledge

Explore the Photo Butter, ice cream, and cheese all start with milk. *How many milk products do you consume each day?*

Reading Guide

Before You Read

Preview Before you read, consider how many of your favorite dishes contain dairy foods. List the dishes and the type of dairy products they include.

Read to Learn

Key Concepts

- **Explain** the nutritional value of dairy foods.
- **List** four different foods that come from milk.
- **Describe** the differences between fresh cheese and ripened cheese.
- **Summarize** reasons for using dairy substitutes.
- **Explain** how to properly store dairy foods.
- **Describe** the effects of heat on milk and cream.

Main Idea

Dairy foods provide many valuable nutrients and come in a variety of flavors and forms. They are an important part of a healthful diet.

Content Vocabulary

- ☐ pasteurized
- ☐ raw milk
- ☐ nonfat milk solids
- ☐ homogenized
- ☐ yogurt
- ☐ curds
- ☐ whey
- ☐ fresh cheese
- ☐ ripened cheese
- ☐ scorching
- ☐ curdling
- ☐ tempering
- ☐ scalded milk
- ☐ foam

Academic Vocabulary

You will find these words in your reading and on your tests. Use the glossary to look up their definitions if necessary.

- require
- concentrated

Graphic Organizer

Use a graphic organizer like the one below to note types of fresh cheese and ripened cheese.

FRESH CHEESE	RIPENED CHEESE

Graphic Organizer Go to this book's Online Learning Center at **glencoe.com** to print out this graphic organizer.

Academic Standards

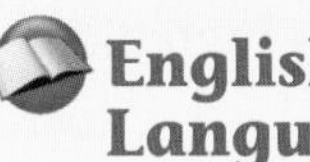

English Language Arts

NCTE 4 Use written language to communicate effectively.

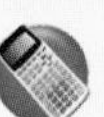

Mathematics

NCTM Algebra Use mathematical models to represent and understand quantitative relationships.

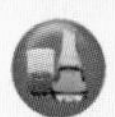

Science

NSES B Develop an understanding of chemical reactions and interactions of energy and matter.

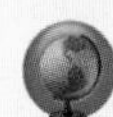

Social Studies

NCSS VII H Production, Distribution and Consumption Apply economic concepts and reasoning when evaluating historical and contemporary social developments and issues.

NCTE *National Council of Teachers of English*
NCTM *National Council of Teachers of Mathematics*
NSES *National Science Education Standards*
NCSS *National Council for the Social Studies*

Looking at Dairy

In the early 1600s, the first dairy cows were brought to the American colonies. The colonists could drink milk fresh from the cow and churn their own butter. After many years and lots of inventiveness, most people now visit supermarkets to choose from a huge array of creamy, refreshing dairy foods and beverages. Milk, cream, butter, yogurt, frozen dairy desserts, and cheese are widely available and ready to eat. Many dairy products are also ready to use as ingredients in dishes.

Nutrients in Dairy Foods

Dairy foods are part of a healthful diet—for good reason. Dairy foods are rich in protein, vitamin A, riboflavin, vitamin B_{12}, calcium, phosphorus, and magnesium. Fortified milk is an excellent source of vitamin D.

Many dairy foods also contain saturated fat and cholesterol. Some, including cheese, are high in sodium. You can manage your nutrition by reading labels and making careful choices.

Health experts recommend three cups of dairy products each day. One cup equals 1 cup of milk or yogurt, 1½ ounces of natural cheese, or 2 ounces of processed cheese. People who choose not to eat dairy should get their calcium from other sources. People who cannot digest lactose, a sugar in milk, should choose lactose-free dairy products.

✓ **Reading Check** **Explain** Why should you read labels and make careful choices about dairy foods?

Milk and Milk Products

According to federal law, all milk must be **pasteurized** (ˈpas-chə-ˌrīzd)—that is, heat-treated to kill enzymes and any harmful bacteria. Pasteurization improves the keeping quality of milk but doesn't change the flavor or nutritional value. UHT (ultra-high temperature) milk is pasteurized at much higher temperatures than usual. As a result, it becomes a shelf-stable product that can be packaged in aseptic containers. Milk that isn't pasteurized is called **raw milk**. Some people believe that raw milk is more nutritious than pasteurized milk. Raw milk may contain harmful bacteria.

Fresh milk contains about 87 percent water and 13 percent solids. **Nonfat milk solids** are substances that contain most of the protein, vitamins, minerals, and lactose (milk sugar) in milk. Another solid in milk is milk fat (sometimes called butterfat). The more milk fat a product has, the higher its calorie count. Milk fat is lighter than other milk fluids and solids, so it separates and rises to the top as cream. To prevent the fat from rising to the top, milk is homogenized. **Homogenized** (hō-ˈmä-jə-ˌnīzd) means processed to make the fat break into small particles and distribute evenly throughout the liquid.

Milk that meets FDA or state standards is labeled "grade A," the highest quality. Only grade-A, pasteurized milk can be shipped between states for retail sale.

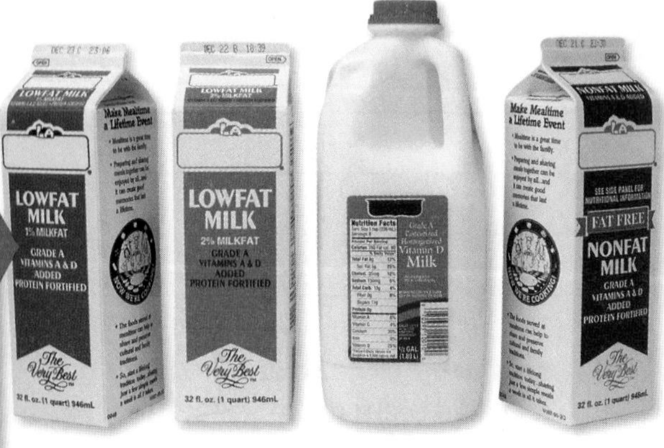

Know Your Milks

Milk comes in many forms, including fresh, canned, and dried. You can even find carbonated milk and milk with orange, strawberry, and caramel flavors. *What forms of milk come in shelf-stable packages?*

Kinds of Milk

Milk is sold in a variety of forms, including low-fat and nonfat. Removing fat from milk also removes most of its vitamin A. By law, vitamin A must be replaced. Most milk producers also fortify milk with vitamin D.

You can find these types of milk at most supermarkets:

Whole Milk Whole milk has the highest amount of fat of any milk. By law, it must have 3.25 percent fat or more.

Reduced-Fat Milk Reduced-fat milk has 2 percent fat.

Low-Fat Milk Low-fat milk has 1 percent fat.

Nonfat Milk Nonfat milk has less than ½ percent fat. It is also called fat-free or skim milk.

Buttermilk Buttermilk has a tangy flavor and a smooth, thick texture. Despite its name, it is not high in fat. Originally, buttermilk was the milk left after making butter. Today, special bacteria are added to pasteurized nonfat milk to produce its flavor and texture. Sometimes flecks of butter are added for flavor and visual appeal. Buttermilk is used in cooking and baking as well as for drinking.

Kefir Kefir is fermented milk with a slightly sour flavor, similar to yogurt. Kefir comes from the Middle East, where it is made from fermented camel's milk. In the United States, kefir is made from cow's milk.

Chocolate Milk Chocolate milk has chocolate or cocoa and sweetener added.

Flavored Milk Like chocolate milk, this is milk with an added flavoring, such as strawberry or vanilla.

Nonfat dry Milk Nonfat dry milk is a powdered form of nonfat milk. It is made by removing the fat and water from pasteurized milk. When dry milk is rehydrated, it can be used like fresh milk and must be refrigerated. Dry milk can be added to recipes to increase nutrients without adding fat. The taste of nonfat dry milk differs slightly from the taste of regular milk.

Evaporated Milk Evaporated milk is canned whole or nonfat milk that contains only half the amount of water in regular milk. It can be used as a cream substitute in beverages.

Nutrition Check

Low-fat Dairy Options

Choose low-fat or nonfat dairy products to obtain valuable nutrients with less fat and calories. Fat-free milk has virtually the same nutrients as whole milk, but 8 fewer grams of fat and 70 fewer calories. Using plain, nonfat yogurt in place of sour cream saves 3 grams of fat per tablespoon. A low-fat variety of ice cream might have 4 fewer grams of fat per serving. Frozen yogurt is another alternative.

Think About It Identify three specific health consequences of eating too much saturated fat. Then write a paragraph giving reasons why it is smart to limit the saturated fat in dairy foods.

Sweetened Condensed Milk Sweetened condensed milk is a concentrated, canned form of milk with sweetener added. It is used to make candy and desserts. Sweetened condensed milk cannot be substituted for evaporated milk or diluted to use as regular milk.

Lactose-Free or Reduced-Lactose Milk These milks are treated to break down lactose. Lactose-free or reduced-lactose milk are used by people who have difficulty digesting or cannot digest lactose.

Acidophilus Milk Acidophilus milk has Lactobacillus acidophilus (ˌlak-tō-bə-ˈsi-ləs ˌa-sə-ˈdä-f(ə-)-ləs) bacteria added to help aid digestion. It tastes and looks like regular milk.

Calcium-Enriched Milk Calcium-enriched milk has 500 milligrams of calcium in one cup. One cup of regular milk has about 300 milligrams.

Cream

Cream is the fatty part of whole milk. Many beverages, cereals, creamy casseroles, soups and sauces, ice cream, baked goods, and sweet syrups contain cream. Federal standards set minimum milk fat for each of these creams:

Half-and-Half This is a homogenized mixture of milk and cream with 10½ to 18 percent milk fat. It is often used in coffee and other beverages.

Light, Coffee, or Table Cream Light cream contains 18 to 30 percent milk fat. It is used in beverages and as a cooking ingredient.

Light Whipping Cream This type of cream has 30 to 36 percent milk fat. It is used in desserts.

Heavy Whipping Cream This type of cream contains more than 36 percent milk fat. It whips easily and is frequently used in desserts.

Sour Cream Thick and rich with a tangy flavor, sour cream is made by adding lactic acid bacteria to light cream. It contains 18 percent milk fat. Sour cream comes plain or with chives, fruit, or other foods added. You can also buy low-fat and nonfat products.

Butter

In colonial times, people made their own butter in large wooden churns. Mechanical means are used today, but churning still separates the fat from the liquid. Federal law **requires**, or mandates, that butter is at least 80 percent milk fat. The rest is buttermilk, which is left for flavor, texture, and appearance. Salt and coloring may also be added.

Butter is graded for quality by the USDA. Grade AA is superior quality. It spreads well and has a delicate, sweet flavor and smooth, creamy texture. Grade A butter is very good quality and has a pleasing flavor with a smooth texture. Grade B butter, made from cream that has gone sour, also has a pleasing flavor.

Butter comes in several forms. Unsalted (sweet) butter has no salt added. Some butter has salt, which adds flavor and acts as a preservative. Butter commonly comes in sticks, usually four to a 1-pound package. Whipped butter, generally unsalted and in tubs, is soft and spreadable. It isn't recommended for baking, however, because added air from whipping changes the density.

Yogurt

Yogurt is a dairy product that is made by adding special harmless bacteria to milk. The result is a thick, creamy product that is like custard and has a tangy flavor. The bacteria added are believed to help keep the digestive system healthy. People eat yogurt from the container, combined with foods in dishes, and in cooking.

Yogurt contains similar nutrients to milk. Because it is more **concentrated**, or dense, however, yogurt has more nutrients than a similar amount of milk. For example, one cup of nonfat yogurt has 452 milligrams of calcium; like regular milk, a cup of nonfat milk contains about 300 milligrams of calcium.

Plain yogurt has no flavorings added. When eating yogurt, you might like a flavored version. Flavored yogurt contains added sugar or sugar substitutes and artificial flavors or real fruits. If you prefer, make your own flavored yogurt by stirring chopped kiwifruit, bananas, or other fruit into plain yogurt.

One cup of yogurt contains 120 to 250 calories, depending on the fat content of the milk used in production. Added sweeteners also affect calories. Check the label for calories and fat.

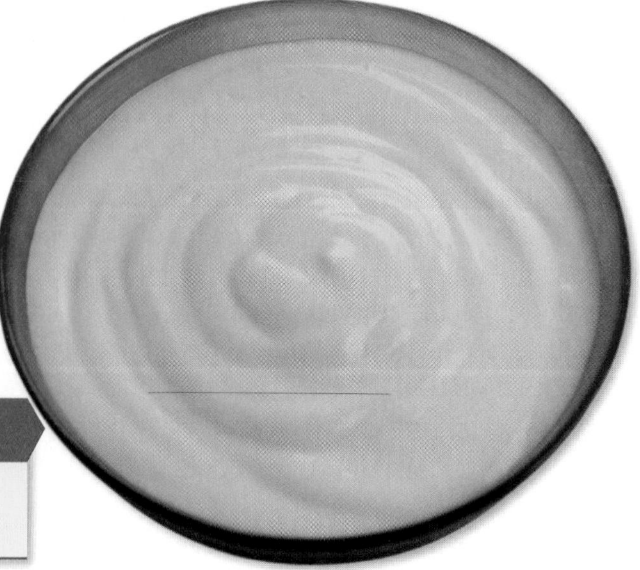

Help For Digestion

Yogurt is made by adding harmless bacteria to milk. *Why is yogurt more nutrient dense than milk?*

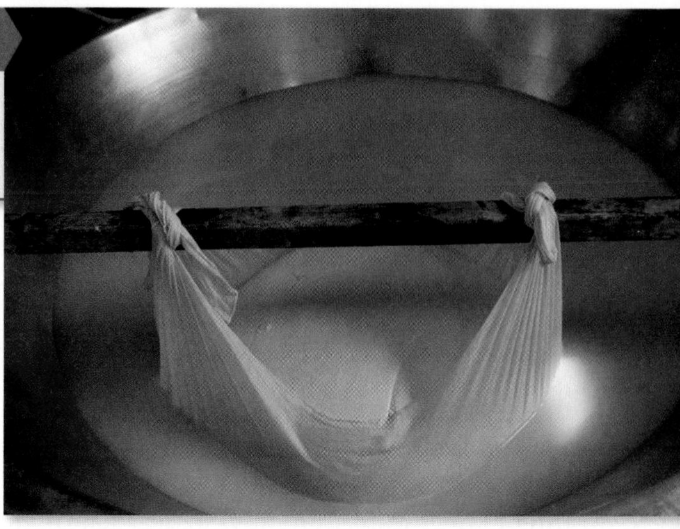

Curds and Whey

Milk can be separated into curds and whey. The curds are used to make cheese, and the whey has many other uses in food processing. *How are the two separated?*

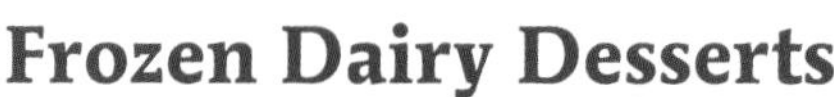

Frozen Dairy Desserts

According to one source, the largest ice cream sundae ever made was 12 feet tall and took over 4,600 gallons of ice cream. That is a sundae to be shared, for sure. A sundae is just one type of frozen dairy dessert you can enjoy.

Ice Cream is a whipped mixture of cream, milk, sugar, flavorings, and stabilizers. It must contain at least 10 percent milk fat. French ice cream has egg yolk solids added. You can buy low-fat, nonfat, and no-sugar-added versions.

Frozen Yogurt varies in fat content depending on the yogurt and other ingredients used. Freezing destroys most of the beneficial bacteria.

Sherbet is made from fruit or juice, sugar, water, flavorings, and milk fat. It generally has less fat but more sugar than ice cream.

Sorbet (sȯr-ˈbā) is the French word for "sherbet." Sorbet is a light dessert made with sweetened fruit, juice, and water, but never milk.

✓ **Reading Check** **Describe** What is yogurt and how is it made?

Types of Cheese

Scan a restaurant menu and you'll probably find cheese in many dishes. Cheese is a concentrated form of milk. When an enzyme such as rennin (ˈre-nən) is added to milk, the milk thickens and separates into solid clusters called **curds** and a thin, bluish liquid called **whey**. The whey is drained from the curds, which become the cheese.

Most cheeses originated in Europe centuries ago. They are made from the milk of such animals as cows, goats, and sheep. Cheeses made in the U.S. are usually made from cows' milk.

Cheese can be divided into two categories: fresh, or unripened, and aged, or ripened. Low-fat and nonfat types are often available.

Fresh Cheese

Fresh cheese is cheese that has not ripened or aged. It is made from pasteurized milk and has a mild flavor. Fresh cheese, which is highly perishable, must be refrigerated and used within a few days. You can snack on fresh cheese or use it in salads, sandwiches, and cooking. These are some fresh cheese favorites:

Cottage Cheese This type of fresh cheese contains large or small curds and has a bland flavor. Fresh cream is added to make creamed cottage cheese. Chives, pineapple, or other flavorings may be added. Cottage cheese does not melt. Both low-fat and nonfat products can be eaten plain or used in salads and other dishes.

Farmer's Cheese With a mild, slightly tangy flavor, this cheese is similar to cottage cheese but drier and usually shaped in a loaf. It can be crumbled or sliced and eaten plain or used in cooking.

Cream Cheese This type of fresh cheese is smooth, creamy, and spreadable, with a mild, slightly tart flavor. Look for low-fat and nonfat varieties. Cream cheese is a spread and an ingredient in many dishes. Seasoned forms are available.

Ricotta (ri-ˈkä-tə) Similar to cottage cheese, Ricotta cheese has a small curd. It has a slightly sweet flavor and is traditional in Italian cuisine.

Ripened Cheese

Ripened cheese, also called aged cheese, is made by adding ripening agents, such as bacteria, mold, yeast, or a combination of these, to the curds. The cheese is then aged under carefully controlled conditions. Aging time depends on the kind of cheese. For example, mild brick cheese ages for two weeks, but extra-sharp Parmesan takes as long as two years. Ripened cheese can be stored longer than fresh cheese.

Hundreds of ripened cheeses are available, each with a distinctive flavor and texture. Flavors vary from mild to very sharp, or strong, and textures range from soft to very hard. **Figure 32.1** describes ripened cheeses. They are grouped according to the following textures:

Firm Cheese with a firm texture can be eaten plain or used in cooking. Most can be grated.

Semisoft Cheese that is semisoft melts smoothly and is eaten plain or used in cooking.

Soft Cheese with a soft texture has a hard, white crust that is edible. It is usually eaten plain.

Blue-Veined Cheese with blue veins has certain molds added during the aging process to create veins or pockets of blue or green edible mold. It can be eaten plain or used in salads, salad dressings, casseroles, and omelets.

Specialty cheeses are made by shredding and blending different ripened cheeses. Sometimes pimientos, pineapples, olives, or other foods are added. These cheeses are semisoft, with a smooth texture. They spread easily and melt quickly.

Specialty cheeses include cold pack cheese, a blend of ripened cheeses processed without heat, and pasteurized process cheese, a blend of ripened cheeses processed with heat. Examples of pasteurized process cheese are American cheese, cheese spread, and cheese food.

✓ Reading Check **Define** What are curds and whey?

Dairy Substitutes

What can you do if you're allergic to the protein in milk or cannot digest lactose? What if you prefer foods that are free of saturated fats and cholesterol? Dairy substitutes provide options.

Margarine Made from hydrogenated vegetable oils and sold in sticks, margarine is similar to butter. Soft margarine blends hydrogenated and liquid vegetable oils to stay soft and spreadable. Liquid margarine is squeezed from pliable plastic bottles. Some margarines have no trans fats, and reduced fat and fat-free margarines are also available. Some of these may have other additives so read Nutrition Facts labels carefully.

Soy Milk The liquid pressed out of soybeans, called soy milk, is high in protein, B vitamins, and iron and low in calcium, fat, and sodium. It has no cholesterol. Choose a brand fortified with calcium and vitamins A, D, and B_{12}.

Soy Cheese Made from soy milk, soy cheese is available in low-fat and nonfat types.

Nondairy Creamer Also called coffee lightener, nondairy creamer is made with partially hydrogenated vegetable oil and corn syrup. It comes as a powder or liquid.

Whipped Toppings These toppings are made from hydrogenated vegetable oils, sweeteners, and nonfat milk solids. They are low in fat but in many cases high in trans fat. You can choose from dry mixes, aerosol cans, or frozen tubs.

Frozen Desserts Non dairy frozen desserts are available as substitutes for ice cream, sorbet sherbet, frozen sandwiches, and fruit pops. They are often made with cooked rice or tofu.

When you buy dairy substitutes, read labels carefully. The products may contain saturated fats, such as coconut or palm oils. As you know, those made with hydrogenated vegetable oils contain trans fats.

✓ Reading Check **List** What are two ingredients that are used to make dairy substitutes?

Figure 32.1 Ripened Cheeses

Cheese Please! Cheese comes in many colors and textures. ***What kind of cheese comes in a deep orange color?***

Cheese	Country of Origin	Description
Firm Ripened Cheeses		
Cheddar	England, United States, and Canada	Pale yellow to deep orange in color; mild to extra-sharp flavor; melts well.
Parmesan/Romano (ˈpär-mə-ˌzän/rə-mä-(ˌ)nō)	Italy	Light yellow color; sharp flavor.
Swiss	Switzerland	Pale yellow with large holes; nutty, slightly sweet flavor; melts well.
Provolone (ˌprō-və-ˈlō-nē)	Italy	Pale yellow with light brown rind; bland to sharp, smoky flavor; melts well.
Semisoft Ripened Cheeses		
Gouda (ˈgü-də)	Netherlands	Creamy yellow with an inedible, yellow or red, wax coating; mild, nut-like flavor; similar to Edam in taste but richer; melts well.
Mozzarella (ˌmät-sə-ˈre-lə)	Italy	Creamy white; elastic texture; sweet, mild flavor; melts easily; also available fresh.
Brick	United States	Light yellow in color; flavor ranges from mild to pungent.
Muenster (ˈmən(t)-stər)	France	Light yellow with orange rind; smooth texture with tiny holes; mild to pungent flavor.
Monterey Jack	United States	Creamy white; smooth texture and tiny cracks; mild flavor; melts well. Jalapeño Jack (ˌhä-lə-ˈpā-(ˌ)nyō) has a spicy-hot flavor.
Edam (ˈē-dəm)	Netherlands	Creamy yellow with an inedible, red wax coating; mild, nutlike flavor; melts well.
Feta (ˈfe-tə)	Greece	Pure white; crumbly texture; salty, sharp, and pickled flavor; must be stored in brine.
Soft Ripened Cheeses		
Brie (ˈbrē)	France	Light yellow; buttery-soft texture; white, edible crust; mild to pungent flavor. When ripe, the interior should be soft enough to ooze.
Neufchâtel (ˌnü-shä-ˈtel)	France	Mild, slightly salty flavor; creamy texture. American version is unripened and sold in bricks like cream cheese but with less fat.
Camembert (ˈka-məm-ˌber)	France	Similar to brie; creamy yellow; buttery texture; edible crust; mild to pungent flavor. When ripe, it should be soft enough to ooze.
Blue-Veined Ripened Cheeses		
Blue cheese	Denmark	Creamy white with blue vein; crumbly texture; salty, tangy flavor.
Roquefort (ˈrōk-fərt)	France	Creamy white with deep blue-green vein; strong, sharp, salty flavor.
Gorgonzola (ˌgȯr-gən-ˈzō-lə)	Italy	Ivory-colored with blue-green vein; rich and creamy; flavor slightly to extremely pungent.
Stilton	England	Pale yellow with blue-green vein; light brown, crusty rind; slightly cheddar flavor; mildest of all blue-veined cheeses.

Buying and Storing Dairy Foods

To be a smart consumer when buying dairy foods, consider fat amounts, container size, and product type. For instance, rich foods generally cost more than low-fat varieties. Large containers are usually a better buy than small ones. Foods with added ingredients, such as flavorings, fruit, and sugar, generally cost more than their plain counterparts.

Always check labels for nutrition and ingredient information. Containers should be tightly sealed and never opened. Also, look for the "sell by" date. Only buy quantities you can use in a relatively short time. Most dairy products must be used within a few days, although yogurt, butter, ripened cheese, and frozen desserts last longer when properly stored.

Dairy foods are highly perishable, so take them home right after purchase and store them properly. It is best to refrigerate all dairy foods in original containers. Since dairy foods can pick up aromas from other foods, make sure containers are tightly closed.

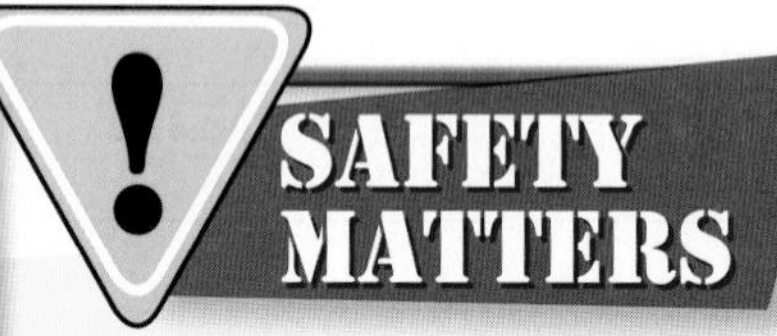

Good Mold, Bad Mold

Typically, people think of mold as something to avoid, especially when it is present in food. Certain molds, however, are carefully selected and added to particular cheeses, including blue cheese, Roquefort, and Gorgonzola. This gives them their characteristic appearance and bold flavor. One type of mold added to cheese is related to penicillin. Because the process is carefully controlled, these cheeses are safe to eat. All cheeses may become moldy if stored improperly or for too long. This new mold that forms on cheese after improper storage is not safe to eat.

What Would You Do? You purchase a flavorful blue-veined cheese, eat some, and store the rest. After two weeks, you pull out the cheese to serve to some friends and notice an unfamiliar white mold on certain areas.

After pouring milk, return the container to the refrigerator immediately. If milk has been sitting out in a serving pitcher, do not pour it back into the original container. Instead, if the milk has been at room temperature for less than two hours, refrigerate it in a separate container and use as soon as possible. Discard milk left at room temperature for more than two hours. Large amounts of harmful bacteria may have developed. Because light destroys the riboflavin in milk, store it away from light.

Keep ripened cheese tightly wrapped so it does not dry out. Firm and semisoft ripened cheeses can be frozen, but the texture changes. Freeze in ½-pound portions and use it crumbled, shredded, or in cooked dishes.

You can refrigerate butter for several weeks and freeze it for up to nine months. Store frozen dairy desserts in tightly covered containers in the freezer.

✓ **Reading Check** **Explain** What is the maximum amount of time you can safely leave milk at room temperature?

Using Dairy Foods

Skillful cooks know how to use dairy products. Whether you make pizza with cheese or pudding with milk, certain knowledge promotes success.

Cooking with Milk and Cream

Milk is not just for drinking and pouring on cereal. It's also used to prepare delicious cooked foods, including cocoa and soups. Since milk contains animal proteins, it is sensitive to heat. Therefore cook at moderate temperatures and for as short a time as possible. Several problems can occur when cooking milk.

Heat turns some milk solids and fat into a tough, rubbery skin that forms on the surface. The skin keeps steam from escaping. Pressure builds until the milk eventually boils over. To prevent skin from forming, cover the pan or stir the milk continuously as it cooks. If a skin does form, beat it into the milk; if you discard the skin, you throw away valuable nutrients.

Scorching can occur if milk overheats. When you heat milk, some solids settle on the sides and some fall to the bottom of the pan. If the milk overheats, the sugar lactose in the solids rapidly caramelizes and burns, or scorches. As a result, the milk develops an off-flavor. To prevent this, use low heat and stir the mixture to keep the solids from settling.

If you cook milk at a temperature that is too high, it separates into curds and whey. This is called **curdling**. Curdling may also occur when you add milk to hot foods, such as gravy, or to acidic foods, such as tomato soup. To prevent curdling, use a method called **tempering**. This technique brings one food to the right temperature or consistency before mixing it completely with another.

1. Pour a small amount of the hot or acidic mixture into the milk first, stirring constantly. Repeat, if needed. By doing this, you raise the temperature or acid level of the milk gradually, so there is less chance of curdling.
2. Slowly add the milk to the remaining mixture, stirring constantly. If you add the milk too quickly, the mixture may curdle.

If the mixture does curdle, you may be able to save it. Beat it vigorously until smooth.

To prevent the problems described, use a double boiler when heating milk. Place water in the bottom pan and milk in the upper one. The heat from the boiling water heats the milk without scorching or curdling.

Some recipes call for **scalded milk**, which is milk heated to just below the boiling point. Use low heat and cook only until bubbles appear around the sides of the pan.

Milk and milk-based recipes can be prepared easily in the microwave oven. Use a low setting to avoid overheating and curdling the milk, and make sure the container is large enough in case the milk foams up.

When choosing cream for whipping, look for heavy cream with a high fat content. This gives greater volume. When cream is whipped, a **foam** forms. As the cream is beaten, air is incorporated. At the same time, beating breaks down the protein, which then forms a fine film around pockets of air. This protein structure holds the air pockets and gives strength, or stability, to the foam. The fat in cream adds rigidity. As air cells multiply and become smaller with continued beating, the foam thickens. Do not over-beat, as cream will turn into butter. When you use cream in a recipe, follow the guidelines for cooking milk.

Science in Action

Aging and Ammonia

Many cheeses obtain their distinctive flavor through aging. The aging period can last days or years. As cheese ages, enzymes and living organisms called microbes intensify its flavor and alter its texture. This transformation results from the breakdown of milk fat and casein proteins into a mixture of fatty acids, amino acids, and amines, which are derived from ammonia.

Procedure Numerous terms are used by cheese connoisseurs to describe the qualities and characteristics of the cheeses they sample. One such term is "ammoniated." This term means that cheese has a strong ammonia odor.

Analysis Do you think "ammoniated" cheese has been aged for a short or a long period? Explain. Express your response in writing, and support it with logical reasoning based on your reading.

NSES B Develop an understanding of interactions of energy and matter.

Making Frozen Dairy Desserts

Special occasions—and even not-so-special occasions—offer a reason to make frozen dairy desserts. Treats like ice cream and mousse ('müs) can be easily made at home.

Ice Cream You can make ice cream with either a hand-operated or electric ice cream maker. Both work the same basic way. The inside container holds the ice cream mixture and a paddle that stirs the mix electrically or by hand. The outer container is filled with ice and salt, which freezes the ice cream mixture as the paddle rotates. (New models don't need ice and salt.) Stirring action prevents ice crystals, making the mixture light and airy.

Mousse A dessert mousse is a soft, creamy dish made with whipped cream and flavored, often with chocolate or fruit. Sometimes gelatin adds body and helps keep the mixture's shape. The dish is chilled or frozen in a mold.

When making frozen dairy desserts, you need to keep ice crystals from forming. One way is to use enough fat since fat prevents crystal formation. The more fat a mixture has, the smoother it will be. That is why ice cream is smoother and richer than sherbet. Another method is to beat the mixture while making it.

Cooking with Yogurt

Yogurt works well as a low-fat substitute for sour cream, cream cheese, and mayonnaise. Yogurt is used in many recipes, including dips, soups, sauces, salads, and main dishes. During storage, the whey may separate from the curd. Stir the whey back into the yogurt before you use it. Cook yogurt at moderate temperatures for only the time needed. Yogurt curdles if overcooked.

Cooking with Cheese

Cheese is a concentrated food, high in protein and fat, so cook with care. If you cook cheese for too long or use a temperature that is too high, the cheese becomes tough and rubbery. If fat separates into globules of grease, food will have an unappetizing appearance.

Cheese should be cooked just until it melts. To reduce cooking time, cut the cheese into small pieces or grate it. To melt cheese by itself, use very low heat or a double boiler. When other foods are combined with cheese, they should either be precooked or need only a short cooking time and moderate temperatures.

Some cheese varieties blend more readily than others during cooking. Processed cheese mixes easily. Cheddar blends well, so it is a favorite for cooking. Fresh cheeses don't blend well unless beaten into the mixture.

Be careful when microwaving dishes with cheese. The fat in the cheese attracts microwaves, so the cheese may be hotter than the rest of the food in the dish.

Light and Healthy Recipe

Tzatziki

Ingredients

- **1** Cucumber
- **1 clove** Garlic
- **1 cup** Plain, lowfat yogurt
- **1 Tbsp.** Lemon juice
- **1 ½ tsp.** Olive oil
- **¼ tsp.** Salt
- **1 tsp.** Chopped mint leaves

Directions

1. Peel and remove the seeds from the cucumber. Dice the cucumber and mince the garlic.
2. Combine all ingredients and mix well. Chill in a refrigerator.
3. Serve cold with pita bread or chips.

Cucumber, fresh mint, and lowfat yogurt make this a light and refreshing snack.

Yield 4 servings

Nutrition Analysis per Serving

■ Calories	77
■ Total fat	3 g
Saturated fat	1 g
Cholesterol	5 mg
■ Sodium	201 mg
■ Carbohydrate	9
Dietary fiber	1 g
Sugars	7 g
■ Protein	5 g

CHAPTER 32 Review & Applications

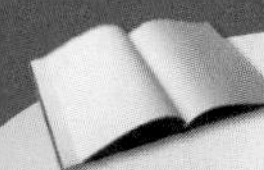

After You Read

Chapter Summary

Dairy foods are flavorful, versatile, and nutritious. They include milk, cream, butter, yogurt, frozen dairy desserts, and cheese. There are many different kinds of milk and cheeses to suit a variety of tastes and purposes. Dairy substitutes are suitable for people who are allergic to dairy foods or prefer foods free of saturated fat and cholesterol. When purchasing dairy foods, consumers should consider fat amounts, container size, and product type. Because dairy foods are perishable, they need to be refrigerated. Special care must be taken when cooking with dairy foods.

Content and Academic Vocabulary Review

1. Create a fill-in-the-blank sentence for each of these content and academic vocabulary words. The sentence should contain enough information to help determine the missing word.

Content Vocabulary

- pasteurized (p. 502)
- raw milk (p. 502)
- nonfat milk solids (p. 502)
- homogenized (p. 502)
- yogurt (p. 504)
- curds (p. 505)
- whey (p. 505)
- fresh cheese (p. 505)
- ripened cheese (p. 506)
- scorching (p. 509)
- curdling (p. 509)
- tempering (p. 509)
- scalded milk (p. 509)
- foam (p. 509)

Academic Vocabulary

- require (p. 504)
- concentrated (p. 504)

Review Key Concepts

2. **Explain** the nutritional value of dairy foods.
3. **List** four different foods that come from milk.
4. **Describe** the differences between fresh cheese and ripened cheese.
5. **Summarize** reasons for using dairy substitutes
6. **Explain** how to properly store dairy products.
7. **Describe** the effects of heat on milk and cream.

Critical Thinking

8. **Explain** how you can still obtain the nutrients milk offers if you do not like the taste of regular milk.
9. **Describe** what should be done with a pitcher of milk that has been sitting on the table during a 90 minute brunch.
10. **Summarize** the reasons why you can burn your tongue on a bite of microwaved pizza but still find the crust comfortably warm to eat.

Foods Lab

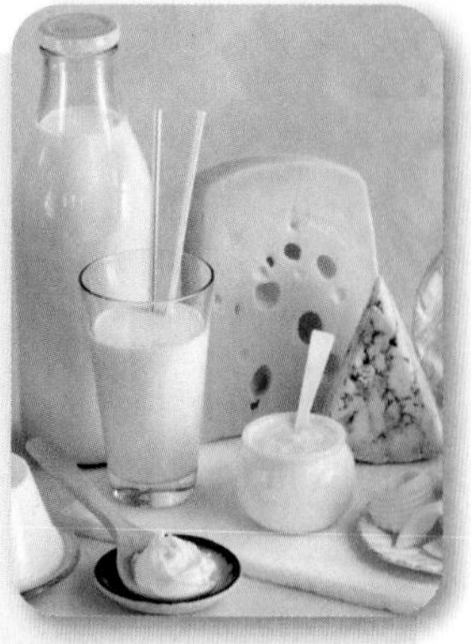

11. Homemade Ice Cream Many people consider ice cream to be a satisfying, sweet treat. It may be even more satisfying, however, if you make it yourself.

Procedure Find recipes for homemade ice cream. Choose one to prepare in the lab, using a hand-crank ice cream maker. Experiment with additions such as chocolate chips, chopped nuts, or dried fruit pieces.

Analysis In an group oral presentation to the class, evaluate your ice cream's taste, texture, and appearance. How does it compare with store-bought versions in quality and cost?

HEALTHFUL CHOICES

12. Maximizing Calcium Janie is a middle-aged woman who maintains a calcium-rich diet to prevent osteoporosis, a degenerative condition that affects bones. She is creating a menu for a lunch that she will eat every day at work. She cannot decide if she should include 1 cup of yogurt or 1 cup of milk with her lunch. Which should she choose and why?

TECH Connection

13. Calcium-Rich Menu Under your teacher's supervision use the Internet to research the amount of calcium teens need per day. How much milk and other dairy foods would you need to get those amounts? What foods besides milk and dairy foods can teens eat to get calcium? Use word processing software to create menus for three days that would provide enough calcium. Write a paragraph summarizing your findings.

Real-World Skills

Problem-Solving Skills

14. Pizza Party Mike wants to have a homemade pizza party and invite several friends to join him in making pizzas. A few of his friends are lactose intolerant. What can Mike do to ensure that all of his guests enjoy the pizza?

Interpersonal and Collaborative Skills

15. Radio Spot Follow your teacher's instructions to form groups. Many teens do not get enough calcium. Work with your group to write an entertaining, two-minute radio spot, or announcement, that promotes milk drinking in teens. Then perform the spot for the class. You may incorporate music, dialogue, funny voices, or other elements.

Financial Literacy Skills

16. Cheap Cheese Visit a supermarket or other business that sells a wide assortment of cheeses. Which cheeses are the least expensive? Which are the most expensive? What qualities seem to set them apart and influence pricing? How can you apply this knowledge in the future? Write your conclusions in a paragraph.

Academic Skills

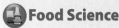

Food Science

17. Curdling Milk The curd proteins in milk will coagulate in acidic conditions. This is what happens when milk gets old and sours or when it is cultured with acid producing bacteria to make yogurt or sour cream.

Procedure Pour 3 ounces of milk in a container. Stir in 1 ounce of white vinegar. Repeat the experiment in a second container, but add water rather than vinegar.

Analysis Write a paragraph explaining how the vinegar affected the milk.

NSES B Develop an understanding of chemical reactions.

Mathematics

18. Kitchen Teamwork Rhonda purchased two pounds of cheddar cheese to be cut into cubes. On her own, Rhonda needs 18 minutes to slice all the cheese into cubes. Rhonda's friend Bianca is a little faster, and needs just 12 minutes to cut up the cheese. If they slice the cheese together, how long will it take?

Math Concept **Combining Rates of Work** Determine the individual rate of work for each worker. Write an algebraic equation with a variable representing the total time needed to complete the job.

Starting Hint If it takes Bianca 12 minutes to cube the cheese, she can complete $1/12$ of the job in one minute. If x represents the total minutes needed for the pair to complete the job together, then $1/x$ represents their combined effort per minute, and you know that $1/12 + 1/18 = 1/x$.

NCTM Algebra Use mathematical models to represent and understand quantitative relationships.

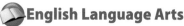

English Language Arts

19. Write a Poem Combine your creative writing skills with your research skills to write a poem about one type of dairy food. Your poem can take a variety of forms, but should express the characteristics of the dairy food that you find appealing. Conduct research about the dairy food you have selected and include your knowledge into the poem. When you are done writing your poem, copy it onto a poster board. Decorate it with illustrations. Share your poem poster with your class.

NCTE 4 Use written language to communicate effectively.

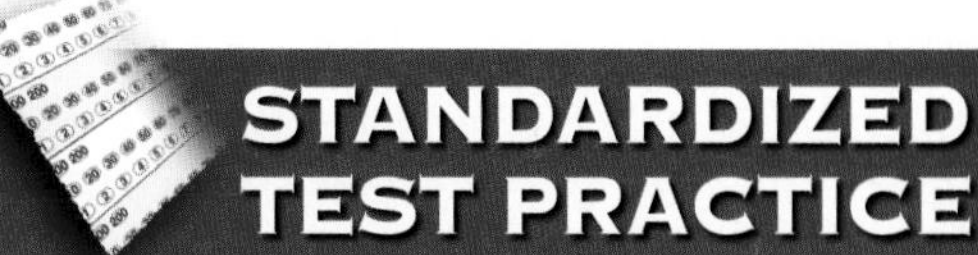

STANDARDIZED TEST PRACTICE

FILL IN THE BLANK

Read the sentence and choose the best word to fill in the blank.

20. Cheese with a ________ texture has a hard, white crust that is edible.

a. soft
b. semisoft
c. firm
d. ripened

Test-Taking Tip When answering a fill-in-the-blank question, silently read the sentence with each of the possible answers in the blank space. This will help you eliminate wrong answers. The best word results in a sentence that is both factual and grammatically correct.

CHAPTER 33

Eggs

Writing Activity 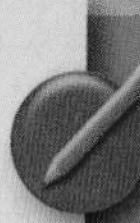 Varied Sentence Structures

Enjoying Eggs Good writing features sentences that have different structures. For example: "Rosie gathered the eggs in a basket" has a different sentence structure than "Using a basket, Rosie gathered the eggs." In what other ways can sentence structures be varied? Write a paragraph that describes eggs or an egg dish you like. Include at least three different sentence structures.

Writing Tips Follow these steps to write a variety of sentences:

- Avoid starting several sentences with the same word.
- Use punctuation correctly to combine some short sentences together.
- Include both long and short sentences in your writing.

Activate Prior Knowledge

Thousands of Uses Eggs are a great source of protein. *What is your favorite recipe that contains eggs?*

Reading Guide

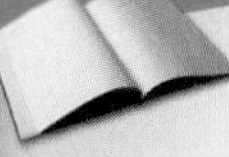

Before You Read

Preview List three questions you have about eggs. As you read, write down the answers to your questions.

Read to Learn

Objectives

- **Identify** and describe three important parts of an egg.
- **Describe** the nutrients found in eggs.
- **Explain** how to safely store eggs.
- **Summarize** why eggs act as a binder.
- **Describe** how beating affects egg whites.
- **Identify** the steps for making an omelet.

Main Idea

Eggs are a nutritious, economical, and versatile food that can be eaten alone and used in many recipes.

Content Vocabulary

You will find definitions for these words in the glossary at the back of this book.

- ☐ air cell
- ☐ albumen
- ☐ yolk
- ☐ chalazae
- ☐ coagulate
- ☐ emulsifier
- ☐ soufflé
- ☐ soft peaks
- ☐ stiff peaks
- ☐ shirred eggs
- ☐ omelet
- ☐ frittata
- ☐ custard
- ☐ quiche
- ☐ meringue
- ☐ weep
- ☐ beading

Academic Vocabulary

You will find these words in your reading and on your tests. Use the glossary to look up their definitions if necessary.

- ruptured
- sieve

Graphic Organizer

Use a graphic organizer like the one below to take notes about the uses and characteristics of grade AA, A, and B eggs.

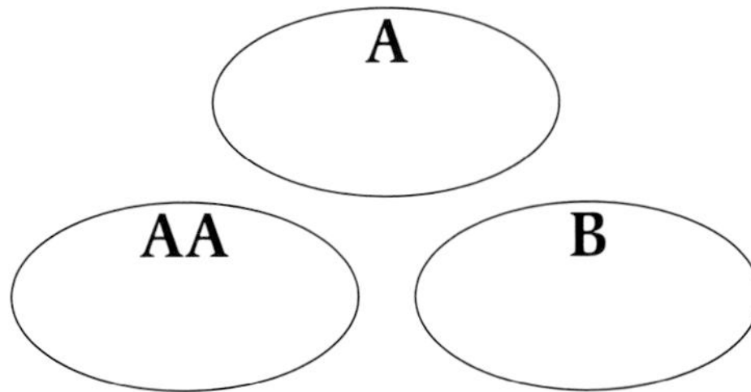

Graphic Organizer Go to this book's Online Learning Center at **glencoe.com** to print out this graphic organizer.

Academic Standards

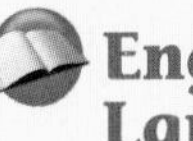

English Language Arts

NCTE 7 Conduct research and gather, evaluate, and synthesize date to communicate discoveries.

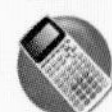

Mathematics

NCTM Data Analysis & Probability Understand and apply basic concepts of probability.

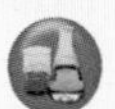

Science

NSES B Develop an understanding of interactions of energy and matter.

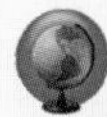

Social Studies

NCSS VII F Production, Distribution, and Consumption Compare how values and beliefs influence economic decisions in different societies.

NCTE *National Council of Teachers of English*
NCTM *National Council of Teachers of Mathematics*
NSES *National Science Education Standards*
NCSS *National Council for the Social Studies*

The Structure of Eggs

Eggs are one of nature's most versatile, nutritious, and economical foods. Besides being tasty, they perform important functions in recipes. Most eggs eaten in the United States come from hens, or female chickens.

An egg has several parts, which are shown in **Figure 33.1**. The hard shell is porous and lined with membranes. A pocket of air, also known as the **air cell**, lies between these membranes at the wide, round end. As an egg ages, this air cell gets larger. The inside of an egg also contains these three parts:

Albumen The thick fluid commonly known as egg white is **albumen** (al-ˈbyü-mən). Albumen gets thinner as an egg ages. Very fresh eggs have cloudy-white albumen.

Yolk The round yellow portion of an egg is the **yolk**. It is encased in a thin membrane and floats within the albumen. The yolk flattens as the egg ages. Its color depends on the hen's diet. Hens that are fed yellow cornmeal or marigold petals produce deeper yellow yolks than those fed white cornmeal. Artificial color additives are not allowed in chicken feeds. Eggs sometimes have a red spot near the yolk, which means that one or more small blood vessels in the yolk have **ruptured**, or broken. The egg is still safe to use.

Chalazae The two, thick, twisted strands of albumen that anchor the yolk in the center of an egg are called the **chalazae** (kə-ˈlā-ˌzē). They are not the beginning of an embryo. The thicker and more prominent the chalazae, the fresher the egg.

✓ **Reading Check** **Explain** What makes some egg yolks a different shade of yellow than others?

Nutrients in Eggs

Eggs are an excellent source of protein and vitamin B_{12}. Both the white and the yolk contain proteins. Eggs also contain other B vitamins as well as vitamins A and D, iron, calcium, phosphorus, and other trace minerals. The egg is one of very few natural sources of Vitamin D. A large hen's eggs are only about 80 calories each.

Figure 33.1 **Parts of an Egg**

Egg Basics These are the basic parts of an egg. *What is the albumen commonly called? What is the purpose of the chalazae?*

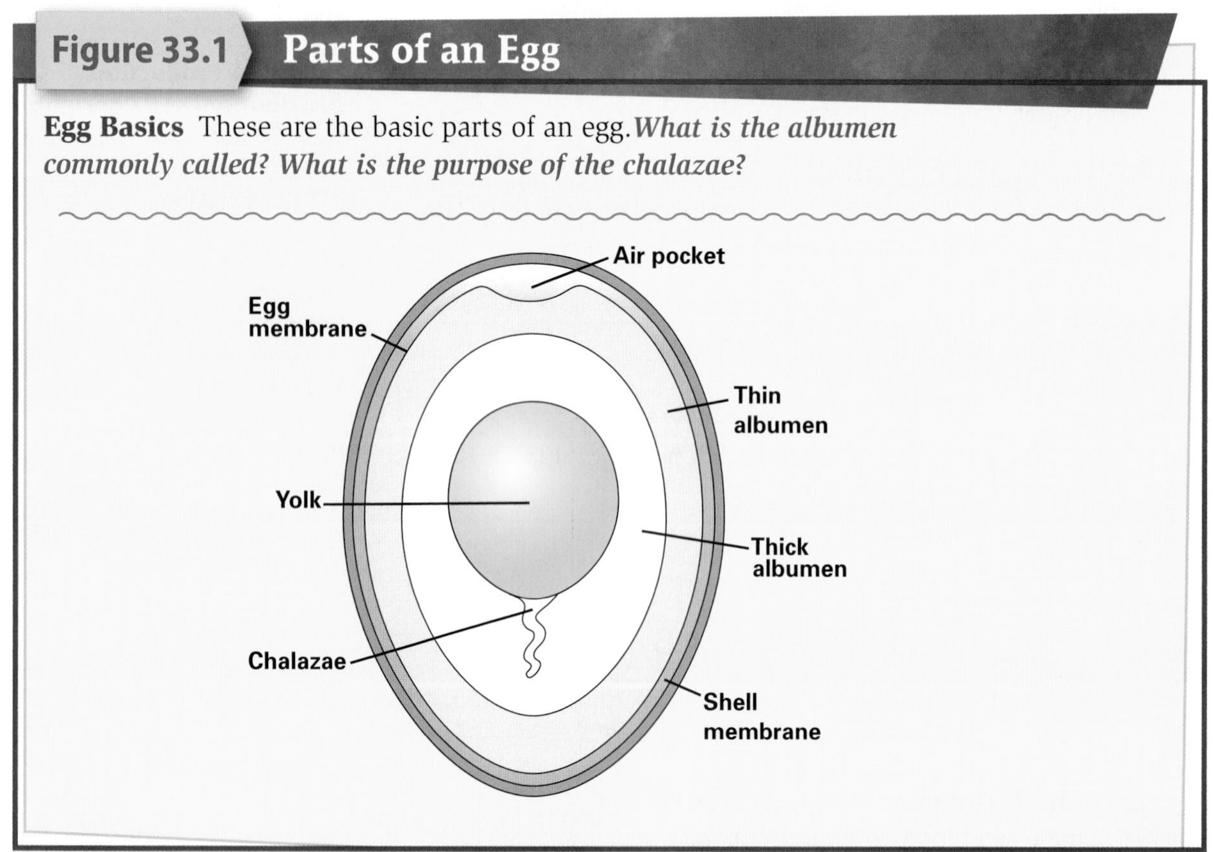

In general, the yolk of an egg contains more vitamins and minerals than the white. Egg yolks are one of the few foods that are a natural source of vitamin D. However, they also contain fats and cholesterol, so health experts recommend eating egg yolks in moderation.

The color of an egg's shell is not related to its nutrients, flavor, or cooking qualities. The breed of hen determines the color of the egg's shell.

✓ **Reading Check** **Identify** Which part of an egg is generally more nutritious?

Selecting and Storing Eggs

Eggs are perishable and breakable, and should be selected and handled with care. Always get refrigerated eggs, and buy them by the sell-by date. Before buying the eggs, open the carton to inspect them. If an egg has an unpleasant odor when opened, it is spoiled. The eggs should be clean and whole, without cracks. They should not be leaking or stuck to the carton.

Eggs are sold according to grade and size standards set by the USDA. The grade and size, which are clearly marked on the package, have no relationship to each other.

Egg Grade

A USDA grade shield on a package means that the eggs have been federally inspected for wholesomeness. The grade is determined by the inner and outer quality of the egg at the time of packaging. Workers examine egg interiors with bright lights in order to sort out unacceptable ones.

The three egg grades are AA, A, and B. Supermarkets typically carry grades AA and A. All grades of egg have the same nutritive value. However, their appearances differ after being cooked. Grades AA and A eggs have a thicker white. Use grades AA and A when appearance is important, as it is in making fried or poached eggs. Grade B eggs can be used in baked goods, when appearance does not matter.

Be a Smart Consumer

A Bacteria Barrier

While the eggshell is essential to the life of an egg, it also plays a role in protecting consumers' health. An eggshell contains up to 17,000 pores, which are protected by a coating called the cuticle, or bloom. The pores grow larger with age, however, increasing the chance for bacterial contamination. To reduce this risk, eggs are gathered soon after laying. They are washed and lightly coated with mineral oil to prevent oxygen from entering the shell. Boiling eggs strips off the oil coat.

Challenge Why do you think hard-cooked eggs must be eaten within a week, while fresh eggs keep for up to four weeks? Write your answer in one or more sentences.

Egg Size

Eggs are classified into sizes by the minimum weight for a dozen, so sizes can vary slightly in the same carton. The sizes most commonly sold are medium, large, extra large, and jumbo. Most recipes assume that large eggs will be used. If you use eggs of another size, you may need more or fewer eggs for the same results.

The price of eggs depends on the size as well as the supply of various sizes. Every time you go shopping, check the unit price to determine which size is the best buy.

Egg Storage

Eggs are highly perishable. Take eggs home right after buying and refrigerate them. Store them in the original carton rather than the egg tray in the refrigerator door, where food is exposed to warm air more often. Eggshells are porous and the eggs may lose quality after too much exposure. They also pick up aromas and flavors from other foods if they are stored uncovered or for too long.

Do not wash eggs before storing them. Washing eggs removes the protective coating that prevents bacteria from getting inside the shell.

Raw eggs stay fresh in the refrigerator for up to four weeks, depending on their freshness when purchased and on the refrigerator temperature. Refrigerate leftover cooked eggs and egg mixtures immediately and use them within three days. Use hard-cooked eggs in the shell within a week.

Some recipes call for only the yolk or the white. You can refrigerate leftover raw yolks, covered with water, for two days. You can refrigerate whites, in a tightly covered container, for four days.

Handle eggs gently to prevent cracking them. Discard dirty, cracked, or leaking eggs.

Freezing Eggs

You can freeze raw egg whites for longer storage. Place each egg white in a separate compartment of an ice cube tray. After freezing, put the frozen cubes in a tightly sealed freezer container and store in the freezer. Use two thawed egg whites to equal one large egg. Do not freeze cooked whites, because this makes them tough and rubbery.

Raw yolks need special treatment for freezing to keep them from getting thick and hard to mix after thawing. For every four yolks, beat in ⅛ teaspoon of salt. If you plan to use the yolks for a dessert, beat in 1½ teaspoons of sugar instead. Mark the container with the number of yolks and whether you added salt or sugar, then freeze them.

Never freeze whole eggs in the shell, because they may burst.

TECHNOLOGY FOR TOMORROW

Egg Laying Technology

The egg may be one of nature's most perfect foods, but nature gets help from technology to keep commercial egg producers in business. Caged hens are served their food by automated feeders set on timers. The light, temperature, and humidity of the indoor environment is monitored to promote egg production. The eggs are automatically gathered by conveyor belts under the cages, and transported to refrigerated holding rooms. Within one or two days, the fresh eggs are available in your supermarket's dairy case. Because the eggs from free-range hens are produced and collected in an environment that is less structured and has less impact on the hens themselves, many consumers choose free-range eggs.

Get Involved Under your teacher's supervision, use the Internet to research how the living conditions of free-range hens differ from those described above. How are the eggs of free-range hens collected? Would you choose to buy free-range eggs? Why or why not?

NCSS VII F Production, Distribution, and Consumption Compare how values and beliefs influence economic decisions in different societies.

Egg Substitutes

Egg substitutes are an alternative to whole eggs. Most are made by combining egg whites with ingredients such as vegetable oils, tofu, nonfat dry milk powder, and chemical additives, including emulsifiers, stabilizers, antioxidants, and artificial colors. You can use egg substitutes much the same as whole eggs. Egg substitutes are available frozen and in refrigerated liquid form.

Because they contain no egg yolks, egg substitutes have no cholesterol or fat and are lower in calories. They are a healthy alternative for people who are trying to reduce fat and cholesterol in their diet. Egg substitutes contain less protein and phosphorus than whole eggs, however, and they may lack some B vitamins. They are also more expensive than whole eggs.

✓ **Reading Check** **Describe** What is one step you should take before buying a carton of eggs?

Egg Science

Eggs have certain special properties that result mostly from their high protein content. Eggs act as a binder, thickener, leavening agent, and emulsifier. You can find eggs in the ingredients list for hamburger, stew, bread and salad dressings. Understanding why they do this can help you cook successfully with eggs.

Coagulation

When you cook eggs, their proteins coagulate, or change from liquid to semisolid. *What causes egg protein to coagulate?*

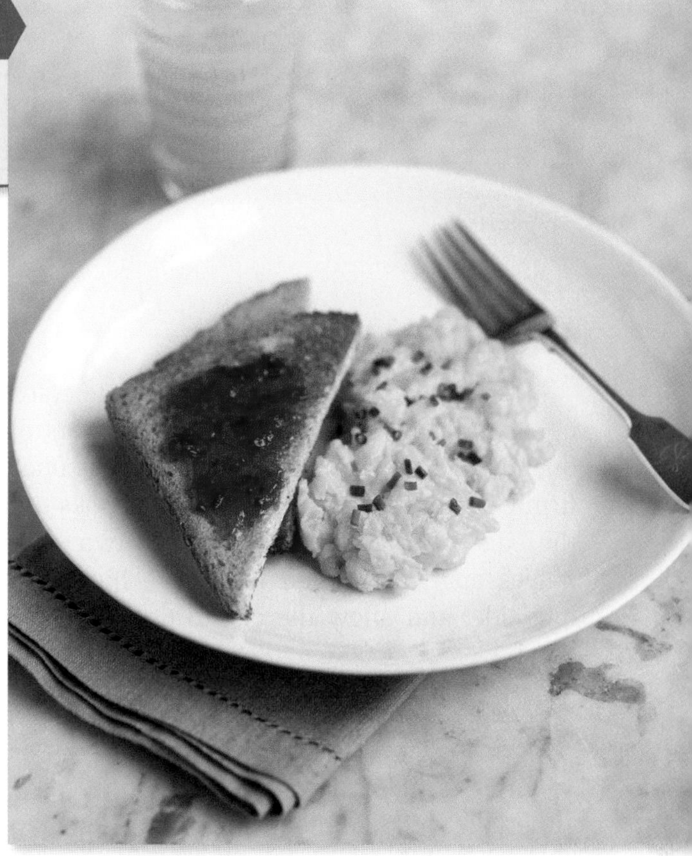

Eggs as a Binder

The proteins in eggs are shaped like coils. When the proteins are heated, the coils unwind and join loosely with other proteins. The new structures form pockets that hold water. When this happens, the egg **coagulates**, or becomes firm, changing from a liquid to a semisolid or solid state. The ability of egg proteins to coagulate is what helps eggs act as a binder in foods like meatloaf, and thicken dishes such as custards and fillings.

High heat and overcooking cause an egg's protein structure to tighten and push out its water. This makes the protein tough and watery. The cooked eggs may be dry and unappetizing. Gentle cooking helps prevents these problems.

Eggs as an Emulsifier

Egg yolks are excellent emulsifiers. An **emulsifier** is a substance that holds together two liquids that normally do not stay mixed, such as water and oil. How does this work? Proteins consist of many linked amino acids. In yolk protein, one end of an amino acid bonds with water, but the other end bonds with oil. This gives egg yolks the power to hold two ingredients together, such as vinegar and oil in salad dressing or lemon juice and oil in mayonnaise.

Eggs as a Leavening Agent

Egg whites act as leavening agents. When you beat egg whites, air enters the mixture and a foam forms. Egg whites have large protein molecules. Beating breaks down the protein. Continued beating thickens the foam.

An egg white foam adds volume and lightness to baked products such as angel food cake and soufflés. A **soufflé** (ˌsü-ˈflā) is a baked dish made by folding stiffly beaten whites into a sauce or puréed food. It is baked in a deep casserole until it puffs up. Beaten egg whites are also used to make meringues.

Preparing Eggs for Cooking

Egg cookery can be simple or complex. You can cook eggs alone or combine them with other ingredients in many recipes.

Some ways of preparing eggs, such as soft-boiling and hard-boiling, do not require any preparation. For most other ways of preparing eggs, such as frying and scrambling, you need to crack open the egg. For baked goods, soufflés, and other more complex dishes that include eggs as an ingredient, you may also need to separate the egg yolk from the white, and sometimes beat the whites.

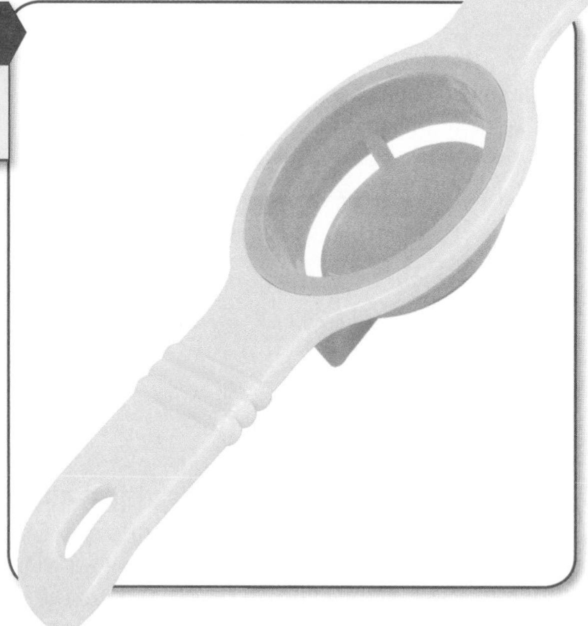

The Art of Separating

Egg separators make it easy to separate whites from yolks. *Why is this method recommended?*

Cracking the Shell

The first step in most egg recipes is to crack open the egg. Hold the egg in the fingers of one hand. Then rap the center of the egg once firmly against a clean surface. Some cooks use the edge of a clean bowl. Pull the two shell halves apart as though they were hinged at one side, and allow the egg to drop into the bowl.

Separating Eggs

Some recipes call for only part of an egg—either the yolk or the white. If you are not using the whole egg, you will need to separate the parts. Yolks are used in custards, sauces, mayonnaise, and pastry. Because beaten egg whites are airy, they add lightness to many baked items.

To separate an egg, carefully break it into an egg separator. An egg separator is a small device that functions like a **sieve**, or strainer, and allows the white to flow through, while leaving the yolk in the separator. An egg separator helps keep the yolk from bursting and running into the white, which can ruin a recipe. Whites that have a bit of yolk in them will not beat properly. Eggs separate more easily when cold. Refrigerate any unused yolk or white for later use.

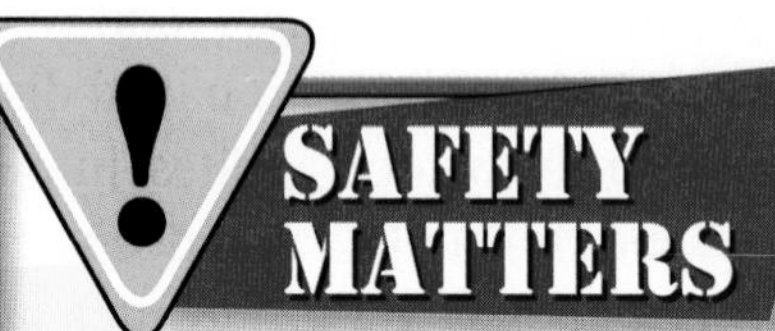

Banish Bacteria

Separate and cook eggs properly to protect yourself from harmful bacteria. Many cooks separate the egg white from the yolk by pouring the yolk back and forth between the two halves of the broken shell, letting the white fall into a bowl. This method is dangerous because bacteria on the shell can get into the egg. An egg separator should be used. To destroy the Salmonella bacteria that lives in some eggs, cook eggs and egg-based dishes to 160°F in the center. Raw eggs and foods that contain them, such as cookie dough, are not safe to eat.

What Would You Do? You prepare a recipe for brownies that calls for two eggs. After you pour the brownie mix into a baking dish, your friend says, "Yum! Let's lick the mixing bowl and spoon!"

Beating Egg Whites

Beaten egg whites are used in many dishes. When you beat whites, the foam should rise well. It should be stable and not collapse when folded with other ingredients and when baked. How can you make this happen?

First, make sure no trace of yolk is in the white. Even a drop of the yolk's fat can keep a foam from reaching full volume. If any yolk falls into the white, refrigerate it for later use and start again with another egg white. Be sure that your beaters and bowls are clean and free of fat. Use only glass or metal bowls. Plastic and wooden bowls absorb fat, and aluminum bowls darken the whites.

If you have time, allow the egg whites to stand at room temperature for up to 20 minutes before beating. This helps the foam reach full volume. If the egg white is cold, the protein does not break down as readily and create foam.

You can add extra ingredients to egg whites before or during beating to keep the foam stable. You can add an acidic ingredient, such as cream of tartar, before beating. Some recipes call for vinegar or lemon juice, which adds flavor. You can also add sugar along with cream of tartar for stabilization. Since sugar increases beating time, however, add it near the end of the beating process. Salt decreases foam stability. If a recipe calls for salt, add it to other ingredients rather than the whites.

Foam, Soft Peaks, and Stiff Peaks

As you beat whites, their texture and color change from thick, colorless, and transparent to fluffy, white, and opaque. You can beat whites to foam, or to soft or stiff peaks. Foam is a soft, airy mass.

Soft peaks gently bend over like waves when you lift the beaters from the mixture. If you continue beating, you will form stiff peaks. **Stiff peaks** stand up straight when the beaters are lifted from the mixture. Stop beating when you reach this stage. Overbeating turns a foam dry, hard, and lumpy, making it fall apart. Once egg whites lose air and moisture, they cannot be used.

Folding In Beaten Egg Whites

When you fold beaten egg whites into another mixture, do so gently. Stirring and beating cause loss of air and volume. Place the beaten whites on top of the mixture. Cut down through the whites with a rubber spatula to the bottom of the bowl. Drag some of the bottom mixture up the side, folding it lightly onto the whites in the middle. Turn the bowl and repeat just until the whites are incorporated.

✓ **Reading Check** **Contrast** When beating egg whites, what is the difference between soft peaks and stiff peaks?

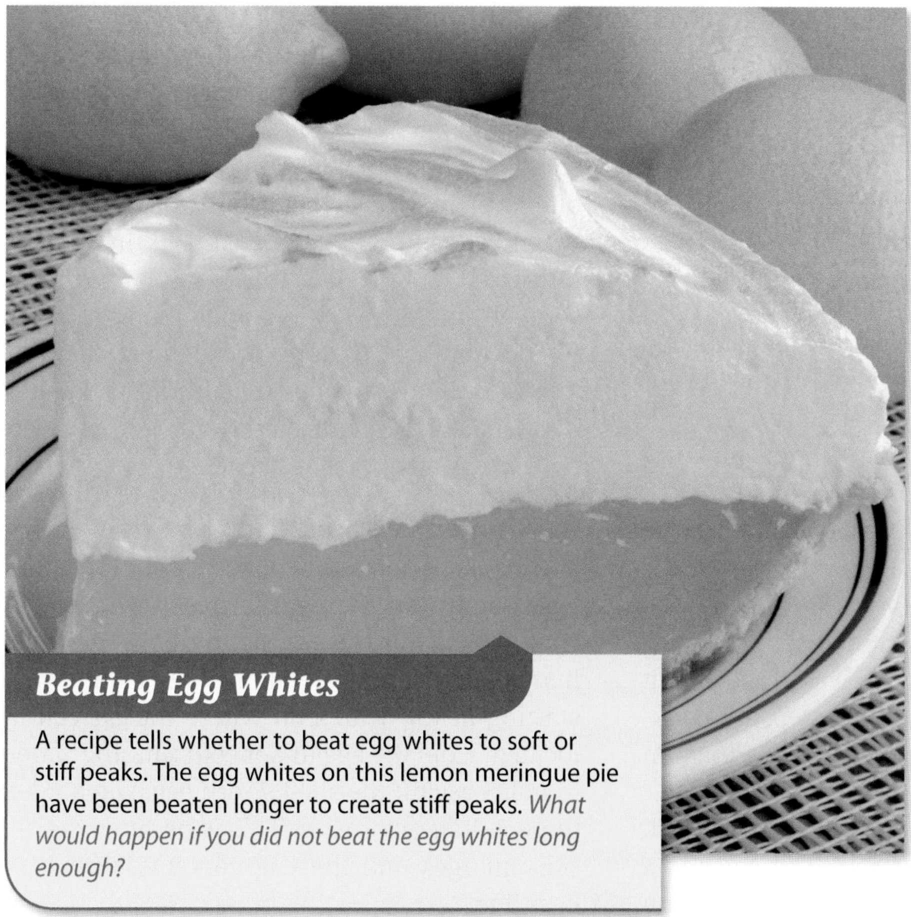

Beating Egg Whites

A recipe tells whether to beat egg whites to soft or stiff peaks. The egg whites on this lemon meringue pie have been beaten longer to create stiff peaks. *What would happen if you did not beat the egg whites long enough?*

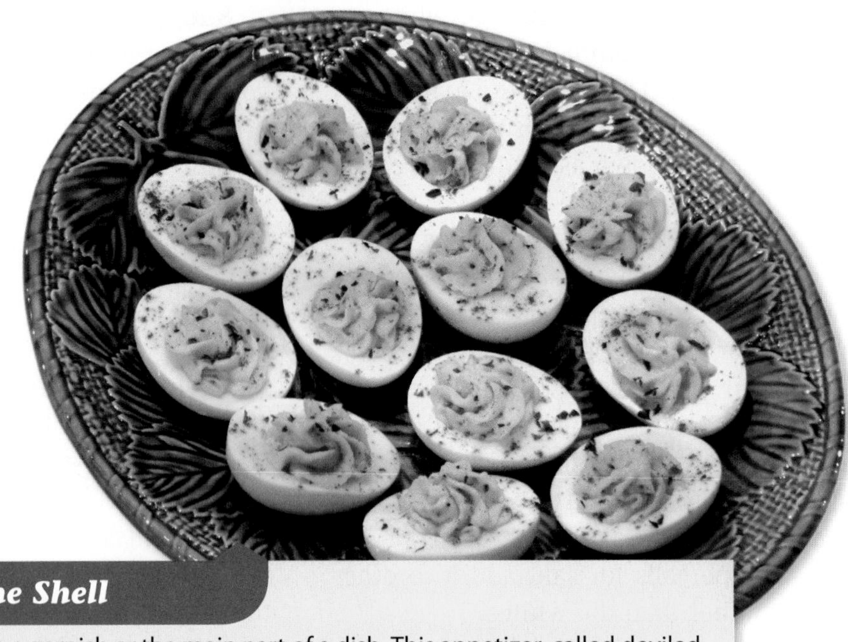

Eggs Cooked in the Shell

Hard-cooked eggs can be a garnish or the main part of a dish. This appetizer, called deviled eggs, uses hard-boiled eggs filled with a filling made from cooked egg yolks, mustard, and mayonnaise, and garnished with paprika. *What is a reliable way to cook eggs in the shell?*

Cooking with Eggs

Egg cookery can be simple or complex. You can cook eggs alone or combine them with other ingredients in many recipes.

Cooking Eggs in the Shell

To cook eggs in the shell, place a single layer of eggs in a saucepan. Add water to at least 1 inch above the eggs. Cover the pan and bring the water to a boil. Turn the heat off as soon as boiling begins. On an electric range, remove the pan from the heating element to prevent further boiling. Let the eggs stand, covered, in the hot water. Allow 12 minutes for medium-size eggs, 15 minutes for large eggs, and 18 minutes for extra large eggs. Do not let the eggs cook for less than 12 minutes, because harmful bacteria may survive.

When eggs are done, immediately pour off the hot water and run cold water over them or place them in ice water to stop the cooking process and cool them. Refrigerate them in their shells until you are ready to serve them.

Have you ever seen a hard-cooked egg yolk that has a gray-green surface? The color is a reaction between sulfur in the white and iron in the yolk. Cook eggs no longer than necessary to prevent this color change

Preventing Cracking

Eggs sometimes crack as they cook because the air inside the eggs expands as it heats. This usually happens when eggs are overheated or cooked for too long. Cooking eggs in more than one layer in a saucepan can also cause cracks when eggs bump together. An egg that cracks during cooking is safe to use, as long as you serve it right away. Never prick the egg with a pin or thumbtack before cooking to release the air. A small hole can create hairline cracks that allow bacteria to enter after the egg has been cooled and saved for later use.

Peeling Eggs Cooked in the Shell

To peel a medium-cooked or hard-cooked egg, gently tap the egg all over to crack the shell. Then roll the egg lightly between your hands to loosen the shell. Peel the shell away, starting at the wide end where the air cell is located. Hold the egg under cold running water to help ease off the shell. Fresh eggs are harder to peel than older eggs. This is because the air cell enlarges and the egg contents shrink as eggs age.

You can use peeled hard-cooked eggs in many ways. You can chop them, slice them, or cut them into wedges. You can add them to salads and casseroles, use them in sandwiches or as a garnish, or make deviled or pickled eggs.

Poaching Eggs

Poaching is one of many ways to cook eggs out of the shell. Poached eggs are cooked in simmering water. Like hard-boiling, this method adds no fat. Using fresh eggs and getting them to set quickly are keys to successful poaching.

To poach eggs, put water, milk, or broth in a saucepan to a depth of about 2 to 3 inches. Heat the liquid to boiling and then reduce it to a gentle simmer. Break one egg at a time into a small dish. Hold the dish close to the surface of the liquid and slip in the egg. Cook each egg until the white is completely set, about 3 to 5 minutes. The yolk should be thickened. Remove cooked eggs, one at a time, with a slotted spoon and drain for a few seconds.

Poached eggs are usually served on toast. You can also spoon cooked vegetables onto toasted English muffins and top them with poached eggs, or pour a flavored sauce, such as a cheese sauce or Hollandaise sauce, over the eggs.

Frying Eggs

Eggs can be fried in oil, margarine, or butter or in a nonstick skillet coated with vegetable oil cooking spray.

First, heat a small amount of fat in a skillet over medium-high heat until hot enough to sizzle a drop of water. Break one egg at a time into a small bowl or custard cup. Then gently slip the egg from the bowl into the heated skillet. This technique helps prevent the yolk from breaking. Cook the eggs until the whites are completely set and the yolks have thickened. To cook the tops, baste them with hot fat, turn the egg over carefully, or cover the skillet with a lid for the last minute or two of cooking.

Careers in Food

Alan Vonderwerth
Wholesale Food Buyer

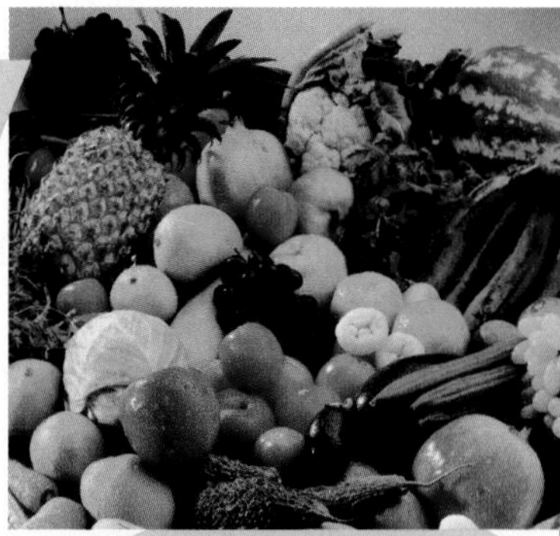

Q: What are your primary responsibilities?

A: My job is to produce a daily summary of the food needed for our culinary classes, generate a shopping list using the computer program ChefTec, and place orders through various vendors. I order from sources throughout the country, but prefer to deal with local companies in order to help the local economy and to keep our freight costs down.

Q: How do you become a wholesale buyer?

A: I got my opportunity through my previous experience in customer service and my management background. I started out as a storeroom clerk. Most companies prefer to promote from within.

Q: What is your favorite part of your job?

A: The challenge of going out and finding things I have not purchased before is a positive of this position.

"If you enjoy working with food, you can be successful."
— Alan Vonderwerth
Purchasing Manager, Professional Culinary Institute, Campbell, CA

Education and Training

A college degree in culinary arts or business. Experience working in the food industry is also helpful.

Qualities and Skills

Computer skills, organization skills, flexibility, and patience are important.

Related Career Opportunities

Other related opportunities include restaurant manager or food and beverage manager at a hotel.

For an interesting variation on fried eggs, make a hole in a slice of bread or frozen waffle and place it in a greased, heated skillet. Break the egg into the hole and fry. Fried eggs can also be served in a sandwich or on top of steak, hash, or vegetables.

Scrambling Eggs

Scrambled eggs are beaten, then fried. To make fluffy scrambled eggs, beat eggs together with water in a bowl. Use 1 tablespoon of water for each egg. Heat a small amount of fat on low in a skillet, or use a vegetable oil cooking spray.

Pour the egg mixture into the heated skillet and let it stand for 30 to 60 seconds. As the mixture starts to thicken, draw an inverted turner gently through the eggs. This forms large curds and allows uncooked egg to flow to the bottom of the skillet. Continue this process until the eggs are thickened and there is no more liquid. Curds should be large and fluffy. Do not stir the eggs constantly. This beats out the air and moisture and creates small, tough curds.

You can also scramble eggs by breaking them directly into the skillet. When the whites begin to set, mix the eggs right in the pan and cook them until they are thickened and there is no more liquid. The eggs will be less fluffy and have streaks of white and yellow.

Baking Eggs

Baked eggs, also known as **shirred eggs**, are eggs baked in a greased, shallow dish and often topped with a small amount of milk.

To make baked eggs, break eggs into a small bowl. Then slip them into a greased, shallow baking dish or a large custard cup. You can use individual dishes or place several eggs in one dish. If you like, top the eggs with a small amount of milk.

Preheat the oven to 325°F. Bake the eggs until the whites are completely set and the yolks thicken, about 12 to 18 minutes.

You can also bake eggs in nests of cooked vegetables, cooked grains, or in hollowed-out rolls.

Making Basic Omelets

An **omelet** is an egg mixture formed into a large, thick pancake, usually filled with ingredients and folded. Unlike scrambled eggs, the eggs in an omelet are not stirred. A **frittata** (frē-ˈtä-tə) is an unfolded omelet with fillings stirred into the egg mixture.

A basic omelet, also called a French omelet, is made as follows:

1. **Mix.** Mix 2 eggs, 2 tablespoons of water, and a dash each of salt and pepper with a fork or whisk until just blended.

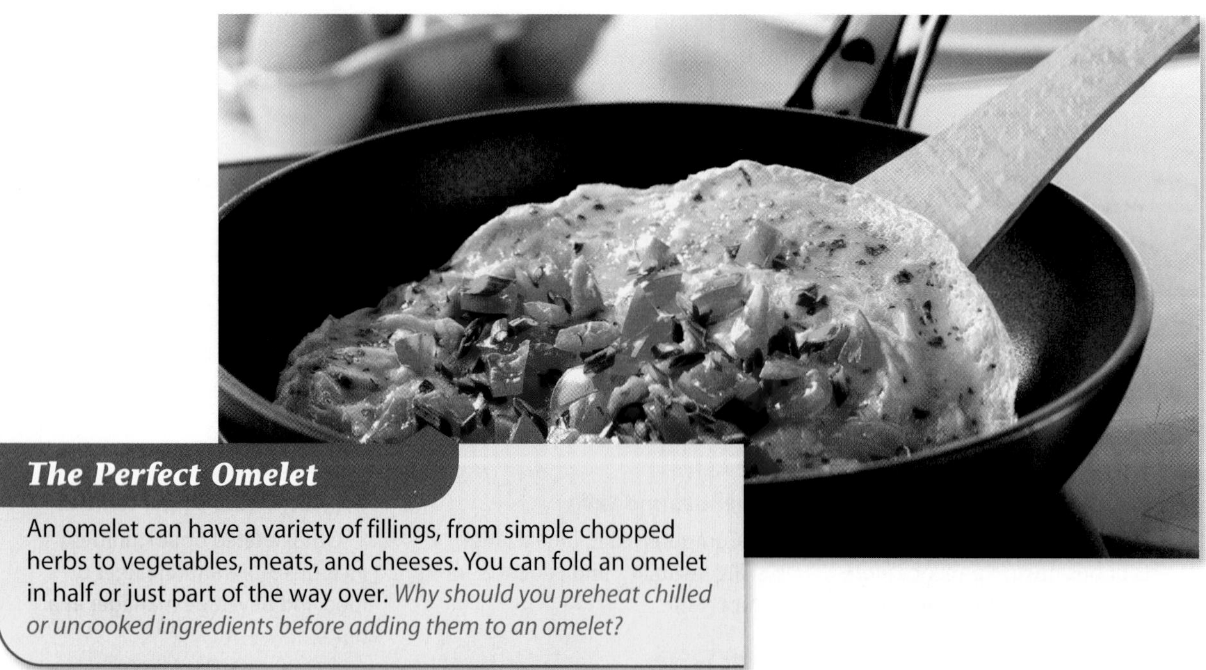

The Perfect Omelet

An omelet can have a variety of fillings, from simple chopped herbs to vegetables, meats, and cheeses. You can fold an omelet in half or just part of the way over. *Why should you preheat chilled or uncooked ingredients before adding them to an omelet?*

2. **Heat.** Heat 1 tablespoon of butter or oil in an omelet pan or a skillet over medium heat until hot enough to sizzle a drop of water.
3. **Pour.** Pour in the egg mixture all at once. Allow it to flow to the edge of the pan, but do not stir. The edge should begin to set right away.
4. **Lift and tilt.** With a turner, lift just a little around the firming edge so that uncooked portions flow beneath to the pan surface. Tilt the pan as needed. Be careful not to break the mixture that has already set. Continue until the top is thickened and no visible liquid egg remains.
5. **Add filling.** Spread filling over half of the omelet.
6. **Fold.** Using the turner, fold the omelet in half or nearly so. Tilting the skillet slightly away from you and folding toward the low side may help.
7. **Serve.** Slide the omelet onto a plate and serve.

Use your imagination when deciding on omelet fillings. You can use cheese, sauces, cooked vegetables, diced or sliced fruit, or cooked diced meat, poultry, or fish. Vegetarian omelets are very popular. Small pieces of filling work best, because they are less likely to tear the omelet. Fillings only have a chance to heat up slightly, so preheat cold fillings and cook raw vegetables and meats before adding them to an omelet.

Making Puffy Omelets

A puffy omelet is made with beaten egg whites and baked in the oven. Separate the eggs and beat the whites and yolks separately. Beating the whites makes the omelet light and fluffy. Fold the stiffly beaten whites into the yolks. Pour the mixture into a skillet with an ovenproof handle.

First, cook the mixture on top of the range, without disturbing it, until it is puffed and lightly browned on the bottom, about 5 minutes. Then move the skillet to an oven preheated to 350°F. Bake for 10 to 12 minutes or until a knife inserted in the center comes out clean.

Science in Action: Denaturation

The protein molecules in egg whites are coiled. Beating them uncoils the molecules. This process results in denaturation, which literally means "changing the nature." When egg whites are beaten into soft peaks, they are partially denatured and retain some elasticity. If they are beaten into stiff peaks, they are fully denatured and have no elasticity.

Procedure Many protein-rich foods undergo denaturation, but not always through beating. Denaturation can also happen through heating, such as when liquid foods become solid. To see denaturation at work, beat the whites of two eggs until they are partially denatured. Then beat them until they are fully denatured.

Analysis Write your observations of how the texture and appearance of the egg whites changed as they became denatured. What is another example of a protein-rich food that undergoes denaturation?

NSES B Develop an understanding of interactions of energy and matter.

You can serve a puffy omelet folded or open-face. To serve it folded, partially cut through the center of the omelet to make it easier to fold. Add fillings and fold. With practice, you can learn to slide half the omelet onto a plate and fold the omelet by lifting the pan as the other half falls out. To serve the omelet open-face, tilt the skillet over a warm plate. Slide the omelet onto the plate. Spoon filling over the top, if desired. Cut the omelet in half or into wedges and serve immediately.

Microwaving Eggs

Cooking eggs in the microwave oven takes special care. Eggs overcook easily, so start with the minimum time suggested and check them frequently. Pierce the yolk before cooking to break the membrane and allow heat and steam to escape. Remove eggs from the microwave while they are still moist and soft. The cooking will finish during the standing time.

You can make eggs in a variety of ways in the microwave oven.

Fried Eggs Break the eggs into a lightly greased dish. Gently pierce the yolks with the tip of a knife or a wooden pick. Cover the eggs and cook them at 50 percent power until they are done, about 2 to 3 minutes. Let stand, covered, until the whites are completely set and the yolks thicken, about 30 seconds to 1 minute.

Scrambled Eggs Pour a beaten egg mixture into a large custard cup. Cook it on full power, stirring once or twice, until almost set, about 1 to 1½ minutes. Stir. If necessary, cover and let stand until the eggs are thick and there is no more liquid, about 1 minute.

Poached Eggs Pour hot water into a large custard cup or a small deep bowl. Break and slip in the eggs. Pierce the yolks with the tip of a knife or a wooden pick. Cook them on full power for 1½ to 3 minutes. If necessary, let stand, covered, until the whites are completely set and the yolks thicken. Lift the eggs out with a slotted spoon, or pour the water off to serve in the custard cup.

Remember that microwave ovens cook unevenly. Make sure the egg or any egg dish is thoroughly cooked before eating.

Never microwave eggs in the shell. Heat and steam build up inside an egg, causing it to explode.

Custards

A **custard** is a thickened blend of milk, eggs, and sugar. It can be a base for many main dishes. Custards come in two types, soft and baked.

Soft Custard

Soft custard, also known as stirred custard, is creamy and pourable. You can serve it as a pudding or as a sauce over cake or fruit. It is used in tarts as the sweet layer between the crust and the fruits. Soft custard is made by beating together eggs, sugar, and salt, if desired, then stirring in nonfat or low-fat milk. The amount of each ingredient determines the custard's thickness.

Cook the mixture over low heat, stirring constantly, until it is just thick enough to coat a metal spoon with a thin film. Remove from the heat to prevent overcooking. If soft custard is overcooked, it curdles. If soft custard is undercooked, it stays thin and watery. Cool cooked custard quickly by setting the pan in a bowl of cold water. Stir for a few minutes, and then stir in vanilla. You can flavor custard at this point. Add chocolate, cinnamon, or flavored syrup. You can also prepare soft custard in a double boiler.

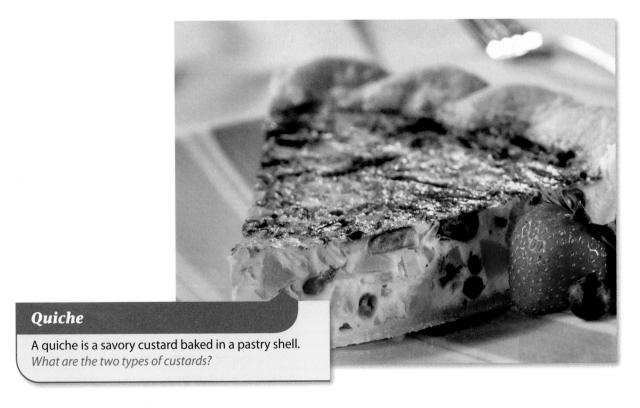

Quiche

A quiche is a savory custard baked in a pastry shell.
What are the two types of custards?

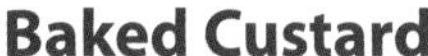

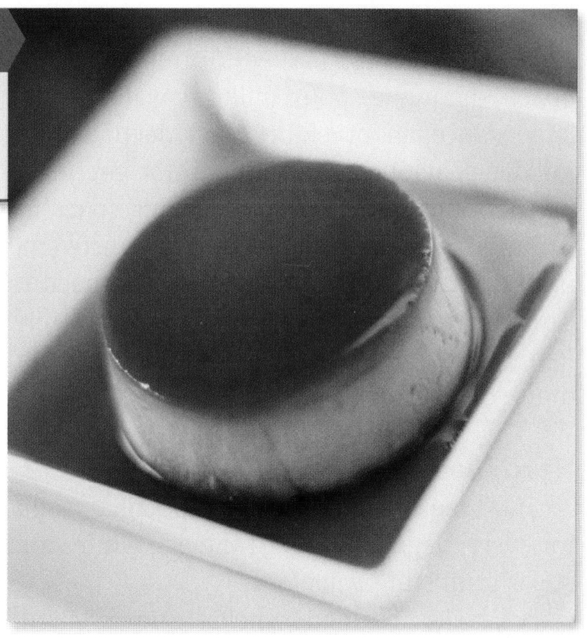

Flan

Flan is a custard that is chilled in a small bowl that has been lined with caramel. *What happens when custard is overbaked?*

Baked Custard

Baked custard has a firm, delicate texture and is cooked in the oven. Many well-known desserts have a baked custard base, including custard pie. Flan is a Spanish custard topped with caramel sauce. Unsweetened, baked custard can be served as a main dish. **Quiche** is a pie with custard filling, containing such foods as chopped vegetables, cheese, and chopped, cooked meat.

To make baked custard, first beat ingredients as you do for soft custard. Then, instead of stirring the mixture over the stove, pour it into lightly greased custard cups or a casserole dish. Set the cups or dish in a large baking pan. Add hot water to the pan to ½ inch below the top of the custard. This insulates the custard so it will not overcook.

If custard is overbaked, it curdles. If custard is underbaked, it will not set. Bake the custard until a knife inserted near the center comes out clean. Remove the custard dish from the hot water and cool it on a wire rack for about 5 to 10 minutes. Serve it warm or refrigerate it for later.

Meringues

Meringue is a foam made of beaten egg whites and sugar and used for baked desserts. Meringues are most frequently used for pie toppings and cake icings. Meringue pies are admired for the lightly browned, white topping that sits tall above a base.

Meringue can be either soft or hard. Soft meringue goes on pies and tarts and is incorporated into rice and bread puddings. Hard meringue is made into cookies and dessert shells.

To make meringue beat egg whites along with cream of tartar until the mixture is foamy. Then gradually beat in sugar, one tablespoon at a time. Continue beating the mixture until the sugar dissolves. If the meringue feels gritty when a little is rubbed between your thumb and forefinger, not all the sugar has dissolved. It takes practice to create a successful meringue.

Soft Meringue

Soft meringue uses 2 tablespoons of sugar for every 1 egg white. You need about 3 egg whites to make enough meringue for a 9-inch pie. Beat the egg whites and sugar only until soft peaks form.

Spread soft meringue over hot, precooked pie filling or pudding. On a pie, the meringue should touch the crust all around the edge. Otherwise, the meringue may shrink during baking. Bake the pie in a preheated oven according to recipe directions until the peaks are lightly browned. If you overbake a meringue, a tough, chewy skin forms.

When liquid accumulates between the meringue and pie filling, the meringue is said to **weep**. This occurs because the meringue was spread on a cool filling. To avoid this, always spread the meringue on a hot filling. **Beading**, brown droplets on the surface of the meringue, may occur if the meringue is overcooked.

You can also poach a soft meringue to serve on puddings or with fruit sauce. To poach meringue, pour milk or water into a large saucepan or skillet, just deep enough for the poaching process. Drop the meringue by spoonfuls into the liquid, leaving space for the meringue to expand. Simmer uncovered until firm, about 5 minutes. You may need to turn larger spoonfuls over to cook completely. Remove the meringue with a slotted spoon and drain. Serve immediately or chill for later.

Hard Meringue

Hard meringue uses 4 tablespoons of sugar for every 1 egg white. Beat the egg whites and sugar until stiff peaks form.

To make meringue shells, line a baking sheet with parchment paper or foil. Use a spoon, spatula, or pastry tube to spread the mixture on the baking sheet to the desired size. Build up the edges to form rims. You can shape small individual shells or a single large one. You can also shape meringue in a pie plate to make a meringue pie crust.

Hard meringue becomes crisp by baking it at a low temperature for a long time. This allows the water to evaporate slowly, leaving the meringue light and crisp. Bake the meringue in a preheated oven at 225°F for 1 to 1½ hours. Then turn off the oven and allow the shells to dry out in the oven for at least one hour. A meringue that does not dry well may be sticky and chewy. Cool the meringue completely and then fill the shells just as you would a pastry shell.

To shape meringue cookies, drop the meringue onto a lightly greased or lined baking sheet with a spoon or pipe it from a pastry bag. When baked, the cookies should be crisp and dry but not browned.

Light and Healthy Recipe

Vegetable Egg White Omelet

Ingredients

- **2** egg whites
- **2 Tbsp.** Water
- **1 tsp.** vegetable oil
- **1 Tbsp.** Julienned onion
- **1 Tbsp.** Julienned red bell pepper
- **1 Tbsp.** Julienned green bell pepper
- **1 Tbsp.** Julienned carrots

Directions

1. Beat the egg whites with the water until light and fluffy.
2. Heat the oil in a small pan on high heat and add the onions. Sauté for one minute.
3. Add the remaining vegetables and sauté for another minute. Remove the vegetables from the heat and set aside.
4. Lower heat to medium and cook the eggs. With a wooden spoon or spatula, lift the eggs so that all can be cooked.
5. Spread the vegetables on one side of the omelet and fold the other side over. Slide the cooked omelet onto a dish and serve.

If served with whole wheat toast and orange juice, this omelet still has all the protein necessary to make a complete meal.

Yield 1 Serving

Nutrition Analysis per Serving

■ Calories	100
■ Total fat	5 g
Saturated fat	0 g
Cholesterol	0 mg
■ Sodium	172 mg
■ Carbohydrate	3 g
Dietary fiber	1 g
Sugars	2 g
■ Protein	11 g

CHAPTER 33 Review & Applications

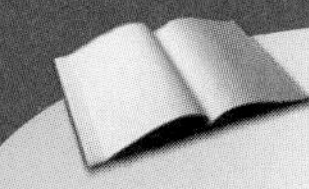

After You Read

Chapter Summary

Eggs are versatile, nutritious, and economic. They are comprised of several parts. Eggs contain many valuable nutrients. They should be selected and handled with care. Eggs are available in different grades and sizes. Proper storage keeps eggs fresh. Egg substitutes are a low-calorie, fat- and cholesterol-free alternative to eggs. Eggs have special properties that allow them to act as binders, emulsifiers, and leavening agents. Some ways of preparing eggs require cracking the shell, separating eggs, or beating egg whites. Egg cookery can be simple or complex. There are numerous methods for cooking eggs.

Content and Academic Vocabulary Review

1. Use each of these content and academic vocabulary words in a sentence.

Content Vocabulary

- air cell (p. 516)
- albumen (p. 516)
- yolk (p. 516)
- chalazae (p. 516)
- coagulate (p. 519)
- emulsifier (p. 519)
- soufflé (p. 519)
- soft peaks (p. 521)
- stiff peaks (p. 521)
- shirred eggs (p. 524)
- omelet (p. 524)
- frittata (p. 524)
- custard (p. 526)
- quiche (p. 527)
- meringue (p. 527)
- weep (p. 527)
- beading (p. 527)

Academic Vocabulary

- ruptured (p. 516)
- sieve (p. 520)

Review Key Concepts

2. **Identify** and describe three important parts of an egg.
3. **Describe** the nutrients found in eggs.
4. **Explain** how to safely store eggs.
5. **Summarize** why eggs act as a binder.
6. **Describe** how beating affects egg whites.
7. **Identify** the steps for making an omelet.

Critical Thinking

8. **Explain** why it is not safe for Gerard to crack eggs on the side of the mixing bowl he is using to combine ingredients.
9. **Conclude** why Vera's cake mix lacks volume even though she quickly stirred in beaten egg whites.
10. **Identify** the reasons why a poached egg dish might be featured on the "Light and Healthy" portion of a restaurant's breakfast menu.

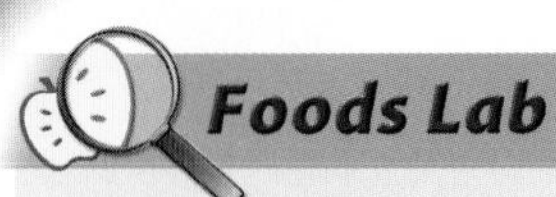

Foods Lab

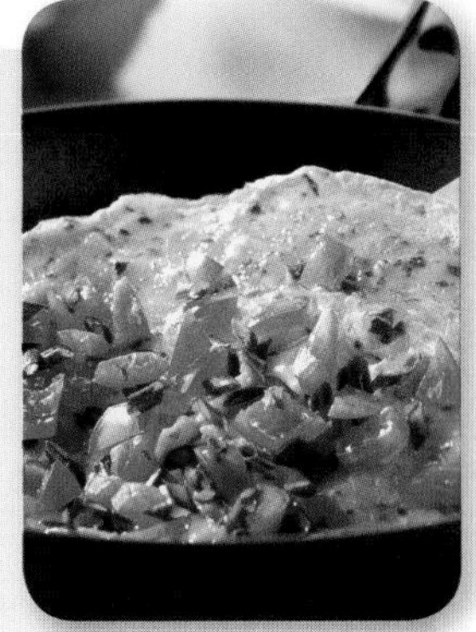

11. Make an Omelet Preparing an omelet is often harder than it looks, and requires care and attention. The end result, however, is usually worth the effort.

Procedure Make a basic omelet. Choose filling and seasoning ingredients. Review the preparation steps and make a list of criteria that you think the finished omelet should meet—such as even browning or warm filling.

Analysis Write one or more paragraphs to answer these questions: How well did the omelet meet the criteria you listed? What was the biggest challenge? How can you make preparation easier in the future? How did the ingredients taste in the cooked omelet?

HEALTHFUL CHOICES

12. The Right Dozen At the supermarket, Rick opens one carton of brown grade AA eggs and finds that two are cracked. A second carton contains white grade A eggs that are crack- and odor-free. A third carton contains grade AA brown eggs, and one is cracked. Which is the most healthful choice?

TECH Connection

13. Eggs Around the World Eggs are regarded as a nutritious food staple around the world. Choose a culture with which you are not familiar. Under your teacher's supervision, use the Internet to research that culture's cuisine and find one interesting dish that is prepared using eggs. Write a summary of your findings and share it with the class. Is the egg used as a main ingredient or a binder, emulsifier, or thickener? Describe the ingredients and preparation method. If possible, show a picture of the egg dish.

Real-World Skills

Problem-Solving Skills

14. Preventing Food Waste Yolanda, a frequent baker, is preparing a dessert that calls for egg yolks. After separating the eggs, Yolanda is left with several egg whites. She does not want to throw them away. How can she store them and use them later?

Interpersonal and Collaborative Skills

15. Egg Examination Follow your teacher's instructions to form pairs. Your teacher will present you with two eggs: one purchased recently, one purchased weeks ago. Crack them open onto separate plates. Take turns examining each. Work together to evaluate the eggs' freshness. What conclusions can you make and why?

Financial Literacy Skills

16. Protein Foods Compare the protein in eggs with three other protein sources. Which of the four foods has the most protein per serving? Compare cost per serving of protein. Which of the four protein sources is the least expensive? Which is the most expensive?

Academic Skills

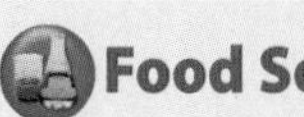

Food Science

17. Egg Thickeners Custard is a liquid thickened or set by gentle coagulation of egg protein. It is usually baked at a moderate temperature in a water bath.

Procedure Combine 3 beaten eggs, 1½ cups milk, ⅓ cup sugar, and 1 teaspoon vanilla in a medium mixing bowl. Combine well, but avoid making air bubbles. Ladle into 6 small bowls. Bake 3 of these in a water bath at 325° for about 35 minutes, or until center is slightly jiggly. Repeat with 2 without a water bath. Bake one in a water bath at 375°. Compare the results.

Analysis Why are temperature and a water bath important in baking custards? What acts as the thickener for the custard?

NCES B Develop an understanding of interactions of energy and matter.

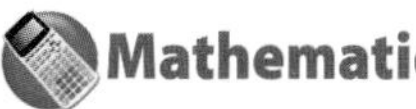

Mathematics

18. Deviled Eggs Wanting to make deviled eggs, Jorge takes six eggs out of a full carton and boils them. Jorge would like them to cool off for a while, so, without thinking, he places them back in the egg carton in the refrigerator. Later, when he goes to take them out, he realizes that he doesn't know which six eggs are hard-boiled, and which six are raw. What is the probability that he will select two hard-boiled eggs from the carton?

Math Concept **Probability** When two events are dependent (i.e., the probability of a second event depends on the outcome of the first), find the probability of each event, and multiply those probabilities together.

Starting Hint For the first egg picked, the probability that it is hard-boiled is 6/12 (or ½). However, when selecting the second egg, there will be one fewer hard-boiled egg, and one fewer egg overall.

NCTM Data Analysis and Probability Understand and apply basic concepts of probability.

English Language Arts

19. Egg Symbology In many cultures, some foods are seen as symbols. Throughout history, eggs have symbolized different things to different people. Research the symbology of the egg in one culture during one time period. Summarize your findings in writing. Present them to the class.

NCTE 7 Conduct research and gather, evaluate, and synthesize data to communicate discoveries.

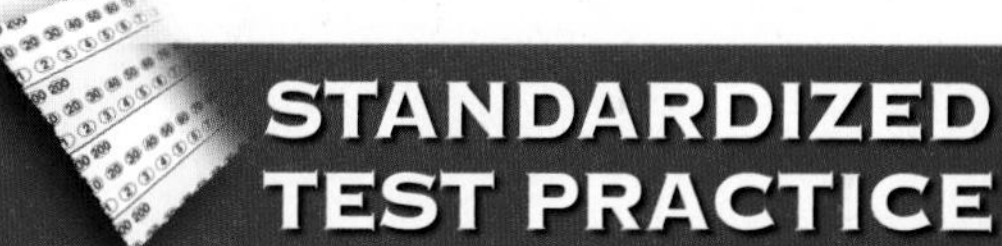

STANDARDIZED TEST PRACTICE

TRUE OR FALSE

Read the statement and determine if it is true or false.

20. Most recipes assume that large eggs will be used.

a. True
b. False

Test-Taking Tip Before deciding whether a statement is true or false, read it carefully, and recall what you have learned from reading the text. Does the statement reflect what you know? Pay close attention to individual words. One word can make the difference between a true statement and a false one.

CHAPTER 34

Meat

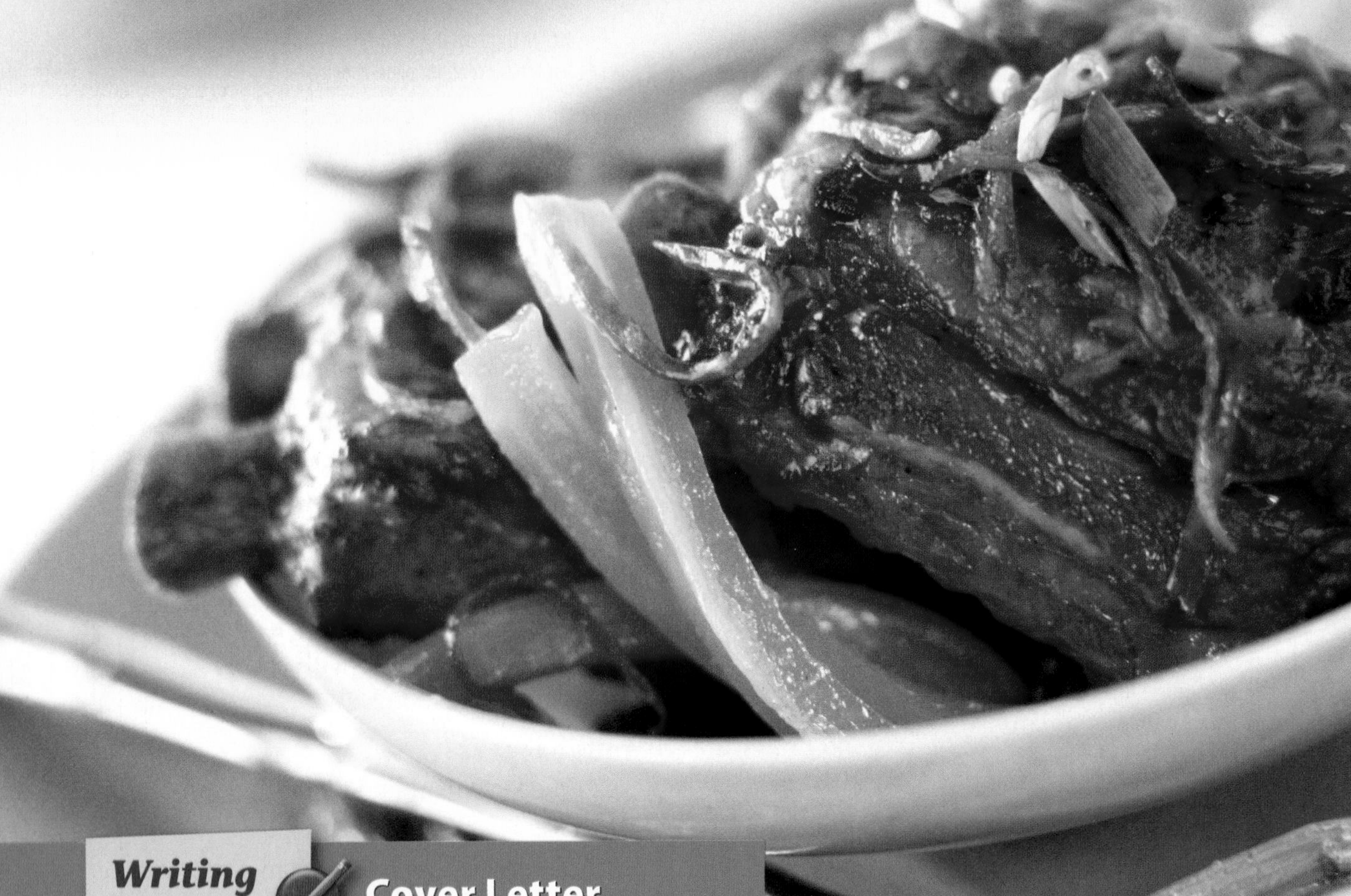

Writing Activity: Cover Letter

Introduce Yourself A new grocery store has opened in your neighborhood. The shop is hiring, and you are interested in a job. Write a cover letter to the shop's manager in which you tell her about yourself and describe the skills you can offer as an employee.

Writing Tips Follow these steps to write a cover letter:

- Include a return-address heading, the date, recipient's address, and salutation, or greeting.
- Make sure your writing has a professional tone.
- End your letter with a closing and your name.
- Proofread the letter to make sure it is free from errors.

Activate Prior Knowledge

Meat as the Centerpiece Meat is the center of many meals. *What is the nutritional benefit of combining a kebab with rice and tomatoes?*

Reading Guide

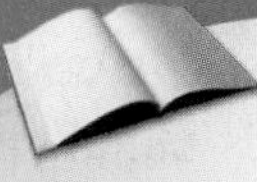

Before You Read

Preview Examine the photos, figures and captions. Consider the variety of meat types, cuts, and cooking methods.

Read to Learn

Key Concepts

- **Explain** the three main parts of meat.
- **Describe** the nutritional value of meat.
- **Identify** and explain the most common grades of beef.
- **Explain** what to look for when buying meat.
- **List** methods for cooking meat.

Main Idea

Meat is a flavorful, versatile, and nutritious food that comes in a variety of forms and can be prepared in many ways.

Content Vocabulary

You will find definitions for these words in the glossary at the back of this book.

- ☐ meat
- ☐ muscle
- ☐ grain
- ☐ connective tissue
- ☐ collagen
- ☐ elastin
- ☐ marbling
- ☐ cut
- ☐ wholesale cut
- ☐ retail cut
- ☐ variety meat
- ☐ processed meat
- ☐ cold cuts
- ☐ doneness

Academic Vocabulary

You will find these words in your reading and on your tests. Use the glossary to look up their definitions if necessary.

- similar
- uniform

Graphic Organizer

Use a graphic organizer like the one below to take notes about the four most common meats sold in the United States.

BEEF	VEAL	LAMB	PORK

Graphic Organizer Go to this book's Online Learning Center at **glencoe.com** to print out this graphic organizer.

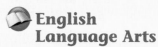

Academic Standards

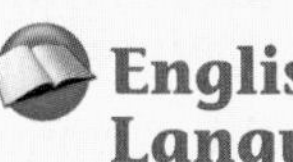

English Language Arts

NCTE 12 Use language to accomplish individual purposes.

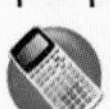

Mathematics

NCTM Number and Operations Understand numbers, ways of representing numbers, relationships among numbers, and number systems.

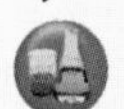

Science

NSES A Develop understandings about scientific inquiry.

NCTE *National Council of Teachers of English*
NCTM *National Council of Teachers of Mathematics*
NSES *National Science Education Standards*
NCSS *National Council for the Social Studies*

Makeup of Meat

Meat is flavorful, versatile, and highly nutritious. **Meat** is the edible muscle of animals, typically cattle, sheep, and pigs.

Meat has three main parts: muscle, connective tissue, and fat. **Figure 34.1** shows the structure of muscle tissue.

Muscle Sometimes called muscle fibers, **muscle** is protein-rich tissue made of long, thin cells grouped together in bundles. As bundles group together, they form individual muscles. The lengthwise direction of muscle is called the **grain**. If you cut meat across the grain, you break up the muscle fibers, making it easier to chew. Most meats sold in retail stores are cut across the grain.

Connective Tissue The protein material that binds muscle together into bundles is called **connective tissue**. This tissue not only holds muscle fibers together but also anchors muscle to bone. Meat has several types of connective tissue, including collagen and elastin. **Collagen** (ˈkä-lə-jən) is the thin, white, transparent connective tissue found in tendons, between muscle cells, and between muscles. When cooked in moist heat, collagen softens and turns into gelatin. **Elastin** (i-ˈlas-tən) is the tough, elastic, and yellowish connective tissue found in ligaments and blood vessel walls. It cannot be softened by heat and is usually cut away before cooking. To tenderize elastin, you must pound, cut, or grind it.

Fat In addition to muscle and connective tissue, meat contains both visible and invisible fat. A layer of visible fat sometimes surrounds the muscle. Small white flecks of fat, called **marbling**, may also appear within the muscle tissue. Invisible fat is part of the chemical composition of meat.

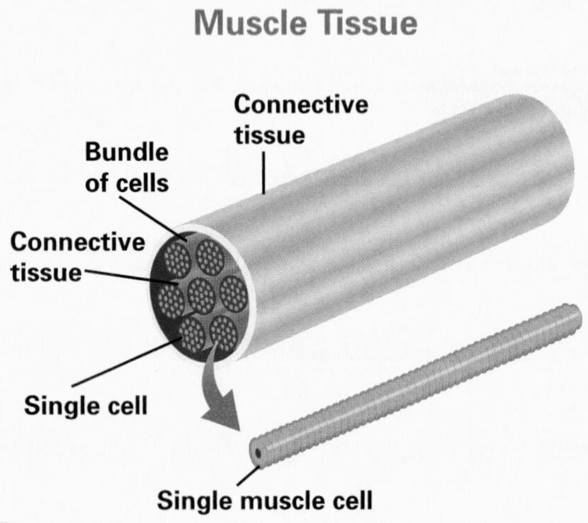

✓ Reading Check **True or False** Cutting meat in the direction of the grain makes it easier to chew.

Figure 34.1 Muscle Fibers

Protein-Rich Tissue Muscle is made of long cells, bundled together with connective tissue. ***What is the major nutrient in muscle?***

Nutrients in Meat

Meat is an excellent source of protein. It is also a major source of iron, zinc, phosphorus, thiamin, riboflavin, niacin, and vitamins B_6 and B_{12}. Meat can be high in saturated fat, however, so choose lean meats when possible.

Meat belongs to the same food group as poultry, fish, dry beans, eggs, and nuts. Teens need 5 to 6 ounces of these protein foods each day. Two to 3 ounces of cooked meat is about the size of your palm.

Types and Cuts of Meat

The four most common meats sold in the United States are beef, veal, lamb, and pork. **Figure 34.2** shows the sources and characteristics of different types of meat.

Cuts of Meat

A **cut** is a specific, edible part of meat, such as a steak, chop, or roast. Meat is first divided into large wholesale cuts, also called primal cuts. A **wholesale cut** is a large cut that is sold to retail stores. **Figure 34.3** shows the wholesale cuts of beef, veal, lamb, and pork. The retailer divides wholesale cuts into retail cuts.

Figure 34.2 Types of Meat

Common Meats Different types of meat come from different animals, as well as animals of different ages. ***How do beef, veal, and baby beef differ in flavor?***

Meat	Source	Characteristics
Beef	Cattle more than one year old.	Hearty flavor; firm texture; bright, deep red color with firm, creamy white fat.
Veal	Calves (young cattle), usually one to three months old.	Mild flavor; firm texture; light, gray-pink color with very little fat.
Baby beef	Calves between six and twelve months old.	Pink-red color; stronger flavor and coarser texture than veal.
Lamb	Sheep less than a year old.	Unique, mild flavor; bright, pink-red color; brittle white fat. Sometimes covered with a fell, a thin membrane under the hide, which helps retain juices during cooking.
Mutton	Sheep over two years old.	Less tender than lamb; stronger flavor.
Pork	Pigs less than a year old.	Tender texture; mild flavor; gray-pink color; soft white fat. Older animals have meat with a darker pink color.

Figure 34.3 Wholesale Cuts of Meat

Primal Cuts Different types of meat are cut into different wholesale cuts. Learning the names of the wholesale cuts can help you buy the right meat for your purpose. ***What is meat from the beef shoulder called? What is meat from the beef leg called?***

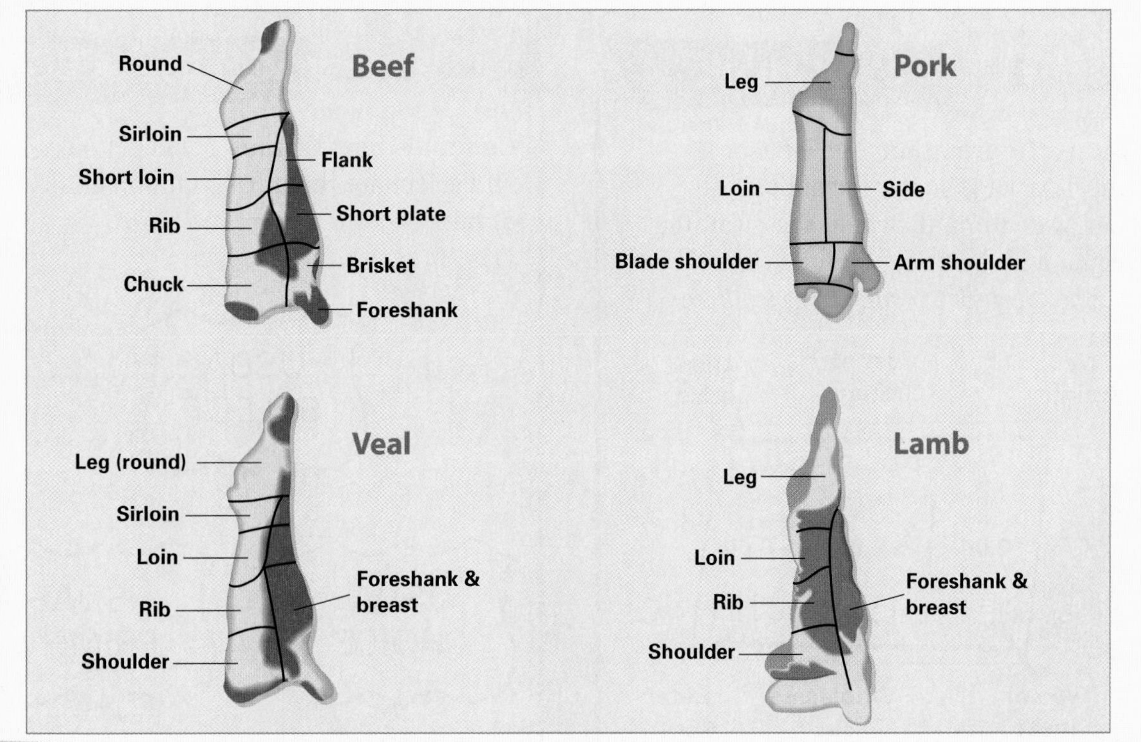

A **retail cut** is the small cut of meat sold to consumers. For example, one wholesale cut of beef is chuck, from the shoulder area. Retail cuts from chuck include blade roast, short ribs, and arm pot roast. Meat cuts from the same location in beef, veal, lamb, and pork are usually **similar**, or alike, in shape but different in size.

The price label on a meat package identifies the cut. The meat type is listed first. The wholesale cut is listed second. This tells you which part of the animal the meat came from. The retail cut is listed third. **Figure 34.4** shows a sample meat label.

Inspection and Grading of Meat

The Federal Meat Inspection Act requires that all meat shipped across state lines be inspected for wholesomeness, or healthfulness before and after the animals are slaughtered. States have similar laws that apply to meat sold within a state. Meat products that pass federal inspection standards are marked with a stamp. The stamp appears in only a few places on the animal.

The USDA also grades meat. Inspection is mandatory, but grading is a voluntary program available to the meat industry, which pays for the service. Meat is graded according to standards that include the amount of meat on the animal, the amount of marbling, the age of the animal, and the texture and appearance of the meat. The grade is stamped on the meat. Both inspection and grade marks are stamped with a harmless vegetable dye, so they do not have to be cut off before cooking.

Lamb, veal, and beef are graded with the same grades with one exception: "good" veal and lamb are the same as "select" beef. Pork is not graded because the meat is more **uniform**, or consistent, in quality.

Prime beef is the highest and most expensive grade. The meat is well marbled, tender, and flavorful. Marbling in meat is valued because it adds to the flavor of the meat. Choice beef has less marbling than prime but is still tender and flavorful. It is the most common grade sold in supermarkets, Select beef has the least amount of marbling and is the least expensive. It is sometimes sold as a store brand. **Figure 34.5** shows what USDA beef stamps look like.

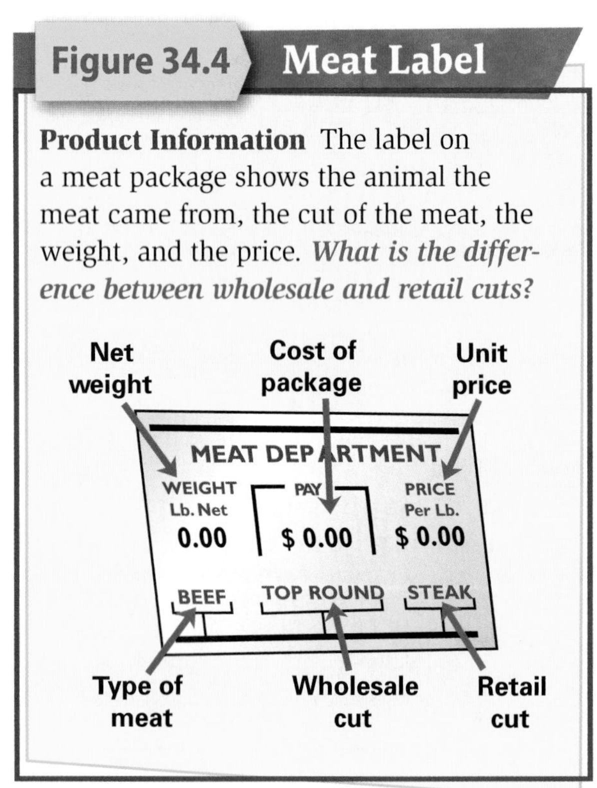

Figure 34.4 Meat Label

Product Information The label on a meat package shows the animal the meat came from, the cut of the meat, the weight, and the price. ***What is the difference between wholesale and retail cuts?***

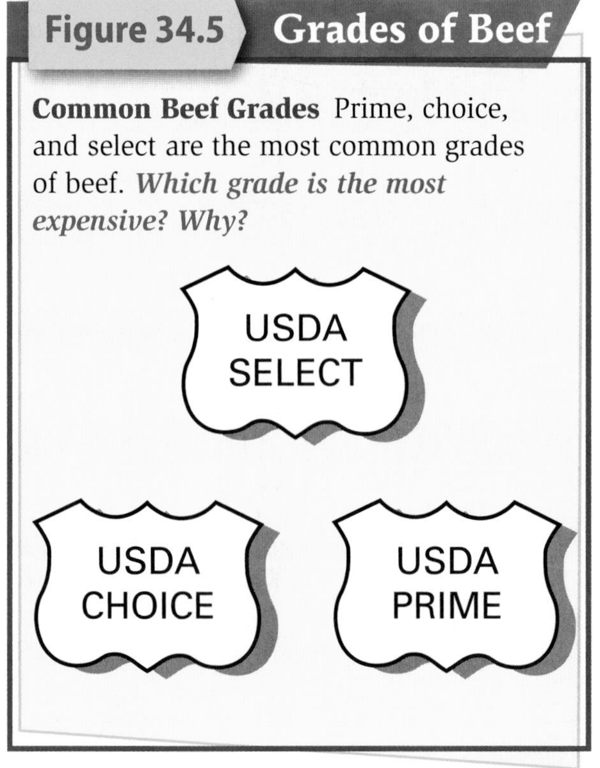

Figure 34.5 Grades of Beef

Common Beef Grades Prime, choice, and select are the most common grades of beef. ***Which grade is the most expensive? Why?***

Figure 34.6 Seven Common Bone Shapes

Clues About Tenderness The areas around the backbone have the tenderest cuts of meat. Look at the shape of the bone as a clue to the tenderness of the cut. ***How can less tender meat be made more tender?***

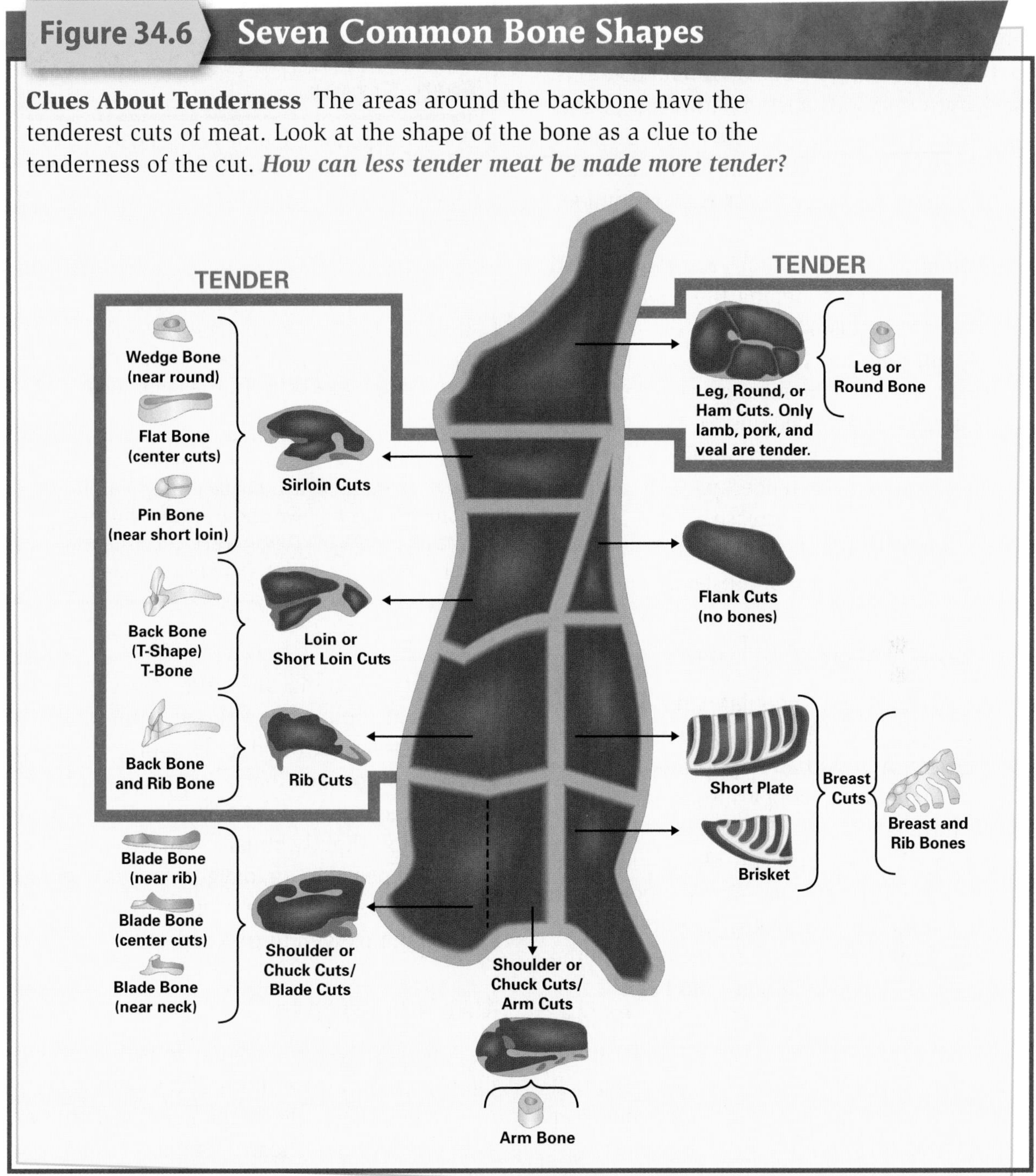

Meat Tenderness

Some cuts of meat are more tender than others. There are two major reasons for this.

Muscle Movement The less a muscle moves, the more tender it is. Muscles along the backbone get very little movement, for example, so meat from that area is more tender than meat from other parts of the animal.

Marbling The amount of marbling affects tenderness. Fat in marbling melts during cooking, releasing juice and flavor. As fat melts, it penetrates the muscle tissue and helps separate muscle fibers, making the meat easier to chew.

Bone shapes give clues about where the meat comes from on the animal and how tender it is. **Figure 34.6** shows the seven common bone shapes. The rib and T-shape bones, which are part of the backbone, indicate that the meat is tender. The meat on a blade bone, which is part of the shoulder, is not as tender.

Tenderizing Meat

Less tender cuts of meat can be tenderized before cooking by one of several methods. Mechanical methods such as grinding, pounding, and cutting tenderize meat by breaking down elastin. Less tender cuts of beef, for example, can be ground into hamburger or pounded with a meat pounder to make cube steaks.

Chemical methods such as adding acid tenderize meat by softening the collagen and breaking down elastin. Tomatoes, sour cream, yogurt, vinegar, and lemon juice can be used to tenderize meat. The meat can be marinated in the mixture before cooking, or the acid mixture can be added during cooking.

Commercial meat tenderizer can also be sprinkled on meat to increase its tenderness. Meat tenderizer contains salt and three papaya enzymes that break down muscle fibers.

Nutrition Check

Fatty Scraps

Due in part to the popularity of hamburgers, ground beef is the top-selling type of beef in the United States. However, there is more to a hamburger than ground beef—namely, fat. As much as 30 percent of the content of meat sold as either "hamburger" or "ground beef" can be fat. The USDA allows any cut of beef to be used to make hamburger or ground beef. Consequently, it is usually made from leftovers—the scraps that remain after sides of beef are cut into steaks and roasts.

Think About It Do you see a connection between U.S. beef and the fact that the United States has the highest obesity rate in the world? What changes can health-conscious consumers make? Write a paragraph explaining your reasoning.

Ground Meat

Ground meat is popular and relatively inexpensive. One of its best known uses is in hamburgers. It is also an important ingredient in meat loaf, tacos, sloppy joes, and tomato-based meat sauces.

Less tender cuts of meat, along with trimmings, are often ground. Ground beef, also called hamburger, is the most popular ground meat. About 45 percent of the beef in the United States is made into ground beef.

Ground beef is available with different amounts of fat. By law, ground beef cannot have more than 30 percent fat by weight. It may contain seasonings, but no extenders or binders. Regular ground beef has the most fat, is the least expensive, and shrinks most when cooked. Ground chuck contains 15 to 20 percent fat, which makes for flavorful and juicy hamburgers. Ground round and ground sirloin have the least fat and are the most expensive. Ground meat that is labeled "lean" must have less than 10 grams of total fat, less than 4.5 grams of saturated fat, and less than 95 milligrams of cholesterol per 3½-ounce serving. Lean ground beef usually costs more than regular ground beef.

You can buy ground beef already packaged or have it ground to order. You can also buy ground lamb, pork, and veal. You can ask to have meat ground for you. A combination of equal parts of ground beef, pork, and veal works well for meatloaf.

Packaged ground beef is often red on the outside and slightly bluish on the inside. When meat is exposed to air, oxygen causes it to turn red. The interior of the ground beef does not get enough oxygen to turn red.

Variety Meats

A **variety meat** is a meat consisting of edible organs and extremities of beef, veal, lamb, or pork. Variety meats include liver, kidney, pigs' feet, brains, heart, tongue, oxtails, and sweetbreads (thymus gland). Variety meats are highly perishable, so they must be fresh when purchased and cooked within 24 hours.

Variety meats are used extensively in Europe and other parts of the world. Andouille (än-ˈdü-ē), for instance, is a French sausage made with chitterlings (pig intestines) and tripe (the stomach lining of cattle). The Cajun version is spicy and is usually made from pork shoulder. Andouille is a major ingredient in jambalaya and gumbo. Variety meats are used less in the United States, so most variety meats produced in the U.S. are exported.

Processed Meats

A **processed meat** is a meat with added flavor and preservatives. Processed meats include ham, bacon, sausage, and cold cuts. **Cold cuts** are processed slices of cold meat and poultry.

About 35 percent of the meat produced in the United States is processed. About 75 percent of all processed meat is pork. The remaining 25 percent is beef.

Three methods are used to process meats: curing, smoking, and cooking. Several methods are often used on one product.

Cured meats Cured meats can be pickle-cured or dry-cured. Pickle-curing involves soaking the meat in a solution of salt, sugar, sodium nitrate, potassium nitrate, ascorbic acid, and water or pumping the solution into the meat. In dry-curing, no water is used. The mixture is rubbed onto the surface of the meat.

Smoked Meats Originally, smoking meat meant exposing it to wood smoke to preserve and flavor it. Today, liquid smoke is used for flavoring.

Cooked Meats Cooked, processed meats are ready to eat. Pasteurization increases the shelf life of the meat.

Convenience Forms of Meat

Convenience forms of meat include canned, frozen, and ready-to cook products. Convenience products cost much more than the same foods prepared from scratch at home.

Careers in Food

Ronnie Huettmann
Butcher

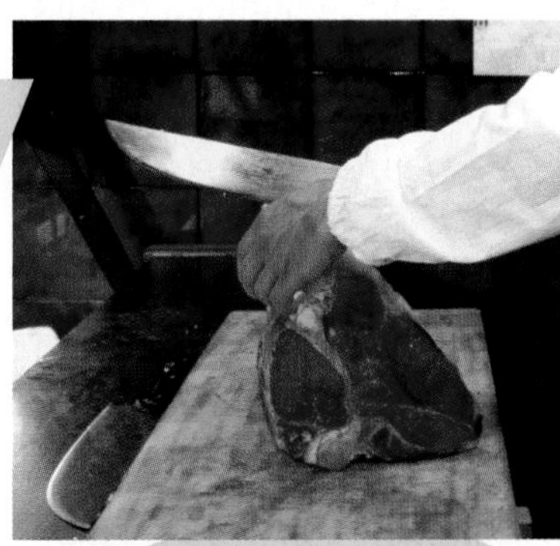

Q: What does a butcher do?

A: A butcher is someone who slaughters and processes meat for retail to the public. Butchers cut up the meat and package it for stores. Meat-cutters cut the meat down into individual portions for customers.

Q: How do you become a butcher?

A: On-the-job training is common among butchers. Simple cutting operations require a few days to learn, while more complicated tasks require several months of training. Trainees learn the proper use and care of tools and equipment, while also learning how to prepare various cuts of meat. After demonstrating skill with various meat cutting tools, trainees learn to divide carcasses into wholesale cuts and wholesale cuts into retail and individual portions. Trainees also may learn to roll and tie roasts, prepare sausage, and cure meat. Those employed in retail food establishments often are taught operations, such as inventory control, meat buying, and recordkeeping.

Q: What type of person typically is best-suited for the profession?

A: People who become butchers usually have a culinary background or an agricultural background.

"It is really important to be the best that you can be at whatever choice you make."
— Ronnie Huettmann,
President, Acre Station Meat Farm – Pinetown, NC

Education and Training

Most butchers learn their skills through on-the-job training. The training period for highly skilled butchers at the retail level may be one or two years.

Qualities and Skills

Knife sharpening skills are very important. Manual dexterity, physical strength, and hand-eye coordination.

Related Career Opportunities

There are career opportunities within the companies that process meat. Butchers in food processing businesses and retail stores may progress to supervisory positions. They may also become meat buyers.

Many canned meat entrées are available, including beef stew and spaghetti and meatballs. Many frozen entrées have meat, along with starches and vegetables. Roast beef, for example, might have side servings of peas and mashed potatoes. Most supermarkets carry ready-to-cook meats, such as ready-made meatloaf that just needs baking.

✓ Reading Check **Identify** What two factors influence meat tenderness?

Buying and Storing Meat

Meat can be one of the most expensive items in the food budget. To get the most for your money, you need to shop wisely and store meat properly.

Buying Meat

Buy only the amount of meat that you need. Calculate how much meat you will need for the recipe you have chosen and the number of people you will serve. Add a little extra if you want leftovers.

Choose the cut that looks the leanest. This saves money because you do not have to pay for extra fat that you will discard. Lean beef roasts and steaks include round, loin, sirloin, and chuck arm. Lean pork roasts and chops include tenderloin, center loin, and ham. Lean lamb roasts and chops include the leg, loin, and foreshank. All veal is lean except ground veal. Tender cuts are usually more expensive than tough cuts. You can save money by learning tasty recipes for tough cuts.

Always compare the cost per serving of different cuts. If you find a bargain that is not on your shopping list, you might decide to change plans. Even small savings add up over time.

Storing Meat

Meat must be refrigerated. Place meat in a plastic bag to keep the juices from dripping on other food. Variety meats should be used within one day, and ground meat should be used within two days. Other fresh meats keep in the refrigerator for three to five days. Freeze meat for longer storage.

If you are refrigerating unopened packages of processed meat, refer to the date on the label for length of storage. If the package has been opened, use the meat within a few days. Read label directions for storing canned meats.

✓ Reading Check **Summarize** How can you save money when buying meat?

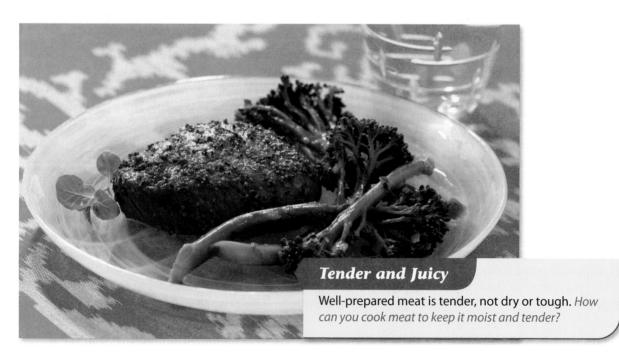

Tender and Juicy

Well-prepared meat is tender, not dry or tough. *How can you cook meat to keep it moist and tender?*

Cooking Meat

Cooking affects meat in several ways. When properly cooked, meat becomes more firm, fat melts, and connective tissues soften. As a result, the meat becomes tender, juicy, and flavorful.

Protein is sensitive to heat, so you must carefully control cooking temperatures and times. Cooking meat for a long time at high temperatures can cause it to shrink significantly. Overcooked meat is tough and dry and may be difficult to cut and digest.

Heat does not usually destroy nutrients in meat. However, water-soluble vitamins, such as B vitamins, may be lost in the meat juices or cooking liquid. To recapture the vitamins, the meat juices or cooking liquid can be added to soups, sauces, or gravies.

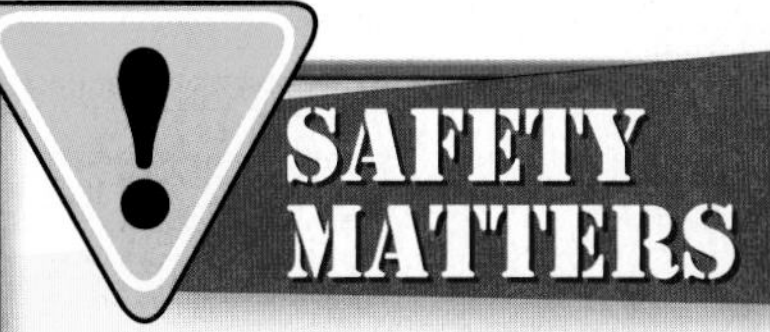

The Threat of Thawing

There are several ways to thaw frozen meat, but not all are safe. Improper thawing leads to the growth of bacteria and threatens food safety. Never thaw meat at room temperature or in warm water. Instead, thaw meat in the refrigerator, where its temperature can decrease slowly and safely. Keep the meat in its orginal packaging with a dish or tray underneath it. You can also thaw meat by putting it in a leakproof bag and immersing it in cold water. Change the water every 30 minutes. Or, use your microwave to quickly thaw meat, following the instructions in the product manual.

What Would You Do? In one hour, you plan to prepare steaks for dinner. However, you forgot to move them from the freezer to the refrigerator to thaw out. You need to have the steaks ready soon.

Preparing Meat

The USDA requires that safe handling instructions be on all packages of raw and partially cooked meat. Make sure to read these instructions when you prepare meat. Here are the basic steps in preparing meat:

Thaw. If the meat is frozen, thaw it before cooking to save time and preserve quality. If you want to cook frozen meat without thawing, increase the cooking time by about 50 percent. For example, if the normal cooking time for a cut is 40 minutes, cook a frozen cut for 60 minutes.

Rinse. Before cooking meat, rinse it under cold water and pat it dry with a paper towel.

Trim fat. Trim any visible fat before cooking so drippings are less fatty. Fat is easier to trim when meat is very cold.

Marinate. Before cooking meat, you can marinate it for added flavor and tenderness. To make a marinade, choose at least one acidic ingredient. Vinegar, yogurt, or fruit juice work well. Add a little cooking oil and season the mix with herbs and spices. Pour the marinade over the meat, cover, and refrigerate. Do not marinate for more than 24 hours or the meat will get mushy.

Marinating works best on thin cuts of meat. Acid pits aluminum, so do not use an aluminum pan for marinating. Marinades can pick up contaminants from raw meat, so do not use leftover marinade for basting unless you boil it first for one minute.

Cook. The tenderness of a meat cut determines its cooking method. Tender cuts, such as steaks, chops, and roasts, can be cooked quickly with dry heat methods, such as roasting and broiling. Less tender cuts, such as arm shoulder chops and short ribs, must be cooked for longer periods with moist heat methods, such as braising and stewing. Moist heat breaks down the collagen in the meat, making it tender. Remember high and fast for tender cuts and low and slow for tough cuts.

Testing for Doneness

Doneness is the point at which meat has cooked enough to make it flavorful and safe to eat. If any part of the meat is not cooked until fully done, it may cause foodborne illness.

Figure 34.7 Temperatures for Meat

Internal Doneness The terms *medium rare, medium,* and *well done* refer to the temperature meat has reached at its thickest point. ***What kind of thermometer would you use to test the temperature of a large piece of precooked ham?***

Food	Temperature in °F
Ground Meat and Meat Mixtures	
Beef, pork, veal, lamb	160
Fresh Beef, Veal, Lamb	
Medium rare	145
Medium	160
Well done	170
Fresh Pork	
Medium	160
Well done	170
Ham	
Fresh (raw)	160
To reheat precooked ham	140
Leftovers and Casseroles	165

Doneness is hard to judge visually. Using a meat thermometer is the safest method. When you roast cuts more than 2 inches thick, insert the meat thermometer into the thickest part. Be sure that the tip of the thermometer does not touch bone or rest in fat, which gives an incorrect reading. You can use an instant-read thermometer or an oven-safe thermometer.

For thin cuts, check the temperature with an instant-read thermometer near the end of the cooking time. Some instant-read thermometers have a dial, and some have a digital display. You can check the accuracy of your thermometer by placing it in a glass of ice water. It should register 37°F.

Meat can be cooked to these basic stages of doneness: medium rare, medium, and well done. Each stage is indicated by a specific internal temperature. **Figure 34.7** shows internal doneness temperatures for various types of meat.

Cooking time depends on the cooking method and the cut of the meat. The cooking time in the recipe is just a guide. Begin testing the meat for doneness about 10 minutes before the end of the expected cooking time.

Broiling Meat

Broiled meat is cooked very close to the heating element. Because it uses high heat, broiled food has an appetizing brown exterior.

Tender cuts of meat such as steaks, chops, ham slices, liver, bacon, and ground beef can be broiled. Steaks and chops should be at least ½ inch thick. Thinner pieces dry out if broiled.

When fat cooks, it melts and shrinks, pulling up the meat. Make slashes through any fat left on the edges of meat before broiling to help keep the meat from curling. You can also add flavor by brushing a sauce on the meat.

Place the broiler pan so the meat is 2 to 5 inches from the heat. Thicker cuts need more time to heat, so they should be placed farther from the heat. Broil until the top is brown and the meat is slightly more than half done inside. Season if desired. Turn and complete the broiling on the other side.

Grilling Meat

Tender cuts of meat can be grilled. You can grill whole cuts or make kebabs. To make kebabs, thread cubes of meat onto skewers, alternating with tomato quarters, mushrooms, green pepper chunks, or other vegetables. Brush with oil, melted butter, or a sauce to keep the foods from drying out.

Heat the grill. Place the meat or kebabs on the grate and turn them regularly to cook through. Brush the meat occasionally with a sauce. Sauces that contain a large amount of sugar, such as barbecue sauce, can cause meat to char. If you want to use a sweet sauce, wait until the last few minutes of cooking to begin basting.

Roasting Meat

Roasting works best with large tender cuts of meat, such as loin, rib, and leg roasts. Follow these steps to roast meat:

1. Place in a pan. Place the meat fat side up on a rack in an open, shallow roasting pan. As the fat melts, it automatically bastes the meat. The rack should hold the roast out of the drippings. For standing rib roasts or crown of pork, the ribs form a natural rack, so the meat can be placed directly on the pan bottom.

2. Season. Season the meat as desired.

3. Insert the thermometer. Insert an oven-safe meat thermometer so the tip is centered in the largest muscle.

4. Roast. Roast at 325°F without preheating the oven. If you wish, add whole small potatoes, onions, and carrots around the roast about an hour before it's done. Do not add water or cover the pan. This causes the meat to cook with moisture rather than dry heat.

5. Test for doneness. Remove the roast from the oven when the meat thermometer registers five degrees lower than the desired internal temperature. The meat continues to cook as it stands.

6. Let stand. Let the roast stand for 15 to 20 minutes after removing it from the oven. This allows the juices to set and makes the roast easier to carve.

Frying Meat

Thin pieces of tender meat can be fried in a small amount of fat. Lean cuts of meat or cuts that are floured or breaded need more fat.

Cook meat uncovered in a skillet preheated to medium. Turn occasionally so both sides brown. Do not cover the skillet or the meat will cook in moist heat and lose crispness and flavor. Season the meat after browning.

Pan-Broiling Meat

Pan-broil tender cuts of meat that are too thin to broil. Use cuts that are 1 inch thick or less. Preheat a heavy skillet. Most cuts have enough fat to prevent sticking without adding oil. If you are using a lean cut, use a nonstick skillet or brush or spray the regular skillet with oil. Use medium heat and do not cover the skillet. Turn the meat occasionally and pour off fat as it accumulates. Cook until brown on both sides, and then season if desired.

Braising Meat

Braising is used to cook large, less tender cuts of meat, such as pot roast and Swiss steak. It also gives flavor to tender cuts.

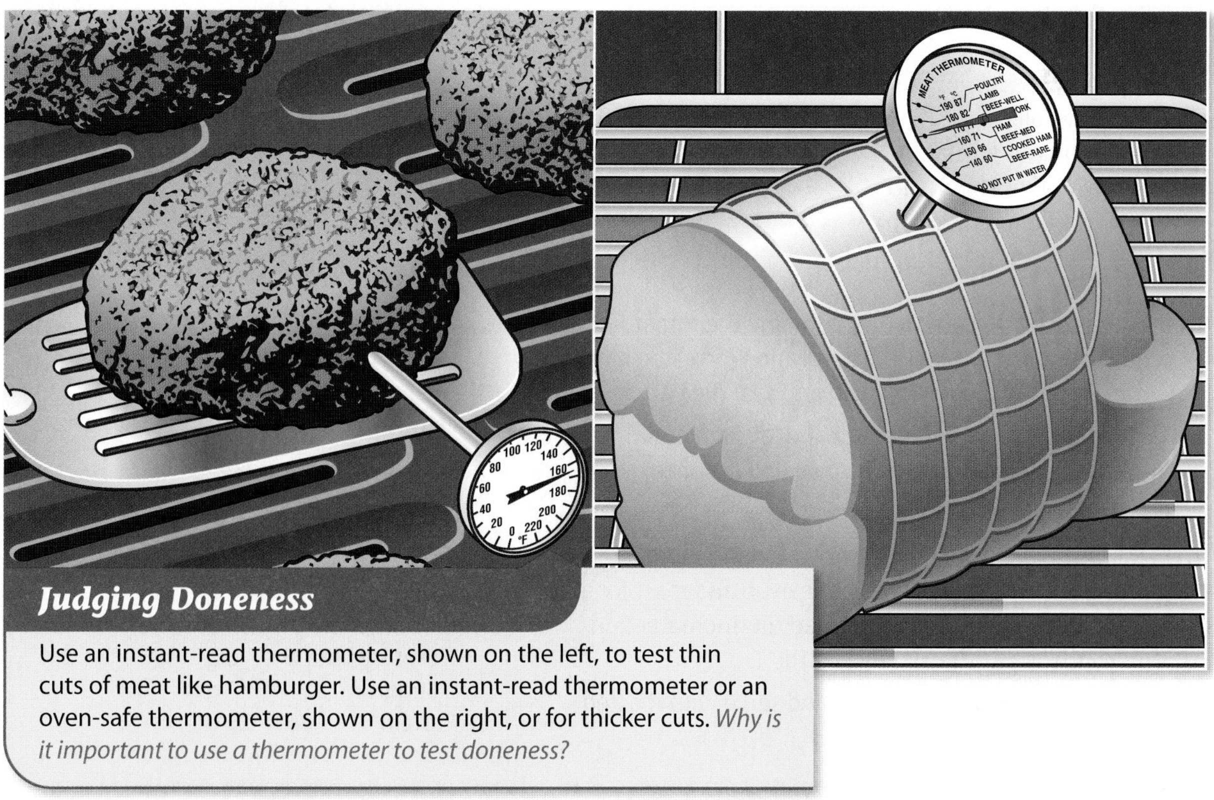

Judging Doneness

Use an instant-read thermometer, shown on the left, to test thin cuts of meat like hamburger. Use an instant-read thermometer or an oven-safe thermometer, shown on the right, or for thicker cuts. *Why is it important to use a thermometer to test doneness?*

Brown the meat on all sides in a large heavy pan, using a little fat if needed to prevent sticking. After browning, drain off excess fat. Add just enough liquid, such as water, tomato juice, meat stock, or another seasoned liquid, to cover the bottom of the pan about ¼ inch deep. The liquid must flow under the food to keep it from sticking to the pan. Add seasonings and cover the pan with a tight-fitting lid.

Simmer on low heat until the meat is tender, or cook in the oven at 325°F. About halfway through the cooking time, you can add carrots, potatoes, and onions.

Pressure-Cooking Meat

Large, less tender cuts of meat can be pressure cooked. This cooks the meat in moist heat and tenderizes it under high pressure within a relatively short time.

Slow-Cooking Meat

A slow cooker uses a low temperature for a long cooking time, which makes it ideal for less tender cuts of meat. A slow cooker allows you to prepare a meal in the morning and have it ready for dinner when you come home from work or school.

Microwaving Meat

Cuts of uniform size are the best choice for microwave cooking. Microwave ovens do not cook evenly, even if they have a turntable. During the standing time, cover the meat loosely with foil to hold in the heat. After the standing time, check the meat in several spots with an instant-read thermometer to be sure it has reached the proper internal temperature throughout.

Light and Healthy Recipe

Pot Roast

Ingredients

- **2 lbs.** Boneless chuck roast
- **1 cup** Tomato juice
- **1 cup** Reduced fat, low-sodium beef broth
- **2 Tbsp.** Olive oil
- **2 Tbsp.** Prepared mustard
- **2 tsp.** Worcestershire sauce
- **1 tsp.** Fresh or dried rosemary

Directions

1. In a large plastic, sealable bag, combine the tomato juice, broth, rosemary, olive oil, mustard, and Worcestershire sauce. Place the meat in the bag and seal the bag.
2. Place the bag in the refrigerator and let sit overnight. After a few hours, turn the bag over at least once.
3. Preheat oven to 350°.
4. Remove the meat from the refrigerator and place it in a roasting pan. Place the meat in the oven and roast for at least two hours. Use an instant-read thermometer and remove the roast when it reaches 160°.
5. Slice the meat against the grain and serve with roasted vegetables.

Though a roast is usually made from a tough piece of meat, that meat is often low in fat. Tenderizing it with a marinade and slowly roasting it creates a savory meal.

Yield 12 servings

Nutrition Analysis per Serving

■ Calories	260
■ Total fat	17 g
Saturated fat	6 g
Cholesterol	72 mg
■ Sodium	198 mg
■ Carbohydrate	2
Dietary fiber	0 g
Sugars	2 g
■ Protein	23 g

CHAPTER 34 Review & Applications

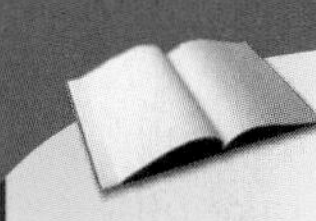

After You Read

Chapter Summary

Meat is made up of muscle, connective tissue, and fat. It provides many nutrients. There are several types and cuts of meat. Meat is inspected for wholesomeness and graded for quality. Some cuts of meat are more tender than others. In addition to meat cuts, there are ground meats, variety meats, processed meats, and convenience forms of meat. Meat should be bought carefully and stored properly. Cooking affects meat in several ways. There are basic steps to prepare meat for cooking. For safety reasons, it is important to check meat for doneness. Meat can be cooked using a variety of methods.

Content and Academic Vocabulary Review

1. Write a sentence using two or more of these content and academic vocabulary words. The sentence should clearly show how the terms are related.

Content Vocabulary

- meat (p. 534)
- muscle (p. 534)
- grain (p. 534)
- connective tissue (p. 534)
- collagen (p. 534)
- elastin (p. 534)
- marbling (p. 534)
- cut (p. 534)
- wholesale cut (p. 534)
- retail cut (p. 536)
- variety meat (p. 538)
- processed meat (p. 539)
- cold cuts (p. 539)
- doneness (p. 541)

Academic Vocabulary

- similar (p. 536)
- uniform (p. 536)

Review Key Concepts

2. **Explain** the three main parts of meat.
3. **Describe** the nutritional value of meat.
4. **Identify** and explain the most common grades of beef.
5. **Explain** what to look for when buying meat.
6. **List** methods for cooking meat.

Critical Thinking

7. **Explain** why a meat label cannot be accurate if it says fat-free.
8. **Infer** why some meat producers keep animals in small confines to prevent too much movement.
9. **Compare and contrast** inspection and grading of meat.
10. **Identify** which tool is absolutely necessary to safely cook meat. Explain why.

Foods Lab

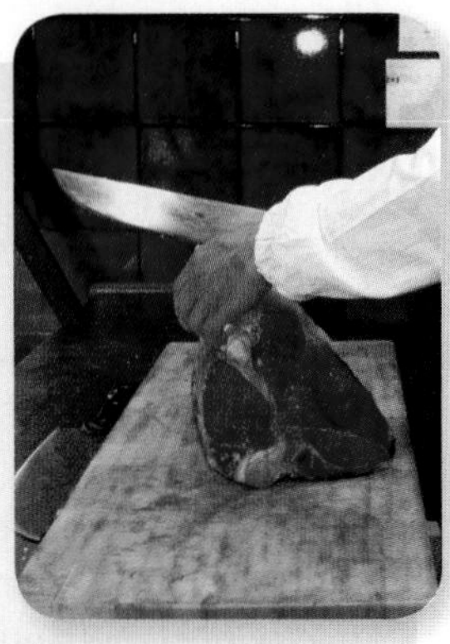

11. Meatball Comparison Meatballs are an easy-to-prepare addition to many dishes. In their convenience form, they require virtually no preparation. Do you prefer homemade or pre-made meatballs?

Procedure Choose a recipe for meatballs and prepare it. Also prepare ready-made meatballs purchased as a convenience food. Follow package directions. Conduct a taste test to sample and compare both products.

Analysis As a team, create a table that compares the taste, texture, appearance, nutrition, and approximate cost per serving of the two forms of meatballs. Share your chart with the class. Explain which form you would choose in the future and why?

HEALTHFUL CHOICES

12. Watching the Fat To maintain a healthy diet, Angela is watching her fat intake. She wants to prepare healthy, low-fat hamburgers topped with roasted vegetables and sandwiched between whole-grain buns. Angela wants to use meat with the lowest amount of fat possible. Should she use ground beef, ground chuck, ground sirloin, or lean ground beef to make her healthy hamburgers?

TECH Connection

13. Nutrition Comparison Compare the protein and fat amounts in four different cuts of beef, such as round, sirloin, rib, and flank. Use spreadsheet or word processing software to create a graph or chart that shows your findings. Then write one or more paragraphs to answer these questions: Which cut provides the least amount of fat? Which cooking method would you choose to use for each of the four different cuts? Explain your answers.

Real-World Skills

Problem-Solving Skills	**14. Managing Meat Juices** Ben, a nutritionist, cooked a lamb roast. He noticed that a lot of meat juices filled the bottom of the roasting pan. Why do you think he viewed this as a problem, and how might he have solved it?
Interpersonal and Collaborative Skills	**15. Meat Cut Display** Follow your teacher's instructions to form pairs. Find an image of the cut of meat your teacher assigns to you. Using the image as a reference, work together to draw an oversized version of the meat cut on a piece of posterboard. Add color and cut it out.
Financial Literacy Skills	**16. Cost Per Serving** Fiona eats two 3-ounce servings of meat per day. She is on a food budget and wants to save money. Each canned meat entrée contains 3 ounces of meat and costs $3.89. Lean lamb chops cost $5.70 per pound. Which choice has the lower cost per 3-ounce serving? By how much is the cost lower?

Academic Skills

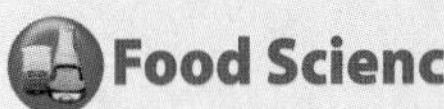

Food Science

17. Browning of Meat Caramelization is the browning of surface sugars on foods such as meat. How can we use this information in cooking meat?

Procedure Cut beef steak into 9 strips $\frac{1}{2}$″ wide and 4″ in length. Divide into 3 groups. Dissolve 2 teaspoons of corn syrup in $\frac{1}{2}$ cup of warm water. Put the first group in this syrup, and marinade for at least an hour or longer. Pat dry. Dip the next group of strips into flour to coat well, shaking off excess. Heat a small amount of vegetable oil in three small skillets, and sauté each group about 5 minutes, turning to brown well on all sides. Use a table to show the results.

Analysis Write a paragraph to describe any differences in browning.

NSES A Develop understandings about scientific inquiry.

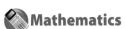

Mathematics

18. Tenderizing Veal Antonia has purchased several veal cutlets, which she would like to bread and fry for use in a veal parmigiana dish. Each cutlet is $\frac{2}{3}$ inch thick when purchased. However, she will need to tenderize the cutlets and reduce their thickness so that they will cook more evenly when frying. Antonia pounds each cutlet to a thickness of $\frac{1}{8}$ inch. What fraction is the new thickness of the original thickness? What percentage is the new thickness of the original thickness?

Math Concept **Convert Fractions to Percents** To convert a fraction into a percent, divide the numerator by the denominator, multiply by 100, and add the percent symbol.

Starting Hint The pounded veal is $(\frac{1}{8})/(\frac{2}{3})$ of the original thickness. Since it is improper to have fractions within a fraction, simplify the fraction by dividing $\frac{1}{8}$ by $\frac{2}{3}$ (which is the same as multiplying $\frac{1}{8}$ by $\frac{3}{2}$). Convert to a percent.

NCTM Number and Operations Understand numbers, ways of representing numbers, relationships among numbers, and number systems.

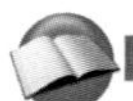

English Language Arts

19. Meat: To Eat or Not to Eat? Vegetarians and meat eaters feel strongly about diets that eliminate or include meat. What is your view? Write a two-minute speech in which you explain why you do or do not eat meat.

NCTE 12 Use language to achieve individual purposes.

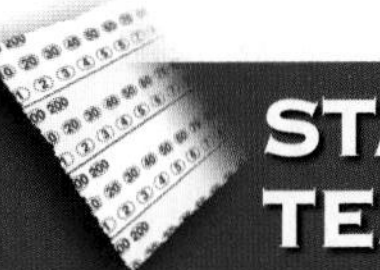

STANDARDIZED TEST PRACTICE

READING COMPREHENSION

Re-read the section about storing meat on page 540. Then select the best answer.

20. How soon after buying should ground meat be used?

a. within one day
b. within two days
c. within three to five days
d. within three days of the sell-by date

Test-Taking Tip Closely read the text to which the question refers. Then read through the question and each of the answer choices. Some answers may seem correct, but they contain subtle errors. Pay attention to every word.

CHAPTER 35

Poultry

Writing Activity — Outlining

Describe a Healthful Diet An outline is a diagram of the main ideas in a document. Outlining helps you organize your thoughts and focus on your most important points. Think about the most important parts of a healthful diet. Then create an outline for a magazine article describing how to make healthy food choices.

Writing Tips Follow these steps to write an outline:

- Write down three to five key points.
- List two or three supporting points or examples under each key point.
- Review the outline. Are the key points arranged in a logical order? Do the supporting points or examples help prove your key points? Make changes as necessary.

Activate Prior Knowledge

Explore the Photo Chicken is a popular food in many cultures. *What dishes do you know that feature chicken?*

Reading Guide

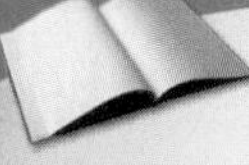

Before You Read

Preview Look at the photos and read their captions. Think about the skills you will need to shop for and cook poultry dishes.

Read to Learn

Key Concepts

- **List** the nutrients found in poultry.
- **Describe** the four most popular types of poultry.
- **List** the common forms of poultry.
- **Explain** how to select and store poultry.
- **Explain** why you should always cook poultry until well done.

Main Idea

Poultry is a healthful and inexpensive source of protein that works well with many cooking methods.

Content Vocabulary

You will find definitions for these words in the glossary at the back of this book.

- ☐ poultry
- ☐ free-range
- ☐ cutlet
- ☐ giblets
- ☐ baste
- ☐ truss
- ☐ stuffing

Academic Vocabulary

You will find these words in your reading and on your tests. Use the glossary to look up their definitions if necessary.

- inspect
- moderate

Graphic Organizer

As you read, take notes about the different types of poultry and the qualities of each.

TYPE OF POULTRY	QUALITIES
Chicken	
Turkey	
Duck	
Goose	

Graphic Organizer Go to this book's Online Learning Center at **glencoe.com** to print out this graphic organizer.

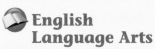

Academic Standards

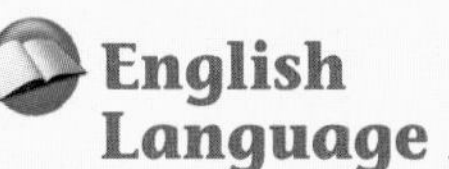

English Language Arts

NCTE 4 Use written language to communicate effectively.

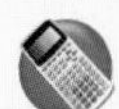

Math

NCTM Number and Operations Compute fluently and make reasonable estimates.

NCTM Measurement Understand measurable attributes of objects and the units, systems, and processes of measurement.

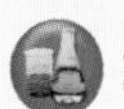

Science

NSES C Develop understanding of organization in living systems and behavior of organisms.

NCTE *National Council of Teachers of English*
NCTM *National Council of Teachers of Mathematics*
NSES *National Science Education Standards*

Nutrients in Poultry

Poultry is any bird raised for food. Poultry is nutritious and easy to prepare. It is also a good value. Americans eat more poultry than any other kind of meat. Because of its mild flavor, poultry lends itself to many different recipes and cooking methods.

Poultry is a good source of protein. It also has niacin, vitamins B_6 and B_{12}, calcium, phosphorus, iron, and other minerals. Poultry is part of the proteins food group. Most teenagers need five or six ounces of protein foods each day. That is about the size of two chicken breasts.

Poultry usually has less fat and calories than red meat. Most of the fat in poultry is attached to the skin. When you cut off the skin, you remove most of the fat.

✓ **Reading Check** **Explain** What nutrients are found in poultry?

Types of Poultry

Chicken, turkey, duck, and goose are the most common types of poultry. Each comes in a variety of types and sizes. **Figure 35.1** shows the qualities of each type of poultry.

Figure 35.1 **Common Types of Poultry**

No-Fly Zone Birds raised as poultry look different than wild game birds. They weigh twice as much and cannot fly. ***Why is this the case?***

Type of Poultry	Class	Age	Weight	Description
Chicken 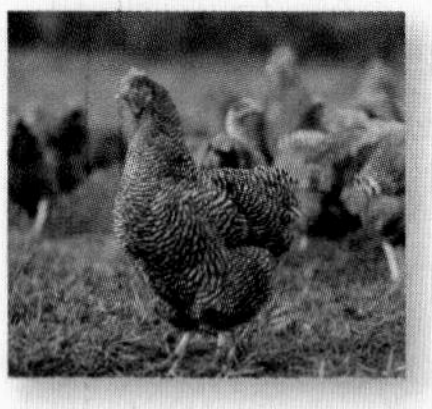	Rock Cornish game hen	5 weeks or under	¾–2 pounds	Breed of small young chicken with tender, delicate meat
	Broiler-fryer	under 7 weeks	3–4 pounds	Young, chicken with tender meat
	Roaster	3–5 months	4–7 pounds	Older, meatier chicken
	Stewing Chickens	over 10 months	4–6 pounds	Large, older birds that need moist heat cooking due to their tougher mature flesh
	Capon	under 10 months	5–8 pounds	Desexed male; tender and flavorful; best when roasted
Turkey 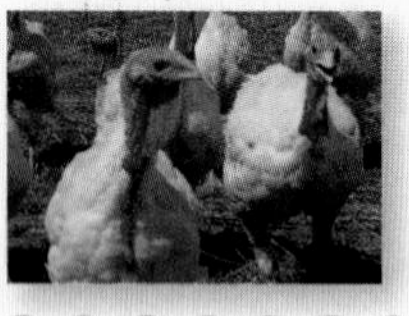	Fryer-roaster	under 16 weeks	4–9 pounds	Young turkey
	Hen turkey	5–7 months	8–16 pounds	Older female turkey
	Tom turkey	5–7 months	8–24 pounds	Older male turkey
Duck 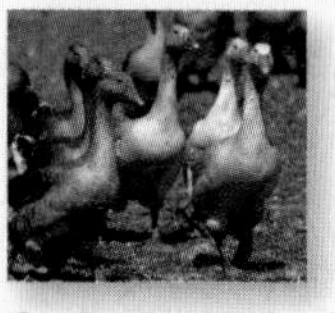	Broilers and fryers	under 8 weeks	3 pounds	Young, tender duck
	Roasters	under 16 weeks	Up to 5½ pounds	Still young, but meatier
Goose 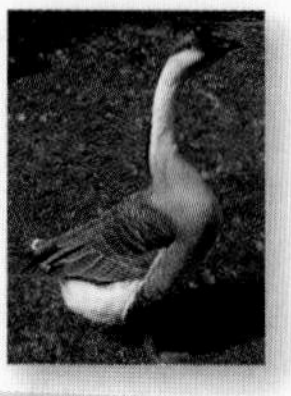	Goose	Under 6 months	5–18 pounds	High in fat but flavorful; Tastes best when roasted

Free-Range and Organic Poultry

Free-range and organic poultry is popular with consumers who care about animal welfare and the environment. Most poultry is kept indoors with little or no space to walk. Free-range is a term given by the U.S.D.A. to birds that have access to the outdoors. Free-range birds can be more flavorful than birds raised on factory farms. They usually have less fat because they move more and are more expensive.

Organic poultry is raised without chemicals that can harm you or the environment. Organic birds eat only organically grown grains and are given fresh air to breathe.

✓ Reading Check **Contrast** How are duck and goose different?

Forms of Poultry

Poultry comes in many forms. You can buy whole birds, or you can choose from pre-cut parts, ground poultry, internal organs, and ready-to-eat products. A cut-up bird costs more than a whole bird. You can save money by buying a whole bird and cutting it up yourself.

Poultry Parts

Poultry is sold whole and in halves and quarters. You can also buy parts, such as breasts, wings, thighs, and drumsticks. Breasts and thighs are sold in several ways: bone-in, boneless and skinless, and in cutlets. A **cutlet** is a thin, tender slice of meat. You can also buy turkey necks and turkey tenderloins, which are cuts from the inside of the breast.

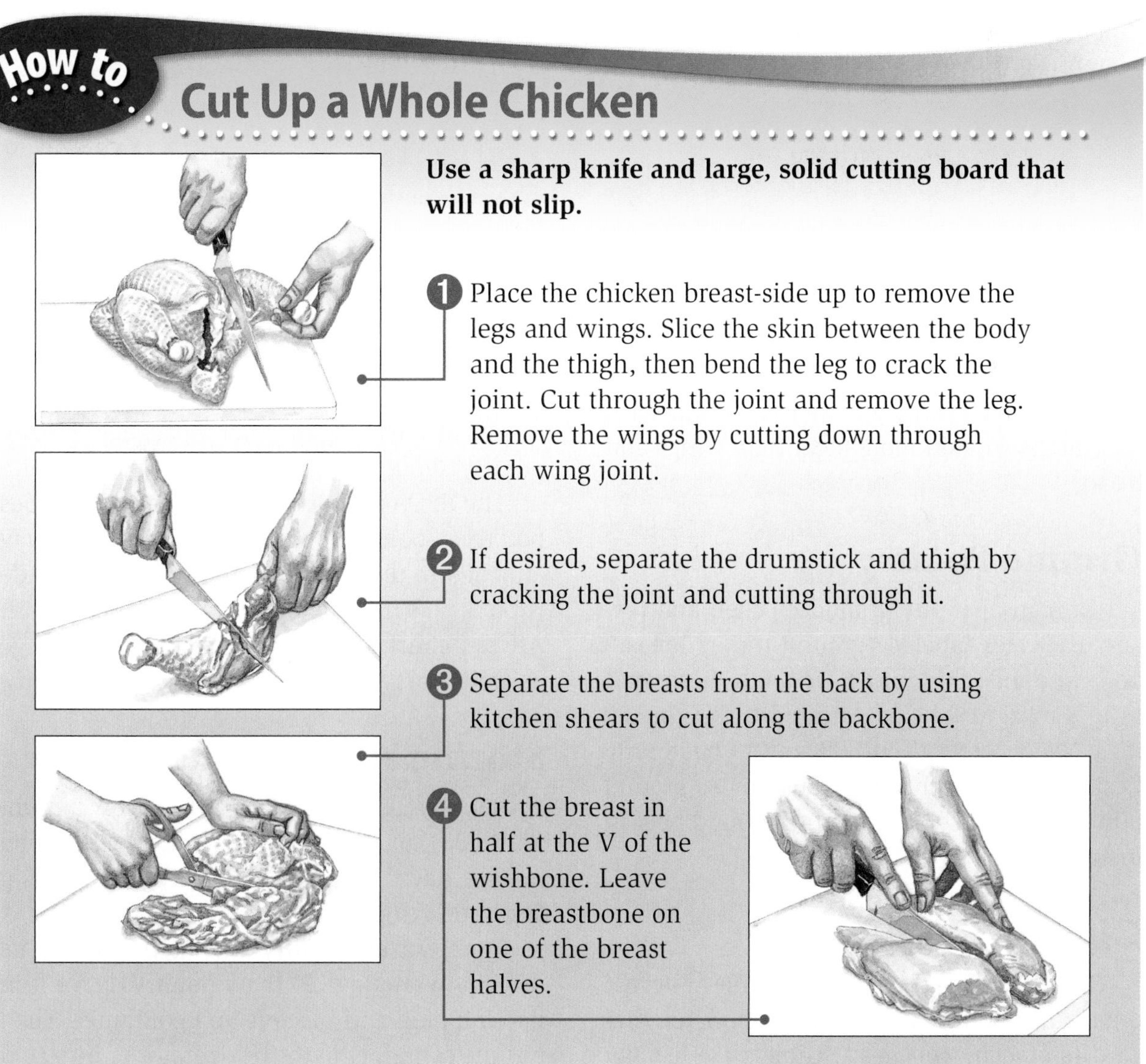

How to
Cut Up a Whole Chicken
Use a sharp knife and large, solid cutting board that will not slip.
1 Place the chicken breast-side up to remove the legs and wings. Slice the skin between the body and the thigh, then bend the leg to crack the joint. Cut through the joint and remove the leg. Remove the wings by cutting down through each wing joint.
2 If desired, separate the drumstick and thigh by cracking the joint and cutting through it.
3 Separate the breasts from the back by using kitchen shears to cut along the backbone.
4 Cut the breast in half at the V of the wishbone. Leave the breastbone on one of the breast halves.

Science in Action

Explaining Dark and Light Meat

Why do chickens and turkeys have light and dark meat? The color depends on the amount of exercise a bird's muscles get. Muscles that work hard use more oxygen. The oxygen is stored in a reddish pigment called myoglobin.

Procedure Conduct research about myoglobin. More myoglobin makes darker meat. Age also affects the amount of myoglobin in poultry. All the meat on a Rock Cornish game hen is light colored because it is too young to have had much exercise. A free range chicken has darker meat because it gets more exercise than a chicken that is not free to roam a farm. Ducks have much more fat than chickens because they live in water and need the fat to keep warm. Since a duck not only walks but flies while carrying extra weight, it must work its muscles harder. That causes darker meat.

Analysis Given what you have learned about myoglobin, write a paragraph to explain why the leg meat from a turkey is among the darkest of poultry meat.

NSES C Develop understanding of matter, energy, and organization in living systems; and behavior of organisms.

Meat on the bone is more tender and flavorful than boneless meat. Breasts, drumsticks, and thighs contain more meat than wings and backs.

Ground Poultry

You can also buy ground chicken and turkey. Packages labeled "ground turkey breast" and "ground chicken" have both flesh and skin. Packages labeled "ground turkey breast meat" and "ground chicken meat" have only flesh and are lower in fat. You can use ground poultry to replace all or part of ground beef in many recipes.

Giblets

Giblets (JIB-litz) are the edible internal organs of poultry. They include the liver, gizzard (stomach) and heart. Giblets are usually included in a package stuffed inside the whole, cleaned bird. They are commonly used to make a flavorful gravy. Chicken livers and gizzards are also sold separately.

Processed and Convenience Forms of Poultry

You can choose from many processed poultry items. Turkey is cured and smoked to make turkey ham, turkey bacon and turkey pastrami.

Ready-to-eat poultry products can help you make a quick meal. You can use canned boneless chicken or turkey in salads, sandwiches and casseroles. Many frozen dinners feature chicken or turkey. Supermarket deli sections often offer ready-to-eat barbecued, roasted and fried chicken as well as turkey and chicken sandwich meat.

✓ **Reading Check** **Summarize** Name four forms of poultry.

How to Select and Store Poultry

Be a smart shopper when buying poultry. Choose poultry that is plump and meaty. It should have smooth, soft skin that is creamy white to yellow. Do not buy poultry that has tiny feathers, has bruised or torn skin, or comes in a leaking or smelly package. Frozen poultry should be frozen solid, with no odor.

The USDA **inspects**, or examines, and grades poultry. Look for the USDA marks on a tag attached to the wing or on the package. Grade A poultry is meaty and has a good appearance. Always check the sell-by date on the package as well.

Storing and Thawing Poultry

Refrigerate poultry at 40°F or lower right after you buy it. Use fresh poultry within one or two days. Refrigerate poultry and stuffing separately to prevent bacteria from growing.

Store frozen poultry in the freezer in its original wrapping. To thaw poultry, leave it in its wrapping and place it in a container. Then put the container in the refrigerator or into cold water. A small bird will thaw in several hours. A large bird will thaw in several days. Never thaw frozen poultry by letting it sit at room temperature. You can defrost poultry in the microwave, but you must cook it right away.

✓ **Reading Check** **Analyze** Why should you not thaw poultry at room temperature?

How to Cook Poultry

You can roast, fry, sauté, stew, and even microwave poultry. Cook poultry at a moderate temperature until well-done. Poultry will dry out and become tough if you cook it for too long or at a temperature that is too high. Bacteria is sometimes found in raw poultry, so you should always handle and cook poultry with care.

Preparing Poultry for Cooking

If you have a whole bird, first remove everything from the cavities (the spaces inside), including the giblets and neck. If you are cooking poultry with a moist-heat method, such as stewing, remove the skin before cooking. If you are using a dry-heat method, such as roasting, leave the skin on. This keeps the poultry from drying.

Nutrition Check

Choosing Between Convenience and Healthfulness

Convenience foods made from poultry are tasty. They also are quick and easy to prepare, but they may not be the most healthful choice. A turkey hot dog and a skinless chicken breast each have about 120 calories, but the hot dog can have 530 mg of sodium. That's 10 times what you will find in the average chicken breast. Also, a hot dog can get 70 percent of its calories from fat. Read the nutrition facts to see whether convenience foods are a good deal for your health.

Think About It Under what circumstances might you choose the hot dog over the skinless chicken breast? When would the chicken breast be the best choice? What factors besides healthfulness might weigh in your decision?

Testing for Doneness

Always cook poultry until well done to avoid becoming sick from bacteria. Use an instant-read thermometer to check the temperature of the meat.

Poultry and stuffing are cooked when they reach an internal temperature of 165°F. Pieces that are too thin or small to test with an instant-read thermometer should be tender, with the juices running clear.

Broiling Poultry

Broiling is one of the quickest ways to cook poultry. To broil a broiler-fryer chicken, first split the chicken in half lengthwise or cut it into quarters or pieces. Place the chicken with the skin side down on a broiler pan. Brush the chicken with oil or melted butter and broil about 15 minutes.

USDA ORGANIC

Go Green

Food products with this stamp are certified organic. Meat, poultry, eggs and dairy products with this seal come from animals that are given no antibiotics or growth hormones. *What factors should you consider when deciding whether to buy organic poultry?*

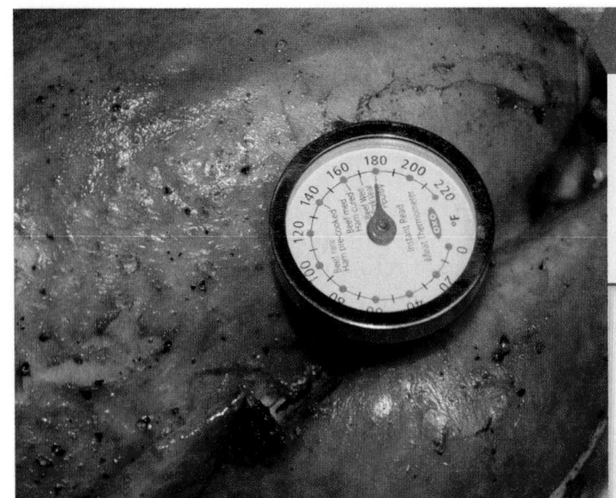

Using an Oven Thermometer

An oven thermometer tells you whether food has reached a safe temperature. The tip of the probe should reach the thickest part of the meat, without touching the bone. *At what temperature is poultry fully cooked?*

Turn the chicken and baste it with oil or melted butter to keep it moist. To **baste** is to pour or brush melted fat, cooking juices, or other liquid over food as it cooks. Continue broiling until the chicken is browned and crisp. Test for doneness with an instant-read thermometer. About two minutes before the chicken is done, you can add flavor by applying a sweetened sauce such as barbecue sauce or sweet-and-sour sauce.

Grilling Poultry

Poultry tastes great grilled. To grill a broiler-fryer chicken, first cut the chicken into halves, quarters, or pieces. Brush the grill grate lightly with oil to keep the chicken from sticking. Place the chicken skin-side up on the grate and brush it with oil or melted butter. Grill the chicken over **moderate**, or less than extreme, heat until the outside is browned and the inside is well-done. Turn the pieces often to avoid burning or overcooking the outside before the inside is done. Brush the chicken with oil or melted butter. As always, test pieces for doneness with an instant-read thermometer.

You can marinate poultry before grilling to add flavor or make kebabs by threading cubes of meat and vegetables onto skewers. You can also add flavor by brushing on a sweetened sauce during the last few minutes of cooking.

✓ Reading Check Why is it important to brush the grill with oil before grilling chicken?

Roasting Poultry

Whole birds are usually cooked by roasting. Turkey, duck, and goose are best roasted. Whole broiler-fryer or roaster chickens also roast well.

Clean the bird and season the cavity with salt, pepper, herbs, and spices. You can insert carrots, onions, celery, or other aromatic vegetables for extra flavor. Many cooks then truss birds before roasting. To **truss** is to hold a roast together with twine or skewers. This makes it easier to handle and more attractive to serve. The photo on page 555 shows an uncooked chicken being trussed with twine.

Kitchen Math: Calculate Roasting Time

At 325° F, an unstuffed turkey needs to roast one minute for every ounce of total weight. How many hours will you need to roast a 12-pound turkey? Round your answer down to a whole number. You round down because when the turkey gets within an hour of being done, you'll check it with a quick-read thermometer.

Math Concept **Multi-Step Problems** This is a multi-step problem since you have make two computations. Think through each step before beginning.

Starting Hint: Remember that there are 16 ounces in a pound. The turkey you need to roast weighs 12 pounds. Multiply 16 times 12. This will give you the number of minutes required and you can divide that number by 60, to get your answer in hours.

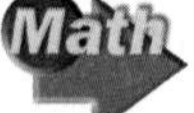
Math Appendix For math help, go to the Math Appendix at the back of the book.

NCTM Number and Operations Compute fluently and make reasonable estimates.

Handling Stuffing Safely

Stuffing is a seasoned mixture of food used to fill meats or vegetables. Bread cubes, vegetables, and eggs are ingredients for stuffing.

It is safest to cook stuffing by itself. Stuffing that is cooked inside a bird can have harmful bacteria. Place the stuffing in a covered, greased casserole dish and bake it for the last forty-five minutes of the bird's roasting time.

If you do stuff a bird, pack the stuffing loosely in the cavity. Use about ¾ cup of stuffing per pound of bird. Wait until roasting time to stuff the bird. Never stuff a bird and store it to roast later, because bacteria will grow inside. Make sure that all the stuffing reaches an internal temperature of 165°F.

Roasting a Whole Bird

After preparing the bird for roasting, follow these steps:

1. Place the bird on a rack in a roasting pan with the breast facing up.
2. Brush the skin of chicken or turkey with a small amount of oil or melted butter. Duck and goose have enough natural fat.
3. Insert an instant-read thermometer into the center of the thigh or the thickest part of the breast. Make sure that the tip does not touch bone or fat. If the bird is stuffed, insert another thermometer into the center of the stuffing.
4. Roast the bird uncovered at 325°F until the meat and stuffing reach 165°F. Baste the bird occasionally. An unstuffed twelve-pound turkey takes about three hours to cook. A stuffed twelve-pound turkey takes about 3½ hours.
5. Remove the turkey and allow it to stand at room temperature for about fifteen minutes. This makes carving easier. Remove any stuffing right after fifteen minutes.

Roasting Poultry Pieces

You can also roast poultry pieces, such as breasts or legs. Place the pieces in a shallow baking pan with the skin facing up and season them. Roast a turkey breast at 350°F until the meat reaches an internal temperature of 165°F. Roast chicken pieces at 400°F for forty-five to fifty-five minutes. Test for doneness with an instant-read thermometer.

Frying Poultry

You can fry cut-up chicken in a skillet, a deep-fryer, or the oven. Bread the chicken or coat it with flour to keep it from drying out.

Pan-Frying Chicken

Pour cooking oil into a large, heavy skillet to a depth of about ½ inch. Heat it until a cube of bread sizzles. Place chicken pieces into the skillet with the skin facing down. Fry uncovered over low heat for thirty to forty-five minutes. Test for doneness with an instant-read thermometer. Remove pieces as they are done, and drain them on paper towels. Keep them warm in the oven.

Deep-Frying Chicken

Heat a deep pan of oil to 350°F. Fry three to four pieces at a time for ten to fifteen minutes or until browned and cooked through. Test for doneness with an instant-read thermometer. Drain the pieces on paper towels.

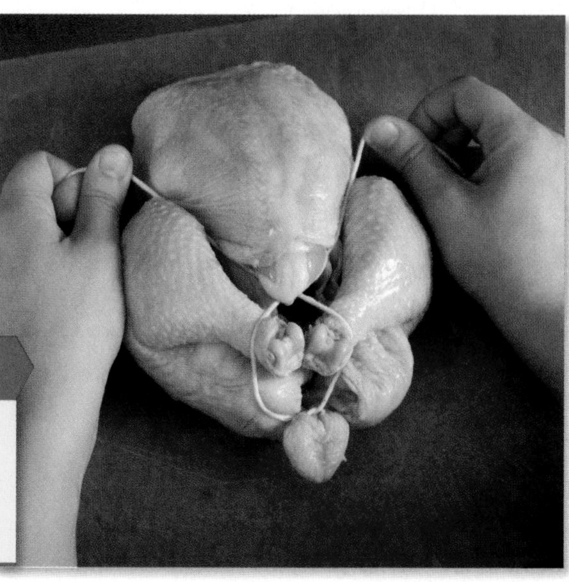

A Trussed Chicken

This whole chicken has been trussed with twine for roasting. The cook wrapped the twine around the legs, then pulled the twine to the opposite side of the bird. *What should you do to prepare the bird before you truss it?*

Oven-Frying Chicken

Put the chicken in a shallow baking pan with the skin facing up. Drizzle with oil or melted butter. Bake uncovered at 350°F about thirty-five to forty-five minutes. Test for doneness with an instant-read thermometer.

Braising Poultry

Braising is a good way to make tough poultry pieces more tender. You can also braise any kind of poultry pieces in sauce to give them flavor.

Brown the poultry pieces and drain off any excess fat. Add seasonings and enough liquid to cover from one half to three quarters the height of the poultry. You can use water, tomato juice or stock. Add vegetables for more flavor. Cover the pan tightly and simmer on the stovetop or in the oven until tender.

Pressure-Cooking and Slow-Cooking Poultry

Pressure-cooking is a good way to cook tough, mature birds. Young, tender birds fall apart in a pressure-cooker. Check the owner's manual for recipes and instructions for using a pressure-cooker.

You can use almost any combination of poultry pieces, liquid, seasonings, and vegetables in a slow cooker. Slow-cooking gives flavors time to develop and blend. It also allows you to prepare dinner ahead of time.

Light and Healthy Recipe

Baked Chicken Nuggets with Baked Sweet Potato "Fries"

Ingredients

Chicken Nuggets

1 pound	chicken breast, cut into bite-size cubes
½ cup	ground bran flakes cereal
1½ cups	ground corn flakes cereal
1 cup	lowfat buttermilk
½ tsp	salt
⅛ tsp	black pepper
⅛ tsp	paprika
⅛ tsp	cayenne

Sweet Potato Fries

2 cups	sweet potato, cut into steak fry-sized rectangles
2 Tbsp.	vegetable oil

These chicken nuggets are made with whole chicken breast pieces and bran flakes. They are baked rather than fried.

Directions

1. Put chicken and milk into a sealable plastic bag, mix well and refrigerate for 15–30 minutes.
2. Toss the sweet potatoes in a mixing bowl with the oil and salt and pepper. Lay out on a sheet tray and bake in a 375°F oven for 25–30 minutes.
3. Mix cereals together with paprika and cayenne. Roll chicken pieces in the ground cereal to coat. Place the chicken in a lightly oiled baking pan and bake in a 375°F oven for 20–25 minutes.

Make It A Meal

Serve with steamed vegetables.

Yield 4 servings

Nutrition Analysis per Serving

■ Calories	363
■ Total fat	10 g
Saturated fat	1 g
Cholesterol	68 mg
■ Sodium	541 mg
■ Carbohydrate	39
Dietary fiber	5 g
Sugars	10 g
■ Protein	31 g

CHAPTER 35 Review & Applications

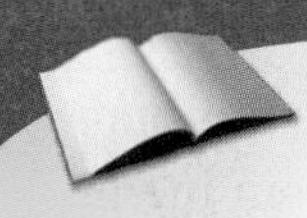

After You Read

Chapter Summary

Poultry is the most popular meat in the United States. It contains protein, vitamins, and minerals and is often low in fat. The most common types of poultry are chicken, turkey, duck, and goose. Poultry comes in many forms, including whole birds, parts, and processed foods. Poultry must be stored in the refrigerator or freezer. Poultry can be cooked in many ways, including grilling, roasting, frying, stewing, and microwaving. Poultry is safe to eat when it reaches an internal temperature of 165°F.

Content and Academic Vocabulary Review

1. Write a fictional story about a special meal using at least four of these content and academic vocabulary words.

Content Vocabulary

- poultry (p. 550)
- free-range (p. 551)
- cutlet (p. 551)
- giblets (p. 552)
- baste (p. 554)
- truss (p. 554)
- stuffing (p. 555)

Academic Vocabulary

- inspect (p. 552)
- moderate (p. 554)

Review Key Concepts

2. **List** the nutrients found in poultry.
3. **Describe** the four most popular types of poultry.
4. **Describe** the common forms of poultry.
5. **Explain** how to select and store poultry.
6. **Explain** why you should always cook poultry until it is well done.

Critical Thinking

7. **Explain** why you would or would not pay more for organic or free-range poultry.
8. **List** several ways to reduce the amount of fat in poultry dishes.
9. **Predict** what might happen if you judged poultry's doneness based on color, rather than temperature.
10. **Evaluate** a recipe for meatloaf that calls for one pound of ground beef. It has many spices and diced celery and onions. Would you replace the ground beef in the recipe with ground turkey? Why or why not? What effect might that have on the finished dish?

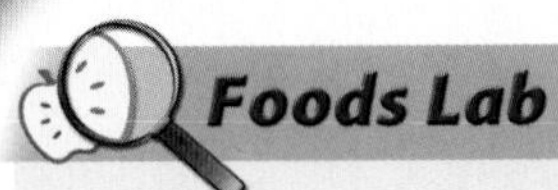

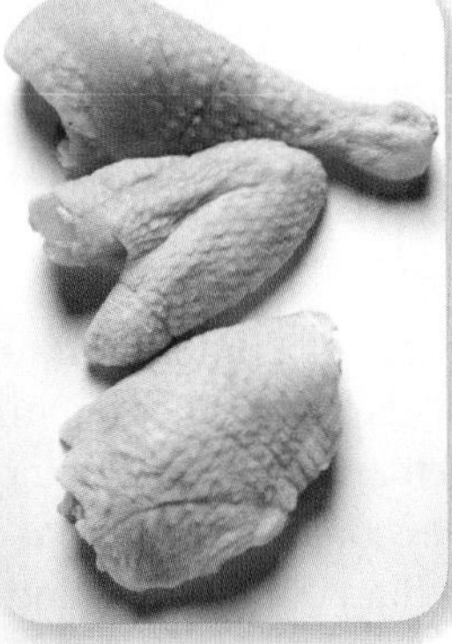

11. Cut Up a Chicken Review the knife safety guidelines in Chapter 20. Then study the directions at the beginning of this chapter on how to cut up a chicken.

Procedure Cut up a whole chicken into parts, including breast halves, wings, thighs and drumsticks. Remember to clean and sanitize your cutting board and work area before you start and when you are finished.

Analysis Write a paragraph about your experience. What parts of the job were difficult? Now that you know how to cut up a whole chicken, would you buy whole chickens instead of chicken parts? Why or why not?

HEALTHFUL CHOICES

12. Adapt a Recipe Conduct research to find a recipe that uses poultry as a main ingredient. Adapt that recipe to make it more healthful. Consider removing skin and fat from the poultry. Consider preparing it in a way that will reduce the amount of fat in the dish. Write out your new recipe and write a paragraph explaining your changes. Discuss how you think your changes will affect the taste of the dish.

TECH Connection

13. Research Ethnic Cuisine Choose a specific culture and research its cuisine. Study that culture's preparation and cooking techniques for poultry. Develop a written outline of key points you want to cover in your presentation. Then use presentation software to develop a seven-slide show for your class. Your presentation should include classic recipes, common spices, photographs, and any special equipment used in the cuisine.

Real-World Skills

Problem-Solving Skills

14. Choose Healthy Foods Meals served at restaurants are usually higher in calories, fat, and salt than meals prepared at home. Brainstorm creative strategies to choose healthy foods and consume moderate portions when eating out.

Interpersonal and Collaborative Skills

15. Plan a Grill Party Follow your teacher's instructions to form into teams. Work together to plan a menu for a grill party featuring grilled chicken, vegetables, salad, beverages, and dessert. Plan the menu by researching healthy, low-fat recipes. Then create a plan to divide the tasks of preparation, cooking, and clean-up among your team.

Financial Literacy Skills

16. Compare Poultry Costs Visit a local supermarket, farmer's market, or meat market. Research the cost per pound of five kinds of chicken, including whole birds, breasts, cutlets, giblets, and processed forms, such as canned or lunchmeat. Compare the costs per pound of the different kinds of poultry. Which is the best value? Why?

Academic Skills

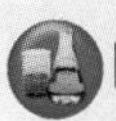

Food Science

17. Understand Bacteria Bacteria called Escherichia coli live in the human intestine and help us digest food. Yet if you eat a piece of poultry contaminated with E. coli, you might get sick.

Procedure Why might E. coli be helpful in one case, and harmful in another? Create a hypothesis, or possible explanation, for this problem.

Analysis Research the topic to see whether your hypothesis is correct. Write one or more paragraphs to explain your answer.

NSES Content Standard C Develop an understanding of organization in living systems and behavior of organisms.

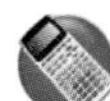

Mathematics

18. Measure Weight and Volume Two types of ounces are used in the United States. A *dry ounce* is a measure of weight. A *fluid ounce* is measure of volume. Fill an eight-ounce measuring cup with flour and weigh it. Now empty the cup, fill it with water, and weigh it. How much does the water weigh, and how much does the flour weigh? As a percentage, how much heavier is the water than the flour?

Math Concept **Transform Fractions into Decimals** Fractions and decimals both represent parts of a whole. Use long division to divide the numerator by the denominator to transform a fraction into a decimal.

Starting Hint Divide the weight of the water by the weight of the flour. Then transform the result from a decimal into a percentage.

NCTM Measurement Understand measurable attributes of objects and the units, systems, and processes of measurement.

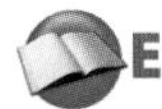

English Language Arts

19. Practice First-Person Writing Write a one-page essay reflecting on how much time and energy you currently devote to healthy eating. To prepare for your essay, keep track of food choices you make during a day and think about your reasons for each choice. Include your thoughts and feelings about foods you eat, or choose not to eat, throughout the day. Remember to make note of snacks you eat. Support points you make in your essay with examples and note healthy alternatives you choose or do not choose. State changes you could make to improve your eating habits and factors that limit your choices.

NCTE 4 Use written language to communicate effectively.

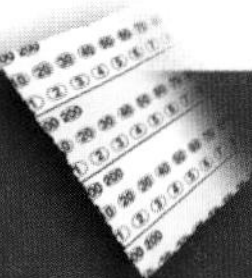

STANDARDIZED TEST PRACTICE

ANALOGY

Select the pair of words that have the same relationship as the pair of words in capitals.

20. POULTRY:PROTEIN

a. safety: seatbelts

b. carbohydrates: fat

c. sleep: alertness

d. carrots: vitamin A

Test-Taking Tip Think about how the two capitalized words relate to one another. Common relationships in analogy questions include cause and effect, part-to-whole, example, and synonym/antonym.

CHAPTER 36

Fish & Shellfish

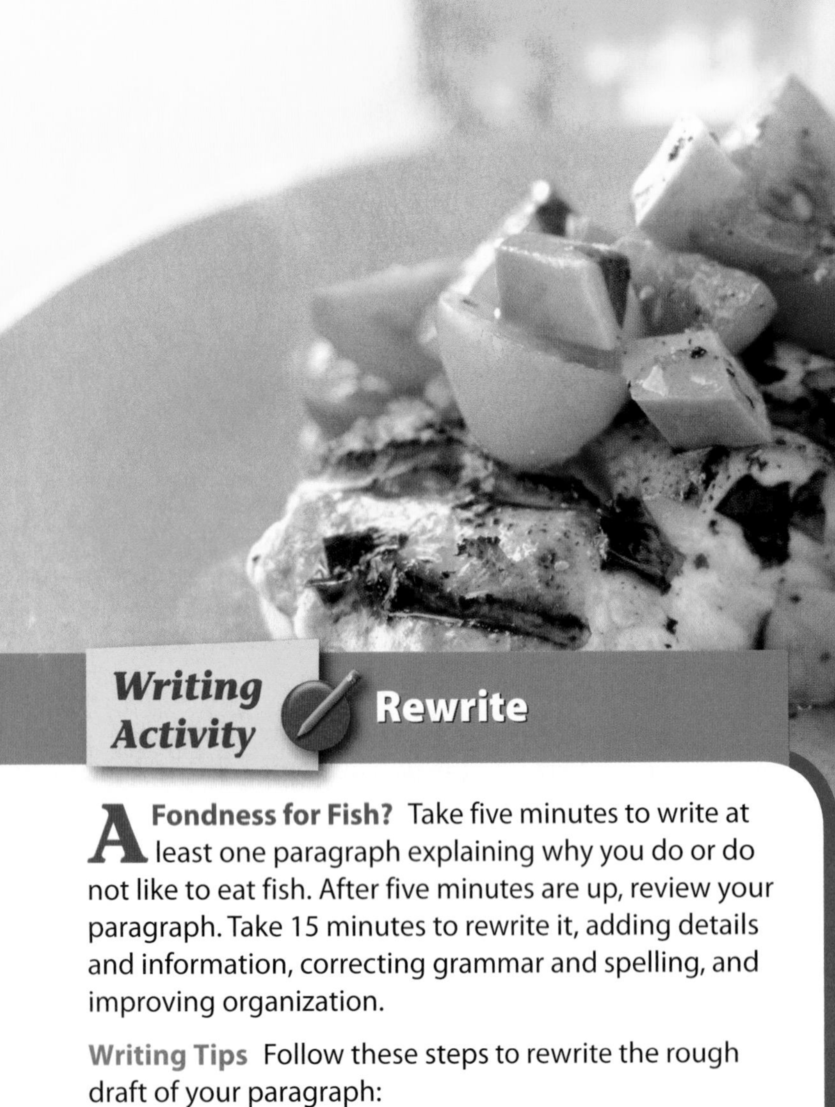

Writing Activity — Rewrite

A Fondness for Fish? Take five minutes to write at least one paragraph explaining why you do or do not like to eat fish. After five minutes are up, review your paragraph. Take 15 minutes to rewrite it, adding details and information, correcting grammar and spelling, and improving organization.

Writing Tips Follow these steps to rewrite the rough draft of your paragraph:

- Circle, underline, and make notes about problems in your paragraph.
- Correct grammar and spelling errors, and improve organization and word choice.
- Add or eliminate words, details, and information where appropriate.

Activate Prior Knowledge

Explore the Photo There are many varieties of fish. *What should you look for when choosing fish?*

Reading Guide

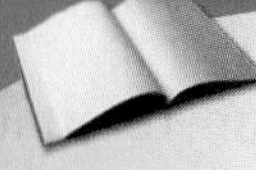

Before You Read

Preview List all the fish cooking methods you can think of. As you read, note the methods you left off your list.

Read to Learn

Key Concepts

- **Describe** the nutrients found in fish and shellfish.
- **Identify** and describe the categories of fish and shellfish.
- **Describe** five market forms of fish.
- **Explain** how to tell when cooked fish is done.

Main Idea

Fish and shellfish are excellent sources of many nutrients, come in numerous forms, and can be prepared using several methods.

Content Vocabulary

You will find definitions for these words in the glossary at the back of this book.

- plankton
- sardines
- overfishing
- fish
- shellfish
- seafood
- low-fat fish
- fatty fish
- whole
- drawn
- dressed
- fillet
- steak
- en papillote

Academic Vocabulary

You will find these words in your reading and on your tests. Use the glossary to look up their definitions if necessary.

- connective
- opaque

Graphic Organizer

Use a graphic organizer like the one below to take notes about the three characteristics you should look for to judge the quality of fresh fish.

JUDGING THE QUALITY OF FRESH FISH		
APPEARANCE	AROMA	TOUCH

Graphic Organizer Go to this book's Online Learning Center at **glencoe.com** to print out this graphic organizer.

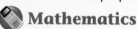

Academic Standards

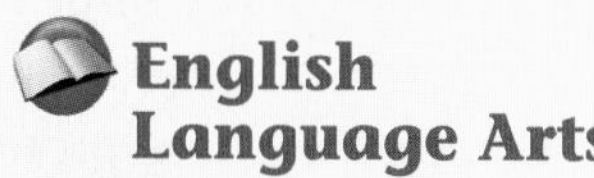

English Language Arts

NCTE 12 Use language to achieve individual purposes.

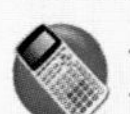

Mathematics

NCTM Number and Operations Compute fluently and make reasonable estimates.

NCTM Data Analysis and Probability Select and use appropriate statistical methods to analyze data.

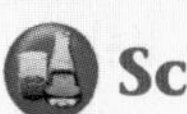

Science

NSES C Develop an understanding of the behavior of organisms.

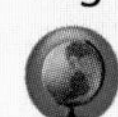

Social Studies

NCSS III G People, Places, and Environments Describe and compare how people create places that reflect culture, human needs, government policy, and current values and ideals as they design and build.

NCTE *National Council of Teachers of English*
NCTM *National Council of Teachers of Mathematics*
NSES *National Science Education Standards*
NCSS *National Council for the Social Studies*

Nutrients in Fish and Shellfish

Fish and shellfish are high in protein, some B vitamins, iron, phosphorus, selenium, zinc, and copper. Fish are one of the few natural sources of vitamin D. Fish, especially salmon, are also good sources of omega-3 fatty acids. Fish and shellfish are low in saturated fat and, except for shrimp and squid, are also low in cholesterol. Saltwater fish are high in iodine.

Fish belong to the same food group as meat, poultry, dry beans, eggs, and nuts. Teens need 5 to 6 ounces of these protein foods each day. Two to 3 ounces of cooked fish is about the size of your palm.

Mercury in Fish

Fish and shellfish can contain mercury. Mercury from factories gets into waterways, where it is absorbed by **plankton**, minute animal and plant life in the water. Small fish eat the plankton and the mercury. The small fish are eaten by larger fish, which are eaten by still larger fish. The most mercury accumulates in the largest fish. Albacore (ˈal-bə-ˌkȯr), or white tuna, is larger than the smaller tuna sold as "chunk light." Albacore tuna may have up to three times the amount of mercury of other tuna.

Besides tuna, other fish that have high mercury levels include shark, swordfish, king mackerel, and tile-fish. Fish that contain low levels of mercury and are safe for most people to eat include canned chunk light tuna, salmon, pollock, catfish, sardines, and herring. **Sardines** is a general term for a variety of small fish with varied characteristics.

Even low levels of mercury are harmful to people in the early years of their life. As a result, the FDA and EPA advise women of childbearing age, pregnant and nursing women, and young children to eat no more than 12 ounces of fish per week. Of that amount, no more than 6 ounces should be albacore tuna.

Sustainable Fisheries

Many fish are becoming increasingly scarce due to overfishing. **Overfishing** means catching too many fish, so that the fish population cannot sustain itself. Some fish are farmed. Unfortunately, fish farms create large amounts of pollution.

Organizations such as the Seafood Choice Alliance recommend fish and shellfish that are safe choices because they are good for health and sustainably harvested or farmed. They also list fish and shellfish that consumers should not buy because their population is in decline, because they are farmed or harvested in a way that hurts the environment, or because they contain toxic materials such as mercury. Types of fish and shellfish to avoid include king crab, flounder, Atlantic halibut, monkfish, rockfish, scallops, shrimp, and red snapper. Good alternatives included Pacific halibut and cod, striped bass, and farmed barramundi and tilapia.

✓ Reading Check **True or False** The smaller the fish, the more mercury it contains.

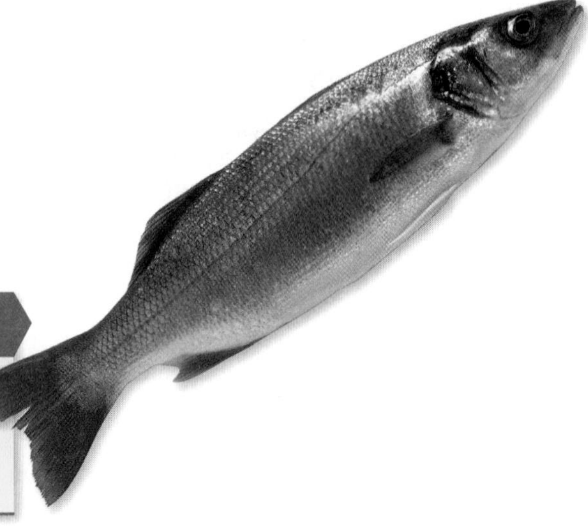

Variety from the Sea

Like meat and poultry, fish and shellfish are rich in protein and can be prepared in a variety of ways, from grilling to microwaving. *What types of fish have you tried? What types of shellfish?*

Types of Fish and Shellfish

What is the difference between fish and shellfish? **Fish** are aquatic animals that have fins and a center spine with bones. **Shellfish** are aquatic animals that have a shell but no spine or bones.

Some fish and shellfish come from freshwater lakes, rivers, streams, and ponds, where water is not salty. These fish are known as freshwater fish. Saltwater fish come from oceans and seas. Some freshwater and saltwater fish and shellfish are raised on fish farms. **Seafood** means saltwater fish and shellfish, but it is often used to mean fish and shellfish from both fresh water and salt water.

Types of Fish

Fish can be divided into two categories: low-fat fish and fatty fish.

Low-fat fish have less than 5 grams of fat per 3½ ounces. The flesh of low-fat fish is white or pale, and it has a delicate texture and a mild flavor. Low-fat fish include barracuda, bass, carp, catfish, cod, haddock, halibut, pike, perch, pollock, red snapper, and whiting. Some of these types of low-fat fish are described in **Figure 36.1**.

Fatty fish have more than 5 grams of fat per 3½ ounces. The flesh of fatty fish is firm, with a deeper color and a stronger flavor than low-fat fish, as well as more calories. Fatty fish include shad as well as the fish described in **Figure 36.2**.

Figure 36.1 A Guide to Low-Fat Fish

Lean Fish Low-fat fish have white or pale flesh, with a delicate texture and a mild flavor. ***How much fat does a 3½-ounce piece of low-fat fish have?***

Type	Characteristics	Common Cooking Method
Carp	Dark flesh. Moderate flavor.	Baked, fried, poached.
Catfish	White flesh; firm yet slightly flaky. Mild flavor with a touch of sweetness.	Fried with cornmeal coating or grilled, broiled, or baked.
Cod*	Opaque flesh; large flakes. Mild, delicate flavor.	Boiled, baked, sautéed, broiled, steamed, or deep-fried.
Haddock	White flesh; firm, tender texture, with fine flake. Delicate, slightly sweet flavor.	Sautéed, poached, pan-fried, or smoked.
Halibut**	Firm flesh. Mild flavor.	Grilled, baked, sautéed, steamed, poached, or broiled.
Perch	Opaque flesh; tender but somewhat firm texture. Mild flavor.	Sautéed, broiled, steamed, baked, or poached.
Pike	Somewhat firm flesh; dry. Moderate flavor.	Grilled, baked, broiled, sautéed, or poached.
Pollock (Alaskan)	Opaque flesh; small flakes; slightly tender. Mild, delicate flavor.	Baked, broiled, steamed, sautéed, or poached.

* Choose Pacific Cod; Atlantic Cod may be unsustainably harvested/raised.

** May be unsustainably harvested/raised.

When preparing fish, you can usually substitute one low-fat fish for another and one fatty fish for another. For example, you could substitute pike for halibut or trout for herring.

Types of Shellfish

Most shellfish have a mild, sweet flavor. Almost all shellfish come from oceans and seas, but a few varieties come from freshwater. There are two types of shellfish, crustaceans and mollusks.

Crustaceans

A crustacean is a type of shellfish with a long body covered by a flexible, jointed shell, or exoskeleton. Shellfish are plentiful and millions of pounds of shellfish are consumed annually. Different kinds of shellfish include:

- **Crabs** Crabs have as many as 10 legs, including the two front arms, which have very strong pinchers for gripping. The meat from a crab comes mainly from the legs. Removing the meat can be difficult as the tough shell surrounding it has to be cracked open.
- **Lobster** Lobster is a much valued shellfish because of its sweet meat. Most of the meat in a lobster is found in the tail and claws. Lobster is usually shipped live and restaurants that serve lobster often keep it in a tank that allows diners to select the one they want. Usually, lobsters are dropped into a pot of boiling water for cooking.
- **Crayfish** Also called crawfish and crawdads, crayfish look like small lobsters and are, in fact, related to lobsters. Crawfish are generally cooked by boiling them

Figure 36.2 A Guide to Fatty Fish

Flavorful Fish Fatty fish have firm flesh, with a deeper color and a stronger flavor than low-fat fish, as well as more calories. ***What other fatty fish has a texture and flakiness similar to that of mackerel?***

Type	Characteristics	Common Cooking Method
Herring	Semi-moist flesh; fine, soft texture. Medium flavor.	Baked, grilled, or sautéed.
Mackerel	Off-white, firm flesh; flaky. May be mild or strong and fishy flavor.	Best grilled or broiled; also baked or poached.
Salmon*	Orange, pink, or red flesh; large, moist flakes. Delicate flavor.	Baked, grilled, broiled, or poached.
Sardines	Sardines is a general term for variety of small fish with varied characteristics. Strong flavor.	Grilled, broiled, or fried. In the U.S., sardines are generally canned, salted, or smoked.
Tuna (Albacore)*	Off-white flesh; firm texture. Mild flavor.	Grilled, broiled, braised.
Tuna (Bluefin)*	Off-white flesh; firm. Distinctive flavor.	Grilled, baked, broiled.
Trout (Rainbow)	Pale white, pink, or orange firm flesh; flaky. Mild, delicate, slightly nutty flavor.	Grilled, broiled, baked, poached, sautéed, deep-fried.

* May contain mercury.

whole. The meat is then pulled or sucked out of the shell.

- **Shrimp** Shrimp, prawns and scampi are different words used interchangeably for shrimp. Grocery stores usually use the word *prawn* for particularly large shrimp but actually they are two different creatures. Prawns have slightly different lung structures. There are thousands of different preparations for shrimp. Tiny bay shrimp are often used in salads. Larger shrimp are prepared by removing the segmented shell and head, then removing the vein that runs along the back of the shrimp.

Mollusks

Mollusks have soft bodies covered by a rigid shell. Clams, mussels, oysters, scallops and squid are all mollusks. Most edible mollusks are prepared in their shells by steaming or boiling.

Inspection and Grading

Several government agencies inspect fish and shellfish. Some state and local government agencies inspect fish. The FDA's food safety system, Hazard Analysis and Critical Control Point (HACCP), identifies and prevents hazards that could cause foodborne illness during stages of fish processing.

The FDA and the National Marine Fisheries Service of the U.S. Department of Commerce work together on a voluntary inspection and grading program for fish. They also inspect fish processing facilities to make sure that food-safety processes are followed. The FDA also has the authority to inspect any fish arriving at ports. It can quarantine fish its inspectors deem dangerous.

✓ Reading Check **Identify** What are the two types of shellfish?

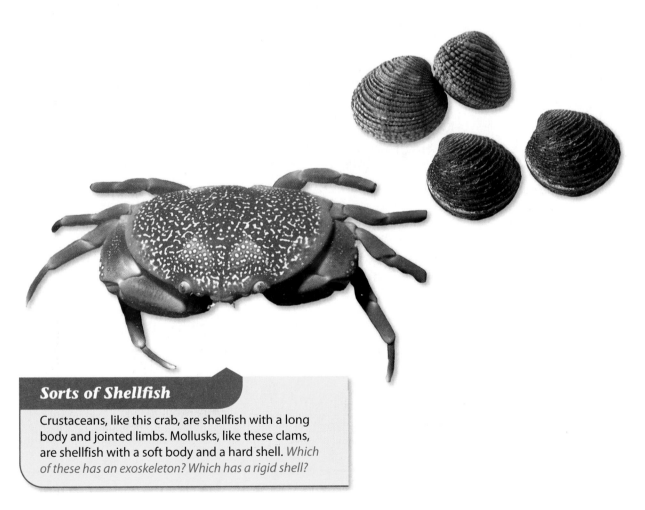

Sorts of Shellfish

Crustaceans, like this crab, are shellfish with a long body and jointed limbs. Mollusks, like these clams, are shellfish with a soft body and a hard shell. *Which of these has an exoskeleton? Which has a rigid shell?*

Buying and Storing Fish and Shellfish

Fish and shellfish retain quality only when they are properly handled from the time they are caught to the time they are cooked. Always start with the freshest fish possible, purchased from a reliable source.

Fish and shellfish should be stored cold. Fresh fish and shellfish are usually packed in ice. If fish are piled too thick, they may be unsafely warm. Do not buy fish or shellfish that are displayed under hot lights. Ready-to-eat fish and shellfish should not be piled next to fresh varieties. Harmful bacteria from the fresh items can transfer to the ready-to-eat products.

Fish and shellfish naturally have a slight fish smell. A strong "fishy" or ammonia odor indicates that the protein in the fish or shellfish has begun to deteriorate.

Buying Fish

You can purchase several market forms of fish, including **whole**, **drawn**, **dressed**, **fillet** (fi-ˈlā), and **steak**. **Figure 36.3** defines these terms. Use appearance, aroma, and touch to judge the quality of fresh fish. Look for shiny skin and glistening color. Whole or drawn fish should have clear, full eyes and bright red or pink gills. Fish should have a mild, fresh aroma like cucumbers or seaweed, not a strong smell.

Fresh fish for sale at a market should be stored on a bed of ice. A fresh fish should have bright, shiny skin, faintly pink gills and bulging eyes. Dull skin, dark gills and eyes that are sunken indicate a fish that is old. Fresh fish smells faintly of the sea. Fish that is too old takes on a foul smell. A fish that is fresh will be firm to the touch. Flesh that is gently pushed will bounce back when released. Soft, mushy flesh indicates a fish that is too old.

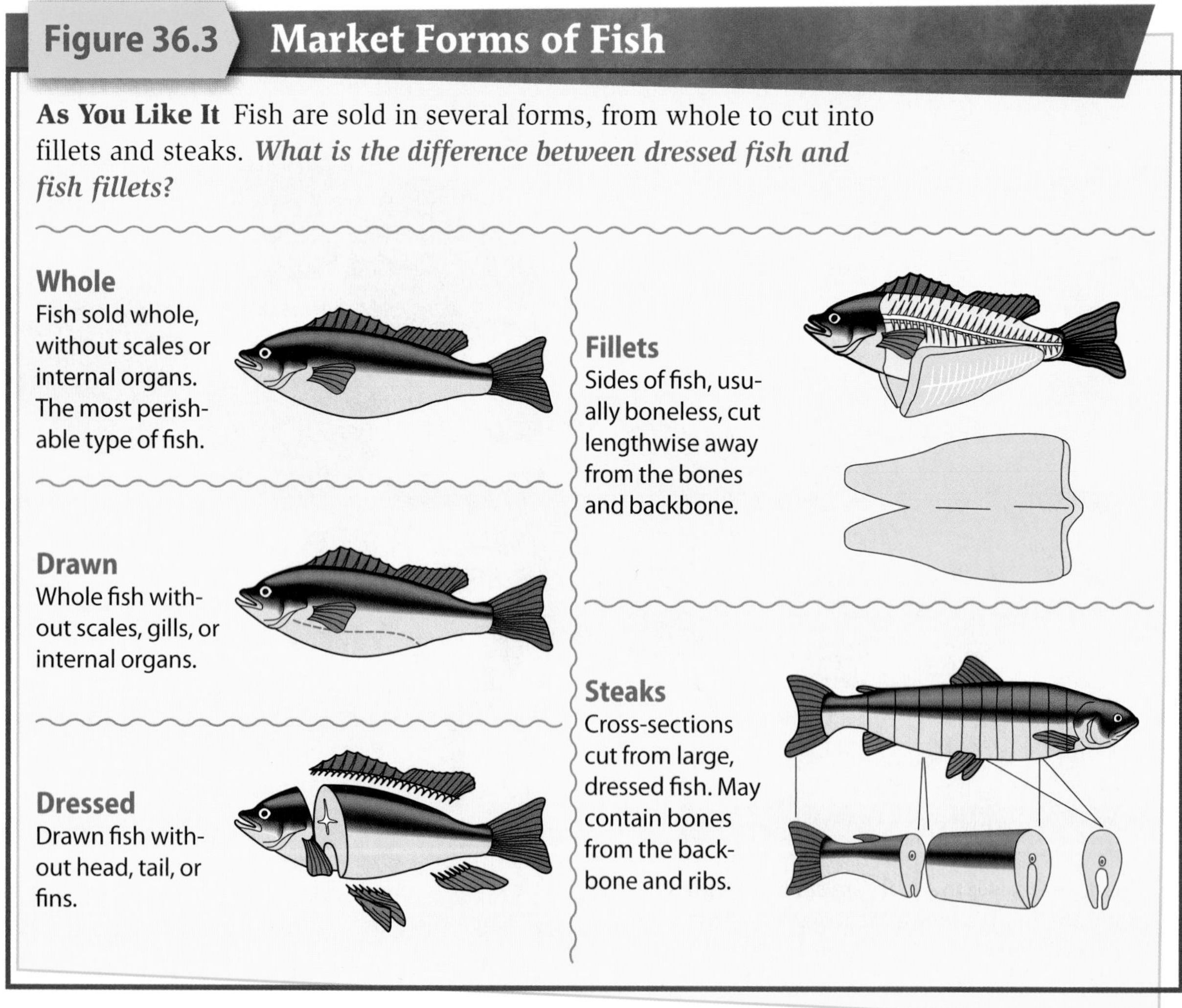

Whole
Fish sold whole, without scales or internal organs. The most perishable type of fish.
Drawn
Whole fish without scales, gills, or internal organs.
Dressed
Drawn fish without head, tail, or fins.
Fillets
Sides of fish, usually boneless, cut lengthwise away from the bones and backbone.
Steaks
Cross-sections cut from large, dressed fish. May contain bones from the backbone and ribs.

Figure 36.3 Market Forms of Fish

As You Like It Fish are sold in several forms, from whole to cut into fillets and steaks. ***What is the difference between dressed fish and fish fillets?***

Buying Shellfish

Some shellfish are sold live because they deteriorate so quickly after they are killed. Look for these signs of quality in shellfish:

Live Clams, Oysters, and Mussels Shells should be tightly closed, moist, and intact, with no cracks, chips, or breaks. If shells are slightly open, tap them with a knife. They should close. If they do not close, discard them. Clams, oysters, and mollusks are also sold without the shell (shucked). Shucked oysters should have a slightly milky or light gray liquid around them.

Scallops Scallops are usually sold without shells. They should look moist but not be in liquid or in direct contact with ice. Scallops should have a fresh sea smell.

Live Lobsters and Crabs Lobsters are dark bluish-green until cooked, when they turn bright red. Look for lobsters and crabs that are active, with legs moving. A lobster's tail should curl under when picked up. Lobsters are usually sold with bands around their claws to prevent them from injuring consumers.

Raw Shrimp Shrimp vary in size and color, and they are sold with or without the shell. Shrimp in the shell should have translucent shells without black spots. Shrimp without the shell should have firm meat. Shrimp should be moist but not in liquid.

Buying Convenience Forms of Fish and Shellfish

You can buy fish and shellfish in several convenience forms, including cooked and ready to eat, canned, frozen, and cured.

Lobster, crab, and shrimp are sold cooked and ready to eat. You can usually buy them by the pound in the fish department.

Canned fish and shellfish are usually ready to eat and are generally used in recipes. Tuna, for instance, is often an ingredient in salads and casseroles. Fish packed in water has fewer calories than fish packed in oil. If you purchase oil-packed fish, drain and rinse it well before using. Canned salmon and sardines are good sources of calcium when eaten with the bones.

Nutrition Check

Tracking Troublesome Mollusks

To prevent widespread foodborne illness, containers of mollusks that arrive at restaurants and supermarkets are labeled with a tag. The tag tells where they were harvested. Sellers are required to keep the tags for 90 days after the containers are emptied. This way, if a consumer gets a foodborne illness from eating the mollusks, the seller can refer to the tags to find out just where the mollusks came from and prevent more from being consumed.

Think About It Because they deteriorate rapidly after harvesting and are sometimes served raw, mollusks commonly cause foodborne illness. In good circumstances, however, they can be a rich source of nutrients. Which two nutrients are they especially rich in?

Many frozen forms of fish are available, including ready-to-cook fillets. Frozen, breaded, fish fillets and fish sticks are usually precooked and only need reheating. Follow the instructions on the label.

Cured fish can be salt-dried, smoked, or pickled. Cod is often salted and dried. Salmon and herring are the most common smoked fish. Herring is often pickled.

Storing Fish and Shellfish

Fish and shellfish are highly perishable. Refrigerate it immediately after purchase and use it within a day or two. Place fish and shellfish in a plastic bag to keep juices from dripping on other foods. Freeze fish for longer storage. Leave already frozen fish in the original wrapping and store it in the freezer immediately. Never store fish that has not been gutted, because organs deteriorate faster than flesh. If you need to store or freeze a fish that has not been gutted, you can easily remove the guts. Cut carefully along the bottom of the fish creating a slit from just below the head to the tail fin. Then scoop out the organs and rinse the cavity with running water.

Refrigerate live shellfish in containers covered with a clean, damp cloth. They need breathing space to stay alive, so do not seal them in a plastic bag. Do not put saltwater shellfish in fresh water, because this will kill them. Properly stored, shellfish live for a few days. If they die in storage, discard them.

Put leftover cooked fish and unused portions of canned fish in a covered container and refrigerate. Use leftovers within three or four days.

✓ Reading Check **Explain** What does a strong, fishy odor indicate in fish?

Cooking Fish and Shellfish

Fish flesh is more tender than meat and poultry flesh and cooks much faster because the muscles are arranged differently. In contrast to the long fibers in meat and poultry, fish flesh has very short fibers arranged in layers. The layers are separated by sheets of very thin, fragile **connective**, or joining, tissue. **Figure 36.4** shows what this structure looks like. When heated, the connective tissue turns into gelatin and the muscle fibers separate. This is why the flesh flakes, or separates into small pieces, when fish is cooked.

Like other high-protein foods, fish must be cooked at low temperatures just until done. If overcooked in dry heat, fish toughens and becomes rubbery. If overcooked in moist heat, the fish falls apart. Fish that is properly cooked flakes when touched with a fork but remains tender.

Dry Heat or Moist Heat?

Because fish is tender, both moist heat and dry heat cook it effectively. Low-fat fish tends to dry out when cooked, however, so moist-heat cooking methods are better. Poaching and steaming are favored techniques for low-fat fish. Low-fat fish cooked in dry heat must be basted generously with oil, melted butter, or a sauce for moisture. Dry-heat methods such as broiling, grilling, and baking are ideal for fatty fish. Moist heat can also be used.

Preparing Fish

Fish must be properly prepared before cooking. Inspect fillets carefully to be sure all bones have been removed. If any bones remain, remove them with clean tweezers. To be sure the fish is clean, wash it under cool, running water and wipe it dry with a paper towel. Thaw frozen fish in the refrigerator and cook it within 24 hours.

Figure 36.4 **Structure of a Fish Muscle**

Flaky Flesh Fish flesh has short fibers arranged in layers, which are separated by sheets of very thin, fragile connective tissue. ***Why does this muscle structure cause fish to flake easily when cooked?***

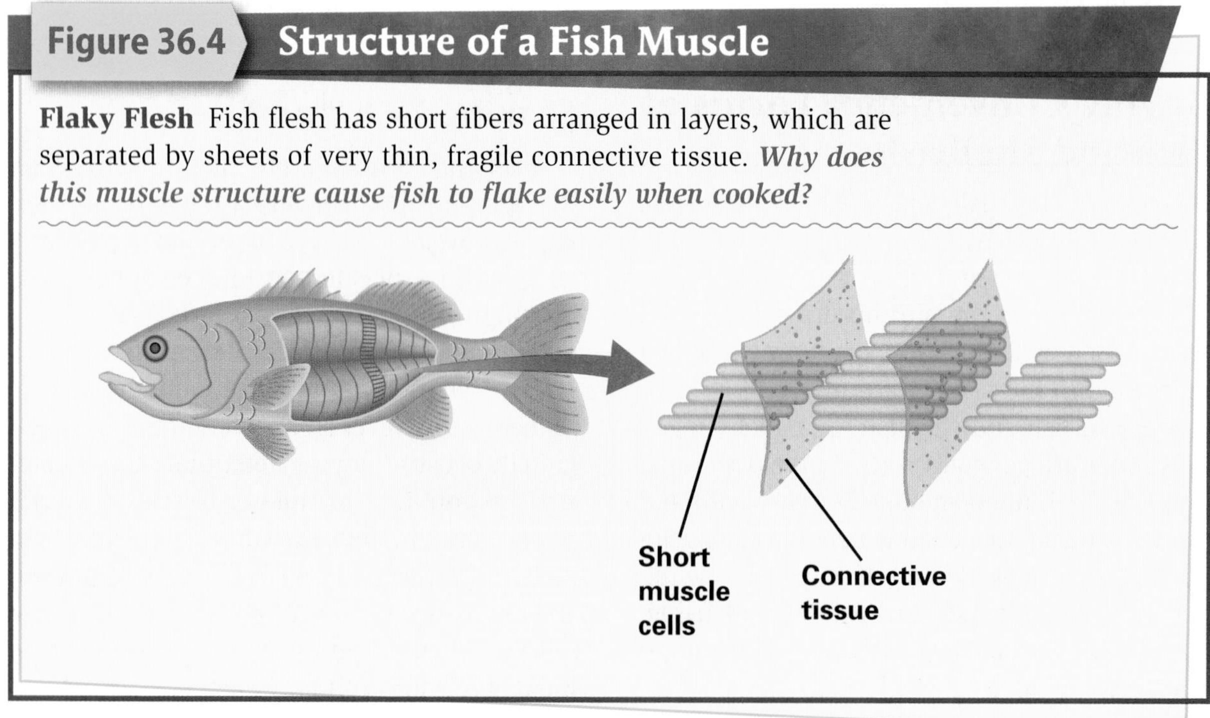

Fish has an unpleasant odor while cooking. Acidic foods help eliminate fish odors, so many fish recipes include an acidic liquid, such as vinegar or a citrus juice. This is why lemon is often served with fish. If fish leaves an odor on your hands, rub your hands with a piece of lemon or rinse them in vinegar.

The 10-Minute Rule

Fish is tender and cooks quickly. The "10-minute rule" can help you cook fish with conventional cooking methods. The rule says to cook fish 10 minutes for every inch of thickness, measured at the thickest part. For example, if a fish fillet is 1 inch thick, cook it for ten minutes (5 minutes on each side).

There are a few exceptions to the 10-minute rule. If fish is baked in a sauce, add about 5 minutes to the cooking time. Also increase cooking time for frozen fish. Some moist-heat recipes need longer cooking times to allow flavors to blend.

Testing for Doneness

Begin to check fish for doneness about 2 or 3 minutes before the cooking time is up. When lifted gently with a fork, the flesh should flake easily. Also look for opaqueness. Raw fish is translucent, because light can pass through individual proteins. Cooked fish is **opaque**, because the proteins coagulate and block light.

Never eat undercooked or raw fish or shellfish. It may be contaminated with harmful bacteria. For example, sushi is a traditional Japanese dish that has become popular in the United States. It is made with various foods, including raw fish. Raw fish may carry harmful parasites, bacteria, and viruses that can cause serious illness. Only specially trained chefs should serve raw fish.

Methods of Cooking Fish

Fish can be cooked in many different ways but because of its delicate structure care and sometimes special equipment is needed. In general, fish cooks quickly and can quickly go from cooked to overcooked so constant attention is necessary.

Kitchen Math

Cooking Fish

For dinner, Sonia is preparing baked Alaskan halibut fillets in a butter, lemon, and garlic sauce. Two of the fillets are thick (about 1¼ inch thick each), while the other two are smaller (at ⅞-inch thickness). If she uses the "10-minute rule," how long should Sonia cook the smaller fillets? The larger fillets?

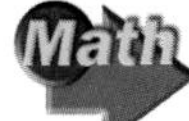

Math Concept **Solving Problems with Proportions** Write two equal ratios (known as a proportion) to relate a quantity you already know to another you are solving for. Use *x* to represent the unknown amount in the second ratio.

Starting Hint The 10-minute rule advises cooking 10 minutes for every inch of thickness. For the smaller fillets, let *x* stand for the total cooking time. Solve for *x* in the proportion 10 minutes / 1 inch = *x* minutes / 0.875 inches. Remember to add additional cooking time to account for the sauce.

Math Appendix For math help, go to the Math Appendix at the back of the book.

NCTM Number and Operations Compute fluently and make reasonable estimates.

Broiling Fish

You can broil fish that is at least 1 inch thick. You can broil drawn and dressed fish under 3 pounds as well as steaks and fillets.

To broil fish, oil the grid of the broiler pan. Place the fish skin-side down in a single layer on the grid, making sure the pieces do not touch each other. Brush with oil, melted butter, or a sauce to prevent drying. Turn the fish halfway through the cooking period. Continue broiling until done, and then baste as needed.

Grilling Fish

Fish must be turned while grilling. Thick cuts of fish grill well because they hold their shape well and can be turned easily. Firm, drawn, and dressed fish also grill well. Avoid grilling a fish that is too large to turn. Thin fillets and small, low-fat, drawn and dressed fish fall apart if you try to turn them. Grill them in a fish basket instead of directly on the grill.

To grill fish, oil the grate lightly. Brush the fish with oil or melted butter to keep it moist. Add seasonings and lemon juice if you wish. Place the fish skin-side down on the grate. Grill it for about half the cooking time, basting frequently with oil or melted butter. Turn the fish and grill it until done, basting frequently.

Baking Fish

Drawn and dressed fish, large steaks, and fillets bake well. For added flavor, season the oil or melted butter for basting. You usually do not need to turn fish while it bakes. You can also prepare fish en papillote. **En papillote** means wrapped, often in parchment paper, and baked.

Choose the baking method based on the type of fish:

Baking Drawn and Dressed Fish Stuff, if desired. Oil a large, shallow baking pan. Place the fish in the pan and brush it with oil or melted butter. Bake it uncovered at 400°F, basting as needed to keep the fish from drying out.

Baking Large Steaks and Fillets Oil a large, shallow, baking pan. Arrange the fish in a single layer, making sure the pieces do not touch each other. Brush with oil or melted butter. Bake at 350°F, basting as needed.

Poaching Fish

Fish is often poached. Many people consider poached fish to be a delicacy, and it is often served in fine restaurants.

You may poach a drawn or dressed fish, fillets, and steaks. The liquid used for poaching can be water, fish or vegetable stock, or milk. Usually the liquid is seasoned to add more flavor to the fish. For example, you can add lemon juice or grapefruit juice. You can also experiment with herbs and spices such as dill or grated fresh ginger, or add sautéed aromatic vegetables such as onions and green peppers.

You can serve hot poached fish with a sauce made from the cooking liquid. After removing the fish from the pan, boil the cooking liquid to thicken it and intensify the flavor.

Choose the poaching method based on the type of fish:

Poaching Fish Fillets Pour the cooking liquid into a large, deep skillet. Bring to a boil and reduce the heat to a simmer. Place the fillets in a single layer in the pan. Add more liquid, if necessary, to cover the fish by at least 1 inch. Cover the pan and simmer gently until the fish is opaque throughout and flakes easily. Do not turn the fillets while poaching.

En Papillote

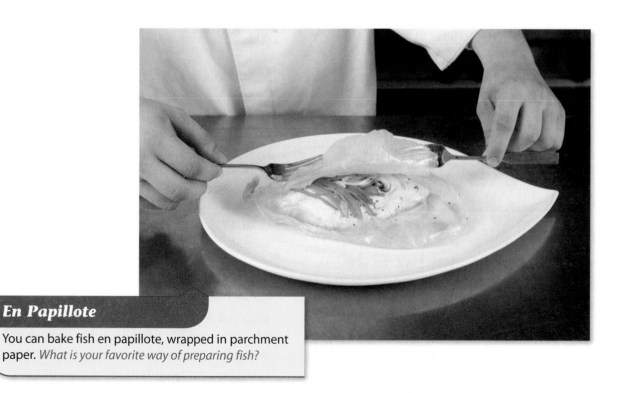

You can bake fish en papillote, wrapped in parchment paper. *What is your favorite way of preparing fish?*

Poaching Drawn and Dressed Fish For easier handling and to help keep the shape of the fish, wrap it in cheesecloth first. Allow enough length at the ends so you can twist and knot the cloth. Use the ends as handles to lower and raise the fish easily. Lower the wrapped fish into simmering liquid in a large pan, making sure the fish is covered by at least 1 inch of liquid. Cover the pan and simmer gently until the fish is opaque and flakes easily. Be careful not to allow the poaching liquid to boil. Boiling can break the fish apart.

Steaming Fish

Drawn and dressed fish, steaks, and large fillets can be steamed. Use a steamer or a large, deep pot fitted with a steaming rack. Pour water into the pot so it is about 1 inch deep but below the level of the rack.

Oil the rack and place the fish on it. Then cover the pot tightly. Heat the water to boiling. Steam the fish over boiling water until the flesh turns opaque and flakes easily.

Braising Fish

Braising is typically used for less tender cuts of meat and poultry, but it also adds flavor and color to fish. The challenge is to cook the fish just long enough for the flavors to blend without overcooking.

Braising is best for a small or medium-size fish that is drawn or dressed. To braise, use a large skillet with a tight-fitting lid. Flour the fish and brown it in the skillet. Add a small amount of liquid, seasonings, and vegetables. Cover and simmer gently just until the fish turns opaque and flakes easily.

Frying Fish

You can fry fillets, small steaks, small drawn or dressed fish, and whole fish, such as trout, in oil, butter, or a mixture of half oil and half butter. The fish is usually floured or breaded first. To fry fish, heat a small amount of fat in a large, heavy skillet over moderate heat. Place the breaded fish in the pan in a single layer, making sure the pieces do not touch. If the pan is crowded, the fish steams and loses crispness. Trout almondine is a traditional fish dish served in which a whole trout is panfried with sliced almonds. Fry on one side for half the cooking time; then turn and fry on the other side until the flesh flakes easily. Drain on paper towels. You may keep the fish warm in the oven until serving.

Breaded fish may also be oven-fried. Grease a large, shallow baking pan. Arrange fish in a single layer, making sure pieces do not touch each other. Drizzle with oil or melted butter and bake, uncovered, at 500°F. Contrary to the general rules for cooking protein, fish is oven-fried at a high temperature. The fish does not dry out or toughen because the crumb coating and high temperature combine to create an attractive, brown crust that holds in juices. Bake without turning or basting until the flesh is golden brown and flakes easily.

TECHNOLOGY FOR TOMORROW

Fish Farming's Flaws

Thanks to technology, it is possible to raise fish in farms and decrease the numbers that are fished from oceans and rivers. Special water purification systems, UV water sterilization, and hydroponic systems that grow algae for fish food are just some of the technologies used in fish farming, or aquaculture. Fish farms, however, have several drawbacks. Thousands of fish are raised together in small spaces. This leads to several forms of pollution. Packed tightly, fish become sickened with infections. Consequently, some fish farms use strong antibiotic drugs to keep the fish alive, which are then consumed by the humans who eat the fish. The waste produced by the fish, along with the drugs, can also affect local waterways. Despite the difficulties of fish farming, it is necessary because a growing number of fish species are becoming endangered because of over fishing. Different fish have natural enemies so the depletion of a particular type of fish can cause havoc with an ocean's entire ecosystem.

Get Involved Research one way that new technology can make aquaculture more environmentally friendly. Write a paragraph.

NCSS III G People, Places, and Environments
Describe and compare how people create places that reflect culture, human needs, government policy, and current values and ideals as they design and build.

Deep-Frying Fish

You can deep-fry small fillets and fish cut into sticks or squares. Bread the pieces first. Then heat a large pot of oil to 375°F and place one layer of breaded fish in a deep-fry basket. Lower it slowly into the fat and fry the fish until golden brown. Remove it and drain on paper towels. Keep warm in the oven while you continue to fry remaining pieces in small batches.

Be careful not to cook too many pieces at a time because the oil may bubble over and ignite. The oil temperature may also go down quickly when several pieces are added, allowing the fish to absorb a great deal of fat. Do not reuse oil used to fry fish. The process of deep frying breaks down the oil and it can become rancid.

Microwaving Fish and Shellfish

Microwaving is ideal for cooking fish and shellfish in moist heat. Cook small amounts at a time, preferably less than a pound, to make sure that the flesh is thoroughly cooked. Place the fish or shellfish in a microwaveable dish. Add a sauce for flavor if you like. Cover with a lid or plastic wrap.

Fish and shellfish cook quickly in the microwave oven, so it is easy to overcook them. Remove them from the oven when the outer edges are opaque and the center is still slightly translucent. Let them stand for five minutes to complete the cooking, then check for doneness. For shellfish, avoid cooking more than six pieces at a time. Brush with melted butter or a sauce before microwaving.

Light and Healthy Recipe

Whitefish en Papillote

Ingredients

- **½ cup** Snap peas
- **1 cup** Julienned carrots
- **½ cup** Shredded napa cabbage
- **1 cup** Onions, sliced in thin circles
- **1 pound** Whitefish fillets (orange roughy, tilapia or other flat fish)
- **1 Tbsp.** Olive oil
- **1 tsp.** Lime zest
- **2 Tbsp.** Lime juice

Directions

1. Preheat oven to 425°. Lay out four pieces of parchment paper or tin foil.
2. Gently toss snap peas, carrots, cabbage and onions in a bowl
3. Using half the vegetables, spread a layer on each piece of paper.
4. Gently brush the fillets with the olive oil.
5. Place a fillet on each bed of vegetables and top with the remaining vegetables.
6. Sprinkle the lime zest and juice over the top of each fish.
7. Fold the paper over and make a seal along all sides. Place the fish in the oven and bake for 10 minutes. Slit the top and serve.

Wrapping the fish and vegetables in paper (you can use aluminum foil if you prefer) allows them to bake in their own juices.

Yield 4 servings

Nutrition Analysis per Serving

Calories	351
Total fat	15 g
Saturated fat	2 g
Cholesterol	119 mg
Sodium	131 mg
Carbohydrate	12
Dietary fiber	3 g
Sugars	5 g
Protein	40 g

CHAPTER 36 Review & Applications

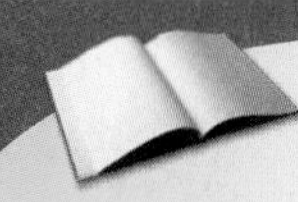

After You Read

Chapter Summary

Fish and shellfish provide many nutrients. Unfortunately, they also contain mercury, which travels to waterways from factories. Many fish are becoming scarce due to overfishing. There are two categories of fish and two categories of shellfish. Government agencies inspect and grade fish and shellfish. There are several qualities to look for when buying fish and shellfish. They are also available in convenience forms. Because they are highly perishable, fish and shellfish must be properly stored. Fish cooks quickly when exposed to dry or moist heat. A variety of methods may be used to cook fish.

Content and Academic Vocabulary Review

1. Arrange these content and academic vocabulary words into groups of related words. Explain why you put the words together.

Content Vocabulary

- plankton (p. 562)
- sardines (p. 562)
- overfishing (p. 562)
- fish (p. 563)
- shellfish (p. 563)
- seafood (p. 563)
- low-fat fish (p. 563)
- fatty fish (p. 563)
- whole (p. 566)
- drawn (p. 566)
- dressed (p. 566)
- fillet (p. 566)
- steak (p. 566)
- en papillote (p. 570)

Academic Vocabulary

- connective (p. 568)
- opaque (p. 569)

Review Key Concepts

2. Describe the nutrients found in fish and shellfish.
3. Identify and describe the categories of fish and shellfish.
4. Describe five market forms of fish.
5. Explain how to tell when cooked fish is done.

Critical Thinking

6. Explain how fish illustrate that the health of the environment directly affects human health.
7. Explain why choosing to eat only sustainably harvested or farmed fish and shellfish can be an ethical decision that is also good for your health.
8. Assess the accuracy of Marie's statement: "I just love to eat oysters. They are my favorite type of crustacean and probably my favorite type of fish."
9. Evaluate whether it is safe for a supermarket to display cooked, ready-to-eat salmon next to fresh whole salmon. Explain your answer.
10. Describe the three most healthful ways to prepare fish and why.

CHAPTER 36 Review & Applications

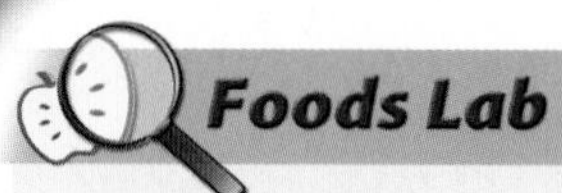

Foods Lab

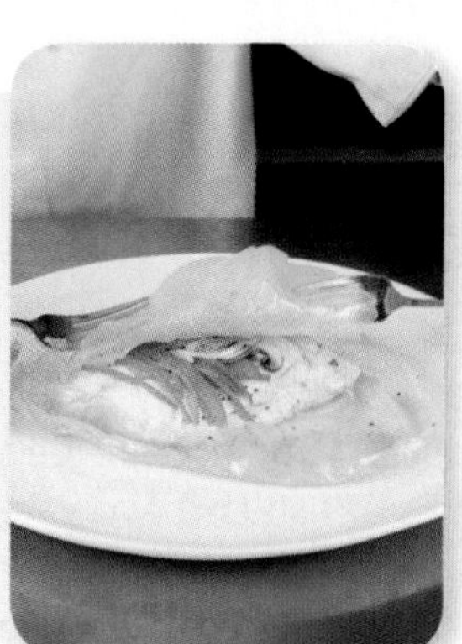

11. Fish Cooking Methods Dry heat and moist heat affect different fish in different ways. Practice with methods that use each type of heat to learn what works.

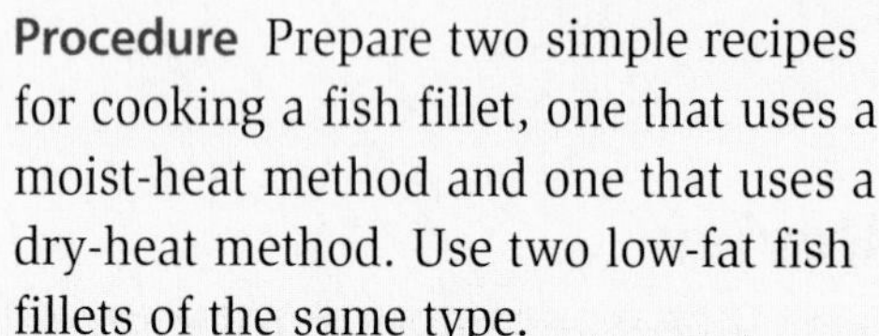

Procedure Prepare two simple recipes for cooking a fish fillet, one that uses a moist-heat method and one that uses a dry-heat method. Use two low-fat fish fillets of the same type.

Analysis Divide a sheet of paper into two columns, and compare the effects of the two cooking methods. Consider ease of preparation and cleanup, as well as appearance and taste of the cooked fish. What do you conclude?

HEALTHFUL CHOICES

12. Monitoring Mercury Talia, who is pregnant, ate 4 ounces of fish on Monday, 3 ounces on Tuesday, and 3 ounces on Wednesday. On Friday, she goes to Bree's house for dinner. Bree offers her a 2-ounce serving of swordfish or a 2-ounce serving of salmon. Can she have either? If so, which one? Why is mercury a concern for Talia?

TECH Connection

13. Ocean Fishing Under your teacher's supervision, use the Internet to research commercial ocean fishing. What methods are used to catch fish and shellfish? Where are many of them caught? How are they stored safely until they are sold? What are the benefits and drawbacks of this industry? What do you think will happen to this industry over the next 10 years? Write a one-page report of your findings.

Real-World Skills

Problem-Solving Skills

14. Safe Storage Dan went fishing and caught several trout. At home, he left them whole, wrapped them, and stored them in the refrigerator. Two days later, they had a rotten smell. What went wrong? How can he solve this problem in the future?

Interpersonal and Collaborative Skills

15. Eating Etiquette Follow your teacher's instructions to form groups. Work together to research the appropriate ways to eat such shellfish as lobster, crab legs, oysters, and clams. Present a skit to the class in which you demonstrate proper and improper shellfish eating techniques.

Financial Literacy Skills

16. Cost of Convenience Visit a supermarket to research the cost per pound of one type of cooked, ready-to-eat fish. Then research the cost per pound of the same type of fish in its uncooked form. What is the price difference? Why is one form more expensive? Do you think the product is worth the extra price?

Academic Skills

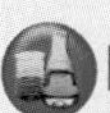

Food Science

17. Perishable Live Shellfish Most mussels are sold live in the shell, but they also come precooked or already shucked. If you are buying them live, they must be tightly closed in order to be safe to eat.

Procedure Select a dozen mussels from a reputable fish supplier. Put the mussels in a bowl and put the bowl in a larger bowl of ice water. Wait 10 minutes and observe the mussels. What happens when you tap the shell gently on the table?

Analysis Write a paragraph recording your observations and conclusions.

NSES C Develop an understanding of behavior of organisms.

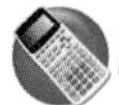

Mathematics

18. Fishy Statistics Jody is going to serve grilled salmon to a group of friends over for a barbecue. She purchases a dozen salmon fillets that weigh, in ounces: 7, 5.5, 6, 8, 6.5, 7.5, 7, 6.5, 9.5, 7.5, 8.5, and 7.5. What is the average (mean) weight of the fillets? What is the median weight? What is the mode?

Math Concept **Mean, Median, and Mode** Given a series of values, the mode is the value that occurs most frequently. The median is the middle number in the series, when the numbers are arranged in order. Add all values together and divide by the number of values to find the mean.

Starting Hint Since there are an even number of weights, there will be two middle numbers. The median is the average of those two numbers.

NCTM Data Analysis and Probability Select and use appropriate statistical methods to analyze data.

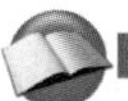

English Language Arts

19. Billboard Create a billboard that will tell passing drivers something about fish. Because people will pass it in a hurry, it can only contain seven words or less. Choose the words carefully. Think of a catchy and memorable slogan or headline. Find an image that expresses an important fact about fish that you think people should know. Use posterboard to design your billboard or use photo editing software to design it. Share your billboard with the class.

NCTE 12 Use language to accomplish individual purposes.

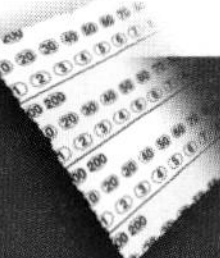

STANDARDIZED TEST PRACTICE

MULTIPLE CHOICE

Read the question and select the best answer from the choices.

20. Which of the following is an example of a fatty fish?
 a. halibut
 b. pike
 c. catfish
 d. salmon

Test-Taking Tip Multiple choice questions may prompt you to select the best answer. They may present you with answers that seem partially true. The best answer is the one that is completely true, and can be supported by information you have read in the text.

CHAPTER 37

Beverages

Writing Activity — Timed Writing

Beverage of Choice Do you like the refreshing simplicity of water, or the sweetness of juice? The bold flavor of coffee, or the creamy texture of a smoothie? In five minutes, write a descriptive paragraph about your favorite beverage. Explain what it is, when you drink it, why you like it, and how you prepare it.

Writing Tips Follow these steps to complete a timed writing:

- Briefly jot down thoughts and details before you begin writing.
- Focus more on the quality of your writing than the quantity.
- If you have time left, make corrections.

Activate Prior Knowledge

Explore the Photo Beverages provide water and nutrients. *Which beverages do you think are the most healthful?*

Reading Guide

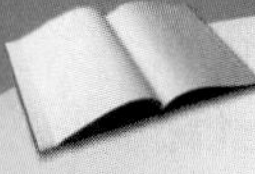

Before You Read

Preview Examine the photos and figure and read their captions. Think about the variety of beverages available.

Read to Learn

Key Concepts

- **Identify** and describe types of bottled waters.
- **List** and describe beverages made with juice.
- **Describe** two types of coffee beans.
- **Explain** how to brew black, oolong, and green tea.
- **Describe** the difference between hot chocolate and hot cocoa.
- **Define** and describe soft drinks and punch.

Main Idea

Beverages provide needed fluids, are refreshing and satisfying, and make meals complete.

Content Vocabulary

You will find definitions for these words in the glossary at the back of this book.

- carbonated
- juice
- juice drink
- fruit-flavored drink
- coffee bean
- caffeine
- decaffeinated
- tea
- steep
- herb tea
- smoothie
- cocoa butter
- cocoa powder
- cocoa
- bloom
- punch
- mulled

Academic Vocabulary

You will find these words in your reading and on your tests. Use the glossary to look up their definitions if necessary.

- contaminate
- originated

Graphic Organizer

Use a graphic organizer like the one below to compare and contrast juice drinks and fruit-flavored drinks.

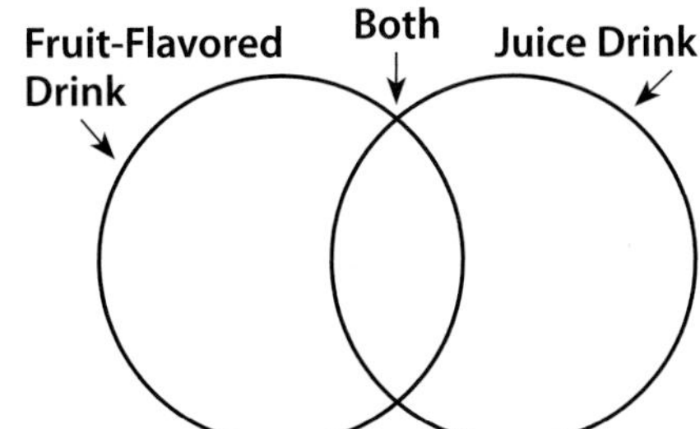

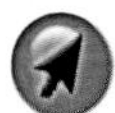

Graphic Organizer Go to this book's Online Learning Center at **glencoe.com** to print out this graphic organizer.

Academic Standards

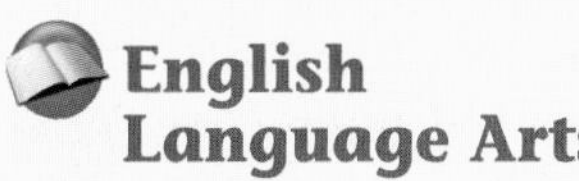

English Language Arts

NCTE 4 Use written language to communicate effectively.

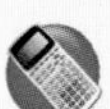

Mathematics

NCTM Number and Operations Compute fluently and make reasonable estimates.

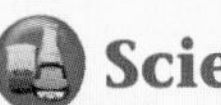

Science

NSES B Develop an understanding of chemical reactions.

NCTE *National Council of Teachers of English*
NCTM *National Council of Teachers of Mathematics*
NSES *National Science Education Standards*
NCSS *National Council for the Social Studies*

Water

Beverages complete meals, are satisfying and refreshing, and are an important source of fluid. Water is one of the main nutrients needed by your body, which makes it one of the most healthful beverages. Tap and bottled water are available almost everywhere. Tap water is more convenient, more economical, and often the safest. Tap water must meet EPA regulations, while bottled water is subject to FDA standards that are not as strict.

If you like to carry bottled water, save money by buying reusable sports bottles and filling them with tap water. You can add a little lemon juice, if you like, for flavor. To minimize the growth of harmful bacteria, wash the bottle thoroughly every day in hot sudsy water. Rinse it well and let it air dry.

Bottled Water

When buying bottled water, read the label and cap carefully. Some bottled water is actually tap water, sometimes with minerals added. If the bottled water comes from a tap, the label will say "from a municipal source or from a community water system."

Bottled water comes in many forms.

Spring Water Spring water comes from an underground spring.

Mineral Water Mineral water contains dissolved minerals such as calcium, magnesium, sodium, and bicarbonates. Some people say mineral water to refer to sparkling water.

Naturally Sparkling Water Often from a spring, this is naturally carbonated water. **Carbonated** means bubbly from dissolved carbon dioxide.

Purified Drinking Water Purified drinking water is processed to remove impurities and to add or remove minerals for health and taste. It is often made with ground water or tap water.

Enhanced Water Enhanced water contains ingredients such as flavorings, sugar, vitamins, minerals, and herbs. If you eat a wide variety of foods or take multivitamin and mineral supplements, avoid enhanced water. It could lead to an overdose of nutrients, which may harm your health.

Potentially Harmful Plastic

Chemicals found in plastic are another reason why bottled water is not always safer than tap. Bisphenol-A, one of several chemicals used to make plastic water bottles, disrupts the human hormone system and is linked to numerous cancers and reproductive disorders. One study found this harmful chemical in the bodies of 95 percent of Americans. To reduce the likelihood that it and other substances will end up in your drinking water, always keep plastic water bottles cool. Heating the bottles encourages the chemicals to leach into the water. Reusing disposable plastic water bottles has a similar effect. Instead, recycle them after each use.

What Would You Do? After unloading several grocery bags from her car on a hot day, Tori said, "I'll leave that box of bottled water in the backseat for now. I'm too tired to carry it inside."

Remember to recycle bottled water containers. Do not reuse them by refilling them with tap water. They are intended for one-time use only. Over time, the plastic could break down and develop cracks or leaks, allowing harmful bacteria to **contaminate**, or pollute, the water.

✓ **Reading Check** **Identify** What form of bottled water is often made with ground water or tap water?

Juices

Fruits and vegetables are converted into a wide array of beverages. Some contain all fruit or vegetable juice. Others have large amounts of added sugar and other ingredients. Read the label to see how much actual juice a drink contains and whether or not it has been pasteurized.

To be labeled **juice**, a product must be 100 percent fruit or vegetable juice. Common fruit juices include orange, apple, grape, pineapple, and grapefruit. Popular vegetable juices include tomato, carrot, and mixed vegetables.

Nutrients in Juices

Juices are among the most nutritious of all beverages. Juices contain all the nutrients found in fruits and vegetables except dietary fiber. Some juices are fortified with nutrients such as vitamins A and D and calcium. Some juices, however, are less nutritious than others. For example, apple and white grape juice are not as nutritious as orange juice.

Fruit juices are concentrated forms of fruit. As a result, they are high in natural sugars and calories. Choose fresh fruits and vegetables more often than juices to get the nutrition without extra calories.

Juice Drinks

Juices are also blended with other ingredients to create juice drinks. A **juice drink**, also also called a "juice cocktail," a blend of 10 to 50 percent juice with water, sweeteners, flavorings, and other additives. The percentage of juice must be listed on the label.

A **fruit-flavored drink** is a drink that tastes like juice but does not have any juice. Fruit-flavored drinks are made with water, sweeteners, and flavorings that give a fruitlike flavor. They are often fortified with vitamins and minerals, but they do not have the nutrition of real juice.

Buying Juices

Juices and drinks are available in the refrigerated section, in cans and bottles in grocery aisles, and as frozen concentrates. Some juices and juice drinks come in powdered form or as liquid concentrates, which must be reconstituted by adding water.

Juices must be pasteurized to destroy harmful bacteria. Juices that are not pasteurized must have a label warning that the juice was not pasteurized and may contain harmful bacteria.

Making Your Own Juice

It is easy to make your own juice with a juicer or blender. The simplest juicer is a hand-operated reamer, which extracts juice from such citrus fruits as oranges, grapefruits, and lemons. You can also buy electric juicers that turn almost any fruit or vegetable into juice.

✓ Reading Check **Explain** When can a product be labeled as a juice?

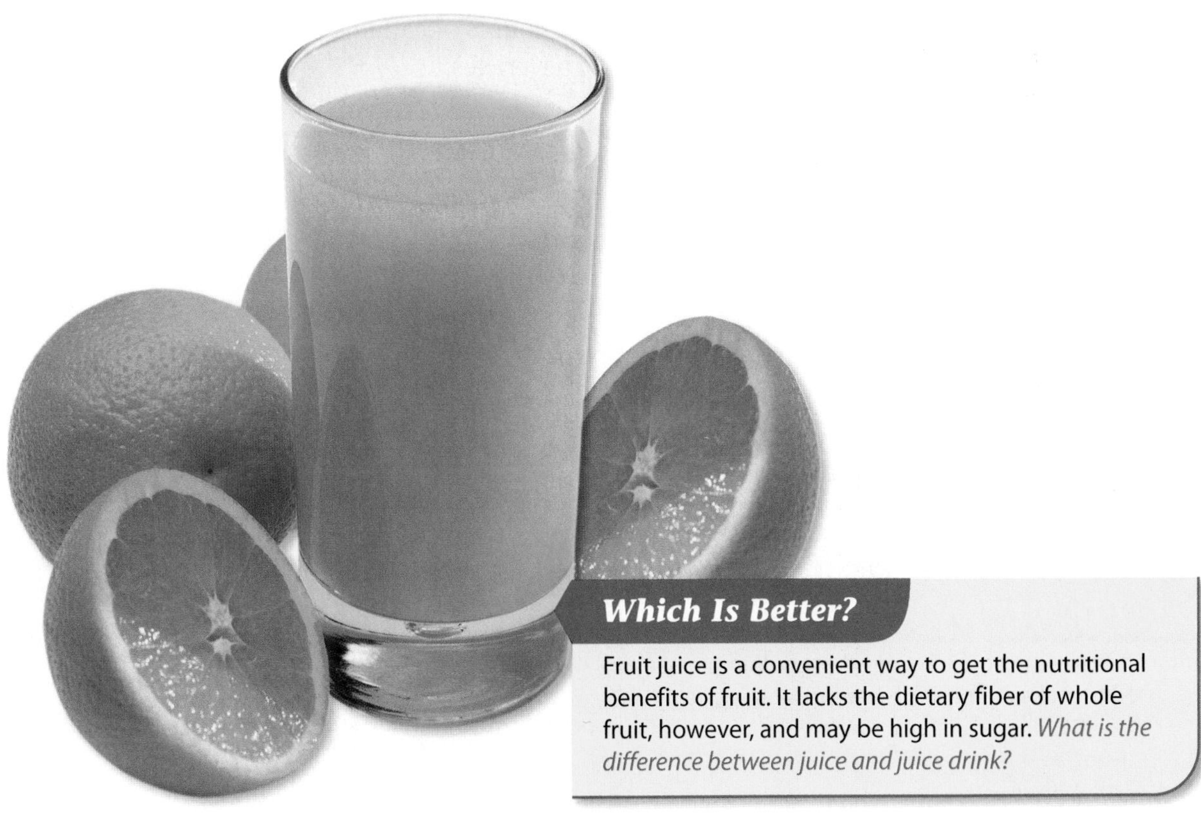

Which Is Better?

Fruit juice is a convenient way to get the nutritional benefits of fruit. It lacks the dietary fiber of whole fruit, however, and may be high in sugar. *What is the difference between juice and juice drink?*

Coffee

People have been drinking coffee for centuries. Coffee is made from the **coffee bean**, the twin seeds of a deep-red fruit produced by the coffee plant. The seeds are fermented, dried, and graded according to size. The beans are then roasted and brewed.

Coffee beans **originated**, or were first discovered, in Ethiopia, but they were first roasted and brewed into a beverage in the Middle East. Coffee spread throughout the world and coffee houses sprang up, providing places for people to gather, drink coffee, and socialize. European colonists introduced coffee to the New World. Today the top coffee producers are Central and South America, Indonesia, Africa, and Hawaii. Coffee, in many flavor combinations, is widely consumed today.

Types of Coffee Beans

Two main types of coffee beans are used in coffee production. Arabica (ə-ˈra-bə-kə) beans produce the finest flavor. Arabica beans are best grown in semitropical climates at high altitudes, so they are often labeled as "mountain-grown." Robusta (rō-ˈbəs-tə) beans grow at low altitudes in tropical climates. They have less flavor than arabicas but twice as much caffeine.

Supermarket coffees usually blend robusta varieties with a little arabica for flavor. Beans sold in specialty coffee shops are usually all arabica.

Hundreds of varieties of these two main beans exist. Usually the region where they are grown gives coffees their name, such as Colombian, Brazilian, Kenyan, or Mocha (after a town in Yemen on the Red Sea). Coffees from different countries and regions have different flavors and levels of acidity.

Caffeine in Coffee

Coffee is one of many beverages that contain caffeine. **Caffeine** is a natural stimulant that affects the nervous system, heart, and kidneys. Caffeine is not harmful in small amounts, but it can produce unwanted side effects such as anxiety and sleeplessness. Coffee, tea, chocolate, and cocoa have naturally occurring caffeine. Many soft drinks and energy drinks have caffeine added during manufacturing.

Coffee, tea, and many other drinks are available **decaffeinated**, with the caffeine removed. Decaffeinated coffee may have a small amount of caffeine, often around 10 percent of the caffeine in regular coffee.

Figure 37.1 shows the approximate amounts of caffeine in coffee and several other beverages.

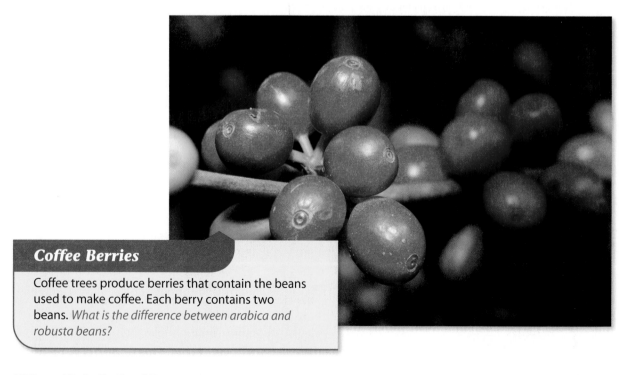

Coffee Berries

Coffee trees produce berries that contain the beans used to make coffee. Each berry contains two beans. *What is the difference between arabica and robusta beans?*

Buying and Storing Coffee

Coffee beans are roasted to bring out the flavor. There are many ways to roast coffee, but the most common is in a cylindrical drum that rotates while being heated from the outside. The length of time coffee is roasted can be varied to make for a lighter or darker roast. A lighter roast of coffee has more caffeine than a darker roast because some caffeine is cooked off in the roasting process.

These are the most popular roasts:

American or Regular Roast American roast is a medium roast that produces a moderate flavor and medium brown color.

French Roast French roast produces a stronger coffee with a dark brown color.

Italian Roast Italian roast is considered the darkest roast for coffee.

Whole and Ground Coffee Beans

Coffee is sold as whole or ground beans. You can often have coffee beans ground to order where you buy them. Grinding the beans just before brewing gives the freshest coffee. Some people prefer to buy whole beans and grind them at home with a coffee grinder.

Ground coffee may be finely or coarsely ground. When finely ground, coffee has a greater surface area exposed to water. As a result, the water takes longer to run through the ground coffee as it brews. When coffee is coarsely ground, less surface area is exposed to water, and the water passes through the ground coffee more quickly.

Regular grind is coarse and is best for electric coffeemakers and percolators. Drip grind is finer and is best for automatic drip coffeemakers. Both work well for vacuum coffeemakers.

Ground coffee comes in cans of various sizes. The label shows the roast and grind, so read carefully to find the right one for your coffeemaker.

Store ground or whole coffee beans in an airtight container in a cool, dry place. You can freeze the beans for longer storage, but the main factors that contribute to coffee going stale are air and light. You can store unopened cans of vacuum-packed ground or whole beans at room temperature for about a year.

Figure 37.1 Caffeine in Coffee and Other Beverages

Limit Caffeine Intake Coffee is not the only beverage with caffeine. Tea, sodas, and energy drinks also have a large amount of caffeine. ***Which of the beverages shown here has the most caffeine per ounce? Which has the least?***

Beverage	Approximate Amount of Caffeine
Coffee (8 oz.)	
Brewed	80 – 150 mg
Instant	65 – 100 mg
Decaffeinated	2 – 5 mg
Espresso (1.5-2 oz.)	60 – 140 mg
Tea (8 oz.)	
Brewed	40 – 100 mg
Instant	25 – 30 mg
Iced (12 oz.)	30 – 75 mg
Caffeinated Soft Drinks (12 oz.)	
Regular	40 – 60 mg
Diet	35 – 45 mg
High-energy drinks	40 – 120 mg
Chocolate milk (8 oz.)	2 – 7 mg
Hot chocolate or cocoa (8 oz.)	3 – 10 mg

Espresso

Though you can buy coffee labeled Espresso Roast, espresso is not a type of roast. Espresso is a thick, syrupy coffee. The word is also used to name the method used to make it. Espresso beans are a blend of mostly dark roasted coffee beans created by a roaster to provide a rich, full-flavor espresso. Coffee roasters creating an espresso blend may use five or more different coffee beans roasted at varying levels of darkness.

Espresso is made with a machine that pumps a small amount of very hot water through finely ground, densely packed coffee under great pressure. A serving size of espresso is 1 to 2 ounces and is usually consumed in two or three sips.

Espresso is combined with steamed milk to make other drinks like cappuccinos and lattes. Cappuccino is made when steamed milk and milk foam is added to espresso. A slightly less foamy milk is used to make a latte.

Espresso combined with chocolate syrup and steamed milk is a mocha. A sugary syrup and seltzer can be added to espresso to make an espresso soda.

Instant Coffee

Instant coffee is prepared coffee in powdered form. You just add hot water to make coffee. Instant coffee powder is made by heat-drying freshly brewed coffee. Freeze-dried coffee is made by freezing and then drying freshly brewed coffee. Freeze-dried coffee is more expensive than coffee powder. Instant and freeze-dried coffees come in jars. Store instant coffee at room temperature in a tightly sealed jar.

You can make instant coffee in the microwave oven. Heat the water in the oven, then add the instant coffee and stir.

Be a *Smart Consumer*

Fair Trade

Much of coffee consumed around the world comes from undeveloped countries, and many of the people who grow and produce it have been unfairly compensated for their product. Fair trade is a consumer trend that seeks to change this. When coffee is certified and labeled Fair Trade, the farmers and workers who grow and produce it get a fair price for their harvest, work in safe and healthy conditions, and earn a decent living wage. They are able to invest in health care, education, environmental conservation and stewardship, and economic independence.

Challenge Research other foods that are part of the fair trade movement, and the pros and cons of fair trade. Write a one-page report on your findings.

Making Coffee

There are many ways to make coffee from ground beans. Most coffee-brewing equipment, including the French press, the percolator, and the stovetop coffeemaker, uses hot water. Espresso machines use hot water under extreme pressure. The cold-brewing technique uses cold water, which is left to sit with ground beans for several hours.

Most Americans use an automatic drip coffeemaker to make coffee. Automatic coffeemakers have four main parts: a water reservoir, a basket that holds a filter and the coffee, a carafe (kə-'raf) that catches the coffee as it brews, and a hot plate that keeps the carafe and coffee warm.

Automatic drip coffeemakers are easy to use. First, put the filter in the coffeemaker basket and place the ground coffee in the filter. Then fill the carafe with the amount of cold water needed and pour the water into the reservoir. Set the carafe in place to catch the coffee, and turn on the controls. You can experiment with the amounts of water and coffee to get the strength you want. Usually 1 to 2 tablespoons are recommended per 6-ounce cup. Coffeemakers usually have convenient markings on the carafe or sides of the reservoir so that you can measure the water easily.

Clean the coffee carafe and basket in hot sudsy water after every use. Coffee contains oils that cling to the inside of the carafe and basket, and they can give the next batch of coffee an unpleasant flavor.

Serving Hot and Cold Coffee

Coffee is best served fresh, right after it is made. Hot coffee should be served piping hot. If held at a high temperature for too long, or reheated, coffee loses it flavor and aroma and may turn bitter. Some people like iced coffee. The coffee is made double strength and poured over ice cubes. Many people enjoy hot and iced coffee with milk, half and half, sweetener, or flavorings such as vanilla or almond.

✓ **Reading Check** **Describe** How do you properly store ground or whole coffee beans?

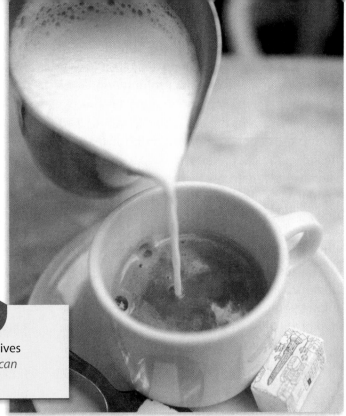

Espresso Drinks

Adding steamed milk and foam to espresso gives you a cappuccino. *What other espresso drinks can you name?*

Tea

Tea is made by soaking the leaves of the tropical tea plant in water. Tea has been used as a beverage in China for centuries. It was not introduced in Europe until the early seventeenth century. Eventually it became the favored beverage among the British. Tea is a popular beverage around the world. Tea is soothing, and studies show that it has health benefits. Tea contains caffeine, although not as much as coffee. It is available decaffeinated.

Buying and Storing Tea

Tea is sold in tea bags and loose leaf. The method of processing determines the tea's appearance and taste.

Black Tea Black tea is made from leaves that are fermented, then heated and dried. This produces a dark brew with a well-developed flavor. Black tea is sometimes flavored with spices, blossoms, or fruits to make different specialty teas.

Green Tea Green tea is made from leaves that are steamed, rolled, and dried but not fermented. This produces a light, greenish-yellow tea with a slightly bitter flavor.

Oolong Tea Oolong tea is made from leaves that are partially fermented. This produces a tea with a color and flavor between those of black and green teas.

Brewing Tea

Tea can be brewed in a pot or in a cup. You can also use an automatic hot tea maker, which works much like an automatic coffeemaker. It preheats the teapot, brews the tea, then holds the tea at serving temperature.

Use a teapot made of ceramic or glass, not metal. Pigments in tea react with metal and give a bitter flavor. They also create a light film over the surface of the tea. As you drink, the film clings to the inside of the cup.

Preheat the teapot or cup by rinsing it out with hot water. Then add 1 teaspoon of tea or one tea bag for each serving. To make loose tea easier to use, put it in an infuser. An infuser is a small container with tiny holes that let water in without allowing the tea leaves to float out into the water. Like tea bags, the infuser is easy to remove at the end of the brewing time. You can make stronger or weaker tea by shortening or lengthening the time you allow the tea to brew.

Brewing Black and Oolong Tea

To make black or oolong tea, heat fresh, cold water in a teakettle to a rolling boil. Pour the boiling water over the tea and let the tea **steep**, or brew, in the hot water for about 3 to 5 minutes, depending on the kind of tea and the strength you prefer. If you like strong tea, use more tea instead of lengthening the steeping time. Tea becomes bitter when it steeps too long.

Brewing Green Tea

The method for making green tea is a little different. The water should be just below the boiling point. Steep green tea for a shorter time than other teas, usually about 1½ minutes. Do not use boiling water or allow the tea to steep longer, because it will turn bitter.

Serving Hot and Cold Tea

Stir tea before pouring or drinking to be sure it is uniformly strong. The color of brewed tea does not always indicate how strong it is. Some varieties have a light color and strong flavor. Others have a dark color and a light flavor. If the brewed tea is too strong, you can add a little hot water. Hot tea is often served with sweetener and milk or lemon. You can make spiced black tea by adding 6 to 8 whole cloves and a cinnamon stick to the teapot when you add the tea.

To make iced tea, brew the tea just like you would for hot tea, but use 50 percent more tea. For example, put 9 teaspoons of tea in the pot to get six servings. After brewing, remove the tea from the pot and pour it over ice, stirring until chilled. Some ice will melt and bring the tea to the correct strength. To prevent the tea from turning cloudy, cool it to room temperature before refrigerating. Adding a little boiling water may remove cloudiness. On a hot summer day, you can make iced tea without boiling water. Place the tea bags and water in a sealable clear glass container and leave it in a place where it will have sunlight for 3 to 5 hours.

Herb Teas

Herb tea is a beverage made from the flowers, leaves, seeds, and roots of herbs and plants other than the tea plant. For example, herb teas may be made from mint, chamomile (ˈka-mə-ˌmī(-ə)l), lemon verbena ((ˌ)vər-ˈbē-nə), valerian, raspberry, or orange peel. Herb teas that are not blended with regular tea are caffeine-free.

To brew herb tea, use 1 tea bag or 1 teaspoon of loose tea for each cup of boiling water. Let steep for no more than 5 minutes. If brewed too long, the tea becomes bitter. Herb tea can be flavored with lemon or honey.

Certain plants used in herb teas can cause allergic reactions for some people. Buy herb teas only from reliable sources. Most supermarkets carry major brands. Avoid teas that make health claims, such as weight loss.

✓ Reading Check **Contrast** What is the difference between black and green tea?

Nutrition Check

Polyphenol Power

Black, green, and oolong teas contain powerful antioxidants called polyphenols that may help keep you healthy and prevent cancer. There are about 8 to 10 times more antioxidants in these types of teas than in fruits and vegetables. Because it is not fermented, green tea contains the most. Scientists suggest drinking 6 cups of tea throughout the day. To limit caffeine consumption, choose decaffeinated teas.

Think About It Scientists believe the high levels of tea consumption in countries like Japan and China have led to lower rates of heart disease and cancer. Write a paragraph explaining why.

Dairy-Based Beverages

Milk provides protein, calcium, phosphorus, and vitamins D and A, making it a wholesome beverage. As a special treat, you can make beverages that combine milk, yogurt, or other dairy products with fruit or flavorings. These beverages are delicious and also contain the nutrients of milk, but they usually have more sugar, fat, and calories.

Smoothies

A **smoothie** is a blend of milk or yogurt and fresh fruit. Smoothies are nutritious and versatile. They are quick and easy to make for a snack or a quick breakfast.

Almost any fruit works in a smoothie. Try combining fruits, such as kiwifruit and melon, or berries and bananas. You can also add foods other than fruit to smoothies, such as peanut butter, wheat germ, or pieces of candied ginger. Ice is sometimes added to smoothies to chill and thicken them, but too much melting ice can dilute the smoothie. Try frozen fruit instead of ice for a thicker mix.

Be careful with serving sizes of smoothies. They are a nutrient-dense beverage, which makes them healthful, but they also can have many calories. Also be sure to check on ingredients added to smoothies you purchase at stores. Avoid consuming smoothies as a meal replacement. Without food in your stomach much of the nutrition in a smoothie can pass through your body before it can be absorbed.

You need a blender to make a smoothie. Small fruits like berries and pitted cherries can be put in the blender whole. Cut larger fruits such as cantaloupe, bananas, and peaches into chunks. Use about 3½ cups of fruit for every cup of liquid.

Pour milk or yogurt into the blender and add the fruit. If you are not using frozen fruit, add a little ice or frozen fruit juice concentrate to chill and thicken the mixture. Blend until the fruit is puréed and the mixture is thick. Serve immediately. Garnish with fruit slices.

Hot Chocolate and Cocoa

Hot chocolate and hot cocoa are the two most popular beverages made with chocolate and milk. Chocolate is a liquid from cacao (kə-ˈkau̇; kə-ˈkā-(ˌ)ō) beans, the seeds from the pods of cacao trees. Chocolate has been popular for centuries. In the 1700s, English chocolate houses, much like coffee houses, provided places to enjoy the beverage.

During the nineteenth century, people learned to separate a fat called **cocoa butter** from the chocolate liquid, leaving solids known as **cocoa powder**. This opened the door to making many chocolate products besides beverages.

Making Hot Chocolate

Hot chocolate is made with solid, unsweetened chocolate. Combine chopped or ground, unsweetened chocolate with milk in a saucepan. Stir it constantly over low heat until the chocolate melts. Add sugar and a pinch of salt and let the mixture simmer for a few minutes without boiling. The cocoa butter found in solid chocolate adds richness to this beverage. You also can heat chocolate syrup with milk.

Making Hot Cocoa

Hot cocoa is made with **cocoa**, a product of cocoa powder. Cocoa has less fat than solid chocolate, so it blends more easily with hot liquid and is less likely to separate. Cocoa comes in unsweetened powder, syrup, and sweetened instant. The powder and syrup forms are mixed with milk. Instant cocoa mixes are combined with milk or water to make hot and cold beverages.

To make hot cocoa, use 1 tablespoon cocoa, 1 tablespoon sugar, and 1 cup of milk for one serving. In a saucepan, mix the cocoa with sugar first for a smooth mixture. Gradually add the milk, stirring well, and cook over low heat. Stir constantly until bubbles appear at the sides, but do not boil. You can use a double boiler to prevent scorching. A lighter version of hot chocolate can be made by combining ground chocolate with steamed milk.

Storing and Serving Cocoa and Chocolate

Cocoa and chocolate should be stored in a cool, dry place in original containers. Cocoa usually keeps better than chocolate. If stored in a hot or humid area, chocolate may develop a bloom. **Bloom** is patches of white caused by cocoa butter that has come to the surface. Bloom also can be caused by the crystallization of sugar. This happens when moisture from humidity accumulates on the surface of the chocolate and reacts with the surface sugars. Bloom does not damage chocolate's flavor.

Chocolate beverages may be served plain or topped with marshmallows, whipped cream, or ground nutmeg. You can also add flavor by stirring with a cinnamon stick. To make mocha, add one ounce of brewed espresso to the chocolate and milk.

Heating Dairy Beverages in the Microwave Oven

Always stir beverages before placing in the oven. When a beverage such as hot cocoa stands for even a short time, it develops a very smooth surface that acts almost like a film or skin. When you stir it, you break up the film. If you heat a beverage without stirring it, the smooth surface could keep steam from escaping and allow it to build up, causing the beverage to spurt out of the container.

✓ **Reading Check** **List** What are three serving ideas for chocolate beverages?

Soft Drinks and Punch

Soft drinks are sweet, carbonated beverages. Soft drinks have few nutrients, if any, and are best consumed sparingly.

Flavored soft drinks are made with water and additives that may include artificial flavorings and colorings, sweeteners, acidifiers for tartness, and sodium. Diet soft drinks are made with sugar substitutes. Cola beverages contain caffeine.

Club soda is carbonated water with added salts and minerals. Seltzer water is carbonated water with no added salts.

Punch

A **punch** is a mixture of fruit juices and tea or a carbonated beverage such as ginger ale or seltzer water. Sherbet, ice cream, or fruit may also be added.

If you are serving punch cold, combine all liquids except the carbonated beverage ahead of time and chill well. Chill the unopened carbonated beverage separately and add just before serving the punch. If added too early, the carbonation is lost.

Punch may also be **mulled**, or served hot and flavored with such spices as cinnamon, nutmeg, or cloves. This is a delicious way to serve cider.

Light and Healthy Recipe

Cranberry Club Soda

In addition to the antioxidants found in the cranberry juice, this refreshing drink has no added sugar.

Ingredients

- **6 oz.** Cranberry juice
- **3 oz.** Orange juice
- **1 oz.** Lime juice
- **12 oz.** Club soda

Directions

1. Pour juices into a large pitcher and stir.
2. Pour the club soda into the juice and stir gently to combine.
3. Serve in glasses over ice.

Yield 4 servings

Nutrition Analysis per Serving

■ Calories	38
■ Total fat	0 g
Saturated fat	0 g
Cholesterol	0 mg
■ Sodium	20 mg
■ Carbohydrate	10 mg
Dietary fiber	0 g
Sugars	9 g
■ Protein	0 g

CHAPTER 37 Review & Applications

After You Read

Chapter Summary

A variety of beverages is available. Water is a healthful beverage and is available bottled or from the tap. Juices are made from fruits and vegetables. Juices and juice drinks can be bought or made at home. Coffee can be bought in many forms and should be stored properly to maintain freshness. Tea comes from a tropical plant, is sold in various forms, and may be brewed and served in different ways. Dairy-based beverages include smoothies, hot chocolate, and hot cocoa. Soft drinks are sweet, carbonated beverages best consumed sparingly. Punch is a mixture of fruit juices and other ingredients.

Content and Academic Vocabulary Review

1. Use each of these content and academic vocabulary words in a sentence.

Content Vocabulary

- ☐ carbonated (p. 578)
- ☐ juice (p. 578)
- ☐ juice drink (p. 579)
- ☐ fruit-flavored drink (p. 579)
- ☐ coffee bean (p. 580)
- ☐ caffeine (p. 580)
- ☐ decaffeinated (p. 580)
- ☐ tea (p. 583)
- ☐ steep (p. 584)
- ☐ herb tea (p. 584)
- ☐ smoothie (p. 585)
- ☐ cocoa butter (p. 585)
- ☐ cocoa powder (p. 585)
- ☐ cocoa (p. 585)
- ☐ bloom (p. 585)
- ☐ punch (p. 586)
- ☐ mulled (p. 586)

Academic Vocabulary

- contaminate (p. 578)
- originated (p. 580)

Review Key Concepts

2. **Identify** and describe types of bottled waters.
3. **List** and describe beverages made with juice.
4. **Describe** two types of coffee beans.
5. **Explain** how to brew black, oolong, and green tea.
6. **Describe** the difference between hot chocolate and hot cocoa.
7. **Define** and describe soft drinks and punch.

Critical Thinking

8. **List** the beverages discussed in this chapter in order of healthfulness. Then write a paragraph explaining your rationale for how you ranked your list.
9. **Explain** why cocoa, coffee, and tea have remained popular beverages throughout history.
10. **Predict** whether soft drinks will remain popular in future centuries the way other beverages have. Explain your reasoning.

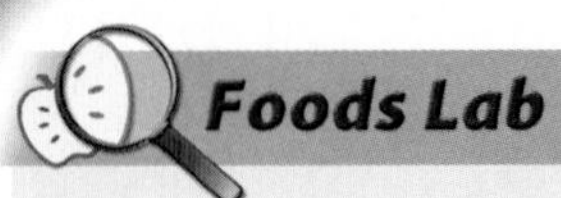

Foods Lab

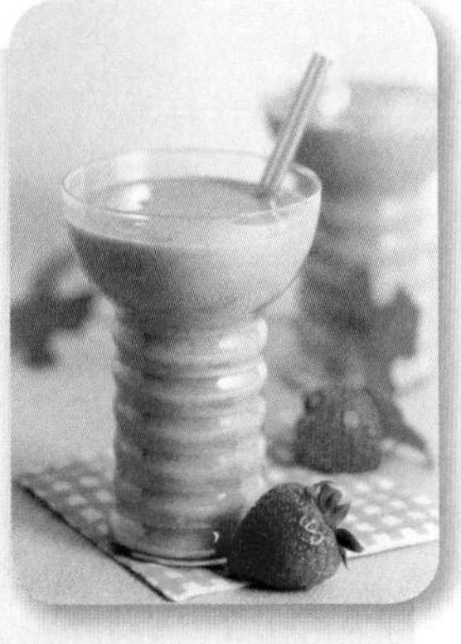

11. Smoothie Recipe Smoothies are satisfying dairy-based beverages that allow room for creativity. Many different ingredients can be combined.

Procedure Develop a recipe for a smoothie. Think of creative ways to add flavor and nutrition. Prepare your smoothie. Offer samples for a taste test and sample the recipes made by different lab groups.

Analysis Create a chart that rates all the smoothie samples, including your own, on appearance, texture, and taste. After tasting other teams' recipes, determine what ingredients you would add to your own. List the ingredients on your chart.

HEALTHFUL CHOICES

12. Fruity Beverages On the juice aisle at the supermarket, Carly examined her options. She could buy a beverage called "Citrus Delight" that contained water, sugar, and orange flavoring but no juice, "Orange Juice," or a "Citrus Cocktail" that contained 40 percent orange juice with water, sugar, and other juice flavorings. Which is the most healthful option and why? What would be the next-best choice? What are the key points to remember about items sold on the juice aisle?

TECH Connection

13. Punch Tasting Under your teacher's supervision, use the Internet to find an appealing punch recipe. Prepare it and serve it to the class. Use word processing software to create evaluation forms for students to fill out after tasting the punch. The forms should have students rate the punch in five categories of your choosing.

Real-World Skills

Problem-Solving Skills	**14. Cutting Out Caffeine** Haley's doctor says she should limit caffeine consumption during her pregnancy because studies have linked it to low birth weight. Haley does not want to lose the health benefits of her regular cups of antioxidant-rich black tea. What can she do?
Interpersonal and Collaborative Skills	**15. High Tea** Follow your teacher's instructions to form groups. Together, research afternoon tea, a tradition that is enjoyed in England. Then have a high tea in the foods lab. How will the tea be prepared and served? What foods will be served with the tea?
Financial Literacy Skills	**16. Cost and Quality** Visit a supermarket. Compare and note the cost per ounce and nutritional quality of six different specific beverages. Include a bottled water, a juice or juice drink, a coffee beverage, a tea drink, a dairy beverage, and a soft drink. Report your findings to the class and make recommendations regarding value and healthfulness.

Academic Skills

Food Science

17. Ginger Ale Fermentation occurs when yeast consumes sugar. It is used to carbonate beverages like soda.

Procedure Pour 1 cup sugar and ¼ teaspoon active dry yeast into a 2 liter plastic bottle through a funnel. Add 2 tablespoons of fresh grated ginger and the juice of 1 lemon. Add water to rinse the funnel until the water comes within an inch of the bottle top. Screw on cap to seal, and shake to dissolve the sugar. Place in a warm location for 24–48 hours, then refrigerate overnight. Open slowly, strain, and enjoy.

Analysis What might happen if you didn't open the bottle slowly?

NCSS B Develop an understanding of chemical reactions.

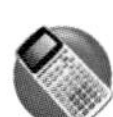

Mathematics

18. Comparing Juice Prices Renee can buy a 64-fluid-ounce carton of orange juice at the grocery store for $3.75, or a 16-fluid-ounce bottle of fresh-squeezed orange juice for $1.99. She can also buy a 12-ounce can of frozen orange juice concentrate for $2.15. If a can of orange juice concentrate makes 48 fl. oz. of juice, which type of juice is cheapest per ounce? How much would a glass of that juice cost?

Math Concept **Calculate Unit Price**

Calculate unit price by dividing the price of an item by the quantity.

Starting Hint Calculate the unit price (price per ounce) of the three containers of orange juice by dividing price by the number of ounces of juice in the container.

NCTM Number and Operations Compute fluently and make reasonable estimates.

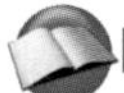

English Language Arts

19. School Beverage Options Conduct research to learn about laws regarding soft drinks sold on school campuses. Then, write a one-page evaluation of the beverage options offered at your school. Are they healthful? Is there room for improvement? Are you satisfied with the choices, their cost, and quality? Why or why not? Make suggestions for changes or substitutions, or explain why changes are not necessary.

NCTE 4 Use written language to communicate effectively.

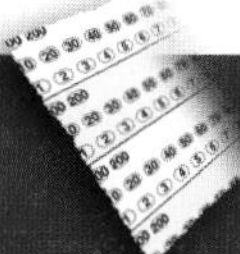

STANDARDIZED TEST PRACTICE

ANALOGY

Read the pairs of terms. Then choose the best term to match.

20. oolong : tea
Arabica: coffee
enhanced water: bottled water
club soda: ___________

a. soft drink
b. carbonated drink
c. punch
d. mineral water

Test-Taking Tip Analogies establish relationships between terms. When you look at the three pairs of terms listed here, identify the relationship that is common to all of them. Then try matching each possible answer with the term club soda. The one that establishes the same type of relationship shared by the other terms is correct.

UNIT 7

Thematic Project

Plan and Prepare a Healthy Meal

Preparing fresh, healthy food from scratch takes planning and practice. In this project you will practice your food-preparation skills by creating and cooking a healthy meal using at least three different preparation methods.

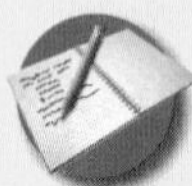

My Journal

If you completed the journal entry from page 429, refer to it to see if your thoughts have changed after reading the unit and completing this project.

Project Assignment

- Create a menu for a low-fat, nutritious breakfast, lunch, or dinner based on fresh, minimally processed ingredients.
- Work with a trusted adult to review and refine your menu and to create a shopping list.
- At the market, select the ingredients for your menu using the food-selection guidelines presented in the unit.

Academic Skills You Will Use

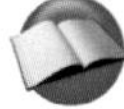

English Language Arts

NCTE 7 Conduct research and gather, evaluate, and synthesize data from a variety of sources to communicate discoveries.

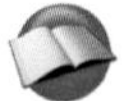

Mathematics

NCTM Measurement Apply appropriate techniques, tools, and formulas to determine measurements.

- Cook your meal using the preparation methods described in the unit and, if possible, photograph various steps of the preparation and cooking process.
- Create a visual presentation that documents what you learned in creating and preparing your meal, and share it with the class.

STEP 1 Plan a Menu

Plan a complete breakfast, lunch, or dinner for two that includes a grain dish, a vegetable or fruit dish, and a protein dish based on dairy, eggs, meat, poultry, or tofu.

- Find recipes using print and Internet resources. Choose recipes with ingredients available in your community.
- Make sure that your meal features at least three different food preparation methods.
- Write a one-page summary of your menu. Name and describe each dish, explain why you chose the dishes, and summarize the food preparation methods you will use.

Writing Skills

- Use complete sentences.
- Use correct spelling and grammar.
- Use a separate paragraph for each idea.
- Write concisely (briefly but completely).

STEP 2 Select Ingredients

Create a shopping list. List alternates (backup options) for ingredients that might be costly or unavailable. Use the guidelines in the unit to select fresh and healthful products.

- Look for fruits and vegetables that are ripe, colorful, and fresh.
- Select whole-grain products rather than products made from refined or processed grains.
- Choose protein foods that are fresh, with no odor. Check the grade marks and sell-by dates.

STEP 3 Connect to Your Community

Work with a friend, mentor, family member, or other adult member of your community to prepare and serve the meal you have planned. Take photographs of each step of your preparations. Eat your meal with your guest. Ask your guest for his or her opinion. Were the foods properly prepared? Did the flavors work well together? Note what you did well and what you would do differently next time.

Food-Preparation Skills

- Follow knife safety rules.
- Handle foods carefully to avoid cross-contamination.
- Test for doneness.

STEP 4 Create Your Presentation

Use the Unit Thematic Project Checklist to plan and complete your project.

STEP 5 Evaluate Your Presentation

Your project will be evaluated based on:

- Thought devoted to planning the menu and choosing recipes.
- Content and organization of your presentation.
- Mechanics—presentation and neatness.

Unit Thematic Project Checklist

Category	Objectives
Plan	☑ Plan a menu and create a list of ingredients.
	☑ Create your menu with an adult community member.
	☑ Make a computer slideshow that documents the process of planning and preparing your menu.
	☑ Organize your slideshow into four parts: planning, selecting, preparing, and lessons learned.
	☑ Include photographs documenting each step of your project.
Present	☑ Make a presentation to the class to share your visual and discuss what you learned.
	☑ Turn in the one-page summary of the menu that you wrote in Step 1 and your electronic presentation to your teacher.
Academic Skills	☑ Organize your presentation so the audience can follow along easily.
	☑ Speak clearly and concisely.
	☑ Thoughtfully express your ideas.

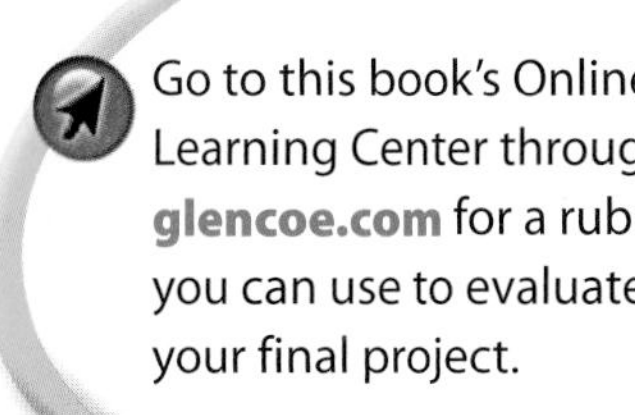

Go to this book's Online Learning Center through **glencoe.com** for a rubric you can use to evaluate your final project.

UNIT 8

Food Combinations

Activate Prior Knowledge

Explore the Photo Individual foods can be combined to make many interesting and tasty dishes. *What is your favorite combination food?*

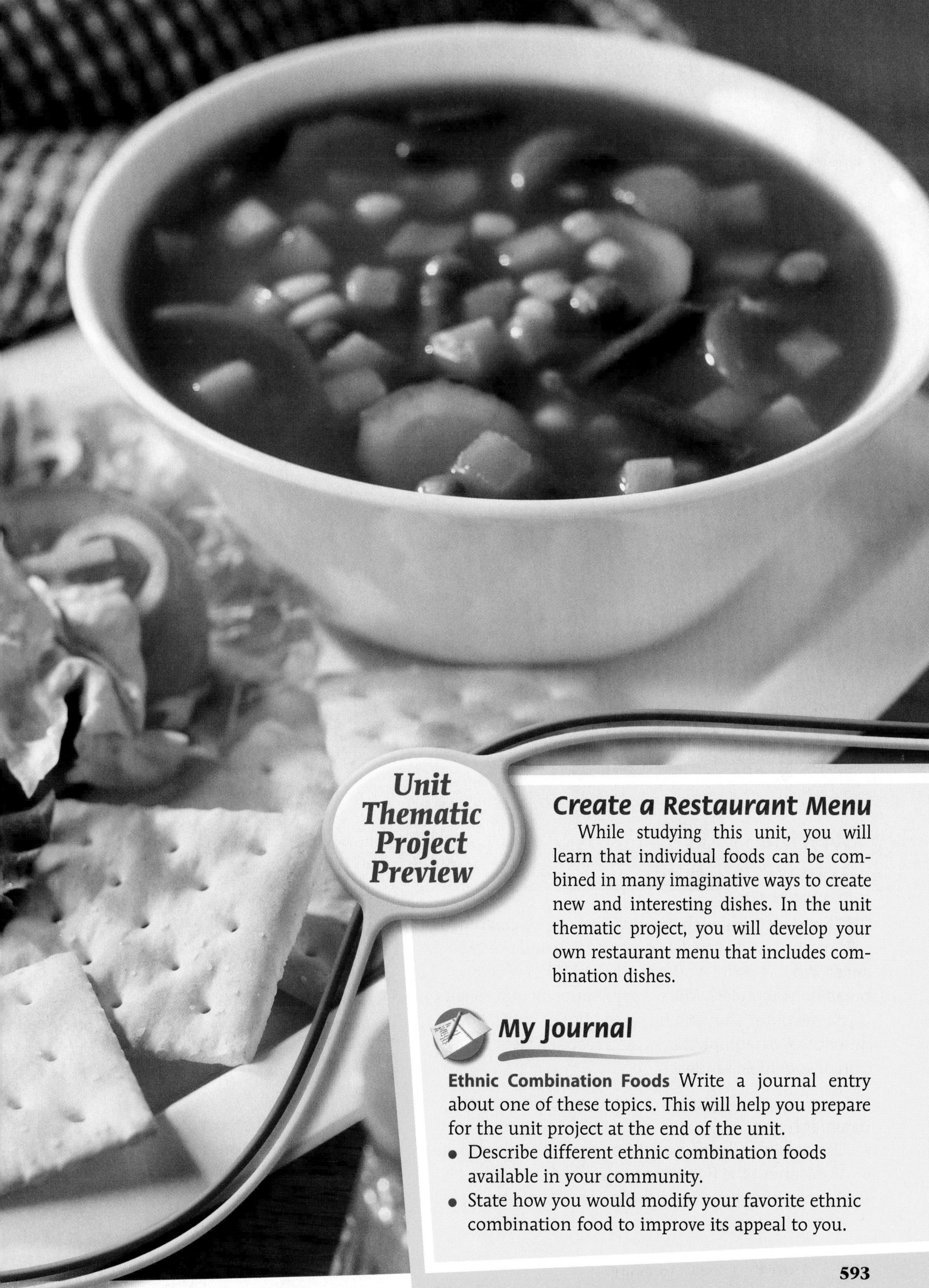

Unit Thematic Project Preview

Create a Restaurant Menu

While studying this unit, you will learn that individual foods can be combined in many imaginative ways to create new and interesting dishes. In the unit thematic project, you will develop your own restaurant menu that includes combination dishes.

My Journal

Ethnic Combination Foods Write a journal entry about one of these topics. This will help you prepare for the unit project at the end of the unit.

- Describe different ethnic combination foods available in your community.
- State how you would modify your favorite ethnic combination food to improve its appeal to you.

CHAPTER 38

Sandwiches & Pizza

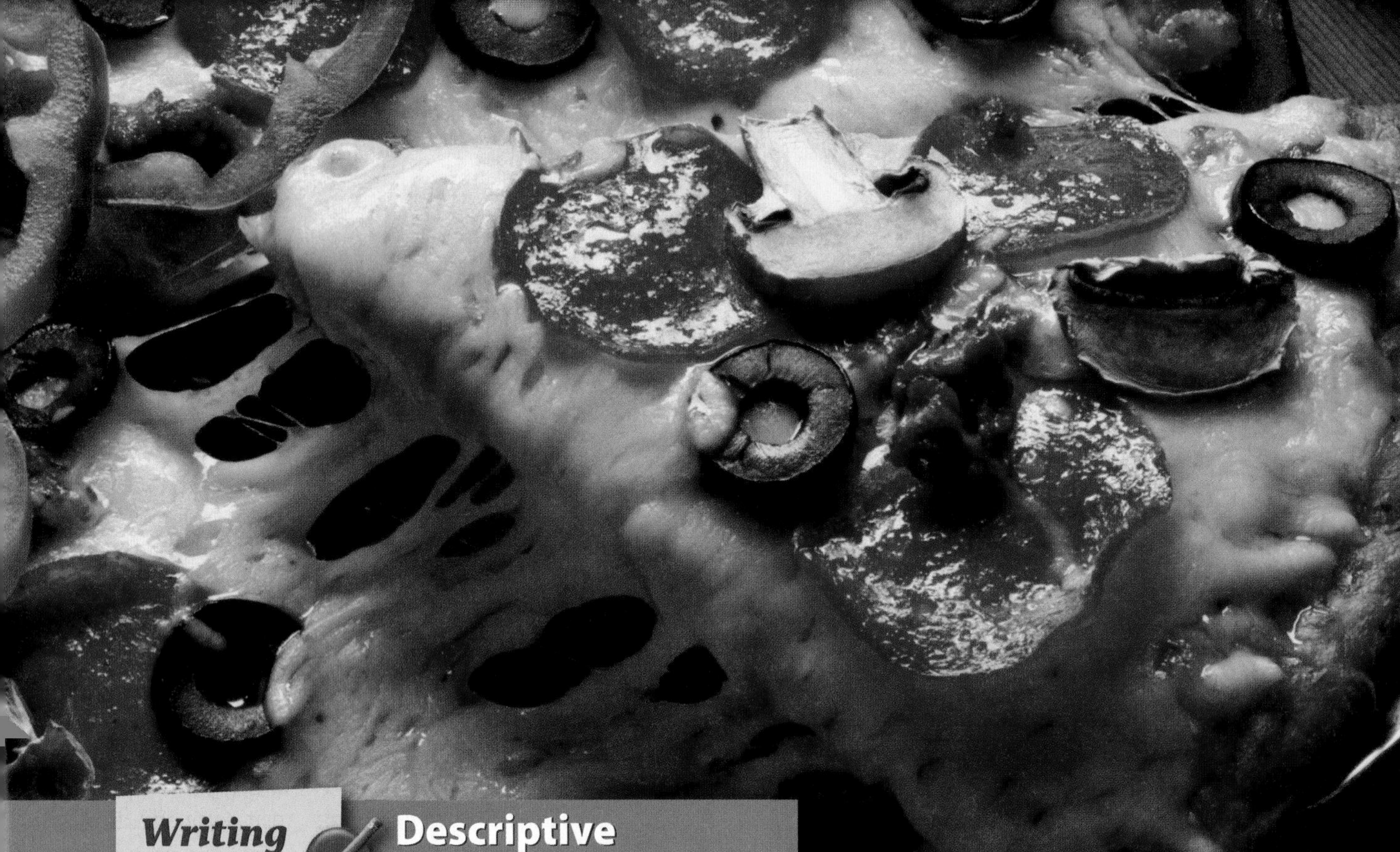

Writing Activity — Descriptive Paragraph

The Ideal Sandwich Sandwiches can be custom made to suit virtually anyone's taste and preferences. What is your favorite sandwich? What type of bread do you prefer? Which combination of ingredients is your favorite? Should it be served hot or cold? Write a descriptive paragraph that gives a reader a clear impression of your ideal sandwich.

Writing Tips Follow these steps to write a descriptive paragraph.

- Use details and adjectives to bring your subject to life.
- Think about the five senses as you write.
- Be specific in your word choices, and avoid being too general or vague.

Activate Prior Knowledge

Global Favorite Sandwiches and pizza combine food groups. *Why are sandwiches so versatile?*

Reading Guide

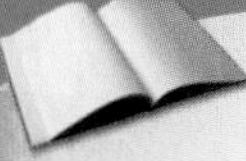

Before You Read

Preview Skim through the chapter. Think about how sandwiches come in many shapes, sizes, forms, and flavors.

Read to Learn

Key Concepts

- **List** three different types of sandwiches and describe how to make them.
- **Describe** how to make pizzas and calzone.

Main Idea

Sandwiches come in many forms. They can be made with a variety of ingredients to suit many different tastes.

Content Vocabulary

You will find definitions for these words in the glossary at the back of this book.

- ☐ sandwich
- ☐ basic sandwich
- ☐ club sandwich
- ☐ open-face sandwich
- ☐ hero
- ☐ wraps
- ☐ pita
- ☐ falafel
- ☐ gyro
- ☐ lavash
- ☐ tortilla
- ☐ fajitas
- ☐ guacamole
- ☐ foccacia
- ☐ tea sandwich
- ☐ pizza
- ☐ calzone

Academic Vocabulary

You will find these words in your reading and on your tests. Use the glossary to look up their definitions if necessary.

- elaborate
- substantial

Graphic Organizer

As you read, take notes about the seven types of sandwiches described in this chapter.

TYPES OF SANDWICHES
1.
2.
3.
4.
5.
6.
7.

Graphic Organizer Go to this book's Online Learning Center at **glencoe.com** to print out this graphic organizer.

Academic Standards

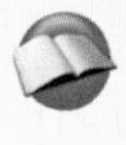

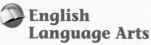

English Language Arts

NCTE 8 Use information resources to gather information and create and communicate knowledge.

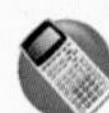

Mathematics

NCTM Geometry Use visualization, spatial reasoning, and geometric modeling to solve problems.

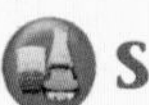

Science

NSES F Develop understanding of personal and community health.

NSES C Develop an understanding of behavior of organisms.

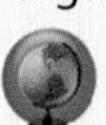

Social Studies

NCSS VII B Production, Distribution, and Consumption Analyze the role that supply and demand, prices, incentives, and profits play in determining what is produced and distributed in a competitive market system.

NCTE *National Council of Teachers of English*
NCTM *National Council of Teachers of Mathematics*
NSES *National Science Education Standards*
NCSS *National Council for the Social Studies*

Types of Sandwiches

A **sandwich** is filling between slices of bread. Sandwiches come in countless forms, and from cultures all over the world. A sandwich can be a simple combination, easy to prepare and ideal for packed lunches and picnics. A sandwich can also be an **elaborate**, or ornate, main dish prepared in an oven and eaten with a knife and fork.

The sandwich takes its name from an 18th-century English lord, John Montagu, the Earl of Sandwich. The popular story is that Montagu frequently played cards for hours and would continue playing through dinner aided by a slice of meat between two pieces of bread. More likely, Montagu frequently worked through dinner because of commitments to the navy, politics, and arts.

Basic Sandwiches

The **basic sandwich** is two slices of bread with a filling in between. It is always served cold. The bread in a basic sandwich is often coated with a fat-based spread, such as butter, margarine, mayonnaise, or cream cheese. The fat adds flavor, helps hold the filling in place, and keeps moist fillings from soaking into the bread.

Here are the steps in making a basic sandwich:

1. Choose bread. Start with firm bread that is easy to cut, handle, and eat. Options include whole wheat, multigrain, rye, and sourdough. You can also use hard rolls, bagels, English muffins, or sandwich buns and rolls. Soft breads can be toasted first to add body.

2. Add filling. Put filling on one slice of bread. You can use almost any filling for sandwiches, including cold cuts, cheese, tuna, shrimp, chicken, egg salad, vegetables, baked tofu, and leftovers. You can use a firm filling or a soft filling. Firm fillings work best with soft breads. To make cutting and eating neater, use several thin slices of meat or cheese rather than one thick slice. Spread soft filling carefully to avoid squashing the bread. Spread soft, chunky fillings like egg salad or tuna or chicken salad thinly just to the edge of the bread to keep them from oozing out. Top fillings with tomato and lettuce.

3. Add spread. Apply spread to the other piece of bread. If you plan to use butter, margarine, or cream cheese, soften it to room temperature for easier spreading. You can also use whipped varieties of butter that spread easily.

4. Cut. Use a sharp, serrated knife to cut sandwiches without smashing or tearing the bread or the filling.

5. Add condiments. Wait until just before serving to add condiments, such as mustard, just before eating. Condiments can make the bread soggy if they sit on the bread too long.

Science in Action

Lunch Meat Preservatives

Lunch meats—such as sausages and molded loafs of meat that are sliced and served cold—are a common filling for sandwiches. Chemical preservatives are added to these meats to prevent bacteria from growing, and sometimes to alter their color. One such preservative is sodium nitrite, a chemical that is protective against harmful bacteria, but can also be toxic to mammals.

Procedure Research health dangers associated with sodium nitrite. What effects can this chemical preservative have on human health? Are lunch meats without preservatives available? Are there safer preservatives that can be used in meats instead of sodium nitrite?

Analysis After researching the answers to the questions above, write your findings in note form. Then share them with the class.

NSES F Develop understanding of personal and community health.

Club Sandwiches

A **club sandwich** is an expanded basic sandwich made with three slices of toasted bread and two layers of different fillings. The classic club has mayonnaise, lettuce, tomato, bacon, and turkey, but you can mix and match ingredients to suit your taste. For example, ham, mustard, and Swiss cheese could be one layer, with sliced roast chicken and tomatoes as the next.

To keep the layers stacked while cutting, secure them with four wooden picks placed in the four corners about an inch from the crust. Cut the sandwich in halves or quarters. Cutting diagonally provides triangular sections. Place the picks accordingly. For a garnish, spear olives or thickly sliced pickle onto the wooden picks.

Open-Face Sandwiches

An **open-face sandwich** has just one slice of bread and a topping. Most any filling can be used, but the bread should be firm enough to support it. Try an open-face sandwich if you like more filling than bread. If you like melted cheese, try topping an open-face sandwich with cheese and melting it in the microwave or toaster oven.

Heroes

A **hero** is a very large sandwich made on a loaf of Italian or French bread or a large hard roll. The sandwich is layered with an assortment of thinly sliced, cooked and cured meats and cheeses with vegetables like onions, lettuce, and tomatoes. The spread is usually mayonnaise or salad dressing. Heroes have different names and recipes in different places. They can be called hoagies, subs, grinders, poor boys, or muffulettas. Meatballs are a popular filling in some places. In others, you might find corned beef and pastrami or fried shrimp.

Unlike the basic sandwich, some heroes improve with "aging." Wrap the hero tightly in foil or plastic and refrigerate for up to four hours to let the flavors blend.

Wraps

Breads do not need to be thick and spongy to hold a filling. In fact, the world's oldest and most popular breads are flat. Sandwiches made by wrapping or rolling a filling in flatbread are called **wraps** or rollups. Wraps are popular around the world, from the Mediterranean to Mexico. Many interesting breads and fillings from world cuisines are available in the United States.

Pita

Pita is a round, leavened flatbread from the Middle East that can be used to make a rollup. Pita forms a pocket when split, so it is also called pocket bread. Pita comes in different sizes and types, including whole wheat.

To make a rollup, spread filling down the center of a pita or over the entire bread, leaving about 1 inch free around the edges. Fold one side partially over the filling and roll the other side over to close the pita. For easier and neater handling, wrap the roll in foil. Peel back the foil as you eat the sandwich.

To use the pocket, cut the pita in half. Gently pull apart the two sides at the cut end to form a pocket. This method makes two sandwiches. You can also slit a whole pita along the seam to make one large pocket.

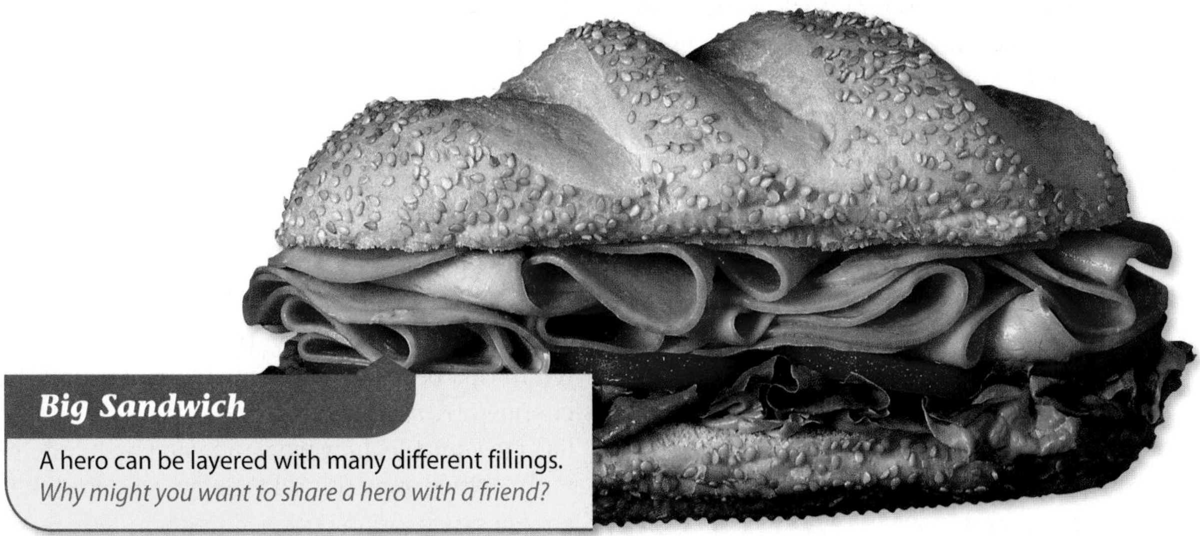

Big Sandwich

A hero can be layered with many different fillings. *Why might you want to share a hero with a friend?*

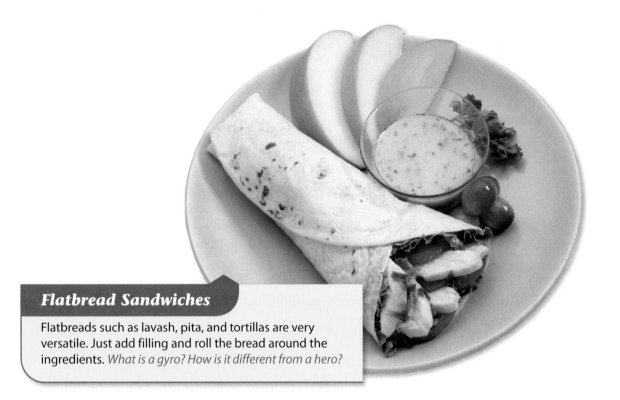

Flatbread Sandwiches

Flatbreads such as lavash, pita, and tortillas are very versatile. Just add filling and roll the bread around the ingredients. *What is a gyro? How is it different from a hero?*

Falafel A favorite Middle Eastern filling for pita is **falafel** (fə-ˈlä-fəl), small, deep-fried patties made with highly seasoned, ground garbanzo beans. Several falafel are placed in each pocket, along with pickled vegetables and hummus, a spread made with mashed, cooked garbanzo beans and ground sesame seeds. You can also fill pita bread with shredded cheese and chopped vegetable salad with ingredients such as fresh mint, tomatoes, bell pepper, radishes, onion, celery, and lettuce. Yogurt makes a tasty dressing.

Gyros Pita bread is also used to make gyros. A **gyro** (ˈyē-ˌrō) is a Greek specialty made with slices of minced roasted lamb that is molded around a spit and vertically roasted, grilled onions, sweet peppers, and a cucumber-yogurt sauce, all wrapped in a pita.

Lavash

Lavash (lä-ˈvȯsh) is an Armenian flatbread that is larger and thinner than pita. Lavash is available crisp or soft and in various flavors, such as spinach or red pepper. The soft version is used for wraps and pockets. Lavash does not have its own pocket, so you spread on the filling and then fold the bottom up and the sides over.

Tortilla

A **tortilla** (tȯr-ˈtē-yə) is a thin, round, unleavened flatbread made with either corn or wheat flour and baked on a griddle. It is a staple in Mexican and Central American cooking.

Tortillas are traditionally made by grinding corn that has been cured in lime juice and water. The curing separates the skin from the corn kernel. The ground corn is precooked then kneaded into a dough that is pressed flat into thin patties and cooked on a very hot griddle. Wheat tortillas are common in the Northwest of Mexico.

Like pita bread, tortillas are the base for several different sandwiches. A large tortilla rolled around a filling is called a burrito. Folded in half, a tortilla forms a soft-shell taco. For a crisper wrap, heat the tortilla for a few minutes in a 400°F oven before filling. You can also deep-fry tortillas briefly and fold them immediately so they hold their shape, or you can buy taco shells ready to use.

In the traditional style, tortillas are filled with combinations of chopped, cooked meat or poultry, refried beans, sour cream, shredded cheese, chopped lettuce and tomatoes, and salsa. Tortillas are versatile, however, and you can fill them with peanut butter and honey, spinach and cheese sauce, or any other filling you like.

Tortillas are also served as fajitas. **Fajitas** (fə-ˈhē-təs) are grilled meat, poultry, fish, or vegetables rolled up in a warm tortilla. They are generally served with other foods such as refried beans, salsa, and **guacamole** (ˌgwä-kə-ˈmō-lē), a Mexican condiment made with mashed avocados, lemon or lime juice, and seasonings.

Tortillas also can be crushed or ground and used as a thickener in soups and sauces. Tortilla soup gets its name from the tortillas used to thicken it.

Spanish Tortilla In Spain and South America, the word *tortilla* has a different meaning. It is not a bread at all, but an unfolded egg omelet, usually made with potatoes and onions.

Hot Sandwiches

You can turn almost any sandwich into a hot sandwich by warming it in a conventional oven, microwave oven, or toaster oven. You can also press the sandwich in a sandwich maker or waffle maker brushed with oil or sprayed with cooking spray. Thick, crusty pieces of bread work well for pressed sandwiches also known as panini. To keep any fresh vegetables or fruits from wilting on the sandwich, add them after heating.

When you microwave a sandwich, wrap it in a paper towel first. The towel absorbs extra moisture. Thirty seconds or less on high power is usually enough.

Cooking is part of the recipe for some sandwiches. In some hot sandwiches, only the filling is hot. A Reuben sandwich is made by heating thin slices of pastrami with Swiss cheese and placing them between two slices of toasted rye bread. In other hot sandwiches, the whole sandwich is grilled.

Careers in Food

Jamee Green
Executive Director

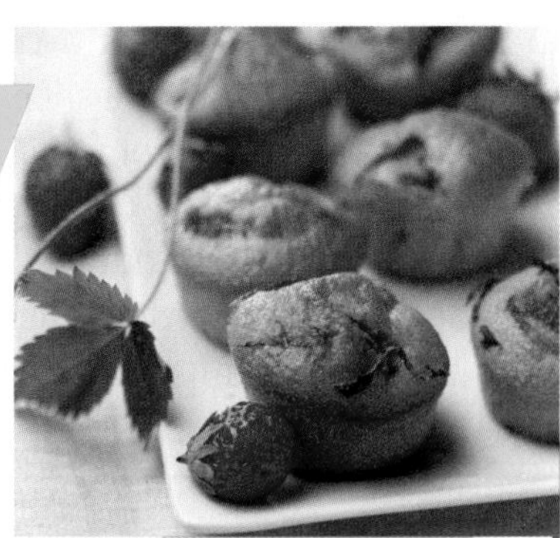

Q: What is the purpose of the Greater Dallas Restaurant Association?

A: The association tries to help growth in the industry by providing educational programs and public awareness campaigns. We're committed to the long-term health of the restaurant industry.

Q: How did you become an executive director?

A: I have worked for six years in management, and four as a lobbyist. I was chosen for my experience working with a board of directors, local media, and different branches of government.

Q: What's your typical day like?

A: I start by holding meetings with members, potential members, members of the media, or elected officials. I spend time returning e-mail and reading industry news and blogs. Afternoons are spent working with staff on related projects.

"The focus is to raise funds for supporting the future of our industry."

— Jamee Green
Greater Dallas Restaurant Association – Dallas, *TX*

Education and Training

An undergraduate degree and a master's degree in marketing are important. When earning degrees it is important to build discipline and skills for success. Experience working with related organizations and understanding of political processes are also important.

Qualities and Skills

Understanding the business and the issues that affect it, the ability to interact with the media, negotiation skills, communication skills, multi-tasking skills and the ability to work within a specific financial budget are all valuable qualities and skills.

Related Career Opportunities

Community Relations Director, Director of Development, or political lobbyist are related occupations.

Sloppy Joe

Ground beef or turkey cooked in chili sauce, ketchup, and Worcestershire sauce makes an appetizing, hot open-face sandwich. *What other hot sandwiches have you eaten?*

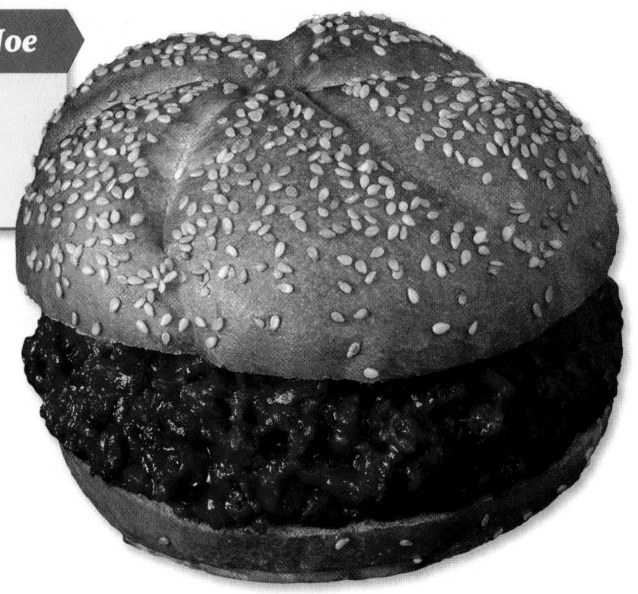

Sandwiches with Cooked Fillings

Sandwiches such as hamburgers, hot dogs, and Sloppy Joes have cooked fillings. The bread or buns may be uncooked or heated in the oven or on the grill.

Hamburgers The traditional hamburger is a ground beef patty seasoned with salt and pepper. Ground poultry is also used. Veggie burgers use grains and vegetables instead of meat. To cook a meat patty by broiling or grilling, make it at least 1 inch thick. Make it thinner to pan-broil or sauté. For a cheeseburger, top the cooked patty with the sliced cheese of your choice and remove from the heat when the cheese starts to melt.

You can serve hamburgers on a bun or roll and top them with a wide range of condiments, such as ketchup, mustard, pickles, sauerkraut, salsa, or chutney. Chutney is a sauce from India made with fruits, sugar, vinegar, and spices.

Nutrition Check

As Healthful As You Make It

A sandwich is as nutritious as the foods that go into it. Read Nutrition Facts panels and ingredient lists to compare the fat, sodium, and sugar content of different bread and filling choices. If a spread is high in fat and calories, balance it with a low-fat filling. Look for fresh foods with less processing, including whole-wheat and multigrain breads.

How does one of your favorite sandwiches fare nutritionally?

Think About It Kevin makes a hamburger using ground beef that contains 30 percent fat. What are some low-fat toppings and spreads he can use to keep the overall fat content of this sandwich low?

Hot Dogs Hot dogs are sold precooked, but they should be heated until steaming for safety. You can add a variety of condiments to hot dogs, just as with hamburgers. Hot dogs topped with chili and cheese are called chili dogs.

Barbecue Sandwiches In a barbecue sandwich, flavor comes in liquid form. Shredded pork or sliced roast beef is heated in a tangy, tomato-based sauce that is seasoned with onions and garlic and sweetened with brown sugar or molasses. For a Sloppy Joe, ground beef is cooked loose-style with chopped onions, chili sauce, ketchup, Worcestershire sauce, and various spices, according to the cook's tastes. The mixture is "slopped" over a split bun. These and other **substantial**, or filling, hot sandwiches may be served open-face and eaten with a knife and fork—and plenty of napkins.

Vegetarian Hot Sandwiches Meat is not the only hot filling for sandwiches. Scrambled eggs on toast or an English muffin is a natural pairing. You can pan-broil patties made of cooked, mashed beans or lentils. Add egg, breadcrumbs, cooked grains, ground nuts, or peanut butter for flavor, body, and nutrition. Explore the increasing variety of frozen soy burgers on the market, or invent your own from textured vegetable protein (TVP). Try a barbecue sandwich with crumbled tofu.

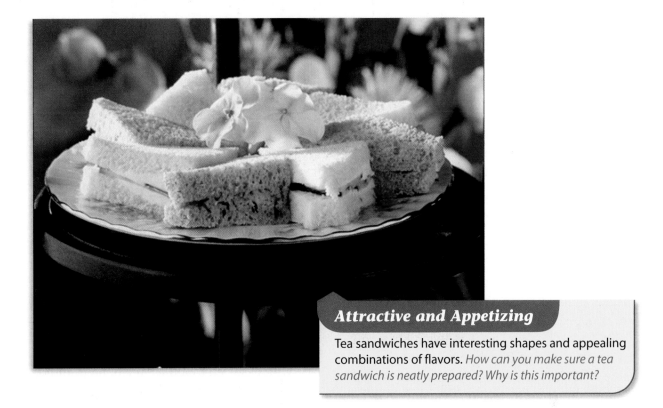

Attractive and Appetizing

Tea sandwiches have interesting shapes and appealing combinations of flavors. *How can you make sure a tea sandwich is neatly prepared? Why is this important?*

Grilled Sandwiches

A true grilled sandwich is made by sautéing filled bread. Some sandwiches have grilled fillings on ungrilled bread.

To make a grilled sandwich, spread both slices of bread on the outside with softened butter or margarine, or melt a little butter or margarine in a heavy skillet. Assemble the sandwich and sauté on both sides until nicely browned. If the filling includes cheese, sauté until the cheese is just melted. Cut the sandwich in half for easier eating.

To keep butter off your hands and the cutting board, you can carefully build the sandwich right in the skillet. Put one slice of bread in the skillet, buttered side down. Add the filling, top with the other slice, buttered side up, and grill.

Grilled cheese is one of the most popular grilled sandwiches. Add sliced tomatoes, crisp cooked bacon, or thinly sliced ham before cooking to make a heartier dish. A Reuben sandwich is a stack of thinly sliced corned beef, sauerkraut, and sliced Swiss cheese pressed between rye bread spread with Russian or Thousand Island dressing.

Broiled Sandwiches

Many sandwiches that can be grilled can also be broiled. Place the sandwich on the broiler pan and brush the outside of the bread with oil or melted butter or margarine. Broil it until lightly browned. Turn the sandwich over and repeat with the other side, or sprinkle the second side with grated cheese and broil it until the cheese melts.

Open-face sandwiches called melts are also made in the broiler. Top the filling with sliced or shredded cheese to keep it from drying out. Broil just long enough to melt the cheese. If you want any ingredients to stay crisp, add them afterward. You can make a tuna melt, tomato melt, and even a peanut butter melt. For variety, build a broiled sandwich on **focaccia** (fō-ˈkä-ch(-ē)ə), a round, herbed, Italian bread that is brushed with olive oil and sometimes topped with herbs.

Tea Sandwiches

A **tea sandwich**, also called a finger sandwich, is a small, attractive, cold type of sandwich often served at receptions and parties.

In tea sandwiches, appearance means as much as taste. Allow six to eight sandwiches per guest, depending on what else will be served. Show your creativity in choosing shapes and fillings. Pay attention to neatness so that the sandwiches are easy to eat with one hand.

Begin with firm, thinly sliced bread or day-old, soft bread that is well chilled. For variety, combine contrasting bread in one sandwich, such as white with whole wheat or pumpernickel.

Choose spreadable fillings such as deviled ham or egg, chicken, or seafood salad. Softened cream cheese also works well. Vary the flavor by adding mixed herbs, grated sharp cheese, drained crushed pineapple, sweet relish, chopped dates, crisp bacon bits, or honey.

To make a basic tea sandwich, trim off the crusts from the bread and cut out shapes, using a sharp knife or cookie cutters. Spread the slices of bread lightly with butter, margarine, or mayonnaise. Then spread a thin layer of filling on half of the slices all the way to the edges. Use just enough to flavor the sandwich. Extra filling will ooze out the edges. Top with a second slice of cut bread.

Tea sandwiches can be prepared several hours ahead of time. Cover them with wax paper and a damp dish towel and refrigerate them until serving time.

✓ Reading Check **Explain** When is the best time to add condiments to a basic sandwich and why?

Pizza

Pizza is an oversized, baked sandwich with a yeast-bread base, usually served open-face with assorted toppings. It can be round or square, shallow or deep, and modestly topped or piled with ingredients.

There is disagreement about the origin of pizza. It is believed that the Ancient Greeks had a flatbread topped with onions and garlic. More than 2,400 years ago, Persian soldiers baked a flatbread on their shields and covered it with cheese and dates. The idea of eating the plate the meal was served on is recorded in ancient Greek poetry. It is believed that the first modern pizza came about when tomatoes were used as a topping in Naples and Italy in the 18th century.

Pizza first appeared in America in the late 19th century, when it was served on the streets of Italian neighborhoods. The first pizzeria is believed to have opened in 1905 in New York City.

Pizza Crusts

Pizzas have toppings on a shell or crust, like pies. In fact, the word *pizza* is Italian for pie. Pizza can have thin or thick crusts. Thin crusts are crispy and crunchy. Thick crusts are softer and chewier. A deep-dish pizza needs a thick crust to support the added filling. Bake deep-dish pizza in a pan that is 2 inches deep. Arrange the dough so that it climbs up the side of the deep pan. Deep-dish pizza also needs to bake longer so that the dough can cook all the way through.

TECHNOLOGY FOR TOMORROW

Pizza Ovens

In the 18th century, people living around Naples, Italy, added tomato sauce to their simple, yeast-based flatbread, and pizza was born. Early pizzas were cooked in wood- or coal-fired ovens made of stone or brick. Over time, technology has caused ovens to evolve. These days, pizza may be baked in a gas oven, a large electric deck oven, or even a special conveyor oven. To use a conveyor oven, cooks place a pizza on one end of a conveyor belt. It passes over and under powerful electric heating elements, and comes out fully cooked. This kind of oven can cook a 12-inch pizza in just 6 ½ minutes.

Get Involved Find out whether some pizza restaurants still use old-fashioned wood- or coal-burning ovens. If so, why do you think this is? Share your insights in a paragraph.

NCSS VII B Production, Distribution, and Consumption Analyze the role that supply and demand, prices, incentives, and profits play in determining what is produced and distributed in a competitive market system.

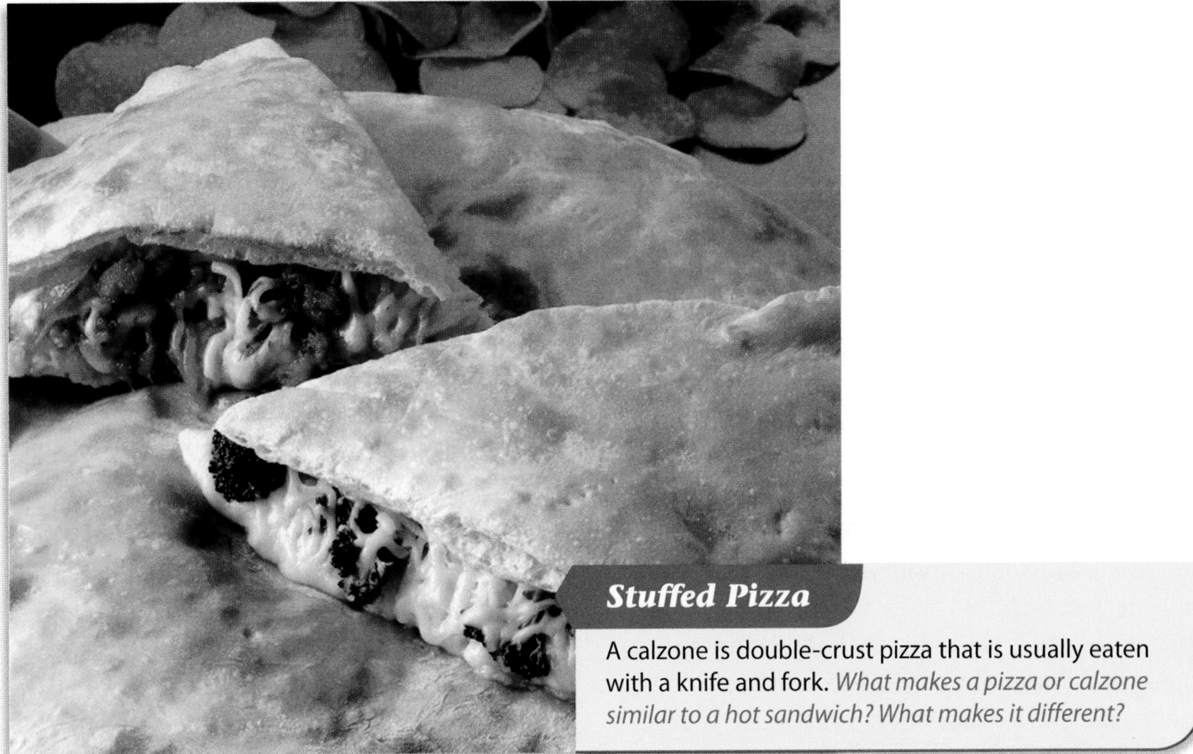

Stuffed Pizza

A calzone is double-crust pizza that is usually eaten with a knife and fork. *What makes a pizza or calzone similar to a hot sandwich? What makes it different?*

Many cooks like to make their own pizza crust. The crust is made with basic yeast dough. Water is used rather than milk for a crispy texture. Punch down and rest the dough, then roll it out on a floured surface to fit the shape of the pan. Place the ball of dough in the center of the pan and alternately press it gently and stretch it to the rim with your fingers. Try to work the dough so that you can leave some extra crust around the outer edge of the pizza. This will bake into a thicker, crustier edge. Pizza dough is usually made with all-purpose flour but a tasty pizza crust can be made by mixing in some whole wheat flour. Some cooks add a small amount of honey to their dough.

Pizza crust can also be stuffed. Roll out the dough so it extends about 1 inch beyond the rim of the pan. About 1 inch from the edge of the dough, place a 1-inch band of cheese, shredded or cut into strips. Fold the overhanging dough over the cheese and press firmly to seal. Top the pizza as desired. Mozzarella is the most common stuffing for pizza crust, but you can experiment with other cheeses that go with the pizza topping.

If you do not want to make dough from scratch, choose a convenience form that is partially or fully prepared. Packaged mixes require oil, water, and kneading. Unbaked frozen dough needs to be thawed. Refrigerated tubes of dough just need to be unrolled and pressed into a pan. Preformed pizza shells are ready to be topped and baked. Pre-made frozen pizzas also are widely available at grocery stores. Some grocery stores offer fresh, ready-to-bake pizzas.

Pizza Toppings

Most pizzas are topped with sauce and cheese. A spicy tomato base comes first. The sauce is much like marinara sauce only it is usually cooked down so that it is thicker and will not run when a slice of pizza is picked up. Mozzarella and Parmesan cheese are traditionally used to top the pizza. Pizza Margherita combines the colors of the Italian flag with red tomato sauce, white mozzarella and green basil leaves. Other traditional toppings include sliced pepperoni, crumbled Italian sausage, and sliced mushrooms, bell peppers, olives, and onions.

Many creative toppings are delicious on pizza. A seafood pizza might feature cooked shrimp, crab, tuna, or salmon in a light white sauce. A vegetarian pizza might feature grilled vegetables, fresh herbs, and olive oil. Pizza might be the first fusion food, because its simple cooking technique can be combined with most any ingredients. A Thai pizza might feature curried chicken. A cheesesteak pizza with thin slices of beef and chopped onions and bell peppers is also common.

After topping the pizza, bake it in a preheated oven at 450°F for 20 minutes or until the crust is golden brown. Deep-dish pizza should be baked at 475°F for 25–30 minutes. Cooks typically bake pizza on a pizza stone, a hard, flat stone that rests on top of the oven rack. The stone prevents the pizza dough from slipping through the rack before it bakes and solidifies. The stone is usually sprinkled generously with cornmeal before the pizza is slid on top. The cornmeal prevents the pizza dough from sticking to the stone. In pizzerias, cooks use a long stick with a wide flat surface called a peel to insert and remove the pizza from the hot oven.

When the pizza is removed, it should be allowed to cool for a few minutes before being sliced and served. This allows the toppings to set. A pizza cutter is a circular knife attached to a handle that allows a cook to cut across the diameter of the pizza. Kitchen shears or a sharp knife can be used instead of a pizza cutter.

Calzone

A **calzone** (kal-ˈzōn) is a double-crust, semicircular pizza. Any dough and fillings that you would put in a pizza can also become a calzone.

Roll the pizza dough out to make a circle about 10 inches in diameter. Spread the filling over one half of the circle to within 1 inch of the edge. Fold the other half of the dough over the filling. Press with your fingertips or the tines of a fork to seal the edges tightly.

Place the calzone on a lightly greased baking sheet and brush it with olive oil. Bake the calzone in a preheated oven at about 400°F for 30 minutes or until golden brown. Cut it into wedges and serve immediately.

Light and Healthy Recipe

Toasted Turkey Sandwich

This sandwich is filling, nutritious and low in fat.

Ingredients

- **4 oz.** Prepared mustard
- **½ tsp.** Celery seed
- **¼ tsp.** Pepper
- **1 Tbsp.** Dried cranberries
- **8 slices** Whole wheat bread
- **8 oz.** Sliced low-fat turkey breast
- **3 oz.** Low-fat, low sodium mozzarella cheese
- **1** Tomato, sliced

Directions

1. Dice the cranberries and put them in a small bowl with the pepper, celery seed and mustard. Mix them and spread lightly on all eight slices of bread.
2. Top four slices of the bread with the turkey and place tomato slices on top. Sprinkle with cheese. Top with tomato slices.
3. Cover with the remaining slices of bread, place in toaster oven and toast.

Yield 4 servings

Nutrition Analysis per Serving

■ Calories	322
■ Total fat	11 g
Saturated fat	3 g
Cholesterol	29 mg
■ Sodium	990 mg
■ Carbohydrate	34 g
Dietary fiber	3 g
Sugars	6 g
■ Protein	22 g

CHAPTER 38 Review & Applications

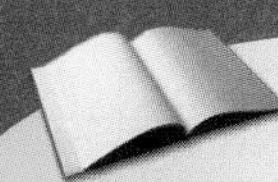

After You Read

Chapter Summary

A sandwich is filling between slices of bread. It is as nutritious as the foods that go into it. Sandwiches can be basic or come in many other forms, including club sandwiches, open-face sandwiches, heroes, and wraps. There are also hot sandwiches, which may have cooked fillings, or can be grilled or broiled. Small, cold tea sandwiches are yet another form. All sandwiches can be prepared using a variety of ingredients. Pizza is a type of oversized, baked sandwich. It consists of fillings on a shell or crust. Many creative toppings are delicious on pizza. A calzone is a double-crust, semicircular pizza.

Content and Academic Vocabulary Review

1. Write four multiple-choice test questions using 16 of these content and academic vocabulary words.

Content Vocabulary

- sandwich (p. 596)
- basic sandwich (p. 596)
- club sandwich (p. 596)
- open-face sandwich (p. 597)
- hero (p. 597)
- wraps (p. 597)
- pita (p. 597)
- falafel (p. 598)
- gyro (p. 598)
- lavash (p. 598)
- tortilla (p. 598)
- fajitas (p. 599)
- guacamole (p. 599)
- focaccia (p. 601)
- tea sandwich (p. 601)
- pizza (p. 602)
- calzone (p. 604)

Academic Vocabulary

- elaborate (p. 596)
- substantial (p. 600)

Review Key Concepts

2. **List** three different types of sandwiches and describe how to make them.
3. **Describe** how to make pizzas and calzones.

Critical Thinking

4. **Design** a sandwich that perfectly suits your taste preferences. Be creative, and use terminology from this chapter to describe your ideal sandwich.
5. **Identify** the basic sandwich-making step that Liz forgot. The cucumber slices she used made the bread soggy.
6. **Describe** a vegetarian wrap that might appeal to a child. Explain your reasoning.
7. **Evaluate** the role sandwiches and pizzas can play in a healthful diet.
8. **Compare and contrast** pita bread and tortillas. How are they similar when used to make sandwiches? How are they different?
9. **Describe** a pizza that contains foods from each of the five food groups.
10. **Explain** why a serving of calzone can be more filling than a serving of pizza made with identical ingredients.

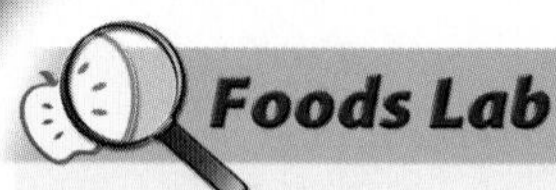

Foods Lab

11. Making Sandwiches Sandwiches can be made with ingredients that suit a variety of tastes, needs, and diets. What kind of sandwich will you make today?

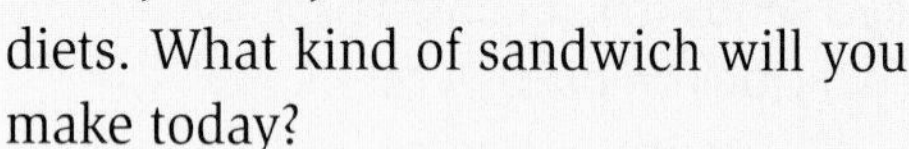

Procedure Choose one of the following kinds of sandwiches to make: basic; club; open-face; hero; flatbread; grilled; broiled. Use ingredients of your choosing, and prepare the sandwich.

Analysis In an oral presentation, explain: What ingredients did you use? How did your sandwich rate on taste, texture, and appearance? What was most challenging about preparing it? What improvements would you make?

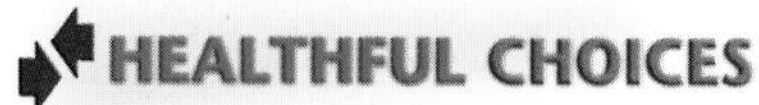

HEALTHFUL CHOICES

12. Hot and Healthful At a build-your-own-sandwich bar, Jess spreads her Parmesan cheese roll with creamy, high-fat dressing and adds cheddar cheese. Now she is looking for a hot filling that will provide nutrients without additional fat. Should she choose ground hamburger, hot dog, shredded barbecued pork, or a patty made of mashed beans and lentils?

TECH Connection

13. Pizza Cost Comparison Compare the cost of delivered pepperoni pizza, frozen pepperoni pizza, and pepperoni pizza made from scratch. Using spreadsheet or word processing software, create a chart with a column that shows the cost per serving of a small pizza of each type. Create columns on the chart where you rate each pizza for taste and quality. Write a summary of your research. In your summary, identify in what situations each pizza type might be the best choice.

Real-World Skills

Problem-Solving Skills

14. Alternative Preparation Methods Kate wants to make a grilled cheese sandwich. After she assembles the sandwich, she prepares to grill it in a skillet, only to find that her range is not working. Her oven, however, is working fine. Can she still make the sandwich? If so, how?

Interpersonal and Collaborative Skills

15. Tea Sandwiches Follow your teacher's instructions to form groups. Work together to create a recipe for a tea sandwich. Recipes should include at least four ingredients. Prepare the sandwiches, and serve them during a class party.

Financial Literacy Skills

16. The Cost of Bread Not all breads taste, or cost, the same. Visit a supermarket and examine four different types of breads, such as potato, whole wheat, focaccia, pita, 7-grain, tortillas, rye, olive, or raisin. Then compare the following: price per serving, calories per serving, nutritional value, and uses. Chart your results. Sort your chart in order of nutritional value.

Academic Skills

Food Science

17. Pizza Dough Science Making a yeast dough requires kneading to make gliadin and glutenin to combine form gluten, the stretchable strands you see when the dough has been worked.

Procedure In a large bowl, dissolve $2\frac{1}{2}$ teaspoons active dry yeast and $\frac{1}{2}$ teaspoon sugar in $\frac{1}{3}$ cup of lukewarm water. Add another $\frac{1}{3}$ cup water, 2 tablespoons olive oil, 2–$2\frac{1}{4}$ cups flour, and $\frac{1}{2}$ teaspoon salt. Blend to form dough. Knead the dough on a floured surface, until it doesn't stick. Continue 5–10 minutes until elastic. Place dough in an oiled bowl, cover with plastic wrap, and let it rise until double in size.

Analysis Why is the yeast added to warm water first? What might happen if the water is too hot? Explain what was going on as the dough doubled in size. Why did we knead the dough?

NSES C Develop an understanding of behavior of organisms.

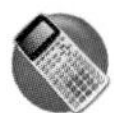

Mathematics

18. Slicing a Pizza Mindy has prepared and cooked an entire pizza from scratch. If the pizza is perfectly round, and she cuts the pizza into 8 equal slices, what is the measure of the angle of each slice? If the pizza is 12 inches in diameter, what is the length (in inches) of one slice? What is the area (in square inches) of one slice?

Math Concept **Circles** When two lines extend inward from a circle's circumference and come together in the center, they form a central angle. The sum of all central angles in a circle is 360°. The radius (r) of a circle is equal to half of its diameter (total width), while the area (A) of a circle is calculated as $A = \pi r^2$. Use 3.14 for π.

Starting Hint The area of one slice will be $\frac{1}{8}$th the area of the entire pizza. The length of one slice will be the pizza's radius, while the angle of one slice will be $\frac{1}{8}$th the number of degrees in the entire pizza.

NCTM Geometry Use visualization, spatial reasoning, and geometric modeling to solve problems.

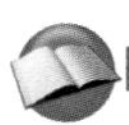

English Language Arts

19. Hot Dog History Use the Internet and at least one book to research the history of the hot dog. Where and when did hot dogs originate? In what circumstances or cultures are they often eaten? Has their safety ever been controversial? Write a one-page report of your findings.

NCTE 8 Use information resources to gather information and create and communicate knowledge.

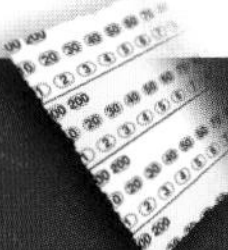

STANDARDIZED TEST PRACTICE

FILL IN THE BLANK

Read the sentence and choose the best word to fill in the blank.

20. Pizza crust is made with a basic ________ dough.

a. white **c.** wheat
b. yeast **d.** unleavened

Test-Taking Tip When answering a fill-in-the-blank question, silently read the sentence with each of the possible answers in the blank space. This will help you eliminate wrong answers. The best word results in a sentence that is both factual and grammatically correct.

CHAPTER 39

Salads & Dressings

Writing Activity 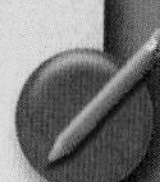 Business Letter

Salad Bar Suggestions A new restaurant featuring an extensive salad bar is opening in your community. The restaurant's owners have asked citizens to suggest foods to include at the salad bar. Write a business letter to the owners in which you introduce yourself and give your suggestions for great salad bar offerings.

Writing Tips Follow these steps to write a business letter:

- Include a return address heading, date, recipient's address, and salutation.
- Use a polite tone.
- End your letter with a closing and your name.
- Key the letter, and proofread the letter to make sure it is free from errors.

Activate Prior Knowledge

Explore the Photo Salads can include foods from all food groups. *What ingredients do you see in this salad? What food groups do they represent?*

Reading Guide

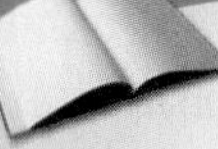

Before You Read

Preview Examine the photos, figure captions, and headings in this chapter. Think about how salads can include foods from all the food groups.

Read to Learn

Key Concepts

- **List** and describe seven types of salads.
- **Explain** how to wash and store salad greens.
- **Identify** different types of salad dressings and explain how to prepare them.
- **Describe** four methods for serving salads.

Main Idea

Salads are mixtures of raw or cooked ingredients that can be creatively prepared to suit a variety of tastes and purposes.

Content Vocabulary

You will find definitions for these words in the glossary at the back of this book.

- ☐ salad
- ☐ crouton
- ☐ tabbouleh
- ☐ molded salad
- ☐ tossed salad
- ☐ salad dressing
- ☐ emulsion
- ☐ temporary emulsion
- ☐ permanent emulsion
- ☐ vinaigrette
- ☐ mayonnaise
- ☐ cooked dressing
- ☐ dairy dressing

Academic Vocabulary

You will find these words in your reading and on your tests. Use the glossary to look up their definitions, if necessary.

- minimal
- restore

Graphic Organizer

Use a graphic organizer like the one below to identify and define types of emulsions.

TEMPORARY EMULSION	PERMANENT EMULSION

Graphic Organizer Go to this book's Online Learning Center at **glencoe.com** to print out this graphic organizer.

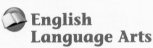

Academic Standards

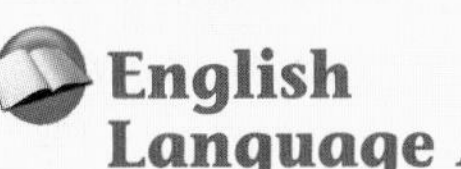

English Language Arts

NCTE 7 Conduct research and gather, evaluate, and synthesize data to communicate discoveries.

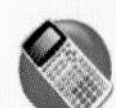

Mathematics

NCTM Data Analysis and Probability Understand and apply basic concepts of probability.

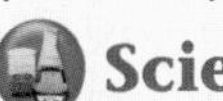

Science

NSES B Develop an understanding of the structure and properties of matter.

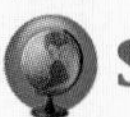

Social Studies

NSES VIII A Science, Technology, and Society Identify and describe both current and historical examples of the interaction and interdependence of science, technology, and society in a variety of cultural settings.

NCTE *National Council of Teachers of English*
NCTM *National Council of Teachers of Mathematics*
NSES *National Science Education Standards*
NCSS *National Council for the Social Studies*

Types of Salads

A **salad** is a mixture of raw or cooked vegetables and other ready-to-eat foods, usually served with a dressing. Salads can be appetizers, entrées, side dishes, and even desserts. Salads made with fresh ingredients and **minimal**, or a small amount of, fat are healthful food choices.

Salads can be made with foods from all of the food groups. Salads come in sweet and savory varieties and can feature vegetables, fruits, grains, and protein foods.

Vegetable Salads

Vegetable salads are made with raw, cooked, or canned vegetables. Vegetable salads usually accompany a meal, but they can sometimes be a main dish.

Cole slaw and potato salad are two well-known vegetable salads. Cole slaw is shredded cabbage mixed with oil and vinegar or a creamy dressing. Potato salad is sliced or cubed cooked potatoes mixed with mayonnaise and seasonings. Both cole slaw and potato salad can be accented with other vegetables, such as carrots, for extra fiber, flavor, crunch, color, and nutrition.

Caesar salad is another popular vegetable salad. It is made from romaine lettuce with a dressing that traditionally consists of olive oil, lemon juice, salt, pepper, Worcestershire sauce, yogurt, and Parmesan cheese. The salad is topped with **croutons**, small pieces of bread made crisp by baking at a low temperature. They are always added to a salad last so they are crisp when served. The salad is named for its creator, Caesar Cardini, and not for the Roman emperor.

Fruit Salads

Fruit salads can provide as much variety as vegetable salads. Ambrosia salad, for example, combines the sweetness of mandarin oranges, bananas, cherries, miniature marshmallows, and flaked coconut with the texture of pecans and tang of pineapple chunks and sour cream. Waldorf salad mixes diced apples, sliced celery, chopped walnuts, and mayonnaise. A refreshing, light dressing can be made with fruit vinegars or spiced citrus juice.

A rich, sweetened dressing turns fruit salad into a dessert. You can mix fruit with cream cheese thinned with evaporated milk or pudding cooked with juice. Frozen fruit salads are usually made with fruits and gelatin, plus mayonnaise, cream cheese, or cream.

Cooked Grain Salads

Any grain can be used in a salad. You can dress grains lightly with oil, vinegar, salt, and pepper or toss them with a creamy dressing. For color and texture contrast, you can add diced bell pepper, sliced olives, or parsley. **Tabbouleh** (tə-ˈbü-lē) is a Middle Eastern salad of cooked bulgur, chopped tomatoes, onions, parsley, mint, olive oil, and lemon juice. Polynesian rice salad features rice mixed with pineapple chunks and orange juice sweetened with honey.

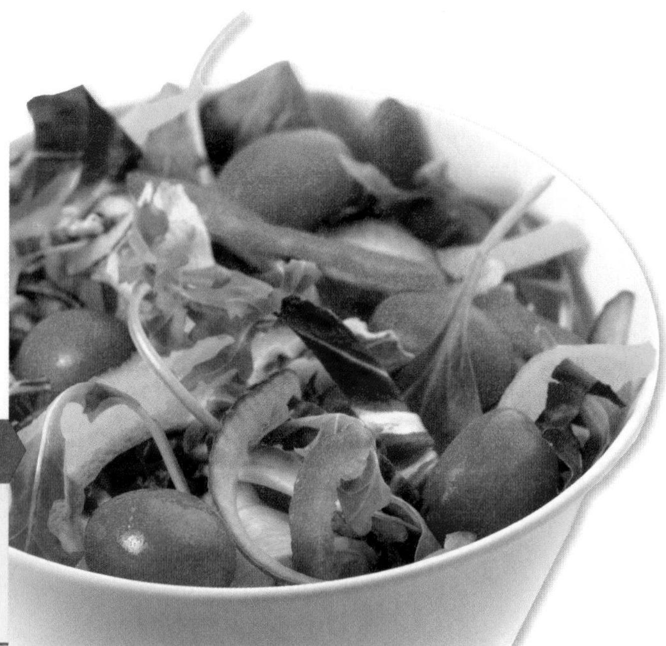

Savory Salad

A salad with varied greens makes a nutritious, tasty meal accompaniment. *What is the benefit of adding additional vegetables, such as carrots or celery, to a salad like the one shown here?*

TECHNOLOGY FOR TOMORROW

Salads in Space

Astronauts must go without fresh fruits and vegetables for most of their stay in space. The practice of space farming, however, could change that. Already, astronauts have grown produce on the International Space Station. One experiment involved growing soybean seeds. The plants thrived in a special growth chamber under conditions monitored and controlled by scientists on earth. The soybeans were the first crops to be sprouted, raised to maturity, and harvested entirely in outer space, and were similar physically and biologically to their earthly counterparts. In the future, scientists hope to grow a variety of crops in space. Someday, astronauts may be able to enjoy fresh salads from their own space gardens.

Get Involved In addition to changing the diets of astronauts, how might space farming affect people on earth? Research this topic and write a paragraph about your findings.

NCSS VIII A Science, Technology, and Society
Identify and describe both current and historical examples of the interaction and interdependence of science, technology, and society in a variety of cultural settings.

Grain salads tend to be more flavorful if prepared warm and then chilled for serving. Hot grains absorb dressings and seasonings better than cold grains. To dry drained, cooked pasta, spread it onto a paper towel-lined baking sheet and roll it gently.

Dry Bean Salads

You can make bean salads with lentils, all kinds of beans, and different seasonings and dressings. You might combine navy and pinto beans with diced tomatoes, sourdough croutons, rice vinegar, and basil. Three-bean salad is a popular mix of common types of beans in oil and vinegar. Seasoned lentils make a tasty cold salad as well. Adding beans to a tossed green salad makes it more filling. There are many recipes for cold salads mixing beans and cold cooked rice with a vinaigrette.

Cooked Meat, Poultry, Fish, and Egg Salads

Chopped salads are made with cooked meat, poultry, fish, or eggs. Chop the main ingredient, then mix it with seasonings and diced vegetables. Onions, celery, and bell peppers are common additions. Most chopped salads are paired with dressing made with sour cream or mayonnaise. You can also try tasty light dressings, including lime juice and honey or rice vinegar and sesame oil.

Combination Salads

A combination salad puts together several different foods. Combination salads can be side dishes or entrées. Greens, tomato wedges, and slices of hard-cooked egg make a filling side salad. Adding strips of ham, turkey, and cheese makes a chef's salad, which is served as a main dish.

Niçoise salad, for example, is a French salad made with tomatoes, anchovies, black olives, green beans, tuna, new potatoes, and hard-boiled eggs, served with an Italian dressing. Other ingredients might include capers, shallots or onions, cucumber, artichoke hearts, or raw peppers.

A wilted salad consists of leafy dark greens and crumbled bacon drizzled with a dressing of hot bacon fat, sugar, and vinegar. The hot fat wilts the greens, warming and softening them. You can also add hard-cooked eggs, tomatoes, mandarin oranges, or cashews.

Leftovers are perfect ingredients for combination salads. Toss cooked vegetables, meat, or eggs with various greens or grains to make interesting combinations.

Molded Salads

A **molded salad** is a salad made with gelatin that thickens and conforms to the shape of a container called a mold. In the past, extracting gelatin from meat and bones was a costly process, and molded salads were rare and expensive. Today, purified gelatin is inexpensive. It is available as an unflavored powder and in sweetened, dry mixes with many different fruit flavors. You can also buy gelatin made from non-animal sources.

Working with Gelatin

Gelatin dissolves in hot water. Like egg protein, gelatin is made of long amino acid chains. Adding hot water breaks the bonds that hold the chains together. As the water and gelatin chill in the refrigerator, these chains reunite in a new structure. Water is trapped in this new protein network, which thickens to hold itself together. Through this process, gelatin can "tie up" as much as 100 times its weight in water. One tablespoon of unflavored gelatin can set 2 cups of liquid.

Before it sets, gelatin traps other foods, such as fruits, vegetables, cooked shrimp, chopped nuts, cottage cheese, or salsa. Lightweight foods, including bananas, apples, pears, and celery, tend to float to the top. Heavier foods, including poultry, fish, grapes, citrus fruits, canned fruits, and many vegetables, drop to the bottom. This can create an attractive layered look. If you would rather distribute foods evenly, fold them in as soon as the mixture has thickened to the consistency of cold egg whites.

A few fruits produce unwelcome results in gelatin salads. Fresh and frozen pineapples, mangoes, kiwifruit, and papayas contain the enzyme bromelin, which digests proteins and keeps the gelatin mixture from setting. Cooked or canned forms of these fruits and juices will work because the heat of cooking or processing deactivates the enzyme.

Molding a Salad

Follow these steps to create a molded salad:

1. Dissolve the gelatin. Mix the gelatin with hot water until it dissolves, according to package directions.

2. Add mix-ins. Mix the salad ingredients into the gelatin.

3. Pour into the mold. Lightly oil the inside of the mold or rinse it with cold water so the salad will be easier to remove later. Then pour in the gelatin mixture. You can choose a ring mold or one with a tiered design or intricate details.

4. Chill. Refrigerate the molded salad until it is completely set.

5. Remove from the mold. Dip the mold almost to the rim in warm (not hot) water for about 10 seconds. Watch a timer so the gelatin does not melt. Lift it from the water, and shake it slightly to loosen the gelatin. Run the tip of a small, pointed knife between the salad and the rim of the mold to loosen the edges of the salad from the mold. Place a serving plate upside down on top of the mold. Invert the plate and mold together so the plate is on the bottom. Shake gently again, and lift off the mold. If necessary, repeat the steps until the salad is released. Slide the salad carefully to center it on the plate. This is easier if you rinse the plate in cold water first.

✓ Reading Check **Explain** How can a salad be made with grains?

Salad Greens

Figure 39.1 shows and defines several popular greens used in salads. Mixing different kinds of greens adds interest to a **tossed salad**. When greens, other chopped or sliced vegetables and a dressing are mixed together, they are a tossed salad.

Selecting Greens

In the supermarket, greens may be sold either in bulk or premixed and packaged. If you keep a home garden, check to see what varieties of greens grow well in your area.

When you buy salad greens, keep in mind that color is the key to nutrition. The greener the greens are, the more vitamin A they contain. Examine greens for brown spotting, called rust, or other signs of disease or spoilage. If you buy packaged greens, look for the sell-by date to get the freshest product.

When buying greens, consider the recipe and dressing you plan to use. Some salad recipes work best with certain greens. Romaine, for example, is typically used for Caesar salad. Iceberg lettuce is often cut into wedges and served with blue cheese dressing. Crisp greens, such as iceberg and romaine, hold up better under thick, creamy dressings than soft greens such as mesclun and watercress.

Figure 39.1 A Guide to Salad Greens

A Variety of Flavors Salad greens have different colors, shapes, textures, and flavors, from mild to sharp. ***Which of the greens shown here have a nutty flavor? Which have a bitter flavor?***

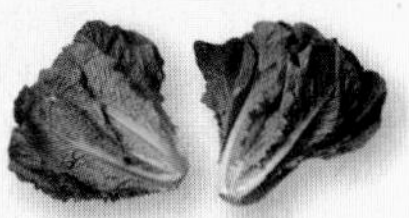

Romaine (rō-'mān)
Long, narrow head of loosely packed leaves. Outer leaves are dark green, and center leaves are pale green. Crisp texture with a sharp, nutty flavor. Most nutritious lettuce.

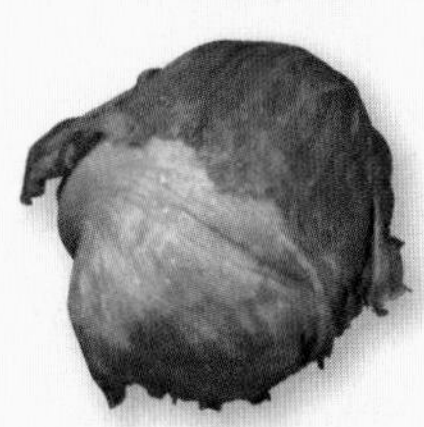

Iceberg Lettuce
Large, round, compact head with pale green, crisp leaves. Mild flavor. Low in nutritional value.

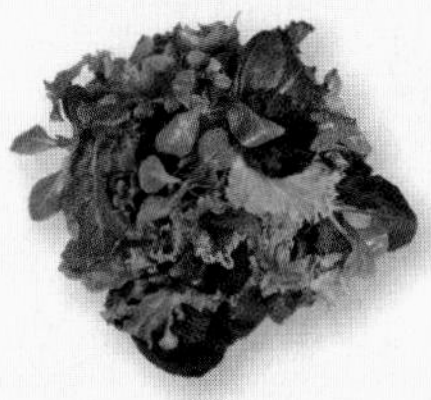

Mesclun ('mes-klən)
A popular mix of various types of young, small greens. Sold in bulk or prepackaged.

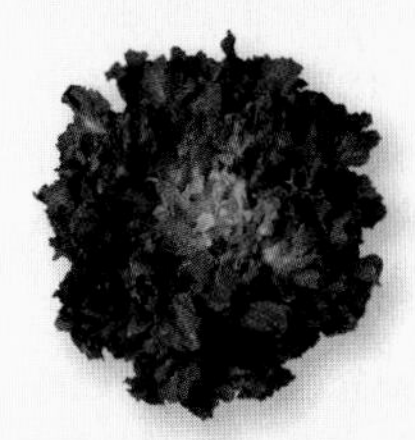

Escarole ('es-kə-ˌrōl)
Flat, loose head of broad, slightly curved leaves. Outer leaves are green, and inner leaves are yellow. Firm texture with a slightly bitter flavor.

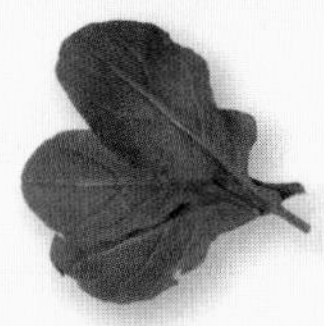

Arugula (ə-'rü-gə-lə)
Small, bright green, smooth leaves. Sold in small bunches. Highly perishable. Tender texture with a pungent, peppery, nutty flavor.

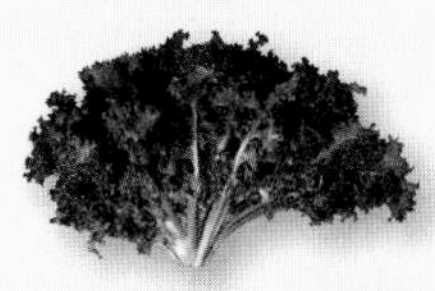

Curly Endive
Sometimes called chicory. Loose head of curled, lacy leaves with bright green edges and an off-white center. Coarse texture with bitter flavor. Best mixed with other greens.

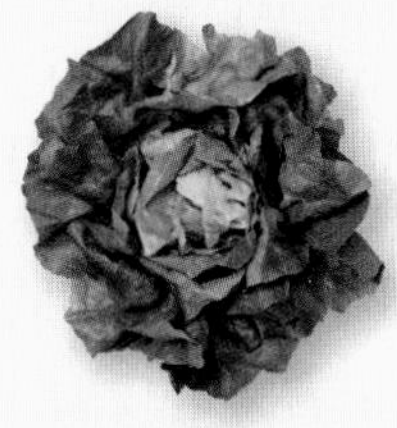

Butterhead Lettuce
Small head with loosely packed leaves. Sweet flavor with a tender, buttery texture. Wash and handle gently to avoid leaf damage. Bibb and Boston are two varieties.

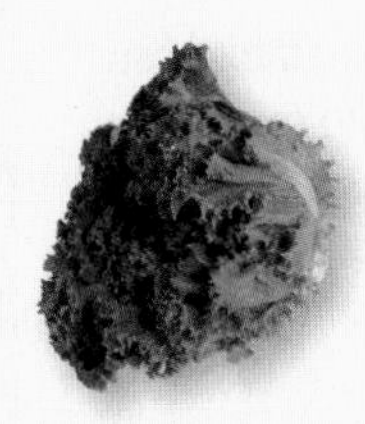

Leaf Lettuce
A loose bunch of crinkly leaves. Crisp texture with a mild flavor. Leaves are usually medium to dark green. Some varieties have red-tipped leaves.

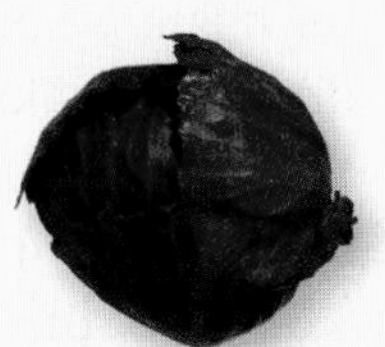

Radicchio (ra-'di-kē-ō)
Small, loose head, either round or long and narrow. Colors vary from deep red with white ribs to streaked with pink, red, or green. Firm texture with slightly bitter flavor.

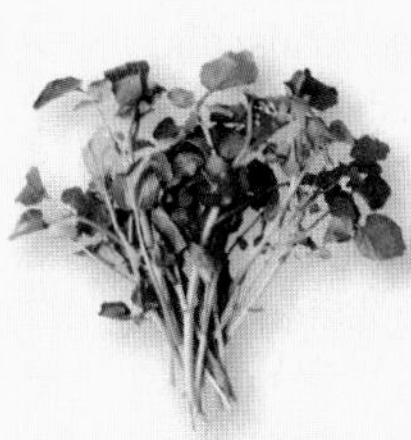

Watercress
Small, dark green leaves. Crisp texture with a slightly bitter, peppery flavor. Grows in running streams.

Coring Iceberg Lettuce

To core iceberg lettuce, strike the core end of the head against the countertop. This loosens the core for easy removal. To wash the lettuce, pour water into the opening and let it drain. *How should you wash greens that come in loose bunches?*

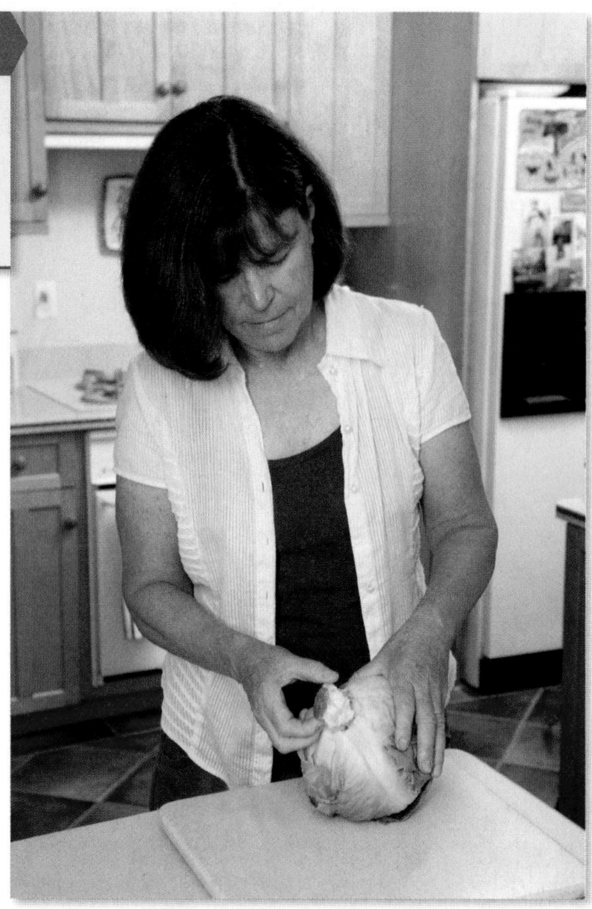

Cleaning Greens

Washing greens rinses away the soil, as well as harmful bacteria. Wash, drain, and refrigerate salad greens as soon as possible after buying to help them stay crisp.

To clean most greens, pull the leaves away from the bunch and wash them individually under cold, running water. You may want to soak them for about ten minutes to rehydrate their cells and **restore**, or renew, crispness. Drain the leaves well, placing each one, stem-side down, in a colander so the water drains off easily. You may need to pat the greens dry with a clean cloth or paper towel before storing them.

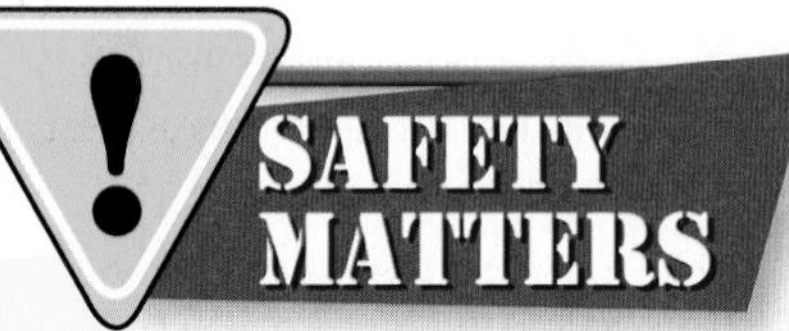

FDA Food Recalls

Like other foods, fresh fruits and vegetables can contain harmful bacteria that lead to cases of foodborne illness, some of them widespread. For example, many people across the country may suffer *Salmonella* poisoning from eating contaminated tomatoes. In such instances, the Food and Drug Administration prevents further illness by issuing a recall of the food or a warning to consumers not to eat it, tracing the tainted tomatoes back to their source and conducting an investigation. In additon to alerting major news outlets, the FDA publishes all food recalls and warnings on its Web site.

What Would You Do? A newspaper reported that some spinach in the United States was contaminated with *E. coli*. You have not heard much about it lately, and want to make a spinach salad. What will you do to be safe?

Iceberg lettuce requires a different cleaning technique. Hold the head of lettuce in your hands, core-side down. Strike the core firmly on a counter to loosen it. Pull out the core and let cold water run into the cavity for a minute, until it pours out between the leaves. Let the head drain in a colander, core-side down.

It is a good idea to wash all greens, even prewashed greens, to get rid of dirt and bacteria. Always wash mixed greens bought in bulk.

Storing Greens

Drain salad greens as thoroughly as possible before storing them. Water hastens spoilage. Water also dilutes salad dressing, making a watery salad.

A salad spinner makes it easy to drain washed greens. This tool has an outer plastic bowl and an inner perforated basket. Pressing a button or turning a handle spins the inner bowl. As it spins, the water flies off the leaves and is caught in the outer bowl.

Keep washed and drained greens wrapped in a dry paper towel and refrigerated in a plastic container or a large plastic bag. Most greens are best when used within one week. Iceberg lettuce holds its quality for about two weeks. If greens look limp, immerse them for a few minutes in ice water and dry them just before making the salad. To prevent enzymatic browning, tear greens or cut them with a plastic lettuce knife rather than a metal knife.

✓ **Reading Check** **Explain** Is it necessary to wash packaged, pre-washed or ready-to-eat greens?

Salad Dressings

Some salads are so flavorful that you could eat them with just a splash of lemon juice and a sprinkling of herbs or seeds. Many people like to add **salad dressing**, a seasoned mixture, often consisting of oil and vinegar, used to flavor a salad. Salad dressing also acts as a binder, holding the salad ingredients together.

Dressings add almost all of the fat and most of the calories in many salads. Use just enough dressing to give flavor, and choose low-fat and nonfat dressings whenever you can. It is polite to offer a variety of dressings at the table so people can choose the type and amount they want.

The dressing you serve should complement the other flavors in the salad. Experiment to find combinations you like.

Look for reduced-fat or fat-free varieties of bottled dressing. Packaged mixes often give directions for low-fat options. Make packaged dressings ahead of time so that the seasonings can blend.

Making your own salad dressing gives the freshest flavor. It also gives you more control over ingredients. You can limit the amount of fat in the dressing and experiment with herbs, spices, and interesting additions.

Most salad dressings are emulsions. An **emulsion** is a mixture of two liquids that normally do not combine, such as oil and vinegar. A mixture of oil and vinegar thickens as the liquids are evenly dispersed in very fine drops.

Science in Action

Unstable and Stable

Emulsions do not form spontaneously. One way to create them is through energy input, such as shaking or stirring. An emulsion created by energy, however, will quickly separate once the motion stops, because it is unstable. Emulsifiers, such as the lecithin found in egg yolks, are substances that cause emulsions to become stable.

Procedure Prepare a salad dressing by combining ½ cup vegetable oil, ½ cup balsamic vinegar, and herbs of your choosing. Emulsify it by shaking, then let it destabilize. Next, add the yolk of one large egg, and shake the dressing.

Analysis In writing, record your observations of how the dressing changes from an unstable to a stable emulsion.

NSES B Develop an understanding of the structure and properties of matter.

However, an oil-and-vinegar blend is only a **temporary emulsion**, an emulsion that quickly separates when not stirred. When mixing stops, the oil and vinegar droplets separate from each other. Eventually, the two liquids separate. That is why it is necessary to shake oil-and-vinegar dressings before using them.

Some dressings are permanent emulsions. A **permanent emulsion** is a mix of liquids that will not separate. To turn a temporary emulsion in to a permanent emulsion, you need an emulsifier, a substance that keeps the oil and vinegar blended. Egg yolk is an effective emulsifier.

Making Vinaigrettes

The simplest salad dressing is vinaigrette (ˌvi-ni-ˈgret), sometimes called French dressing. A **vinaigrette** is a mixture of oil, vinegar or lemon juice, and seasonings.

The basic recipe for vinaigrette is 3 parts oil to 1 part vinegar or juice. Whisk the oil steadily into the other ingredients until the two liquids thicken and blend. Add seasonings, such as salt and pepper, to taste. A vinaigrette is a temporary emulsion, so it requires shaking before use.

Making Mayonnaise

Mayonnaise is a thick, creamy dressing that is a permanent emulsion of oil, vinegar or lemon juice, egg yolks, and seasonings. It is vinaigrette with egg yolks added as an emulsifier. To make mayonnaise, very slowly drizzle and blend the oil into the other ingredients with a whisk. The oil must break down into tiny droplets and be coated with yolk so this is a gradual process. Mustard, both the spice and the condiment, is a secondary emulsifier in many mayonnaise recipes and in some vinaigrettes.

Due to concerns about *Salmonella* contamination, some new recipes for making mayonnaise call for cooking the egg mixture before adding the oil. If you want to make a recipe that calls for raw eggs, use egg substitutes or pasteurized eggs, which are safe to eat uncooked.

Making Cooked Dressings

A **cooked dressing** is made by cooking fat and water with starch paste, which serves as an emulsifier. Fat and water do not separate when they are cooked with a dissolved starch like flour or cornstarch. Traditional German potato salad, for instance, is made with a cooked dressing of bacon drippings, flour, sugar, and cider vinegar.

Commercially prepared mayonnaise and cooked dressings, which by law are called salad dressings, are emulsified with both proteins and starches. Starches are useful as egg yolk replacers in reduced-fat dressings. They appear on ingredient lists as cellulose gel, maltodextrin, xanthan (ˈzan-thən) gum, and gum arabic.

Making Dairy Dressings

A **dairy dressing** is a dressing made with buttermilk, yogurt, sour cream, or cottage cheese, and seasonings. Dairy dressings are usually enhanced with other ingredients. Ranch dressing, for example, includes chopped green onion, ground pepper, thyme, and garlic. A blend of yogurt, brown sugar, cinnamon, and frozen juice concentrate makes a creamy dressing for fruit salad.

✓ Reading Check **Describe** What is the basic recipe for vinaigrette?

Nutrition Check

Drenched or Drizzled

A few tablespoons of salad dressing can contain substantial fat and calories. On a salad dressing label, 2 grams of saturated fat per tablespoon may seem minimal, but if you pour on 5 tablespoons, that is nearly half a day's recommended limit of saturated fat. Pay attention to the quantity you use. Salads drizzled in a little dressing often taste better than those that are drenched in a lot of dressing. You can also have dressings served on the side.

Think About It What is the fat and calorie content of a dressing you typically use? How much fat and calories are in the amount you usually add to your salad?

Making and Serving Salads

Creativity and presentation help make salads taste good and look appetizing. Choose fresh ingredients that complement each other and the rest of the meal in flavor, color, texture, and nutrients. Chilling the bowl or plate in the refrigerator or freezer beforehand helps the salad stay cold for serving and eating. Salads can be served tossed, arranged, layered, or bound.

Tossed Salads A tossed salad is usually a mixture of greens and a dressing, often mixed with other vegetables. Tossed salads are mixed well, with ingredients distributed throughout.

Arranged Salads An arranged salad is a salad with ingredients placed in an attractive pattern. For example, you could place wedges of tomato in a fan around a scoop of chicken salad on a bed of lettuce.

Layered Salads A layered salad is like an arranged salad, except that ingredients are placed in layers one on top of the other, rather than in a flat pattern on the plate. Serve a layered salad in a glass bowl for the best visual effect.

Bound Salads A bound salad is held together tightly by a thick, usually creamy dressing. Coleslaw is a popular bound salad.

CHAPTER 39 Review & Applications

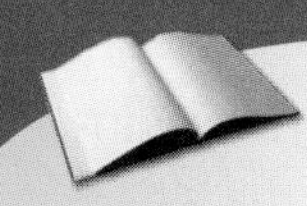

After You Read

Chapter Summary

Salads are mixtures of raw or cooked vegetables and other ready-to-eat foods. There are several types of salads suitable for different tastes, meals, and occasions. Many salads include greens. Greens should be selected with care, cleaned thoroughly, and stored properly. Salad greens vary in taste, texture, and appearance. Dressings are seasoned mixtures that are often used to flavor salads. They should be chosen to complement other flavors. Many types of salad dressing can also be made at home. Creativity and presentation help make salads tasty and appealing. Salads can be served in different styles.

Content and Academic Vocabulary Review

1. Use each of these content and academic vocabulary terms to create a crossword puzzle on graph paper. Use the definitions as clues.

Content Vocabulary

- salad (p. 610)
- crouton (p. 610)
- tabbouleh (p. 610)
- molded salad (p. 611)
- tossed salad (p. 612)
- salad dressing (p. 615)
- emulsion (p. 615)
- temporary emulsion (p. 615)
- permanent emulsion (p. 615)
- vinaigrette (p. 615)
- mayonnaise (p. 616)
- cooked dressing (p. 616)
- dairy dressing (p. 616)

Academic Vocabulary

- minimal (p. 610)
- restore (p. 614)

Review Key Concepts

2. **List** and describe seven different types of salads.
3. **Explain** how to wash and store salad greens.
4. **Identify** different types of salad dressings and explain how to prepare them.
5. **Describe** four methods for serving salads.

Critical Thinking

6. **Evaluate** Marisa's claim that all salads are healthful.
7. **Identify** whether a cook who mixes canned tuna with onions, chives, olives, walnuts, mayonnaise, and herbs has made a salad or a sandwich filling.
8. **Create** a recipe for a dry bean salad that contains a food from the following food groups: meat and beans, milk, vegetable, grains.
9. **Explain** how the tropical molded salad that Sam made could have turned out watery, even though he chilled it for two days.
10. **Describe** the best salad serving style to use with picky eaters who may not like every ingredient.

Foods Lab

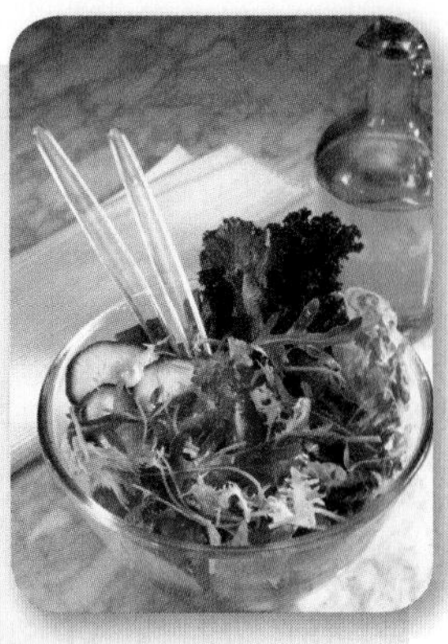

11. Ethnic Salads Thousands of different salads are enjoyed all over the world. The cuisine of virtually every culture features its own type of salad.

Procedure Explore ethnic salad recipes, and choose one to prepare. You might select a recipe from the culture of one of your classmates. Prepare the recipe, and share samples in class.

Analysis In an oral presentation, answer these questions: What is the ethnic origin of the salad you prepared? Is the salad authentic, or has it been modified to suit American taste? How did it taste? Did your classmates like it? What improvements would you make?

HEALTHFUL CHOICES

12. Salad Bar Selection Joni wants to assemble a nutrient-packed salad from the salad bar at her school cafeteria. She knows she will pile an assortment of colorful vegetables, dry beans, and cooked grains on a bed of lettuce. But what type of lettuce should she choose? The salad bar offers iceberg lettuce, pale green butterhead lettuce, or dark green romaine lettuce. Which is the most nutritious option and why?

TECH Connection

13. Grow Your Own Choose a vegetable that you enjoy in salads, such as lettuce, carrots, or beets. Use the Internet to research how to grow the vegetable in a garden in your region. What type of soil and sunlight does the vegetable require? When is the best time of year to plant it? When should it be harvested? Is it best grown from seeds or from small plants? How can it be used in salads? Write a one-page report of your findings, and share it in a presentation to the class.

Real-World Skills

Problem-Solving Skills

14. Choose a Dressing For a special meal with his grandmother, Leo made a salad of cooked, chilled artichoke hearts. He thought they would taste great drizzled with vinaigrette dressing, and used oil and vinegar to make some. Then he remembered his grandmother liked to eat artichoke hearts with mayonnaise. What can he do?

Interpersonal and Collaborative Skills

15. Demonstrate Skills Follow your teacher's instructions to form pairs. Choose one of the following tasks to demonstrate to the class: 1. unmolding gelatin, 2. washing salad greens, 3. making vinaigrette, 4. making mayonnaise. During your demonstration, you and your partner should make sure to show and to verbally explain your actions.

Financial Literacy Skills

16. Homemade or Store-Bought Store-bought buttermilk salad dressing costs $4.79. To make an equal amount of the same dressing at home, Beau can buy a container of buttermilk for $1.89, three types of seasonings for $2.49 each, and a lemon for 69 cents. Which is the more economical option? Do you think this is always the case? Explain.

Academic Skills

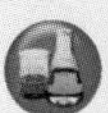

Food Science

17. Vinaigrette Emulsions Emulsions contain two liquids that do not dissolve in each other. An emulsifier is an agent that helps the two liquids stay blended.

Procedure Add 3 ounces vegetable oil and 1 ounce vinegar to each of 3 glass jars. Pour the first sample into a blender; process 3 minutes before returning to the jar. Place the lid on the second jar, shaking vigorously 3 minutes. Observe both jars for 5 minutes. Beat an egg yolk, then slowly pour in the third sample, processing for 3 minutes. Observe all jars after 10 minutes.

Analysis Which of the first two jars separated faster? What happened with the third jar? What ingredient acted as an emulsifier? Which is a stable emulsion?

NSES B Develop an understanding of structure and properties of matter.

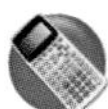

Mathematics

18. Selecting Salad Dressing Monica has purchased seven different bottles of salad dressing, which she keeps lined up in a single-file row on a shelf in her refrigerator door. How many different ways can Monica arrange these dressings on the shelf? If Monica has a buffet-style dinner and wants to pick three of the dressings to place on the counter next to a salad, how many different ways can she pick and arrange three dressings in a row?

Math Concept **Permutations** A permutation is an ordered arrangement of a group of items. If there are n total items, the number of ways to arrange all n of them is $n!$. If you select r of the items, then the number of permutations is equal to $n! / [(n-r)!]$.

Starting Hint The "!" above stands for *factorial*. $n!$ is the product of all sequential integers between 1 and n. For example, $4! = 1 \times 2 \times 3 \times 4$.

NCTM Data Analysis and Probability Understand and apply basic concepts of probability.

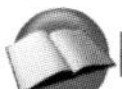

English Language Arts

19. Salad Stories Some of the most popular salads have interesting stories behind how they were invented. Choose a famous salad, such as the Cobb, Caesar, Crab Louie, Waldorf, or Salad Niçoise. Research when, where, and how this salad got started, and who was responsible. Then tell your salad story to the class.

NCTE 7 Conduct research and gather, evaluate, and synthesize data to communicate discoveries.

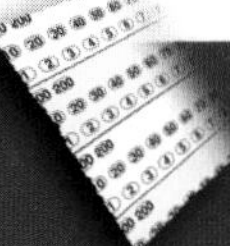

STANDARDIZED TEST PRACTICE

TRUE OR FALSE

Read the statement and determine if it is true or false.

20. A slightly bitter flavor is normal in some salad greens.

a. True

b. False

Test-Taking Tip Before deciding whether a statement is true or false, read it carefully and recall what you have learned from reading the text. Pay close attention to individual words. One word can make the difference between a true statement and a false one.

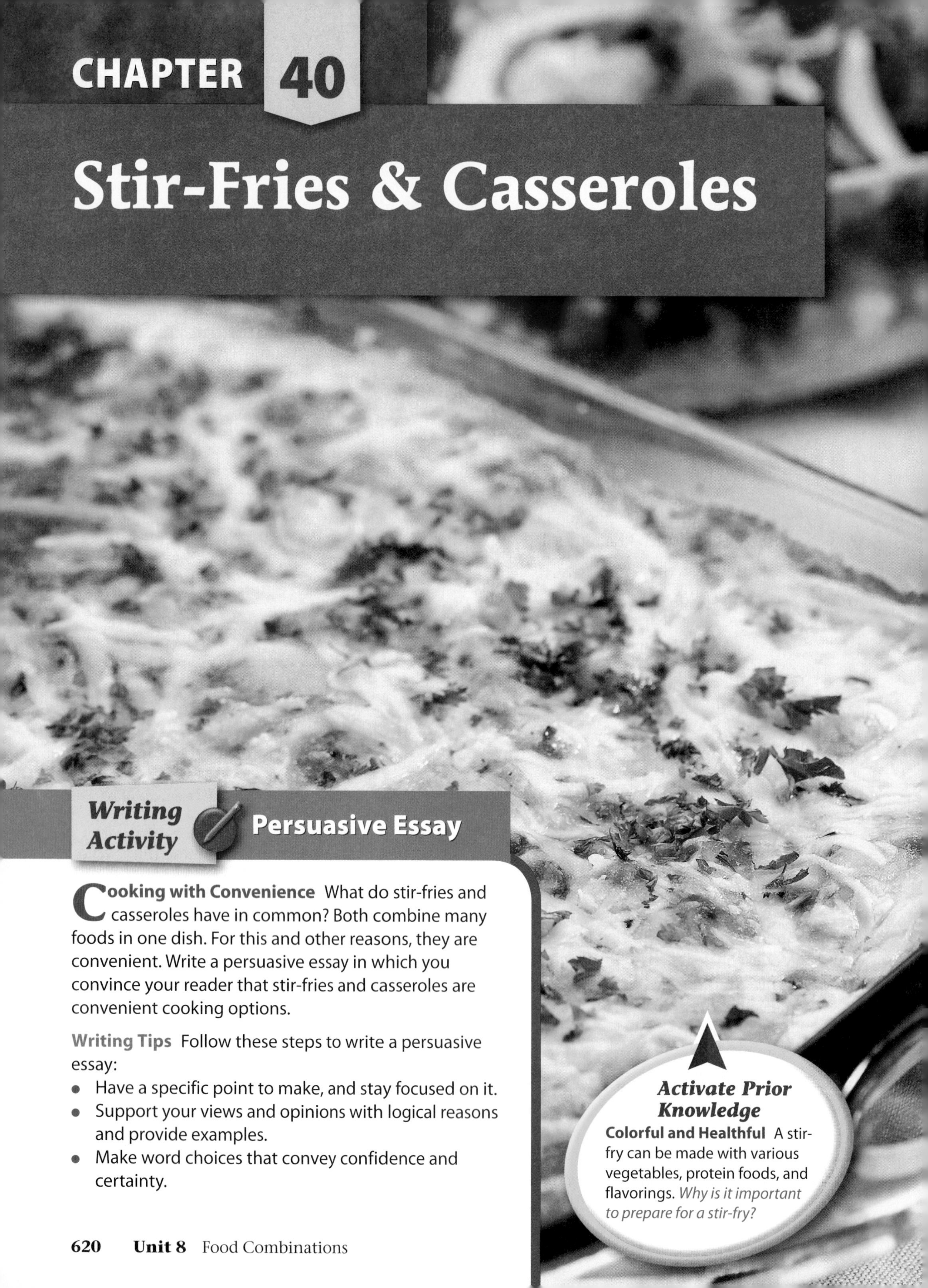

CHAPTER 40

Stir-Fries & Casseroles

Writing Activity — Persuasive Essay

Cooking with Convenience What do stir-fries and casseroles have in common? Both combine many foods in one dish. For this and other reasons, they are convenient. Write a persuasive essay in which you convince your reader that stir-fries and casseroles are convenient cooking options.

Writing Tips Follow these steps to write a persuasive essay:

- Have a specific point to make, and stay focused on it.
- Support your views and opinions with logical reasons and provide examples.
- Make word choices that convey confidence and certainty.

Activate Prior Knowledge

Colorful and Healthful A stir-fry can be made with various vegetables, protein foods, and flavorings. *Why is it important to prepare for a stir-fry?*

Reading Guide

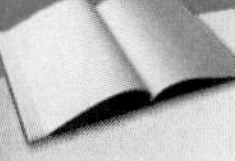

Before You Read

Preview Jot down ingredients you have eaten in stir-fries or casseroles. Skim through the chapter to learn about other possibilities.

Read to Learn

Key Concepts

- **Summarize** the basic steps of stir-frying.
- **Explain** the roles of basic ingredients in a casserole.

Main Idea

Stir-fries and casseroles are economical combination dishes that are easy to prepare and serve.

Content Vocabulary

You will find definitions for these words in the glossary at the back of this book.

- stir-fry
- mise en place
- wok
- casserole
- binder
- au gratin

Academic Vocabulary

You will find these words in your reading and on your tests. Use the glossary to look up their definitions if necessary.

- coordinate
- continuously

Graphic Organizer

Use a graphic organizer like the one below to note the seven common ingredients in a stir-fry.

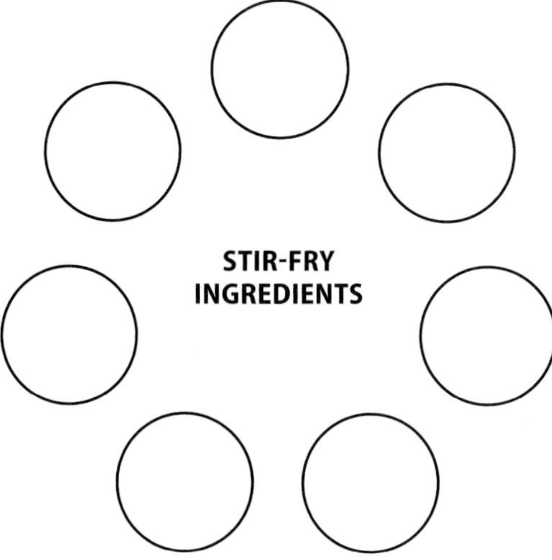

Graphic Organizer Go to this book's Online Learning Center at **glencoe.com** to print out this graphic organizer.

Academic Standards

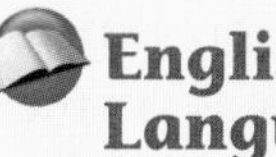

English Language Arts

NCTE 8 Use information resources to gather information and create and communicate knowledge.

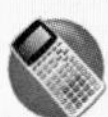

Mathematics

NCTM Measurement Apply appropriate techniques, tools, and formulas to determine measurements.

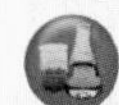

Science

NSES B Develop an understanding of the structure and properties of matter.

NCTE *National Council of Teachers of English*
NCTM *National Council of Teachers of Mathematics*
NSES *National Science Education Standards*
NCSS *National Council for the Social Studies*

Stir-Fries

A **stir-fry** is a combination dish of bite-size pieces of food that are stirred constantly while frying in a small amount of oil over high heat. Stir-fried vegetables are tender on the outside, yet crisp on the inside. They are cooked at high temperatures for a short time, between 30 seconds and 5 minutes, depending on the ingredients. Stir-frying helps foods retain nutrients while absorbing little fat.

Stir-fries usually feature a combination of vegetables and protein foods. Meat, poultry, or seafood is one of the ingredients, rather than the center of the recipe. Stir-fried dishes include a light, flavorful sauce. Add a cooked grain and a side salad and this is a nutritious, appealing meal.

The keys to a good stir-fry are preparation and organization. This is true because all the ingredients need special treatment.

Science in Action: Reducing Sauces

A thin or watery sauce can become thicker and more substantial when it is heated. Why? The thickening is a result of evaporation. The water in the sauce evaporates over heat, while the more solid components of the sauce remain behind and become more concentrated in flavor. A term to describe this is reduction.

Procedure Combine ¼ cup of soy sauce with ¼ cup of water, along with 1 teaspoon of herbs or spices. Pour the sauce into a saucepan, and note its appearance. Then heat and simmer the sauce. Stir it, and pay attention to how it changes.

Analysis In a paragraph, describe how the sauce tasted and appeared before its reduction, how long it took to become noticeably thicker, and how it tasted and appeared after being reduced.

NSES B Develop an understanding of the structures and properties of matter.

Preparing Stir-Fries

Prepare well before you start a stir-fry. Review the recipe steps several times before beginning cooking. Cook the grain, cut the ingredients, mix the sauce, and arrange all of the ingredients in the order you will add them to the pan. Once the oil is hot, you will not have time to hunt for missing ingredients or do last-minute prep work.

Cook the Grain

Most stir-fries are served with a cooked grain. The grain should be ready and waiting when the stir-fry is finished. **Coordinate**, or synchronize, tasks so that the grain cooks while you prepare the other foods. Rice is a traditional accompaniment, but other options include barley, brown rice, couscous, millet, or pasta. To save time, reheat precooked grain or use packaged chow mein noodles.

Each grain has its own characteristic flavor and texture. Choose a grain that complements the stir-fry sauce and ingredients. Different grains have different cooking times as well, so adjust the timetable as needed. In the time it takes to cook rice, you can usually complete all of your other preparations.

Prepare the Vegetables

Cut vegetables into pieces of similar size to promote even cooking. Slice large vegetables into pieces ¼ inch thick or less. Cut dense or fibrous vegetables, such as green beans, green onions, and carrots, on the diagonal. This exposes a larger area to the heat. It also adds visual interest.

Remove the midrib, or "backbone," and the stem ends from cabbage and leafy greens before slicing them. Finely chop the midrib and stem ends separately. Coarsely chop greens, bell peppers, and onions.

Keep the vegetables separate after cutting them. Vegetables that cook quickly, such as spinach, will need to go into the stir-fry later than vegetables that take longer to cook, such as carrots.

Prepare Protein Foods

If using raw meat or poultry, cut it across the grain into very thin strips about 1½ inches long. Use a large, sharp knife and a secure cutting board. Cutting meat and poultry is easier when the food is slightly frozen.

Fresh fish should also be cut into strips. Choose a firm-fleshed variety such as tuna, halibut, mahi-mahi, or bass. Fresh shrimp and scallops are perfectly sized for stir-frying. Cut tofu or tempeh into cubes. To add flavor and to protect against drying out, marinate protein foods before adding them to the stir-fry.

It is also possible to use slices or cubes of cooked meat, poultry, and seafood, either canned or left over. These foods are usually added last, because they only need to be heated through.

Mix the Sauce

Sauce is the thing that brings all the flavors in a stir fry together. Use a base of water, broth, or juice seasoned with soy, tamari, Worcestershire sauce, or fish sauce along with herbs and spices. Common ingredients in a stir fry sauce also include rice vinegar, sugar, honey, prepared mustards, and sesame seeds. Put the mixture, along with cornstarch as the thickener, into a small bowl and whisk it to blend. Set it aside until needed. Cornstarch will settle in the bottom of the bowl as it sits, so you may need to give the mixture a quick whisk again before you add it to your stir fry.

When a sauce is added to the stir-fry, heat thickens it. Some recipes call for additional water or broth to cook vegetables that need more moisture. Other recipes have you remove the meat and vegetables from the wok or push them to the sides of it so that the sauce can combine by itself and then be mixed into the food. It is best to let the sauce cook for a minute or two to mellow the taste of the cornstarch. Keep the recipe close by for easy reference.

Arranging the Ingredients

In stir-frying, the sequence of adding ingredients is important. The goal is thorough, even cooking. Begin by adding foods that take the longest to cook, and end by adding foods that cook most quickly. Keep the food moving. If pieces stay in one place too long they will burn.

Careers in Food

John Kessler
Food Writer

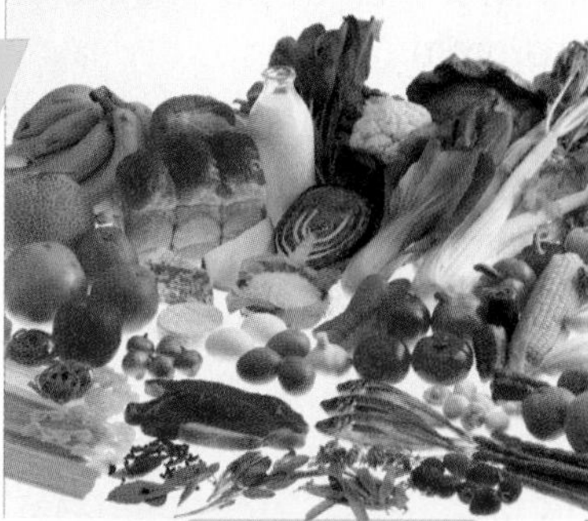

Q: How do you come up with ideas to write about?

A: My topics are about working in the home kitchen and cooking. I listen to readers, do some looking on the Internet, and I get out of the office as much as I can.

Q: Do you also write restaurant reviews?

A: Many papers have a restaurant reviewer in addition to food writers. My focus is on writing about cooking and food in general, although eating in restaurants is also part of the job. If I am writing about chicken wings, I might end up eating chicken wings at eight different places in one day! When I eat in restaurants, I want to try as many different things as possible.

"If you can both inform and entertain readers, you have done your job."
— John Kessler
Columnist, Atlanta Journal-Constitution – Atlanta, GA

Education and Training

Experience with food is very important. Being a trained chef with a degree from a cooking school gives you credibility when you talk with professionals.

Qualities and Skills

You have to be willing to express critical opinions when it is called for. You need to be able to express humor and criticism in your writing.

Related Career Opportunities

In addition to the job of food writer, there is restaurant critic, food editor, lifestyles features writer, and general assignment features writer.

When cooking ingredients that each need different cooking times, chefs use a practice called mise en place. **Mise en place** (ˌmē-ˌzän-pläs) means arranging ingredients in the order in which they will be cooked. Mise en place is French for "put in place." Assemble the ingredients in separate bowls on a countertop, a large tray, or a cart close to the cooktop.

When making a stir-fry, ingredients should be easy to reach, and they should be arranged in this order:

1. **Oil** Any oil with a smoking point of about 400°F can take the heat of stir-frying. That includes almost all commercially available types. Peanut oil adds a rich flavor.
2. **Seasonings** Fresh ginger and minced garlic are usually added at the beginning of stir-frying to flavor the oil and the meat. You can add other seasonings, such as ground spices, later in cooking.
3. **Raw Meat, Poultry, and Seafood** Cook meat, poultry, fish, and most shellfish before the other ingredients. Add scallops with the vegetables to avoid toughening their delicate protein.
4. **Vegetables** Add sturdy vegetables such as carrots and broccoli stems before tender vegetables such as cabbage and spinach. Check the recipe to see whether vegetables should be added in a certain order.
5. **Cooked Meat, Poultry, Seafood, and Tofu** Precooked, ready-to-eat foods only need to be heated, so they are added near the end of the cooking time.
6. **Fruits** Stir-fry recipes occasionally include such tropical fruits as pineapples and mangoes that contrast with spicy or sour ingredients. You can cook these with the tender vegetables or add them just before serving.
7. **Sauce** Add sauce a few minutes before cooking is complete.

Cooking the Stir-Fry

The right equipment and technique can help you create a successful stir-fry.

Woks and Stir-Fry Tools

A stir-fry is traditionally prepared in a **wok**, which is a roomy, bowl-shaped pan. Many different sizes and kinds of woks are available. Food in the rounded bottom is nearest to the heat, where it cooks quickly. Food up the sides of the pan stays warm without overcooking. The curved sides of a wok also let you briskly stir and lightly toss food with a wooden spoon or tongs without tossing it out of the pan. Using a wok skillfully takes practice.

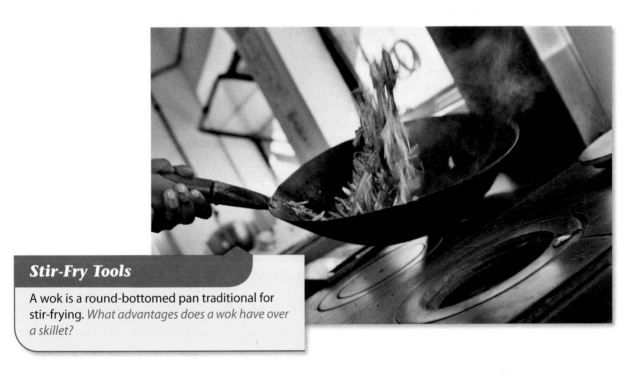

Stir-Fry Tools

A wok is a round-bottomed pan traditional for stir-frying. *What advantages does a wok have over a skillet?*

Special tools can also help you make a stir-fry. A stir-fry spatula has an angled edge that conforms to the wok's sloping sides, where food might escape a straight-edge spatula. A shallow, wide-mesh strainer helps drain oil when removing food. If you feel more comfortable cooking with conventional cookware, use a large, deep skillet and a wide spatula instead of a wok.

Stir-Fry Technique

When stir-frying, work quickly and in small batches, stirring and tossing food as you go. To fry rather than steam, foods must directly touch the pan. The water released by cooking needs room to evaporate. Be ready to add a tablespoon of water if the pan or food seems to be burning.

Compared to the advance preparation, stir-frying itself goes quickly. Most recipes follow these basic steps:

1. **Heat the wok.** Heat the wok on high until a few water drops sizzle and evaporate immediately.
2. **Add oil.** Add 1 to 2 tablespoons of oil to the wok. Tilt the pan to coat the entire surface. In some recipes, half the oil is used to brown the meat, and the other half is added before cooking the vegetables.
3. **Add seasonings.** Add seasonings, such as salt, ginger, or soy sauce, as directed in the recipe.
4. **Add raw protein.** Add raw meat, poultry, or seafood. Stir constantly, and gently tumble the food to brown all sides. Some recipes call for these foods to be completely cooked and then removed or pushed up the side of the wok. Others instruct cooking to finish with the vegetables.
5. **Add vegetables in order.** Add the vegetables according to cooking time. To prevent burning, stir them **continuously**, or constantly, until they are softened on the outside but still firm inside. It is better to undercook vegetables than to overcook them. Undercooked food can always be returned to the heat.

Working with the Wok

To work safely with a wok requires care and patience. Because woks are used over high heat, severe burns can happen easily. Use long-handled, heat-resistant utensils to stir food and avoid contact with the wok. Even steam can cause serious burns, so do not hover your hands over the wok for long periods, and stand back when removing the lid. Wear oven mitts while stirring to protect yourself from burns. Be careful when tossing food in a wok. Hot food, oil, and sauce can fly out and burn skin. Practice tossing cold food in a cold wok. Do not use a wok unsupervised until you are used to using a wok.

What Would You Do? While you prepare a stir fry in a hot wok, your friends are having a food fight behind you. One of them accidentally tosses a potato chip into your stir fry. What will you do?

6. **Add cooked protein.** Add cooked meat, poultry, seafood, or tofu to the pan. If protein was cooked and removed earlier, now is the time to return it to the pan.
7. **Add sauce.** Shake or mix the sauce to recombine the ingredients. Stir it into the wok and cook the mixture with the other ingredients, stirring, until the sauce thickens.
8. **Cover.** Cover the pan briefly, if needed, to steam the vegetables until done. Some vegetables have enough natural moisture to create sufficient steam. Others may need an extra spoonful or two of hot broth or water.
9. **Serve.** Serve the stir-fry immediately on a bed of hot grain. Stir-fries are best when piping hot and fresh from the heat.

✓ Reading Check **Identify** What combination of foods do stir-fries usually feature?

What Makes a Casserole?

A **casserole** is a flavorful combination of precooked or quick-cooking foods in a one-dish meal. The word casserole is French for a baking dish, but American casseroles draw on many influences, from the Asian one-pot meal to medieval pies made with a mashed rice crust.

Casseroles gained popularity in the United States in the early and mid-20th century. The effects of the Great Depression, two world wars, and women increasingly joining the workforce left families needing nourishing, easy-to-prepare meals that made use of ingredients that were on hand. Casseroles are still a great way to use leftover cooked meat, poultry, grains, dried beans, and vegetables. They make a little go a long way.

In some ways, casseroles are the oppostite of stir-fries. Casseroles bake for up to an hour and are often reheated after cooking, while stir-fries are quickly sautéed and served right away. Both dishes, however, turn varied and creative ingredients into economical, appealing meals. Both dishes require preparation tasks to be done in advance, and both use certain types of ingredients.

Main Casserole Ingredients

The main ingredient in a casserole provides the dominant flavor. Main-dish casseroles may include cooked meat or poultry, canned fish or shellfish, or tofu. Cooked ground meat is first drained of fat. Meat is usually browned before going into a casserole. Browning brings out the flavor and helps seared or roasted meat and poultry stand out when combined with other foods.

A main ingredient in a casserole can also be a vegetable, grain, or legume. Cassoulet is a French casserole based on beans. A casserole based on sweet potatoes, brown rice, or lentils makes a hearty side dish or a meatless entrée.

Vegetables

Any cooked, canned, fresh, or frozen vegetables that cook quickly can go into a casserole. Chopped aromatic vegetables, such as celery, onions, bell peppers, and garlic, bring color and flavor.

Broccoli, pasta, sliced mushrooms, and toasted almonds baked in a cream soup serve more people than broccoli alone. You can add ingredients that go well with other dishes. For example, you could add brown sugar and apples to a sweet potato casserole to complement the flavor of baked ham.

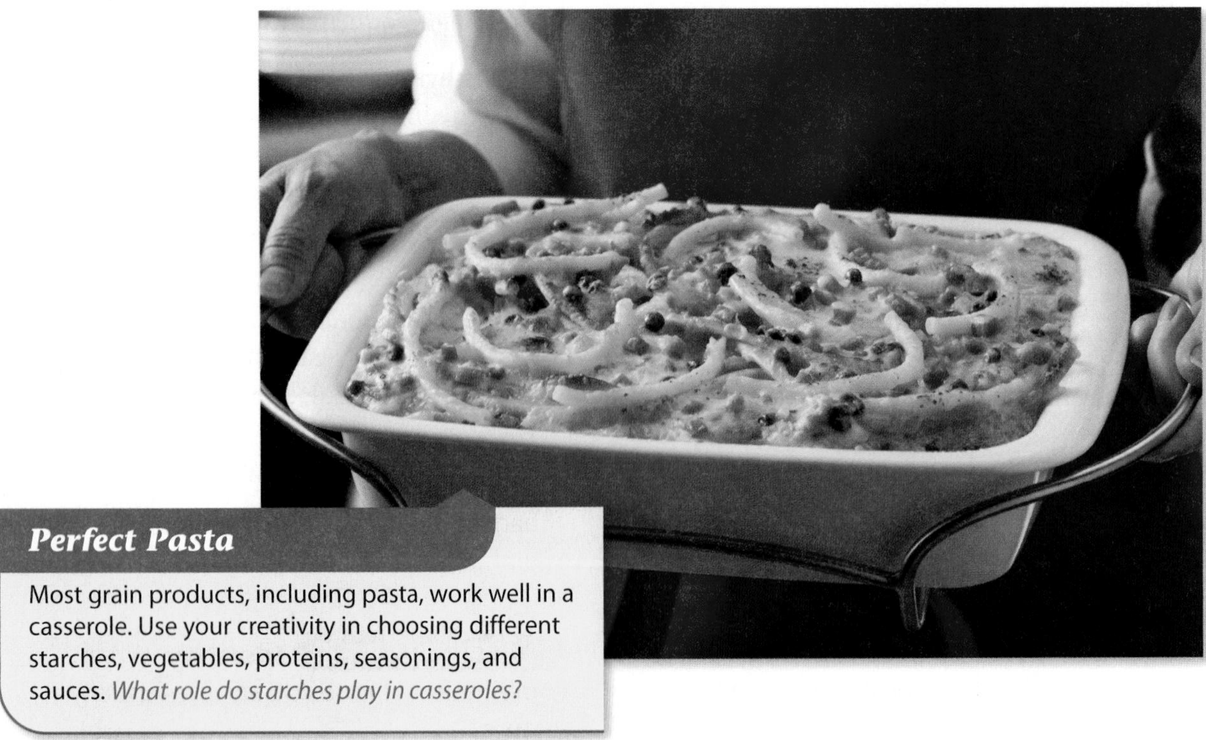

Perfect Pasta

Most grain products, including pasta, work well in a casserole. Use your creativity in choosing different starches, vegetables, proteins, seasonings, and sauces. *What role do starches play in casseroles?*

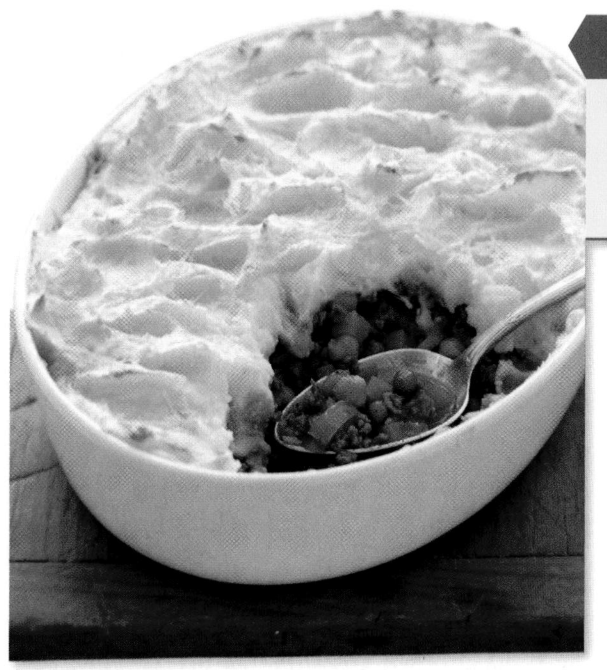

Tempting Topping

A shepherd's pie is a type of casserole with a topping of mashed potatoes over a blend of ground meat, onion, corn, green beans, and seasonings. *What other ingredients can be used to top casseroles?*

Starches

Starches thicken a casserole by absorbing liquids. They also add flavor and nutrients. You can use starches such as cooked dry beans, potatoes, and cooked grain products including pasta, rice, and barley. You might also try something new, such as quinoa or wild rice.

Bread also works well in casseroles. A brunch casserole might include cubes of bread, cheese, and ham in a custard of beaten eggs and milk. Poultry stuffing uses coarse, fresh, or dry bread cubes.

Binders

A **binder** is a liquid that helps hold a mixture together. Binders come in different textures and flavors. Milk, cream soup, and pasta sauce work well as binders in casseroles and can help to thicken the mixture. A baked macaroni and cheese casserole, for example, gets body from eggs, cheese, and milk.

Seasonings

Countless seasonings are used in casseroles. Herbs and spices such as oregano, basil, tarragon, black pepper, and marjoram bring out a food's savory qualities. For a sweet accent, try ginger, nutmeg, cinnamon, or allspice. In casseroles, dried herbs work better than fresh. Fresh herbs lose their flavor during long cooking times.

Casseroles can also be seasoned by bottled sauces such as soy, Worcestershire, tamari, barbecue, or hot pepper sauce. You can also add mustards and other condiments.

Some binders add seasonings as well. Canned, condensed soups are often highly salted. A pasta sauce may contribute garlic or Romano cheese. Canned beans often include spices. If you are adding a sauce or a soup, make sure not to add too much salt or other seasonings.

Toppings

Like dressings on salads, casserole toppings add flavor, color, and texture and keep the mixture from drying out. Crunchy toppings include croutons, cracker crumbs, and chow mein noodles.

Be a *Smart Consumer*

Convenient Casseroles

Due to consumers' increasing demand for convenience, the one-dish casserole has evolved into the one-hand meal. Common casseroles are widely available as frozen convenience foods. They make quick meals or snacks and can be heated in the microwave in a matter of minutes. Nutritionally, however, these convenient casseroles may not measure up to their traditional counterparts. They are often high in fat, calories, sodium, and additives.

Challenge Evaluate a frozen convenience casserole. How might a homemade casserole have better nutritional values? The trend of turning traditional foods into convenient forms has affected more than just casseroles. What other foods or meals are now available in convenient forms?

A casserole described as **au gratin** (ō-ˈgrä-tən) is topped with buttered breadcrumbs or grated cheese. It may be browned under the broiler after baking. Mashed potatoes and unbaked biscuits provide a fluffy topping texture.

You can top a casserole before it goes in the oven or a few minutes before it comes out. Some toppings need time to cook, while others brown quickly. Frozen onion rings need to bake with the casserole, for example, while cheese strips only need to melt for a few minutes.

Baking Casseroles

Most casseroles are baked in the oven. Prepare all the casserole ingredients, then mix them together, place them in a casserole dish, and cover them with topping. A casserole dish is about two to four inches deep and usually has a lid. Most are designed for both baking and serving.

Some casseroles are constructed in layers. Lasagne, for example, has several layers of cooked noodles, cooked ground meat or vegetables, ricotta or cottage cheese, and tomato sauce, with grated cheese as a topping.

Casseroles are typically baked for 30 to 45 minutes in an oven preheated to about 350°F. They may be covered at the beginning and uncovered toward the end of the cooking time to thicken the mixture or brown the crust. Casseroles should rest for about 10 minutes before serving so that the ingredients can set.

Casseroles can be microwaved, too. Combine all ingredients except the topping in an ungreased baking dish. Cover and cook the casserole at 100 percent power for 6 to 18 minutes, depending on the ingredients. Stir once or twice during cooking, or rotate large layered casseroles through the cooking time. Add the topping and brown the casserole under the broiler to achieve a crisp, browned surface.

Light and Healthy Recipe

Baked Ziti

This is a nutritious dish that can be prepared early, then placed in the oven to finish shortly before dinner time.

Ingredients

4 tsp. Olive oil
1 cup Diced onions
½ pound Ground turkey
1 pound Dried ziti or penne pasta
1 jar (26 oz.) Prepared low-sodium spaghetti sauce
8 oz. Shredded lowfat mozzarella cheese

Directions

1. Fill a large pot with water and bring to a boil.
2. Heat the olive oil in a pan on medium heat and add the onions. Cook until tender. Add the ground turkey and continue cooking until it is done.
3. Preheat the oven to 350°. Cook the pasta in the boiling water.
4. Drain the pasta and return it to the pot. Add the sauce, ground turkey and onions and mix well.
5. Pour the mixture evenly into a baking pan. Top with the cheese and cover with aluminum foil. Bake for 25 minutes. Remove the foil and bake uncovered an additional 10 minutes.

Yield 8 servings

Nutrition Analysis per Serving

■ Calories	418
■ Total fat	9 g
Saturated fat	3 g
Cholesterol	23 mg
■ Sodium	245 mg
■ Carbohydrate	56 g
Dietary fiber	4 g
Sugars	11 g
■ Protein	24 g

CHAPTER 40 Review & Applications

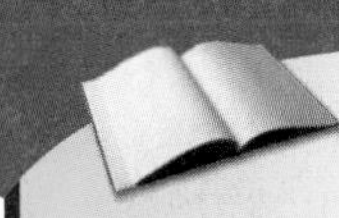

After You Read

Chapter Summary

A stir-fry is a combination dish of bite-sized pieces of food. Preparation and organization are needed to cook a stir-fry. Stir-fries usually contain grains, vegetables, protein, and sauce. The ingredients should be arranged in a certain order and cooked using the proper kitchen tools. A casserole is a flavorful combination of foods in a one-dish meal. They usually contain a main ingredient, vegetables, starches, binders, seasonings, and toppings. Casseroles are easy to assemble and bake. Both stir-fries and casseroles can be nutritious, economical, and convenient dishes.

Content and Academic Vocabulary Review

1. Use six of these content and academic vocabulary words in a short story about making a meal.

Content Vocabulary

- ☐ stir-fry (p. 622)
- ☐ mise en place (p. 624)
- ☐ wok (p. 624)
- ☐ casserole (p. 626)
- ☐ binder (p. 627)
- ☐ au gratin (p. 628)

Academic Vocabulary

- coordinate (p. 622)
- continuously (p. 625)

Review Key Concepts

2. **Summarize** the basic steps of stir-frying.
3. **Explain** the roles of basic ingredients in a casserole.

Critical Thinking

4. **Explain** why a stir-fry is a good meal for a single person who lives alone.
5. **Predict** what will happen if Eli stir-fries leftover chicken and then adds vegetables.
6. **Evaluate** Phil's plan to cut dime-sized bell peppers, quarter-sized zucchinis, and slivered carrots for his stir-fry.
7. **Create** an original stir-fry combination that balances taste, color, and texture. Explain why you think these ingredients will work well together.
8. **Evaluate** Molly's decision to make her broccoli-chicken-cheese casserole lower in fat by adding only ½ cup of cheese instead of the 1 cup that the recipe requires.
9. **Explain** why Ben's mixed vegetable and cheese casserole turned out watery. What can he do to prevent this in the future?
10. **Analyze** why many people regard casseroles as comfort food.

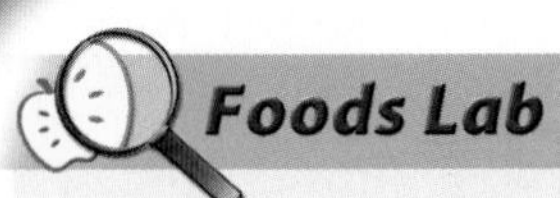

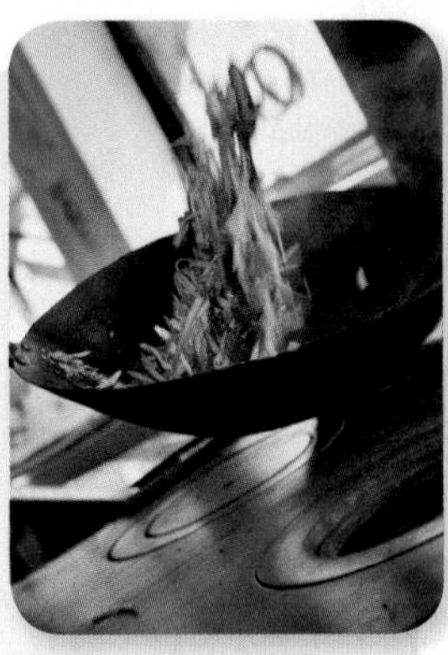

11. Stir-Fry Recipes Stir-fries are fun to cook because they allow room for creativity. The possible combinations of foods are virtually limitless.

Procedure Develop a recipe for a stir-fry. Use grains, vegetables, a protein food, seasonings, and a simple sauce. Prepare the recipe, and ask three other lab teams to sample it.

Analysis Develop an evaluation form that asks other lab teams to assess the flavor, texture, and appearance of your recipe, and to make suggestions for improvement. Collect the forms, and use them to determine three specific ways to improve your recipe.

HEALTHFUL CHOICES

12. Low-Calorie Combination Myra is hosting a dinner party. She wants to provide a low-calorie combination dish as an option for people who are watching their calorie intake. She is deciding between a rice, mixed vegetable, and seafood stir-fry, or a potato, mixed vegetable, shredded beef, and cheese casserole. Which should she prepare and why? Do you think one type of combination dish is generally lower in calories than the other type? Explain.

TECH Connection

13. From Side Dish to One-Dish Choose a vegetable or fruit that is often used in side dishes for a meal. Apples, sweet potatoes, and green beans are examples. Find and compare recipes for three casseroles that use the food as a main ingredient. Which one is the most nutritious? Use word processing software to type the recipe, and contribute it to a cookbook for the foods lab.

Real-World Skills

Problem-Solving Skills

14. Strong Sauce Diedre used herbs and spices, juice, and soy sauce to make a sauce for her stir fry. Before she cooked the sauce, it tasted just right. After she cooked it, it was too strong and overwhelmed the other the ingredients. Explain why. Note how she can prevent it next time.

Interpersonal and Collaborative Skills

15. Quiz Show Follow your teacher's instructions to form groups. Work together to develop ten quiz questions about stir-fries and casseroles. Develop a format for a TV quiz show, or imitate the format of an existing quiz show. Invite another team to come on your "show" and answer the questions you have developed.

Financial Literacy Skills

16. Vegetable Comparison Your stir-fry calls for a half-pound of each vegetable. Half-pound packages of pre-cut carrots, sweet potatoes, and zucchini sell for $3.29 each. Carrots are $1.88 per pound, sweet potatoes cost $1.69 per pound, and zucchinis cost $2.09 per pound. Is it more economical to buy the whole vegetables and cut them up yourself, or should you buy the pre-cut vegetables?

Academic Skills

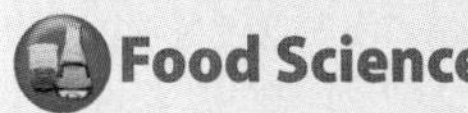

Food Science

17. Casseroles A casserole is both a baking dish and a one-dish meal.

Procedure Cook 1 cup of elbow macaroni in boiling water about 10 minutes. Drain. Make a roux in a separate pan with 1 tablespoon each of butter and flour. Whisk in 1¼ cups milk, and cook until slightly thickened. Season. Add 1½ cups of grated cheddar cheese, stirring until melted. Stir in the cooked macaroni, and transfer to a 1-quart casserole. Bake at 350°F about 25 minutes.

Analysis What is the purpose of the roux?

NSES B Develop an understanding of structure and properties of matter.

Mathematics

18. Measuring Circles A wok has a flat, circular bottom that is 5½ inches in diameter. The top of the wok is much wider, at 10¾ inches in diameter. The base of the casserole dish has a diameter of 9 inches, while the top of the casserole dish is 11 inches in diameter. For each dish, calculate the ratio of the circumference of the top to the circumference of the base.

Math Concept Circumference The distance around a circle is its circumference. Calculate circumference (C) as $C = \pi d$, where d = the circle's diameter and $\pi = 3.14$. If you know the radius (r), use $C = 2\pi r$.

Starting Hint Calculate all four circumferences, rounded to the nearest inch. For each dish, write a fraction with the top circumference as the numerator and the bottom circumference as the denominator. Reduce to lowest terms.

NCTM Measurement Apply appropriate techniques, tools, and formulas to determine measurements.

English Language Arts

19. Wok Poster Using knowledge you have gained from this chapter, combine words and images to create an educational poster about cooking with a wok and the utensils used with woks. Name and describe the purpose of each tool. Be sure your poster teaches basic concepts about wok cooking. Make sure every item on your poster is properly labeled.

NCTE 8 Use information resources to gather information and create and communicate knowledge.

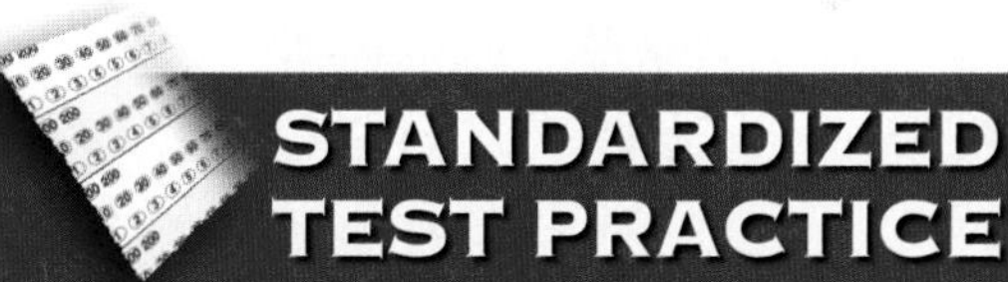

STANDARDIZED TEST PRACTICE

READING COMPREHENSION

Re-read the paragraph about binders on page 627. Then select the best answer to the question.

20. Binders are ____________.

a. usually made with dairy foods.

b. available in different textures and flavors.

c. important because they absorb excess liquid.

d. the most important ingredient in a casserole.

Test-Taking Tip Before you answer a reading comprehension question, closely read the text to which the question refers. Then read through the question and each of the answer choices. Next, take a second look at the text to confirm which answer is correct. Some answers may seem identical, but they contain subtle differences. Pay attention to every word.

CHAPTER 41

Soups, Stews, & Sauces

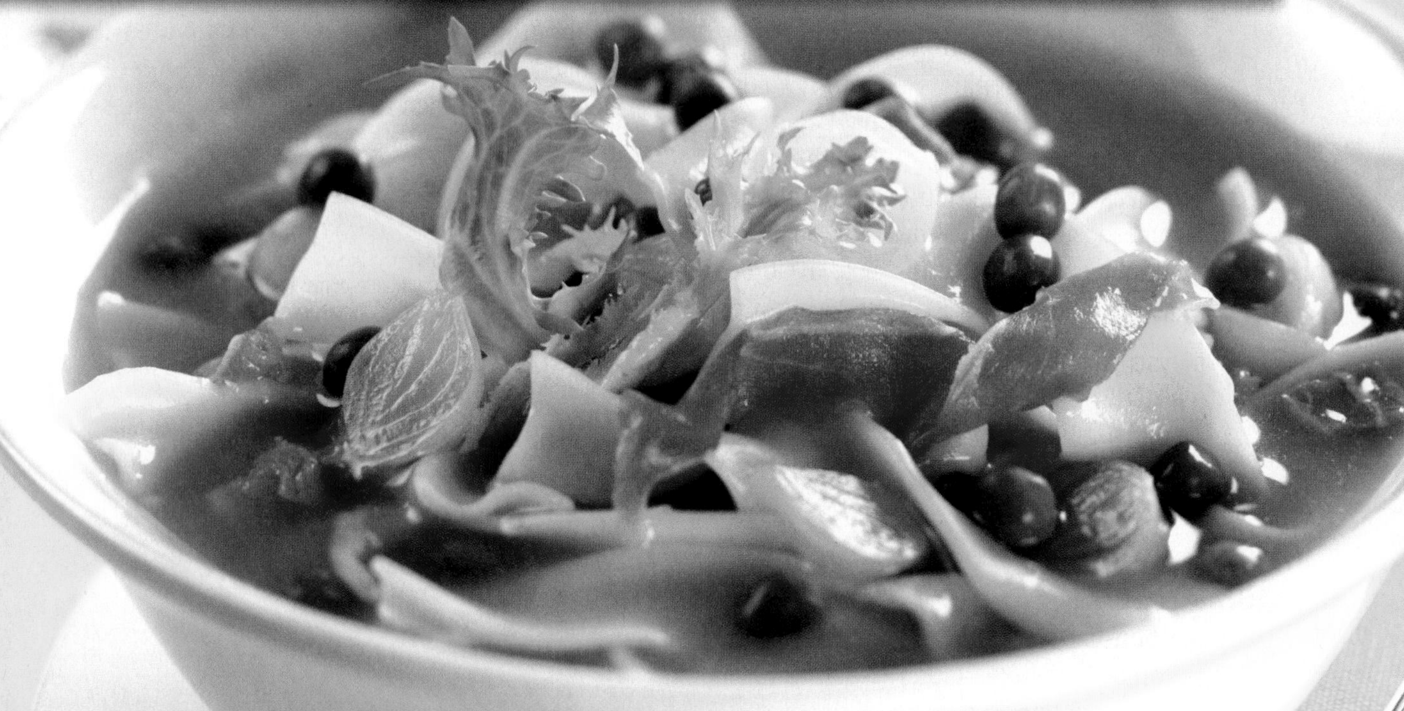

Writing Activity 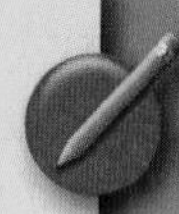 Dialogue

The Scoop on Soup Write a dialogue between two people, an adult and a young child. Imagine the child is about to try soup for the first time. What questions will the child have? What will the adult tell the child about soup? What comments will the child make after tasting the soup?

Writing Tips Follow these steps to write a dialogue:

- Indicate clearly who is speaking.
- Convey characters' ages and personalities through their speech.
- Use quotation marks before and after the speaker's words.

Activate Prior Knowledge

Explore the Photo Soup comes in many different forms and flavors, from rich and creamy to light and fruity. *What is your favorite soup?*

Reading Guide

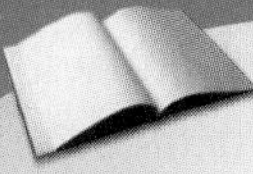

Before You Read

Preview Write the first three words that come to your mind when you think of soups, stews, and sauces. Then skim through the chapter and think about the variety among these foods.

Read to Learn

Key Concepts

- **Explain** how to make broth and stock.
- **List** ways to thicken a liquid.
- **Summarize** how to make a basic chicken vegetable soup.
- **Describe** how to make a basic meat stew.
- **Describe** six types of sauces.

Main Idea

Soups, stews, and sauces are flavorful and versatile creations that can be made using a variety of ingredients.

Content Vocabulary

You will find definitions for these words in the glossary at the back of this book.

- ☐ broth
- ☐ stock
- ☐ bouillon
- ☐ reduction
- ☐ cornstarch
- ☐ gelatinization
- ☐ roux
- ☐ soup
- ☐ consommé
- ☐ bisque
- ☐ stew
- ☐ sauce
- ☐ au jus
- ☐

Academic Vocabulary

You will find these words in your reading and on your tests. Use the glossary to look up their definitions if necessary.

- originated
- associated

Graphic Organizer

Use a graphic organizer like the one below to take notes about the four basic steps for making soup.

Making Soup

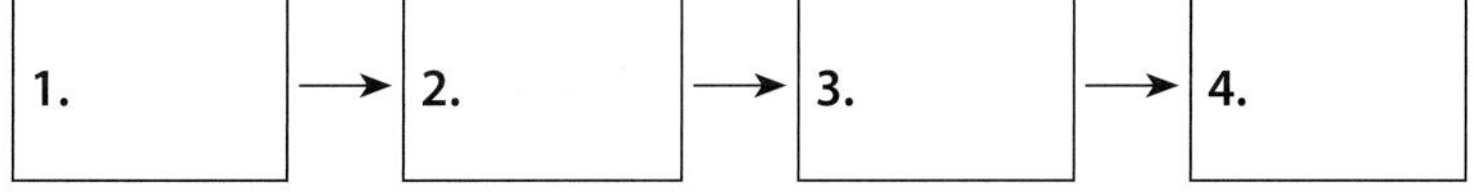

Graphic Organizer Go to this book's Online Learning Center at **glencoe.com** to print out this graphic organizer.

Academic Standards

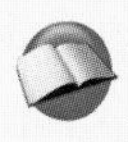

English Language Arts

NCTE 12 Use language to accomplish individual purposes.

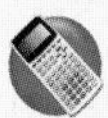

Mathematics

NCTM Problem Solving Apply and adapt a variety of appropriate strategies to solve problems.

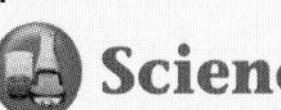

Science

NSES B Develop an understanding of the structure and properties of matter.

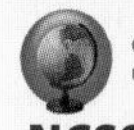

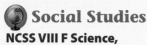

Social Studies

NCSS VIII F Science, Technology, and Society Formulate strategies and develop policies for influencing public discussions associated with technology-society issues.

NCTE *National Council of Teachers of English*
NCTM *National Council of Teachers of Mathematics*
NSES *National Science Education Standards*
NCSS *National Council for the Social Studies*

Base Liquids

Stews, sauces, and soups have two basic ingredients: a liquid and a thickener. The liquid is often broth or stock. **Broth** is the flavorful liquid made by simmering meat, poultry, fish, animal bones, or vegetables in water. **Stock** is similar to broth, but is made with vegetables and sometimes animal bones, and not meat. These liquids form the foundation of sauces and soups. A beef stew might start with beef broth, while a pumpkin soup might start with vegetable stock. A mild soup based on one vegetable can also use juice as a base. Tomato soup, for example, might start with tomato juice.

Making Broth and Stock

Making broth and stock can be time-consuming, but it often gives a richer flavor than store-bought broths and stocks. Making broth or stock at home also lets you create exactly the flavor you like.

Broth or stock is a great use for food scraps such as seafood shells, vegetable trimmings or peels, and animal bones. Bones with some meat attached give the richest flavor. The gelatin in bones from raw meat and poultry adds richness. Aromatic vegetables, such as onions, leeks, carrots, and celery, lend a complex flavor.

Rinse the bones in cold water to remove any impurities. Place the ingredients in a large pot with herbs and cover the ingredients with cold water. Bring the water to a boil, then turn down the heat and let the mixture simmer for several hours. Simmering slowly allows the ingredients to release their full flavor. Add water if necessary so that the solid ingredients remain submerged. As a final step, strain the broth or stock and discard the solid ingredients.

Harmful bacteria can multiply in broth or stock as it cools, especially if it has fat or protein from meat. Pour the broth into shallow containers and chill it quickly. Any fat will set and rise to the surface. When the stock has cooled, suction the fat off with a baster or skim it off with a spoon and discard it. Transfer the stock to a plastic container with a tight-fitting lid. Use homemade broth or stock within about four days, or freeze it in recipe-size portions for up to three months.

Buying Prepared Broth and Stock

If you do not have the time or ingredients to make homemade broth or stock, you can choose from convenience forms. Canned or boxed ready-to-use broth and stock come in several varieties, including reduced-sodium, fat-free, vegetarian, and organic. Concentrated stocks are also available. These come in cubes or granules that are dissolved in hot water. This form is often labeled **bouillon** (ˈbü(l)-ˌyän), which is another name for broth or stock. Convenience broths are sometimes flavored with animal fat and dehydrated meat, poultry, or vegetables, but their main ingredient is usually salt.

✓ Reading Check **Explain** What is the difference between broth and stock?

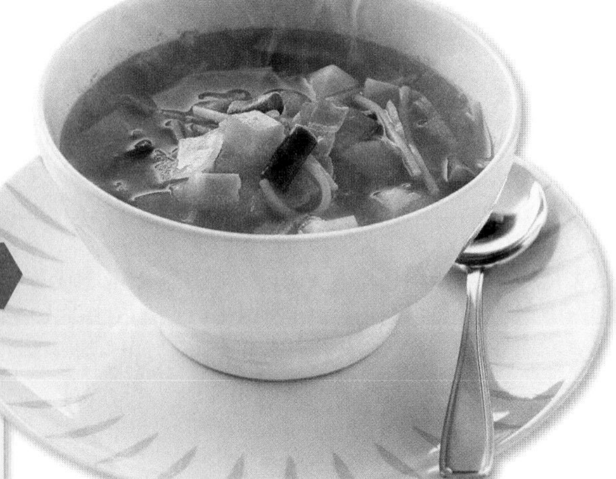

Super Soup

Every cuisine features some type of soup. Soup is both elegant and economical, and comes in many different flavors. *How much soup should you make for a dinner party with 12 guests, if you plan to serve it as an appetizer?*

Figure 41.1 Using Flour or Cornstarch for Thickening

Starch Amounts It takes about twice as much flour as cornstarch to thicken a cup of liquid. ***What effect do flour and cornstarch have on a liquid's appearance?***

Degree of Thickness	Cornstarch	Flour
Thin	1 ½ tsp.	1 Tbsp.
Medium	1 Tbsp.	2 Tbsp.
Thick	1 ½ Tbsp.	3 Tbsp.

Thickening Methods

In many soups, stews, and sauces, the liquid is thickened. This gives a richer flavor and consistency. This is done by using a thickening agent. A thickening agent is an ingredient that adds body to the soup, stew, or sauce. There are two ways to thicken a soup, stew, or sauce: decrease the amount of liquid or add starch or protein to absorb liquid.

As you thicken soups, stews, and sauces, cook them over low or medium heat. High heat speeds evaporation, and the food may get too thick or burn. Evaporation continues as the mixture cools, often leaving an unsightly skin of concentrated proteins on the surface. To prevent this, lightly press a piece of wax paper or plastic wrap onto the surface and leave it in place until serving time.

Reduction

A simple thickening technique is **reduction**, the process of simmering an uncovered mixture until some of the liquid evaporates. Cook the liquid until it reaches the volume and consistency you prefer. Reduction is often used to thicken liquids used in cooking meat or vegetables. For example, you might poach fish in fish stock and then simmer it down into a sauce after the fish is done cooking. A liquid can be cooked down to one-half or one-fourth of its original amount.

Reduction concentrates flavors because the amount of water is reduced, so wait until the liquid is reduced to season it to taste.

Grain Products

Another way to thicken soups, stews, and sauces is to use the starch in grain products.

Prepared Grain Products

Whole grains and baked products thicken soups and stews by absorbing water and releasing starch as they cook. They also contribute texture and nutrients. Many European cuisines use grain products in soups and stews. Oats are popular in some Irish stews. The German beef dish sauerbraten is served with gravy thickened with ground gingersnap cookies.

Add grains such as barley and rice to a soup or stew according to their cooking time. If rice takes 20 minutes to cook, add it when the soup has 20 minutes of cooking time left. You can also soak bread slices or crumbs with water to make a paste and then stir in the paste during the last 10 minutes of cooking.

Flour and Cornstarch

Flour is the most common thickener for soups, stews, and sauces. Any flour works, but all-purpose flour works best because it has more starch than other types. Flour can also be combined with butter that has just been melted as a quick way to thicken. A liquid thickened with flour turns opaque, like gravy.

Cornstarch is another popular thickener. **Cornstarch** is a fine, white powder of pure starch made from the endosperm of the corn kernel. Cornstarch is often used to thicken desserts and Asian stir-fries. Cornstarch has twice the thickening power of flour, as seen in **Figure 41.1**.

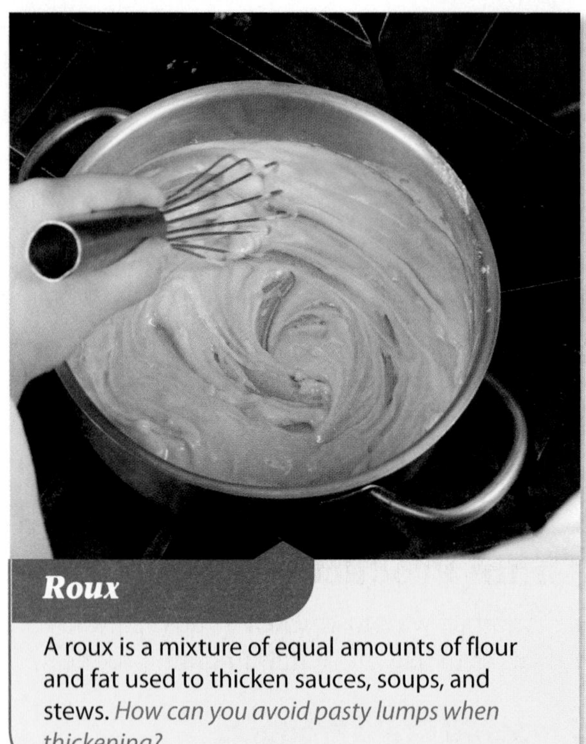

Roux

A roux is a mixture of equal amounts of flour and fat used to thicken sauces, soups, and stews. *How can you avoid pasty lumps when thickening?*

Unappetizing lumps form if you add flour or cornstarch directly to hot liquid. If caught in time, these pasty lumps can be mashed against the sides of the pan or strained out. To avoid lumps, follow these three steps:

1. Mix starch and cold water. Mix one part starch with two parts cold water in a jar or small bowl. This separates the starch granules so they will not clump together when they make contact with the hot liquid. This mixture is called a slurry. You can vary how much starch you use to get different consistencies. A medium thickness is enough to coat the back of a spoon. To thicken 1 cup of liquid to medium thickness, you need 2 tablespoons of flour. Mix that amount with twice as much cold water, or 4 tablespoons (¼ cup), before adding it to the hot liquid.

2. Pour slowly and stir. Slowly pour the cool starch mixture into the hot liquid, stirring gently all the while.

3. Simmer and stir. Simmer the hot liquid over medium heat until it thickens, stirring constantly to keep the starch granules separated. You need to simmer a flour mixture for several minutes to get rid of the raw flour taste.

Thickened mixtures are sensitive. If you overcook them, freeze them, or stir them too much, they can become runny again. To avoid this problem, add starch during the last minutes of cooking and simmer the mixture very gently. Freeze soup or stew unthickened, and stir in the starch when you reheat it for serving.

Gelatinization The chemical process that takes place as starch thickens liquid is called **gelatinization** (jə-ˌla-tə-nə-ˈzā-shən). Energized by heat, the starch granules absorb water and swell. Eventually, the granules burst and the starch that rushes out thickens the liquid very quickly. Wait for this thickening process to occur before deciding you need to add extra starch. Adding more starch too soon might make your dish too thick. Acids interfere with gelatinization. If you plan to add an ingredient such as lemon juice, wait until the liquid has thickened.

Making a Roux

Another way to use flour to thicken a liquid is to make a roux. A **roux** (ˈrü) is a mixture of equal amounts of flour and fat. You can use butter, margarine, or fat drippings from cooked foods. Use Figure 41.1 to figure out how much flour you need for the thickness you want and the amount of liquid you have.

Measure out the amount of flour and fat you need. If necessary, melt the fat over medium heat to liquefy it. Then stir in the flour. Keep stirring until the fat coats the starch granules and a smooth paste forms. Cook and stir the roux only until it bubbles. Gradually stir the roux into the liquid that you want to thicken. Stirring constantly, continue to cook it over low heat until the mixture is smooth and thick.

Some recipes call for a roux that is beige to dark brown in color. You create a darker roux by cooking it longer, as long as 20 minutes or more. This creates a nutty flavor but lessens the roux's thickening power. Constant attention and frequent stirring is necessary when making a dark roux because it can burn easily. You need more flour in proportion to fat, depending on how much you plan to brown the roux.

You can refrigerate or freeze uncooked roux by the tablespoon, and use it when you need to fix a runny sauce.

Legumes and Vegetables

Cooked legumes and vegetables thicken in the same way that grain products do. Beans, split peas, and other high-starch foods thicken best. Broccoli, squash, and carrots thicken less well because they have less starch, but they add more color and flavor. Mash or purée the ingredients and stir them into the soup or stew. Simmer a few minutes to let them blend, release their starch, and heat through.

You can thicken 1 cup of liquid with 3 tablespoons of grated raw potato. Add the potato about 15 to 20 minutes before the end of the cooking time.

Eggs

Eggs are less effective than starch at thickening liquids, but they add richness and flavor. Generally, 1 large egg or 2 yolks thicken 1 cup of liquid, depending on the other foods in the mixture.

Eggs curdle easily when added to a hot liquid or an acidic food, so they must be tempered. First beat the eggs lightly. Then stir in a small amount of the hot or acidic liquid. Pour the diluted egg mixture a little at a time into the rest of the liquid, stirring constantly. If the mixture starts to curdle, strenuous beating and straining can sometimes save it.

✓ **Reading Check** **Describe** How do prepared grain products thicken soups and stews?

Soup Types and Cooking Method

A **soup** is a dish made by cooking solid foods in liquid. Soups often contain broth or stock as the liquid, along with meat, poultry, seafood, grains, or vegetables.

All cultures have recipes for soup, and some recipes go back for thousands of years. The ancient Greeks, for example, ate white beans in beef broth and garbanzo beans with spinach. Borscht, a beet soup that can be served cold or hot, was first served in Eastern Europe in the 5th century. Certain international soups, such as French onion, have become mainstream in the U.S.

Soups can be highly nutritious, especially when they are filled with vegetables. Long cooking destroys vitamin C and some of the B vitamins, but other water-soluble vitamins remain in the liquid.

Soups can be served as a starter or a main dish. As a rule, one quart of soup serves six as an appetizer or three as an entrée. Refrigerate leftover soups immediately. Use leftover soup within three or four days or freeze it for up to three months.

Types of Soup

Soup comes in five basic types: clear, cream, chunky, fruit, and cold. Most soups, except fruit soups, are savory.

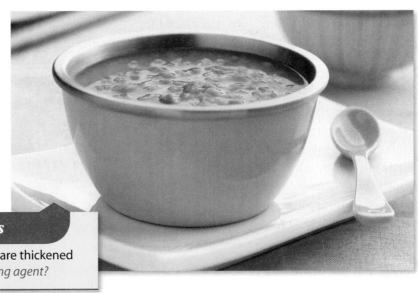

Legumes as Thickeners

Some soups, like split pea soup, are thickened with legumes. *What is a thickening agent?*

Clear Soups

Broth provides a base for more complex soups and sauces, but it is also served as a clear, thin soup. **Consommé** is a clarified broth, completely strained of all particles and sediment. A broth or stock is clarified by cooking it with egg whites, finely chopped vegetables and herbs. As the egg white cooks, it absorbs the fats and other impurities in the stock. Once the stock is strained, it is a clear consommé. It is often served warm as an appetizer. A favorite breakfast food in Japan is a clear soup made from miso (ˈmē-(ˌ)sō), a fermented soybean paste.

Cream Soups

Cream soups are smooth but thick. Many cream soups are made with some form of milk. Because cream soups are made with milk, it is best to eat them soon after preparing them. A smooth cream soup typically begins with vegetables and seasonings that are cooked in a liquid such as broth. The mixture is puréed in a blender, food processor, or food mill and thickened with flour and milk or cream. Low-fat recipes use evaporated milk or nonfat dry milk powder.

Almost any vegetable can be used as the base for a cream soup. Broccoli, squash, and asparagus are popular choices. A **bisque** (ˈbisk) is a rich cream soup that uses shellfish as the base.

Soups made with starchy foods such as potatoes and legumes become creamy without puréeing or adding milk or thickeners. Split pea soup, for instance, is made by cooking green split peas in liquid with seasonings and puréeing the mixture. You can make black bean soup by cooking black beans in water, puréeing the mixture, and adding seasonings, including hot pepper sauce and liquid smoke.

Chunky Soups

Chunky soups brim with chunks of vegetables, meat, poultry, seafood, legumes, and pasta in assorted combinations. A chunky soup, some crusty bread, and a salad make a simple but nourishing meal.

Here are a few of the most popular chunky soups:

Chowder Chowders are made with fish, meat, or vegetables and thickened with potatoes or cream. Some chowders are thickened with roux. The classic New England clam chowder is thick with cream, chunky with potatoes, and flavored with bacon. Manhattan clam chowder is lighter and features chunks of potatoes and tomatoes.

Mulligatawny (ˌmə-lə-gə-ˈtȯ-nē) Mulligatawny means "pepper water" in southern India, where this soup **originated**, or came into existence. It starts with a chicken broth, highly seasoned with chiles, curry powder, and other spices. Some versions include poultry or meat, a variety of vegetables, rice, eggs or cream.

Minestrone (ˌmi-nə-ˈstrō-nē; mi-nə-ˈstrōn) Minestrone is a hearty Italian soup made with vegetables, beans, and pasta and topped with grated Parmesan cheese.

Fruit Soups

Fruit soups have their origins in Scandinavia and Eastern Europe. They are served hot or cold and can be made with fresh seasonal fruits or with dried, canned, or frozen fruits.

To make fruit soup, fruits are puréed, flavored with spices or grated peel, and thickened with cornstarch, gelatin, buttermilk, or yogurt. Dry fruits, and sometimes fresh, are simmered first in water or juice. Richer recipes call for light cream or sour cream.

Cold Soups

Fruit soups are not the only soups that can be served cold. Cold vegetable soups make a refreshing beginning to a meal, especially in hot weather. Cold soups are either cooked and chilled, or they are not cooked at all. Vichyssoise and gazpacho are two of the most common cold soups.

Vichyssoise (ˌvi-shī-ˈswäz) One of the most popular cooked cold soups is vichyssoise. An elegant purée of cooked leeks and potatoes in heavy cream, vichyssoise is usually garnished with chives.

Gazpacho (gəz-ˈpä-(ˌ)-chō) Dry bread is soaked and puréed with fresh tomatoes, bell peppers, onions, celery, cucumbers, olive oil, and vinegar to create gazpacho. This well-seasoned, uncooked soup originated in southern Spain.

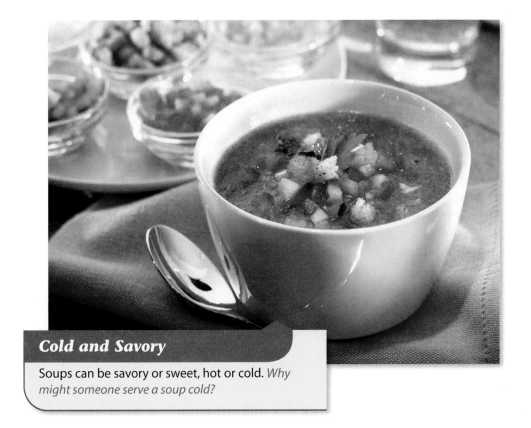

Cold and Savory

Soups can be savory or sweet, hot or cold. *Why might someone serve a soup cold?*

Making Soup

The way you start a soup depends on the result you want. For a hot, simmered soup, such as chicken vegetable soup, follow these four basic steps.

1. Sauté aromatic vegetables. Sauté chopped onions, carrots, celery, garlic, and other aromatic vegetables in a pot or slow cooker.

2. Add liquid and solids. Add the liquid and main ingredients to the pot. You can add flavor and color by using three or four different vegetables such as tomatoes, potatoes, carrots, and corn. Add ingredients at different times, if needed, depending on how long each one takes to cook. For a chicken, rice, and vegetable soup, raw chicken nuggets go in first, followed by rice, sliced fresh vegetables, and cooked vegetables. As an alternative, you can sauté the chicken first to bring out the flavor. You can also put in whole pieces of chicken, remove the flesh from the bones after cooking, and return the chicken to the pot.

3. Season and simmer. Season and simmer the soup until all ingredients are tender. Thicken the broth if needed. Finally, taste the soup and adjust the seasonings before serving.

4. Garnish. Soup can be garnished to enhance appearance, complement flavor, and add texture. You might top a thin onion soup with crisp croutons or finish a seafood chowder with a sprinkle of chopped, fresh parsley. You can place toppings in each bowl before serving or arrange them as an assortment to let guests choose their own.

Soups with Convenience

Homemade soups take time. A microwave oven can help with some steps, but not with the slow simmering needed to tenderize meats or bring out flavors. Many people make a large pot of soup when time permits and refrigerate or freeze servings for later meals. Frozen soup stored in individual containers is easy to reheat in the microwave.

Packaged soup starters speed preparation. You can also make your own soup starter. Stir together grains, legumes, seasonings, and bouillon granules. Store the mix in a cool, dry place. To prepare, add liquid and fresh ingredients to the mix and simmer it until done.

✓ **Reading Check** **Identify** What are two types of cold soups?

Stew Types and Cooking Method

A **stew** is any dish prepared by stewing, or simmering, pieces of food in a tightly covered pan. Most stews include vegetables and meat, poultry, or fish. Stews usually contain less liquid than soups. Most stews are made with water, but broth, tomato or vegetable juice, or fruit juice can also be used. Stew ingredients are usually cut into larger pieces than soup ingredients. This helps them to retain their individual flavors. Stews are more likely to be served as main courses than soups.

Stews have several names, with subtle differences in meaning. A ragout (ra-ˈgü) is thick, meaty, and highly seasoned. Fricassee (ˈfri-kə-ˌsē) usually refers to a chicken stew. To fricassee is to sauté in butter without browning, which is the first step in the recipe.

Many world cuisines have special stews, including:

Goulash Goulash is a Hungarian dish made with beef cubes, onions, bell peppers, water, vinegar, and lots of paprika. It is usually served over buttered noodles or a pasta called spaetzle, which is made from flour and eggs.

Irish Stew A traditional Irish stew is made with lamb, water, potatoes, onions, and parsley. Turnips, carrots, and barley are sometimes added as well.

Dovi (dō-ˈvē) Started in Zimbabwe, dovi is a stew with tomatoes, sweet potatoes, okra, and other vegetables simmered with chicken in a stock thickened with peanut butter. Dovi is traditionally scooped from a communal pot with flatbread or served with cornmeal mush.

Israeli Wheat Berry Stew This hearty vegetarian stew uses the entire wheat kernel, or berry, along with beans and potatoes. It is seasoned with garlic and onions.

Posole (pō-ˈsō-(ˌ)lā) Many Mexican homes serve the pork stew posole as a Christmas tradition. Authentic recipes use posole corn kernels that have been soaked and dried. Hominy, the flaked inner kernel, is a common replacement. Posole is seasoned with chiles, garlic, and cilantro, and topped with thinly sliced lettuce, cabbage, or radishes.

Burgoo (ˈbər-ˌgü) A meat stew that originated in the South, burgoo traditionally featured game such as squirrel or deer. Modern versions feature beef and chicken along with carrots, tomatoes, potatoes, cabbage, celery, and onions.

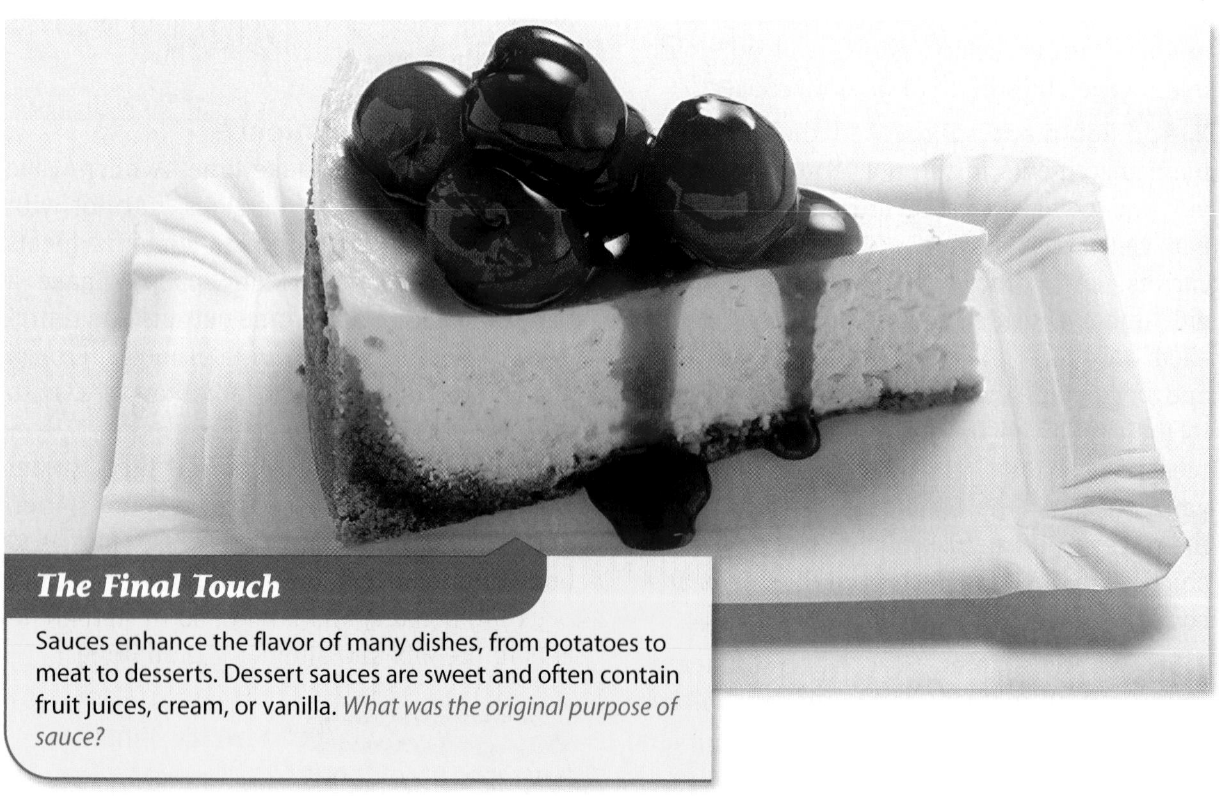

The Final Touch

Sauces enhance the flavor of many dishes, from potatoes to meat to desserts. Dessert sauces are sweet and often contain fruit juices, cream, or vanilla. *What was the original purpose of sauce?*

Making a Stew

Stew is an ideal way to prepare inexpensive cuts of meat and poultry. The slow simmering tenderizes tough cuts and releases juices that flavor the liquid. There is a basic method for making a meat stew.

1. Prepare the meat. Cut meat for stewing into 1- to 2-inch cubes. Cut chicken into parts. Since the chicken cooks in liquid, removing the skin reduces fat. Dredge the meat in flour and brown it in a small amount of fat in a large pot or skillet. Chicken may be browned or not, as you like. After cooking, transfer the meat to a clean plate. Drain any excess fat from the pan.

2. Sauté the vegetables. Sauté aromatic vegetables, such as onions, carrots, and celery, in the fat remaining in the pan. Because stews simmer for long periods, stews usually include large chunks or quarters of carrots, potatoes, parsnips, and other root vegetables and tubers. More delicate vegetables like baby corn can be added later during cooking.

3. Add water and simmer. Return the meat to the pan. Add seasonings and enough liquid to cover the meat. Cover the pan and simmer until the meat is tender. Beef may need to simmer for 2 to 3 hours. Poultry may cook in less than an hour. Fish may need as little as 10 minutes and is often added after other ingredients.

Stews can also be prepared in an oven or a slow cooker. Meat or poultry may be browned or simply added with other ingredients. Browning produces an even, attractive color for the meat. Stew cooks at a low temperature, usually around 300°F, for up to 5 hours.

As with soups, it is important to refrigerate leftover stews immediately. Use them within three or four days or freeze them for up to three months.

Stew Variations

There are countless recipes for stews. To vary the flavor, consider adding fruit or juice to a stew. Some suitable combinations include pork with fresh apples, beef with dried plums or apricots, and poultry with pineapple or orange juice.

Science in Action

Thickening with Cornstarch

How does cornstarch thicken sauces? Heat causes the starch to bind to water molecules. The starch cells absorb liquid and swell. When a sauce nears boiling, the starch granules are about ten times their size at room temperature. Too much heat or stirring will cause the starch cells to rupture and the sauce to thin again.

Procedure Mix 2 tablespoons of cornstarch in ¼ cup of cold water. Add this slurry to some already-cooking pasta sauce. Heat the sauce to near boiling, and observe how it thickens. Then boil the sauce for several minutes while stirring. Watch what happens.

Analysis Verbally share your observations with the class. How did cornstarch affect the sauce? How did extra heat and motion affect the cornstarch?

NSES B Develop an understanding of the structure and properties of matter.

You can make a vegetarian stew by cooking virtually any vegetables with seasonings in vegetable broth. You might try carrots, tomatoes, bell peppers, leeks, turnips, okra, acorn squash, Brussels sprouts, or green beans.

A stew can be served over noodles, hot biscuits, mashed potatoes, or brown rice.

✓ **Reading Check** **Define** What are ragout and fricassee?

Sauce Types and Cooking Methods

A **sauce** is a flavored liquid that is often thickened and that is served to enhance the flavor of another food. Sauces come in many forms, from the ketchup served with french fries to the fruit sauce served on a pie.

Sauces go back to the days before refrigeration. They literally covered up the taste of foods that were going bad. Inspired by Italian chefs, the French elevated sauce making to an art by the 1800s. In fact, one principle of French cuisine states that "the sauce is everything."

Sauces come in several basic types: hollandaise, basic white, stock-based, and tomato-based.

Like soups and stews, leftover sauces should be refrigerated immediately. Some sauces may be frozen, but mixtures thickened with flour or cornstarch may separate when thawed.

Hollandaise Sauce

Hollandaise sauce is made by whisking egg yolks with melted butter and lemon juice over a double boiler. The texture of hollandaise sauce is smooth and creamy. The taste is rich and buttery. The yolks act as an emulsifier to hold the mixture together. Hollandaise sauce turns poached eggs, ham, and an English muffin into eggs Benedict. The sauce is also a favorite on asparagus or fish.

Hollandaise is the foundation for béarnaise (ˌbā-är-ˈnāz) sauce, which features white vinegar, green onions, and tarragon. Puréed tomatoes turn hollandaise into Choron (shō-ˈrän) sauce.

Basic White Sauce

White sauce is milk or cream thickened with a butter-and-flour roux. It is also called cream sauce or béchamel (ˌbā-shə-ˈmel). Make the roux according to the thickness you want. Cook the roux only until it bubbles, without browning it. Gradually stir in the milk and cook it over low heat, stirring constantly until thickened. Season as desired.

White sauce has a mild flavor that works well in many different classic recipes. Add heavy cream and Parmesan cheese to make Alfredo sauce to toss with pasta. Add cream and paprika to make a rich Newburg sauce for a lobster dish. White sauce is also the base for that great American classic, macaroni and cheese.

Stock-Based Sauces

A stock-based sauce is made like a white sauce, with animal fat and meat juices replacing the butter and milk. Poultry drippings and a white roux produce a light sauce. Red meat juices and a brown roux produce a brown sauce.

Pan or "country" gravy is a popular stock-based sauce. After cooking meat or poultry, remove it from the pan and pour the juices from the pan into a measuring cup. Skim off the fat and reserve it. Make a roux in the roasting pan, using 2 tablespoons each of flour and reserved fat for each cup of juice. Add beef or chicken broth if you do not have enough juice. For a richer flavor, scrape the bottom of the pan to loosen browned bits of meat or poultry. Use a wooden spoon to scrape. Never scrape a metal pan with a metal spoon.

Like white sauce, stock-based sauces can be expanded into different recipes. Chicken gravy reduced with heavy cream is called supreme sauce. Deviled sauce is a brown sauce made with vinegar or Worcestershire sauce and cayenne pepper.

TECHNOLOGY FOR TOMORROW

Sauce Stabilizers

In the past, certain types of sauces could not be sold in supermarkets because their ingredients would cause them to have a strange appearance and short shelf life. They would appear lumpy, or the oils in them would separate. Such sauces were best reserved for home cooking. Now, thanks to sauce stabilizers, a wide variety of sauces line supermarket shelves, ready to be heated and served. Stabilizers are additives that help sauces to maintain a uniform texture and consistency. They can also stabilize emulsions that would otherwise separate. Examples of stabilizers include guar gum, which is extract from beans, pectin, which comes from the cells of certain plants, and agar and carrageen, which are seaweed derivatives.

What do you think? Identify a supermarket product that uses a stabilizer and conduct research about the stabilizer. Prepare a presentation in which you use your research to argue for or against the use of the stabilizer.

NCSS VIII F Formulate strategies and develop policies for influencing public discussions associated with technology-society issues.

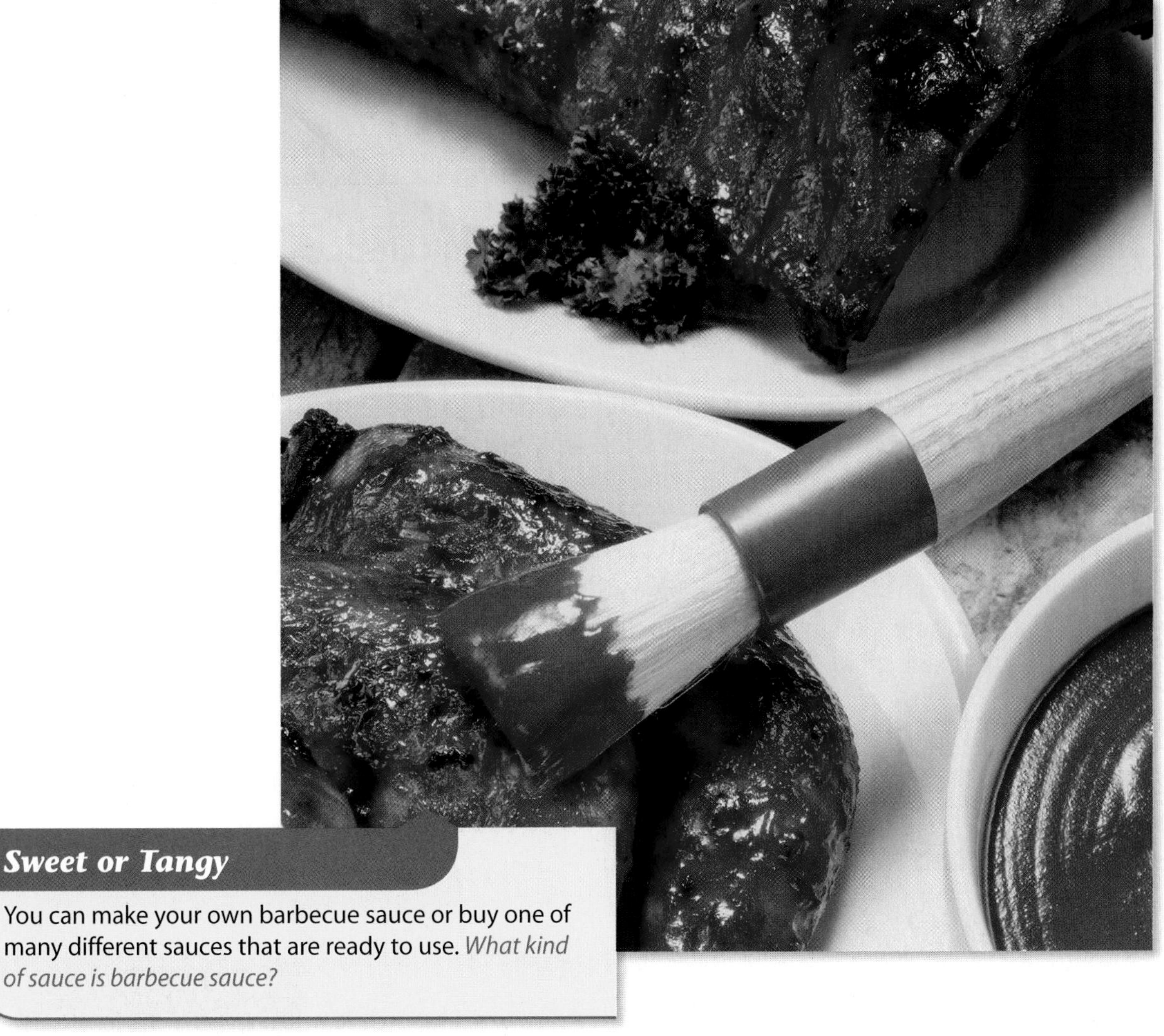

Sweet or Tangy

You can make your own barbecue sauce or buy one of many different sauces that are ready to use. *What kind of sauce is barbecue sauce?*

Tomato-Based Sauces

A basic tomato sauce takes nothing more than sautéed aromatic vegetables and a tomato product. The thickness, flavor, and color depend on the ingredients you choose. Tomatoes have a rich flavor, soft flesh, and high water content, so they cook into a sauce well.

The simplest tomato sauce consists of chopped tomatoes, simmered and seasoned with salt. Traditional Italian sauces start with onions and garlic sautéed in olive oil or butter. To maintain a smooth texture, stir in canned tomato paste or purée diluted with hot water or broth. Simmer and reduce to the desired thickness, adding herbs and spices in the last 10 minutes of cooking.

Tomato sauces are usually **associated** with, or connected to, pasta, but they complement other dishes as well. Slices of eggplant are breaded, fried, and covered with tomato sauce for eggplant Parmesan. You can serve rice with a hot Creole tomato sauce made with celery and bell pepper. Barbecue sauce is also a tomato-based sauce. Sweet barbecue sauce has brown sugar or molasses, and tangy barbecue sauce has mustard, onions, and garlic.

Oil-and-Vinegar Sauces

Oil-and-vinegar sauces use the same basic ingredients as vinaigrettes: oil, acidic liquids, and seasonings. Oil-and-vinegar sauces, however, use more vinegar than salad dressings do. An Asian sweet and sour sauce, for example, is made with a few tablespoons of peanut oil to a cup of rice vinegar, along with garlic, ginger, and ketchup.

Marinades are also oil-and-vinegar sauces. Marinades add flavor and tenderize less costly cuts of meat by breaking down connective tissue. To prevent eating contaminants picked up from raw meat, poultry, or fish, marinades should be discarded after use. You can make extra marinade to serve as a sauce. To make marinades, use any type of cooking oil and substitute other acidic ingredients for the vinegar, such as cider or buttermilk. For seasonings, try such aromatic vegetables as onions and garlic along with your choice of herbs and spices.

To use a marinade, shake the ingredients in a tightly closed jar. Place the food in a pan made of glass, stainless steel, or enamel. Pour the marinade over the food and refrigerate it. You can also marinate food in a plastic bag that zips securely closed. Place it in a container. For even coverage, turn or stir the food at least once while marinating.

Marinating time depends on the food. Fish fillets may get mushy after 30 minutes. Some meats can be marinated for up to 24 hours.

Quick Sauces

When time or other resources are short, you can make sauces by diluting cream soups with a little milk or stock. Yogurt is a common sauce base in Mediterranean cuisines. Tailor convenience sauces to fit your recipe by adding seasonings, mustard, honey, citrus juice, or relishes. The simplest, lightest option when preparing roasts is to serve them **au jus** (ō-ˈzhü(s)), with the natural meat juices, unthickened and skimmed of fat. For a quick marinade, try a salad dressing.

Light and Healthy Recipe

Marinara Sauce

Ingredients

- **¼ cup** Olive oil
- **2 cups** Onions, finely chopped
- **1 cup** Carrots, finely chopped
- **1 cup** Celery, finely chopped
- **3 cloves** Garlic, minced
- **3½ cups** Crushed tomatoes, canned
- **2 cups** Vegetable stock
- **1 tsp.** Ground basil
- **1 tsp.** Ground oregano

Directions

1. In a pan, warm the olive oil over medium heat.
2. Add the onions, carrots, and celery and cook until tender. Add the garlic. Carefully pour the sautéed vegetables into a blender. Cover and blend until liquified.
3. Return the puréed vegetables to the pan and add the crushed tomatoes.
4. Allow the vegetables to simmer until the tomatoes break down. Add the vegetable stock and spices.
5. Stir the mixture and allow it to simmer 20 minutes.
6. Serve over fresh-cooked pasta.

This is a vegetarian sauce containing no cholesterol. The only fat comes from the olive oil.

Yield 6 servings

Nutrition Analysis per Serving

Calories	194
Total fat	11 g
Saturated fat	2 g
Cholesterol	2 mg
Sodium	333 mg
Carbohydrate	21 g
Dietary fiber	5 g
Sugars	5 g
Protein	5 g

CHAPTER 41 Review & Applications

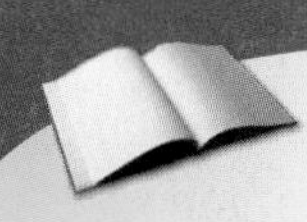

After You Read

Chapter Summary

Soups, stews, and sauces all contain a base liquid, often broth or stock. Broth and stock can be homemade or bought. There are several ways to thicken soups, stews, and sauces. Soup comes in five basic types. The cooking methods used to prepare soups vary. A stew is prepared by simmering food in a covered pan. Many cuisines around the world have their own stews. There is a basic method to making a stew, but the possibilities for stew recipes are countless. Sauces enhance other foods. There are several basic types of sauces, each with its own recipe and preparation method.

Content and Academic Vocabulary Review

1. Create a fill-in-the-blank sentence using each of these content and academic vocabulary words. The sentence should contain enough information to help determine the missing word.

Content Vocabulary

- broth (p. 634)
- stock (p. 634)
- bouillon (p. 634)
- reduction (p. 635)
- cornstarch (p. 635)
- gelatinization (p. 636)
- roux (p. 636)
- soup (p. 637)
- consommé (p. 638)
- bisque (p. 638)
- stew (p. 640)
- sauce (p. 641)
- au jus (p. 644)

Academic Vocabulary

- originated (p. 638)
- associated (p. 643)

Review Key Concepts

2. Explain how to make broth and stock.
3. List ways to thicken a liquid.
4. Summarize how to make a basic chicken vegetable soup.
5. Explain how to make a basic meat stew.
6. Describe six types of sauces.

Critical Thinking

7. Explain the value of knowing how to make broth and stock. How might having this skill save you money?

8. Analyze this scenario. The pan gravy you have made has lumps in it. What might you have done wrong?

9. Evaluate Trey's plan to serve soup at an outdoor lunch on a 90°F summer day. What kind of soup would you suggest Trey serve and why?

10. Determine what Jasmine can do. She meant to prepare a special mint sauce to serve with her roasted lamb, but forgot. She wants to serve some kind of sauce. What can she do?

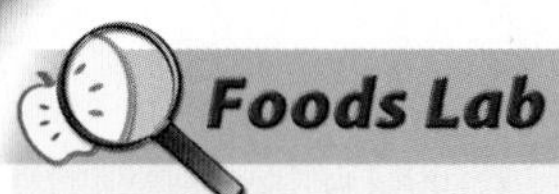

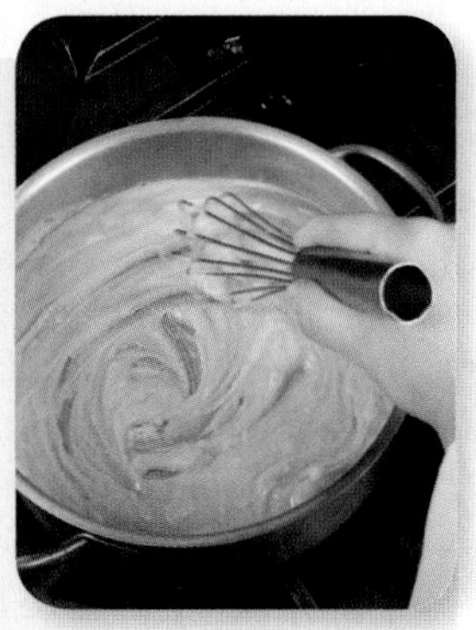

11. Comparing Thickeners There are many ways to thicken a soup, stew, or sauce. Some work better than others, depending on the circumstances.

Procedure Prepare a sauce recipe provided by your teacher. Then, separate half of the sauce into a different pan and thicken it using reduction. Thicken the other half with 2 Tbsp. cornstarch dissolved in ¼ cup water.

Analysis After sampling and comparing each sauce, write answers to the following: How did each method affect the sauce's appearance, taste, and texture? Which method do you think gave better results? Why?

HEALTHFUL CHOICES

12. Sauce Selection Tess orders roast beef and mashed potatoes from a restaurant menu. She wants to enhance their flavors with a sauce. Because she is maintaining a heart-healthy diet, she wants a sauce that will add as little additional fat and calories as possible. The waiter gives her the sauce options: pan gravy, au jus, or white sauce. Which should she choose and why?

TECH Connection

13. Create a Menu Use word processing software to create an appealing, one-page menu for a shop where soups and sandwiches are served together. What kinds of soups will the shop sell? What types of sandwiches will the soups complement? Include at least one ethnic soup on the menu. In addition to choosing precise and descriptive words to tell about your food offerings, think carefully about font choices, color, and spacing when creating your menu.

Real-World Skills

Problem-Solving Skills

14. A Soup with Skin After she finished cooking a vegetable beef soup, Julia served it, but was disappointed to notice that an unattractive skin had formed on the surface. Why did this happen, and what can she do to prevent it from happening in the future?

Interpersonal and Collaborative Skills

15. Stew Across Cultures Follow your teacher's instructions to form groups. Your teacher will assign one of the following stews to your group: goulash, Irish stew, dovi, Israeli wheat berry stew, posole, or burgoo. Work together to research how to make it. Then explain the recipe in a presentation to the class.

Financial Literacy Skills

16. Cost Comparison Zach spends $16 each month on canned chicken stock. He buys a whole chicken for $6 and roasts it. After eating the meat, he uses the bones to make enough homemade stock to last three weeks. Find the difference in cost of three weeks' worth of homemade stock and three weeks' worth of storebought stock.

Academic Skills

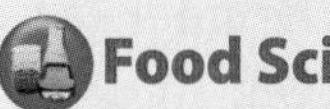

Food Science

17. Mayonnaise Unlike sauces thickened by starches, proteins, or solids, emulsions tend to be unstable, so are more challenging to make. Mayonnaise is an example of a cold emulsion sauce.

Procedure Place a room temperature egg yolk and ⅛ teaspoon salt in a food processor or blender. Pulse to combine. Add 1-2 tablespoons of lemon juice and ½ teaspoon Dijon mustard, blending well. With the motor running, gradually add ¾ cup vegetable oil, drop by drop. Do not rush this, or the sauce may separate. Add water as needed if too thick.

Analysis What are the 2 incompatible liquids? What turns this emulsion into a permanent stable sauce? Make a table comparing the ingredients of commercial mayonnaise with this one.

NSES B Develop an understanding of the structure and properties of matter.

Mathematics

18. Thickening a Sauce Beverly would like to make a large batch of sweet and sour sauce to store. She cooks 2 quarts of sauce, which needs to be thickened. How many cups of corn starch and water should she add to the sauce to bring it to a "thin" level of thickness? Remember, she will need to mix 1½ teaspoons of corn starch and 3 teaspoons of water for every cup of sauce.

Math Concept **Equivalent Volume Measurements** There are 3 teaspoons in 1 tablespoon. There are 16 tablespoons in 1 cup. There are 4 cups in 1 quart. When converting from a smaller unit to a larger unit, divide by the conversion factor. When converting from larger to smaller, multiply.

Starting Hint Start by converting the 2 quarts of sauce into cups by multiplying by 4. Determine the teaspoons of corn starch and water she will need, and convert to cups.

NCTM Problem Solving Apply and adapt a variety of appropriate strategies to solve problems.

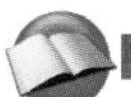

English Language Arts

19. Demonstration Write and prepare an oral presentation to the class in which you will combine words and actions to demonstrate how to make one of the following in the foods lab: roux; white sauce; lemon sauce with cornstarch; homemade stock; cold fruit soup.

NCTE 12 Use language to accomplish individual purposes.

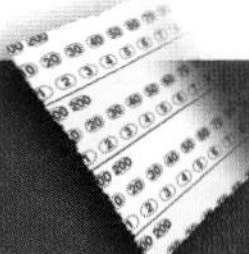

STANDARDIZED TEST PRACTICE

MULTIPLE CHOICE

Read the question and select the best answer from the choices.

20. What is the most common thickener for soups, stews, and sauces?

a. flour
b. cornstarch
c. gelatin
d. eggs

Test-Taking Tip Multiple-choice questions may prompt you to select the "best" answer. They may present you with answers that seem partially true. The best answer is the one that is completely true, and can be supported by information you have read in the text.

UNIT 8

Thematic Project

Create a Restaurant Menu

Combination foods can take a variety of different forms and can include almost any combination of ingredients imaginable. In this project, you will use what you learned in the unit to choose a menu concept and create a restaurant menu that includes combination dishes such as pizza, sandwiches, salads, soups, and so on. Your menu will include dishes for lunch and dinner.

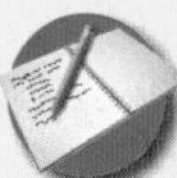

My Journal

If you completed the journal entry from page 593, refer to it to see if your thoughts have changed after reading the unit and completing this project.

Project Assignment

- Select a menu concept for a restaurant and create a menu.
- Write a list of interview questions to ask a restaurant manager or owner about how he or she chooses the dishes on his or her restaurant's menu.
- Interview a restaurant manager or owner in your community.
- Arrange, take notes, and type the interview with the restaurant manager.
- Make a presentation to your class about your menu.

Academic Skills You Will Use

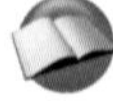

English Language Arts

NCTE 12 Use language to accomplish individual purposes.

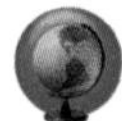

Social Studies

NCSS IV E Examine the interaction of ethnic, national, or cultural influences in specific situations or events.

STEP 1 Select a Menu Concept and Create a Menu

Imagine that you are going to open your own restaurant. What kind of menu would you choose to serve? You could design a menu based on a type of ethnic food, like Italian or Mexican, or you could choose a menu concept based on lifestyle choices, like sugar-free, fat-free, or vegetarian. Choose a menu concept, then create a menu for your restaurant. Include categories on your menu for all of the combination foods you learned about in this unit: sandwiches, pizzas, salads, stir-fries, casseroles, soups, and stews. Make sure the items you choose to feature on your menu match the restaurant concept you choose. Write a brief description of your menu concept and menu.

Writing Skills

- Use complete sentences.
- Use correct spelling and grammar.
- Use examples to illustrate your points.

STEP 2 Write Interview Questions

Arrange to interview a chef or restaurant manager or owner. Then, write a list of interview questions. Ask what criteria were used to determine what items would be on the menu. Also ask if ethnic or cultural influences affected the choice of items on the menu. Find out how often the menu is updated, and reasons why it needs to be updated.

STEP 3 Connect to Your Community

Interview a member of your community who manages or owns an independent restaurant. Do not interview the manager or owner of a chain restaurant because menus for chain restaurants are generally not set by local chefs and managers. Share your menu with the chef or manager. Ask the questions you wrote in Step 2.

Interview Skills

- Take notes during the interview.
- When you transcribe your notes, write in complete sentences and use correct spelling and grammar.
- Send a thank you note to the manager after the interview.

STEP 4 Make a Presentation About Your Menu

Use the Unit Thematic Project Checklist to plan and complete your project and evaluate your work.

STEP 5 Evaluate Your Presentation

Your project will be evaluated based on:

- Content of the menu.
- Layout and design of the menu.
- Mechanics — presentation and neatness.

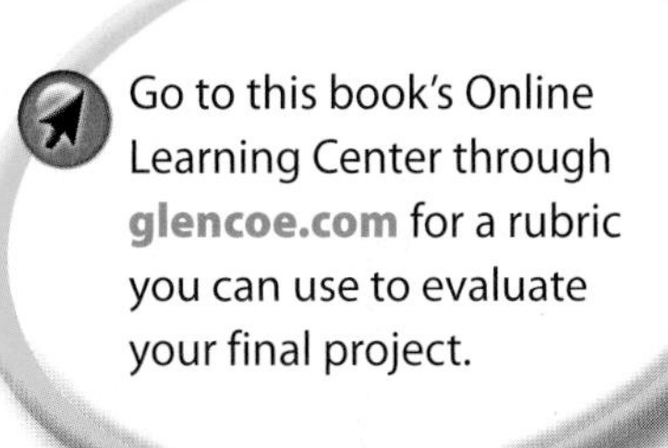

Go to this book's Online Learning Center through **glencoe.com** for a rubric you can use to evaluate your final project.

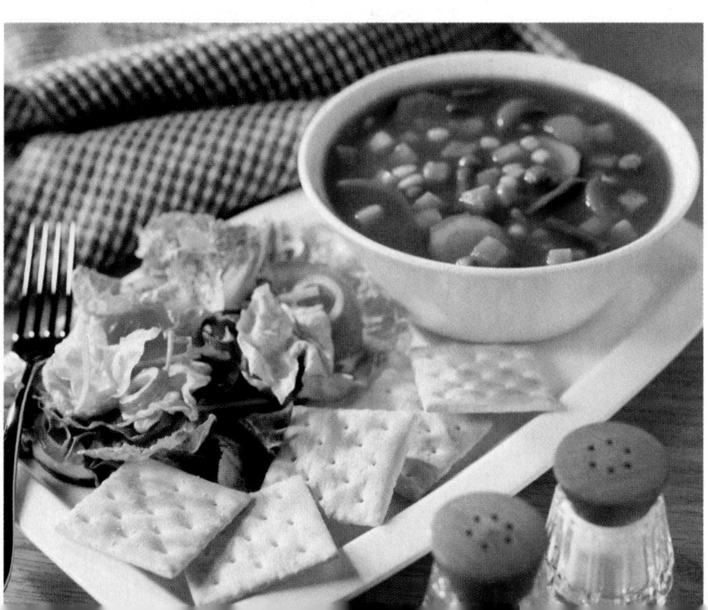

Unit Thematic Project Checklist

Category	Objectives for Your Visual
Plan	☑ Use word processing software to design and create a menu.
	☑ In your menu, include categories for all of the combination dishes you learned about in this unit. Include dishes for lunch and dinner on your menu.
	☑ Create a presentation about your menu to give to your class.
Present	☑ Make a presentation to your class to share your menu and discuss what you learned.
	☑ Invite the students in your class to ask you any questions they may have. Answer three questions.
	☑ When students ask you questions, demonstrate in your answers that you respect their perspectives.
	☑ Turn in the paragraph describing your menu concept, your menu, and the notes from your interview to your teacher.
Academic Skills	☑ Be sensitive to the needs of different audiences.
	☑ Adapt and modify language to suit different purposes.
	☑ Thoughtfully express your ideas.

UNIT 9

The Art of Baking

Activate Prior Knowledge

Explore the Photo Quick breads and yeast breads are some of the many types of baked goods. *What is your favorite baked good?*

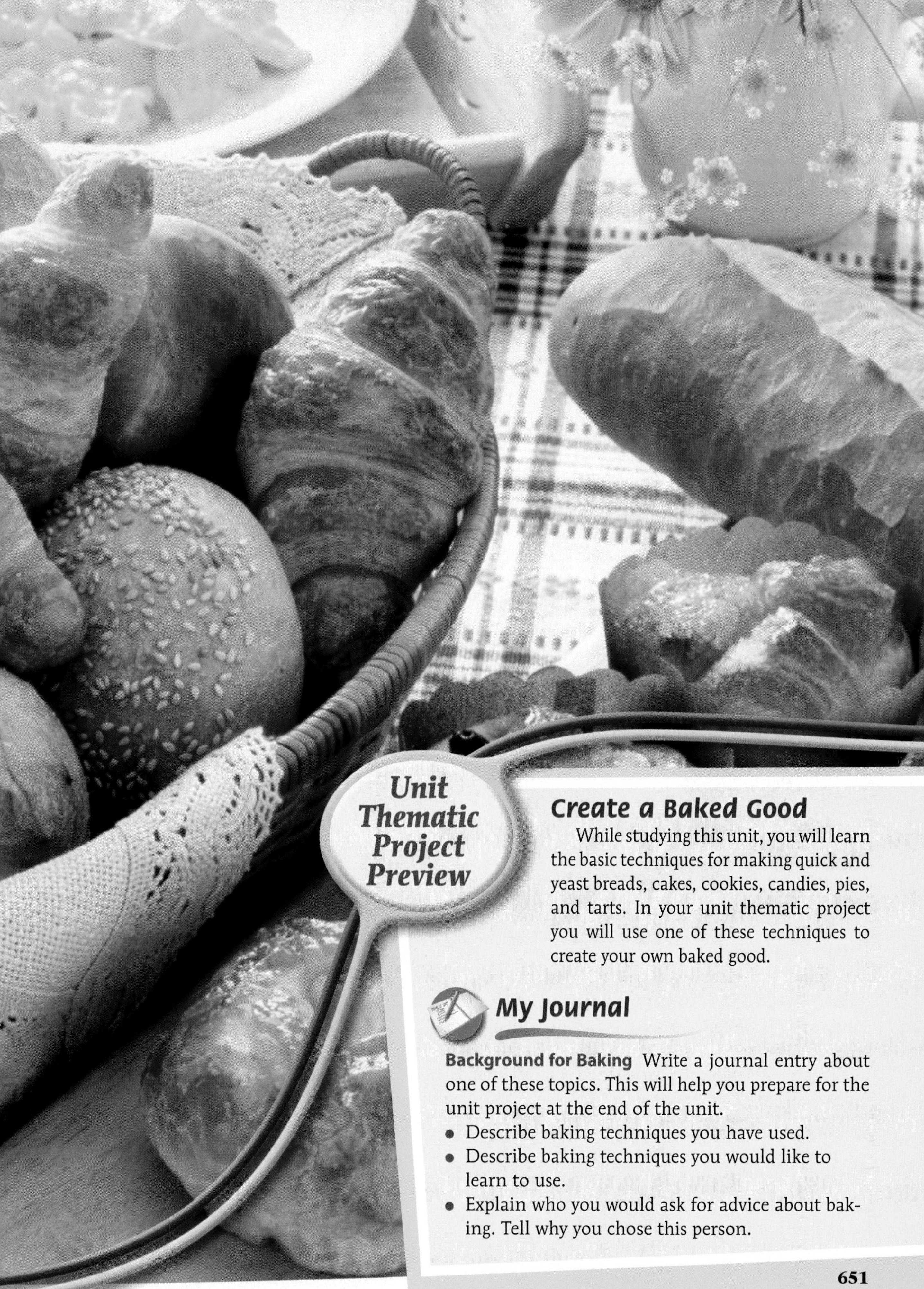

Unit Thematic Project Preview

Create a Baked Good

While studying this unit, you will learn the basic techniques for making quick and yeast breads, cakes, cookies, candies, pies, and tarts. In your unit thematic project you will use one of these techniques to create your own baked good.

My Journal

Background for Baking Write a journal entry about one of these topics. This will help you prepare for the unit project at the end of the unit.

- Describe baking techniques you have used.
- Describe baking techniques you would like to learn to use.
- Explain who you would ask for advice about baking. Tell why you chose this person.

CHAPTER 42

Baking Basics

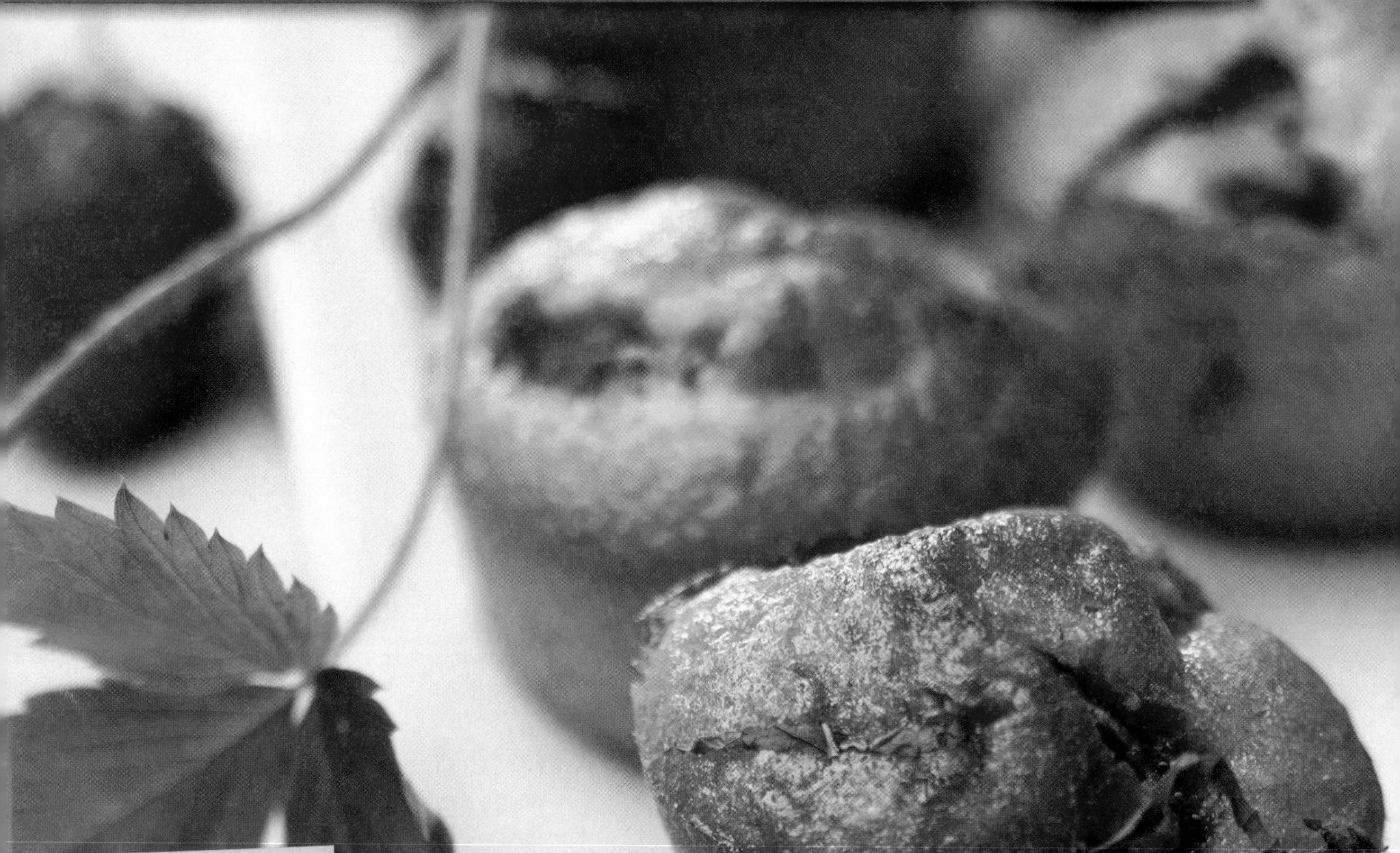

Writing Activity — Cover Letter

A Bakery Job To apply for an after-school job at a bakery in your neighborhood, you must create a resume and submit it to the bakery along with a cover letter. Write a cover letter that explains what specific qualities, knowledge, and experience you can offer as an employee at a bakery.

Writing Tips Follow these steps to write a cover letter:

- Use a business letter format.
- Do not exceed one page.
- Detail what you can offer as an employee.
- Describe your background and future goals.

Activate Prior Knowledge

Explore the Photo Baking is more science than art. It requires precise measuring. *What baked items do you enjoy most?*

Reading Guide

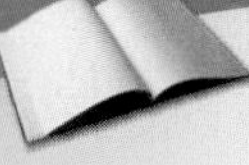

Before You Read

Preview What ingredients and equipment do you think are needed for baking? List three. Then skim through the chapter to see if they are discussed.

Read to Learn

Key Concepts

- **List** the basic ingredients for baking and explain their roles.
- **Describe** how to prepare and place pans for baking.
- **Explain** why it is important to store baked goods properly, and how to do so.

Main Idea

Baking is an art that allows you to combine ingredients to create delicious and nutritious foods with different tastes, textures, nutrients, and visual appeal.

Content Vocabulary

You will find definitions for these words in the glossary at the back of this book.

- ☐ gluten
- ☐ bleached flour
- ☐ unbleached flour
- ☐ self-rising flour
- ☐ leavening agent
- ☐ active dry yeast
- ☐ quick-rising yeast
- ☐ compressed yeast
- ☐ proofing
- ☐ granulated sugar
- ☐ confectioners' sugar
- ☐ brown sugar
- ☐ preheat
- ☐ hot spot

Academic Vocabulary

You will find these words in your reading and on your tests. Use the glossary to look up their definitions if necessary.

- neutralize
- framework

Graphic Organizer

Use a graphic organizer like the one below to note the five basic steps of the baking process.

THE BAKING PROCESS

STEP	NOTES
1.	
2.	
3.	
4.	
5.	

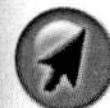

Graphic Organizer Go to this book's Online Learning Center at **glencoe.com** to print out this graphic organizer.

Academic Standards

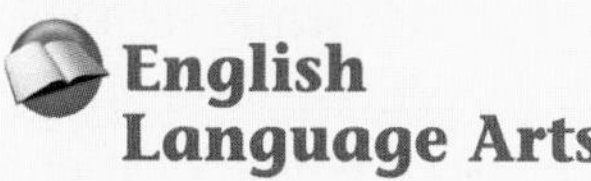

English Language Arts

NCTE 4 Use written language to communicate effectively.

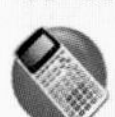

Mathematics

NCTM Measurement Apply appropriate techniques, tools, and formulas to determine measurements.

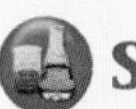

Science

NSES B Develop an understanding of chemical reactions and interactions of energy and matter.

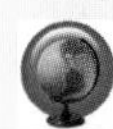

Social Studies

NCSS VIII B Science, Technology, and Society Make judgments about how science and technology can transform the physical world and human society.

NCTE *National Council of Teachers of English*
NCTM *National Council of Teachers of Mathematics*
NSES *National Science Education Standards*
NCSS *National Council for the Social Studies*

Ingredients for Baking

The basic ingredients for baking are simple: flour, liquid, leavening agents, fat, sweeteners, eggs, and flavoring. Yet baking is a complex art. You can combine ingredients in many creative ways to create baked goods with different flavors, textures, nutrients, and visual appeal.

Flours

Standard white flour is made of ground wheat kernels, minus the bran and germ. White flour is made of endosperm, so it contains starch and proteins that give structure to baked goods. Starch absorbs some of the liquid in the recipe. Some of the proteins in wheat flour combine with liquid to create an elastic substance called **gluten** (ˈglü-tən). The more gluten a baked product has, the chewier its texture will be.

The Role of Gluten

Gluten develops when you mix flour with liquid. Gluten forms strong, elastic strands that crisscross in a springy weave of tiny cells. These cells trap gas. As the food bakes, cells expand with heated gas, much like bubble gum stretches to hold air without bursting. The gas bubbles are trapped in the gluten bonds.

The longer you mix a dough or batter, the stronger gluten becomes. Cake batter is mixed quickly, so the gluten remains weak and the cells remain small. The result is a silky, melt-in-the-mouth texture.

The dough of yeast breads, by contrast, is kneaded for up to ten minutes to develop the gluten. This creates a very elastic **framework**, or structure, that expands easily. Air bubbles grow larger, which gives yeast breads a chewy texture.

Kinds of Wheat

The wheat flour used for most baking in the United States comes from two varieties of wheat, hard wheat and soft wheat.

Hard Wheat Hard wheat is high in protein and forms very strong gluten. The word "hard" refers to this wheat's high protein content. Commercial bakers prefer hard-wheat flour for making bread.

Soft Wheat Soft wheat is lower in protein and forms weak gluten. Soft-wheat flour is ideal when you want a tender, delicate texture.

Flour is also made from a third type of wheat, called durum wheat. Durum wheat is the hardest type of wheat. It is too hard for baked products, but it is milled into semolina, a grainy flour that gives pasta its sturdy structure.

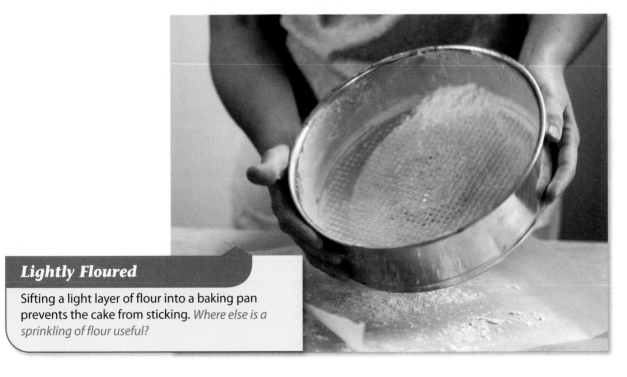

Lightly Floured

Sifting a light layer of flour into a baking pan prevents the cake from sticking. *Where else is a sprinkling of flour useful?*

Kinds of Flour

Different types of flours have different protein content, which affects gluten strength and therefore the texture of the baked product. The five most common types of flours are:

All-Purpose Flour All-purpose flour is the most-used flour in American kitchens. It is blended from hard and soft wheat and has a moderate protein content. All-purpose flour is sometimes **bleached**, or chemically treated, to **neutralize**, or counteract, the pigment and break down gluten. **Unbleached flour** has its natural color and is slightly less white than bleached flour. Unbleached flour does not have additives. **Self-rising flour** contains added baking powder and salt.

Whole-Wheat Flour Whole-wheat flour is made from the whole grain, including the germ and the bran. Bran limits gluten formation, so baked goods made from whole-wheat flour are denser and heavier than those made with all-purpose flour. When you use whole-wheat flour, you usually mix it with an equal or greater amount of all-purpose flour.

Bread Flour Bread flour is made from a combination of unbleached hard-wheat flour and barley flour. Bread flour has high gluten potential and works well for making yeast bread.

Cake and Pastry Flours Cake and pastry flours are made from soft wheat. They create less gluten and therefore produce baked goods with a fine, tender texture. Cake flour is bleached. Pastry flour is available in white and whole-wheat varieties.

Gluten Flour Gluten flour is a high-protein flour made from hard wheat, with protein solids added and most starch removed. The protein forms a strong gluten. Gluten flour is never used alone. It is mixed with low-protein flour, such as rye flour, to raise the gluten content. Bagels and hearty breads are sometimes strengthened with gluten flour.

Specialty Flours Flour is made from other grains as well, including buckwheat, oats, and rice. Nuts and legumes can also be milled into flour. Specialty flours lack the right combination of proteins to form gluten, however, so most recipes call for mixing them with wheat flour.

Buying and Storing Flour

Most home bakers buy wheat flour in 5-pound paper bags. Most specialty flours come in smaller bags. Check that the bag is well sealed and undamaged. Handle bags carefully because they tear easily.

Store flour in a cool, dry place. Transfer flour from an opened bag to a tightly covered container to keep it free from dirt, moisture, and pests. Refrigerate opened packages of whole-grain flour, which contains oils that could turn rancid at room temperature.

Liquids

Liquids help develop gluten and make possible many of the physical and chemical changes that add structure and texture to baked goods. Some recipes call for water, milk, fruit juice, buttermilk, sour cream, or yogurt. Different liquids create different results. The proteins in milk, for instance, add richness and increase browning. Some breads get their thick crust from ice placed into the oven just as the bread is put in to bake.

Doughs and Batters

Baked goods are made from either batter or dough. Batters have more liquid and less flour than doughs. Doughs have less liquid and more flour than batters. The types of batters and doughs are:

Pour Batters Pour batters are thin and are made from nearly equal amounts of liquid and flour. Cakes, pancakes, and waffles are made with pour batter.

Drop Batters Drop batters are thicker mixtures that contain twice as much flour as liquid. They are usually dropped by the spoonful onto baking pans or sheets for quick breads and cookies.

Soft Doughs Soft doughs have a ratio of one part liquid to three parts flour. Soft dough is sticky but moldable. It is the basis for many yeast breads and rolled biscuits.

Stiff Doughs Stiff doughs have a ratio of one part liquid to six to eight parts flour. Stiff doughs are the easiest to handle. Piecrusts and some rolled cookies are made from stiff dough.

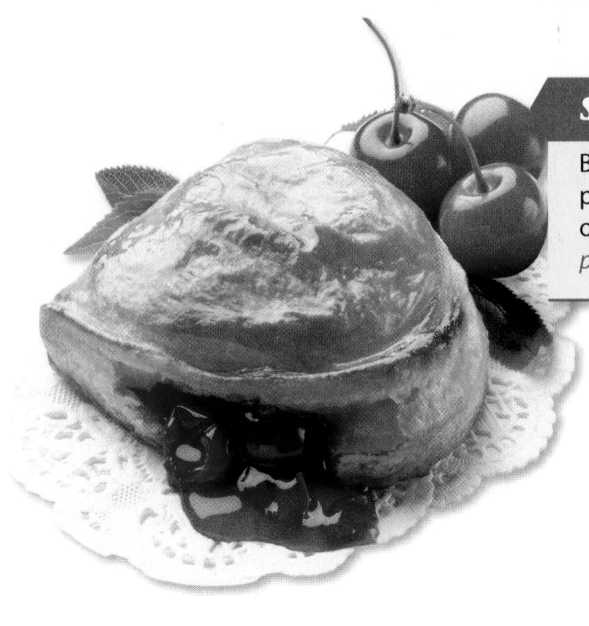

Steam Power

Baked products can be leavened in several ways. The popover shown here is leavened through the action of air and steam. *How do baking soda and baking powder leaven?*

Leavening Agents

A **leavening agent**, or leavener, is a substance that triggers a chemical reaction that makes a baked product grow larger, or rise. Many recipes use a combination of leaveners to adding volume and height. Leavening agents come in many forms:

Air Air is added to batters and doughs as you combine ingredients, for example when you sift flour, cream fat and sugar, and beat batter. When the mixture is heated, the trapped air expands and raises the product. Angel food cake is leavened mainly by the air in beaten egg whites.

Steam Steam leavens baked goods that contain large amounts of liquid. The heat of baking turns the liquid into steam. As the steam expands and rises, so does the food. Popovers and cream puffs are leavened by steam.

Baking Soda Baking soda leavens chemically. It reacts with acidic liquids, such as buttermilk, to produce carbon dioxide gas that expands when heated. Baking soda reacts with acidic liquid instantly. Mix it first with dry ingredients and then with the liquid to prevent gas from escaping before baking.

Baking Powder Baking powder is a combination of baking soda and a dry acid such as cream of tartar. It does not need acidic liquid to work. The most common type of baking powder, double-acting baking powder, releases some carbon dioxide when first mixed with liquid. More releases during baking.

Recipes that use an acidic liquid such as buttermilk or yogurt often call for baking powder as well as baking soda. The baking powder leavens the food, and the baking soda neutralizes the excess acid.

Yeast Yeast also leavens using carbon dioxide. Yeast is a fungus that thrives on moisture and warmth. It feeds on the simple sugars in flour and sweeteners. Yeast gives off carbon dioxide as it grows. Other yeast by-products give food a distinctive flavor and aroma. **Active dry yeast** is partially dormant yeast contained in flour granules. It comes in packets and jars. **Quick-rising yeast** works twice as fast as regular yeast. **Compressed yeast** is a moist combination of yeast and starch that comes in small, individually wrapped cakes that are very perishable.

Buying and Storing Leavening Agents

Baking soda and baking powder and active dry yeast are grouped with baking supplies in the supermarket. Store these ingredients in a cool, dry cabinet. Keep the baking powder container tightly sealed. Moisture can ruin it.

Compressed yeast is found in the refrigerated section of the supermarket. Store it in the refrigerator. Compressed yeast is a light gray when fresh but turns brown as it ages.

All leaveners lose their potency over time, so observe the sell-by and use-by dates on labels. To test baking soda for freshness, add 1 teaspoon of soda to 2 tablespoons of white vinegar. Fresh baking soda will fizz and froth. To test baking powder, mix 1 teaspoon of powder with ⅓ cup of hot water. It should bubble.

You can test yeast by a process called **proofing**. Place the yeast in a small bowl with a pinch of sugar and enough warm water to dissolve. Set it aside for 5 to 10 minutes. If the mixture puffs and foams, the yeast is alive.

Fats

Fats add richness and flavor to baked goods. They help crusts brown and create tender textures. Solid fats add volume by trapping air. Common solid fats used for baking include butter, margarine, vegetable shortening, and lard. Butter and margarine add flavor and sometimes include additives such as salt and coloring. Vegetable shortening is an oil that has been hydrogenated, or chemically altered to make it solid. It does not add flavor or color. Lard is purified pork fat. It makes very flaky piecrusts and biscuits but is used less in home baking than in commercial baking.

You can replace one solid fat with another in most recipes or create a blend. Different fats create different flavors. Do not substitute whipped butter and soft margarines for solid fats.

Solid fats and oils work differently in baking. Oils add moistness and density, not volume. If a recipe calls for oil, always use oil and not solid fat. Any mild-flavored cooking oil can be used, and one can be substituted for another. Corn, canola, and vegetable oil are common choices. Olive oil has a distinctive flavor and is not usually used for baking.

Buying and Storing Fat

Keep butter and margarine in the coldest part of the refrigerator, usually toward the rear of the middle shelf. Be sure they are well wrapped, because they tend to absorb flavors and aromas from other foods. Use butter within one month of purchase and margarine within two months, or freeze them in their original containers for up to four months.

Vegetable shortening and oils usually keep well in a cool, dry area. They may need refrigeration, especially if you need to keep them longer than one month. Check labels for storage instructions and freshness dates.

Sweeteners

Just like fats, sweeteners add flavor and tenderness and help with browning. Different sweeteners have different types of sugar and different amounts of liquid, so they create different results.

The following sweeteners are commonly used in baking:

Sugar **Granulated sugar** is highly refined sucrose crystals made by boiling the juice of sugarcane or sugar beets. When creamed with a solid fat, granulated sugar adds air and volume. **Confectioners' sugar**, or powdered sugar, is pulverized granulated sugar with a trace of added cornstarch. It dissolves easily and is most often used for frostings. **Brown sugar** is granulated sugar coated with molasses. Molasses adds moisture and a caramel flavor but reduces sugar's ability to trap air. A light or dark color reflects the amount of molasses and intensity of flavor.

Honey Honey is produced by bees from flower nectar. Different flowers give honey different colors and flavors. Mild clover honey is most popular in baking. Honey contains fructose, which is much sweeter than sucrose. Honey also attracts and holds more moisture than sugar, so baked goods stay fresh longer.

Science in Action: Yeast at Work

Today, commercial yeast manufacturers grow yeast on molasses. Then they process, package, and sell it in convenient forms. Before the commercial production of yeast in the 1880s, people leavened the bread that they baked by simply leaving it exposed to the yeast organisms present in the air. They prepared a dough and left it uncovered. Yeasts landed on it and began the fermentation process.

Procedure With your teacher's guidance, conduct an experiment with two batches of dough. To one batch, add commercially produced yeast from the supermarket. Leave the other batch uncovered in an undisturbed place. Record your observations of each batch of dough over a period of days.

Analysis In a paragraph, explain the changes you observed in both batches of dough, and when they occurred. Also answer this question: How has commercially produced yeast changed the nature and process of baking?

NSES B Develop an understanding of chemical reactions and interactions of energy and matter.

Molasses Molasses is a syrup that forms when sugarcane juice is boiled to make crystallized sugar. It is less sweet than sugar. Light molasses is extracted first and is highest in sugar and sweetness. Dark molasses is less sweet. It is made later in the sugar-manufacturing process, after boiling has extracted more raw sugar from the sugarcane juice.

Corn Syrup Corn syrup is made by breaking down the starch in corn into dextrose and water. Dark corn syrup has added caramel flavoring. Corn syrup is often used in frostings and candies. Small amounts of corn syrup can make baked goods soft and chewy.

Buying and Storing Sweeteners

Most sweeteners keep best in tightly sealed containers in a cool, dry area. Check the label to be sure. After using liquid sweeteners, wipe the containers with a damp cloth to remove drips. Traces of sugar attract insects.

Confectioners' sugar often cakes, even when properly stored. Remove lumps by sifting. Brown sugar can also harden. Soften it by putting a piece of fresh bread in the container or microwaving the sugar with a few drops of water in a glass bowl for 10 to 15 seconds.

Be a Smart Consumer

Low-Fat Baking

More varieties of margarine are available now than ever, but not every margarine is suited for every recipe. A vegetable spread used for baking should be at least 60 percent fat. Thus, any item labeled margarine should be suitable for baking. However, diet and light margarines may not produce the same browning and texture in baked goods. Low-fat spreads contain more water. Cookies may spread and run together. Pastry dough will be sticky and hard to handle. If limiting fats is a concern, look for specially formulated, low-fat recipes.

Challenge As a consumer, what are three resources you would use to find low-fat baking recipes? Explain your ideas in a paragraph.

Honey can crystallize, especially when refrigerated. To liquefy crystallized honey, remove the lid and set the container in about two inches of warm water.

Eggs

Eggs are another key ingredient in many baked products. The fats in eggs add flavor, color, richness, and tenderness. Fats in the yolk create an emulsion, binding liquids and fats in the recipe to keep batters from separating. Beating egg whites adds air and volume to batters. Heating egg whites helps set their structure.

Flavorings

Seasonings and flavorings add variety to baked products. Recipes often include spices or liquid extracts, such as maple, almond, or vanilla. Some recipes call for dried fruit, chopped nuts, citrus peel, or flavored syrups. Chocolate flavor is sometimes combined with unsweetened baking chocolate for more flavor. Flavorings change the texture and color of baked goods as well as their flavor.

✓ **Reading Check** **Describe** What is the difference between hard and soft wheat?

The Baking Process

Once you choose a recipe and ingredients, it is time to begin baking. First you need to prepare the oven, the pans, and the batter or dough. Then you need to bake the food at the right temperature and time, and remove it carefully from the pan. There are five basic steps to the baking process.

Choose Oven Temperature

Baking takes precise timing. Consider how a biscuit rises in a hot oven. As the surface absorbs heat, moisture evaporates and a crust forms. The crust temperature rises, and the crust begins to brown. At the same time, heat reaches the inside of the biscuit, activating leavening agents that push against the crust to raise the biscuit.

Correct oven temperatures help baked goods rise properly. If the oven is too hot, the crust forms too quickly. The biscuit struggles to expand, and the crust sometimes cracks. The crust may brown while the inside is only half baked. If the oven is not hot enough, the biscuit rises too quickly. The leavening gas escapes before the gluten and starch in the flour can form the framework to trap it. Your biscuit comes out dry and fallen.

To avoid these problems, always use the temperature given in the recipe. Make sure the oven racks are properly positioned before you turn on the oven. For one pan, place the rack near the middle of the chamber. Preheat the oven unless the recipe says not to. To **preheat** is to turn the oven on about 10 minutes before using so it will be at the desired temperature when the food is placed inside.

Choose Pans

Recipes are developed for specific pan sizes. Use the type and size of pan listed in the recipe. If you need to substitute a different pan, make sure both pans have a similar volume. You can compare volume by measuring the amount of water each pan holds.

Use a pan that is the right depth. If you use a pan that is too deep or too shallow, the food may not rise properly. Avoid pans with warps and dents that will ruin the shape of the baked item.

Different materials transfer heat at different rates. Most recipes assume the use of shiny metal pans. Pans made of glass or dark metal retain more heat and can create a thick crust. Lower the oven temperature by about 10 degrees when using dark metal pans and by 25 degrees when using glass. If you are using cast iron or other materials, follow the manufacturer's directions. When using a glass pan, it is best to monitor the baking closely and judge doneness by sight.

Prepare the Pans

Most recipes tell you how to prepare the pan so the product can be easily removed after baking. Prepare the pan before mixing ingredients.

TECHNOLOGY FOR TOMORROW

Cryogenics in the Kitchen

Baking ingredients that get too hot in storage or during mixing can affect the final product. Overheated butter becomes unworkable. Overheated flour can damage the quality of dough. To cool things down, chefs may add ice to recipes, but then must adjust the other ingredients to compensate for the extra moisture. A solution can be found in cryogenics, a technology that can be used to cool storage and mixing equipment. Cryogenic cooling systems change liquid nitrogen and solid carbon dioxide (dry ice) to gases, a process that absorbs heat and lowers the surrounding temperature. These systems cool more efficiently than conventional refrigeration systems and are programmed to maintain the desired temperature.

Get Involved List and briefly explain three specific circumstances or places in which this type of technology would be most beneficial.

NCSS VIII B Science, Technology, and Society Make judgments about how science and technology can transform the physical world and human society.

Do not grease the pan when making a high-fat recipe or when cooking in a microwave oven. Also, do not grease the pan when making cakes with beaten egg white, such as angel food cake. These cakes need to cling to the sides of the pan to rise.

Common methods for preparing pans include:

Grease and flour. To grease and flour means to coat a pan lightly with solid fat and then dust it with flour. Do not use salted butter or margarine for greasing a pan, because salt creates a darkened crust that sticks to the pan. Use wax paper to spread the fat. Thoroughly grease the corners and the crease between the sides and bottom, where foods are most likely to stick. Sprinkle the pan with a little all-purpose flour. Tilt and shake the pan to distribute the flour evenly. Turn the pan upside down over the sink, and tap it to remove any excess flour.

Spray with cooking spray. Cooking spray coats a pan easily but may leave a sticky film on pans. Spray may not work for all pans or recipes, so follow label or recipe directions.

Line with paper. You can also line a pan with cooking parchment (parchment paper). Do not use ordinary brown paper or wax paper. Brown paper may transfer chemicals to food, and wax paper may transfer wax. Cut a piece of parchment the same shape and size as the bottom of the pan. Grease the pan and line the bottom with the parchment. Peel the paper off the food after you remove it from the pan. Aluminum foil can be used instead of parchment paper.

Bake the Food

To bake evenly, food must be placed in the oven so that heated air can circulate around it freely. Allow at least 1 inch of space between pans on a rack and between pans and oven walls. Crowded pans may create a **hot spot**, an area of concentrated heat that can cause uneven baking and browning.

If you are using one pan, place it in the center of the oven. If you are using two pans, place them on separate racks in diagonally opposite corners. If you are using three or four pans, stagger them so that they are not directly above one another. See **Figure 42.1**. Rotate the pans halfway during baking to help guarantee even baking.

As soon as the pans are in the oven, set a timer. Start checking for doneness about 5 minutes before the time is up. To prevent heat loss, avoid opening the oven door until then.

Baking in a Convection Oven

Most recipes for baked products are developed for conventional ovens but adapt well to convection ovens. A convection oven creates a continuous current of hot air that speeds some chemical reactions in foods. Products brown faster and lose less moisture. Some baked goods also rise more quickly. When baking in a convection oven, reduce temperatures by 25 to 50 degrees and reduce baking time by one-third. Check the owner's manual for more detailed conversions. You can also use a convection oven cookbook to find recipes similar to your own as a guide to making adjustments.

Baking in a Microwave Oven

Microwave ovens do not bake. They cook with moist heat. Foods cooked in a microwave oven do not brown or develop a crust. They stay very tender and moist, however, because less water evaporates.

It can be difficult to adapt recipes for baked goods to microwave ovens. Factors such as rapid cooking rates and pale color can lead to overbaking. For best results, use a recipe developed for microwaving.

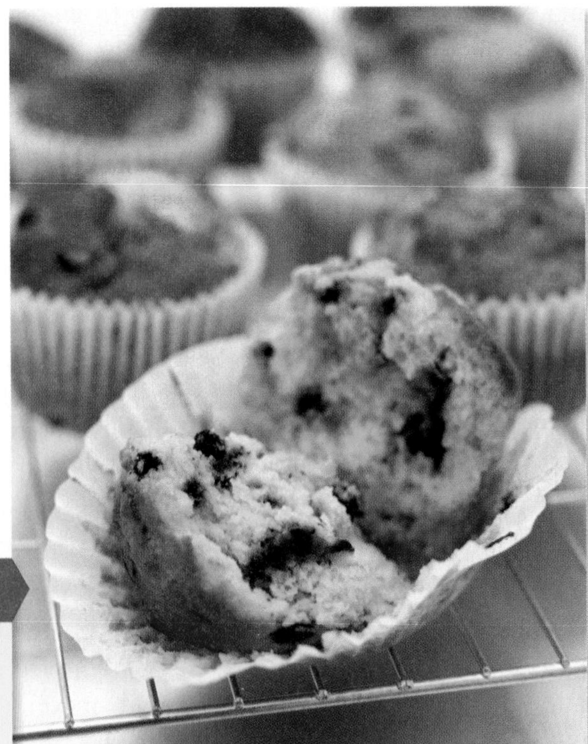

Cupcake Liners

You can use paper or foil liners in muffin tins and cupcake pans to make cleanup easier. *What other problem will using liners prevent?*

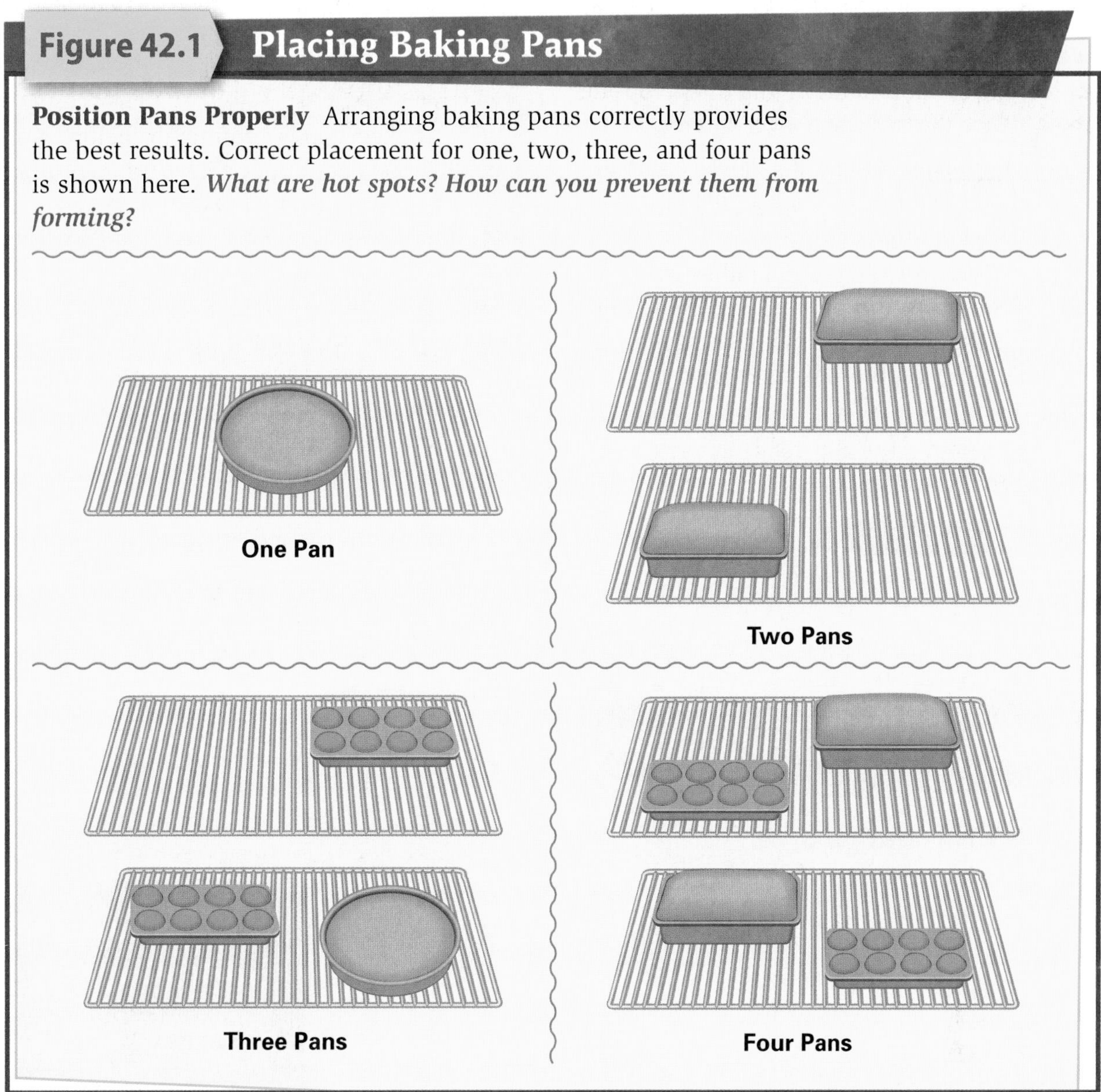

Figure 42.1 Placing Baking Pans

Position Pans Properly Arranging baking pans correctly provides the best results. Correct placement for one, two, three, and four pans is shown here. ***What are hot spots? How can you prevent them from forming?***

Removing Baked Products from Pans

Follow recipe directions for removing baked goods from the pan to get the best results.

Most cookies and muffins should be removed from the pan immediately. This prevents cookies from sticking and muffins from overbaking. Some cookies need to cool for just a minute to firm up before you remove them. Most cakes and some breads need to cool partially in the pan to prevent them from cracking or tearing when you remove them. Cakes made without fat need to cool completely in the pan. Some items can be served directly from the baking pan.

Use wire cooling racks to promote quick cooling. A countertop or other solid surface does not work well for cooling because it holds the heated air, which collects moisture and makes the food soggy.

Gently remove cookies from baking sheets with a wide spatula and gentle handling. To remove yeast bread from a pan, turn the pan on its side on a wire rack. Ease the bread out with a clean pot holder or dish towel. Place the bread right side up on the wire rack.

Use this technique to remove cakes and quick breads from the pan:

1. **Loosen.** Gently run a spatula along the sides of the pan, if needed, to eliminate sticking points.

2. Flip. Place a wire cooling rack over the top of the cake or bread. Holding the pan and rack securely with pot holders, flip them upside down. Place the rack on a level surface.

3. Lift. Continue using pot holders and carefully lift the pan off the cake or bread, which is now upside down.

4. Flip again. Quickly place another wire rack on the bottom of the baked item. Using both hands, grasp both racks without squeezing. Flip the racks so the baked product is right side up.

5. Cool. Remove the top rack and allow the item to cool completely.

✓ **Reading Check** **Explain** Can you bake foods in a microwave?

Storing Baked Products

Cool baked goods thoroughly before storing. This prevents trapped heat from producing moisture that can make the food soggy and prone to spoilage. If baked goods are not going to be consumed, it is important to store them immediately because baked goods begin to lose quality the moment they finish baking.

Most cookies, cakes, and breads can be kept at room temperature in a sealed container for up to three days. They usually freeze well also. Refrigerate perishable products, including foods with custard, cream, or fruit fillings and frostings. Do not freeze filled foods, because fillings tend to separate when they thaw.

Light and Healthy Recipe

Banana Nut Muffins

Ingredients

- **1 cup** Flour
- **½ cup** Sugar
- **2 tsp.** Baking powder
- **¼ tsp.** Salt
- **½ tsp.** Baking soda
- 1 Beaten egg
- **3 Tbsp.** Butter
- **½ cup** Buttermilk
- 2 Mashed bananas
- **½ cup** Chopped walnuts

Directions

1. Preheat oven to 375°.
2. In a large bowl, combine the flour, sugar, baking powder, salt, and baking soda.
3. Melt two tablespoons of the butter and, in a separate bowl, combine it with the egg and buttermilk. Mix well and combine with the dry ingredients. Do not overmix.
4. Use the remaining butter to grease a muffin tin. Fold in bananas and walnuts, and pour batter into muffin tins. Fill tins three-quarters full.
5. Place in oven and bake for 35 minutes.

Bananas and nuts provide energy to get you started in the morning and minerals that keep you going later in the day.

Yield 10 servings

Nutrition Analysis per Serving

■ Calories	188
■ Total fat	8 g
Saturated fat	3 mg
Cholesterol	33 mg
■ Sodium	240 mg
■ Carbohydrate	27 g
Dietary fiber	1 g
Sugars	14 g
■ Protein	4 g

CHAPTER 42 Review & Applications

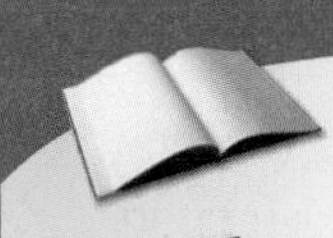

After You Read

Chapter Summary

Baking is a complex art in which ingredients can be combined in different ways to create many types of baked goods. There are several basic ingredients required for baking, each with its own role and guidelines for buying and storing. The right types of ingredients must be chosen and used correctly for the best outcome. The baking process is comprised of a series of steps, including choosing oven temperature and pans, preparing pans, baking the food, and removing it once cooked. Baked products must be stored properly to retain their quality, freshness, and taste.

Content and Academic Vocabulary Review

1. Write a sentence using at least two of these content and academic vocabulary words. The sentence should clearly show how the terms are related.

Content Vocabulary

- ☐ gluten (p. 654)
- ☐ bleached (p. 655)
- ☐ unbleached flour (p. 655)
- ☐ self-rising flour (p. 655)
- ☐ leavening agent (p. 656)
- ☐ active dry yeast (p. 656)
- ☐ quick-rising yeast (p. 656)
- ☐ compressed yeast (p. 656)
- ☐ proofing (p. 656)
- ☐ granulated sugar (p. 657)
- ☐ confectioners' sugar (p. 657)
- ☐ brown sugar (p. 657)
- ☐ preheat (p. 659)
- ☐ hot spot (p. 660)

Academic Vocabulary

- framework (p. 654)
- neutralize (p. 655)

Review Key Concepts

2. **List** the basic ingredients for baking and explain their roles.
3. **Describe** how to prepare and place pans for baking.
4. **Explain** why it is important to store baked goods properly, and how to do so.

Critical Thinking

5. **Describe** how you envision the texture of a special gluten-free bread that is consumed by some people with allergies to gluten.
6. **Explain** which questions you would ask if your homemade croissants did not turn out as light and delicate as you had hoped.
7. **Compare and contrast** doughs and batters. How does the ratio of flour to liquid affect the thickness?
8. **Evaluate** Barry's plan to cook his homemade bread faster by increasing the oven temperature.
9. **Infer** why one cake cooked completely and another cooked only partially if they were baked in the same oven at the same time.
10. **Explain** whether you should wrap a loaf of banana bread in aluminum foil immediately after removing it from the oven.

CHAPTER 42 Review & Applications

Foods Lab

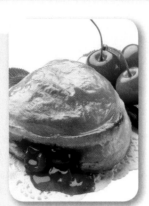

11. Testing Leaveners Several products make effective leaveners. Before using one of them, however, it is important to test its potency. Then you can be confident your baked goods will rise.

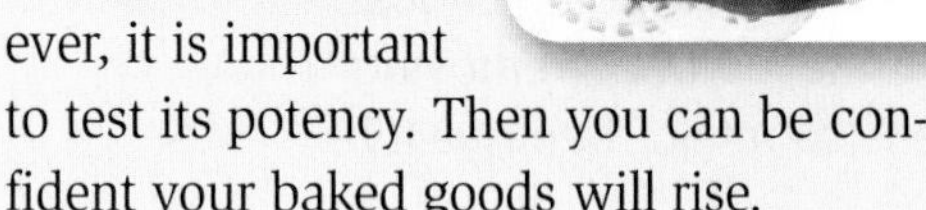

Procedure Use the procedures described in this chapter to test the potency of samples of baking soda, baking powder, and yeast provided by your teacher. Make sure to mark the samples. Record your observations.

Analysis Answer the following questions: What did you observe when you tested each sample? Which leavener[s] would you use for baking angel food cake?

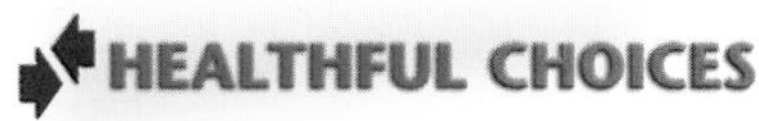

HEALTHFUL CHOICES

12. Avoiding Additives Ellen is concerned about the possible health risks associated with some food additives. She chooses to avoid them as much as possible in her diet. At the supermarket, she shops for ingredients to make some appealing recipes for homemade breads and biscuits. She decides an all-purpose flour would be best, but should she choose unbleached or bleached? State and explain your answer in a paragraph.

TECH Connection

13. Gluten Balls What are gluten balls? Under your teacher's supervision, use the Internet to find instructions on how to make them. Then conduct an experiment to make the gluten balls. If possible, use a digital camera to take photos during different stages of your experiment, and upload the photos onto a computer to show the class. Verbally explain what you learned about gluten from this activity.

Real-World Skills

Problem-Solving Skills

14. Decreasing Saturated Fat Lily found an appealing recipe for cookies. However, it calls for 4 cups of butter. Lily thinks the cookies will contain too much saturated fat and cholesterol. Can she modify the recipe to solve the problem and make the cookies more health-friendly? If so, how? How might your solution affect the taste and texture of the cookies?

Interpersonal and Collaborative Skills

15. Flour Display Follow your teacher's instructions to form groups. Work together to make a display of five different kinds of flours. Label them with descriptions, protein levels, and storage hints. Include visuals that show how each flour type is used in baking.

Financial Literacy Skills

16. Flour Cost Comparison Visit the supermarket and compare the costs of 5 flour types (not necessarily 5 brands) of your choosing. Types may include organic, whole grain, unbleached, or oat flour. Create a chart that shows the types of flours and their costs, and share your findings with the class, giving an example of when each type may be used.

Academic Skills

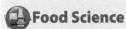

Food Science

17. Chemical Leaveners Both baking soda and baking powder are bases that react with acids to produce carbon dioxide. The difference between the two is that the soda needs an acid to react with, and the powder comes already packaged with an acid mixed in.

Procedure Place a teaspoon of baking soda and baking powder in two separate small bowls. Mix in 2 teaspoons of water to each bowl, and record results. Now add 2-3 teaspoons of vinegar to each bowl, and record results. Finally, microwave each for 30 seconds on high. Record the results.

Analysis Research double-acting baking powder, then use this information along with the results of your experiments to write a paragraph explaining what you learned.

NSES B Develop an understanding of chemical reactions and interactions of energy and matter.

Mathematics

18. Comparing Pan Volume A lemon pound cake recipe calls for the cake to be baked in a 9 inch × 5 inch × 3 inch loaf pan. However, you do not have a pan with those dimensions. You have a square pan that measures 8 inches × 8 inches × 2 inches and an 8-inch (in diameter) cylindrical springform pan that is 3 inches deep. Which is the best substitute?

Math Concept **Calculate Volume** Volume is the amount of space inside an object. The volume of a rectangular three-dimensional shape (or box) equals length × width × height. The volume of a cylinder equals $\pi \times$ radius^2 × height.

Starting Hint Find the pan with the closest volume to the one called for by the recipe. For the springform pan, use $r = ½$ of the diameter. Use 3.14 for π.

NCTM Measurement Apply appropriate techniques, tools, and formulas to determine measurements.

English Language Arts

19. Comic Strip It is possible to have a sense of humor about baking mishaps. Create a comic strip that shows an example of baking gone wrong.

NCTE 4 Use written language to communicate effectively.

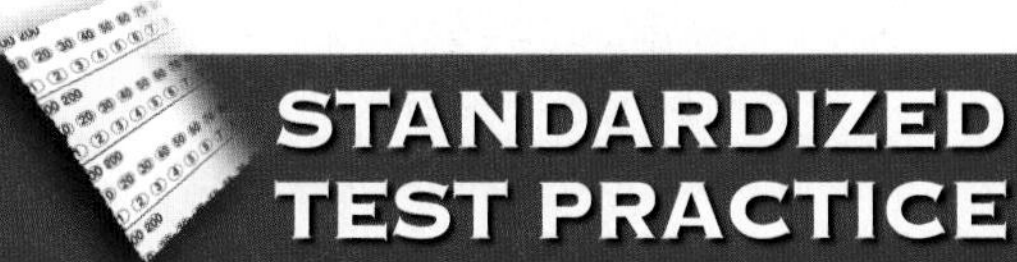

STANDARDIZED TEST PRACTICE

ANALOGY

Read the three pairs of terms. Then choose the best word to match with the term leavening agent.

20. oven: cook

molasses: sweeten

egg: bind

a. baking soda

b. yeast

c. rise

d. air

Test-Taking Tip Analogies establish relationships between terms. When you look at the three pairs of terms listed here, identify the relationship that is common to all of them. Then try matching each possible answer with the term leavening agent. The one that establishes the same type of relationship as the other terms is correct.

CHAPTER 43

Quick & Yeast Breads

Writing Activity: Editorial

Bread Ban Imagine that you have a friend who has decided to stop eating bread in order to help maintain a healthy weight. Write an editorial for the school newspaper in response to this approach to weight loss. An editorial is a newspaper column that gives an author's opinion or perspective on a topic without using the first person.

Writing Tips Follow these steps to write an editorial:

- Analyze and interpret information, and express your perspective.
- Do not write in the first person.
- If possible, strengthen your perspective with data and statistics.

Activate Prior Knowledge

Explore The Photo There are two main types of bread. *What nutrients are found in bread?*

Reading Guide

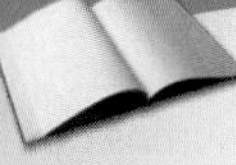

Before You Read

Preview Think about the role that bread plays in your diet. Then skim through the chapter and consider what ingredients and methods are used to make it.

Read to Learn

Key Concepts

- **Describe** methods for making quick breads.
- **Describe** methods for making yeast breads.

Main Idea

The two major types of breads are yeast breads and quick breads, which are prepared using different methods.

Content Vocabulary

You will find definitions for these words in the glossary at the back of this book.

- ☐ quick bread
- ☐ muffin method
- ☐ biscuit method
- ☐ cut in
- ☐ rolled biscuit
- ☐ knead
- ☐ drop biscuit
- ☐ yeast bread
- ☐ fermentation
- ☐ conventional method
- ☐ quick-mix method
- ☐ score

Academic Vocabulary

You will find these words in your reading and on your tests. Use the glossary to look up their definitions if necessary.

- symmetrical
- pliable

Graphic Organizer

Use a graphic organizer like the one below to note how yeast causes bread to rise, to form more gluten, and to be more flavorful.

CAUSE	EFFECT

Graphic Organizer Go to this book's Online Learning Center at **glencoe.com** to print out this graphic organizer.

Academic Standards

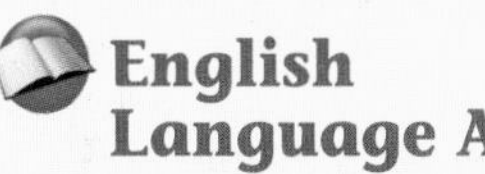

English Language Arts

NCTE 12 Use language to achieve individual purposes.

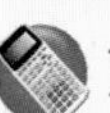

Mathematics

NCTM Number and Operations Compute fluently and make reasonable estimates.

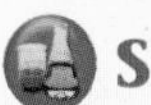

Science

NSES B Develop an understanding of chemical reactions.

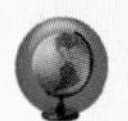

Social Studies

NCSS VIII B Science, Technology, and Society Make judgments about how science and technology can transform the physical world and human society.

NCTE *National Council of Teachers of English*
NCTM *National Council of Teachers of Mathematics*
NSES *National Science Education Standards*
NCSS *National Council for the Social Studies*

Making Quick Breads

Breads come in two major types: quick breads, such as biscuits and muffins, and yeast breads, such as sandwich breads. A **quick bread** is a bread leavened by agents that allow speedy baking, such as air, steam, baking soda, and baking powder.

Two basic mixing methods are used for quick bread batter: the muffin method and the biscuit method.

Kitchen Math

Changing Portion Size

Sylvia has a new recipe for blueberry muffins that she would like to try. The recipe yields 8 large muffins, but Sylvia prefers to use her mini-muffin baking pan to make 24 smaller muffins. If the recipe indicates that a large muffin has 383 calories and 16.1 grams of fat, how many calories and fat grams will each smaller-sized muffins have?

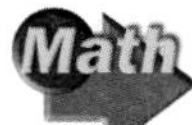

Multi-Step Problems Think through the steps before you start. If you calculate the calories and fat grams for all muffins combined, you can then divide by 24 to find the per-muffin amounts.

Starting Hint Determine the total calories in a batch of muffins by multiplying 383 by 8. All of the smaller muffins combined will have this same number of total calories. Divide by 24 to find the calories per small muffin. Perform similar calculations to find fat grams in the smaller muffins.

Math **Appendix** For math help, go to the Math Appendix at the back of the book.

NCTM Number and Operations Compute fluently and make reasonable estimates.

Muffin Method

The **muffin method** is a method of making quick breads in which liquid ingredients are lightly mixed into dry ingredients to create a batter with a slightly coarse yet tender texture. Use the muffin method to make a pour batter or a drop batter for pancakes, muffins, some coffeecakes, fruit and nut loaves, and a soft cornbread casserole called spoon bread.

The challenge with the muffin method is to avoid over mixing. Recipes that use the muffin method contain little fat, so beating the ingredients produces a chewy, heavy texture. Muffins end up with air spaces, or tunnels, on the inside and peaks on top.

To get a tender texture, follow these steps:

1. **Measure ingredients.** Measure all ingredients accurately.
2. **Mix the dry ingredients.** Sift the dry ingredients together in a mixing bowl. If you are using whole-grain flour, blend ingredients thoroughly with a spoon or whisk instead.
3. **Mix the liquid ingredients.** In a small bowl, beat all liquid ingredients—eggs, milk or water, oil or melted fat, and flavorings—until well blended.
4. **Make a well.** Using the back of a spoon, make a well in the center of the dry mixture.
5. **Pour and fold.** Pour the liquid all at once into the well in the dry ingredients. Fold in the dry ingredients just until they are moistened. Use as few strokes as possible. A few floury streaks can remain, and the batter should be lumpy.

For muffins or bread, gently spoon the batter into greased muffin tins or loaf pans. You can also line muffin pans with paper baking cups. Fill cups no more than two-thirds full to avoid overflows.

For pancakes, pour small amounts of the batter onto a hot, greased skillet or griddle, making a few at a time. Bake waffles in a waffle iron according to the owner's manual.

Testing for Doneness

Learn to spot the signs of doneness in different types of quick breads made using the muffin method.

Muffins Finished muffins will be lightly browned with rounded, pebbly tops. Remove them from the tins immediately unless the recipe states otherwise. A well-made muffin has a **symmetrical**, or balanced, shape and is fine, light, and tender on the inside.

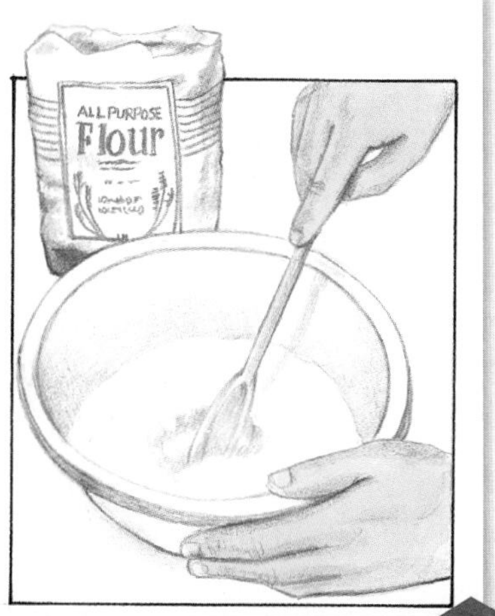

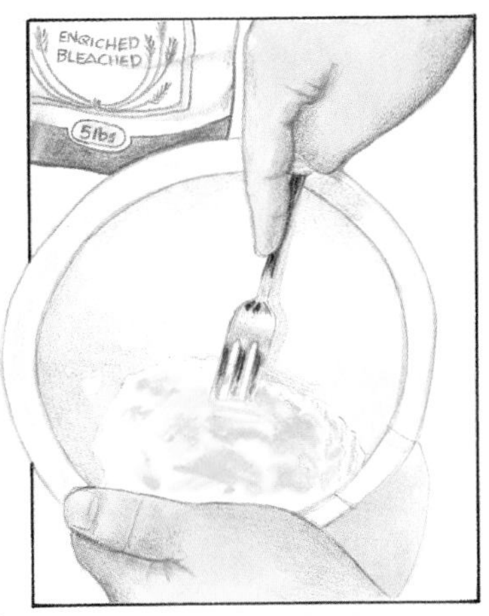

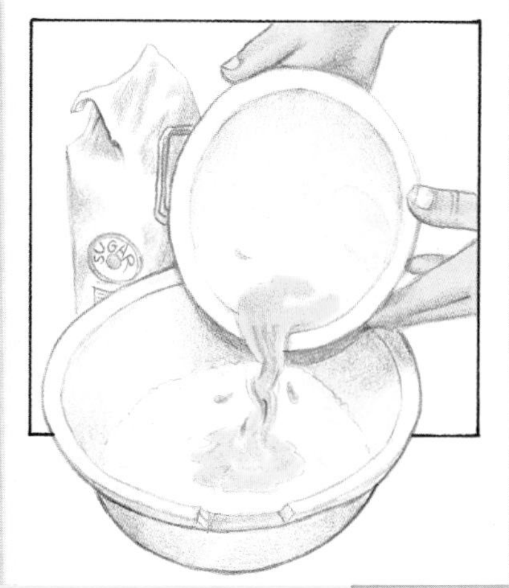

The Muffin Method

To make quick breads using the muffin method, sift dry ingredients together and make a well in the center (left). Beat the liquid ingredients in a separate bowl (center). Pour the liquid mixture into the well all at once (right). Fold together without over mixing. *What happens to quick bread batter if you over mix it?*

Loaf Breads Finished loaf breads will be lightly browned and have pulled away slightly from the sides of the pan. They should have a center crack and feel firm when tapped. Follow recipe directions for removing loaf breads from the pan.

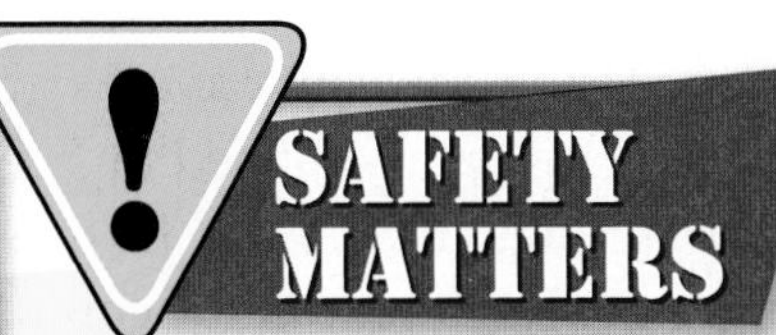

Safe Work Surfaces

To ensure food safety and quality, always clean the work surface on which you will mix baking ingredients. Invisible bacteria and other debris, such as leftover food crumbs, can get on your mixing utensil each time you rest it on the counter, and end up in your mix. A clean work surface is also very important for bakers who mix their liquid and dry ingredients right on a table or countertop, rather than in a bowl. Before baking, use a clean sponge or cloth, hot water, and non toxic cleanser or dish soap to wipe down work surfaces and dry them thoroughly.

What Would You Do? You are about to mix bread ingredients on a countertop in the foods lab. The team that used the lab before you was supposed to have cleaned it, and you see no signs of dirt.

Pancakes To know when pancakes are ready to turn, look for dry edges and bubbles starting to break on top. Cook until the underside is golden.

Muffins and pancakes are best served fresh and warm, though they can also be reheated. Allow loaf breads to cool completely before serving. During cooling, the flavors blend and the texture firms, making the loaf easier to slice.

Biscuit Method

The **biscuit method** gives a flaky layering and is used for making biscuits, scones, and shortcakes. To use the biscuit method, cut solid fat into the dry ingredients before lightly mixing in the liquids. To **cut in** means to mix solid fat and flour using a pastry blender or two knives and a cutting motion. Cutting in disperses fine fat particles in the dough. During baking, the fat melts between layers of flour, and its liquid content turns to steam, giving rise to a flaky biscuit.

Biscuits use a higher ratio of flour to liquid than muffins, making a dough rather than a batter. Roll them out and cut them or drop them onto a cookie sheet, depending on the amount of liquid in the recipe.

Follow these steps when using the biscuit method:

1. Measure ingredients. Make sure measurements are accurate.

2. Combine the dry ingredients. Sift together the dry ingredients in a large mixing bowl.

3. Combine the liquids. Mix the wet ingredients in a separate bowl until well blended.

4. Cut in the fat. Cut the fat into the flour until the particles are the size of peas or coarse bread crumbs. Use cold fat, which cuts in more quickly and makes a lighter texture.

5. Make a well. Using the back of a spoon, make a well in the center of the dry mixture.

6. Pour and mix. Pour the liquid all at once into the well. Using a fork, mix until the dry ingredients are just moistened.

Rolled Biscuits

A **rolled biscuit** is a biscuit that is lightly kneaded, rolled out to an even thickness, and cut to biscuit size before baking. To **knead** means to work dough with the hands to combine ingredients and develop gluten. In order to create a light, flaky product, very little kneading is done with rolled biscuits.

Science in Action: Pre-fermenting

Rather than simply dissolving yeast and adding it directly to a bread recipe, some bakers use a starter, also known as a pre-ferment or sponge. A starter is a mix of flour, water, and yeast that has already fermented together in a bowl for a period of time.

Procedure Conduct research to answer these questions: Why do starter ingredients combined in a container rise to three times their size? How does using a starter affect the flavor of bread? Why is sourdough bread often made with starter rather than conventional yeast?

Analysis Using what you know of yeast and fermentation, as well as critical thinking skills, write at least one sentence to answer each of the questions.

NSES B Develop an understanding of chemical reactions.

The dough for rolled biscuits should "clean" the sides of the bowl, which means that it holds together in a ball and no longer sticks to the bowl. After the dough reaches this stage, follow these steps:

1. Turn out the dough onto a board. Sprinkle just enough flour on the dough to keep it from sticking to the board. Too much flour toughens the texture.

2. Knead and fold the dough. Make sure to knead the dough lightly, using only your fingertips. This keeps the fat from melting in the dough. If necessary to avoid sticking, dust your hands with a little flour. Gently fold the dough in half toward you and give it a quarter turn. Continue to knead gently, fold, and turn as directed in the recipe, usually six turns or fewer. The dough should lose its stickiness. Overworking the dough creates tough, compact biscuits.

3. Roll the dough. Roll out the dough gently to about ½-inch thickness using a lightly floured rolling pin on a clean, lightly floured surface. Keep the dough circular to avoid waste when cutting. Maintain an even thickness so that the biscuits bake evenly. Dust the board and rolling pin with flour only as needed to prevent sticking.

4. Cut the dough. Using a biscuit cutter or the rim of a beverage glass lightly dipped in flour, cut straight down through the dough. (A twisting or turning motion can pull the biscuit out of shape.) You can cut square biscuits with a sharp knife dipped in flour. Work carefully to avoid tearing or pulling the dough. You can use cookie cutters, if they are deep enough to cut without flattening the dough. Scones are usually cut into wedges.

5. Gather leftover dough. Pat together leftover dough, roll it again, and cut it. Handle it as little as possible so that it remains tender and flaky.

6. Place and bake. Use a wide spatula to place the biscuits about 1 inch apart on an ungreased baking sheet. Bake as the recipe directs. Some cooks place the baking sheet in the refrigerator for 10–15 minutes before baking so that the butter will be firm when the biscuits go into the oven.

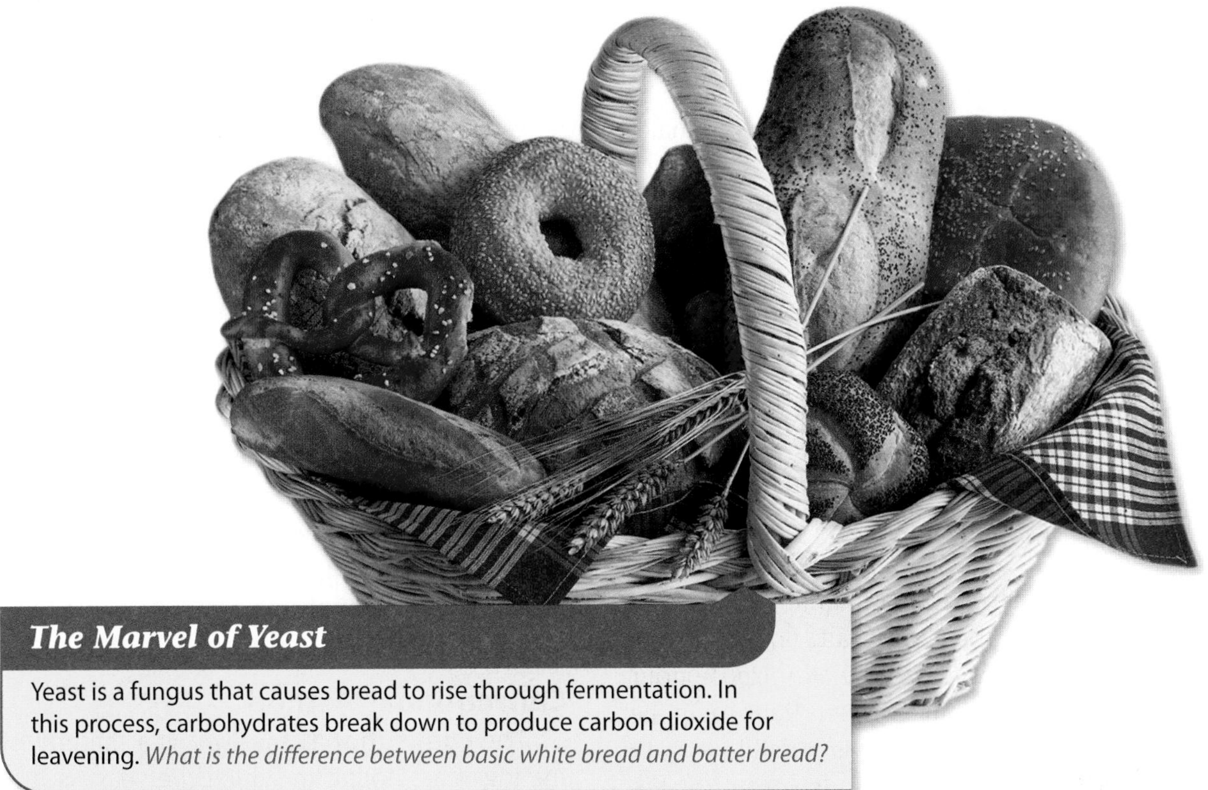

The Marvel of Yeast

Yeast is a fungus that causes bread to rise through fermentation. In this process, carbohydrates break down to produce carbon dioxide for leavening. *What is the difference between basic white bread and batter bread?*

Drop Biscuits

A **drop biscuit** is a biscuit made with more liquid in proportion to flour than a rolled biscuit. You can turn a rolled biscuit into a drop biscuit by increasing its liquid content. The sticky dough holds its shape when mounded but does not clean the sides of the bowl. It is not kneaded or rolled. Oil sometimes replaces solid fat, and the muffin method may be used for mixing. These differences make drop biscuits more mealy than flaky.

To form drop biscuits, place large spoonfuls of dough about 1 inch apart on a greased cookie sheet, or use muffin tins for a more symmetrical shape. Bake according to recipe directions. You can also spoon drop biscuits onto a casserole as a topping or onto a fruit filling to make a cobbler.

Testing for Doneness

Both rolled and drop biscuits double in size when they bake. Rolled biscuits have golden brown tops and straight, cream-colored sides. Drop biscuits have golden brown, irregular contours.

✓ **Reading Check** **Explain** How do you cut in ingredients?

Making Yeast Breads

A **yeast bread** is a bread leavened with yeast. Yeast is used in many kinds of bread, including sandwich bread, pizza crusts, pita bread, rolls, pretzels, pastries, and bagels.

The dough for yeast bread must be well kneaded and allowed to rise before baking. It takes longer to make yeast breads than quick breads, but the process is not difficult. "Hands-on" steps of kneading and shaping dough alternate with "hands-off" stages of letting dough rise. Some recipes can be started one day and finished the next.

How Yeast Works

How does yeast make bread rise? Yeast, and the enzymes in yeast, produce alcohols and carbon dioxide gas by breaking down carbohydrates, a process called **fermentation**. As the gas leavens the bread, it moves protein and water molecules, enabling them to form more gluten. In addition to causing rising, fermentation creates by-products such as alcohols, amino acids, and fatty acids, that add flavor.

Types of Yeast Breads

Yeast breads fall into five basic categories:

Basic White Bread Basic white bread is made with all-purpose flour, yeast, salt, sugar, fat, and water or milk.

Batter Bread Additional liquid and beating instead of kneading differentiates batter bread from basic white bread. The result is a lighter texture.

Sweet White Bread Basic white bread ingredients plus butter, eggs, extra sugar, and sometimes nuts and fruits, create a sweet white bread. Pecan rolls and coffeecakes are examples.

Whole-Grain Bread Whole-grain bread is always made with whole-grain flour, but this may replace part or all of the all-purpose flour in basic white bread. Gluten flour may be added to lighten the loaf. It is possible to substitute whole-grain flour for up to half of the total flour in most recipes.

Sourdough Bread Leavened with a well-fermented mixture of yeast, water, and flour, sourdough bread has a tangy flavor and a chewy texture.

Be a *Smart Consumer*

Bread Machines

Thanks to bread machines, consumers can have fresh, hot bread without much effort. To use a bread machine, simply put the ingredients in the appropriate compartment, program the machine, and let it handle the rest. These appliances come in a variety of forms and offer several different functions. They can produce round, square, and rectangular loaves, operate at different cycles, and be adjusted to enhance crustiness or work with different flours. Some include removable bread pans, a "keep warm" feature, and a delayed start function.

Challenge List the pros and cons you perceive in bread machines. What are the positive aspects of using one and what, if any, are the drawbacks?

Mixing Yeast Dough

Mixing is the first step in making yeast bread. Mixing both combines the ingredients and activates the yeast. When yeast produces carbon dioxide, gluten in the flour stretches and dough rises. Gluten traps carbon dioxide, forming tiny pockets in the dough. Bread flour is an excellent gluten producer, which makes it ideal for making yeast dough. All-purpose flour is a less expensive, satisfying substitute.

You can choose from two methods for mixing yeast dough: the conventional method and the quick-mix method. For both methods, bring all ingredients to room temperature to promote yeast growth.

Conventional Method

The **conventional method** is a method of mixing yeast dough in which the yeast is first dissolved in warm water to activate growth. Dissolving yeast is also a method of testing yeast, called proofing. Temperature is critical. Yeast will not grow if the water is too cool. Yeast will die if the water is too hot. Check the water temperature with a candy thermometer if you have one. Otherwise, let a drop fall on the inside of your forearm. It should feel pleasantly warm.

The steps in the conventional method are:

1. Dissolve the yeast in water. Use water that is about 105° to 115° and let the mixture stand for 5 to 10 minutes.

2. Heat the liquid. Heat the fat, sugar, and liquid until the fat melts. Cool the mixture to lukewarm.

3. Mix in the yeast. Add the dissolved yeast to the liquid, along with any eggs in the recipe.

4. Mix in the flour. Add enough flour to make a soft or stiff dough, as the recipe indicates. Recipes may give a range for the amount of flour rather than an exact amount. This is because flour varies in how much liquid it can absorb. On humid days, for instance, flour absorbs less liquid because it has already taken in some moisture from the air. There is enough flour when the dough cleans the sides of the bowl.

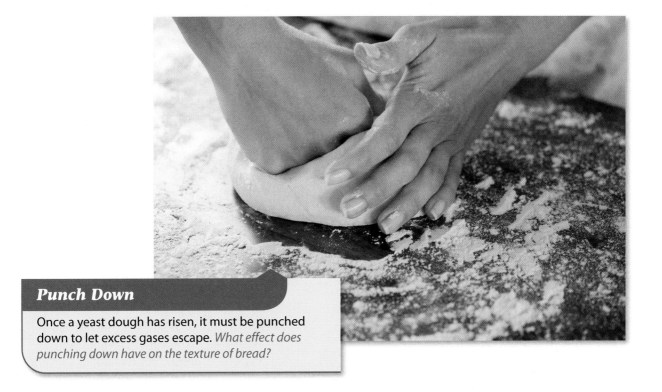

Punch Down

Once a yeast dough has risen, it must be punched down to let excess gases escape. *What effect does punching down have on the texture of bread?*

Quick-Mix Method

The **quick-mix method** is a method of mixing yeast dough in which dry yeast is combined with the dry ingredients and then with a liquid. The liquids must be warmer than in the conventional method because the dry ingredients absorb some of the heat. You can use a standard electric mixer until the dough thickens and becomes too heavy. Then switch to a sturdy spoon. The mixer develops gluten, cutting down on kneading time later. Some mixers have paddles that allow you to mix the dough fully.

The steps in the quick-mix method are:

1. **Mix the dry ingredients.** Combine part of the flour with the undissolved yeast, sugar, and salt in a large bowl.
2. **Heat the liquid.** Heat the liquid and fat to between 120° and 130°.
3. **Beat the dough.** Add the liquid to the dry ingredients and beat until well blended. Make sure all the flour is incorporated.
4. **Add flour.** Add just enough of the remaining flour to make the kind of dough specified in the recipe. Pay attention to recipe directions that explain how wet or dry a dough should be.

Kneading Yeast Dough

Except for batter breads, most yeast doughs must be kneaded to develop a strong gluten structure that holds up when the dough rises. You can use your hands or a food processor or heavy-duty mixer with a dough hook, which saves a few minutes and some labor.

Follow these steps to knead yeast dough:

1. **Turn out the dough.** Sprinkle a clean work surface and your hands with just enough flour to keep the dough from sticking. If the dough absorbs too much extra flour, the bread will be dry and tough. Turn the ball of dough out on the surface and flatten it slightly.
2. **Push the dough.** With the heels of both hands, press the top of the dough and push away from you.
3. **Fold the dough.** Pull the far side of the dough toward you, folding the dough in half.
4. **Turn the dough.** Rotate the dough one quarter turn.
5. **Knead the dough until glossy.** Continue the push, fold, and turn technique for 8 to 10 minutes, using a steady rhythm. When the rough, sticky mass becomes a smooth, glossy, elastic ball, it is ready to let rise.

Letting Yeast Dough Rise

The next step after kneading is to let the dough rise. Rising allows yeast colonies to multiply and flavors to develop. Recipes that use quick-rise yeast can be baked after only one rise. Recipes that use regular yeast must rise twice, once after kneading and again after the dough is shaped.

For the first rising, place the ball-shaped dough in a large, lightly greased bowl. The bowl must be large enough to allow the dough to double in size. Turn the dough over so the greased surface is on top, and press plastic wrap lightly onto it. This helps keep the dough from forming a crust or drying out, both of which limit yeast growth. Cover the bowl with a clean, dry dish towel or another sheet of plastic wrap stretched tightly to the edges of the bowl. You can put batter breads directly into the baking pan to rise.

TECHNOLOGY FOR TOMORROW

Mass-Produced Breads

Although there has been a resurgence in the popularity of artisanal breads—which are prepared in small batches using old-fashioned recipes and methods—most Americans also consume mass-produced breads. Technology has made it possible for factories to make a quarter of a million loaves of such breads daily, but some quality is lost in producing such large quantities. Because mass-produced breads are baked at temperatures up to 400°, many nutrients in the flour are depleted. Most mass-produced breads have a softer texture than their artisanal counterparts. They also contain chemical additives, including preservatives, which allow them to be shipped long distances to supermarkets and remain on shelves without spoiling.

Get Involved Go to your local supermarket. See if you can find any mass-produced breads that are high in nutrients and free of chemical preservatives. Share your findings with the class.

NCSS VIII B Science, Technology, and Society Make judgments about how science and technology can transform the physical world and human society.

Choose a warm place for the dough to rise. A temperature of 75° to 85° is ideal. Avoid drafts, which cool the dough, as well as radiators and furnace vents, which cook it. If you cannot find a suitable spot, make one by filling a large bowl two-thirds full of hot water and setting the dough on a wire rack over the water. Replace water as it cools with hot water. You can also use a microwave oven, but check the owner's manual for specific instructions. In most microwaves, you warm the oven, leave it off for a time, then warm it again.

Let the dough rise until it doubles in bulk, usually about 1 to 1½ hours. Stiff doughs and doughs made with whole-grain flour or nuts and fruits take longest to rise. Allow extra time for refrigerated dough. If you use quick-rising yeast, check the package to estimate rising time.

To test the dough, gently poke two fingers about ½ inch into the surface. If a dent remains, the dough is ready to shape. If the dent springs back, let the dough rise a little longer and then test it again.

Punching Down Yeast Dough

Once dough has risen, it must be punched down. Punching down lets excess gases escape, making the dough easier to shape. It gives the bread a fine texture by eliminating large air bubbles, which would leave large holes during baking. Punching down also redistributes yeast cells, giving them fresh sugar and starch molecules to feed on as fuel for the second rising.

To punch down, thrust your fist into the center of the dough with one quick punch. Then pull the dough away from the sides of the bowl and press it down toward the center to form a ball. Turn the dough out on a lightly floured surface. To make it more flexible, you can let the dough rest for about 10 minutes after punching down.

After it is punched down, the dough is ready to be shaped. Cover and refrigerate it overnight if needed. The dough will rise slowly.

Batter breads are stirred down rather than punched down. Stir the batter with a sturdy spoon until it is close to its original size. Spread the dough in the baking pan for the second rising.

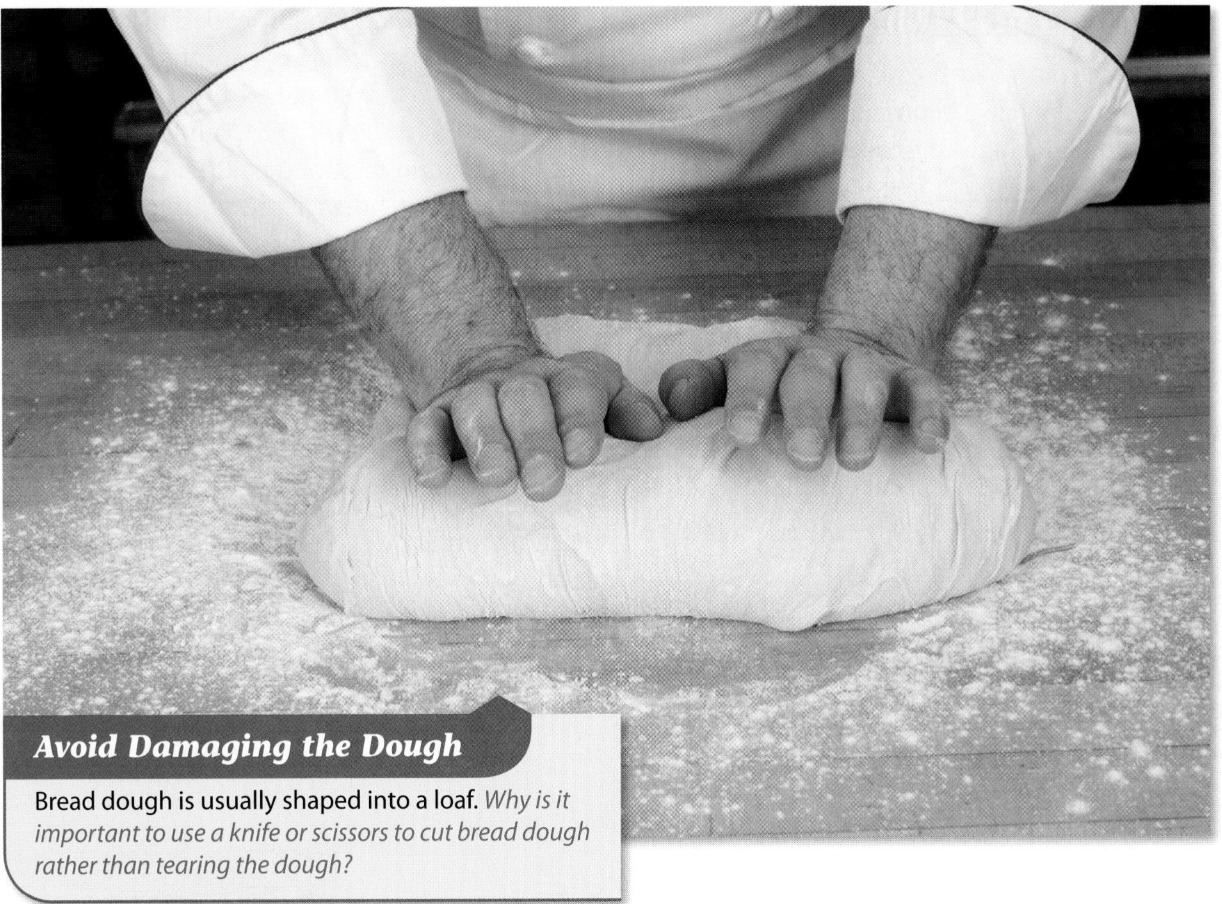

Avoid Damaging the Dough

Bread dough is usually shaped into a loaf. *Why is it important to use a knife or scissors to cut bread dough rather than tearing the dough?*

Shaping Yeast Dough and the Second Rise

Bread dough is usually shaped into a loaf. Some breads are baked free-form on a baking sheet. Some doughs are cut and rolled into several small balls. Other breads are placed in pans to set their shape. Usually the dough is cut in half before baking. Use kitchen shears, a sharp knife, or a bench scraper to cut the dough. Do not tear the dough, because this stretches, weakens, and damages the strands of gluten.

Follow these steps to shape a loaf for baking:

1. Flatten the dough. Flour the work surface lightly. With a rolling pin, roll the dough into an 8 × 10 inch rectangle. Make sure the dough is the same thickness throughout. Roll out the bubbles in the edges.

2. Roll up the dough. Starting at one of the short ends, roll up the dough tightly. This helps press out air.

3. Pinch and seal the roll. Turn the roll so the seam is on top. With your fingers, pinch the seam edge to the roll so it stays closed. Turn the roll seam-side down. Hold your hands with palms pressed together. With the bottom edge of your hands, press down on both ends of the roll, about ¼ inch inside the edge, to pinch and seal the ends. Tuck the flattened ends under the roll. Then turn the roll upside down and pinch the ends into it. Place the roll seam-side down in a greased loaf pan.

Yeast dough is very **pliable**, or supple, and accepts many different shapes. You can make a braid, a wreath, or a braided wreath. Twist rolls into figure-eights, cloverleaves, sailor's knots, or crescents. Challah is a traditional Jewish bread made by braiding as many as six strands of dough. Stick smaller balls on larger ones for bunny heads or teddy bears.

Place the shaped dough in the baking pans. Cover it with a dry dish towel and let it rise again until it doubles in size. The second rising usually takes less time than the first rising.

Baking Yeast Dough

Preheat the oven before the bread finishes rising. You may also choose to score the loaves just before baking. To **score** means to make slashes about ½ inch deep across the top of the bread. Scoring prevents the crust from cracking as the dough rises. Diagonal scoring adds a decorative touch.

The heat of the oven gives yeast one last burst of activity, resulting in a sudden rising called oven spring. This indicates a good start, and a nicely browned crust indicates the bread is nearly finished baking. Baking times vary considerably, however, so always bake as directed in the recipe. To check for doneness, remove the loaf from its pan and tap the bottom and sides. Well-baked bread sounds hollow. If you hear a dull thud, put the bread back in the pan and continue baking.

As soon as bread is done, remove it from the pan and place it on a wire cooling rack. Keep the bread away from drafts, because rapid cooling can crack the crust top. Let loaves stand about 20 minutes for easier slicing. Always use a serrated knife to cut bread. A well-baked loaf is smooth, rounded, and nicely browned. Inside, the bread has a soft and springy texture that is consistently fine throughout.

Light and Healthy Recipe

Buttermilk Biscuits

This easy-to-make biscuit recipe includes whole wheat flour, adding texture and fiber.

Ingredients

1 ½ cups All-purpose flour
½ cup Whole wheat flour
1 tsp. Salt
1 tsp. Baking powder
½ tsp. Baking soda
¼ cup Butter
¾ cup Buttermilk

Directions

1. Preheat oven to 450°F.
2. In a large mixing bowl, combine the two flours with the salt, baking powder and baking soda. Mix well.
3. Cut in the butter. It may be easier to work the butter into the flour with your hands until the butter is reduced to pea-sized bits.
4. Add the buttermilk and mix with your hands just until the dough can be put out on a table.
5. Roll out the dough and with a cutter or a wide glass, cut out circles of dough. When you cannot cut out any more circles, push the dough together. Do not roll out again. Cut out more circles.
6. Place the circles on a baking sheet and bake in the oven until golden brown.
7. Biscuits are best when served hot.

Yield 8 servings

Nutrition Analysis per Serving

■ Calories	171
■ Total fat	6 g
Saturated fat	4 g
Cholesterol	16 mg
■ Sodium	316 mg
■ Carbohydrate	24 g
Dietary fiber	2 g
Sugars	1 g
■ Protein	4 g

CHAPTER 43 Review & Applications

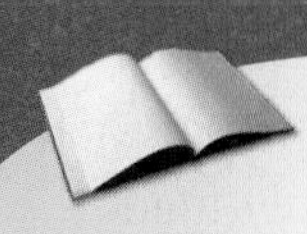

After You Read

Chapter Summary

The two major types of breads are quick breads and yeast breads. A quick bread is leavened by agents that allow speedy baking, such as air, steam, baking soda, and baking powder. A yeast bread is leavened by yeast. These two types of bread are prepared using different methods. Two basic methods are used to make quick bread batter, the muffin method and the biscuit method. The biscuit method has variations that result in different appearances and textures. There are five basic categories of yeast breads. Each kind of yeast bread can be made by following a series of steps.

Content and Academic Vocabulary Review

1. Write each of these content and academic vocabulary words on an index card, and the definitions on separate index cards. Work in pairs or small groups to match each term to its definition.

Content Vocabulary

- quick bread (p. 668)
- muffin method (p. 668)
- biscuit method (p. 669)
- cut in (p. 669)
- rolled biscuit (p. 670)
- knead (p. 670)
- drop biscuit (p. 671)
- yeast bread (p. 671)
- fermentation (p. 671)
- conventional method (p. 672)
- quick-mix method (p. 673)
- score (p. 676)

Academic Vocabulary

- symmetrical (p. 668)
- pliable (p. 675)

Review Key Concepts

2. **Describe** the two methods for making quick breads.
3. **Describe** methods for making yeast breads.

Critical Thinking

4. **Decide** what you would do if you were making bread from scratch. Would you prefer to make quick bread or yeast bread? Give three specific reasons for your answer.
5. **Predict** what would happen if you made muffins by stirring the dry and liquid ingredients together in a bowl until you had a thoroughly wet mix.
6. **Evaluate** the consequences of over-kneading dough for rolled biscuits.
7. **Identify** which type of biscuits you would make if you wanted them to have a slightly rustic, imperfect appearance. Explain your reasoning.
8. **Explain** what you could do if you wanted to make a yeast bread, but wanted to avoid too much kneading.
9. **Analyze** what would happen to dough that was left to rise near a refrigerator that was repeatedly opened and closed.
10. **Describe** three original, creative, and realistic possibilities for shaping yeast dough.

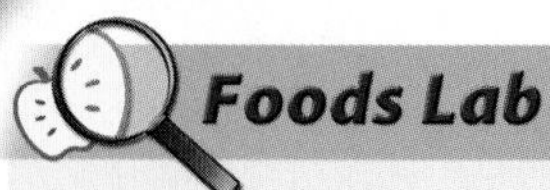

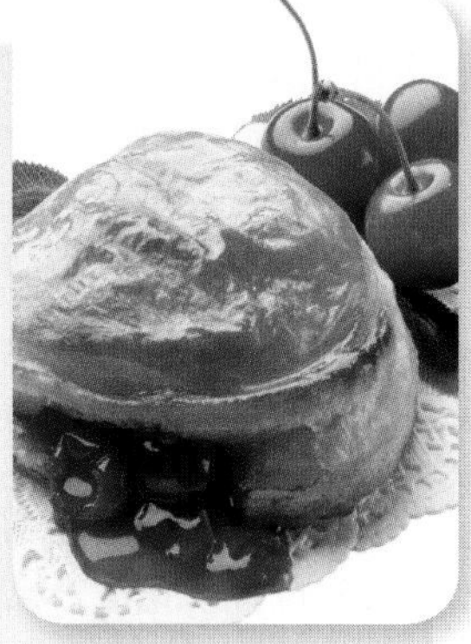

11. Fun Quick Breads Popovers and cream puffs are two popular varieties of quick bread that use leavening in different ways to create cavities for fun fillings.

Procedure Follow your teacher's instructions to form teams. Find and prepare a recipe for popovers or cream puffs, as assigned by your teacher. Print or copy the recipe you used, and display it with the baked goods for a class evaluation.

Analysis Sample and evaluate all teams' popovers and/or cream puffs, including your own. List the differences and similarities between the two varieties of bread.

HEALTHFUL CHOICES

12. At the Bakery Ravi visits his neighborhood bakery in search of a loaf of freshly made yeast bread. He is looking for bread that will be low in sugar and as rich in nutrients as possible. The bakery has the following options available: basic white, sweet white, sourdough, and whole grain. Which should Ravi choose and why?

TECH Connection

13. Muffin Ingredients Imagine you need six dozen assorted muffins for a brunch. Use technology to help you get organized. Under your teacher's supervision, use the Internet to find six appealing and varied muffin recipes. Then use spreadsheet software to create an ingredient list for all of the supplies and ingredients you will need to make each of the six recipes. Then combine all six ingredient lists into one shopping list.

Real-World Skills

Problem-Solving Skills

14. From Simple to Sweet Greg assembles the ingredients to make a basic white bread for dinner. When he learns that his dinner guests will bring children, he decides that a sweet white bread would be appealing to the children. Can he use the ingredients he has to make sweet white bread, or must he add additional ingredients? Explain your answer.

Interpersonal and Collaborative Skills

15. Water Temperature Test Follow your teacher's instructions to form pairs. One person should pour a water sample and privately take its temperature with a thermometer. The other person should determine if the water is the right temperature to dissolve yeast. Take turns.

Financial Literacy Skills

16. Mass-Produced or Made with Care Visit a supermarket and a bakery in your neighborhood. Find out how much a loaf of pre-sliced, packaged, mass-produced sourdough bread costs at the supermarket. Then find out how much the same sized loaf of freshly made sourdough bread costs at the bakery. What is the difference in cost?

Academic Skills

Food Science

17. Quick Breads Because these breads have chemical leaveners and do not rely on yeast, they are quick to prepare and bake.

Procedure Mix together 1 3/4 cup flour, 1/3 cup of sugar, 2 teaspoons baking powder, and 1/4 teaspoon of salt. Make a well in the center. In a separate bowl, mix together 1 beaten egg, 3/4 cup of milk, and 1/4 cup vegetable oil. Then pour into the well of the first bowl. Fold together just until moistened. Spoon batter into paper lined muffin cups until 2/3 full. Bake at 400° for 20 minutes.

Analysis Which ingredients provide the leavening in this recipe? What would happen if you substituted baking soda for the powder? What if buttermilk were used instead?

NSES B Develop an understanding of chemical reactions.

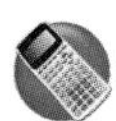

Mathematics

18. Changing Recipe Yield Beatrice needs to prepare 30 biscuits for a large upcoming brunch. However, the biscuit recipe she is using has a yield of just 12 biscuits. If the biscuit recipe calls for 2 1/2 cups of flour, 1 Tbsp. of baking powder, 1/2 tsp. of salt, 1 Tbsp. of sugar, 1/2 cup of butter, 3/4 cup of milk, and 1 egg, rewrite the recipe to yield 30 biscuits.

Math Concept **Multiplying Fractions** To multiply fractions, first convert any mixed or whole numbers to improper fractions. Then multiply all numerators to get the new numerator, and multiply the denominators to get the new denominator. Reduce to lowest terms.

Starting Hint You will need to multiply each ingredient amount by the ratio of the new yield to the old yield, written as a fraction in lowest terms.

NCTM Number and Operations Compute fluently and make reasonable estimates.

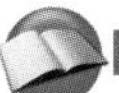

English Language Arts

19. Bread Song Write a song to educate children about the two major types of bread. Your song may have an original tune or may be set to a familiar tune. Make your song informative, factual, and fun. Include all the steps involved in baking bread in your lyrics. Include four verses and a chorus that is repeated between them.

NCTE 12 Use language to accomplish individual purposes.

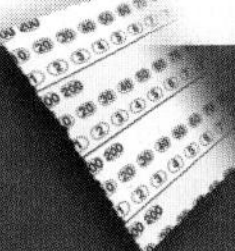

STANDARDIZED TEST PRACTICE

TRUE OR FALSE

Read the statement and determine if it is true or false.

20. To punch down dough, thrust your fist into the center of the dough 3 to 5 times.

a. True

b. False

Test-Taking Tip Before deciding whether a statement is true or false, read it carefully, and recall what you have learned from reading the text. Does the statement reflect what you know? Pay close attention to individual words. One word can make the difference between a true statement and a false one.

CHAPTER 44

Cakes, Cookies, & Candies

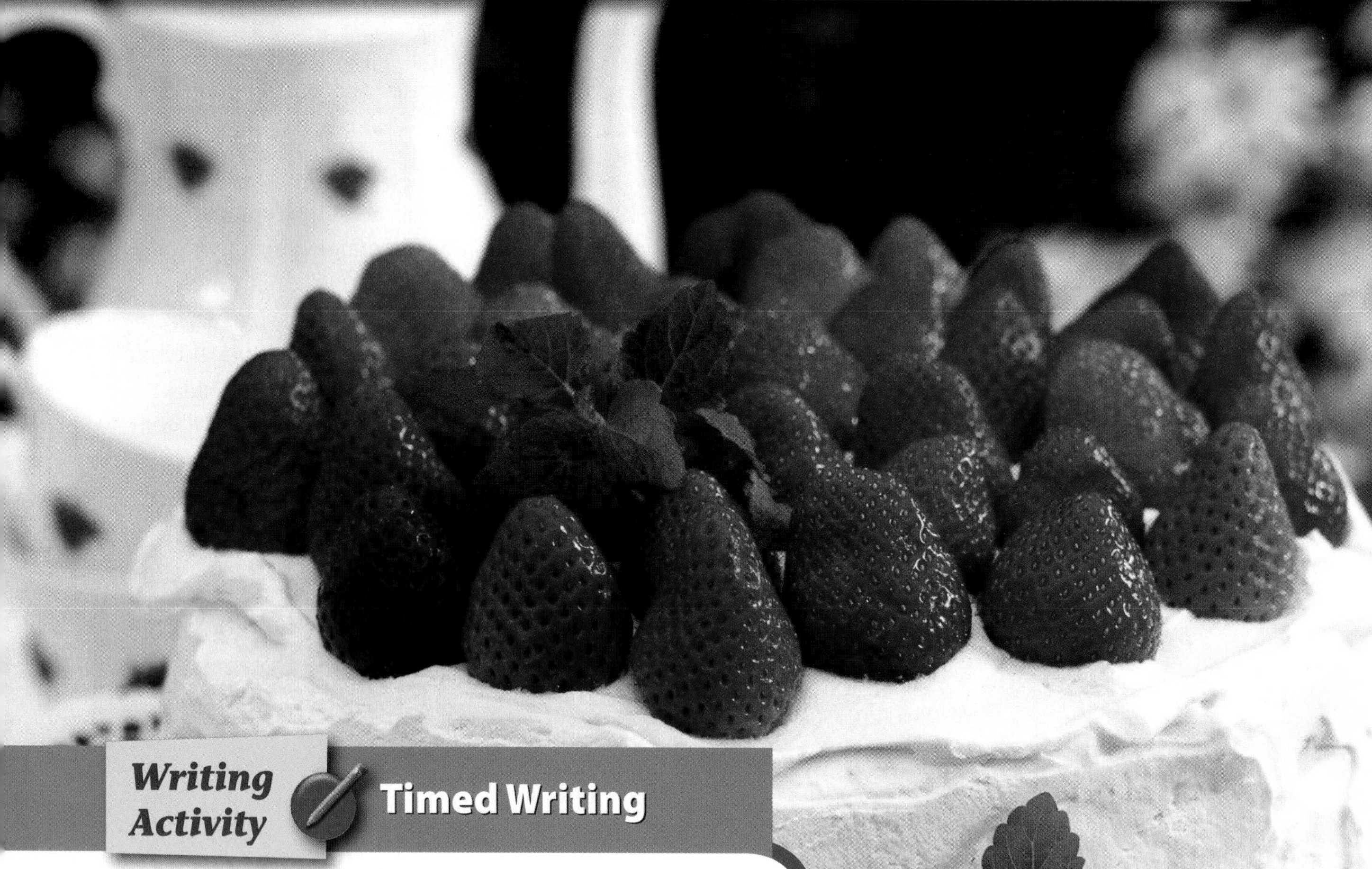

Writing Activity — Timed Writing

Celebratory Foods Some foods, including cakes, cookies, and candies, are associated with celebrations, gatherings, and holidays. Take 20 minutes to compose a one-page essay on the topic of celebratory foods. Why are specific foods eaten during certain occasions? What are some examples of foods and occasions? Which is your favorite and why?

Writing Tips Follow these steps to complete a timed writing:

- Plan your essay's organization before you begin writing by creating an outline.
- Take a few minutes to jot down notes and ideas in your outline.
- Focus more on the quality of content than the quantity.

Activate Prior Knowledge

Treats Cakes, cookies, and candies often look as good as they taste. *What are some ways to make cakes and cookies look special?*

Reading Guide

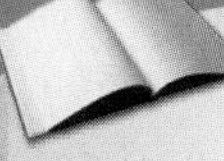

Before You Read

Preview Examine the photos and read their captions. Think about methods you may have used to prepare cakes, cookies, or candy.

Read to Learn

Key Concepts

- **Describe** methods for making and decorating cakes.
- **List** and describe the six types of cookies.
- **Explain** the impact of temperature and crystallization in candy making.

Main Idea

Cakes, cookies, and candies are flavorful and appealing treats that can be made by carefully and precisely following recipes.

Content Vocabulary

You will find definitions for these words in the glossary at the back of this book.

- ☐ shortened cake
- ☐ conventional method
- ☐ one-bowl method
- ☐ foam cake
- ☐ bar cookie
- ☐ drop cookie
- ☐ rolled cookie
- ☐ molded cookie
- ☐ refrigerator cookie
- ☐ pressed cookie
- ☐ cold water test
- ☐ crystallization
- ☐ interfering agent

Academic Vocabulary

You will find these words in your reading and on your tests. Use the glossary to look up their definitions, if necessary.

- precision
- induce

Graphic Organizer

Use a graphic organizer like the one below to take notes about the six types of cookies.

TYPE	DESCRIPTION
bar cookie	
drop cookie	
rolled cookie	
molded cookie	
refrigerator cookie	
pressed cookie	

Graphic Organizer Go to this book's Online Learning Center at **glencoe.com** to print out this graphic organizer.

Academic Standards

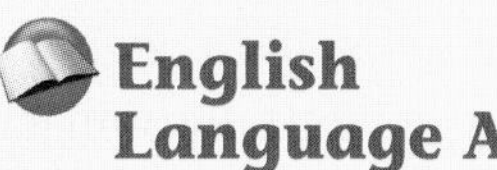

English Language Arts

NCTE 8 Use information resources to gather information and create and communicate knowledge.

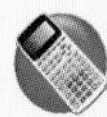

Mathematics

NCTM Geometry Use visualization, spatial reasoning, and geometric modeling to solve problems.

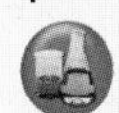

Science

NSES B Develop an understanding of chemical reactions.

NSES B Develop an understanding of the interactions of energy and matter.

NCTE *National Council of Teachers of English*
NCTM *National Council of Teachers of Mathematics*
NSES *National Science Education Standards*
NCSS *National Council for the Social Studies*

Making Cakes

To make a cake successfully, it is important to follow a recipe very carefully. Ingredient amounts, mixing techniques, and baking times are developed to work together with scientific **precision**, or exactness. Always check a reliable guide before making ingredient substitutions. Remember that mixing directions are calculated to incorporate the right amount of air to give a cake batter the best volume and texture.

Ingredients should usually be at room temperature before you begin to make a cake batter. Using ingredients at room temperature makes fat easier to mix and prevents eggs from curdling.

Shortened Cakes

The two basic types of cakes are shortened cakes and foam cakes. A **shortened cake** contains a solid fat such as butter, margarine, or shortening, as well as flour, salt, sugar, eggs, and liquid. The main leavening agent is baking powder or baking soda. Shortened cakes are sometimes called butter cakes.

A quality shortened cake has good volume and a moist, tender texture. It has been mixed thoroughly, yet quickly, to control the amount of gluten and air. The result is grain that is fine and even, without tunnels. Shortened cake usually requires what is known as the conventional mixing method, but some recipes call for the faster, one-bowl method.

Conventional Method

In the **conventional method** for making shortened cakes, fat and sugar are creamed together. Sugar crystals grate against the fat, creating holes that fill with air. This builds volume into the batter.

Follow these steps to make a shortened cake with the conventional method:

1. Sift the dry ingredients. All of the dry ingredients should be sifted together.

2. Cream the fat and sugar. The solid fat and the sugar mixture should be combined until it has a light and fluffy consistency resembling whipped cream.

3. Beat the eggs. If eggs are to be beaten into the creamed mixture, pour them into the mixture according to the recipe. Recipes usually call for the eggs to be added one at a time.

4. Mix the liquid ingredients. The liquid ingredients should be combined in a separate bowl.

5. Blend dry and moist ingredients. Add one-fourth of the dry ingredients to the creamed mixture. Then add one-third of the liquids. Repeat, ending with the dry ingredients. This method helps keep the fat from separating, which could allow air to escape. Beat just enough to mix the ingredients after each addition. The batter should be thick and smooth. Overbeating causes a coarse texture and smaller volume.

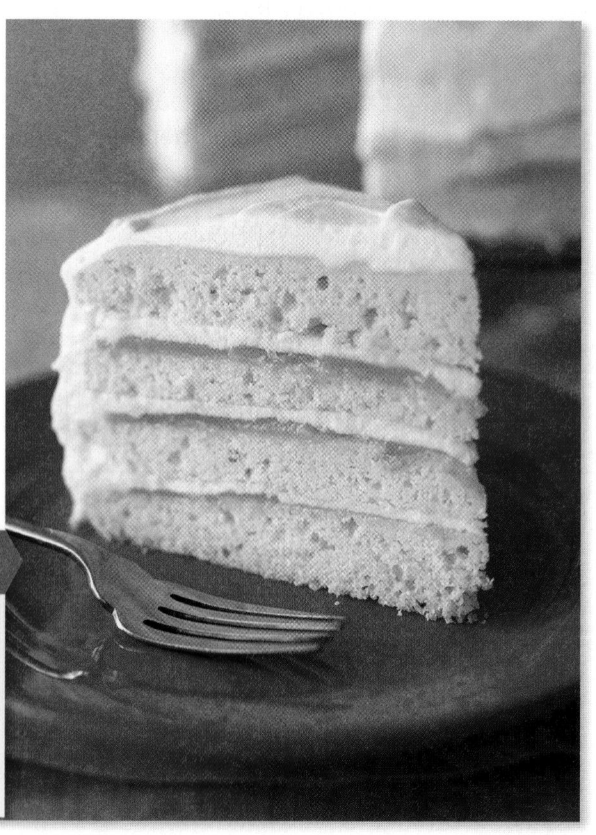

Foam Cake

Different cakes have different textures. A foam cake, like this angel food cake, is leavened by air trapped in beaten egg whites. A shortened cake is higher in fat with a more tender texture. *What is the purpose of creaming fat and sugar when making a shortened cake using the conventional method?*

Figure 44.1 Baking Pan Equivalents

Pan Sizes Using the right size pan gives a cake that is tender, not overcooked or undercooked. Leave room for cakes to rise by filling the pan only about half full with batter. ***About how much cake batter does it take to fill a single muffin cup?***

Batter Amounts	Pan Sizes to Use
4 cups of batter	8 × 1½ inch round cake or pie pan; 12-cup muffin pan
6 cups of batter	8 × 2 inch round cake pan; 9 × 1½ inch round cake pan; 8 × 8 inch square cake pan; 7½-inch Bundt pan
8 cups of batter	9 × 2 inch round cake or pie pan; 8 × 8 inch square cake pan; 5 × 3 inch loaf pan; 9-inch Bundt pan

One-Bowl Method

The **one-bowl method** is a quick way to mix ingredients for a shortened cake. In this method, combine dry ingredients first and then add moist ingredients. Some cakes made with the one-bowl method use oil instead of solid fat. Use the quick method only when a recipe calls for it. Cakes made using this method generally have a coarser texture. If you prefer a light and airy cake, do not use this method.

Follow these steps to make a shortened cake with the one-bowl method:

1. **Mix the dry ingredients.** Combine the dry ingredients in a large mixing bowl.
2. **Add fat and liquid.** Add to the dry ingredient mixture the fat, flavoring, and part of the liquid. Mix to make batter.
3. **Add eggs and liquid.** Add the unbeaten eggs and the remaining liquid and beat until thick and smooth. This can be done by hand or with an electric mixer. Scrape down the sides of the bowl several times to catch traces of unmixed ingredients.

Baking Shortened Cakes

Shortened cakes can be baked in a variety of pans, including muffin pans, sheet pans, and bundt pans in all types of shapes. Use the pan size specified in the recipe. If this is not possible, choose a pan in which the batter fills no more than about one half. Adjust the baking time accordingly. **Figure 44.1** shows what size pan to use for various amounts of batter.

Cakes continue to bake even after they have risen to full size. When a cake is done, it has a thin, shiny crust, is nicely browned, and slightly rounded. The sides start to pull away from the pan and the top feels firm but springy. To test for doneness, insert a wooden toothpick in the center. If it comes out free of moist batter, the cake is done.

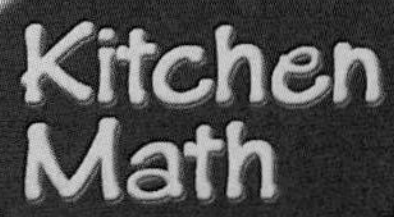

Novelty Baking Pans

At a garage sale, Kevin picks out a triangular baking pan, thinking that it will be fun to bake triangular cakes. Unfortunately, when he gets home, he realizes that he has no idea how much the pan holds. If the pan is 9 in. wide, 9 in. tall, and 3 in. deep, how many cups of batter will it hold?

Math Concept **Volume of a Prism** A prism is a solid that has two parallel, equal-sized, polygonal bases. To calculate volume, find the area of one of the bases, and multiply by the height of the prism.

Starting Hint Think of the pan as a prism with a triangular base. You will need to calculate the area of the triangle by multiplying ½ × base × height (½ in. × 9 in. × 9 in.). Then multiply by the depth of the pan to find the total volume in cubic inches. Divide by 14.4 to convert to cups, and round to the nearest cup.

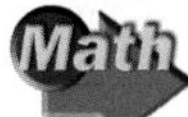

Appendix For math help, go to the Math Appendix at the back of the book.

NCTM Geometry Use visualization, spatial reasoning, and geometric modeling to solve problems.

Foam Cakes

A **foam cake** is leavened by air trapped in a protein foam of stiffly beaten egg whites. Foam cakes have a light, spongy texture and high volume. They come in three types: angel food, sponge, and chiffon.

Angel Food Cakes Containing no fat, angel-food cakes are made by beating egg whites with sugar until the mixture is stiff and glossy. Flour is sifted and gently folded in.

Sponge Cakes Named for their springy consistency, sponge cakes include egg yolks that are beaten until pale and thick, then mixed with the liquid ingredients. Flour is sifted and folded into the beaten egg whites, and the two mixtures are folded together.

Chiffon Cakes It takes four mixing steps to create a chiffon cake. First, flour, sugar, and baking powder are sifted together. Second, egg yolks are beaten with oil and liquids. Third, the liquid ingredients are stirred into the dry ingredients. Fourth, beaten egg whites are gradually folded into the batter.

Baking Foam Cakes

A tube pan is traditional for foam cakes because it gives the airy batter plenty of support to rise. Two-piece tube pans have a separate bottom for removing the cake more easily. A one-piece pan can be lined with parchment paper to help prevent sticking.

To test for doneness, touch the top lightly. It should spring back. Cool the cake upside down in the pan to keep its fragile structure from collapsing. Some pans have legs on the rim for this purpose. You may also invert the cake on an empty glass bottle with a slender neck or on a large funnel turned upside down.

When the cake is cool, gently loosen it from the sides of the pan with a spatula. If the pan has a removable bottom, push it upward and use the spatula to free the cake. Invert the pan and the cake onto a serving plate.

Decorating Cakes

Frostings can be cooked or uncooked. Cooked frosting is heated to a certain temperature that is measured with a candy thermometer. The frosting is then cooled slightly and beaten until creamy. Frosting can also be cooked in a double boiler while being beaten with a mixer until it stands in soft peaks.

Uncooked frosting is easier to make. Cream confectioners' sugar with butter, margarine, or cream cheese. Blend in milk to make it easier to spread. Extracts, such as chocolate or vanilla, can be added to add flavor. Thin glazes are made the same way.

When making frosting, cover the container as you work to keep the mixture from drying out and forming a crust. Dry frosting is difficult to use, and flakes of crust are unattractive.

Frosting is high in fat, sugar, and calories. One alternative is a drizzling of glaze made with confectioners' sugar and fruit juice. Another option is to stencil a decorative design onto the cake using confectioners' sugar or another powder such as cocoa.

✓ **Reading Check** **Explain** How can you prevent a foam cake from sticking to a one-piece pan?

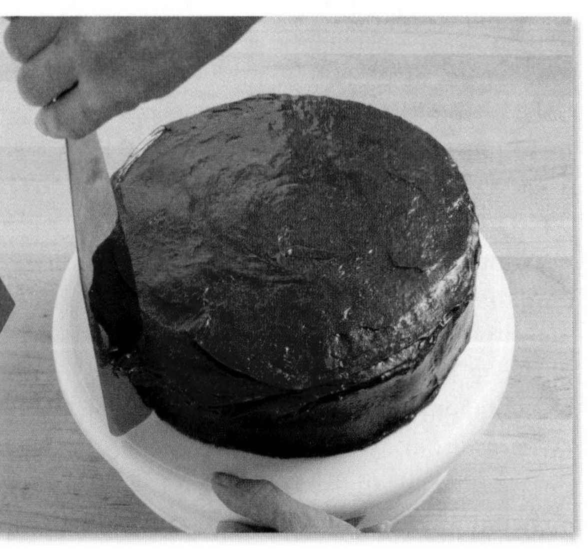

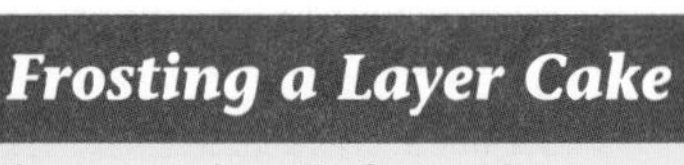

Frosting a Layer Cake

Frosting holds layer cakes together. To frost a layer cake, first brush off crumbs carefully. Frost the tops of the lower layers, but not their sides. Stack the layers and put the top layer in place. Frost the sides and top of the cake. *How is uncooked frosting made?*

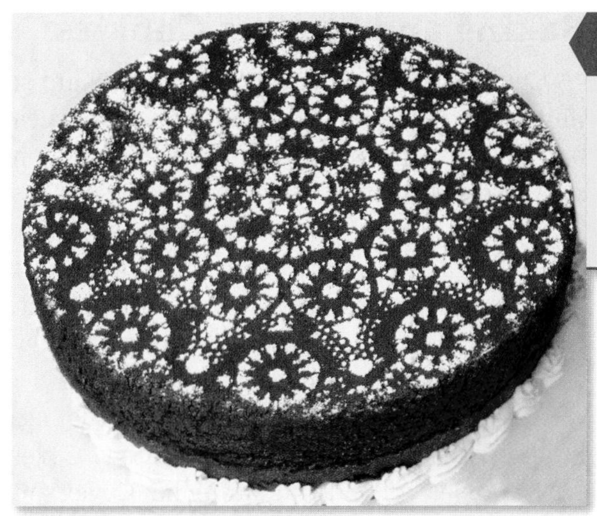

Finishing Touches

To stencil a cake, place a stencil or doily on top and sprinkle with confectioners' sugar, cocoa, ground cinnamon, grated chocolate, or finely ground nuts. Remove the stencil carefully. *What is the nutritional benefit of using this decorative method?*

Making Cookies

Cakes and cookies are made with similar ingredients. The main difference is that cookies have relatively little liquid, which gives them a thicker texture.

Cookies come in countless varieties, from crunchy butter wafers to soft, jam-filled rings. There are six basic types of cookies, based on how they are formed. These are bar cookies, drop cookies, rolled cookies, molded cookies, refrigerator cookies, and pressed cookies.

Bar Cookies

Baked in a shallow pan and then cut into a bar or square, a **bar cookie** can be soft, firm or layered with different bases, fillings, and toppings. Brownies are a popular type of bar cookie.

Bar cookies are usually cut when cool. Use a sharp, thin-bladed knife to make clean, even cuts. Removing a corner piece first makes others easier to lift out.

Drop Cookies

A **drop cookie** is made from soft dough dropped onto a cookie sheet. Chocolate chip cookies are popular drop cookies.

A small cookie scoop is handy for forming drop cookies. You can also scoop a rounded portion of the dough on a teaspoon and then push it onto the sheet with a rubber scraper or another teaspoon. Allow at least 2 inches between cookies on the sheet, since they spread and flatten during baking.

Rolled Cookies

Made from stiff dough, a **rolled cookie** has been cut into different shapes with cookie cutters before baking. Chill rolled cookie dough to make it easier to handle. Work with a small amount of dough at a time, leaving the rest in the refrigerator. On a lightly floured surface, roll the dough to about ⅛ inch in thickness. Use as little flour as possible to avoid drying out the cookies.

Before cutting rolled cookies, dip the cookie cutter in flour and shake off the excess. Work efficiently by positioning cutters to minimize excess scraps of dough. These can be rolled and cut again, but they get a little tougher in texture each time. Use a spatula to place the cookies on a baking sheet about 1 inch apart.

Molded Cookies

Shaped by hand, a **molded cookie** can be rolled in chopped nuts or other coatings before baking. Some are flattened with the bottom of a glass. Others are patterned with cookie stamps or tiles. Peanut butter cookies are pressed with a fork, creating their characteristic ridges. You can also make crescents, pretzels, logs, or twists.

Chill molded cookie dough to make it easier to shape. Pinch off walnut-size pieces of dough and form them quickly. Overworking makes cookies tough. Press the dough together so the cookies hold their shape.

Place molded cookies about 1 inch apart on a cookie sheet, or 3 inches apart if you are going to flatten them. If using a glass or fork for pressing, dip it in flour or granulated sugar to keep it from sticking to the dough. If using cookie stamps, oil them lightly before use and flour them between cookies.

Raw Cookie Dough

Many people love to eat raw cookie dough, which has all the sweetness and flavor of a cookie, but with an appealing, soft, and gooey texture. For safety reasons, however, you should resist the temptation to nibble on even small amounts of raw, homemade cookie dough while baking. It nearly always contains raw eggs, which can carry a dangerous bacterium called *Salmonella*, one of the leading causes of food-borne illness-related deaths in the United States. Are you wondering about your favorite flavor of ice cream? Cookie dough ice cream contains specially made and pasteurized cookie dough, so it is safe to eat.

What Would You Do? Kenny loves to eat cookie dough, but knows it is unsafe. Instead, he undercooks his cookies by about 5 minutes so they will have a soft and gooey texture. Would you eat Kenny's cookies?

Refrigerator Cookies

A **refrigerator cookie** starts with dough formed into long, even rolls about 1½ to 2 inches in diameter. Wrap the rolls well in wax paper, foil, or plastic wrap, and chill them as the recipe directs. The dough can be prepared several days in advance.

To cut, slice the roll by encircling it with heavy thread and pulling the ends. Place slices about 1 inch apart on the cookie sheet.

Pressed Cookies

Dough can be forced through a cookie press and directly onto a baking sheet. The result is a **pressed cookie**. Spritz cookies, made with a basic butter dough, are a popular type of pressed cookie. Cookie presses include disks for making an array of shapes, from clovers to camels.

The pressed cookie dough must be soft enough to press but firm enough to hold its shape. Work quickly for best results. Pressed cookies have a stiff dough that spreads very little, so you need only about ½ inch between cookies on the sheet.

Baking and Storing Cookies

Cookies bake more evenly when they are of uniform size. Let cookie sheets cool between batches. Dough softens and loses its shape on a hot baking sheet.

Cookies are delicately browned when done. To test drop and bar cookies, lightly press one with your finger. You should see a slight imprint. Remove cookies from the sheet as soon as they are done unless the recipe states otherwise.

Store cookies in a container after cooling. Store crisp and soft cookies separately. Cover crisp cookies with a loose-fitting lid. Cover soft cookies with a tight-fitting lid. You can also freeze cookies for longer storage.

Convenience Cakes and Cookies

Cake and cookie mixes are prepared mixes that you combine with water, oil, and eggs. Some mixes rival homemade recipes in taste and quality. Many boxes list recipe variations. Frostings are also sold in mixes and ready-to-use forms.

You can make cookies from cake mix by reducing the amount of liquid in the recipe. You can also find ready-to-use cookie dough in the store's refrigerator case.

✓ **Reading Check** **Describe** How can you tell when cookies are done baking?

Making Candies

Candies are sweet, chewy, or crunchy desserts made from sugar, liquid, flavorings, and sometimes other ingredients such as egg whites, fat, and cream. Candy making is an even more exact art and science than baking. You cannot substitute ingredients in a candy recipe as you might in a cookie.

You must also pay attention to temperature and time. Thirty seconds can mean the difference between success and failure.

Increasing or decreasing the yields in candy recipes is tricky. If the yield of a recipe is too small, make additional batches rather than doubling the recipe.

Types of Candies

Like cakes and cookies, candy comes in many forms, including:

Nougat Chewy or crunchy, nougat is made by beating hot sugar syrup into beaten egg whites.

Fondant Smooth and pliable, fondant is usually a base for other candies, including mint patties and chocolate-covered cherries. Fondant is extremely sweet because it is made by cooking large amounts of sugar into water. Cooking the sugar allows it to form tiny crystals that come out smooth. Fondant is so smooth in texture that it is used for attractive cakes, including wedding cakes.

Divinity The soft, sweet, and puffy qualities of divinity come from its stiffly beaten egg whites, sugar, corn syrup, and flavoring.

Taffy Pulled and twisted into long strands to incorporate air, taffy is a soft, chewy candy that is made in many colors.

Caramel Rich and chewy, caramel is formed by cooking butter, milk or cream, and sugar.

If you are new to making candy, it is a good idea to build your skills by starting with easy-to-prepare candies that need little or no cooking.

Principles of Candy Making

In candy making, chemical processes transform the ingredients from liquid to solid. To master the art, you need to understand its two most important aspects: temperature and crystallization.

The Role of Temperature

Why do candy recipes call for such unusual temperatures, such as 248°F? As you cook a candy mixture, the mixture starts to boil. As liquid evaporates, the mixture thickens and its boiling point rises. The boiling point continues to rise as more liquid escapes. Therefore, the longer candy boils and the drier it becomes, the hotter it gets. Temperature is a measure of how much liquid is left in the mixture.

To monitor the temperature of candy-in-progress, place a candy thermometer in the pan so it can be read at any time. Make sure the bulb of the thermometer does not touch the bottom of the pan.

If you do not have a thermometer, you can use the **cold water test**, a way to estimate syrup temperature based on how it acts in cold water. This test is less reliable than a thermometer, but it is still effective.

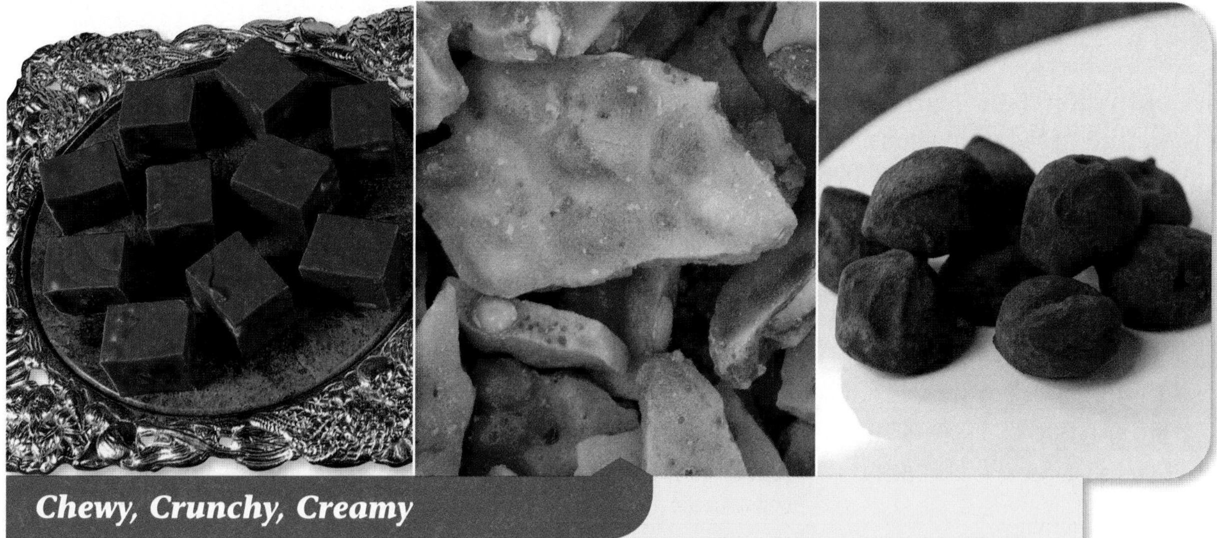

Chewy, Crunchy, Creamy

Different candies have different textures. Creamy, semisoft fudge (left) is made with sugar, corn syrup, butter, and cream. Crunchy brittle (center) is made with caramelized sugar and nuts. Rich, creamy truffles (right) are made with chocolate, sugar, butter or cream, and flavorings. They are rolled into balls and coated with chocolate. *What are the ingredients in caramel?*

To perform the cold water test, follow these steps:

1. Drop syrup into water. With a clean wooden spoon, drop about ½ teaspoon of the hot syrup into a cup of cold, not icy, water.

2. Form the syrup into a ball. Use your fingertips to form the drops of syrup into a ball in the water.

3. Test for firmness. Remove the ball from the water and note its firmness. Hotter syrups form harder balls. If the syrup does not behave as the recipe directs, it has not reached the proper temperature. Cook it a few minutes longer and test again. **Figure 44.2** shows how to estimate the temperature of syrup based on its consistency.

Crystallization

Crystallization is the formation of sugar crystals in syrup. It happens when molecules of glucose and fructose that are dissolved in syrup reunite and turn back into granulated sugar. Crystallization can happen as a mixture boils, when less water is available to keep the molecules dissolved. Sometimes a solid sugar crystal or bit of lint falls into the mixture, starting a chain reaction of crystallization. Crystallization can also occur as candy cools and is less able to hold dissolved sugar.

Science in Action: The Role of Humidity in Candy Making

Humidity in the air impacts candy making. Why? Sugar attracts moisture. On hot and humid days, candy absorbs water vapor from the air and stays softer than desired. That is why many people make candy only in dry weather. At higher altitudes, mixtures boil at lower temperatures, which can also affect the candy making process.

Procedure High altitudes are usually less humid than lower ones. So why and how do you think candy is affected if syrup mixtures boil at lower temperatures in high altitudes? Use the Internet to research what can be done to ensure a good outcome when making candy at high altitudes.

Analysis Write a list of suggestions you have found for making candy at high altitudes.

NSES B Develop an understanding of the interactions of energy and matter.

Small crystals create the smooth, silky texture that marks a superior candy. Large crystals, however, feel gritty on the tongue. That is why controlling crystallization is the key to candy making.

Figure 44.2 Estimating Candy Temperature

Cold Water Test The cold water test is a way to estimate a candy's temperature based on its consistency. As candy cooks, it passes through the stages shown in this chart, from loose and sticky to brittle. ***If a recipe calls for candy to reach 245°F, how should it behave during the cold water test?***

Stage	Temperature	Consistency
Thread stage	230–233°F	Forms a loose, sticky thread that will not form into a ball.
Soft-ball stage	234–240°F	Forms a soft ball that flattens.
Firm-ball stage	244–248°F	Forms a ball that holds its shape, is pliable, and does not flatten.
Hard-ball stage	250–266°F	Forms a hard, compact ball that holds its shape but flattens when pressed between the fingers.
Soft-crack stage	270–290°F	Forms firm threads that are pliable when removed from water.
Hard-crack stage	300–310°F	Forms brittle threads that break or snap easily when removed from water.
Caramel stage	320–338°F	Forms brittle threads, and liquid turns brown.

Molding Candy

You can pour many types of candies into molds. The candy cools in the mold, taking on a decorative shape. *What kind of pan should you use for making candy? Why?*

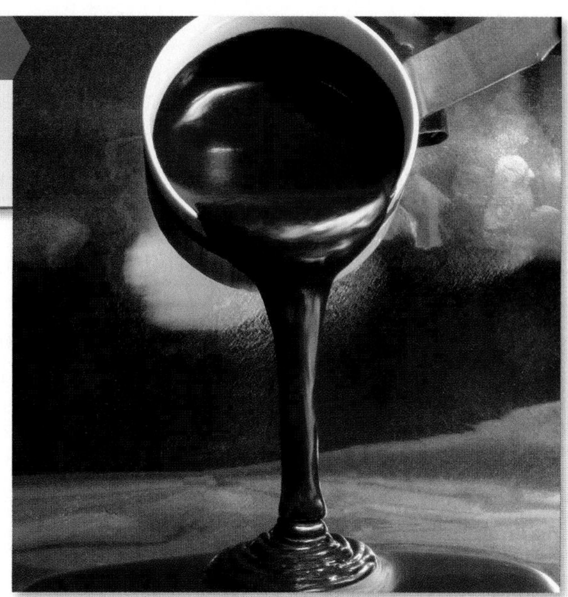

To keep sugar crystals small, recipes often include ingredients called interfering agents. An **interfering agent** is an ingredient that breaks down sugar crystals or keeps them from forming. Cream of tartar is an acid that breaks down sugar crystals. Fat gets between sugar molecules and keeps them apart. Corn syrup adds extra glucose to the syrup, which helps to block excessive crystallization.

You can also manage crystals by mixing. You can **induce**, or bring about, crystallization by starting to beat the mixture when it has cooled. Continue to beat the mixture to produce more small crystals. If you keep beating until crystallization stops, you will create a creamy, velvety texture. Some candies, such as toffee and caramel, should not have any crystals at all. These candies have a large amount of butter and are cooled without stirring.

Preventing Unwanted Crystallization The following guidelines can help you prevent unwanted crystallization:

- Have all ingredients at room temperature.
- Use only clean pans, spoons, and thermometers. Wash and dry equipment before reusing it. Dip cold utensils in warm water to warm them.
- Rub the sides of the pan with butter to prevent sugar from sticking.
- Put sugar in the pan first. Wash the sides with the liquid used in the recipe.
- Dissolve crystals on pan sides with a pastry brush dipped in hot water while cooking. Watch for crystals that start to slide into the syrup.
- Work quickly when pouring out the mixture. Be careful not to scrape the sides or the bottom of the pan.
- Save syrup that starts to crystallize by adding a small amount of water. You will have to cook the mixture again.

Steps in Candy Making

Most candy is made by heating ingredients in a pan, stirring and beating the mixture, and then molding or cutting it to shape. Candy making requires exact timing, so pre-preparation is essential.

Preparing to Cook Candy

Read the entire candy recipe before beginning to cook. Measure and arrange all ingredients so they will be at hand when needed. Assemble the equipment you will need, such as a baking sheet and cooling racks. Some candies, such as nougat and divinity, require a sturdy, free-standing electric mixer. Portable mixers do not have enough power. Some candies also require specialized equipment, such as candy molds and dipping forks.

For most candy recipes you will need:

- A candy thermometer.
- A heavy, deep pan with straight sides. Choose a pan that holds about three times the volume of the ingredients. If the pan is too small, the syrup can foam up and boil over, making a mess and possibly causing burns. If the pan is too large, the mixture may not be deep enough to cover the bulb of the thermometer.
- A wooden or silicone spoon with a long handle. Sugar syrups reach very high temperatures. Metal spoons get too hot to hold, and plastic spoons may melt.

Cooking Candy

Different candies are made using different methods. Most candies require quick action, so read recipes through before beginning. One process found in many recipes involves these steps:

1. Attach the thermometer. Clip the candy thermometer to the side of the pan.

2. Add ingredients to the pan. Add the basic ingredients, such as sugars, liquids, and butter.

3. Heat and stir. Place the pan over low heat and stir until the sugar is completely dissolved. Stir constantly but carefully to minimize splashing. Avoid scraping the sides, which could trigger crystallization.

4. Boil. Add other ingredients as called for in the recipe, and bring the mixture to the correct temperature. Stir as the recipe instructs. You may need to stir the boiling mixture occasionally or stop stirring once the sugar dissolves.

5. Remove from heat. After moving the pan away from the heat, stir in extracts, nuts, or other flavorings, as directed.

6. Let cool. Let the mixture cool undisturbed to the temperature indicated. Some recipes advise placing the pan in water to speed cooling and encourage fine crystals to grow.

7. Beat. Beat the mixture according to the recipe. Pour or drop the candy onto baking sheets or pans, which are usually prepared by buttering or lining with wax paper.

Storing Candies

Allow candies to cool completely before storing them. Keep them in a cool place in a tightly covered container, layered between sheets of wax paper, plastic, or foil. You can also wrap them individually. Most candies can keep this way for up to three weeks. Many candies can be frozen for up to one year.

Light and Healthy Recipe

Orange-Almond Biscotti

This biscotti recipe is a low-sugar, low-fat treat.

Ingredients

- **1½ cup** Flour
- **½ cup** Sugar
- **1 tsp.** Orange zest
- **¼ tsp.** Salt
- **2** Eggs
- **¼ cup** Olive oil
- **1 tsp.** Vanilla extract

Directions

1. Preheat oven to 450°F.
2. In a large mixing bowl, combine the flour, sugar, orange zest, and salt. Mix well. In a separate bowl, beat the eggs and add the olive oil and vanilla extract.
3. Mix the dry ingredients with the wet ingredients.
4. Pour the batter onto a baking sheet lined with parchment. Pour in a straight line across the middle of the baking sheet so that the center is higher than the edges.
5. Bake for 25 minutes.
6. Remove from the oven and let cool.
7. Slice lengthwise into 1-inch pieces and lay the pieces on their sides on a baking sheet. Bake again for 20 minutes.

Yield 16 servings

Nutrition Analysis per Serving

■ Calories	100
■ Total fat	4 g
Saturated fat	1 g
Cholesterol	30 mg
■ Sodium	83 mg
■ Carbohydrate	14 g
Dietary fiber	0 g
Sugars	5 g
■ Protein	2 g

CHAPTER 44 Review & Applications

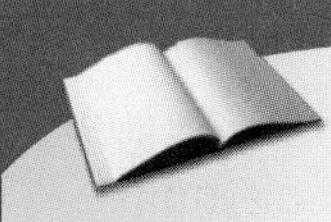

After You Read

Chapter Summary

Cakes, cookies, and candies are flavorful treats. The two basic types of cakes are shortened cakes and foam cakes, which are made using different methods. Cakes can be decorated using frosting, icing, or other toppings. Cookies have a thicker texture than cakes, but are made using similar ingredients. There are several types of cookies, each with its own taste, texture, appearance, and preparation method. Cookies must be baked and stored properly. Cakes, cookies, and frostings are available in convenience forms. Candies also come in many forms, and are made through a chemical process. They should be stored properly to retain their flavor and freshness.

Content and Academic Vocabulary Review

1. Use each of these content and academic vocabulary words in a sentence.

Content Vocabulary

- ▫ shortened cake (p. 682)
- ▫ conventional method (p. 682)
- ▫ one-bowl method (p. 683)
- ▫ foam cake (p. 684)
- ▫ bar cookie (p. 685)
- ▫ drop cookie (p. 685)
- ▫ rolled cookie (p. 685)
- ▫ molded cookie (p. 685)
- ▫ refrigerator cookie (p. 686)
- ▫ pressed cookie (p. 686)
- ▫ cold water test (p. 687)
- ▫ crystallization (p. 688)
- ▫ interfering agent (p. 689)

Academic Vocabulary

- precision (p. 682)
- induce (p. 689)

Review Key Concepts

2. **Describe** methods for making and decorating cakes.
3. **List** and describe the six types of cookies.
4. **Explain** the impact of temperature and crystallization in candy making.

Critical Thinking

5. **Evaluate** whether you should bake a cake without a recipe, even if you remember most of the ingredients.
6. **Predict** the consequences if Jorge uses the one-bowl method to prepare a cake recipe that calls for the conventional method.
7. **Compare and contrast** cakes and cookies. How are they similar? How are they different?
8. **Explain** two reasons why candy might come out softer than desired, even if you carefully follow the recipe instructions.
9. **Evaluate** whether a bit of lint that fell from Elsa's sweater into her candy mixture started a chain reaction of crystallization.
10. **Infer** why there is no category for cakes and cookies in MyPyramid.

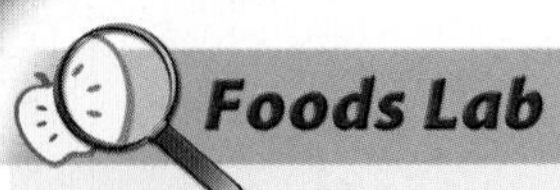

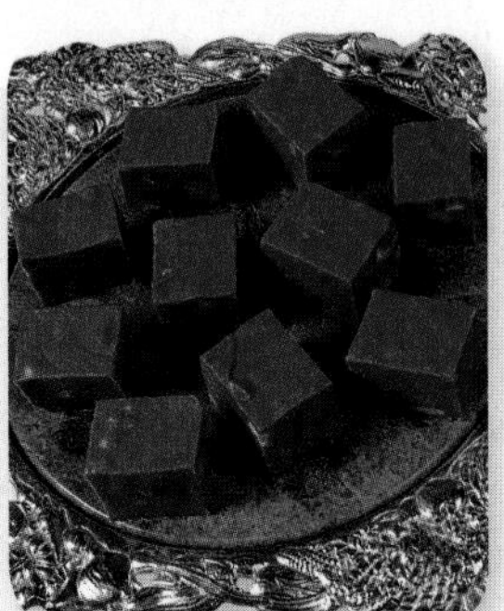

11. Reduced-Fat Brownies Special low-fat recipes can make treats like brownies more healthful. How does the reduction of fat content affect taste?

Procedure Prepare the full-fat or a reduced-fat brownie recipe assigned by your teacher. Serve samples of your recipe for a class taste test. Label your samples with a code, such as Team A.

Analysis Taste all samples, including your own. List them by their code names in order of preference. Which sample had the most appealing taste and appearance? The least?

HEALTHFUL CHOICES

12. Low-Fat Decorating Daphne is baking and decorating a cake for her friend's birthday party. The cake is made with a large quantity of butter, and has a high fat content. Daphne wants to decorate the cake, but is hesitant to add more fat. She does not want the cake to be left plain. What method of decorating can she choose?

TECH Connection

13. Cake Decorating Slideshow Under your teacher's supervision, use the Internet to find at least five creative ideas for cake decorating. They may involve unique ingredients, methods of application, or handy tools. Use slide show software to translate these ideas into an informative presentation for your classmates, so that they can try them in the future. If possible, add pictures to illustrate the decorating ideas.

Real-World Skills

Problem-Solving Skills

14. Broken Thermometer Enrique was in the middle of making a batch of candy. He was using a thermometer to monitor the temperature of his candy as it cooked, until the thermometer broke. Can Enrique still monitor the temperature of his candy mixture? If so, by what method?

Interpersonal and Collaborative Skills

15. Cookie Sale Follow your teacher's instructions to form groups. Then participate in a teacher-led, classwide discussion to plan a cookie sale. Decide on a worthy cause for which you would like to earn funds, and determine what type of cookies each group will prepare. Work with your group to find a recipe for the cookies you will make and sell.

Financial Literacy Skills

16. Cookie Sale Costs Work with the same group as in the interpersonal and collaborative activity above. Determine the cost of making 36 cookies using the recipe your group has chosen for the cookie sale. If you want to make a 75 percent profit, how much will you charge for each cookie?

Academic Skills

Food Science

17. Leavening Actions Baking soda and baking powder are two leavening agents frequently used in cakes and cookies.

Procedure Pour ½ cup of cold water into each of two bowls. Dissolve ½ teaspoon of baking soda into one bowl and ½ teaspoon of baking powder into the other. Observe and record the results. Add a teaspoon of vinegar to each bowl and observe and record the results.

Analysis Write a paragraph explaining what you have learned about baking soda and baking powder from this experiment.

NSES B Develop an understanding of chemical reactions.

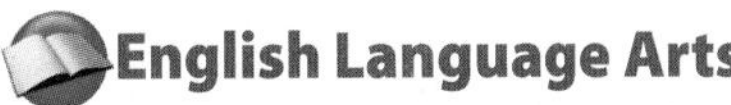

English Language Arts

19. History of Famous Cakes Research the history of cakes, learning about different famous types, such as Lady Baltimore cake, which is thought to have originated in the late 19th century, or Red Velvet cake, the deep red color of which camouflages the mild chocolate flavor it contains. Write a one-page report explaining the history or origins of one type of famous cake, as well as its ingredients, flavor, and appearance.

NCTE 8 Use information resources to gather information and create and communicate knowledge.

Mathematics

18. Frosting a Layer Cake Marie is making a circular, three-layer yellow cake. Each layer of cake is 2 inches tall and 8 inches in diameter. She would like to put a layer of chocolate frosting on top of each layer of cake, and would also like to cover the sides in the same chocolate frosting. If the frosting will be ½-inch thick in each location, what is the total surface area to be frosted?

Math Concept **Area and Circumference of Circles** Calculate circumference (C) as $C = \pi d$, where d = the circle's diameter and $\pi = 3.14$. Calculate the area (A) of a circle as $A = \pi r^2$, where the radius $r = (½)d$.

Starting Hint Calculate the area on the top of one circular layer of cake. Then multiply by 3 (since there are three layers). Find the area of the sides of the cake by multiplying the circumference of the cake by the total height (3 cake layers + 3 frosting layers) of the cake.

NCTM Geometry Use visualization, spatial reasoning, and geometric modeling to solve problems.

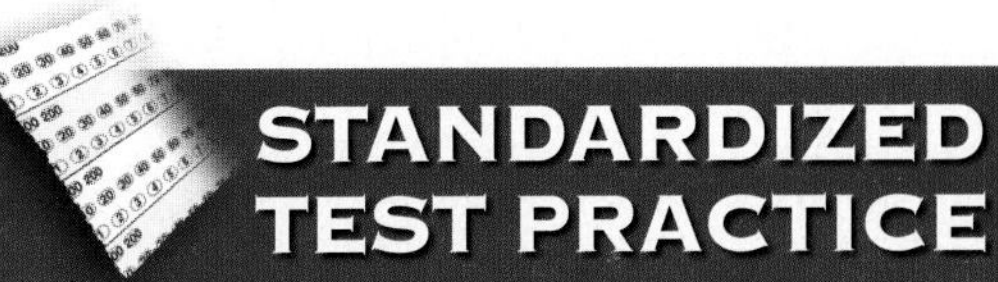

STANDARDIZED TEST PRACTICE

FILL IN THE BLANK

Read the sentence and choose the best phrase to fill in the blank.

20. A[n] __________ breaks down sugar crystals or keeps them from forming.

a. high elevation
b. humid environment
c. bit of lint
d. interfering agent

Test-Taking Tip When answering a fill-in-the-blank question, silently read the sentence with each of the possible answers in the blank space. This will help you eliminate wrong answers. The best word results in a sentence that is both factual and grammatically correct.

CHAPTER 45

Pies & Tarts

Writing Activity 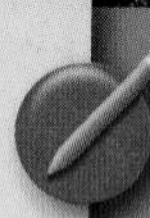 Evaluation

Read a Recipe Read a recipe for a pie or tart. Does the recipe appeal to you? Why or why not? Write a half-page evaluation of the recipe. Assess ingredients, preparation methods, the nutritional value, and other qualities. Explain why you would or would not choose to prepare this recipe.

Writing Tips Follow these steps to write an evaluation:

- Carefully examine a recipe and form opinions about it.
- Explain your perception of the recipe's strengths and weaknesses.
- Imagine that others will use your evaluation to decide whether to make the recipe.

Activate Prior Knowledge

Explore the Photo A pie is any dish that has a crust with a filling. *What kind of pies have you tried?*

Reading Guide

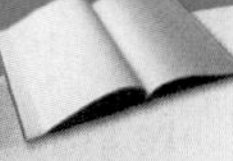

Before You Read

Preview Describe or draw the first image that comes to your mind when you think of pie. Then skim through the chapter. Think about the variety of pies and tarts you can make.

Read to Learn

Key Concepts

- **List** the four types of pies and give examples.
- **Describe** how to prepare and roll pastry dough.
- **Identify** ways that tarts and turnovers differ from pies.
- **Explain** how to prevent problems while baking pies and tarts.

Main Idea

Pies and tarts are dishes made with pastry crust and a variety of sweet or savory fillings, and may be served as appetizers, entrees, or desserts.

Content Vocabulary

You will find definitions for these words in the glossary at the back of this book.

- ☐ pie
- ☐ fluted edge
- ☐ lattice crust
- ☐ pie shell
- ☐ docking
- ☐ crumb crust
- ☐ streusel
- ☐ tart
- ☐ flan
- ☐ galette
- ☐ turnover

Academic Vocabulary

You will find these words in your reading and on your tests. Use the glossary to look up their definitions, if necessary.

- tendency
- coarse

Graphic Organizer

As you read, use a graphic organizer like the one below to take notes about four popular types of pies.

FRUIT PIES	CREAM PIES	CUSTARD PIES	SAVORY PIES

Graphic Organizer Go to this book's Online Learning Center at **glencoe.com** to print out this graphic organizer.

Academic Standards

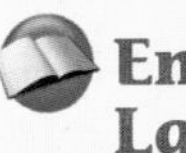

English Language Arts

NCTE 4 Use written language to communicate effectively.

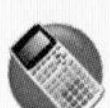

Mathematics

NCTM Problem Solving Solve problems that arise in mathematics and in other contexts.

NCTM Geometry Analyze characteristics and properties of two- and three-dimensional geometric shapes and develop mathematical arguments about geometric relationships.

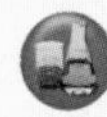

Science

NSES B Develop an understanding of the structure and properties of matter.

NCTE *National Council of Teachers of English*
NCTM *National Council of Teachers of Mathematics*
NSES *National Science Education Standards*
NCSS *National Council for the Social Studies*

Types of Pies

A **pie** is any dish that has a crust with a filling. Popular types of pies include:

Fruit Pies In fruit pies, whole or sliced fruit is combined with sugar and a starch thickener. The ratio of sugar to thickener varies depending on the fruit. The sugar and the fruit juices form into syrup. The thickener congeals the syrup to firm up the filling as it bakes. Common fruit pie thickeners include flour, cornstarch, and tapioca starch. Some pie makers blend thickeners to get the best qualities of each one, adding body and gloss but no color or flavor.

Cream Pies The "cream" in cream pies is usually a pudding. It has eggs, milk, cornstarch, and flavoring. The mixture is cooked until thick, then cooled and poured into a baked, cooled crust. Popular cream pie flavors include lemon, banana, coconut, butterscotch, and chocolate.

Custard Pies Custard pies are similar in texture to cream pies. They are made by baking uncooked custard along with the crust. Pumpkin pie and pecan pie are popular custard pies.

Savory Pies Savory pies contain cooked meat, poultry, seafood, or vegetables in a thickened sauce. Savory pies are usually served as a main course. The first pies ever made were probably savory.

✓ **Reading Check** **Identify** What type of pie contains meat?

Making Piecrust

The foundation of any pie is its crust. A tender and flaky pastry crust makes for the most appealing pie.

Pastry Dough Ingredients

Basic pastry dough has four ingredients: flour, water, fat, and salt. Flour and water form the structure. Fat tenderizes and adds flavor. Ice-cold water helps keep the fat from melting during mixing, which ensures a flaky texture. Some recipes include a little sugar and vinegar, which bind with flour proteins to limit the formation of gluten.

Most recipes for piecrust call for all-purpose flour. Some bakers use equal parts of all-purpose and cake flour. The resulting dough is softer and requires quick, skilled handling.

Vegetable shortening and lard are pure fat and make the flakiest crust. Butter, margarine, and cream cheese contain a little water, which creates a slightly crumbly texture like a butter cookie. These flavorful crusts are often used for tarts.

Piecrust can also be made with oil instead of solid fat, and with hot water instead of cold water. These changes require slightly different mixing methods and produce crusts with a different texture. Piecrusts made with oil are tender, but are more dry and grainy than flaky.

Preparing Pastry Dough

Preparing piecrust is similar to preparing biscuits. Cut the fat into the flour with a pastry blender or two knives until the mixture resembles coarse crumbs or small peas. Add water one tablespoon at a time, mixing lightly with a fork each time. Form a ball of dough that is neither crumbly nor sticky. You may need less water in humid weather.

Mix and handle piecrust as little as possible to keep particles of fat separated by moistened flour. If you mix the pastry too much, the particles break down. Overmixing overdevelops the gluten, changing texture from feathery to leathery.

After mixing, let the dough rest to relax the gluten. This keeps the dough from shrinking as it bakes. Cover the dough with wax paper and a towel so it stays moist. While the dough rests, you can work on the filling. If you handle the pastry too much, the particles melt from the heat in your hands.

Rolling Pastry Dough

After the dough rests, it is time to roll it out. You can roll piecrust on any clean, washable surface that is at a comfortable height. Follow these steps to roll crust:

1. Prepare the surface. Use one of two methods: Sprinkle your work surface and rolling pin with flour, or place the dough between two pieces of wax paper or plastic wrap. You do not need flour if you use wax paper.

2. Roll out the dough evenly. Press the ball of dough to flatten it slightly. Gently roll the dough out from the center in all directions, giving it an occasional quarter-turn to maintain a circular shape. Roll out the dough evenly to a thickness of about ⅛ inch and a diameter that measures 2 inches larger than the pie pan. Flour the rolling pin and surface only if the dough sticks.

3. Move the dough to the pan. Once you have the size and shape you want, brush any excess flour off the dough. Place the pie pan nearby and transfer the dough to the pan by one of two methods: Fold the dough in half or quarters, lift it into the pan, and gently unfold it; or wind the dough loosely around the rolling pin, hold the rolling pin over the far edge of the pie pan, and unwind the dough into the pan.

4. Press the dough into the pan. Carefully center the dough in the pan. Push it gently onto the bottom and up the sides. Avoid stretching the dough, which increases its **tendency**, or inclination, to shrink.

Handling Cracked Pastry Dough

Avoid starting over with the dough. Overkneading can make the dough tough and chewy instead of flaky and crisp. As you roll out piecrust, it may crack or lose its shape. Patch or reshape the dough by cutting off a piece from an area where you have extra dough. Use cold water to slightly moisten the area that you need to repair. Place the patch on the dough and press firmly. Sprinkle with a little flour and roll with the pin to even out the patched spot. Save any extra piecrust to make designs to place on the edges of the pie.

Careers in Food

Thomas Huebner
Pastry Chef

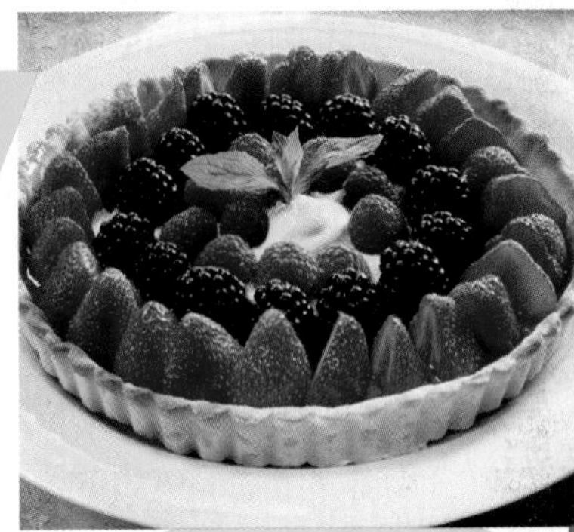

Q: What does a pastry chef do?

A: A pastry chef prepares pies, tarts, cakes, and other desserts. Sometimes pastry chefs are also in charge of preparing and baking the bread served at a restaurant.

Q: What are the biggest challenges with the job?

A: It is a challenge to make and prepare different pastry, pie, and tart doughs. It takes planning and effort to get all the necessary tasks done on time. Working with weights and measurements takes care and attention to detail.

Q: What do you enjoy about being a pastry chef?

A: It is rewarding because desserts complete a meal and they are the thing people remember as they leave a restaurant.

"You can use a lot of creativity and talent. It is a very artistic job!"
—Thomas Huebner
Master Pastry Chef,
The Arizona Biltmore
– Phoenix, AZ

Education and Training

A culinary school is a good place to learn about being a pastry chef, but it takes years of practice to become good at the job. A complete understanding of weights and measures is extremely important.

Qualities and Skills

A pastry chef has many things to accomplish in limited time each day, so organization and the ability to design and stick to a work plan are important. Patience is important because working with dough and chocolate takes care. The ability to critique the look and taste of your work is also important.

Related Career Opportunities

The skills used for careers in baking and being a chocolatier are related. Another related career is cake decorating. Artistic careers are also related.

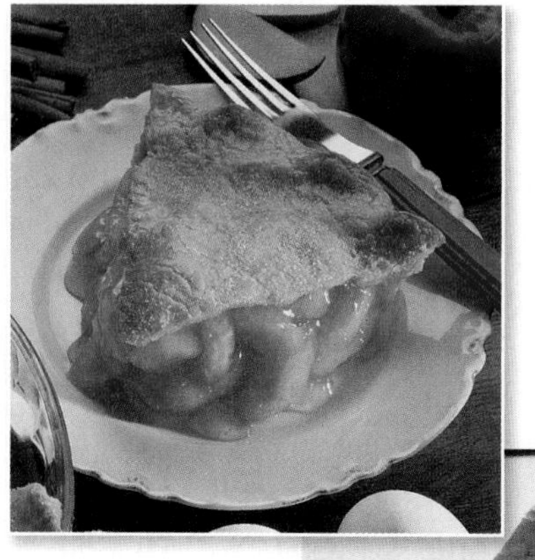

Finishing Touches

Some pies have a top crust, often with decorative cutouts or additions. *How do you make a fluted edge on a piecrust?*

Decorating the Edge of the Piecrust

A piecrust should have a fluted edge. A **fluted edge** is a ridged edge made with the tines of a fork or with your thumbs and index fingers.

Two-Crust Pies

To make a two-crust pie, divide the dough into two portions, one slightly larger than the other. Roll out the larger portion and fit it into the pan. Then make the top crust using these steps:

1. Trim the bottom dough. Use scissors or a knife to make it even with the edge of the pan.

2. Roll the top dough. Roll out the second ball of dough. Cover it to keep it from drying out.

3. Add the pie filling. Pour the filling over the bottom dough.

4. Place the top dough. Position the top dough on the filled pie.

5. Trim the top dough. Trim the top dough to about ½ inch larger than the pie pan.

6. Press top and bottom together. Slightly moisten the edge of the bottom dough. Tuck the overhanging top dough under the edge of the bottom dough. Press both together. This forms a seal to keep in juices. Flute the edge.

7. Cut slits in the top dough. Use a knife to cut slits in the top dough so steam can escape.

8. Glaze and decorate. You can glaze the top dough before baking by brushing it with milk and a light sprinkle of sugar, or with beaten egg mixed with water. You can also use a cookie cutter to cut shapes from dough and place them on the top dough.

Lattice Crusts

A **lattice crust**, or a crust that is woven, makes an eye-catching top on a two-crust pie, especially when the pie has a colorful filling that contrasts with the color of the crust. To make a lattice crust, cut strips and weave them as shown in **Figure 45.1**. Use a ruler to measure the strips so that they are all the same width. You can use leftover bits of crust to cut out leaves for a decoration.

Kitchen Math

Decorative Crust

Linda is preparing the crust for an apple pie, and would like to make a forked edge, which requires pressing the tines of a fork repeatedly around the edge of the crust. The fork she would like to use is ¾-inch wide. How many times will she need to press the fork into the crust if the pie is 9 ½ inches in diameter?

Math Concept **Dividing Decimals** To divide decimals, convert the divisor to a whole number by multiplying by a power of 10. Multiply the dividend by the same power of 10.

Starting Hint Find the answer by dividing the circumference of the pie by 0.75 inches (the width of the fork). Remember, circumference equals π times diameter. Use 3.14 for π. Round your answer to the nearest whole number.

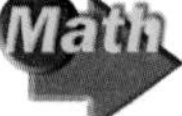

Math Appendix For math help, go to the Math Appendix at the back of the book.

NCTM Problem Solving Solve problems that arise in mathematics and in other contexts.

Figure 45.1 How to Make a Lattice Piecrust

Woven Top Crust Follow these steps to weave an attractive lattice piecrust. ***What is the purpose of a lattice crust?***

4
3
2
1

Step 1 Add Horizontal Strips

Lay half of the strips across the pie.

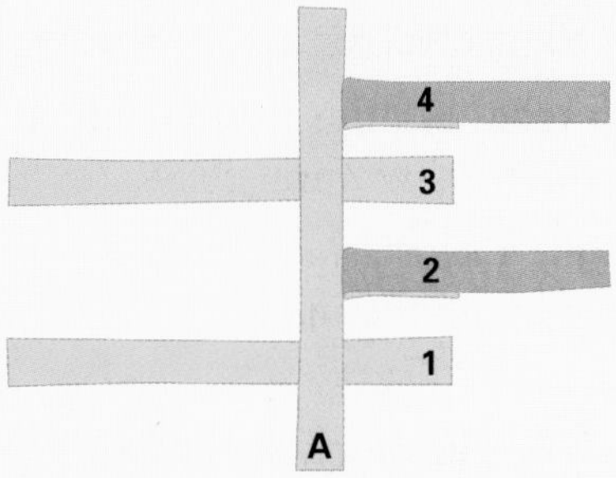

4
3
2
1
A

Step 2 Fold Back and Add a Vertical Strip

Fold back alternating horizontal strips (2 and 4) so the folds are near the edge of the pie. Add a vertical strip (A) close to the folds.

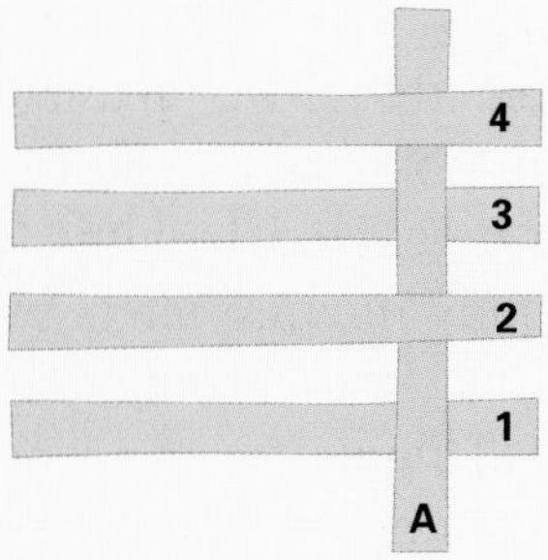

4
3
2
1
A

Step 3 Unfold

Unfold horizontal strips 2 and 4.

4
3
2
1
B A

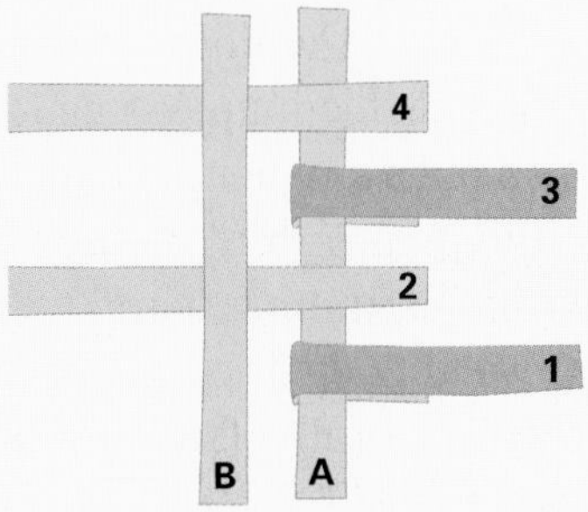

Step 4 Fold Back and Add Another Vertical Strip

Fold back the other alternating strips (1 and 3) as far as they will go. Add vertical strip B.

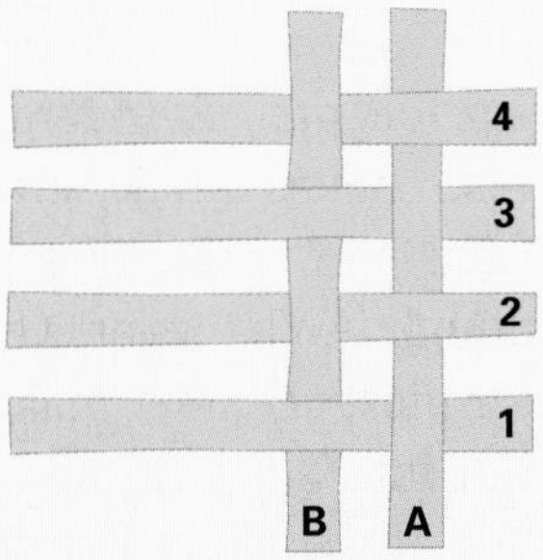

4
3
2
1
B A

Step 5 Unfold Again

Unfold strips 1 and 3.

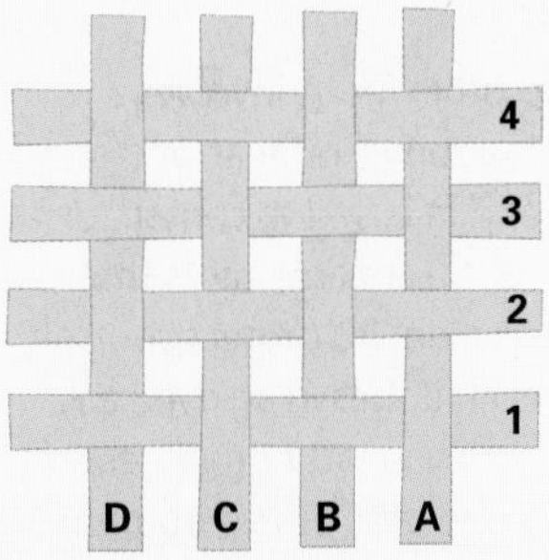

4
3
2
1
D C B A

Step 6 Repeat Until Finished

Repeat steps 2–5 until all the strips are woven.

One-Crust Pies

For some one-crust pies, the crust and filling are baked together. For others, the crust is baked empty, or blind, and a prepared filling is added later. A bottom crust baked before filling is called a **pie shell**.

To prepare rolled piecrust for a one-crust pie:

1. **Let the dough rest.** Let the bottom dough rest in the pie pan for a few minutes.
2. **Trim the dough.** Use scissors or a sharp knife to trim the dough ½ inch beyond the edge of the pan.
3. **Tuck the dough under.** Tuck the overhanging dough under to form a double-thick edge.
4. **Flute.** Flute the edge of the dough.
5. **Bake.** Bake the shell blind, or fill it as directed and then bake.

Sometimes pie shells puff up while baking. To keep this from happening, use a fork to poke small holes all over the dough before putting it in the oven. This technique is called **docking**. You can also put a smaller pie pan on top of the dough in the pan. A third method is to line the dough with aluminum foil and then fill the foil with pie weights or dried beans or peas. Lift them out with the foil a few minutes before the crust is done.

SAFETY MATTERS

Beat the Heat

Baking pies, tarts, and other foods involves a lot of heat. The oven is a source of heat, and so are the pans, dishes, and foil used to contain or cover the pies and tarts. Steam and juices that escape from pies are also hot. To protect yourself, wear oven mitts. To reach dishes in an oven easily, slide the rack closer to you rather than reaching in far. Cooked pies and tarts pulled from the oven stay hot for a long time, so handle them with care.

What Would You Do? While your pie is baking, you notice the edges turning brown at a faster rate than the rest of the pie. Quickly, you grab a few strips of aluminum foil to cover the edges. What should you do next?

Crumb Crusts

A **crumb crust** is a piecrust made of crushed crackers or cookies instead of pastry dough. It is a sweeter, simpler alternative for a one-crust pie. Graham cracker crusts are traditional for cheesecakes, cream pies, and frozen pies. You can also make crumb crusts from gingersnaps, sandwich cookies, shortbread, vanilla wafers, macaroons, or a combination of these.

Use fine crumbs to make a crust. **Coarse**, or large, fresh crumbs do not hold together well. Some recipes call for the crust to be baked before the filling is added. For variety, add chopped nuts, oats, coconut, or spices. Stir in melted butter or margarine and mix well. Then press the mixture into the pan. Make sure the crust is spread evenly. You can bake a crumb crust or chill it to make it firmer.

Crumbs can also be used for the top of the pie. Try scattering the top of a one-crust pie with crumbs from the crust mixture or with buttered breadcrumbs. For a sweet topping on a fruit pie, cover it generously with a **streusel** (ˈstrü-səl), a crumbly mixture made by cutting butter into flour, sugar, and sometimes spices. Use spices in small amounts so they add flavor without overwhelming the taste of the pie. Spices like cinnamon, cardamom and nutmeg work best.

Convenience Piecrust

Piecrust mixes and ready-made crumb crusts are sold in the baking aisle. Pastry crusts are sold in the refrigerator or freezer case, often in their own foil pan. Refrigerated crescent roll dough also makes a flaky crust. For a dessert pie, line the pan with slices of refrigerated cookie dough. Whenever you make your own crust for pies, consider making extra crust, rolling it out into a pie tin and freezing it for later use.

You can also buy prepared fillings for pies. You can use canned fruit, prepared cream fillings, or pudding mixes. Garnish with fresh fruit, chocolate curls, or other creative touches.

✓ **Reading Check** **Explain** How can you repair cracked pastry dough?

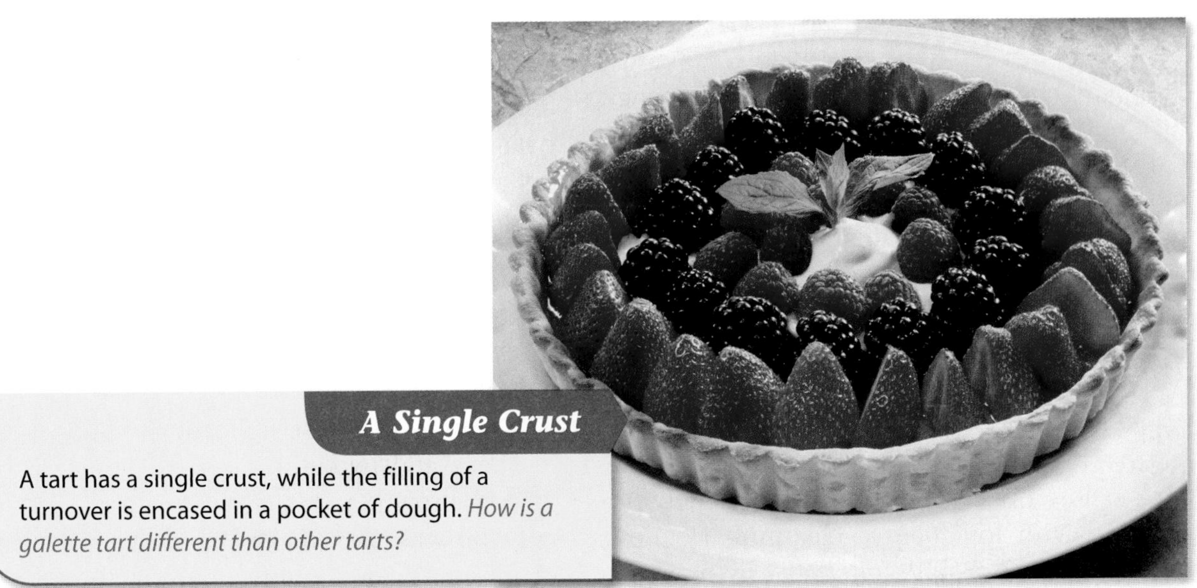

A Single Crust

A tart has a single crust, while the filling of a turnover is encased in a pocket of dough. *How is a galette tart different than other tarts?*

Tarts and Turnovers

Tarts and turnovers are variations on pies. Both use pastry crust and fillings, but in different ways.

Tarts

A **tart** is a filled dessert with a single crust. Like pies, tarts can be appetizers, entrées, or desserts. Unlike pies, tarts are always removed from the pan before serving.

A full-size tart, also called a **flan**, is made in a two-piece flan pan. A flan pan has a removable bottom and a straight, fluted edge about 1 inch deep. You can also use a flan ring, a bottomless metal rim that is set on a cookie sheet to form a pan, or a standard pie pan. A **galette** (gə-ˈlet) is a hand-shaped tart made by folding and pleating the edge of the dough to form the sides.

Miniature tarts are made individually in deeper pans that are similar to small muffin or pie pans. You can buy inexpensive miniature tart pans made of foil, or you can use muffin pans and baking cups.

Be a Smart Consumer

Prepackaged Pie Crusts

Prepackaged pie crusts are a good option for consumers who want to prepare pies and tarts but lack the time or expertise to make crusts from scratch. These convenient crusts usually come frozen, with two per package. Prepackaged crusts are available in white, wheat, whole-grain, and even gluten-free forms. Some are even free of trans-fats, making them a more healthful option than a homemade crust made with shortening.

Challenge Do you think using prepackaged pie crusts might limit a cook's creativity? Write two sentences to explain your thoughts.

Turnovers

A **turnover** is a square or circle of pastry dough folded over a sweet or savory filling. Bite-size turnovers are sometimes served as appetizers or snacks. Large turnovers are a tasty way to serve individual servings of entrées or desserts. Turnovers may be baked or deep-fried.

To make a turnover, roll out pastry dough and cut it into squares or circles. Add the filling and brush a little water along the edge of the dough. Fold the dough over and press the edges together with the tines of a fork. Put one or two slits in the top.

✓ Reading Check **Contrast** How is a turnover different from a tart?

Baking Pies and Tarts

Baking times and temperatures vary among pie and tart recipes. Pie shells are usually baked at 425°F or 450°F for about 20 minutes. Filled pies are baked at 425°F or 450°F for the first 10 minutes, and then at around 350°F to cook the filling.

Preventing Baking Problems

Some juicy pie fillings bubble over during baking. Put a shallow pan on the oven rack below the pie to catch the juices. Line the pan with foil to ease clean-up. Do not line the oven rack with foil, because this prevents hot air from circulating evenly around the pan.

Soggy bottom crusts can be another problem when baking pies. To keep crusts flaky, add the filling just before baking. You can also bake the shell blind and then seal it with a light egg wash. Then fill the pie and continue baking it. Warm jelly or melted chocolate also makes a tasty, functional seal for a baked and cooled shell.

Judging Doneness

Color is the best indication of doneness in shells and two-crust pies. They should be golden brown and slightly blistered. If the edge browns too quickly, cover it with strips of aluminum foil to protect it during the rest of the cooking time. Test filled pies for doneness as the recipe directs.

Light and Healthy Recipe

Strawberry Pie

Ingredients

For crust

- **2½ cups** Flour
- **1 tsp** Salt
- **⅔ cup** Vegetable oil
- **¼ cup** Nonfat milk

For the filling

- **2 Tbsp** Lemon juice
- **3 Tbsp** Cornstarch
- **¼ cup** Sugar
- **1 pound** Whole, fresh strawberries

Directions

1. Preheat oven to 450°.
2. Combine the flour and salt in a mixing bowl. In another bowl, mix the vegetable oil and milk. Combine the dry ingredients with the wet ingredients and mix.
3. When the pie crust dough is well mixed, roll it into a ball and turn it out on a lightly floured table.
4. With a rolling pin, roll the dough into a ¼-inch thin sheet and lay it over a pie tin. Fill the tin with weights and bake for 20 minutes, or until golden brown on the edges.
5. While the crust bakes, combine lemon juice, cornstarch, and sugar. Mix well. Pour the mixture over the strawberries and gently mix. Pour the mixture into the baked, cooled pie crust and put in the refrigerator to set.
6. Serve cold.

With a healthy crust and fresh berries, this pie is a delicious and healthy desert.

Yield 8 servings

Nutrition Analysis per Serving

■ Calories	356
■ Total fat	19 g
Saturated fat	1 g
Cholesterol	0 mg
■ Sodium	305 mg
■ Carbohydrate	43 g
Dietary fiber	2 g
Sugars	9 g
■ Protein	5 g

CHAPTER 45 Review & Applications

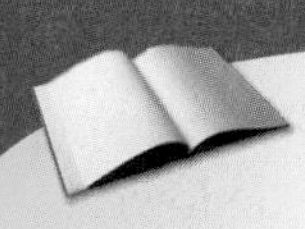

After You Read

Chapter Summary

Pies and tarts are made with pastry crust and sweet or savory fillings. There are four popular types of pies. Crust is the foundation of any pie. The right ingredients and preparation are required to make crusts for one- and two-crust pies. Convenience piecrusts and fillings are available. Tarts and turnovers are variations on pies. Tarts have a single crust and are always removed from the pan before serving. Turnovers consist of pastry dough folded over fillings. When baking pies and tarts, it is important to use the correct oven temperature, prevent baking problems, and make sure pies are thoroughly cooked.

Content and Academic Vocabulary Review

1. Write your own definition for each of these content and academic vocabulary words.

Content Vocabulary

- pie (p. 696)
- fluted edge (p. 698)
- lattice crust (p. 698)
- pie shell (p. 700)
- docking (p. 700)
- crumb crust (p. 700)
- streusel (p. 700)
- tart (p. 701)
- flan (p. 701)
- galette (p. 701)
- turnover (p. 701)

Academic Vocabulary

- tendency (p. 697)
- coarse (p. 700)

Review Key Concepts

2. **List** the four types of pies and give examples.
3. **Describe** how to prepare and roll pastry dough.
4. **Identify** ways that tarts and turnovers differ from pies.
5. **Explain** how to prevent problems while baking pies and tarts.

Critical Thinking

6. **Describe** the types of pie you would serve for breakfast, lunch, dinner, and dessert if you owned an all-pie restaurant.
7. **Explain** why might a pie turn out heavy and leathery rather than light and flaky even if it is not overcooked.
8. **Identify** which types of crust you would choose for these pies and explain why: banana cream; cherry; pumpkin; apple; and chicken pot pie.
9. **Explain** how Nuala can use the pastry dough and pie filling she prepared even if she does not have a pie dish.
10. **Predict** what might happen if Toni, who must make 12 pies for a bake sale, adds the fillings to the prepared shells one day before baking them.

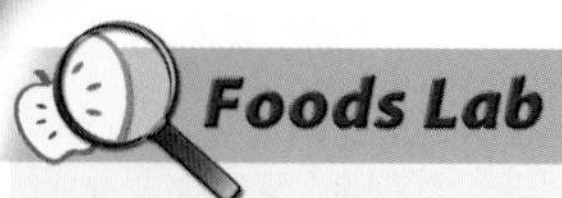

Foods Lab

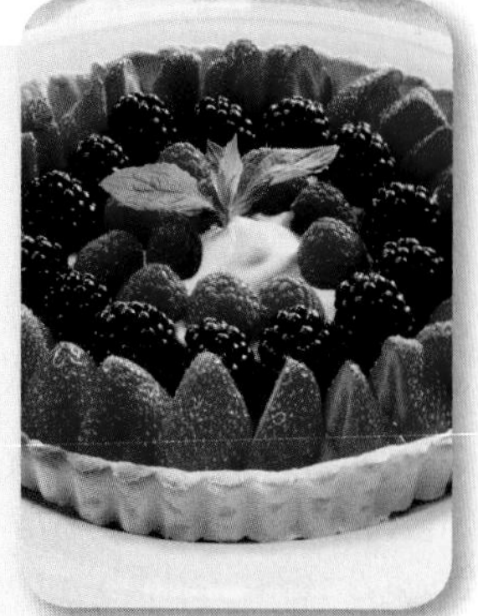

11. Pies and Tarts There are nearly endless variations of pies and tarts, each with their own taste, texture, and appearance. Which type will be the most highly rated in your class and why?

Procedure Prepare one of the following pies: fruit pie; cream pie; custard pie; pie made with convenience products; and fruit tart. Serve samples for a class taste test.

Analysis Create a chart on which you rate each of the samples on a scale of 1 to 5 in the following categories: crust texture; filling texture; filling flavor; visual appeal. Which is the highest-rated? Which is the lowest-rated?

HEALTHFUL CHOICES

12. Crust Choices At the cafeteria, Paola wants to choose the pie that is likely to be lowest in fat. Her choices are: a one-crust peach pie; a lattice-crust cherry pie; a one-crust butterscotch cream pie; and a two-crust peach pie. Identify the pie that Paola should choose by explaining which is likely to be lowest in fat and why.

TECH Connection

13. Recipe Booklet Under your teacher's supervision, use the Internet to find one recipe to represent each of the four types of pies. Then use word processing software to create a 5-page pie recipe booklet. Neatly type each recipe on one page, considering spacing, margins, font choices, and color. Create a cover page, and give your recipe booklet a title. Print and bind the booklet using staples or a three-hole punch and string.

Real-World Skills

Problem-Solving Skills

14. Manage Pie Juices Every time Vera bakes one of her favorite two-crust fruit pies, juices bubble out and fall to the bottom of her oven, where they make a hard, sticky mess that is difficult to clean. What are two measures that Vera can take to prevent this problem in the future?

Interpersonal and Collaborative Skills

15. Creative Crust Demonstrations Follow your teacher's instructions to form pairs. Using dough or clay made for children's play, work together to practice creating one of these types of pie crust: A lattice crust; A fluted crust; A crust featuring decorative shapes. Display your crust to the class.

Financial Literacy Skills

16. Pie Crust Costs Nancy must make 16 pies for a sale. A package of two pre-made pie crusts costs $4.99. To buy the supplies to make 16 pie crusts at home, Nancy would need to buy a bag of flour for $2.99, a container of shortening for $2.09, and a container of salt for $1.95. How much can Nancy save if she makes homemade crusts?

Academic Skills

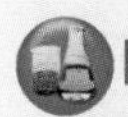

Food Science

17. Working with Chocolate The two biggest problems in working with chocolate are moisture and excess heat. If a small amount of water is added to already melted chocolate, the chocolate will seize into a grainy paste. If too high a temperature is used, the chocolate will burn.

Procedure Heat ¼ cup chocolate semi-sweet morsels until melted in three different ways: directly in a pan on the stovetop, in a microwave safe dish at 50% power, and over a double boiler. Once melted, compare your results. Now stir in a teaspoon of water to each to see what happens.

Analysis Which proved the best way to melt the chocolate? What happened when water was added?

NSES B Develop an understanding of the structure and properties of matter.

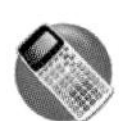

Mathematics

18. Triangular Turnovers After making her apple pie, Linda has some extra pie filling and pie crust dough left over, and starts to make turnovers. She rolls out her dough and cuts it into squares measuring 4 inches by 4 inches. Linda scoops some pie filling into the squares, and folds each one in half diagonally, forming a triangle. What is the length of the diagonal side of each turnover?

Math Concept **Pythagorean Theorem** If you know the lengths of two sides of a right triangle, you can determine the third length using the Pythagorean Theorem, which states that $a^2 + b^2 = c^2$ (where c is the length of the hypotenuse, or side opposite the right angle, and a and b are the other two sides).

Starting Hint Insert the two known side lengths for a and b, and solve for c by calculating the square root of $a^2 + b^2$.

NCTM Geometry Analyze characteristics and properties of two- and three-dimensional geometric shapes and develop mathematical arguments about geometric relationships.

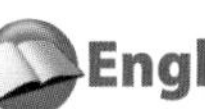

English Language Arts

19. Brochure Fold an 8½ by 11 inch sheet of paper into thirds. Use it to create a brochure for a bakery that sells homemade pies and tarts. Combine text and images with captions to attract customers and inform them of your offerings.

NCTE 4 Use written language to communicate effectively.

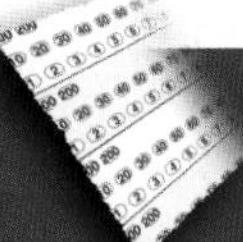

STANDARDIZED TEST PRACTICE

READING COMPREHENSION

Re-read the section about turnovers on page 701. Then select the best answer:

20. Which of the following is a way to cook turnovers?

a. roasting
b. deep-frying
c. sautéing
d. steaming

Test-Taking Tip Before you answer a reading comprehension question, closely read the text to which the question refers. Then read through the question and each of the answer choices. Next, take a second look at the text to confirm which answer is correct. Some answers may seem identical, but they contain subtle differences. Pay attention to every word.

UNIT 9

Thematic Project

Create a Baked Good

Baked goods are a favorite of many people. Breads, cakes, cookies, pies and other baked goods smell wonderful and taste good, too. In this unit, you have learned the basics of baking different types of foods. In this project, you will talk with an adult of your community who bakes. Then you will use what you learned in this unit and from your interview to create a baked good.

My Journal

If you completed the journal entry from page 651, refer to it to see if your thoughts have changed after reading the unit and completing this project.

Project Assignment

- Select a type of baked good that you would like to prepare.
- Find a recipe to prepare. The recipe should be affordable and fit with your skill level.
- Talk to someone in your community about the recipe you have chosen.
- Prepare the recipe and, if possible, take photos of various steps of the preparation process.
- Create a presentation using the photos.

Academic Skills You Will Use

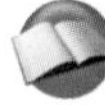

English Language Arts

NCTE 12 Use language to accomplish individual purposes.

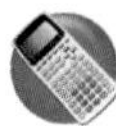

Mathematics

NCTM Measurement Understand measurable attributes of objects and the units, systems, and processes of measurement.

STEP 1 Select a Baked Good to Prepare

Select one of these types of baked goods to prepare and then write a paragraph to explain why you selected the type of baked good.

- Quick bread
- Yeast bread
- Cake
- Cookie
- Candy
- Pie
- Tart

Writing Skills

- Use complete sentences.
- Use correct spelling and grammar.
- Type your paragraph on a computer or use neat handwriting.

STEP 2 Find a Recipe

Look through cookbooks, talk with friends or relatives, or search the Internet to find a recipe for the type of baked good you selected in Step 1. Then make a list of the ingredients you will need to prepare this recipe.

STEP 3 Connect to Your Community

Talk to someone in your community about your baked good. The person you choose to talk to about your recipe should have experience or expertise in baking. Ask for advice and feedback. Discuss the process you will need to follow and the techniques you will use. Take notes, and transcribe the notes after the interview.

Interviewing Skills

- Listen attentively.
- Make eye contact and respond appropriately and with interest to feedback.
- Be aware of nonverbal communication.
- Ask additional questions if you do not understand.
- Send a thank-you note after the interview.

STEP 4 Create Your Recipe and Presentation

Use the Unit Thematic Project Checklist to plan and complete your project, and then prepare and give your presentation.

STEP 5 Evaluate Presentation

Your project will be evaluated based on:

- How the baked good turns out.
- List of ingredients and nutritional value.
- Audio and visual components of your presentation.

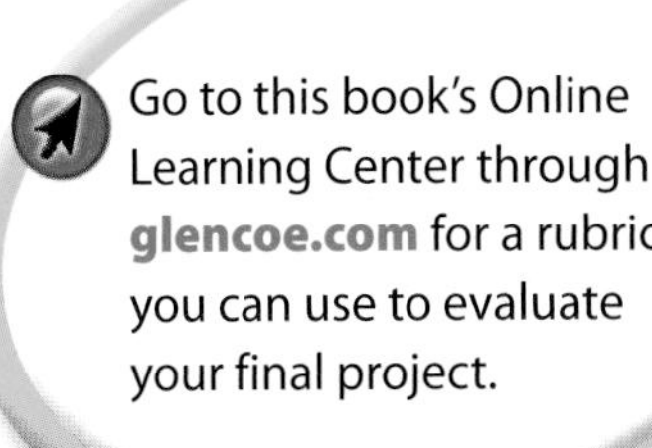

Go to this book's Online Learning Center through **glencoe.com** for a rubric you can use to evaluate your final project.

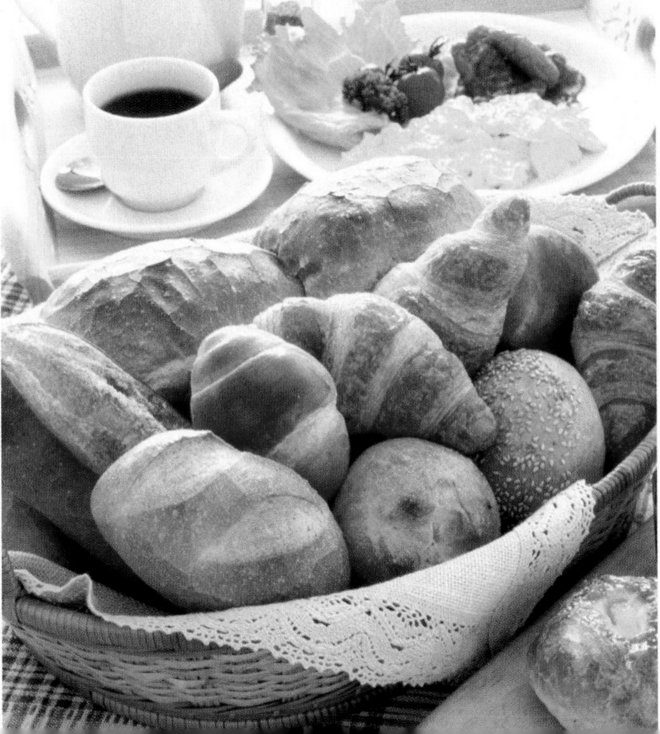

Unit Thematic Project Checklist

Category	Objectives
Plan	☑ Choose a recipe and interview someone about it.
	☑ Under adult supervision, make your recipe and take photos of each step of the process.
	☑ Use presentation software to create a presentation showing the process you used during the preparation of your baked good.
Present	☑ Make a presentation to your class to share your recipe and your presentation and to discuss what you learned.
	☑ Invite the students in your class to ask you any questions they may have. Answer three questions.
	☑ When students ask you questions, demonstrate in your answers that you respect their perspectives.
	☑ Turn in the paragraph about why you choose your recipe, the notes from your interview, and your presentation to your teacher.
Academic Skills	☑ Organize your visual and your presentation for sense and flow.
	☑ Adapt and modify language to suit your audience.
	☑ Speak clearly and concisely.

UNIT 10

Global Foods

CHAPTER **46** **Foods of the United States & Canada**

CHAPTER **47** **Foods of South America, Latin America, & the Caribbean**

CHAPTER **48** **Foods of Western, Northern, & Southern Europe**

CHAPTER **49** **Foods of Eastern Europe & Russia**

CHAPTER **50** **Foods of South, East, & Southeast Asia**

CHAPTER **51** **Foods of Southwest Asia, the Middle East, & Africa**

Activate Prior Knowledge

Explore the Photo In different countries and in different cultures, people have their own foods. *What are some ways you can learn about foods from around the world?*

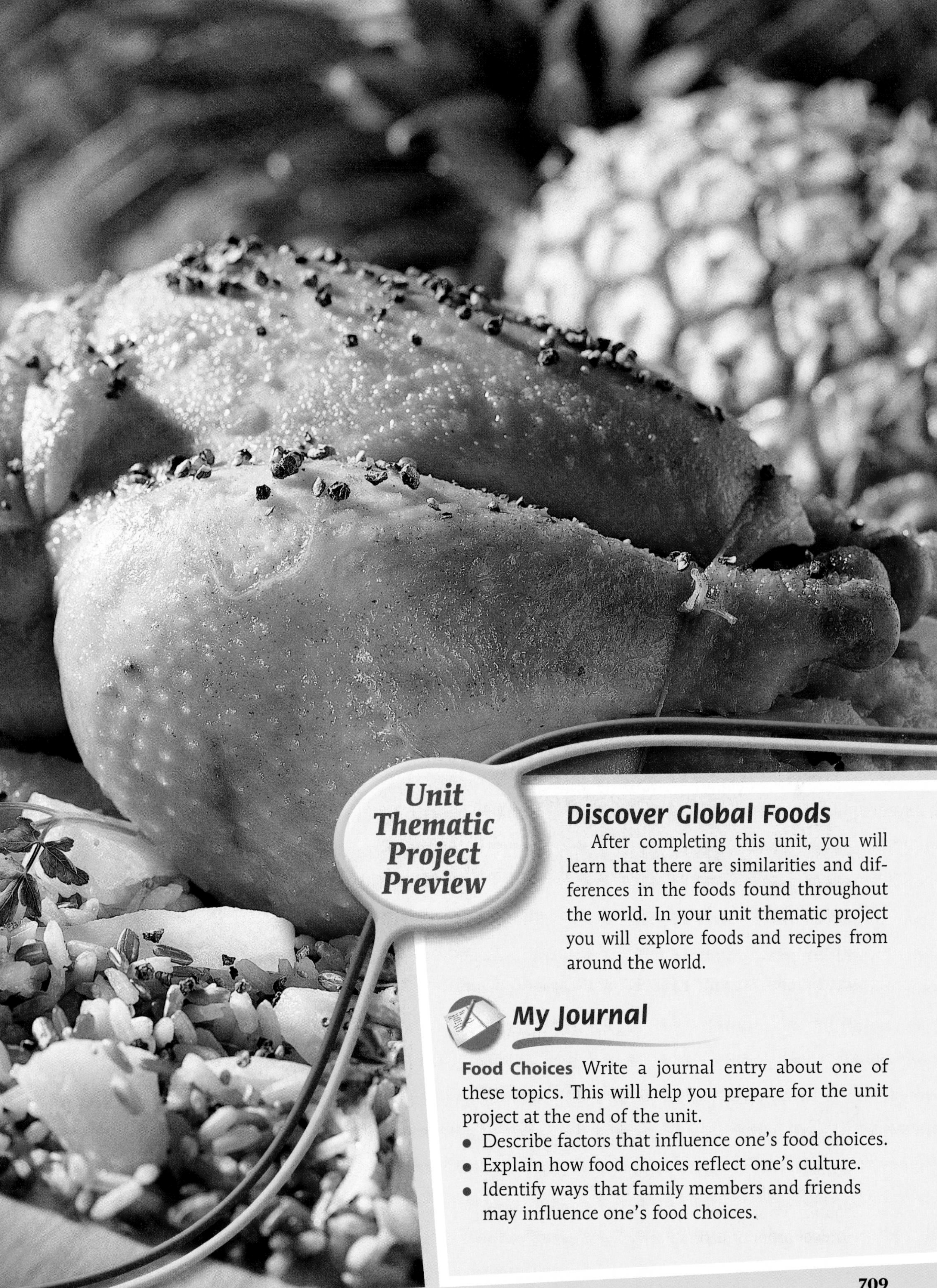

Unit Thematic Project Preview

Discover Global Foods

After completing this unit, you will learn that there are similarities and differences in the foods found throughout the world. In your unit thematic project you will explore foods and recipes from around the world.

My Journal

Food Choices Write a journal entry about one of these topics. This will help you prepare for the unit project at the end of the unit.

- Describe factors that influence one's food choices.
- Explain how food choices reflect one's culture.
- Identify ways that family members and friends may influence one's food choices.

CHAPTER 46

Foods of the United States & Canada

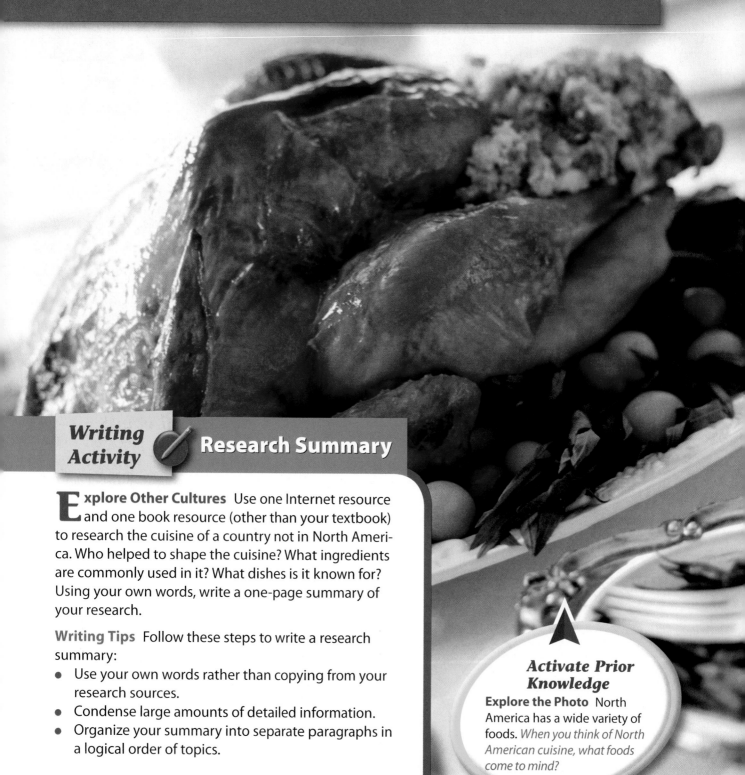

Writing Activity — Research Summary

Explore Other Cultures Use one Internet resource and one book resource (other than your textbook) to research the cuisine of a country not in North America. Who helped to shape the cuisine? What ingredients are commonly used in it? What dishes is it known for? Using your own words, write a one-page summary of your research.

Writing Tips Follow these steps to write a research summary:

- Use your own words rather than copying from your research sources.
- Condense large amounts of detailed information.
- Organize your summary into separate paragraphs in a logical order of topics.

Activate Prior Knowledge

Explore the Photo North America has a wide variety of foods. *When you think of North American cuisine, what foods come to mind?*

Reading Guide

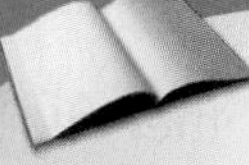

Before You Read

Preview Brainstorm two styles of American cuisine with which you are familiar. Then skim through the contents of this chapter, taking note of any cuisines you are not familiar with. Which cuisines are new to you?

Read to Learn

Key Concepts

- **Describe** the main food regions of the United States and give examples of regional ingredients and dishes.
- **Identify** the main food regions of Canada and give examples of regional ingredients and dishes.

Main Idea

The United States and Canada are home to many regional cuisines that reflect a variety of influences from around the globe.

Content Vocabulary

You will find definitions for these words in the glossary at the back of this book.

- ☐ succotash
- ☐ scrapple
- ☐ goulash
- ☐ jambalaya
- ☐ gumbo
- ☐ étouffée
- ☐ cioppino
- ☐ poke
- ☐ taro root
- ☐ bannock
- ☐ croquettes

Academic Vocabulary

You will find these words in your reading and on your tests. Use the glossary to look up their definitions if necessary.

- regional
- thrive

Graphic Organizer

Use a graphic organizer like the one below to note examples of dishes from the main regions of the United States.

REGION	REGIONAL SPECIALTIES
Northeast	
Midwest	
South	
Southwest	
West	

Graphic Organizer Go to this book's Online Learning Center at **glencoe.com** to print out this graphic organizer.

Academic Standards

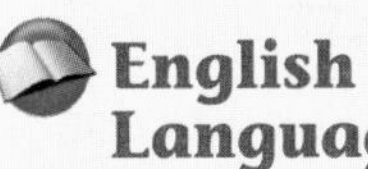

English Language Arts

NCTE 7 Conduct research and gather, evaluate, and synthesize data to communicate discoveries.

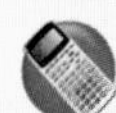

Mathematics

NCTM Geometry Use visualization, spatial reasoning, and geometric modeling to solve problems.

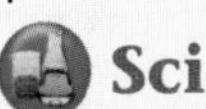

Science

NSES B Develop an understanding of the structure and properties of matter.

Social Studies

NCSS IX D Global Connections Analyze the causes, consequences, and potential solutions to persistent, contemporary, and emerging global issues.

NCTE *National Council of Teachers of English*
NCTM *National Council of Teachers of Mathematics*
NSES *National Science Education Standards*
NCSS *National Council for the Social Studies*

The United States

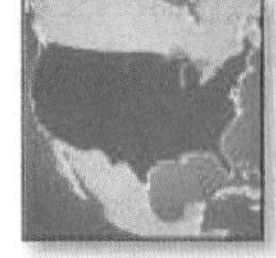

The United States is home to several cuisines. Many cultures have contributed new flavors and foods to American cuisine. The United States also has many of its own **regional**, or local, dishes that reflect the history of the different regions. **Figure 46.1** shows the main regions of the United States and its northern neighbor, Canada.

Northeast

The Northeast region of the United States stretches along the northeastern seacoast from New England, which consists of the states of Maine, New Hampshire, Vermont, Massachusetts, Rhode Island, and Connecticut, to the mid-Atlantic region.

Many recipes from the Northeast, such as the famous New England clam chowder, feature seafood such as lobster, clams, salmon, and other fish.

Another New England dish, the one-pot boiled dinner, or "potboiler," has a British origin. Cast-iron pots filled with corned beef or brisket, mutton, or pork, carrots, onions, and squash, were traditionally cooked over open fireplaces. Red flannel hash is another New England classic. The name and color come from beets added to finely chopped corned beef, potatoes, carrots, and onions. **Succotash**, a dish of beans and corn adopted from Native Americans, is one of the most well-established dishes from New England. Codfish cakes and codfish balls mixed with mashed potatoes are traditional in Rhode Island. Maple sugar and maple syrup are Vermont specialties.

Figure 46.1 United States and Canada

North American Regions The United States has 50 states, which are traditionally divided into the six regions shown here. Canada is divided into 10 provinces and three territories, which are traditionally broken into five regions. ***In which region do you live?***

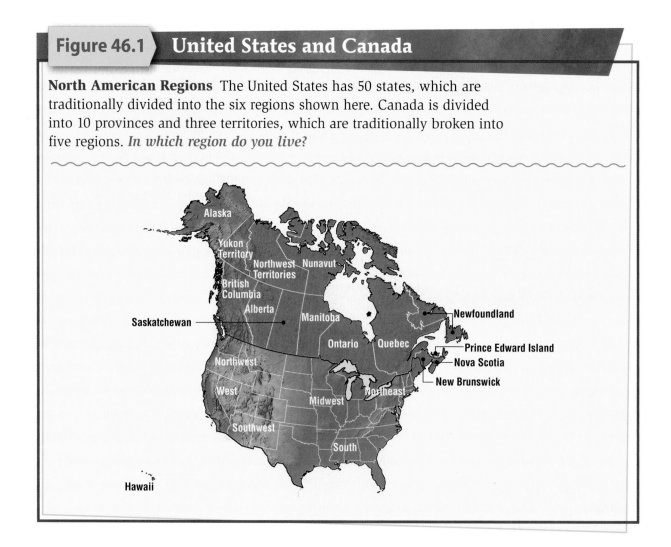

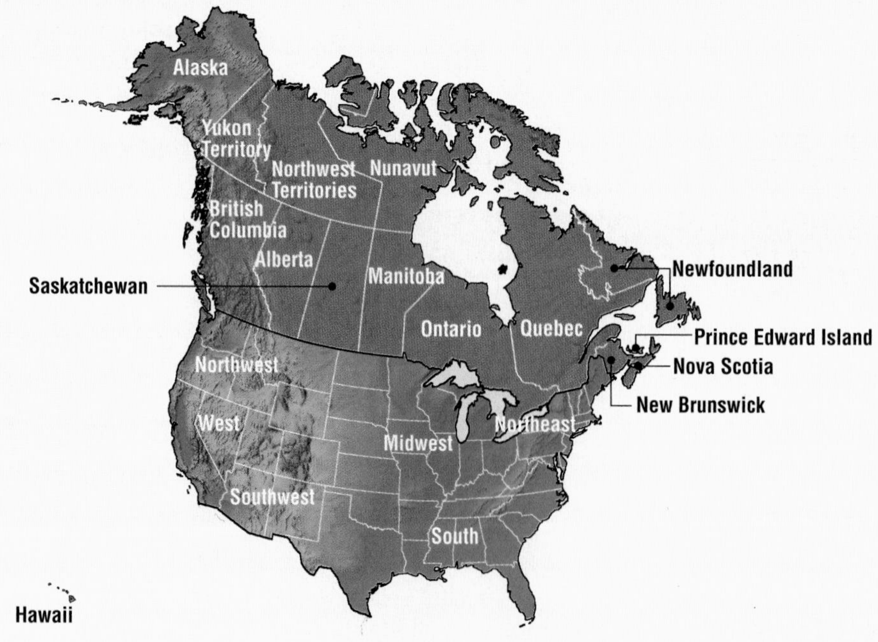

New England Clam Chowder

Chowder is a hearty milk-based soup, often made with fish. Chowders get their name from chaudière, French for the fisherman's cooking cauldron. *What is the difference between New England clam chowder and Manhattan clam chowder?*

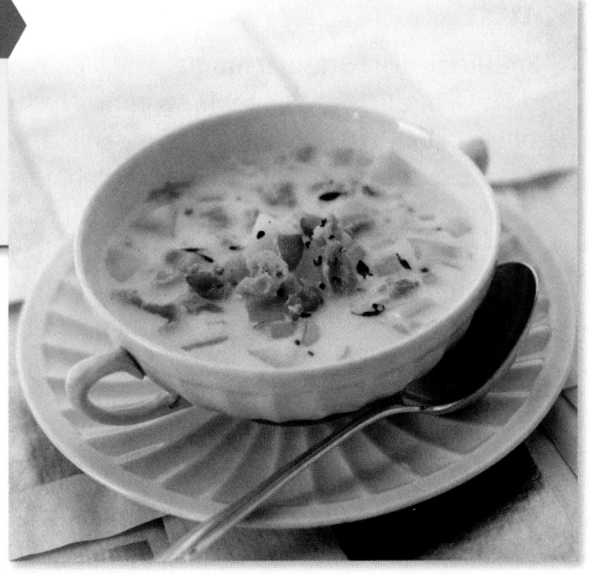

New York City

New York City, New York, is the ultimate melting pot. This is where millions of immigrants over many generations created vibrant neighborhoods dotted with ethnic markets, delis, and restaurants that keep their cooking styles alive. Chinatown and Little Italy are two of the city's best-known ethnic neighborhoods.

New York City lends its name to several foods, such as New York cheesecake and New York chowder. New York cheesecake is a dense cheesecake with eggs, cream, and cream cheese. Unlike New England clam chowder, Manhattan clam chowder has a tomato-based broth.

Boston

The city of Boston, Massachusetts, where many Irish settled, contributes its name to several foods. Boston brown bread is dark, sweet, steamed bread made with rye and wheat flours, cornmeal, and molasses. Boston cream pie is a dessert with two layers of sponge cake, a custard filling, and a topping of chocolate or powdered sugar. Boston baked beans are slow-cooked beans sweetened with molasses. Molasses is also featured in New England Indian pudding, which is made of pumpkin, molasses, cornmeal, raisins, and spices. Some call this the first pumpkin pie.

Pennsylvania Dutch

The Germans who settled in Pennsylvania are called the Pennsylvania Dutch. Their cooking features many German dishes, such as sausages, also known as wursts, made from pork and beef, as well as sauerkraut and pretzels. Shoofly pie, a very sweet pie made with molasses, is another Pennsylvania Dutch recipe.

German immigrants were thrifty in their cooking, reusing leftovers and scraps. **Scrapple**, for example, is a bake of pork scraps with cornmeal, flavored with thyme and sage. It is served cut into slices and fried.

Midwest

The Midwest, which generally includes Illinois, Indiana, Iowa, Kansas, Michigan, Minnesota, Missouri, Ohio, Nebraska, North Dakota, South Dakota, and Wisconsin, is known for its hearty cooking that features meat and potatoes. Beef and pork are typical star players in dishes served in the Midwest. In Minnesota, beef is made into Swedish meatballs, which are cooked in sour cream. Corn and soybeans are grown throughout the Midwest, especially in Iowa, Illinois, and Kansas. These crops are used for livestock feed and cooking oil.

In the mid-1800s, Germans, Estonians, Ukrainians, Latvians, Scandinavians, and Hungarians immigrated to the Midwest, bringing their cuisine with them. Kielbasa, a Polish sausage, is a midwestern favorite. Many Swiss and Germans settled in Wisconsin to raise milk cows and produce cheese. Today, Wisconsin is renowned for its cheeses and other dairy products. Hungarian dishes found in the Midwest include chicken paprika and stuffed bell peppers. **Goulash** is a Hungarian stew made with beef and vegetables and flavored with paprika. Sour cream is part of many Hungarian dishes.

South

Southern dishes are at home in Alabama, Florida, Georgia, Kentucky, Mississippi, North Carolina, South Carolina, Tennessee, and Virginia. Southern cooking often incorporates rice, corn, peanuts, sesame seeds, sweet potatoes, and pork. African-American culture has influenced many dishes in the South.

Grits are a Southern specialty made from ground dried corn called hominy. Grits are often served for breakfast. Hushpuppies are deep-fried corn fritters typically served with catfish. Ham hocks, bacon, and salted pork are used to flavor pots of beans and greens. Pork is also made into sausages and ham.

In Florida, peanuts are often boiled. In North Carolina, they are added to stuffing for roast chicken. In Alabama and Mississippi, peanuts are used in soups. Dumplings, biscuits, and cornbread are popular breads in the South. Fried foods, such as fried chicken and fried catfish, are also popular in Southern cooking. Brunswick stew, originally made from squirrel and now usually made with chicken, is a classic stew from Kentucky to Alabama.

Sweet Southern dishes include peanut brittle and sweet potato pie. Georgia is famous for peaches, which are often made into cobbler, an upside-down pie with a biscuit-like crust on top. In the Florida Keys, where limes are grown, Key lime pie is a regional specialty.

Be a Smart Consumer

Saving Money with Spice Blends

Spices and herbs are sold individually and in mixtures known as blends. People can buy individual containers of oregano, basil, and red pepper, or buy an "Italian Blend" that contains them all, plus others. Blends are especially useful in cuisines that feature many herbs and spices, such as Cajun. They also can save money. Still, some people prefer to have more control and creativity when they cook, and develop their own blends.

Challenge What is one drawback to having more blends than individual spices and herbs in your kitchen?

Louisiana

Creole, or mixed heritage, cooking began in the 1700s in Louisiana when the French settled in New Orleans. Africans who worked in the kitchens of plantation owners blended African, French, Spanish, Caribbean, and Native American ingredients and techniques to create Louisiana Creole cuisine. Creole cooking is a true original American cuisine.

Jambalaya is the perfect example of Creole cooking. This rice dish features ham, seafood, chicken, and sausages with rice, vegetables, and seasonings. Another well-known Creole dish is **gumbo**, which combines the Spanish custom of mixing seafood and meat with French-style andouille sausages. Filé, a powder made from the sassafras plant, is used to season gumbo. Gumbo also uses a classic Louisiana base, a chocolate-colored roux. Shrimp or crawfish, also called "mud bugs," are cooked **étouffée** (ˌā-tü-ˈfā), a French word that means smothered. This is a typical Southern method of cooking food covered in liquid or sauce.

Around 1755, the Acadians from Canada settled in Louisiana. Their descendants, the Cajuns, settled along the swampy bayous. Cajun cooking combines the cuisines of France and the South.

Southwest

The American Southwest includes New Mexico, Oklahoma, Texas, and parts of Arizona and Colorado. Southwestern cooking includes Spanish, Mexican, and Pueblo influences. Spaniards introduced cattle to the area in the sixteenth century. The bison that roamed the region provided a ready meat source. By the 1800s, ranches dotted the Texas plains, with cowboys tending large herds of longhorn cattle.

Long before the Spaniards arrived, Pueblo peoples such as the Zuni and Hopi were raising corn, beans, pumpkins, chiles, and squash. Other native peoples, including Apache, Comanche, and Navajo, cooked pumpkins and seasoned stews with local juniper berries. Pine nuts, the nutritious seeds of pinecones, were also staples. Later, Native Americans used European wheat to make fry bread. Sopaipillas are a sweet fry bread topped with honey.

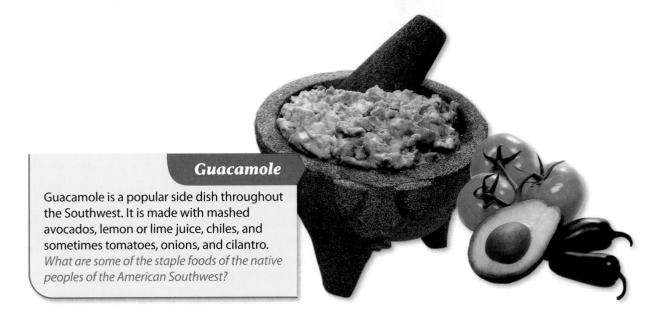

Guacamole

Guacamole is a popular side dish throughout the Southwest. It is made with mashed avocados, lemon or lime juice, chiles, and sometimes tomatoes, onions, and cilantro. *What are some of the staple foods of the native peoples of the American Southwest?*

Tex-Mex Cooking

Corn, tomatoes, chiles, and beans are mainstays in Texas and much of New Mexico. The cuisine of Texas is often called Tex-Mex, referring to the important influence of Mexican cooking. In many areas outside of Texas, Tex-Mex is synonymous with Southwestern cuisine. Tex-Mex cuisine is known for its use of melted cheese, beef, beans, spices, and tortillas. The ultimate Tex-Mex dish is chili con carne, which includes chile peppers, meat, and often beans and tomatoes. A Southwestern breakfast dish, huevos rancheros, is eggs topped with spicy tomato and pepper sauce. Another breakfast dish, called migas, is scrambled eggs with cheese, peppers, and tortillas. Chips and salsa is a classic Tex-Mex appetizer.

Beef barbecue in Texas is legendary. Settlers built huge smokers to infuse beef with a smoky flavor. Like chili, barbecue recipes vary from cook to cook. Most Texas cooks agree that the meat in a true barbecue should be seasoned only with a dry rub of spices, rather than a sauce.

West

The cuisine of the West, which generally includes California, Nevada, Utah, and parts of Colorado, Idaho, Montana and Wyoming, has many Spanish and Mexican influences. A region of immigrants, the West also features food traditions from all corners of the globe, especially Central America and Asia.

California

The Spanish settled in California in the 1700s and divided the land into ranchos, or small ranches, that covered some of the most fertile land in California. Rancho cooking combined Spanish, Mexican, and Native American ingredients and techniques. Rancho cooking is still a major culinary influence in California.

Plum, apple, and pear trees grow in Northern California. Oranges, olives, and avocados grow in Southern California. Grapes **thrive**, or flourish, throughout the state. Rice grows in the delta around Sacramento.

The Central Valley, which runs through the middle of the state, produces most of California's produce. Farmers grow grains, fruits, nuts, garlic, tomatoes, and more. Artichokes, asparagus, and apples grow closer to the coast. The Pacific Ocean provides many different kinds of seafoods, including crab, salmon, rockfish, shrimp, and tuna.

Different regions of California have different cuisines and specialty dishes. **Cioppino** (chə-pē-(ˌ)nō) is fish stew originally made at Fisherman's Wharf in San Francisco. The Brown Derby Restaurant in Los Angeles contributed the Cobb salad, pictured on the next page.

Many immigrant groups have influenced California's cooking. Basques, for example, settled in the Sierra foothills in California, bringing dishes such as grilled lamb chops and roasts, pots of beans and chewy sheepherder bread. Immigrants from Asia, Africa, and Central America have also influenced California cuisine.

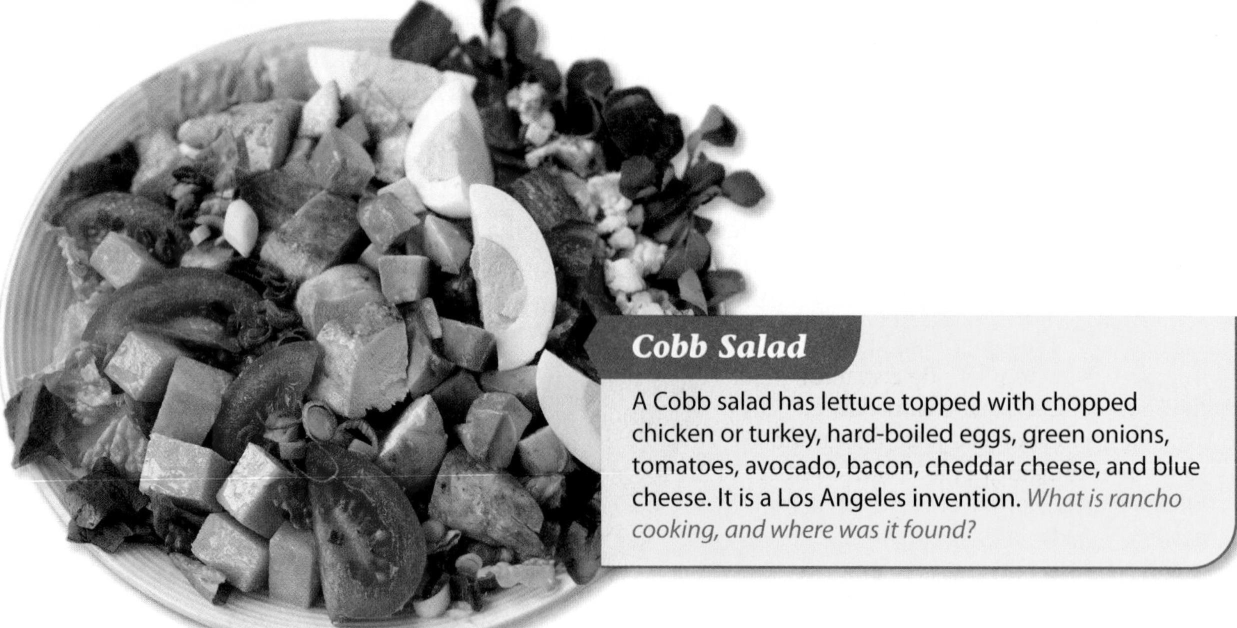

Cobb Salad

A Cobb salad has lettuce topped with chopped chicken or turkey, hard-boiled eggs, green onions, tomatoes, avocado, bacon, cheddar cheese, and blue cheese. It is a Los Angeles invention. *What is rancho cooking, and where was it found?*

Northwest

Oregon, Washington, and Alaska are renowned for their seafood dishes. The Pacific Ocean provides a wide variety of seafood, including clams, mussels, shrimp, giant halibut, salmon, and tiny Olympic oysters.

Washington leads the country in apple production, but also provides crops of sweet Walla Walla onions, pears, hazelnuts, cherries, vegetables (including potatoes), herbs, and wheat. Aplets and cotlets are Washington's famous candies made from apples and apricots plus sugar and walnuts. Seattle, like many places along the Pacific Coast, has adopted many elements of Asian cuisines.

Alaska is the largest and coldest state of the American Northwest. During the summer, sunlight lasts for 84 straight days in the northern part of the state. The nonstop sunlight allows vegetables to thrive. Much of the crop has to be canned, frozen, or otherwise preserved for the long, cold winter. Alaskan food often features seafood, such as king crab and salmon.

Hawaii

The South Pacific islands of Hawaii have a tropical climate, perfect for growing pineapples, papayas, coconuts, macadamia nuts, and other tropical produce. Both the Pacific Ocean and freshwater inland streams provide flavorful fish, which are featured in many Hawaiian recipes. **Poke** is sliced raw fish mixed with seaweed, onions, chiles, and soy sauce.

Native Hawaiians maintain many traditional Polynesian foodways. The famous luau is a celebratory meal cooked in a pit on the beach. Typically, a whole pig is injected with brine and then cooked for hours. An accompaniment might be poi, which is mashed, cooked **taro root**, the large tuber of the tropical taro plant. Other Hawaiian dishes include lomi lomi, salmon cut into pieces and mixed with tomatoes and onions, and haupia, a coconut-flavored pudding.

✓ Reading Check **List** List foods that are often incorporated in Southern cooking.

Canada

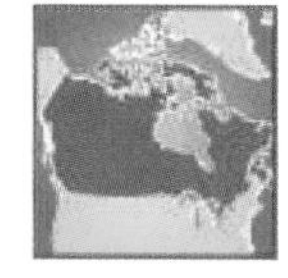

Canada is the second largest country in the world. Most Canadians live along the coasts and in cities toward the warmer southern parts of the country. As in the United States, Canadian foods reflect the nation's natural resources and rich history and cultural diversity.

Only about five percent of Canada's land can be used for growing crops. Native ingredients include wild rice, maple syrup, Saskatoon berries, Jerusalem artichokes, wild mushrooms, reindeer, turkey, duck, trout, buffalo, fiddlehead ferns, and a wide range of freshwater fish and seafood. Two of Canada's most important crops are wheat and rapeseed, the seeds used to make canola oil.

Canadian food reflects the cuisines of its many immigrants. Scottish immigrants, for example, brought **bannock**, a flat, biscuit-like bread made with flour or oats and cooked on a cast iron surface over a hot grill. Classic Canadian desserts include raisin pie and butter tarts. A butter tart is a pie pastry filled with a mixture of brown sugar, corn syrup, butter, and vanilla. Date squares, known as matrimonial cakes, are common in western Canada.

Canada is divided into provinces, each with distinctive foods and dishes. Immigrant food traditions have melded with local ingredients and native traditions to form varied regional cuisines.

Northeast

Newfoundland, Nova Scotia, New Brunswick, and Prince Edward Island are the provinces that make up northeastern Canada. Newfoundland has a beautiful terrain, with inland fjords and towering icebergs. Many people here make their living from the sea. Cod is the foundation of "Newfie" cuisine, which also features tuna, herring, mackerel, squid, shrimp, snow crab, and lobster. Blueberries and golden-colored cloudberries also grow well in Newfoundland.

Fish and oyster farming is an important industry in coastal Nova Scotia. Prince Edward Island is renowned for cultured (farmed) mussels. Seafood chowders are made with scallops, swordfish, cod, salmon, mussels, and clams.

New Brunswick is surrounded by the Atlantic Ocean. It is best known for farming and fishing. Potatoes are the most valuable crop, and the most valuable seafood catches are scallops and lobster.

East

Quebec and Ontario are the two provinces of Canada's East. Quebec has strong French roots. French is its official language, and French culinary influences abound. Quebec is home to excellent fresh and aged cheeses from the milk of cows, goats, and sheep.

In Quebec, seafood is broiled, baked, and made into **croquettes** (krō-ˈkets), puréed seafood that is bound with a thick sauce, formed into small shapes, then breaded and deep-fried. While smoking has been a meat preservation method for thousands of years, Montreal's unique smoked meat sandwiches can be traced to Eastern European Jewish communities. A popular fast food dish in Quebec, poutine, consists of French fries and cheese curds topped with hot chicken gravy.

Quebec produces about 90 percent of Canada's maple syrup. The sugar season, called temps des sucres in French, is one of Quebec's oldest culinary traditions. During spring, places called sugar shacks serve a traditional meal of eggs, baked beans, fried pork, and bacon, all covered in maple syrup.

Ontario has a fertile southern region, where apples, peaches, and plums are grown. Farmers in Ontario raise beef, pork, quail, pheasant, and partridge. Cheddar cheese is also a specialty.

Midwest

The Midwestern provinces of Manitoba, Saskatchewan, and Alberta are known as Canada's "market basket." Vast fields of wheat, corn, rye, millet, and sunflowers span this prairie land. Cattle and bison graze on the range.

TECHNOLOGY FOR TOMORROW

Lobster Traps

Until the early 1800s, people simply collected lobsters by hand along the shoreline. Then, fishermen caught lobsters by placing fragile, wooden traps on the sea floor. These were replaced by metal or wire traps. Most modern traps are made with plastic. The ease with which lobsters can be trapped has led to concern about overharvesting of lobsters.

Get Involved Examine the concept of overharvesting of lobsters. What steps are governments and other organizations taking to prevent overharvesting? Use the Internet to research, and write a paragraph about your findings.

NCSS IX D Global Connections Analyze the causes, consequences, and potential solutions to persistent, contemporary, and emerging global issues.

Manitoba is known for its excellent wild rice. A variety of fish thrive in the lakes of Manitoba, including Winnipeg goldeye, pickerel, northern pike, trout, carp, and Arctic char.

Saskatchewan has a thriving agricultural industry. The largest city, Saskatoon, is named for the native Cree word for the local Saskatoon berry, which is made into pies and preserves. Wild rice also grows in Saskatchewan, where it is often served as a stuffing.

Alberta is cattle country. Beans and potatoes grow here, as do Jerusalem artichokes, which are native to this part of the world. Also called sunchokes, these small tubers with bumpy skins are peeled, then eaten raw in salads or sautéed.

West

British Columbia, like the rest of Canada, has rich culinary traditions from its first peoples. Native peoples of British Columbia practice a tradition known as the potlatch, part of which is a feast with dancing and eating. Traditional potlatch foods include salmon, venison, moose, clams, huckleberries, and blackberries.

North

The territories of Yukon, Northwest, and Nunavut have abundant lakes and rivers with Alaskan salmon, halibut, trout, Arctic Grayling, and Kokanee salmon. Popular meat dishes include caribou steak, venison, and buffalo.

Light and Healthy Recipe

Cajun-Style Gumbo

Ingredients

- **4 oz.** Butter
- **4 oz.** Flour
- **¼ pound** Diced andouille sausage
- **1 cup** Diced onion
- **½ cup** Diced green bell pepper
- **½ cup** Diced celery
- **1 cup** Sliced okra
- **2 cups** Rice
- **8 oz.** Grilled, chopped chicken breast
- **6 cups** Chicken stock
- **3 Tbsp.** Cajun spice blend
- **1 Tbsp.** Gumbo filé

Directions

1. Melt the butter on low heat and add the flour. Stir the flour into the butter continuously to break up the clumps and begin making a roux. The roux will need to cook until it is a very dark brown. Stir it continuously and cook it under low heat for at least 20 minutes. Do not let it burn.
2. In a separate pan, saute the sausage until it is completely cooked. Remove the sausage and set it aside. Lower the heat in the pan and cook the onions, green peppers, and celery in the fat left from the sausage until all the vegetables are tender.
3. When the roux is done, add the cooked sausage and chicken to the pot. Add the vegetables. Pour in the chicken stock and the spice blend.
4. Let the gumbo mixture cook, covered, on low heat, for at least an hour. Cook the rice 25 minutes before serving time.
5. Add the gumbo filé five minutes before serving.
6. At serving time, scoop rice into bowls and pour the gumbo over the top. This is a soup so serve it piping hot.

Most Cajun and Creole dishes are made with a trio of healthy vegetables: onions, green peppers, and celery.

Yield 8 servings

Nutrition Analysis per Serving

■ Calories	378
■ Total fat	17 g
Saturated fat	9 g
Cholesterol	59 mg
■ Sodium	916 mg
■ Carbohydrate	39 g
Dietary fiber	2 g
Sugars	4 g
■ Protein	17 g

CHAPTER 46 Review & Applications

After You Read

Chapter Summary

The United States and Canada are home to many regional cuisines that reflect a variety of influences from around the globe. Many cultures have put down roots in the United States, contributing new flavors and foods. The six regions of the United States are characterized by their unique cuisines. Canadian food also reflects the cuisines of its many immigrants. Each of its provinces has distinctive foods and dishes. In both the United States and Canada, the food traditions of native people blended with those of settlers.

Content and Academic Vocabulary Review

1. Use each of these key terms and academic vocabulary words to create a crossword puzzle on graph paper. Use the definitions as clues.

Content Vocabulary

- succotash (p. 712)
- scrapple (p. 713)
- goulash (p. 713)
- jambalaya (p. 714)
- gumbo (p. 714)
- étouffée (p. 714)
- cioppino (p. 715)
- poke (p. 716)
- taro root (p. 716)
- bannock (p. 717)
- croquettes (p. 717)

Academic Vocabulary

- regional (p. 712)
- thrive (p. 715)

Review Key Concepts

2. **Describe** the main food regions of the United States and give examples of regional ingredients and dishes.
3. **Identify** the main food regions of Canada and give examples of regional ingredients and dishes.

Critical Thinking

4. **Explain** whether you agree or disagree with this statement: "Food boundaries in the various regions of the United States are less clear than they once were."
5. **Compare and contrast** Creole cuisine and Cajun cuisine.
6. **Explain** whether you think any American foods are truly American. Give examples to support your ideas.
7. **Assess** the affect of climate on a region's cuisine. Give examples.
8. **Describe** how Canadian cuisine is affected by the fact that most Canadians live along the coasts and in southern cities.
9. **Evaluate** Whitney's statement: "My parents wanted to experience French culture and cuisine on their vacation, but they went to Canada!"
10. **Identify** which areas of Canada have cuisine similar to the Northwest region in the United States. Explain why.

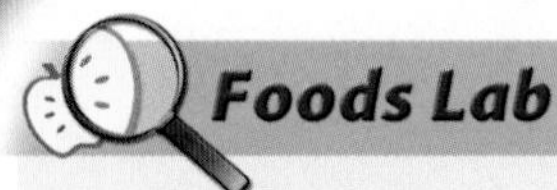

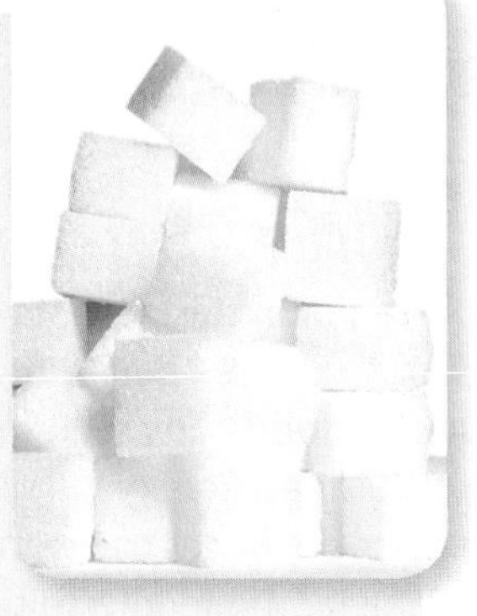

11. Contrast Sweeteners Different natural sweeteners are associated with cuisines in different areas of United States, such as maple sugar in Vermont, molasses in Massachusetts and Pennsylvania, and honey in the Southwest.

Procedure Do a taste test of maple sugar or syrup, molasses, and honey. Sample the sweeteners alone. Then pair each one with available foods, such as squares of bread or fruit slices.

Analysis In writing, describe the taste of each sweetener. Suggest one use for each sweetener that is not already mentioned in the text.

HEALTHFUL CHOICES

12. Regional and Healthful At a regional foods fair celebrating cuisines from around the United States, Nate wants to choose a lunch dish that is high in nutrients and low in fat and calories. He has narrowed down his options to the following: succotash, scrapple, kielbasa, or a Cobb salad. Which option do you think Nate should choose and why?

TECH Connection

13. Mapping Influences Select a regional dish mentioned in the chapter. Which cultures influenced the dish? Where did those cultures originate? Use the Internet to find maps that show each of the countries whose culture influenced the dish. If possible, find an image of the dish, as well. Print the images, cut them out, and create a collage that visually depicts a dish and the countries that influenced it.

Real-World Skills

Problem-Solving Skills

14. Plan a Menu Imagine your class is having a regional foods festival this Saturday and Sunday. The plan is to serve breakfast, lunch, and dinner on both days, with each meal representing cuisine from a different region in the United States. Write out a menu for the weekend that will accomplish this goal.

Interpersonal and Collaborative Skills

15. Canada Study Follow your teacher's instructions to form groups. Together, choose one region of Canada to study. Using at least four research resources, learn more about the history, geography, foods, and dishes of the region. Using such visual aids as photos, drawings, and handouts, work together to give a class presentation.

Financial Literacy Skills

16. Adjusting a Recipe Marcus wants to prepare enough jambalaya to serve at a party for 24 people. The dish requires many different ingredients, and the cost of buying enough ham, seafood, chicken, sausages, rice, vegetables, and seasonings to prepare a recipe that serves 8 is $21. How much will Marcus spend to prepare enough to serve 24?

Academic Skills

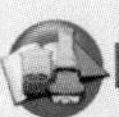

Food Science

17. Raw Hamburger The color of raw meat is due to myoglobin. If oxygenated, it is bright red in color; if not, it is grayish purple. Fresh meat is not spoiled when it looks purplish—it just lacks oxygen.

Procedure Observe the surface color of a package of ground beef. Open the package, and divide the ground beef into three equal parts, observing the cut interior color. Form a large patty with the first sample. For the second sample, mix in juice from 1 lemon. Leave the third sample in its original form, without shaping. Record any color changes after 5–10 minutes.

Analysis Research deoxymyoglobin, oxymyoglobin, and metmyoglobin then write a paragraph explaining your results.

NSES B Develop an understanding of the structure and properties of matter.

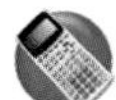

Mathematics

18. Ranching A ranch occupies 1,000 acres of land, and is shaped in an exact square. How many yards of fencing would it take to surround the perimeter of the ranch?

Math Concept Perimeter and Area of Squares If s is the length of one side of a square, then the area of the square equals $s \times s$, or s^2. The perimeter, or distance around the outside of the square, equals $4s$.

Starting Hint One acre equals 4,840 square yards. Multiply the area of the ranch (1,000 acres) by 4,840 to convert from acres to square yards. Take the square root of that area to find the length of s, in yards. Multiply s by 4 to find the perimeter.

NCTM Geometry Use visualization, spatial reasoning, and geometric modeling to solve problems.

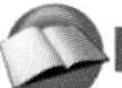

English Language Arts

19. Research and Report Write a one-page research report on one of the following topics: the history of African-American soul food; Hawaiian luaus; the Native American influence on North American cuisine. Visit the library and conduct thorough research on your topic. Examine at least three books or articles. When you use your research in your paper, cite the articles you use. Properly cite the books and articles you used for your research on a separate sheet of paper.

NCTE 7 Conduct research and gather, evaluate, and synthesize data to communicate discoveries.

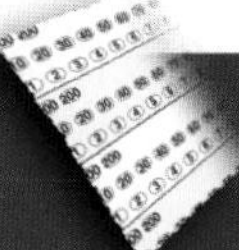

STANDARDIZED TEST PRACTICE

MULTIPLE CHOICE

Read the question and select the best answer from the choices.

20. What percentage of Canada's land cannot be used for growing crops?

a. 5 percent
b. 95 percent
c. 90 percent
d. 10 percent

Test-Taking Tip Multiple-choice questions may prompt you to select the "best" answer. They may present you with answers that seem partially true. The best answer is the one that is completely true, and can be supported by information you have read in the text.

CHAPTER 47

Foods of South America, Latin America, & the Caribbean

Writing Activity — Report

Andean Cuisine Research and write a one-page report about one of the following Andean countries and its cuisine: Colombia, Ecuador, Peru, or Chile. Use at least two resources besides your textbook. Find out about common ingredients and popular dishes in the country you chose. Explain how the country's people and climate have shaped its cuisine.

Writing Tips Follow these steps to write a report:

- Use more than one resource to conduct your research.
- Report your most interesting and relevant research findings.
- Write in your own words and quote others correctly.

Activate Prior Knowledge

Explore the Photo Many foods from Latin America and the Caribbean have elements of European and African cuisine. *What foods can you name that come from Latin America?*

Reading Guide

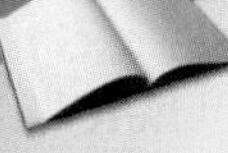

Before You Read

Preview Examine the photos and figures and read their captions. Think about the flavorful foods found in Latin America and the Caribbean.

Read to Learn

Key Concepts

- **Describe** four common Latin American dishes.
- **Identify** ingredients that play a role in Caribbean cuisine.

Main Idea

The cuisines of Latin America and the Caribbean are flavorful, diverse, and influenced by many different cultures.

Content Vocabulary

You will find definitions for these words in the glossary at the back of this book.

- ☐ cassava
- ☐ salsa
- ☐ empanada
- ☐ chorizo
- ☐ ceviche
- ☐ sopa
- ☐ masa
- ☐ frijoles
- ☐ mole
- ☐ jerk

Academic Vocabulary

You will find these words in your reading and on your tests. Use the glossary to look up their definitions if necessary.

- native
- province

Graphic Organizer

Use a graphic organizer like the one below to note the nations that comprise Central America, South America, and the Caribbean.

CENTRAL AMERICA	SOUTH AMERICA	THE CARIBBEAN

Graphic Organizer Go to this book's Online Learning Center at **glencoe.com** to print out this graphic organizer.

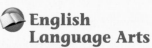

Academic Standards

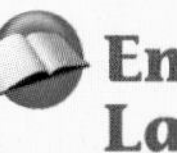

English Language Arts

NCTE 4 Use written language to communicate effectively.

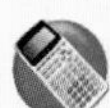

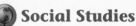

Mathematics

NCTM Number and Operations Understand numbers, ways of representing numbers, relationships among numbers, and number systems.

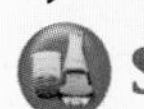

Science

NSES B Develop an understanding of the structure and properties of matter.

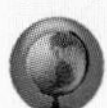

Social Studies

NCSS VIII A Identify and describe both current and historical examples of the interaction and interdependence of science, technology, and society in a variety of cultural settings.

NCTE *National Council of Teachers of English*
NCTM *National Council of Teachers of Mathematics*
NSES *National Science Education Standards*
NCSS *National Council for the Social Studies*

Learning Latin American Cuisine

Latin America boasts dramatic contrasts in climate and geography, from rugged mountain ranges to tropical rain forests. **Figure 47.1** shows a map of Latin America.

Three **native**, or local, cultures have dominated the history of Latin America: the Aztecs in Mexico, the Mayas in Central America, and the Incas in South America. All three cultures cultivated corn, beans, chiles, squash, potatoes, tomatoes, avocados, and a starchy root vegetable called **cassava** (kə-'sä-və).

European colonists introduced their own staple foods. The Portuguese, for example, brought wheat and hogs. Pork became the most important meat in Latin America, except in Argentina and northern Mexico, where Spaniards introduced beef cattle. The Spanish also introduced rice, goats, sheep, and chickens. The French brought herbs, including thyme and chives. Europeans also introduced coffee, which now grows across Latin America.

Chiles are native to Latin America and are central to Latin American cuisine. Chiles provide seasoning and spiciness and are the basis for **salsa**, or sauce. Some salsas are chunky

Figure 47.1 **Latin America**

Cultural Influences South of Mexico is Central America, which extends from Belize and Guatemala to Panama. East of Central America are the islands in the Caribbean Sea. ***What three native cultures are most important in Latin American history?***

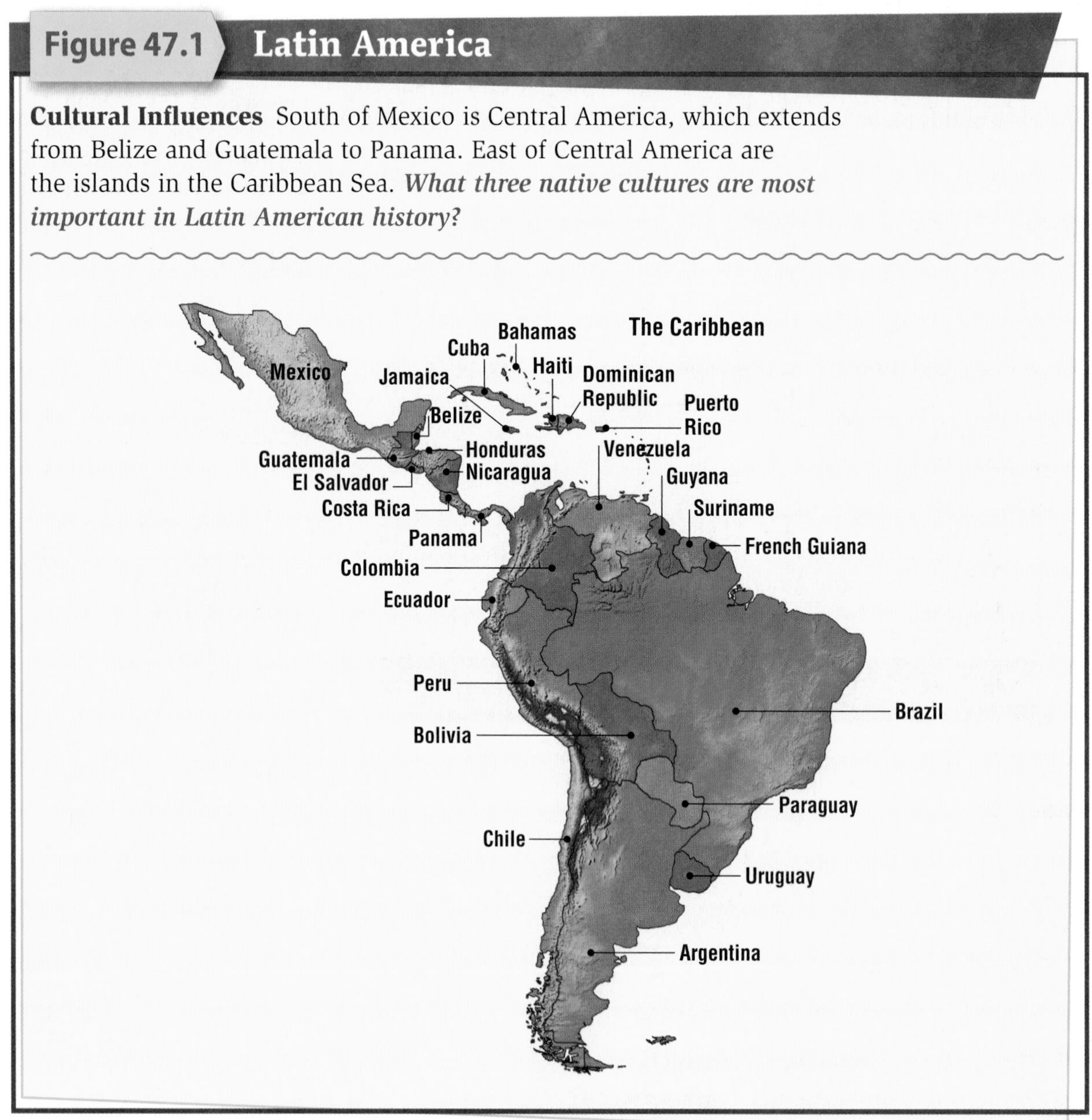

mixtures with added tomatoes, onions, garlic, and spices. Mexican, Brazilian, and Caribbean salsas, however, can be as simple as chopped chiles, salt, and lime juice. Adobo is a spicy vinegar salsa used as a rub or serving sauce for meats. Escabèche, originally a Spanish pickling sauce, is a marinade for cooked fish, chicken, and vegetables. The annatto seed is ground with chiles, onions, and herbs to make achiote sauce.

Latin American Dishes

Latin American cuisine has many dishes featuring corn, rice, and beans, which together provide complete protein. Rice is paired with chicken in pollo con arroz, for example, and rice pudding is a popular dessert.

Barbecuing and grilling are popular ways to serve meat. Leftovers may be chopped with onions, garlic, and herbs and used in an **empanada** (ˌem-pə-ˈnä-də), a turnover filled with meat, vegetables, fruit, or all three. Empanadas were introduced by the Spanish, as were albondigas, meatballs that are sometimes made with rice. **Chorizo** (chə-rē-(ˌ)zō), a spicy sausage, flavors many stews.

Seafood is important in the cuisine of coastal areas, from the Gulf of Mexico to Chile's Cape Horn. Each region has a recipe for **ceviche** (sə-vē-(ˌ)chā), an appetizer of raw fish marinated in citrus juice until firm and opaque. The fish is drained and served with chiles, tomatoes, and onions.

Latin American soup, or **sopa**, features meat as the main ingredient. Peanuts and squash are also used. Toasted cassava meal, cornmeal, ground nuts, and potatoes are used to thicken soups.

Mexico

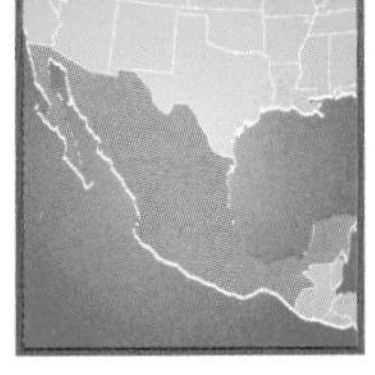

Mexican cuisine uses local foods in creative ways. Corn, beans, wheat, and rice are grown in Mexico, as well as coffee, vegetables, fruit, and livestock. The hilly landscape of the north is well suited to ranching, while coffee and sugarcane come from the south.

Mexican cuisine reflects Aztec influence. The Aztecs considered corn sacred, and corn is still central to Mexican cooking. About 60 varieties of corn are grown. Corn is enjoyed in soups and fresh on the cob. Mainly, however, corn is dried, cooked, soaked in limewater, and then ground into dough, or **masa** (ˈmä-sə). Dried, ground masa is sold as masa harina, a coarse-grained corn flour. People use masa to make tortillas, a flatbread that is part of many Mexican meals.

Avocados and squash are two other native foods that are important in Mexican cooking. Avocado is added to salads and chilled soups and mashed into guacamole. Squash and squash blossoms are used for soups, fritters, and empanada fillings.

Chocolate came to Mexico from trade with the Maya in Central America. The Aztecs used it in a hot, frothy beverage that they enriched with corn milk and seasoned with chiles, vanilla, and other spices. Hot chocolate, sometimes thickened with cornstarch or flavored with vanilla, is still a favorite. Chocolate is also used to season sauces and main dishes.

In many Mexican recipes, tortillas are filled with combinations of meat, poultry, beans, fish, and cheese and then prepared in different ways. Small tortillas are simply folded to make tacos. Tortillas are folded around cheese and grilled to make quesadillas. Tortillas are dipped in chile sauce, then filled and baked to make enchiladas. Deep-fried stuffed tortillas are called flautas. Uncooked masa is wrapped in cornhusks and steamed to make tamales.

Beans, called **frijoles** (frē-ˈhō-lēs) in Spanish, are a versatile ingredient in Mexican dishes. Frijoles refritos, for example, is a side dish of red or pinto beans, mashed and fried in lard. Like other Latin American countries, Mexico has regional recipes for bean stew, or cocido.

Tortilla soup is made with tomatoes, onions, garlic, chiles, and tortilla strips and served as a first course. Posole is a main-course soup of pork or chicken and dried corn. Menudo combines tripe (the lining of a cow's stomach), hominy, and chiles. In the northern Mexican state of Sonora, a favorite dish is potato soup (sopa de papas) laced with melted cheese.

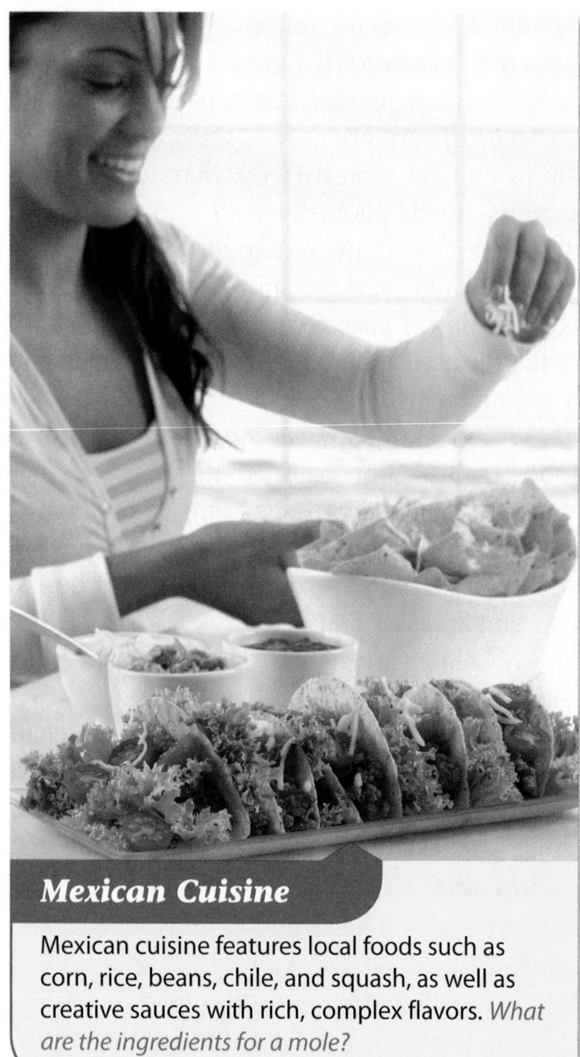

Mexican Cuisine

Mexican cuisine features local foods such as corn, rice, beans, chile, and squash, as well as creative sauces with rich, complex flavors. *What are the ingredients for a mole?*

Salsas are an everyday condiment in Mexico. In Guadalajara, a salsa is made with chipotle chiles (smoked jalapeños) and tomatillos (Mexican green tomatoes). A **mole** (ˈmō-lā) is a thick blend of chiles, ground pumpkin or sesame seeds, onions, unsweetened chocolate, and spices. Some variations include tomatoes, bananas, sugar, or raisins. The best-known version of mole, mole poblano, traditionally accompanies turkey or chicken.

Mexican seafood recipes feature local fish and shellfish, such as shrimp from the Gulf of Mexico. Shrimp is often prepared with puréed plantains (a starchy banana), onion, tomato, and salsa. On the Yucatan peninsula, shrimp is served chilled en escabèche or grilled in an achiote paste.

Central America

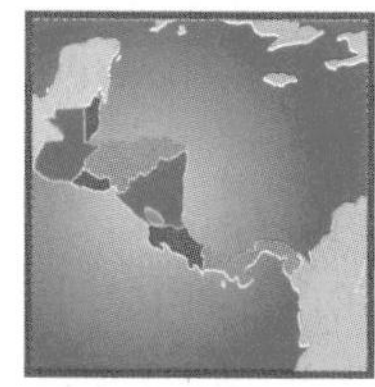

The tropical countries of Central America join the continents of North and South America. These countries share several food traditions. The native berry allspice flavors many sweet and savory dishes. Chicken is a popular ingredient and is sometimes flavored with pineapple, tomatoes, or raisins. Chayote, a native squashlike fruit, is eaten raw or cooked and stuffed with cheese.

Each country also has its own food specialties. For example, oysters are popular in Guatemalan cooking. Pollo pepian is a Guatemalan dish of chicken in a spicy sauce with sesame and pumpkin seeds. The signature dish of El Salvador is the pupusa, a corn cake filled with refried beans, cheese, and pork and served with a cabbage, onion, and carrot slaw.

A popular dish in Nicaragua is nacatamal, made from cabbage, plantain, and pork steamed in banana leaves. Popular dishes in Costa Rica include gallo pinto (fried black beans and rice) and arroz con tuna (rice with tuna). A Panamanian breakfast tortilla is a thick corn pastry, deep-fried and topped with cheese and eggs.

South America

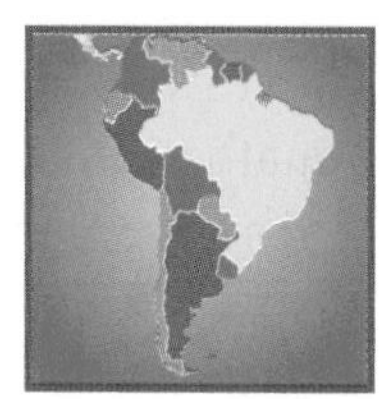

Thirteen countries make up South America, a continent about three times the size of the United States. It is a vast land with a wide variety of ingredients and cooking styles. Potatoes and quinoa are big plant crops, particularly on the west coast of the continent.

Brazil

Brazil is a country of many ethnicities and cultural groups, where cuisine varies greatly from region to region. The Portuguese once ruled Brazil, bringing slaves from Africa to work on local sugar plantations. Brazilian cooking therefore shows Portuguese and African influences, as well as influences of native cultures.

Dende oil, a bright orange palm oil, is the fat of choice for many recipes. It is used in the national dish of Brazil, an Afro-Brazilian specialty, called feijoada completa. The elaborate meal features the main dish of black beans and various meats simmered in a well-seasoned stock. Fresh and dried beef, chorizo, pig's feet, and other cuts of pork may be used. The stew is often prepared over a low fire in a thick clay pot. Simple side dishes such as orange slices, rice, and vegetables round out the meal. A pot of hot pepper sauce may be provided on the side.

The African influence on Brazilian cooking also shows in its many seafood stews. Moqueca, for example, has a variety of seafood, from swordfish to shrimp, in a base of coconut milk, palm oil, and tomatoes. Vatapa is a paste made with bread, shrimp, coconut milk and palm oil. It is often eaten with rice.

Other popular Brazilian dishes include greens sautéed in dende oil and a crumbly dish called farofa made from sautéed cassava meal, nuts, and raisins. Shrimp caruru is traditional in the **province**, or state, of Bahia. The guarana fruit, whose seeds contain caffeine, is made into a popular soft drink, a powder, and a syrup.

For desserts, figs, papayas, oranges, pears, peaches, and pumpkins are served with solid fresh cheese. Pudim de päo is a pie made from day-old bread submerged in milk and thickened with eggs and sugar. Dried orange slices and cloves add additional flavor.

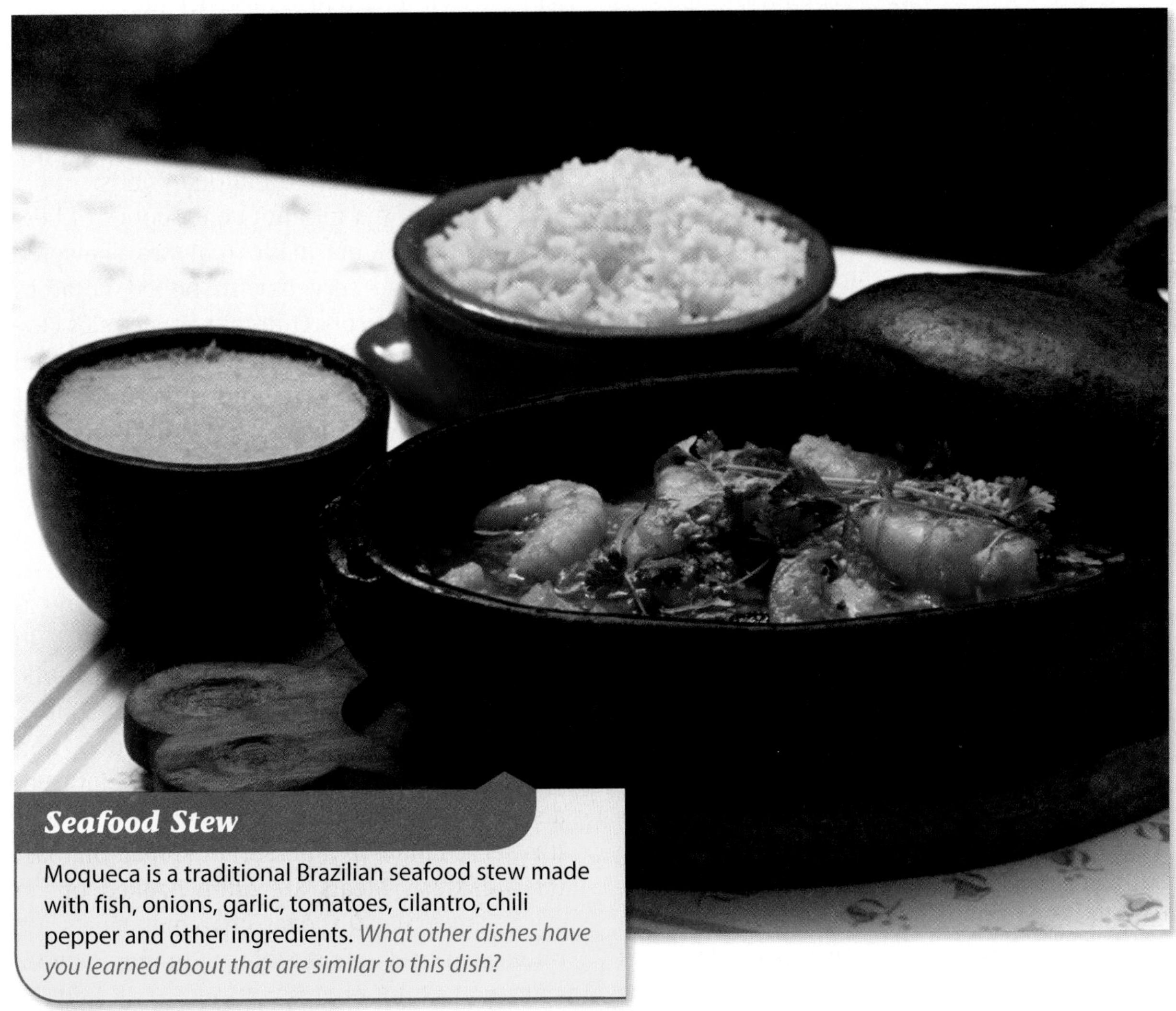

Seafood Stew

Moqueca is a traditional Brazilian seafood stew made with fish, onions, garlic, tomatoes, cilantro, chili pepper and other ingredients. *What other dishes have you learned about that are similar to this dish?*

TECHNOLOGY FOR TOMORROW

Jerky Production

Did you know the native people of the Andes began making jerky centuries ago? The English word jerky comes from the term charqui, a Quechua word that means dried meat. Traditionally, native South Americans cut thin slices of meat from the animals they hunted or raised. They dried it for days in the sun and wind beside a smoky fire, which repelled insects and preserved the jerky from spoiling. In present-day America, most jerky is mass-produced in factories. Large ovens made of insulated panels feature heaters and special fans that remove moisture from the air. The combination of fast moving air and low heat dries the meat within just a few hours.

Get Involved How is modern-day, mass-produced jerky typically preserved? Write your findings in a paragraph.

NCSS VIII A Identify and describe both current and historical examples of the interaction and interdependence of science, technology, and society in a variety of cultural settings.

Argentina

Argentinian cuisine shows many Western and Eastern European influences, reflecting the many Europeans who immigrated there. Seasonings include milder, Old World herbs as well as spicy chiles. Pastas are popular, and yeast breads are as common as tortillas. Many Argentineans take afternoon tea with a South American beverage, yerba mate, brewed from holly leaves.

Argentina has vast grasslands, or pampas, that support cattle. Beef is the major industry and national food. Beef is often grilled outdoors and served with Argentina's signature sauce, chimichurri, a blend of vinegar, olive oil, and seasonings including garlic, parsley, onion, and oregano. Meats are also combined with local fruits and vegetables to make carbonada criolla, or mixed stew. Another popular stew is locro, made with corn, beef, a spicy Spanish sausage, and vegetables. Onions, pumpkin, and beans may be included.

Andean Countries

In the Andean nations of Colombia, Ecuador, Peru, and Chile, the geography is dominated by mountains, seacoasts, and tropical rainforests. These features also influence the local cooking, which is usually less spicy than that of Mexico and Central America.

Corn, beans, chile peppers, and potatoes grow in the cool, dry climate of the fertile Andean foothills. Potatoes, in fact, may have originated there.

The Pacific Ocean provides seafood, from sea bass to sea urchin. Cassava and chiles thrive in tropical areas. Grazing land is limited, so meat often comes from chickens, guinea pigs, and llamas. Llama meat is salted and dried to make charqui (jerky).

The Andean countries have several foods in common. Arepa is a small griddlecake made with cooked cracked corn. Aji, a local chile, is used for seasoning and is made into a hot sauce. Each nation also has specialties.

Colombia is known for ajiaco, a soup of chicken, potatoes, and corn. Arepa, a thick flatbread made from corn, and sancocho, a soup featuring large pieces of meat and vegetables in a broth, are traditional foods.

Peru is known for anticucho, cubes of beef heart in an aji marinade that are skewered and grilled and served with boiled potatoes and corn on the cob. Different versions of ceviche, made with fish or shellfish, are found throughout the many regions of Peru. Butifarras is a sandwich made on a long bread roll with ham and a spicy sauce with chili peppers and lime.

Uruguay

Located south of Brazil and east of Argentina, Uruguay features many foods common to its neighbors. The sweet and syrupy dulce de leche is used in many deserts. Milk is cooked with sugar slowly at low temperatures and develops a taste like caramel. Dulce Membrillo, a sweet paste made of quince, also is popular. It is served plain as a dessert or spread on toast for breakfast. Meats are often cooked on an open flame, usually over charcoal. Meats are often skewered before grilling. Hungara, a very spicy sort of hot dog, is a popular grill item.

Paraguay

Much like Argentina, its neighbor to the south, Paraguayan cuisine favors meats cooked on an open grill, called parrillada. Mazamorra is a corn mush eaten with many meals. Mandioca is a local staple root crop. It is combined with cornmeal and cheese to create chipa, a bagel-like bread. Sopa paraguaya is a cornbread made with cheese and onions. A special cheese called Paraguay cheese is made by a process that includes soaking curds in sour orange and lemon juice. It is one of the most often-used ingredients in Paraguayan cuisine.

Mate, a hot caffeinated beverage made by steeping the dried leaves of the yerba mate plant in water, is the national drink of Argentina, Paraguay, and Uruguay. Terere is a cold version of mate.

✓ **Reading Check** **Identify** What three common ingredients make many Latin American dishes sources of complete protein?

Learning Caribbean Cuisine

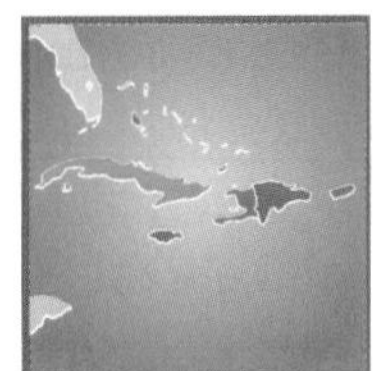

Hundreds of tropical islands dot the Caribbean Sea. The earliest known inhabitants of these islands were the Caribs and the Arawaks. Spanish, French, British, and Dutch colonists, as well as Africans, came later, creating a lively fusion of cuisines.

Seafood is a staple in the Caribbean. Conch, a prized shellfish, is saved for special occasions. Chicken is often served in main dishes, as are pork and goat on some islands. Rice and legumes are central to meals, especially black and red beans, black-eyed peas, and pigeon peas.

Tropical fruits are important in Caribbean cooking. Mangoes, figs, pomegranates, and coconuts are eaten raw, cooked in side dishes, and used to flavor meats.

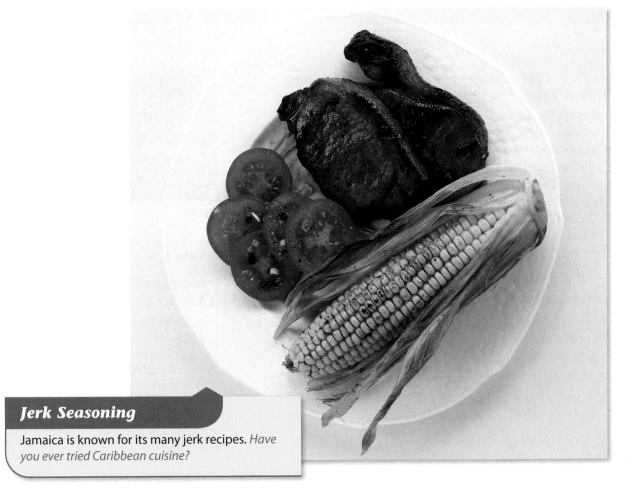

Jerk Seasoning

Jamaica is known for its many jerk recipes. *Have you ever tried Caribbean cuisine?*

Caribbean Dishes

Each Caribbean country has a different history and combination of cultural influences. African culture is important in Jamaica. Fish, vegetables and beans are mainstays of the diet. Meat is used in a limited manner. Ackee and saltfish, the Jamaican national dish combines two West African imports: saltfish, or dried cod, and ackee, a tropical fruit that resembles scrambled eggs when it is cooked.

Jamaica is known for its many jerk recipes. **Jerk** is a blend of chiles, onions, garlic, allspice, and other herbs and spices used to season meat, poultry, and fish. Marinades are made by adding oil, citrus juice, and molasses to the jerk spice blend.

Haitian cooking shows a French influence. Rice and beans are the native dish. Mais Moulu is a popular dish consisting of a cornmeal mash, similar to polenta, and a sauce made from mashed beans. A griot is made with cubes of meat marinated in citrus juice, salt, pepper, and thyme, then simmered and fried. Chicken is very common in Haitian cuisine. Flattened plantain slices, cooked in oil like potato chips, are a common snack food.

Cuban cuisine has strong Spanish and African influences. Many main dishes start with a sofrito, a sauté of onion, garlic, and bell pepper in olive oil that is also used in the Creole cooking of New Orleans. Sandwiches in Cuba are usually made with a long loaf of bread made with lard and water. The Cuban sandwich, a popular export, features bread, thin slices of roast pork and ham, mustard and sweet pickles. It is toasted like a panini. Cuba has regions where distinct methods and ingredients are used, but all regions make use of beans and rice. Meat is limited.

Light and Healthy Recipe

Gallo Pinto

Ingredients

- **3 Tbsp.** Olive oil
- **1 cup** Diced onion
- **1 clove** Minced garlic
- **½ cup** Diced red bell pepper
- **½ cup** Diced green bell pepper
- **1 pound** Black beans
- **2 cups** Cooked rice
- **2 Tbsp.** Chopped cilantro
- **½ tsp.** Salt
- **½ tsp.** Pepper

Directions

1. Heat the olive oil in a large pot and add the onion. Fry the onion until it begins to take on color. Then add the garlic and fry two minutes more.
2. Add the bell pepper and cook until tender.
3. Add the beans and rice and cook until both are heated through.
4. Add the cilantro and season with salt and pepper.
5. Garnish with cilantro leaf and serve hot.

This simple dish of beans, rice, and vegetables is the national dish of Costa Rica and Nicaragua.

Yield 6 servings

Nutrition Analysis per Serving

■ Calories	325
■ Total fat	12 g
Saturated fat	2 g
Cholesterol	0 mg
■ Sodium	644 mg
■ Carbohydrate	45 g
Dietary fiber	8 g
Sugars	4 g
■ Protein	9 g

CHAPTER 47 Review & Applications

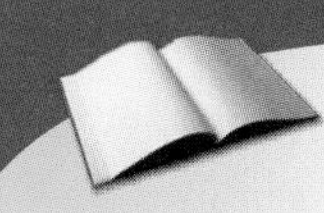

After You Read

Chapter Summary

The cuisines of Latin America and the Caribbean are flavorful, diverse, and influenced by many different cultures. Three native cultures of Latin America—the Aztecs, Mayas, and Incas—had their own cuisines based on the foods they cultivated. Later, their food traditions blended with those of European colonists. Mexico, Central America, and South America are all parts of Latin America. Each has its own distinctive cuisine. The Caribbean is comprised of hundreds of islands. Many people—including Caribs, Arawaks, Spanish, French, British, Dutch, and Africans—created a fusion of cuisines. Each Caribbean country, such as Jamaica, Haiti, and Cuba, has a unique history and cuisine.

Content and Academic Vocabulary Review

1. Use each of these content and academic vocabulary words in a sentence.

Content Vocabulary

- cassava (p. 724)
- salsa (p. 724)
- empanada (p. 725)
- chorizo(p. 725)
- ceviche (p. 725)
- sopa (p. 725)
- masa (p. 725)
- frijoles (p. 725)
- mole (p. 726)
- jerk (p. 730)

Academic Vocabulary

- native (p. 724)
- province (p. 727)

Review Key Concepts

2. **Describe** four common Latin American dishes.
3. **Identify** ingredients that play a role in Caribbean cuisine.

Critical Thinking

4. **Explain** whether you think food would be different worldwide if cultures did not intermingle. If so, how?
5. **Describe** how understanding the influences on a country's cuisine can help you to understand the country's history. Give examples.
6. **Explain** why Mexican dishes are more known in the United States than dishes from South America.
7. **Identify** two characteristics that Latin American cuisines have in common with U.S. cuisine.
8. **Describe** two specific, food-related things that you think Caribbean natives may have taught European colonists.
9. **Evaluate** the consequences of assuming that all Caribbean countries have the same cuisine.
10. **Explain** which areas of Latin America or the Caribbean you would visit on a culinary journey. Give three reasons why.

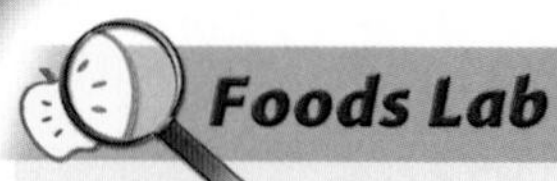

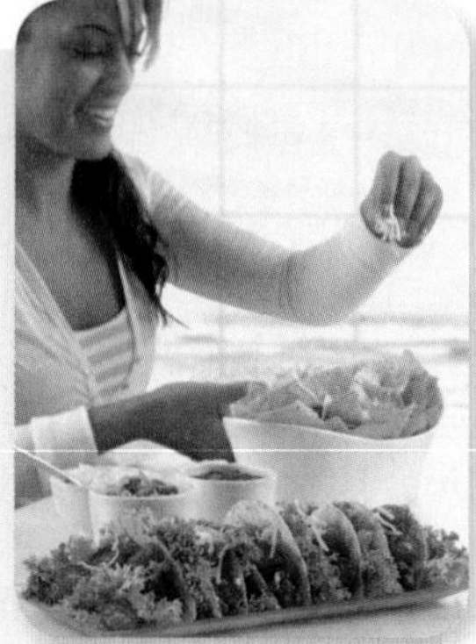

11. Making Salsa Salsa figures prominently in the cuisine of Latin America, yet recipes for it differ widely among countries, and even among individuals.

Procedure Develop and prepare a recipe for tomato-based salsa. Refer to existing recipes and to this chapter for ideas about ingredients and techniques. Then experiment with your own seasonings and proportions.

Analysis In an oral presentation, explain the following: What ingredients did you use? Is your salsa hot, medium, or mild? What makes your recipe unique? After tasting it, would you alter it in any way? If so, how?

HEALTHFUL CHOICES

12. High Protein Dip Karl, a teen, tries to consume the daily recommended amount of protein each day. Today, however, he has not eaten enough. After school, he prepares a snack of baked tortilla chips and dip. There are two kinds of dip to choose from: a salsa made of chopped tomatoes, peppers, and onions, or a dip made of mashed frijoles and spices. Which should he choose and why?

TECH Connection

13. Mexican Holiday Despite its name, the Mexican holiday known as the Day of the Dead is a festive occasion. During this holiday, family and friends honor and remember friends and relatives who have died. Under your teacher's supervision, use the Internet to research this holiday, including its origins, date, and information about the foods that are part of the festivities. Then use word processing software to write a one-page report.

Real-World Skills

Problem-Solving Skills

14. Plan a Buffet Imagine your class is having a Latin American-themed party. You have been assigned the job of planning a buffet that will contain the following: a seafood option, a beef option, a vegetarian option, and two kinds of salsas. What Latin American dishes or foods will the buffet offer? Write them in list form.

Interpersonal and Collaborative Skills

15. Chile Pepper Display Follow your teacher's instructions to form pairs. Work together to research a type of chile pepper assigned to you by your teacher. Draw and color an image of it at least 8 inches tall. Write facts about it, including its uses and degree of spiciness, on the image. Then add it to a classroom chile pepper display.

Financial Literacy Skills

16. Avoiding Waste The Garcia family grilled $54 worth of meat and poultry during a party. When the party was over, they still had half of the meat and poultry left over, which they plan to throw away. What traditional Latin American dish can they make with the leftover meat, and how much money will they avoid wasting if they do?

Academic Skills

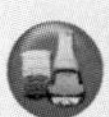

Food Science

17. Heat Transfer Potatoes are useful in showing heat transfer in food, because as they cook, they go from opaque to translucent. They cook from the outside inwards, and show an ever increasing ring width of translucence.

Procedure Bring a pot of water to a boil. Add 4 small potatoes all at once. Set timers for 1, 4, 8, and 12 minutes. Remove a potato from the pot at each time interval. Cut the potatoes in half to observe the rings that are translucent or cooked.

Analysis What can you conclude about the relationship of the cooked areas to the time?

NSES B Develop an understanding of the structure and properties of matter.

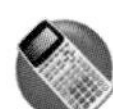

Mathematics

18. Chile Peppers Frequently used in Latin American cuisines, chile peppers vary greatly in spiciness, due to varying amounts of a chemical known as capsaicin. The amount of capsaicin found in a chile is measured on the Scoville scale, with higher numbers indicating spicier peppers. A habanero pepper can rate up to 580,000 Scoville heat units, while a serrano can hit 23,000. Write each number in scientific notation.

Math Concept **Scientific Notation** Scientific notation uses powers of 10 as shorthand for writing very large numbers. Start by moving the decimal point so that just one digit is to the left of the decimal. Count the number of places you moved the decimal. Remove all of the ending zeros, and write the number multiplied by 10 to the power of the number of decimal places moved.

Starting Hint For example, to write 7,365,000 in scientific notation, move the decimal point so that just one digit is to its left, and remove all trailing zeros, resulting in 7.365. Since we moved the decimal point six places to the left, we rewrite the number as 7.365×10^6.

NCTM Number and Operations Understand numbers, ways of representing numbers, relationships among numbers, and number systems.

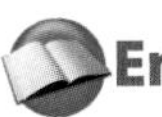

English Language Arts

19. Write a Letter Write a letter to an imaginary pen pal who lives in a specific country in Latin America or the Caribbean. In the letter, share three things that you have learned about your pen pal's cuisine.

NCTE 4 Use written language to communicate effectively.

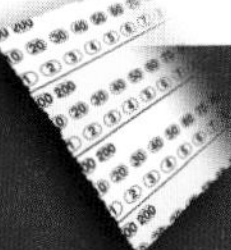

STANDARDIZED TEST PRACTICE

TRUE OR FALSE

Read the statement and determine if it is true or false.

20. There are hundreds of islands in the Caribbean Sea, but they are all part of one country.
    a. True
    b. False

Test-Taking Tip Before deciding whether a statement is true or false, read it carefully, and recall what you have learned from reading the text. Pay close attention to individual words. One word can make the difference between a true statement and a false one.

CHAPTER 48

Foods of Western, Northern, & Southern Europe

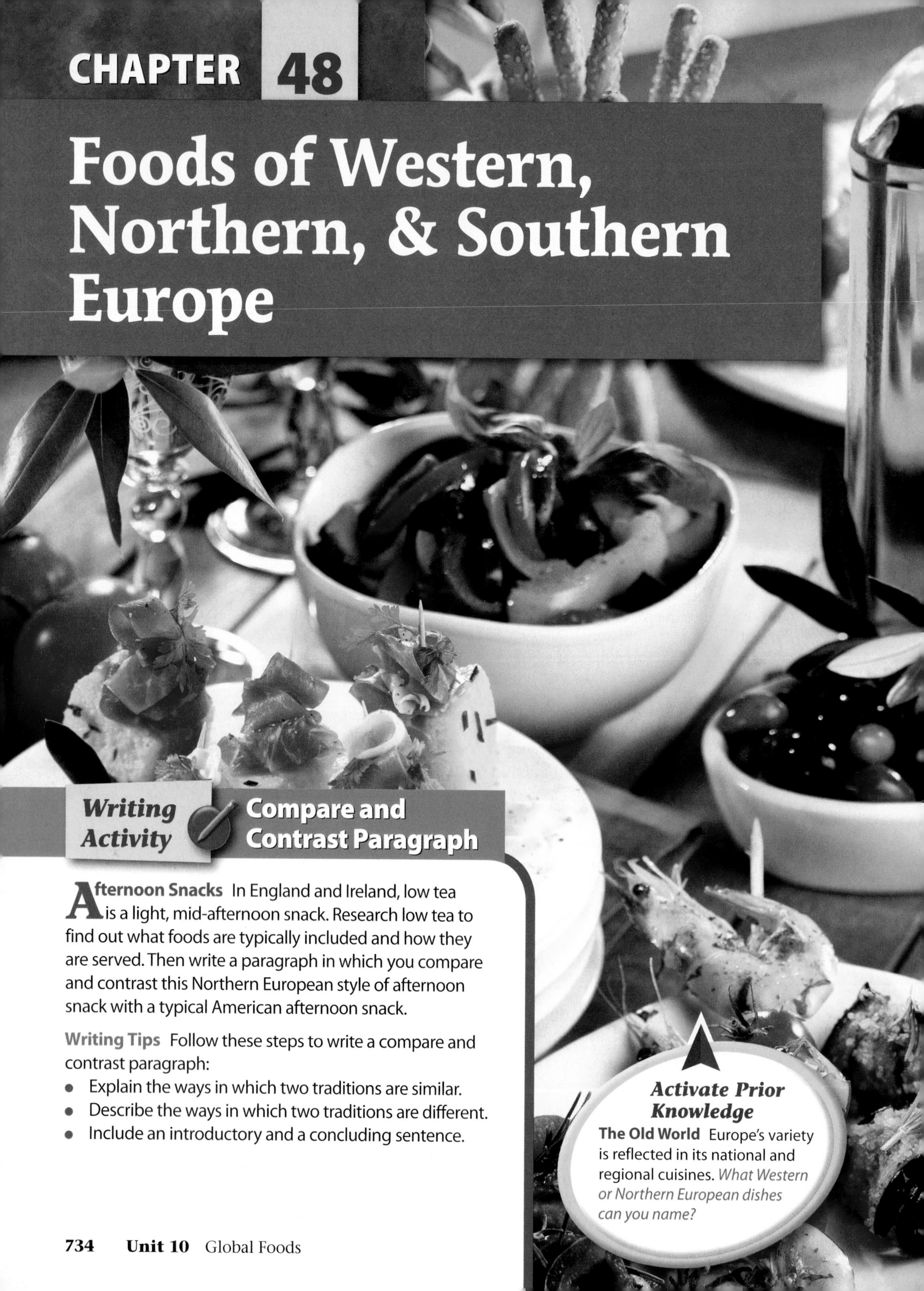

Writing Activity — Compare and Contrast Paragraph

Afternoon Snacks In England and Ireland, low tea is a light, mid-afternoon snack. Research low tea to find out what foods are typically included and how they are served. Then write a paragraph in which you compare and contrast this Northern European style of afternoon snack with a typical American afternoon snack.

Writing Tips Follow these steps to write a compare and contrast paragraph:

- Explain the ways in which two traditions are similar.
- Describe the ways in which two traditions are different.
- Include an introductory and a concluding sentence.

Activate Prior Knowledge

The Old World Europe's variety is reflected in its national and regional cuisines. *What Western or Northern European dishes can you name?*

Reading Guide

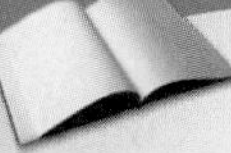

Before You Read

Preview List three facts you know or assumptions you have about Western, Northern, and Southern European cuisine. As you read, check your knowledge.

Read to Learn

Key Concepts

- **Describe** popular dishes from Western Europe.
- **Describe** how Northern Europe's geography and climate affect its cuisine.
- **Explain** why the Mediterranean diet is lighter than the cuisine of Western and Northern Europe.

Main Idea

Western, Northern, and Southern Europe are home to diverse cuisines that use a variety of ingredients and cooking methods.

Content Vocabulary

You will find definitions for these words in the glossary at the back of this book.

- ☐ Yorkshire pudding
- ☐ fool
- ☐ haggis
- ☐ laverbread
- ☐ colcannon
- ☐ baguette
- ☐ haute cuisine
- ☐ sauerbraten
- ☐ stollen
- ☐ torte
- ☐ smorgasbord
- ☐ lutefisk
- ☐ marzipan
- ☐ paella
- ☐ tapas
- ☐ pancetta
- ☐ antipasto
- ☐ pesto
- ☐ gnocchi
- ☐ polenta
- ☐ cannoli
- ☐ biscotti
- ☐ moussaka
- ☐ dolma
- ☐ baklava

Academic Vocabulary

You will find these words in your reading and on your tests. Use the glossary to look up their definitions if necessary.

- immigration
- elaborate

Graphic Organizer

Use a graphic organizer like the one below to take notes about Western, Northern, and Southern European cuisine.

Western European Cuisine	Northern European Cuisine	Southern European Cuisine

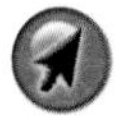

Graphic Organizer Go to this book's Online Learning Center at **glencoe.com** to print out this graphic organizer.

Academic Standards

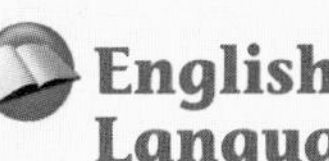

English Language Arts

NCTE 8 Use information resources to gather information and create and communicate knowledge.

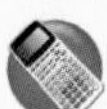

Mathematics

NCTM Measurement Understand measurable attributes of objects and the units, systems, and processes of measurement.

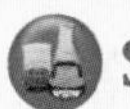

Science

NSES B Develop an understanding of the structure and properties of matter.

NCTE *National Council of Teachers of English*
NCTM *National Council of Teachers of Mathematics*
NSES *National Science Education Standards*
NCSS *National Council for the Social Studies*

Western European Cuisine

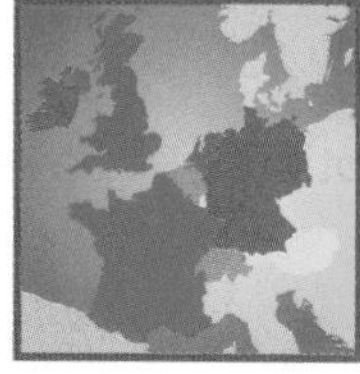

Western Europe has a long and sophisticated culinary tradition. It has a temperate, wet climate that supports abundant agriculture and livestock such as sheep, cattle, chicken, and pigs. Seafood is important in coastal areas, although even landlocked nations are not far from an ocean or sea. The United Kingdom, Germany, and France are the largest countries of Western Europe. **Figure 48.1** shows the geography of Western and Northern Europe.

The United Kingdom and Ireland

The United Kingdom is made up of England, Scotland, Wales, and Northern Ireland. Northern Ireland and the Republic of Ireland share the island of Ireland.

Separated from continental Europe by the North Sea and the English Channel, the United Kingdom and Ireland have developed a cuisine that is unique in all of Europe. Traditional cooking here is simple, substantial, and nourishing.

Tea is the national beverage of Britain and Ireland. The word tea is also used for the afternoon snack or evening meal. Low tea is a light, mid-afternoon snack of small sandwiches, bread and jam, or scones and clotted (thickened) cream. It is called low tea because it is usually served in a sitting room on low tables. Scones may also be topped with lemon curd. Low tea is followed by a larger late dinner. High tea is a hearty early evening dinner, often with meats, fish, cheeses, bread and butter, pastries, and tea.

Fish and chips are also popular throughout the United Kingdom and Ireland. Deep-fried fillets, usually of haddock, cod, or sole, are served with french-fried potatoes, sprinkled with salt and splashed with malt vinegar.

Figure 48.1 Western and Northern Europe

Cultural Influences Western and Northern Europe includes the western part of the continent of Europe, the Scandinavian peninsula, and the islands of the United Kingdom, Ireland, and Iceland. ***What are the largest countries in Western Europe?***

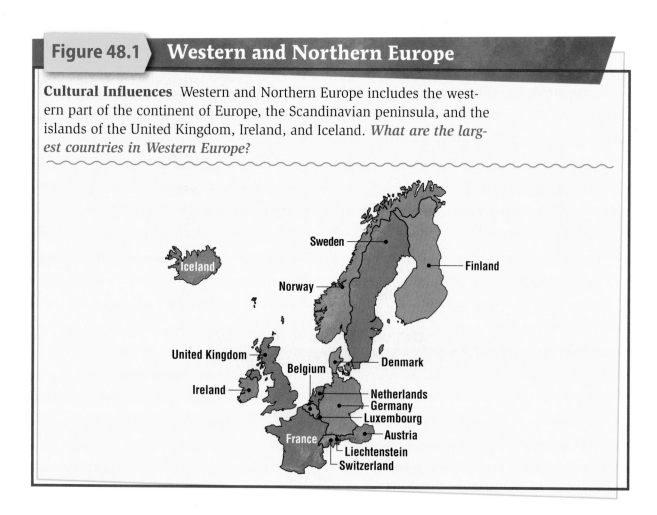

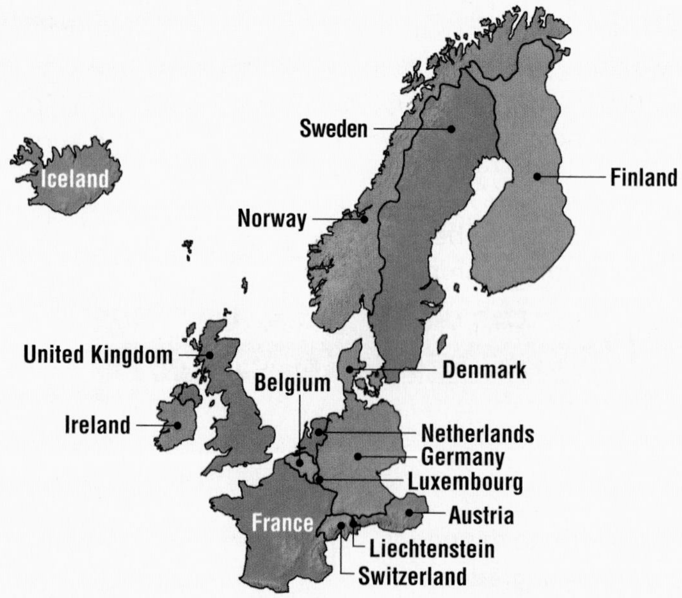

Sweden
Iceland
Finland
Norway
United Kingdom
Belgium
Denmark
Ireland
Netherlands
Germany
Luxembourg
Austria
France
Liechtenstein
Switzerland

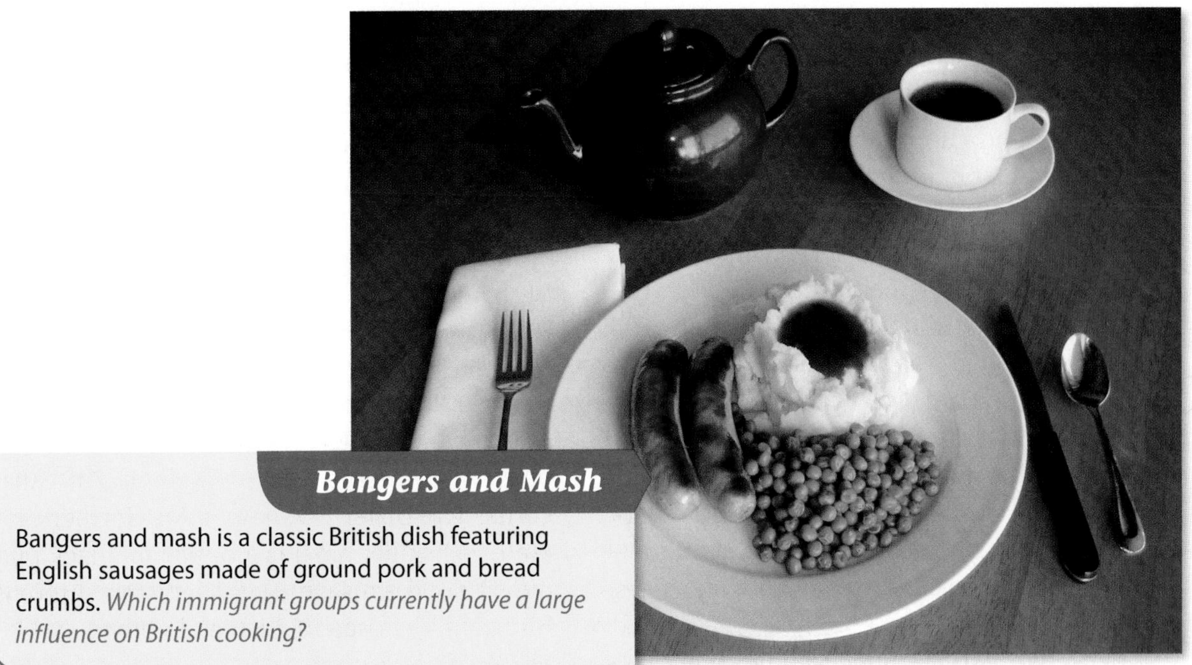

Bangers and Mash

Bangers and mash is a classic British dish featuring English sausages made of ground pork and bread crumbs. *Which immigrant groups currently have a large influence on British cooking?*

England

The English standard dinner consists of meat and two vegetables. One vegetable is usually potatoes. A typical example is bangers and mash (sausage and mashed potatoes) served with peas.

Meat pies are a popular main dish in England. Shepherd's pie features lamb or beef with diced carrots and peas under a mashed potato crust. Steak and kidney pie may include oysters or mushrooms. Cornish pasties are handheld turnovers filled with meat and root vegetables and shaped like a half moon.

The classic Sunday dinner is roast beef and **Yorkshire pudding**, a popover baked in the hot pan drippings from the roast beef. A popover is a puffy, muffin-size bread with a crisp brown crust and a hollow, moist interior.

English desserts include fruit cobbler, shortbread biscuits, and bread-and-butter pudding. Special occasions might call for a trifle, with varied layers of sponge cake, jam, gelatin, custard, and whipped cream, or a **fool**, puréed fruit folded into whipped cream.

Recent **immigration**, or movement from one place to another, from India, Pakistan, and East Asia has brought new foods to English cuisine. Today, Indian curries are one of the area's most popular foods. Chinese "takeaways" (take-out restaurants) are common.

Scotland

Oats are a dietary staple in Scotland. Oat porridge is eaten at breakfast, and sweet oatcakes are offered at tea. Toasted oats are folded into whipped cream and layered with fresh fruit in a dessert called cranachan.

Angus cattle and Blackface sheep are important sources of meat in Scotland. Steak and meat pies are popular. So is stovies, a hash of fried onion, chunks of potato, and beef or lamb. Chicken and leeks are used in cock-a-leekie soup.

The North Sea and Atlantic Ocean provide swordfish and mackerel. Salmon from Scotland is among the best in the world and is widely exported. Smoked herring, called kippers, and potted (pickled) herring are enjoyed at breakfast and tea. Finnan haddie is lightly smoked haddock. It is often poached and served with potatoes in seasoned milk or over toast in a white sauce.

Scotland's most famous dish is haggis. **Haggis** is made by stuffing a sheep's stomach with a mixture of oats, organ meats, onions, and beef or lamb suet, and then boiling it. Suet is the solid white fat found around the kidneys. It lends richness. Traditional side dishes are bashed neeps (mashed turnips) and chappit tatties (mashed potatoes).

Wales

Traditional Welsh cooking is simple and hearty and often features lamb, beef, seafood, leeks, and cabbage. A typical breakfast is bacon, eggs, and a stack of crempog (buttermilk pancakes) layered with butter. Cawl is a lamb stew with root vegetables, usually leeks, potatoes, and turnips. Leftover meat and vegetables are used to fill oggies (turnovers).

Tea breads such as bara brith ("speckled bread") are flavored with currants or cinnamon. Cakes are sprinkled with fine-grained caster sugar. Teisen sinamon (cinnamon cake) is spread with meringue and jam. Lemon marmalade sweetens a steamed dish called Snowdon pudding. Gooseberries and loganberries are popular in pies.

The Welsh harvest herring, mackerel, and oysters from the ocean, and salmon and sea trout from rivers. Cockles, or heart clams, are also popular in Wales. They are used in appetizers and savory pies, often served with **laverbread**, or processed seaweed. Griddlecakes of laverbread and oatmeal, called bara lawr, are a traditional breakfast food.

Ireland

The potato has been a staple in Irish cooking since the 1600s. Sheep, pigs, and cattle are raised across Ireland, and fish are caught along the coasts. Oats, barley, carrots, cabbage, and onions are widely grown.

Irish stew combines lamb or mutton, potatoes, and onions. Other stews feature a medley of root vegetables in a barley-thickened broth. Fish pies are filled with cod, scallops, and oysters in a thick white sauce. Corned beef, a form of brined brisket, goes back to a time when beef was preserved with pellets of salt called corns. The Ulster Fry, named for Northern Ireland, is a skillet breakfast of bacon, black pudding (blood sausage), eggs, and mushrooms. Buttermilk is used in Irish soda bread and oat bread.

The potato has nearly endless uses. Potatoes are mashed with leeks and mixed with chopped, cooked cabbage in **colcannon**. Potatoes are also mashed and fried with cabbage and leftover meat in butter or bacon fat to make bubble and squeak. The name comes from the sound the mixture makes as it cooks.

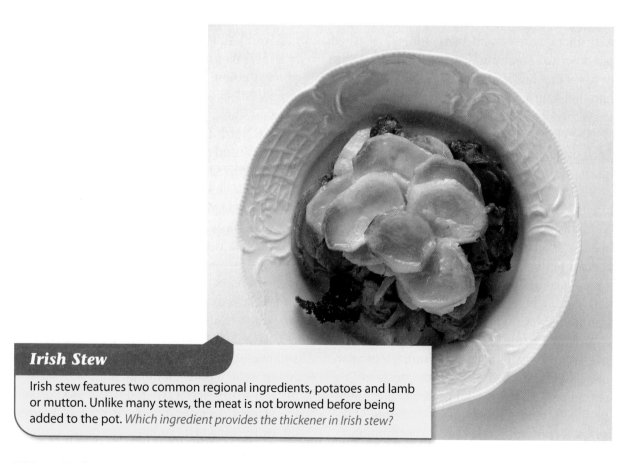

Irish Stew

Irish stew features two common regional ingredients, potatoes and lamb or mutton. Unlike many stews, the meat is not browned before being added to the pot. *Which ingredient provides the thickener in Irish stew?*

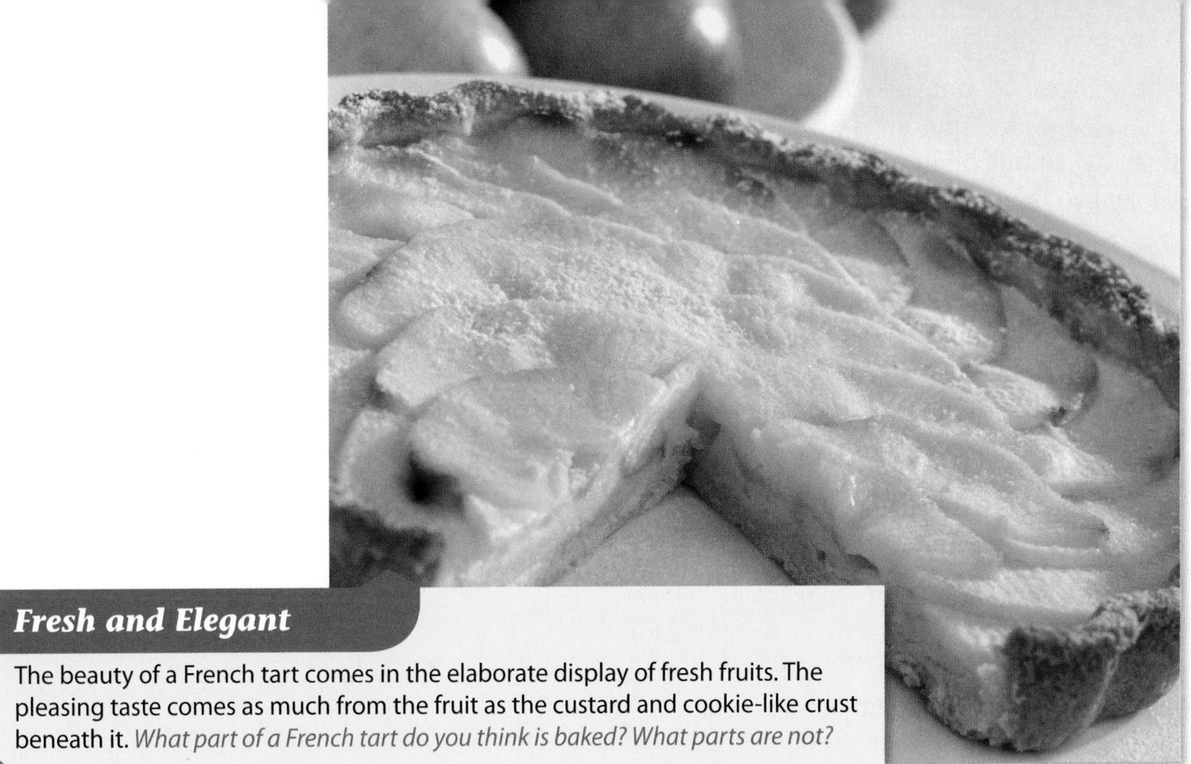

Fresh and Elegant

The beauty of a French tart comes in the elaborate display of fresh fruits. The pleasing taste comes as much from the fruit as the custard and cookie-like crust beneath it. *What part of a French tart do you think is baked? What parts are not?*

France

France's location is responsible for its remarkably varied cuisine. Mountains in the east and southwest, alternating with coastlines, create a range of climates. Vegetables, grains, and fruits thrive in the rich soil of the Alpine valley.

Regional French Cooking

France has many regional cuisines that use local ingredients, including local fats and oils. Olive oil is used in southeastern France, near the Mediterranean Sea, in such dishes as the fish stew bourride. Olive oil is also the base of an accompanying hot pepper and breadcrumb sauce, rouille. In the southwest, duck or goose fat flavors such dishes as cassoulet, a casserole of white beans, duck, and sausage.

In the northwest, cooks use butter and cream. Shellfish is sautéed in butter and served in a cream-based béchamel sauce. Caramelized sugar and cream are gently cooked into crème caramel. Apples fill the buttery crust of a galette des pommes (apple tart).

Eastern France shares a hearty, meat-heavy cuisine with neighboring Germany. Lard seasons dishes such as choucroute garni, a platter of sauerkraut with sausage and ham. Baeckeoffe is a braised dish with meat, potatoes, and onions.

Types of French Cuisines

French home cooking is known as cuisine paysanne, or country cooking. Provincial is another term for this cuisine. In home cooking, the main meal might include seafood stew or roast chicken, mixed greens, and seasonal vegetables. Recipes are prepared simply and seasoned with sage, tarragon, rosemary, and other common herbs. Bread is part of every meal. A long, crusty **baguette** (ba-ˈget) is bought or baked fresh daily. Leftovers are used for pain perdu, or "lost bread," called French toast by Americans.

Cheeses and fruits end the meal. France produces more than 400 different kinds of cheese. Brie, Camembert, and chèvre (goat cheese) are among the best known.

In contrast to cuisine paysanne is **haute cuisine** (ōt-kwi-ˈzēn), the classic French cuisine known for high-quality ingredients, expertly prepared and artistically presented. Dishes in haute cuisine are complicated and often rich, featuring Hollandaise and béchamel sauces.

In the 1970s, a new style of cuisine called nouvelle cuisine arose in reaction to traditional heavy dishes. Nouvelle cuisine, which means new cooking, emphasizes food's natural flavor and uses small portions, fresh foods, light cooking techniques, and less butter and cream.

The sauces of nouvelle cuisine are lighter because they are thickened by reduction rather than by adding flour. Vegetables are quickly cooked so they are tender yet crisp.

Germany

German cooking is hearty and features many different meats, especially wurst (sausage), schnitzel (cutlets), and braten (roasts). Bratwurst is a sausage of veal and pork seasoned with ginger and caraway seed, a common spice in German cuisine. Wiener Schnitzel (Viennese cutlet) is a breaded, fried veal cutlet. A beef roast marinated in vinegar with cloves, bay leaves, and peppercorns is **sauerbraten**. When the beef is finished the marinade is made into a gravy thickened with ginger snaps.

Cured meats are as common as fresh meats. Braunschweiger is a smoked, spreadable sausage made with pork liver. Acorn-fed pigs produce the famous Westphalian ham. Smoked eel and herring are popular in northern Germany.

Dishes made with root vegetables are also popular in Germany. Examples are Kartoffelklösse (potato dumplings) and Himmel und Erde (heaven and earth), potatoes and applesauce topped with fried onions and bacon. Red cabbage is also used in several dishes.

Germany has a great tradition of baking. Breads range from plain hard rolls to **stollen**, a yeast bread filled with dried fruit. Layers of chocolate cake, cherries, and whipped cream create Schwarzwälderkirschtorte, the celebrated Black Forest cake.

Belgium

Three foods are considered national dishes:

- Carbonnade flamande is beef stewed in a thickened broth made with onions and brown sugar.
- Endive, a white lettuce called "white gold," is added to cream soups or braised with a sauce of lemon juice and sugar.
- Potatoes are stuffed, mashed for pancakes and croquettes, or fried as pommes frites (french-fried potatoes), which are served with béarnaise sauce.

Seafood, especially mussels, is also popular in Belgium. A thick stew called waterzooi van tarbot combines monkfish, cod, or other whitefish in a broth enriched with egg yolks and cream. Belgian waffles, topped with fruit or jam and cream, are a favorite street food. Some of the world's finest chocolates also come from Belgium.

The Netherlands

The Netherlands, also known as Holland, borders the North Sea. Street vendors sell fresh mussels and oysters, baked fish, and seafood salads. Herring is eaten both raw and salted.

As in Germany and Belgium, Dutch cuisine features root vegetables, cabbage, and sausage. Stamppot is a mix of mashed potatoes or leeks with kale or cabbage. Plate-size yeast pancakes are served with sausage or vegetables as a main dish or topped with apples and whipped cream as dessert.

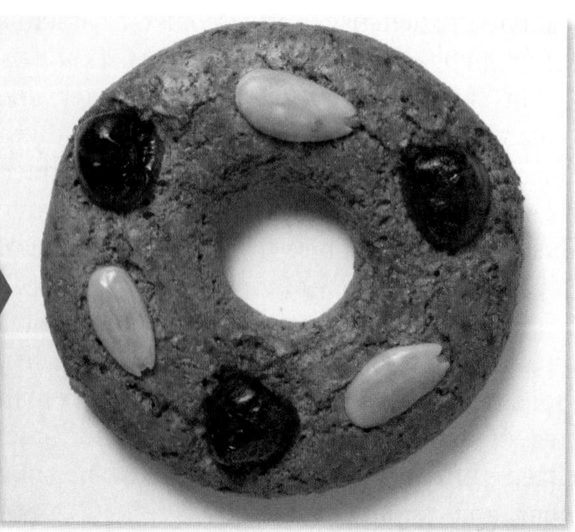

Sweet Treats

Lebkuchen, a German cookie baked on top of unleavened bread, is made of a soft, spiced gingerbread cookie topped with nuts and cinnamon or chocolate. *Why do you think unleavened bread is placed at the bottom of the cookie?*

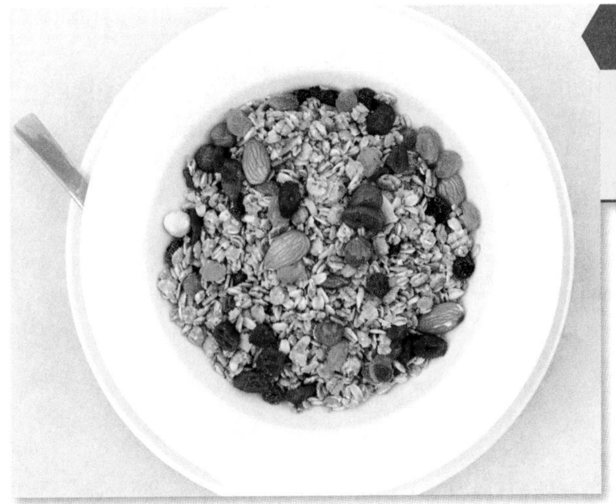

What's for Breakfast?

In Switzerland, muesli is a popular breakfast. It is a cereal made of uncooked, rolled oats, fruit, and nuts. *Why is this combination a good choice for breakfast?*

Dairy foods are a staple at most meals, especially such cheeses as Gouda, Edam, and quark, an unripened cheese similar to sour cream. Vla, a custard, is a common dessert.

Trade with the West Indies brought new foods to the Netherlands. The Dutch adapted an Indonesian custom, calling it rijsttafel, or "rice table." This is a buffet of rice and a variety of highly seasoned sauces, meats, and vegetables. From the West Indies, the Dutch also imported cinnamon, cloves, and ginger. It was the Dutch who found a way to process the cacao bean into cocoa powder, leading to the creation of chocolate candy.

Switzerland, Liechtenstein, and Luxembourg

The cuisines of Switzerland, Liechtenstein, and Luxembourg are influenced by the cuisines of Germany and France. Roesti, pan-fried, shredded potatoes and onions, is a common side dish. In Liechtenstein, Roesti is a main dish. It is seasoned with bacon, topped with Gruyère, and served with a fried egg. Zürcher Geschnetzeltes, strips of veal in a mushroom cream sauce, is a specialty of Zurich, the largest city in the German-speaking part of Switzerland. Smoked pork and broad beans, or Judd mat Gaardebounen, is a national dish in Luxembourg.

Meats are often smoked and dried throughout the region. People enjoy a small but varied crop of local produce, including apples, berries, carrots, beans, and potatoes.

Swiss dairy cows give rich milk that makes superior dairy products, including chocolates and cheeses. Cheese fondue is traditionally made by melting Emmentaler and Gruyère with white wine and seasonings. Diners use long forks to dip chunks of bread into the hot mixture. Râclette is a dish of melted cheese smothered over individual potatoes and served with gherkin pickles. The Swiss were the first to powder milk and add it to chocolate, creating milk chocolate.

Austria

Austria draws culinary influences from many parts of Europe. Tafelspitz, beef brisket boiled with carrots and onions, is from the Eastern European tradition. Austrians enjoy many of the same dishes as Germans, including sauerkraut, wurst, hearty breads, and strudel. Weiner Schnitzel (Viennese cutlet), named for the Austrian capital, is Austria's most famous dish.

Dumplings, or Knödel, come in many variations in Austrian cooking. Speckknödel are bacon-filled potato dumplings. Semmelknödel are made from stale bread cubes soaked in beaten eggs and milk.

Austrian pastries are internationally known. Strudel is made from layers of paper-thin pastry rolled with a sweet or savory filling, such as fruit, cheese, or nuts. A **torte** is a rich cake made with a small amount of flour and often with ground nuts or bread crumbs. Sachertorte is a dense chocolate layer cake, thinly spread with apricot jam and a glossy chocolate glaze. Dobos Torte is a six-layer vanilla sponge cake filled with chocolate cream. From the city of Linz comes Linzer Torte, a hazelnut crust filled with raspberry jam.

✓ **Reading Check** **Identify** What is the name of a new style of lighter, healthier French haute cuisine?

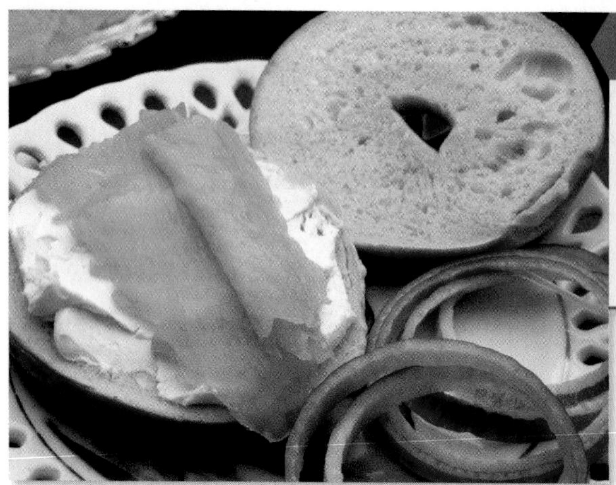

Gravlax

Cured fish is popular throughout Scandinavia. Gravlax is a Swedish cured fish made with salmon, salt, and sugar. It is related to the lox shown here, which is often served with cream cheese and bagels in the United States. *In Sweden, what sauce is traditionally served with gravlax?*

Northern European Cuisine

Northern Europe includes Scandinavia—Denmark, Sweden, Norway, Finland, and Iceland. The northernmost part of this area extends into the Arctic Circle. Foods tend to be filling, yet creative. They often include fish, cured meats, and dairy foods.

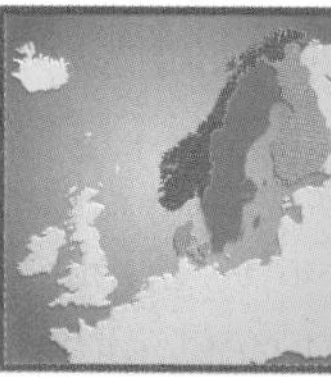

Denmark

Denmark is the southernmost country in Scandinavia and shares a border with Germany. The island of Greenland is a province of Denmark. Salmon, cod, and herring are staples here. Eel is served baked, pickled, or stuffed. Frikadeller are flat, fried dumplings of minced meat.

Denmark has the greenest terrain in Scandinavia. Most farmland is used to raise cattle and hogs. Many meat dishes, such as frickadeller (meatballs), are sharpened with sour cream and horseradish.

Carrots, cabbage, potatoes, and kale are popular in side dishes and soups. They are often served creamed or glazed in sugar and vinegar.

At least one meal each day is a smorrebrod, or open-face sandwich. Whole-wheat and rye breads are topped with a variety of spreads and toppings, including herbed butter, anchovy paste, meats, cheeses, slices of hard-cooked egg, and sweet pickles.

Sweden

The best-known Swedish dish is the **smorgasbord**, a buffet laden with cured fish, cold meats, cheeses, salads, and vegetables. A typical spread might feature smoked salmon, herring salad, cheese-stuffed eggs, spiced gooseberries, and pickled beets. A smorgasbord can be simple or elaborate and can consist of only appetizers or make up the entire meal.

Swedish foods offer an interesting mix of flavors. Köttbullar (Swedish meatballs) are spiced with nutmeg and served in sour cream gravy. A mustard sauce with dill traditionally accompanies gravlax, salmon cured in salt and sugar.

Potatoes are used in side dishes, including pancakes and bacon-filled dumplings called kroppkaker. Jannsons frestelse (Jannson's temptation) is a casserole of potatoes, onions, anchovies, and cream.

Fruits have many uses in Swedish cuisine. The chilled soup fruktsoppa features dried fruits. Lingonberry preserves, a favorite in Sweden, accompany small, thin pancakes called plattar.

Norway

Small family farms are traditional in Norway. The country is dominated by mountains, wilderness and the ocean that surrounds it on three sides. Fish is a major element of the national diet and smoked salmon is a traditional dish, as is gravlax, a smoked salmon cured with salt and sugar. Farm products supplement fish dishes such as herring burgers and **lutefisk**, dried cod soaked in culinary ash and water. Herring is a factor in many dishes. It is served pickled, in a tomato-based sauce, or in a curry sauce.

Ground beef and pork are often seasoned with ginger, nutmeg, and black pepper to make cabbage rolls. Beef is pounded very thin and rolled with chopped bacon and onions and simmered in a covered pot to make a dish called boneless birds. Lefse is a traditional soft potato flatbread made from kneaded rolled dough and cooked on a griddle. It is used in a variety of ways, including sweetened and rolled as a desert.

Dairy products are used in many dishes. Cream enriches dishes ranging from fiskepudding (fish pudding) to lefse. Jarlsberg cheese is exported throughout the world.

Whipped cream is the usual filling for layer cakes and for krumkake, wafer-thin waffle cookies that are rolled into a cone. Krumkake are traditionally made during the holidays. Cardamom is a popular spice used in baking, adding flavor to coffee cakes and pastries. Other bakery treats include tortes, fruit pastries, and decorative, cardamom-spiced cookies. Due to the cold climate, berries grow in smaller volume but with intense taste. Strawberries, blueberries, lingonberries, and raspberries are common.

Finland and Iceland

Despite a short growing season, Finnish farmers raise almost all food eaten in the country. Karelian hot pot is a stew of beef, pork, and lamb, often served with potatoes or turnips. Fish and meat are seasoned and baked in pastry dough to make kalakukko. Cold smoked fish is also a common dinner centerpiece. Carrots, potatoes, and beets are mixed with a creamy sweet-and-sour dressing to make roselli. Breakfast often consists of buttered bread topped with hard cheese or cold cuts.

Iceland, in the far North Atlantic, has a wide range of foods, including mutton and lamb, fish, game, and dairy foods, and potatoes, rutabagas, cabbage, and rhubarb. Among the most widely consumed fish are haddock, plaice, halibut, herring and shrimp. Skyr, a fresh, strained cheese is popular. Dairy foods are an important element of Icelandic cuisine. Hot springs warm greenhouses, enabling farmers to grow tomatoes, peas, and even bananas.

✓ **Reading Check** **Describe** Sweden's best-known dish.

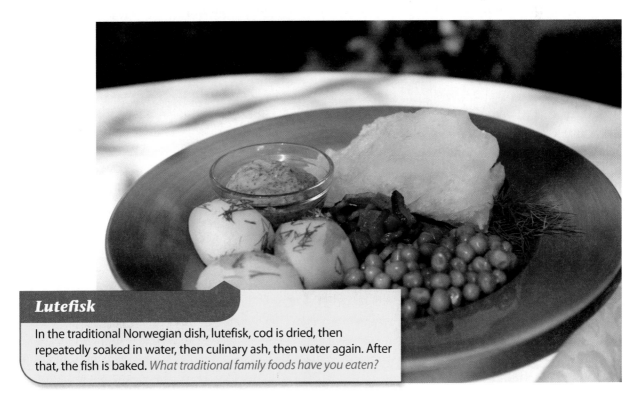

Lutefisk

In the traditional Norwegian dish, lutefisk, cod is dried, then repeatedly soaked in water, then culinary ash, then water again. After that, the fish is baked. *What traditional family foods have you eaten?*

Mediterranean Cuisine

Cooking in Southern Europe is lighter than cooking in Northern and Western Europe. The Mediterranean diet is based on whole grains, fresh fruits and vegetables, fish, and poultry, with smaller amounts of meat and dairy foods. Sauces are usually light, and olive oil is the main cooking fat. **Figure 48.2** shows the Mediterranean Sea and several of the countries surrounding it. These countries are collectively referred to as the Mediterranean.

Spain

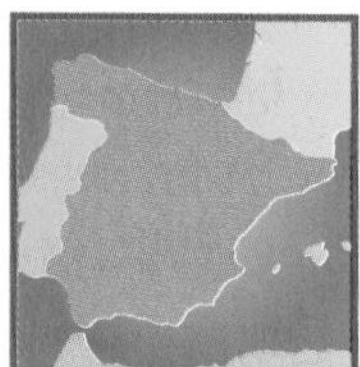

Spain covers most of the Iberian Peninsula of southwestern Europe, the gateway between the Mediterranean Sea and the Atlantic Ocean.

Spanish Ingredients

Phoenicians from the Middle East settled in Spain some 3,000 years ago. Their diet included fish, shellfish, pigs, and sheep, as well as salt cod and garlic. The Romans colonized Spain about a thousand years later, bringing olive trees. The Romans also brought hams and treasured the fava beans native to Spain. Cabbages were also appreciated and thought to be a cure for various sicknesses.

The Moors of North Africa ruled most of Spain from the 7th to the 13th century BCE. They added eggplants, artichokes, tropical fruits, nuts, rice, and spices, most notably saffron, to Spain's cuisine. They also brought new dishes, such as meats spiced with cinnamon, rice cooked with dates, and pastries sweetened with honey, enriched with egg yolks, and leavened by egg whites. The Moors also introduced **marzipan** (ˈmärt-sə-ˌpän), a confection made of almond paste and sugar.

Figure 48.2 The Mediterranean

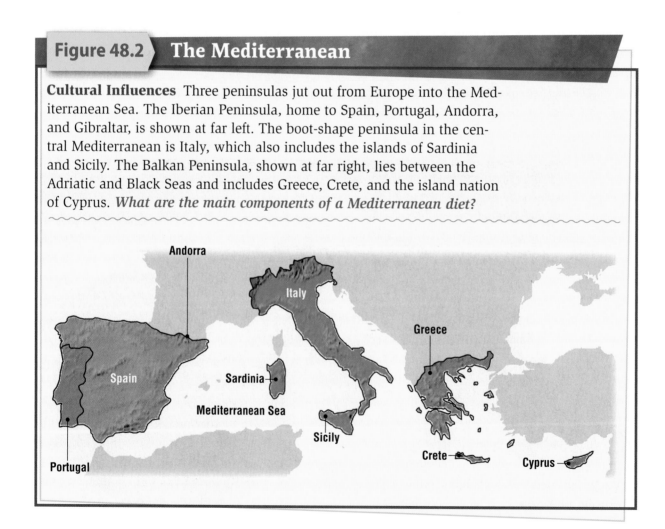

Cultural Influences Three peninsulas jut out from Europe into the Mediterranean Sea. The Iberian Peninsula, home to Spain, Portugal, Andorra, and Gibraltar, is shown at far left. The boot-shape peninsula in the central Mediterranean is Italy, which also includes the islands of Sardinia and Sicily. The Balkan Peninsula, shown at far right, lies between the Adriatic and Black Seas and includes Greece, Crete, and the island nation of Cyprus. ***What are the main components of a Mediterranean diet?***

Andorra
Italy
Greece
Spain
Sardinia
Mediterranean Sea
Sicily
Crete
Cyprus
Portugal

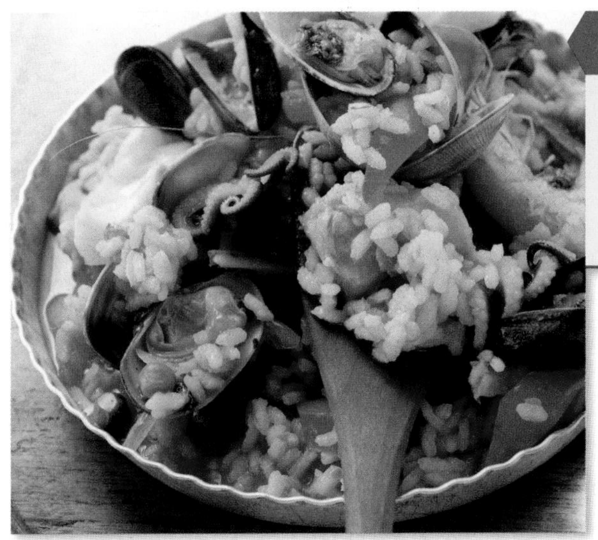

Paella

Paella is a Spanish dish with many variations, often with poultry and seafood. It takes its name from the broad, shallow pan in which it is traditionally cooked. *What three cultural groups have played an important role in Spanish cuisine over the centuries?*

Spanish cuisine was also enriched by foods brought back by European explorers, such as potatoes, tomatoes, peppers, beans, vanilla, and chocolate.

Spanish Dishes

Garlic and olive oil are prominent in savory dishes of Spain, along with pinches of saffron and sprinkles of parsley. Spain is the world's largest producer of olive oil, supplying ⅓ of all the olive oil world-wide. Flan and custard-filled sponge cakes, part of the Moorish pastry tradition, are favorite desserts.

Spain's national dish, **paella** (pä-ˈe-lə), is rice seasoned with saffron and mixed with a purée of onions, red bell peppers and tomatoes, meat and seafood. Its ingredients vary from region to region. Paella in Valencia, on the southeastern coast, uses only shellfish. Paella in Catalonia, in the north of Spain, often includes sausage and chicken, reflecting food traditions from Germany and France.

Another popular Spanish dish is cocido, an **elaborate**, or lavish, stew of beans, mixed meats, vegetables, and a starch cooked in one pot. Madrid's well-known cocido madrileño includes garbanzo beans, bacon, beef, chicken, chorizo, and rice or fine noodles. A Catalan cocido may use pig's feet, lamb shank, a local sausage called butifarra, and potatoes.

Small snacks or appetizers, called **tapas** (ˈtä-pəs), are extremely popular. Different regions have different specialties. In Andalusia, in the south, you might find battered and fried olives. In Galicia, in the northwest, you might find grilled squid or octopus.

Regional Spanish Cuisine

Each region of Spain has signature dishes. Catalonia's adventurous cooks make zarzuelas, stews of a half-dozen kinds of fish and shellfish plus almonds and hazelnuts. Andalusia is home to gazpacho, a cold soup of dry bread soaked and puréed with tomatoes, other vegetables, and garlic. Chopped tomatoes, cucumbers, sweet peppers, and onions may be passed at the table.

Lamb and suckling pig roasted in wood-burning brick ovens are regional dishes of the central Castile region. The area just north of Castile, called Asturia, is known for fabada, a casserole of white beans, chorizo, ham, and blood sausage. It resembles the cassoulet found across the bay in France. In Galicia, Celtic influence shows in the form of fish and meat pies, including empanadas.

Basque Cuisine

The Basques are a cultural group that lives on both sides of the Spanish-French border. They are sheepherders by tradition. Meals are traditionally large and hearty. Salsa is commonly served as a condiment added to soups. Basque cooking features seafood, pork, and beans as well as lamb and mutton. Specialties include young eel and smoked cheese from sheep's milk. In bacalao pil-pil, salt cod is gently heated in olive oil and garlic, releasing the gelatin to thicken the sauce.

Portuguese Soup

Sopa Alentejana is a soup from Portugal. It's made with mashed cilantro, garlic, olive oil, and salt and served with lots of crusty bread in the broth, topped by poached eggs. *What nutrients does the poached egg supply in this soup?*

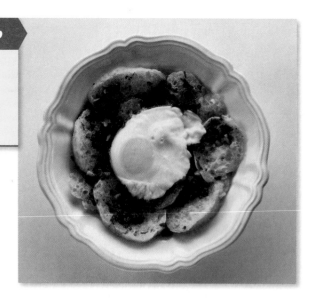

Portugal

Portugal has a unique cuisine, with a food history and tradition all its own, although it shares some of its culinary roots with Spain.

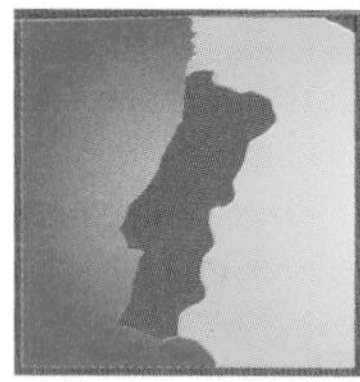

Portuguese Ingredients

Celts, early settlers of the land that is now Portugal, raised cattle and pigs in the north. The Romans brought herbs and vegetables such as cilantro, parsley, and fava beans. The Moors grew rice in the marshy south and brought irrigation systems that turned dry land into groves of almonds, figs, lemons, and oranges. The Moors also introduced a cooking technique called na cataplana. This technique uses a cataplana, a copper vessel with rounded sides and a hinged, domed lid, to simmer seafood or small pieces of meat until tender and flavorful.

In the 1500s, traders in Indian and Indonesian spices brought cinnamon, black pepper, and curry powder to Portugal. New World colonies supplied green beans, tomatoes, and potatoes. From Africa came fiery piri-piri chiles, the base of numerous hot sauces. Portuguese sailors helped inspire the popularity of salt cod. They caught and preserved the fish in great quantities on long voyages.

Portuguese Dishes

Traditional Portuguese dishes are thrifty, nourishing, and creative. Salt cod, or bacalhau, is a good example. The Portuguese are said to have 365 ways to prepare cod, one for each day of the year. Cod may be grilled, fried into fish cakes, or made into bacalhau à Gomes de Sá, a layered casserole of salt cod, sliced potatoes, and sautéed onion and garlic garnished with hard-cooked eggs and black olives.

Pork is a favorite meat in Portugal. Linguiça is a smoked sausage seasoned with garlic, paprika, and pepper. It flavors stews, beans, and egg dishes. A smoked ham, presunto, is thinly sliced and served with figs as an appetizer.

Many Portuguese dishes pair meat with seafood. Marinated pork cubes and clams, for example, are browned and simmered to make porco a alentejana.

Chicken is often paired with the piri-piri chile. Another popular dish is roasted chicken marinated in paprika and garlic and stuffed with ground pork, onions, olives, and hard-cooked eggs.

Soups are also popular in Portuguese cuisine. A simple chicken soup, canja, is flavored with lemon and mint. The more elaborate caldeirada de peixe is a layered stew, in which a variety of fish alternates with sliced tomatoes, onions, and peppers. "Dry" soups called açordas are thickened with bread, using a technique similar to making gazpacho. The best-known vegetable soup is the deep green caldo verde, made with finely shredded kale and mashed potatoes in a broth seasoned with garlic and pepper. Rice is the most popular grain. It is paired with seafood and chicken in many recipes. In paelha (Portuguese paella), rice is spiced up with linguiça and piri-piri sauce. Breads range from pao doce, a light, slightly sweet loaf, to broa, a "peasant" bread made heavy by stone-ground cornmeal.

Italy

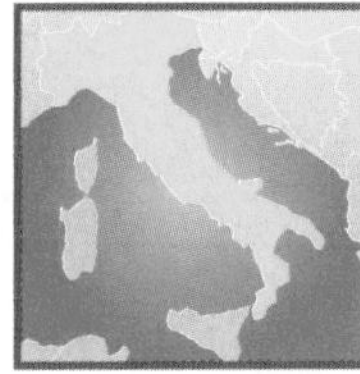

Italian cuisine is the best known European cuisine in the United States. The Italian food served in American restaurants, however, is often different from the food served in a home in Italy. Italy has a great range of regional cuisines, with different dishes and cooking styles in the north and south.

Italian Ingredients

Italy has a long coastline, and seafood therefore features in many recipes. Olives, artichokes, fennel, lettuce, and chard grow in the rich volcanic soil in southern Italy. Spinach and eggplant were introduced by the Moors, and squash and tomatoes came from the New World. Goats and sheep are raised in Italy's foothills.

Staples such as wheat, rice, corn, beans, peppers, and radicchio, a form of chicory, grow in the northern river valleys of Italy. Dairy cows produce the butter and cream used in regional dishes. Cured meats such as Parma ham, Genoa salami, and sausages like pepperoni and **pancetta** ((ˌ)pan-ˈche-tə) are popular.

Garlic, onions, basil, oregano, rosemary, sage, and saffron are the most popular herbs and aromatic vegetables in Italian cooking.

Italian Dishes

Italian meals are often served in courses, beginning with soup or an appetizer, continuing with a serving of pasta, and finishing with a meat, poultry, or seafood dish. The first course is often a light soup, or a variety of appetizers called antipasto. **Antipasto** is Italian for before the meal.

Pasta appears in hundreds of shapes and sizes, depending on region and recipe. Northern Italians favor meatier sauces and **pesto**, a sauce of ground fresh basil, pine nuts, garlic, Parmesan cheese, and olive oil, often served with fettucini, a thick, flat pasta. Southern Italians often serve capelli d'angelo (angel hair pasta), a very thin spaghetti that is often tossed with crushed tomatoes sautéed in olive oil and garlic.

In northern Italy, pasta is often replaced by rice, by tender, boiled potato dumplings called **gnocchi** (ˈnȯ-kē), or by a thick cornmeal porridge called **polenta** (pō-ˈlen-tə). Gnocchi and polenta are served with meat and tomato sauce. Polenta is the usual accompaniment to rabbit stew. Risotto comes in many variations, such as risotto alla milanese made with chicken broth and saffron. Parma ham or bacon is combined with rice and peas to make risi e bisi.

Meats are cooked differently in different regions of Italy. In the far south, pork is used in various ways, from stews to stuffed pork rinds. A festive occasion in central Italy and Sardinia might feature roast suckling lamb. In Milan, in northern Italy, a special meal might include osso bucco (braised veal shanks) garnished with gremolata, a mixture of parsley, garlic, and lemon peel.

Seafood is common on the coast. Sicilians bake swordfish with chopped tomatoes, olives, raisins, and pine nuts. Their northern neighbors in Tuscany prepare cacciuco, a soup of fish, shellfish, and squid.

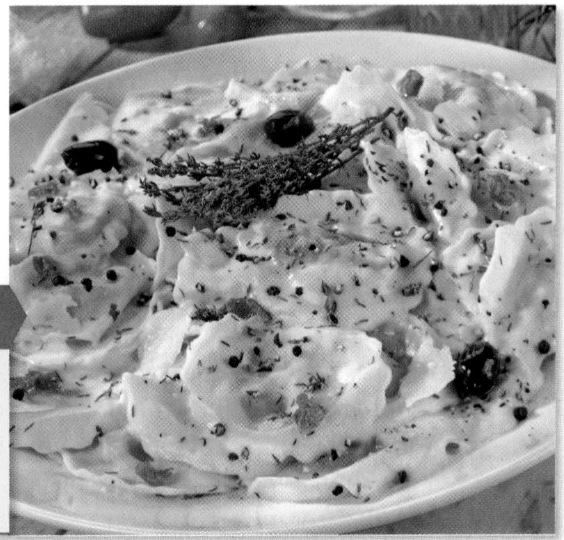

Pasta Carbonara

Pasta carbonara is believed to have originated as a hearty dish that coal miners ate before going into the mines. It is made with pasta, pancetta, eggs, romano cheese, and lots of black pepper. *Why would this dish provide lots of energy?*

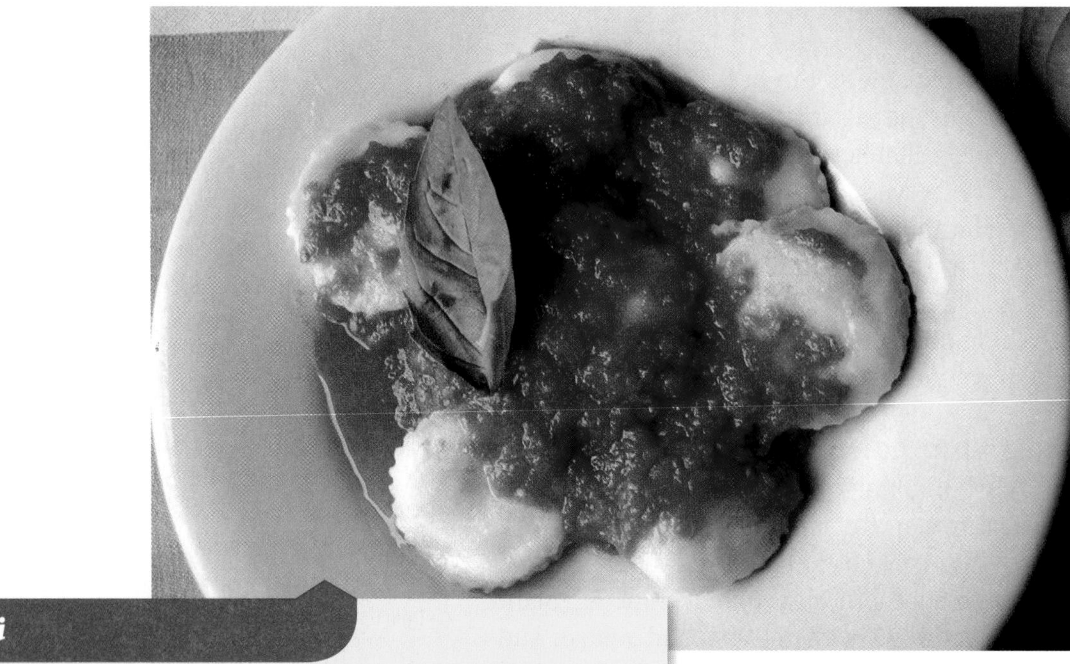

Ravioli

Ravioli is a type of pasta with filling sealed between two thin layers of pasta dough. *What is a typical first course in a traditional Italian meal?*

Vegetables are used in numerous dishes besides soups and antipasto. Fresh green salads are common. Peppers, onions, and eggplant are used in sauces or roasted in olive oil and tossed with basil. Raw vegetables and bagna cauda, a warm anchovy and garlic dip, are served as an appetizer.

In Italy, cheese is not only used as an ingredient, but also served as a course in a meal. Asiago and blue-veined Gorgonzola are made from cow's milk. Pecorino is made with sheep's milk. Mozzarella is traditionally made from the milk of the water buffalo, although cow's milk is also used.

Fresh fruits are served as a light dessert. Apricots, plums, and melons are summer fruits. Apples, pears, oranges, and grapes are plentiful in fall and winter.

Breads and Pastries

Breads are important in Italian cooking and come in a wide range of shapes and flavors. A simple breakfast might feature a small, loaf-shaped roll, or panino, with butter or jam, along with coffee or hot chocolate. Panino with a chunk of cheese or walnuts is an afternoon snack. A chewy Tuscan loaf complements soup.

Pizza began as focaccia, a yeast flatbread drizzled with olive oil and sprinkled with herbs. In 1889, a pizza chef in Naples topped his creation with red tomatoes, white mozzarella cheese, and green basil. The colors represented the Italian flag to impress an honored customer, Italian Queen Margherita. Pizza Margherita remains a specialty in Naples. Other regions have their own versions of pizza, using combinations of fresh herbs, olives, peppers, onions, mushrooms, sausage, and seafood. Crust thickness varies from place to place, but all traditional pizza is baked in a wood-fired brick oven.

Italy also has a well-known pastry tradition, which was begun by the Moors. Panforte, a chewy Christmas confection, is made with honey and dried fruits. Deep-fried pastry tubes called **cannoli** and the sponge cake cassata have a mixture of sweetened ricotta cheese, citrus peel, pistachios, and shaved chocolate. Crunchy, anise-flavored **biscotti** ("twice-baked" cookies) are excellent for dipping in coffee. Biscotti is made by pouring batter across the length of a long pan. After baking, the loaf is sliced. Pieces are turned on their side and baked again.

Greece

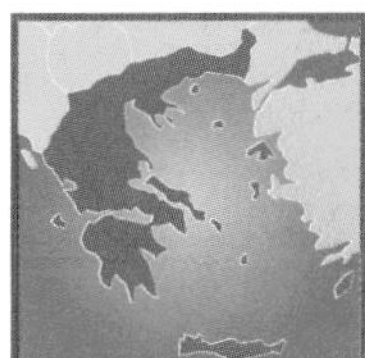

Greece has an ancient civilization with a long culinary history. Ancient Greek traditions have blended with those of Italy, Turkey, and the Middle East to form contemporary Greek cuisine.

Greek Ingredients

Greece's sunny climate is excellent for growing grains and vegetables such as rice, wheat, beans, tomatoes, eggplant, onions, and garlic. Orchards yield olives, nuts, figs, oranges, apricots, and lemons. Oregano, rosemary, mint, and thyme grow wild in the hills. Sheep and pigs produce meat, while sheep and goats supply milk for the yogurt and the many cheeses that are basic to Greek cuisine. Seafood is also a staple.

Greek Dishes

Greek main dishes are characterized by zesty seasonings. **Moussaka** is a casserole with lamb, eggplant, and tomatoes in a custard or white sauce seasoned with herbs and spices such as oregano, thyme, black pepper, allspice, and cinnamon. Souvlaki is marinated, grilled meat served with tzatziki, a yogurt sauce flavored with lemon, mint, and garlic. Souvlaki is served on a skewer or in pita bread, garnished with tomatoes and onions. Bourtheto, a specialty on the island of Corfu, is whitefish baked in a sauce of grated tomatoes, cayenne, and black pepper.

Dolma is a stuffed vegetable dish served in many nations including Greece. One popular version features herbs, rice, and sometimes cheese or meat wrapped in grape leaves.

Seasonal vegetables feature in a variety of cooked and raw salads. Shredded cabbage and boiled beets are traditional in winter. Horiatiki, a traditional Greek salad of tomatoes, peppers, cucumbers, onions, and olives with oregano and olive oil, is popular in summer. Phyllo is filled with spinach and feta cheese to make spanakopita. Greece's famed **baklava** (ˈbä-klə-ˌvä) is a sweet dessert made with layers of phyllo with finely chopped walnuts or almonds mixed with sugar and cinnamon. It is baked, cut into diamonds, and steeped in warm honey syrup. Another dessert, halva, combines ground sesame seeds and honey. This candy-like confection is popular across a large area of southeast Europe, the Balkans, and the Middle East.

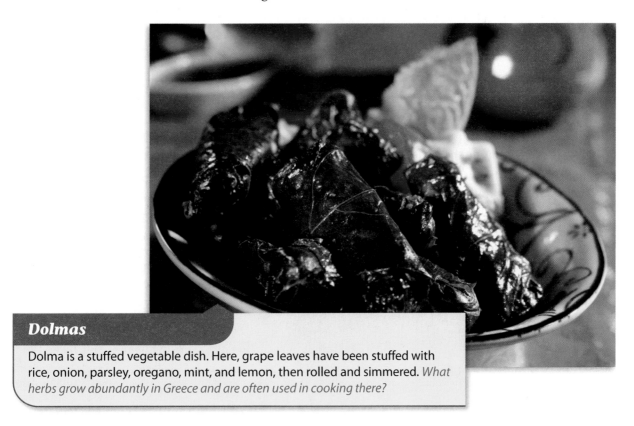

Dolmas

Dolma is a stuffed vegetable dish. Here, grape leaves have been stuffed with rice, onion, parsley, oregano, mint, and lemon, then rolled and simmered. *What herbs grow abundantly in Greece and are often used in cooking there?*

Light and Healthy Recipe

Homemade Pasta with Pomodoro Sauce

Fresh pasta is easy to make and, served with pomodoro sauce, makes a great treat.

Ingredients

For the pasta

- **2** Eggs
- **¼ cup** Olive oil
- **1½ cups** All-purpose flour
- **1½ cups** Semolina flour
- **½ tsp.** Salt

For the sauce

- **4** Diced tomatoes
- **1** Small diced onion
- **3 cloves** Minced garlic
- **3 Tbsp.** Diced fresh basil leaves (or 1½ Tbsp. dried basil)
- **1 Tbsp.** Olive oil

Directions

1. Make the pasta by first beating the eggs and then combining them with the olive oil, flours, and salt. Knead the dough only enough to combine the ingredients well. Once combined, roll the dough into a ball. Wrap the dough in plastic wrap and refrigerate for at least one hour.
2. Roll out the pasta dough on a lightly floured surface until it is very thin (about ⅛ of an inch). A pasta machine works best for rolling out fresh pasta, but you can use a rolling pin or dowel to roll out the pasta dough. If you do not have a pasta machine, you can still make attractive, even cuts with the dough using a pizza cutter or a sharp knife. Whatever size width you make the pasta, keep it consistent.
3. After cutting the pasta, dust it thoroughly with flour to keep the pieces from sticking together. If you need to set it aside, place it on a piece of lightly floured parchment or tin foil and lay another sheet over the top. Keep the pasta cool until you are ready to cook it.
4. Begin cooking the sauce by pouring the olive oil into a wide pan. When the oil is warm, add the onions and cook them on low heat until tender.
5. Put a pot of water on to boil.
6. Add the tomatoes and garlic and turn the heat up to medium. Continue cooking until the tomatoes start to break down. The sauce should be wet but chunky.
7. Add the fresh basil and stir to mix it in 5-10 minutes before serving time.
8. Meanwhile, put the pasta into the boiling water and cook it. Fresh pasta will sink to the bottom of the pot when it is put in. About one minute after it rises to the top of the pot, it will be finished cooking. Taste it to be sure, then drain the pasta.
9. Scoop pasta onto dishes and top with the hot sauce. Another option is to put the pasta back into the empty pot, add the sauce and gently mix everything together. Do this carefully, so that you don't break or mash the noodles.

Yield 6 servings

Nutrition Analysis per Serving

■ Calories	425
■ Total fat	14 g
Saturated fat	2 g
Cholesterol	79 mg
■ Sodium	229 mg
■ Carbohydrate	61
Dietary fiber	4 g
Sugars	5 g
■ Protein	12 g

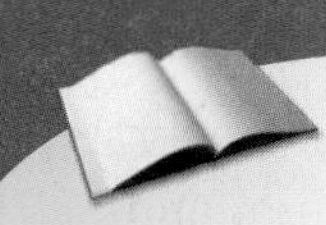

After You Read

Chapter Summary

Western, Northern, and Southern Europe are home to diverse cuisines that use a variety of flavorful ingredients and cooking methods. Each of these three regions of Europe offers unique cuisines influenced by climate, geography, and different cultures.

Content and Academic Vocabulary Review

1. Use each of these content and academic vocabulary words in a sentence.

Content Vocabulary

- Yorkshire pudding (p. 737)
- fool (p. 737)
- haggis (p. 737)
- laverbread (p. 738)
- colcannon (p. 738)
- baguette (p. 739)
- haute cuisine (p. 739)
- sauerbraten (p. 740)
- stollen (p. 740)
- torte (p. 741)
- smorgasbord (p. 742)
- lutefisk (p. 742)
- marzipan (p. 744)
- paella (p. 745)
- tapas (p. 745)
- pancetta (p. 747)
- antipasto (p. 747)
- pesto (p. 747)
- gnocchi (p. 747)
- polenta (p. 747)
- cannoli (p. 748)
- biscotti (p. 748)
- moussaka (p. 749)
- dolma (p. 749)
- baklava (p. 749)

Academic Vocabulary

- immigration (p. 737)
- elaborate (p. 745)

Review Key Concepts

2. **Describe** popular dishes from Western Europe.
3. **Describe** how Northern Europe's geography and climate affects its cuisine.
4. **Explain** why the Mediterranean diet is lighter than the cuisine of Western and Northern Europe.

Critical Thinking

5. **Examine** why the cuisines of so many Western European countries feature root vegetables as opposed to other types of vegetables.
6. **Contrast** cuisine paysanne with haute cuisine.
7. **Evaluate** Gilda's plan to serve a smorgasbord at her upcoming party. Is this a good idea? Give reasons to support your evaluation.
8. **Contrast** northern and southern Italian cuisine
9. **List** several geographical factors that account for the differences between Greek and Finnish cuisine.
10. **Identify** which region or country you think has the most healthful, nutrient-rich cuisine. Explain your answer.

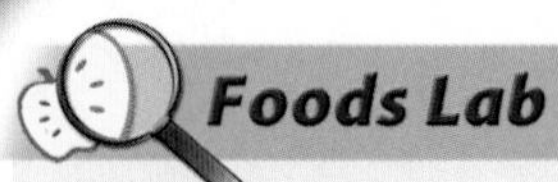

Foods Lab

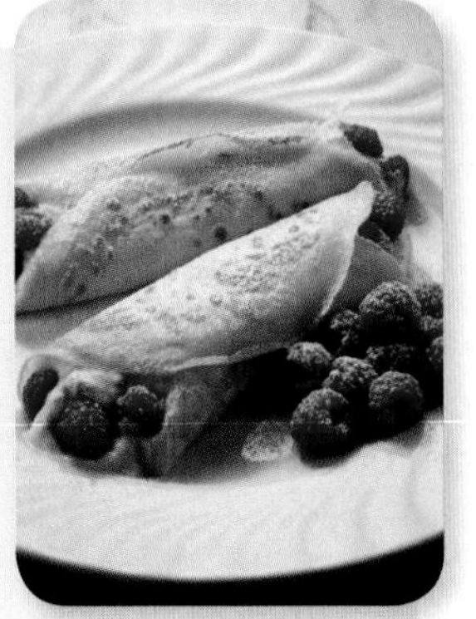

11. Making Crepes Crepes, delicate wraps made of eggs and flour surrounding a variety of sweet and savory fillings, are a popular feature of French cuisine.

Procedure Find and prepare a recipe for crepes. Fill them with your choice of fruits, meats, cheeses, vegetables, or other ingredients to create a dessert or main dish.

Analysis In a class discussion, give feedback to the following questions: How do crepes differ from pancakes? How well did the taste of eggs combine with a sweet or savory filling? What challenges did you encounter? How could these be managed?

HEALTHFUL CHOICES

12. Food Fair At a European food fair celebrating cuisines from Northern, Western, and Southern Europe, Ben wants to eat a dish that is high in nutrients and low in fat and calories. His choices are haggis, a torte, marzipan, or vegetarian dolmas. Which option do you think Ben should choose and why?

TECH Connection

13. Dinners from Europe You are in charge of planning a weeks' worth of dinners for your family. Each dinner should feature an appetizer, entrée, or dessert from a different country in Northern, Western, or Southern Europe. Use spreadsheet software to create a chart that shows seven days and seven dinners. Color code the entries blue for Western European dishes, green for Northern European dishes, and red for Southern European dishes. Include the national origin for each dish.

Real-World Skills

Problem-Solving Skills

14. Vegetarian Options Kelsey is opening a new restaurant that specializes in German cuisine, which emphasizes many different meats and hearty meat-based dishes. She wants her restaurant to be a place where vegetarians can eat, too. Can she offer any meatless dishes that are traditionally German? If so, what are they?

Interpersonal and Collaborative Skills

15. Country Study Follow your teacher's instructions to form groups. Work together to research the Northern, Western, or Southern European country that has been assigned to your group. Learn about the country's history, geography, and culture, and find out more about its cuisine. Using visual aids and speech, give a class presentation.

Financial Literacy Skills

16. Find the Best Value At Michaela's neighborhood Greek restaurant, her favorite dish, a plate of 6 dolmas, costs 9 dollars. She visits the restaurant twice a week. For 7 dollars, she can make 12 dolmas. How much money will she save per week if she makes her own dolmas rather than visiting the restaurant?

Academic Skills

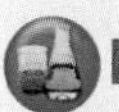

Food Science

17. Purées as Thickeners As part of nouvelle cuisine, chefs turned to letting the main ingredient serve as its own thickener, creating a coulis, a purée served as a sauce.

Procedure Sauté 1 seeded and chopped red bell pepper and 1 chopped shallot in olive oil until soft. Add ¼ cup chicken broth, and simmer for a few minutes. Puree in a blender. Strain. Adjust consistency with more chicken broth as needed. Season to taste.

Analysis Based on what you know about sauces and thickness, how is a coulis different?

NSES B Develop an understanding of the structure and properties of matter.

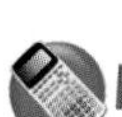

Mathematics

18. Comparing Baguettes One baguette is 84 centimeters in length. A second baguette is 0.9 meters long. A third measures 942 millimeters in length. Which baguette is longest? Which is shortest?

Math Concept **Metric Length Equivalents** The metric system of measurement is based on powers of ten. Prefixes are placed in front of unit names to indicate these powers of ten. The prefix milli means one-thousandth, while the prefix centi means one-hundredth. Thus, one millimeter is $\frac{1}{1000}$ of a meter, or 0.001 meter. One centimeter is similarly $\frac{1}{100}$ of a meter, or 0.01 meter.

Starting Hint To convert millimeters to meters, divide by 1000. To convert centimeters to meters, divide by 100. If converting from meters to centimeters or millimeters, multiply instead of divide.

NCTM Measurement Understand measurable attributes of objects and the units, systems, and processes of measurement.

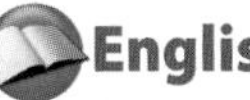

English Language Arts

19. Rates of Obesity Study Research the rates of obesity in five of the countries mentioned in this chapter. Then create a chart that shows each country and its obesity rate. Which has the highest rate of obesity? The lowest? In an oral presentation to the class, share your findings and chart, give possible reasons for differences you found. What staple foods might contribute to a nation's obesity rate? Are preparation techniques a factor? Does climate have an effect?

NCTE 8 Use information resources to gather information and create and communicate knowledge.

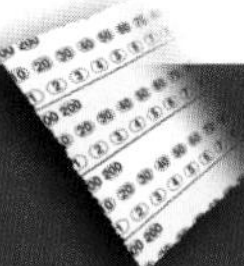

STANDARDIZED TEST PRACTICE

ANALOGY

Read the pairs of terms. Then choose the best word to match the term Italy.

20. stollen : Germany
laverbread : Wales
baguette : France
_______ : Italy

a. panino
b. cannoli
c. biscotti
d. gnocchi

Test-Taking Tip Analogies establish relationships between terms. Match each possible answer with the term Italy. The one that establishes the same type of relationship as the other terms is correct.

CHAPTER 49

Foods of Eastern Europe & Russia

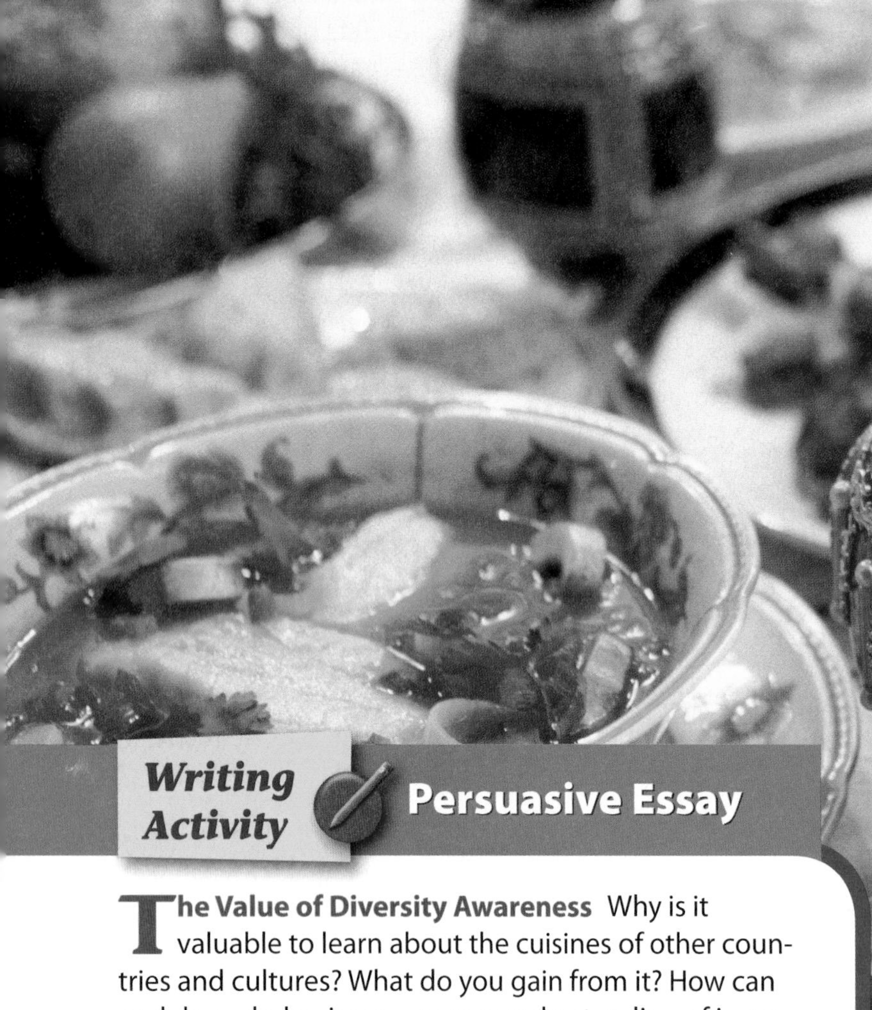

Writing Activity — Persuasive Essay

The Value of Diversity Awareness Why is it valuable to learn about the cuisines of other countries and cultures? What do you gain from it? How can such knowledge improve your understanding of ingredients and cooking methods? How can it change your relationships with others? Write a persuasive, one-page essay explaining the value of diversity awareness.

Writing Tips Follow these steps to write a persuasive essay:

- Appeal to readers' logic and emotions.
- Give specific facts, details, and examples to support your views.
- Consider reasons why readers may not agree, and address them.

Activate Prior Knowledge

Explore the Photo Eastern European cuisine offers many delicious discoveries. *What foods or dishes from Eastern Europe or Russia can you name?*

Reading Guide

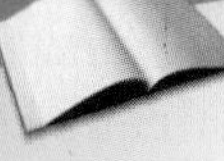

Before You Read

Preview Skim through the chapter to locate the names of several Eastern European countries. Think about the diversity among each of their cuisines.

Read to Learn

Key Concepts

- **List** the six subregions of Eastern Europe.
- **Describe** the roles that bread and tea play in Russian cuisine, and give examples of each.

Main Idea

The cuisines of Eastern Europe and Russia reflect the influences of many different cultures and feature hearty ingredients and flavorful dishes.

Content Vocabulary

You will find definitions for these words in the glossary at the back of this book.

- kringel
- pierogis
- bigos
- kielbasa
- kolache
- pilaf
- blini
- caviar
- pelmeni

Academic Vocabulary

You will find these words in your reading and on your tests. Use the glossary to look up their definitions if necessary.

- hearty
- multitude

Graphic Organizer

Use a graphic organizer like the one below to list the nations that make up Eastern Europe.

The Baltic Countries	
The Central Countries	
The Balkan Countries	
The Caucasus	
Central Asian Countries	
Other	

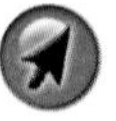

Graphic Organizer Go to this book's Online Learning Center at **glencoe.com** to print out this graphic organizer.

Academic Standards

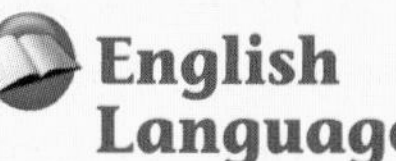

English Language Arts

NCTE 12 Use language to accomplish individual purposes.

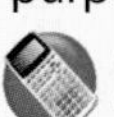

Mathematics

NCTM Number and Operations Compute fluently and make reasonable estimates.

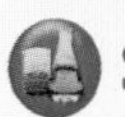

Science

NSES G Develop an understanding of science as a human endeavor.

NCTE *National Council of Teachers of English*
NCTM *National Council of Teachers of Mathematics*
NSES *National Science Education Standards*
NCSS *National Council for the Social Studies*

Cuisines of Eastern Europe

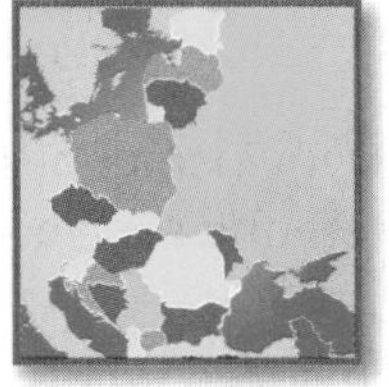

Cooking traditions of North and South meet in the countries of Eastern Europe. The Norse tradition of pickling and salting foods to stretch them through a short growing season lives on in countries of northeast Europe, such as Estonia, Latvia, Lithuania, and Belarus. Many food customs of the Mediterranean are found in countries of southeast Europe, such as Croatia, Slovenia, and Yugoslavia.

Eastern Europe stretches across a vast area, from Estonia to southern Albania. Russia stretches from Europe in the west to Asia in the east. **Figure 49.1** shows the countries of Eastern Europe as well as the vast country of Russia.

The Baltic Countries

Estonia, Latvia, and Lithuania are countries in northeast Europe on the Baltic Sea. Cooking in these countries is heavy on meat and potatoes. Potatoes are so basic that they are called "second bread." They are grated or mashed for puddings, pancakes, and dumplings and for small, savory tarts called sklandu rausi.

Figure 49.1 **Eastern Europe and Russia**

Cultural Influences Eastern Europe was under the control or influence of the Soviet Union during the second half of the 20th century. ***What culinary influences would you guess to be important in Eastern Europe?***

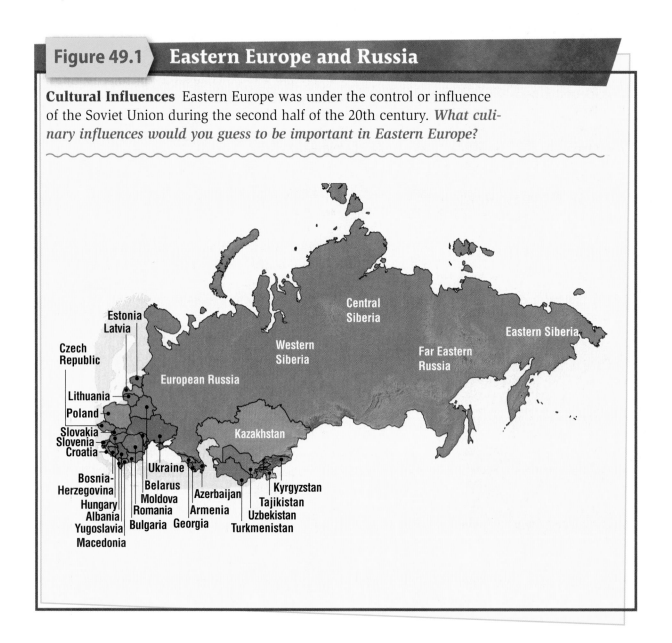

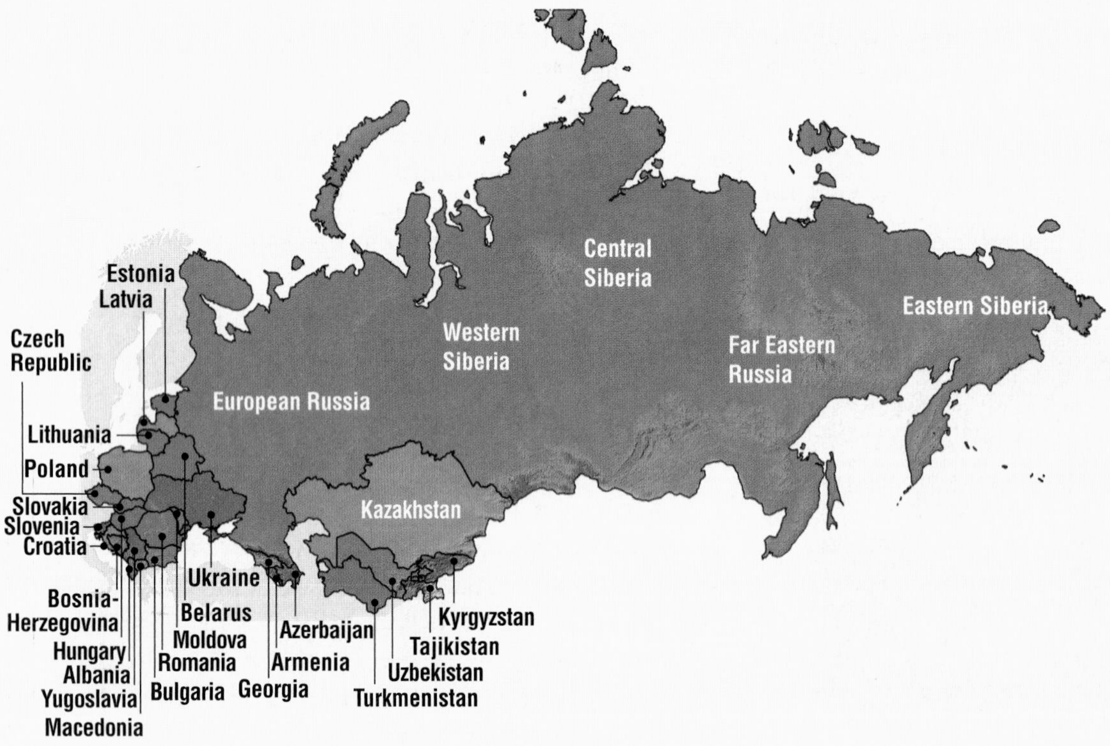

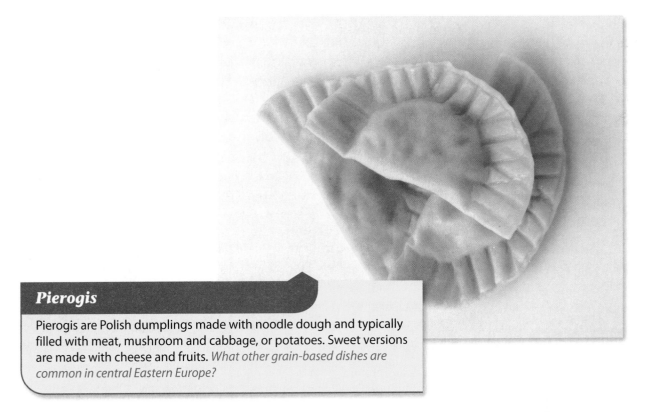

Pierogis

Pierogis are Polish dumplings made with noodle dough and typically filled with meat, mushroom and cabbage, or potatoes. Sweet versions are made with cheese and fruits. *What other grain-based dishes are common in central Eastern Europe?*

Sturdy vegetables, such as fresh and pickled beets and cabbage, are used in soups and tossed with cooked eggs in salads. Grains are a staple of most meals. The daily bread is a dark rye sourdough, often dotted with caraway seeds. Special occasions call for lighter breads. Lithuanians bake a **hearty**, or filling, dish of barley groats (hulled kernels) and onions fried with bacon. Cooked farina is leavened with beaten eggs to make Latvia's most famous dessert, buberts. Farina is a bland flour made from cereal grains. Sour milk thickened with cooked barley is a traditional cold beverage.

A range of dairy products is used in cooking. Sour cream dresses salads and garnishes soups, pancakes, and desserts. Farmer's cheese fills potato dumplings and is also cooked with beaten eggs to make Janu siers, a cheese served in Latvia for the summer solstice. Butter is used in many sweet and savory pastries.

Pork is the most popular meat. An Estonian favorite, sült, is shredded pork and veal jellied in their drippings. Pirags, bacon-stuffed turnovers, often accompany soup in Latvia. Perch, pike, and eel are popular freshwater fish, and herring and cod are popular saltwater fish. Pheasant and other game are eaten during the fall hunting season.

Smoked foods are traditional in the Baltic region. A juniper-smoked sausage called skilandis, for example, is a Lithuanian specialty. Smoked lamprey eel is a delicacy throughout the region.

Many desserts feature fruits. A purée of cooked apples, plums, and rhubarb is thickened with potato starch to make Latvian kîsêlis. Blueberry dumplings are served with sour cream. Birthdays in Latvia are celebrated with festively decorated **kringel**, a rich, yeast oval-shaped or pretzel-shaped coffee cake. Some kringels are made with nuts or fruit filling.

The Central Countries

Like much of Eastern Europe, Poland, the Czech Republic, Slovakia, and Hungary show a strong Slavic influence in their cuisine. However, a warmer climate and proximity to Western Europe influence the cuisine of these countries as well. Smoked herring and pickled beets are eaten here, just as in the North, but so is paraszt-saláta, a Hungarian salad with fresh tomatoes, bell peppers, chopped parsley, and vinaigrette that shows Mediterranean influences. Ground paprika, a red pepper, adds varying degrees of sweetness and heat to Hungarian and Slovakian cooking.

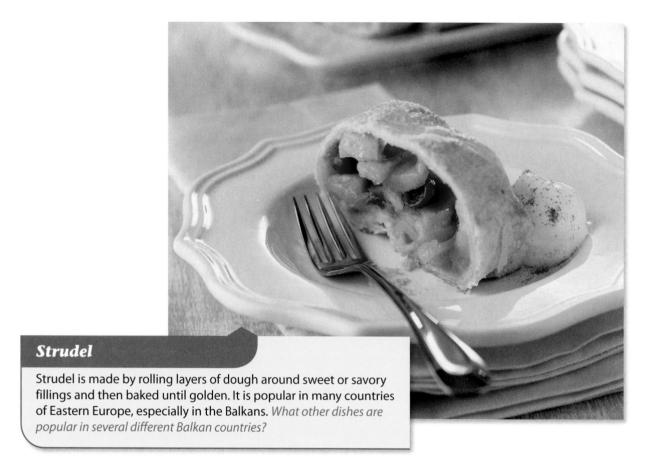

Strudel

Strudel is made by rolling layers of dough around sweet or savory fillings and then baked until golden. It is popular in many countries of Eastern Europe, especially in the Balkans. *What other dishes are popular in several different Balkan countries?*

Grains are made into breads, noodles, dumplings, and side dishes. Wheat flour is more common than rye flour in baking, so lighter breads are more common. Noodles are sometimes added to stews, such as in Hungarian goulash. Dumplings, such as Polish **pierogis** (pə-ˈrō-gēs), are made with noodle dough. Rice is as popular as potatoes as a side dish in Slovakia.

Breaded and fried pork cutlets are popular, reflecting German influence. The sweet-and-sour Polish stew **bigos** (bē-ˈgōs) includes sauerkraut as well as pork, apples, cabbage, and **kielbasa**, a Polish smoked sausage. Bigos is considered the Polish national dish.

Poland, the Czech Republic, Slovakia, and Hungary share a long baking tradition. Polish mazurek is a shortbread made with fruit and nuts and served on Easter. Czech **kolache** (kə-ˈlä-chē) is a type of pastry with fillings such as fruits, cheeses, fruit butter, nuts, or poppy seed paste. Hungarian diós bukta, a Christmas treat, is a spiral of rich yeast dough filled with ground walnuts, dates, raisins, apples, apricot jam, and chocolate.

The Balkan Countries

The Balkan Peninsula extends to the south from Central Europe into the Mediterranean Sea. Slovenia, Croatia, Yugoslavia, Bosnia and Herzegovina, Serbia, Bulgaria, Macedonia, and Albania occupy the Balkan Peninsula, which lies between the Adriatic Sea and the Black Sea in southeastern Europe.

Balkan cuisine, just like Balkan society, combines many different cultural influences from north and south. Slovenians and Croatians enjoy Austrian-style sausages, potato dumplings, and jota, a soup of sauerkraut, potatoes, and smoked pork. They also eat typical Italian dishes, such as minestrone, risotto, and zlinkrofi (meat dumplings much like ravioli). The consumption of meat is an important part of the Balkan diet.

Balkan cooking, especially in the south, has a strong Mediterranean influence. Lamb, eggplant, tomatoes, peppers, and yogurt are common ingredients. Yogurt is a daily part of the Bulgarian diet. Lemon, garlic, and parsley are favored seasonings.

Many dishes are popular across all countries of the Balkans. Grilled meatballs and stuffed grape leaves, for example, are found throughout the region. Phyllo dough layered with cheese or spinach is known as banitsa in Bulgaria and byrek in Albania. It is called burek in Yugoslavia, where a meat-filled version is eaten for breakfast. Turkish coffee, a strong coffee made by boiling finely ground beans, is brewed throughout the region.

Romania, which is adjacent to the Balkan Peninsula, uses a blend of many cuisines. Mamaliga is a cornmeal porridge like Italian polenta. It is served with meat stew, sauerkraut, or sour cream and Greek feta cheese. Samarle can use grape or cabbage leaves, stuffed with a mixture of ground pork and beef or lamb along with sour cream or yogurt. Ciorba is a soup made with sour cream. It may also include chicken, lemon, and parsley.

Ukraine, Belarus, and Moldova

Northeast of the Balkans and west of Russia lie numerous independent republics that were once part of the Soviet Union. Ukraine and Belarus are the largest of these.

The center of the original Russian state, which came into existence in the ninth century, Ukraine is a leading wheat producer and is sometimes called "the breadbasket of Europe." Bakers in this region prepare a **multitude**, or large number, of light breads in numerous shapes. Artistically presented breads are served on holidays and other special occasions. A wedding bread might be ornamented with doves, for example. Another specialty is kutia, boiled wheat groats mixed with poppy seeds, honey, and nuts. It is served chilled on Christmas Eve.

Careers in Food

Kim Cross
Online Editor

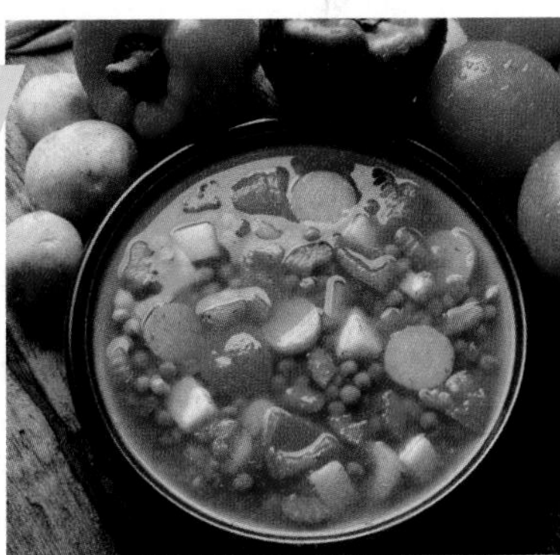

"I wear many hats in a job that changes daily!"
— Kim Cross
Editor, CookingLight.com
Birmingham, AL

Q: What are your primary responsibilities?

A: My regular tasks include keeping the Web site humming with fresh and timely content, writing and taking photos for our blog, editing a newsletter that is mailed to 170,000 subscribers, and moderating our online community of readers who chat on the bulletin boards. I also work with our in-house film crew to help direct videos for the Web.

Q: How is being an online editor different from being a print editor?

A: The roles are different at each publication. The food editors of *Cooking Light Magazine* take a story from inception to print, which involves many steps. They develop story concepts, work with recipe developers, and collaborate with the test kitchen. The magazine's success depends on my collaboration with different groups, including the print editors, on multimedia projects and timely stories that cannot be covered with the magazine's four-month lead time.

Q: Do you spend a lot of time cooking?

A: Of course! I learn something about cooking every day, and I take those lessons home and apply them in my kitchen.

Education and Training

Some editors come from a journalism or technical background, while others have a strong background in food, with a culinary education or certification.

Qualities and Skills

Strong writing, editing, and organization skills, plus a working knowledge of food, are necessary skills. Technical skills such as Web design are also helpful.

Related Career Opportunities

Writer, journalist, advertising, marketing, project manager.

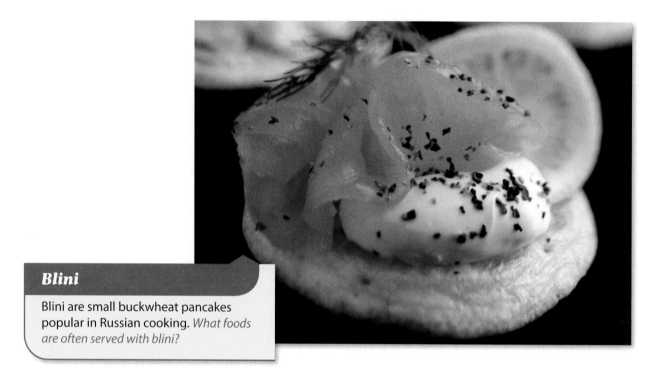

Blini

Blini are small buckwheat pancakes popular in Russian cooking. *What foods are often served with blini?*

Kitchen Math — Exchange Rates

While on vacation in Moscow, the capital of Russia, Anna decided that she would like to have a late night snack of tea and apple dumplings. The restaurant by her hotel sells a samovar of tea for 18 rubles (the Russian currency), and it sells the apple dessert Anna wants for 30 rubles. If the current exchange rate is 25.2 rubles per dollar, how much will Anna's meal cost in dollars?

Math Concept **Solving Problems with Proportions** Write two equal ratios (known as a proportion) to relate a quantity you already know to another quantity you are solving for. Use x to represent the unknown amount in the second ratio.

Starting Hint Anna will spend a total of $18 + 30 = 48$ rubles on the meal. Follow these directions to figure how much 48 rubles equals in American dollars. Write two ratios of dollars to rubles, and set them equal to each other: $1/25.2 = x/48$. Solve for x, which represents the total meal price in dollars.

Math Appendix For math help, go to the Math Appendix at the back of the book.

NCTM Number and Operations Compute fluently and make reasonable estimates.

Cabbage and root vegetables are also popular in Ukraine, Belarus, and Moldova. Ukrainian borscht, a soup with beets as the main ingredient, is served hot, not cold as in Russia. In Ukraine borscht is usually made with meat. Nakypliak is a steamed cabbage soufflé.

Belarusian cooking also has German and Polish accents. Grated potatoes are fried into draniki (pancakes) and folded with eggs in babkas (puffy casseroles). Pork is a favorite meat, and lightly smoked salt pork is a common flavoring. Both fresh and salt pork are used in machanka, a stew of pork ribs and sausage.

Moldova lies between Ukraine and Romania and shows elements of both cuisines. Poultry is more popular than pork in Moldovan cooking, and some borscht recipes use chicken. One recipe for Moldovan ciorba (sour soup) combines chicken giblets and cabbage.

The Caucasus

Georgia, Armenia, and Azerbaijan make up the Caucasus, a region named for the Caucasus Mountains that separate Europe from Asia. These countries lie just south of Russia, but their cuisine has Mediterranean influences.

An Armenian appetizer, imom bayeldi, is eggplant slices under sautéed onions, peppers, and tomatoes, seasoned with garlic, mint, basil, and parsley. Dovga is a chilled Azerbaijani soup of yogurt and cucumber, sometimes with eggs and garbanzo beans, or raisins and walnuts. Plum and pomegranate sauces are popular on meat and poultry in Georgian cooking. Satvisi is chicken with a walnut and garlic sauce, flavored with cinnamon and cilantro.

In western Georgia, cooks serve stews with ghomi, a millet porridge. Armenians often serve lavash, a thin, blistered flatbread. Rice and bulgur are stuffed into grape leaves or cooked in a **pilaf** (pi-ˈläf), sautéed grains cooked in a seasoned liquid with dried fruit and nuts or strips of meat.

Central Asian Countries

Kazakhstan, Uzbekistan, Turkmenistan, Kyrgyzstan, and Tajikistan are part of Asia, but their cuisine shares many features with the cuisine of Eastern Europe and Russia.

Flatbreads, called nan or chorek, are essential to meals. Some breads are leavened with yeast, others with sour milk. Mutton fat is sometimes added for tenderness. In rural areas, bread is baked in the traditional way, on the inner wall of a brick oven.

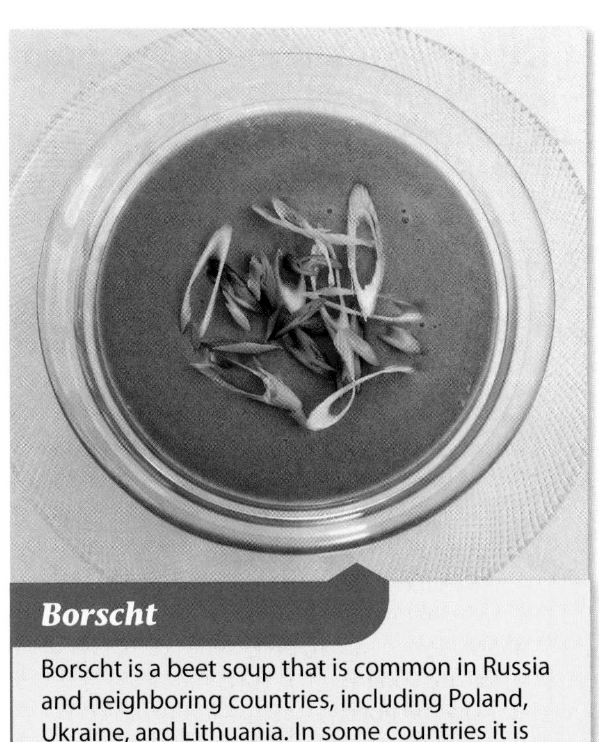

Borscht

Borscht is a beet soup that is common in Russia and neighboring countries, including Poland, Ukraine, and Lithuania. In some countries it is served hot, in others cold. *What are two Russian dishes that show a French influence?*

Sheep provide meat for many main dishes. Cubes of lamb, marinated in lemon juice or vinegar, are grilled and served with raw onion as shashlyk. Mutton is ground to fill large, steamed meat dumplings called manty. Mutton is also stewed with turnips, carrots, tomatoes, and garbanzo beans in shurpa.

✓ **Reading Check** **Explain** Why does Central Asian cuisine have so many Russian influences?

Cuisine of Russia

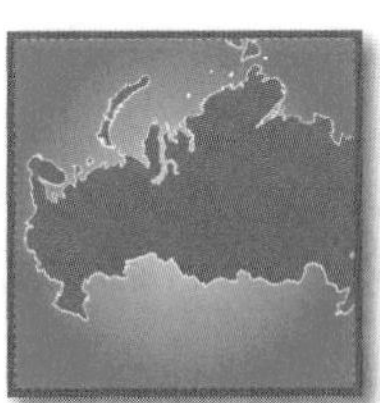

Russia is the world's largest country. It stretches from Europe in the west to Asia in the East. With six and a half million square miles, it is almost twice the size of the United States. Farmland is limited, however, and the growing season is short and cool. Traditional meals rely on grains, beef, pork, dairy foods, and hearty vegetables such as potatoes, cabbage, and beets. Mushrooms are used in many dishes, and fish are eaten near rivers and along the coasts.

Many Russian dishes reflect the practical cooking of the Slavs, the Vikings, and the Mongols. Russian cuisine also shows French influence, in large part because of Russian emperor Peter the Great. In the 1700s, he adopted Western ideas and technology and introduced French customs to the upper classes.

Grains are basic to Russian cuisine. Bread is eaten at every meal. Choices include flatbread, wheat rolls, and Russian black bread. Russian black bread is a moist rye loaf flavored with chocolate, caraway, coffee, and molasses. A sweet, cold beverage, kvas, is made by soaking black bread fermented with yeast.

Kasha is a versatile porridge made with buckwheat groats, or sometimes with oats, barley, rice, or millet. Kasha cooked with milk is eaten at breakfast. Kasha with meat is served as a main dish. Rice kasha with honey and raisins is eaten as a dessert.

Blini (ˈblē-nē) are small, yeast-leavened, buckwheat pancakes. Most people enjoy them with jam or sour cream.

Blini are sometimes served as elegant zakuski (hors d'oeuvres) with smoked salmon or sour cream and **caviar** (ˈka-vē-ˌär), the salted eggs of the sturgeon, a large fish. Caviar is a major export of Russia. A zakuska is an hors d'oeuvre table inspired by the Scandinavian smorgasbord.

Both hot and cold soups are common. Okroshka is a cool summer soup of diced raw vegetables, boiled potatoes, eggs, and ham. Shchi, a soup made with cabbage, root vegetables, and broth, is served warm.

Main dishes in Russia often include ground meat. Pork and beef fill cabbage rolls and **pelmeni** (pȧl-ˈmenē) dumplings. Kulebiaka is a festive dish that features salmon layered with sauteed mushrooms, slices of hard-boiled egg, onions, and rice. The food is then wrapped in a buttery bread dough in the shape of a fish and baked.

Chicken Kiev is a breaded, fried chicken breast enfolding a square of seasoned butter. Beef stroganoff is beef strips browned and simmered with mushrooms in a sour cream sauce, served over egg noodles.

Russian tea (zavarka) is brewed strong and is traditionally served in a samovar urn. It is poured into the cup, diluted with hot water, and sweetened with sugar, honey, or jam.

Russian desserts include fruit dumplings, teacakes (butter cookies), and sweet cheese dishes. Traditional Easter sweets include pashka, a pyramid of cream, sugar, and eggs cooked and blended with cottage cheese, raisins, and almonds. Kulich, a yeast bread with raisins and almonds baked in a round mold, has alternating white and brown shortcake layers with caramel and icing.

Light and Healthy Recipe

Hungarian Goulash

Ingredients

- **1 tbsp.** Canola oil
- **1 pound** Cubed beef chuck roast
- **2 cups** Chopped onions
- **2 cups** Diced potatoes
- **5 cups** Low-sodium beef broth
- **2 tbsp.** Paprika

Directions

1. Pour the oil into a large pot and sauté the meat until the pieces are just browned on all sides. Remove the meat and set it aside.
2. Lower the heat and cook the onions until tender.
3. Return the meat to the pot and add the potatoes, broth, and paprika. Cover the pot and let cook on low heat for one hour.
4. Serve hot.

This thick stew is made with tough meat, potatoes and paprika. The collagen in the meat and the starch in the potatoes are the only thickeners it needs.

Yield 6 servings

Nutrition Analysis per Serving

■ Calories	343
■ Total fat	18 g
Saturated fat	6 g
Cholesterol	72 mg
■ Sodium	101 mg
■ Carbohydrate	16
Dietary fiber	3 g
Sugars	22 g
■ Protein	28 g

CHAPTER 49 Review & Applications

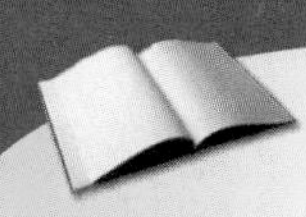

After You Read

Chapter Summary

The cuisines of Eastern Europe and Russia reflect the influences of many different cultures and feature hearty ingredients and flavorful dishes. Eastern Europe is divided into several regions: the Baltic countries; the Central countries; the Balkan countries; the Ukraine, Belarus, and Moldova; the Caucasus; and the Central Asian countries. Each of these regions is characterized by a certain style of cuisine, common ingredients, and popular dishes. Once controlled by the Soviet Union, today their native traditions are re-emerging. Russia's cuisine features grains, beef, pork, dairy foods, and hearty vegetables, as well as mushrooms and fish.

Content and Academic Vocabulary Review

1. Create two multiple-choice test questions using eight of these content and academic vocabulary words.

Content Vocabulary

- kringel (p. 757)
- pierogis (p. 758)
- bigos (p. 758)
- kielbasa (p. 758)
- kolache (p. 758)
- pilaf (p. 761)
- blini (p. 761)
- caviar (p. 762)
- pelmeni (p. 762)

Academic Vocabulary

- hearty (p. 757)
- multitude (p. 759)

Review Key Concepts

2. **List** the six regions of Eastern Europe.
3. **Describe** the roles that bread and tea play in Russian cuisine, and give examples of each.

Critical Thinking

4. **Explain** why the cuisine in Baltic countries is rich in carbohydrates.
5. **Describe** three dishes from the Balkans that are similar to each other.
6. **Identify** which region of Eastern Europe Peter should visit if he wants to eat Austrian-, Italian-, and Mediterranean-style cuisine. Explain why.
7. **Evaluate** Tameesha's comment: "There are probably many good bakeries in the Ukraine."
8. **Compare and contrast** Latvian kringel, Polish mazurek, and Czech kolache. How are they similar? How are they different?
9. **Compare and contrast** Estonian pirags, Lithuanian skilandis, Polish bigos, Belarusian machanka, and Russian pelmeni. How are they similar? How are they different?
10. **Infer** how Russia's climate has affected its cuisine. It is a northern country with long-lasting cold winters. The essential components of Russian cuisine provide more carbohydrates and fat rather than proteins, and fresh fruits and vegetables are not usually used in food.

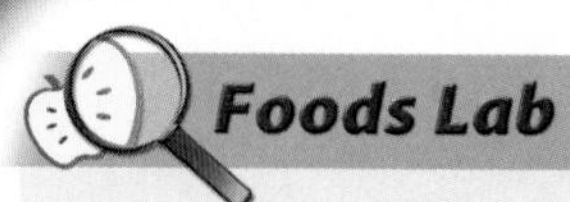

Foods Lab

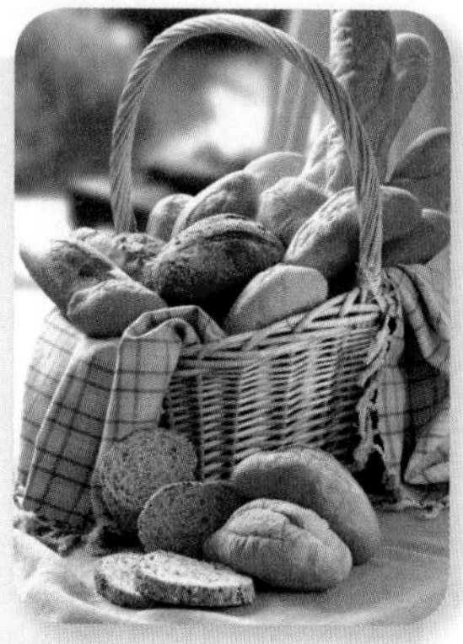

11. Breads of Eastern Europe and Russia Many varieties of bread are available in Eastern Europe and Russia, each with its own taste, texture, and appearance.

Procedure Sample different types of breads that are popular in Eastern Europe and Russia, such as black bread, potato bread, sesame seed, pumpernickel, and varieties of rye bread. Try them with different spreads, meats, or cheeses.

Analysis In a class discussion, offer feedback on the following: How do the taste, texture, and appearance of these breads compare to typical American breads?

HEALTHFUL CHOICES

12. A Taste of the Mediterranean While on a tour of Eastern Europe, Braden has enjoyed a variety of flavorful and filling cuisines, many of them rich in meat and potatoes. Braden is aware that Mediterranean cuisine is one of the most healthful cuisines in the world. He is craving its flavors as well as its health benefits. Where in Eastern Europe can Braden go to eat this type of healthful cuisine?

TECH Connection

13. News Update Under your teacher's supervision, use the Internet to research recent news in one of the countries discussed in this chapter. Write notes about your findings. In an oral presentation to the class, explain what current events are shaping this part of the world, and describe possible ways that food or cuisine might be affected. Prepare a list of talking points you wish to cover in your presentation.

Real-World Skills

Problem-Solving Skills	**14. Plan an Ethnic Meal** You must prepare a dish from Eastern Europe or Russia by 3 p.m. tomorrow. Find a recipe for one of the dishes mentioned in this chapter. Make a list of ingredients you will need to buy. Then write out a timeline explaining when you will complete each preparation step to have the dish ready in time.
Interpersonal and Collaborative Skills	**15. Country Study** Follow your teacher's instructions to form groups. Work together to research Russia or the country in Eastern Europe that has been assigned to your group. Learn about the country's history, geography, and culture, and find out more about its cuisine. Using visual aids and speech, give a class presentation.
Financial Literacy Skills	**16. Bite-Sized Samples** Imagine you are preparing 100 bite-sized samples of Bulgarian banitsa to offer to your fellow students. Your recipe for banitsa serves 10. It costs $16 to purchase all the ingredients necessary to make the recipe. One serving equals 10 bite-sized samples. How much is each sample worth?

Academic Skills

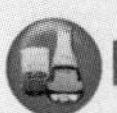

Food Science

17. Global Pancakes While Russians revere blini as being "truly Russian," they have many counterparts among world cultures. In Russia, blini are made from wheat or buckwheat flour, yeast, butter, eggs and milk.

Procedure What are some foods from around the world that are similar to Russian blini? Conduct research on different types of flatbreads made from sweet batter from around the world. Find out how they are similar and how they are different.

Analysis Write a paragraph to describe blini and five other types of flatbreads made from sweet batter from around the world. Explain how each is similar to and different from blini. Explain what can you do to make sure that your blini are not pancakes or crepes. What is it that sets Russian blini apart from most of their counterparts?

NSES G Develop an understanding of science as a human endeavor.

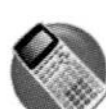

Mathematics

18. Travel Distance While on vacation in Eastern Europe, Alexis drives 515 kilometers from Prague, Czech Republic, to Warsaw, Poland. She then goes another 475 kilometers from Warsaw to Minsk, Belarus. From there, she hops on a train that takes her 403 kilometers to Riga, Latvia. Alexis then travels into Russia, going 485 kilometers to St. Petersburg and another 632 kilometers to Moscow. What is the total distance traveled by Alexis in miles?

Math Concept **Converting Distance Units** While the customary system of measurement uses the mile as a unit for large distances, the metric system uses kilometers. One kilometer (km) equals 0.621 mile, while one mile equates to 1.61 kilometers.

Starting Hint Add up all the kilometers traveled by Alexis on her vacation. Convert to miles by multiplying by 0.621.

NCTM Measurement Understand measurable attributes of objects and the units, systems, and processes of measurement.

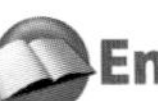

English Language Arts

19. First-Hand Experience Invite a guest speaker to speak with your class about a nation or region covered in this chapter. The person you invite should have lived in or visited the nation or region. He or she should be familiar with the region's food and culture. Write five questions to ask the speaker, including questions about foods. Ask the questions clearly, and take note of the answers you receive.

NCTE 12 Use language to accomplish individual purposes.

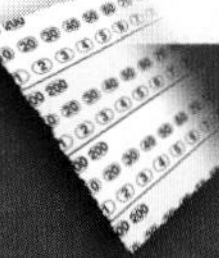

STANDARDIZED TEST PRACTICE

FILL IN THE BLANK

Read the sentence and choose the best word to fill in the blank.

20. In Russia, the growing season is _________.

a. long and warm
b. short and cool
c. from January to February
d. year-round

Test-Taking Tip When answering a fill-in-the-blank question, silently read the sentence with each of the possible answers in the blank space. This will help you eliminate wrong answers. The best word results in a sentence that is both factual and grammatically correct.

CHAPTER 50

Foods of South, East, & Southeast Asia

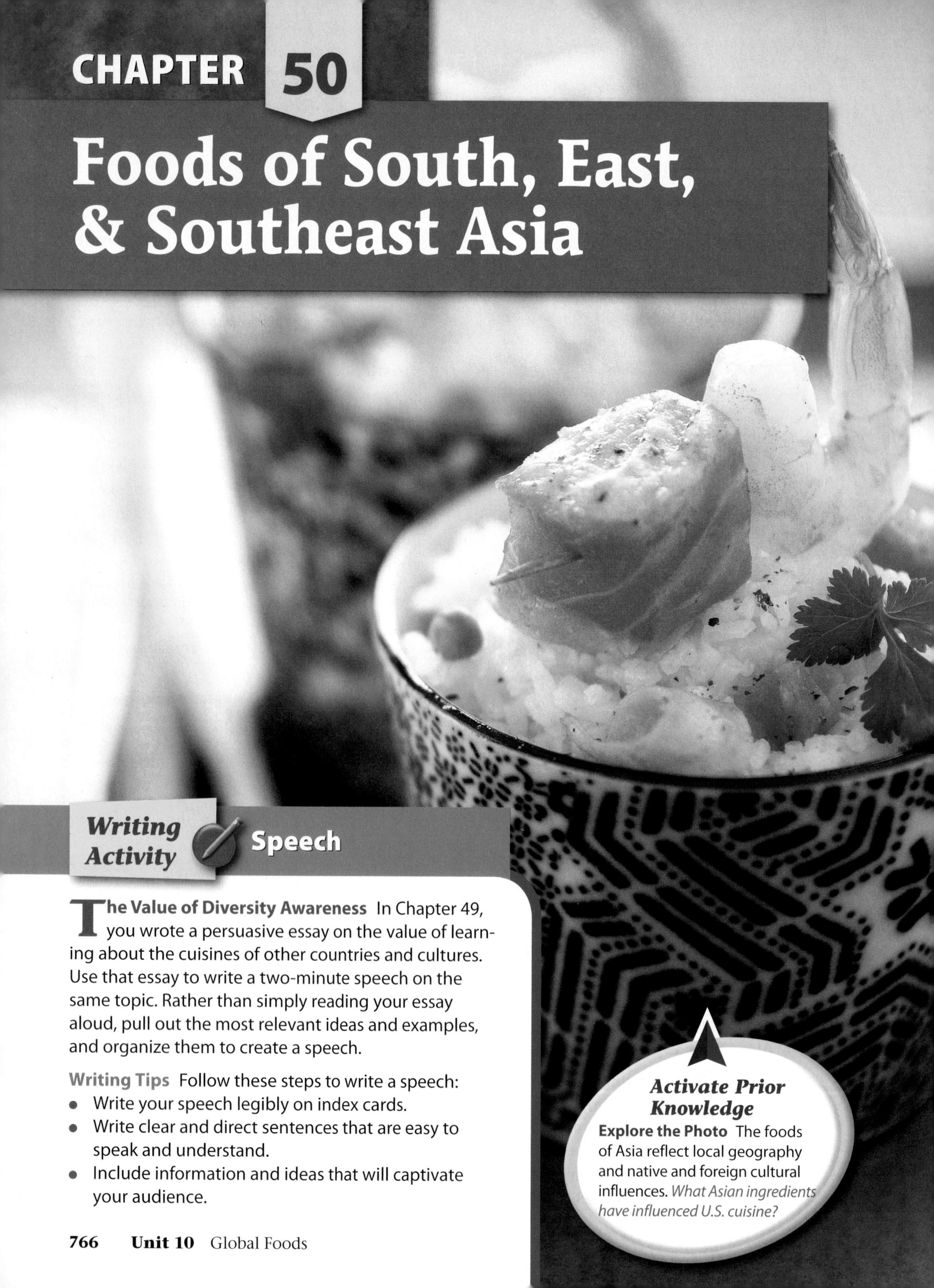

Writing Activity — Speech

The Value of Diversity Awareness In Chapter 49, you wrote a persuasive essay on the value of learning about the cuisines of other countries and cultures. Use that essay to write a two-minute speech on the same topic. Rather than simply reading your essay aloud, pull out the most relevant ideas and examples, and organize them to create a speech.

Writing Tips Follow these steps to write a speech:

- Write your speech legibly on index cards.
- Write clear and direct sentences that are easy to speak and understand.
- Include information and ideas that will captivate your audience.

Activate Prior Knowledge

Explore the Photo The foods of Asia reflect local geography and native and foreign cultural influences. *What Asian ingredients have influenced U.S. cuisine?*

Reading Guide

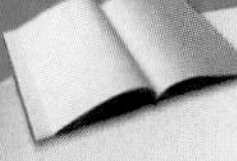

Before You Read

Preview Recall ingredients and flavors you may have tasted while eating Asian food. As you read the chapter, see if any of them are mentioned.

Read to Learn

Key Concepts

- **Compare and contrast** Northern Indian and Southern Indian cuisine.
- **Describe** popular dishes from China, Japan, and Korea.
- **Identify** popular dishes from Laos, Thailand, Cambodia, and Vietnam.

Main Idea

The cuisines of South, East, and Southeast Asia are diverse, vibrant, and flavorful, and include a variety of colorful ingredients and tasty dishes.

Content Vocabulary

You will find definitions for these words in the glossary at the back of this book.

- ☐ curry
- ☐ dal
- ☐ chutney
- ☐ tandoor
- ☐ daikon
- ☐ hoisin
- ☐ dim sum
- ☐ sashimi
- ☐ sushi
- ☐ nori
- ☐ kimchi

Academic Vocabulary

You will find these words in your reading and on your tests. Use the glossary to look up their definitions if necessary.

- tailor
- signature

Graphic Organizer

As you read, use a graphic organizer like the one below to list the Asian nations that make up South Asia, East Asia, and Southeast Asia.

SOUTH ASIA	EAST ASIA	SOUTHEAST ASIA

Graphic Organizer Go to this book's Online Learning Center at **glencoe.com** to print out this graphic organizer.

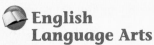

Academic Standards

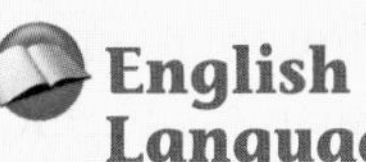

English Language Arts

NCTE 4 Use written language to communicate effectively.

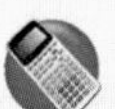

Mathematics

NCTM Algebra Use mathematical models to represent and understand quantitative relationships.

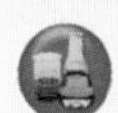

Science

NSES B Develop an understanding of the structure and properties of matter.

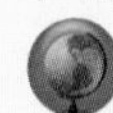

Social Studies

NCSS VIII B Make judgments about how science and technology can transform the physical world and human society.

NCTE *National Council of Teachers of English*
NCTM *National Council of Teachers of Mathematics*
NSES *National Science Education Standards*
NCSS *National Council for the Social Studies*

Cuisine of South Asia

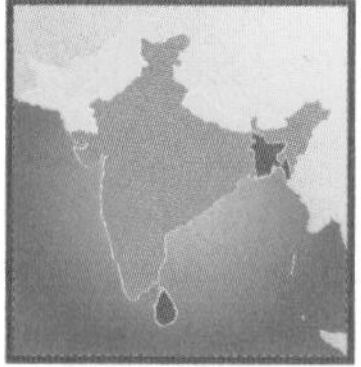

South Asia centers on the Indian subcontinent, home to India, Pakistan, Bangladesh, Nepal, Bhutan, and Sri Lanka. South Asia is bordered by East Asia to the east and Southeast Asia. **Figure 50.1** shows the Indian subcontinent and surrounding Asian countries.

India is the largest and most populous country in South Asia, and many elements of Indian cuisine are found throughout the region, with national and regional variations. Cooks in Sri Lanka, for example, prepare curries and lentil dishes just as cooks in India do, but they often use coconut oil instead of ghee (clarified butter).

Indian Ingredients

Farming is a major industry in South Asia. The Indus and Ganges rivers deposit rich soil in the central plains of Pakistan and India, and in Bangladesh's Ganges Delta. Southern India and Sri Lanka have tropical climates. The geography of South Asia is ideal for growing rice, wheat, legumes, chiles, coconuts, mangoes, tamarinds, almonds, pistachios, and tea.

Figure 50.1 **Asia**

Cultural Influences Asia is the world's largest continent. ***What is the most influential cuisine in South Asia? Speculate why.***

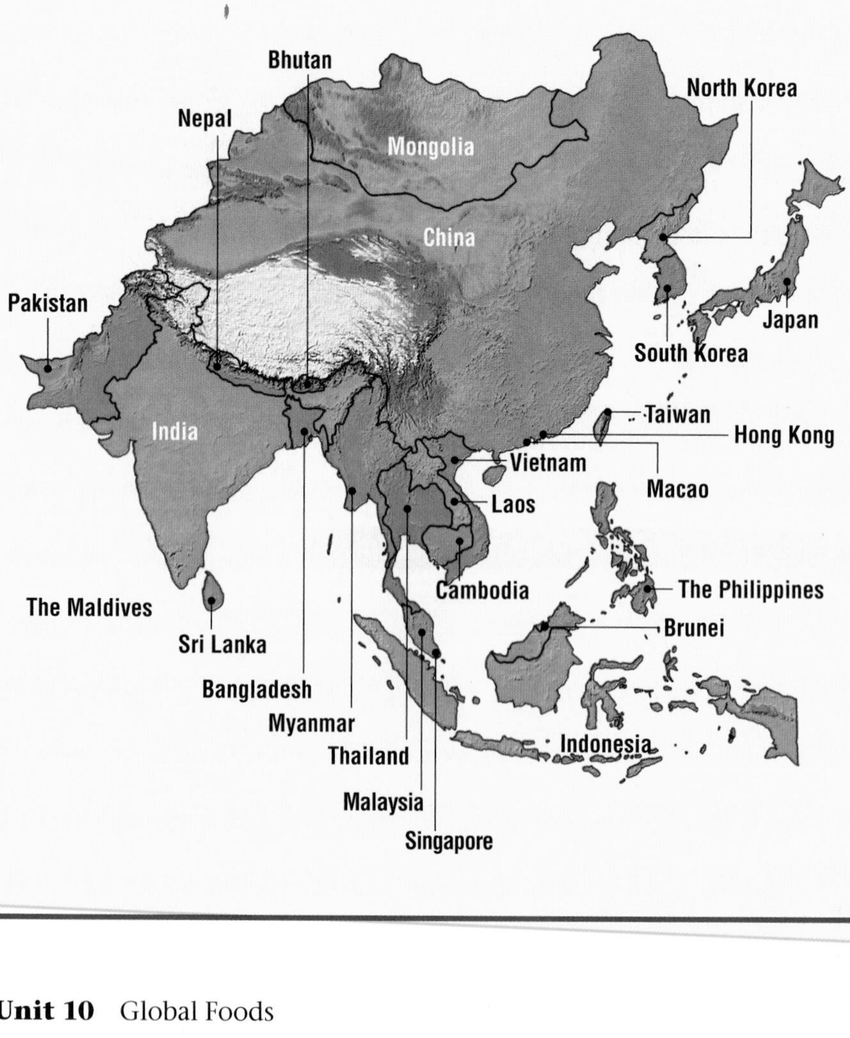

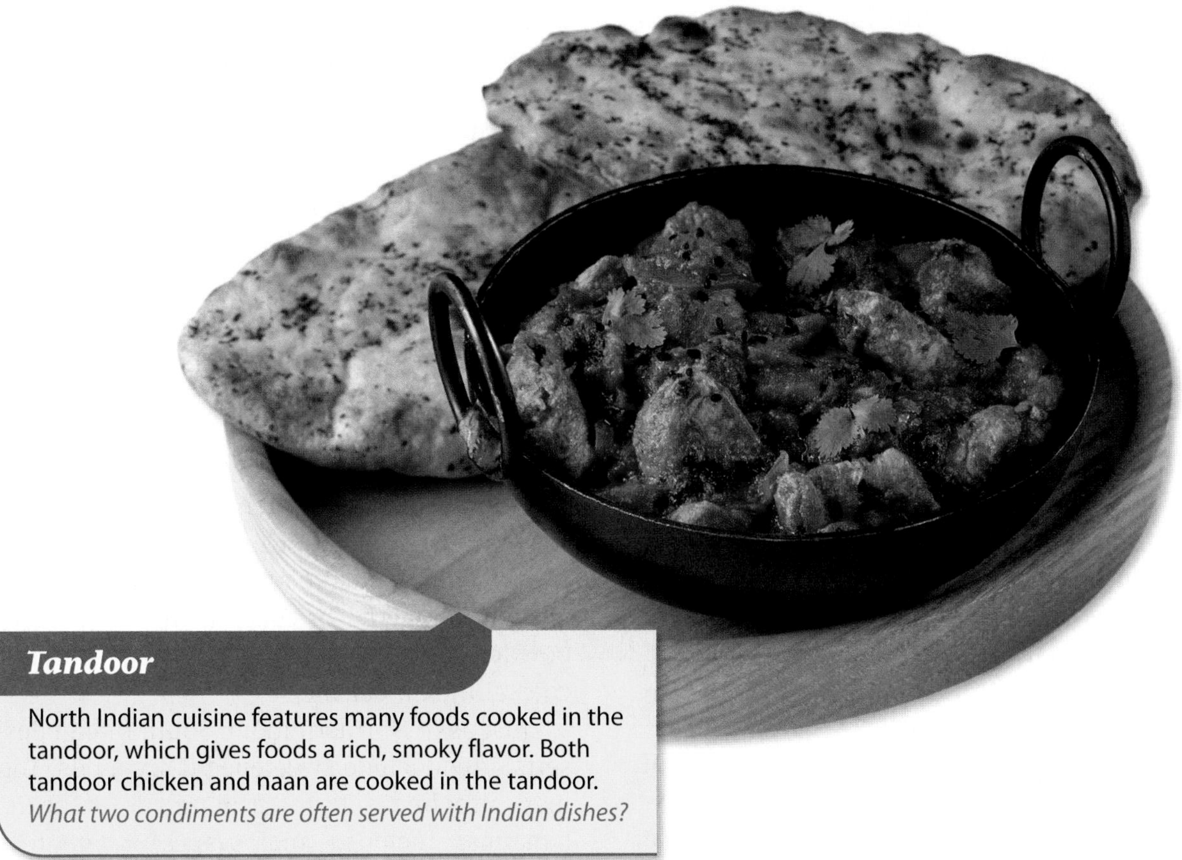

Tandoor

North Indian cuisine features many foods cooked in the tandoor, which gives foods a rich, smoky flavor. Both tandoor chicken and naan are cooked in the tandoor. *What two condiments are often served with Indian dishes?*

Cattle, sheep, and goats are raised in hilly northern pastures. Oceans and rivers supply a variety of seafood, especially in the south.

Indian cuisine is known for its creative use of spices. Cinnamon, cumin, cardamom, cloves, ginger, pepper, turmeric, garlic, cilantro, fenugreek, and mint are among the most common herbs and spices. Garam masala is a flavoring blend made by mixing and grinding whole seeds, pods, and buds. Indian cooks have their own recipes for garam masala, which they **tailor**, or adjust, for each dish.

Indian Dishes

Indian dishes offer amazing variety, thanks to the diversity of seasonings and ingredients. India is renowned for its curries. A **curry** is a dish of vegetables, legumes, and sometimes meat in hot, highly seasoned sauces. Seafood curries are popular in coastal areas. **Dal** (ˈdäl) is a mixture or purée of legumes—mung beans, garbanzo beans, split peas, and more—as well as onions, chiles, and tomatoes.

Chutney is served with most meals. **Chutney** is a zesty condiment made from fruit, sugar, spices, and vinegar. Chutneys come in mild, hot, and sweet varieties that often combine contrasting flavors, such as sweet peppers with hot peppers or mangoes with pepper. A yogurt condiment called raita often includes cucumber, onion, mint, or garlic.

Northern Indian Dishes

Indian cuisine has many regional variations, featuring different ingredients and recipes in the south and the north.

Both bread and rice are common in Northern India. Both may be found in the same meal. Naan, the traditional flatbread, is usually leavened with yogurt. Naan is cooked in a **tandoor**, a rounded, clay, charcoal-burning oven. Chapati is an unleavened round bread of whole-wheat flour and water. Breads serve as a scoop for main dishes. Eating with the fingertips of the right hand is a traditional North Indian custom.

Main dishes in North India often include meat. Murgh tikka masala is chicken kebabs marinated in seasoned yogurt. Rogan josh is lamb simmered in a yogurt sauce and served over rice. Biryani is a casserole of meat sautéed in ghee, then cooked with rice and flavored with fried onions.

Desserts often feature sweetened dairy foods. Cardamom, cinnamon, and nutmeg are often used in sweet dishes. Northeastern India is known for "burned milk" dishes such as sandesh. In this dish, condensed milk is cooked with paneer, a firm yogurt cheese similar to ricotta. Gajar halwa, a custard of grated carrots cooked with milk and sugar, is garnished with raisins and nuts. Shredded coconut is moistened with condensed milk and wrapped around ground pistachios to make coco pista pasand.

Southern Indian Dishes

South Indian cooking has more vegetarian dishes than North Indian cuisine. Many devout Hindus follow a vegetarian diet. South Indian cooking features more vegetables and legumes than North Indian cuisine, and often substitutes sesame oil for ghee. Aloo gobhi matar, a dish made of cauliflower, potatoes, peas, and tomatoes, is fried in a heavy mixture of cumin, coriander, turmeric, and red pepper flakes.

Rice is the staple grain in the south. Parboiled rice and soaked beans are ground to make the batter for dosa. These large, crisp crepes are filled and rolled. Filling is often spiced potatoes, another staple starch. A special meal might include puffy, deep-fried rounds of bread called poori. Sauces often accompany meals. Popular sauces include tamarind sauce, mint sauce, and coconut sauce.

South Indian dishes tend to be spicier than North Indian dishes. Chiles are used abundantly and are often paired with coconut milk. Shrimp simmered in coconut milk and curry powder, served over rice, is typical of southern coastal Indian cuisine.

Just as in Northern India, South Indian desserts often include sweetened dairy foods. You may also find colorful fruit salads of pears, bananas, melons, and grapes, sometimes served with honey and orange juice and garnished with nuts.

Be a Smart Consumer

Salty Soy Sauce

In addition to adding flavor to a variety of Asian cuisines, soy sauce may also add nutritional benefits. For example, one study showed that Chinese dark soy sauce is extremely high in antioxidants, and can help prevent cardiovascular disease. This is good news for health-conscious consumers. However, consumers who follow a low-sodium diet should think twice before slathering their food with soy sauce, because it can be very high in sodium. Although it is impossible to make soy sauce without using some salt, low-sodium varieties are offered at most supermarkets and restaurants.

Challenge Find out the difference in sodium content between regular and low-sodium soy sauce. How much of the daily recommended value for sodium is in one serving of each variety?

✓ **Reading Check** **List** What are three characteristics of Southern Indian cooking that distinguish it from Northern Indian cooking?

Cuisine of East Asia

The cuisines of China, Mongolia, Japan, and Korea feature a balance of flavors, textures, and techniques. Something sweet may be balanced with something sour, or salty. Despite some similarities, however, Chinese, Japanese, and Korean cuisines each have distinctive ingredients and dishes.

China

Chinese cuisine involves a mix of different styles. Different cultural groups and geographic regions contribute varying ingredients and techniques. Szechuan in the south is known for its hot, peppery dishes, for example, while Shandong in the east is known for its many seafood recipes.

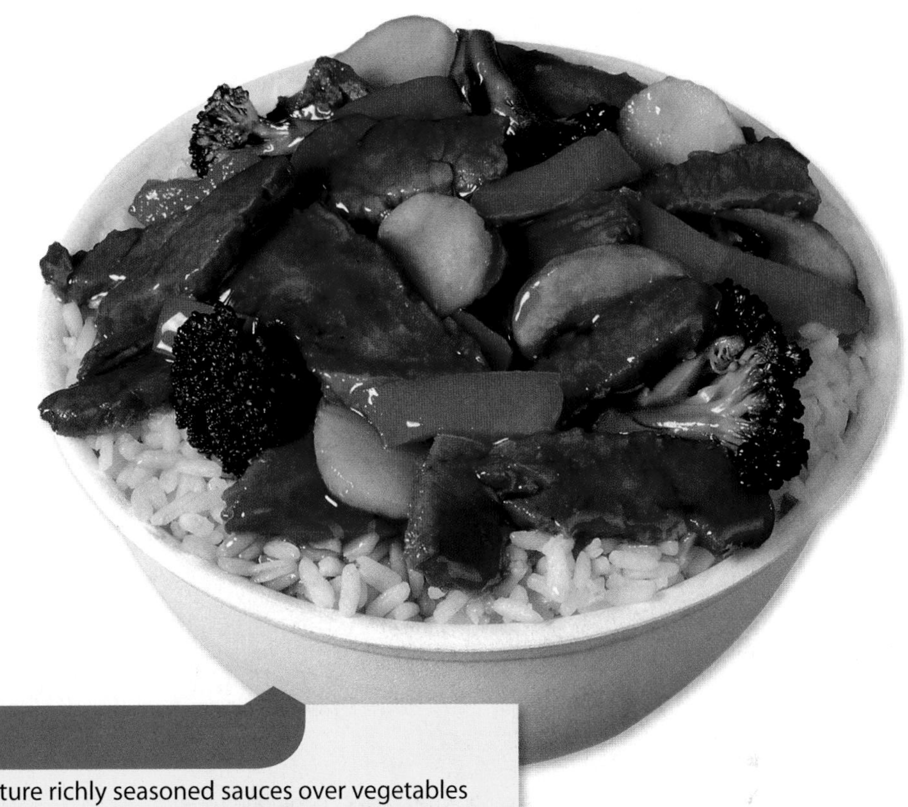

Sweet and Spicy

Many Chinese dishes feature richly seasoned sauces over vegetables and meat, poultry, or seafood. Hoisin sauce, sometimes called Chinese barbecue sauce, gives foods a sweet, salty, and slightly spicy flavor. *What are the uses of soy in Chinese cooking?*

Chinese Ingredients

Chinese farmers supply almost all of the food needs of China's 1.3 billion residents.

Vegetables and long-grain rice are the mainstays of Chinese cooking. Onions, scallions, broccoli, spinach, cabbage, eggplant, peppers, green beans, bean sprouts, and mushrooms are used in many recipes. Carrots, **daikon** (a large white radish with a mild flavor), and other root vegetables are also common. Pork, chicken, beef, and duck have been popular meats since the second century BCE. Lamb is popular in the far north of the country. Fish is usually served whole with the head and tail on. Diners pull pieces from the whole fish with chopsticks.

Meals in China are typically served family style, and each diner is given his or her own bowl of rice. Wheat is a common grain in North China, while rice is more common in South China. Preserved and pickled food are popular in North China because winters make growing seasons short.

Wheat, rice flour, and bean starch are used to make noodles and dumplings. Soybeans are the base of soy sauce, a staple seasoning. The Chinese are credited with inventing tofu, which they use in both savory and sweet dishes. Mushrooms provide both texture and flavor.

Chinese condiments add sweetness and spice. In addition to soy sauce, cooks use plum sauce, oyster sauce, and **hoisin** sauce, a thick, sweet and salty paste made with fermented soy, chiles, vinegar, and garlic. Black and red beans and dried shrimp are also mashed into seasoning pastes. Spicy Chinese mustard is used alone or mixed with other condiments. Sesame and peanut oil are used in stir fries to give foods a slightly nutty flavor.

Stir-frying is a typical cooking method in China. Steaming and deep-frying are also common. Some foods are deep-fried first to develop a crispy crust, then steamed to finish cooking.

Unlike many other cuisines, Chinese cuisine shows little outside influence. Different styles developed in different regions within China, often using the same basic ingredients.

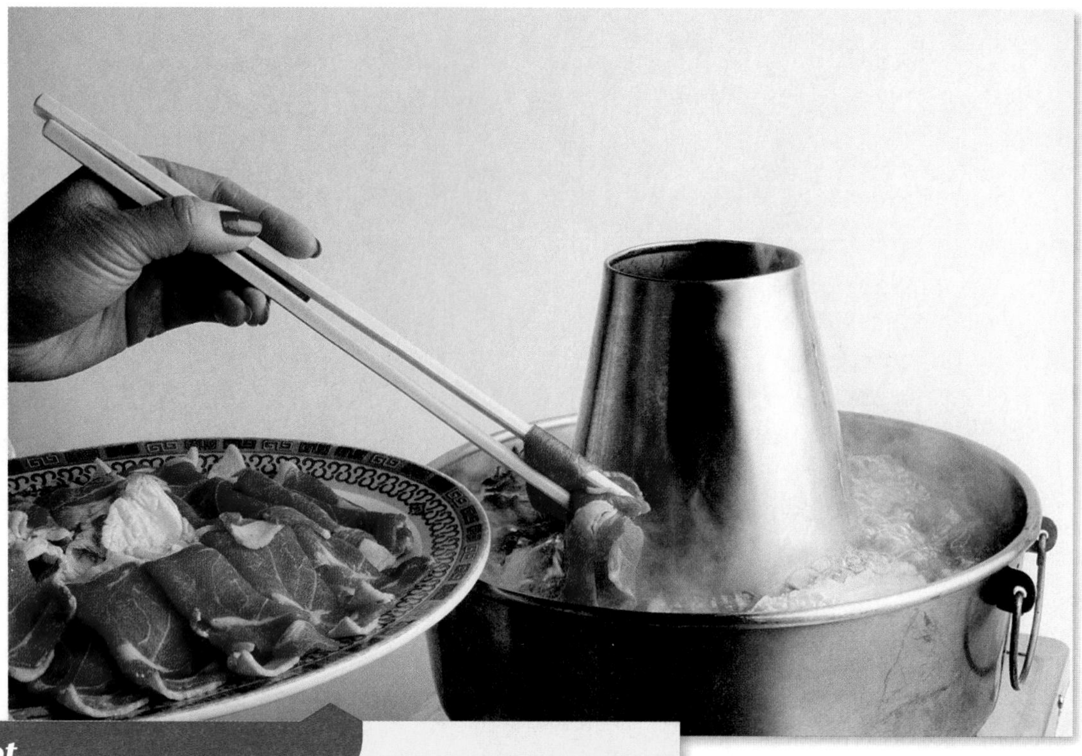

Hot Pot

Hot pot is sometimes called Chinese fondue. Diners cook raw meat and vegetables in broth that is kept boiling at the table. *Does rice grow in North China? Why or why not?*

South Coastal Chinese Dishes

Cantonese cuisine is influenced by the tropical climate and an abundant supply of fresh food, especially seafood.

Cantonese foods are mildly seasoned and lightly cooked. They are often steamed or stir-fried. Bass steamed with ginger, onion, and soy sauce is a popular dish. Spring rolls, which are similar to egg rolls but smaller and more delicate, are popular. Buddha's delight, a stir-fried medley of carrots, mushrooms, snow peas, water chestnuts, and other vegetables, may be tossed with noodles or bean curd sticks. Almonds and peanuts are often added.

Cantonese cuisine is also known for **dim sum**, bite-size dishes eaten at tea or between courses of a banquet. Dim sum morsels are meant to delight the eye as well as the tongue with their artistry and variety. A tray may include small plates of steamed dumplings filled with meat or vegetables, deep-fried sesame balls, custard tarts, and fried chicken feet flavored with star anise and ginger.

North Chinese and Mongolian Dishes

Natural resources are scarcer in North China than elsewhere in the country. Because this region is dry, wheat and millet, rather than rice, grow here. Cabbage is the main vegetable. Much of the food in North China is prepared simply. Noodle soups are made with sliced meat and vegetables, grilled lamb or mutton, and a minimum of seasoning.

Beijing, the capital of China, has a cuisine that is simple but refined. Peking duck is the most famous dish of the north. This dish, which takes two days to prepare, is duck that is moist inside, with crispy, golden skin outside. Peking duck is coated with a honey mixture and hung until the skin is dry and hard; then it is roasted. Another specialty is called Lotus buns or Beijing flower rolls, steamed dumplings filled with minced green onion and ham.

Cooking at the dining table is a specialty in Northern China and neighboring Mongolia. To make Mongolian Hot Pot, a cook sets a special brass vessel on the table, fills it with broth, and brings the liquid to a boil. Diners drop wafer-thin slices of meat (lamb, beef, fish, and poultry) and vegetables into the boiling broth and retrieve them with chopsticks when they are cooked. They then dip the slices of meat in a selection of condiments and eat it.

Central and Western Chinese Dishes

The cooking of the Szechuan, Hunan, and Yunnan provinces is famous for intense seasoning. The traits of chiles and sesame oil are used frequently, as is the Szechuan peppercorn. Su ch'un chuan are crisply fried vegetarian spring rolls served with sweet and sour sauce. Carp from the Yellow River is served with bean sauce or sweet and sour sauce. Hot and sour soup made with tofu, pork, and black mushrooms is a specialty. Kung pao chicken is made with diced chicken, peanuts, and chili peppers.

East Coastal Chinese Dishes

In Hangchow, Soochow, and Shanghai, dishes are marked by a careful blend of sweet and sour flavors. Cooks prepare steamed dumplings and thick round noodles. Seafood and fish from the Yangtze River are used in many recipes. A rice dish called juk often accompanies meals. Many dishes are braised, and the **signature**, or specialty, sauce is a rich brown sauce. Bird's nest soup comes from this area.

Japan

Japan has four large islands and about 3,000 small islands. The islands are mountainous. Only twelve to fifteen percent of the land is fertile enough for raising crops. The climate varies from cold in the north to very hot in the south. Foods from the sea, including seafood and sea vegetables, play a large role in Japanese cuisine.

Japanese cuisine is known for its emphasis on the quality of its ingredients and delicacy of its preparation. It features native ingredients and techniques, as well as influences from nations near and far. Beautiful visual presentation is an important part of traditional Japanese cuisine. Presentation is marked by simplicity, subtlety, and seasonality. Because of the limited land, eating foods that are in season is a necessity.

Japanese Ingredients

The soybean is essential to Japanese cuisine. Soy was brought from China by Buddhist monks in the seventh century. Soy sauce is a primary seasoning ingredient. Tofu is sautéed, broiled, and deep-fried for use in dishes. Miso, a fermented bean paste, comes in a variety of flavors and colors. It flavors and thickens broths, marinades, sauces, and salad dressings. A simple broth made from miso is considered a refreshing start to a meal. Raw soybeans, called edamame, are also used creatively.

The Japanese harvest fish, shellfish, and sea vegetables, and cultivate rice, soybeans, fruit, and mushrooms. Rice is a staple in Japan, as it is throughout Asia.

Though noodles originated in China, they are an essential part of Japanese cuisine. There are four popular types of noodles: soba, made of buckwheat; udon, made from wheat flour; soma, very thin noodles made from wheat; and somen, wheat noodles made by repeatedly pulling and stretching dough.

TECHNOLOGY FOR TOMORROW

Commercial Fishing Technology

Overfishing is a major environmental problem. It results in a decline in fish populations, the possible extinction of certain species, the death of accidentally caught marine animals, and the destruction of marine ecosystems. Japan is the world's biggest consumer of ocean fish. Commercial fishers in Japan catch as many as five million tons of fish each year. Some species, such as bluefin tuna, are so overfished they are at risk of becoming extinct. In an effort to fish more conservatively, Japan has scaled back on the technology that made it possible to catch so many fish. It has reduced the size of its fleet of commercial fishing boats by a quarter, and also reduced the number of its factory ships.

Get Involved How have modern commercial fishing boats and factory ships made it easier for people to catch and sell large quantities of fish? Write your findings in a paragraph.

NCSS VIII B Make judgments about how science and technology can transform the physical world and human society.

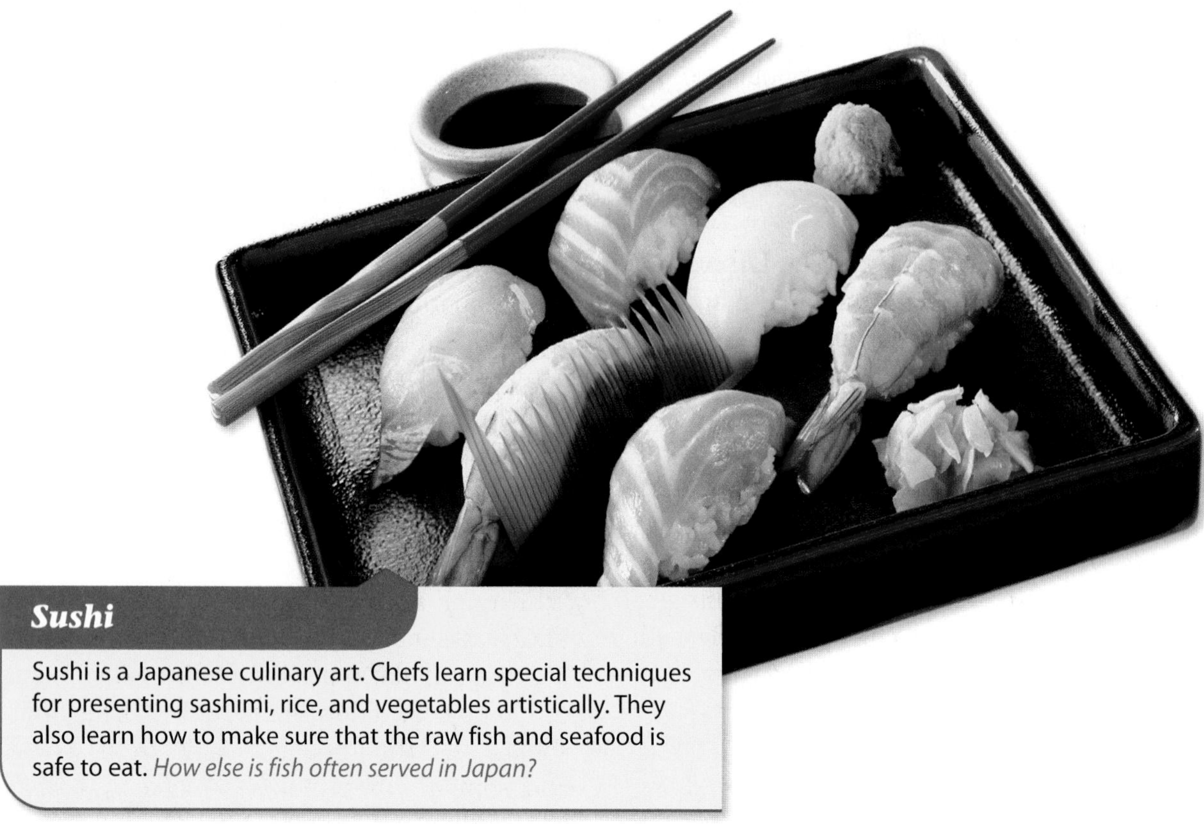

Sushi

Sushi is a Japanese culinary art. Chefs learn special techniques for presenting sashimi, rice, and vegetables artistically. They also learn how to make sure that the raw fish and seafood is safe to eat. *How else is fish often served in Japan?*

Japanese Dishes

The Japanese are famous for Kobe beef, a particularly tender and flavorful variety of meat from cattle raised on a special diet in Kobe, Japan. Traditionally, meat in Japanese dishes is cut into small pieces and then grilled. Sukiyaki consists of uniformly thin slices of seasoned beef and vegetables that are quickly grilled, sometimes at the table. Its counterpart, teriyaki, is small, marinated slices of chicken or fish that are grilled or broiled to a shiny glaze.

Japanese dishes use a variety of mushrooms. Shiitake, oyster, and enoki mushrooms are cultivated in Japan.

Foods from the sea are featured in many of the country's dishes. Fish is often cooked whole, with the skin on, to keep the flesh moist. Tuna is dried into bonito flakes to make dashi, a stock for soup or for flavoring other dishes. Tempura is a dish of crisp, batter-fried vegetable and fish morsels. Fish and shellfish are also served raw with condiments, such as in the dish **sashimi**. **Sushi** is the name of the vinegar-dressed rice that is combined with sashimi or rolled in **nori** (seaweed wrapper).

Fruit is often a simple dessert. Citrus fruits like kumquats, a bitter orange called daidai, and a small seedless orange called mikan are prized. Persimmons are also widely eaten.

North and South Korea

Korea occupies a peninsula between China and Japan. The peninsula is currently divided into two countries: the Democratic People's Republic of Korea, better known as North Korea, and the Republic of Korea, better known as South Korea.

Korean cuisine is based largely on rice, vegetables, fish, seaweed, and tofu. Korea is renowned for a traditional dish called **kimchi**, made by a unique process of preserving vegetables by fermentation. Cabbage, daikon radish, or cucumbers are seasoned with salt, pepper, garlic, and chiles, and packed with water into jars. The mix is then left until the vegetables ferment. Kimchi is served as a side dish or cooked into soups and rice dishes. Traditionally, Koreans would make enough kimchi to last throughout winter.

Chiles and peppers season most Korean dishes. Garlic, soy sauce, salt, and ginger are also used. Sesame seeds are used toasted, as oil, and as a paste. Abalone, crayfish, scallops, clams, shrimp, squid, and octopus are among the Korean seafood dishes cooked with noodles or rice.

Korean barbecue is known as bulgogi. For bulgogi, diners grill their own paper-thin slices of beef on a small grill in the middle of the dining table and then dip it in a hot pepper sauce. The meat is marinated with a mixture of soy sauce, sugar, and other ingredients before it is cooked.

Desserts is often tteok, a chewy rice cake sweetened with bean paste. Hangwa is a candy made of flour, sugar, and fruit.

✓ **Reading Check** **Identify** What ingredient is essential to cuisine in Japan, and how did it get there?

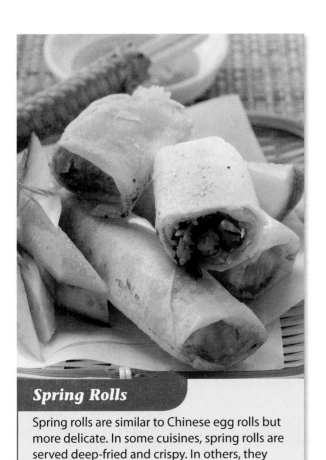

Spring Rolls

Spring rolls are similar to Chinese egg rolls but more delicate. In some cuisines, spring rolls are served deep-fried and crispy. In others, they are served steamed and soft. *What seasoning is widely used in the cooking of Laos, Thailand, Cambodia, and Vietnam?*

Cuisine of Southeast Asia

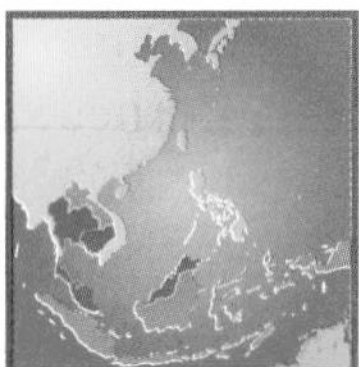

Southeast Asia is south of China and east of India. This diverse area includes a peninsula and thousands of islands with fascinating cuisines.

Laos, Thailand, Cambodia, and Vietnam

The cuisines of Laos, Thailand, Cambodia, and Vietnam feature fresh, intense flavors with vivid herbs and spices. The most important seasoning in the region is fish sauce, an intensely flavored, salty sauce made from fermented fish. It is called nam pla in Thailand and nuoc nam in Vietnam.

In Laos, Cambodia, and Vietnam, cooks often wrap ingredients in leaves. For example, ground pork is seasoned with herbs and spices, grilled, and served wrapped in crisp lettuce leaves.

Thai food features colorful green, yellow, and red curries made with fish, pork, duck, and vegetables. Thai cuisine is centered around the idea of balancing five flavors: spicy hot, sour, sweet, salty, and bitter. Rice is the featured grain, and Jasmine rice is native to Thailand. Key spices are lemongrass, basil garlic, and ginger. Spring rolls are made with soft rice papers wrapped around crab, pork, mushrooms, bean threads, and bean sprouts. A favorite dessert in Thailand is kha ya khoo, green tea ice cream.

Vietnam's national dish is pho, a beef and noodle soup. Pho is often served for breakfast. Another regional specialty is chao tom. A length of sugarcane stalk is peeled, coated with a layer of pounded shrimp, and grilled. It is dipped in a fish-based sauce and served with fried shrimp wafers. Nuoc man, a fish sauce, is used in many dishes. Soy sauce is also used. Fried bananas on custard is a typical Vietnamese dessert.

Wild mushrooms grow in Laos, where the national dish is larb, a meat salad made with meat and ground toasted rice mixed with minced chili peppers, mint, and vegetables, and seasoned with fish sauce and lime.

Indonesia

Indonesia spans more than 15,000 islands in the Pacific Ocean covering nearly 800,000 square miles. The major islands are Java, Bali, Borneo, Sumatra, and Celebes. Indonesia crosses the equator and lies between Australia and the Asian mainland. Turmeric, cloves, nutmeg, mace, and cinnamon thrive in this tropical zone. Fruits such as oranges, mandarins, grapefruits, mangoes, bananas, pineapples, papayas, avocados, and coconuts are plentiful. Coffee is a major crop.

A condiment unique to Indonesia and other parts of Southeast Asia is a soy sauce called ketjap manis. It is thick, syrupy, and sweet because sugar is added. Other typical seasonings include coconut, lemongrass, shrimp paste, and chiles.

The Philippines

The cuisine of the Philippines shows a blend of influences, including native Malay influences and Chinese and Spanish influences from the colonial era. Rice is eaten at most meals, and seafood is the most important ingredient. Kinilaw is fish preserved in a vinegar-and-salt mixture.

Filipino noodles, called pansit, are made with rice flour and typically sautéed with garlic. Lumpia are spring rolls dipped in a soy sauce, vinegar, and garlic mixture. The main vegetables used are sweet potatoes, tomatoes, cabbage, and eggplant. Spanish influence shows in dishes such as paellas, Spanish sausage, and tortas. Coconuts, tomatoes, and bananas are frequent additions to meals.

Light and Healthy Recipe

Beef and Broccoli with Hoisin Sauce

Served with rice, this is a complete, low-calorie dinner that is high in fiber and antioxidants.

Ingredients

- **3 Tbsp.** Soy sauce
- **1 Tbsp.** Peanut butter
- **1 Tbsp.** Honey
- **1 Tbsp.** Rice vinegar
- **1 tsp.** Minced garlic
- **2 tsp.** Canola oil
- **¼ tsp.** Black pepper
- **1 Pound** Lean beef, sliced thin
- **1 Pound** Broccoli
- **2 cups** Rice

Directions

1. In a small bowl, mix the soy sauce, peanut butter, honey, rice vinegar, minced garlic, and black pepper. Mix briskly and chill for at least one hour.
2. Put the rice in a pot and pour in four cups of water. Bring to a boil, reduce to a simmer and let the rice cook, covered for 20 minutes on low.
3. In a large skillet or wok, stir fry the beef in the canola oil until browned on all sides. Add the broccoli and continue stir-frying until it is tender-crisp.
4. Add the sauce and mix with the broccoli and beef until the sauce is warmed through.
5. Serve over the rice.

Yield 6 servings

Nutrition Analysis per Serving

■ Calories	383
■ Total fat	16 g
Saturated fat	6 g
Cholesterol	66 mg
■ Sodium	395 mg
■ Carbohydrate	33 g
Dietary fiber	3 g
Sugars	4 g
■ Protein	26 g

CHAPTER 50 Review & Applications

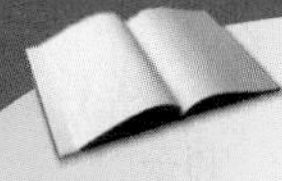

After You Read

Chapter Summary

The cuisines of South, East, and Southeast Asia are diverse, vibrant, and flavorful, and include a variety of colorful ingredients and tasty dishes. The cuisine in South Asia features many elements of Indian cooking, including common Indian ingredients and popular Northern and Southern Indian dishes. East Asia includes China, Japan, and Korea. The cuisine in this region features a balance of tastes, textures, and techniques, but each nation has its own distinctive ingredients and dishes. Southeast Asia includes Laos, Thailand, Cambodia, Vietnam, Indonesia, and the Philippines. The cuisines of these nations show a blend of influences.

Content and Academic Vocabulary Review

1. Create a fill-in-the-blank sentence for each of these content and academic vocabulary words. The sentence should contain enough information to help determine the missing word.

Content Vocabulary

- curry (p. 769)
- dal (p. 769)
- chutney (p. 769)
- tandoor (p. 769)
- daikon (p. 771)
- hoisin (p. 771)
- dim sum (p. 772)
- sashimi (p. 774)
- sushi (p. 774)
- nori (p. 774)
- kimchi (p. 774)

Academic Vocabulary

- tailor (p. 769)
- signature (p. 773)

Review Key Concepts

2. Compare and contrast Northern Indian cuisine and Southern Indian cuisine.
3. Describe popular dishes from China, Japan, and Korea.
4. Identify popular dishes from Laos, Thailand, Cambodia, and Vietnam.

Critical Thinking

5. Describe how spices have the power to make cuisine diverse, and give examples.
6. Explain how spiritual beliefs can influence the cuisine in an entire region, and give one example.
7. Infer at least one reason why Chinese cuisine, unlike other cuisines, shows little outside influence.
8. List three advantages of cooking at the table in a hot pot.
9. Identify one reason why Japan is the world's largest consumer of seafood, and explain your reasoning.
10. Explain why Javier, a resident of Spain, ate food while on vacation in Southeast Asia and said, "Mmm…this reminds me of home!"

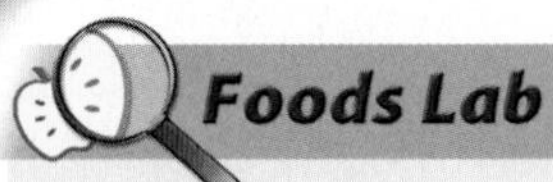

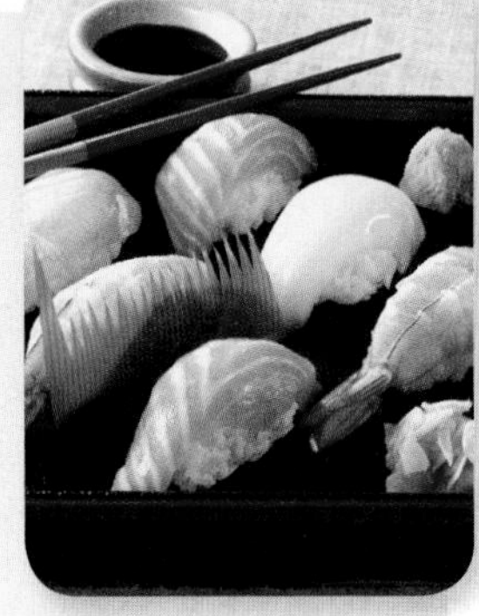

11. Traditional Serving Styles Foods in the cuisines of South, East, and Southeast Asia are often served in a particular style or arrangment to maximize their appeal.

Procedure Learn how a particular dish described in the chapter is traditionally served. Demonstrate this technique for the class. If possible, use authentic foods, serving pieces, and table settings.

Analysis Discuss how this method of serving compares to that used in typical American meals. How do you think this way of serving reflects the culture's philosophy of cooking or sharing meals?

HEALTHFUL CHOICES

12. Choosing a Cooking Method Gina is eating dinner at a Chinese restaurant. The menu offers a variety of foods that may be prepared using one of three common Chinese cooking methods: stir-frying, steaming, or deep-frying. Gina would like to order bass, because it is nutritious, high in protein, and low in fat. Which cooking method should she choose to avoid adding any additional fat to her fish?

TECH Connection

13. Menu Interpretation Obtain a menu from a restaurant that serves cuisine from one of the countries described in the chapter. For example, you may use a menu from an restaurant that serves Indian food. Choose five unfamiliar terms from the menu that are related to dishes, such as korma and vindaloo. Use the Internet to research what the terms mean. Find out how they are made and what ingredients they are made of. Explain the terms to the class.

Real-World Skills

Problem-Solving Skills

14. Avoiding Meat Pia wants to share her Indian culture with her date, a strict vegetarian, by taking him out to dinner for some Indian food. Their community has two Indian restaurants. One specializes in Southern Indian cuisine. The other specializes in Northern Indian cusine. Which restaurant should Pia take her date to and why?

Interpersonal and Collaborative Skills

15. Country Study Follow your teacher's instructions to form groups. Work together to research a country in South, East, or Southeast Asia that has been assigned to your group. Create a posterboard display to educate others about the country's history, geography, culture, and aspects of its cuisine, including some that are not mentioned in the chapter.

Financial Literacy Skills

16. Calculate Cost Yuri is selling coco pista pasands, an Indian dessert, for $2.50 each. In order to make a profit, he has priced each coco pista pasand at 100 percent higher than it cost him to make. How much did it cost Yuri to make a recipe for 12 coco pista pasands?

Academic Skills

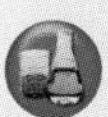

Food Science

17. Steeping and Extraction Making a tea infusion comes from extracting chemicals from tea leaves into water by steeping. The concentration of water soluble chemicals is dependent on time and temperature.

Procedure Bring a pot of water to a boil. Set up three Styrofoam cups, each with a tea bag. Ladle in boiling water to each cup until ¾ full. Remove the tea bag from one cup after one minute. Remove the second tea bag after three minutes and the third after five minutes. Compare color, aroma, and taste. Now add a squirt of lemon to each, and compare.

Analysis Write one or more paragraphs to explain the effect of infusion time on the tea strength. Include details about how each sample looks, tastes, and smells.

NSES B Develop an understanding of the structure and properties of matter, motions, and forces.

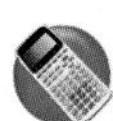

Mathematics

18. Food Fair Along with several of her classmates, Serena organized an Asian food fair at her school, where students made and shared a variety of Asian delicacies. Tickets to the event cost $2.50 each for students, and $5 each for everyone else. The event was a success, with 224 people purchasing tickets. If Serena collected a total of $775 from ticket sales, how many student tickets were sold, and how many regular tickets were sold?

Math Concept **Distributive Property of Multiplication** Multiplying a sum by a number is the equivalent of multiplying each addend by that same number, and then adding the two products. For example, $7(4 + 2)$ is the same as $(7 \times 4) + (7 \times 2)$.

Starting Hint Let s stand for the number of student tickets sold. Then, the number of regular tickets sold must equal $(224 - s)$. Solve for s in the equation $(\$2.50)(s) + (\$5)(224 - s) = \$775$.

NCTM Algebra Use mathematical models to represent and understand quantitative relationships.

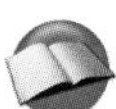

English Language Arts

19. Travel Advertisement Write a magazine advertisement that will encourage readers to travel to one of the countries mentioned in the chapter. The advertisement should highlight the country's cuisine and explain why it is appealing for adventurous travelers.

NCTE 4 Use written language to communicate effectively.

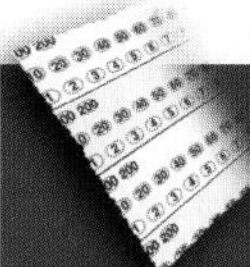

STANDARDIZED TEST PRACTICE

READING COMPREHENSION

Re-read the section about North and South Korea on pages 774–775. Then select the best answer to the question.

20. During bulgogi, what do diners dip their slices of beef in after grilling it?

a. a hot pot
b. boiling water
c. hot pepper sauce
d. kimchi

Test-Taking Tip Before you answer a reading comprehension question, closely read the text to which the question refers. Some answers may seem identical, but they contain subtle differences. Pay attention to every word.

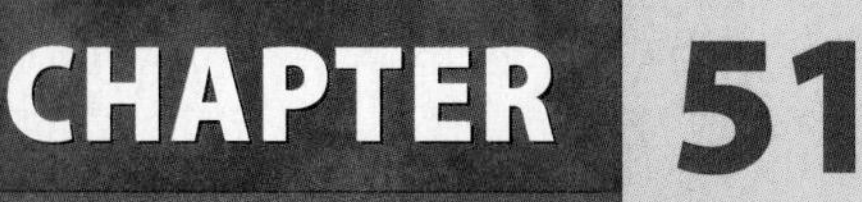

CHAPTER 51

Foods of Southwest Asia, the Middle East, & Africa

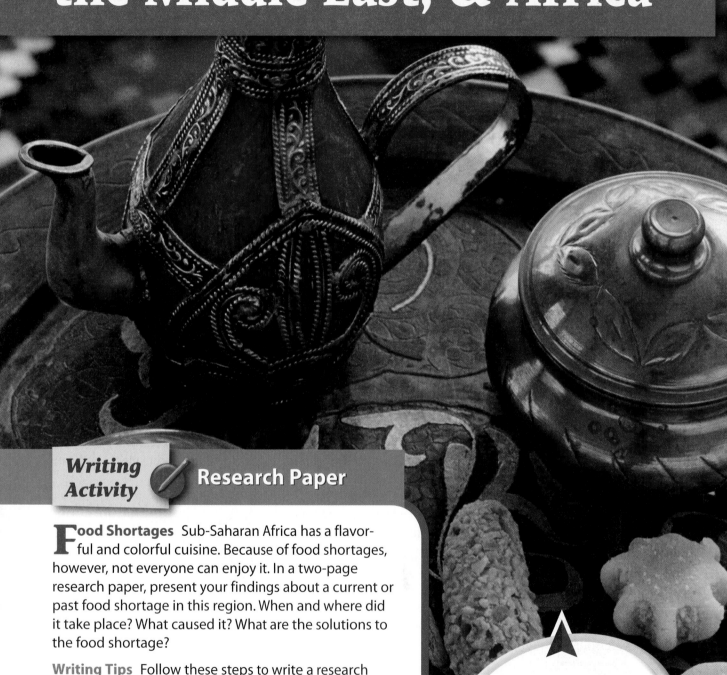

Writing Activity — Research Paper

Food Shortages Sub-Saharan Africa has a flavorful and colorful cuisine. Because of food shortages, however, not everyone can enjoy it. In a two-page research paper, present your findings about a current or past food shortage in this region. When and where did it take place? What caused it? What are the solutions to the food shortage?

Writing Tips Follow these steps to write a research paper:

- Use a variety of research sources.
- Present findings in your own words and/or quote sources correctly.
- Include a bibliography.

Activate Prior Knowledge

Explore the Photo Almonds are a basic ingredient in many Tunisian pastries. *What African nations can you name?*

Reading Guide

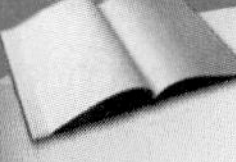

Before You Read

Preview Examine the photos and figures and read their captions. Think about the possible similarities between cuisines in Southwest Asia, North Africa, and sub-Saharan Africa.

Read to Learn

Key Concepts

- **Describe** ingredients common to the cuisine of Southwest Asia.
- **Explain** how access to multiple water sources affects the cuisine of North Africa.
- **List** spices typical to sub-Saharan African cuisine.

Main Idea

The cuisines of Southwest Asia, North Africa, and sub-Saharan Africa are bold, flavorful, and colorful, with diverse ingredients and dishes.

Content Vocabulary

You will find definitions for these words in the glossary at the back of this book.

- ☐ tahini
- ☐ sumac
- ☐ saffron
- ☐ meze
- ☐ tagine
- ☐ injera

Academic Vocabulary

You will find these words in your reading and on your tests. Use the glossary to look up their definitions if necessary.

- interconnected
- essential

Graphic Organizer

Use a graphic organizer like the one below to note grains, spices, meats, fruits and vegetables common to Southwest Asia, the Middle East, and Africa.

	GRAINS	SPICES	MEATS	FRUITS	VEGETABLES
SOUTHWEST ASIA AND THE MIDDLE EAST					
NORTH AFRICA					
SUB-SAHARAN AFRICA					

Graphic Organizer Go to this book's Online Learning Center at **glencoe.com** to print out this graphic organizer.

Academic Standards

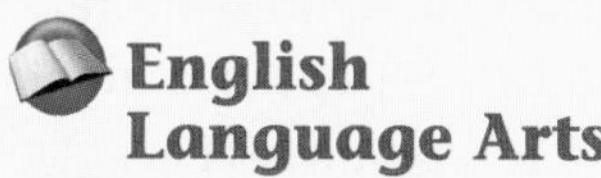

English Language Arts

NCTE 4 Use written language to communicate effectively.

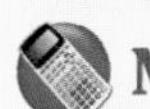

Mathematics

NCTM Number and Operations Compute fluently and make reasonable estimates.

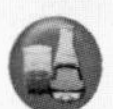

Science

NSES B Develop an understanding of chemical reactions.

NCTE *National Council of Teachers of English*
NCTM *National Council of Teachers of Mathematics*
NSES *National Science Education Standards*
NCSS *National Council for the Social Studies*

Southwest Asia and the Middle East

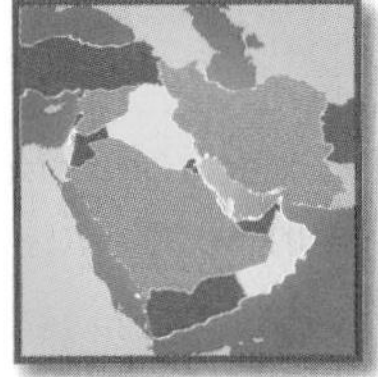

Southwest Asia includes the Middle East and neighboring countries such as Turkey, Afghanistan, and Armenia. The Middle East lies across the Black Sea from Eastern Europe and across the Red Sea from Africa. Most of the countries in the Middle East share an Arab heritage and a Muslim religious tradition. Saudia Arabia, Iran, and Iraq are the largest countries in the Middle East. The area also includes many smaller countries, including Lebanon, Syria, Qatar, Oman, Yemen, and Israel. Israel is a Jewish state in which many Arabs also reside. Egypt, in Africa, is sometimes also considered part of the Middle East. **Figure 51.1** shows the **interconnected**, or related, regions of Southwest Asia and Africa.

People have lived in the Middle East since at least 10,000 BCE Farming began here, and it continues along the great rivers of the region: the Tigris, the Euphrates, the Nile, and the Jordan, as well as in Lebanon's Bekaa Valley. Wheat and barley were among the region's earliest crops. Rice, sugarcane, and olives were grown later. Today, irrigated fields and hothouses produce a wide range of vegetables and fruits, from cabbage and potatoes to bananas and watermelon.

Figure 51.1 Africa and Southwest Asia

Cultural Influences The culture of Africa is influenced by the many countries that colonized it, including France, Britain, Portugal, Germany, Belgium, and Italy. Southwest Asian countries are influenced by the Muslim culture. ***What geographical factor might explain the close ties between the cuisine of the Middle East and the cuisine of North Africa?***

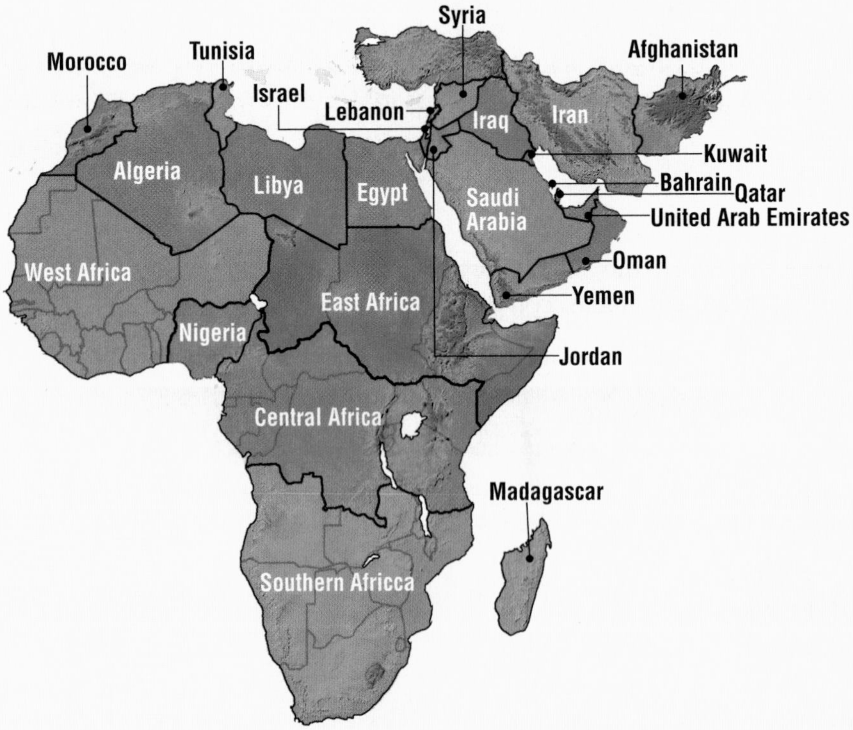

Southwest Asian Ingredients

Ingredients in Southwest Asian dishes draw on food traditions from around the Mediterranean and Asia. Lamb and chicken are favored for main dishes, and goat is often served, as well. Seafood is served both fresh and preserved in olive oil. Fish and shellfish, including grouper, snapper, tuna, sea bream, shrimp, and prawns, are caught in the Mediterranean Sea and Persian Gulf. Nile perch from East Africa is served both fresh and dried.

Yogurt, called laban or labneh, is a main ingredient in many Southwest Asian dishes. Many cooks make their own. Yogurt is eaten plain or with cucumbers and raisins. It is sometimes stirred into dishes and served as a sauce. A diluted, lightly salted yogurt drink is served throughout this region. Iranians call it abdug. Afghanis call it dugh and serve it with mint.

Grains are crucial to Southwest Asian cooking. Wheat is used for baking, and rice and bulgur are used in many dishes. Arab cooks often prepare basmati rice, a long-grain, aromatic variety from Pakistan and India.

Favorite fruits include lemons, oranges, dates, figs, grapes, raisins, and quince. Eggplant, spinach, zucchini, artichokes, tomatoes, and okra are popular vegetables in this region. Legumes such as garbanzo beans, fava beans, and lentils are frequently served. Sesame seeds are used whole, pressed for oil, and ground into a thick paste called **tahini**. Almonds, walnuts, and pistachios also have many uses in Southwest Asian recipes.

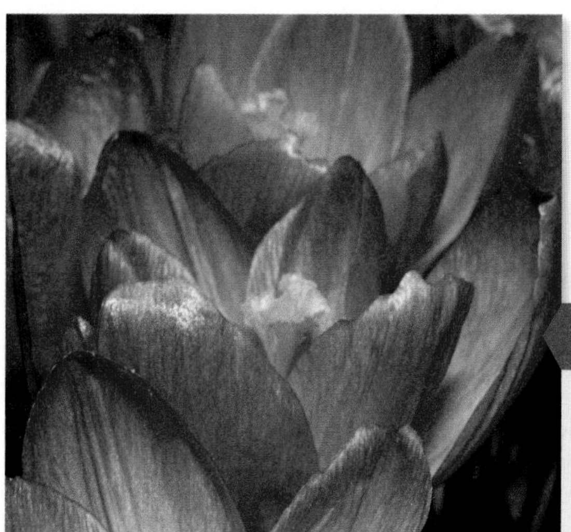

A Flower with Spice

Because of the labor involved in separating and drying the spice saffron from the crocus flower, saffron is the most expensive spice in the world by weight. *What dishes have you had that contain saffron?*

Be a Smart Consumer

Splurging on Saffron

For several decades, saffron has been the world's most expensive spice by weight. Why? Saffron crocus flowers bloom for only 1 to 2 weeks, and it takes 150 flowers to yield 1 gram of dry saffron threads. Saffron prices can range from 500 to 5,000 dollars per pound. Cost is also determined by the quality of the spice. Saffron is graded on a scale of one to four according to the quality of its taste, color, and fragrance.

Challenge Find three examples of saffron for sale from online retailers. Find the average cost per gram.

Southwest Asian Seasonings

Seasonings are as important as main ingredients in Southwest Asian cooking. Vegetables, rice, beans, and meat are often spiced with coriander, cardamom, cinnamon, ginger, turmeric, and allspice. **Sumac**, a deep-red native berry usually used ground, adds a fruity tartness. **Saffron**, the thread-like center of the crocus flower, turns rice a brilliant yellow and adds a pungent flavor. Pastries are made aromatic with rose water, orange blossom water, or mahleb, the almond-flavored ground kernel of sour cherry pits.

Mint, parsley, dill, and cilantro are among the most common herbs. Many cooks create their own combinations of zatar, a seasoning blend that includes marjoram, thyme, sumac, and salt. Olive oil flavors salads and cooked dishes. Honey, nuts, and fruits are also used as seasonings in dishes.

Southwest Asian Dishes

Breakfast is a light meal in the Southwest Asian diet, often consisting of labneh (a strained yogurt with the consistency of soft cheese) on a flatbread. Marcook, a dome-shaped flatbread, is baked on the surface of a rounded pan. Taboun, a thick Palestinian loaf, is traditionally baked on hot rocks in a round oven of the same name. Watermelon seeds are eaten as a snack. Kanafeh is a common dessert, made with finely shredded pastry noodles with honey-sweetened cheese. Many desserts are filled with nuts, including almonds, walnuts, and pistachios. A Lebanese favorite is the zatar-topped manakeesh, a flat tart with various savory spices.

The midday meal is the main meal of the day in Southwest Asia. It often starts with **meze** (me-ˈzā), or appetizers. Common appetizers include hummus, puréed garbanzo beans seasoned with tahini and sometimes garlic, and baba ghannoush, a seasoned purée of eggplant. Hummus and baba ghannoush are both served with strips of pita bread. You might find falafel (fə-ˈlä-fəl), fried patties of seasoned ground garbanzo beans, served with tahini or yogurt dipping sauce. Fatayer is a turnover filled with a combination of foods, including minced meat, cheese, cooked onions, pine nuts, and spinach. Sesame seeds are used in flatbreads and tarts. The most commonly used meat in the area is lamb.

Vegetables and legumes appear in side dishes as well as meze. Fresh salads are built around cucumbers, tomatoes, and onions. Tabbouleh (tə-ˈbü-lə) combines chopped parsley, tomatoes, onions, and bulgur with mint, lemon juice, and olive oil. Eggplant, cabbage, grape leaves, and zucchini are stuffed with rice, nuts, and other vegetables to make dolmas. Vegetables are also sliced, breaded, and fried. Lentils are added to soups and pilafs. Often-used spices include mint, black pepper, cinnamon, and allspice.

Careers in Food

Allan Borgen
Radio Host

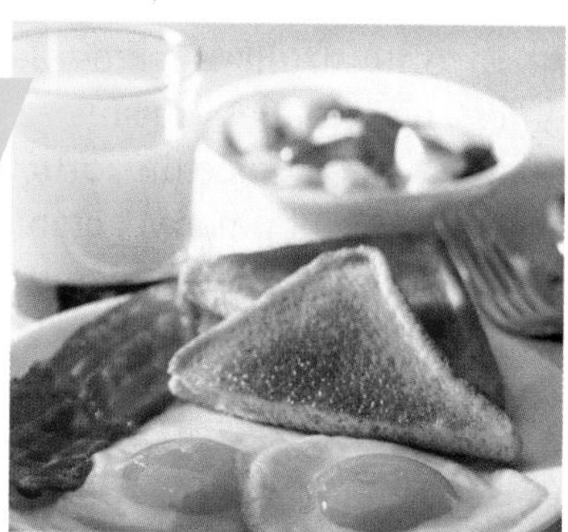

Q: What was your career path?

A: I have always had an interest in food and culture. I worked at various restaurants through high school, and I took chef training at a trade school in Los Angeles. At one point, I was offered the chance to write a weekly review. I was given $100 per week and paid for my food, and I thought it was the ideal opportunity. I had an idea to do a TV show and convinced the local station to do it. It ran for 18 years. I needed another outlet, so I started the radio show.

Q: What background do you need to host a radio show about food besides just knowing about food?

A: Every business has little things you have to know. The big thing is knowing about food, if you want to do a food show. You learn the other stuff as you go.

"Food brings people together no matter what their background or culture."
—Allan Borgen
Host of "Let's Dine Out," KTIE-590 A.M.
– San Bernardino, CA

Education and Training

It is important to have education or training in a culinary environment. An understanding of the language of food, and the ability to speak clearly are required. Formal training in broadcasting is an asset.

Qualities and Skills

To be a professional food critic, you have to be so passionate about it that you can tell people about it in a way that makes them want to watch or listen to you to learn more.

Related Career Opportunities

Work in other aspects of radio, as a producer or copy writer are related jobs. Food writers for newspapers, magazines, and Web sites write about food instead of talking about it.

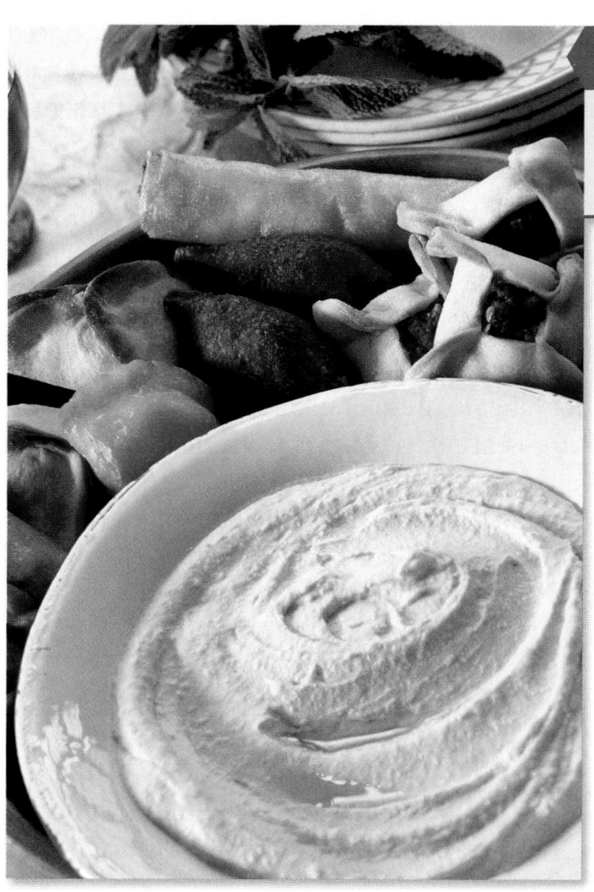

Hummus

Hummus is a Southwest Asian dish made of puréed garbanzo beans seasoned with tahini and sometimes garlic. *What is a typical breakfast in Southwest Asia?*

Many main dishes balance meats with grain and vegetables. Kebabs are small pieces or patties of meat, fish, or shellfish threaded on skewers and grilled. Kebabs are usually served over rice. Kibbeh, the national dish of Lebanon and Syria, is a baked dish made by layering mixtures of ground lamb or beef with onions. Some recipes use bulgur, and others use pine nuts. Iranian cooks combine meat with fruits in zerkeshk polo, rice with chicken, raisins, and bright red barberries.

Fish is eaten in coastal regions. Whitefish is baked with tahini and pine nuts. Shrimp kebabs are basted with a garlic-seasoned yogurt marinade. Chebeh rubyan is a dish made up of balls of ground shrimp and rice, stuffed with onions and simmered in a sauce of tomato and tamarind.

Coffee (kahwah) symbolizes hospitality throughout the Arab world. Coffee is often made in the Turkish style: boiled three times, sweetened, and sometimes spiced with cardamom.

Desserts include fresh and dried fruit and halvah, bars of candy made with ground sesame seeds, honey, and sometimes nuts. Katayef contains sweetened cheese or cream custard between shredded pastry dough, sweetened with syrup. Mamoul, nut-filled semolina cookies, are a tradition on the Islamic holiday Eid al-Fitr.

Israeli Cuisine

Israeli cuisine features many dishes that are served throughout the Middle East. Falafel, for example, is as common in Israel as it is in Jordan and Lebanon. Falafel is a small croquette of mashed chickpeas or fava beans seasoned with sesame seeds. Other Israeli dishes were brought by Jewish immigrants from other parts of the world, especially Eastern Europe. The knish, a turnover filled with potatoes, cheese, kasha, or chicken liver, is similar to a Polish pierogi. Bourekas are cheese-filled pastries similar to Serbia's burek. They are a popular street food. Ethiopian immigrants have introduced curry powder and chiles to Israeli cuisine. Pita bread is sometimes referred to as the national bread of Israel. It is used to scoop dips or it is filled.

Foods that can be prepared in advance are **essential**, or necessary, for the Jewish Sabbath (sundown Friday to sundown Saturday), when work is prohibited. Cholent, a stew of beans, potatoes, barley, and sometimes meat, is started Friday and cooked overnight. Lokshen kugel (noodle pudding) is often baked at the same time.

✓ **Reading Check** **Identify** Which is the main meal of the day in Southwest Asia?

North Africa

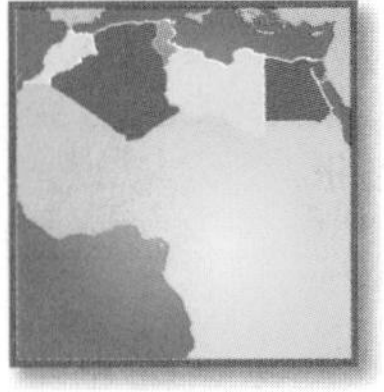

The hot and dry Sahara Desert sweeps across most of North Africa, prompting people to live by the Mediterranean coast or along rivers. The countries of North Africa, including Egypt, Libya, Tunisia, Algeria, and Morocco, share many Middle Eastern food traditions. The Nile River stretches through Egypt and Sudan, providing water for crops such as wheat, barley, dates, nuts, olives, potatoes, and citrus fruits. Chickens, sheep, cattle, and goats are raised throughout North Africa, and seafood is caught in the Atlantic Ocean and the Mediterranean Sea.

North African Dishes

North African foods show the influence of the Arab culture. The main grain is couscous, which is cooked by steaming. Traditionally, it is set over a simmering meat or vegetable stew to absorb moisture and flavor. Couscous is also sweetened with sugar and dried fruit to make breakfast cereal.

North African cooks use a variety of hot spices. Harissa, a garlic-seasoned red pepper paste, is a common ingredient and condiment, especially in Morocco and Tunisia. Harissa is sometimes used in merguez, a spicy Tunisian lamb sausage.

National Specialties

Each nation has its own specialties. The best-known Moroccan dish is the **tagine**, a well-seasoned stew made in a covered pot, also called a tagine. Meat and fruit combinations, such as lamb with prunes, are popular. A b'stilla is a pie filled with cooked, spiced chicken in a curdled egg sauce and topped with sugar and cinnamon-coated almonds. Preserved lemons are used in many recipes.

Fava beans, called ful, are favorites in Egypt. Egyptian falafel uses locally grown, small, brown fava beans rather than garbanzo beans. Ful mesdames, a thick stew of lightly mashed beans garnished with cooked eggs, is eaten at many different meals.

Libya was an Italian colony in the early 20th century, and its cuisine features several macaroni dishes. In Tunisia, a turnover called brik has a filling that includes a whole egg, which is soft-cooked while the pastry surrounding it fries. In Algeria, a sweet lamb stew called el ham lahlou is made with raisins, almonds, and cinnamon. Eggs are poached over sautéed tomatoes, peppers, and onions to make chakchouka.

✓ Reading Check **Explain** Why does Libyan cuisine feature macaroni dishes?

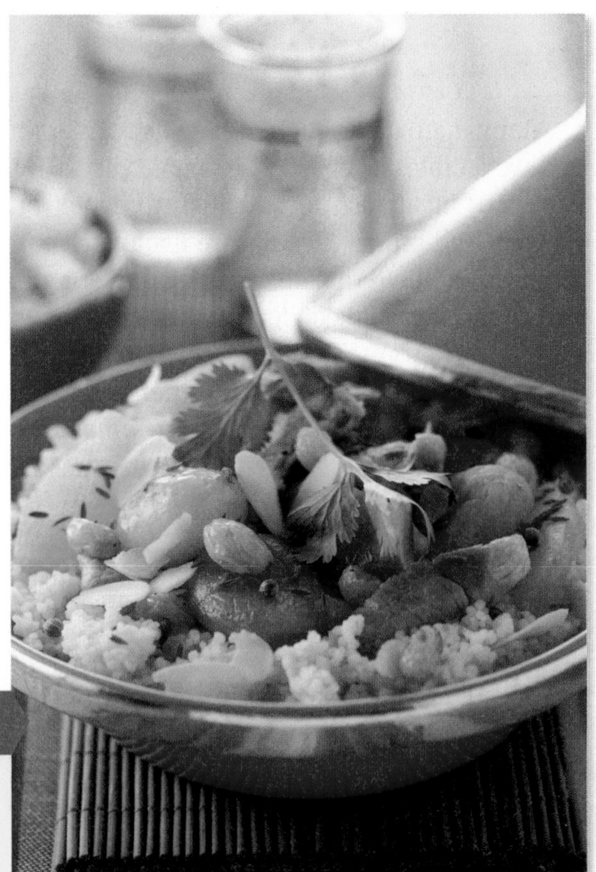

Tajine

A tajine is a dish named for the special dish in which it is cooked. *From what nation does the tajine originate?*

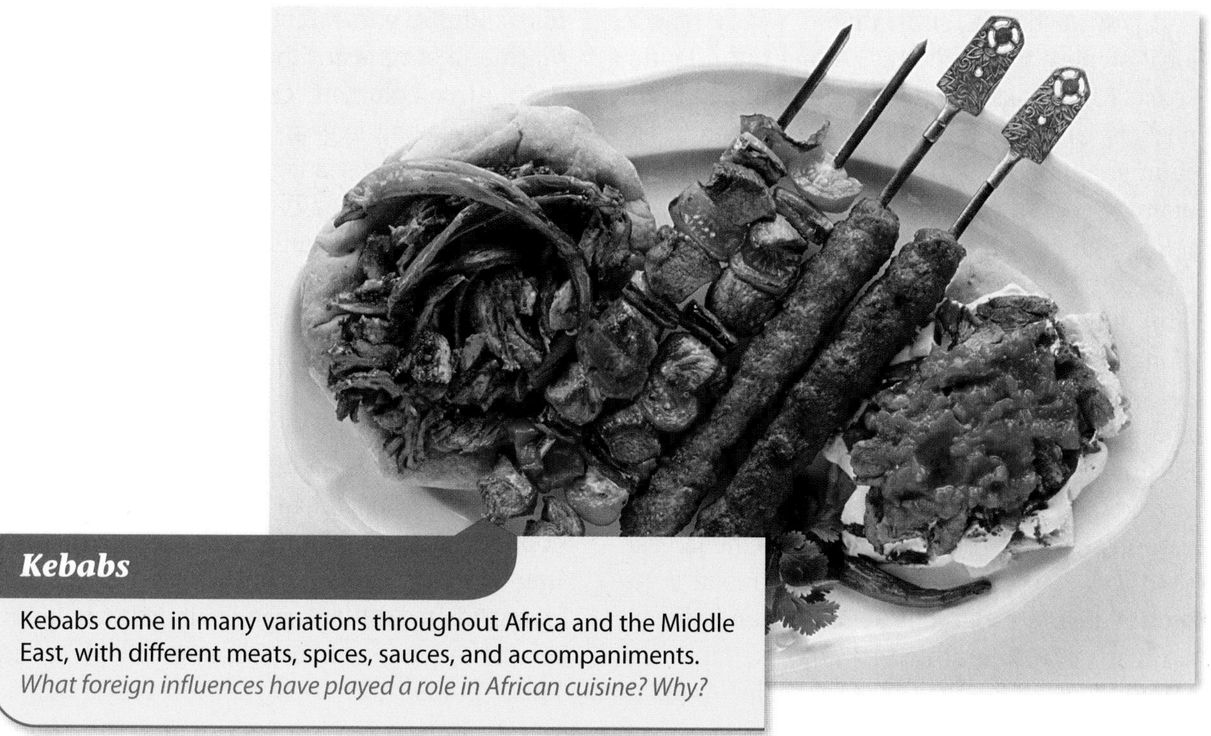

Kebabs

Kebabs come in many variations throughout Africa and the Middle East, with different meats, spices, sauces, and accompaniments. *What foreign influences have played a role in African cuisine? Why?*

Sub-Saharan Africa

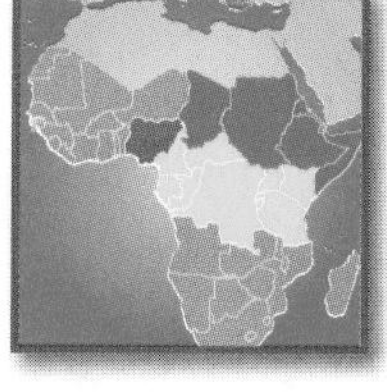

The African countries south of the Sahara Desert are known as sub-Saharan Africa. They have an enormous diversity of landscape, culture, language, and cuisine.

Sub-Saharan African cooking is bold in flavor and color. Staple starches include rice, corn, millet, plantains, cassava, and yams. Common legumes and vegetables include black-eyed peas, groundnuts (peanuts), tomatoes, sweet peppers, squash, okra, and greens of all types, from beet leaves to spinach. Meatless meals are common, but so are meals with chicken, guinea fowl, beef, fish, or goat. Chiles, red and black pepper, onions, garlic, cinnamon, nutmeg, ginger, peanut butter, and coconut milk add sweetness and heat. Banana, guava, papaya, and other tropical fruits are grown in many areas of sub-Saharan Africa.

Sub-Saharan Dishes

Ingredients and recipes vary greatly among the regions of sub-Saharan Africa. Customs and ingredients sometimes blend local crops and traditions with French, English, Dutch, Belgian, German, Spanish, Italian, or Portuguese influences, due to a long history of colonization by European countries.

Stew with grains is a typical main meal. A common stew base is moambé, a broth made of palm nut pulp seasoned with sauce. In central Africa, stews sometimes feature the peppery egusi sauce, a blend of ground roasted squash seeds and tomato paste. In Ethiopia, a popular seasoning is berberé paste, which includes red pepper, fenugreek, allspice, cloves, cardamom, and turmeric.

Rice often accompanies stew in African meals. Mashed cassava is common in Central Africa, as are mashed yams in West Africa. Both foods are locally known as fufu. East Africa's ugali and Southern Africa's mealie meal both refer to a mound of fine cornmeal porridge, shaped and used as an edible scoop. Ethiopians use injera at many meals. **Injera** is a thin, spongy, flatbread made from a hardy grain called teff. The bread is torn into bits and used to scoop meats, legumes and vegetables. Ethiopia is the birthplace of coffee, and an elaborate ceremony for preparing and serving coffee is often performed. Kenyans serve stew in a ring of irio, a mash of peas, potatoes, corn, and greens.

Many dishes in sub-Saharan Africa reflect local staples and traditions. Along the Atlantic coast, fish steaks or fillets are often filled with pockets of peppery stuffing, fried, and then simmered in a tomato broth. Senegal's thiebou dienn, a rice and fish stew, is made this way. In other regions, grasshoppers, ants, and caterpillars are used in cooking. Peanuts are a primary crop in Senegal. They are used in many meals, along with couscous, bananas, and black-eyed peas. For example, they are fried with onions and peppers in a peanut sauce. Central African cuisine features plantains and cassava. The cassava root is one of the most widely consumed carbohydrates in the world. Africa is the largest producer. A popular dish is a stew made from ground peanuts with chicken, okra, and ginger.

Just as in Southwest Asia, kebabs are popular in sub-Saharan Africa. In Angola, for example, you might find beef kebabs in a marinade of piri-piri, the fiery chile brought by Portuguese colonists. On Africa's east coast, a common kebab is goat with garlic, ginger, and curry powder. In Madagascar, a large island off Africa's east coast, a typical meal features rice topped with a seasonal vegetable, such as peas flavored with pork.

South African cuisine shows influences of the Dutch, German, and French settlers who created the nation's Afrikaner ethnic group. Typical South African dishes include boerewors, a sausage made with beef and spices, and hoender pastei, a pie of chicken, hard-cooked eggs, and ham, seasoned with pickling spices. A cuisine known as Cape Dutch is found in South Africa. It is known for its use of spices such as nutmeg, allspice, and hot peppers.

Light and Healthy Recipe

Injera

Ingredients

- **1 ½ cups** Warm water
- **¼ tsp.** Dry active yeast
- **¼ cup** Teff or wheat flour
- **¾ cup** All-purpose flour
- **1 tsp.** Plain yogurt
- **¼ tsp.** Salt
- **1 Tbsp.** Vegetable oil

Teff is a grain rich in iron and fiber. Teff flour gives injera a slightly sour taste.

Directions

1. Add the yeast to the warm water and mix gently until the yeast is dissolved.
2. In a large bowl, combine the flours, yogurt, and salt with the yeast and water and mix. Cover the mixture and allow it to ferment overnight.
3. Heat a wide pan on high until a drop of water will sizzle on it. Then coat the pan with oil and add enough of the batter to just cover the bottom of the pan in a thin layer.
4. When the dough has changed colors and starts to curl at the edges, it is finished. Remove it from the pan with a spatula and repeat until all the batter is cooked.

Yield 6 servings

Nutrition Analysis per Serving

Calories	97
Total fat	3 g
Saturated fat	0 g
Cholesterol	0 mg
Sodium	101 mg
Carbohydrate	16 g
Dietary fiber	1 g
Sugars	0 g
Protein	2 g

CHAPTER 51 Review & Applications

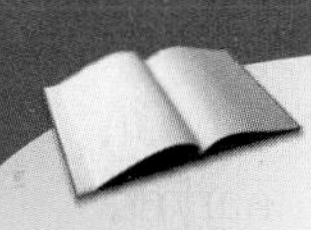

After You Read

Chapter Summary

The cuisines of Southwest Asia, North Africa, and sub-Saharan Africa are bold, flavorful, and colorful, with diverse ingredients and dishes. Southwest Asia includes the Middle East and neighboring countries. Its cuisine consists of a variety of ingredients and seasonings, as well as Israeli traditions. North African cuisine is influenced by Arab cultures. Each North African nation has its own specialties. The countries in sub-Saharan Africa have an enormous diversity of cuisine. Many dishes reflect the influence of countries that have colonized sub-Saharan Africa, while others reflect local staples and traditions.

Content and Academic Vocabulary Review

1. Use each of these content and academic vocabulary words in a sentence.

Content Vocabulary

- tahini (p. 783)
- sumac (p. 783)
- saffron (p. 783)
- meze (p. 784)
- tagine (p. 786)
- injera (p. 787)

Academic Vocabulary

- interconnected (p. 782)
- essential (p. 785)

Review Key Concepts

2. **Describe** ingredients common to the cuisine of Southwest Asia.
3. **Explain** how access to multiple water sources affects the cuisine of North Africa.
4. **List** spices typical to sub-Saharan African cuisine.

Critical Thinking

5. **Determine** three characteristics of Southwest Asian cuisine that you think make it a healthful cuisine, and explain why.
6. **Explain** why Josepha will probably eat foods with origins in Europe while on her trip to Israel.
7. **Assess** the nutritional advantages of cooking couscous by steaming, as North Africans do, rather than the typical method of cooking grains by simmering them in water.
8. **Compare** one of the national specialties of the North African region and a dish you learned about in a different chapter of this book. Explain their similarities and differences.
9. **Evaluate** whether berbere paste, a popular seasoning in Ethiopia, probably has a cool, mild taste. Do you agree? Why or why not?
10. **Identify** a food that you read about in Chapter 50 that is used similarly to the way injera is used in Ethiopia.

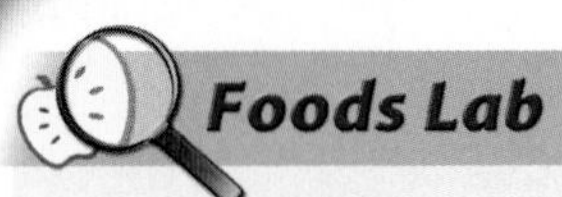

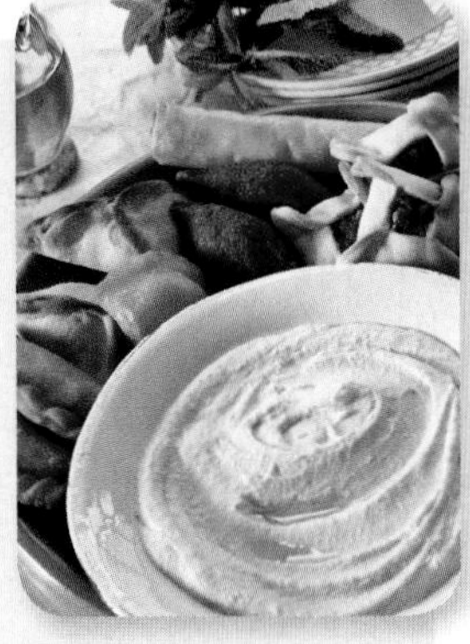

11. Hummus Recipes Hummus plays a significant role in Middle-Eastern cuisine. Different ingredients and seasonings are added to puréed garbanzo beans to create various hummus recipes.

Procedure Find and prepare a recipe for hummus. Experiment and create a dish using hummus as a spread, filling, or dip. Share samples of your hummus with the class.

Analysis Write a paragraph answering the following question: What ingredients made your hummus distinctive? How did the taste, texture, and appearance of your hummus compare to that of other lab teams? What makes your hummus healthful?

HEALTHFUL CHOICES

12. Sweet Bars Will is craving a sweet treat, such as a candy bar. At the supermarket, he is torn between a candy bar made of milk chocolate and caramel, which contains added sugar, or a Middle Eastern-style bar called a halvah that he has never tried. Research halvah and how it is made. Identify which bar is the healthier choice for Will.

TECH Connection

13. Recipe Book Use the Internet or cookbooks to find recipes for five dishes mentioned in this chapter. Use word processing software to neatly type the recipes. Decide on a standard set of style rules and stick to them as you type all of the recipes. Consider font style, size, and color, as well as spacing, and make recipes clear and easy to read. Arrange your selected recipes in alphabetical order, type a table of contents for the recipe book, and print it.

Real-World Skills

Problem-Solving Skills

14. Middle Eastern Meal Imagine you are going to host a dinner party for eight people. The theme is Middle Eastern foods. Plan the menu. Find recipes for each dish. Ensure that each recipe serves eight, or adjust it accordingly. Make a shopping list of ingredients. Then develop a work plan for preparing the meal.

Interpersonal and Collaborative Skills

15. Country Study Follow your teacher's instructions to form groups. Work together to research a country in Southwest Asia, North Africa, or sub-Saharan Africa that has been assigned to your group. Create a 5-minute video that will educate others about the country's history, geography, and culture, and aspects of its cuisine not mentioned in the chapter.

Financial Literacy Skills

16. Serving Cost Lilah prepared a kibbeh in a large baking dish. The cost of ingredients required to prepare enough kibbeh to fill the dish was $12. Lilah then cut the kibbeh into 36 small pieces to be served at a party. Jerome, a party guest, took 4 pieces. How much money was his portion of kibbeh worth?

Academic Skills

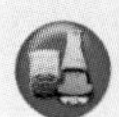

Food Science

Yogurt as Thickener Yogurt is used in many Southwest Asian and Middle Eastern dishes. Yogurt is a fermented milk product that can be used as a thickener because the casein (protein) has already been coagulated, and the whey drained.

Procedure Combine 1 tablespoon olive oil, 1 teaspoon vinegar, and 1 clove of crushed garlic, beating well in a mixing bowl. Add 1 peeled, finely diced cucumber, 1 tablespoon fresh chopped mint, ½ teaspoon salt, and 8 ounces of plain yogurt. Mix well, and chill before serving as a dipping sauce.

Analysis Conduct research to find out how an emulsion can be stabilized by a protein thickener. Write a paragraph on your finding and the results of your food science experiment.

NSES B Develop an understanding of chemical reactions.

Mathematics

18. **Making Falafel** Courtney is attempting to prepare a falafel dinner for her family, which consists of five people (including Courtney). She has a recipe that will produce about 40 falafel balls, each 1 inch in diameter. Courtney would like to make larger falafel that are 2 inches in diameter. She would also like each person to get at least 3 falafel. Will the existing recipe yield enough to meet Courtney's needs?

Math Concept **Volume of a Sphere** The volume (V) of a sphere (or ball) is calculated using the formula $V = \frac{4}{3}\pi r^3$, where r is the radius (or ½ of the diameter) of the sphere. Use 3.14 for π.

Starting Hint Use the volume formula to find the volume of a 2-inch falafel, using $r = 1$. Since Courtney needs 3 falafel per person, multiply the volume by 15 (3×5 people) to find the total volume needed. Determine if this amount is less than the total volume produced by the original recipe.

NCTM Measurement Apply appropriate techniques, tools, and formulas to determine measurements.

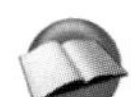

English Language Arts

19. **Recipe Book Introduction** Write a one-page introduction to the recipe book you created during the Tech Connection activity in this chapter review. Your introduction should share interesting information about the cuisines featured in your cookbook.

NCTE 4 Use written language to communicate effectively.

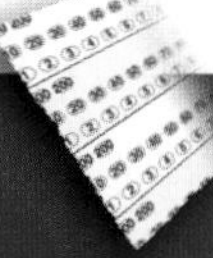

STANDARDIZED TEST PRACTICE

MULTIPLE CHOICE

Read the question and select the best answer from the choices.

20. What is the main grain in North Africa?
    - **a.** couscous
    - **b.** wheat
    - **c.** brown rice
    - **d.** tagine

Test-Taking Tip Multiple-choice questions may prompt you to select the "best" answer. They may present you with answers that seem partially true. The best answer is the one that is completely true.

UNIT 10

Thematic Project

Discover Global Foods

In this unit you have learned about foods from various regions around the world. Each country has distinct dishes and there are many variations within each country. You have also learned that different factors influence the types of foods that people eat. Geography, trade, and agriculture all influence eating patterns and food preparation practices. People living in coastal regions, for example, may eat more seafood than their inland neighbors. The crops grown in each region also offer their unique influence to the flavors of the food eaten by people of the region. In this project, you will research a cuisine from a part of the world that you are curious about and you will create a presentation about it.

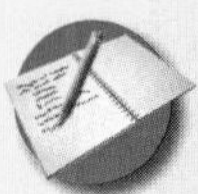

My Journal

If you completed the journal entry from page 709, refer to it to see if your thoughts have changed after reading the unit and completing this project.

Academic Skills You Will Use

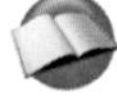

English Language Arts

NCTE 8 Use information resources to gather information and create and communicate knowledge.

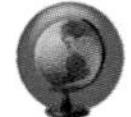

Social Studies

NCSS I A Analyze and explain the ways groups, societies, and cultures address human needs and concerns.

Project Assignment

- Conduct research about the cuisine of another culture.
- Create an outline as you conduct your research.
- Write a summary of your research.
- Collect images of ingredients, dishes, and preparation methods used in the culture you choose to research.
- Interview someone who is qualified to discuss the cuisine you choose to research.
- Use what you learn during your research to create an electronic slide show presentation.

STEP 1 Choose a Country to Research

Select an ethnic cuisine that you are interested in learning about. You can choose a cuisine you have tried before, or you can choose one you would like to try. Conduct research about the cuisine. Find out about the agriculture, geography, and culture of the place from which the cuisine originates. While you conduct your research, save electronic files of photos of maps, people, ingredients, and dishes from that cuisine. You will need them when you create your slide show presentation.

Research Skills

- Organize information from multiple sources.
- Create an outline to help organize your presentation.
- Cite your sources.

STEP 2 Write Interview Questions

Use the information you gathered in your research to write interview questions. Arrange to interview someone in your community who is qualified to discuss ingredients and preparation of the foods from the culture that you have researched. Qualified people may include a chef at a restaurant that serves the type of cuisine that you are researching, someone who comes from that region, or a teacher who is knowledgeable about the geography and customs of that area.

Writing Skills

- Use complete sentences.
- Use correct spelling and grammar.
- Organize your questions in the order you want to ask them.

STEP 3 Connect to Your Community

Use your list of interview questions and the knowledge that you have acquired through research to discuss your project with someone in your community who is qualified to offer you new information.

Interviewing Skills

- Record responses and take notes.
- Listen attentively.
- Transcribe your notes in complete sentences using correct grammar and spelling.

STEP 4 Create Your Presentation

Use the Unit Thematic Project Checklist to plan and complete your project and evaluate your work.

STEP 5 Evaluate Your Presentation

Your project will be evaluated based on:

- Logical sequence of your report.
- Content of your presentation.
- Mechanics — presentation and neatness.

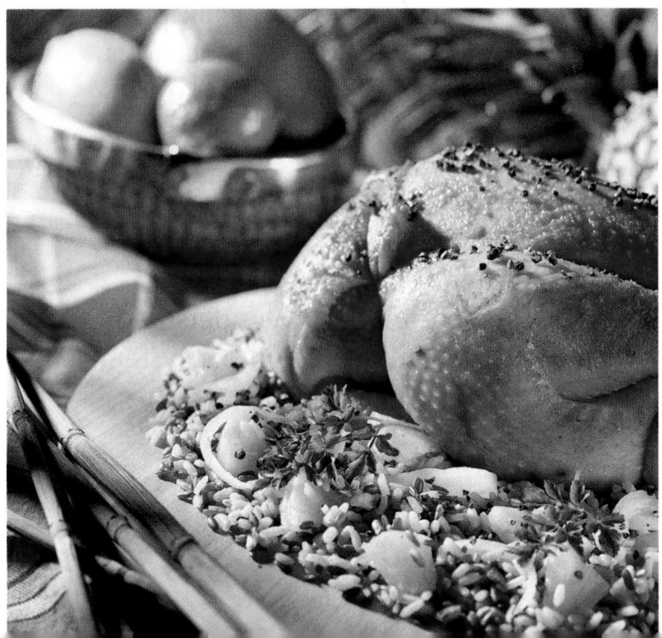

Unit Thematic Project Checklist

Category	Objectives for Your Visual
Plan	☑ Conduct research to gather information.
	☑ Write an outline of your research to help organize your presentation.
	☑ Create a slide show presentation that describes and illustrates the cusine and dishes, ingredients, and preparation methods unique to the cuisine.
Present	☑ Make a presentation to your class to share your research.
	☑ Invite the students in your class to ask you any questions that they might have.
	☑ When students ask you questions, demonstrate that you respect their perspectives.
	☑ Turn in the notes from your interview and your slide show presentation to your teacher.
Academic Skills	☑ Be sensitive to the needs of different audiences.
	☑ Adapt and modify language to suit different purposes.
	☑ Thoughtfully express your ideas.

Go to this book's Online Learning Center through **glencoe.com** for a rubric you can use to evaluate your final project.

Number and Operations

Understand numbers, ways of representing numbers, relationships among numbers, and number systems

Fraction, Decimal, and Percent

A percent is a ratio that compares a number to 100. To write a percent as a fraction, drop the percent sign, and use the number as the numerator in a fraction with a denominator of 100. Simplify, if possible. For example, 76% = $\frac{76}{100}$, or $\frac{19}{25}$. To write a fraction as a percent, convert it to an equivalent fraction with a denominator of 100. For example, $\frac{3}{4} = \frac{75}{100}$, or 75%. A fraction can be expressed as a percent by first converting the fraction to a decimal (divide the numerator by the denominator) and then converting the decimal to a percent by moving the decimal point two places to the right.

Comparing Numbers on a Number Line

In order to compare and understand the relationship between real numbers in various forms, it is helpful to use a number line. The zero point on a number line is called the origin; the points to the left of the origin are negative, and those to the right are positive. The number line below shows how numbers in fraction, decimal, percent, and integer form can be compared.

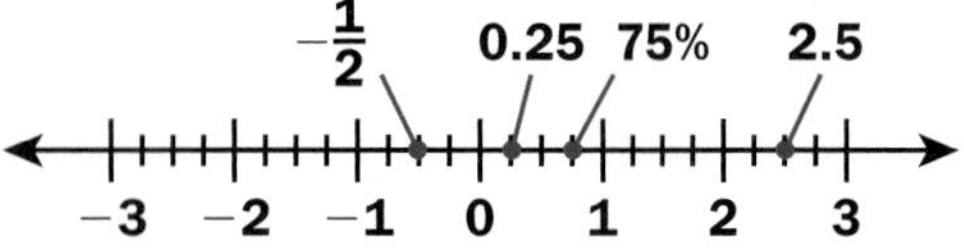

Percents Greater Than 100 and Less Than 1

Percents greater than 100% represent values greater than 1. For example, if the weight of an object is 250% of another, it is 2.5, or $2\frac{1}{2}$, times the weight.

Percents less than 1 represent values less than $\frac{1}{100}$. In other words, 0.1% is one tenth of one percent, which can also be represented in decimal form as 0.001, or in fraction form as $\frac{1}{1,000}$. Similarly, 0.01% is one hundredth of one percent or 0.0001 or $\frac{1}{10,000}$.

Ratio, Rate, and Proportion

A ratio is a comparison of two numbers using division. If a basketball player makes 8 out of 10 free throws, the ratio is written as 8 to 10, 8:10, or $\frac{8}{10}$. Ratios are usually written in simplest form. In simplest form, the ratio "8 out of 10" is 4 to 5, 4:5, or $\frac{4}{5}$. A rate is a ratio of two measurements having different kinds of units—cups per gallon, or miles per hour, for example. When a rate is simplified so that it has a denominator of 1, it is called a unit rate. An example of a unit rate is 9 miles per hour. A proportion is an equation stating that two ratios are equal. $\frac{3}{18} = \frac{13}{78}$ is an example of a proportion. The cross products of a proportion are also equal. $\frac{3}{18} = \frac{13}{78}$ and $3 \times 78 = 18 \times 13$.

Representing Large and Small Numbers

In order to represent large and small numbers, it is important to understand the number system. Our number system is based on 10, and the value of each place is 10 times the value of the place to its right.

The value of a digit is the product of a digit and its place value. For instance, in the number 6,400, the 6 has a value of six thousands and the 4 has a value of four hundreds. A place value chart can help you read numbers. In the chart, each group of three digits is called a period. Commas separate the periods: the ones period, the thousands period, the millions period, and so on. Values to the right of the ones period are decimals. By understanding place value you can write very large numbers like 5 billion and more, and very small numbers that are less than 1, like one-tenth.

Scientific Notation

When dealing with very large numbers like 1,500,000, or very small numbers like 0.000015, it is helpful to keep track of their value by writing the numbers in scientific notation. Powers of 10 with positive exponents are used with a decimal between 1 and 10 to express large numbers. The exponent represents the number of places the decimal point is moved to the right. So, 528,000 is written in scientific notation as 5.28×10^5. Powers of 10 with negative exponents are used with a decimal between 1 and 10 to express small numbers. The exponent represents the number of places the decimal point is moved to the left. The number 0.00047 is expressed as 4.7×10^{-4}.

Factor, Multiple, and Prime Factorization

Two or more numbers that are multiplied to form a product are called factors. Divisibility rules can be used to determine whether 2, 3, 4, 5, 6, 8, 9, or 10 are factors of a given number. Multiples are the products of a given number and various integers. For example, 8 is a multiple of 4 because $4 \times 2 = 8$. A prime number is a whole number that has exactly two factors: 1 and itself. A composite number is a whole number that has more than two factors. Zero and 1 are neither prime nor composite. A composite number can be expressed as the product of its prime factors. The prime factorization of 40 is $2 \times 2 \times 2 \times 5$, or $2^3 \times 5$. The numbers 2 and 5 are prime numbers.

Integers

A negative number is a number less than zero. Negative numbers like −8, positive numbers like +6, and zero are members of the set of integers. Integers can be represented as points on a number line. A set of integers can be written {..., −3, −2, −1, 0, 1, 2, 3, ...} where ... means "continues indefinitely."

Real, Rational, and Irrational Numbers

The real number system is made up of the sets of rational and irrational numbers. Rational numbers are numbers that can be written in the form a/b where a and b are integers and $b \neq 0$. Examples are 0.45, $\frac{1}{2}$, and $\sqrt{36}$. Irrational numbers are non-repeating, non-terminating decimals. Examples are $\sqrt{71}$, π, and 0.020020002....

Complex and Imaginary Numbers

A complex number is a mathematical expression with a real number element and an imaginary number element. Imaginary numbers are multiples of i, the "imaginary" square root of −1. Complex numbers are represented by $a + bi$, where a and b are real numbers and i represents the imaginary element. When a quadratic equation does not

MATH APPENDIX

have a real number solution, the solution can be represented by a complex number. Like real numbers, complex numbers can be added, subtracted, multiplied, and divided.

Vectors and Matrices

A matrix is a set of numbers or elements arranged in rows and columns to form a rectangle. The number of rows is represented by m and the number of columns is represented by n. To describe the number of rows and columns in a matrix, list the number of rows first using the format $m \times n$. Matrix A below is a 3×3 matrix because it has 3 rows and 3 columns. To name an element of a matrix, the letter i is used to denote the row and j is used to denote the column, and the element is labeled in the form $a_{i,j}$. In matrix A below, $a_{3,2}$ is 4.

$$\text{Matrix A} = \begin{pmatrix} 1 & 3 & 5 \\ 0 & 6 & 8 \\ 3 & 4 & 5 \end{pmatrix}$$

A vector is a matrix with only one column or row of elements. A transposed column vector, or a column vector turned on its side, is a row vector. In the example below, row vector b' is the transpose of column vector b.

$$b = \begin{pmatrix} 1 \\ 2 \\ 3 \\ 4 \end{pmatrix}$$

$$b' = \begin{pmatrix} 1 & 2 & 3 & 4 \end{pmatrix}$$

Understand meanings of operations and how they relate to one another

Properties of Addition and Multiplication

Properties are statements that are true for any numbers. For example, $3 + 8$ is the same as $8 + 3$ because each expression equals 11. This illustrates the Commutative Property of Addition. Likewise, $3 \times 8 = 8 \times 3$ illustrates the Commutative Property of Multiplication.

When evaluating expressions, it is often helpful to group or associate the numbers. The Associative Property says that the way in which numbers are grouped when added or multiplied does not change the sum or product. The following properties are also true:

- **Additive Identity Property:** When 0 is added to any number, the sum is the number.
- **Multiplicative Identity Property:** When any number is multiplied by 1, the product is the number.
- **Multiplicative Property of Zero:** When any number is multiplied by 0, the product is 0.

Rational Numbers

A number that can be written as a fraction is called a rational number. Terminating and repeating decimals are rational numbers because both can be written as fractions.

Decimals that are neither terminating nor repeating are called irrational numbers because they cannot be written as fractions. Terminating decimals can be converted to fractions by placing the number (without the decimal point) in the numerator. Count the number of places to the right of the decimal point, and in the denominator, place a 1 followed by a number of zeros equal to the number of places that you counted. The fraction can then be reduced to its simplest form.

Writing a Fraction as a Decimal

Any fraction $\frac{a}{b}$, where $b \neq 0$, can be written as a decimal by dividing the numerator by the denominator. So, $\frac{a}{b} = a \div b$. If the division ends, or terminates, when the remainder is zero, the decimal is a terminating decimal. Not all fractions can be written as terminating decimals. Some have a repeating decimal. A bar indicates that the decimal repeats forever. For example, the fraction $\frac{4}{9}$ can be converted to a repeating decimal, $0.\overline{4}$

Adding and Subtracting Like Fractions

Fractions with the same denominator are called like fractions. To add like fractions, add the numerators and write the sum over the denominator. To add mixed numbers with like fractions, add the whole numbers and fractions separately, adding the numerators of the fractions, then simplifying if necessary. The rule for subtracting fractions with like denominators is similar to the rule for adding. The numerators can be subtracted and the difference written over the denominator. Mixed numbers are written as improper fractions before subtracting. These same rules apply to adding or subtracting like algebraic fractions. An algebraic fraction is a fraction that contains one or more variables in the numerator or denominator.

Adding and Subtracting Unlike Fractions

Fractions with different denominators are called unlike fractions. The least common multiple of the denominators is used to rename the fractions with a common denominator. After a common denominator is found, the numerators can then be added or subtracted. To add mixed numbers with unlike fractions, rename the mixed numbers as improper fractions. Then find a common denominator, add the numerators, and simplify the answer.

Multiplying Rational Numbers

To multiply fractions, multiply the numerators and multiply the denominators. If the numerators and denominators have common factors, they can be simplified before multiplication. If the fractions have different signs, then the product will be negative. Mixed numbers can be multiplied in the same manner, after first renaming them as improper fractions. Algebraic fractions may be multiplied using the same method described above.

MATH APPENDIX

Dividing Rational Numbers

To divide a number by a rational number (a fraction, for example), multiply the first number by the multiplicative inverse of the second. Two numbers whose product is 1 are called multiplicative inverses, or reciprocals. $\frac{7}{4} \times \frac{4}{7} = 1$. When dividing by a mixed number, first rename it as an improper fraction, and then multiply by its multiplicative inverse. This process of multiplying by a number's reciprocal can also be used when dividing algebraic fractions.

Adding Integers

To add integers with the same sign, add their absolute values. The sum takes the same sign as the addends. An addend is a number that is added to another number (the augend). The equation $-5 + (-2) = -7$ is an example of adding two integers with the same sign. To add integers with different signs, subtract their absolute values. The sum takes the same sign as the addend with the greater absolute value.

Subtracting Integers

The rules for adding integers are extended to the subtraction of integers. To subtract an integer, add its additive inverse. For example, to find the difference $2 - 5$, add the additive inverse of 5 to 2: $2 + (-5) = -3$. The rule for subtracting integers can be used to solve real-world problems and to evaluate algebraic expressions.

Additive Inverse Property

Two numbers with the same absolute value but different signs are called opposites. For example, -4 and 4 are opposites. An integer and its opposite are also called additive inverses. The Additive Inverse Property says that the sum of any number and its additive inverse is zero. The Commutative, Associative, and Identity Properties also apply to integers. These properties help when adding more than two integers.

Absolute Value

In mathematics, when two integers on a number line are on opposite sides of zero, and they are the same distance from zero, they have the same absolute value. The symbol for absolute value is two vertical bars on either side of the number. For example, $|-5| = 5$.

Multiplying Integers

Since multiplication is repeated addition, $3(-7)$ means that -7 is used as an addend 3 times. By the Commutative Property of Multiplication, $3(-7) = -7(3)$. The product of two integers with different signs is always negative. The product of two integers with the same sign is always positive.

Dividing Integers

The quotient of two integers can be found by dividing the numbers using their absolute values. The quotient of two integers with the same sign is positive, and the quotient of two integers with a different sign is negative. $-12 \div (-4) = 3$ and $12 \div (-4) = -3$. The division of integers is used in statistics to find the average, or mean, of a set of data. When finding the mean of a set of numbers, find the sum of the numbers, and then divide by the number in the set.

Adding and Multiplying Vectors and Matrices

In order to add two matrices together, they must have the same number of rows and columns. In matrix addition, the corresponding elements are added to each other. In other words $(a + b)_{ij} = a_{ij} + b_{ij}$. For example,

$$\begin{pmatrix} 1 & 2 \\ 2 & 1 \end{pmatrix} + \begin{pmatrix} 3 & 6 \\ 0 & 1 \end{pmatrix} = \begin{pmatrix} 1+3 & 2+6 \\ 2+0 & 1+1 \end{pmatrix} = \begin{pmatrix} 4 & 8 \\ 2 & 2 \end{pmatrix}$$

Matrix multiplication requires that the number of elements in each row in the first matrix is equal to the number of elements in each column in the second. The elements of the first row of the first matrix are multiplied by the corresponding elements of the first column of the second matrix and then added together to get the first element of the product matrix. To get the second element, the elements in the first row of the first matrix are multiplied by the corresponding elements in the second column of the second matrix then added, and so on, until every row of the first matrix is multiplied by every column of the second. See the example below.

$$\begin{pmatrix} 1 & 2 \\ 3 & 4 \end{pmatrix} \times \begin{pmatrix} 3 & 6 \\ 0 & 1 \end{pmatrix} = \begin{pmatrix} (1\times3)+(2\times0) & (1\times6)+(2\times1) \\ (3\times3)+(4\times0) & (3\times6)+(4\times1) \end{pmatrix} = \begin{pmatrix} 3 & 8 \\ 9 & 22 \end{pmatrix}$$

Vector addition and multiplication are performed in the same way, but there is only one column and one row.

Permutations and Combinations

Permutations and combinations are used to determine the number of possible outcomes in different situations. An arrangement, listing, or pattern in which order is important is called a permutation. The symbol P(6, 3) represents the number of permutations of 6 things taken 3 at a time. For P(6, 3), there are $6 \times 5 \times 4$ or 120 possible outcomes. An arrangement or listing where order is not important is called a combination. The symbol C(10, 5) represents the number of combinations of 10 things taken 5 at a time. For C(10, 5), there are $(10 \times 9 \times 8 \times 7 \times 6) \div (5 \times 4 \times 3 \times 2 \times 1)$ or 252 possible outcomes.

Powers and Exponents

An expression such as $3 \times 3 \times 3 \times 3$ can be written as a power. A power has two parts, a base and an exponent. $3 \times 3 \times 3 \times 3 = 3^4$. The base is the number that is multiplied (3). The exponent tells how many times the base is used as a factor (4 times). Numbers and variables can be written using exponents. For example, $8 \times 8 \times 8 \times m \times m \times m \times m \times m$ can be expressed 8^3m^5. Exponents also can be used with place value to express numbers in expanded form. Using this method, 1,462 can be written as $(1 \times 10^3) + (4 \times 10^2) + (6 \times 10^1) + (2 \times 10^0)$.

Squares and Square Roots

The square root of a number is one of two equal factors of a number. Every positive number has both a positive and a negative square root. For example, since $8 \times 8 = 64$, 8 is a square root of 64. Since $(-8) \times (-8) = 64$, -8 is also a square root of 64. The notation $\sqrt{\ }$ indicates the positive square root, $-\sqrt{\ }$ indicates the negative square root, and $\pm\sqrt{\ }$ indicates both square roots. For example, $\sqrt{81} = 9$, $-\sqrt{49} = -7$, and $\pm\sqrt{4} = \pm2$. The square root of a negative number is an imaginary number because any two factors of a negative number must have different signs, and are therefore not equivalent.

Logarithm

A logarithm is the inverse of exponentiation. The logarithm of a number x in base b is equal to the number n. Therefore, $b^n = x$ and $\log bx = n$. For example, $\log_4(64) = 3$ because $4^3 = 64$. The most commonly used bases for logarithms are 10, the common logarithm; 2, the binary logarithm; and the constant e, the natural logarithm (also called $ln(x)$ instead of $\log_e(x)$). Below is a list of some of the rules of logarithms that are important to understand if you are going to use them.

$\log_b(xy) = \log_b(x) + \log_b(y)$

$\log_b(x/y) = \log_b(x) - \log_b(y)$

$\log_b(1/x) = -\log_b(x)$

$\log_b(x)y = y\log_b(x)$

Compute fluently and make reasonable estimates

Estimation by Rounding

When rounding numbers, look at the digit to the right of the place to which you are rounding. If the digit is 5 or greater, round up. If it is less than 5, round down. For example, to round 65,137 to the nearest hundred, look at the number in the tens place. Since 3 is less than 5, round down to 65,100. To round the same number to the nearest ten thousandth, look at the number in the thousandths place. Since it is 5, round up to 70,000.

Finding Equivalent Ratios

Equivalent ratios have the same meaning. Just like finding equivalent fractions, to find an equivalent ratio, multiply or divide both sides by the same number. For example, you can multiply 7 by both sides of the ratio 6:8 to get 42:56. Instead, you can also divide both sides of the same ratio by 2 to get 3:4. Find the simplest form of a ratio by dividing to find equivalent ratios until you can't go any further without going into decimals. So, 160:240 in simplest form is 2:3. To write a ratio in the form *1:n,* divide both sides by the left-hand number. In other words, to change 8:20 to *1:n,* divide both sides by 8 to get 1:2.5.

Front-End Estimation

Front-end estimation can be used to quickly estimate sums and differences before adding or subtracting. To use this technique, add or subtract just the digits of the two highest place values, and replace the other place values with zero. This will give you an estimation of the solution of a problem. For example, 93,471 – 22,825 can be changed to 93,000 – 22,000 or 71,000. This estimate can be compared to your final answer to judge its correctness.

Judging Reasonableness

When solving an equation, it is important to check your work by considering how reasonable your answer is. For example, consider the equation $9\frac{3}{4} \times 4\frac{1}{3}$. Since $9\frac{3}{4}$ is between 9 and 10 and $4\frac{1}{3}$ is between 4 and 5, only values that are between 9×4 or 36 and 10×5 or 50 will be reasonable. You can also use front-end estimation, or you can round and estimate a reasonable answer. In the equation 73×25, you can round and solve to estimate a reasonable answer to be near 70×30 or 2,100.

Algebra

▶ *Understand patterns, relations, and functions*

Relation

A relation is a generalization comparing sets of ordered pairs for an equation or inequality such as $x = y + 1$ or $x > y$. The first element in each pair, the x values, forms the domain. The second element in each pair, the y values, forms the range.

Function

A function is a special relation in which each member of the domain is paired with exactly one member in the range. Functions may be represented using ordered pairs, tables, or graphs. One way to determine whether a relation is a function is to use the vertical line test. Using an object to represent a vertical line, move the object from left to right across the graph. If, for each value of x in the domain, the object passes through no more than one point on the graph, then the graph represents a function.

Linear and Nonlinear Functions

Linear functions have graphs that are straight lines. These graphs represent constant rates of change. In other words, the slope between any two pairs of points on the graph is the same. Nonlinear functions do not have constant rates of change. The slope changes along these graphs. Therefore, the graphs of nonlinear functions are *not* straight lines. Graphs of curves represent nonlinear functions. The equation for a linear function can be written in the form $y = mx + b$, where m represents the constant rate of change, or the slope. Therefore, you can determine whether a function is linear by looking at the equation. For example, the equation $y = \frac{3}{x}$ is nonlinear because x is in the denominator and the equation cannot be written in the form $y = mx + b$. A nonlinear function does not increase or decrease at a constant rate. You can check this by using a table and finding the increase or decrease in y for each regular increase in x. For example, if for each increase in x by 2, y does not increase or decrease the same amount each time, the function is nonlinear.

Linear Equations in Two Variables

In a linear equation with two variables, such as $y = x - 3$, the variables appear in separate terms and neither variable contains an exponent other than 1. The graphs of all linear equations are straight lines. All points on a line are solutions of the equation that is graphed.

Quadratic and Cubic Functions

A quadratic function is a polynomial equation of the second degree, generally expressed as $ax^2 + bx + c = 0$, where a, b, and c are real numbers and a is not equal to zero. Similarly, a cubic function is a polynomial equation of the third degree, usually expressed as $ax^3 + bx^2 + cx + d = 0$. Quadratic functions can be graphed using an equation or a table of values. For example, to graph $y = 3x^2 + 1$, substitute the values −1, −0.5, 0, 0.5, and 1 for x to yield the point coordinates (−1, 4), (−0.5, 1.75), (0, 1), (0.5, 1.75), and (1, 4).

Plot these points on a coordinate grid and connect the points in the form of a parabola. Cubic functions also can be graphed by making a table of values. The points of a cubic function form a curve. There is one point at which the curve changes from opening upward to opening downward, or vice versa, called the point of inflection.

Slope

Slope is the ratio of the rise, or vertical change, to the run, or horizontal change of a line: slope = rise/run. Slope (m) is the same for any two points on a straight line and can be found by using the coordinates of any two points on the line:

$$m = \frac{y_2 - y_1}{x_2 - x_1}, \text{ where } x_2 \neq x_1$$

Asymptotes

An asymptote is a straight line that a curve approaches but never actually meets or crosses. Theoretically, the asymptote meets the curve at infinity. For example, in the function $f(x) = \frac{1}{x}$, two asymptotes are being approached: the line $y = 0$ and $x = 0$. See the graph of the function below.

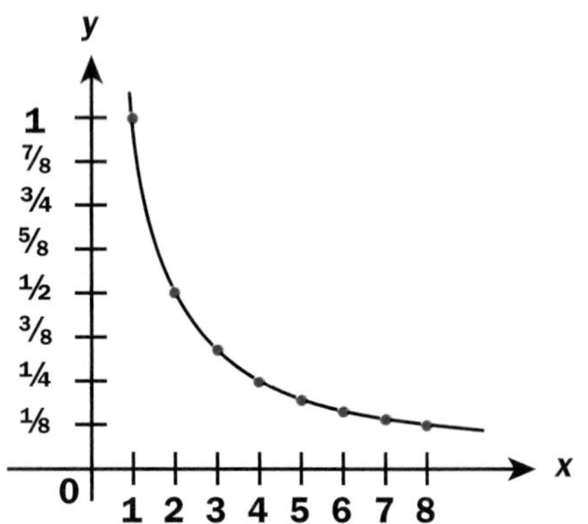

▶ Represent and analyze mathematical situations and structures using algebraic symbols

Variables and Expressions

Algebra is a language of symbols. A variable is a placeholder for a changing value. Any letter, such as x, can be used as a variable. Expressions such as $x + 2$ and $4x$ are algebraic expressions because they represent sums and/or products of variables and numbers. Usually, mathematicians avoid the use of i and e for variables because they have other mathematical meanings ($i = \sqrt{-1}$ and e is used with natural logarithms). To evaluate an algebraic expression, replace the variable or variables with known values, and then solve using order of operations. Translate verbal phrases into algebraic expressions by first defining a variable: Choose a variable and a quantity for the variable to represent. In this way, algebraic expressions can be used to represent real-world situations.

Constant and Coefficient

A constant is a fixed value unlike a variable, which can change. Constants are usually represented by numbers, but they can also be represented by symbols. For example, π is a symbolic representation of the value 3.1415.... A coefficient is a constant by which a variable or other object is multiplied. For example, in the expression $7x^2 + 5x + 9$, the coefficient of x^2 is 7 and the coefficient of x is 5. The number 9 is a constant and not a coefficient.

Monomial and Polynomial

A monomial is a number, a variable, or a product of numbers and/or variables such as 3×4. An algebraic expression that contains one or more monomials is called a polynomial. In a polynomial, there are no terms with variables in the denominator and no terms with variables under a radical sign. Polynomials can be classified by the number of terms contained in the expression. Therefore, a polynomial with two terms is called a binomial ($z^2 - 1$), and a polynomial with three terms is called a trinomial ($2y^3 + 4y^2 - y$). Polynomials also can be classified by their degrees. The degree of a monomial is the sum of the exponents of its variables. The degree of a nonzero constant such as 6 or 10 is 0. The constant 0 has no degree. For example, the monomial $4b^5c^2$ had a degree of 7. The degree of a polynomial is the same as that of the term with the greatest degree. For example, the polynomial $3x^4 - 2y^3 + 4y^2 - y$ has a degree of 4.

Equation

An equation is a mathematical sentence that states that two expressions are equal. The two expressions in an equation are always separated by an equal sign. When solving for a variable in an equation, you must perform the same operations on both sides of the equation in order for the mathematical sentence to remain true.

Solving Equations with Variables

To solve equations with variables on both sides, use the Addition or Subtraction Property of Equality to write an equivalent equation with the variables on the same side. For example, to solve $5x - 8 = 3x$, subtract $3x$ from each side to get $2x - 8 = 0$. Then add 8 to each side to get $2x = 8$. Finally, divide each side by 2 to find that $x = 4$.

Solving Equations with Grouping Symbols

Equations often contain grouping symbols such as parentheses or brackets. The first step in solving these equations is to use the Distributive Property to remove the grouping symbols. For example $5(x + 2) = 25$ can be changed to $5x + 10 = 25$, and then solved to find that $x = 3$.

Some equations have no solution. That is, there is no value of the variable that results in a true sentence. For such an equation, the solution set is called the null or empty set, and is represented by the symbol $\varnothing$ or $\{\}$. Other equations may have every number as the solution. An equation that is true for every value of the variable is called the identity.

Inequality

A mathematical sentence that contains the symbols $<$ (less than), $>$ (greater than), $\leq$ (less than or equal to), or $\geq$ (greater than or equal to) is called an inequality. For example, the statement that it is legal to drive 55 miles per hour or slower on a stretch of the highway can be shown by the sentence $s \leq 55$. Inequalities with variables are called open sentences. When a variable is replaced with a number, the inequality may be true or false.

Solving Inequalities

Solving an inequality means finding values for the variable that make the inequality true. Just as with equations, when you add or subtract the same number from each side of an inequality, the inequality remains true. For example, if you add 5 to each side of the inequality $3x < 6$, the resulting inequality $3x + 5 < 11$ is also true. Adding or subtracting the same number from each side of an inequality does not affect the inequality sign. When multiplying or dividing each side of an inequality by the same positive number, the inequality remains true. In such cases, the inequality symbol does not change. When multiplying or dividing each side of an inequality by a negative number, the inequality symbol must be reversed. For example, when dividing each side of the inequality $-4x \geq -8$ by -2, the inequality sign must be changed to $\leq$ for the resulting inequality, $2x \leq 4$, to be true. Since the solutions to an inequality include all rational numbers satisfying it, inequalities have an infinite number of solutions.

Representing Inequalities on a Number Line

The solutions of inequalities can be graphed on a number line. For example, if the solution of an inequality is $x < 5$, start an arrow at 5 on the number line, and continue the arrow to the left to show all values less than 5 as the solution. Put an open circle at 5 to show that the point 5 is *not* included in the graph. Use a closed circle when graphing solutions that are greater than or equal to, or less than or equal to, a number.

Order of Operations

Solving a problem may involve using more than one operation. The answer can depend on the order in which you do the operations. To make sure that there is just one answer to a series of computations, mathematicians have agreed upon an order in which to do the operations. First simplify within the parentheses, often called graphing symbols, and then evaluate any exponents. Then multiply and divide from left to right, and finally add and subtract from left to right.

Parametric Equations

Given an equation with more than one unknown, a statistician can draw conclusions about those unknown quantities through the use of parameters, independent variables that the statistician already knows something about. For example, you can find the velocity of an object if you make some assumptions about distance and time parameters.

Recursive Equations

In recursive equations, every value is determined by the previous value. You must first plug an initial value into the equation to get the first value, and then you can use the first value to determine the next one, and so on. For example, in order to determine what the population of pigeons will be in New York City in three years, you can use an equation with the birth, death, immigration, and emigration rates of the birds. Input the current population size into the equation to determine next year's population size, then repeat until you have calculated the value for which you are looking.

Use mathematical models to represent and understand quantitative relationships

Solving Systems of Equations

Two or more equations together are called a system of equations. A system of equations can have one solution, no solution, or infinitely many solutions. One method for solving a system of equations is to graph the equations on the same coordinate plane. The coordinates of the point where the graphs intersect is the solution. In other words, the solution of a system is the ordered pair that is a solution of all equations. A more accurate way to solve a system of two equations is by using a method called substitution. Write both equations in terms of y. Replace y in the first equation with the right side of the second equation. Check the solution by graphing. You can solve a system of three equations using matrix algebra.

Graphing Inequalities

To graph an inequality, first graph the related equation, which is the boundary. All points in the shaded region are solutions of the inequality. If an inequality contains the symbol $\leq$ or $\geq$, then use a solid line to indicate that the boundary is included in the graph. If an inequality contains the symbol $<$ or $>$, then use a dashed line to indicate that the boundary is not included in the graph.

Analyze change in various contexts

Rate of Change

A change in one quantity with respect to another quantity is called the rate of change. Rates of change can be described using slope:

$$\text{slope} = \frac{\textit{change in } y}{\textit{change in } x}$$

You can find rates of change from an equation, a table, or a graph. A special type of linear equation that describes rate of change is called a direct variation. The graph of a direct variation always passes through the origin and represents a proportional situation. In the equation $y = kx$, k is called the constant of variation. It is the slope, or rate of change. As x increases in value, y increases or decreases at a constant rate k, or y varies directly with x. Another way to say this is that y is directly proportional to x. The direct variation $y = kx$ also can be written as $k = \frac{y}{x}$. In this form, you can see that the ratio of y to x is the same for any corresponding values of y and x.

Slope-Intercept Form

Equations written as $y = mx + b$, where m is the slope and b is the y-intercept, are linear equations in slope-intercept form. For example, the graph of $y = 5x - 6$ is a line that has a slope of 5 and crosses the y-axis at $(0, -6)$. Sometimes you must first write an equation in slope-intercept form before finding the slope and y-intercept. For example, the equation $2x + 3y = 15$ can be expressed in slope-intercept form by subtracting $2x$ from each side and then dividing by 3: $y = -\frac{2}{3}x + 5$, revealing a slope of $-\frac{2}{3}$ and a y-intercept of 5. You can use the slope-intercept form of an equation to graph a line easily. Graph the y-intercept and use the slope to find another point on the line, then connect the two points with a line.

MATH APPENDIX

Geometry

Analyze characteristics and properties of two- and three-dimensional geometric shapes and develop mathematical arguments about geometric relationships

Angles

Two rays that have the same endpoint form an angle. The common endpoint is called the vertex, and the two rays that make up the angle are called the sides of the angle. The most common unit of measure for angles is the degree. Protractors can be used to measure angles or to draw an angle of a given measure. Angles can be classified by their degree measure. Acute angles have measures less than 90° but greater than 0°. Obtuse angles have measures greater than 90° but less than 180°. Right angles have measures of 90°.

Triangles

A triangle is a figure formed by three line segments that intersect only at their endpoints. The sum of the measures of the angles of a triangle is 180°. Triangles can be classified by their angles. An acute triangle contains all acute angles. An obtuse triangle has one obtuse angle. A right triangle has one right angle. Triangles can also be classified by their sides. A scalene triangle has no congruent sides. An isosceles triangle has at least two congruent sides. In an equilateral triangle all sides are congruent.

Quadrilaterals

A quadrilateral is a closed figure with four sides and four vertices. The segments of a quadrilateral intersect only at their endpoints. Quadrilaterals can be separated into two triangles. Since the sum of the interior angles of all triangles totals 180°, the measures of the interior angles of a quadrilateral equal 360°. Quadrilaterals are classified according to their characteristics, and include trapezoids, parallelograms, rectangles, squares, and rhombuses.

Two-Dimensional Figures

A two-dimensional figure exists within a plane and has only the dimensions of length and width. Examples of two-dimensional figures include circles and polygons. Polygons are figures that have three or more angles, including triangles, quadrilaterals, pentagons, hexagons, and many more. The sum of the angles of any polygon totals at least 180° (triangle), and each additional side adds 180° to the measure of the first three angles. The sum of the angles of a quadrilateral, for example, is 360°. The sum of the angles of a pentagon is 540°.

Three-Dimensional Figures

A plane is a two-dimensional flat surface that extends in all directions. Intersecting planes can form the edges and vertices of three-dimensional figures or solids. A polyhedron is a solid with flat surfaces that are polygons. Polyhedrons are composed of faces, edges, and vertices and are differentiated by their shape and by their number of bases. Skew lines are lines that lie in different planes. They are neither intersecting nor parallel.

Congruence

Figures that have the same size and shape are congruent. The parts of congruent triangles that match are called corresponding parts. Congruence statements are used to identify corresponding parts of congruent triangles. When writing a congruence statement, the letters must be written so that corresponding vertices appear in the same order. Corresponding parts can be used to find the measures of angles and sides in a figure that is congruent to a figure with known measures.

Similarity

If two figures have the same shape but not the same size they are called similar figures. For example, the triangles below are similar, so angles *A*, *B*, and *C* have the same measurements as angles *D*, *E*, and *F*, respectively. However, segments *AB*, *BC*, and *CA* do not have the same measurements as segments *DE*, *EF*, and *FD* , but the measures of the sides are proportional.

For example, $\frac{\overline{AB}}{\overline{DE}} = \frac{\overline{BC}}{\overline{EF}} = \frac{\overline{CA}}{\overline{FD}}$.

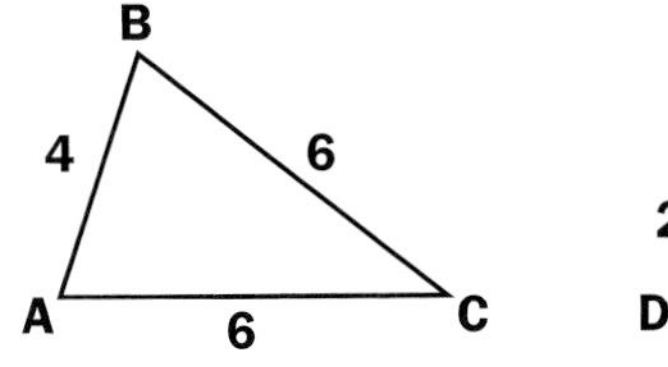

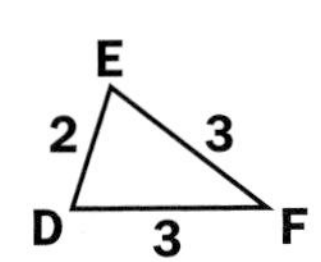

Solid figures are considered to be similar if they have the same shape and their corresponding linear measures are proportional. As with two-dimensional figures, they can be tested for similarity by comparing corresponding measures. If the compared ratios are proportional, then the figures are similar solids. Missing measures of similar solids can also be determined by using proportions.

The Pythagorean Theorem

The sides that are adjacent to a right angle are called legs. The side opposite the right angle is the hypotenuse.

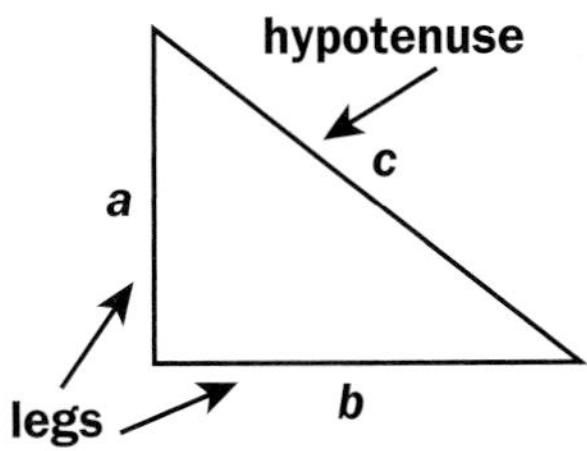

The Pythagorean Theorem describes the relationship between the lengths of the legs a and b and the hypotenuse c. It states that if a triangle is a right triangle, then the square of the length of the hypotenuse is equal to the sum of the squares of the lengths of the legs. In symbols, $c^2 = a^2 + b^2$.

Sine, Cosine, and Tangent Ratios

Trigonometry is the study of the properties of triangles. A trigonometric ratio is a ratio of the lengths of two sides of a right triangle. The most common trigonometric ratios are the sine, cosine, and tangent ratios. These ratios are abbreviated as *sin*, *cos*, and *tan*, respectively.

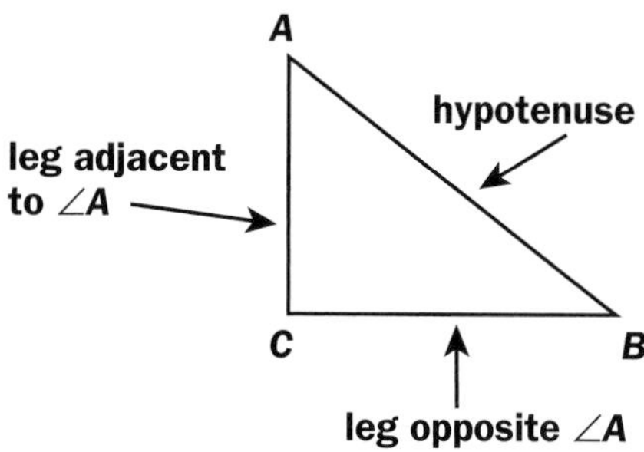

If $\angle A$ is an acute angle of a right triangle, then

$$\sin \angle A = \frac{\text{measure of leg opposite } \angle A}{\text{measure of hypotenuse}},$$

$$\cos \angle A = \frac{\text{measure of leg adjacent to } \angle A}{\text{measure of hypotenuse}}, \text{ and}$$

$$\tan \angle A = \frac{\text{measure of leg opposite } \angle A}{\text{measure of leg adjacent to } \angle A}.$$

Specify locations and describe spatial relationships using coordinate geometry and other representational systems

Polygons

A polygon is a simple, closed figure formed by three or more line segments. The line segments meet only at their endpoints. The points of intersection are called vertices, and the line segments are called sides. Polygons are classified by the number of sides they have. The diagonals of a polygon divide the polygon into triangles. The number of triangles formed is two less than the number of sides. To find the sum of the measures of the interior angles of any polygon, multiply the number of triangles within the polygon by 180. That is, if n equals the number of sides, then $(n - 2)\ 180$ gives the sum of the measures of the polygon's interior angles.

Cartesian Coordinates

In the Cartesian coordinate system, the y-axis extends above and below the origin and the x-axis extends to the right and left of the origin, which is the point at which the x- and y-axes intersect. Numbers below and to the left of the origin are negative. A point graphed on the coordinate grid is said to have an x-coordinate and a y-coordinate. For example, the point (1,–2) has as its x-coordinate the number 1, and has as its y-coordinate the number –2. This point is graphed by locating the position on the grid that is 1 unit to the right of the origin and 2 units below the origin.

The x-axis and the y-axis separate the coordinate plane into four regions, called quadrants. The axes and points located on the axes themselves are not located in any of the quadrants. The quadrants are labeled I to IV, starting in the upper right and proceeding counterclockwise. In quadrant I, both coordinates are positive. In quadrant II, the x-coordinate is negative and the y-coordinate is positive. In quadrant III, both coordinates are negative. In quadrant IV, the x-coordinate is positive and the y-coordinate is negative. A coordinate graph can be used to show algebraic relationships among numbers.

Apply transformations and use symmetry to analyze mathematical situations

Similar Triangles and Indirect Measurement

Triangles that have the same shape but not necessarily the same dimensions are called similar triangles. Similar triangles have corresponding angles and corresponding sides. Arcs are used to show congruent angles. If two triangles are similar, then the corresponding angles have the same measure, and the corresponding sides are proportional. Therefore, to determine the measures of the sides of similar triangles when some measures are known, proportions can be used.

Transformations

A transformation is a movement of a geometric figure. There are several types of transformations. In a translation, also called a slide, a figure is slid from one position to another without turning it. Every point of the original figure is moved the same distance and in the same direction. In a reflection, also called a flip, a figure is flipped over a line to form a mirror image. Every point of the original figure has a corresponding point on the other side of the line of symmetry. In a rotation, also called a turn, a figure is turned around a fixed point. A figure can be rotated 0°–360° clockwise or counterclockwise. A dilation transforms each line to a parallel line whose length is a fixed multiple of the length of the original line to create a similar figure that will be either larger or smaller.

Use visualizations, spatial reasoning, and geometric modeling to solve problems

Two-Dimensional Representations of Three-Dimensional Objects

Three-dimensional objects can be represented in a two-dimensional drawing in order to more easily determine properties such as surface area and volume. When you look at the triangular prism, you can see the orientation of its three dimensions, length, width, and height. Using the drawing and the formulas for surface area and volume, you can easily calculate these properties.

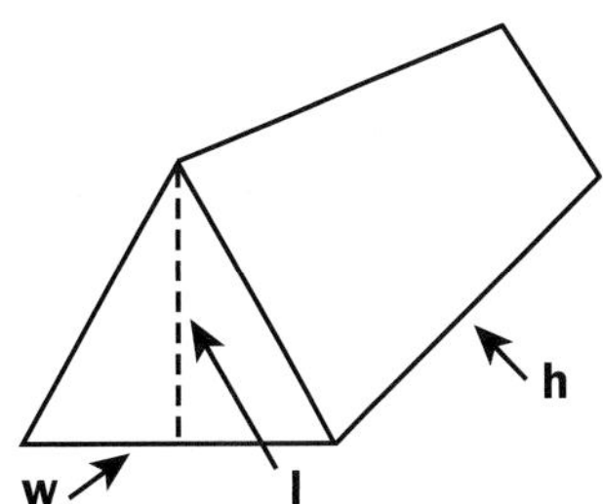

Another way to represent a three-dimensional object in a two-dimensional plane is by using a net, which is the unfolded representation. Imagine cutting the vertices of a box until it is flat then drawing an outline of it. That's a net. Most objects have more than one net, but any one can be measured to determine surface area. Below is a cube and one of its nets.

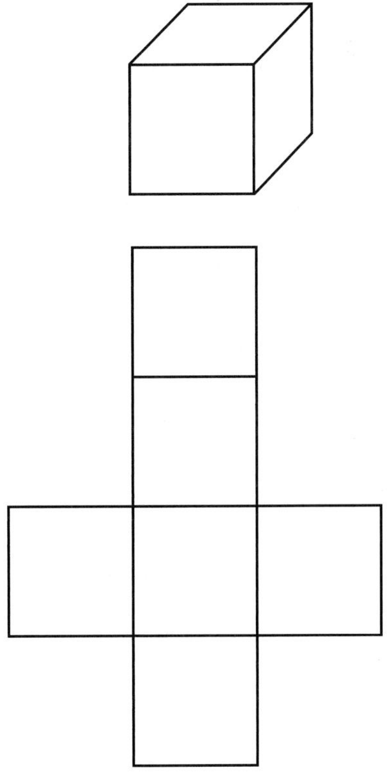

Measurement

▶ *Understand measurable attributes of objects and the units, systems, and processes of measurement*

Customary System

The customary system is the system of weights and measures used in the United States. The main units of weight are ounces, pounds (1 equal to 16 ounces), and tons (1 equal to 2,000 pounds). Length is typically measured in inches, feet (1 equal to 12 inches), yards (1 equal to 3 feet), and miles (1 equal to 5,280 feet), while area is measured in square feet and acres (1 equal to 43,560 square feet). Liquid is measured in cups, pints (1 equal to 2 cups), quarts (1 equal to 2 pints), and gallons (1 equal to 4 quarts). Finally, temperature is measured in degrees Fahrenheit.

Metric System

The metric system is a decimal system of weights and measurements in which the prefixes of the words for the units of measure indicate the relationships between the different measurements. In this system, the main units of weight, or mass, are grams and kilograms. Length is measured in millimeters, centimeters, meters, and kilometers, and the units of area are square millimeters, centimeters, meters, and kilometers. Liquid is typically measured in milliliters and liters, while temperature is in degrees Celsius.

Selecting Units of Measure

When measuring something, it is important to select the appropriate type and size of unit. For example, in the United States it would be appropriate when describing someone's height to use feet and inches. These units of height or length are good to use because they are in the customary system, and they are of appropriate size. In the customary system, use inches, feet, and miles for lengths and perimeters; square inches, feet, and miles for area and surface area; and cups, pints, quarts, gallons or cubic inches and feet (and less commonly miles) for volume. In the metric system use millimeters, centimeters, meters, and kilometers for lengths and perimeters; square units millimeters, centimeters, meters, and kilometers for area and surface area; and milliliters and liters for volume. Finally, always use degrees to measure angles.

▶ *Apply appropriate techniques, tools, and formulas to determine measurements*

Precision and Significant Digits

The precision of measurement is the exactness to which a measurement is made. Precision depends on the smallest unit of measure being used, or the precision unit. One way to record a measure is to estimate to the nearest precision unit. A more precise method is to include all of the digits that are actually measured, plus one estimated digit. The digits recorded, called significant digits, indicate the precision of the measurement. There are special rules for determining significant digits. If a number contains a decimal point, the number of significant digits is found by counting from left to right, starting with the first nonzero digit. If the number does not contain a decimal point, the number of significant digits is found by counting the digits from left to right, starting with the first digit and ending with the last nonzero digit.

Surface Area

The amount of material needed to cover the surface of a figure is called the surface area. It can be calculated by finding the area of each face and adding them together. To find the surface area of a rectangular prism, for example, the formula $S = 2lw + 2lh + 2wh$ applies. A cylinder, on the other hand, may be unrolled to reveal two circles and a rectangle. Its surface area can be determined by finding the area of the two circles, $2\pi r^2$, and adding it to the area of the rectangle, $2\pi rh$ (the length of the rectangle is the circumference of one of the circles), or $S = 2\pi r^2 + 2\pi rh$. The surface area of a pyramid is measured in a slightly different way because the sides of a pyramid are triangles that intersect at the vertex. These sides are called lateral faces and the height of each is called the slant height. The sum of their areas is the lateral area of a pyramid. The surface area of a square pyramid is the lateral area $\frac{1}{2}bh$ (area of a lateral face) times 4 (number of lateral faces), plus the area of the base. The surface area of a cone is the area of its circular base (πr^2) plus its lateral area (πrl, where l is the slant height).

Volume

Volume is the measure of space occupied by a solid region. To find the volume of a prism, the area of the base is multiplied by the measure of the height, $V = Bh$. A solid containing several prisms can be broken down into its component prisms. Then the volume of each component can be found and the volumes added. The volume of a cylinder can be determined by finding the area of its circular base, πr^2, and then multiplying by the height of the cylinder. A pyramid has one-third the volume of a prism with the same base and height. To find the volume of a pyramid, multiply the area of the base by the pyramid's height, and then divide by 3. Simply stated, the formula for the volume of a pyramid is $V = \frac{1}{3}bh$. A cone is a three-dimensional figure with one circular base and a curved surface connecting the base and the vertex. The volume of a cone is one-third the volume of a cylinder with the same base area and height. Like a pyramid, the formula for the volume of a cone is $V = \frac{1}{3}bh$. More specifically, the formula is $V = \frac{1}{3}\pi r^2h$.

Upper and Lower Bounds

Upper and lower bounds have to do with the accuracy of a measurement. When a measurement is given, the degree of accuracy is also stated to tell you what the upper and lower bounds of the measurement are. The upper bound is the largest possible value that a measurement could have had before being rounded down, and the lower bound is the lowest possible value it could have had before being rounded up.

Data Analysis and Probability

Formulate questions that can be addressed with data and collect, organize, and display relevant data to answer them

Histograms

A histogram displays numerical data that have been organized into equal intervals using bars that have the same width and no space between them. While a histogram does not give exact data points, its shape shows the distribution of the data. Histograms also can be used to compare data.

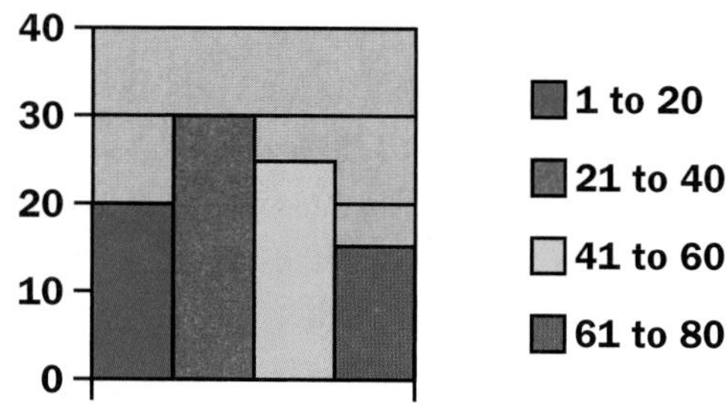

Box-and-Whisker Plot

A box-and-whisker plot displays the measures of central tendency and variation. A box is drawn around the quartile values, and whiskers extend from each quartile to the extreme data points. To make a box plot for a set of data, draw a number line that covers the range of data. Find the median, the extremes, and the upper and lower quartiles. Mark these points on the number line with bullets, then draw a box and the whiskers. The length of a whisker or box shows whether the values of the data in that part are concentrated or spread out.

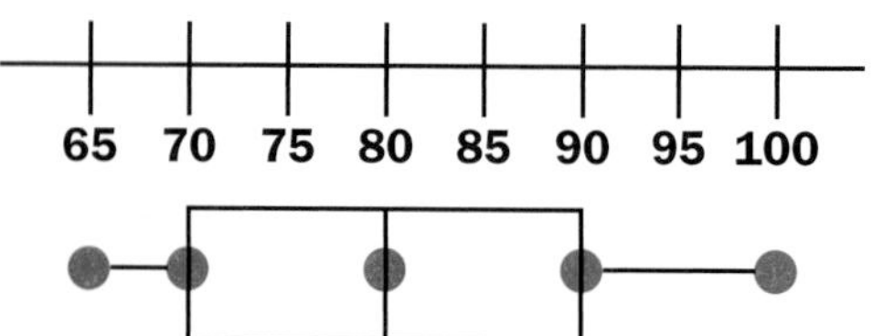

Scatter Plots

A scatter plot is a graph that shows the relationship between two sets of data. In a scatter plot, two sets of data are graphed as ordered pairs on a coordinate system. Two sets of data can have a positive correlation (as x increases, y increases), a negative correlation (as x increases, y decreases), or no correlation (no obvious pattern is shown). Scatter plots can be used to spot trends, draw conclusions, and make predictions about data.

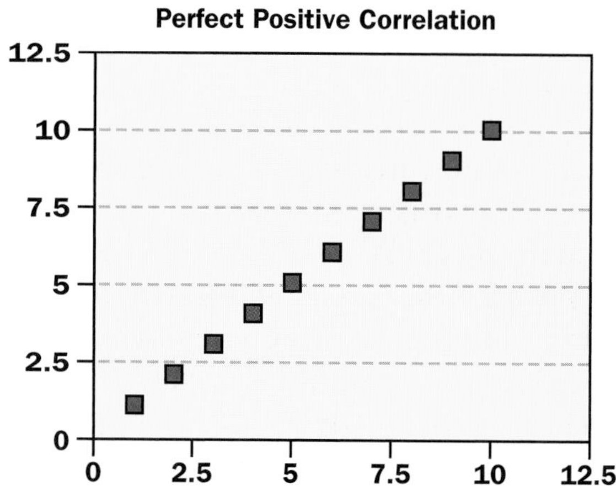

Randomization

The idea of randomization is a very important principle of statistics and the design of experiments. Data must be selected randomly to prevent bias from influencing the results. For example, you want to know the average income of people in your town but you can only use a sample of 100 individuals to make determinations about everyone. If you select 100 individuals who are all doctors, you will have a biased sample. However, if you chose a random sample of 100 people out of the phone book, you are much more likely to accurately represent average income in the town.

Statistics and Parameters

Statistics is a science that involves collecting, analyzing, and presenting data. The data can be collected in various ways—for example through a census or by making physical measurements. The data can then be analyzed by creating summary statistics, which have to do with the distribution of the data sample, including the mean, range, and standard error. They can also be illustrated in tables and graphs, like boxplots, scatter plots, and histograms. The presentation of the data typically involves describing the strength or validity of the data and what they show. For example, an analysis of ancestry of people in a city might tell you something about immigration patterns, unless the data set is very small or biased in some way, in which case it is not likely to be very accurate or useful.

Categorical and Measurement Data

When analyzing data, it is important to understand if the data is qualitative or quantitative. Categorical data is qualitative and measurement, or numerical, data is quantitative. Categorical data describes a quality of something and can be placed into different categories. For example, if you are analyzing the number of students in different grades in a school, each grade is a category. On the other hand, measurement data is continuous, like height, weight, or any other measurable variable. Measurement data can be converted into categorical data if you decide to group the data. Using height as an example, you can group the continuous data set into categories like under 5 feet, 5 feet to 5 feet 5 inches, over 5 feet five inches to 6 feet, and so on.

Univariate and Bivariate Data

In data analysis, a researcher can analyze one variable at a time or look at how multiple variables behave together. Univariate data involves only one variable, for example height in humans. You can measure the height in a population of people then plot the results in a histogram to look at how height is distributed in humans. To summarize univariate data, you can use statistics like the mean, mode, median, range, and standard deviation, which is a measure of variation. When looking at more than one variable at once, you use multivariate data. Bivariate data involves two variables. For example, you can look at height and age in humans together by gathering information on both variables from individuals in a population. You can then plot both variables in a scatter plot, look at how the variables behave in relation to each other, and create an equation that represents the relationship, also called a regression. These equations could help answer questions such as, for example, does height increase with age in humans?

Select and use appropriate statistical methods to analyze data

Measures of Central Tendency

When you have a list of numerical data, it is often helpful to use one or more numbers to represent the whole set. These numbers are called measures of central tendency. Three measures of central tendency are mean, median, and mode. The mean is the sum of the data divided by the number of items in the data set. The median is the middle number of the ordered data (or the mean of the two middle numbers). The mode

MATH APPENDIX

is the number or numbers that occur most often. These measures of central tendency allow data to be analyzed and better understood.

Measures of Spread

In statistics, measures of spread or variation are used to describe how data are distributed. The range of a set of data is the difference between the greatest and the least values of the data set. The quartiles are the values that divide the data into four equal parts. The median of data separates the set in half. Similarly, the median of the lower half of a set of data is the lower quartile. The median of the upper half of a set of data is the upper quartile. The interquartile range is the difference between the upper quartile and the lower quartile.

Line of Best Fit

When real-life data are collected, the points graphed usually do not form a straight line, but they may approximate a linear relationship. A line of best fit is a line that lies very close to most of the data points. It can be used to predict data. You also can use the equation of the best-fit line to make predictions.

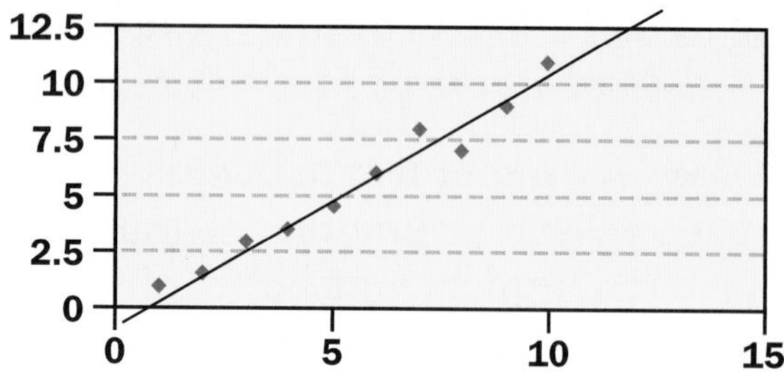

Stem and Leaf Plots

In a stem and leaf plot, numerical data are listed in ascending or descending order. The greatest place value of the data is used for the stems. The next greatest place value forms the leaves. For example, if the least number in a set of data is 8 and the greatest number is 95, draw a vertical line and write the stems from 0 to 9 to the left of the line. Write the leaves to the right of the line, with the corresponding stem. Next, rearrange the leaves so they are ordered from least to greatest. Then include a key or explanation, such as 1|3 = 13. Notice that the stem-and-leaf plot below is like a histogram turned on its side.

```
0|8
1|3 6
2|5 6 9
3|0 2 7 8
4|0 1 4 7 9
5|1 4 5 8
6|1 3 7
7|5 8
8|2 6
9|5
```

Key: **1|3 = 13**

Develop and evaluate inferences and predictions that are based on data

Sampling Distribution

The sampling distribution of a population is the distribution that would result if you could take an infinite number of samples from the population, average each, and then average the averages. The more normal the distribution of the population, that is, how closely the distribution follows a bell curve, the more likely the sampling distribution will also follow a normal distribution. Furthermore, the larger the sample, the more likely it will accurately represent the entire population. For instance, you are more likely to gain more representative results from a population of 1,000 with a sample of 100 than with a sample of 2.

Validity

In statistics, validity refers to acquiring results that accurately reflect that which is being measured. In other words, it is important when performing statistical analyses, to ensure that the data are valid in that the sample being analyzed represents the population to the best extent possible. Randomization of data and using appropriate sample sizes are two important aspects of making valid inferences about a population.

▶ *Understand and apply basic concepts of probability*

Complementary, Mutually Exclusive Events

To understand probability theory, it is important to know if two events are mutually exclusive, or complementary: the occurrence of one event automatically implies the non-occurrence of the other. That is, two complementary events cannot both occur. If you roll a pair of dice, the event of rolling 6 and rolling doubles have an outcome in common (3, 3), so they are not mutually exclusive. If you roll (3, 3), you also roll doubles. However, the events of rolling a 9 and rolling doubles are mutually exclusive because they have no outcomes in common. If you roll a 9, you will not also roll doubles.

Independent and Dependent Events

Determining the probability of a series of events requires that you know whether the events are independent or dependent. An independent event has no influence on the occurrence of subsequent events, whereas, a dependent event does influence subsequent events. The chances that a woman's first child will be a girl are $\frac{1}{2}$,and the chances that her second child will be a girl are also $\frac{1}{2}$ because the two events are independent of each other. However, if there are 7 red marbles in a bag of 15 marbles, the chances that the first marble you pick will be red are $\frac{7}{15}$ and if you indeed pick a red marble and remove it, you have reduced the chances of picking another red marble to $\frac{6}{14}$.

Sample Space

The sample space is the group of all possible outcomes for an event. For example, if you are tossing a single six-sided die, the sample space is {1, 2, 3, 4, 5, 6}. Similarly, you can determine the sample space for the possible outcomes of two events. If you are going to toss a coin twice, the sample space is {(heads, heads), (heads, tails), (tails, heads), (tails, tails)}.

Computing the Probability of a Compound Event

If two events are independent, the outcome of one event does not influence the outcome of the second. For example, if a bag contains 2 blue and 3 red marbles, then the probability of selecting a blue marble, replacing it, and then selecting a red marble is $P(A) \times P(B) = \frac{2}{5} \times \frac{3}{5}$ or $\frac{6}{25}$.

If two events are dependent, the outcome of one event affects the outcome of the second. For example, if a bag contains 2 blue and 3 red marbles, then the probability of selecting a blue and then a red marble without replacing the first marble is $P(A) \times P(B \text{ following } A) = \frac{2}{5} \times \frac{3}{4}$ or $\frac{3}{10}$. Two events that cannot happen at the same time are mutually exclusive. For example, when you roll two number cubes, you cannot roll a sum that is both 5 and even. So, $P(A \text{ or } B) = \frac{4}{36} + \frac{18}{36}$ or $\frac{11}{18}$.

MATH APPENDIX

Career Skills

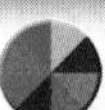 MAKING CAREER CHOICES

A career differs from a job in that it is a series of progressively more responsible jobs in one field or a related field. You will need to learn some special skills to choose a career and to help you in your job search. Choosing a career and identifying career opportunities require careful thought and preparation. To aid you in making important career choices, follow these steps.

STEPS TO MAKING A CAREER DECISION

1. Conduct a self-assessment to determine your:
   - values
   - lifestyle goals
   - interests
   - skills and aptitudes
   - personality
   - work environment preferences
   - relationship preferences
2. Identify possible career choices based on your self-assessment.
3. Gather information on each choice, including future trends.
4. Evaluate your choices based on your self-assessment.
5. Make your decision.

After you make your decision, plan how you will reach your goal. It is best to have short-term, medium-term, and long-term goals. In making your choices, explore the future opportunities in this field or fields over the next several years. What impact will new technology and automation have on job opportunities in the next few years? Remember, if you plan, you make your own career opportunities.

PERSONAL CAREER PORTFOLIO

You will want to create and maintain a personal career portfolio. In it you will keep all the documents you create and receive in your job search:

- Contact list
- Résumé
- Letters of recommendation
- Employer evaluations
- Awards
- Evidence of participation in school, community, and volunteer activities
- Notes about your job search
- Notes made after your interviews

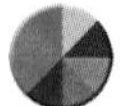 CAREER RESEARCH RESOURCES

In order to gather information on various career opportunities, there are a variety of sources to research:

- **Libraries.** Your school or public library offers good career information resources. Here you will find books, magazines, pamphlets, films, videos, and special reference materials on careers. In particular, the U.S. Department of Labor publishes three reference books that are especially helpful: the *Dictionary of Occupational Titles (DOT),* which describes about 20,000 jobs and their relationships with data, people, and things; the *Occupational Outlook Handbook (OOH),* with information on more than 200 occupations; and the *Guide for Occupational Exploration (GOE),* a reference that organizes the world of work into 12 interest areas that are subdivided into work groups and subgroups.
- **The Internet.** The Internet is becoming a primary source of research on any topic. It is especially helpful in researching careers.
- **Career Consultations.** Career consultation, an informational interview with a professional who works in a career that interests you, provides an opportunity to learn about the day-to-day realities of a career.
- **On-the-Job Experience.** On-the-job experience can be valuable in learning firsthand about a job or career. You can find out if your school has a work-experience program, or look into a company or organization's internship opportunities. Interning gives you direct work experience and often allows you to make valuable contacts for future full-time employment.

THE JOB SEARCH

To aid you in your actual job search, there are various sources to explore. You should contact and research all the sources that might produce a job lead, or information about a job. Keep a contact list as you proceed with your search. Some of these resources include:

- **Networking with family, friends, and acquaintances.** This means contacting people you know personally, including school counselors, former employers, and professional people.
- **Cooperative education and work-experience programs.** Many schools have such programs in which students work part-time on a job related to one of their classes. Many also offer work-experience programs that are not limited to just one career area, such as marketing.
- **Newspaper ads.** Reading the Help Wanted advertisements in your local papers will provide a source of job leads, as well as teach you about the local job market.
- **Employment agencies.** Most cities have two types of employment agencies, public and private. These employment agencies match workers with jobs. Some private agencies may charge a fee, so be sure to know who is expected to pay the fee and what the fee is.
- **Company personnel offices.** Large and medium-sized companies have personnel offices to handle employment matters, including the hiring of new workers. You can check on job openings by contacting the office by telephone or by scheduling a personal visit.
- **Searching the Internet.** Cyberspace offers multiple opportunities for your job search. Web sites, such as Hotjobs.com or Monster.com, provide lists of companies offering employment. There are tens of thousands of career-related Web sites, so the challenge is finding those that have jobs that interest you and that are up-to-date in their listings. Companies that interest you may have a Web site, which will provide valuable information on their benefits and opportunities for employment.

APPLYING FOR A JOB

When you have contacted the sources of job leads and found some jobs that interest you, the next step is to apply for them. You will need to complete application forms, write letters of application, and prepare your own résumé. Before you apply for a job, you will need to have a work permit if you are under the age of 18 in most states. Some state and federal labor laws designate certain jobs as too dangerous for young workers. Laws also limit the number of hours of work allowed during a day, a week, or the school year. You will also need to have proper documentation, such as a green card if you are not a U.S. citizen.

JOB APPLICATION

You can obtain the job application form directly at the place of business, by requesting it in writing, or over the Internet. It is best if you can fill the form out at home, but some businesses require that you fill it out at the place of work.

Fill out the job application forms neatly and accurately, using standard English, the formal style of speaking and writing you learned in school. You must be truthful and pay attention to detail in filling out the form.

PERSONAL FACT SHEET

To be sure that the answers you write on a job application form are accurate, make a personal fact sheet before filling out the application:

- Your name, home address, and phone number
- Your Social Security number
- The job you are applying for
- The date you can begin work
- The days and hours you can work
- The pay you want
- Whether or not you have been convicted of a crime
- Your education
- Your previous work experience
- Your birth date
- Your driver's license number if you have one
- Your interests and hobbies, and awards you have won
- Your previous work experience, including dates
- Schools you have attended
- Places you have lived
- Accommodations you may need from the employer
- A list of references—people who will tell an employer that you will do a good job, such as relatives, students, former employers, and the like

LETTERS OF RECOMMENDATION

Letters of recommendation are helpful. You can request teachers, counselors, relatives, and other acquaintances who know you well to write these letters. They should be short, to the point, and give a brief overview of your assets. A brief description of any of your important accomplishments or projects should follow. The letter should end with a brief description of your character and work ethic.

LETTER OF APPLICATION

Some employees prefer a letter of application, rather than an application form. This letter is like writing a sales pitch about yourself. You need to tell why you are the best person for the job, what special qualifications you have, and include all the information usually found on an application form. Write the letter in standard English, making certain that it is neat, accurate, and correct.

RÉSUMÉ

The purpose of a résumé is to make an employer want to interview you. A résumé tells prospective employers what you are like and what you can do for them. A good résumé summarizes you at your best in a one- or two-page outline. It should include the following information:

1. **Identification.** Include your name, address, telephone number, and e-mail address.
2. **Objective.** Indicate the type of job you are looking for.
3. **Experience.** List experience related to the specific job for which you are applying. List other work if you have not worked in a related field.
4. **Education.** Include schools attended from high school on, the dates of attendance, and diplomas or degrees earned. You may also include courses related to the job you are applying for.
5. **References.** Include up to three references or indicate that they are available. Always ask people ahead of time if they are willing to be listed as references for you.

A résumé that you put online or send by e-mail is called an electronic résumé. Some Web sites allow you to post them on their sites without charge. Employers access these sites to find new employees. Your electronic résumé should follow the guidelines for a regular one. It needs to be accurate. Stress your skills and sell yourself to prospective employers.

COVER LETTER

If you are going to get the job you want, you need to write a great cover letter to accompany your résumé. Think of a cover letter as an introduction: a piece of paper that conveys a smile, a confident hello, and a nice, firm handshake. The cover letter is the first thing a potential employer sees, and it can make a powerful impression. The following are some tips for creating a cover letter that is professional and gets the attention you want:

- **Keep it short.** Your cover letter should be one page, no more.
- **Make it look professional.** These days, you need to type your letter on a computer and print it on a laser printer. Do not use an inkjet printer unless it produces extremely crisp type. Use white or buff-colored paper; anything else will draw the wrong kind of attention. Type your name, address, phone number, and e-mail address at the top of the page.
- **Explain why you are writing.** Start your letter with one sentence describing where you heard of the opening. "Joan Wright suggested I contact you regarding a position in your marketing department," or "I am writing to apply for the position you advertised in the Sun City Journal."
- **Introduce yourself.** Give a short description of your professional abilities and background. Refer to your attached résumé: "As you will see in the attached résumé, I am an experienced editor with a background in newspapers, magazines, and textbooks." Then highlight one or two specific accomplishments.

- **Sell yourself.** Your cover letter should leave the reader thinking, "This person is exactly what we are looking for." Focus on what you can do for the company. Relate your skills to the skills and responsibilities mentioned in the job listing. If the ad mentions solving problems, relate a problem you solved at school or work. If the ad mentions specific skills or knowledge required, mention your mastery of these in your letter. (Also be sure these skills are included on your résumé.)
- **Provide all requested information.** If the Help Wanted ad asked for "salary requirements" or "salary history," include this information in your cover letter. However, you do not have to give specific numbers. It is okay to say, "My wage is in the range of $10 to $15 per hour." If the employer does not ask for salary information, do not offer any.
- **Ask for an interview.** You have sold yourself, now wrap it up. Be confident, but not pushy. "If you agree that I would be an asset to your company, please call me at [insert your phone number]. I am available for an interview at your convenience." Finally, thank the person. "Thank you for your consideration. I look forward to hearing from you soon." Always close with a "Sincerely," followed by your full name and signature.
- **Check for errors.** Read and re-read your letter to make sure each sentence is correctly worded and there are no errors in spelling, punctuation, or grammar. Do not rely on your computer's spell checker or grammar checker. A spell check will not detect if you typed "tot he" instead of "to the." It is a good idea to have someone else read your letter, too. He or she might notice an error you overlooked.

INTERVIEW

Understanding how to best prepare for and follow up on interviews is critical to your career success. At different times in your life, you may interview with a teacher or professor, a prospective employer, a supervisor, or a promotion or tenure committee. Just as having an excellent résumé is vital for opening the door, interview skills are critical for putting your best foot forward and seizing the opportunity to clearly articulate why you are the best person for the job.

RESEARCH THE COMPANY

Your ability to convince an employer that you understand and are interested in the field you are interviewing to enter is important. Show that you have knowledge about the company and the industry. What products or services does the company offer? How is it doing? What is the competition? Use your research to demonstrate your understanding of the company.

PREPARE QUESTIONS FOR THE INTERVIEWER

Prepare interview questions to ask the interviewer. Some examples include:

- "What would my responsibilities be?"
- "Could you describe my work environment?"
- "What are the chances to move up in the company?"
- "Do you offer training?"
- "What can you tell me about the people who work here?"

DRESS APPROPRIATELY

You will never get a second chance to make a good first impression. Nonverbal communication is 90 percent of communication, so dressing appropriately is of the utmost importance. Every job is different, and you should wear clothing that is appropriate for the job for which you are applying. In most situations, you will be safe if you wear clean, pressed, conservative business clothes in neutral colors. Pay special attention to grooming. Keep makeup light and wear very little jewelry. Make certain your nails and hair are clean, trimmed, and neat. Do not carry a large purse, backpack, books, or coat. Simply carry a pad of paper, a pen, and extra copies of your résumé and letters of reference in a small folder.

EXHIBIT GOOD BEHAVIOR

Conduct yourself properly during an interview. Go alone; be courteous and polite to everyone you meet. Relax and focus on your purpose: to make the best possible impression.

- Be on time.
- Be poised and relaxed.
- Avoid nervous habits.
- Avoid littering your speech with verbal clutter such as "you know," "um," and "like."
- Look your interviewer in the eye and speak with confidence.
- Use nonverbal techniques to reinforce your confidence, such as a firm handshake and poised demeanor.
- Convey maturity by exhibiting the ability to tolerate differences of opinion.
- Never call anyone by a first name unless you are asked to do so.
- Know the name, title, and the pronunciation of the interviewer's name.
- Do not sit down until the interviewer does.
- Do not talk too much about your personal life.
- Never bad-mouth your former employers.

BE PREPARED FOR COMMON INTERVIEW QUESTIONS

You can never be sure exactly what will happen at an interview, but you can be prepared for common interview questions. There are some interview questions that are illegal. Interviewers should not ask you about your age, gender, color, race, or religion. Employers should not ask whether you are married or pregnant, or question your health or disabilities.

Take time to think about your answers now. You might even write them down to clarify your thinking. The key to all interview questions is to be honest, and to be positive. Focus your answers on skills and abilities that apply to the job you are seeking. Practice answering the following questions with a friend:

- "Tell me about yourself."
- "Why do you want to work at this company?"
- "What did you like/dislike about your last job?"
- "What is your biggest accomplishment?"
- "What is your greatest strength?"
- "What is your greatest weakness?"
- "Do you prefer to work with others or on your own?"
- "What are your career goals?" or "Where do you see yourself in five years?"
- "Tell me about a time that you had a lot of work to do in a short time. How did you manage the situation?"
- "Have you ever had to work closely with a person you didn't get along with? How did you handle the situation?"

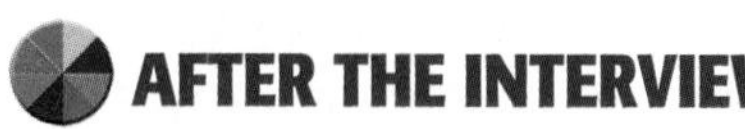

AFTER THE INTERVIEW

Be sure to thank the interviewer after the interview for his or her time and effort. Do not forget to follow up after the interview. Ask, "What is the next step?" If you are told to call in a few days, wait two or three days before calling back.

If the interview went well, the employer may call you to offer you the job. Find out the terms of the job offer, including job title and pay. Decide whether you want the job. If you decide not to accept the job, write a letter of rejection. Be courteous and thank the person for the opportunity and the offer. You may wish to give a brief general reason for not accepting the job. Leave the door open for possible employment in the future.

FOLLOW UP WITH A LETTER

Write a thank-you letter as soon as the interview is over. This shows your good manners, interest, and enthusiasm for the job. It also shows that you are organized. Make the letter neat and courteous. Thank the interviewer. Sell yourself again.

ACCEPTING A NEW JOB

If you decide to take the job, write a letter of acceptance. The letter should include some words of appreciation for the opportunity, written acceptance of the job offer, the terms of employment (salary, hours, benefits), and the starting date. Make sure the letter is neat and correct.

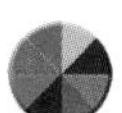

STARTING A NEW JOB

Your first day of work will be busy. Determine what the dress code is and dress appropriately. Learn to do each task assigned properly. Ask for help when you need it. Learn the rules and regulations of the workplace.

You will do some paperwork on your first day. Bring your personal fact sheet with you. You will need to fill out some forms. Form W-4 tells your employer how much money to withhold for taxes. You may also need to fill out Form I-9. This shows that you are allowed to work in the United States. You will need your Social Security number and proof that you are allowed to work in the United States. You can bring your U.S. passport, your Certificate of Naturalization, or your Certificate of U.S. Citizenship. If you are not a permanent resident of the United States, bring your green card. If you are a resident of the United States, you will need to bring your work permit on your first day. If you are under the age of 16 in some states, you need a different kind of work permit.

You might be requested to take a drug test as a requirement for employment in some states. This could be for the safety of you and your coworkers, especially when working with machinery or other equipment.

IMPORTANT SKILLS AND QUALITIES

You will not work alone on a job. You will need to learn skills for getting along and being a team player. There are many good qualities necessary to get along in the workplace. They include being positive, showing sympathy, taking an interest in others, tolerating differences, laughing a little, and showing respect. Your employer may promote you or give you a raise if you show good employability skills.

There are several qualities necessary to be a good employee and get ahead in your job:

- be cooperative
- possess good character
- be responsible
- finish what you start
- work fast but do a good job
- have a strong work ethic
- work well without supervision
- work well with others
- possess initiative
- show enthusiasm for what you do
- be on time
- make the best of your time
- obey company laws and rules
- be honest
- be loyal
- exhibit good health habits

LEAVING A JOB

If you are considering leaving your job or are being laid off, you are facing one of the most difficult aspects in your career. The first step in resigning is to prepare a short resignation letter to offer your supervisor at the conclusion of the meeting you set up with him or her. Keep the letter short and to the point. Express your appreciation for the opportunity you had with the company. Do not try to list all that was wrong with the job.

You want to leave on good terms. Do not forget to ask for a reference. Do not talk about your employer or any of your coworkers. Do not talk negatively about your employer when you apply for a new job.

If you are being laid off or face downsizing, it can make you feel angry or depressed. Try to view it as a career-change opportunity. If possible, negotiate a good severance package. Find out about any benefits you may be entitled to. Perhaps the company will offer job-search services or consultation for finding new employment.

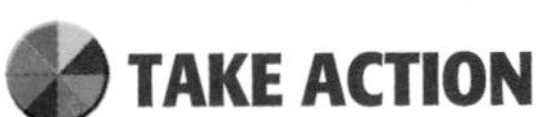

It is time for action. Remember the networking and contact lists you created when you searched for this job. Reach out for support from friends, family, and other acquaintances. Consider joining a job-search club. Assess your skills. Upgrade them if necessary. Examine your attitude and your vocational choices. Decide the direction you wish to take and move on!

MyPyramid Serving Amounts: Food Group Equivalencies

GRAIN GROUP

One ounce (28 g) equals:

1 regular slice enriched or whole grain bread
1 6-inch (15-cm) tortilla
½ burger bun, mini bagel, pita, or English muffin
1 cup (250 mL) ready-to-eat cereal (flakes or rounds)
½ cup (125 mL) cooked cereal, pasta, rice or other cooked grain
1 4½-inch (11-cm) pancake or waffle
5 whole wheat crackers
1 ounce (28 g) pretzels
3 cups (750 mL) popped corn

VEGETABLE GROUP

One cup (250 mL) equals:

2 cups (500 mL) raw leafy greens
1 cup (250 mL) cooked or chopped raw vegetables
1 cup (250 mL) cooked dry beans, peas, or lentils*
1 medium potato
1 cup (250 mL) vegetable juice

FRUIT GROUP

One cup (250 mL) equals:

1 small whole apple
1 medium grapefruit
1 cup (250 mL) berries or cut-up canned, frozen, or cooked fruit
1 large banana, orange or peach
1 cup (250 mL) fruit juice
½ cup (125 mL) dried fruit

MILK GROUP

One cup (250 mL) equals:

1 cup (250 mL) milk, buttermilk, yogurt, or pudding made with milk
1½ ounces (42 g) hard cheese, such as cheddar, Swiss, Monterey Jack, or mozzarella
2 ounces (56 g) process cheese, such as American
⅓ cup (75 mL) shredded cheese
2 cups (500 mL) cottage cheese
1 cup (250 mL) frozen yogurt
1½ cups (375 mL) ice cream

MEAT & BEANS GROUP

One ounce (28 g) equals:

1 ounce (28 g) cooked lean meat, poultry, or fish
¼ cup (50 mL) cooked dry beans, peas, or lentils*
1 egg
1 tablespoon (15 mL) peanut butter
¼ cup (50 mL) egg substitute
½ ounce (14 g) nuts
¼ cup (50 mL) tofu
2 tablespoons (30 mL) hummus

* Count dry beans, peas, or lentils toward either the Vegetable Group or the Meat & Beans Group but not both.

Daily Values and DRIs for Teens

The Daily Values are standard values developed by the Food and Drug Administration (FDA) for use on food labels. Dietary Reference Intakes (DRIs) are used by nutrition professionals. They give nutrient reference amounts for specific ages and genders. Only the amounts for teens are included here. You may find it interesting to compare the DRIs for your age and gender to the Daily Values.

The DRIs include four types of nutrient reference values. Most of the values listed below are Recommended Dietary Allowances (RDAs). An RDA is the daily amount of a nutrient that will meet the needs of nearly all healthy people. For some nutrients, there is not yet enough data to establish an RDA. In the case, the value listed is an Adequate Intake (AI), an amount believed to be adequate.

		Dietary Reference Intake (RDA or AI)			
Nutrient	**Daily Value**	**Males 9–13**	**Males 14–18**	**Females 9–13**	**Females 14–18**
Protein	50 g	34 g	52 g	34 g	46 g
Carbohydrate (total)	300 g	130 g	130 g	130 g	130 g
Fiber	25 g	31 g	38 g	26 g	26 g
Fat (total)	65 g	**	**	**	**
Saturated fat	20 g	**	**	**	**
Cholesterol	300 mg	**	**	**	**
Vitamin A	5,000 IU (875 μg RE)	600 μg RAE	900 μg RAE	600 μg RAE	700 μg RAE
Thiamin	1.5 mg	0.9 mg	1.2 mg	0.9 mg	1.0 mg
Riboflavin	1.7 mg	0.9 mg	1.3 mg	0.9 mg	1.0 mg
Niacin	20 mg NE	12 mg NE	16 mg NE	12 mg NE	14 mg NE
Vitamin B6	2 mg	1.0 mg	1.3 mg	1.0 mg	1.2 mg
Vitamin B12	6 μg	1.8 μg	2.4 μg	1.8 μg	2.4 μg
Folate	400 μg	300 μg DFE	400 μg DFE	300 μg DFE	400 μg DFE
Biotin	300 μg	20 μg	25 μg	20 μg	25 μg
Pantothenic acid	10 mg	4 mg	5 mg	4 mg	5 mg
Vitamin C	60 mg	45 mg	75 mg	45 mg	65 mg
Vitamin D	400 IU (6.5 μg)	5 μg	5 μg	5 μg	5 μg
Vitamin E	30 IU (9 mg α-TE)	11 mg α-TE	15 mg α-TE	11 mg α-TE	15 mg α-TE
Vitamin K	80 mg	60 μg	75 μg	60 μg	75 μg
Calcium	1,000 mg	1,300 mg	1,300 mg	1,300 mg	1,300 mg
Chloride	3,400 mg	2,300 mg	2,300 mg	2,300 mg	2,300 mg
Copper	2 mg	700 μg	890 μg	700 μg	890 μg
Iodine	150 μg	120 μg	150 μg	120 μg	150 μg
Iron	18 mg	8 mg	11 mg	8 mg	15 mg
Magnesium	400 mg	240 mg	410 mg	240 mg	360 mg
Phosphorus	1,000 mg	1,250 mg	1,250 mg	1,250 mg	1,250 mg
Potassium	3,500 mg	4,500 mg	4,700 mg	4,500 mg	4,700 mg
Selenium	70 μg	40 μg	55 μg	45 μg	55 μg
Sodium	2,400 mg	1,500 mg	1,500 mg	1,500 mg	1,500 mg
Zinc	15 mg	8 mg	11 mg	8 mg	9 mg
Water	**	2.4 L	3.3 L	2.1 L	2.3 L

*Based on a diet of 2,000 calories per day **No value established

Key to nutrient measures

g gram
mg milligram (1000 mg = 1 g)
μg microgram (1000 μg = 1 mg; 1,000,000 μg = 1 g)
IU International Unit (an old measurement of vitamin activity)
RAE retinol activity equivalents (a measure of Vitamin A activity)
NE niacin equivalents (a measure of niacin activity)
DFE dietary folate equivalents (a measure of folate activity
α-TE alpha-tocopherol equivalents (a measure of Vitamin E activity)
L liter

NUTRITIVE VALUE OF FOODS APPENDIX

Item No.	Food Description	Approximate Measure	Weight	Food energy	Protein	Fat	Cholesterol	Calcium	Iron	Sodium	Vitamin A value*	Vitamin C
				Nutrients in Indicated Quantity								
			Grams	Calories	Grams	Grams	Milligrams	Milligrams	Milligrams	Milligrams	Retinol equivalents	Milligrams
	Beverages											
9	Club soda	12 fl oz	355	0	0	0	0	18	Tr	75	0	0
10	Regular cola	12 fl oz	369	137	Tr	Tr	0	7	0.4	15	0	0
11	Diet, artificially sweetened cola	12 fl oz	355	7	Tr	Tr	0	11	0.4	28	0	0
20	Fruit punch drink	8 fl oz	248	119	0	0	0	20	0.2	25	0	1
	Dairy Product											
	Natural Cheese											
32	Cheddar, cut pieces	1 oz	28	114	7	9	30	205	0.2	176	75	0
38	Cottage cheese, lowfat (2%)	1 cup	226	163	28	2	9	138	0.3	918	25	0
43	Mozzarella, part skim milk	1 oz	28	86	7	6	15	208	Tr	150	39	0
46	Parmesan, grated	1 tbsp	5	22	2	1	4	55	Tr	76	6	0
52	Pasteurized process American cheese	1 oz	28	105	6	9	26	155	Tr	417	71	0
	Milk, fluid:											
78	Whole (3.3% fat)	1 cup	244	146	8	8	24	276	Tr	98	68	0
79	Reduced fat (2%)	1 cup	244	122	8	5	20	285	Tr	100	134	1
83	Nonfat (skim)	1 cup	247	86	8	Tr	5	504	0.1	128	338	3
85	Buttermilk	1 cup	245	98	8	2	10	284	0.1	257	17	2
88	Evaporated skim milk	1 cup	245	100	10	Tr	5	372	0.4	149	149	2
91	Dried, nonfat, instantized	1 cup	245	81	8	Tr	5	284	Tr	130	162	1
	Milk beverages:											
94	Chocolate milk, low-fat (1%)	1 cup	250	158	8	3	8	288	0.6	152	145	2
105	Shakes, thick; Vanilla	10 oz	283	379	8	13	48	275	0.3	133	133	8
	Milk desserts, frozen:											
	Ice cream, vanilla, regular (about 11% fat):											
107	Hardened	1 cup	133	267	5	14	53	168	0.2	98	146	1
109	Frozen yogurt	1 cup	200	214	9	3	10	318	0.5	120	24	1
	Ice cream, vanilla, low-fat:											
113	Hardened (about 4% fat)	1 cup	131	216	6	6	35	211	0.3	97	168	2
116	Sherbet (about 2% fat)	1 cup	193	278	2	4	0	104	0.3	89	19	11
	Yogurt, made with low-fat milk:											
117	Fruit-flavored	8 oz	245	250	11	3	10	372	0.2	142	24	2
118	Plain	8 oz	245	154	13	4	15	448	0.2	172	34	2

Eggs												
	Eggs, large (24 oz. per dozen):											
124	Fried in margarine	1 egg	46	89	6	7	210	26	1.9	238	88	0
125	Hard-cooked, shell removed	1 egg	50	77	6	5	211	25	0.6	139	84	0
Fats and Oils												
129	Butter (4 sticks per lb) (⅛ stick)	1 tbsp	14	102	Tr	12	31	3	0.0	82	97	0
138	Margarine (⅛ stick)	1 tbsp	14	100	Tr	11	0	0	Tr	93	116	0
147	Corn oil	1 cup	218	1,927	0	218	0	0	0.0	0	0	0
	Salad dressings, commercial:											
162	French, Regular	1 tbsp	16	60	Tr	6	1	3	Tr	197	2	0
163	French, Low calorie	1 tbsp	16	24	Tr	2	1	3	0.1	179	2	0
Fish and Shellfish												
177	Fish sticks, frozen, reheated (stock, 4 by 1 by ½ in.)	1 fish stick	28	70	3	4	9	7	0.3	118	9	0
181	Haddock, breaded, fried	3 oz	85	151	16	7	57	44	1.2	105	14	0
182	Halibut, broiled, with butter and lemon juice	3 oz	85	113	19	4	48	19	0.4	354	34	3
195	Tuna, canned, oil packed, chunk light	3 oz	85	168	25	7	15	11	1.2	301	20	0
196	Tuna, canned, water-pack, solid white	3 oz	85	99	22	1	26	9	1.3	287	14	0
Fruits and Fruit Juices												
198	Apples, raw, unpeeled, 2¾-in. diam.	1 apple	138	72	Tr	Tr	0	8	0.2	1	4	6
202	Apple juice, bottled or canned	1 cup	248	117	Tr	Tr	0	17	1.0	7	0	28
204	Applesauce, canned, unsweetened	1 cup	244	105	Tr	Tr	0	7	0.3	5	2	3
215	Bananas, raw, without peel, whole	1 banana	118	105	1	Tr	0	7	0.3	1	4	10
229	Fruit cocktail, canned, juice pack	1 cup	237	109	1	Tr	0	19	0.5	9	36	6
230	Grapefruit, raw, without peel, 3¾-in. diam.	½ grapefruit	128	41	1	Tr	0	15	0.1	0	59	44
233	Grapefruit juice, canned, unsweetened	1 cup	247	94	1	Tr	0	17	0.5	2	0	72
237	Grapes, Thompson Seedless	10 grapes	50	30	Tr	Tr	0	0	Tr	0	0	15
239	Grape juice, canned or bottled	1 cup	253	154	1	Tr	0	23	0.6	8	0	0.3
242	Kiwi fruit, raw, without skin	1 kiwifruit	76	46	1	Tr	0	26	0.2	2	3	71
250	Mangos, raw, without skin and seed	1 mango	207	135	1	1	0	21	0.3	4	79	57
251	Cantaloupe	1 melon	814	277	7	2	0	73	1.7	130	1,376	300
253	Nectarines, raw, without pits	1 nectarine	136	60	1	Tr	0	8	0.4	0	23	7
254	Oranges, raw, whole	1 orange	131	62	1	Tr	0	52	0.1	0	14	70
260	Orange juice, frozen concentrate, diluted	1 cup	249	112	2	Tr	0	27	0.3	5	12	98
262	Papayas, raw, ½-in. cubes	1 cup	140	55	1	Tr	0	34	0.1	4	77	87
263	Peaches, raw, whole, 2½-in.diam.	1 peach	98	38	1	Tr	0	6	0.2	0	16	7
273	Pears, raw, with skin, cored, Bartlett, 2½-in. diam.	1 pear	166	96	1	1	0	15	0.3	2	2	7
283	Pineapple, chunks or tidbits, juice pack	1 cup	249	149	1	Tr	0	35	0.7	2	5	24

Item No.	Food Description	Approximate Measure	Weight	Nutrients in Indicated Quantity								
				Food energy	Protein	Fat	Cholesterol	Calcium	Iron	Sodium	Vitamin A value*	Vitamin C
			Grams	Calories	Grams	Grams	Milligrams	Milligrams	Milligrams	Milligrams	Retinol equivalents	Milligrams
287	Plantains, without peel, cooked, boiled, sliced	1 cup	190	220	2	Tr	0	4	1.1	10	86	21
288	Plums, raw, 2⅛-in. diam.	1 plum	66	30	Tr	Tr	0	4	0.1	0	11	6
297	Raisins, seedless, cup, not pressed down	1 cup	145	434	5	Tr	0	72	2.7	16	0	3
303	Strawberries, raw, capped, whole	1 cup	144	46	1	Tr	0	23	0.6	1	1	85
309	Watermelon, 4 by 8 in. wedge	1 piece	286	86	2	Tr	0	20	0.7	3	80	23
Grain Products												
311	Bagels, plain or water, enriched	1 bagel	69	177	7	1	0	61	4.1	309	0	1
314	Biscuits, from mix, 2 in. diameter	1 biscuit	30	97	2	4	2	54	0.6	274	7	Tr
	Breads:											
319	Cracked-wheat bread (18 per loaf)	1 slice	26	68	2	1	0	27	0.9	138	0	0
332	Pita bread, enriched, white, 6½-in. diam.	1 pita	85	234	8	1	0	73	2.2	456	0	0
346	White bread, enriched (18 per loaf)	1 slice	26	69	2	1	0	39	0.9	177	0	0
353	Whole-wheat bread (16 per loaf)	1 slice	29	80	3	1	0	23	1.1	172	0	0
355	Bread stuffing, dry type, from mix	1 cup	140	246	4	12	0	41	1.5	720	109	0
	Breakfast cereals:											
359	Cream of Wheat®, cooked	1 cup	241	106	3	Tr	0	94	8.0	431	0	0
367	Cheerios®	1 oz	30	111	4	2	0	122	10.3	213	150	6
368	Kellogg's® Corn Flakes	1 oz	25	90	2	Tr	0	15	6.7	197	136	5
383	Shredded Wheat	1 oz	25	84	3	1	0	12	0.7	2	0	3
386	Sugar Frosted Flakes, Kellogg's®	1 oz	31	114	1	Tr	0	2	4.5	148	160	6
390	Wheaties®	1 oz	30	106	3	1	0	0	8.1	218	150	6
	Cakes prepared from cake mixes:											
394	Angelfood, 1⁄12 of cake	1 piece	57	143	3	Tr	0	47	0.1	283	0	0
396	Coffeecake, crumb, 1⁄12 of 8" cake	1 piece	42	136	3	4	40	47	0.7	181	15	0
398	Devil's food with chocolate frosting, 1⁄12 of cake	1 piece	109	405	4	16	31	102	2.7	289	61	0
	Cookies, commercial:											
424	Brownies with nuts and frosting	1 brownie	34	129	2	5	12	11	1.1	50	2	0
426	Chocolate chip, 2¼ in. diam.	4 cookies	30	147	2	7	0	10	1.1	89	0	0
429	Fig bars, square, 1⅝-in. square	4 cookies	64	224	2	2	0	40	1.8	224	0	4
430	Oatmeal with raisins, 2⅝-in. diam.	4 cookies	30	135	2	5	0	11	0.7	115	2	Tr
437	Corn chips	1-oz pkg.	28	145	2	8	0	46	0.4	172	0	0

	Crackers:											
444	Graham, plain, 2½-in. square	2 crackers	14	59	1	1	0	3	0.5	85	0	0
448	Snack-type, standard	1 cracker	3	15	Tr	1	0	4	0.1	25	0	0
449	Wheat, thin	4 crackers	8	36	1	2	0	4	Tr	64	0	0
	Doughnuts, made with enriched flour:											
456	Cake type, plain, 3¼-in. diam.	1 doughnut	25	105	1	6	9	11	0.5	136	10	0
457	Yeast-leavened, glazed, 3¾-in. diam.	1 doughnut	60	242	4	14	4	26	1.2	205	2	Tr
458	English muffins, plain, enriched	1 muffin	58	132	5	1	0	95	2.3	246	0	1
461	Macaroni, enriched, cooked	1 cup	140	220	8	1	0	10	1.9	325	0	0
	Muffins, 2½-in. diam., commercial mix:											
467	Blueberry	1 muffin	66	183	4	4	20	38	1.1	295	15	1
468	Bran	1 muffin	58	127	5	1	0	54	3.1	183	39	0
470	Noodles (egg noodles), enriched, cooked	1 cup	160	219	7	3	46	19	2.3	378	10	0
	Pancakes, 4-in. diam.:											
474	Plain mix (with enriched flour), egg, milk, oil added	1 pancake	29	65	2	2	5	21	0.6	146	19	Tr
	Pies, 9-in. diam.:											
478	Apple, ⅛ of pie	1 piece	150	356	3	17	0	16	0.7	399	48	5
488	Lemon meringue, ⅛ of pie	1 piece	137	367	2	12	62	77	0.8	200	70	4
494	Pumpkin, ⅛ of pie	1 piece	155	316	2	14	65	146	1.9	349	660	3
	Popcorn, popped:											
497	Air-popped, unsalted	1 cup	8	31	1	Tr	0	1	0.3	1	1	0
498	Popped in vegetable oil, salted	1 cup	11	55	1	3	0	1	0.3	97	0	0
499	Sugar syrup coated	1 cup	35	135	2	1	0	2	0.5	Tr	3	0
500	Pretzels	10 twists	60	229	5	2	0	22	1.0	1,029	0	0
	Rice:											
503	Brown, cooked, served hot	1 cup	195	214	5	2	0	20	0.8	587	0	0
505	White, enriched, cooked, served hot	1 cup	158	204	4	Tr	0	16	1.9	577	0	0
	Rolls, enriched, commercial:											
509	Dinner, 2½-in.diam.	1 roll	28	87	3	2	1	50	1.0	150	0	Tr
510	Frankfurter and hamburger	1 roll	43	120	4	2	0	59	1.4	206	0	0
514	Spaghetti, enriched, cooked	1 cup	140	220	8	1	0	10	1.9	325	0	0
	Legumes, Nuts, and Seeds											
526	Almonds, shelled, whole	1 oz	28	162	6	14	0	69	1.2	0	0	0
	Beans, dry, cooked, drained:											
527	Black	1 cup	177	312	12	15	0	64	2.3	414	0	0
528	Great Northern	1 cup	180	356	16	15	0	149	6.1	356	0	0
531	Pinto	1 cup	178	313	12	15	0	57	2.4	352	0	2

Item No.	Food Description	Approximate Measure	Weight	Food energy	Protein	Fat	Cholesterol	Calcium	Iron	Sodium	Vitamin A value*	Vitamin C
				Nutrients in Indicated Quantity								
			Grams	Calories	Grams	Grams	Milligrams	Milligrams	Milligrams	Milligrams	Retinol equivalents	Milligrams
536	Black-eyed peas, dry, cooked (with cooking liquid)	1 cup	224	419	11	20	20	36	3.6	844	0	Tr
544	Chickpeas, cooked, drained	1 cup	169	399	15	18	0	74	3.8	409	2	2
550	Lentils, dry, cooked, with peanuts	1 cup	196	323	16	13	0	35	6.1	431	0	3
553	Mixed nuts, dry roasted, salted	1 oz	28	173	5	16	0	30	0.9	111	0	1
555	Peanuts, roasted in oil, salted	1 cup	144	863	40	76	0	88	2.2	461	0	1
557	Peanut butter	1 tbsp	16	94	4	8	0	7	0.3	73	0	0
564	Refried beans, canned	1 cup	253	367	16	13	15	96	4.2	711	0	10
	Soy Products:											
567	Miso	1 cup	275	547	32	17	0	157	6.9	10,252	11	0
568	Tofu, piece 2¼ by 2¾ by 1 in.	1 piece	124	76	8	5	0	138	1.4	10	0	Tr
569	Sunflower seeds, dry, hulled	1 oz	28	162	7	14	0	33	1.9	1	1	Tr
570	Tahini	1 tbsp	15	89	3	8	0	64	1.3	17	0	0
	Meat and Meat Products											
	Beef, cooked:											
	Braised or pot roasted:											
575	Chuck blade. lean and fat, piece	3 oz	85	258	24	17	80	10	2.5	189	0	0
577	Round, bottom, lean and fat piece	3 oz	85	190	29	8	84	7	2.3	37	0	0
578	Lean only from item 577	3 oz	85	144	24	5	61	5	2.0	32	0	0
580	Ground beef, regular, broiled, patty	4 oz	85	235	22	16	75	26	2.0	340	0	0
585	Round, eye of, lean and fat, roasted	3 oz	85	143	25	4	46	6	2.0	32	0	0
587	Sirloin, steak, broiled, lean and fat	3 oz	85	214	23	13	70	14	1.6	317	0	0
590	Beef, dried, chipped	2.5 oz	71	109	22	1	56	4	2.1	1,981	0	0
	Lamb:											
593	Chops, loin, broiled, lean and fat	4 oz	72	226	16	18	68	14	1.4	281	0	0
	Pork, cured, cooked:											
599	Bacon, regular	3 slices	16	87	6	7	18	2	0.2	370	2	0
601	Ham, light cure, roasted, lean and fat	3 oz	85	137	17	7	54	7	0.6	936	9	0
	Luncheon meat:											
605	Chopped ham (8 slices per 6-oz pkg.)	1 slice	28	45	5	2	15	2	0.3	358	0	0
	Pork, fresh, cooked:											
610	Chop, loin, pan fried, lean and fat	3 oz	44	123	12	8	35	10	0.4	169	1	Tr
614	Rib, roasted, lean and fat	3 oz	85	279	20	22	78	21	0.9	44	3	Tr

No.	Food	Measure	Weight (g)									
	Sausages:											
618	Bologna, slice (8 per 8-oz pkg.)	1 slice	28	86	4	7	17	24	0.3	206	7	Tr
620	Brown and serve, browned	1 link	13	44	2	4	7	2	0.2	150	0	0
621	Frankfurter, cooked (reheated)	1	57	176	8	15	43	28	1.0	712	5	0
Mixed Dishes												
629	Beef and vegetable stew, home recipe	1 cup	249	182	25	5	42	47	2.5	817	271	7
631	Chicken a la king, home recipe	1 cup	241	460	25	33	190	142	1.9	952	323	5
642	Spaghetti in tomato sauce with cheese, home recipe	1 cup	248	293	10	4	0	40	2.7	563	32	4
Fast Foods												
645	Cheeseburger, regular	1 sandwich	107	317	17	15	46	164	2.8	547	29	0
648	English muffin, egg, cheese, bacon	1 sandwich	135	382	21	19	247	258	3.7	932	140	1
649	Fish sandwich, regular, with cheese	1 sandwich	207	596	27	30	72	286	4.2	1,176	43	Tr
651	Hamburger, regular	1 sandwich	93	270	15	11	34	86	2.7	369	0	0
653	Pizza, cheese, 1/8 of 12-in. diam.	1 slice	86	237	11	10	21	181	1.6	462	68	Tr
654	Roast beef sandwich	1 sandwich	136	341	27	14	67	86	4.3	602	0	0
655	Taco	1 taco	76	98	7	3	50	64	0.9	306	9	3
Poultry and Poultry Products												
	Chicken:											
	Fried, flesh, with skin and bones:											
656	Breast, ½ breast, batter dipped	4.9 oz	140	365	34	19	102	27	1.9	396	35	0
657	Drumstick, batter dipped	2.5 oz	112	280	31	17	133	16	1.5	473	47	0
	Roasted, flesh only:											
660	Breast, ½ breast	3.0 oz	86	162	25	6	76	13	1.0	351	14	0
662	Stewed, flesh only, light and dark meat	1 cup	140	332	43	17	116	18	2.0	109	48	0
	Turkey, roasted, flesh only:											
665	Dark meat, piece, 2½ by 1⅝ by ½ in.	4 pieces	78	145	22	6	66	25	1.8	188	0	0
666	Light meat, piece, 4 by 2 by ¼ in.	2 pieces	75	117	22	2	52	14	1.0	170	0	0
667	Chopped or diced	1 cup	135	279	38	13	111	35	2.4	310	0	0
Soups, Sauces, and Gravies												
	Soups, condensed:											
	Canned, prepared with milk:											
679	Cream of mushroom	1 cup	248	169	6	10	10	159	1.4	861	67	0
680	Tomato	1 cup	248	136	6	3	10	159	1.4	742	82	16
	Canned, prepared with water:											
681	Bean with bacon	1 cup	253	172	8	6	3	83	2.0	954	46	2
682	Beef broth, bouillon, consomme	1 cup	240	17	3	1	0	14	0.4	782	0	0
684	Chicken noodle	1 cup	241	65	3	2	14	14	1.7	868	51	0
693	Vegetarian	1 cup	241	72	2	2	0	24	1.1	827	174	1

Item No.	Food Description	Approximate Measure	Weight	Nutrients in Indicated Quantity								
				Food energy	Protein	Fat	Cholesterol	Calcium	Iron	Sodium	Vitamin A value*	Vitamin C
			Grams	Calories	Grams	Grams	Milligrams	Milligrams	Milligrams	Milligrams	Retinol equivalents	Milligrams
	Dehydrated, prepared with water:											
697	Onion	1 pkt	100	349	9	Tr	0	257	1.6	21	1	75
	Sauces, ready to serve:											
703	Barbecue	2 tbsp	35	52	0	Tr	0	4	0.1	392	4	Tr
704	Soy	1 tbsp	16	8	1	Tr	0	3	0.3	902	0	0
	Gravies:											
708	Brown, from dry mix	1 cup	233	123	9	6	7	14	1.6	1,305	2	0
709	Chicken, from dry mix	1 serving	8	30	1	1	2	12	0.1	332	3	0
	Sugars and Sweets											
	Candy:											
711	Chocolate, milk, plain	1 oz	28	150	2	8	6	53	0.6	22	14	0
712	Chocolate, milk, with almonds	1 oz	41	216	4	14	8	92	0.7	30	18	Tr
717	Fondant, uncoated (mints, other)	1 oz	22	82	0	0	0	0	0.0	4	0	0
720	Hard candy	1 oz	28	112	0	Tr	0	1	Tr	11	0	0
723	Custard, baked	1 cup	244	232	12	9	198	271	0.9	215	159	0
724	Gelatin dessert	½ cup	120	74	1	0	0	4	Tr	90	0	0
726	Honey, strained or extracted	1 tbsp	21	64	Tr	0	0	1	0.1	1	0	Tr
727	Jams and preserves	1 tbsp	21	55	Tr	Tr	0	4	0.1	8	2	2
739	Pudding, vanilla, instant	1 cup	267	358	7	10	13	238	0.9	352	21	2
	Sugars:											
741	Brown, pressed down	1 cup	220	829	0	0	0	187	4.2	86	0	0
742	White, granulated	1 tsp	4.2	16	0	0	0	0	0.0	0	0	0
745	White, powdered, sifted	1 cup	120	467	0	Tr	0	1	Tr	1	0	0
	Syrups:											
748	Molasses, cane, blackstrap	2 tbsp	40	116	0	Tr	0	82	1.9	15	0	0
749	Table syrup (corn and maple)	2 tbsp	41	106	0	Tr	0	3	Tr	34	0	0
	Vegetables and Vegetable Products											
750	Alfalfa sprouts, raw	1 cup	33	10	1	Tr	0	11	0.3	2	3	3
761	Beans, string, cooked, drained, from frozen (cut)	1 cup	140	83	3	4	0	59	0.9	433	88	13
771	Broccoli, raw	1 spear	31	11	1	Tr	0	15	0.2	10	10	28
772	Broccoli, cooked	1 spear	38	21	1	1	0	15	0.3	110	37	24
778	Cabbage, common variety, raw, coarsely shredded	1 cup	89	21	1	Tr	0	42	0.5	16	8	29

780	Cabbage, Chinese, Pak-choi, cooked, drained	1 cup	175	66	2	5	0	145	1.4	612	304	41
784	Carrots, whole, 7½ by 1⅛ in.	1 carrot	72	30	1	Tr	0	24	0.2	50	606	4
786	Carrots, cooked, sliced, drained, from raw	1 cup	151	82	1	4	0	44	0.5	462	1,290	5
792	Celery, pascal type, raw, stalk, lrg. outer, 8 by 1½ in.	1 stalk	40	6	Tr	Tr	0	16	Tr	32	9	1
795	Collards, cooked, drained, from frozen (chopped)	1 cup	175	94	5	4	0	355	1.9	486	1,012	45
796	Corn, sweet, cooked, drained, raw ear 5 by 1¾ in.	1 ear	89	110	3	3	0	2	0.5	226	31	5
798	Corn, sweet, cooked, drained, from frozen kernels	1 cup	164	133	4	1	0	5	0.8	372	16	6
799	Corn, sweet, canned, cream style	1 cup	256	184	5	1	0	8	0.9	730	0	12
800	Corn, sweet, canned, whole kernel, vacuum pack	½ cup	128	82	3	1	0	5	0.5	273	0	7
801	Cucumber, with peel, slices	½ cup	52	8	Tr	Tr	0	8	0.2	1	3	2
806	Kale, cooked, drained, from raw	1 cup	135	119	3	4	0	93	1.2	339	921	53
813	Lettuce, raw, crisp head, as iceberg, chopped	1 cup	55	8	1	Tr	0	10	0.2	6	14	2
814	Lettuce, raw, loose leaf, chopped or shredded	1 cup	55	7	1	Tr	0	19	0.7	3	91	2
830	Peas, green, frozen, cooked, drained	1 cup	165	157	8	4	0	38	2.4	516	206	16
832	Peppers, sweet, raw	1 pepper	74	15	1	Tr	0	7	0.2	2	13	60
834	Potatoes, baked, with skin	1 potato	178	194	4	4	0	27	1.9	418	41	17
838	Potatoes, french fried, strip, frozen, oven heated	10 strips	50	70	1	3	0	6	0.4	194	0	7
839	Potatoes, french fried, strip, frozen, fried in veg. oil	10 strips	50	160	2	9	0	6	0.7	96	0	1
849	Potato chips	1 oz	28	155	2	11	0	7	0.5	149	0	5
852	Radishes, raw	½ cup	58	9	Tr	Tr	0	14	0.2	23	0	9
856	Spinach, raw, chopped	1 cup	30	7	1	Tr	0	30	0.8	24	141	8
858	Spinach, cooked, drained, from frozen (leaf)	1 cup	210	101	8	5	0	313	4.0	630	1,270	4
861	Squash, summer, sliced, cooked, drained	1 cup	185	68	2	4	0	48	0.7	496	57	10
862	Squash, winter, cubes, baked	1 cup	210	151	2	4	0	52	1.0	384	538	19
863	Sweet potatoes, baked in skin, peeled	1 potato	119	134	2	4	0	44	0.8	441	1,128	22
868	Tomatoes, raw, 2⅗-in. diam.	1 tomato	123	22	1	Tr	0	12	0.3	6	52	16
869	Tomatoes, canned, solids and liquid	1 cup	240	46	2	Tr	0	72	1.3	24	17	34
870	Tomato juice, canned	1 cup	243	41	2	Tr	0	24	1.0	654	56	45
877	Vegetable juice cocktail, canned	1 cup	242	44	2	Tr	0	24	1.0	653	121	56
Miscellaneous Items												
885	Catsup	1 cup	240	233	4	1	0	43	1.2	2,674	113	36
894	Mustard, prepared, yellow	1 tsp	5	3	Tr	Tr	0	4	0.1	56	0	Tr
895	Olives, canned, green, medium	4 olives	13	19	Tr	1	0	7	Tr	202	3	0
	Pickles, cucumber:											
901	Dill, medium, whole, 33/4 in.	1 cup	65	12	Tr	Tr	0	6	0.3	833	6	1
903	Sweet, small, whole, 21/2 in. long	1 cup	37	7	Tr	Tr	0	3	0.2	474	3	Tr

NOTE: Nutritive values of most packaged foods may be obtained from the "Nutrition Facts" panel on the container.

Glossary

How to Use This Glossary

- Content vocabulary terms in this glossary are words that relate to this book's content. They are **highlighted yellow** in your text.
- Words in this glossary that have an asterisk (*) are academic vocabulary terms. They help you understand your school subjects and are used on tests. They are **boldfaced blue** in your text.
- Some of the vocabulary words in this book include pronunciation symbols to help you sound out the words. Use the pronunciation key to help you pronounce the words.

Pronunciation Key		
a . . . . **a**t	**ô** . . . . f**o**rk, **a**ll	**th** . . . **th**in
ā . . . . **a**pe	**oo** . . . w**oo**d, p**u**t	**th** . . . **th**is
ä . . . . f**a**ther	**o͞o** . . . f**oo**l	**zh** . . . trea**s**ure
e . . . . **e**nd	**oi** . . . **oi**l	**ə** . . . . **a**go, tak**e**n, penc**i**l, lem**o**n, circ**u**s
ē . . . . m**e**	**ou** . . . **ou**t	**ˈ** . . . . indicates primary stress (symbol in front of and *above* letter)
i . . . . **i**t	**u** . . . . **u**p	**ˌ** . . . . indicates secondary stress (symbol in front of and *below* letter)
ī . . . . **i**ce	**ü** . . . . **u**se	
o . . . . h**o**t	**ü** . . . . r**u**le	
ō . . . . h**o**pe	**u̲** . . . . p**u**ll	
ȯ . . . . s**a**w	**ŋ** . . . . si**ng**	

20-second scrub Using soap and warm water to scrub your hands for 20 seconds. (p. 281)

à la carte Listed and priced individually. (p. 269)

absorption The process by which nutrients move into the bloodstream. (p. 67)

* **abundant** Plentiful. (p. 212)

* **accelerate** Speed up. (p. 43)

active dry yeast Partially dormant yeast contained in flour granules. (p. 656)

added sugar A sugar that is extracted from plants and used to sweeten foods is an added sugar. (p. 78)

* **adequate** Sufficient. (p. 79)

Adequate Intake (AI) A nutrient standard that is used when a lack of scientific information makes it impossible to establish the RDA for a particular nutrient. (p. 61)

* **advocate** Push for. (p. 211)

aerobic exercise (ˌer-ˈō-bik) An activity that increases the heart and breathing rate for at least 20 minutes. (p. 155)

* **affect** Change. (p. 374)

agroforestry An ancient practice of raising shade-loving crops, such as mushrooms and cocoa, under the shelter of trees. (p. 37)

air cell A pocket of air. (p. 516)

al dente (äl-den-ˌtā) Cooked so that the pasta is firm to the bite, rather than soft and mushy. (p. 478)

albumen (al-ˈbyü-mən) The thick fluid commonly known as egg white. (p. 516)

amino acid A molecule that combines with other amino acid molecules to make proteins. (p. 88)

anaerobic exercise (ˌa-nə-ˈrō-bik) Involving short, intense bursts of activity "without oxygen." (p. 155)

analogs (ˈa-nə-ˌlȯgs) Foods made to imitate other foods. (p. 45)

anemia (ə-ˈnē-mē-ə) A blood disorder that causes lack of energy, weakness, shortness of breath, and cold hands and feet. (p. 60)

annual percentage rate (APR) The yearly rate of interest that you must pay on the principal. (p. 322)

anorexia nervosa (ˌa-nəh-ˈrek-sē-ə ˌ nər-ˈvō-sə) An intense fear of gaining weight that leads to unhealthy eating and dangerous weight loss. (p. 168)

antioxidants (ˌan-tē-ˈäk-sə-dənts) Substances that protect cells and the immune system from damage by harmful chemicals. (p. 103)

antipasto A variety of appetizers. Italian word for before the meal. (p. 747)

appetizer A small portion of food served at the beginning of a meal to whet the appetite. (p. 260)

aquaculture A method of raising seafood in enclosed areas of water. (p. 37)

arcing The production of electrical sparks that can damage the oven or start a fire. (p. 395)

aromatic vegetables Vegetables that have their flavor brought out by sautéing. (p. 462)

* **aseptic** Preventing infection. (p. 492)

aseptic packages (ˌā-ˈsep-tik) Consisting of layers of plastic, paperboard, and aluminum foil. (p. 46)

* **assess** Evaluate. (p. 319)

* **associated** Related. (p. 643)

au gratin (ō-ˈgrä-tən) Topped with buttered breadcrumbs or grated cheese. (p. 628)

au jus (ō-ˈzhü(s)) With the natural meat juices, unthickened and skimmed of fat. (p. 644)

B

baguette (ba-ˈget) A long, crusty loaf of bread. (p. 739)

bakeware Equipment for cooking food in an oven. (p. 326)

baklava (ˈbä-klə-ˌvä) A sweet dessert made with layers of phyllo with finely chopped walnuts or almonds mixed with sugar and cinnamon. (p. 749)

bannock A flat, biscuit-like bread made with flour or oats and cooked on cast iron over a hot grill. (p. 717)

bar cookie Baked in a shallow pan and then cut into a bar or square; it can be soft, firm or layered with different bases, fillings, and toppings. (p. 685)

basal metabolism (ˈbā-səl mə-ˈta-bə-ˌli-zəm) The energy you need to maintain automatic processes. (p. 68)

basic sandwich Two slices of bread with a filling in between. (p. 596)

baste To pour or brush melted fat, cooking juices, or other liquid over food as it cooks. (p. 554)

beading Brown droplets on the surface of the meringue, occurring if the meringue is overcooked. (p. 527)

behavior modification Making gradual, permanent changes in eating and activity habits. (p. 153)

beta-carotene (ˈbā-tə-ˈkar-ə-ˌtēn) An orange or red phytochemical found in dark green and orange vegetables and fruits, such as carrots. (p. 122)

bigos (bē-ˈgōs) Sweet-and-sour Polish stew that includes sauerkraut as well as pork, apples, cabbage, and kielbasa. (p. 758)

binder A liquid that helps hold a mixture together. (p. 627)

binge eating disorder An eating disorder that causes people to binge, or eat enormous amounts of food in a short time. It is the most common eating disorder. (p. 169)

biodegradable Materials that can be broken down by microorganisms. (p. 344)

biodiversity A wide variety of species. (p. 30)

biscotti Crunchy, anise-flavored, twice baked cookies. (p. 748)

biscuit method Gives a flaky layering and is used for making biscuits, scones, and shortcakes. (p. 669)

bisque (ˈbisk) A rich cream soup that uses shellfish as the base. (p. 638)

blanching Brief cooking in boiling water. (p. 292)

bleached Chemically-treated to counteract the pigment and break down gluten. (p. 655)

blini (ˈblē-nē) Small, yeast-leavened, buckwheat pancakes. (p. 761)

bloom Patches of white caused by cocoa butter that has come to the surface. (p. 585)

body fat percentage A comparison of the amount of fat and muscle in a person's body. (p. 152)

Body Mass Index (BMI) A measurement of body fat that uses a ratio of weight to height. (p. 151)

boiling-water bath A large, deep kettle with a tight-fitting lid. (p. 293)

bouillon (ˈbü(l)-ˌyän) Concentrated cubes or granules dissolved in hot water, broth or stock. (p. 634)

bouquet garni (bō-ˈkā gärˈnē) A bundled or bagged collection of herbs that flavors foods while cooking and is later removed. (p. 414)

bran The edible, outer layer of the kernel. (p. 470)

broth The flavorful liquid made by simmering meat, poultry, fish, animal bones, or vegetables in water. (p. 634)

brown sugar Granulated sugar coated with molasses. (p. 657)

budget A plan for managing money. (p. 223)

buffet A method of serving food in which people help themselves to food set out on a table. (p. 259)

bulimia nervosa (bü-ˈlē-mē-ə ˌnər-ˈvō-sə) An eating disorder that combines bingeing with purging, or ridding the body of the food to prevent weight gain. (p. 169)

bulk foods Shelf-stable foods sold loose in covered bins or barrels. (p 227)

C

caffeine A natural stimulant that affects the nervous system, heart, and kidneys. (p. 580)

calorie The amount of energy needed to raise the temperature of 1 kilogram of water (a little more than 4 cups) by 1 degree Celsius. (p. 68)

calzone (kal-ˈzōn) A double-crust, semicircular pizza. (p. 604)

canapé (ˈka-nə-pā) An hors d'oeuvre consisting of a small piece of bread in an interesting shape with flavorful toppings. (p. 260)

cannoli Deep-fried pastry tubes. (p. 748)

carbohydrates (ˌkär-bō-ˈhī-ˌdrāts) The body's main source of energy. (p. 76)

carbon monoxide An odorless, highly poisonous gas. (p. 308)

carbonated Bubbly from dissolved carbon dioxide. (p. 578)

cardiopulmonary resuscitation (CPR) (ˌkär-dē-ō-ˈpu̇lmə-ˌner-ē ri-ˌsə-sə-ˈtā-shən) A technique used to revive a person whose breathing and heartbeat have stopped. (p. 310)

* **career** A long-term job a person pursues. (p. 10)

carnivore (ˈkär-nə-ˌvor) An organism that feeds almost entirely on other animals. (p. 30)

carotenoid (kə-ˈrä-tə-ˌnȯid) A yellow, orange, or red phytochemical that gives color to fruits and vegetables, such as carrots and red peppers. (p. 119)

cassava (kə-ˈsä-və) A starchy root vegetable. (p. 724)

casserole A flavorful combination of precooked or quick-cooking foods in a one-dish meal. (p. 626)

caviar (ˈka-vē-ˌär) The salted eggs of sturgeon. (p. 762)

ceviche (sə-vē-ˌchā) An appetizer of raw fish marinated in citrus juice until firm and opaque. (p. 725)

chalazae (kə-ˈlā-ˌzē) The two, thick, twisted strands of albumen that anchor the yolk in the center of an egg. (p. 516)

* **characteristic** A distinguishing trait. (p. 438)

chlorophyll (ˈklȯr-ə-ˌfil) The green pigment in plants, necessary for photosynthesis. (p. 76)

cholesterol (kə-ˈles-tə-ˌrōl) A fatlike substance in cells that is needed for many body processes. (p. 93)

chorizo (chə-rē-(ˌ)zō) A spicy sausage. (p. 725)

* **chronic** Recurring or taking place over a long period of time. (p. 157, 166)

* **chronological** Organized according to time. (p. 404)

chutney A condiment made from fruit, sugar, spices, and vinegar. (p. 769)

chyme A thick liquid churned by the stomach through peristalsis. (p. 66)

cioppino (chə-pē-ˌnō) A specialty fish stew originally made at Fisherman's Wharf in San Francisco. (p. 715)

clone A genetic copy of an organism. (p. 47)

club sandwich An expanded basic sandwich made with three slices of toasted bread and two layers of different fillings. (p. 596)

coagulate Become firm, changing from a liquid to a semisolid or solid state. (p. 519)

* **coarse** Made of large particles. (p. 700)

coating Adding a thin layer of food on top of another food. (p. 378)

cocoa A product of cocoa powder. (p. 585)

cocoa butter A separated fat from the chocolate liquid. (p. 585)

cocoa powder The non-fat solids in chocolate liquid. (p. 585)

code dating The use of a series of numbers or letters that indicate where and when the product was packaged. (p. 244)

coffee bean The twin seeds of a deep-red fruit produced by the coffee plant. (p. 580)

colcannon Potatoes mashed with leeks and mixed with chopped, cooked cabbage. (p. 738)

cold cuts Processed slices of cold meat and poultry. (p. 539)

cold water test A way to estimate syrup temperature based on how it acts in cold water. (p. 687)

collagen (ˈkä-lə-jən) The thin, white, transparent connective tissue found in tendons, between muscle cells and muscles. (p. 534)

colostrum (kə-ˈläs-trəm) A thick, yellowish fluid that a mother produces for about three days after birth and that is rich in nutrients and antibodies. (p. 180)

comfort foods Familiar foods that make people feel good. (p. 8)

commodity A product of agriculture, often surplus food purchased from farmers. (p. 224)

comparison shopping Matching prices and characteristics of similar items to determine which offers the best value. (p. 246)

* **compensate** Make up for. (p. 364)

* **complement** Enhance. (p. 229, 257, 420)

complete protein A food that contains all nine essential amino acids. (p. 89)

complex carbohydrate A carbohydrate that requires more work for the body to digest. (p. 78)

* **component** Element or ingredient of something. (p. 91)

* **compound** A combination of two or more substances. (p. 457)

compressed yeast A moist combination of yeast and starch that comes in small, individually wrapped cakes that are very perishable. (p. 656)

* **concentrated** Dense. (p. 504)

condiment A liquid or semi-liquid accompaniment to food. (p. 419)

conduction A method of transferring heat by direct contact. (p. 386)

confectioners' sugar Powdered sugar; pulverized granulated sugar with a trace of added cornstarch. (p. 657)

connective tissue The protein material that binds muscle into bundles. (p. 534)

* **connective** Joining. (p. 568)

* **consecutive** Following one after another. (p. 223)

conservation The protection of the environment to preserve it for the future. (p. 342)

* **considerable** Large amounts. (p. 473)

consommé A clarified broth, completely strained of all particles and sediment. (p. 638)

* **consumption** The amount of resources you use. (p. 344)

contaminant A substance, such as a chemical or organism, that makes food unsafe to eat. (p. 280)

* **contaminate** Pollute. (p. 578)

* **continuous, continuously** Uninterrupted, constantly. (p. 89, 625)

convection A method of transferring heat through the movement of molecules in air or liquid. (p. 386)

convection oven An oven with a fan that circulates heated air to equalize temperatures throughout. (p. 323)

convenience foods Foods that have been processed to make them easier and faster to use. (p. 226)

conventional method A method of mixing yeast dough in which the yeast is first dissolved in warm water to activate growth. (p. 672)

conventional method A method for making shortened cakes in which fat and sugar are creamed together. (p. 682)

cooked dressing Made by cooking fat and water with starch paste, which serves as an emulsifier. (p. 616)

cooking greens Leafy greens that are eaten cooked. (p. 451)

cooking power The amount of energy the microwave oven uses to generate microwaves. (p. 395)

cookware Equipment for cooking food on top of the range. (p. 326)

* **coordinate** Synchronize. (p. 622)

cornstarch A fine, white powder of pure starch made from the endosperm of the corn kernel. (p. 635)

cover The area containing each person's tableware. (p. 257)

credit A financial arrangement that delays payment for an item. (p. 321)

critical thinking Analyzing and evaluating what you hear and read. (p. 11)

croquettes (krō-ˈkets) Puréed seafood that is bound with a thick sauce, formed into small shapes, then breaded and deep fried. (p. 717)

cross-contamination The spread of harmful bacteria from one food to another. (p. 283)

croutons Small pieces of bread made crisp by baking or sautéing. (p. 610)

cruciferous vegetable A vegetable from the cabbage family, such as cabbage, broccoli, brussels sprouts, cauliflower, kale, Swiss chard, and bok choy. (p. 123)

crudités Sliced or small whole vegetables served raw, often with dip, as an appetizer. (p. 459)

crumb crust A piecrust made of crushed crackers or cookies instead of pastry dough. (p. 700)

crystal A type of glassware that contains lead, which gives clarity and sparkle. (p. 256)

crystallization The formation of sugar crystals in syrup. (p. 688)

cuisine (kwi-ˈzēn) A culture's foods and styles of cooking. (p. 18)

culture A set of customs, traditions, and beliefs shared by a large group of people. (p. 18)

curdling When milk separates into curds and whey. (p. 509)

curds Milk-solid clusters. (p. 505)

curry A dish of vegetables, legumes, and sometimes meat, in hot, highly seasoned sauces. (p. 769)

custard A thickened blend of milk, eggs, and sugar. (p. 526)

custom A group's specific way of doing things. (p. 18)

customary system Also called U.S. standard or English, a system of measurement used in the United States. (p. 359)

* **customize** Tailor. (p. 241)

cut in To mix solid fat and flour using a pastry blender or two knives and a cutting motion. (p. 669)

cut A specific, edible part of meat, such as a steak, chop, or roast. (p. 534)

cutlet A thin, tender slice of meat. (p. 551)

cutting Dividing a food into smaller parts by using a tool with a sharp blade. (p. 375)

D

daikon A large white radish with a mild flavor. (p. 771)

Daily Value (DV) The needed amount of a nutrient based on current nutrition recommendations for a 2,000-calorie diet. (p. 140)

* **dainty** Delicate and small. (p. 451)

dairy dressing A dressing based on buttermilk, yogurt, sour cream, or cottage cheese, with seasonings added. (p. 616)

dal (ˈdäl) A mixture or purée of legumes, onions, chiles, and tomatoes. (p. 769)

decaffeinated The caffeine removed. (p. 580)

* **defuse** Make it less harmful. (p. 165)

dehydration A condition in which the body has too little water. (p. 119)

developing nations Countries that are not yet industrialized or that are just beginning that process. (p. 34)

diabetes A condition in which the body cannot control blood sugar levels. (p. 167)

dietary fiber Plant material that cannot be digested. (p. 78)

Dietary Reference Intake (DRI) The recommended daily amount of nutrients for people of a certain age and gender group. (p. 61)

dietary supplement A nutrient substance taken to supplement, or add to, nutrients in the food you eat. (p. 141)

digestion The mechanical and chemical process of breaking down food and changing nutrients into forms your body can use. (p. 65)

* **dilemma** Problem. (p. 185)

disaccharide (ˌdī-ˈsa-kə-ˌrīd) A sugar made of two monosaccharides; a combination of glucose and another sugar. (p. 77)

dim sum Bite-sized dishes eaten at tea or between courses of a banquet. (p. 772)

docking The process of using a fork to poke small holes all over the dough before putting it in the oven as a way of preventing the shells from puffing (p. 700)

dolma A stuffed vegetable dish. (p. 749)

*** domestic** For use in one's own country. (p. 31)

doneness The point at which meat has cooked enough to make it flavorful and safe to eat. (p. 541)

dovetail To fit different tasks together to make good use of time. (p. 404)

down payment A portion of the purchase price that you must pay before you take the item home. (p. 321)

drawn Whole fish without scales, gills, or internal organs. (p. 566)

dressed Drawn fish without head, tail, or fins. (p. 566)

drop biscuit A biscuit made with more liquid in proportion to flour than a rolled biscuit. (p. 671)

drop cookie Made from soft dough dropped onto a cookie sheet. (p. 685)

drupe A fruit with a single hard seed, also called a pit or stone, and soft inner flesh covered by a tender, edible skin. (p. 432)

dry-heat cooking Cooking food uncovered without added liquid or fat. (p. 392)

dry legume A seed or seed pod from a mature plant that has been left in the field to dry. (p. 486)

dry-pack method The technique of freezing fruit directly in freezer containers. (p. 292)

E

eating disorder A condition marked by extreme emotions, attitudes, and behaviors related to food, eating, and weight. (p. 168)

eating patterns A mix of food customs and habits that include when, what, and how much people eat. (p. 198)

ecosystem An environment and its community of organisms, which all depend upon each other for survival. (p. 30)

*** effect** Result. (p. 376)

*** elaborate** Ornate. (p. 596, 745)

elastin (i-ˈlas-tən) The tough, elastic, and yellowish connective tissue found in ligaments and blood vessel walls. (p. 534)

electrolyte mineral A mineral that helps form particles called electrolytes, which help cells function. (p. 110)

emotional eating Using food to relieve negative feelings. (p. 154)

empanada (ˌem-pə-ˈnä-də) A turnover filled with meat, vegetables, fruit, or all three. (p. 725)

emulsifier A substance that holds together two liquids that normally do not stay mixed, such as water and oil. (p. 519)

emulsion A mixture of two liquids that normally do not combine, such as oil and vinegar. (p. 615)

en papillote Wrapped, often in parchment paper, and baked. (p. 570)

endosperm The largest part of the kernel, which is made of proteins and starches that supply the plant with food. (p. 470)

EnergyGuide label A yellow label on large appliances that shows the average cost per year of using the appliance. (p. 320)

enrichment Restoring nutrients that were lost in processing. (p. 48)

entrée (ˈän-ˌtrā) Main dish. (p. 202)

enzymatic browning A chemical reaction in which oxygen in the air reacts with an enzyme in the fruit and turns it brown. (p. 440)

enzyme A special protein that helps a chemical reaction take place. (p. 65, 440)

equivalent Equal to. (p. 360)

ergonomics (ˌər-gə-ˈnä-miks) The study of ways to make space and equipment easier and more comfortable to use. (p. 49)

esophagus (i-ˈsä-fə-gəs) The part of the digestive tract that connects the mouth and the stomach. (p. 66)

*** essential** Necessary. (p. 121, 785)

essential amino acid An amino acid that your body needs but cannot make. (p. 89)

ethnic Relating to a specific culture. (p. 18)

etiquette The courtesy you show to others by using good manners. (p. 265)

étouffée (ˌā-tü-ˈfā) French for "smothered" describing a typical Southern method of cooking food covered in liquid or sauce. (p. 714)

F

fad diet A popular weight-loss method that is not based on sound nutrition principles. (p. 156)

fajitas (fə-ˈhē-təs) Grilled meat, poultry, fish, or vegetables rolled up in a warm tortilla. (p. 599)

falafel (fə-ˈlä-fəl) Small, deep-fried patties made with highly seasoned, ground garbanzo beans. (p. 598)

family service A way of serving meals in which food is placed in serving dishes and passed around the table. (p. 258)

famine The most severe form of a food shortage, which can last for months or years and cause thousands of deaths. (p. 34)

fasting Abstaining from some or all foods for a period of time; a practice in many religions. (p. 21)

fat-soluble vitamin A vitamin that is absorbed and transported by fat. (p. 106)

fatty acid The basic building block of fats. (p. 92)

fatty fish Fish with more than 5 grams of fat per 3½ ounces. (p. 563)

fermentation A process in which yeast and the enzymes in yeast produce alcohols and carbon dioxide gas by breaking down carbohydrates (p. 671)

fetus (ˈfē-təs) An unborn baby from the age of eight weeks to birth. (p. 176)

fillet (fi-ˈlā) Sides of fish, usually boneless, cut lengthwise away from the bones and backbone. (p. 566)

finance charge Fees plus interest; the total amount you pay for borrowing. (p. 322)

fish Aquatic animals that have fins and a center spine with bones. (p. 563)

flan A full-size tart. (p. 701)

flatbread Any bread that is unleavened, or made without leavenings. (p. 477)

flatware Eating and serving utensils, such as knives, forks, spoons, ladles, and cake servers. (p. 256)

fluted edge A ridged edge that creates an attractive, shaped finish. (p. 698)

foam A light mass of bubbles formed in or on the surface of liquid. (p. 509)

foam cake A cake leavened by air trapped in a protein foam of stiffly beaten egg whites. (p. 684)

focaccia (fō-ˈkä-ch-ēə) A round, herbed, Italian bread that is brushed with olive oil and sometimes topped with herbs. (p. 601)

food additive A substance added to food for a specific reason during processing. (p. 32)

food allergy An abnormal response to certain foods by the body's immune system. (p. 167)

food chain The flow of food energy from simpler to more complex organisms. (p. 30)

food cooperative or co-op A food distribution business owned and operated by its members. (p. 239)

food intolerance A negative physical reaction to food that does not involve the immune system. (p. 167)

food safety Keeping food safe to eat by following proper food handling and cooking practices. (p. 280)

food science The study of all aspects of food, including processing, storage, and preparation. It is an applied science utilizing the natural sciences, such as biology, chemistry, and physics, to solve practical problems. (p. 44)

food waste Edible food that is discarded; represented by the loss of food and of the resources used to produce it. (p. 346)

foodborne illness Sickness caused by eating food that contains a contaminant. (p. 280)

fool Puréed fruit folded into whipped cream. (p. 737)

formal service The most elaborate style of serving food. Banquets in restaurants and hotels often use formal service. (p. 260)

formed products Foods made from an inexpensive source and processed to imitate a more expensive food. (p. 45)

fortification Added nutrients that are not normally found in a food. (p. 48)

* **framework** Structure. (p. 654)

fraud When people gain something of value, often money, by deceiving others. (p. 144)

free-range A term for birds that have access to the outdoors. (p. 551)

free radical An unstable substance that can damage body cells. (p. 103)

freezer burn Moisture loss caused by improper packaging or overly long storage in the freezer. (p. 287)

fresh cheese Cheese that has not ripened or aged. (p. 505)

fresh legume A seed or seed pod from a young plant, sold as a vegetable. (p. 486)

fricassee (ˈfri-kə-ˌsē) To sauté in butter without browning. (p. 640)

frijoles (frē-ˈhō-lēs) The Spanish word for beans. (p. 725)

frittata (frē-ˈtä-tə) An unfolded omelet with fillings stirred into the egg mixture. (p. 524)

fritter Cut-up fruit dipped in batter and fried until golden brown. (p. 443)

fruit The part of a plant that holds the seeds. (p. 432)

fruitarian One who eats only the ripe fruits of plants and trees, such as grains, nuts, fruits, and some vegetables and who tries to choose foods that can be harvested without killing the plant. (p. 210)

fruit-flavored drink A drink that tastes like juice but does not have any juice. (p. 579)

functional foods Foods with ingredients that offer specific health benefits. (p. 48)

fusion cuisine The practice of creating new recipes by mixing the influences and preparation techniques of different food traditions. (p. 23)

G

galette (gə-ˈlet) A hand-shaped tart made by folding and pleating the edge of the dough to form the sides. (p. 701)

garnish A small, decorative piece of food used to enhance the appearance of a dish. (p. 420)

gelatinization (jə-ˌla-tə-nə-ˈzā-shən) A process in which, energized by heat, the starch granules absorb water and swell. (p. 636)

genetic engineering Genes are removed from one organism, such as a plant, animal, or microorganism, and transferred to another organism with the desired outcome of a new, distinct organism. (p. 47)

germ The seed that grows into a new plant. (p. 470)

giblets (ˈjib-ləts) The edible internal organs of poultry. (p. 552)

glucose (ˈglü-ˌkōs) Blood sugar; the body's basic fuel. (p. 67)

gluten (ˈglü-tən) An elastic substance created when some of the proteins in wheat flour combine with liquid. (p. 654)

glycogen (ˈglī-kə-jən) A storage form of glucose. (p. 67)

gnocchi Tender, boiled potato dumplings. (p. 747)

goulash A Hungarian stew made with beef and vegetables and flavored with paprika. (p. 713)

grain The lengthwise direction of muscle. (p. 534)

grains Plants in the grass family cultivated for their fruits or seeds. (p. 470)

granulated sugar Highly-refined sucrose crystals made by boiling the juice of sugarcane or sugar beets. (p. 657)

GRAS The Generally Recognized as Safe list. (p. 296)

gratuity (grə-ˈtü-ə-tē) A tip, or extra money, in appreciation for service. (p. 269)

grazing Eating five or more small meals throughout the day instead of three large ones. (p. 200)

greenhouse gas A gas that traps heat in the earth's atmosphere and contributes to global warming. (p. 342)

grounding The process of providing a path for electrical current to travel back through the electrical system, rather than through your body. (p. 319)

groundwater Water beneath the earth's surface, in the cracks and spaces between rocks and sediment. (p. 37)

guacamole (ˌgwä-kə-ˈmō-lē) A Mexican condiment made of mashed avocados, lemon or lime juice, and seasonings. (p. 599)

gumbo Combines the Spanish custom of mixing seafood and meat with French-style andouille sausages. (p. 714)

gyro (ˈyē-ˌrō) A Greek specialty made with minced roasted lamb, grilled onions, sweet peppers, and a cucumber-yogurt sauce, all wrapped in a pita. (p. 598)

H

haggis A dish made by stuffing a sheep's stomach with a mixture of oats, organ meats, onions, and beef or lamb suet, and then boiling it. (p. 737)

haute cuisine (ōt-kwi-ˈzēn) A classic French cuisine known for high-quality ingredients, expertly prepared and artistically presented. (p. 739)

headspace Room left in a container for food to expand. (p. 292)

* **hearty** Filling. (p. 757)

heating unit An energy source in the range. (p. 322)

Heimlich maneuver A way to dislodge an object from the throat of a person who is choking by using a series of upward thrusts on the abdomen. (p. 310)

hemoglobin (ˈhē-mə-ˌglō-bən) A protein that transports oxygen in the blood to all the cells in your body. (p. 88)

herb The flavorful leaf or stem of a soft, fleshy and moisture-rich plant that grows in a temperate climate. (p. 414)

herb tea A beverage made from the flowers, leaves, seeds, and roots of herbs and plants other than the tea plant. (p. 584)

herbal A plant used for medicinal purposes. (p. 142)

herbivore (ˈ(h)ərbə-ˌvor) An organism that eats only plants. (p. 30)

hero A very large sandwich made on a loaf of Italian or French bread or a large hard roll. (p. 597)

high-altitude Adjusting for higher elevations. (p. 364)

hilum (ˈhī-ləm) The scar on the bean where it was attached to the stem in the pod. (p. 489)

HIV/AIDS A disorder that weakens the immune system. (p. 167)

hoisin A thick, sweet and salty paste made with fermented soy, chiles, vinegar, and garlic. (p. 771)

homogenized (hō-ˈmä-jə-ˌnīzd) Processed to make the fat break into small particles and distribute evenly throughout the liquid. (p. 502)

hors d'oeuvres (ȯr-ˈdərvs) A small serving of hot or cold food served as an appetizer. (p. 260)

hospitality Kindness in welcoming guests or strangers. (p. 8)

hot spot An area of concentrated heat that can cause uneven baking and browning. (p. 660)

hot-pack method The technique of canning simmered foods. (p. 293)

hull An inedible outer coat that covers some grains. (p. 470)

hydration (hī-ˈdrā-shən) Getting enough water to meet all the body's needs. (p. 119)

hydrogenation (hī-ˌdrä-jə-ˈnā-shən) A chemical process that turns vegetable oils into solids. (p. 94)

hydroponics (ˈhi-drə-ˈpä-niks) Growing plants without soil. (p. 37)

hypertension High blood pressure linked to high salt intake. (p. 110)

I

immature fruit Fruit that is still growing and is not yet mature. (p. 437)

* **immigration** Movement from one place to another. (p. 737)

* **impact** Effect. (p. 21)

impulse buying Buying items you did not plan to purchase and do not really need. (p. 241)

incomplete protein A food that lacks one or more essential amino acids. (p. 89)

* **induce** Bring about. (p. 689)

industrialized nation A country with a developed economy and a high standard of living. (p. 34)

injera A thin, spongy flatbread made from a hardy grain. (p. 787)

* **inspect** Carefully examine. (p. 305, 552)

* **interconnected** Related. (p. 782)

interest A fee for the loan expressed as a percentage of the amount borrowed. (p. 322)

interfering agent An ingredient that breaks down sugar crystals or keeps them from forming. (p. 689)

internal temperature The temperature deep inside the thickest part of the food. (p. 284)

iron-deficiency anemia Too little iron leads to having too few red blood cells, causing people to become tired, weak, short of breath, pale, and cold. (p. 111)

irradiation The process of exposing food to high-intensity energy waves to increase its shelf life and kill harmful microorganisms. (p. 297)

island A freestanding counter that is open on all sides and is often placed in the center of the kitchen. (p. 316)

J

jambalaya A Creole rice dish featuring ham, seafood, chicken, and sausages with rice, vegetables, and seasonings. (p. 714)

jerk A blend of chiles, onions, garlic, allspice, and other herbs and spices used to season meat, poultry, and fish. (p. 730)

juice A beverage that is 100 percent fruit or vegetable juice. (p. 578)

juice drink Called a "juice cocktail," a blend of 10 to 50 percent juice with water, sweeteners, flavorings, and other additives. (p. 579)

K

kernels Small, separate dry fruits produced by some grains. (p. 470)

kielbasa A Polish smoked sausage. (p. 758)

kimchi Preserved fermented vegetables. (p. 774)

knead Working dough with the hands to combine ingredients and develop gluten. (p. 670)

kolache (kə-ˈlä-chē) A sweet roll filled with fruit butter, nuts, or poppy seed paste. (p. 758)

kringel A rich, yeast oval-shaped or pretzel-shaped coffee cake. (p. 757)

L

lactation Breast milk production. (p. 180)

lacto-ovo-vegetarian Eats foods from plant sources, plus dairy products and eggs. (p. 210)

lacto-vegetarian Eats foods from plant sources, plus dairy products. (p. 210)

lattice crust A crust that is woven. (p. 698)

lavash (lä-ˈvȯsh) An Armenian flatbread that is larger and thinner than pita. (p. 598)

laverbread Processed seaweed. (p. 738)

leadership The ability to guide or direct people. (p. 12)

leavened bread (ˈle-və-niŋd) Bread made with a leavening agent, such as yeast or baking powder, which makes the bread rise. (p. 477)

leavening agent A substance that triggers a chemical reaction that makes a baked product grow larger, or rise. (p. 656)

legume A plant with seed pods that split along both sides when ripe. (p. 486)

life span All the stages of growth and development throughout life, from before birth to old age. (p. 176)

lipoprotein (lī-pō-ˈprō-ˌtēn) A fat-protein unit. (p. 93)

low-fat fish Fish with less than 5 grams of fat per 3½ ounces. (p. 563)

lutefisk Dried cod soaked in culinary ash and water. (p. 742)

M

macaroni A pasta made from durum, wheat flour and water. (p. 474)

macrobiotics A diet that includes only unprocessed foods, mostly whole grains, beans, and organically grown fruits and vegetables. (p. 210)

Maillard reaction Browning that occurs when heat provokes a series of chemical reactions between certain sugars and proteins in the food; named for the person who discovered it, Dr. L.C. Maillard. (p. 387)

* **maintain** Keep and preserve. (p. 60)

major mineral A mineral that you need in the amount of 100 mg or more a day. (p. 108)

malnutrition Poor nourishment resulting from a lack of nutrients. (p. 60)

management Handling resources wisely to reach goals. (p. 12)

manufactured food A product developed as a substitute for another food. (p. 45)

MAP (modified atmosphere packaging) MAP packaging uses carbon dioxide, oxygen, and nitrogen to slow bacterial growth. (p. 44)

marbling Small white flecks of fat. (p. 534)

marzipan (ˈmärt-sə-ˌpän) A confection made of almond paste and sugar. (p. 744)

masa (ˈmä-sə) Corn that has been dried, cooked, soaked in limewater, and then ground into dough. (p. 725)

mature fruit A fruit that has reached its full size and color. (p. 437)

mayonnaise A thick, creamy dressing that is a permanent emulsion of oil, vinegar or lemon juice, egg yolks, and seasonings. (p. 616)

meat The edible muscle of animals, typically cattle, sheep, and pigs. (p. 534)

* **membrane** A thin layer of tissue. (p. 432)

meringue A foam made of beaten egg whites and sugar and used for baked desserts. (p. 527)

metabolism (mə-ˈta-bə-ˌli-zəm) The use of nutrients to provide energy. (p. 68)

metric system A system of measurement based on multiples of ten. (p. 359)

meze (me-ˈzā) Appetizers. (p. 784)

microorganism A living thing so small that it can only be seen through a microscope. (p. 280)

microwave cooking Cooking food with energy in the form of electrical waves. (p. 394)

microwave time The time the food needs to cook with microwave energy. (p. 397)

* **minimal** Small amount. (p. 610)

* **minimize** Lessen. (p. 151)

mise en place (ˌmē-ˌzän-pläs) French for "put in place," means arranging ingredients in the order in which they will be cooked. (p. 624)

mixing Combining two or more ingredients thoroughly. (p. 377)

* **moderate** Not extreme. (p. 137, 554)

GLOSSARY

modified English service A more formal way of serving a meal for a small group. (p. 259)

moist-heat cooking A method of cooking food in hot liquid, steam, or both. (p. 388)

molded cookie A cookie that can be rolled in chopped nuts or other coatings before baking. (p. 685)

molded salad A salad made with gelatin that thickens and conforms to the shape of a container called a mold. (p. 611)

mole (ˈmō-lā) A thick blend of chiles, ground pumpkin or sesame seeds, onions, unsweetened chocolate, and spices. (p. 726)

monosaccharide (ˌmä-nə-ˈsa-kə-ˌrīd) A sugar with a single chemical unit. (p. 77)

moussaka A casserole with lamb, eggplant, and tomatoes in a custard or white sauce seasoned with herbs and spices such as oregano, thyme, black pepper, allspice, and cinnamon. (p. 749)

muffin method A method of making quick breads in which liquid ingredients are lightly mixed into dry ingredients to create a batter with a slightly coarse yet tender texture. (p. 668)

mulled Served hot and flavored with such spices as cinnamon, nutmeg, or cloves. (p. 586)

* **multitude** A large number. (p. 759)

muscle Protein-rich tissue made of long, thin cells grouped together in bundles. (p. 534)

N

* **native** Local. (p. 724)

natural food A food that has been minimally processed and has few additives, such as dyes and added sugars. (p. 238)

* **neutralize** Counteract. (p. 655)

nonfat milk solids Substances that contain most of the protein, vitamins, minerals, and lactose in milk. (p. 502)

nonrenewable resource Resource that cannot be replaced once it is used. (p. 342)

nonverbal communication Sending and receiving information, thoughts, and feelings without words. (p. 11)

noodles A pasta made from wheat flour and water, and egg solids added for tenderness. (p. 474)

nori Seaweed wrapper. (p. 774)

nut An edible kernel surrounded by a hard shell. (p. 493)

nutrient density The relationship between nutrients and calories in a food. (p. 137)

nutrient A chemical substance, such as protein, carbohydrate, fat, or fiber, that your body needs to function, grow, repair itself, and create energy. (p. 6)

Nutrition Facts panel A label with easy-to-read information about the calories and nutrients of foods sold in containers. (p.140)

nutrition The study of nutrients and how the body uses them. (p. 6)

O

obese Having a Body Mass Index of over 30. (p. 151)

* **observe** Look at or study. (p. 79)

obstetrician (ˌäb-stə-ˈtri-shən) A physician who specializes in the care of women during pregnancy and childbirth. (p. 177)

omelet A egg mixture formed into a large, thick pancake, usually filled with ingredients and folded. (p. 524)

* **omit** To leave out. (p 362)

omnivore (ˈäm-ni-ˌvor) An organism that eats both plants and animals. (p. 30)

one-bowl method A quick way to mix ingredients for a shortened cake. (p. 683)

* **opaque** Light-shielding. (p. 418, 569)

open dating The use of a day, month, and sometimes a year to indicate a product's freshness. (p. 244)

open-face sandwich Just one slice of bread and a topping. (p. 597)

organic farming A way of farming that protects the environment and does not use pesticides or artificial fertilizers. (p. 37)

organic food A food produced without the use of pesticides, artificial fertilizers, growth hormones, or antibiotics, and without genetic modification or irradiation. (p. 239)

* **organization** An ordered manner of doing things. (p. 12)

* **originated** Came into existence; was first discovered (p. 580, 638)

osteoporosis A condition in which bones become fragile and break easily. (p. 177)

overfishing Catching too many fish, so that the fish population cannot sustain itself. (p. 562)

overweight Having a Body Mass Index of between 25 and 29.9. (p. 151)

ovo-vegetarian Eats foods from plant sources, plus eggs. (p. 210)

oxidation A chemical reaction in which molecules combine with oxygen. (p. 68)

P

paella (pä-ˈe-lə) Rice seasoned with saffron and mixed with a purée of onions, red bell peppers and tomatoes, and meat and seafood. (p. 745)

palate A person's ability to taste and judge food. (p. 9)

pancetta (ˌpan-ˈche-tə) An Italian sausage. (p. 747)

pancreas (ˈpaŋ-krē-əs) A gland connected to the small intestine. (p. 66)

pasta An Italian word meaning paste, referring to dough made from flour and water. (p. 474)

pasteurized (ˈpas-chə-ˌrīzd) Heat-treated to kill enzymes and any harmful bacteria. (p. 502)

pediatrician A physician who cares for infants and children. (p. 181)

peer pressure The influence of people in your age group. (p. 183)

pelmeni (pėl-ˈmenē) Russian dumplings. (p 762)

peninsula A countertop extension that is open on two sides and on one end. (p. 316)

* **periodic** From time to time. (p. 35)

perishable food Food that can spoil quickly. (p. 198, 240)

peristalsis (ˌper-əh-ˈstȯl-səs) Rhythmic movements of muscles. (p. 66)

permanent emulsion A mix of liquids that will not separate. (p. 615)

personal hygiene Thoroughly washing your body, face, and hands. (p. 281)

pesto A sauce of ground fresh basil, pine nuts, garlic, Parmesan cheese, and olive oil. (p. 747)

pescatarian One who eats fish and shellfish and foods from plant sources. (p. 210)

photosynthesis (ˈfō-tō-ˈsin(t)-thə-səs) The process by which plants use the sun's energy to convert carbon dioxide and water into oxygen and glucose. (p. 76)

phytochemical A chemical compound that occurs naturally in plants. (p. 120)

pica An unusual appetite for ice, clay, or other nonfood items; a craving for things that are not normally eaten. (p. 112)

pie Any dish that has a crust with a filling. (p. 696)

pie shell A bottom crust baked before filling. (p. 700)

pierogis (pə-ˈrō-gēs) Polish dumplings made with noodle dough. (p. 758)

pilaf (pi-ˈläf) Sautéed grains cooked in a seasoned liquid with dried fruit and nuts or strips of meat. (p. 761)

pita A round, leavened flatbread from the Middle East that can be used to make a rollup. (p. 597)

pizza An oversized, baked sandwich with a yeast-bread base, usually served open face with assorted toppings. (p. 602)

place setting The tableware needed by one person to eat a meal. (p. 256)

plankton Minute animal and plant life in the water. (p. 562)

plate service A way of serving meals in which food is portioned out on individual plates in the kitchen and brought to the table. (p. 258)

* **pliable** Supple. (p. 675)

poke Sliced raw fish mixed with seaweed, onions, chiles, and soy sauce. (p. 716)

polarized plug A plug that has one blade wider than the other and can reduce the risk of shock if used with a polarized outlet. (p. 307)

polenta (pō-ˈlen-tə) A thick cornmeal porridge. (p. 747)

polysaccharide (ˈpä-lē-ˈsa-kə-ˌrīd) A sugar made of several monosaccharides. (p. 75)

pome A fruit with several small seeds and thick, firm flesh with a tender, edible skin. (p. 432)

poultry Any bird raised for food. (p. 550)

* **precision** Exactness. (p. 682)

preheat To turn the oven on about 10 minutes before using so it will be at the desired temperature when the food is placed inside. (p. 659)

pre-preparation Includes tasks that can be done before you begin to put the recipes together. (p. 404)

preserve To prepare food in a way that allows it to be safely stored for later use. (p. 291)

pressed cookie Dough forced through a cookie press and directly onto a baking sheet. (p. 686)

pressure canning Canning using a pressure canner, which is like a large pressure cooker. (p. 293)

principal The purchase price minus the down payment. (p 321)

* **principle** A basic rule. (p 270)

processed meat Meat with added flavor and preservatives. (p. 539)

produce Fresh fruits and vegetables. (p. 437)

proofing A process by which you can test yeast. (p. 656)

* **provide** Give. (p. 19)

province A country or region. (p. 727)

punch A mixture of fruit juices and tea or a carbonated beverage such as ginger ale or seltzer water. (p. 586)

Q

quiche A pie with custard filling, containing such foods as chopped vegetables, cheese, and chopped, cooked meat. (p. 527)

quick bread A bread leavened by agents that allow speedy baking, such as air, steam, baking soda, and baking powder. (p. 668)

quick-mix method A method of mixing yeast dough in which dry yeast is combined with the dry ingredients and then with a liquid. (p. 673)

quick-rising yeast Works twice as fast as regular yeast. (p. 656)

quorn (ˈkwȯrn) A meat substitute made of protein from a type of fungus. (p. 214)

R

radiation A method of transferring heat as waves of energy. (p. 386)

rancidity (ran-ˈsi-də-tē) Spoilage due to the breakdown of fats. (p. 287)

raw milk Milk that is not pasteurized. (p. 502)

raw-pack method The technique of canning raw foods. (p. 293)

raw vegan A vegan who eats only unprocessed vegan foods that have not been heated above 115°F. (p. 210)

rebate Partial refund from the maker of an item. (p. 247)

recall The immediate removal of a product from store shelves. (p. 297)

recipe A set of directions for making a food or beverage. (p. 358)

Recommended Dietary Allowance (RDA) The amount of a nutrient needed by 98 percent of the people in a given age and gender group.(p. 61)

* **reconstitute** To restore a dried food to its former condition by adding water. (p. 442, 492)

recycle To reprocess discarded products so they can be used again. (p. 347)

reduction The process of simmering an uncovered mixture until some of the liquid evaporates. (p. 635)

refrigerator cookie A cookie that starts with dough formed into long, even rolls about 1½ to 2 inches in diameter; then the rolls are wrapped in wax paper, foil, or plastic wrap, and chilled. (p. 686)

* **regional** Localized. (p. 712)

regreening The return of chlorophyll, the greening substance in plants, to the skin of ripe oranges during warm weather or under bright light. (p. 438)

* **regulate** Control and maintain. (p. 110)

rehydrate Absorb water and become soft again. (p. 295)

* **reinforce** Strengthen. (p. 202)

* **reliable** Trustworthy. (p. 134)

renewable resource A resource that can be replaced once it is used. (p. 342)

* **replenish** Replace. (p. 184)

* **representative** Sample. (p. 240)

* **requires** Mandates. (p. 504)

reservation An arrangement made ahead of time by phone or on the Web for a table at a restaurant. (p. 268)

* **reserve** To set aside. (p. 283)

* **resistance** Does not go along easily. (p. 121)

resources People, things, and qualities that can help you reach a goal. (p. 196)

* **restore** Renew. (p. 614)

retail cut The small cut of meat sold to consumers. (p. 536)

retort pouches Flexible packages made of aluminum foil and plastic film. (p. 46)

rice The starchy seed of plants grown in flooded fields in warm climates. (p. 472)

ripe fruit When a mature fruit reaches its peak of flavor and is ready to eat. (p. 437)

ripened cheese Aged cheese; is made by adding ripening agents, such as bacteria, mold, yeast, or a combination of these, to the curds. (p. 506)

role A set of responsibilities based on your different relationships to others. (p. 222)

rolled biscuit A biscuit that is lightly kneaded, rolled out to an even thickness, and cut to biscuit size before baking. (p. 670)

rolled cookie Made from stiff dough, it can be cut into different shapes with cookie cutters before baking. (p. 685)

roux (ˈrü) A mixture of equal amounts of flour and fat. (p. 636)

* **ruptured** Broken. (p. 516)

S

saffron Thread-like center of the crocus flower; turns rice a brilliant yellow and adds a pungent flavor. (p. 783)

salad A mixture of raw or cooked vegetables and other ready-to-eat foods, usually served with a dressing. (p. 610)

salad dressing A seasoned mixture, often consisting of oil and vinegar, used to flavor a salad. (p. 615)

salad greens Leafy greens that are eaten raw. (p. 451)

salsa A chili-based sauce. (p. 724)

sandwich Filling between slices of bread. (p. 596)

sanitary landfill A landfill insulated with clay and plastic liner, where trash is thinly spread, compacted, and covered with a layer of soil. (p. 345)

sanitation The prevention of illness through cleanliness. (p. 281)

sardines A general term for a variety of small fish with varied characteristics. (p. 562)

sashimi Fish and shellfish served raw with condiments. (p 774)

saturated fatty acid (ˈsa-chə-ˌrā-ted) A fatty acid that contains all the hydrogen it can chemically hold. (p. 92)

sauce A flavored liquid that is often thickened and that is served to enhance the flavor of another food. (p. 641)

sauerbraten A beef roast marinated in vinegar with cloves, bay leaves, and peppercorns. (p. 740)

savory Flavorful but not sweet. (p. 432)

scalded milk Milk heated to just below the boiling point. (p. 509)

science The study of the physical world. (p. 44)

scorching Occurs if milk overheats and some solids settle on the sides and some fall to the bottom of the pan. (p. 509)

score Make slashes about ½ inch deep across the top of the bread. (p. 676)

scrapple A bake of pork scraps with cornmeal, flavored with thyme and sage. (p. 713)

scratch cooking Preparing a dish from basic ingredients. (p. 226)

sea vegetables Seaweeds used as vegetables. (p. 456)

seafood Saltwater fish and shellfish, but it is often used to mean fish and shellfish from both fresh water and salt water. (p. 563)

sear Brown quickly over high heat. (p. 391)

seasoning blend A pre-mixed combination of herbs and spices. (p. 414)

seed The edible dried kernel of certain plants. (p. 495)

seitan (ˈsā-tän) Wheat gluten with seasonings. (p. 214)

self-esteem The feeling that you are a worthwhile, capable person. (p. 11)

self-rising flour Contains added baking powder and salt. (p. 655)

sell-by date The last day the product should remain on the store shelf. (p. 244)

semi-vegetarian Avoids certain kinds of meat, poultry, or fish. (p. 210)

service contract An insurance that covers repair and maintenance of a product for a specific length of time. (p. 321)

service plate A large, often beautifully decorated plate that holds other plates. (p. 260)

shelf life The length of time food holds its flavor and quality. (p. 31)

shelf-stable Able to be stored at room temperature for weeks or months in the original, unopened containers. (p. 31)

shellfish Aquatic animals that have a shell but no spine or bones. (p. 563)

shirred eggs Eggs baked in a greased, shallow dish and often topped with a small amount of milk. (p. 524)

shortened cake Cake made with a solid fat such as butter, margarine, or shortening, as well as flour, salt, sugar, eggs, and liquid. (p. 682)

* **sieve** A strainer. (p. 520)

* **signature** Specialty. (p. 773)

* **significant** Important. (p. 198)

* **similar** Alike. (p. 536)

simple carbohydrate A carbohydrate with a simple chemical structure. (p. 77)

smoking point The temperature at which a fat begins to break down and burn. (p. 391)

smoothie A blend of milk or yogurt and fresh fruit. (p. 585)

smorgasbord A buffet laden with cured fish, cold meats, cheeses, salads, and vegetables. (p. 742)

soft peaks Peaks that gently bend over like waves when you lift the beaters from the mixture. (p. 521)

solanine A bitter, toxic compound. (p. 457)

sopa Latin American soup. (p. 725)

soufflé (ˌsü-ˈflā) A baked dish made by folding stiffly beaten whites into a sauce or puréed food. (p. 519)

soup A dish made by cooking solid foods in liquid. (p. 637)

speed-scratch cooking An approach to cooking that uses a few convenience foods along with basic ingredients for easier meal preparation. (p. 227)

spice The dried form of various buds, bark, fruits, seeds, stems, or roots, typically from an aromatic plant or tree that grows in a tropical or subtropical region. (p. 414)

spore A protected cell that develops into a bacterium when it has the right conditions of food, warmth, and moisture. (p. 280)

* **stabilize** To hold steady. (p. 106, 167)

* **stagger** To alternate or overlap. (p. 406)

* **standing time** The time after microwave time during which foods continue to cook on their own. (p. 397)

staple food The most widely produced and eaten food in an area. (p. 19)

staples Basic items that are used on a regular basis, such as milk, cereal, eggs, and bread. (p. 224)

starch A carbohydrate with a more complex chemical structure than a sugar. (p. 77)

steak Cross-sections cut from large, dressed fish and may contain bones from the backbone and ribs. (p. 566)

steep Brew. (p. 584)

stew Any dish prepared by stewing, or simmering, pieces of food in a tightly covered pan. (p. 640)

stiff peaks Peaks that stand up straight when the beaters are lifted from the mixture. (p. 521)

stir-fry A combination dish of bite-size pieces of food that are stirred constantly while frying in a small amount of oil over high heat. (p. 622)

stock Similar to broth, but made with vegetables and sometimes animal bones, and not meat. (p. 634)

stollen A yeast bread filled with dried fruit. (p. 740)

store brand A line of food produced and packaged for a specific store chain. (p. 248)

stress A physical or mental tension caused by a person's reaction to a situation. (p. 164)

stress hormones Hormones released by the body in times of stress. (p. 8)

streusel (ˈstrü-səl) A crumbly mixture made by cutting butter into flour, sugar, and sometimes spices. (p. 700)

stuffing A seasoned mixture of food used to fill meats or vegetables. (p. 555)

subsistence farming A practice of raising one's own food on a small plot of land. (p. 34)

* **substantial** Filling. (p. 600)

succotash A dish of beans and corn. (p. 712)

sugar The form of carbohydrate that supplies energy to the body. (p. 74)

sugar substitute A substance that tastes sweet but has few or no calories. (p. 81)

sugar-pack method The technique of freezing fruit coated in sugar. (p. 292)

sumac A deep-red native berry usually used ground; adds a fruity tartness. (p. 783)

* **supplemental** Additional. (p. 225)

sushi Vinegar-dressed rice that is combined with sashimi or rolled in nori. (p. 774)

sustainable living The alternative life choice to meet your own needs while still protecting the environment. (p. 38)

* **symmetrical** Balanced. (p. 668)

* **synthetic** Not naturally occurring. (p. 345)

syrup-pack method The technique of freezing fruit in sugar water. (p. 292)

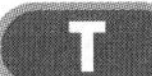

T

tabbouleh (tə-ˈbü-lē) A Middle Eastern salad of cooked bulgur, chopped tomatoes, onions, parsley, mint, olive oil, and lemon juice. (p. 610)

tableware Any item used to serve or eat food. (p. 256)

tagine A well-seasoned stew made in a covered pot. (p. 786)

tahini Sesame seeds ground into a thick paste. (p. 783)

* **tailor** Adjust. (p. 769)

tandoor A rounded, clay, charcoal-burning oven. (p. 769)

tapas Small snacks or appetizers. (p. 745)

taring Subtracting the weight of the container from the total weight in order to find the weight of the food. (p. 374)

taro root The large tuber of the tropical taro plant. (p. 716)

tart A filled dessert with a single crust. (p. 701)

task lighting Bright, shadow-free light over specific work areas. (p. 319)

tea Made by soaking the leaves of the tropical tea plant in water. (p. 583)

tea sandwich Called a finger sandwich, a small, attractive, cold type of sandwich often served at receptions and parties. (p. 601)

teamwork Combining individual efforts to reach a shared goal. (p. 407)

technology The practical application of scientific knowledge. (p. 44)

tempeh (ˈtem-ˌpā) A pressed cake of fermented, cooked soybeans mixed with a grain, usually rice. (p. 213)

tempering A technique that brings one food to the right temperature or consistency before mixing it completely with another. (p. 509)

temporary emulsion An emulsion that quickly separates when not stirred. (p. 615)

* **tendency** Inclination. (p. 697)

* **thrive** Flourish. (p. 715)

timetable Shows the amount of time you will need to complete preparation tasks and lists when you should start each task. (p. 404)

tofu A custard-like product made from soybeans. (p. 492)

tolerance A maximum safe level in food. (p. 298)

* **tolerate** Allow. (p. 280)

torte A rich cake made with a small amount of flour and often with ground nuts or bread crumbs. (p. 741)

tortilla (tȯr-ˈtē-yə) A thin, round, unleavened flatbread made with either corn or wheat flour and baked on a griddle. (p. 598)

tossed salad When greens, chopped or sliced vegetables, and a dressing are mixed together. (p. 612)

toxicity Poisoning from too much of a substance. (p. 106)

toxin Poison. (p. 280)

trace mineral A mineral that you need in the amount of less than 100 mg a day; sometimes called micro-minerals. (p. 111)

* **trait** Characteristic. (p. 47)

trans fats The hydrogenation of fatty acids; also called trans fats. (p. 94)

* **translucent** Clear or transparent. (p. 476)

tray-pack method The technique of freezing fruit whole on a tray. (p. 292)

trifle (ˈtrī-fəl) A refrigerated dessert with layers that may include cake, jam or jelly, fruit, custard, and whipped cream. (p. 440)

triglyceride (ˌtrī-ˈgli-sə-ˌrīd) A basic fat molecule. (p. 91)

truss To hold a roast together with twine or skewers. (p. 554)

tuber A large underground stem that stores nutrients. (p. 451)

turnover A square or circle of pastry dough folded over a sweet or savory filling. (p. 701)

U

unbleached flour Flour that has its natural color, is slightly less white than bleached flour, and does not have additives. (p. 655)

under ripe fruit A very firm mature fruit that lacks flavor and has not reached top eating quality. (p. 437)

* **uniform** The same or consistent. (p. 388, 536)

unit price The cost per ounce, quart, pound, or other unit of an item. (p. 246)

universal design A way of making objects and spaces easy to use by everyone, regardless of age or physical ability. (p. 317)

universal product code (UPC) A bar code that can be read by a scanner, which makes checkout faster and more accurate. (p. 244)

use-by date The last day on which the product will still have high quality. (p. 44)

V

values Beliefs and concepts that a person holds as important. (p. 197)

variety meat A meat consisting of edible organs and extremities of beef, veal, lamb, or pork. (p. 538)

vegan (ˈvē-gən) A person who eats only foods from plant sources. (p. 210)

vegetarian A person who does not eat meat, poultry, or fish. (p. 210)

verbal communication The use of words to send and receive information, thoughts, and feelings. (p. 11)

* **versatile** Variable. (p. 325)

villi (ˈvi-ˌlī) Billions of tiny, finger-like projections covering the inner wall of the small intestine. (p. 67)

vinaigrette (ˌvi-ni-ˈgret) A mixture of oil, vinegar or lemon juice, and seasonings. (p. 615)

* **vital** Essential. (p. 68)

volume The amount of space an ingredient takes up. (p. 359)

* **vulnerable** Susceptible to harm. (p. 309)

W

warranty A manufacturer's guarantee that a product will perform as advertised. (p. 321)

water-soluble vitamin A vitamin that dissolves in water and passes easily into the bloodstream during digestion. (p. 103)

weep When liquid accumulates between the meringue and pie filling (p. 527)

weight The heaviness of an ingredient. (p. 359)

wellness Good health and positive well-being, including physical, mental, and emotional health. (p. 6)

wheat One of the oldest cereal grains. (p. 471)

whey A thin, bluish liquid derived from milk. (p. 505)

whole fish Fish sold whole, without scales or internal organs. The most perishable type of fish. (p. 566)

whole grain Made of the entire grain kernel and containing most of the original nutrients. (p. 471)

whole wheat Made from the whole wheat grain. (p. 477)

wholesale cut A large cut that is sold to retail stores. (p. 534)

* **withstand** Resist. (p. 395)

wok A roomy, bowl-shaped pan. (p. 392, 624)

work center An area designed for performing specific kitchen tasks. (p. 316)

work flow All the steps involved in removing food from storage, preparing it, and serving it. (p. 316)

work plan A list of all the tasks you need to do in order to prepare a meal. (p. 404)

work triangle The arrangement of the three main work centers in a kitchen. (p. 316)

wraps Sandwiches made by wrapping or rolling a filling in flatbread. (p. 597)

Y

yeast bread A bread leavened with yeast. (p. 671)

yield The amount or the number of servings that the recipe makes. (p. 358)

yogurt A dairy product that is made by adding special harmless bacteria to milk. (p. 504)

yolk The round yellow portion of an egg. (p. 516)

Yorkshire pudding A popover baked in the hot pan drippings from the roast beef. (p. 737)

Index

A

B

INDEX

D

INDEX

INDEX

INDEX

I

J

K

L

INDEX

N

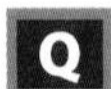

S

T

INDEX

Z

Photography Credits

Cover Ed-Imaging; **v** Comstock/Corbis RF; **vii** DEA/G.UMMARINO/Getty Images; **viii** BananaStock/age fotostock RF; **ix** Maximilian Stock Ltd/photocuisine/Corbis; **x** Photolibrary; **xi** Jerzyworks/Masterfile; **xiii** Masterfile |Royalty Free (RF); **xiv** Cultura Limited/Superstock RF; **xv** Mary Kate Denny/PhotoEdit; **2–3** Getty Images RF; **4–5** Edward Pond/Masterfile; **6** BananaStock/age fotostock RF; **7** Blend Images/age fotostock; **9** Cindy Charles/PhotoEdit; **10** Envision/Corbis; **11** age fotostock RF; **14** Cindy Charles/PhotoEdit; **16–17** Studio Eye/Corbis RF; **18** Food And Drink Photos/age fotostock; **19** Richard Heinzen/Superstock; **20** FoodCollection/SuperStock; **23** Tim Mantoani/Masterfile; **26** Richard Heinzen/Superstock; **28–29** David Sanger/Getty Images; **31** Corbis; **33b** PureStock/age fotostock; **33m** Thinkstock/Corbis; **33t** age fotostock; **35** Wojtek Buss/age fotostock; **36** Spence Inga/age fotostock; **40** age fotostock; **42–43** Javier Larrea/age fotostock; **45** Photodisc/SuperStock; **46m** Banana/SuperStock; **46r** Amy Etra/PhotoEdit; **46l** David Young-Wolff/PhotoEdit; **48** age fotostock/SuperStock; **49** Japack/age fotostock; **52** Photodisc/SuperStock; **55** Getty Images RF; **56–57** Japack/age fotostock; **58–59** Corbis/SuperStock RF; **61** Masterfile Royalty Free; **65** Onoky/SuperStock; **69b** Michael Newman/PhotoEdit; **69m** Getty Images RF; **69l** PhotoAlto/SuperStock; **72** Onoky/SuperStock; **77** Photocuisine/age fotostock; **771** Brand X/SuperStock RF; **79** Pixtal/age fotostock; **80** fStop/SuperStock; **84** Pixtal/age fotostock; **86–87** Brand X/SuperStock RF; **88** Masterfile Royalty Free; **90** Jeff Greenberg/PhotoEdit; **91** Pixtal/age fotostock; **92** Stockbyte/Getty Images; **98** Pixtal/age fotostock; **100–101** Begsteiger/age fotostock; **102t** Steve Shott/Getty Images; **105** Zia Soleil/Getty Images; **106** RubberBall/SuperStock; **107** David Young-Wolff/PhotoEdit; **108** Creatas/age fotostock; **111** Image Source/SuperStock; **116–117** J Silver/SuperStock; **118** WP Simon/Getty Images; **121** Steve Lupton/Corbis; **123** Studio Eye/Corbis RF; **126** WP Simon/Getty Images; **129** Japack/age fotostock; **130–131** RubberBall/SuperStock RF; **132–133** Mauritius/Superstock; **143** David Young-Wolff/PhotoEdit; **146** Mauritius/Superstock; **148–149** Jerzyworks/Masterfile; **151l** Masterfile Royalty Free; **151r** Masterfile Royalty Free; **154** Masterfile Royalty Free; **156** PureStock/age fotostock; **157** Thomas Northcut/Getty Images; **160** Masterfile Royalty Free; **162–163** Terry Vine/Getty Images; **164** Masterfile Royalty Free; **166** Brand X/Superstock; **167** Tony Latham/Getty Images; **172** Brand X/Superstock; **174–175** Allana Wesley White/Corbis; **176** Blend Images/Superstock; **179** Digital Vision/age fotostoock; **180** Camille Tokerud/Getty Images; **182** Masterfile Royalty Free; **184** Marshall Gordon/Cole Group/Getty Images RF; **185** Blend Images/Superstock RF; **188** PureStock/age fotostock; **192–193**, Cultura Limited/SuperStock RF; **194–195** Mary Kate Denny/PhotoEdit; **200** LWA-Sharie Kennedy/Corbis; **201** Corbis/Superstock; **208–209** Mark Tomalty/Masterfile; **211** Mitch Hrdlicka/Getty Images; **213** Photodisc/Superstock; **214** Andrew Bret Wallis/Superstock; **218** Mitch Hrdlicka/Getty Images; **220–221** Cultura Limited/Superstock RF; **225** Comstock/Corbis RF; **228** FoodCollection/Superstock; **229** Creatas/SuperStock RF; **234** J.Riou/photocuisine/Corbis; **236–237** Masterfile Royalty Free (RF); **238** Envision/Corbis; **243** Tony Freeman/PhotoEdit; **244** Noel Hendrickson/Getty Images; **246** Bonnie Kamin/PhotoEdit; **248** Patti McConville/Getty Images; **252** Amy Etra/PhotoEdit; 254–255 Asia Images Group/age fotostock; **256** Digital Vision Ltd./Superstock; **258** Masterfile Royalty Free (RF); **259** Pixtal/Superstock; **261** Studio Eye/Corbis; **262** Brand X/Superstock; **263** Ingram Publishing/SuperStock RF; **264** Philip J Brittan/Getty Images; **630** Lew Robertson/Getty Images; **265** BananaStock/Superstock; **266** Ryuhei Shindo/Getty Images; **267** Floresco Productions/Corbis; **272** Studio Eye/Corbis; **275** Cultura Limited/SuperStock RF; **276–277** Corbis/Jupiter Images RF; **278–279** Don Farrall/Getty Images; **280** age fotostock/Superstock; **282** Sean Justice/Corbis; **283** Michael Newman/PhotoEdit; **286** George D. Lepp/Corbis; **290** age fotostock RF; **302–303** Getty Images RF; **305** Image Source/Corbis; **306** Ingram Publishing/Superstock; **307** Photodisc/Superstock; **309** Image Source/Superstock; **312** Image Source/Corbis; **314–315** James Baigrie/Getty Images; **320** Bill Aron/PhotoEdit; **323** Raymond Forbes/Masterfile; **324** InsideOut Pix/Superstock; **325br** Amy Erta/PhotoEdit; **325tm** Richard Hutchings/PhotoEdit; **328b** Bill Aron/PhotoEdit; **328b** PhotoSpin/age fotostock RF; **328t** David Murray/Getty Images; **328t** Mike Randolph/Masterfile; **329b** PhotoSpin/age fotostock RF; **329ml** Felicia Martinez Photography/PhotoEdit; **329tr** Getty Images RF; **333** Dave King/Getty Images; **334** Digital Vision Ltd./SuperStock; **335ml** Lauren Burke/Getty Images; **335tl** Image Source/SuperStock RF; **340–341** Brian Sytnyk/Masterfile; **344** Photodisc/Superstock; **346** Polka Dot Images/SuperStock RF; **347** Peter Dazeley/Getty Images; **350** Photodisc/Superstock; **353** Corbis/Jupiter Images RF; **354–355** Foodfolio/age fotostock; **356–357** Andersen Ross/Getty Images; **358** FoodCollection/SuperStock RF; **364** Corbis/SuperStock RF; **365l** Getty Images Royalty Free; **365r** Paul Poplis/Getty Images; **368** Paul Poplis/Getty Images; **370–371** David Young-Wolff/PhotoEdit; **374** Envision/Corbis; **375** Image Source/SuperStock RF; **376** FoodCollection/SuperStock RF; **376** Image Source/SuperStock RF; **377l** Howard Shooter/Getty Images RF; **377r** Dorling Kindersley/Getty Images; **378** FoodCollection/SuperStock RF; **379** KAZUNORI YOSHIKAWA/amanaimages/Corbis; **382** Polka Dot Images/SuperStock RF; **384–385** Vance Fox/Getty Images; **389** Jonathan Nourok/PhotoEdit; **390** Bernard Radvaner/Getty Images; **393** Getty Images Royalty Free; **394** Masterfile Royalty Free (RF); **396** Mary Kate Denny/PhotoEdit; **397** Steven Mark Needham/Envision/Corbis RF; **400** Getty Images Royalty Free; **402–403** Getty Images RF; **407** Jose Luis Pelaez/Blend Images/Corbis; **410 630** Lew Robertson/Getty Images; Jose Luis Pelaez/Blend Images/Corbis; **412–413** J. Rynio/Getty Images; **415** David Murray and Jules Selmes/Getty Images; **416** Foodfolioage fotostock; **416** Image Source/Getty Images RF; **416** Image Source/SuperStock RF; **416** Lew Robertson/Getty Images; **417** Image Source/Getty Images RF; **417** Image Source/SuperStock RF; **417** Lew Robertson/Getty Images; **417** Lew Robertson/Getty Images; **420l** FoodCollection/SuperStock RF; **420m** FoodCollection/SuperStock RF; **420r** Stockbyte/SuperStock RF;

421 Brand X/SuperStock RF; **427** Foodfolio/age fotostock; **428-429** Jerzyworks/Masterfile; **430–431** Imageshop/SuperStock RF; **441l** Ryman Cabannes/photocuisine/Corbis; **441r** Masterfile Royalty Free (RF); **443** Ryman Cabannes/photocuisine/Corbis; **446** Ryman Cabannes/photocuisine/Corbis; **448–449** Jeff Greenberg/PhotoEdit; **460** Jeff Greenberg/PhotoEdit; **463** Brand X/SuperStock RF; **468–469** Dennis Gottlie/FooodPix/Jupiter Images; **475** FoodCollection/SuperStock RF; **475** Franco Pizzochero/age fotostock; **476** age fotostock/SuperStock; **484–485** Thomas Del Brase/Getty Images; **486** Kevin Summers/Getty Images; **489** Javier Ortega/Corbis; **491** James Baigrie/Getty Images; **494** FoodCollection/SuperStock RF; **494** Image Source/SuperStock RF; **500–501** Maximilian Stock Ltd/photocuisine/Corbis; **502** Felicia Martinez/PhotoEdit; **505** Masterfile Royalty Free; **512** Maximilian Stock Ltd/photocuisine/Corbis; **519** Envision/Corbis; **520** Hemera/age fotostock RF; **522** Bill Arce/Getty Images; **523** Corbis/SuperStock RF; **524** Klaus Arras/Getty Images; **526** Colin Cooke/Getty Images; **527** Photodisc/SuperStock RF; **530** Klaus Arras/Getty Images; **532–533** Desgrieux/SoFood/Corbis; **539** Atlantide Phototravel/Corbis; **540** Brand X/SuperStock RF; **546** Atlantide Phototravel/Corbis; **548–549** Masterfile Royalty Free; **550** Joel Sartore/Getty Images RF; **550** John A. Rizzo/Getty Images RF; **550** Martial Colomb/Getty Images RF; **558** FoodCollection/Stockfood; **560–561** Leigh Beisch/Getty Images; **562** Image Source/SuperStock RF; **563** FoodCollection/SuperStock RF; **576–577** Duncan Smith/Corbis RF; **579** Polka Dot Images/SuperStock RF; **580** age fotostock/SuperStock; **583** Fogstock LLC/SuperStock; **591** Jerzyworks/Masterfile; **592–593,** Acme Food Arts/Getty Images; **597** Brand X/SuperStock; **598, 606** Brand X/SuperStock RF; **599** Photolibrary; **601** Corbis/SuperStock RF; **603** Corbis/SuperStock RF; **608–609** Pixtal/age fotostock RF; **610** Purestock/Getty Images RF; **614** David Young-Wolff/PhotoEdit; **620–621,** Lew Robertson/Getty Images; **623** RubberBall/SuperStock RF; **624** Image Source/SuperStock RF; **626** FoodCollection/SuperStock RF; **627** Louise Lister/Getty Images; **630** Lew Robertson/Getty Images; **632–633** Thomas Firak/Getty Images; **634** Masterfile Royalty Free (RF); **637** Brand X/SuperStock RF; **639** FoodCollection/SuperStock RF; **640** Foodcollection/etty Images RF; **643** BlueMoon Stock/SuperStock RF; **649** Acme Food Arts/Getty Images; **650–651** apack Company/Corbis; **652–653** Photolibrary; **654** Envision/Corbis; **656** FoodCollection/SuperStock RF; **660** Polka Dot Images/SuperStock RF; **664** FoodCollection/SuperStock RF; **666–667** Masterfile Royalty Free (RF); **671** Mauritius/SuperStock; **680–681** NordicPhotos/age fotostock; **682** Masterfile Royalty Free (RF); **684** Marshall Gordon/Cole Group/Getty Images RF; **685** Steven Mark Needham/Envision/Corbis RF; **687l,** Brand X/SuperStock RF; **687m** Getty Images Royalty Free; **687r** Masterfile Royalty Free (RF); **689** Ginet-drin/photocuisine/Corbis; **692** Brand X/SuperStock RF; **694–695** FoodCollection/SuperStock RF; **697** SoFood/age fotostock RF; **698b** Envision/Corbis; **698t** Photodisc/SuperStock RF; **701** SoFood/age fotostock RF; **704** SoFood/age fotostock RF; **708–709** Agence Images/Jupiter Images; **710–711** Rick Barrentine/Corbis; **713** Quentin Bacon/Getty Images; **715** Javier Ortega/Corbis; **716** Envision/Corbis; **720** fStop/SuperStock; **722–723** Brand X/SuperStock RF; **726** Blend Images/SuperStock RF; **727** Estudio Boccato/Getty Images; **727** PunchStock; **729** Dorling Kindersley/DK Images; **732** Blend Images/SuperStock RF; **734–735** B. Marielle/photocuisine/Corbis; **738** Dorling Kindersley/DK Images; **739** Corbis/age fotostock RF; **74–75** DEA/G.UMMARINO/Getty Images; **740** FoodCollection/age fotostock RF; **741** Getty Images RF; **742** age fotostock/SuperStock; **745** Masterfile Royalty Free (RF); **746** Dorling Kindersley/DK Images; **747** Foodfolio/age fotostock; **748** age fotostock/SuperStock; **749** Getty Images Royalty Free; **752** Photodisc/SuperStock RF; **754–755** Envision/Corbis; **757** FoodCollection/SuperStock RF; **758** Michael Alberstat/Masterfile; **759** Mark Tomalty/Masterfile; **760** Ingram Publishing/SuperStock RF; **761** Masterfile Royalty Free (RF); **764** Masterfile Royalty Free (RF); **766–767** B.Radvaner/photocuisine/Corbis; **769** Ingram Publishing/SuperStock RF; **772** Photodisc/SuperStock RF; **774** Hall/photocuisine/Corbis; **775** FoodCollection/SuperStock RF; **778** Hall/photocuisine/Corbis; **780–781** Ludovic Maisant/Corbis; **785, 790** PhotoAlto/SuperStock RF; **786** Riou/photocuisine/Corbis; **787** Canan Silay/Getty Images; **793** Agence Images/Jupiter Images.

Of course, if we showed more decimal places, the average velocities before and after $t = 1$ would no longer agree. To calculate the velocity at $t = 1$ to more decimal places of accuracy, we take smaller and smaller intervals on either side of $t = 1$ until the average velocities agree to the number of decimal places we want. In this way, we can estimate the velocity at $t = 1$ to any accuracy.

Defining Instantaneous Velocity Using the Idea of a Limit

When we take smaller intervals near $t = 1$, it turns out that the average velocities for the grapefruit are always just above or just below 68 ft/sec. It seems natural, then, to define velocity at the instant $t = 1$ to be 68 ft/sec. This is called the *instantaneous velocity* at this point. Its definition depends on our being convinced that smaller and smaller intervals provide average velocities that come arbitrarily close to 68. This process is referred to as *taking the limit.*

> The **instantaneous velocity** of an object at time t is defined to be the limit of the average velocity of the object over shorter and shorter time intervals containing t.

Notice that the instantaneous velocity seems to be exactly 68, but what if it were 68.000001? How can we be sure that we have taken small enough intervals? Showing that the limit is exactly 68 requires more precise knowledge of how the velocities were calculated and of the limiting process; see the Focus on Theory section.

Instantaneous Rate of Change

We can define the *instantaneous rate of change* of any function $y = f(t)$ at a point $t = a$. We mimic what we did for velocity and look at the average rate of change over smaller and smaller intervals.

> The **instantaneous rate of change** of f at a, also called the **rate of change** of f at a, is defined to be the limit of the average rates of change of f over shorter and shorter intervals around a.

Since the average rate of change is a difference quotient of the form $\Delta y/\Delta t$, the instantaneous rate of change is a limit of difference quotients. In practice, we often approximate a rate of change by one of these difference quotients.

Example 1 The quantity (in mg) of a drug in the blood at time t (in minutes) is given by $Q = 25(0.8)^t$. Estimate the rate of change of the quantity at $t = 3$ and interpret your answer.

Solution We estimate the rate of change at $t = 3$ by computing the average rate of change over intervals near $t = 3$. We can make our estimate as accurate as we like by choosing our intervals small enough. Let's look at the average rate of change over the interval $3 \leq t \leq 3.01$:

$$\text{Average rate of change} = \frac{\Delta Q}{\Delta t} = \frac{25(0.8)^{3.01} - 25(0.8)^3}{3.01 - 3.00} = \frac{12.7715 - 12.80}{3.01 - 3.00} = -2.85.$$

A reasonable estimate for the rate of change of the quantity at $t = 3$ is -2.85. Since Q is in mg and t in minutes, the units of $\Delta Q/\Delta t$ are mg/minute. Since the rate of change is negative, the quantity of the drug is decreasing. After 3 minutes, the quantity of the drug in the body is decreasing at 2.85 mg/minute.

In Example 1, we estimated the rate of change using an interval to the right of the point ($t = 3$ to $t = 3.01$). We could use an interval to the left of the point, or we could average the rates of change to the left and the right. In this text, we usually use an interval to the right of the point.

The Derivative at a Point

The instantaneous rate of change of a function f at a point a is so important that it is given its own name, the *derivative of f at a*, denoted $f'(a)$ (read "f-prime of a"). If we want to emphasize that $f'(a)$ is the rate of change of $f(x)$ as the variable x increases, we call $f'(a)$ the derivative of f *with respect to x* at $x = a$. Notice that the derivative is just a new name for the rate of change of a function.

> The **derivative of f at a**, written $f'(a)$, is defined to be the instantaneous rate of change of f at the point a.

A definition of the derivative using a formula is given in the Focus on Theory section.

Example 2 Estimate $f'(2)$ if $f(x) = x^3$.

Solution Since $f'(2)$ is the derivative, or rate of change, of $f(x) = x^3$ at 2, we look at the average rate of change over intervals near 2. Using the interval $2 \le x \le 2.001$, we see that

$$\begin{array}{c}\text{Average rate of change}\\ \text{on } 2 \le x \le 2.001\end{array} = \frac{(2.001)^3 - 2^3}{2.001 - 2} = \frac{8.0120 - 8}{0.001} = 12.0.$$

The rate of change of $f(x)$ at $x = 2$ appears to be approximately 12, so we estimate $f'(2) = 12$.

Visualizing the Derivative: Slope of the Graph and Slope of the Tangent Line

Figure 2.2 shows the average rate of change of a function represented by the slope of the secant line joining points A and B. The derivative is found by taking the average rate of change over smaller and smaller intervals. In Figure 2.3, as point B moves toward point A, the secant line becomes the tangent line at point A. Thus, the derivative is represented by the slope of the tangent line to the graph at the point.

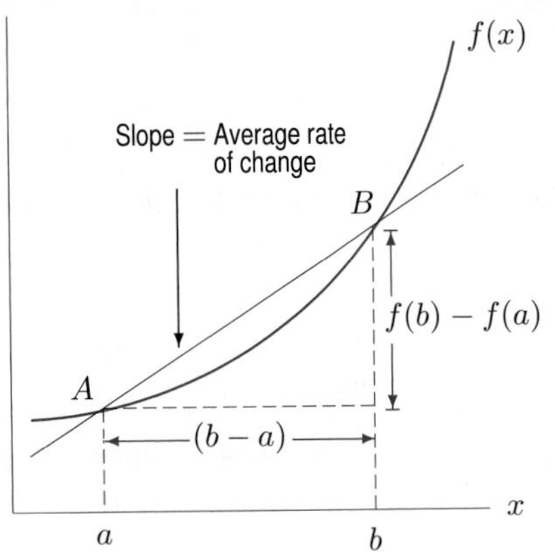

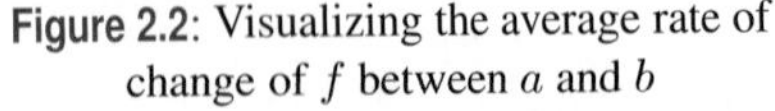

Figure 2.2: Visualizing the average rate of change of f between a and b

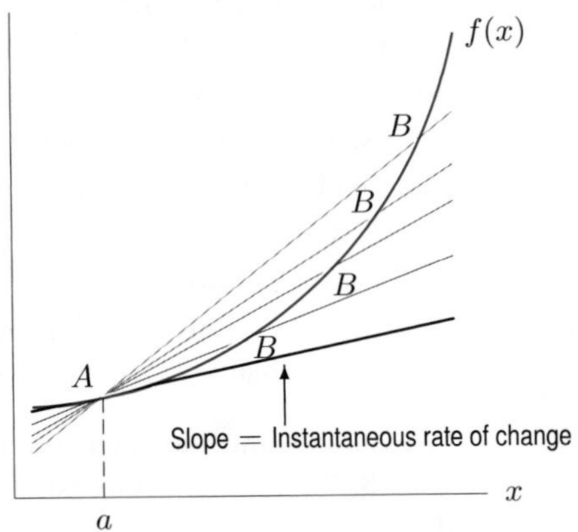

Figure 2.3: Visualizing the instantaneous rate of change of f at a

Alternatively, take the graph of a function around a point and "zoom in" to get a close-up view. (See Figure 2.4.) The more we zoom in, the more the graph appears to be straight. We call the slope of this line the *slope of the graph* at the point; it also represents the derivative.

> The derivative of a function at the point A is equal to
>
> - The slope of the graph of the function at A.
> - The slope of the line tangent to the curve at A.

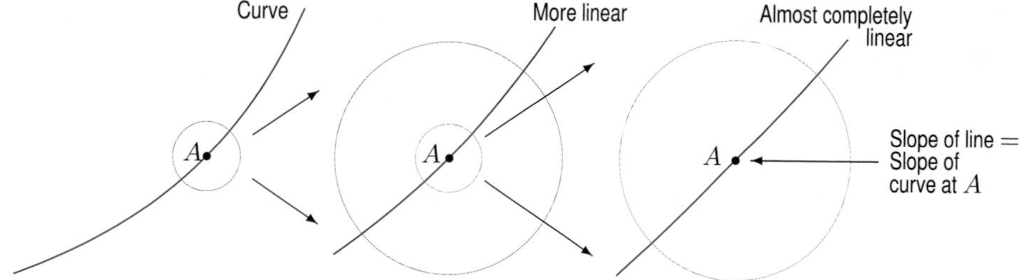

Figure 2.4: Finding the slope of a curve at a point by "zooming in"

The slope interpretation is often useful in gaining rough information about the derivative, as the following examples show.

Example 3 Use a graph of $f(x) = x^2$ to determine whether each of the following quantities is positive, negative, or zero: (a) $f'(1)$ (b) $f'(-1)$ (c) $f'(2)$ (d) $f'(0)$

Solution Figure 2.5 shows tangent line segments to the graph of $f(x) = x^2$ at the points $x = 1$, $x = -1$, $x = 2$, and $x = 0$. Since the derivative is the slope of the tangent line at the point, we have:

(a) $f'(1)$ is positive.
(b) $f'(-1)$ is negative.
(c) $f'(2)$ is positive (and larger than $f'(1)$).
(d) $f'(0) = 0$ since the graph has a horizontal tangent at $x = 0$.

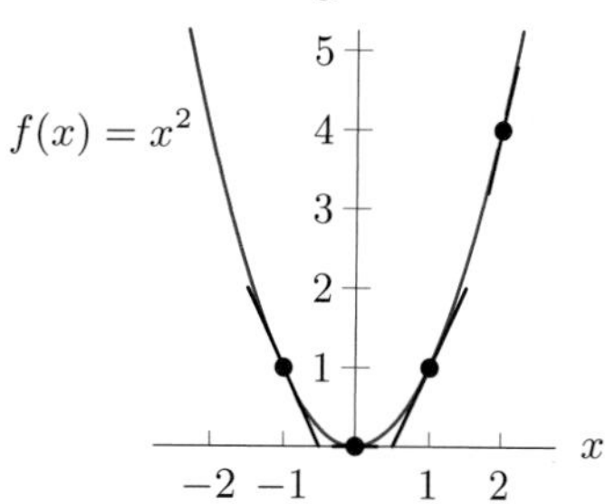

Figure 2.5: Tangent lines showing sign of derivative of $f(x) = x^2$

Example 4 Estimate the derivative of $f(x) = 2^x$ at $x = 0$ graphically and numerically.

Solution Graphically: If we draw a tangent line at $x = 0$ to the exponential curve in Figure 2.6, we see that it has a positive slope between 0.5 and 1.

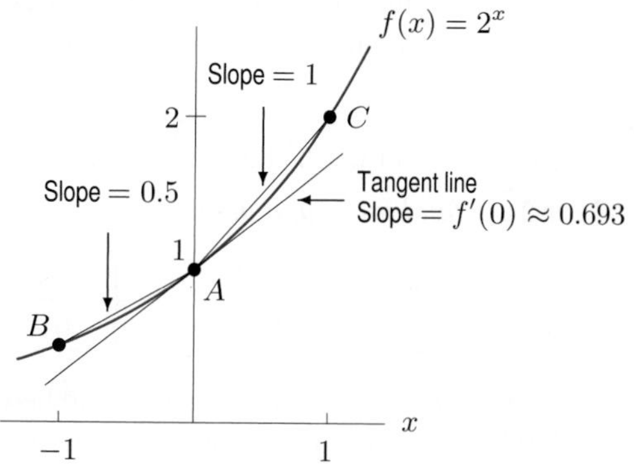

Figure 2.6: Graph of $f(x) = 2^x$ showing the derivative at $x = 0$

Numerically: To estimate the derivative at $x = 0$, we compute the average rate of change on an interval around 0.

$$\begin{array}{l}\text{Average rate of change}\\ \text{on } 0 \le x \le 0.0001\end{array} = \frac{2^{0.0001} - 2^0}{0.0001 - 0} = \frac{1.000069317 - 1}{0.0001} = 0.69317.$$

Since using smaller intervals gives approximately the same values, it appears that the derivative is approximately 0.69317; that is, $f'(0) \approx 0.693$.

Example 5 The graph of a function $y = f(x)$ is shown in Figure 2.7. Indicate whether each of the following quantities is positive or negative, and illustrate your answers graphically.

(a) $f'(1)$ (b) 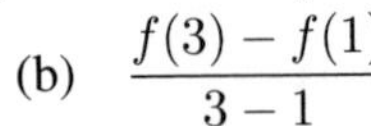 $\dfrac{f(3) - f(1)}{3 - 1}$ (c) $f(4) - f(2)$

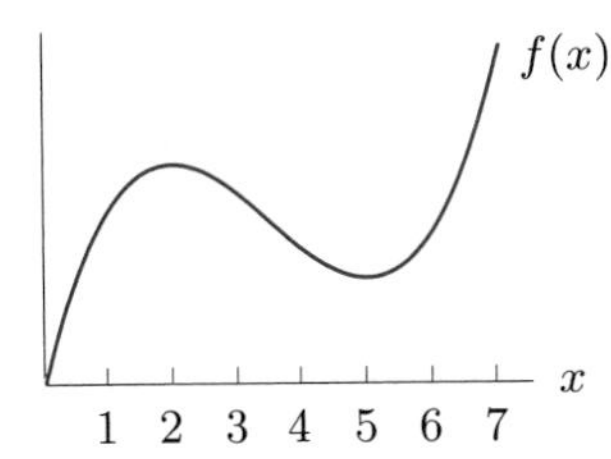

Figure 2.7

Solution (a) Since $f'(1)$ is the slope of the graph at $x = 1$, we see in Figure 2.8 that $f'(1)$ is positive.

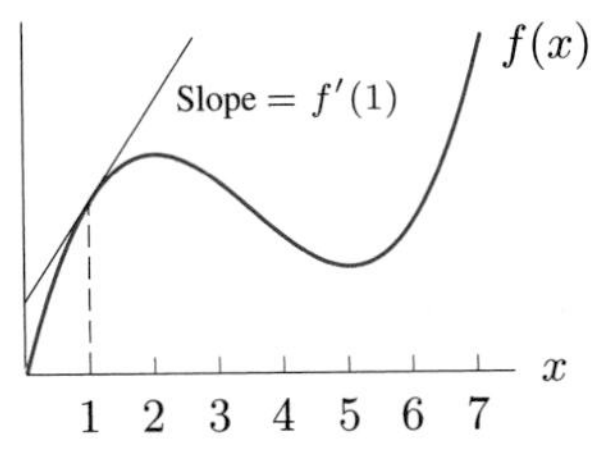

Figure 2.8

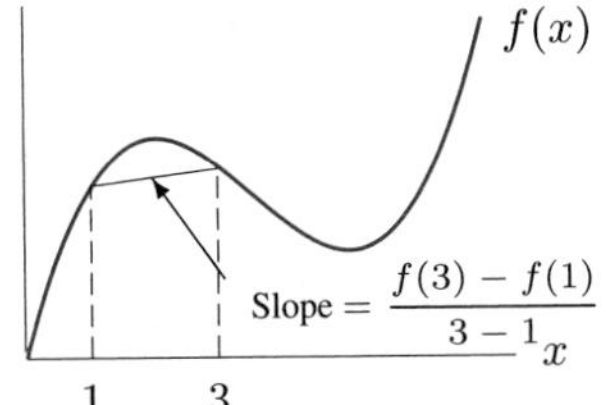

Figure 2.9

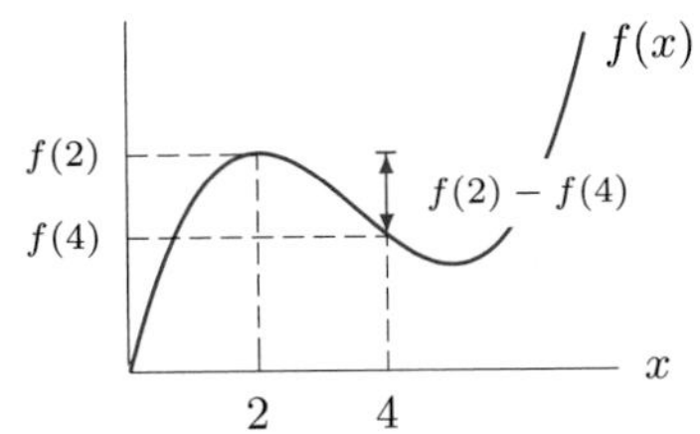

Figure 2.10

(b) The difference quotient $(f(3) - f(1))/(3 - 1)$ is the slope of the secant line between $x = 1$ and $x = 3$. We see from Figure 2.9 that this slope is positive.

(c) Since $f(4)$ is the value of the function at $x = 4$ and $f(2)$ is the value of the function at $x = 2$, the expression $f(4) - f(2)$ is the change in the function between $x = 2$ and $x = 4$. Since $f(4)$ lies below $f(2)$, this change is negative. See Figure 2.10.

Estimating the Derivative of a Function Given Numerically

If we are given a table of values for a function, we can estimate values of its derivative. To do this, we have to assume that the points in the table are close enough together that the function does not change wildly between them.

Example 6 The total acreage of farms in the US[1] has decreased since 1980. See Table 2.2.

Table 2.2 *Total farm land in million acres*

Year	1980	1985	1990	1995	2000
Farm land (million acres)	1039	1012	987	963	945

(a) What was the average rate of change in farm land between 1980 and 2000?
(b) Estimate $f'(1995)$ and interpret your answer in terms of farm land.

---

[1] *Statistical Abstracts of the United States 2004–2005*, Table 796.

Solution (a) Between 1980 and 2000,

$$\text{Average rate of change} = \frac{945 - 1039}{2000 - 1980} = \frac{-94}{20} = -4.7 \text{ million acres per year.}$$

Between 1980 and 2000, the amount of farm land was decreasing at an average rate of 4.7 million acres per year.

(b) We use the interval from 1995 to 2000 to estimate the instantaneous rate of change at 1995:

$$f'(1995) = \begin{array}{c}\text{Rate of change}\\ \text{in 1995}\end{array} \approx \frac{945 - 963}{2000 - 1995} = \frac{-18}{5} = -3.6 \text{ million acres per year.}$$

In 1995, the amount of farm land was decreasing at a rate of approximately 3.6 million acres per year.

Problems for Section 2.1

1. Use the graph in Figure 2.7 to decide if each of the following quantities is positive, negative or approximately zero. Illustrate your answers graphically.

(a) The average rate of change of $f(x)$ between $x = 3$ and $x = 7$.

(b) The instantaneous rate of change of $f(x)$ at $x = 3$.

2. Figure 2.11 shows $N = f(t)$, the number of farms in the US[2] between 1930 and 2000 as a function of year, t.

(a) Is $f'(1950)$ positive or negative? What does this tell you about the number of farms?

(b) Which is more negative: $f'(1960)$ or $f'(1980)$? Explain.

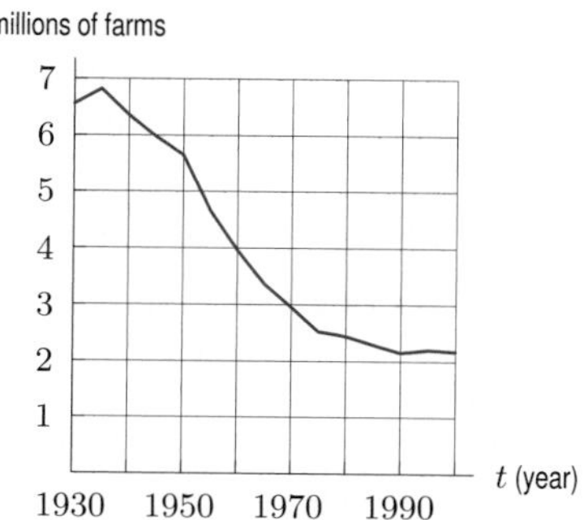

Figure 2.11

3. In a time of t seconds, a particle moves a distance of s meters from its starting point, where $s = 3t^2$.

(a) Find the average velocity between $t = 1$ and $t = 1 + h$ if:

(i) $h = 0.1$, (ii) $h = 0.01$, (iii) $h = 0.001$.

(b) Use your answers to part (a) to estimate the instantaneous velocity of the particle at time $t = 1$.

4. Find the average velocity over the interval $0 \le t \le 0.8$, and estimate the velocity at $t = 0.2$ of a car whose position, s, is given by the following table.

t (sec)	0	0.2	0.4	0.6	0.8	1.0
s (ft)	0	0.5	1.8	3.8	6.5	9.6

5. The distance (in feet) of an object from a point is given by $s(t) = t^2$, where time t is in seconds.

(a) What is the average velocity of the object between $t = 3$ and $t = 5$?

(b) By using smaller and smaller intervals around 3, estimate the instantaneous velocity at time $t = 3$.

6. Figure 2.12 shows the cost, $y = f(x)$, of manufacturing x kilograms of a chemical.

(a) Is the average rate of change of the cost greater between $x = 0$ and $x = 3$, or between $x = 3$ and $x = 5$? Explain your answer graphically.

(b) Is the instantaneous rate of change of the cost of producing x kilograms greater at $x = 1$ or at $x = 4$? Explain your answer graphically.

(c) What are the units of these rates of change?

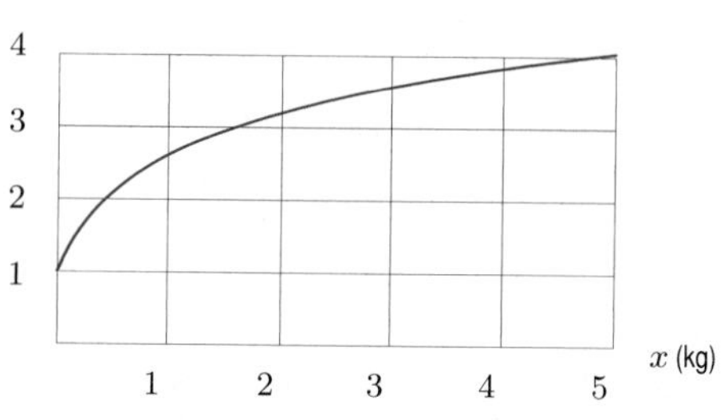

Figure 2.12

[2]www.nass.usda.gov:81/ipedb/farmnum.htm, accessed April 11, 2005.

7. The size, S, of a tumor (in cubic millimeters) is given by $S = 2^t$, where t is the number of months since the tumor was discovered. Give units with your answers.

(a) What is the total change in the size of the tumor during the first six months?
(b) What is the average rate of change in the size of the tumor during the first six months?
(c) Estimate the rate at which the tumor is growing at $t = 6$. (Use smaller and smaller intervals.)

8. (a) Using Table 2.3, find the average rate of change in the world's population between 1975 and 2005. Give units.
(b) If $P = f(t)$ with t in years, estimate $f'(2005)$ and give units.

Table 2.3 *World population, in billions of people*

Year	1975	1980	1985	1990	1995	2000	2005
Population	4.08	4.45	4.84	5.27	5.68	6.07	6.45

9. Let $f(x) = 5^x$. Use a small interval to estimate $f'(2)$. Now improve your accuracy by estimating $f'(2)$ again, using an even smaller interval.

10. (a) Let $g(t) = (0.8)^t$. Use a graph to determine whether $g'(2)$ is positive, negative, or zero.
(b) Use a small interval to estimate $g'(2)$.

11. (a) The function f is given in Figure 2.13. At which of the labeled points is $f'(x)$ positive? Negative? Zero?
(b) At which labeled point is f' largest? At which labeled point is f' most negative?

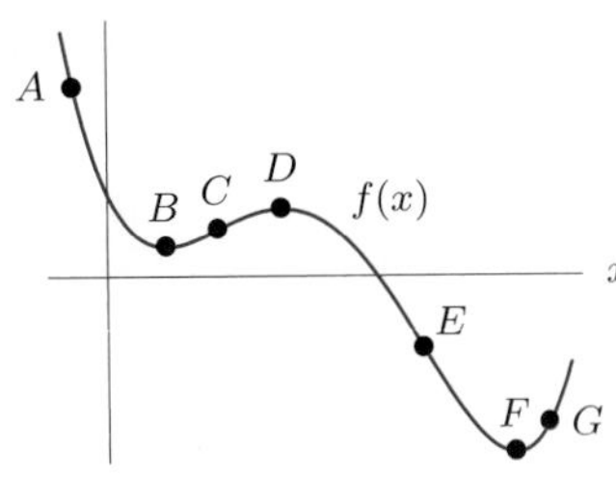

Figure 2.13

12. Estimate $f'(2)$ for $f(x) = 3^x$. Explain your reasoning.

13. Figure 2.14 shows the graph of f. Match the derivatives in the table with the points a, b, c, d, e.

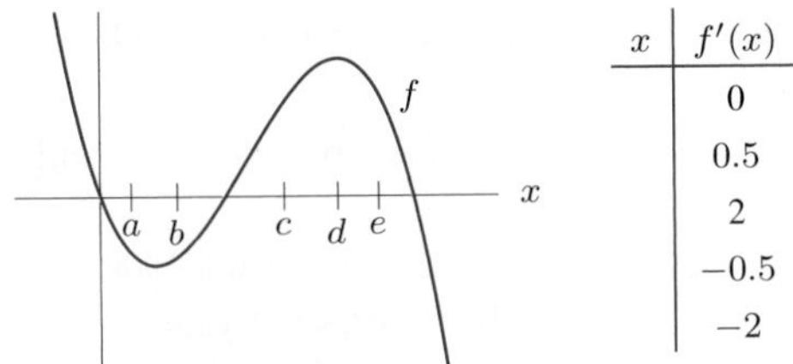

x	$f'(x)$
	0
	0.5
	2
	−0.5
	−2

Figure 2.14

14. The following table gives the percent of the US population living in urban areas as a function of year.[3]

Year	1800	1830	1860	1890	1920
Percent	6.0	9.0	19.8	35.1	51.2
Year	**1950**	**1980**	**1990**	**2000**	
Percent	**64.0**	**73.7**	**75.2**	**79.0**	

(a) Find the average rate of change of the percent of the population living in urban areas between 1890 and 1990.
(b) Estimate the rate at which this percent is increasing at the year 1990.
(c) Estimate the rate of change of this function for the year 1830 and explain what it is telling you.
(d) Is this function increasing or decreasing?

15. (a) Graph $f(x) = x^2$ and $g(x) = x^2 + 3$ on the same axes. What can you say about the slopes of the tangent lines to the two graphs at the point $x = 0$? $x = 1$? $x = 2$? $x = a$, where a is any value?
(b) Explain why adding a constant to any function will not change the value of the derivative at any point.

16. Table 2.4 gives $P = f(t)$, the percent of households in the US with cable television t years since 1990.[4]

(a) Does $f'(6)$ appear to be positive or negative? What does this tell you about the percent of households with cable television?
(b) Estimate $f'(2)$. Estimate $f'(10)$. Explain what each is telling you, in terms of cable television.

Table 2.4

t (years since 1990)	0	2	4	6	8	10	12
P (% with cable)	59.0	61.5	63.4	66.7	67.4	67.8	68.9

17. Estimate $P'(0)$ if $P(t) = 200(1.05)^t$. Explain how you obtained your answer.

---

[3] *Statistical Abstracts of the US*, 1985, US Department of Commerce, Bureau of the Census, p. 22, and *World Almanac and Book of Facts 2005*, p. 624 (New York).
[4] *The World Almanac and Book of Facts 2005*, p. 310 (New York).

18. The function in Figure 2.15 has $f(4) = 25$ and $f'(4) = 1.5$. Find the coordinates of the points A, B, C.

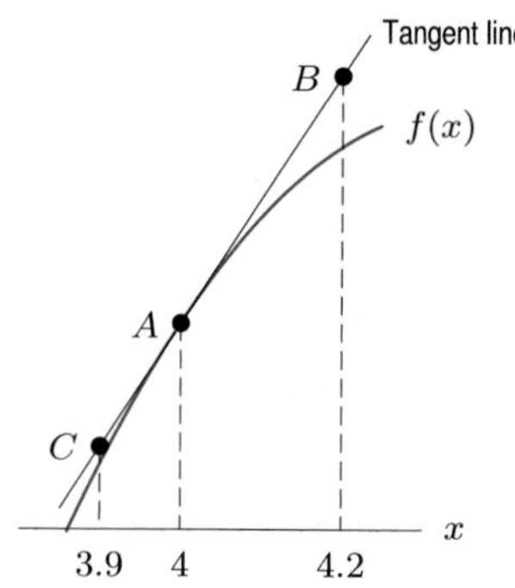

Figure 2.15

19. Use Figure 2.16 to fill in the blanks in the following statements about the function g at point B.

(a) $g(\_\_) = \_\_$ **(b)** $g'(\_\_) = \_\_$

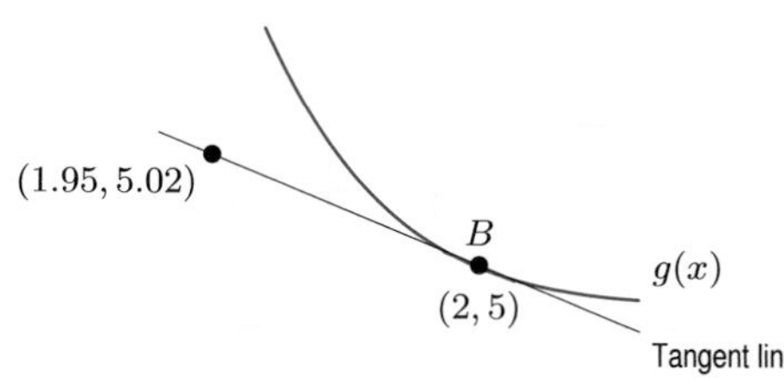

Figure 2.16

20. Show how to represent the following on Figure 2.17.

(a) $f(4)$ **(b)** $f(4) - f(2)$

(c) $\dfrac{f(5) - f(2)}{5 - 2}$ **(d)** $f'(3)$

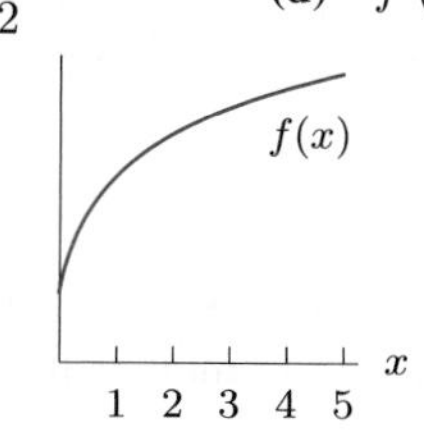

Figure 2.17

21. For each of the following pairs of numbers, use Figure 2.17 to decide which is larger. Explain your answer.

(a) $f(3)$ or $f(4)$?

(b) $f(3) - f(2)$ or $f(2) - f(1)$?

(c) $\dfrac{f(2) - f(1)}{2 - 1}$ or $\dfrac{f(3) - f(1)}{3 - 1}$?

(d) $f'(1)$ or $f'(4)$?

22. Estimate the instantaneous rate of change of the function $f(x) = x \ln x$ at $x = 1$ and at $x = 2$. What do these values suggest about the concavity of the graph between 1 and 2?

23. On October 17, 2006, in an article called "US Population Reaches 300 Million," the BBC reported that the US gains 1 person every 11 seconds. If $f(t)$ is the US population in millions t years after October 17, 2006, find $f(0)$ and $f'(0)$.

24. The following table shows the number of hours worked in a week, $f(t)$, hourly earnings, $g(t)$, in dollars, and weekly earnings, $h(t)$, in dollars, of production workers as functions of t, the year.[5]

(a) Indicate whether each of the following derivatives is positive, negative, or zero: $f'(t)$, $g'(t)$, $h'(t)$. Interpret each answer in terms of hours or earnings.

(b) Estimate each of the following derivatives, and interpret your answers:

(i) $f'(1970)$ and $f'(1995)$

(ii) $g'(1970)$ and $g'(1995)$

(iii) $h'(1970)$ and $h'(1995)$

t	1970	1975	1980	1985	1990	1995	2000
$f(t)$	37.0	36.0	35.2	34.9	34.3	34.3	34.3
$g(t)$	3.40	4.73	6.84	8.73	10.09	11.64	14.00
$h(t)$	125.80	170.28	240.77	304.68	349.29	399.53	480.41

2.2 THE DERIVATIVE FUNCTION

In Section 2.1 we looked at the derivative of a function at a point. In general, the derivative takes on different values at different points and is itself a function. Recall that the derivative is the slope of the tangent line to the graph at the point.

Finding the Derivative of a Function Given Graphically

Example 1 Estimate the derivative of the function $f(x)$ graphed in Figure 2.18 at $x = -2, -1, 0, 1, 2, 3, 4, 5$.

[5] *The World Almanac and Book of Facts 2005,* p. 151 (New York). Production workers includes nonsupervisory workers in mining, manufacturing, construction, transportation, public utilities, wholesale and retail trade, finance, insurance, real estate, and services.

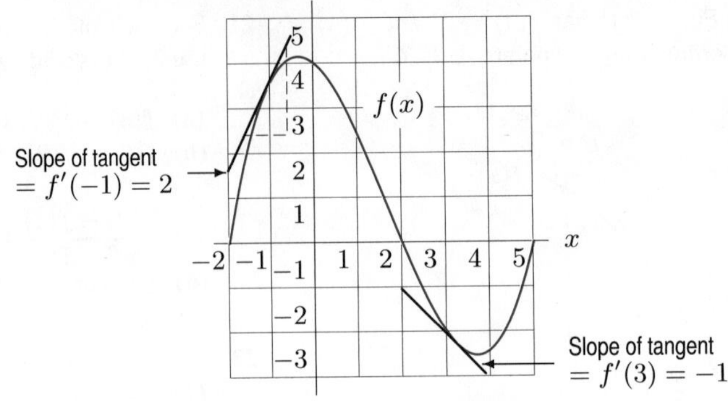

Figure 2.18: Estimating the derivative graphically as the slope of a tangent line

Solution From the graph, we estimate the derivative at any point by placing a straightedge so that it forms the tangent line at that point, and then using the grid to estimate the slope of the tangent line. For example, the tangent at $x = -1$ is drawn in Figure 2.18, and has a slope of about 2, so $f'(-1) \approx 2$. Notice that the slope at $x = -2$ is positive and fairly large; the slope at $x = -1$ is positive but smaller. At $x = 0$, the slope is negative, by $x = 1$ it has become more negative, and so on. Some estimates of the derivative, to the nearest integer, are listed in Table 2.5. You should check these values yourself. Is the derivative positive where you expect? Negative?

Table 2.5 *Estimated values of derivative of function in Figure 2.18*

x	-2	-1	0	1	2	3	4	5
Derivative at x	6	2	-1	-2	-2	-1	1	4

The important point to notice is that for every x-value, there is a corresponding value of the derivative. The derivative, therefore, is a function of x.

> For a function f, we define the **derivative function**, f', by
>
> $$f'(x) = \text{Instantaneous rate of change of } f \text{ at } x.$$

Example 2 Plot the values of the derivative function calculated in Example 1. Compare the graphs of f' and f.

Solution Graphs of f and f' are in Figures 2.19 and 2.20, respectively. Notice that f' is positive (its graph is above the x-axis) where f is increasing, and f' is negative (its graph is below the x-axis) where f is decreasing. The value of $f'(x)$ is 0 where f has a maximum or minimum value (at approximately $x = -0.4$ and $x = 3.7$).

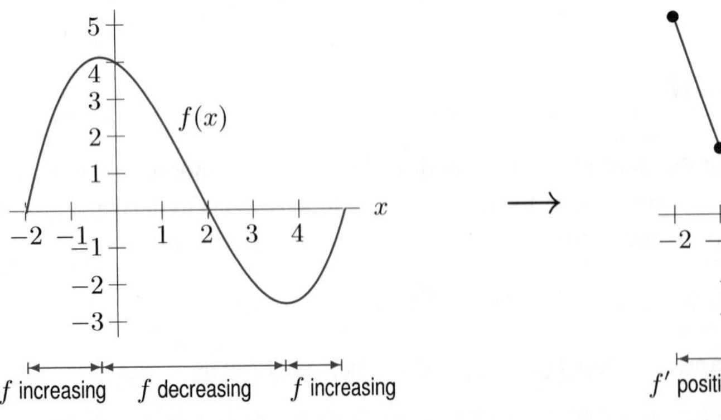

Figure 2.19: The function f

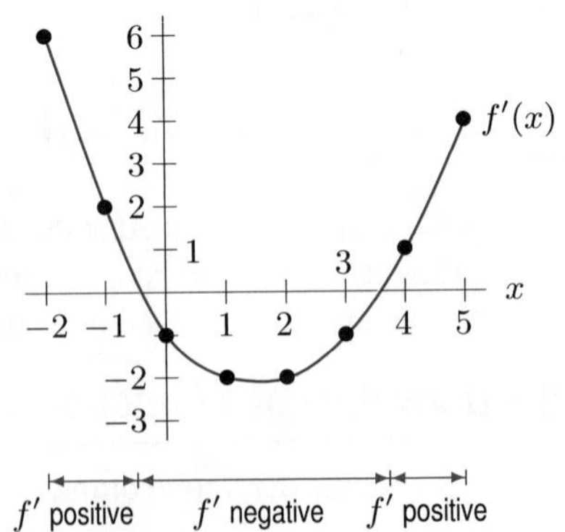

Figure 2.20: Estimates of the derivative, f'

Example 3 The graph of f is in Figure 2.21. Which of the graphs (a)–(c) is a graph of the derivative, f'?

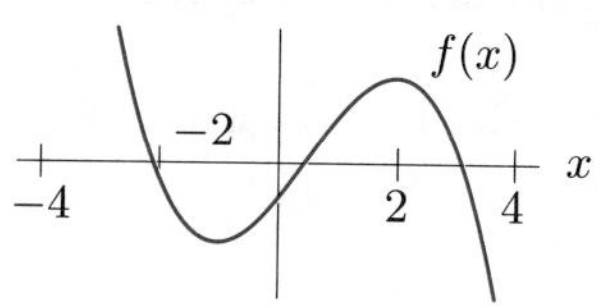

Figure 2.21

(a)

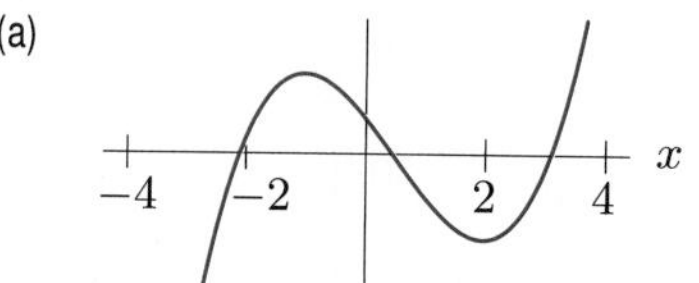

(b)

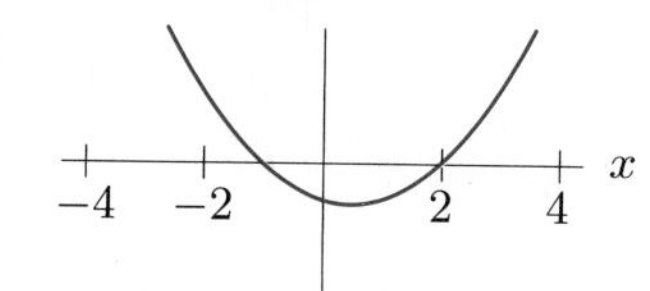

(c)

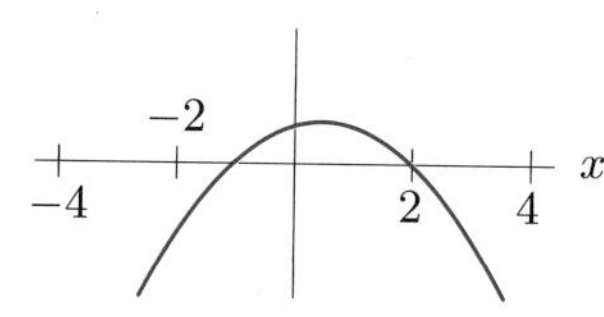

Solution Since the graph of $f(x)$ is horizontal at $x = -1$ and $x = 2$, the derivative is zero there. Therefore, the graph of $f'(x)$ has x-intercepts at $x = -1$ and $x = 2$.

The function f is decreasing for $x < -1$, increasing for $-1 < x < 2$, and decreasing for $x > 2$. The derivative is positive (its graph is above the x-axis) where f is increasing, and the derivative is negative (its graph is below the x-axis) where f is decreasing. The correct graph is (c).

What Does the Derivative Tell Us Graphically?

Where the derivative, f', of a function is positive, the tangent to the graph of f is sloping up; where f' is negative, the tangent is sloping down. If $f' = 0$ everywhere, then the tangent is horizontal everywhere and so f is constant. The sign of the derivative f' tells us whether the function f is increasing or decreasing.

> If $f' > 0$ on an interval, then f is *increasing* over that interval.
> If $f' < 0$ on an interval, then f is *decreasing* over that interval.
> If $f' = 0$ on an interval, then f is *constant* over that interval.

The magnitude of the derivative gives us the magnitude of the rate of change of f. If f' is large in magnitude, then the graph of f is steep (up if f' is positive or down if f' is negative); if f' is small in magnitude, the graph of f is gently sloping.

Estimating the Derivative of a Function Given Numerically

If we are given a table of function values instead of a graph of the function, we can estimate values of the derivative.

Example 4 Table 2.6 gives values of $c(t)$, the concentration (mg/cc) of a drug in the bloodstream at time t (min). Construct a table of estimated values for $c'(t)$, the rate of change of $c(t)$ with respect to t.

Table 2.6 *Concentration of a drug as a function of time*

t (min)	0	0.1	0.2	0.3	0.4	0.5	0.6	0.7	0.8	0.9	1.0
$c(t)$ (mg/cc)	0.84	0.89	0.94	0.98	1.00	1.00	0.97	0.90	0.79	0.63	0.41

Solution To estimate the derivative of c using the values in the table, we assume that the data points are close enough together that the concentration does not change wildly between them. From the table, we see that the concentration is increasing between $t = 0$ and $t = 0.4$, so we expect a positive derivative there. From $t = 0.5$ to $t = 1.0$, the concentration starts to decrease, and the rate of decrease gets larger and larger, so we would expect the derivative to be negative and of greater and greater magnitude.

We estimate the derivative for each value of t using a difference quotient. For example,

$$c'(0) \approx \frac{c(0.1) - c(0)}{0.1 - 0} = \frac{0.89 - 0.84}{0.1} = 0.5 \text{ (mg/cc) per minute.}$$

Similarly, we get the estimates

$$c'(0.1) \approx \frac{c(0.2) - c(0.1)}{0.2 - 0.1} = \frac{0.94 - 0.89}{0.1} = 0.5$$
$$c'(0.2) \approx \frac{c(0.3) - c(0.2)}{0.3 - 0.2} = \frac{0.98 - 0.94}{0.1} = 0.4$$

and so on. These values are tabulated in Table 2.7. Notice that the derivative has small positive values up until $t = 0.4$, and then it gets more and more negative, as we expected.

Table 2.7 *Derivative of concentration*

t	0	0.1	0.2	0.3	0.4	0.5	0.6	0.7	0.8	0.9
$c'(t)$	0.5	0.5	0.4	0.2	0.0	−0.3	−0.7	−1.1	−1.6	−2.2

Improving Numerical Estimates for the Derivative

In the previous example, our estimate for the derivative of $c(t)$ at $t = 0.2$ used the point to the right. We found the average rate of change between $t = 0.2$ and $t = 0.3$. However, we could equally well have gone to the left and used the rate of change between $t = 0.1$ and $t = 0.2$ to approximate the derivative at 0.2. For a more accurate result, we could average these slopes, getting the approximation

$$c'(0.2) \approx \frac{1}{2}\left(\begin{array}{c}\text{Slope to left}\\ \text{of } 0.2\end{array} + \begin{array}{c}\text{Slope to right}\\ \text{of } 0.2\end{array} \right) = \frac{0.5 + 0.4}{2} = 0.45.$$

Each of these methods of approximating the derivative gives a reasonable answer. We will usually estimate the derivative by going to the right.

Finding the Derivative of a Function Given by a Formula

If we are given a formula for a function f, can we come up with a formula for f'? Using the definition of the derivative, we often can. Indeed, much of the power of calculus depends on our ability to find formulas for the derivatives of all the familiar functions. This is explained in detail in Chapter 3. In the next example, we see how to guess a formula for the derivative.

Example 5 Guess a formula for the derivative of $f(x) = x^2$.

Solution We use difference quotients to estimate the values of $f'(1)$, $f'(2)$, and $f'(3)$. Then we look for a pattern in these values which we use to guess a formula for $f'(x)$.

Near $x = 1$, we have

$$f'(1) \approx \frac{1.001^2 - 1^2}{0.001} = \frac{1.002 - 1}{0.001} = \frac{0.002}{0.001} = 2.$$

Similarly,

$$f'(2) \approx \frac{2.001^2 - 2^2}{0.001} = \frac{4.004 - 4}{0.001} = \frac{0.004}{0.001} = 4$$
$$f'(3) \approx \frac{3.001^2 - 3^2}{0.001} = \frac{9.006 - 9}{0.001} = \frac{0.006}{0.001} = 6.$$

Knowing the value of f' at specific points cannot tell us the formula for f', but it can be suggestive: knowing $f'(1) \approx 2$, $f'(2) \approx 4$, $f'(3) \approx 6$ suggests that $f'(x) = 2x$. In Chapter 3, we show that this is indeed the case.

Problems for Section 2.2

1. The graph of $f(x)$ is given in Figure 2.22. Draw tangent lines to the graph at $x = -2$, $x = -1$, $x = 0$, and $x = 2$. Estimate $f'(-2)$, $f'(-1)$, $f'(0)$, and $f'(2)$.

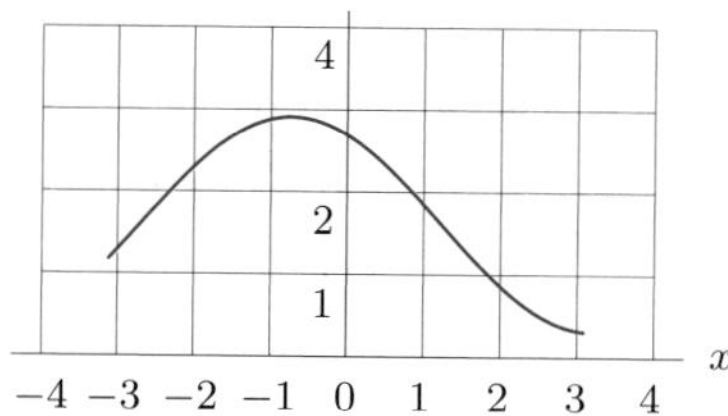

Figure 2.22

For Problems 2–7, graph the derivative of the given functions.

2.
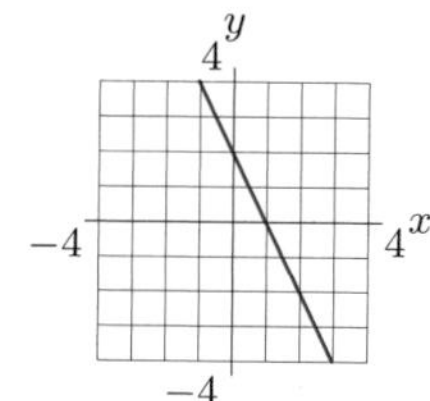

3.
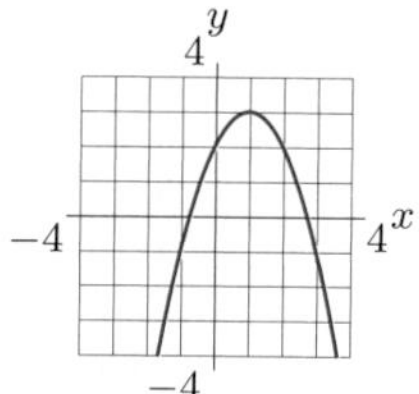

4.
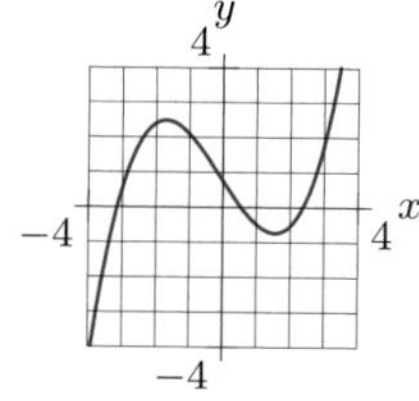

5.
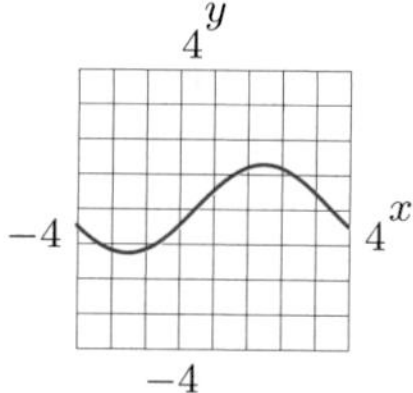

6.
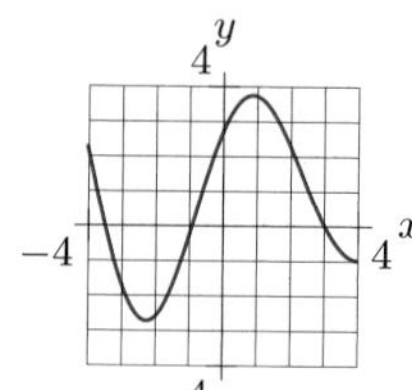

7.
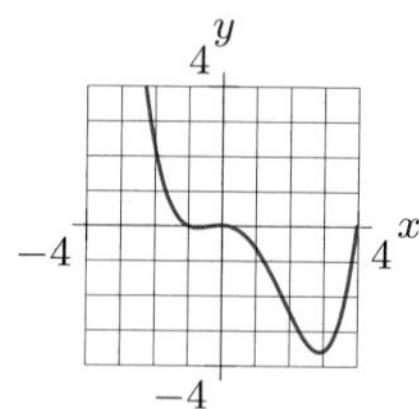

8. Given the numerical values shown, find approximate values for the derivative of $f(x)$ at each of the x-values given. Where is the rate of change of $f(x)$ positive? Where is it negative? Where does the rate of change of $f(x)$ seem to be greatest?

x	0	1	2	3	4	5	6	7	8
$f(x)$	18	13	10	9	9	11	15	21	30

9. Find approximate values for $f'(x)$ at each of the x-values given in the following table.

x	0	5	10	15	20
$f(x)$	100	70	55	46	40

10. In the graph of f in Figure 2.23, at which of the labeled x-values is

(a) $f(x)$ greatest?
(b) $f(x)$ least?
(c) $f'(x)$ greatest?
(d) $f'(x)$ least?

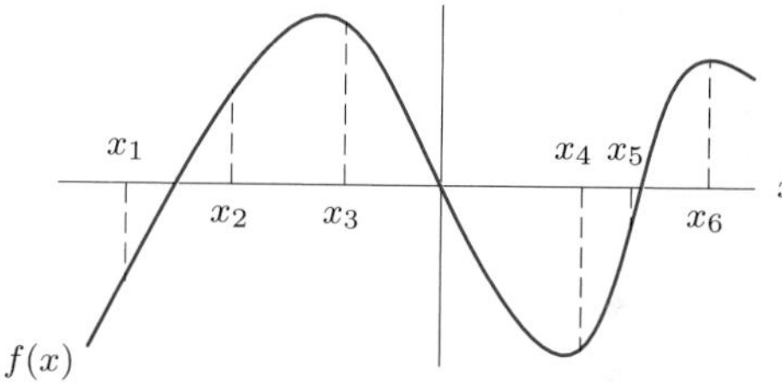

Figure 2.23

Sketch the graphs of the derivatives of the functions shown in Problems 11–18. Be sure your sketches are consistent with the important features of the graphs of the original functions.

11.
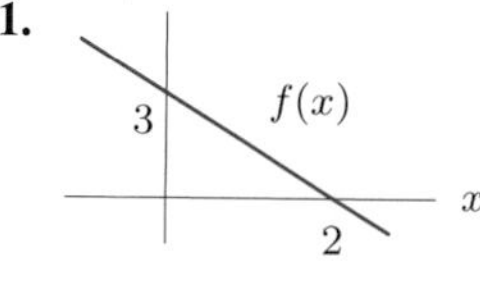

12.
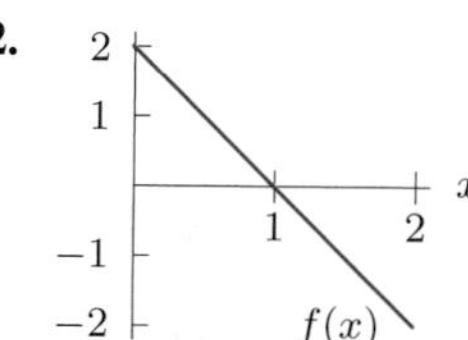

13.
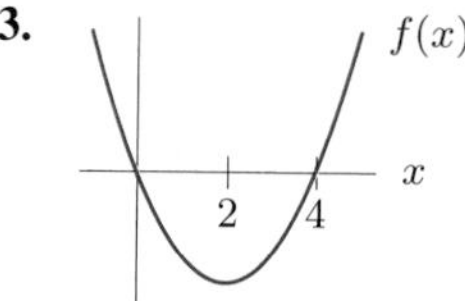

14.
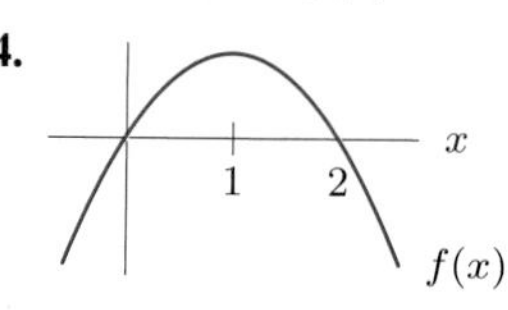

15.
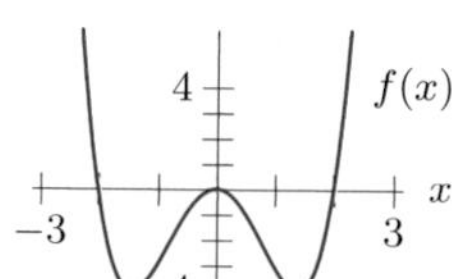

16.
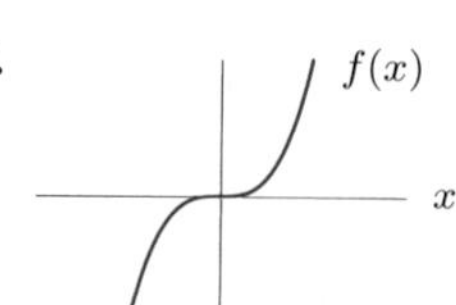

17.
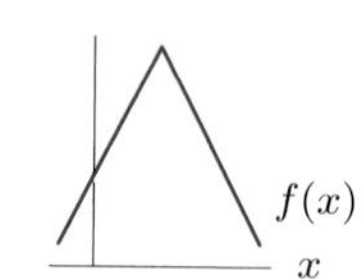

18.
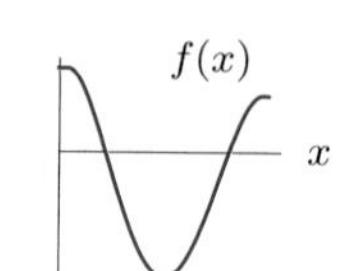

19. A city grew in population throughout the 1980s. The population was at its largest in 1990, and then shrank throughout the 1990s. Let $P = f(t)$ represent the population of the city t years since 1980. Sketch graphs of $f(t)$ and $f'(t)$, labeling the units on the axes.

20. Values of x and $g(x)$ are given in the table. For what value of x does $g'(x)$ appear to be closest to 3?

x	2.7	3.2	3.7	4.2	4.7	5.2	5.7	6.2
$g(x)$	3.4	4.4	5.0	5.4	6.0	7.4	9.0	11.0

Match the functions in Problems 21–24 with one of the derivatives in Figure 2.24.

(I)

(II)

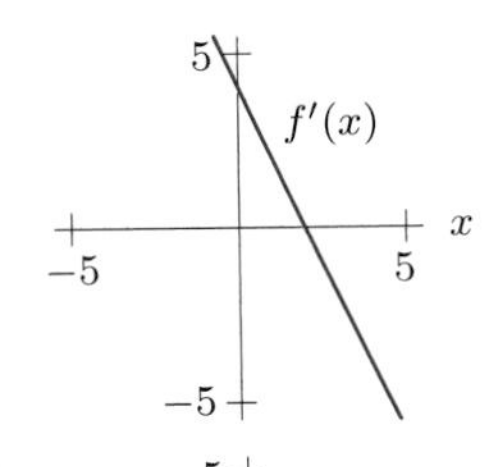

(III)

(IV)

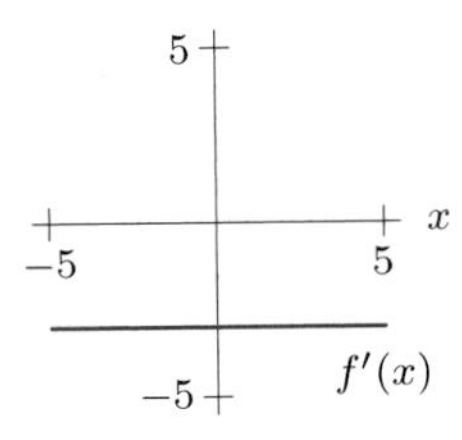

(V)

(VI)

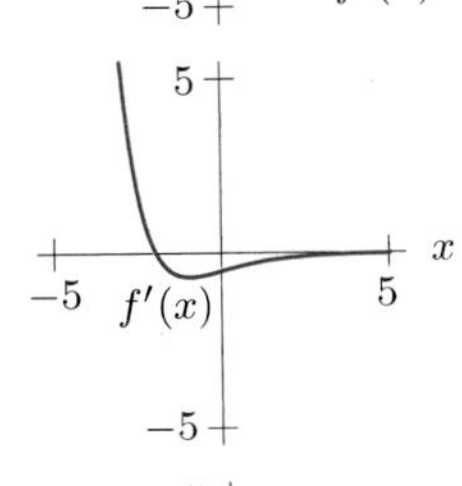

(VII)

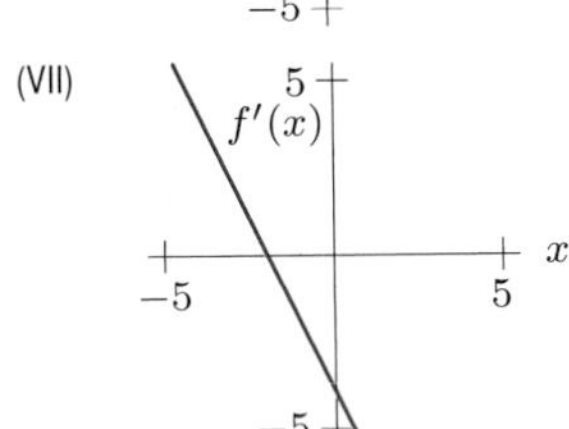

(VIII)

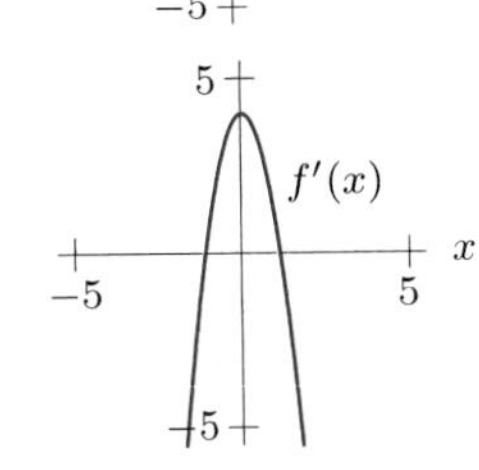

Figure 2.24

21.

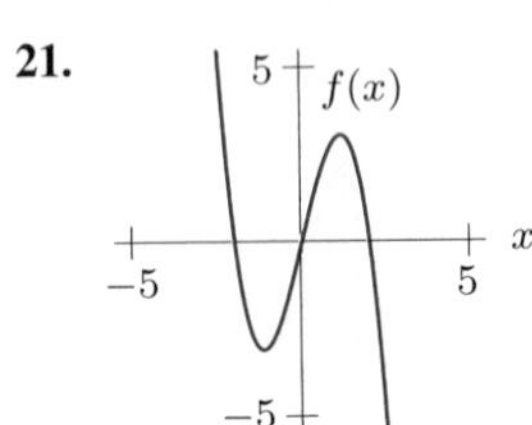

22.

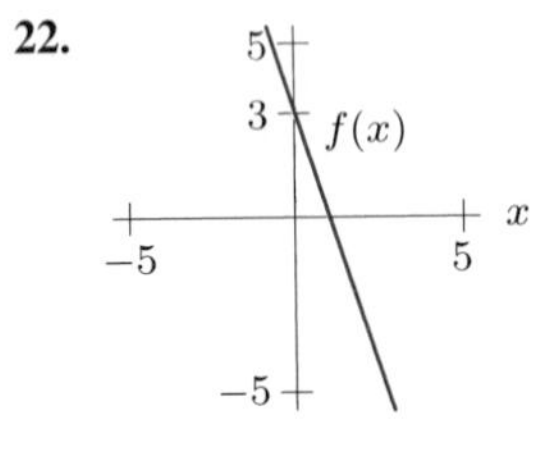

23.

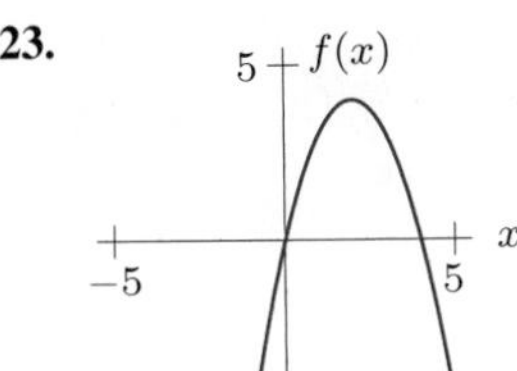

24.

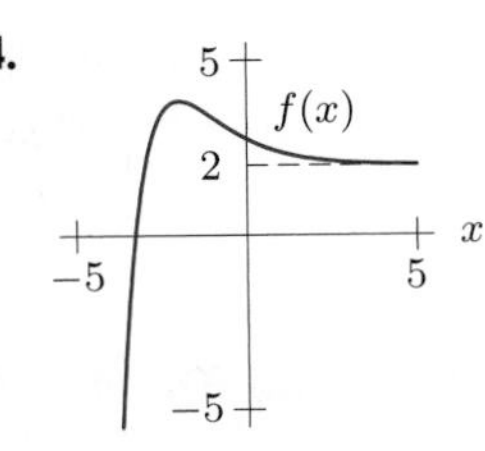

25. Draw a possible graph of $y = f(x)$ given the following information about its derivative.

- $f'(x) > 0$ for $x < -1$
- $f'(x) < 0$ for $x > -1$
- $f'(x) = 0$ at $x = -1$

26. Draw the graph of a continuous function $y = f(x)$ that satisfies the following three conditions:

- $f'(x) > 0$ for $1 < x < 3$
- $f'(x) < 0$ for $x < 1$ and $x > 3$
- $f'(x) = 0$ at $x = 1$ and $x = 3$

27. A vehicle moving along a straight road has distance $f(t)$ from its starting point at time t. Which of the graphs in Figure 2.25 could be $f'(t)$ for the following scenarios? (Assume the scales on the vertical axes are all the same.)

(a) A bus on a popular route, with no traffic
(b) A car with no traffic and all green lights
(c) A car in heavy traffic conditions

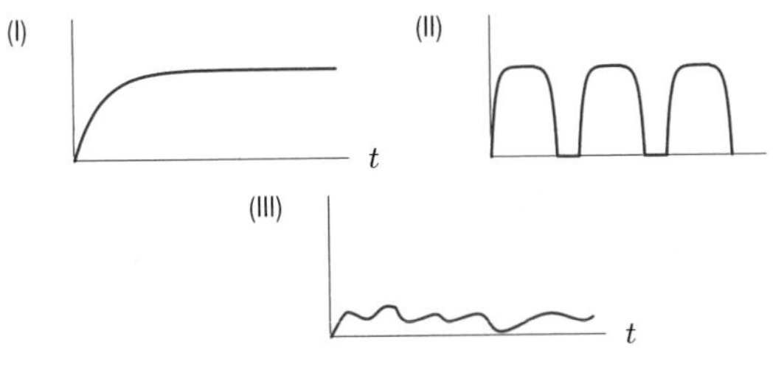

Figure 2.25

28. **(a)** Let $f(x) = \ln x$. Use small intervals to estimate $f'(1)$, $f'(2)$, $f'(3)$, $f'(4)$, and $f'(5)$.
(b) Use your answers to part (a) to guess a formula for the derivative of $f(x) = \ln x$.

29. Suppose $f(x) = \frac{1}{3}x^3$. Estimate $f'(2)$, $f'(3)$, and $f'(4)$. What do you notice? Can you guess a formula for $f'(x)$?

30. Match each of the following descriptions of a function with one of the following graphs.

(a) $f'(1) > 0$ and f' is always decreasing
(b) $f'(1) > 0$ and f' is always increasing
(c) $f'(1) < 0$ and f' is always decreasing
(d) $f'(1) < 0$ and f' is always increasing

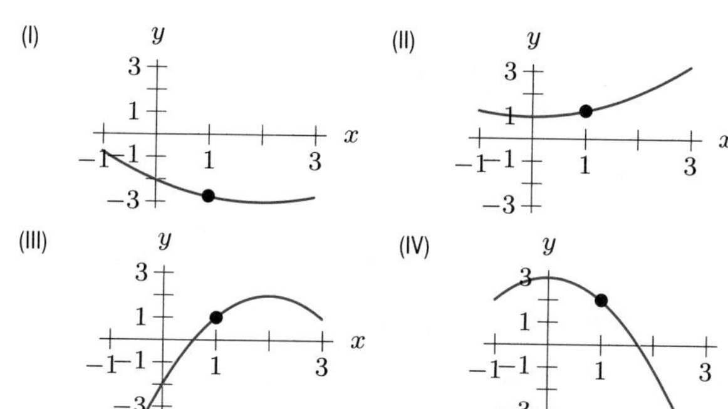

31. A child inflates a balloon, admires it for a while and then lets the air out at a constant rate. If $V(t)$ gives the volume of the balloon at time t, then Figure 2.26 shows $V'(t)$ as a function of t. At what time does the child:

(a) Begin to inflate the balloon?
(b) Finish inflating the balloon?
(c) Begin to let the air out?
(d) What would the graph of $V'(t)$ look like if the child had alternated between pinching and releasing the open end of the balloon, instead of letting the air out at a constant rate?

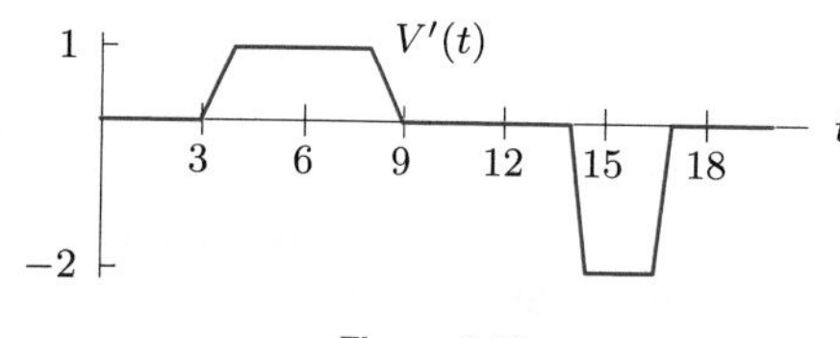

Figure 2.26

2.3 INTERPRETATIONS OF THE DERIVATIVE

We have seen the derivative interpreted as a slope and as a rate of change. In this section, we see other interpretations. The purpose of these examples is not to make a catalog of interpretations but to illustrate the process of obtaining them. There is another notation for the derivative that is often helpful.

An Alternative Notation for the Derivative

So far we have used the notation f' to stand for the derivative of the function f. An alternative notation for derivatives was introduced by the German mathematician Gottfried Wilhelm Leibniz (1646–1716) when calculus was first being developed. We know that $f'(x)$ is approximated by the average rate of change over a small interval. If $y = f(x)$, then the average rate of change is given by $\Delta y/\Delta x$. For small Δx, we have

$$f'(x) \approx \frac{\Delta y}{\Delta x}.$$

Leibniz's notation for the derivative, dy/dx, is meant to remind us of this. If $y = f(x)$, then we write

$$f'(x) = \frac{dy}{dx}.$$

Leibniz's notation is quite suggestive, especially if we think of the letter d in dy/dx as standing for "small difference in . . . ." The notation dy/dx reminds us that the derivative is a limit of ratios of the form

$$\frac{\text{Difference in } y\text{-values}}{\text{Difference in } x\text{-values}}.$$

The notation dy/dx is useful for determining the units for the derivative: the units for dy/dx are the units for y divided by (or "per") the units for x.

The separate entities dy and dx officially have no independent meaning: they are part of one notation. In fact, a good formal way to view the notation dy/dx is to think of d/dx as a single symbol meaning "the derivative with respect to x of . . .". Thus, dy/dx could be viewed as

$$\frac{d}{dx}(y), \quad \text{meaning "the derivative with respect to } x \text{ of } y\text{."}$$

On the other hand, many scientists and mathematicians really do think of dy and dx as separate entities representing "infinitesimally" small differences in y and x, even though it is difficult to say exactly how small "infinitesimal" is. It may not be formally correct, but it is very helpful intuitively to think of dy/dx as a very small change in y divided by a very small change in x.

For example, recall that if $s = f(t)$ is the position of a moving object at time t, then $v = f'(t)$ is the velocity of the object at time t. Writing

$$v = \frac{ds}{dt}$$

reminds us that v is a velocity since the notation suggests a distance, ds, over a time, dt, and we know that distance over time is velocity. Similarly, we recognize

$$\frac{dy}{dx} = f'(x)$$

as the slope of the graph of $y = f(x)$ by remembering that slope is vertical rise, dy, over horizontal run, dx.

The disadvantage of the Leibniz notation is that it is awkward to specify the value at which a derivative is evaluated. To specify $f'(2)$, for example, we have to write

$$\left.\frac{dy}{dx}\right|_{x=2}.$$

Using Units to Interpret the Derivative

Suppose a body moves along a straight line. If $s = f(t)$ gives the position in meters of the body from a fixed point on the line as a function of time, t, in seconds, then knowing that

$$\frac{ds}{dt} = f'(2) = 10 \text{ meters/sec}$$

tells us that when $t = 2$ sec, the body is moving at a velocity of 10 meters/sec. If the body continues to move at this velocity for a whole second (from $t = 2$ to $t = 3$), it would move an additional 10 meters.

In other words, if Δs represents the change in position during a time interval Δt, and if the body continues to move at this velocity, we have $\Delta s = 10\Delta t$, so

$$\Delta s = f'(2)\,\Delta t = 10\,\Delta t.$$

If the velocity is varying, this relationship is no longer exact. For small values of Δt, we have the *Tangent Line Approximation*

$$\Delta s \approx f'(t)\Delta t.$$

(See also Local Linear Approximation in this section.)Notice that, for a given positive Δt, a large derivative gives large change in s; a small derivative gives small change in s. In general:

- The units of the derivative of a function are the units of the dependent variable divided by the units of the independent variable. In other words, the units of dA/dB are the units of A divided by the units of B.
- If the derivative of a function is not changing rapidly near a point, then the derivative is approximately equal to the change in the function when the independent variable increases by 1 unit.

The following examples illustrate how useful units can be in suggesting interpretations of the derivative.

Example 1 The cost C (in dollars) of building a house A square feet in area is given by the function $C = f(A)$. What are the units and the practical interpretation of the function $f'(A)$?

Solution In the Leibniz notation,

$$f'(A) = \frac{dC}{dA}.$$

This is a cost divided by an area, so it is measured in dollars per square foot. You can think of dC as the extra cost of building an extra dA square feet of house. So if you are planning to build a house with area A square feet, $f'(A)$ is approximately the cost per square foot of the *extra* area involved in building a slightly larger house, and is called the *marginal cost*.

Example 2 The cost of extracting T tons of ore from a copper mine is $C = f(T)$ dollars. What does it mean to say that $f'(2000) = 100$?

Solution In the Leibniz notation,

$$f'(2000) = \left.\frac{dC}{dT}\right|_{T=2000}.$$

Since C is measured in dollars and T is measured in tons, dC/dT is measured in dollars per ton. You can think of dC as the extra cost of extracting an extra dT tons of ore. So the statement

$$\left.\frac{dC}{dT}\right|_{T=2000} = 100$$

says that when 2000 tons of ore have already been extracted from the mine, the cost of extracting the next ton is approximately \$100. Another way of saying this is that it costs about \$100 to extract the 2001st ton.

Example 3 If $q = f(p)$ gives the number of thousands of tons of zinc produced when the price is p dollars per ton, then what are the units and the meaning of

$$\left.\frac{dq}{dp}\right|_{p=900} = 0.2?$$

Solution The units of dq/dp are the units of q over the units of p, or thousands of tons per dollar. You can think of dq as the extra zinc produced when the price increases by dp. The statement

$$\left.\frac{dq}{dp}\right|_{p=900} = f'(900) = 0.2 \text{ thousand tons per dollar}$$

tells us that the instantaneous rate of change of q with respect to p is 0.2 when $p = 900$. This means that when the price is \$900, the quantity produced increases by about 0.2 thousand tons, or 200 tons for a one-dollar increase in price.

Example 4 The time, L (in hours), that a drug stays in a person's system is a function of the quantity administered, q, in mg, so $L = f(q)$.

(a) Interpret the statement $f(10) = 6$. Give units for the numbers 10 and 6.
(b) Write the derivative of the function $L = f(q)$ in Leibniz notation. If $f'(10) = 0.5$, what are the units of the 0.5?
(c) Interpret the statement $f'(10) = 0.5$ in terms of dose and duration.

Solution

(a) We know that $f(q) = L$. In the statement $f(10) = 6$, we have $q = 10$ and $L = 6$, so the units are 10 mg and 6 hours. The statement $f(10) = 6$ tells us that a dose of 10 mg lasts 6 hours.
(b) Since $L = f(q)$, we see that L depends on q. The derivative of this function is dL/dq. Since L is in hours and q is in mg, the units of the derivative are hours per mg. In the statement $f'(10) = 0.5$, the 0.5 is the derivative and the units are hours per mg.
(c) The statement $f'(10) = 0.5$ tells us that, at a dose of 10 mg, the instantaneous rate of change of duration is 0.5 hour per mg. In other words, if we increase the dose by 1 mg, the drug stays in the body approximately 30 minutes longer.

In the previous example, notice that $f'(10) = 0.5$ tells us that a 1 mg increase in dose leads to about a 0.5-hour increase in duration. If, on the other hand, we had had $f'(10) = 20$, we would have known that a 1-mg increase in dose leads to about a 20-hour increase in duration. Thus the derivative is the multiplier relating changes in dose to changes in duration. The magnitude of the derivative tells us how sensitive the time is to changes in dose.

We define the derivative of velocity, dv/dt, as *acceleration*.

Example 5 If the velocity of a body at time t seconds is measured in meters/sec, what are the units of the acceleration?

Solution Since acceleration, dv/dt, is the derivative of velocity, the units of acceleration are units of velocity divided by units of time, or (meters/sec)/sec, written meters/sec^2.

Using the Derivative to Estimate Values of a Function

Since the derivative tells us how fast the value of a function is changing, we can use the derivative at a point to estimate values of the function at nearby points.

Example 6 Fertilizers can improve agricultural production. A Cornell University study[6] on maize (corn) production in Kenya found that the average value, $y = f(x)$, in Kenyan shillings of the yearly maize production from an average plot of land is a function of the quantity, x, of fertilizer used in kilograms. (The shilling is the Kenyan unit of currency.)

(a) Interpret the statements $f(5) = 11{,}500$ and $f'(5) = 350$.
(b) Use the statements in part (a) to estimate $f(6)$ and $f(10)$.
(c) The value of the derivative, f', is increasing for x near 5. Which estimate in part (b) is more reliable?

Solution

(a) The statement $f(5) = 11{,}500$ tells us that $y = 11{,}500$ when $x = 5$. This means that if 5 kg of fertilizer are applied, maize worth 11,500 Kenyan shillings is produced. Since the derivative is dy/dx, the statement $f'(5) = 350$ tells us that

$$\frac{dy}{dx} = 350 \quad \text{when } x = 5.$$

This means that if the amount of fertilizer used is 5 kg and increases by 1 kg, then maize production increases by about 350 Kenyan shillings.

(b) We want to estimate $f(6)$, that is the production when 6 kg of fertilizer are used. If instead of 5 kg of fertilizer, one more kilogram is used, giving 6 kg altogether, we expect production, in Kenyan shillings, to increase from 11,500 by about 350. Thus,

$$f(6) \approx 11{,}500 + 350 = 11{,}850.$$

Similarly, if 5 kg more fertilizer is used, so 10 kg are used altogether, we expect production to increase by about $5 \cdot 350 = 1750$ Kenyan shillings, so production is approximately

$$f(10) \approx 11{,}500 + 1750 = 13{,}250.$$

(c) To estimate $f(6)$, we assume that production increases at rate of 350 Kenyan shillings per kilogram between $x = 5$ and $x = 6$ kg. To estimate $f(10)$, we assume that production continues to increase at the same rate all the way from $x = 5$ to $x = 10$ kg. Since the derivative is increasing for x near 5, the estimate of $f(6)$ is more reliable.

[6] "State-conditional fertilizer yield response on western Kenyan farms", by P. Marenya, C. Barrett, Social Science Research Network, abstract = 1141937.

In Example 6, representing the change in y by Δy and the change in x by Δx, we used the result introduced earlier in this section:

Local Linear Approximation

If $y = f(x)$ and Δx is near 0, then $\Delta y \approx f'(x)\Delta x$. Then for x near a and $\Delta x = x - a$,

$$f(x) \approx f(a) + f'(a)\Delta x.$$

This is called the Tangent Line Approximation.

Relative Rate of Change

In Section 1.5, we saw that an exponential function has a constant percent rate of change. Now we link this idea to derivatives. Analogous to the relative change, we look at the rate of change as a fraction of the original quantity.

The **relative rate of change** of $y = f(t)$ at $t = a$ is defined to be

$$\text{Relative rate of change of } y \text{ at } a = \frac{dy/dt}{y} = \frac{f'(a)}{f(a)}.$$

We see in Section 3.3 that an exponential function has a constant relative rate of change. If the independent variable is time, the relative rate is often given as a percent change per unit time.

Example 7 Annual world soybean production, $W = f(t)$, in million tons, is a function of t years since the start of 2000.

(a) Interpret the statements $f(8) = 253$ and $f'(8) = 17$ in terms of soybean production.
(b) Calculate the relative rate of change of W at $t = 8$; interpret it in terms of soybean production.

Solution (a) The statement $f(8) = 253$ tells us that 253 million tons of soybeans were produced in the year 2008. The statement $f'(8) = 17$ tells us that in 2008 annual soybean production was increasing at a rate of 17 million tons per year.

(b) We have

$$\text{Relative rate of change of soybean production} = \frac{f'(8)}{f(8)} = \frac{17}{253} = 0.067.$$

In 2008, annual soybean production was increasing at a rate of 6.7% per year.

Example 8 Solar photovoltaic (PV) cells are the world's fastest growing energy source.[7] Annual production of PV cells, S, in megawatts, is approximated by $S = 277e^{0.368t}$, where t is in years since 2000. Estimate the relative rate of change of PV cell production in 2010 using

(a) $\Delta t = 1$ (b) $\Delta t = 0.1$ (c) $\Delta t = 0.01$

Solution Let $S = f(t)$. The relative rate of change of f at $t = 10$ is $f'(10)/f(10)$. We estimate $f'(10)$ using a difference quotient.

(a) Estimating the relative rate of change using $\Delta t = 1$ at $t = 10$, we have

$$\frac{dS/dt}{S} = \frac{f'(10)}{f(10)} \approx \frac{1}{f(10)}\frac{f(11) - f(10)}{1} = 0.445 = 44.5\% \text{ per year}$$

[7] *Vital Signs 2007-2008*, The Worldwatch Institute, W.W. Norton & Company, 2007, p. 38.

(b) With $\Delta t = 0.1$ and $t = 10$, we have

$$\frac{dS/dt}{S} = \frac{f'(10)}{f(10)} \approx \frac{1}{f(10)} \frac{f(10.1) - f(10)}{0.1} = 0.375 = 37.5\% \text{ per year}$$

(c) With $\Delta t = 0.01$ and $t = 10$, we have

$$\frac{dS/dt}{S} = \frac{f'(10)}{f(10)} \approx \frac{1}{f(10)} \frac{f(10.01) - f(10)}{0.01} = 0.369 = 36.9\% \text{ per year}$$

The relative rate of change is approximately 36.9% per year. From Section 1.6, we know that the exponential function $S = 277e^{0.368t}$ has a continuous rate of change for all t of 36.8% per year, which is the exact relative rate of change of this function.

Example 9 In April 2009, the US Bureau of Economic Analysis announced that the US gross domestic product (GDP) was decreasing at an annual rate of 6.1%. The GDP of the US at that time was 13.84 trillion dollars. Calculate the annual rate of change of the US GDP in April 2009.

Solution The Bureau of Economic Analysis is reporting the relative rate of change. In April 2009, the relative rate of change of GDP was -0.061 per year. To find the rate of change, we use:

$$\begin{aligned}
\text{Relative rate of change in April 2009} &= \frac{\text{Rate of change in April 2009}}{\text{GDP in April 2009}} \\
-0.061 &= \frac{\text{Rate of change}}{13.84} \\
\text{Rate of change in April 2009} &= -0.061 \cdot 13.84 = -0.84424 \text{ trillion dollars per year.}
\end{aligned}$$

The GDP of the US was decreasing at a rate of 844.24 billion dollars per year in April 2009.

Problems for Section 2.3

In Problems 1–4, write the Leibniz notation for the derivative of the given function and include units.

1. The cost, C, of a steak, in dollars, is a function of the weight, W, of the steak, in pounds.

2. The distance to the ground, D, in feet, of a skydiver is a function of the time t in minutes since the skydiver jumped out of the airplane.

3. An employee's pay, P, in dollars, for a week is a function of the number of hours worked, H.

4. The number, N, of gallons of gas left in a gas tank is a function of the distance, D, in miles, the car has been driven.

5. The cost, $C = f(w)$, in dollars of buying a chemical is a function of the weight bought, w, in pounds.

   (a) In the statement $f(12) = 5$, what are the units of the 12? What are the units of the 5? Explain what this is saying about the cost of buying the chemical.

   (b) Do you expect the derivative f' to be positive or negative? Why?

   (c) In the statement $f'(12) = 0.4$, what are the units of the 12? What are the units of the 0.4? Explain what this is saying about the cost of buying the chemical.

6. The time for a chemical reaction, T (in minutes), is a function of the amount of catalyst present, a (in milliliters), so $T = f(a)$.

   (a) If $f(5) = 18$, what are the units of 5? What are the units of 18? What does this statement tell us about the reaction?

   (b) If $f'(5) = -3$, what are the units of 5? What are the units of -3? What does this statement tell us?

7. An economist is interested in how the price of a certain item affects its sales. At a price of \$$p$, a quantity, q, of the item is sold. If $q = f(p)$, explain the meaning of each of the following statements:

   (a) $f(150) = 2000$ **(b)** $f'(150) = -25$

8. Figure 2.27 shows the length, L, in cm, of a sturgeon (a type of fish) as a function of the time, t, in years.[8] Estimate $f'(10)$. Give units and interpret your answer.

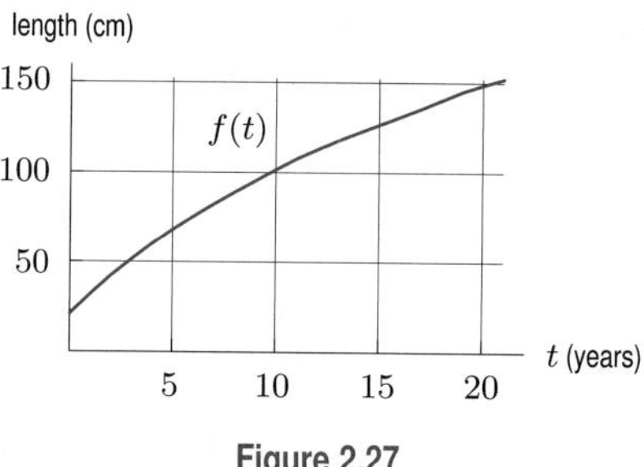

Figure 2.27

9. The temperature, T, in degrees Fahrenheit, of a cold yam placed in a hot oven is given by $T = f(t)$, where t is the time in minutes since the yam was put in the oven.

(a) What is the sign of $f'(t)$? Why?
(b) What are the units of $f'(20)$? What is the practical meaning of the statement $f'(20) = 2$?

10. On May 9, 2007, CBS Evening News had a 4.3 point rating. (Ratings measure the number of viewers.) News executives estimated that a 0.1 drop in the ratings for the CBS Evening News corresponds to a \$5.5 million drop in revenue.[9] Express this information as a derivative. Specify the function, the variables, the units, and the point at which the derivative is evaluated.

11. When you breathe, a muscle (called the diaphragm) reduces the pressure around your lungs and they expand to fill with air. The table shows the volume of a lung as a function of the reduction in pressure from the diaphragm. Pulmonologists (lung doctors) define the *compliance* of the lung as the derivative of this function.[10]

(a) What are the units of compliance?
(b) Estimate the maximum compliance of the lung.
(c) Explain why the compliance gets small when the lung is nearly full (around 1 liter).

Pressure reduction (cm of water)	Volume (liters)
0	0.20
5	0.29
10	0.49
15	0.70
20	0.86
25	0.95
30	1.00

12. Meteorologists define the temperature lapse rate to be $-dT/dz$ where T is the air temperature in Celsius at altitude z kilometers above the ground.

(a) What are the units of the lapse rate?
(b) What is the practical meaning of a lapse rate of 6.5?

13. Investing \$1000 at an annual interest rate of $r\%$, compounded continuously, for 10 years gives you a balance of $\$B$, where $B = g(r)$. Give a financial interpretation of the statements:

(a) $g(5) \approx 1649$.
(b) $g'(5) \approx 165$. What are the units of $g'(5)$?

14. Let $f(x)$ be the elevation in feet of the Mississippi River x miles from its source. What are the units of $f'(x)$? What can you say about the sign of $f'(x)$?

15. The average weight, W, in pounds, of an adult is a function, $W = f(c)$, of the average number of Calories per day, c, consumed.

(a) Interpret the statements $f(1800) = 155$ and $f'(2000) = 0$ in terms of diet and weight.
(b) What are the units of $f'(c) = dW/dc$?

16. The cost, C (in dollars), to produce g gallons of a chemical can be expressed as $C = f(g)$. Using units, explain the meaning of the following statements in terms of the chemical:

(a) $f(200) = 1300$ **(b)** $f'(200) = 6$

17. The weight, W, in lbs, of a child is a function of its age, a, in years, so $W = f(a)$.

(a) Do you expect $f'(a)$ to be positive or negative? Why?
(b) What does $f(8) = 45$ tell you? Give units for the numbers 8 and 45.
(c) What are the units of $f'(a)$? Explain what $f'(a)$ tells you in terms of age and weight.
(d) What does $f'(8) = 4$ tell you about age and weight?
(e) As a increases, do you expect $f'(a)$ to increase or decrease? Explain.

18. Let G be annual US government purchases, T be annual US tax revenues, and Y be annual US output of all goods and services. All three quantities are given in dollars. Interpret the statements about the two derivatives, called fiscal policy multipliers.

(a) $dY/dG = 0.60$ **(b)** $dY/dT = -0.26$

19. A recent study reports that men who retired late developed Alzheimer's at a later stage than those who stopped work earlier. Each additional year of employment was associated with about a six-week later age of onset. Express these results as a statement about the derivative of a function. State clearly what function you use, including the units of the dependent and independent variables.

[8] Data from von Bertalanffy, L., *General System Theory*, p. 177 (New York: Braziller, 1968).
[9] OC Register, May 9, 2007; *The New York Times*, May 14, 2007.
[10] Adapted from John B. West, *Respiratory Physiology*, 4th Ed. (New York: Williams and Wilkins, 1990).

20. The thickness, P, in mm, of pelican eggshells depends on the concentration, c, of PCBs in the eggshell, measured in ppm (parts per million); that is, $P = f(c)$.

(a) The derivative $f'(c)$ is negative. What does this tell you?
(b) Give units and interpret $f(200) = 0.28$ and $f'(200) = -0.0005$ in terms of PCBs and eggs.

Problems 21–24 concern $g(t)$ in Figure 2.28, which gives the weight of a human fetus as a function of its age.

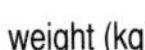

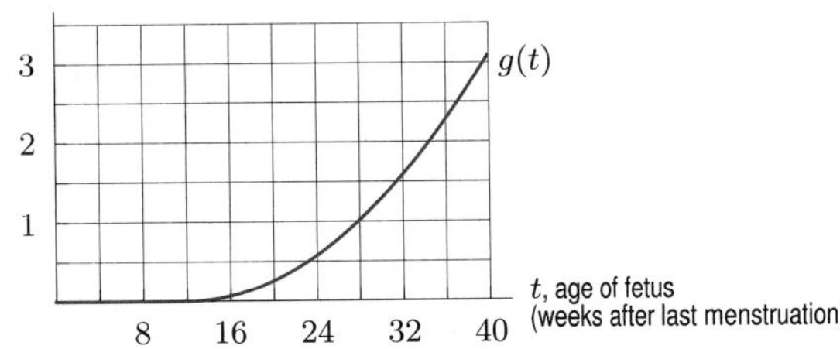

Figure 2.28

21. **(a)** What are the units of $g'(24)$?
(b) What is the biological meaning of $g'(24) = 0.096$?

22. **(a)** Which is greater, $g'(20)$ or $g'(36)$?
(b) What does your answer say about fetal growth?

23. Is the instantaneous weight growth rate greater or less than the average rate of change of weight over the 40-week period

(a) At week 20? **(b)** At week 36?

24. Estimate **(a)** $g'(20)$ **(b)** $g'(36)$
(c) The average rate of change of weight for the entire 40-week gestation.

25. Suppose that $f(t)$ is a function with $f(25) = 3.6$ and $f'(25) = -0.2$. Estimate $f(26)$ and $f(30)$.

26. Suppose that $f(x)$ is a function with $f(20) = 345$ and $f'(20) = 6$. Estimate $f(22)$.

27. Annual net sales, in billion of dollars, for the Hershey Company, the largest US producer of chocolate, is a function $S = f(t)$ of time, t, in years since 2000.

(a) Interpret the statements $f(8) = 5.1$ and $f'(8) = 0.22$ in terms of Hershey sales.[11]
(b) Estimate $f(12)$ and interpret it in terms of Hershey sales.

28. World meat[12] production, $M = f(t)$, in millions of metric tons, is a function of t, years since 2000.

(a) Interpret $f(5) = 249$ and $f'(5) = 6.5$ in terms of meat production.
(b) Estimate $f(10)$ and interpret it in terms of meat production.

29. For some painkillers, the size of the dose, D, given depends on the weight of the patient, W. Thus, $D = f(W)$, where D is in milligrams and W is in pounds.

(a) Interpret the statements $f(140) = 120$ and $f'(140) = 3$ in terms of this painkiller.
(b) Use the information in the statements in part (a) to estimate $f(145)$.

30. The quantity, Q mg, of nicotine in the body t minutes after a cigarette is smoked is given by $Q = f(t)$.

(a) Interpret the statements $f(20) = 0.36$ and $f'(20) = -0.002$ in terms of nicotine. What are the units of the numbers 20, 0.36, and -0.002?
(b) Use the information given in part (a) to estimate $f(21)$ and $f(30)$. Justify your answers.

31. A mutual fund is currently valued at \$80 per share and its value per share is increasing at a rate of \$0.50 a day. Let $V = f(t)$ be the value of the share t days from now.

(a) Express the information given about the mutual fund in term of f and f'.
(b) Assuming that the rate of growth stays constant, estimate and interpret $f(10)$.

32. Figure 2.29 shows how the contraction velocity, $v(x)$, of a muscle changes as the load on it changes.

(a) Find the slope of the line tangent to the graph of contraction velocity at a load of 2 kg. Give units.
(b) Using your answer to part (a), estimate the change in the contraction velocity if the load is increased from 2 kg by adding 50 grams.
(c) Express your answer to part (a) as a derivative of $v(x)$.

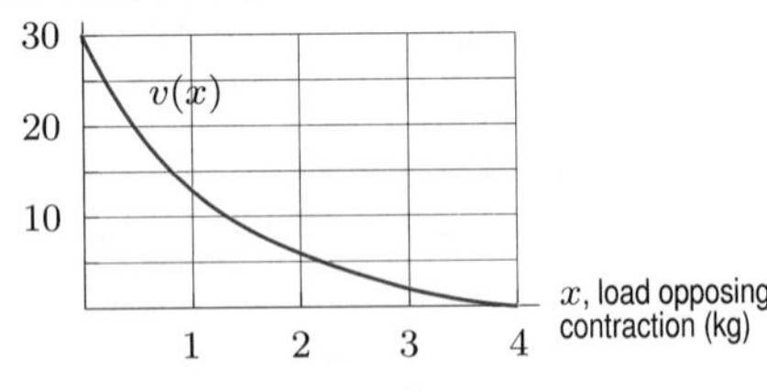

Figure 2.29

[11] 2008 Annual Report to Stockholders, accessed at www.thehersheycompany.com.
[12] *FAO Statistical Yearbook 2007–2008*, Food and Agriculture Organization of the United Nations, http://www.fao.org/economic/ess/publications-studies/statistical-yearbook/fao-statistical-yearbook-2007-2008.

33. Figure 2.30 shows how the pumping rate of a person's heart changes after bleeding.

(a) Find the slope of the line tangent to the graph at time 2 hours. Give units.
(b) Using your answer to part (a), estimate how much the pumping rate increases during the minute beginning at time 2 hours.
(c) Express your answer to part (a) as a derivative of $g(t)$.

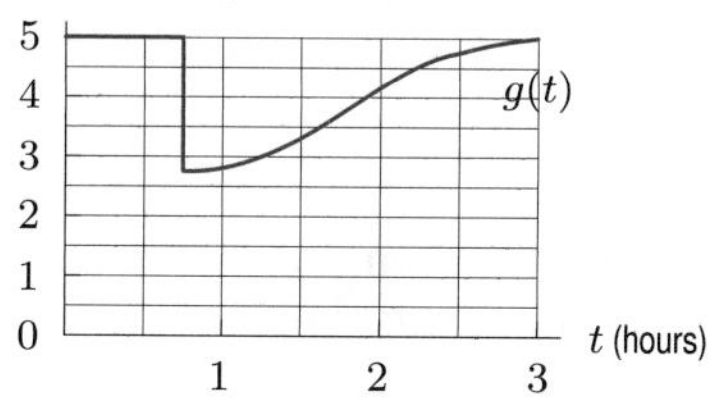

Figure 2.30

34. Suppose $C(r)$ is the total cost of paying off a car loan borrowed at an annual interest rate of $r\%$. What are the units of $C'(r)$? What is the practical meaning of $C'(r)$? What is its sign?

35. A company's revenue from car sales, C (in thousands of dollars), is a function of advertising expenditure, a, in thousands of dollars, so $C = f(a)$.

(a) What does the company hope is true about the sign of f'?
(b) What does the statement $f'(100) = 2$ mean in practical terms? How about $f'(100) = 0.5$?
(c) Suppose the company plans to spend about \$100,000 on advertising. If $f'(100) = 2$, should the company spend more or less than \$100,000 on advertising? What if $f'(100) = 0.5$?

36. A person with a certain liver disease first exhibits larger and larger concentrations of certain enzymes (called SGOT and SGPT) in the blood. As the disease progresses, the concentration of these enzymes drops, first to the predisease level and eventually to zero (when almost all of the liver cells have died). Monitoring the levels of these enzymes allows doctors to track the progress of a patient with this disease. If $C = f(t)$ is the concentration of the enzymes in the blood as a function of time,

(a) Sketch a possible graph of $C = f(t)$.
(b) Mark on the graph the intervals where $f' > 0$ and where $f' < 0$.
(c) What does $f'(t)$ represent, in practical terms?

Problems 37–41 refer to Figure 2.31, which shows the depletion of food stores in the human body during starvation.

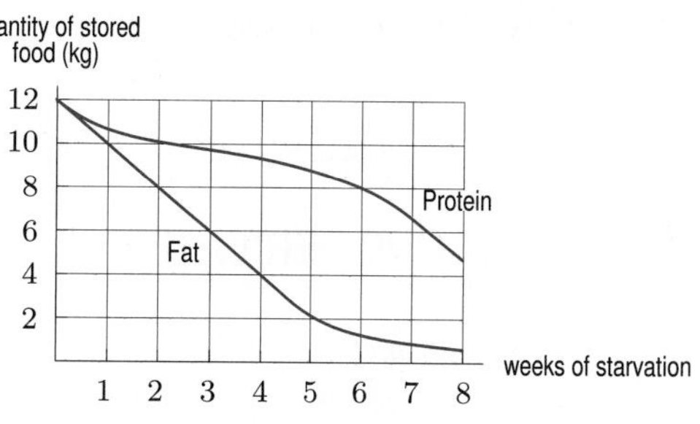

Figure 2.31

37. Which is being consumed at a greater rate, fat or protein, during the

(a) Third week? **(b)** Seventh week?

38. The fat storage graph is linear for the first four weeks. What does this tell you about the use of stored fat?

39. Estimate the rate of fat consumption after

(a) 3 weeks **(b)** 6 weeks **(c)** 8 weeks

40. What seems to happen during the sixth week? Why do you think this happens?

41. Figure 2.32 shows the derivatives of the protein and fat storage functions. Which graph is which?

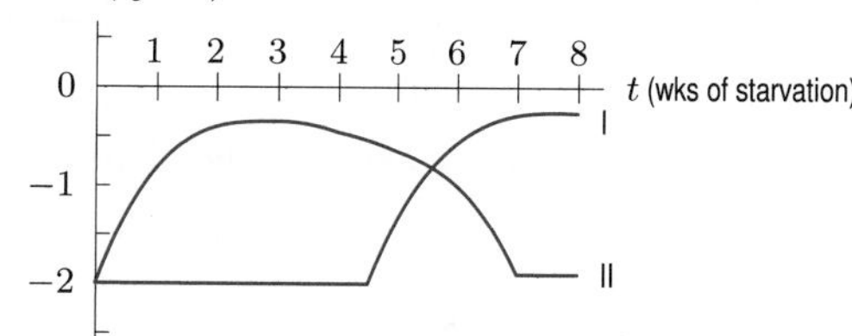

Figure 2.32

42. The area of Brazil's rain forest, $R = f(t)$, in million acres, is a function of the number of years, t, since 2000.

(a) Interpret $f(9) = 740$ and $f'(9) = -2.7$ in terms of Brazil's rain forests.[13]
(b) Find and interpret the relative rate of change of $f(t)$ when $t = 9$.

43. The number of active Facebook users hit 175 million at the end of February 2009 and 200 million[14] at the end of April 2009. With t in months since the start of 2009, let $f(t)$ be the number of active users in millions. Estimate $f(4)$ and $f'(4)$ and the relative rate of change of f at $t = 4$. Interpret your answers in terms of Facebook users.

44. The weight, w, in kilograms, of a baby is a function $f(t)$ of her age, t, in months.

(a) What does $f(2.5) = 5.67$ tell you?
(b) What does $f'(2.5)/f(2.5) = 0.13$ tell you?

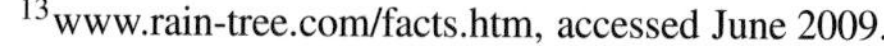

[13] www.rain-tree.com/facts.htm, accessed June 2009.
[14] www.facebook.com/press, accessed June 2009.

45. Estimate the relative rate of change of $f(t) = t^2$ at $t = 4$. Use $\Delta t = 0.01$.

46. The population, P, of a city (in thousands) at time t (in years) is $P = 700e^{0.035t}$. Estimate the relative rate of change of the population at $t = 3$ using

(a) $\Delta t = 1$ **(b)** $\Delta t = 0.1$ **(c)** $\Delta t = 0.01$

2.4 THE SECOND DERIVATIVE

glabelsec:2second-derivative

Since the derivative is itself a function, we can calculate its derivative. For a function f, the derivative of its derivative is called the *second derivative*, and written f''. If $y = f(x)$, the second derivative can also be written as $\frac{d^2y}{dx^2}$, which means $\frac{d}{dx}\left(\frac{dy}{dx}\right)$, the derivative of $\frac{dy}{dx}$.

What Does the Second Derivative Tell Us?

Recall that the derivative of a function tells us whether the function is increasing or decreasing:

If $f' > 0$ on an interval, then f is increasing over that interval.
If $f' < 0$ on an interval, then f is decreasing over that interval.

Since f'' is the derivative of f', we have

If $f'' > 0$ on an interval, then f' is increasing over that interval.
If $f'' < 0$ on an interval, then f' is decreasing over that interval.

So the question becomes: What does it mean for f' to be increasing or decreasing? The case in which f' is increasing is shown in Figure 2.33, where the graph of f is bending upward, or is *concave up*. In the case when f' is decreasing, shown in Figure 2.34, the graph is bending downward, or is *concave down*.

> $f'' > 0$ on an interval means f' is increasing, so the graph of f is concave up there.
> $f'' < 0$ on an interval means f' is decreasing, so the graph of f is concave down there.

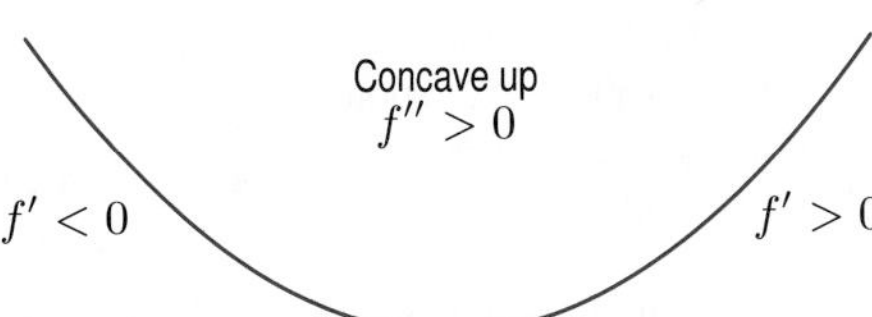

Figure 2.33: Meaning of f'': The slope increases from negative to positive as you move from left to right, so f'' is positive and f is concave up

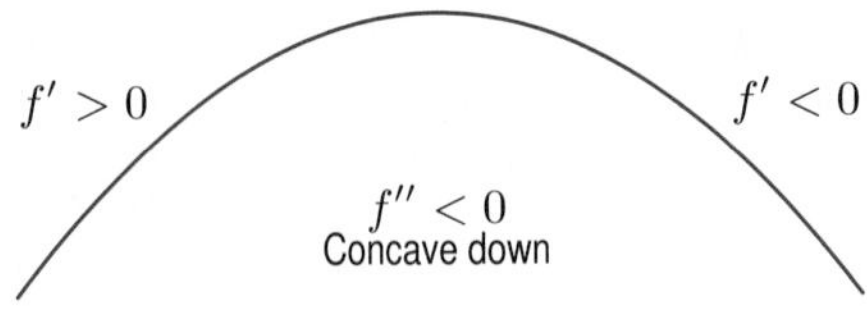

Figure 2.34: Meaning of f'': The slope decreases from positive to negative as you move from left to right, so f'' is negative and f is concave down

---

Example 1 For the functions whose graphs are given in Figure 2.35, decide where their second derivatives are positive and where they are negative.

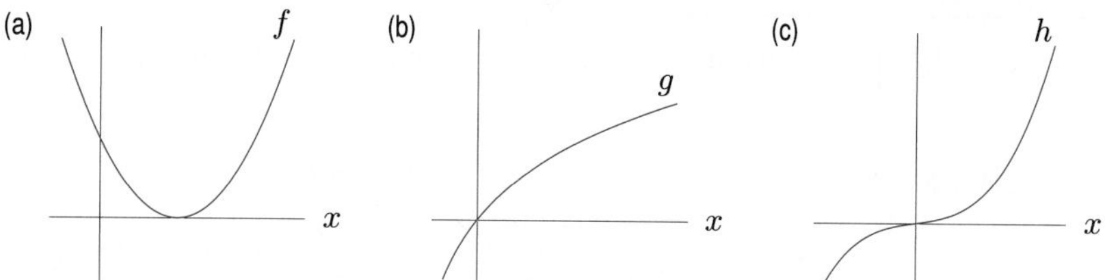

Figure 2.35: What signs do the second derivatives have?

Solution From the graphs it appears that

(a) $f'' > 0$ everywhere, because the graph of f is concave up everywhere.
(b) $g'' < 0$ everywhere, because the graph is concave down everywhere.
(c) $h'' > 0$ for $x > 0$, because the graph of h is concave up there; $h'' < 0$ for $x < 0$, because the graph of h is concave down there.

Interpretation of the Second Derivative as a Rate of Change

If we think of the derivative as a rate of change, then the second derivative is a rate of change of a rate of change. If the second derivative is positive, the rate of change is increasing; if the second derivative is negative, the rate of change is decreasing.

The second derivative is often a matter of practical concern. In 1985 a newspaper headline reported the Secretary of Defense as saying that Congress and the Senate had cut the defense budget. As his opponents pointed out, however, Congress had merely cut the rate at which the defense budget was increasing.[15] In other words, the derivative of the defense budget was still positive (the budget was increasing), but the second derivative was negative (the budget's rate of increase had slowed).

Example 2 A population, P, growing in a confined environment often follows a *logistic* growth curve, like the graph shown in Figure 2.36. Describe how the rate at which the population is increasing changes over time. What is the sign of the second derivative d^2P/dt^2? What is the practical interpretation of t^* and L?

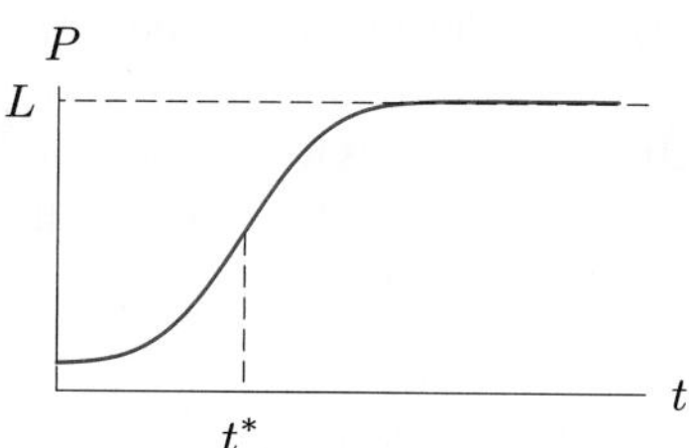

Figure 2.36: Logistic growth curve

Solution Initially, the population is increasing, and at an increasing rate. So, initially dP/dt is increasing and $d^2P/dt^2 > 0$. At t^*, the rate at which the population is increasing is a maximum; the population is growing fastest then. Beyond t^*, the rate at which the population is growing is decreasing, so $d^2P/dt^2 < 0$. At t^*, the graph changes from concave up to concave down and $d^2P/dt^2 = 0$.

The quantity L represents the limiting value of the population that is approached as t tends to infinity; L is called the *carrying capacity* of the environment and represents the maximum population that the environment can support.

[15] In the *Boston Globe*, March 13, 1985, Representative William Gray (D–Pa.) was reported as saying: "It's confusing to the American people to imply that Congress threatens national security with reductions when you're really talking about a reduction in the increase."

Example 3 Table 2.8 shows the number of abortions per year, A, reported in the US[16] in the year t.

Table 2.8 *Abortions reported in the US (1972–2000)*

Year, t	1972	1975	1980	1985	1990	1995	2000	2005
1000s of abortions reported, A	587	1034	1554	1589	1609	1359	1313	1206

(a) Calculate the average rate of change for the time intervals shown between 1972 and 2005.
(b) What can you say about the sign of d^2A/dt^2 during the period 1972–1995?

Solution (a) For each time interval we can calculate the average rate of change of the number of abortions per year over this interval. For example, between 1972 and 1975

$$\text{Average rate of change} = \frac{\Delta A}{\Delta t} = \frac{1034 - 587}{1975 - 1972} = \frac{447}{3} = 149.$$

Thus, between 1972 and 1975, there were approximately 149,000 more abortions reported each year. Values of $\Delta A/\Delta t$ are listed in Table 2.9.

Table 2.9 *Rate of change of number of abortions reported*

Time	1972–75	1975–80	1980–85	1985–90	1990–95	1995–2000	2000–05
Average rate of change, $\Delta A/\Delta t$ (1000s/year)	149	104	7	4	-50	-9.2	-21.4

(b) We assume the data lies on a smooth curve. Since the values of $\Delta A/\Delta t$ are decreasing dramatically for 1975–1995, we can be pretty certain that dA/dt also decreases, so d^2A/dt^2 is negative for this period. For 1972–1975, the sign of d^2A/dt^2 is less clear; abortion data from 1968 would help. Figure 2.37 confirms this; the graph appears to be concave down for 1975–1995. The fact that dA/dt is positive during the period 1972–1980 corresponds to the fact that the number of abortions reported increased from 1972 to 1980. The fact that dA/dt is negative during the period 1990–2005 corresponds to the fact that the number of abortions reported decreased from 1990 to 2005. The fact that d^2A/dt^2 is negative for 1975–1995 reflects the fact that the rate of increase slowed over this period.

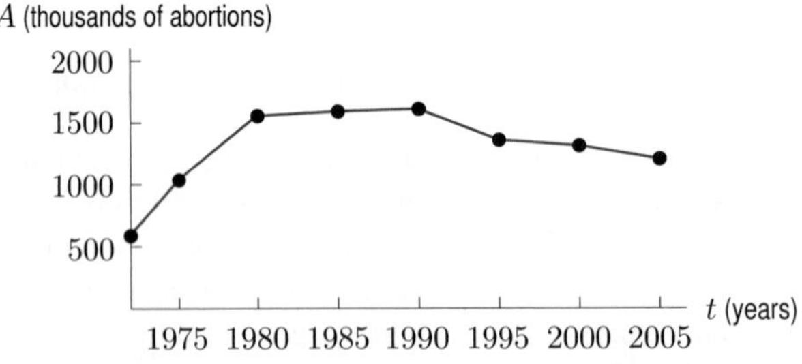

Figure 2.37: How the number of reported abortions in the US is changing with time

[16] *Statistical Abstracts of the United States 2004–2009*, Table 99.

Problems for Section 2.4

1. For the function graphed in Figure 2.38, are the following nonzero quantities positive or negative?

(a) $f(2)$ **(b)** $f'(2)$ **(c)** $f''(2)$

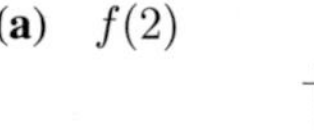
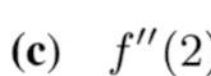

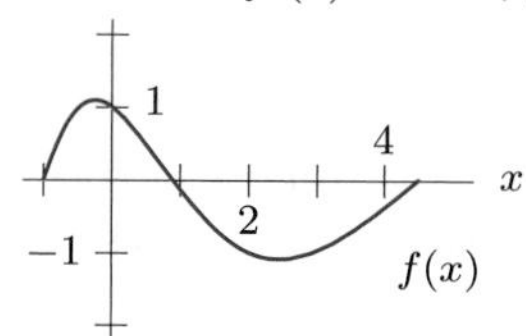

Figure 2.38

2. At one of the labeled points on the graph in Figure 2.39 both dy/dx and d^2y/dx^2 are positive. Which is it?

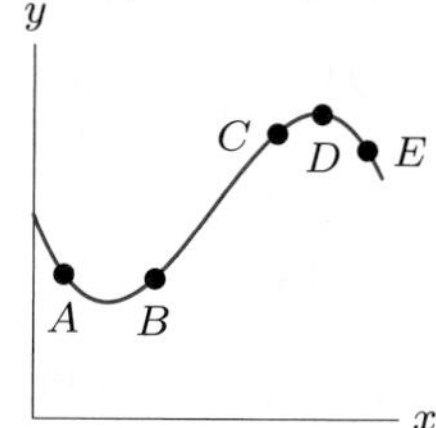

Figure 2.39

For Problems 3–8, give the signs of the first and second derivatives for the following functions. Each derivative is either positive everywhere, zero everywhere, or negative everywhere.

3.

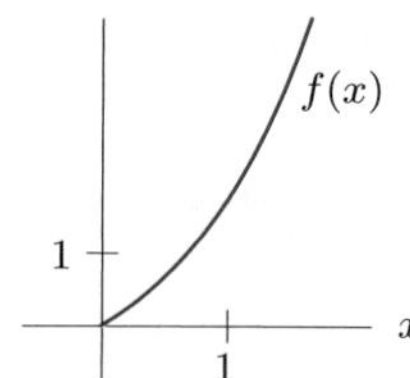

4.

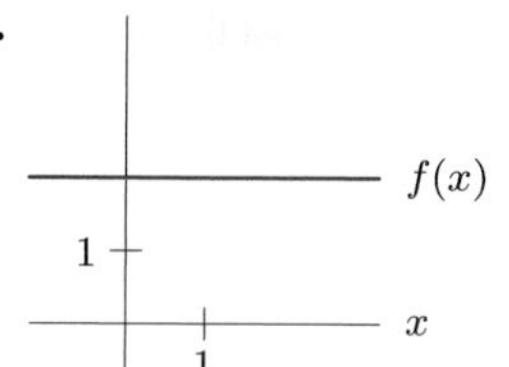

5.

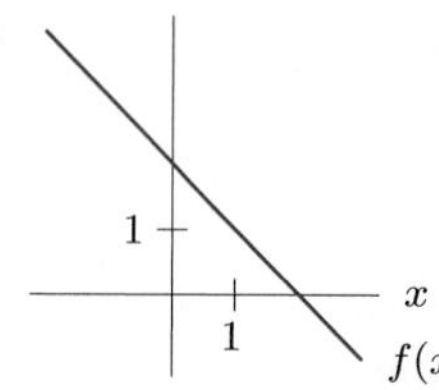

6.

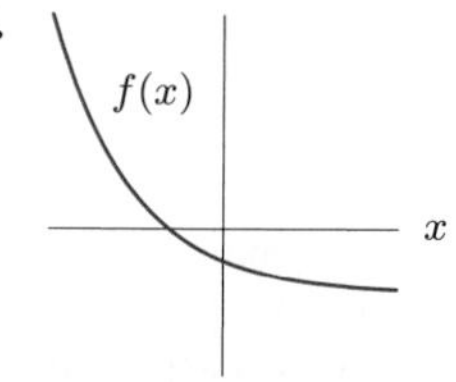

7.

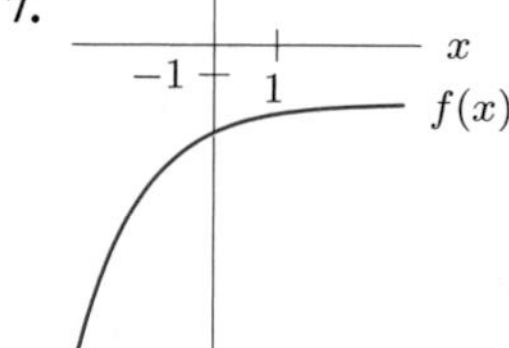

8.

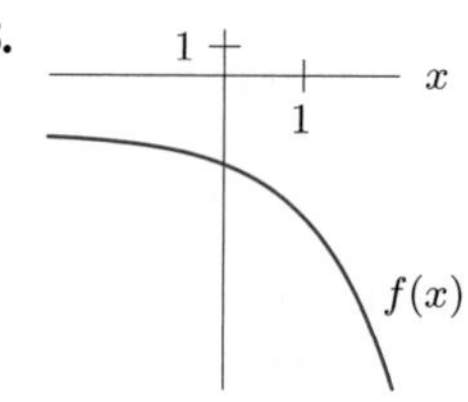

9. Graph the functions described in parts (a)–(d).

(a) First and second derivatives everywhere positive.
(b) Second derivative everywhere negative; first derivative everywhere positive.
(c) Second derivative everywhere positive; first derivative everywhere negative.
(d) First and second derivatives everywhere negative.

In Problems 10–11, use the values given for each function.

(a) Does the derivative of the function appear to be positive or negative over the given interval? Explain.
(b) Does the second derivative of the function appear to be positive or negative over the given interval? Explain.

10.

t	100	110	120	130	140
$w(t)$	10.7	6.3	4.2	3.5	3.3

11.

t	0	1	2	3	4	5
$s(t)$	12	14	17	20	31	55

12. Sketch the graph of a function whose first derivative is everywhere negative and whose second derivative is positive for some x-values and negative for other x-values.

13. IBM-Peru uses second derivatives to assess the relative success of various advertising campaigns. They assume that all campaigns produce some increase in sales. If a graph of sales against time shows a positive second derivative during a new advertising campaign, what does this suggest to IBM management? Why? What does a negative second derivative suggest?

14. Values of $f(t)$ are given in the following table.

(a) Does this function appear to have a positive or negative first derivative? Second derivative? Explain.
(b) Estimate $f'(2)$ and $f'(8)$.

t	0	2	4	6	8	10
$f(t)$	150	145	137	122	98	56

15. The table gives the number of passenger cars, $C = f(t)$, in millions,[17] in the US in the year t.

(a) Do $f'(t)$ and $f''(t)$ appear to be positive or negative during the period 1940–1980?
(b) Estimate $f'(1975)$. Using units, interpret your answer in terms of passenger cars.

t	1940	1950	1960	1970	1980	1990	2000
C	27.5	40.3	61.7	89.2	121.6	133.7	133.6

[17] www.bts.gov/publications/national_transportation_statistics/html/table_01_11.html. Accessed June 22, 2008.

In Problems 16–17, use the graph given for each function.

(a) Estimate the intervals on which the derivative is positive and the intervals on which the derivative is negative.

(b) Estimate the intervals on which the second derivative is positive and the intervals on which the second derivative is negative.

16.

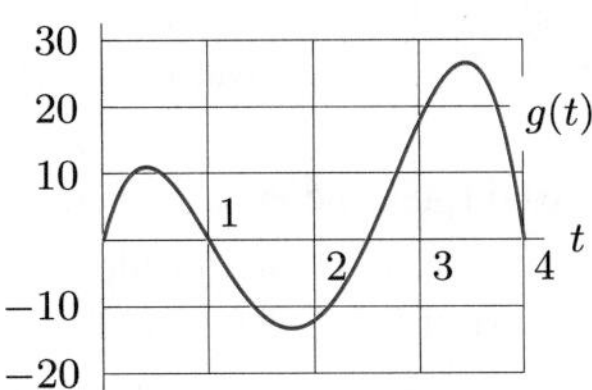

17.

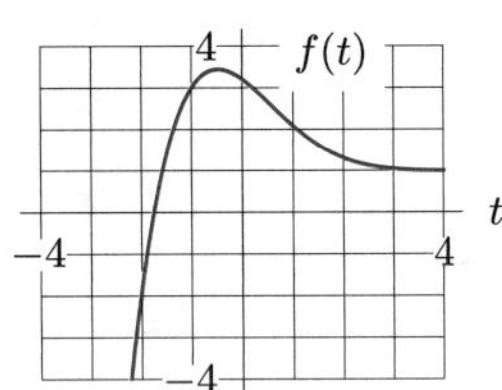

18. Sketch a graph of a continuous function f with the following properties:

- $f'(x) > 0$ for all x
- $f''(x) < 0$ for $x < 2$ and $f''(x) > 0$ for $x > 2$.

19. At exactly two of the labeled points in Figure 2.40, the derivative f' is 0; the second derivative f'' is not zero at any of the labeled points. On a copy of the table, give the signs of f, f', f'' at each marked point.

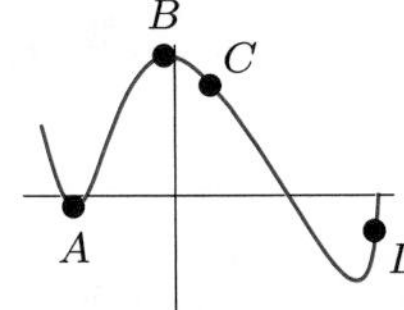

Point	f	f'	f''
A			
B			
C			
D			

Figure 2.40

20. For three minutes the temperature of a feverish person has had positive first derivative and negative second derivative. Which of the following is correct?

(a) The temperature rose in the last minute more than it rose in the minute before.
(b) The temperature rose in the last minute, but less than it rose in the minute before.
(c) The temperature fell in the last minute but less than it fell in the minute before.
(d) The temperature rose two minutes ago but fell in the last minute.

21. Yesterday's temperature at t hours past midnight was $f(t)$ °C. At noon the temperature was 20°C. The first derivative, $f'(t)$, decreased all morning, reaching a low of 2°C/hour at noon, then increased for the rest of the day. Which one of the following must be correct?

(a) The temperature fell in the morning and rose in the afternoon.
(b) At 1 pm the temperature was 18°C.
(c) At 1 pm the temperature was 22°C.
(d) The temperature was lower at noon than at any other time.
(e) The temperature rose all day.

22. Sketch the graph of a function f such that $f(2) = 5$, $f'(2) = 1/2$, and $f''(2) > 0$.

23. A function f has $f(5) = 20$, $f'(5) = 2$, and $f''(x) < 0$, for $x \geq 5$. Which of the following are possible values for $f(7)$ and which are impossible?

(a) 26 **(b)** 24 **(c)** 22

24. An industry is being charged by the Environmental Protection Agency (EPA) with dumping unacceptable levels of toxic pollutants in a lake. Over a period of several months, an engineering firm makes daily measurements of the rate at which pollutants are being discharged into the lake. The engineers produce a graph similar to either Figure 2.41(a) or Figure 2.41(b). For each case, give an idea of what argument the EPA might make in court against the industry and of the industry's defense.

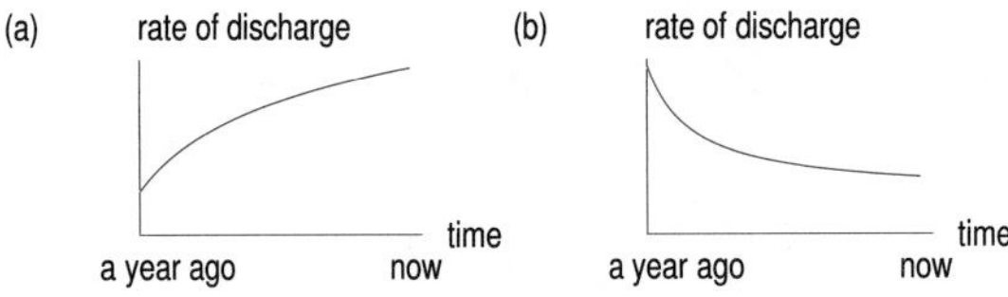

Figure 2.41

25. "Winning the war on poverty" has been described cynically as slowing the rate at which people are slipping below the poverty line. Assuming that this is happening:

(a) Graph the total number of people in poverty against time.
(b) If N is the number of people below the poverty line at time t, what are the signs of dN/dt and d^2N/dt^2? Explain.

26. Let $P(t)$ represent the price of a share of stock of a corporation at time t. What does each of the following statements tell us about the signs of the first and second derivatives of $P(t)$?

(a) "The price of the stock is rising faster and faster."
(b) "The price of the stock is close to bottoming out."

27. In economics, *total utility* refers to the total satisfaction from consuming some commodity. According to the economist Samuelson:[18]

> As you consume more of the same good, the total (psychological) utility increases. However, ...with successive new units of the good, your total utility will grow at a slower and slower rate because of a fundamental tendency for your psychological ability to appreciate more of the good to become less keen.

(a) Sketch the total utility as a function of the number of units consumed.
(b) In terms of derivatives, what is Samuelson saying?

28. Each of the graphs in Figure 2.42 shows the position of a particle moving along the x-axis as a function of time, $0 \le t \le 5$. The vertical scales of the graphs are the same. During this time interval, which particle has

(a) Constant velocity?
(b) The greatest initial velocity?
(c) The greatest average velocity?
(d) Zero average velocity?
(e) Zero acceleration?
(f) Positive acceleration throughout?

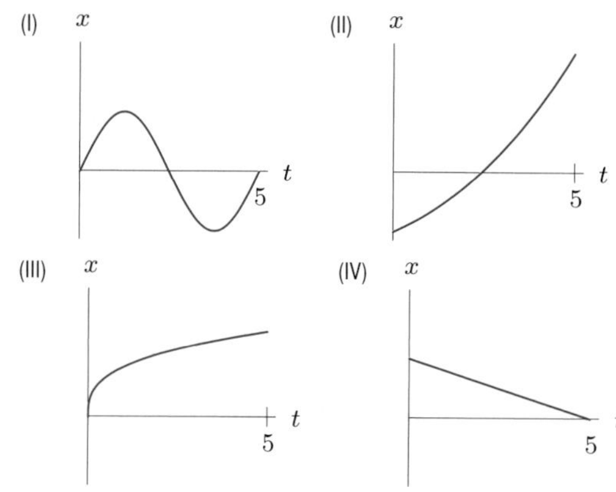

Figure 2.42

2.5 MARGINAL COST AND REVENUE

Management decisions within a particular firm or industry usually depend on the costs and revenues involved. In this section we look at the cost and revenue functions.

Graphs of Cost and Revenue Functions

The graph of a cost function may be linear, as in Figure 2.43, or it may have the shape shown in Figure 2.44. The intercept on the C-axis represents the fixed costs, which are incurred even if nothing is produced. (This includes, for instance, the cost of the machinery needed to begin production.) In Figure 2.44, the cost function increases quickly at first and then more slowly because producing larger quantities of a good is usually more efficient than producing smaller quantities—this is called *economy of scale*. At still higher production levels, the cost function increases faster again as resources become scarce; sharp increases may occur when new factories have to be built. Thus, the graph of a cost function, C, may start out concave down and become concave up later on.

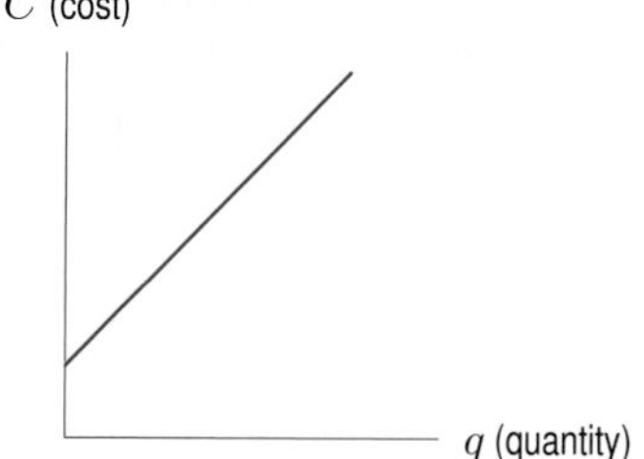

Figure 2.43: A linear cost function

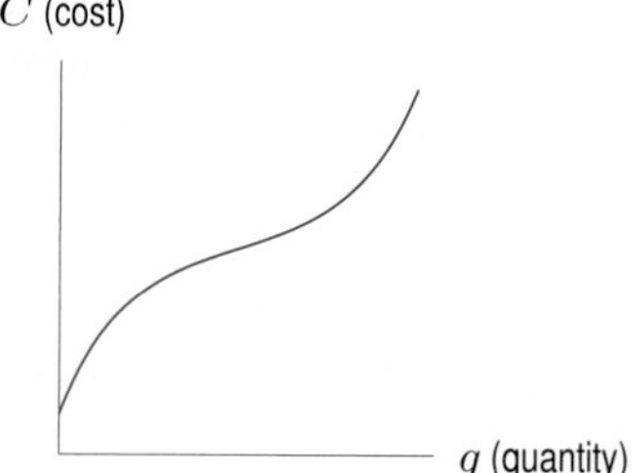

Figure 2.44: A nonlinear cost function

The revenue function is $R = pq$, where p is price and q is quantity. If the price, p, is a constant, the graph of R against q is a straight line through the origin with slope equal to the price. (See

[18]From Paul A. Samuelson, *Economics*, 11th edition (New York: McGraw-Hill, 1981).

Figure 2.45.) In practice, for large values of q, the market may become glutted, causing the price to drop and giving R the shape in Figure 2.46.

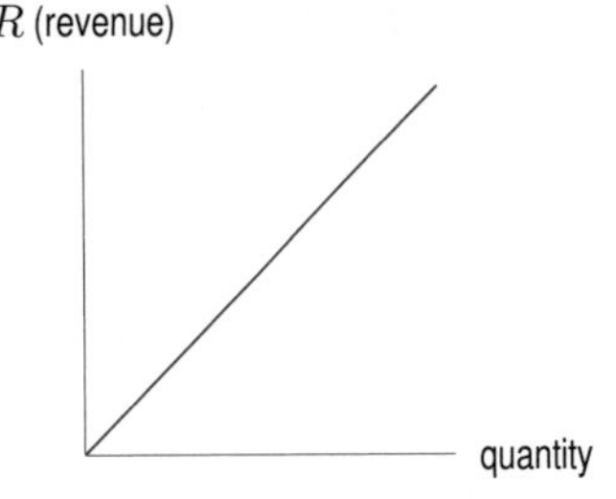

Figure 2.45: Revenue: Constant price

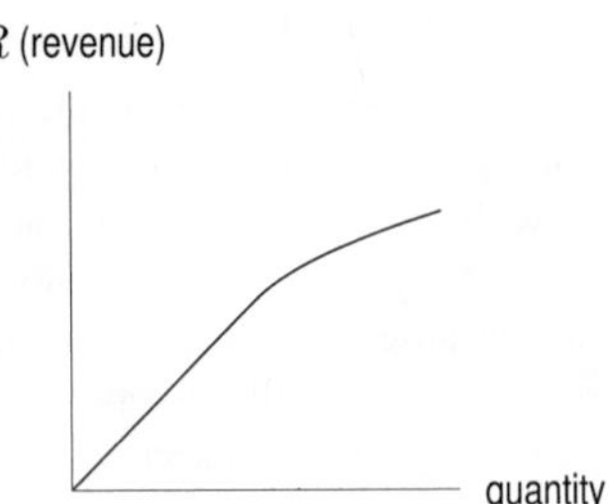

Figure 2.46: Revenue: Decreasing price

Example 1 If cost, C, and revenue, R, are given by the graph in Figure 2.47, for what production quantities does the firm make a profit?

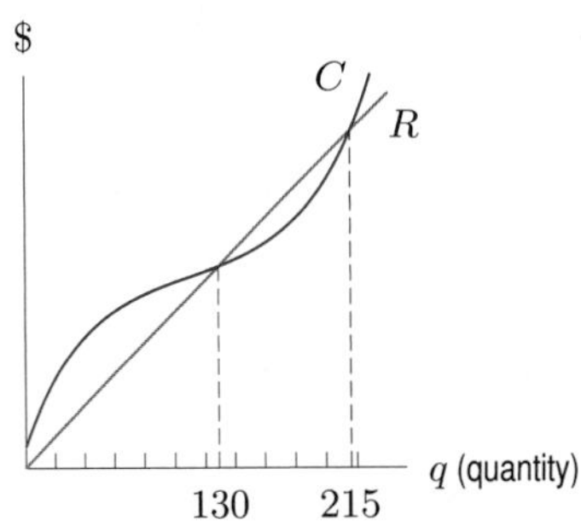

Figure 2.47: Costs and revenues for Example 1

Solution The firm makes a profit whenever revenues are greater than costs, that is, when $R > C$. The graph of R is above the graph of C approximately when $130 < q < 215$. Production between 130 units and 215 units will generate a profit.

Marginal Analysis

Many economic decisions are based on an analysis of the costs and revenues "at the margin." Let's look at this idea through an example.

Suppose you are running an airline and you are trying to decide whether to offer an additional flight. How should you decide? We'll assume that the decision is to be made purely on financial grounds: if the flight will make money for the company, it should be added. Obviously you need to consider the costs and revenues involved. Since the choice is between adding this flight and leaving things the way they are, the crucial question is whether the *additional costs* incurred are greater or smaller than the *additional revenues* generated by the flight. These additional costs and revenues are called *marginal costs* and *marginal revenues*.

Suppose $C(q)$ is the function giving the cost of running q flights. If the airline had originally planned to run 100 flights, its costs would be $C(100)$. With the additional flight, its costs would be $C(101)$. Therefore,

$$\text{Additional cost "at the margin"} = C(101) - C(100).$$

Now

$$C(101) - C(100) = \frac{C(101) - C(100)}{101 - 100},$$

and this quantity is the average rate of change of cost between 100 and 101 flights. In Figure 2.48 the average rate of change is the slope of the secant line. If the graph of the cost function is not curving too fast near the point, the slope of the secant line is close to the slope of the tangent line

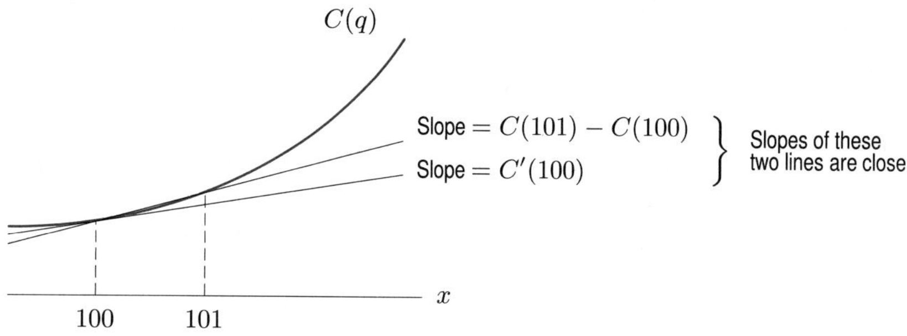

Figure 2.48: Marginal cost: Slope of one of these lines

there. Therefore, the average rate of change is close to the instantaneous rate of change. Since these rates of change are not very different, many economists choose to define marginal cost, MC, as the instantaneous rate of change of cost with respect to quantity:

> Marginal cost $= MC = C'(q)$ so Marginal cost $\approx C(q+1) - C(q)$.

Marginal cost is represented by the slope of the cost curve.

Similarly if the revenue generated by q flights is $R(q)$ and the number of flights increases from 100 to 101, then

$$\text{Additional revenue “at the margin”} = R(101) - R(100).$$

Now $R(101) - R(100)$ is the average rate of change of revenue between 100 and 101 flights. As before, the average rate of change is approximately equal to the instantaneous rate of change, so economists often define

> Marginal revenue $= MR = R'(q)$ so Marginal revenue $\approx R(q+1) - R(q)$.

Example 2 If $C(q)$ and $R(q)$ for the airline are given in Figure 2.49, should the company add the 101st flight?

Solution The marginal revenue is the slope of the revenue curve at $q = 100$. The marginal cost is the slope of the graph of C at $q = 100$. Figure 2.49 suggests that the slope at point A is smaller than the slope at B, so $MC < MR$ for $q = 100$. This means that the airline will make more in extra revenue than it will spend in extra costs if it runs another flight, so it should go ahead and run the 101st flight.

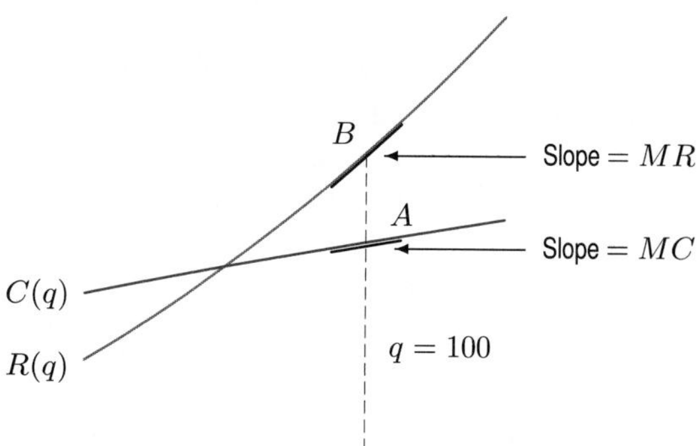

Figure 2.49: Cost and revenue for Example 2

Example 3 The graph of a cost function is given in Figure 2.50. Does it cost more to produce the 500th item or the 2000th? Does it cost more to produce the 3000th item or the 4000th? At approximately what production level is marginal cost smallest? What is the total cost at this production level?

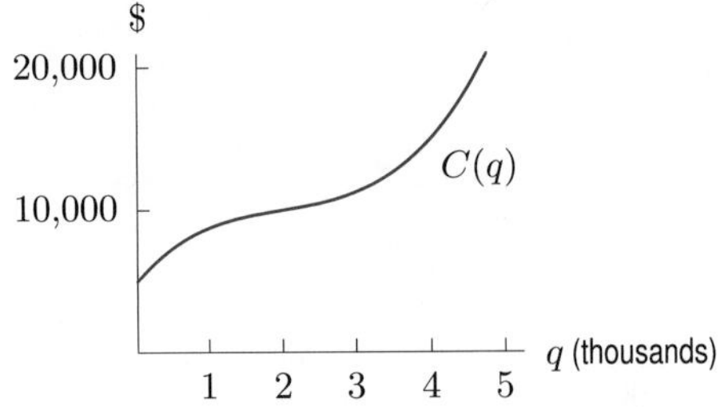

Figure 2.50: Estimating marginal cost: Where is marginal cost smallest?

Solution The cost to produce an additional item is the marginal cost, which is represented by the slope of the cost curve. Since the slope of the cost function in Figure 2.50 is greater at $q = 0.5$ (when the quantity produced is 0.5 thousand, or 500) than at $q = 2$, it costs more to produce the 500th item than the 2000th item. Since the slope is greater at $q = 4$ than $q = 3$, it costs more to produce the 4000th item than the 3000th item.

The slope of the cost function is close to zero at $q = 2$, and is positive everywhere else, so the slope is smallest at $q = 2$. The marginal cost is smallest at a production level of 2000 units. Since $C(2) \approx 10{,}000$, the total cost to produce 2000 units is about $10,000.

Example 4 If the revenue and cost functions, R and C, are given by the graphs in Figure 2.51, sketch graphs of the marginal revenue and marginal cost functions, MR and MC.

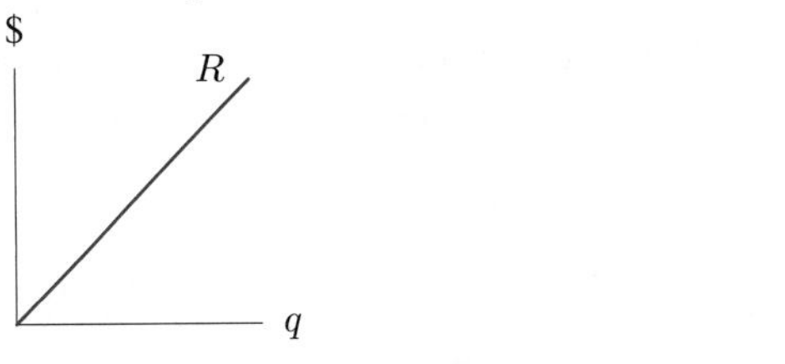

Figure 2.51: Total revenue and total cost for Example 4

Solution The revenue graph is a line through the origin, with equation

$$R = pq$$

where p represents the constant price, so the slope is p and

$$MR = R'(q) = p.$$

The total cost is increasing, so the marginal cost is always positive. For small q values, the graph of the cost function is concave down, so the marginal cost is decreasing. For larger q, say $q > 100$, the graph of the cost function is concave up and the marginal cost is increasing. Thus, the marginal cost has a minimum at about $q = 100$. (See Figure 2.52.)

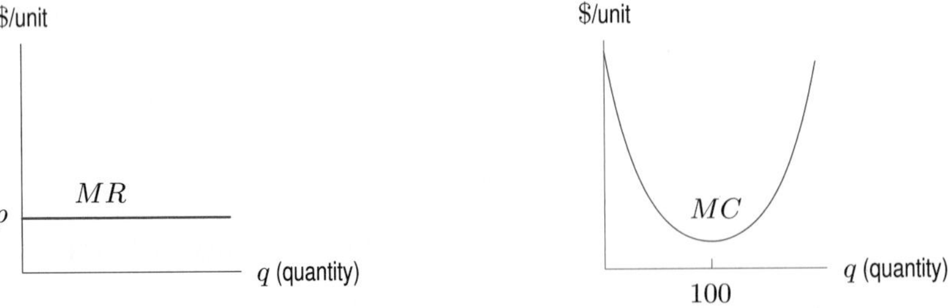

Figure 2.52: Marginal revenue and costs for Example 4

Problems for Section 2.5

1. The function $C(q)$ gives the cost in dollars to produce q barrels of olive oil.

(a) What are the units of marginal cost?
(b) What is the practical meaning of the statement $MC = 3$ for $q = 100$?

2. It costs $4800 to produce 1295 items and it costs $4830 to produce 1305 items. What is the approximate marginal cost at a production level of 1300 items?

3. In Figure 2.53, is marginal cost greater at $q = 5$ or at $q = 30$? At $q = 20$ or at $q = 40$? Explain.

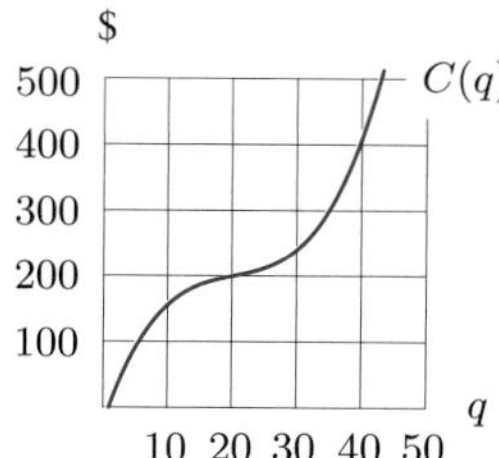

Figure 2.53

4. In Figure 2.54, estimate the marginal cost when the level of production is 10,000 units and interpret it.

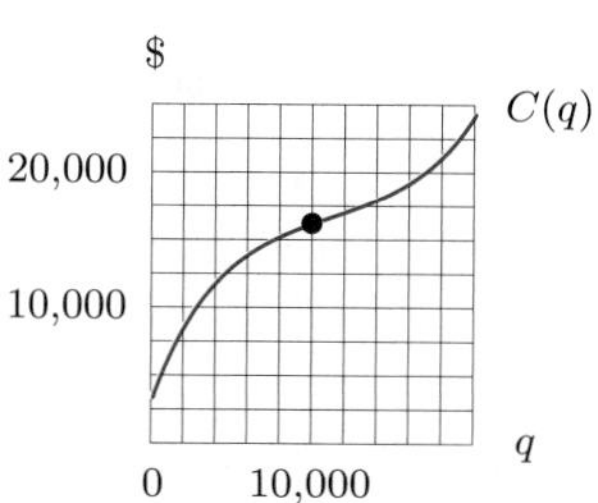

Figure 2.54

5. In Figure 2.55, estimate the marginal revenue when the level of production is 600 units and interpret it.

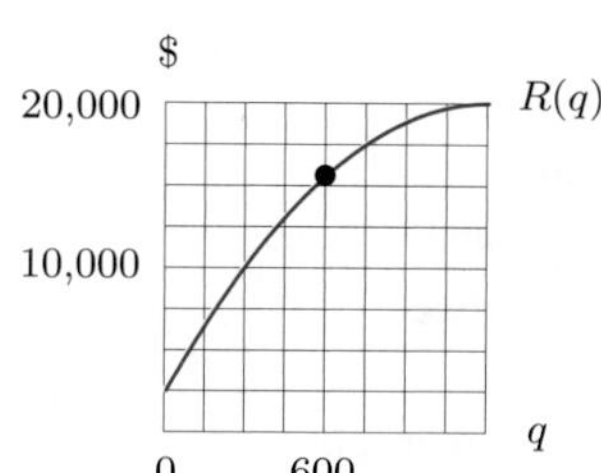

Figure 2.55

6. For q units of a product, a manufacturer's cost is $C(q)$ dollars and revenue is $R(q)$ dollars, with $C(500) = 7200$, $R(500) = 9400$, $MC(500) = 15$, and $MR(500) = 20$.

(a) What is the profit or loss at $q = 500$?
(b) If production is increased from 500 to 501 units, by approximately how much does profit change?

7. The cost of recycling q tons of paper is given in the following table. Estimate the marginal cost at $q = 2000$. Give units and interpret your answer in terms of cost. At approximately what production level does marginal cost appear smallest?

q (tons)	1000	1500	2000	2500	3000	3500
$C(q)$ (dollars)	2500	3200	3640	3825	3900	4400

8. Figure 2.56 shows part of the graph of cost and revenue for a car manufacturer. Which is greater, marginal cost or marginal revenue, at

(a) q_1? **(b)** q_2?

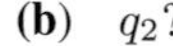

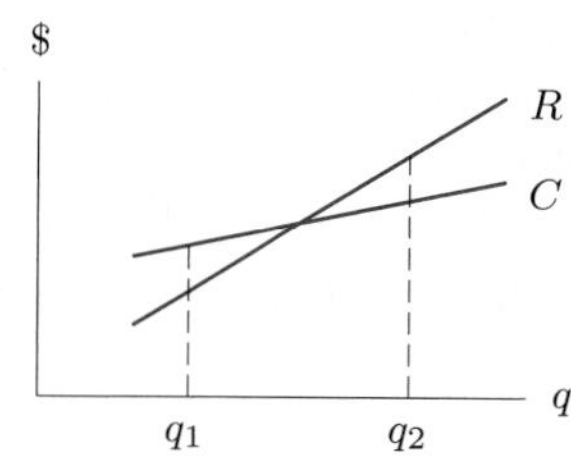

Figure 2.56

9. Let $C(q)$ represent the total cost of producing q items. Suppose $C(15) = 2300$ and $C'(15) = 108$. Estimate the total cost of producing: **(a)** 16 items **(b)** 14 items.

10. To produce 1000 items, the total cost is $5000 and the marginal cost is $25 per item. Estimate the costs of producing 1001 items, 999 items, and 1100 items.

11. Let $C(q)$ represent the cost and $R(q)$ represent the revenue, in dollars, of producing q items.

(a) If $C(50) = 4300$ and $C'(50) = 24$, estimate $C(52)$.
(b) If $C'(50) = 24$ and $R'(50) = 35$, approximately how much profit is earned by the 51st item?
(c) If $C'(100) = 38$ and $R'(100) = 35$, should the company produce the 101st item? Why or why not?

12. Cost and revenue functions for a charter bus company are shown in Figure 2.57. Should the company add a 50th bus? How about a 90th? Explain your answers using marginal revenue and marginal cost.

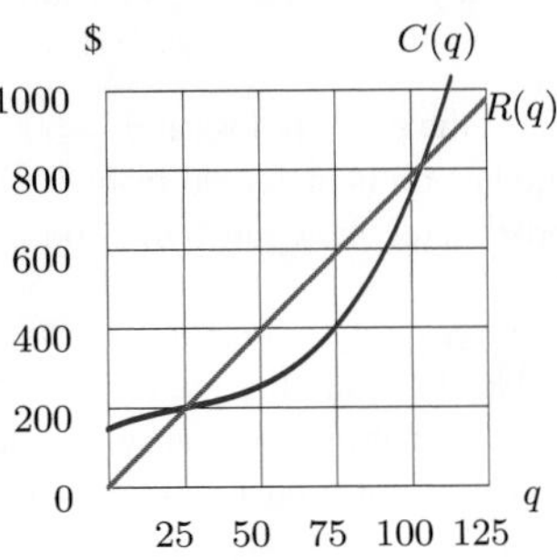

Figure 2.57

13. A company's cost of producing q liters of a chemical is $C(q)$ dollars; this quantity can be sold for $R(q)$ dollars. Suppose $C(2000) = 5930$ and $R(2000) = 7780$.

(a) What is the profit at a production level of 2000?
(b) If $MC(2000) = 2.1$ and $MR(2000) = 2.5$, what is the approximate change in profit if q is increased from 2000 to 2001? Should the company increase or decrease production from $q = 2000$?
(c) If $MC(2000) = 4.77$ and $MR(2000) = 4.32$, should the company increase or decrease production from $q = 2000$?

14. An industrial production process costs $C(q)$ million dollars to produce q million units; these units then sell for $R(q)$ million dollars. If $C(2.1) = 5.1$, $R(2.1) = 6.9$, $MC(2.1) = 0.6$, and $MR(2.1) = 0.7$, calculate

(a) The profit earned by producing 2.1 million units
(b) The approximate change in revenue if production increases from 2.1 to 2.14 million units.
(c) The approximate change in revenue if production decreases from 2.1 to 2.05 million units.
(d) The approximate change in profit in parts (b) and (c).

15. Let $C(q)$ be the total cost of producing a quantity q of a certain product. See Figure 2.58.

(a) What is the meaning of $C(0)$?
(b) Describe in words how the marginal cost changes as the quantity produced increases.
(c) Explain the concavity of the graph (in terms of economics).
(d) Explain the economic significance (in terms of marginal cost) of the point at which the concavity changes.
(e) Do you expect the graph of $C(q)$ to look like this for all types of products?

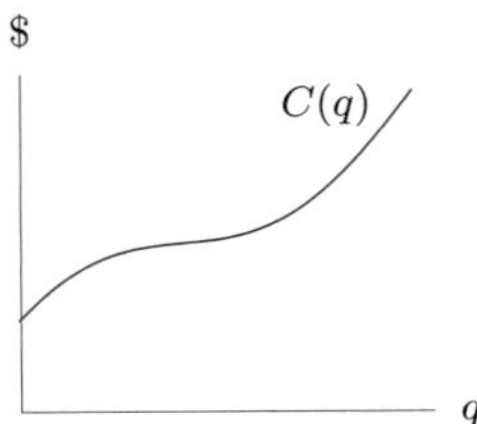

Figure 2.58

CHAPTER SUMMARY

- **Rate of change**
  Average, instantaneous
- **Estimating derivatives**
  Estimate derivatives from a graph, table of values, or formula
- **Interpretation of derivatives**
  Rate of change, slope, using units, instantaneous velocity
- **Relative rate of change**
  Calculation and interpretation
- **Marginality**
  Marginal cost and marginal revenue
- **Second derivative**
  Concavity
- **Derivatives and graphs**
  Understand relation between sign of f' and whether f is increasing or decreasing. Sketch graph of f' from graph of f. Marginal analysis

REVIEW PROBLEMS FOR CHAPTER TWO

1. In a time of t seconds, a particle moves a distance of s meters from its starting point, where $s = 4t^2 + 3$.
   (a) Find the average velocity between $t = 1$ and $t = 1 + h$ if:
   (i) $h = 0.1$, (ii) $h = 0.01$, (iii) $h = 0.001$.
   (b) Use your answers to part (a) to estimate the instantaneous velocity of the particle at time $t = 1$.

2. Match the points labeled on the curve in Figure 2.59 with the given slopes.

Slope	Point
-3	
-1	
0	
1/2	
1	
2	

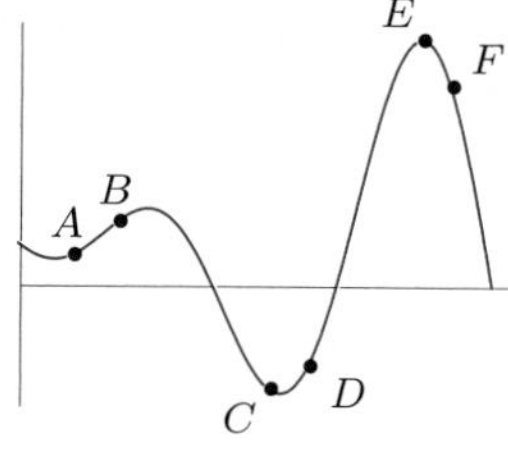

Figure 2.59

3. **(a)** Use a graph of $f(x) = 2 - x^3$ to decide whether $f'(1)$ is positive or negative. Give reasons.
   (b) Use a small interval to estimate $f'(1)$.

4. For the function $f(x) = 3^x$, estimate $f'(1)$. From the graph of $f(x)$, would you expect your estimate to be greater than or less than the true value of $f'(1)$?

5. For the function shown in Figure 2.60, at what labeled points is the slope of the graph positive? Negative? At which labeled point does the graph have the greatest (i.e., most positive) slope? The least slope (i.e., negative and with the largest magnitude)?

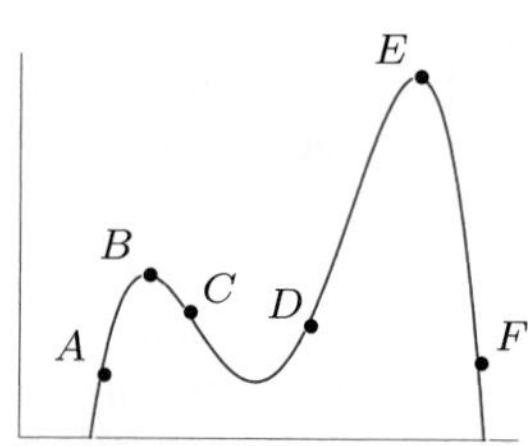

Figure 2.60

6. Use Figure 2.61 to fill in the blanks in the following statements about the function f at point A.
   (a) $f(\_\_) = \_\_$ **(b)** $f'(\_\_) = \_\_$

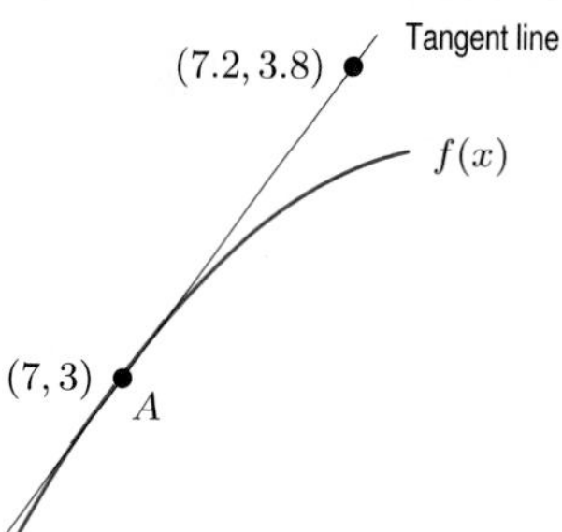

Figure 2.61

7. In a time of t seconds, a particle moves a distance of s meters from its starting point, where $s = \sin(2t)$.
   (a) Find the average velocity between $t = 1$ and $t = 1 + h$ if:
   (i) $h = 0.1$, (ii) $h = 0.01$, (iii) $h = 0.001$.
   (b) Use your answers to part (a) to estimate the instantaneous velocity of the particle at time $t = 1$.

For Problems 8–13, sketch the graph of $f'(x)$.

8. 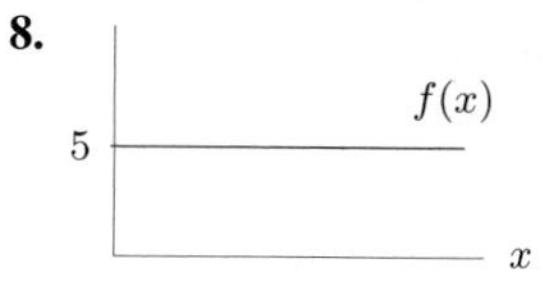

9. 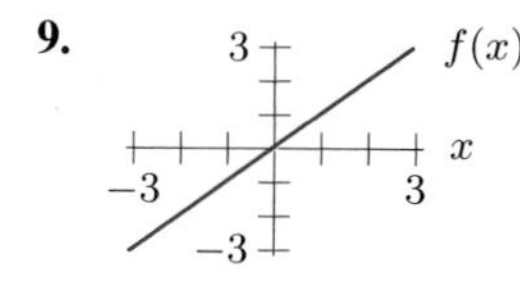

10. 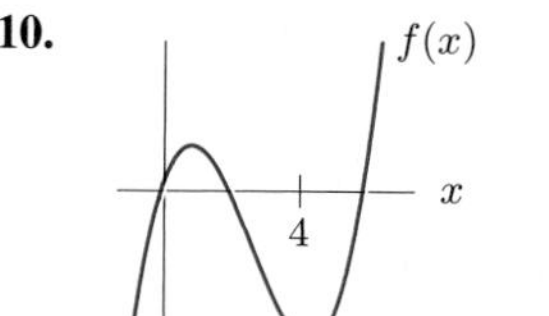

11. 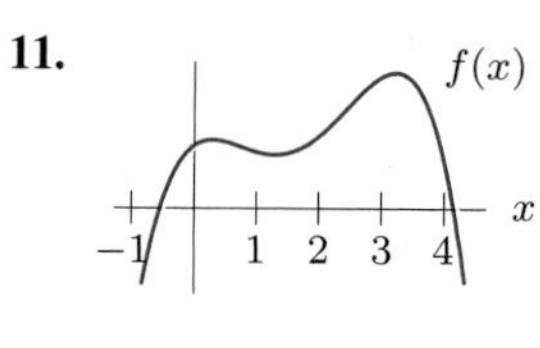

12. 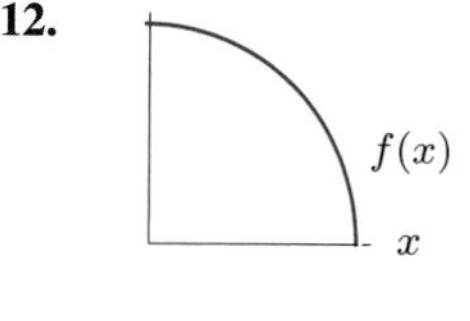

13. 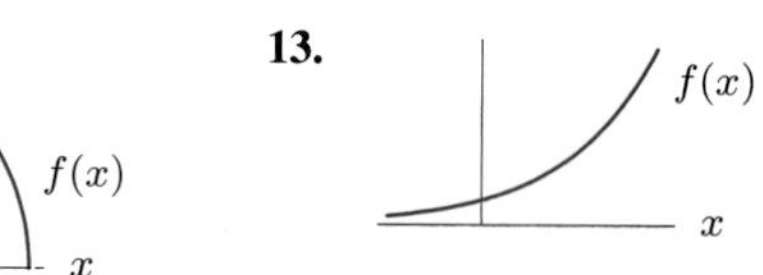

14. **(a)** Estimate $f'(2)$ using the values of f in the table.
    (b) For what values of x does $f'(x)$ appear to be positive? Negative?

x	0	2	4	6	8	10	12
$f(x)$	10	18	24	21	20	18	15

15. Figure 2.62 is the graph of f', the derivative of a function f. On what interval(s) is the function f

(a) Increasing? **(b)** Decreasing?

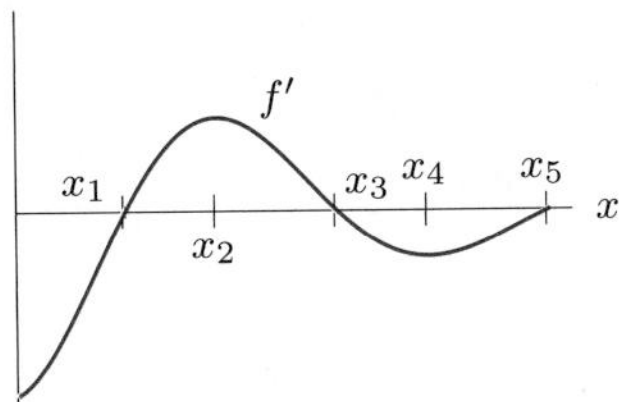

Figure 2.62: Graph of f', not f

16. The average weight W of an oak tree in kilograms that is x meters tall is given by the function $W = f(x)$. What are the units of measurement of $f'(x)$?

17. The percent, P, of US households with a personal computer is a function of the number of years, t, since 1982 (when the percent was essentially zero), so $P = f(t)$. Interpret the statements $f(20) = 57$ and $f'(20) = 3$.

18. A yam has just been taken out of the oven and is cooling off before being eaten. The temperature, T, of the yam (measured in degrees Fahrenheit) is a function of how long it has been out of the oven, t (measured in minutes). Thus, we have $T = f(t)$.

(a) Is $f'(t)$ positive or negative? Why?
(b) What are the units for $f'(t)$?

19. The quantity sold, q, of a certain product is a function of the price, p, so $q = f(p)$. Interpret each of the following statements in terms of demand for the product:

(a) $f(15) = 200$ **(b)** $f'(15) = -25$.

20. Figure 2.63 shows world solar energy output, in megawatts, as a function of years since 1990.[19] Estimate $f'(6)$. Give units and interpret your answer.

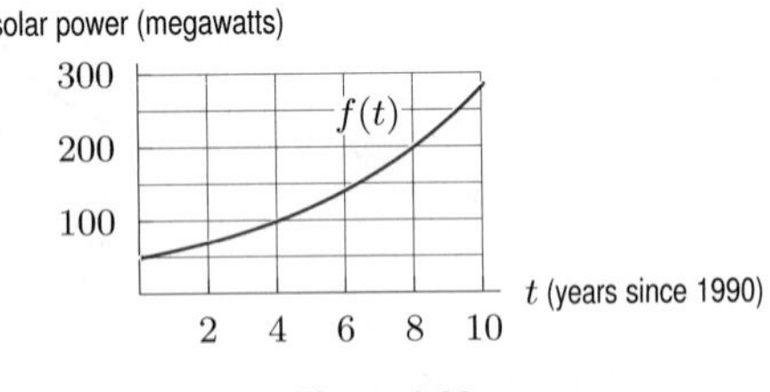

Figure 2.63

21. For a function $f(x)$, we know that $f(20) = 68$ and $f'(20) = -3$. Estimate $f(21)$, $f(19)$ and $f(25)$.

22. Table 2.10 shows world gold production,[20] $G = f(t)$, as a function of year, t.

(a) Does $f'(t)$ appear to be positive or negative? What does this mean in terms of gold production?
(b) In which time interval does $f'(t)$ appear to be greatest?
(c) Estimate $f'(2002)$. Give units and interpret your answer in terms of gold production.
(d) Use the estimated value of $f'(2002)$ to estimate $f(2003)$ and $f(2010)$, and interpret your answers.

Table 2.10 *World gold production*

t (year)	1990	1993	1996	1999	2002
G (mn troy ounces)	70.2	73.3	73.6	82.6	82.9

23. The wind speed W in meters per second at a distance x kilometers from the center of a hurricane is given by the function $W = h(x)$. What does the fact that $h'(15) > 0$ tell you about the hurricane?

24. You drop a rock from a high tower. After it falls x meters its speed S in meters per second is $S = h(x)$. What is the meaning of $h'(20) = 0.5$?

25. If t is the number of years since 2003, the population, P, of China, in billions, can be approximated by the function

$$P = f(t) = 1.291(1.006)^t.$$

Estimate $f(6)$ and $f'(6)$, giving units. What do these two numbers tell you about the population of China?

26. After investing \$1000 at an annual interest rate of 7% compounded continuously for t years, your balance is \$$B$, where $B = f(t)$. What are the units of dB/dt? What is the financial interpretation of dB/dt?

27. Let $f(t)$ be the depth, in centimeters, of water in a tank at time t, in minutes.

(a) What does the sign of $f'(t)$ tell us?
(b) Explain the meaning of $f'(30) = 20$. Include units.
(c) Using the information in part (b), at time $t = 30$ minutes, find the rate of change of depth, in meters, with respect to time in hours. Give units.

28. A climber on Mount Everest is 6000 meters from the start of a trail and at elevation 8000 meters above sea level. At x meters from the start, the elevation of the trail is $h(x)$ meters above sea level. If $h'(x) = 0.5$ for x near 6000, what is the approximate elevation another 3 meters along the trail?

29. Let $f(v)$ be the gas consumption (in liters/km) of a car going at velocity v (in km/hr). In other words, $f(v)$ tells you how many liters of gas the car uses to go one kilometer at velocity v. Explain what the following statements tell you about gas consumption:

$$f(80) = 0.05 \quad \text{and} \quad f'(80) = 0.0005.$$

[19] The Worldwatch Institute, *Vital Signs* 2001, p. 47 (New York: W.W. Norton, 2001).
[20] *The World Almanac and Book of Facts 2005*, p. 135 (New York).

30. To study traffic flow, a city installs a device which records $C(t)$, the total number of cars that have passed by t hours after 4:00 am. The graph of $C(t)$ is in Figure 2.64.

(a) When is the traffic flow the greatest?
(b) Estimate $C'(2)$.
(c) What does $C'(2)$ mean in practical terms?

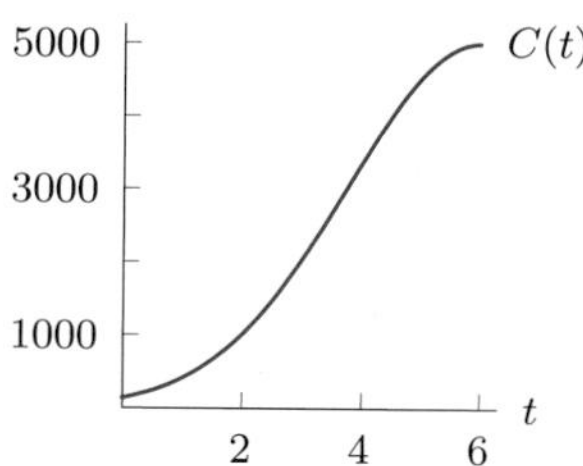

Figure 2.64

31. The temperature, H, in degrees Celsius, of a cup of coffee placed on the kitchen counter is given by $H = f(t)$, where t is in minutes since the coffee was put on the counter.

(a) Is $f'(t)$ positive or negative? Give a reason for your answer.
(b) What are the units of $f'(20)$? What is its practical meaning in terms of the temperature of the coffee?

32. Suppose that $f(x)$ is a function with $f(100) = 35$ and $f'(100) = 3$. Estimate $f(102)$.

33. Suppose $P(t)$ is the monthly payment, in dollars, on a mortgage which will take t years to pay off. What are the units of $P'(t)$? What is the practical meaning of $P'(t)$? What is its sign?

34. The table[21] shows $f(t)$, total sales of music compact discs (CDs), in millions, and $g(t)$, total sales of music cassettes, in millions, as a function of year t.

(a) Estimate $f'(2002)$ and $g'(2002)$. Give units with your answers and interpret each answer in terms of sales of CDs or cassettes.
(b) Use $f'(2002)$ to estimate $f(2003)$ and $f(2010)$. Interpret your answers in terms of sales of CDs.

Year, t	1994	1996	1998	2000	2002
CD sales, $f(t)$	662.1	778.9	847.0	942.5	803.3
Cassette sales, $g(t)$	345.4	225.3	158.5	76.0	31.1

35. For each part below, sketch a graph of a function that satisfies the given conditions. There are many possible correct answers.

(a) $f' > 0$ and $f'' > 0$.
(b) $f' > 0$ and $f'' < 0$.
(c) $f' < 0$ and $f'' > 0$.
(d) $f' < 0$ and $f'' < 0$.

36. For each function, do the signs of the first and second derivatives of the function appear to be positive or negative over the given interval?

(a)

x	1.0	1.1	1.2	1.3	1.4	1.5
f(x)	10.1	11.2	13.7	16.0	21.2	27.7

(b)

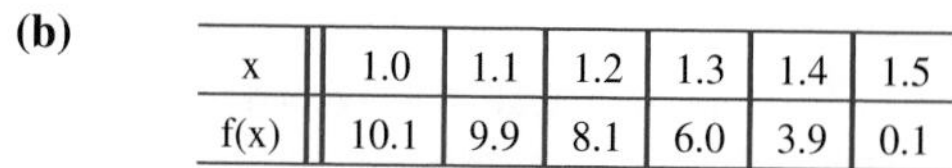

x	1.0	1.1	1.2	1.3	1.4	1.5
f(x)	10.1	9.9	8.1	6.0	3.9	0.1

(c)

x	1.0	1.1	1.2	1.3	1.4	1.5
f(x)	1000	1010	1015	1018	1020	1021

37. The length L of the day in minutes (sunrise to sunset) x kilometers north of the equator on June 21 is given by $L = f(x)$. What are the units of

(a) $f'(3000)$? **(b)** $f''(3000)$?

38. Sketch the graph of a function whose first and second derivatives are everywhere positive.

39. At which of the marked x-values in Figure 2.65 can the following statements be true?

(a) $f(x) < 0$
(b) $f'(x) < 0$
(c) $f(x)$ is decreasing
(d) $f'(x)$ is decreasing
(e) Slope of $f(x)$ is positive
(f) Slope of $f(x)$ is increasing

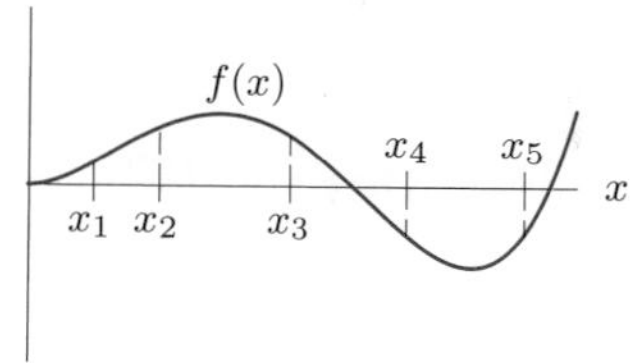

Figure 2.65

40. Sketch the graph of the height of a particle against time if velocity is positive and acceleration is negative.

41. Figure 2.66 gives the position, $f(t)$, of a particle at time t. At which of the marked values of t can the following statements be true?

(a) The position is positive
(b) The velocity is positive
(c) The acceleration is positive
(d) The position is decreasing
(e) The velocity is decreasing

[21] *The World Almanac and Book of Facts 2005*, p. 309 (New York).

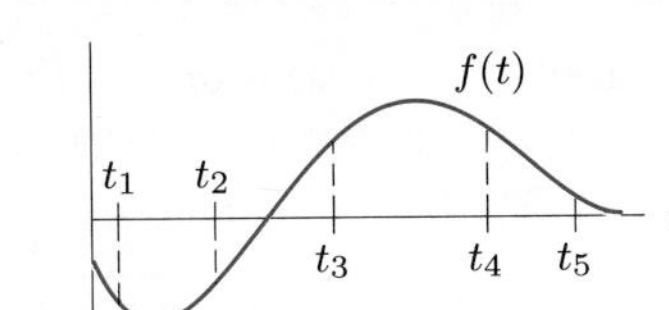

Figure 2.66

42. A high school principal is concerned about the drop in the percentage of students who graduate from her school, shown in the following table.

Year entered school, t	1992	1995	1998	2001	2004
Percent graduating, P	62.4	54.1	48.0	43.5	41.8

(a) Calculate the average rate of change of P for each of the three-year intervals between 1992 and 2004.
(b) Does d^2P/dt^2 appear to be positive or negative between 1992 and 2004?
(c) Explain why the values of P and dP/dt are troublesome to the principal.
(d) Explain why the sign of d^2P/dt^2 and the magnitude of dP/dt in the year 2001 may give the principal some cause for optimism.

43. Students were asked to evaluate $f'(4)$ from the following table which shows values of the function f:

x	1	2	3	4	5	6
$f(x)$	4.2	4.1	4.2	4.5	5.0	5.7

- Student A estimated the derivative as $f'(4) \approx \frac{f(5)-f(4)}{5-4} = 0.5$.
- Student B estimated the derivative as $f'(4) \approx \frac{f(4)-f(3)}{4-3} = 0.3$.
- Student C suggested that they should split the difference and estimate the average of these two results, that is, $f'(4) \approx \frac{1}{2}(0.5+0.3) = 0.4$.

(a) Sketch the graph of f, and indicate how the three estimates are represented on the graph.
(b) Explain which answer is likely to be best.

44. Figure 2.67 shows the rate at which energy, $f(v)$, is consumed by a bird flying at speed v meters/sec.

(a) What rate of energy consumption is needed by the bird to keep aloft, without moving forward?
(b) What does the shape of the graph tell you about how birds fly?
(c) Sketch $f'(v)$.

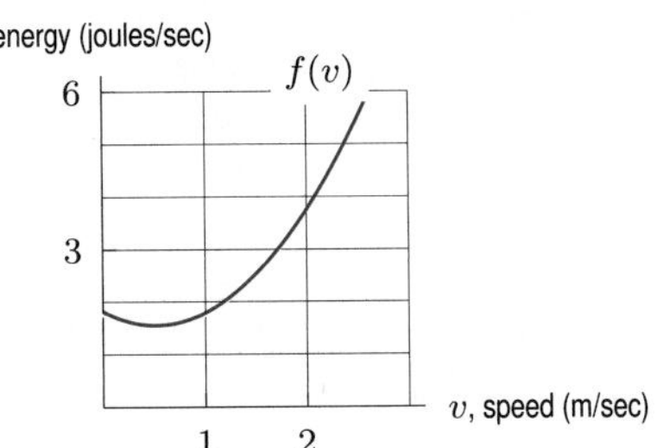

Figure 2.67

CHECK YOUR UNDERSTANDING

In Problems 1–55, indicate whether the statement is true or false.

1. The derivative of f at a is the instantaneous rate of change of f at the point a.

2. If $f(x) = x^2$ then $f'(1)$ is positive.

3. If $g(t) = 2^t$ then $g'(1) \approx (2^{1.001} - 2^1)/(1.001 - 1)$.

4. The slope of the graph of $H(x) = \sqrt{x}$ is negative at $x = 2$.

5. A function f cannot have both $f(a) = 0$ and $f'(a) = 0$.

6. The average rate of change of f between 0 and 1 is always less than the slope of the graph of f at 0.

7. The function r in the following table appears to have a negative derivative at $t = 0.5$:

t	0.3	0.5	0.7	0.9
$r(t)$	1.2	6.5	9.7	13.4

8. The derivative of f at 3 is given by the difference quotient $(f(3) - f(0))/(3 - 0)$.

9. If $R(w) = w^3$ then $R'(-2)$ is negative.

10. A function can have more than one point where the derivative is 0.

11. If $f' > 0$ on an interval, then f is increasing on that interval.

12. The f is negative on an interval, then the derivative of f is decreasing on that interval.

13. If f is always increasing, then f' is always increasing.

14. If $f(2) > g(2)$ then $f'(2) > g'(2)$.
15. The derivative of the constant function $q(x) = 5$ is $q'(x) = 0$.
16. The derivative of a function that is always decreasing is also always decreasing.
17. The function $g(t) = \ln(t)$ has $g'(1) < 0$.
18. If f is a function with $f(3) = 0$ then $f'(3) = 0$.
19. If f' is zero at all points in an interval, then the graph of f is a horizontal line on that interval.
20. If f' is negative at all points in an interval, then f is decreasing on that interval.
21. If the cost C (in dollars) of feeding x students in the dining center is given by $C = f(x)$, then the units of dC/dx are dollars per student.
22. If $y = f(x)$ then dy/dx and $f'(x)$ mean the same thing.
23. If the cost C (in dollars) of extracting T tons of ore is given by $C = f(T)$ then $f'(2000)$ is the approximate cost to extract the 2001st ton.
24. If $f(10) = 20$ and $f'(10) = 3$, then 23 is a reasonable approximation of $f(11)$.
25. The units of dA/dB are the units of A divided by the units of B.
26. If $A = f(B)$ then the units of $f'(B)$ are the units of B divided by the units of A.
27. If $f'(100) = 2$ and the derivative of f is not changing rapidly, then $f(101) - f(100) \approx 2$.
28. If t (in minutes) is the time that a dose of D milligrams of morphine is effective as a painkiller, so that $t = f(D)$, then the units of $f'(D)$ are minutes per milligram.
29. If $h = f(a)$ gives height h (in inches) of a child aged a years, then dh/da is positive when $0 < a < 10$.
30. If $W = f(R)$ and $f'(R)$ is negative, then we expect W to decrease as R increases.
31. If $f'' > 0$ on an interval, then f is increasing on that interval.
32. If $f'' < 0$ on an interval, then f is concave down on that interval.
33. If $f'' > 0$ on an interval, then $f' > 0$ on that interval.
34. If f' is decreasing on an interval, then f is concave down on that interval.
35. If a car is slowing down, then the second derivative of its distance as a function of time is negative.
36. There is a function with $f > 0$ and $f' > 0$ and $f'' > 0$ everywhere.
37. There is a function with $f > 0$ and $f' < 0$ and $f'' > 0$ everywhere.
38. There is a function with $f'' = 0$ everywhere.
39. The function $f(x) = e^x$ has $f'' > 0$ everywhere.
40. The function $f(x) = \ln(x)$ has $f'' > 0$ for $x > 0$.
41. Marginal cost is the instantaneous rate of change of cost with respect to quantity.
42. Marginal revenue is the derivative of the revenue function with respect to quantity.
43. If marginal revenue is greater than marginal cost when quantity is 1000, then increasing the quantity to 1001 will increase the profit.
44. Marginal cost is always greater than or equal to zero.
45. If the revenue function is linear with slope 5, then marginal revenue is always zero.
46. The units of marginal cost are quantity per dollar.
47. The units of marginal revenue are the same as the units of marginal cost.
48. Marginal cost is never equal to marginal revenue.
49. If the graphs of the cost and revenue functions $C(q)$ and $R(q)$ cross at q^*, then marginal revenue is equal to marginal cost at q^*.
50. If the graphs of the marginal cost and marginal revenue functions $C'(q)$ and $R'(q)$ cross at q^*, then marginal revenue is equal to marginal cost at q^*.
51. If P is a function of t, then the relative rate of change of P is $(1/P)(dP/dt)$.
52. If $f(25) = 10$ gallons and $f'(25) = 2$ gallons per minute, then at $t = 25$, the function f is changing at a rate of 20% per minute.
53. If a quantity is 100 and has relative rate of change -3% per minute, we expect the quantity to be about 97 one minute later.
54. If a population of animals changes from 500 to 400 in one month, then the relative rate of change is about -100 animals per month.
55. Linear functions have constant rate of change and exponential functions have constant relative rate of change.

PROJECTS FOR CHAPTER TWO

1. Estimating the Temperature of a Yam

Suppose you put a yam in a hot oven, maintained at a constant temperature of 200°C. As the yam picks up heat from the oven, its temperature rises.[22]

[22]From Peter D. Taylor, *Calculus: The Analysis of Functions* (Toronto: Wall & Emerson, Inc., 1992).

(a) Draw a possible graph of the temperature T of the yam against time t (minutes) since it is put into the oven. Explain any interesting features of the graph, and in particular explain its concavity.

(b) Suppose that, at $t = 30$, the temperature T of the yam is 120° and increasing at the (instantaneous) rate of 2°/min. Using this information, plus what you know about the shape of the T graph, estimate the temperature at time $t = 40$.

(c) Suppose in addition you are told that at $t = 60$, the temperature of the yam is 165°. Can you improve your estimate of the temperature at $t = 40$?

(d) Assuming all the data given so far, estimate the time at which the temperature of the yam is 150°.

2. Temperature and Illumination

Alone in your dim, unheated room, you light a single candle rather than curse the darkness. Depressed with the situation, you walk directly away from the candle, sighing. The temperature (in degrees Fahrenheit) and illumination (in % of one candle power) decrease as your distance (in feet) from the candle increases. In fact, you have tables showing this information.

Distance (feet)	Temperature (°F)
0	55
1	54.5
2	53.5
3	52
4	50
5	47
6	43.5

Distance (feet)	Illumination (%)
0	100
1	85
2	75
3	67
4	60
5	56
6	53

You are cold when the temperature is below 40°. You are in the dark when the illumination is at most 50% of one candle power.

(a) Two graphs are shown in Figures 2.68 and 2.69. One is temperature as a function of distance and one is illumination as a function of distance. Which is which? Explain.

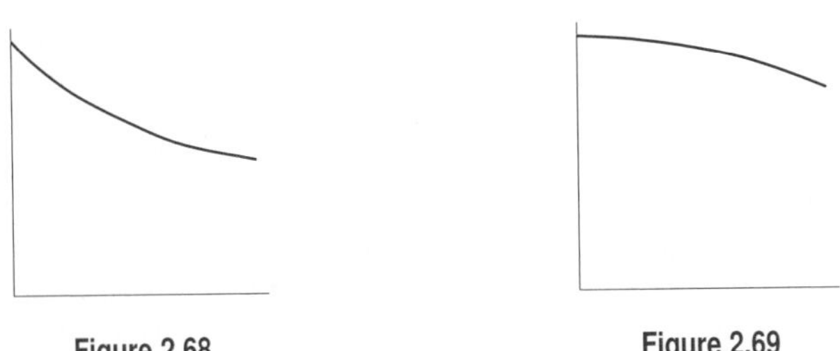

Figure 2.68　　Figure 2.69

(b) What is the average rate at which the temperature is changing when the illumination drops from 75% to 56%?

(c) You can still read your watch when the illumination is about 65%. Can you still read your watch at 3.5 feet? Explain.

(d) Suppose you know that at 6 feet the instantaneous rate of change of the temperature is -4.5°F/ft and the instantaneous rate of change of illumination is -3% candle power/ft. Estimate the temperature and the illumination at 7 feet.

(e) Are you in the dark before you are cold, or vice versa?

FOCUS ON THEORY

LIMITS, CONTINUITY, AND THE DEFINITION OF THE DERIVATIVE

The velocity at a single instant in time is surprisingly difficult to define precisely. Consider the statement "At the instant it crossed the finish line, the horse was traveling at 42 mph." How can such a claim be substantiated? A photograph taken at that instant will show the horse motionless—it is no help at all. There is some paradox in trying to quantify the property of motion at a particular instant in time, since by focusing on a single instant we stop the motion!

A similar difficulty arises whenever we attempt to measure the rate of change of anything—for example, oil leaking out of a damaged tanker. The statement "One hour after the ship's hull ruptured, oil was leaking at a rate of 200 barrels per second" seems not to make sense. We could argue that at any given instant *no* oil is leaking.

Problems of motion were of central concern to Zeno and other philosophers as early as the fifth century BC. The approach that we took, made famous by Newton's calculus, is to stop looking for a simple notion of speed at an instant, and instead to look at speed over small intervals containing the instant. This method sidesteps the philosophical problems mentioned earlier but brings new ones of its own.

Definition of the Derivative Using Average Rates

In Section 2.1, we defined the derivative as the instantaneous rate of change of a function. We can estimate a derivative by computing average rates of change over smaller and smaller intervals. We use this idea to give a symbolic definition of the derivative. Letting h represent the size of the interval, we have

$$\begin{array}{c}\text{Average rate of change}\\ \text{between } x \text{ and } x+h\end{array} = \frac{f(x+h)-f(x)}{(x+h)-x} = \frac{f(x+h)-f(x)}{h}.$$

To find the derivative, or instantaneous rate of change at the point x, we use smaller and smaller intervals. To find the derivative exactly, we take the limit as h, the size of the interval, shrinks to zero, so we say

$$\text{Derivative} = \text{Limit, as } h \text{ approaches zero, of } \frac{f(x+h)-f(x)}{h}.$$

Finally, instead of writing the phrase "limit, as h approaches 0," we use the notation $\lim\limits_{h\to 0}$. This leads to the following symbolic definition:

For any function f, we define the **derivative function**, f', by

$$f'(x) = \lim_{h\to 0} \frac{f(x+h)-f(x)}{h},$$

provided the limit exists. The function f is said to be **differentiable** at any point x at which the derivative function is defined.

Notice that we have replaced the original difficulty of computing velocity at a point by an argument that the average rates of change approach a number as the time intervals shrink in size. In a sense, we have traded one hard question for another, since we don't yet have any idea how to be certain what number the average velocities are approaching.

The Idea of a Limit

We used a limit to define the derivative. Now we look a bit more at the idea of the limit of a function at the point c. Provided the limit exists:

> We write $\lim_{x\to c} f(x)$ to represent the number approached by $f(x)$ as x approaches c.

Example 1 Investigate $\lim_{x\to 2} x^2$.

Solution Notice that we can make x^2 as close to 4 as we like by taking x sufficiently close to 2. (Look at the values of 1.9^2, 1.99^2, 1.999^2, and 2.1^2, 2.01^2, 2.001^2 in Table 2.11; they seem to be approaching 4.) We write

$$\lim_{x\to 2} x^2 = 4,$$

which is read "the limit, as x approaches 2, of x^2 is 4." Notice that the limit does not ask what happens *at* $x = 2$, so it is not sufficient to substitute 2 to find the answer. The limit describes behavior of a function *near* a point, not *at* the point.

Table 2.11 *Values of x^2 near $x = 2$*

x	1.9	1.99	1.999	2.001	2.01	2.1
x^2	3.61	3.96	3.996	4.004	4.04	4.41

Example 2 Use a graph to estimate $\lim_{x\to 0} \dfrac{2^x - 1}{x}$.

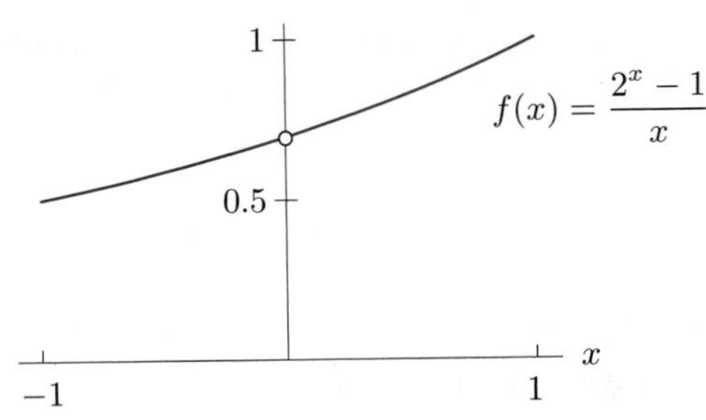

Figure 2.70: Find the limit as $x \to 0$ of $\dfrac{2^x - 1}{x}$

Solution Notice that the expression $\dfrac{2^x - 1}{x}$ is undefined at $x = 0$. To find out what happens to this expression as x approaches 0, look at a graph of $f(x) = \dfrac{2^x - 1}{x}$. Figure 2.70 shows that as x approaches 0 from either side, the value of $\dfrac{2^x - 1}{x}$ appears to approach 0.7. If we zoom in on the graph near $x = 0$, we can estimate the limit with greater accuracy, giving

$$\lim_{x\to 0} \frac{2^x - 1}{x} \approx 0.693.$$

Example 3 Estimate $\lim_{h\to 0} \frac{(3+h)^2-9}{h}$ numerically.

Solution The limit is the value approached by this expression as h approaches 0. The values in Table 2.12 seem to be approaching 6 as $h \to 0$. So it is a reasonable guess that

$$\lim_{h\to 0} \frac{(3+h)^2-9}{h} = 6.$$

However, we cannot be sure that the limit is *exactly* 6 by looking at the table. To calculate the limit exactly requires algebra.

Table 2.12 *Values of* $\left((3+h)^2-9\right)/h$

h	-0.1	-0.01	-0.001	0.001	0.01	0.1
$\left((3+h)^2-9\right)/h$	5.9	5.99	5.999	6.001	6.01	6.1

Example 4 Use algebra to find $\lim_{h\to 0} \frac{(3+h)^2-9}{h}$.

Solution Expanding the numerator gives

$$\frac{(3+h)^2-9}{h} = \frac{9+6h+h^2-9}{h} = \frac{6h+h^2}{h}.$$

Since taking the limit as $h \to 0$ means looking at values of h near, but not equal, to 0, we can cancel a common factor of h, giving

$$\lim_{h\to 0} \frac{(3+h)^2-9}{h} = \lim_{h\to 0} \frac{6h+h^2}{h} = \lim_{h\to 0}(6+h).$$

As h approaches 0, the values of $(6+h)$ approach 6, so

$$\lim_{h\to 0} \frac{(3+h)^2-9}{h} = \lim_{h\to 0}(6+h) = 6.$$

Continuity

Roughly speaking, a function is said to be *continuous* on an interval if its graph has no breaks, jumps, or holes in that interval. A continuous function has a graph that can be drawn without lifting the pencil from the paper.

Example: The function $f(x) = 3x^2 - x^2 + 2x + 1$ is continuous on any interval. (See Figure 2.71.)

Example: The function $f(x) = 1/x$ is not defined at $x = 0$. It is continuous on any interval not containing the origin. (See Figure 2.72.)

Example: Suppose $p(x)$ is the price of mailing a first-class letter weighing x ounces. It costs 34¢ for one ounce or less, 57¢ between the first and second ounces, and so on. So the graph (in Figure 2.73) is a series of steps. This function is not continuous on intervals such as $(0, 2)$ because the graph jumps at $x = 1$.

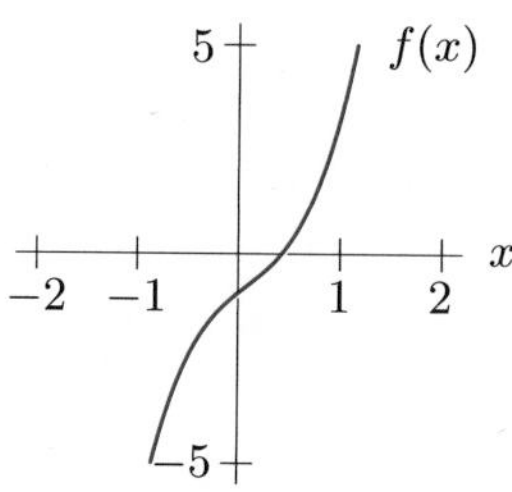

Figure 2.71: The graph of $f(x) = 3x^3 - x^2 + 2x - 1$

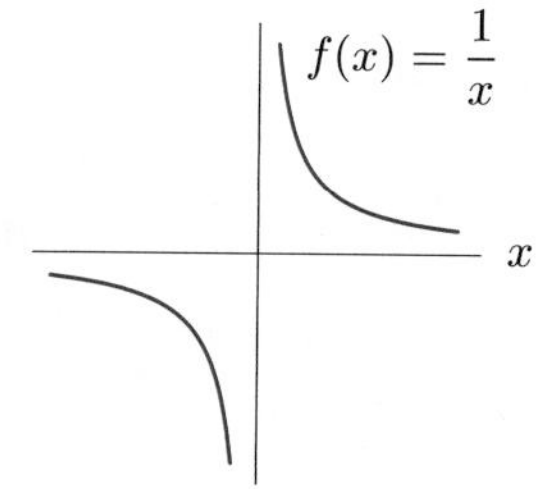

Figure 2.72: Graph of $f(x) = 1/x$: Not defined at 0

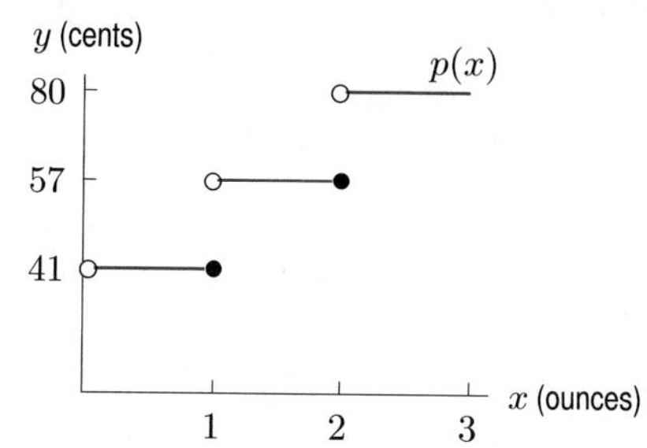

Figure 2.73: Cost of mailing a letter

What Does Continuity Mean Numerically?

Continuity is important in practical work because it means that small errors in the independent variable lead to small errors in the value of the function.

Example: Suppose that $f(x) = x^2$ and that we want to compute $f(\pi)$. Knowing f is continuous tells us that taking $x = 3.14$ should give a good approximation to $f(\pi)$, and that we can get a better approximation to $f(\pi)$ by using more decimals of π.

Example: If $p(x)$ is the cost of mailing a letter weighing x ounces, then $p(0.99) = p(1) = 34$¢, whereas $p(1.01) = 57$¢, because as soon as we get over 1 ounce, the price jumps up to 57¢. So a small difference in the weight of a letter can lead to a significant difference in its mailing cost. Hence p is not continuous at $x = 1$.

Definition of Continuity

We now define continuity using limits. The idea of continuity rules out breaks, jumps, or holes by demanding that the behavior of a function *near* a point be consistent with its behavior *at* the point:

> The function f is **continuous** at $x = c$ if f is defined at $x = c$ and
>
> $$\lim_{x \to c} f(x) = f(c).$$
>
> The function is **continuous on an interval** (a, b) if it is continuous at every point in the interval.

Which Functions Are Continuous?

Requiring a function to be continuous on an interval is not asking very much, as any function whose graph is an unbroken curve over the interval is continuous. For example, exponential functions, polynomials, and sine and cosine are continuous on every interval. Functions created by adding, multiplying, or composing continuous functions are also continuous.

Using the Definition to Calculate Derivatives

By estimating the derivative of the function $f(x) = x^2$ at several points, we guessed in Example 5 of Section 2.2 that the derivative of x^2 is $f'(x) = 2x$. In order to show that this formula is correct, we have to use the symbolic definition of the derivative given earlier in this section.

In evaluating the expression

$$\lim_{h \to 0} \frac{f(x+h) - f(x)}{h},$$

we simplify the difference quotient first, and then take the limit as h approaches zero.

Example 5 Show that the derivative of $f(x) = x^2$ is $f'(x) = 2x$.

Solution Using the definition of the derivative with $f(x) = x^2$, we have

$$\begin{aligned} f'(x) &= \lim_{h \to 0} \frac{f(x+h) - f(x)}{h} = \lim_{h \to 0} \frac{(x+h)^2 - x^2}{h} \\ &= \lim_{h \to 0} \frac{x^2 + 2xh + h^2 - x^2}{h} = \lim_{h \to 0} \frac{2xh + h^2}{h} \\ &= \lim_{h \to 0} \frac{h(2x + h)}{h}. \end{aligned}$$

To take the limit, look at what happens when h is close to 0, but do not let $h = 0$. Since $h \neq 0$, we cancel the common factor of h, giving

$$f'(x) = \lim_{h \to 0} \frac{h(2x+h)}{h} = \lim_{h \to 0} (2x+h) = 2x,$$

because as h gets close to zero, $2x + h$ gets close to $2x$. So

$$f'(x) = \frac{d}{dx}(x^2) = 2x.$$

Example 6 Show that if $f(x) = 3x - 2$, then $f'(x) = 3$.

Solution Since the slope of the linear function $f(x) = 3x - 2$ is 3 and the derivative is the slope, we see that $f'(x) = 3$. We can also use the definition to get this result:

$$\begin{aligned} f'(x) &= \lim_{h \to 0} \frac{f(x+h) - f(x)}{h} = \lim_{h \to 0} \frac{(3(x+h) - 2) - (3x - 2)}{h} \\ &= \lim_{h \to 0} \frac{3x + 3h - 2 - 3x + 2}{h} = \lim_{h \to 0} \frac{3h}{h}. \end{aligned}$$

To find the limit, look at what happens when h is close to, but not equal to, 0. Simplifying, we get

$$f'(x) = \lim_{h \to 0} \frac{3h}{h} = \lim_{h \to 0} 3 = 3.$$

Problems on Limits and the Definition of the Derivative

1. On Figure 2.74, mark lengths that represent the quantities in parts (a) – (e). (Pick any h, with $h > 0$.)

   (a) $a + h$ **(b)** h **(c)** $f(a)$
   (d) $f(a+h)$ **(e)** $f(a+h) - f(a)$

   (f) Using your answers to parts (a)–(e), show how the quantity $\dfrac{f(a+h) - f(a)}{h}$ can be represented as the slope of a line on the graph.

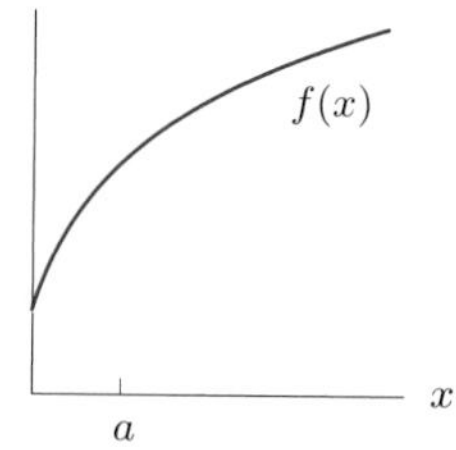

Figure 2.74

2. On Figure 2.75, mark lengths that represent the quantities in parts (a)–(e). (Pick any h, with $h > 0$.)

   (a) $a + h$ **(b)** h **(c)** $f(a)$
   (d) $f(a+h)$ **(e)** $f(a+h) - f(a)$

   (f) Using your answers to parts (a)–(e), represent the quantity $\dfrac{f(a+h) - f(a)}{h}$ as the slope of a line on the graph.

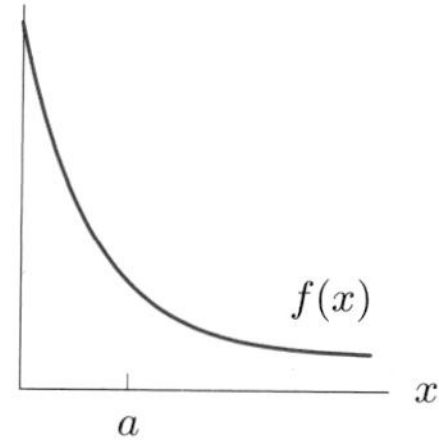

Figure 2.75

Use a graph to estimate the limits in Problems 3–4.

3. $\lim_{x\to 0} \frac{\sin x}{x}$ (with x in radians)

4. $\lim_{x\to 0} \frac{5^x - 1}{x}$

Estimate the limits in Problems 5–8 by substituting smaller and smaller values of h. For trigonometric functions, use radians. Give answers to one decimal place.

5. $\lim_{h\to 0} \frac{(3+h)^3 - 27}{h}$

6. $\lim_{h\to 0} \frac{7^h - 1}{h}$

7. $\lim_{h\to 0} \frac{e^{1+h} - e}{h}$

8. $\lim_{h\to 0} \frac{\cos h - 1}{h}$

In Problems 9–12, does the function $f(x)$ appear to be continuous on the interval $0 \le x \le 2$? If not, what about on the interval $0 \le x \le 0.5$?

9.

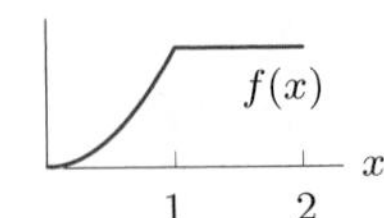

10.

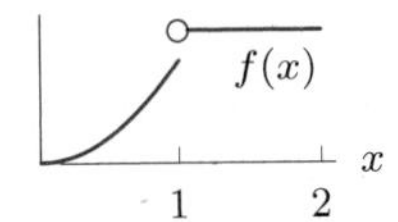

11.

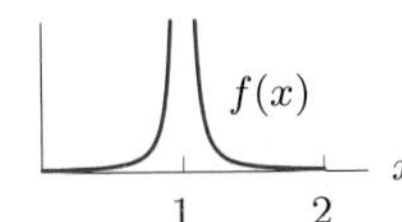

12.

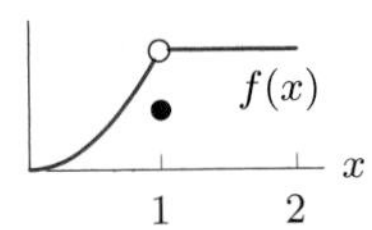

Are the functions in Problems 13–18 continuous on the given intervals?

13. $f(x) = x + 2$ on $-3 \le x \le 3$

14. $f(x) = 2^x$ on $0 \le x \le 10$

15. $f(x) = x^2 + 2$ on $0 \le x \le 5$

16. $f(x) = \frac{1}{x-1}$ on $2 \le x \le 3$

17. $f(x) = \frac{1}{x-1}$ on $0 \le x \le 2$

18. $f(x) = \frac{1}{x^2+1}$ on $0 \le x \le 2$

Which of the functions described in Problems 19–23 are continuous?

19. The number of people in a village as a function of time.

20. The weight of a baby as a function of time during the second month of the baby's life.

21. The number of pairs of pants as a function of the number of yards of cloth from which they are made. Each pair requires 3 yards.

22. The distance traveled by a car in stop-and-go traffic as a function of time.

23. You start in North Carolina and go westward on Interstate 40 toward California. Consider the function giving the local time of day as a function of your distance from your starting point.

Use the definition of the derivative to show how the formulas in Problems 24–33 are obtained.

24. If $f(x) = 5x$, then $f'(x) = 5$.

25. If $f(x) = 3x - 2$, then $f'(x) = 3$.

26. If $f(x) = x^2 + 4$, then $f'(x) = 2x$.

27. If $f(x) = 3x^2$, then $f'(x) = 6x$.

28. If $f(x) = -2x^3$, then $f'(x) = -6x^2$.

29. If $f(x) = x - x^2$, then $f'(x) = 1 - 2x$.

30. If $f(x) = 1 - x^3$, then $f'(x) = -3x^2$.

31. If $f(x) = 5x^2 + 1$, then $f'(x) = 10x$.

32. If $f(x) = 2x^2 + x$, then $f'(x) = 4x + 1$.

33. If $f(x) = 1/x$, then $f'(x) = -1/x^2$.

Chapter Three

SHORTCUTS TO DIFFERENTIATION

Contents

3.1 DERIVATIVE FORMULAS FOR POWERS AND POLYNOMIALS

The derivative of a function at a point represents a slope and a rate of change. In Chapter 2, we learned how to estimate values of the derivative of a function given by a graph or by a table. Now, we learn how to find a formula for the derivative of a function given by a formula.

Derivative of a Constant Function

The graph of a constant function $f(x) = k$ is a horizontal line, with a slope of 0 everywhere. Therefore, its derivative is 0 everywhere. (See Figure 3.1.)

> If $f(x) = k$, then $f'(x) = 0$.

For example, $\frac{d}{dx}(5) = 0$.

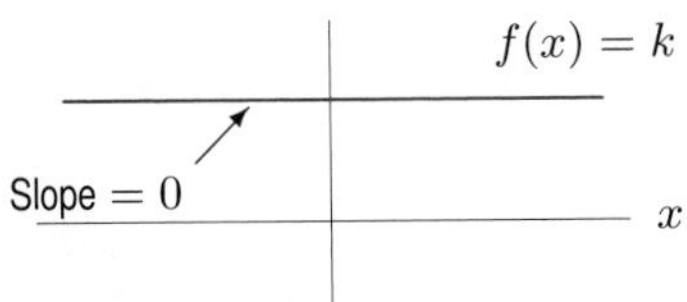

Figure 3.1: A constant function

Derivative of a Linear Function

We already know that the slope of a line is constant. This tells us that the derivative of a linear function is constant.

> If $f(x) = b + mx$, then $f'(x) =$ Slope $= m$.

For example, $\frac{d}{dx}(5 - \frac{3}{2}x) = -\frac{3}{2}$.

Derivative of a Constant Times a Function

Figure 3.2 shows the graph of $y = f(x)$ and of three multiples: $y = 3f(x)$, $y = \frac{1}{2}f(x)$, and $y = -2f(x)$. What is the relationship between the derivatives of these functions? In other words, for a particular x-value, how are the slopes of these graphs related?

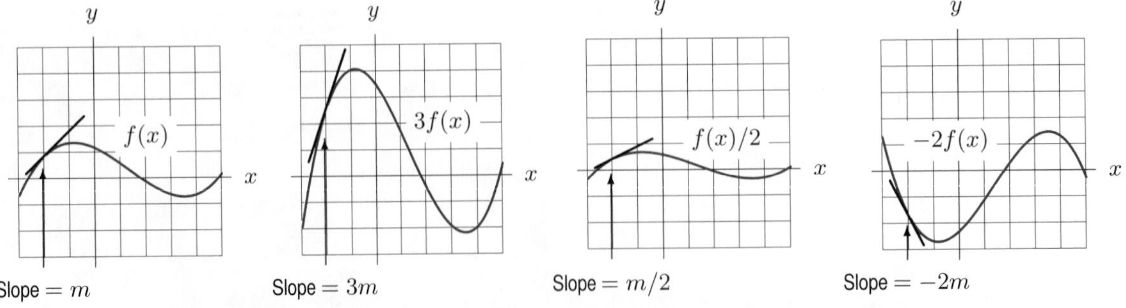

Figure 3.2: A function and its multiples: Derivative of multiple is multiple of derivative

Multiplying by a constant stretches or shrinks the graph (and reflects it about the x-axis if the constant is negative). This changes the slope of the curve at each point. If the graph has been stretched, the "rises" have all been increased by the same factor, whereas the "runs" remain the same. Thus, the slopes are all steeper by the same factor. If the graph has been shrunk, the slopes are all smaller by the same factor. If the graph has been reflected about the x-axis, the slopes will all have their signs reversed. Thus, if a function is multiplied by a constant, c, so is its derivative:

Derivative of a Constant Multiple

If c is a constant,

$$\frac{d}{dx}[cf(x)] = cf'(x).$$

Derivatives of Sums and Differences

Values of two functions, $f(x)$ and $g(x)$, and their sum $f(x) + g(x)$, are listed in Table 3.1.

Table 3.1 *Sum of functions*

x	$f(x)$	$g(x)$	$f(x)+g(x)$
0	100	0	100
1	110	0.2	110.2
2	130	0.4	130.4
3	160	0.6	160.6
4	200	0.8	200.8

We see that adding the increments of $f(x)$ and the increments of $g(x)$ gives the increments of $f(x) + g(x)$. For example, as x increases from 0 to 1, $f(x)$ increases by 10 and $g(x)$ increases by 0.2, while $f(x)+g(x)$ increases by $110.2 - 100 = 10.2$. Similarly, as x increases from 3 to 4, $f(x)$ increases by 40 and $g(x)$ by 0.2, while $f(x) + g(x)$ increases by $200.8 - 160.6 = 40.2$.

From this example, we see that the rate at which $f(x)+g(x)$ is increasing is the sum of the rates at which $f(x)$ and $g(x)$ are increasing. Similar reasoning applies to the difference, $f(x) - g(x)$. In terms of derivatives:

Derivative of Sum and Difference

$$\frac{d}{dx}[f(x) + g(x)] = f'(x) + g'(x) \quad \text{and} \quad \frac{d}{dx}[f(x) - g(x)] = f'(x) - g'(x).$$

Powers of x

We start by looking at $f(x) = x^2$ and $g(x) = x^3$. We show in the Focus on Theory section at the end of this chapter that

$$f'(x) = \frac{d}{dx}(x^2) = 2x \quad \text{and} \quad g'(x) = \frac{d}{dx}(x^3) = 3x^2.$$

The graphs of $f(x) = x^2$ and $g(x) = x^3$ and their derivatives are shown in Figures 3.3 and 3.4. Notice $f'(x) = 2x$ has the behavior we expect. It is negative for $x < 0$ (when f is decreasing), zero for $x = 0$, and positive for $x > 0$ (when f is increasing). Similarly, $g'(x) = 3x^2$ is zero when $x = 0$, but positive everywhere else, as g is increasing everywhere else. These examples are special cases of the power rule.

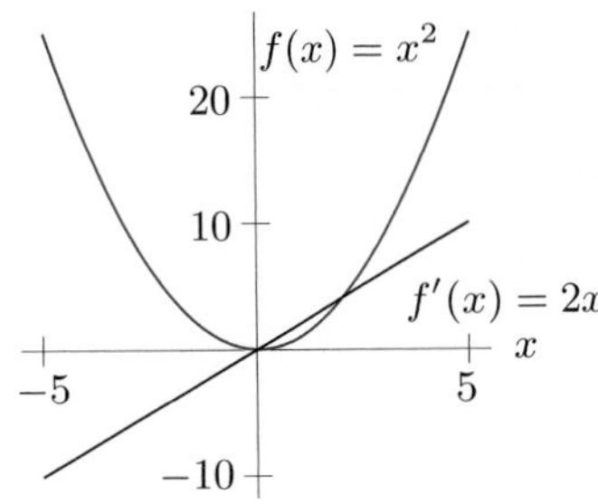

Figure 3.3: Graphs of $f(x) = x^2$ and its derivative $f'(x) = 2x$

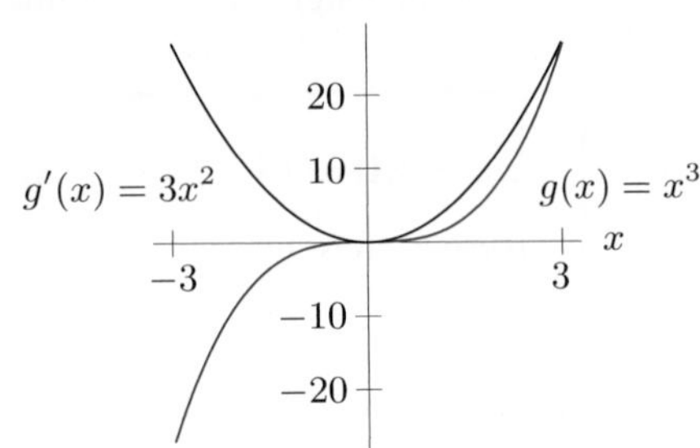

Figure 3.4: Graphs of $g(x) = x^3$ and its derivative $g'(x) = 3x^2$

The Power Rule

For any constant real number n,

$$\frac{d}{dx}(x^n) = nx^{n-1}.$$

Example 1 Find the derivative of (a) $h(x) = x^8$ (b) $P(t) = t^7$.

Solution (a) $h'(x) = 8x^7$. (b) $P'(t) = 7t^6$.

Derivatives of Polynomials

Using the derivatives of powers, constant multiples, and sums, we can differentiate any polynomial.

Example 2 Differentiate:

(a) $A(t) = 3t^5$ (b) $r(p) = p^5 + p^3$

(c) $f(x) = 5x^2 - 7x^3$ (d) $g(t) = \dfrac{t^2}{4} + 3$

Solution (a) Using the constant multiple rule: $A'(t) = \frac{d}{dt}(3t^5) = 3\frac{d}{dt}(t^5) = 3 \cdot 5t^4 = 15t^4$.

(b) Using the sum rule: $r'(p) = \frac{d}{dp}(p^5 + p^3) = \frac{d}{dp}(p^5) + \frac{d}{dp}(p^3) = 5p^4 + 3p^2$.

(c) Using both rules together:

$$\begin{aligned} f'(x) = \frac{d}{dx}(5x^2 - 7x^3) &= \frac{d}{dx}(5x^2) - \frac{d}{dx}(7x^3) && \text{Derivative of difference} \\ &= 5\frac{d}{dx}(x^2) - 7\frac{d}{dx}(x^3) && \text{Derivative of multiple} \\ &= 5(2x) - 7(3x^2) = 10x - 21x^2. \end{aligned}$$

(d) Using both rules:

$$g'(t) = \frac{d}{dt}\left(\frac{t^2}{4} + 3\right) = \frac{1}{4}\frac{d}{dt}(t^2) + \frac{d}{dt}(3)$$
$$= \frac{1}{4}(2t) + 0 = \frac{t}{2}.$$

Since the derivative of a constant, $\frac{d}{dt}(3)$, is zero.

We can use the power rule to differentiate negative and fractional powers.

Example 3 Use the power rule to differentiate (a) $\frac{1}{x^3}$ (b) $\sqrt{x}$ (c) $2t^{4.5}$.

Solution (a) For $n = -3$: $\frac{d}{dx}\left(\frac{1}{x^3}\right) = \frac{d}{dx}(x^{-3}) = -3x^{-3-1} = -3x^{-4} = -\frac{3}{x^4}.$

(b) For $n = 1/2$: $\frac{d}{dx}(\sqrt{x}) = \frac{d}{dx}\left(x^{1/2}\right) = \frac{1}{2}x^{(1/2)-1} = \frac{1}{2}x^{-1/2} = \frac{1}{2\sqrt{x}}.$

(c) For $n = 4.5$: $\frac{d}{dt}\left(2t^{4.5}\right) = 2\left(4.5t^{4.5-1}\right) = 9t^{3.5}.$

Using the Derivative Formulas

Since the slope of the tangent line to a curve is given by the derivative, we use differentiation to find the equation of the tangent line.

Example 4 Find an equation for the tangent line at $x = 1$ to the graph of

$$y = x^3 + 2x^2 - 5x + 7.$$

Sketch the graph of the curve and its tangent line on the same axes.

Solution Differentiating gives

$$\frac{dy}{dx} = 3x^2 + 2(2x) - 5(1) + 0 = 3x^2 + 4x - 5,$$

so the slope of the tangent line at $x = 1$ is

$$m = \left.\frac{dy}{dx}\right|_{x=1} = 3(1)^2 + 4(1) - 5 = 2.$$

When $x = 1$, we have $y = 1^3 + 2(1^2) - 5(1) + 7 = 5$, so the point $(1, 5)$ lies on the tangent line. Using the formula $y - y_0 = m(x - x_0)$ gives

$$y - 5 = 2(x - 1)$$
$$y = 3 + 2x.$$

The equation of the tangent line is $y = 3 + 2x$. See Figure 3.5.

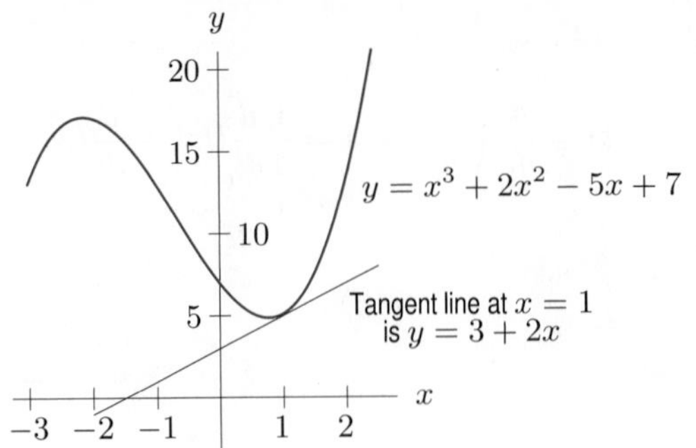

Figure 3.5: Find the equation for this tangent line

Example 5 Find and interpret the second derivatives of (a) $f(x) = x^2$ (b) $g(x) = x^3$.

Solution

(a) Differentiating $f(x) = x^2$ gives $f'(x) = 2x$, so $f''(x) = \dfrac{d}{dx}(2x) = 2$. Since f'' is always positive, the graph of f is concave up, as expected for a parabola opening upward. (See Figure 3.6.)

(b) Differentiating $g(x) = x^3$ gives $g'(x) = 3x^2$, so $g''(x) = \dfrac{d}{dx}(3x^2) = 3\dfrac{d}{dx}(x^2) = 3 \cdot 2x = 6x$. This is positive for $x > 0$ and negative for $x < 0$, which means that the graph of $g(x) = x^3$ is concave up for $x > 0$ and concave down for $x < 0$. (See Figure 3.7.)

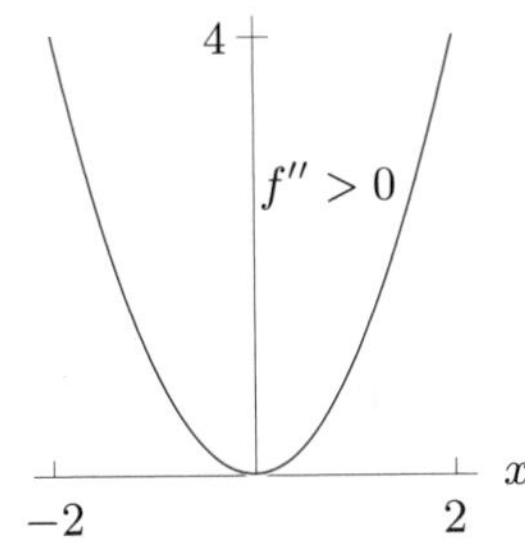

Figure 3.6: Graph of $f(x) = x^2$ with $f''(x) = 2$

Figure 3.7: Graph of $g(x) = x^3$ with $g''(x) = 6x$

Example 6 The revenue (in dollars) from producing q units of a product is given by

$$R(q) = 1000q - 3q^2.$$

Find $R(125)$ and $R'(125)$. Give units and interpret your answers.

Solution We have

$$R(125) = 100 \cdot 125 - 3 \cdot 125^2 = 78{,}125 \text{ dollars}.$$

Since $R'(q) = 1000 - 6q$, we have

$$R'(125) = 1000 - 6 \cdot 125 = 250 \text{ dollars per unit}.$$

If 125 units are produced, the revenue is 78,125 dollars. If one additional unit is produced, revenue increases by about $250.

Example 7 Figure 3.8 shows the graph of a cubic polynomial. Both graphically and algebraically, describe the behavior of the derivative of this cubic.

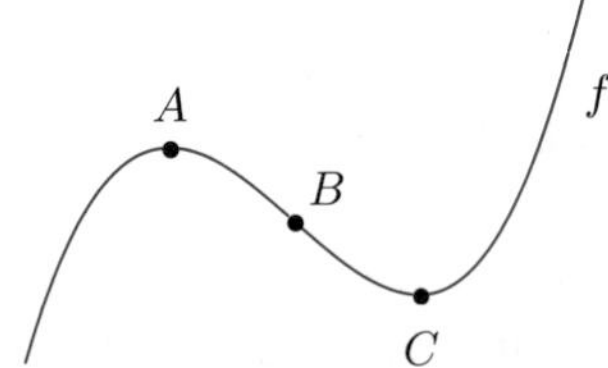

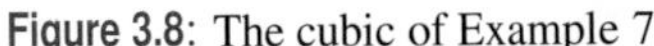

Figure 3.8: The cubic of Example 7

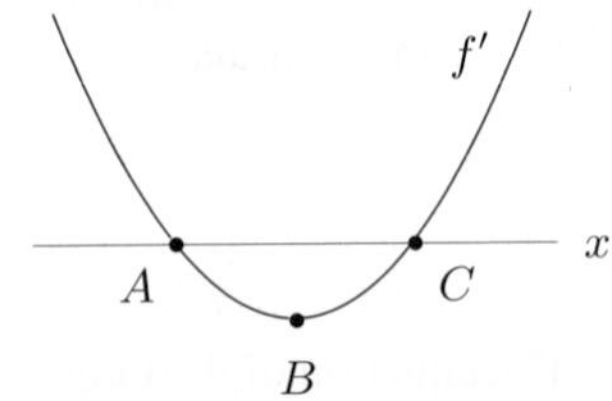

Figure 3.9: Derivative of the cubic of Example 7

Solution

Graphical approach: Suppose we move along the curve from left to right. To the left of A, the slope is positive; it starts very positive and decreases until the curve reaches A, where the slope is 0. Between A and C the slope is negative. Between A and B the slope is decreasing (getting more negative); it is most negative at B. Between B and C the slope is negative but increasing; at C the slope is zero. From C to the right, the slope is positive and increasing. The graph of the derivative function is shown in Figure 3.9.

Algebraic approach: f is a cubic that goes to $+\infty$ as $x \to +\infty$, so

$$f(x) = ax^3 + bx^2 + cx + d$$

with $a > 0$. Hence,

$$f'(x) = 3ax^2 + 2bx + c,$$

whose graph is a parabola opening upward, as in Figure 3.9.

Problems for Section 3.1

For Problems 1–36, find the derivative. Assume a, b, c, k are constants.

1. $y = 5$

2. $y = 3x$

3. $y = x^{12}$

4. $y = x^{-12}$

5. $y = x^{4/3}$

6. $y = 8t^3$

7. $y = 3t^4 - 2t^2$

8. $y = 5x + 13$

9. $f(x) = \dfrac{1}{x^4}$

10. $f(q) = q^3 + 10$

11. $y = x^2 + 5x + 9$

12. $y = 6x^3 + 4x^2 - 2x$

13. $y = 3x^2 + 7x - 9$

14. $y = 8t^3 - 4t^2 + 12t - 3$

15. $y = 4.2q^2 - 0.5q + 11.27$

16. $y = -3x^4 - 4x^3 - 6x + 2$

17. $g(t) = \dfrac{1}{t^5}$

18. $f(z) = -\dfrac{1}{z^{6.1}}$

19. $y = \dfrac{1}{r^{7/2}}$

20. $y = \sqrt{x}$

21. $h(\theta) = \dfrac{1}{\sqrt[3]{\theta}}$

22. $f(x) = \sqrt{\dfrac{1}{x^3}}$

23. $y = 3t^5 - 5\sqrt{t} + \dfrac{7}{t}$

24. $y = z^2 + \dfrac{1}{2z}$

25. $y = 3t^2 + \dfrac{12}{\sqrt{t}} - \dfrac{1}{t^2}$

26. $h(t) = \dfrac{3}{t} + \dfrac{4}{t^2}$

27. $y = \sqrt{x}(x + 1)$

28. $h(\theta) = \theta(\theta^{-1/2} - \theta^{-2})$

29. $f(x) = kx^2$

30. $y = ax^2 + bx + c$

31. $Q = aP^2 + bP^3$

32. $v = at^2 + \dfrac{b}{t^2}$

33. $P = a + b\sqrt{t}$

34. $V = \frac{4}{3}\pi r^2 b$

35. $w = 3ab^2 q$

36. $h(x) = \dfrac{ax + b}{c}$

37. **(a)** Use a graph of $P(q) = 6q - q^2$ to determine whether each of the following derivatives is positive, negative, or zero: $P'(1)$, $P'(3)$, $P'(4)$. Explain.
(b) Find $P'(q)$ and the three derivatives in part (a).

38. Let $f(x) = x^3 - 4x^2 + 7x - 11$. Find $f'(0)$, $f'(2)$, $f'(-1)$.

39. Let $f(t) = t^2 - 4t + 5$.

(a) Find $f'(t)$.
(b) Find $f'(1)$ and $f'(2)$.
(c) Use a graph of $f(t)$ to check that your answers to part (b) are reasonable. Explain.

40. Find the rate of change of a population of size $P(t) = t^3 + 4t + 1$ at time $t = 2$.

41. The height of a sand dune (in centimeters) is represented by $f(t) = 700 - 3t^2$, where t is measured in years since 2005. Find $f(5)$ and $f'(5)$. Using units, explain what each means in terms of the sand dune.

42. Zebra mussels are freshwater shellfish that first appeared in the St. Lawrence River in the early 1980s and have spread throughout the Great Lakes. Suppose that t months after they appeared in a small bay, the number of zebra mussels is given by $Z(t) = 300t^2$. How many zebra mussels are in the bay after four months? At what rate is the population growing at that time? Give units.

43. The quantity, Q, in tons, of material at a municipal waste site is a function of the number of years since 2000, with

$$Q = f(t) = 3t^2 + 100.$$

Find $f(10)$, $f'(10)$, and the relative rate of change f'/f at $t = 10$. Interpret your answers in terms of waste.

44. The number, N, of acres of harvested land in a region is given by

$$N = f(t) = 120\sqrt{t},$$

where t is the number of years since farming began in the region. Find $f(9)$, $f'(9)$, and the relative rate of change f'/f at $t = 9$. Interpret your answers in terms of harvested land.

45. If $f(t) = 2t^3 - 4t^2 + 3t - 1$, find $f'(t)$ and $f''(t)$.

46. If $f(t) = t^4 - 3t^2 + 5t$, find $f'(t)$ and $f''(t)$.

47. The time, T, in seconds for one complete oscillation of a pendulum is given by $T = f(L) = 1.111\sqrt{L}$, where L is the length of the pendulum in feet. Find the following quantities, with units, and interpret in terms of the pendulum.

(a) $f(100)$ **(b)** $f'(100)$.

48. Kleiber's Law states that the daily calorie requirement, $C(w)$, of a mammal is proportional to the mammal's body weight w raised to the 0.75 power.[1] If body weight is measured in pounds, the constant of proportionality is approximately 42.

(a) Give formulas for $C(w)$ and $C'(w)$.
(b) Find and interpret
(i) $C(10)$ and $C'(10)$
(ii) $C(100)$ and $C'(100)$
(iii) $C(1000)$ and $C'(1000)$

49. Find the equation of the line tangent to the graph of f at $(1, 1)$, where f is given by $f(x) = 2x^3 - 2x^2 + 1$.

50. **(a)** Find the equation of the tangent line to $f(x) = x^3$ at the point where $x = 2$.
(b) Graph the tangent line and the function on the same axes. If the tangent line is used to estimate values of the function, will the estimates be overestimates or underestimates?

51. Find the equation of the line tangent to the graph of $f(t) = 6t - t^2$ at $t = 4$. Sketch the graph of $f(t)$ and the tangent line on the same axes.

52. If you are outdoors, the wind may make it feel a lot colder than the thermometer reads. You feel the windchill temperature, which, if the air temperature is 20°F, is given in °F by $W(v) = 48.17 - 27.2v^{0.16}$, where v is the wind velocity in mph for $5 \leq v \leq 60$.[2]

(a) If the air temperature is 20°F, and the wind is blowing at 40 mph, what is the windchill temperature, to the nearest degree?
(b) Find $W'(40)$, and explain what this means in terms of windchill.

53. **(a)** Use the formula for the area of a circle of radius r, $A = \pi r^2$, to find dA/dr.
(b) The result from part (a) should look familiar. What does dA/dr represent geometrically?
(c) Use the difference quotient to explain the observation you made in part (b).

54. Suppose W is proportional to r^3. The derivative dW/dr is proportional to what power of r?

55. The cost to produce q items is $C(q) = 1000 + 2q^2$ dollars. Find the marginal cost of producing the 25th item. Interpret your answer in terms of costs.

56. The demand curve for a product is given by $q = 300 - 3p$, where p is the price of the product and q is the quantity that consumers buy at this price.

(a) Write the revenue as a function, $R(p)$, of price.
(b) Find $R'(10)$ and interpret your answer in terms of revenue.
(c) For what prices is $R'(p)$ positive? For what prices is it negative?

57. The yield, Y, of an apple orchard (measured in bushels of apples per acre) is a function of the amount x of fertilizer in pounds used per acre. Suppose

$$Y = f(x) = 320 + 140x - 10x^2.$$

(a) What is the yield if 5 pounds of fertilizer is used per acre?
(b) Find $f'(5)$. Give units with your answer and interpret it in terms of apples and fertilizer.
(c) Given your answer to part (b), should more or less fertilizer be used? Explain.

58. The demand for a product is given, for $p, q \geq 0$, by

$$p = f(q) = 50 - 0.03q^2.$$

(a) Find the p- and q-intercepts for this function and interpret them in terms of demand for this product.
(b) Find $f(20)$ and give units with your answer. Explain what it tells you in terms of demand.
(c) Find $f'(20)$ and give units with your answer. Explain what it tells you in terms of demand.

59. The cost (in dollars) of producing q items is given by $C(q) = 0.08q^3 + 75q + 1000$.

(a) Find the marginal cost function.
(b) Find $C(50)$ and $C'(50)$. Give units with your answers and explain what each is telling you about costs of production.

60. A ball is dropped from the top of the Empire State Building. The height, y, of the ball above the ground (in feet) is given as a function of time, t, (in seconds) by

$$y = 1250 - 16t^2.$$

(a) Find the velocity of the ball at time t. What is the sign of the velocity? Why is this to be expected?
(b) When does the ball hit the ground, and how fast is it going at that time? Give your answer in feet per second and in miles per hour (1 ft/sec = 15/22 mph).

61. Let $f(x) = x^3 - 6x^2 - 15x + 20$. Find $f'(x)$ and all values of x for which $f'(x) = 0$. Explain the relationship between these values of x and the graph of $f(x)$.

62. Show that for any power function $f(x) = x^n$, we have $f'(1) = n$.

63. If the demand curve is a line, we can write $p = b + mq$, where p is the price of the product, q is the quantity sold at that price, and b and m are constants.

(a) Write the revenue as a function of quantity sold.
(b) Find the marginal revenue function.

[1] Strogatz, S., "Math and the City", *The New York Times*, May 20, 2009.
[2] www.weather.gov/om/windchill/index.shtml Accessed on 4/21/09.

3.2 EXPONENTIAL AND LOGARITHMIC FUNCTIONS

The Exponential Function

What do we expect the graph of the derivative of the exponential function $f(x) = a^x$ to look like? The graph of an exponential function with $a > 1$ is shown in Figure 3.10. The function increases slowly for $x < 0$ and more rapidly for $x > 0$, so the values of f' are small for $x < 0$ and larger for $x > 0$. Since the function is increasing for all values of x, the graph of the derivative must lie above the x-axis. In fact, the graph of f' resembles the graph of f itself. We will see how this observation holds for $f(x) = 2^x$ and $g(x) = 3^x$.

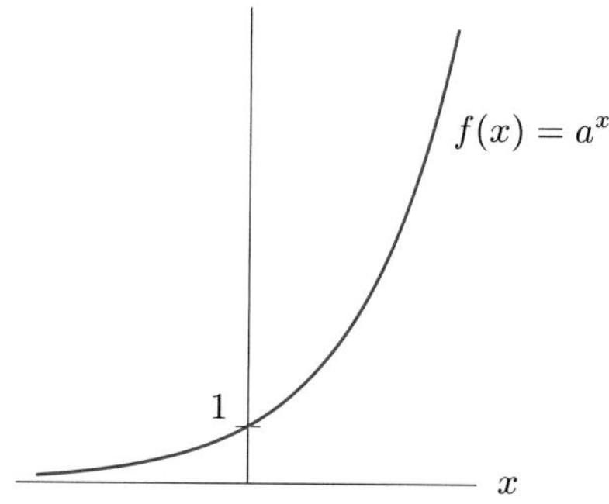

Figure 3.10: $f(x) = a^x$, with $a > 1$

The Derivatives of 2^x and 3^x

In Section 2.1,we estimated the derivative of $f(x) = 2^x$ at $x = 0$:

$$f'(0) \approx 0.693.$$

By estimating the derivative at other values of x, we obtain the graph in Figure 3.11. Since the graph of f' looks like the graph of f stretched vertically, we assume that f' is a multiple of f. Since $f'(0) \approx 0.693 = 0.693 \cdot 1 = 0.693f(0)$, the multiplier is approximately 0.693, which suggests that

$$\frac{d}{dx}(2^x) = f'(x) \approx (0.693)2^x.$$

Similarly, in Figure 3.12, the derivative of $g(x) = 3^x$ is a multiple of g, with multiplier $g'(0) \approx 1.0986$. So

$$\frac{d}{dx}(3^x) = g'(x) \approx (1.0986)3^x.$$

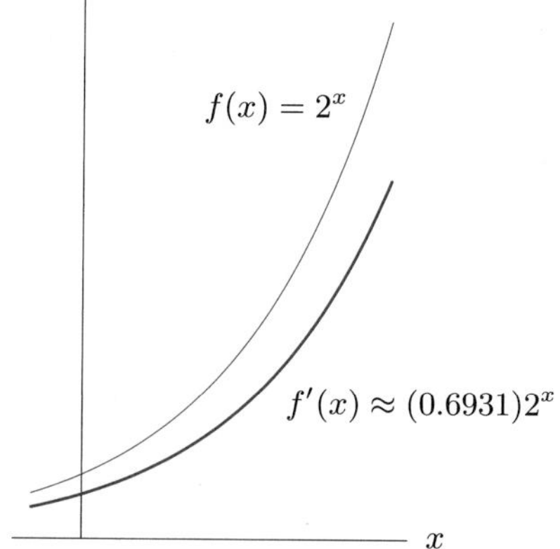

Figure 3.11: Graph of $f(x) = 2^x$ and its derivative

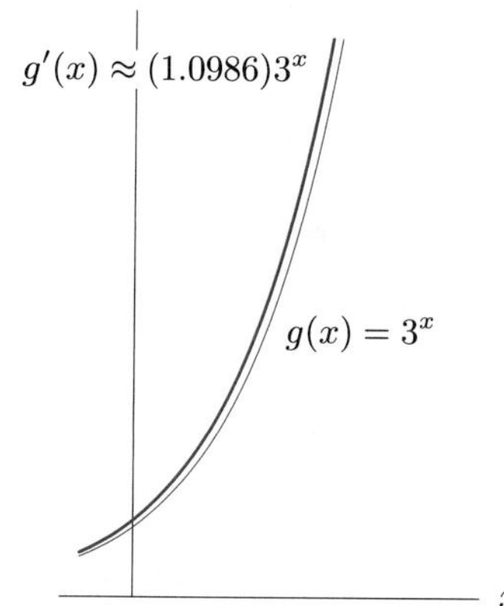

Figure 3.12: Graph of $g(x) = 3^x$ and its derivative

The Derivative of a^x and the Number e

The calculation of the derivative of $f(x) = a^x$, for $a > 0$, is similar to that of 2^x and 3^x. The derivative is again proportional to the original function. When $a = 2$, the constant of proportionality (0.6931) is less than 1, and the derivative is smaller than the original function. When $a = 3$, the constant of proportionality (1.0986) is more than 1, and the derivative is greater than the original function. Is there an in-between case, when derivative and function are exactly equal? In other words:

$$\text{Is there a value of } a \text{ that makes } \frac{d}{dx}(a^x) = a^x?$$

The answer is yes: the value is $a \approx 2.718\ldots$, the number e introduced in Chapter 1. This means that the function e^x is its own derivative:

$$\boxed{\frac{d}{dx}(e^x) = e^x.}$$

It turns out that the constants involved in the derivatives of 2^x and 3^x are natural logarithms. In fact, since $0.6931 \approx \ln 2$ and $1.0986 \approx \ln 3$, we (correctly) guess that

$$\frac{d}{dx}(2^x) = (\ln 2)2^x \quad \text{and} \quad \frac{d}{dx}(3^x) = (\ln 3)3^x.$$

In the Focus on Theory section at the end of this chapter, we show that, in general:

The Exponential Rule

For any positive constant a,

$$\frac{d}{dx}(a^x) = (\ln a)a^x.$$

Since $\ln a$ is a constant, the derivative of a^x is proportional to a^x. Many quantities have rates of change that are proportional to themselves; for example, the simplest model of population growth has this property. The fact that the constant of proportionality is 1 when $a = e$ makes e a particularly useful base for exponential functions.

Example 1 Differentiate $2 \cdot 3^x + 5e^x$.

Solution We have $\frac{d}{dx}(2 \cdot 3^x + 5e^x) = 2\frac{d}{dx}(3^x) + 5\frac{d}{dx}(e^x) = 2\ln 3 \cdot 3^x + 5e^x$.

The Derivative of e^{kt}

Since functions of the form e^{kt} where k is a constant are often useful, we calculate the derivative of e^{kt}. Since $e^{kt} = (e^k)^t$, the derivative is $(\ln(e^k))(e^k)^t = (k\ln e)(e^{kt}) = ke^{kt}$. Thus, if k is a constant,

$$\boxed{\frac{d}{dt}(e^{kt}) = ke^{kt}.}$$

Example 2 Find the derivative of $P = 5 + 3x^2 - 7e^{-0.2x}$.

Solution The derivative is

$$\frac{dP}{dx} = 0 + 3(2x) - 7(-0.2e^{-0.2x}) = 6x + 1.4e^{-0.2x}.$$

The Derivative of ln x

What does the graph of the derivative of the logarithmic function $f(x) = \ln x$ look like? Figure 3.13 shows that $\ln x$ is increasing, so its derivative is positive. The graph of $f(x) = \ln x$ is concave down, so the derivative is decreasing. Furthermore, the slope of $f(x) = \ln x$ is very large near $x = 0$ and very small for large x, so the derivative tends to $+\infty$ for x near 0 and tends to 0 for very large x. See Figure 3.14. It turns out that

$$\frac{d}{dx}(\ln x) = \frac{1}{x}.$$

We give an algebraic justification for this rule in the Focus on Theory section.

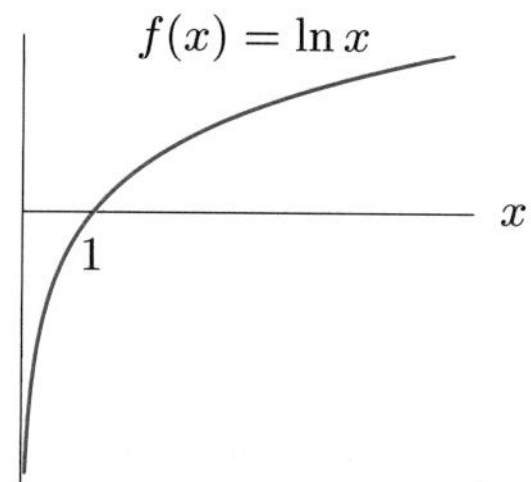

Figure 3.13: Graph of $f(x) = \ln x$

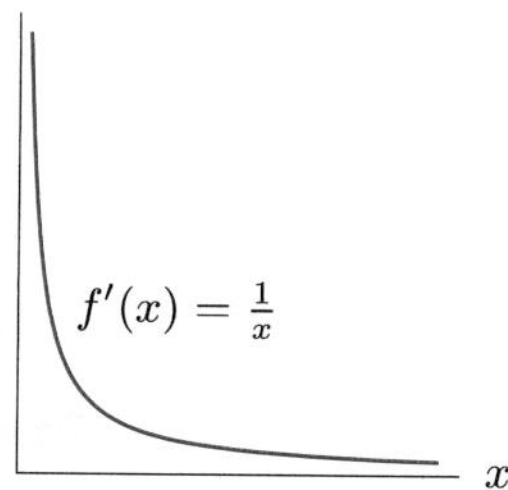

Figure 3.14: Graph of the derivative of $f(x) = \ln x$

Example 3 Differentiate $y = 5\ln t + 7e^t - 4t^2 + 12$.

Solution We have

$$\begin{aligned}\frac{d}{dt}(5\ln t + 7e^t - 4t^2 + 12) &= 5\frac{d}{dt}(\ln t) + 7\frac{d}{dt}(e^t) - 4\frac{d}{dt}(t^2) + \frac{d}{dt}(12) \\ &= 5\left(\frac{1}{t}\right) + 7(e^t) - 4(2t) + 0 \\ &= \frac{5}{t} + 7e^t - 8t.\end{aligned}$$

Using the Derivative Formulas

Example 4 In Chapter 1, we saw that the population of Nevada, P, in millions, can be approximated by

$$P = 2.020(1.036)^t,$$

where t is years since the start of 2000. At what rate was the population growing at the beginning of 2009? Give units with your answer.

Solution The instantaneous rate of growth is the derivative, so we want dP/dt when $t = 9$. We have:

$$\frac{dP}{dt} = \frac{d}{dt}(2.020(1.036)^t) = 2.020(\ln 1.036)(1.036)^t = 0.0714(1.036)^t.$$

Substituting $t = 9$ gives

$$0.0714(1.036)^9 = 0.0982.$$

The population of Nevada was growing at a rate of about 0.0982 million, or 98,200, people per year at the start of 2009.

Example 5 Find the equation of the tangent line to the graph of $f(x) = \ln x$ at the point where $x = 2$. Draw a graph with $f(x)$ and the tangent line on the same axes.

Solution Since $f'(x) = 1/x$, the slope of the tangent line at $x = 2$ is $f'(2) = 1/2 = 0.5$. When $x = 2$, $y = \ln 2 = 0.693$, so a point on the tangent line is $(2, 0.693)$. Substituting into the equation for a line, we have:

$$y - 0.693 = 0.5(x - 2)$$
$$y = -0.307 + 0.5x.$$

The equation of the tangent line is $y = -0.307 + 0.5x$. See Figure 3.15.

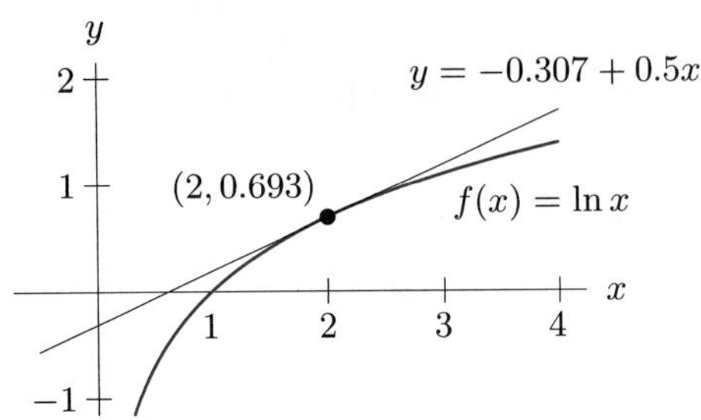

Figure 3.15: Graph of $f(x) = \ln x$ and a tangent line

Example 6 Suppose $1000 is deposited into a bank account that pays 8% annual interest, compounded continuously.

(a) Find a formula $f(t)$ for the balance t years after the initial deposit.
(b) Find $f(10)$ and $f'(10)$ and explain what your answers mean in terms of money.

Solution (a) The balance is $f(t) = 1000e^{0.08t}$.
(b) Substituting $t = 10$ gives

$$f(10) = 1000e^{(0.08)(10)} = 2225.54.$$

This means that the balance is $2225.54 after 10 years.

To find $f'(10)$, we compute $f'(t) = 1000(0.08e^{0.08t}) = 80e^{0.08t}$. Therefore,

$$f'(10) = 80e^{(0.08)(10)} = 178.04.$$

This means that after 10 years, the balance is growing at the rate of about $178 per year.

Problems for Section 3.2

Differentiate the functions in Problems 1–28. Assume that A, B, and C are constants.

1. $f(x) = 2e^x + x^2$

2. $P = 3t^3 + 2e^t$

3. $y = 5t^2 + 4e^t$

4. $f(x) = x^3 + 3^x$

5. $y = 2^x + \dfrac{2}{x^3}$

6. $y = 5 \cdot 5^t + 6 \cdot 6^t$

7. $f(x) = 2^x + 2 \cdot 3^x$

8. $y = 4 \cdot 10^x - x^3$

9. $y = 3x - 2 \cdot 4^x$

10. $y = 5 \cdot 2^x - 5x + 4$

11. $f(t) = e^{3t}$

12. $y = e^{0.7t}$

13. $y = e^{-4t}$

14. $P = e^{-0.2t}$

15. $P = 50e^{-0.6t}$

16. $P = 200e^{0.12t}$

17. $P(t) = 3000(1.02)^t$

18. $P(t) = 12.41(0.94)^t$

19. $P(t) = Ce^t$.

20. $y = B + Ae^t$

21. $f(x) = Ae^x - Bx^2 + C$

22. $y = 10^x + \dfrac{10}{x}$

23. $R = 3\ln q$

24. $D = 10 - \ln p$

25. $y = t^2 + 5\ln t$

26. $R(q) = q^2 - 2\ln q$

27. $y = x^2 + 4x - 3\ln x$

28. $f(t) = Ae^t + B\ln t$

29. For $f(t) = 4-2e^t$, find $f'(-1)$, $f'(0)$, and $f'(1)$. Graph $f(t)$, and draw tangent lines at $t = -1$, $t = 0$, and $t = 1$. Do the slopes of the lines match the derivatives you found?

30. Find the equation of the tangent line to the graph of $y = 3^x$ at $x = 1$. Check your work by sketching a graph of the function and the tangent line on the same axes.

31. Find the equation of the tangent line to $y = e^{-2t}$ at $t = 0$. Check by sketching the graphs of $y = e^{-2t}$ and the tangent line on the same axes.

32. Find the equation of the tangent line to $f(x) = 10e^{-0.2x}$ at $x = 4$.

33. A fish population is approximated by $P(t) = 10e^{0.6t}$, where t is in months. Calculate and use units to explain what each of the following tells us about the population:

(a) $P(12)$ **(b)** $P'(12)$

34. The world's population is about $f(t) = 6.8e^{0.012t}$ billion,[3] where t is time in years since 2009. Find $f(0)$, $f'(0)$, $f(10)$, and $f'(10)$. Using units, interpret your answers in terms of population.

35. The demand curve for a product is given by

$$q = f(p) = 10{,}000e^{-0.25p},$$

where q is the quantity sold and p is the price of the product, in dollars. Find $f(2)$ and $f'(2)$. Explain in economic terms what information each of these answers gives you.

36. Worldwide production of solar power, in megawatts, can be modeled by $f(t) = 1040(1.3)^t$, where t is years[4] since 2000. Find $f(0)$, $f'(0)$, $f(15)$, and $f'(15)$. Give units and interpret your answers in terms of solar power.

37. A new DVD is available for sale in a store one week after its release. The cumulative revenue, $\$R$, from sales of the DVD in this store in week t after its release is

$$R = f(t) = 350 \ln t \quad \text{with} \quad t > 1.$$

Find $f(5)$, $f'(5)$, and the relative rate of change f'/f at $t = 5$. Interpret your answers in terms of revenue.

38. In 2009, the population of Hungary[5] was approximated by

$$P = 9.906(0.997)^t,$$

where P is in millions and t is in years since 2009. Assume the trend continues.

(a) What does this model predict for the population of Hungary in the year 2020?

(b) How fast (in people/year) does this model predict Hungary's population will be decreasing in 2020?

39. With t in years since January 1, 2010, the population P of Slim Chance is predicted by

$$P = 35{,}000(0.98)^t.$$

At what rate will the population be changing on January 1, 2023?

40. Some antique furniture increased very rapidly in price over the past decade. For example, the price of a particular rocking chair is well approximated by

$$V = 75(1.35)^t,$$

where V is in dollars and t is in years since 2000. Find the rate, in dollars per year, at which the price is increasing at time t.

41. Find the value of c in Figure 3.16, where the line l tangent to the graph of $y = 2^x$ at $(0, 1)$ intersects the x-axis.

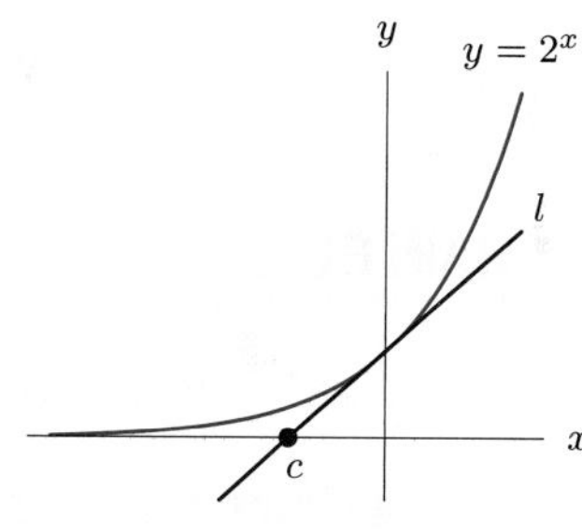

Figure 3.16

42. At a time t hours after it was administered, the concentration of a drug in the body is $f(t) = 27e^{-0.14t}$ ng/ml. What is the concentration 4 hours after it was administered? At what rate is the concentration changing at that time?

43. The cost of producing a quantity, q, of a product is given by

$$C(q) = 1000 + 30e^{0.05q} \quad \text{dollars.}$$

Find the cost and the marginal cost when $q = 50$. Interpret these answers in economic terms.

44. With time, t, in minutes, the temperature, H, in degrees Celsius, of a bottle of water put in the refrigerator at $t = 0$ is given by

$$H = 4 + 16e^{-0.02t}.$$

How fast is the water cooling initially? After 10 minutes? Give units.

[3] www.census/gov/ipc/www/popclockworld.html and www.cia.gov/library/publications/the-world-factbook/print/xx.html.

[4] https://www.solarbuzz.com/FastFactsIndustry.htm, accessed 4/14/09.

[5] https://www.cia.gov/library/publications/the-world-factbook/print/hu.html, accessed 4/14/09.

45. Carbon-14 is a radioactive isotope used to date objects. If A_0 represents the initial amount of carbon-14 in the object, then the quantity remaining at time t, in years, is

$$A(t) = A_0 e^{-0.000121t}.$$

(a) A tree, originally containing 185 micrograms of carbon-14, is now 500 years old. At what rate is the carbon-14 decaying?
(b) In 1988, scientists found that the Shroud of Turin, which was reputed to be the burial cloth of Jesus, contained 91% of the amount of carbon-14 in freshly made cloth of the same material. [6] According to this data, how old was the Shroud of Turin in 1988?

46. For the cost function $C = 1000 + 300 \ln q$ (in dollars), find the cost and the marginal cost at a production level of 500. Interpret your answers in economic terms.

47. In 2009, the population, P, of India was 1.166 billion and growing at 1.5% annually.[7]

(a) Give a formula for P in terms of time, t, measured in years since 2009.
(b) Find $\frac{dP}{dt}$, $\left.\frac{dP}{dt}\right|_{t=0}$, and $\left.\frac{dP}{dt}\right|_{t=25}$. What do each of these represent in practical terms?

48. In 2009, the population of Mexico was 111 million and growing 1.13% annually, while the population of the US was 307 million and growing 0.975% annually.[8] If we measure growth rates in people/year, which population was growing faster in 2009?

49. **(a)** Find the equation of the tangent line to $y = \ln x$ at $x = 1$.
(b) Use it to calculate approximate values for $\ln(1.1)$ and $\ln(2)$.
(c) Using a graph, explain whether the approximate values are smaller or larger than the true values. Would the same result have held if you had used the tangent line to estimate $\ln(0.9)$ and $\ln(0.5)$? Why?

50. Find the quadratic polynomial $g(x) = ax^2 + bx + c$ which best fits the function $f(x) = e^x$ at $x = 0$, in the sense that

$$g(0) = f(0), \text{ and } g'(0) = f'(0), \text{ and } g''(0) = f''(0).$$

Using a computer or calculator, sketch graphs of f and g on the same axes. What do you notice?

3.3 THE CHAIN RULE

We now see how to differentiate composite functions such as $f(t) = \ln(3t)$ and $g(x) = e^{-x^2}$.

The Derivative of a Composition of Functions

Suppose $y = f(z)$ with $z = g(t)$ for some inside function g and outside function f, where f and g are differentiable. A small change in t, called Δt, generates a small change in z, called Δz. In turn, Δz generates a small change in y, called Δy. Provided Δt and Δz are not zero, we can say

$$\frac{\Delta y}{\Delta t} = \frac{\Delta y}{\Delta z} \cdot \frac{\Delta z}{\Delta t}.$$

Since the derivative $\frac{dy}{dt}$ is the limit of the quotient $\frac{\Delta y}{\Delta t}$ as Δt gets smaller and smaller, this suggests

The Chain Rule

If $y = f(z)$ and $z = g(t)$ are differentiable, then the derivative of $y = f(g(t))$ is given by

$$\frac{dy}{dt} = \frac{dy}{dz} \cdot \frac{dz}{dt}.$$

In words, the derivative of a composite function is the derivative of the outside function times the derivative of the inside function:

$$\frac{d}{dt}(f(g(t))) = f'(g(t)) \cdot g'(t).$$

[6] The New York Times, October 18, 1988.
[7] https: //www.cia.gov/library/publications/the-world-factbook/print/in.html, accessed 4/14/09.
[8] https:/www.cia.gov/library/publications/the-world-factbook/print/ms.html and https://www.cia.gov/library/publications/the-world-factbook/print/us.html, accessed 4/14/09.

The following example shows us how to interpret the chain rule in practical terms.

Example 1 The amount of gas, G, in gallons, consumed by a car depends on the distance traveled, s, in miles, and s depends on the time, t, in hours. If 0.05 gallons of gas is consumed for each mile traveled, and the car is traveling at 30 miles/hr, how fast is gas being consumed? Give units.

Solution We expect the rate of gas consumption to be in gallons/hr. We are told that

$$\begin{array}{rl} \text{Rate gas is consumed with respect to distance} & = \dfrac{dG}{ds} = 0.05 \text{ gallons/mile} \\ \text{Rate distance is increasing with respect to time} & = \dfrac{ds}{dt} = 30 \text{ miles/hr.} \end{array}$$

We want to calculate the rate at which gas is being consumed with respect to time, or dG/dt. We think of G as a function of s, and s as a function of t. By the chain rule we know that

$$\frac{dG}{dt} = \frac{dG}{ds} \cdot \frac{ds}{dt} = \left(0.05 \frac{\text{gallons}}{\text{mile}}\right) \cdot \left(30 \frac{\text{miles}}{\text{hour}}\right) = 1.5 \text{ gallons/hour.}$$

Thus, gas is being consumed at a rate of 1.5 gallons/hour.

The Chain Rule for Functions Given by Formulas

In order to use the chain rule to differentiate a composite function, we first rewrite the function using a new variable z to represent the inside function:

$$y = (t+1)^4 \quad \text{is the same as} \quad y = z^4 \quad \text{where} \quad z = t+1.$$

Example 2 Use a new variable z for the inside function to express each of the following as a composite function:
(a) $y = \ln(3t)$ (b) $P = e^{-0.03t}$ (c) $w = 5(2r+3)^2$.

Solution (a) The inside function is $3t$, so we have $y = \ln z$ with $z = 3t$.
(b) The inside function is $-0.03t$, so we have $P = e^z$ with $z = -0.03t$.
(c) The inside function is $2r+3$, so we have $w = 5z^2$ with $z = 2r+3$.

Example 3 Find the derivative of the following functions: (a) $y = (4t^2+1)^7$ (b) $P = e^{3t}$.

Solution (a) Here $z = 4t^2+1$ is the inside function; $y = z^7$ is the outside function. Since $dy/dz = 7z^6$ and $dz/dt = 8t$, we have

$$\frac{dy}{dt} = \frac{dy}{dz} \cdot \frac{dz}{dt} = (7z^6)(8t) = 7(4t^2+1)^6(8t) = 56t(4t^2+1)^6.$$

(b) Let $z = 3t$ and $P = e^z$. Then $dP/dz = e^z$ and $dz/dt = 3$, so

$$\frac{dP}{dt} = \frac{dP}{dz} \cdot \frac{dz}{dt} = e^z \cdot 3 = e^{3t} \cdot 3 = 3e^{3t}.$$

Notice that the derivative formula for e^{kt} introduced in Section 3.2 is just a special case of the chain rule.

The derivative rules give us

$$\frac{d}{dt}(t^n) = nt^{n-1} \qquad \frac{d}{dt}(e^t) = e^t \qquad \frac{d}{dt}(\ln t) = \frac{1}{t}.$$

Using the chain rule in addition, we have the following results.

If z is a differentiable function of t, then

$$\frac{d}{dt}(z^n) = nz^{n-1}\frac{dz}{dt}, \qquad \frac{d}{dt}(e^z) = e^z\frac{dz}{dt}, \qquad \frac{d}{dt}(\ln z) = \frac{1}{z}\frac{dz}{dt}$$

Example 4 Differentiate (a) $(3t^3 - t)^5$ (b) $\ln(q^2 + 1)$ (c) e^{-x^2}.

Solution (a) Let $z = 3t^3 - t$, giving

$$\frac{d}{dt}(3t^3 - t)^5 = \frac{d}{dt}(z^5) = 5z^4\frac{dz}{dt} = 5(3t^3 - t)^4(9t^2 - 1).$$

(b) We have $z = q^2 + 1$, so

$$\frac{d}{dq}(\ln(q^2 + 1)) = \frac{d}{dq}(\ln z) = \frac{1}{z}\frac{dz}{dq} = \frac{1}{q^2 + 1}(2q).$$

(c) Since $z = -x^2$, the derivative is

$$\frac{d}{dx}(e^{-x^2}) = \frac{d}{dx}(e^z) = e^z\frac{dz}{dx} = e^{-x^2}(-2x) = -2xe^{-x^2}.$$

As we see in the following example, it is often faster to use the chain rule without introducing the new variable, z.

Example 5 Differentiate
(a) $(x^2 + 4)^3$ (b) $5\ln(2t^2 + 3)$ (c) $\sqrt{1 + 2e^{5t}}$

Solution (a) We have

$$\begin{aligned}\frac{d}{dx}\left((x^2 + 4)^3\right) &= 3(x^2 + 4)^2 \cdot \frac{d}{dx}\left(x^2 + 4\right)\\ &= 3(x^2 + 4)^2 \cdot 2x\\ &= 6x(x^2 + 4)^2.\end{aligned}$$

(b) We have

$$\begin{aligned}\frac{d}{dt}\left(5\ln(2t^2 + 3)\right) &= 5 \cdot \frac{1}{2t^2 + 3} \cdot \frac{d}{dt}\left(2t^2 + 3\right)\\ &= 5 \cdot \frac{1}{2t^2 + 3} \cdot 4t\\ &= \frac{20t}{2t^2 + 3}.\end{aligned}$$

(c) Here we use the chain rule twice, giving

$$\begin{aligned}\frac{d}{dt}\left((1 + 2e^{5t})^{1/2}\right) &= \frac{1}{2}(1 + 2e^{5t})^{-1/2} \cdot \frac{d}{dt}\left(1 + 2e^{5t}\right)\\ &= \frac{1}{2}(1 + 2e^{5t})^{-1/2} \cdot 2e^{5t} \cdot \frac{d}{dt}\left(5t\right)\\ &= \frac{1}{2}(1 + 2e^{5t})^{-1/2} \cdot 2e^{5t} \cdot 5\\ &= \frac{5e^{5t}}{\sqrt{1 + 2e^{5t}}}.\end{aligned}$$

Example 6 Let $h(x) = f(g(x))$ and $k(x) = g(f(x))$. Use Figure 3.17 to estimate: (a) $h'(1)$ (b)$k'(2)$

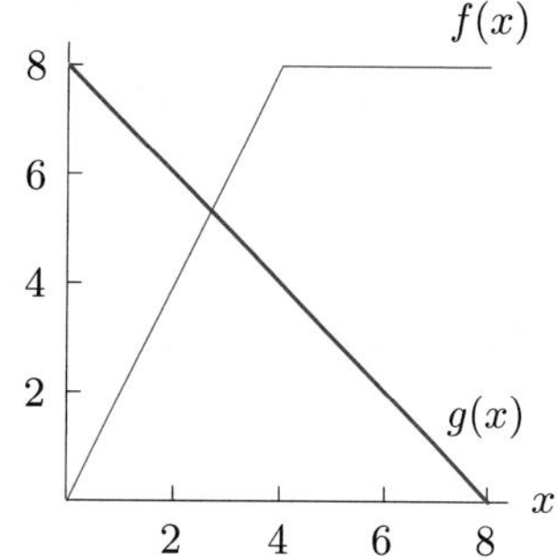

Figure 3.17: Graphs of f and g for Example 6

Solution (a) The chain rule tells us that $h'(x) = f'(g(x)) \cdot g'(x)$, so

$$\begin{aligned} h'(1) &= f'(g(1)) \cdot g'(1) \\ &= f'(7) \cdot g'(1) \\ &= 0 \cdot (-1) \\ &= 0. \end{aligned}$$

We use the slopes of the lines in Figure 3.17 to find the derivatives $f'(7) = 0$ and $g'(1) = -1$.

(b) The chain rule tells us that $k'(x) = g'(f(x)) \cdot f'(x)$, so

$$\begin{aligned} k'(2) &= g'(f(2)) \cdot f'(2) \\ &= g'(4) \cdot f'(2) \\ &= (-1) \cdot 2 \\ &= -2. \end{aligned}$$

We use slopes to compute the derivatives $g'(4) = -1$ and $f'(2) = 2$.

Relative Rates and Logarithms

In Section 2.3 we defined the relative rate of change of a function $z = f(t)$ to be

$$\text{Relative rate of change} = \frac{f'(t)}{f(t)} = \frac{1}{z}\frac{dz}{dt}.$$

Since

$$\frac{d}{dt}(\ln z) = \frac{1}{z}\frac{dz}{dt},$$

we have the following result:

> For any positive function $f(t)$,
>
> $$\begin{matrix}\text{Relative rate of change} \\ \text{of } f(t)\end{matrix} = \frac{d}{dt}(\ln f(t)).$$

Just as linear functions have constant rates of change, in the following example we see that exponential functions have constant relative rates of change.

Example 7 Find the relative rate of change of the exponential function $z = P_0e^{kt}$.

Solution Since

$$\ln z = \ln(P_0e^{kt}) = \ln P_0 + \ln(e^{kt}) = \ln P_0 + kt,$$

we have

$$\frac{d}{dt}(\ln z) = k.$$

The relative rate of change of the exponential function P_0e^{kt} is the constant k.

Example 8 The surface area S of a mammal, in cm^2, is a function of the body mass, M, of the mammal, in kilograms, and is given by $S = 1095 \cdot M^{2/3}$. Find the relative rate of change of S with respect to M and evaluate for a human with body mass 70 kilograms. Interpret your answer.

Solution We have

$$\ln S = \ln(1095 \cdot M^{2/3}) = \ln(1095) + \ln(M^{2/3}) = \ln(1095) + \frac{2}{3}\ln M.$$

Thus,

$$\begin{aligned}\text{Relative rate of change} &= \frac{d}{dM}(\ln S)\\ &= \frac{d}{dM}\left(\ln(1095) + \frac{2}{3}\ln M\right)\\ &= \frac{2}{3}\cdot\frac{1}{M}.\end{aligned}$$

For a human with body mass $M = 70$ kilograms, we have

$$\text{Relative rate} = \frac{2}{3}\frac{1}{70} = 0.0095 = 0.95\%.$$

The surface area of a human with body mass 70 kilograms increases by about 0.95% if body mass increases by 1 kilogram.

Problems for Section 3.3

Find the derivative of the functions in Problems 1–28.

1. $(4x^2+1)^7$

2. $f(x) = (x+1)^{99}$

3. $R = (q^2+1)^4$

4. $w = (t^2+1)^{100}$

5. $w = (t^3+1)^{100}$

6. $w = (5r-6)^3$

7. $y = \sqrt{s^3+1}$

8. $y = 12 - 3x^2 + 2e^{3x}$

9. $C = 12(3q^2-5)^3$

10. $f(x) = 6e^{5x} + e^{-x^2}$

11. $y = 5e^{5t+1}$

12. $w = e^{-3t^2}$

13. $w = e^{\sqrt{s}}$

14. $y = \ln(5t+1)$

15. $f(x) = \ln(1-x)$

16. $f(t) = \ln(t^2+1)$

17. $f(x) = \ln(1-e^{-x})$

18. $f(x) = \ln(e^x+1)$

19. $f(t) = 5\ln(5t+1)$

20. $g(t) = \ln(4t+9)$

21. $y = 5 + \ln(3t+2)$

22. $Q = 100(t^2+5)^{0.5}$

23. $y = 5x + \ln(x+2)$

24. $y = (5+e^x)^2$

25. $P = (1+\ln x)^{0.5}$

26. $\sqrt{e^x+1}$

27. $f(x) = \sqrt{1-x^2}$

28. $f(\theta) = (e^\theta + e^{-\theta})^{-1}$

In Problems 29–34, find the relative rate of change, $f'(t)/f(t)$, of the function $f(t)$.

29. $f(t) = 10t+5$

30. $f(t) = 15t+12$

31. $f(t) = 8e^{5t}$

32. $f(t) = 30e^{-7t}$

33. $f(t) = 6t^2$

34. $f(t) = 35t^{-4}$

In Problems 35–38, find the relative rate of change of $f(t)$ using the formula $\frac{d}{dt}\ln f(t)$.

35. $f(t) = 5e^{1.5t}$

36. $f(t) = 6.8e^{-0.5t}$

37. $f(t) = 3t^2$

38. $f(t) = 4.5t^{-4}$

39. Find the equation of the tangent line to $f(x) = (x-1)^3$ at the point where $x = 2$.

40. A firm estimates that the total revenue, R, received from the sale of q goods is given by

$$R = \ln(1 + 1000q^2).$$

Calculate the marginal revenue when $q = 10$.

41. The distance, s, of a moving body from a fixed point is given as a function of time by $s = 20e^{t/2}$. Find the velocity, v, of the body as a function of t.

42. If you invest P dollars in a bank account at an annual interest rate of $r\%$, then after t years you will have B dollars, where

$$B = P\left(1 + \frac{r}{100}\right)^t.$$

(a) Find dB/dt, assuming P and r are constant. In terms of money, what does dB/dt represent?
(b) Find dB/dr, assuming P and t are constant. In terms of money, what does dB/dr represent?

43. The distance traveled, D in feet, is a function of time, t, in seconds, with $D = f(t) = \sqrt{t^3+1}$. Find $f(10)$, $f'(10)$, and the relative rate of change f'/f at $t = 10$. Interpret your answers in terms of distance traveled.

In Problems 44–47, use Figure 3.18 to evaluate the derivative.

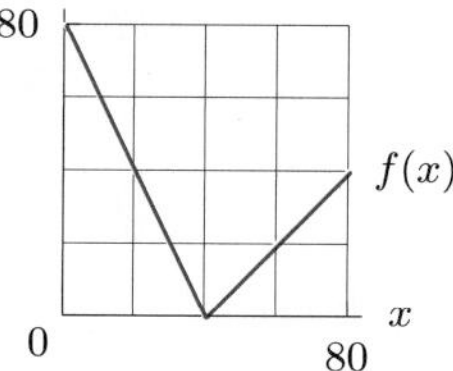

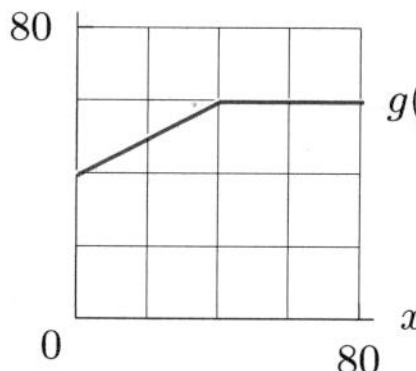

Figure 3.18

44. $\frac{d}{dx}f(g(x))|_{x=30}$

45. $\frac{d}{dx}f(g(x))|_{x=70}$

46. $\frac{d}{dx}g(f(x))|_{x=30}$

47. $\frac{d}{dx}g(f(x))|_{x=70}$

For Problems 48–51, let $h(x) = f(g(x))$ and $k(x) = g(f(x))$. Use Figure 3.19 to estimate the derivatives.

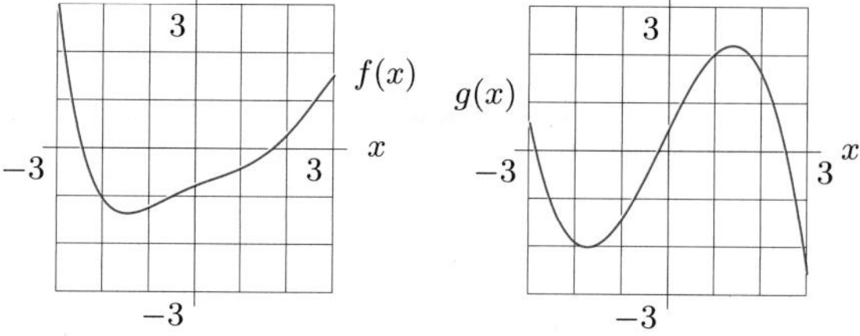

Figure 3.19

48. $h'(1)$

49. $k'(1)$

50. $h'(2)$

51. $k'(2)$

52. Some economists suggest that an extra year of education increases a person's wages, on average, by about 14%. Assume you could make \$10 per hour with your current level of education and that inflation increases wages at a continuous rate of 3.5% per year.

(a) How much would you make per hour with four additional years of education?
(b) What is the difference between your wages in 20 years' time with and without the additional four years of education?
(c) Is the difference you found in part (b) increasing with time? If so, at what rate? (Assume the number of additional years of education stays fixed at four.)

53. Show that if the graphs of $f(t)$ and $h(t) = Ae^{kt}$ are tangent at $t = a$, then k is the relative rate of change of f at $t = a$.

3.4 THE PRODUCT AND QUOTIENT RULES

This section shows how to find the derivatives of products and quotients of functions.

The Product Rule

Suppose we know the derivatives of $f(x)$ and $g(x)$ and want to calculate the derivative of the product, $f(x)g(x)$. We start by looking at an example. Let $f(x) = x$ and $g(x) = x^2$. Then

$$f(x)g(x) = x \cdot x^2 = x^3,$$

so the derivative of the product is $3x^2$. Notice that the derivative of the product is *not* equal to the product of the derivatives, since $f'(x) = 1$ and $g'(x) = 2x$, so $f'(x)g'(x) = (1)(2x) = 2x$. In general, we have the following rule, which is justified in the Focus on Theory section at the end of this chapter.

The Product Rule

If $u = f(x)$ and $v = g(x)$ are differentiable functions, then

$$(fg)' = f'g + fg'.$$

The product rule can also be written

$$\frac{d(uv)}{dx} = \frac{du}{dx} \cdot v + u \cdot \frac{dv}{dx}.$$

In words:

The derivative of a product is the derivative of the first times the second, plus the first times the derivative of the second.

We check that this rule gives the correct answers for $f(x) = x$ and $g(x) = x^2$. The derivative of $f(x)g(x)$ is

$$f'(x)g(x) + f(x)g'(x) = 1(x^2) + x(2x) = x^2 + 2x^2 = 3x^2.$$

This is the answer we expect for the derivative of $f(x)g(x) = x \cdot x^2 = x^3$.

Example 1 Differentiate (a) x^2e^{2x} (b) $t^3\ln(t+1)$ (c) $(3x^2+5x)e^x$.

Solution (a) Using the product rule, we have

$$\begin{aligned}\frac{d}{dx}(x^2e^{2x}) &= \frac{d}{dx}(x^2)\cdot e^{2x} + x^2\frac{d}{dx}(e^{2x})\\ &= (2x)e^{2x} + x^2(2e^{2x})\\ &= 2xe^{2x} + 2x^2e^{2x}.\end{aligned}$$

(b) Differentiating using the product rule gives

$$\begin{aligned}\frac{d}{dt}(t^3\ln(t+1)) &= \frac{d}{dt}(t^3)\cdot\ln(t+1) + t^3\frac{d}{dt}(\ln(t+1))\\ &= (3t^2)\ln(t+1) + t^3\left(\frac{1}{t+1}\right)\\ &= 3t^2\ln(t+1) + \frac{t^3}{t+1}.\end{aligned}$$

(c) The product rule gives

$$\begin{aligned}\frac{d}{dx}((3x^2+5x)e^x) &= \left(\frac{d}{dx}(3x^2+5x)\right)e^x + (3x^2+5x)\frac{d}{dx}(e^x)\\ &= (6x+5)e^x + (3x^2+5x)e^x\\ &= (3x^2+11x+5)e^x.\end{aligned}$$

Example 2 Find the derivative of $C = \dfrac{e^{2t}}{t}$.

Solution We write $C = e^{2t}t^{-1}$ and use the product rule:

$$\begin{aligned}\frac{d}{dt}(e^{2t}t^{-1}) &= \frac{d}{dt}(e^{2t})\cdot t^{-1} + e^{2t}\frac{d}{dt}(t^{-1})\\ &= (2e^{2t})\cdot t^{-1} + e^{2t}(-1)t^{-2}\\ &= \frac{2e^{2t}}{t} - \frac{e^{2t}}{t^2}.\end{aligned}$$

Example 3 A demand curve for a product has the equation $p = 80e^{-0.003q}$, where p is price and q is quantity.

(a) Find the revenue as a function of quantity sold.
(b) Find the marginal revenue function.

Solution (a) Since Revenue = Price × Quantity, we have $R = pq = (80e^{-0.003q})q = 80qe^{-0.003q}$.

(b) The marginal revenue function is the derivative of revenue with respect to quantity. The product rule gives

$$\begin{aligned}\text{Marginal Revenue} &= \frac{d}{dq}(80qe^{-0.003q}) \\ &= \left(\frac{d}{dq}(80q)\right)e^{-0.003q} + 80q\left(\frac{d}{dq}(e^{-0.003q})\right) \\ &= (80)e^{-0.003q} + 80q(-0.003e^{-0.003q}) \\ &= (80 - 0.24q)e^{-0.003q}.\end{aligned}$$

The Quotient Rule

Suppose we want to differentiate a function of the form $Q(x) = f(x)/g(x)$. (Of course, we have to avoid points where $g(x) = 0$.) We want a formula for Q' in terms of f' and g'. We have the following rule, which is justified in the Focus on Theory section at the end of this chapter.

The Quotient Rule

If $u = f(x)$ and $v = g(x)$ are differentiable functions, then

$$\left(\frac{f}{g}\right)' = \frac{f'g - fg'}{g^2},$$

or equivalently,

$$\frac{d}{dx}\left(\frac{u}{v}\right) = \frac{\frac{du}{dx}\cdot v - u\cdot\frac{dv}{dx}}{v^2}.$$

In words:

The derivative of a quotient is the derivative of the numerator times the denominator minus the numerator times the derivative of the denominator, all over the denominator squared.

Example 4 Differentiate (a) $\dfrac{5x^2}{x^3+1}$ (b) $\dfrac{1}{1+e^x}$ (c) $\dfrac{e^x}{x^2}$.

Solution (a) Using the quotient rule

$$\begin{aligned}\frac{d}{dx}\left(\frac{5x^2}{x^3+1}\right) &= \frac{\left(\frac{d}{dx}(5x^2)\right)(x^3+1) - 5x^2\frac{d}{dx}(x^3+1)}{(x^3+1)^2} = \frac{10x(x^3+1) - 5x^2(3x^2)}{(x^3+1)^2} \\ &= \frac{-5x^4 + 10x}{(x^3+1)^2}.\end{aligned}$$

(b) Differentiating using the quotient rule yields

$$\frac{d}{dx}\left(\frac{1}{1+e^x}\right) = \frac{\left(\frac{d}{dx}(1)\right)(1+e^x) - 1\frac{d}{dx}(1+e^x)}{(1+e^x)^2} = \frac{0(1+e^x) - 1(0+e^x)}{(1+e^x)^2}$$

$$= \frac{-e^x}{(1+e^x)^2}.$$

(c) The quotient rule gives

$$\frac{d}{dx}\left(\frac{e^x}{x^2}\right) = \frac{\left(\frac{d}{dx}(e^x)\right)x^2 - e^x\left(\frac{d}{dx}(x^2)\right)}{(x^2)^2} = \frac{e^x x^2 - e^x(2x)}{x^4}$$

$$= e^x\left(\frac{x^2-2x}{x^4}\right) = e^x\left(\frac{x-2}{x^3}\right).$$

Problems for Section 3.4

1. If $f(x) = (2x+1)(3x-2)$, find $f'(x)$ two ways: by using the product rule and by multiplying out. Do you get the same result?

2. If $f(x) = x^2(x^3+5)$, find $f'(x)$ two ways: by using the product rule and by multiplying out before taking the derivative. Do you get the same result? Should you?

For Problems 3–33, find the derivative. Assume that a, b, c, and k are constants.

3. $f(x) = xe^x$

4. $f(t) = te^{-2t}$

5. $y = 5xe^{x^2}$

6. $y = t^2(3t+1)^3$

7. $y = x\ln x$

8. $y = (t^2+3)e^t$

9. $z = (3t+1)(5t+2)$

10. $y = (t^3 - 7t^2 + 1)e^t$

11. $P = t^2 \ln t$

12. $R = 3qe^{-q}$

13. $f(t) = \frac{5}{t} + \frac{6}{t^2}$

14. $f(x) = \frac{x^2+3}{x}$

15. $y = te^{-t^2}$

16. $f(z) = \sqrt{z}e^{-z}$

17. $g(p) = p\ln(2p+1)$

18. $f(t) = te^{5-2t}$

19. $f(w) = (5w^2+3)e^{w^2}$

20. $y = x \cdot 2^x$

21. $w = (t^3+5t)(t^2-7t+2)$

22. $z = (te^{3t} + e^{5t})^9$

23. $f(x) = \frac{x}{e^x}$

24. $w = \frac{3z}{1+2z}$

25. $z = \frac{1-t}{1+t}$

26. $y = \frac{e^x}{1+e^x}$

27. $w = \frac{3y+y^2}{5+y}$

28. $y = \frac{1+z}{\ln z}$

29. $f(x) = \frac{ax+b}{cx+k}$

30. $f(x) = (ax^2+b)^3$

31. $f(x) = axe^{-bx}$

32. $f(t) = ae^{bt}$

33. $g(\alpha) = e^{\alpha e^{-2\alpha}}$

34. If $f(x) = (3x+8)(2x-5)$, find $f'(x)$ and $f''(x)$.

35. Find the equation of the tangent line to the graph of $f(x) = x^2e^{-x}$ at $x = 0$. Check by graphing this function and the tangent line on the same axes.

36. Find the equation of the tangent line to the graph of $f(x) = \frac{2x-5}{x+1}$ at the point at which $x = 0$.

37. The quantity of a drug, Q mg, present in the body t hours after an injection of the drug is given is

$$Q = f(t) = 100te^{-0.5t}.$$

Find $f(1)$, $f'(1)$, $f(5)$, and $f'(5)$. Give units and interpret the answers.

38. A drug concentration curve is given by $C = f(t) = 20te^{-0.04t}$, with C in mg/ml and t in minutes.

(a) Graph C against t. Is $f'(15)$ positive or negative? Is $f'(45)$ positive or negative? Explain.
(b) Find $f(30)$ and $f'(30)$ analytically. Interpret them in terms of the concentration of the drug in the body.

39. For positive constants c and k, the *Monod growth curve* describes the growth of a population, P, as a function of the available quantity of a resource, r:

$$P = \frac{cr}{k+r}.$$

Find dP/dr and interpret it in terms of the growth of the population.

40. If p is price in dollars and q is quantity, demand for a product is given by

$$q = 5000e^{-0.08p}.$$

(a) What quantity is sold at a price of \$10?
(b) Find the derivative of demand with respect to price when the price is \$10 and interpret your answer in terms of demand.

41. The demand for a product is given in Problem 40. Find the revenue and the derivative of revenue with respect to price at a price of \$10. Interpret your answers in economic terms.

42. The quantity demanded of a certain product, q, is given in terms of p, the price, by

$$q = 1000e^{-0.02p}$$

(a) Write revenue, R, as a function of price.
(b) Find the rate of change of revenue with respect to price.
(c) Find the revenue and rate of change of revenue with respect to price when the price is \$10. Interpret your answers in economic terms.

43. If $\frac{d}{dt}(tf(t)) = 1 + f(t)$, what is $f'(t)$?

44. The quantity, q, of a certain skateboard sold depends on the selling price, p, in dollars, so we write $q = f(p)$. You are given that $f(140) = 15{,}000$ and $f'(140) = -100$.

(a) What do $f(140) = 15{,}000$ and $f'(140) = -100$ tell you about the sales of skateboards?
(b) The total revenue, R, earned by the sale of skateboards is given by $R = pq$. Find $\left.\frac{dR}{dp}\right|_{p=140}$.
(c) What is the sign of $\left.\frac{dR}{dp}\right|_{p=140}$? If the skateboards are currently selling for \$140, what happens to revenue if the price is increased to \$141?

45. Show that the relative rate of change of a product fg is the sum of the relative rates of change of f and g.

46. Show that the relative rate of change of a quotient f/g is the difference between the relative rates of change of f and g.

47. If $h = f^n$, show that

$$\frac{(f^n)'}{f^n} = n\frac{f'}{f}.$$

3.5 DERIVATIVES OF PERIODIC FUNCTIONS

Since the sine and cosine functions are periodic, their derivatives must be periodic also. (Why?) Let's look at the graph of $f(x) = \sin x$ in Figure 3.20 and estimate the derivative function graphically.

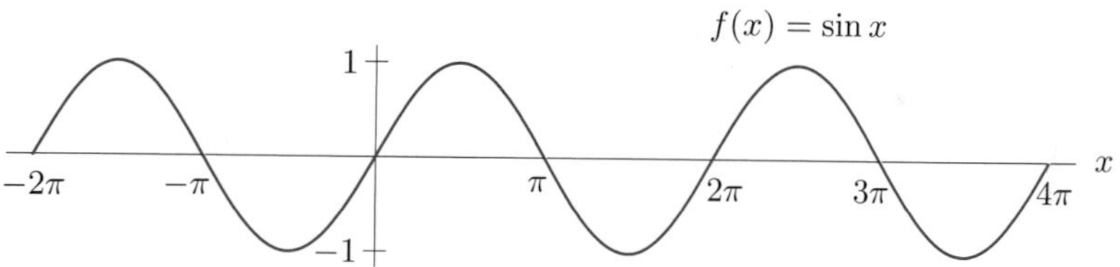

Figure 3.20: The sine function

First we might ask ourselves where the derivative is zero. (At $x = \pm\pi/2, \pm 3\pi/2, \pm 5\pi/2$, etc.) Then ask where the derivative is positive and where it is negative. (Positive for $-\pi/2 < x < \pi/2$; negative for $\pi/2 < x < 3\pi/2$, etc.) Since the largest positive slopes are at $x = 0, 2\pi$, and so on, and the largest negative slopes are at $x = \pi, 3\pi$, and so on, we get something like the graph in Figure 3.21.

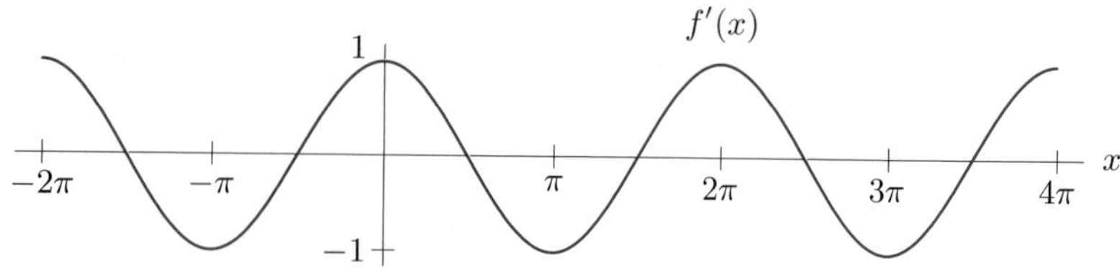

Figure 3.21: Derivative of $f(x) = \sin x$

The graph of the derivative in Figure 3.21 looks suspiciously like the graph of the cosine function. This might lead us to conjecture, quite correctly, that the derivative of the sine is the cosine.

Of course, we cannot be sure, just from the graphs, that the derivative of the sine really is the cosine. However, this is in fact true.

One thing we can do is to check that the derivative function in Figure 3.21 has amplitude 1 (as it must if it is the cosine). That means we have to convince ourselves that the derivative of $f(x) = \sin x$ is 1 when $x = 0$. The next example suggests that this is true when x is in radians.

Example 1 Using a calculator, estimate the derivative of $f(x) = \sin x$ at $x = 0$. Make sure your calculator is set in radians.

Solution We use the average rate of change of $\sin x$ on the small interval $0 \le x \le 0.01$ to compute

$$f'(0) \approx \frac{\sin(0.01) - \sin(0)}{0.01 - 0} = \frac{0.0099998 - 0}{0.01} = 0.99998 \approx 1.0.$$

The derivative of $f(x) = \sin x$ at $x = 0$ is approximately 1.0.

Warning: It is important to notice that in the previous example x was in *radians*; any conclusions we have drawn about the derivative of $\sin x$ are valid *only* when x is in radians.

Example 2 Starting with the graph of the cosine function, sketch a graph of its derivative.

Solution The graph of $g(x) = \cos x$ is in Figure 3.22(a). Its derivative is 0 at $x = 0, \pm\pi, \pm 2\pi$, and so on; it is positive for $-\pi < x < 0$, $\pi < x < 2\pi$, and so on, and it is negative for $0 < x < \pi$, $2\pi < x < 3\pi$, and so on. The derivative is in Figure 3.22(b).

(a)

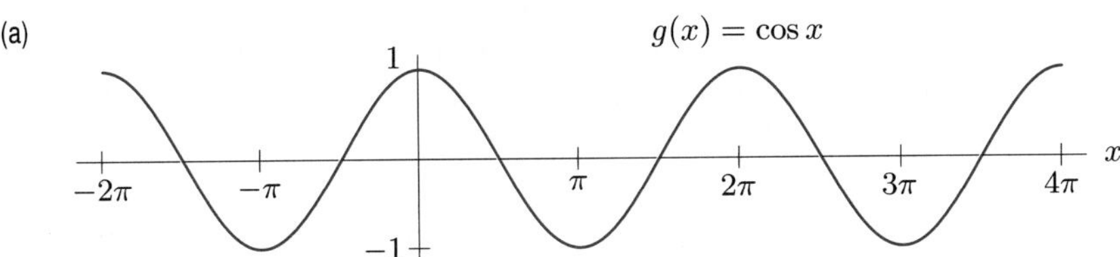

(b)

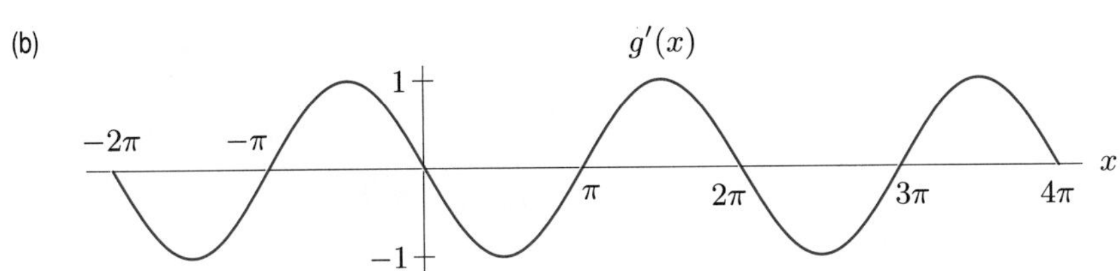

Figure 3.22: $g(x) = \cos x$ and its derivative, $g'(x)$

As we did with the sine, we'll use the graphs to make a conjecture. The derivative of the cosine in Figure 3.22(b) looks exactly like the graph of sine, except reflected about the x-axis. It turns out that the derivative of $\cos x$ is $-\sin x$.

For x in radians,

$$\frac{d}{dx}(\sin x) = \cos x \quad \text{and} \quad \frac{d}{dx}(\cos x) = -\sin x.$$

Example 3 Differentiate (a) $5\sin t - 8\cos t$ (b) $5 - 3\sin x + x^3$

Solution (a) Differentiating gives

$$\frac{d}{dt}(5\sin t - 8\cos t) = 5\frac{d}{dt}(\sin t) - 8\frac{d}{dt}(\cos t) = 5(\cos t) - 8(-\sin t) = 5\cos t + 8\sin t$$

(b) We have

$$\frac{d}{dx}(5-3\sin x+x^3) = \frac{d}{dx}(5)-3\frac{d}{dx}(\sin x)+\frac{d}{dx}(x^3) = 0-3(\cos x)+3x^2 = -3\cos x+3x^2.$$

The chain rule tells us how to differentiate composite functions involving the sine and cosine. Suppose $y = \sin(3t)$, so $y = \sin z$ and $z = 3t$, so

$$\frac{dy}{dt} = \frac{dy}{dz}\cdot\frac{dz}{dt} = \cos z\frac{dz}{dt} = \cos(3t)\cdot 3 = 3\cos(3t).$$

In general,

> If z is a differentiable function of t, then
>
> $$\frac{d}{dt}(\sin z) = \cos z\frac{dz}{dt} \quad \text{and} \quad \frac{d}{dt}(\cos z) = -\sin z\frac{dz}{dt}$$

In many applications, $z = kt$ for some constant k. Then we have:

> If k is a constant, then
>
> $$\frac{d}{dt}(\sin kt) = k\cos kt \quad \text{and} \quad \frac{d}{dt}(\cos kt) = -k\sin kt$$

Example 4 Differentiate:

(a) $\sin(t^2)$ (b) $5\cos(2t)$ (c) $t\sin t$.

Solution (a) We have $y = \sin z$ with $z = t^2$, so

$$\frac{d}{dt}(\sin(t^2)) = \frac{d}{dt}(\sin z) = \cos z\frac{dz}{dt} = \cos(t^2)\cdot 2t = 2t\cos(t^2).$$

(b) We have $y = 5\cos z$ with $z = 2t$, so

$$\frac{d}{dt}(5\cos(2t)) = 5\frac{d}{dt}(\cos(2t)) = 5(-2\sin(2t)) = -10\sin(2t).$$

(c) We use the product rule:

$$\frac{d}{dt}(t\sin t) = \frac{d}{dt}(t)\cdot\sin t + t\frac{d}{dt}(\sin t) = 1\cdot\sin t + t(\cos t) = \sin t + t\cos t.$$

Problems for Section 3.5

Differentiate the functions in Problems 1–20. Assume that A and B are constants.

1. $y = 5\sin x$
2. $P = 3 + \cos t$
3. $y = t^2 + 5\cos t$
4. $y = B + A\sin t$
5. $R(q) = q^2 - 2\cos q$
6. $y = 5\sin x - 5x + 4$
7. $f(x) = \sin(3x)$
8. $R = \sin(5t)$
9. $W = 4\cos(t^2)$
10. $y = 2\cos(5t)$
11. $y = \sin(x^2)$
12. $y = A\sin(Bt)$
13. $z = \cos(4\theta)$
14. $y = 6\sin(2t) + \cos(4t)$
15. $f(x) = x^2\cos x$
16. $f(x) = 2x\sin(3x)$
17. $f(\theta) = \theta^3\cos\theta$
18. $z = \dfrac{e^{t^2} + t}{\sin(2t)}$
19. $f(t) = \dfrac{t^2}{\cos t}$
20. $f(\theta) = \dfrac{\sin\theta}{\theta}$

21. Find the equation of the tangent line to the graph of $y = \sin x$ at $x = \pi$. Graph the function and the tangent line on the same axes.

22. If t is the number of months since June, the number of bird species, N, found in an Ohio forest oscillates approximately according to the formula

$$N = f(t) = 19 + 9\cos\left(\frac{\pi}{6}t\right).$$

(a) Graph $f(t)$ for $0 \le t \le 24$ and describe what it shows. Use the graph to decide whether $f'(1)$ and $f'(10)$ are positive or negative.
(b) Find $f'(t)$.
(c) Find and interpret $f(1)$, $f'(1)$, $f(10)$, and $f'(10)$.

23. Is the graph of $y = \sin(x^4)$ increasing or decreasing when $x = 10$? Is it concave up or concave down?

24. Find equations of the tangent lines to the graph of $f(x) = \sin x$ at $x = 0$ and at $x = \pi/3$. Use each tangent line to approximate $\sin(\pi/6)$. Would you expect these results to be equally accurate, since they are taken equally far away from $x = \pi/6$ but on opposite sides? If the accuracy is different, can you account for the difference?

25. A company's monthly sales, $S(t)$, are seasonal and given as a function of time, t, in months, by

$$S(t) = 2000 + 600\sin\left(\frac{\pi}{6}t\right).$$

(a) Graph $S(t)$ for $t = 0$ to $t = 12$. What is the maximum monthly sales? What is the minimum monthly sales? If $t = 0$ is January 1, when during the year are sales highest?
(b) Find $S(2)$ and $S'(2)$. Interpret in terms of sales.

26. A boat at anchor is bobbing up and down in the sea. The vertical distance, y, in feet, between the sea floor and the boat is given as a function of time, t, in minutes, by

$$y = 15 + \sin(2\pi t).$$

(a) Find the vertical velocity, v, of the boat at time t.
(b) Make rough sketches of y and v against t.

27. The depth of the water, y, in meters, in the Bay of Fundy, Canada, is given as a function of time, t, in hours after midnight, by the function

$$y = 10 + 7.5\cos(0.507t).$$

How quickly is the tide rising or falling (in meters/hour) at each of the following times?

(a) 6:00 am **(b)** 9:00 am
(c) Noon **(d)** 6:00 pm

28. The average adult takes about 12 breaths per minute. As a patient inhales, the volume of air in the lung increases. As the patient exhales, the volume of air in the lung decreases. For t in seconds since start of the breathing cycle, the volume of air inhaled or exhaled since $t = 0$ is given [9], in hundreds of cubic centimeters, by

$$A(t) = -2\cos\left(\frac{2\pi}{5}t\right) + 2.$$

(a) How long is one breathing cycle?
(b) Find $A'(1)$ and explain what it means.

29. On July 7, 2009, there was a full moon in the Eastern time zone.[10] If t is the number of days since July 7th, the percent of moon illuminated can be represented by

$$H(t) = 50 + 50\cos\left(\frac{\pi}{15}t\right).$$

(a) Find $H'(t)$. Explain what this tells about the moon.
(b) For $0 \le t \le 30$, when is $H'(t) = 0$? What does this tell us about the moon?
(c) For $0 \le t \le 30$, when is $H'(t)$ negative? When is it positive? Explain what positive and negative values of $H'(t)$ tell us about the moon.

30. Paris, France, has a latitude of approximately 49° N. If t is the number of days since the start of 2009, the number of hours of daylight in Paris can be approximated by

$$D(t) = 4\cos\left(\frac{2\pi}{365}(t - 172)\right) + 12.$$

(a) Find $D(40)$ and $D'(40)$. Explain what this tells about daylight in Paris.
(b) Find $D(172)$ and $D'(172)$. Explain what this tells about daylight in Paris.

[9]Based upon information obtained from Dr. Gadi Avshalomov on August 14, 2008.
[10]www.aa.usno.navy.mil/feq/docs/moon_phases.php, accessed on April 14, 2009.

CHAPTER SUMMARY

- **Derivatives of elementary functions**
  Powers, polynomials, exponential functions, logarithms, periodic functions
- **Derivatives of sums, differences, constant multiples**
- **Chain rule**
- **Product and quotient rules**
- **Relative rates of change**
  Using logarithms
- **Tangent line approximation**
- **Interpreting derivatives found using formulas**

REVIEW PROBLEMS FOR CHAPTER THREE

Find the derivatives for the functions in Problems 1–40. Assume k is a constant.

1. $f(t) = 6t^4$

2. $f(x) = x^3 - 3x^2 + 5x$

3. $P(t) = e^{2t}$

4. $W = r^3 + 5r - 12$

5. $C = e^{0.08q}$

6. $y = 5e^{-0.2t}$

7. $y = xe^{3x}$

8. $s(t) = (t^2 + 4)(5t - 1)$

9. $g(t) = e^{(1+3t)^2}$

10. $f(x) = x^2 + 3\ln x$

11. $Q(t) = 5t + 3e^{1.2t}$

12. $g(z) = (z^2 + 5)^3$

13. $f(x) = 6(5x - 1)^3$

14. $f(z) = \ln(z^2 + 1)$

15. $h(x) = (1 + e^x)^{10}$

16. $q = 100e^{-0.05p}$

17. $y = x^2 \ln x$

18. $s(t) = t^2 + 2\ln t$

19. $P = 4t^2 + 7\sin t$

20. $R(t) = (\sin t)^5$

21. $h(t) = \ln\left(e^{-t} - t\right)$

22. $f(x) = \sin(2x)$

23. $g(x) = \dfrac{25x^2}{e^x}$

24. $h(t) = \dfrac{t+4}{t-4}$

25. $y = x^2 \cos x$

26. $h(x) = \ln(1 + e^x)$

27. $h(w) = e^{\ln w + 1}$

28. $h(x) = \ln(x^3 + x)$

29. $q(x) = \dfrac{1+e^x}{1-e^{-x}}$

30. $q(x) = \dfrac{x}{1+x}$

31. $f(x) = xe^x$

32. $h(x) = \sin(e^x)$

33. $h(x) = \cos(x^3)$

34. $z = \dfrac{3t+1}{5t+2}$

35. $z = \dfrac{t^2 + 5t + 2}{t+3}$

36. $h(p) = \dfrac{1+p^2}{3+2p^2}$

37. $y = \dfrac{3^x}{3} + \dfrac{33}{\sqrt{x}}$

38. $f(t) = \sin\sqrt{e^t + 1}$

39. $g(y) = e^{2e^{(y^3)}}$

40. $g(t) = \dfrac{\ln(kt) + t}{\ln(kt) - t}$

41. Let $f(x) = x^2 + 1$. Compute the derivatives $f'(0)$, $f'(1)$, $f'(2)$, and $f'(-1)$. Check your answers graphically.

42. Let $f(x) = x^2 + 3x - 5$. Find $f'(0)$, $f'(3)$, $f'(-2)$.

43. Find the equation of the line tangent to the graph of $f(x) = 2x^3 - 5x^2 + 3x - 5$ at $x = 1$.

In Problems 44–47, find the relative rate of change $f'(t)/f(t)$ of the function at the given value of t. Assume t is in years and give your answer as a percent.

44. $f(t) = 3t + 2;\quad t = 5$

45. $f(t) = 2e^{0.3t};\quad t = 7$

46. $f(t) = 2t^3 + 10;\quad t = 4$

47. $f(t) = \ln(t^2 + 1);\quad t = 2$

48. With a yearly inflation rate of 5%, prices are given by

$$P = P_0(1.05)^t,$$

where P_0 is the price in dollars when $t = 0$ and t is time in years. Suppose $P_0 = 1$. How fast (in cents/year) are prices rising when $t = 10$?

49. According to the US Census, the world population P, in billions, was approximately [11]

$$P = 6.8e^{0.012t}$$

where t is in years since January 1, 2009. At what rate was the world's population increasing on that date? Give your answer in millions of people per year.

50. Let $f(x) = x^2 - 4x + 8$. For what x-values is $f'(x) = 0$?

51. A football player kicks a ball at an angle of 30° from the ground with an initial velocity of 64 feet per second. Its height t seconds later is $h(t) = 32t - 16t^2$.

(a) Graph the height of the ball as a function of the time.
(b) Find $v(t)$, the velocity of the ball at time t.
(c) Find $v(1)$, and explain what is happening to the ball at this time. What is the height of the ball at this time?

[11] www.census.gov/ipc/www/popclockworld.html and www.cia.gov/library/publications/the-world-factbook/print/xx.html.

52. The graph of $y = x^3 - 9x^2 - 16x + 1$ has a slope of 5 at two points. Find the coordinates of the points.

53. (a) Find the slope of the graph of $f(x) = 1 - e^x$ at the point where it crosses the x-axis.
(b) Find the equation of the tangent line to the curve at this point.

54. Find the equation of the tangent line to the graph of $P(t) = t \ln t$ at $t = 2$. Graph the function $P(t)$ and the tangent line $Q(t)$ on the same axes.

55. The balance, $\$B$, in a bank account t years after a deposit of \$5000 is given by $B = 5000e^{0.08t}$. At what rate is the balance in the account changing at $t = 5$ years? Use units to interpret your answer in financial terms.

56. If a cup of coffee is left on a counter top, it cools off slowly. The temperature in degrees Fahrenheit t minutes after it was left on the counter is given by

$$C(t) = 74 + 103e^{-0.033t}.$$

(a) What was the temperature of the coffee when it was left on the counter?
(b) If the coffee was left on the counter for a long time, what is the lowest temperature the coffee would reach? What does that temperature represent?
(c) Find $C(5)$ and $C'(5)$. Explain what this tells about the temperature of the coffee.
(d) Without calculation, decide if the magnitude of $C'(50)$ is greater or less than the magnitude of $C'(5)$? Why?

57. With length, l, in meters, the period T, in seconds, of a pendulum is given by

$$T = 2\pi\sqrt{\frac{l}{9.8}}.$$

(a) How fast does the period increase as l increases?
(b) Does this rate of change increase or decrease as l increases?

58. One gram of radioactive carbon-14 decays according to the formula

$$Q = e^{-0.000121t},$$

where Q is the number of grams of carbon-14 remaining after t years.

(a) Find the rate at which carbon-14 is decaying (in grams/year).
(b) Sketch the rate you found in part (a) against time.

59. The temperature, H, in degrees Fahrenheit (°F), of a can of soda that is put into a refrigerator to cool is given as a function of time, t, in hours, by

$$H = 40 + 30e^{-2t}.$$

(a) Find the rate at which the temperature of the soda is changing (in °F/hour).
(b) What is the sign of dH/dt? Explain.
(c) When, for $t \geq 0$, is the magnitude of dH/dt largest? In terms of the can of soda, why is this?

60. Explain for which values of a the function a^x is increasing and for which values it is decreasing. Use the fact that, for $a > 0$,

$$\frac{d}{dx}(a^x) = (\ln a)a^x.$$

61. The value of an automobile purchased in 2009 can be approximated by the function $V(t) = 25(0.85)^t$, where t is the time, in years, from the date of purchase, and $V(t)$ is the value, in thousands of dollars.

(a) Evaluate and interpret $V(4)$.
(b) Find an expression for $V'(t)$, including units.
(c) Evaluate and interpret $V'(4)$.
(d) Use $V(t)$, $V'(t)$, and any other considerations you think are relevant to write a paragraph in support of or in opposition to the following statement: "From a monetary point of view, it is best to keep this vehicle as long as possible."

62. The temperature Y in degrees Fahrenheit of a yam in a hot oven t minutes after it is placed there is given by

$$Y(t) = 350(1 - 0.7e^{-0.008t}).$$

(a) What was the temperature of the yam when it was placed in the oven?
(b) What is the temperature of the oven?
(c) When does the yam reach 175° F?
(d) Estimate the rate at which the temperature of the yam is increasing when $t = 20$.

63. Kepler's third law of planetary motion states that, $P^2 = kd^3$, where P represents the time, in earth days, it takes a planet to orbit the sun once, d is the planet's average distance, in miles, from the sun, and k is a constant.[12]

(a) If $k = 1.65864 \cdot 10^{-19}$, write P as a function of d.
(b) Mercury is approximately 36 million miles from the sun. How long does it take Mercury to orbit the sun?
(c) Find $P'(d)$. What does the sign of the derivative tell us about the time it takes a planet to orbit the sun? Why does this make sense from a practical viewpoint?

64. Imagine you are zooming in on the graph of each of the following functions near the origin:

$y = x$ $\quad y = \sqrt{x}$ $\quad y = x^2$

$y = x^3 + \frac{1}{2}x^2$ $\quad y = x^3$ $\quad y = \ln(x+1)$

$y = \frac{1}{2}\ln(x^2+1)$ $\quad y = \sqrt{2x - x^2}$

Which of them look the same? Group together those functions which become indistinguishable near the origin, and give the equations of the lines they look like.

[12] www.exploratorium.edu/ronh/age/index.html, accessed on 5/3/09.

65. Given a power function of the form $f(x) = ax^n$, with $f'(2) = 3$ and $f'(4) = 24$, find n and a.

66. Given $r(2) = 4$, $s(2) = 1$, $s(4) = 2$, $r'(2) = -1$, $s'(2) = 3$, and $s'(4) = 3$, compute the following derivatives, or state what additional information you would need to be able to compute the derivative.

(a) $H'(2)$ if $H(x) = r(x) + s(x)$
(b) $H'(2)$ if $H(x) = 5s(x)$
(c) $H'(2)$ if $H(x) = r(x) \cdot s(x)$
(d) $H'(2)$ if $H(x) = \sqrt{r(x)}$

67. Given $F(2) = 1, F'(2) = 5, F(4) = 3, F'(4) = 7$ and $G(4) = 2, G'(4) = 6, G(3) = 4, G'(3) = 8$, find:

(a) $H(4)$ if $H(x) = F(G(x))$
(b) $H'(4)$ if $H(x) = F(G(x))$
(c) $H(4)$ if $H(x) = G(F(x))$
(d) $H'(4)$ if $H(x) = G(F(x))$
(e) $H'(4)$ if $H(x) = F(x)/G(x)$

68. A dose, D, of a drug causes a temperature change, T, in a patient. For C a positive constant, T is given by

$$T = \left(\frac{C}{2} - \frac{D}{3}\right) D^3.$$

(a) What is the rate of change of temperature change with respect to dose?
(b) For what doses does the temperature change increase as the dose increases?

69. A yam is put in a hot oven, maintained at a constant temperature 200°C. At time $t = 30$ minutes, the temperature T of the yam is 120° and is increasing at an (instantaneous) rate of 2°/min. Newton's law of cooling (or, in our case, warming) implies that the temperature at time t is given by

$$T(t) = 200 - ae^{-bt}.$$

Find a and b.

For Problems 70–75, let $h(x) = f(x) \cdot g(x)$, and $k(x) = f(x)/g(x)$, and $l(x) = g(x)/f(x)$. Use Figure 3.23 to estimate the derivatives.

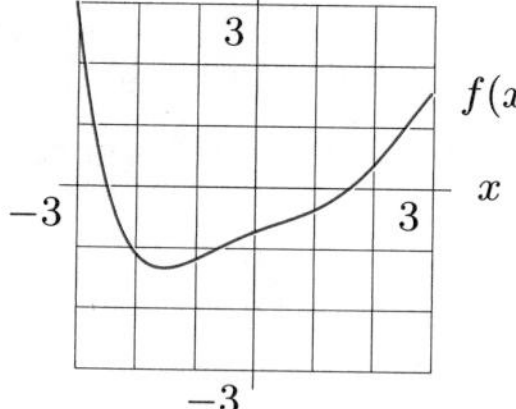

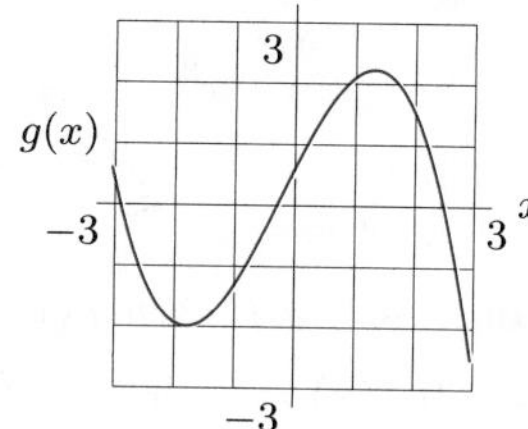

Figure 3.23

70. $h'(1)$ **71.** $k'(1)$
72. $h'(2)$ **73.** $k'(2)$
74. $l'(1)$ **75.** $l'(2)$

76. On what intervals is the function $f(x) = x^4 - 4x^3$ both decreasing and concave up?

77. Given $p(x) = x^n - x$, find the intervals over which p is a decreasing function when:

(a) $n = 2$ **(b)** $n = \frac{1}{2}$ **(c)** $n = -1$

78. Using the equation of the tangent line to the graph of e^x at $x = 0$, show that

$$e^x \geq 1 + x$$

for all values of x. A sketch may be helpful.

79. In Section 1.10 the depth, y, in feet, of water in Portland, Maine is given in terms of t, the number of hours since midnight, by

$$y = 4.9 + 4.4 \cos\left(\frac{\pi}{6}t\right).$$

(a) Find dy/dt. What does dy/dt represent, in terms of water level?
(b) For $0 \leq t \leq 24$, when is dy/dt zero? (Figure 1.98 may be helpful.) Explain what it means (in terms of water level) for dy/dt to be zero.

80. Using a graph to help you, find the equations of all lines through the origin tangent to the parabola

$$y = x^2 - 2x + 4.$$

Sketch the lines on the graph.

81. A museum has decided to sell one of its paintings and to invest the proceeds. If the picture is sold between the years 2000 and 2020 and the money from the sale is invested in a bank account earning 5% interest per year compounded annually, then $B(t)$, the balance in the year 2020, depends on the year, t, in which the painting is sold and the sale price $P(t)$. If t is measured from the year 2000 so that $0 < t < 20$ then

$$B(t) = P(t)(1.05)^{20-t}.$$

(a) Explain why $B(t)$ is given by this formula.
(b) Show that the formula for $B(t)$ is equivalent to

$$B(t) = (1.05)^{20} \frac{P(t)}{(1.05)^t}.$$

(c) Find $B'(10)$, given that $P(10) = 150{,}000$ and $P'(10) = 5000$.

82. Find the mean and variance of the normal distribution of statistics using parts (a) and (b) with $m(t) = e^{\mu t + \sigma^2 t^2/2}$.

(a) Mean $= m'(0)$
(b) Variance $= m''(0) - (m'(0))^2$

83. Given a number $a > 1$, the equation

$$a^x = 1 + x$$

has the solution $x = 0$. Are there any other solutions? How does your answer depend on the value of a? [Hint: Graph the functions on both sides of the equation.]

84. Suppose that f is a positive function such that $f(t_0) = P_0$ and $f(t_1) = P_1$. If $h(t) = Ae^{kt}$ is the exponential function taking the same values as f at $t = t_0$ and $t = t_1$, show that $k = (\ln P_1 - \ln P_0)/(t_1 - t_0)$.

85. Figure 3.24 shows the number of gallons, G, of gasoline used on a trip of M miles.

(a) The function f is linear on each of the intervals $0 < M < 70$ and $70 < M < 100$. What is the slope of these lines? What are the units of these slopes?

(b) What is gas consumption (in miles per gallon) during the first 70 miles of this trip? During the next 30 miles?

(c) Figure 3.25 shows distance traveled, M (in miles), as a function of time t, in hours since the start of the trip. Describe this trip in words. Give a possible explanation for what happens one hour into the trip. What do your answers to part (b) tell you about the trip?

(d) If we let $G = k(t) = f(h(t))$, estimate $k(0.5)$ and interpret your answer in terms of the trip.

(e) Find $k'(0.5)$ and $k'(1.5)$. Give units and interpret your answers.

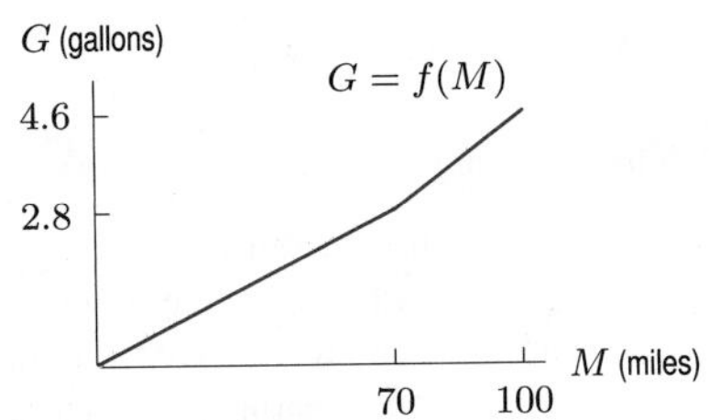

Figure 3.24

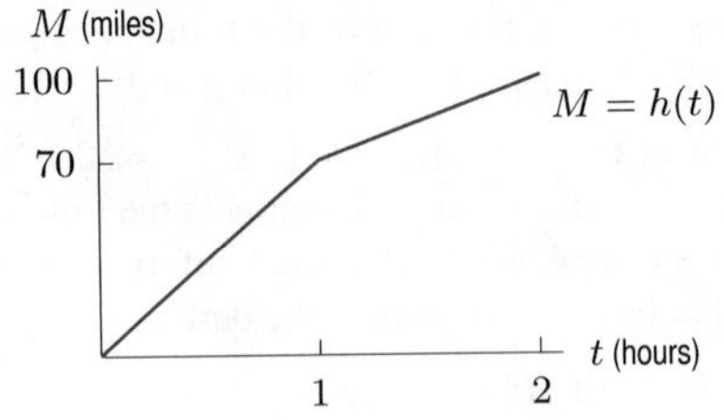

Figure 3.25:

86. On October 17, 2006, the US population was 300 million and growing exponentially. If the population was increasing at a rate of 2.9 million a year on that date, find a formula for the population as a function of time, t, in years since that date.

87. The speed of sound in dry air is

$$f(T) = 331.3\sqrt{1 + \frac{T}{273.15}} \text{ meters/second}$$

where T is the temperature in ° Celsius. Find a linear function that approximates the speed of sound for temperatures near 0°C.

CHECK YOUR UNDERSTANDING

In Problems 1–50, indicate whether the statement is true or false.

1. If $f(x) = 5x^2 + 1$ then $f'(-1) = -10$.

2. The two functions $f(x) = 3x^5$ and $g(x) = 3x^5 + 7$ have the same derivative.

3. The derivative of $h(t) = (3t^2 + 1)(2t)$ is $h'(t) = (6t)(2) = 12t$.

4. If $k(s) = \sqrt{s^3}$ then $k'(s) = \sqrt{3s^2}$.

5. The equation of the line tangent to $f(x) = x^5 + 5$ at $x = 1$ is $y = 9x - 3$.

6. The derivative of $f(r) = 1/r^5$ is $f'(r) = 1/5r^4$.

7. The function $g(w) = w^3 - 3w$ has exactly two places where $g'(w) = 0$.

8. If $f(x) = 3x^3 - x^2 + 2x$ then f is decreasing at $x = 1$.

9. If $f(x) = 3x^3 - x^2 + 2x$ then the graph of f is concave up at $x = 1$.

10. If $g(t) = t^\pi$ then $g'(1) = \pi$.

11. If $f(x) = e^x$ then $f'(x) = xe^{x-1}$.

12. If $g(s) = 5\ln(s)$ then $g'(2) = 5/2$.

13. The function $f(x) = 3e^x + x$ has tangent line at $x = 0$ with equation $y = 4x + 3$.

14. The function $h(x) = 2\ln x - x^2$ is decreasing at $x = 1$.

15. The graph of $h(x) = 2\ln x - x^2$ is concave down at $x = 1$.

16. If $f(x) = \ln 2$ then $f'(x) = 1/2$.

17. If $f(x) = e^{2x}$ then $f'(x) = e^{2x}$.

18. If $w(q) = 10^q$ then $w'(q) = \log(10) \cdot 10^q$.

19. If $k(p) = 5 \cdot e^p$ then $k'(p) = \ln 5 \cdot e^p$.

20. If $f(x) = 3e^{5x}$ then $f'(x) = 15e^{5x}$.

21. The derivative of $f(t) = e^{t^2}$ is $f'(t) = 2e^{2t}$.

22. If $y = (x + x^2)^5$ then $dy/dx = 5(1 + 2x)^4$.

23. If $y = \ln(x^2 + 4)$ then $dy/dx = (2x)/(x^2 + 4)$.

24. If $y = \sqrt{1 - 2t}$ then $y' = 1/(2\sqrt{1 - 2t})$.

25. If $y = e^{-x}$ then $dy/dx = -e^{-x}$.

26. The chain rule says $d/dt(f(g(t))) = f(g'(t)) \cdot g(t)$.

27. If $g(x) = \ln(x^2 + 3x)$ then $g'(x) = (1/x)(2x + 3)$.

28. The function $f(x) = e^{1-x}$ is decreasing at $x = 1$.

29. The graph of $f(x) = e^{1-x}$ is concave up at $x = 1$.

30. If $B = 30(1 + 2r)^5$ then $dB/dr = 150(1 + 2r)^4$.

31. If $y = e^x \ln(x)$ then $y' = e^x/x$.

32. If $y = (x^2 + 1)2^x$ then $y' = 2x(\ln 2)2^x$.

33. If $y = x/e^x$ then $y' = (e^x - xe^x)/e^{2x} = (1 - x)/e^x$.

34. If $z = 2/(1 + t^2)$ then $z' = -4t/(1 + t^2)^2$.

35. If $s = w^2 e^w$ then $s' = 2we^w$.

36. If $P = q\ln(q^2 + 1)$ then $P' = q/(q^2 + 1) + \ln(q^2 + 1)$.

37. If $y = e^{x \ln x}$ then $y' = e^{x \ln x}(1 + \ln x)$.

38. Using the product rule to differentiate $x^2 \cdot x^2$ gives the same result as differentiating x^4 directly.

39. The derivative of the product of two functions is the product of their derivatives.

40. The derivative of the quotient of two functions is the quotient of their derivatives.

41. The derivative of $\sin t + \cos t$ is $\cos t - \sin t$.

42. The second derivative of $f(t) = \sin t$ is $f''(t) = \sin t$.

43. The second derivative of $g(t) = \cos t$ is $g''(t) = -\cos t$.

44. If $y = \sin 2t$ then $y' = \cos 2t$.

45. If $y = \cos t^2$ then $y' = -\sin 2t$.

46. If $z = (\sin 2t)\cos 3t$ then $z' = -6(\cos 2t)\sin 3t$.

47. If $y = \sin(\cos t)$ then $y' = \cos(\cos t) + \sin(-\sin t)$.

48. If $P = 1/\sin q$ then $dP/dq = 1/\cos q$.

49. If $Q = \cos(\pi - t)$ then $dQ/dt = \sin(\pi - t)$.

50. If $Q = \sin(\pi t + 1)$ then $dQ/dt = \pi\cos(\pi t + 1)$.

PROJECTS FOR CHAPTER THREE

1. Coroner's Rule of Thumb

Coroners estimate time of death using the rule of thumb that a body cools about 2°F during the first hour after death and about 1°F for each additional hour. Assuming an air temperature of 68°F and a living body temperature of 98.6°F, the temperature $T(t)$ in °F of a body at a time t hours since death is given by

$$T(t) = 68 + 30.6e^{-kt}.$$

(a) For what value of k will the body cool by 2°F in the first hour?
(b) Using the value of k found in part (a), after how many hours will the temperature of the body be decreasing at a rate of 1°F per hour?
(c) Using the value of k found in part (a), show that, 24 hours after death, the coroner's rule of thumb gives approximately the same temperature as the formula.

2. Air Pressure and Altitude

Air pressure at sea level is 30 inches of mercury. At an altitude of h feet above sea level, the air pressure, P, in inches of mercury, is given by

$$P = 30e^{-3.23\times10^{-5}h}$$

(a) Sketch a graph of P against h.
(b) Find the equation of the tangent line at $h = 0$.
(c) A rule of thumb used by travelers is that air pressure drops about 1 inch for every 1000-foot increase in height above sea level. Write a formula for the air pressure given by this rule of thumb.
(d) What is the relation between your answers to parts (b) and (c)? Explain why the rule of thumb works.
(e) Are the predictions made by the rule of thumb too large or too small? Why?

3. Relative Growth Rates: Population, GDP, and GDP per capita

(a) Let Y be the world's annual production (GDP). The world GDP per capita is given by Y/P where P is world population. Figure 3.26 shows relative growth rate of GDP and GDP per capita for 1952–2000.[13]

(i) Explain why the vertical distance between the two curves gives the relative rate of growth of the world population.

(ii) Estimate the relative rate of population growth in 1970 and 2000.

(b) In 2006 the relative rate of change of the GDP in developing countries was 4.5% per year, and the relative rate of change of the population was 1.2%. What was the relative rate of change of the per capita GDP in developing countries?

(c) In 2006 the relative rate of change of the world's total production (GDP) was 3.8% per year, and the relative rate of change of the world's per capita production was 2.6% per year. What was the relative rate of change of the world population?

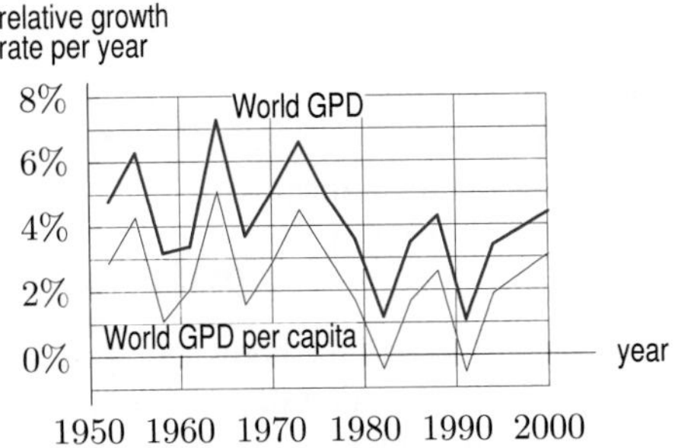

Figure 3.26

[13] Angus Maddison, *The World Economy: Historical Statistics*, OECD, 2003.

FOCUS ON THEORY

ESTABLISHING THE DERIVATIVE FORMULAS

The graph of $f(x) = x^2$ suggests that the derivative of x^2 is $f'(x) = 2x$. However, as we saw in the Focus on Theory section in Chapter 2, to be sure that this formula is correct, we have to use the definition:

$$f'(x) = \lim_{h \to 0} \frac{f(x+h) - f(x)}{h}.$$

As in Chapter 2, we simplify the difference quotient and then take the limit as h approaches zero.

Example 1 Confirm that the derivative of $g(x) = x^3$ is $g'(x) = 3x^2$.

Solution Using the definition, we calculate $g'(x)$:

$$g'(x) = \lim_{h \to 0} \frac{g(x+h) - g(x)}{h} = \lim_{h \to 0} \frac{(x+h)^3 - x^3}{h}$$

Multiplying out $\longrightarrow$
$$= \lim_{h \to 0} \frac{x^3 + 3x^2h + 3xh^2 + h^3 - x^3}{h}$$

$$= \lim_{h \to 0} \frac{3x^2h + 3xh^2 + h^3}{h}$$

Simplifying $\longrightarrow$
$$= \lim_{h \to 0} (3x^2 + 3xh + h^2) = 3x^2.$$

$\nwarrow$ Looking at what happens as $h \to 0$

So $g'(x) = \dfrac{d}{dx}(x^3) = 3x^2$.

Example 2 Give an informal justification that the derivative of $f(x) = e^x$ is $f'(x) = e^x$.

Solution Using $f(x) = e^x$, we have

$$f'(x) = \lim_{h \to 0} \frac{f(x+h) - f(x)}{h} = \lim_{h \to 0} \frac{e^{x+h} - e^x}{h}$$

$$= \lim_{h \to 0} \frac{e^x e^h - e^x}{h} = \lim_{h \to 0} e^x \left(\frac{e^h - 1}{h} \right).$$

What is the limit of $\dfrac{e^h - 1}{h}$ as $h \to 0$? The graph of $\dfrac{e^h - 1}{h}$ in Figure 3.27 suggests that $\dfrac{e^h - 1}{h}$ approaches 1 as $h \to 0$. In fact, it can be proved that the limit equals 1, so

$$f'(x) = \lim_{h \to 0} e^x \left(\frac{e^h - 1}{h} \right) = e^x \cdot 1 = e^x.$$

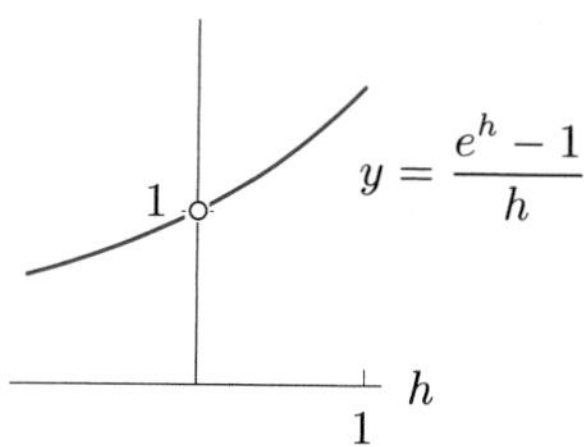

Figure 3.27: What is $\lim_{h \to 0} \frac{e^h - 1}{h}$?

Example 3 Show that if $f(x) = 2x^2 + 1$, then $f'(x) = 4x$.

Solution We use the definition of the derivative with $f(x) = 2x^2 + 1$:

$$f'(x) = \lim_{h\to 0} \frac{f(x+h) - f(x)}{h} = \lim_{h\to 0} \frac{(2(x+h)^2 + 1) - (2x^2 + 1)}{h}$$
$$= \lim_{h\to 0} \frac{2(x^2 + 2xh + h^2) + 1 - 2x^2 - 1}{h} = \lim_{h\to 0} \frac{2x^2 + 4xh + 2h^2 + 1 - 2x^2 - 1}{h}$$
$$= \lim_{h\to 0} \frac{4xh + 2h^2}{h} = \lim_{h\to 0} \frac{h(4x + 2h)}{h}$$

To find the limit, look at what happens when h is close to 0, but $h \neq 0$. Simplifying, we have

$$f'(x) = \lim_{h\to 0} \frac{h(4x + 2h)}{h} = \lim_{h\to 0} (4x + 2h) = 4x$$

because as h gets close to 0, we know that $4x + 2h$ gets close to $4x$.

Using the Chain Rule to Establish Derivative Formulas

We use the chain rule to justify the formulas for derivatives of $\ln x$ and of a^x.

Derivative of $\ln x$

We'll differentiate an identity that involves $\ln x$. In Section 1.6, we have $e^{\ln x} = x$. Differentiating gives

$$\frac{d}{dx}(e^{\ln x}) = \frac{d}{dx}(x) = 1.$$

On the left side, since e^x is the outside function and $\ln x$ is the inside function, the chain rule gives

$$\frac{d}{dx}(e^{\ln x}) = e^{\ln x} \cdot \frac{d}{dx}(\ln x).$$

Thus, as we said in Sections 3.2,

$$\frac{d}{dx}(\ln x) = \frac{1}{e^{\ln x}} = \frac{1}{x}.$$

Derivative of a^x

Graphical arguments suggest that the derivative of a^x is proportional to a^x. Now we show that the constant of proportionality is $\ln a$. For $a > 0$, we use the identity from Section 1.6:

$$\ln(a^x) = x \ln a.$$

On the left side, using $\frac{d}{dx}(\ln x) = \frac{1}{x}$ and the chain rule gives

$$\frac{d}{dx}(\ln a^x) = \frac{1}{a^x} \cdot \frac{d}{dx}(a^x).$$

Since $\ln a$ is a constant, differentiating the right side gives

$$\frac{d}{dx}(x \ln a) = \ln a.$$

Since the two sides are equal, we have

$$\frac{1}{a^x}\frac{d}{dx}(a^x) = \ln a.$$

Solving for $\frac{d}{dx}(a^x)$ gives the result of Section 3.2. For $a > 0$,

$$\frac{d}{dx}(a^x) = (\ln a)a^x.$$

The Product Rule

Suppose we want to calculate the derivative of the product of differentiable functions, $f(x)g(x)$, using the definition of the derivative. Notice that in the second step below, we are adding and subtracting the same quantity: $f(x)g(x+h)$.

$$\begin{aligned}\frac{d[f(x)g(x)]}{dx} &= \lim_{h\to 0}\frac{f(x+h)g(x+h)-f(x)g(x)}{h}\\ &= \lim_{h\to 0}\frac{f(x+h)g(x+h)-f(x)g(x+h)+f(x)g(x+h)-f(x)g(x)}{h}\\ &= \lim_{h\to 0}\left[\frac{f(x+h)-f(x)}{h}\cdot g(x+h)+f(x)\cdot\frac{g(x+h)-g(x)}{h}\right]\end{aligned}$$

Taking the limit as $h \to 0$ gives the product rule:

$$(f(x)g(x))' = f'(x)\cdot g(x) + f(x)\cdot g'(x).$$

The Quotient Rule

Let $Q(x) = f(x)/g(x)$ be the quotient of differentiable functions. Assuming that $Q(x)$ is differentiable, we can use the product rule on $f(x) = Q(x)g(x)$:

$$f'(x) = Q'(x)g(x) + Q(x)g'(x).$$

Substituting for $Q(x)$ gives

$$f'(x) = Q'(x)g(x) + \frac{f(x)}{g(x)}g'(x).$$

Solving for $Q'(x)$ gives

$$Q'(x) = \frac{f'(x) - \dfrac{f(x)}{g(x)}g'(x)}{g(x)}.$$

Multiplying the top and bottom by $g(x)$ to simplify gives the quotient rule:

$$\left(\frac{f(x)}{g(x)}\right)' = \frac{f'(x)g(x) - f(x)g'(x)}{(g(x))^2}.$$

Problems on Establishing the Derivative Formulas

For Problems 1–7, use the definition of the derivative to obtain the following results.

1. If $f(x) = 2x+1$, then $f'(x) = 2$.
2. If $f(x) = 5x^2$, then $f'(x) = 10x$.
3. If $f(x) = 2x^2+3$, then $f'(x) = 4x$.
4. If $f(x) = x^2+x$, then $f'(x) = 2x+1$.
5. If $f(x) = 4x^2+1$, then $f'(x) = 8x$.
6. If $f(x) = x^4$, then $f'(x) = 4x^3$. [Hint: $(x+h)^4 = x^4+4x^3h+6x^2h^2+4xh^3+h^4$.]
7. If $f(x) = x^5$, then $f'(x) = 5x^4$. [Hint: $(x+h)^5 = x^5+5x^4h+10x^3h^2+10x^2h^3+5xh^4+h^5$.]
8. **(a)** Use a graph of $g(h) = \dfrac{2^h-1}{h}$ to explain why we believe that $\lim\limits_{h\to 0}\dfrac{2^h-1}{h} \approx 0.6931$.

   (b) Use the definition of the derivative and the result from part (a) to explain why, if $f(x) = 2^x$, we believe that $f'(x) \approx (0.6931)2^x$.
9. Use the definition of the derivative to show that if $f(x) = C$, where C is a constant, then $f'(x) = 0$.
10. Use the definition of the derivative to show that if $f(x) = b + mx$, for constants m and b, then $f'(x) = m$.
11. Use the definition of the derivative to show that if $f(x) = k\cdot u(x)$, where k is a constant and $u(x)$ is a function, then $f'(x) = k\cdot u'(x)$.
12. Use the definition of the derivative to show that if $f(x) = u(x)+v(x)$, for functions $u(x)$ and $v(x)$, then $f'(x) = u'(x)+v'(x)$.

FOCUS ON PRACTICE

Find derivatives for the functions in Problems 1–63. Assume a, b, c, and k are constants.

1. $f(t) = t^2 + t^4$
2. $g(x) = 5x^4$
3. $y = 5x^3 + 7x^2 - 3x + 1$
4. $s(t) = 6t^{-2} + 3t^3 - 4t^{1/2}$
5. $f(x) = \dfrac{1}{x^2} + 5\sqrt{x} - 7$
6. $P(t) = 100e^{0.05t}$
7. $f(x) = 5e^{2x} - 2 \cdot 3^x$
8. $P(t) = 1{,}000(1.07)^t$
9. $D(p) = e^{p^2} + 5p^2$
10. $y = t^2 e^{5t}$
11. $y = x^2\sqrt{x^2+1}$
12. $f(x) = \ln\left(x^2+1\right)$
13. $s(t) = 8\ln(2t+1)$
14. $g(w) = w^2 \ln(w)$
15. $f(x) = 2^x + x^2 + 1$
16. $P(t) = \sqrt{t^2+4}$
17. $C(q) = (2q+1)^3$
18. $g(x) = 5x(x+3)^2$
19. $P(t) = be^{kt}$
20. $f(x) = ax^2 + bx + c$
21. $y = x^2 \ln(2x+1)$
22. $f(t) = \left(e^t + 4\right)^3$
23. $f(x) = 5\sin(2x)$
24. $W(r) = r^2 \cos r$
25. $g(t) = 3\sin(5t) + 4$
26. $y = e^{3t}\sin(2t)$
27. $y = 2e^x + 3\sin x + 5$
28. $f(t) = 3t^2 - 4t + 1$
29. $y = 17x + 24x^{1/2}$
30. $g(x) = -\frac{1}{2}(x^5 + 2x - 9)$
31. $f(x) = 5x^4 + \dfrac{1}{x^2}$
32. $y = \dfrac{e^{2x}}{x^2+1}$
33. $f(x) = \dfrac{x^2+3x+2}{x+1}$
34. $y = \left(\dfrac{x^2+2}{3}\right)^2$
35. $g(x) = \sin(2-3x)$
36. $f(z) = \dfrac{z^2+1}{3z}$
37. $q(r) = \dfrac{3r}{5r+2}$
38. $y = x\ln x - x + 2$
39. $j(x) = \ln(e^{ax} + b)$
40. $g(t) = \dfrac{t-4}{t+4}$
41. $h(w) = (w^4 - 2w)^5$
42. $h(w) = w^3 \ln(10w)$
43. $f(x) = \ln(\sin x + \cos x)$
44. $w(r) = \sqrt{r^4+1}$
45. $h(w) = -2w^{-3} + 3\sqrt{w}$
46. $h(x) = \sqrt{\dfrac{x^2+9}{x+3}}$
47. $v(t) = t^2 e^{-ct}$
48. $f(x) = \dfrac{x}{1+\ln x}$
49. $g(\theta) = e^{\sin\theta}$
50. $p(t) = e^{4t+2}$
51. $j(x) = \dfrac{x^3}{a} + \dfrac{a}{b}x^2 - cx$
52. $f(z) = \dfrac{z^2+1}{\sqrt{z}}$
53. $h(r) = \dfrac{r^2}{2r+1}$
54. $g(x) = 2x - \dfrac{1}{\sqrt[3]{x}} + 3^x - e$
55. $f(t) = 2te^t - \dfrac{1}{\sqrt{t}}$
56. $w = \dfrac{5-3z}{5+3z}$
57. $f(x) = \dfrac{x^3}{9}(3\ln x - 1)$
58. $g(x) = \dfrac{x^2+\sqrt{x}+1}{x^{3/2}}$
59. $y = \left(x^2+5\right)^3\left(3x^3-2\right)^2$
60. $f(x) = \dfrac{a^2-x^2}{a^2+x^2}$
61. $w(r) = \dfrac{ar^2}{b+r^3}$
62. $H(t) = (at^2+b)e^{-ct}$
63. $g(w) = \dfrac{5}{(a^2-w^2)^2}$

Chapter Four

USING THE DERIVATIVE

Contents

4.1 LOCAL MAXIMA AND MINIMA

What Derivatives Tell Us About a Function and Its Graph

When we graph a function on a computer or calculator, we often see only part of the picture. Information given by the first and second derivatives can help identify regions with interesting behavior.

Example 1 Use a computer or calculator to sketch a useful graph of the function

$$f(x) = x^3 - 9x^2 - 48x + 52.$$

Solution Since f is a cubic polynomial, we expect a graph that is roughly S-shaped. Graphing this function with $-10 \leq x \leq 10$, $-10 \leq y \leq 10$ gives the two nearly vertical lines in Figure 4.1. We know that there is more going on than this, but how do we know where to look?

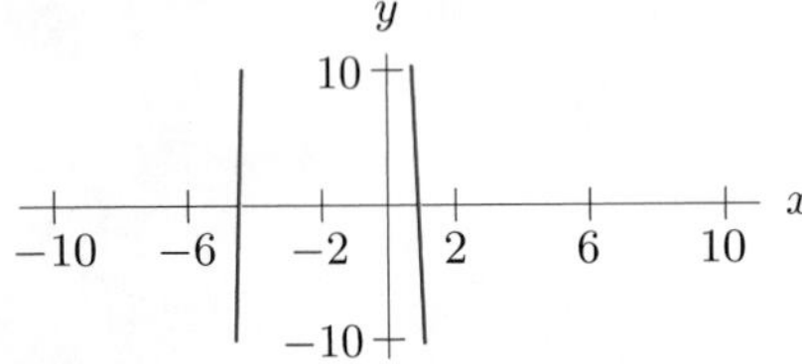

Figure 4.1: Unhelpful graph of $f(x) = x^3 - 9x^2 - 48x + 52$

We use the derivative to determine where the function is increasing and where it is decreasing. The derivative of f is

$$f'(x) = 3x^2 - 18x - 48.$$

To find where $f' > 0$ or $f' < 0$, we first find where $f' = 0$, that is, where $3x^2 - 18x - 48 = 0$. Factoring gives $3(x-8)(x+2) = 0$, so $x = -2$ or $x = 8$. Since $f' = 0$ *only* at $x = -2$ and $x = 8$, and since f' is continuous, f' cannot change sign on any of the three intervals $x < -2$, or $-2 < x < 8$, or $8 < x$. How can we tell the sign of f' on each of these intervals? The easiest way is to pick a point and substitute into f'. For example, since $f'(-3) = 33 > 0$, we know f' is positive for $x < -2$, so f is increasing for $x < -2$. Similarly, since $f'(0) = -48$ and $f'(10) = 72$, we know that f decreases between $x = -2$ and $x = 8$ and increases for $x > 8$. Summarizing:

	$x = -2$		$x = 8$		
f increasing ↗		f decreasing ↘		f increasing ↗	x
$f' > 0$	$f' = 0$	$f' < 0$	$f' = 0$	$f' > 0$	

We find that $f(-2) = 104$ and $f(8) = -396$. Hence, on the interval $-2 < x < 8$ the function decreases from a high of 104 to a low of -396. (Now we see why not much showed up in our first calculator graph.) One more point on the graph is easy to get: the y-intercept, $f(0) = 52$. With just these three points we can get a much more helpful graph. By setting the plotting window to $-10 \leq x \leq 20$ and $-400 \leq y \leq 400$, we get Figure 4.2, which gives much more insight into the behavior of $f(x)$ than the graph in Figure 4.1.

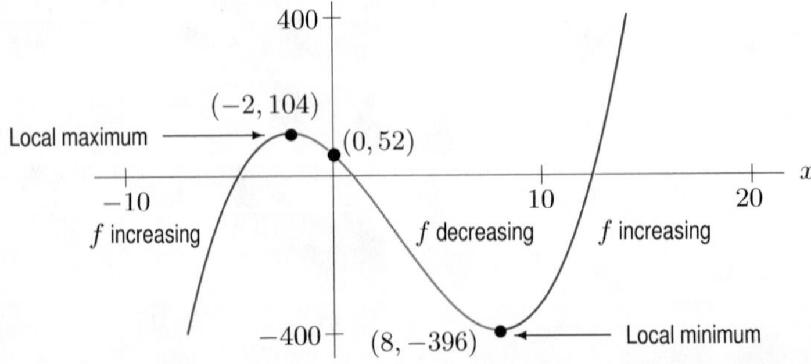

Figure 4.2: Useful graph of $f(x) = x^3 - 9x^2 - 48x + 52$. Notice that the scales on the x-and y-axes are different

Local Maxima and Minima

We are often interested in points such as those marked local maximum and local minimum in Figure 4.2. We have the following definition:

Suppose p is a point in the domain of f:

- f has a **local minimum** at p if $f(p)$ is less than or equal to the values of f for points near p.
- f has a **local maximum** at p if $f(p)$ is greater than or equal to the values of f for points near p.

We use the adjective "local" because we are describing only what happens near p.

How Do We Detect a Local Maximum or Minimum?

In the preceding example, the points $x = -2$ and $x = 8$, where $f'(x) = 0$, played a key role in leading us to local maxima and minima. We give a name to such points:

For any function f, a point p in the domain of f where $f'(p) = 0$ or $f'(p)$ is undefined is called a **critical point** of the function. In addition, the point $(p, f(p))$ on the graph of f is also called a critical point. A **critical value** of f is the value, $f(p)$, of the function at a critical point, p.

Notice that "critical point of f" can refer either to points in the domain of f or to points on the graph of f. You will know which meaning is intended from the context.

Geometrically, at a critical point where $f'(p) = 0$, the line tangent to the graph of f at p is horizontal. At a critical point where $f'(p)$ is undefined, there is no horizontal tangent to the graph—there is either a vertical tangent or no tangent at all. (For example, $x = 0$ is a critical point for the absolute value function $f(x) = |x|$.) However, most of the functions we will work with will be differentiable everywhere, and therefore most of our critical points will be of the $f'(p) = 0$ variety.

The critical points divide the domain of f into intervals on which the sign of the derivative remains the same, either positive or negative. Therefore, if f is defined on the interval between two successive critical points, its graph cannot change direction on that interval; it is either going up or it is going down. We have the following result:

If a function, continuous on an interval (its domain), has a local maximum or minimum at p, then p is a critical point or an endpoint of the interval.

A function may have any number of critical points or none at all. (See Figures 4.3–4.5.)

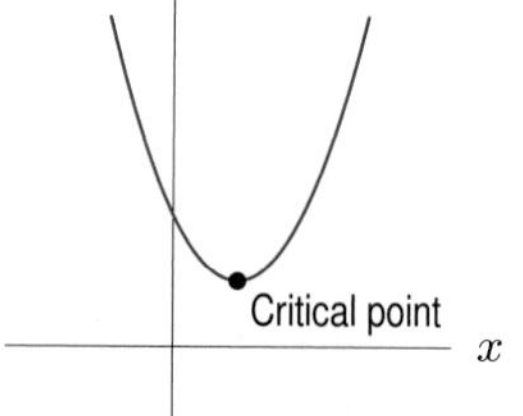

Figure 4.3: A quadratic: One critical point

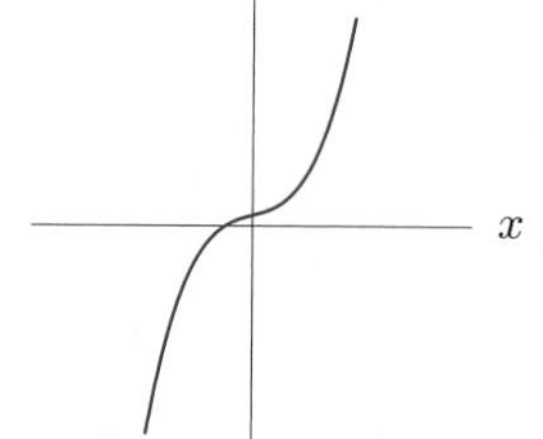

Figure 4.4: $f(x) = x^3 + x + 1$: No critical points

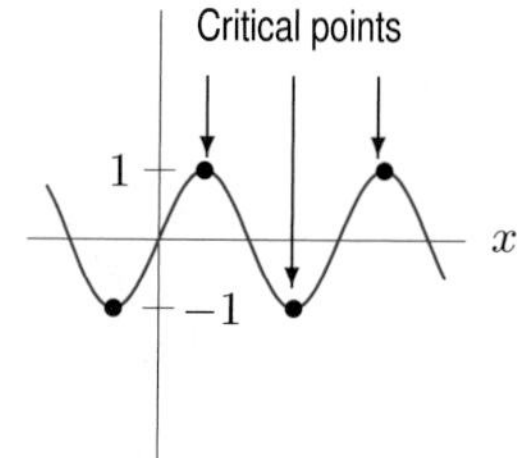

Figure 4.5: Many critical points

Testing For Local Maxima and Minima

If f' has different signs on either side of a critical point p with $f'(p) = 0$, then the graph changes direction at p and looks like one of those in Figure 4.6. We have the following criteria:

> **First Derivative Test for Local Maxima and Minima**
>
> Suppose p is a critical point of a continuous function f. Then, as we go from left to right:
> - If f changes from decreasing to increasing at p, then f has a local minimum at p.
> - If f changes from increasing to decreasing at p, then f has a local maximum at p.

Alternatively, the concavity of the graph of f gives another way of distinguishing between local maxima and minima:

> **Second Derivative Test for Local Maxima and Minima**
>
> Suppose p is a critical point of a continuous function f, and $f'(p) = 0$.
> - If f is concave up at p, then f has a local minimum at p.
> - If f is concave down at p, then f has a local maximum at p.

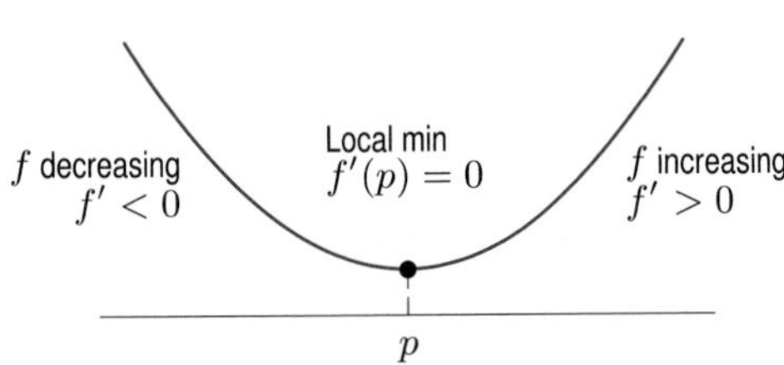

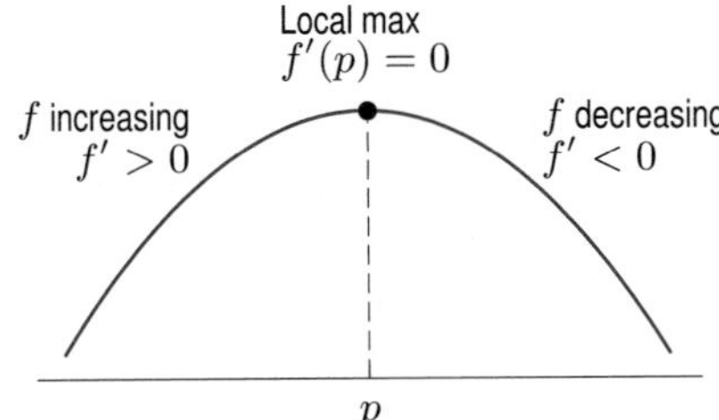

Figure 4.6: Changes in direction at a critical point, p: Local maxima and minima

---

Example 2 Use the second derivative test to confirm that $f(x) = x^3 - 9x^2 - 48x + 52$ has a local maximum at $x = -2$ and a local minimum at $x = 8$.

Solution In Example 1, we calculated $f'(x) = 3x^2 - 18x - 48 = 3(x - 8)(x + 2)$, so $f'(8) = f'(-2) = 0$. Differentiating again gives $f''(x) = 6x - 18$. Since $f''(8) = 6 \cdot 8 - 18 = 30$ and $f''(-2) = 6(-2) - 18 = -30$, the second derivative test confirms that $x = 8$ is a local minimum and $x = -2$ is a local maximum.

Example 3
(a) Graph a function f with the following properties:
- $f(x)$ has critical points at $x = 2$ and $x = 5$;
- $f'(x)$ is positive to the left of 2 and positive to the right of 5;
- $f'(x)$ is negative between 2 and 5.

(b) Identify the critical points as local maxima, local minima, or neither.

Solution
(a) We know that $f(x)$ is increasing when $f'(x)$ is positive, and $f(x)$ is decreasing when $f'(x)$ is negative. The function is increasing to the left of 2 and increasing to the right of 5, and it is decreasing between 2 and 5. A possible sketch is given in Figure 4.7.

(b) We see that the function has a local maximum at $x = 2$ and a local minimum at $x = 5$.

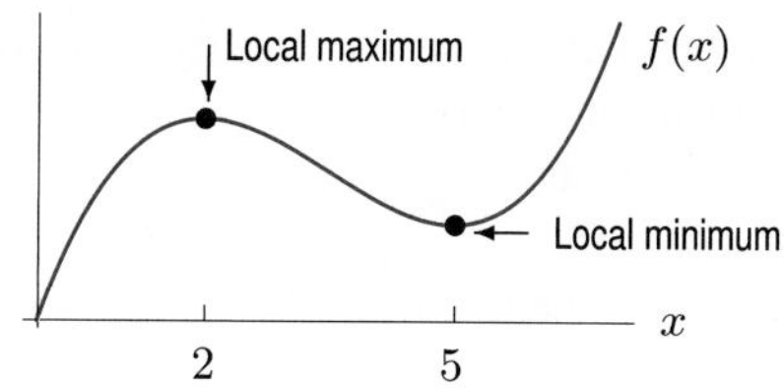

Figure 4.7: A function with critical points at $x = 2$ and $x = 5$

Warning!

Not every critical point of a function is a local maximum or minimum. For instance, consider $f(x) = x^3$, graphed in Figure 4.8. The derivative is $f'(x) = 3x^2$ so $x = 0$ is a critical point. But $f'(x) = 3x^2$ is positive on both sides of $x = 0$, so f increases on both sides of $x = 0$. There is neither a local maximum nor a local minimum for $f(x)$ at $x = 0$.

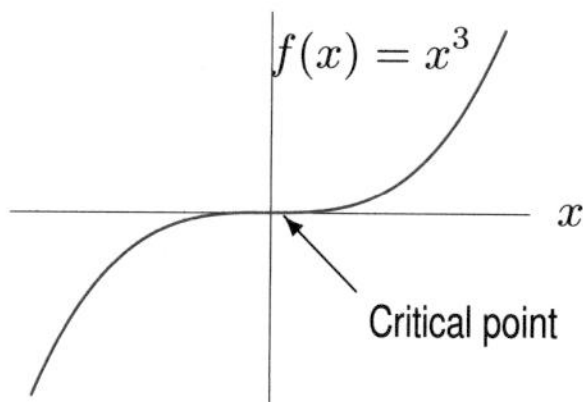

Figure 4.8: A critical point which is neither a local maximum nor minimum.

Example 4 The value of an investment at time t is given by $S(t)$. The rate of change, $S'(t)$, of the value of the investment is shown in Figure 4.9.

(a) What are the critical points of the function $S(t)$?
(b) Identify each critical point as a local maximum, a local minimum, or neither.
(c) Explain the financial significance of each of the critical points.

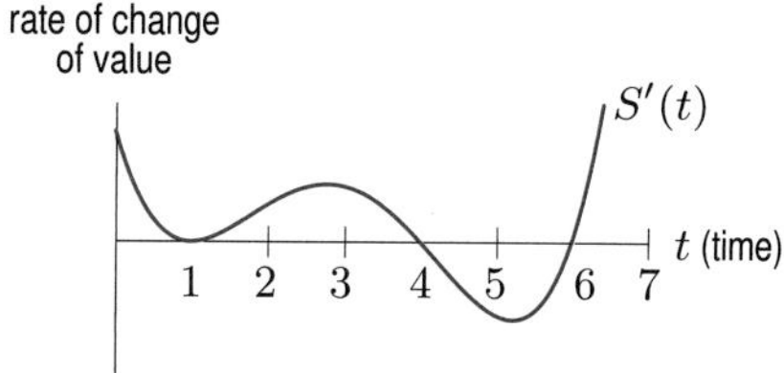

Figure 4.9: Graph of $S'(t)$, the rate of change of the value of the investment

Solution

(a) The critical points of S occur at times t when $S'(t) = 0$. We see in Figure 4.9 that $S'(t) = 0$ at $t = 1$, 4, and 6, so the critical points occur at $t = 1$, 4, and 6.
(b) In Figure 4.9, we see that $S'(t)$ is positive to the left of 1 and between 1 and 4, that $S'(t)$ is negative between 4 and 6, and that $S'(t)$ is positive to the right of 6. Therefore $S(t)$ is increasing to the left of 1 and between 1 and 4 (with a slope of zero at 1), decreasing between 4 and 6, and increasing again to the right of 6. A possible sketch of $S(t)$ is given in Figure 4.10. We see that S has neither a local maximum nor a local minimum at the critical point $t = 1$, but that it has a local maximum at $t = 4$ and a local minimum at $t = 6$.

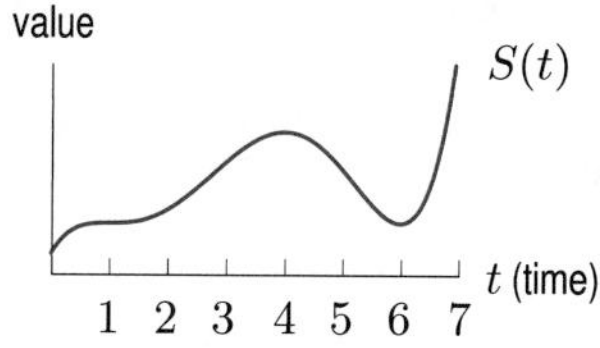

Figure 4.10: Possible graph of the function representing the value of the investment at time t

(c) At time $t = 1$ the investment momentarily stopped increasing in value, though it started increasing again immediately afterward. At $t = 4$, the value peaked and began to decline. At $t = 6$, it started increasing again.

Example 5 Find the critical point of the function $f(x) = x^2 + bx + c$. What is its graphical significance?

Solution Since $f'(x) = 2x + b$, the critical point x satisfies the equation $2x + b = 0$. Thus, the critical point is at $x = -b/2$. The graph of f is a parabola and the critical point is its vertex. See Figure 4.11.

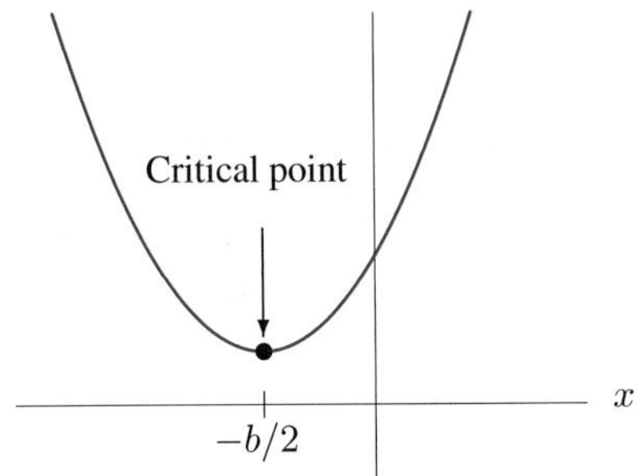

Figure 4.11: Critical point of the parabola $f(x) = x^2 + bx + c$. (Sketched with $b, c > 0$)

Problems for Section 4.1

In Problems 1–4, indicate all critical points of the function f. How many critical points are there? Identify each critical point as a local maximum, a local minimum, or neither.

1. 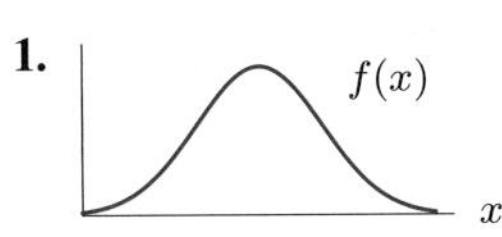

2. 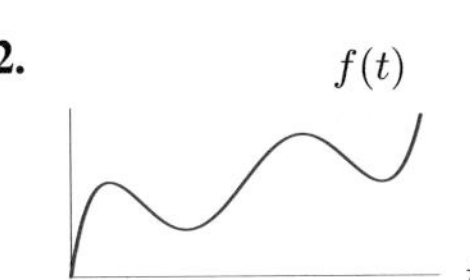

3. 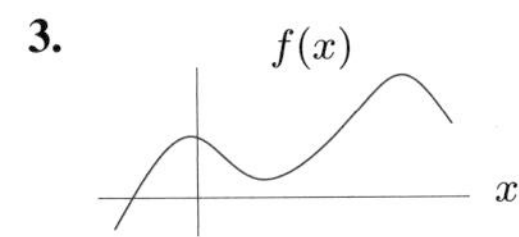

4. 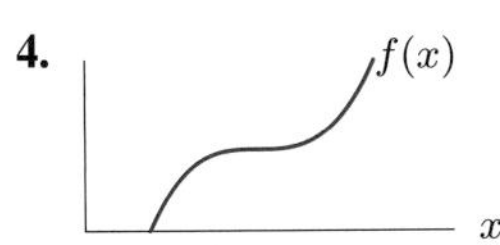

5. **(a)** Graph a function with two local minima and one local maximum.

(b) Graph a function with two critical points. One of these critical points should be a local minimum, and the other should be neither a local maximum nor a local minimum.

6. During an illness a person ran a fever. His temperature rose steadily for eighteen hours, then went steadily down for twenty hours. When was there a critical point for his temperature as a function of time?

7. Graph two continuous functions f and g, each of which has exactly five critical points, the points A–E in Figure 4.12, and which satisfy the following conditions:

(a) $f(x) \to \infty$ as $x \to -\infty$ and
$f(x) \to \infty$ as $x \to \infty$

(b) $g(x) \to -\infty$ as $x \to -\infty$ and
$g(x) \to 0$ as $x \to \infty$

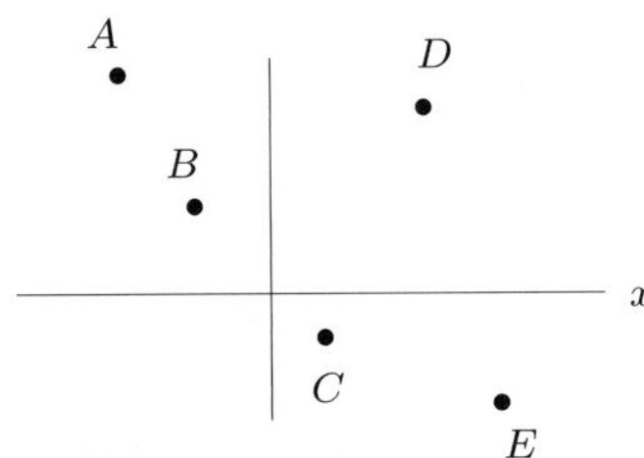

Figure 4.12

Problems 8–9 show the graph of a derivative function f'. Indicate on a sketch the x-values that are critical points of the function f itself. Identify each critical point as a local maximum, a local minimum, or neither.

8. **9.**

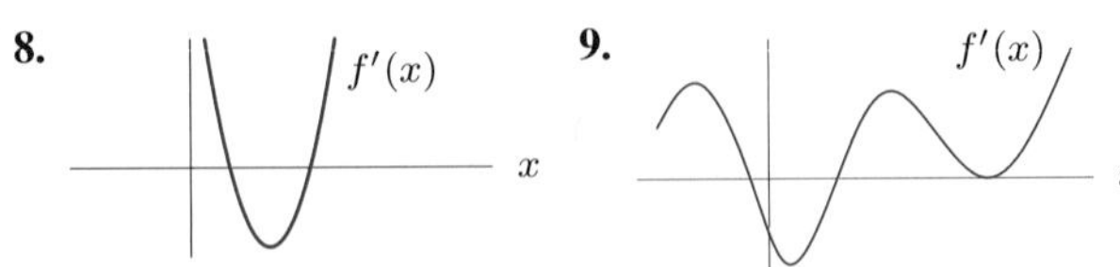

Using a calculator or computer, graph the functions in Problems 10–15. Describe in words the interesting features of the graph, including the location of the critical points and where the function is monotonic (that is, increasing or decreasing). Then use the derivative and algebra to explain the shape of the graph.

10. $f(x) = x^3 - 6x + 1$

11. $f(x) = x^3 + 6x + 1$

12. $f(x) = 3x^5 - 5x^3$

13. $f(x) = e^x - 10x$

14. $f(x) = x \ln x, \quad x > 0$

15. $f(x) = x + 2\sin x$

16. Figure 4.13 is a graph of f'. For what values of x does f have a local maximum? A local minimum?

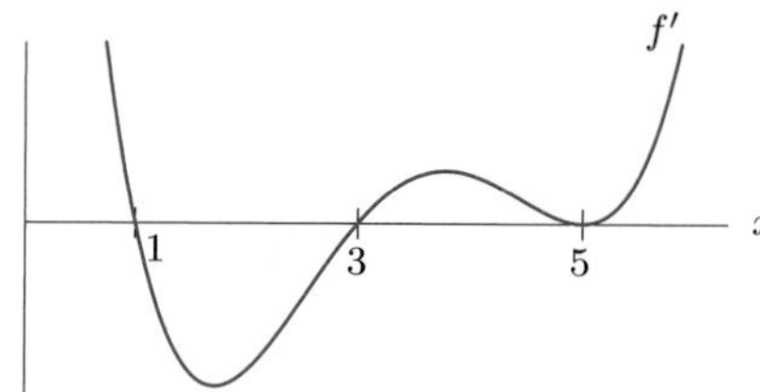

Figure 4.13: Graph of f' (not f)

17. On the graph of f' in Figure 4.14, indicate the x-values that are critical points of the function f itself. Are they local maxima, local minima, or neither?

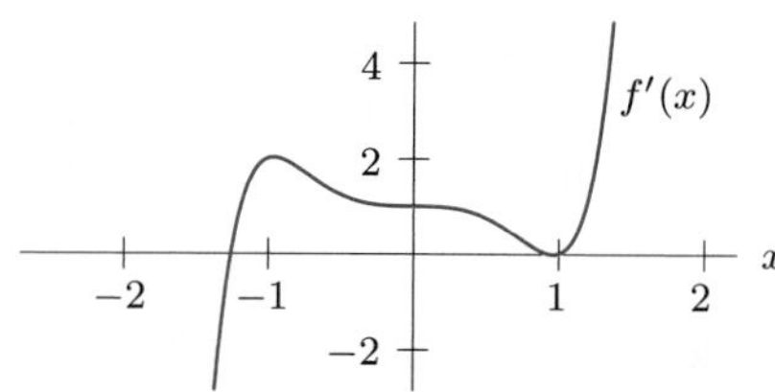

Figure 4.14: Graph of f' (not f)

18. The derivative of $f(t)$ is given by $f'(t) = t^3 - 6t^2 + 8t$ for $0 \le t \le 5$. Graph $f'(t)$, and describe how the function $f(t)$ changes over the interval $t = 0$ to $t = 5$. When is $f(t)$ increasing and when is it decreasing? Where does $f(t)$ have a local maximum and where does it have a local minimum?

19. If U and V are positive constants, find all critical points of

$$F(t) = Ue^t + Ve^{-t}.$$

20. Consumer demand for a certain product is changing over time, and the rate of change of this demand, $f'(t)$, in units/week, is given, in week t, in the following table.

t	0	1	2	3	4	5	6	7	8	9	10
$f'(t)$	12	10	4	−2	−3	−1	3	7	11	15	10

(a) When is the demand for this product increasing? When is it decreasing?

(b) Approximately when is demand at a local maximum? A local minimum?

21. Suppose f has a continuous derivative whose values are given in the following table.

(a) Estimate the x-coordinates of critical points of f for $0 \le x \le 10$.

(b) For each critical point, indicate if it is a local maximum of f, local minimum, or neither.

x	0	1	2	3	4	5	6	7	8	9	10
$f'(x)$	5	2	1	−2	−5	−3	−1	2	3	1	−1

22. The function $f(x) = x^4 - 4x^3 + 8x$ has a critical point at $x = 1$. Use the second derivative test to identify it as a local maximum or local minimum.

23. Find and classify the critical points of $f(x) = x^3(1-x)^4$ as local maxima and minima.

In Problems 24–26, investigate the one-parameter family of functions. Assume that a is positive.

(a) Graph $f(x)$ using three different values for a.

(b) Using your graph in part (a), describe the critical points of f and how they appear to move as a increases.

(c) Find a formula for the x-coordinates of the critical point(s) of f in terms of a.

24. $f(x) = (x - a)^2$

25. $f(x) = x^3 - ax$

26. $f(x) = x^2 e^{-ax}$

In Problems 27–28, find constants a and b so that the minimum for the parabola $f(x) = x^2 + ax + b$ is at the given point. [Hint: Begin by finding the critical point in terms of a.]

27. $(3, 5)$

28. $(-2, -3)$

29. Sketch several members of the family $y = x^3 - ax^2$ on the same axes. Discuss the effect of the parameter a on the graph. Find all critical points for this function.

30. For what values of a and b does $f(x) = a(x - b\ln x)$ have a local minimum at the point $(2, 5)$? Figure 4.15 shows a graph of $f(x)$ with $a = 1$ and $b = 1$.

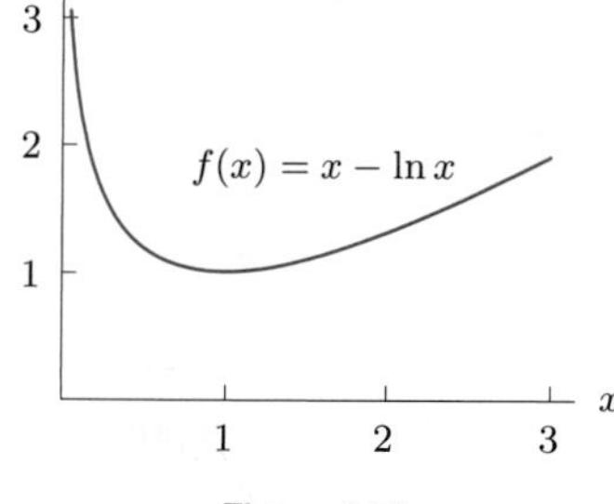

Figure 4.15

31. Find the value of a so that the function $f(x) = xe^{ax}$ has a critical point at $x = 3$.

32. **(a)** If b is a positive constant and $x > 0$, find all critical points of $f(x) = x - b\ln x$.
(b) Use the second derivative test to determine whether the function has a local maximum or local minimum at each critical point.

33. **(a)** For a a positive constant, find all critical points of $f(x) = x - a\sqrt{x}$.
(b) What value of a gives a critical point at $x = 5$? Does $f(x)$ have a local maximum or a local minimum at this critical point?

34. Let $g(x) = x - ke^x$, where k is any constant. For what value(s) of k does the function g have a critical point?

35. If a and b are nonzero constants, find the domain and all critical points of

$$f(x) = \frac{ax^2}{x-b}.$$

36. Assume f has a derivative everywhere and has just one critical point, at $x = 3$. In parts (a)–(d), you are given additional conditions. In each case decide whether $x = 3$ is a local maximum, a local minimum, or neither. Explain your reasoning. Sketch possible graphs for all four cases.

(a) $f'(1) = 3$ and $f'(5) = -1$
(b) $f(x) \to \infty$ as $x \to \infty$ and as $x \to -\infty$
(c) $f(1) = 1$, $f(2) = 2$, $f(4) = 4$, $f(5) = 5$
(d) $f'(2) = -1$, $f(3) = 1$, $f(x) \to 3$ as $x \to \infty$

37. **(a)** On a computer or calculator, graph $f(\theta) = \theta - \sin\theta$. Can you tell whether the function has any zeros in the interval $0 \le \theta \le 1$?
(b) Find f'. What does the sign of f' tell you about the zeros of f in the interval $0 \le \theta \le 1$?

4.2 INFLECTION POINTS

Concavity and Inflection Points

A study of the points on the graph of a function where the slope changes sign led us to critical points. Now we will study the points on the graph where the concavity changes, either from concave up to concave down, or from concave down to concave up.

> A point at which the graph of a function f changes concavity is called an **inflection point** of f.

The words "inflection point of f" can refer either to a point in the domain of f or to a point on the graph of f. The context of the problem will tell you which is meant.

How Do You Locate an Inflection Point?

Since the concavity of the graph of f changes at an inflection point, the sign of f'' changes there: it is positive on one side of the inflection point and negative on the other. Thus, at the inflection point, f'' is zero or undefined. (See Figure 4.16.)

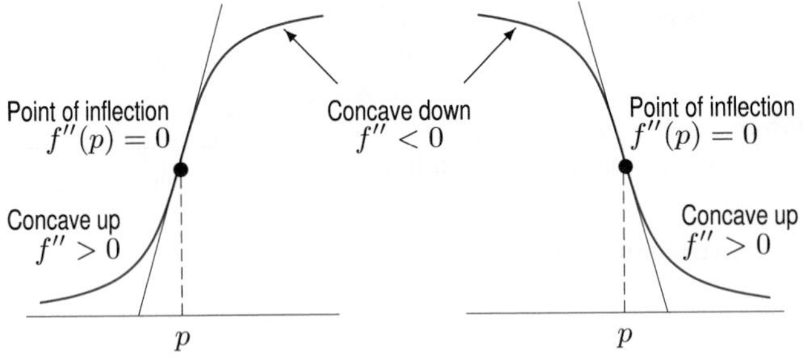

Figure 4.16: Change in concavity (from positive to negative or vice versa) at point p

---

Example 1 Find the inflection points of $f(x) = x^3 - 9x^2 - 48x + 52$.

Solution In Figure 4.17, part of the graph of f is concave up and part is concave down, so the function must have an inflection point. However, it is difficult to locate the inflection point accurately by examining the graph. To find the inflection point exactly, calculate where the second derivative is zero.[1] Since $f'(x) = 3x^2 - 18x - 48$,

[1] For a polynomial, the second derivative cannot be undefined.

$$f''(x) = 6x - 18 \quad \text{so} \quad f''(x) = 0 \quad \text{when} \quad x = 3.$$

The graph of $f(x)$ changes concavity at $x = 3$, so $x = 3$ is an inflection point.

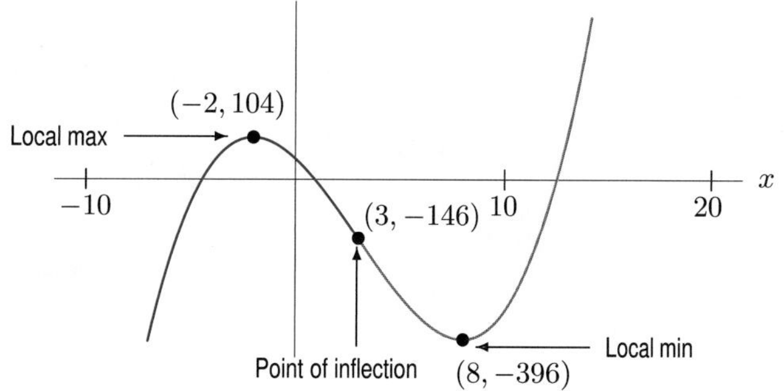

Figure 4.17: Graph of $f(x) = x^3 - 9x^2 - 48x + 52$ showing the inflection point at $x = 3$

Example 2 Graph a function f with the following properties: f has a critical point at $x = 4$ and an inflection point at $x = 8$; the value of f' is negative to the left of 4 and positive to the right of 4; the value of f'' is positive to the left of 8 and negative to the right of 8.

Solution Since f' is negative to the left of 4 and positive to the right of 4, the value of $f(x)$ is decreasing to the left of 4 and increasing to the right of 4. The values of f'' tell us that the graph of $f(x)$ is concave up to the left of 8 and concave down to the right of 8. A possible sketch is given in Figure 4.18.

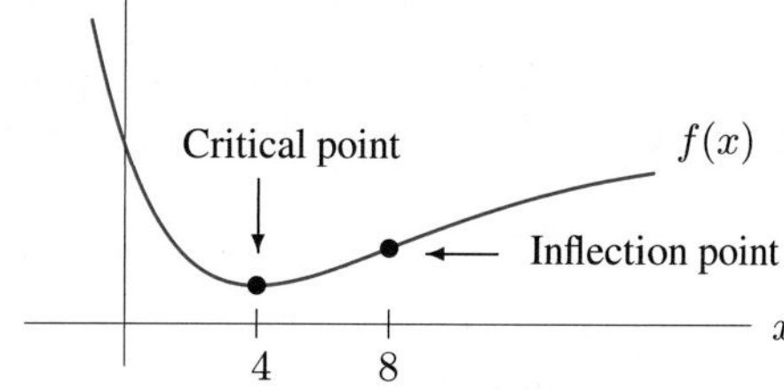

Figure 4.18: A function with a critical point at $x = 4$ and an inflection point at $x = 8$

Example 3 Figure 4.19 shows a population growing toward a limiting population, L. There is an inflection point on the graph at the point where the population reaches $L/2$. What is the significance of the inflection point to the population?

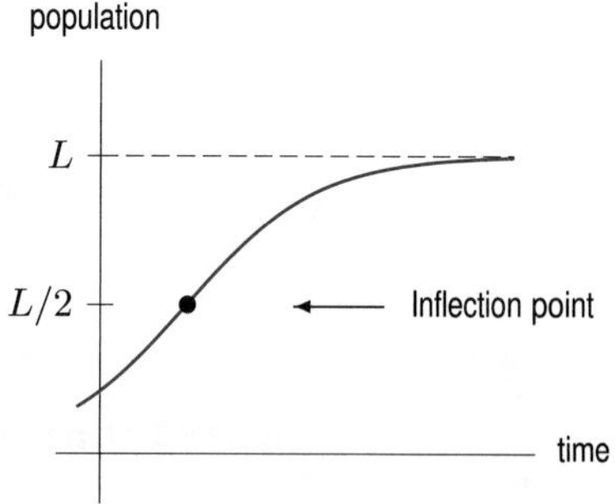

Figure 4.19: Inflection point on graph of a population growing toward a limiting population, L

Solution At times before the inflection point, the population is increasing faster every year. At times after the inflection point the population is increasing slower every year. At the inflection point, the population is growing fastest.

Example 4 (a) How many critical points and how many inflection points does the function $f(x) = xe^{-x}$ have?
(b) Use derivatives to find the critical points and inflection points exactly.

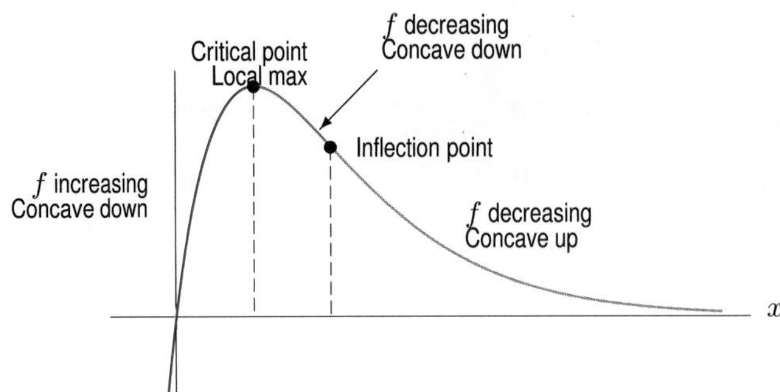

Figure 4.20: Graph of $f(x) = xe^{-x}$

Solution (a) Figure 4.20 shows the graph of $f(x) = xe^{-x}$. It appears to have one critical point, which is a local maximum. Are there any inflection points? Since the graph of the function is concave down at the critical point and concave up for large x, the graph of the function changes concavity, so there must be an inflection point to the right of the critical point.

(b) To find the critical point, find the point where the first derivative of f is zero or undefined. The product rule gives

$$f'(x) = x(-e^{-x}) + (1)(e^{-x}) = (1-x)e^{-x}.$$

We have $f'(x) = 0$ when $x = 1$, so the critical point is at $x = 1$. To find the inflection point, we find where the second derivative of f changes sign. Using the product rule on the first derivative, we have

$$f''(x) = (1-x)(-e^{-x}) + (-1)(e^{-x}) = (x-2)e^{-x}.$$

We have $f''(x) = 0$ when $x = 2$. Since $f''(x) > 0$ for $x > 2$ and $f''(x) < 0$ for $x < 2$, the concavity changes sign at $x = 2$. So the inflection point is at $x = 2$.

Warning!

Not every point x where $f''(x) = 0$ (or f'' is undefined) is an inflection point (just as not every point where $f' = 0$ is a local maximum or minimum). For instance, $f(x) = x^4$ has $f''(x) = 12x^2$ so $f''(0) = 0$, but $f'' > 0$ when $x > 0$ and when $x < 0$, so the graph of f is concave up on both sides of $x = 0$. There is *no* change in concavity at $x = 0$. (See Figure 4.21.)

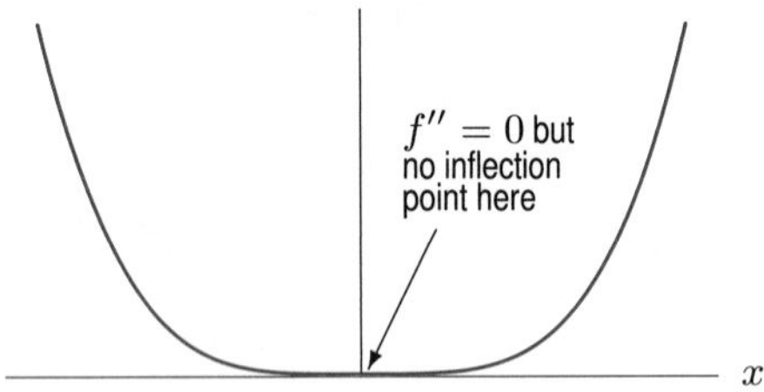

Figure 4.21: Graph of $f(x) = x^4$

Example 5 Suppose that water is being poured into the vase in Figure 4.22 at a constant rate measured in liters per minute. Graph $y = f(t)$, the depth of the water against time, t. Explain the concavity, and indicate the inflection points.

Solution Notice that the volume of water in the vase increases at a constant rate.

At first the water level, y, rises quite slowly because the base of the vase is wide, and so it takes a lot of water to make the depth increase. However, as the vase narrows, the rate at which the water level rises increases. This means that initially y is increasing at an increasing rate, and the graph is concave up. The water level is rising fastest, so the rate of change of the depth y is at a maximum, when the water reaches the middle of the vase, where the diameter is smallest; this is an inflection point. (See Figure 4.23.) After that, the rate at which the water level changes starts to decrease, and so the graph is concave down.

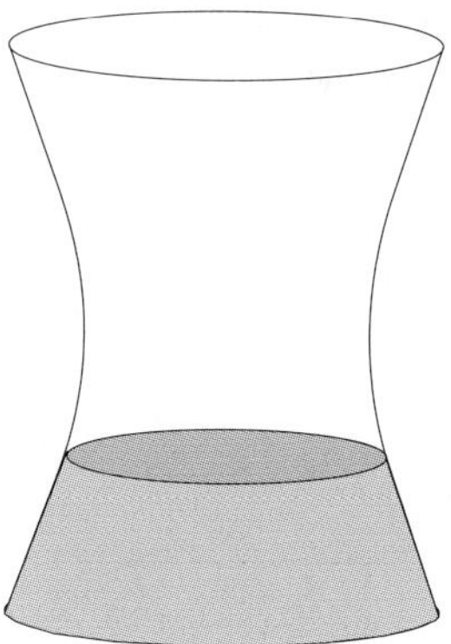

Figure 4.22: A vase

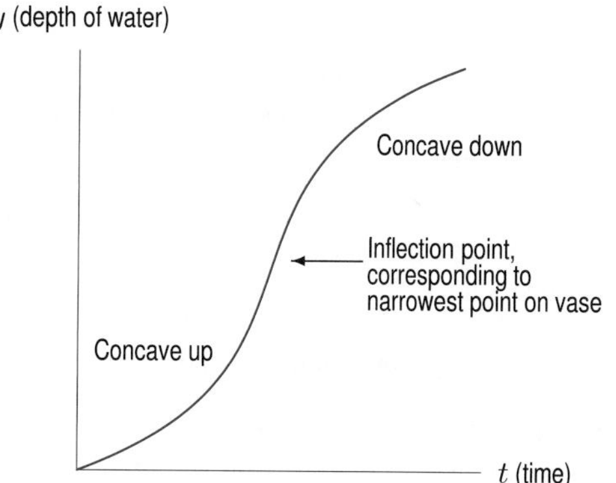

Figure 4.23: Graph of depth of water in the vase, y, against time, t

---

Example 6 What is the concavity of the graph of $f(x) = ax^2 + bx + c$?

Solution We have $f'(x) = 2ax + b$ and $f''(x) = 2a$. The second derivative of f has the same sign as a. If $a > 0$, the graph is concave up everywhere, an upward-opening parabola. If $a < 0$, the graph is concave down everywhere, a downward-opening parabola. (See Figure 4.24.)

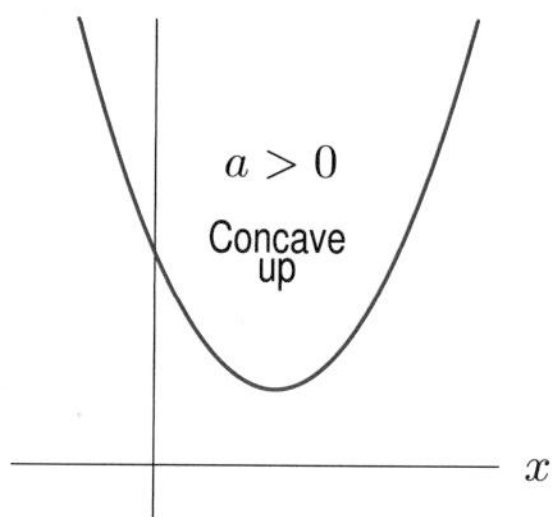

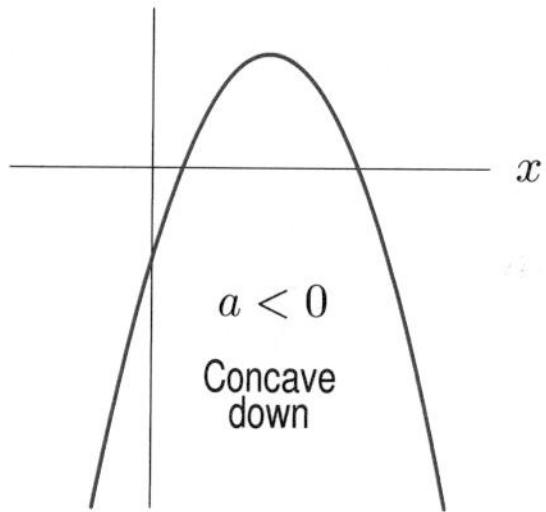

Figure 4.24: Concavity of $f(x) = ax^2 + bx + c$

Problems for Section 4.2

In Problems 1–4, indicate the approximate locations of all inflection points. How many inflection points are there?

1.

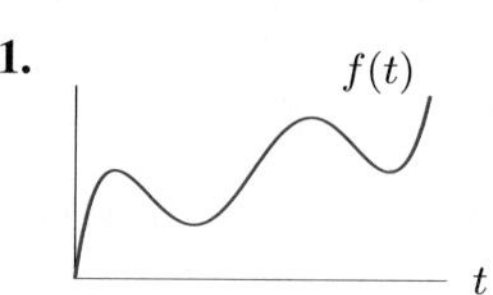

2.

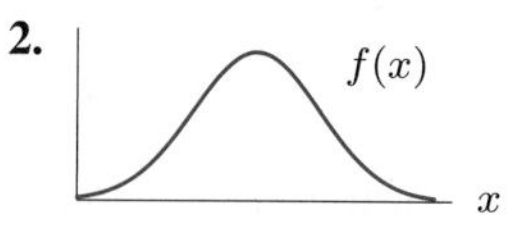

3.

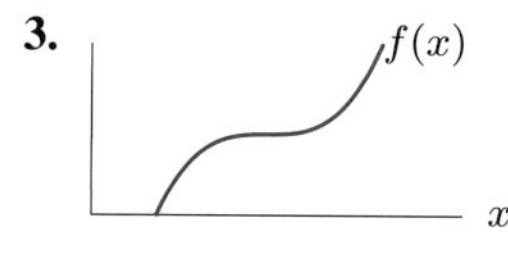

4.

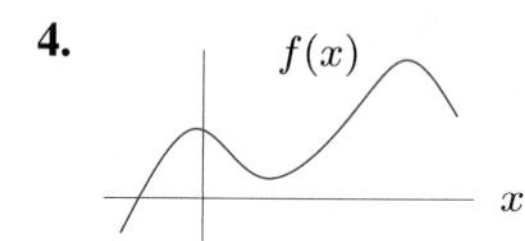

5. **(a)** Graph a polynomial with two local maxima and two local minima.

(b) What is the least number of inflection points this function must have? Label the inflection points.

6. Graph a function with only one critical point (at $x = 5$) and one inflection point (at $x = 10$). Label the critical point and the inflection point on your graph.

7. Graph a function which has a critical point and an inflection point at the same place.

8. During a flood, the water level in a river first rose faster and faster, then rose more and more slowly until it reached its highest point, then went back down to its pre-flood level. Consider water depth as a function of time.

(a) Is the time of highest water level a critical point or an inflection point of this function?

(b) Is the time when the water first began to rise more slowly a critical point or an inflection point?

9. When I got up in the morning I put on only a light jacket because, although the temperature was dropping, it seemed that the temperature would not go much lower. But I was wrong. Around noon a northerly wind blew up and the temperature began to drop faster and faster. The worst was around 6 pm when, fortunately, the temperature started going back up.

(a) When was there a critical point in the graph of temperature as a function of time?

(b) When was there an inflection point in the graph of temperature as a function of time?

10. For $f(x) = x^3 - 18x^2 - 10x + 6$, find the inflection point algebraically. Graph the function with a calculator or computer and confirm your answer.

In each of Problems 11–20, use the first derivative to find all critical points and use the second derivative to find all inflection points. Use a graph to identify each critical point as a local maximum, a local minimum, or neither.

11. $f(x) = x^2 - 5x + 3$

12. $f(x) = x^3 - 3x + 10$

13. $f(x) = 2x^3 + 3x^2 - 36x + 5$

14. $f(x) = \dfrac{x^3}{6} + \dfrac{x^2}{4} - x + 2$

15. $f(x) = x^4 - 2x^2$

16. $f(x) = 3x^4 - 4x^3 + 6$

17. $f(x) = x^4 - 8x^2 + 5$

18. $f(x) = x^4 - 4x^3 + 10$

19. $f(x) = x^5 - 5x^4 + 35$

20. $f(x) = 3x^5 - 5x^3$

21. Find the inflection points of $f(x) = x^4 + x^3 - 3x^2 + 2$.

22. **(a)** Find all critical points and all inflection points of the function $f(x) = x^4 - 2ax^2 + b$. Assume a and b are positive constants.

(b) Find values of the parameters a and b if f has a critical point at the point $(2, 5)$.

(c) If there is a critical point at $(2, 5)$, where are the inflection points?

For Problems 23–26, sketch a possible graph of $y = f(x)$, using the given information about the derivatives $y' = f'(x)$ and $y'' = f''(x)$. Assume that the function is defined and continuous for all real x.

23.

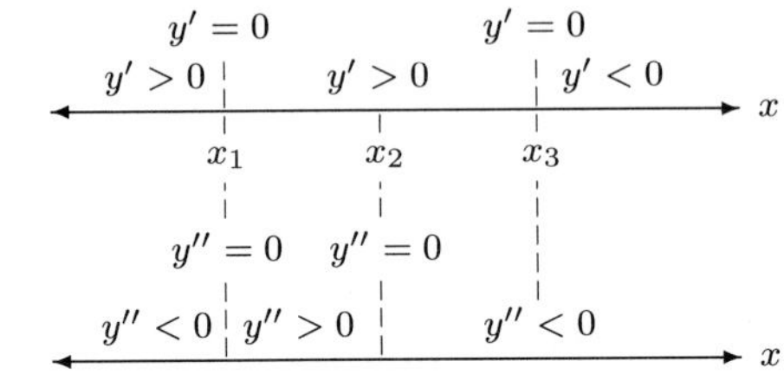

24.

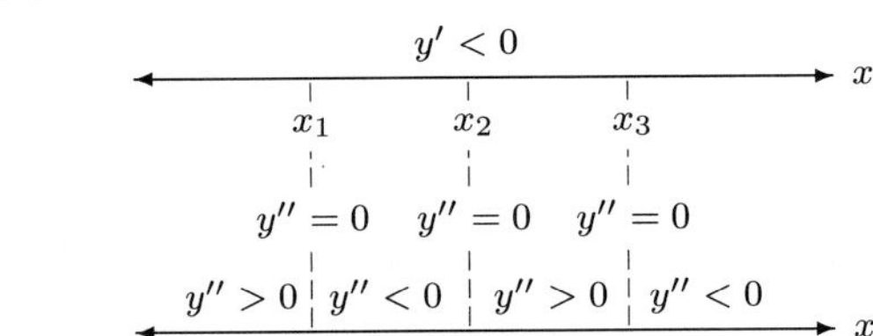

25.

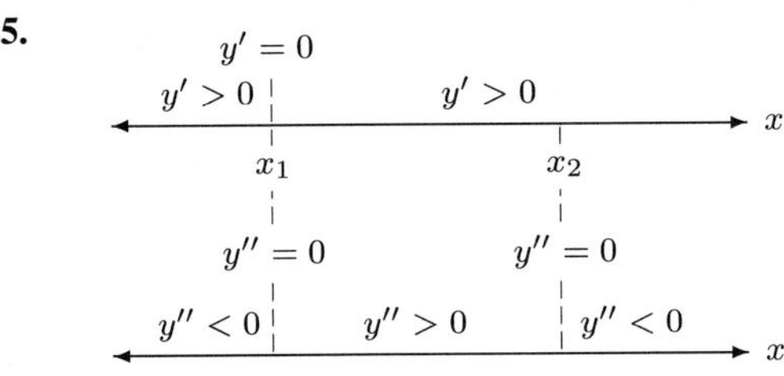

26.

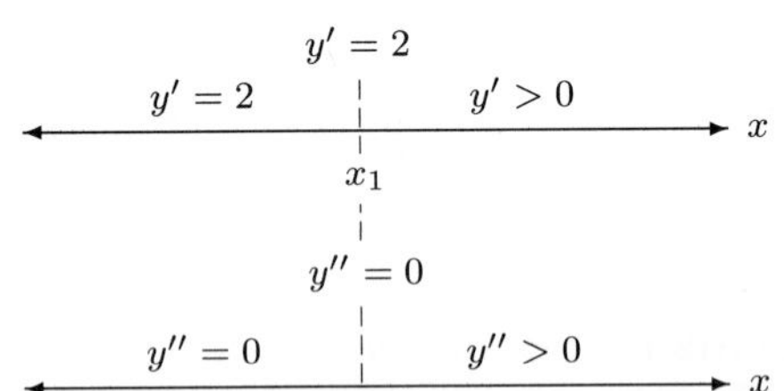

27. In 1774, Captain James Cook left 10 rabbits on a small Pacific island. The rabbit population is approximated by

$$P(t) = \frac{2000}{1 + e^{5.3 - 0.4t}}$$

with t measured in years since 1774. Using a calculator or computer:

(a) Graph P. Does the population level off?

(b) Estimate when the rabbit population grew most rapidly. How large was the population at that time?

(c) Find the inflection point on the graph and explain its significance for the rabbit population.

(d) What natural causes could lead to the shape of the graph of P?

28. (a) Water is flowing at a constant rate (i.e., constant volume per unit time) into a cylindrical container standing vertically. Sketch a graph showing the depth of water against time.

(b) Water is flowing at a constant rate into a cone-shaped container standing on its point. Sketch a graph showing the depth of the water against time.

29. If water is flowing at a constant rate (i.e., constant volume per unit time) into the Grecian urn in Figure 4.25, sketch a graph of the depth of the water against time. Mark on the graph the time at which the water reaches the widest point of the urn.

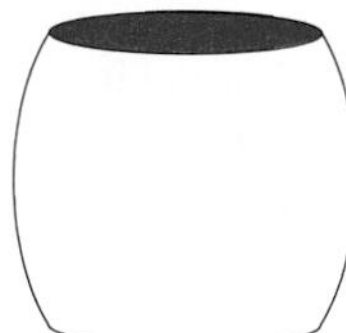

Figure 4.25

30. If water is flowing at a constant rate (i.e., constant volume per unit time) into the vase in Figure 4.26, sketch a graph of the depth of the water against time. Mark on the graph the time at which the water reaches the corner of the vase.

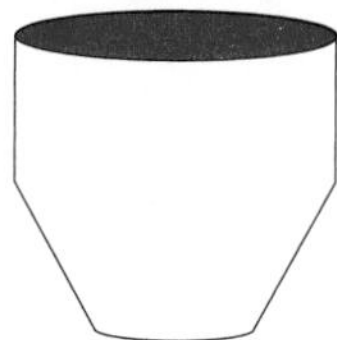

Figure 4.26

31. Water flows at a constant rate into the left side of the W-shaped container in Figure 4.27. Sketch a graph of the height, H, of the water in the left side of the container as a function of time, t. The container starts empty.

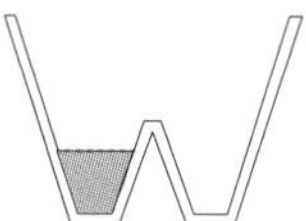

Figure 4.27

32. The vase in Figure 4.28 is filled with water at a constant rate (i.e., constant volume per unit time).

(a) Graph $y = f(t)$, the depth of the water, against time, t. Show on your graph the points at which the concavity changes.

(b) At what depth is $y = f(t)$ growing most quickly? Most slowly? Estimate the ratio between the growth rates at these two depths.

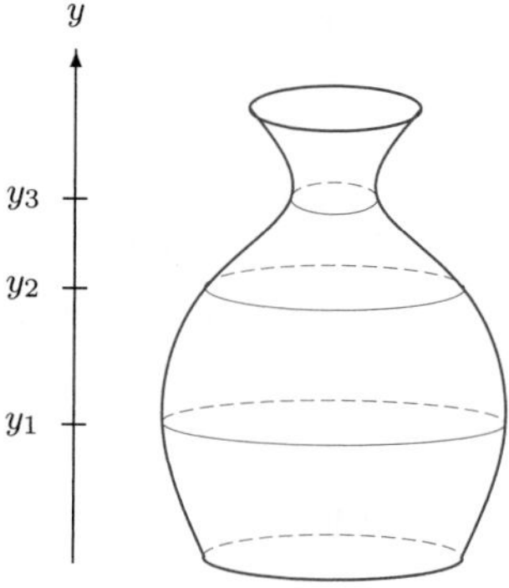

Figure 4.28

Find formulas for the functions described in Problems 33–34.

33. A cubic polynomial, $ax^3 + bx^2 + cx + d$, with a critical point at $x = 2$, an inflection point at $(1, 4)$, and a leading coefficient of 1.

34. A function of the form $y = bxe^{-ax}$ with a local maximum at $(3, 6)$.

35. Indicate on Figure 4.29 approximately where the inflection points of $f(x)$ are if the graph shows

(a) The function $f(x)$ (b) The derivative $f'(x)$

(c) The second derivative $f''(x)$

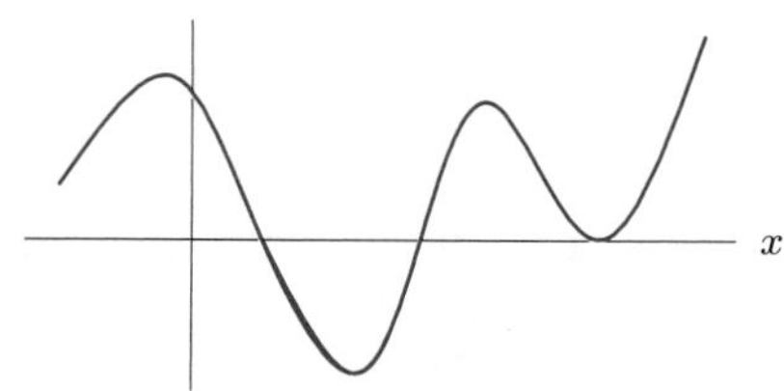

Figure 4.29

36. Assume that the polynomial f has exactly two local maxima and one local minimum, and that these are the only critical points of f.

(a) Sketch a possible graph of f.

(b) What is the largest number of zeros f could have?

(c) What is the least number of zeros f could have?

(d) What is the least number of inflection points f could have?

(e) What is the smallest degree f could have?

(f) Find a possible formula for $f(x)$.

4.3 GLOBAL MAXIMA AND MINIMA

Global Maxima and Minima

The techniques for finding maximum and minimum values make up the field called *optimization*. Local maxima and minima occur where a function takes larger or smaller values than at nearby points. However, we are often interested in where a function is larger or smaller than at all other points. For example, a firm trying to maximize its profit may do so by minimizing its costs. We make the following definition:

For any function f:

- f has a **global minimum** at p if $f(p)$ is less than or equal to all values of f.
- f has a **global maximum** at p if $f(p)$ is greater than or equal to all values of f.

How Do We Find Global Maxima and Minima?

If f is a continuous function defined on an interval $a \leq x \leq b$ (including its endpoints), Figure 4.30 illustrates that the global maximum or minimum of f occurs either at a local maximum or a local minimum, respectively, or at one of the endpoints, $x = a$ or $x = b$, of the interval.

To find the global maximum and minimum of a continuous function on an interval including endpoints: Compare values of the function at all the critical points in the interval and at the endpoints.

What if the continuous function is defined on an interval $a < x < b$ (excluding its endpoints), or on the entire real line which has no endpoints? The function graphed in Figure 4.31 has no global maximum because the function has no largest value. The global minimum of this function coincides with one of the local minima and is marked. A function defined on the entire real line or on an interval excluding endpoints may or may not have a global maximum or a global minimum.

To find the global maximum and minimum of a continuous function on an interval excluding endpoints or on the entire real line: Find the values of the function at all the critical points and sketch a graph.

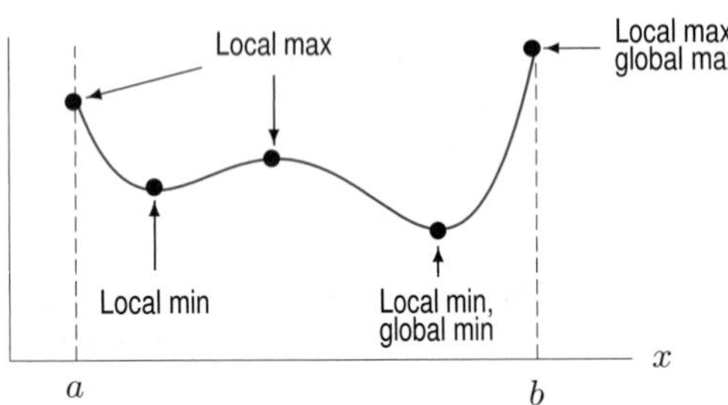

Figure 4.30: Global maximum and minimum on an interval domain, $a \leq x \leq b$

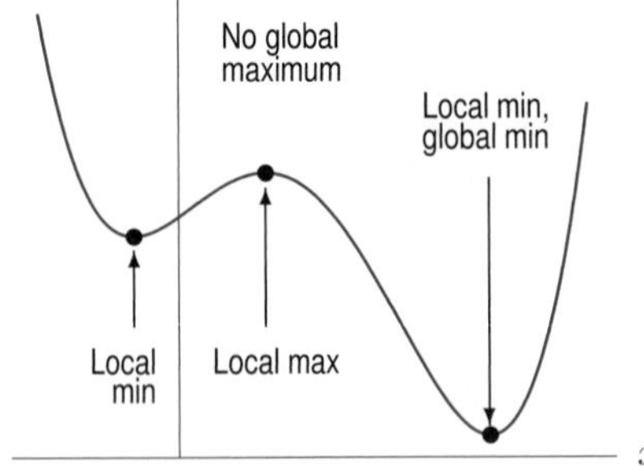

Figure 4.31: Global maximum and minimum on the entire real line

Example 1 Find the global maximum and minimum of $f(x) = x^3 - 9x^2 - 48x + 52$ on the interval $-5 \le x \le 14$.

Solution We have calculated the critical points of this function previously using

$$f'(x) = 3x^2 - 18x - 48 = 3(x+2)(x-8),$$

so $x = -2$ and $x = 8$ are critical points. Since the global maxima and minima occur at a critical point or at an endpoint of the interval, we evaluate f at these four points:

$$f(-5) = -58, \qquad f(-2) = 104, \qquad f(8) = -396, \qquad f(14) = 360.$$

Comparing these four values, we see that the global maximum is 360 and occurs at $x = 14$, and that the global minimum is -396 and occurs at $x = 8$. See Figure 4.32.

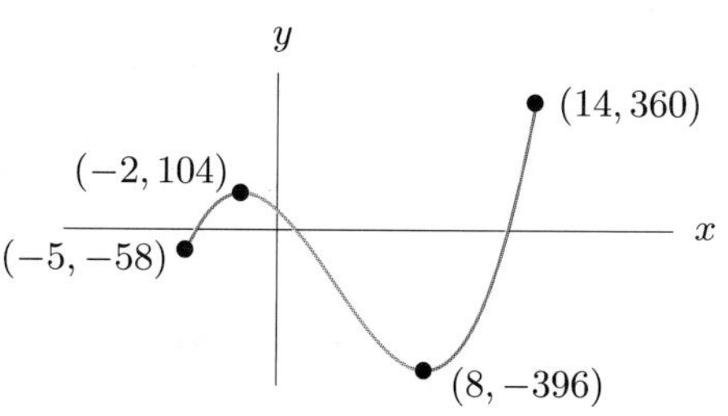

Figure 4.32: Global maximum and minimum on the interval $-5 \le x \le 14$

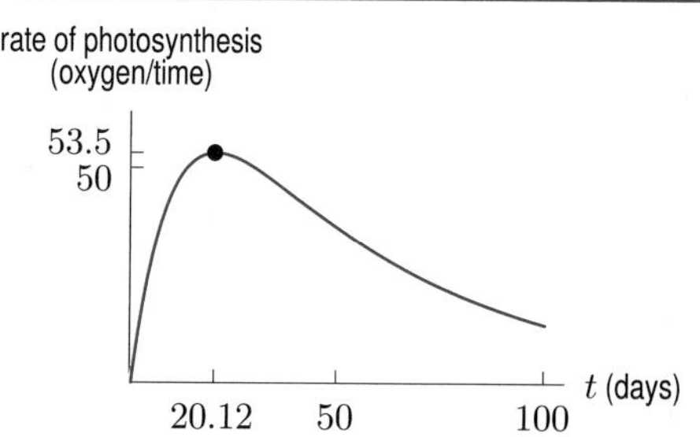

Figure 4.33: Maximum rate of photosynthesis

Example 2 For time, $t \ge 0$, in days, the rate at which photosynthesis takes place in the leaf of a plant, represented by the rate at which oxygen is produced, is approximated by[2]

$$p(t) = 100(e^{-0.02t} - e^{-0.1t}).$$

When is photosynthesis occurring fastest? What is that rate?

Solution To find the global maximum value of $p(t)$, we first find critical points. We differentiate, set equal to zero, and solve for t:

$$\begin{aligned}
p'(t) = 100(-0.02e^{-0.02t} + 0.1e^{-0.1t}) &= 0 \\
-0.02e^{-0.02t} &= -0.1e^{-0.1t} \\
\frac{e^{-0.02t}}{e^{-0.1t}} &= \frac{0.1}{0.02} \\
e^{-0.02t+0.1t} &= 5 \\
e^{0.08t} &= 5 \\
0.08t &= \ln 5 \\
t &= \frac{\ln 5}{0.08} = 20.12 \text{ days.}
\end{aligned}$$

Differentiating again gives

$$p''(t) = 100(0.0004e^{-0.02t} - 0.01e^{-0.1t})$$

and substituting $t = 20.12$ gives $p''(20.12) = -0.107$, so $t = 20.12$ is a local maximum. However, there is only one critical point, so this local maximum is the global maximum. See Figure 4.33.

When $t = 20.12$ days, the rate, in units of oxygen per unit time, is

$$p(20.12) = 100\left(e^{-0.02(20.12)} - e^{-0.1(20.12)}\right) = 53.50.$$

[2]Examples adapted from Rodney Gentry, *Introduction to Calculus for the Biological and Health Sciences* (Reading: Addison-Wesley, 1978).

A Graphical Example: Minimizing Gas Consumption

Next we look at an example in which a function is given graphically and the optimum values are read from a graph. You already know how to estimate the optimum values of $f(x)$ from a graph of $f(x)$—read off the highest and lowest values. In this example, we see how to estimate the optimum value of the quantity $f(x)/x$ from a graph of $f(x)$ against x.

The question we investigate is how to set driving speeds to maximize fuel efficiency.[3] We assume that gas consumption, g (in gallons/hour), as a function of velocity, v (in mph) is as shown in Figure 4.34. We want to minimize the gas consumption per *mile*, not the gas consumption per hour. Let $G = g/v$ represent the average gas consumption per mile. (The units of G are gallons/mile.)

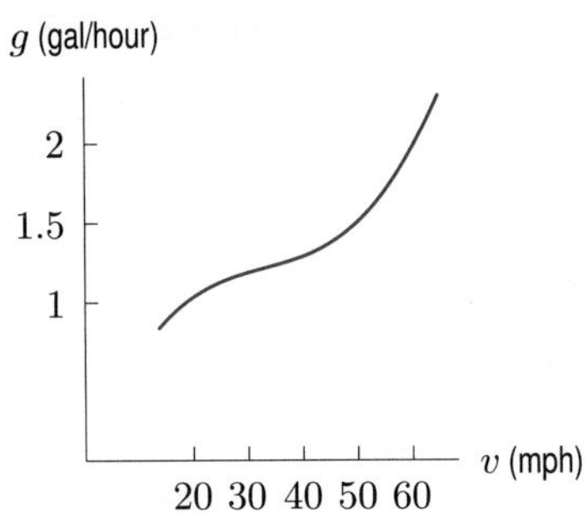

Figure 4.34: Gas consumption versus velocity

Example 3 Using Figure 4.34, estimate the velocity which minimizes $G = g/v$.

Solution We want to find the minimum value of $G = g/v$ when g and v are related by the graph in Figure 4.34. We could use Figure 4.34 to sketch a graph of G against v and estimate a critical point. But there is an easier way. Figure 4.35 shows that g/v is the slope of the line from the origin to the point P. Where on the curve should P be to make the slope a minimum? From the possible positions of the line shown in Figure 4.35, we see that the slope of the line is both a local and global minimum when the line is tangent to the curve. From Figure 4.36, we can see that the velocity at this point is about 50 mph. Thus to minimize gas consumption per mile, we should drive about 50 mph.

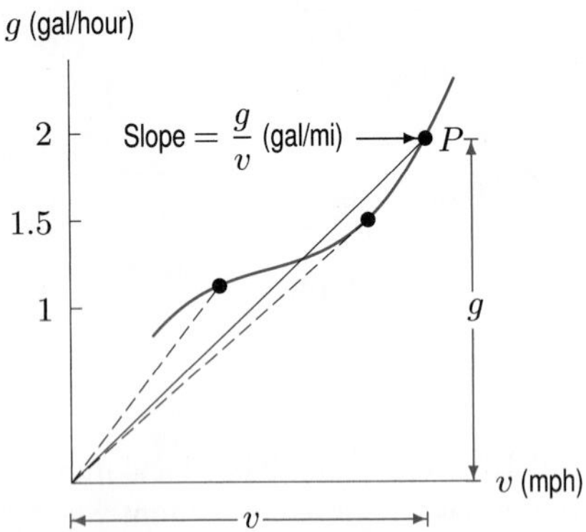

Figure 4.35: Graphical representation of gas consumption per mile, $G = g/v$

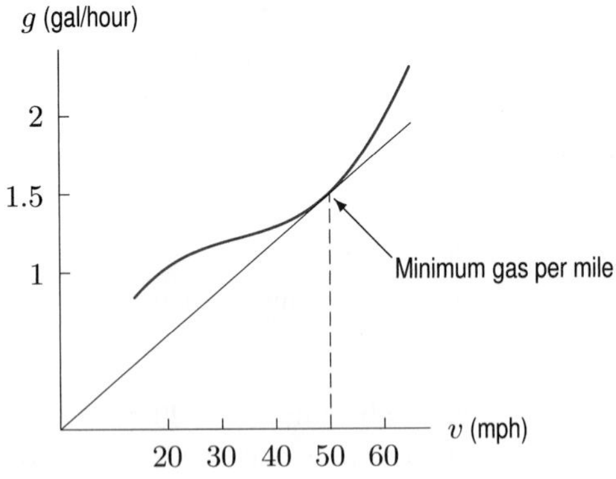

Figure 4.36: Velocity for maximum fuel efficiency

[3]Adapted from Peter D. Taylor, *Calculus: The Analysis of Functions* (Toronto: Wall & Emerson, 1992).

Problems for Section 4.3

For Problems 1–2, indicate all critical points on the given graphs. Which correspond to local minima, local maxima, global maxima, global minima, or none of these? (Note that the graphs are on closed intervals.)

1. **2.**

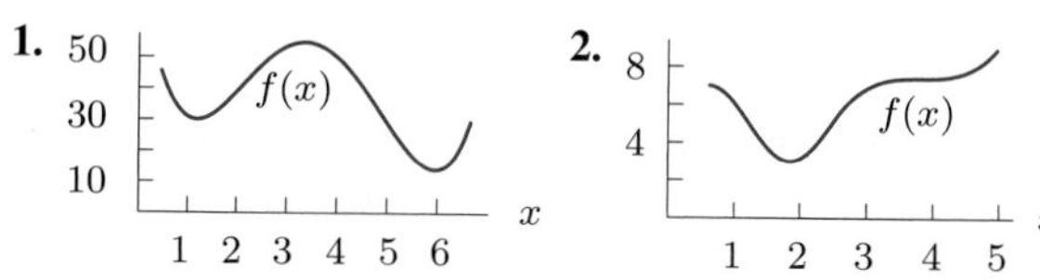

3. For each interval, use Figure 4.37 to choose the statement that gives the location of the global maximum and global minimum of f on the interval.

(a) $4 \leq x \leq 12$ **(b)** $11 \leq x \leq 16$
(c) $4 \leq x \leq 9$ **(d)** $8 \leq x \leq 18$

(I) Maximum at right endpoint, minimum at left endpoint.
(II) Maximum at right endpoint, minimum at critical point.
(III) Maximum at left endpoint, minimum at right endpoint.
(IV) Maximum at left endpoint, minimum at critical point.

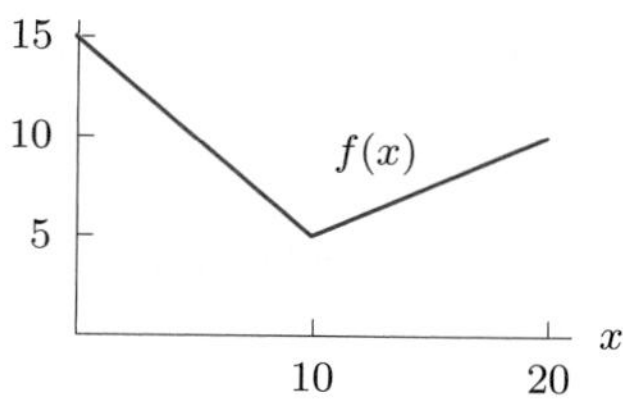

Figure 4.37

In Problems 4–7, graph a function with the given properties.

4. Has local minimum and global minimum at $x = 3$ but no local or global maximum.

5. Has local minimum at $x = 3$, local maximum at $x = 8$, but no global maximum or minimum.

6. Has local and global minimum at $x = 3$, local and global maximum at $x = 8$.

7. Has no local or global maxima or minima.

8. True or false? Give an explanation for your answer. The global maximum of $f(x) = x^2$ on every closed interval is at one of the endpoints of the interval.

In Problems 9–12, sketch the graph of a function on the interval $0 \leq x \leq 10$ with the given properties.

9. Has local minimum at $x = 3$, local maximum at $x = 8$, but global maximum and global minimum at the endpoints of the interval.

10. Has local and global maximum at $x = 3$, local and global minimum at $x = 10$.

11. Has local and global minimum at $x = 3$, local and global maximum at $x = 8$.

12. Has global maximum at $x = 0$, global minimum at $x = 10$, and no other local maxima or minima.

13. A grapefruit is tossed straight up with an initial velocity of 50 ft/sec. The grapefruit is 5 feet above the ground when it is released. Its height at time t is given by

$$y = -16t^2 + 50t + 5.$$

How high does it go before returning to the ground?

14. Find the value of x that maximizes $y = 12 + 18x - 5x^2$ and the corresponding value of y, by

(a) Estimating the values from a graph of y.
(b) Finding the values using calculus.

15. Plot the graph of $f(x) = x^3 - e^x$ using a graphing calculator or computer to find all local and global maxima and minima for: **(a)** $-1 \leq x \leq 4$ **(b)** $-3 \leq x \leq 2$

16. Figure 4.38 shows the rate at which photosynthesis is taking place in a leaf.

(a) At what time, approximately, is photosynthesis proceeding fastest for $t \geq 0$?
(b) If the leaf grows at a rate proportional to the rate of photosynthesis, for what part of the interval $0 \leq t \leq 200$ is the leaf growing? When is it growing fastest?

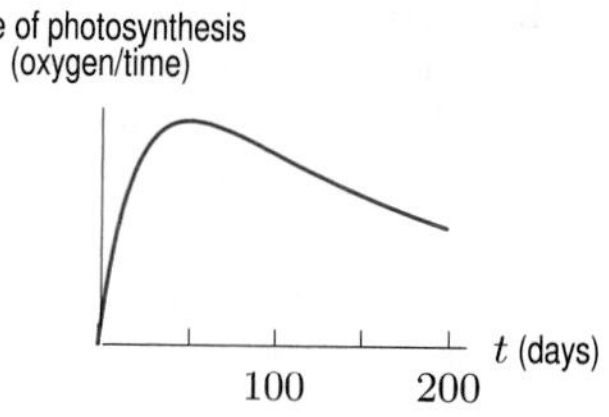

Figure 4.38

17. For some positive constant C, a patient's temperature change, T, due to a dose, D, of a drug is given by

$$T = \left(\frac{C}{2} - \frac{D}{3}\right) D^2.$$

(a) What dosage maximizes the temperature change?
(b) The sensitivity of the body to the drug is defined as dT/dD. What dosage maximizes sensitivity?

For the functions in Problems 18–22, do the following:

(a) Find f' and f''.

(b) Find the critical points of f.
(c) Find any inflection points of f.
(d) Evaluate f at its critical points and at the endpoints of the given interval. Identify local and global maxima and minima of f in the interval.
(e) Graph f.

18. $f(x) = x^3 - 3x^2 \quad (-1 \le x \le 3)$

19. $f(x) = 2x^3 - 9x^2 + 12x + 1 \, (-0.5 \le x \le 3)$

20. $f(x) = x^3 - 3x^2 - 9x + 15 \quad (-5 \le x \le 4)$

21. $f(x) = x + \sin x \quad (0 \le x \le 2\pi)$

22. $f(x) = e^{-x} \sin x \quad (0 \le x \le 2\pi)$

In Problems 23–28, find the exact global maximum and minimum values of the function. The domain is all real numbers unless otherwise specified.

23. $g(x) = 4x - x^2 - 5$

24. $f(x) = x + 1/x$ for $x > 0$

25. $g(t) = te^{-t}$ for $t > 0$

26. $f(x) = x - \ln x$ for $x > 0$

27. $f(t) = \dfrac{t}{1 + t^2}$

28. $f(t) = (\sin^2 t + 2) \cos t$

29. Find the value(s) of x that give critical points of $y = ax^2 + bx + c$, where a, b, c are constants. Under what conditions on a, b, c is the critical value a maximum? A minimum?

30. What value of w minimizes S if $S - 5pw = 3qw^2 - 6pq$ and p and q are positive constants?

31. Figure 4.39 gives the derivative of $g(x)$ on $-2 \le x \le 2$.

(a) Write a few sentences describing the behavior of $g(x)$ on this interval.
(b) Does the graph of $g(x)$ have any inflection points? If so, give the approximate x-coordinates of their locations. Explain your reasoning.
(c) What are the global maxima and minima of g on $[-2, 2]$?
(d) If $g(-2) = 5$, what do you know about $g(0)$ and $g(2)$? Explain.

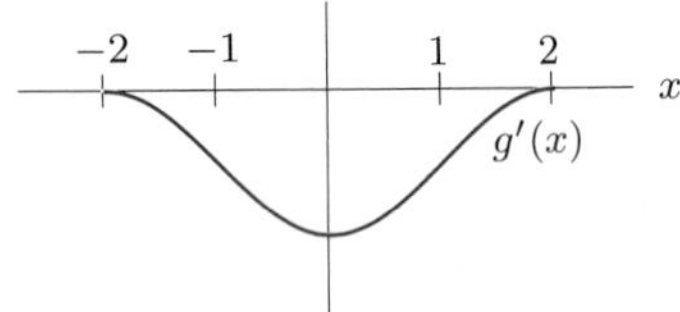

Figure 4.39

32. The energy expended by a bird per day, E, depends on the time spent foraging for food per day, F hours. Foraging for a shorter time requires better territory, which then requires more energy for its defense.[4] Find the foraging time that minimizes energy expenditure if

$$E = 0.25F + \frac{1.7}{F^2}.$$

33. If you have 100 feet of fencing and want to enclose a rectangular area up against a long, straight wall, what is the largest area you can enclose?

34. A closed box has a fixed surface area A and a square base with side x.

(a) Find a formula for its volume, V, as a function of x.
(b) Sketch a graph of V against x.
(c) Find the maximum value of V.

35. On the west coast of Canada, crows eat whelks (a shellfish). To open the whelks, the crows drop them from the air onto a rock. If the shell does not smash the first time, the whelk is dropped again.[5] The average number of drops, n, needed when the whelk is dropped from a height of x meters is approximated by

$$n(x) = 1 + \frac{27}{x^2}.$$

(a) Give the total vertical distance the crow travels upward to open a whelk as a function of drop height, x.
(b) Crows are observed to drop whelks from the height that minimizes the total vertical upward distance traveled per whelk. What is this height?

36. During a flu outbreak in a school of 763 children, the number of infected children, I, was expressed in terms of the number of susceptible (but still healthy) children, S, by the expression[6]

$$I = 192 \ln\left(\frac{S}{762}\right) - S + 763.$$

What is the maximum possible number of infected children?

37. An apple tree produces, on average, 400 kg of fruit each season. However, if more than 200 trees are planted per km^2, crowding reduces the yield by 1 kg for each tree over 200.

(a) Express the total yield from one square kilometer as a function of the number of trees on it. Graph this function.
(b) How many trees should a farmer plant on each square kilometer to maximize yield?

[4] Adapted from Graham Pyke, reported by J. R. Krebs and N. B. Davis in *An Introduction to Behavioural Ecology* (Oxford: Blackwell, 1987).

[5] Adapted from Reto Zach, reported by J. R. Krebs and N. B. Davis in *An Introduction to Behavioural Ecology* (Oxford: Blackwell, 1987).

[6] Data from Communicable Disease Surveillance Centre (UK), reported in "Influenza in a Boarding School", *British Medical Journal*, March 4, 1978.

38. The number of offspring in a population may not be a linear function of the number of adults. The Ricker curve, used to model fish populations, claims that $y = axe^{-bx}$, where x is the number of adults, y is the number of offspring, and a and b are positive constants.

(a) Find and classify all critical points of the Ricker curve.
(b) Is there a global maximum? What does this imply about populations?

39. The oxygen supply, S, in the blood depends on the hematocrit, H, the percentage of red blood cells in the blood:

$$S = aHe^{-bH} \quad \text{for positive constants } a, b.$$

(a) What value of H maximizes the oxygen supply? What is the maximum oxygen supply?
(b) How does increasing the value of the constants a and b change the maximum value of S?

40. The quantity of a drug in the bloodstream t hours after a tablet is swallowed is given, in mg, by

$$q(t) = 20(e^{-t} - e^{-2t}).$$

(a) How much of the drug is in the bloodstream at time $t = 0$?
(b) When is the maximum quantity of drug in the bloodstream? What is that maximum?
(c) In the long run, what happens to the quantity?

41. When birds lay eggs, they do so in clutches of several at a time. When the eggs hatch, each clutch gives rise to a brood of baby birds. We want to determine the clutch size which maximizes the number of birds surviving to adulthood per brood. If the clutch is small, there are few baby birds in the brood; if the clutch is large, there are so many baby birds to feed that most die of starvation. The number of surviving birds per brood as a function of clutch size is shown by the benefit curve in Figure 4.40.[7]

(a) Estimate the clutch size which maximizes the number of survivors per brood.
(b) Suppose also that there is a biological cost to having a larger clutch: the female survival rate is reduced by large clutches. This cost is represented by the dotted line in Figure 4.40. If we take cost into account by assuming that the optimal clutch size in fact maximizes the vertical distance between the curves, what is the new optimal clutch size?

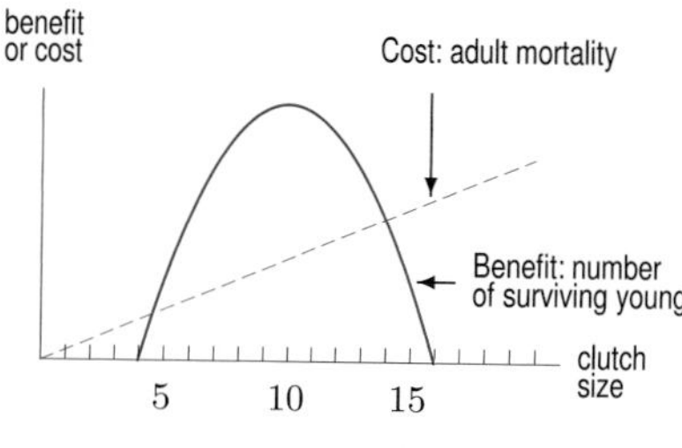

Figure 4.40

42. Let $f(v)$ be the amount of energy consumed by a flying bird, measured in joules per second (a joule is a unit of energy), as a function of its speed v (in meters/sec). Let $a(v)$ be the amount of energy consumed by the same bird, measured in joules per meter.

(a) Suggest a reason (in terms of the way birds fly) for the shape of the graph of $f(v)$ in Figure 4.41.
(b) What is the relationship between $f(v)$ and $a(v)$?
(c) Where is $a(v)$ a minimum?
(d) Should the bird try to minimize $f(v)$ or $a(v)$ when it is flying? Why?

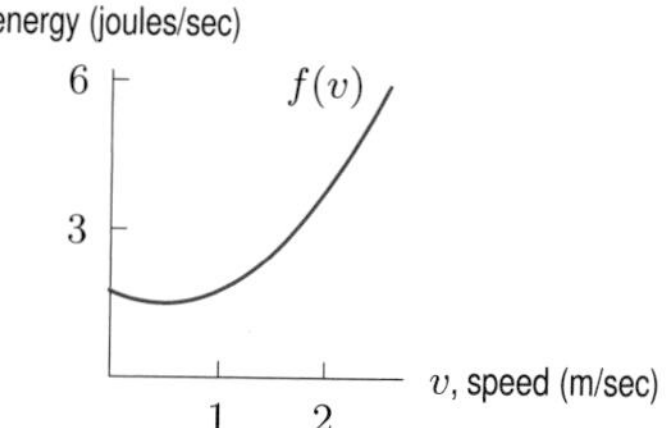

Figure 4.41

43. As an epidemic spreads through a population, the number of infected people, I, is expressed as a function of the number of susceptible people, S, by

$$I = k \ln\left(\frac{S}{S_0}\right) - S + S_0 + I_0, \quad \text{for } k, S_0, I_0 > 0.$$

(a) Find the maximum number of infected people.
(b) The constant k is a characteristic of the particular disease; the constants S_0 and I_0 are the values of S and I when the disease starts. Which of the following affects the maximum possible value of I? Explain.

- The particular disease, but not how it starts.
- How the disease starts, but not the particular disease.
- Both the particular disease and how it starts.

44. The hypotenuse of a right triangle has one end at the origin and one end on the curve $y = x^2e^{-3x}$, with $x \geq 0$. One of the other two sides is on the x-axis, the other side is parallel to the y-axis. Find the maximum area of such a triangle. At what x-value does it occur?

[7]Data from C. M. Perrins and D. Lack, reported by J. R. Krebs and N. B. Davies in *An Introduction to Behavioural Ecology* (Oxford: Blackwell, 1987).

45. A person's blood pressure, p, in millimeters of mercury (mm Hg) is given, for t in seconds, by

$$p = 100 + 20\sin(2.5\pi t).$$

(a) What are the maximum and minimum values of blood pressure?
(b) What is the interval between successive maxima?
(c) Show your answers on a graph of blood pressure against time.

46. A chemical reaction converts substance A to substance Y; the presence of Y catalyzes the reaction. At the start of the reaction, the quantity of A present is a grams. At time t seconds later, the quantity of Y present is y grams. The rate of the reaction, in grams/sec, is given by

$$\text{Rate} = ky(a-y), \quad k \text{ is a positive constant.}$$

(a) For what values of y is the rate nonnegative? Graph the rate against y.
(b) For what values of y is the rate a maximum?

47. In a chemical reaction, substance A combines with substance B to form substance Y. At the start of the reaction, the quantity of A present is a grams, and the quantity of B present is b grams. At time t seconds after the start of the reaction, the quantity of Y present is y grams. Assume $a < b$ and $y \leq a$. For certain types of reactions, the rate of the reaction, in grams/sec, is given by

$$\text{Rate} = k(a-y)(b-y), \quad k \text{ is a positive constant.}$$

(a) For what values of y is the rate nonnegative? Graph the rate against y.
(b) Use your graph to find the value of y at which the rate of the reaction is fastest.

4.4 PROFIT, COST, AND REVENUE

Maximizing Profit

A fundamental issue for a producer of goods is how to maximize profit. For a quantity, q, the profit $\pi(q)$ is the difference between the revenue, $R(q)$, and the cost, $C(q)$, of supplying that quantity. Thus, $\pi(q) = R(q) - C(q)$. The marginal cost, $MC = C'$, is the derivative of C; marginal revenue is $MR = R'$.

Now we look at how to maximize total profit, given functions for revenue and cost. The next example suggests a criterion for identifying the optimal production level.

Example 1 Estimate the maximum profit if the revenue and cost are given by the curves R and C, respectively, in Figure 4.42.

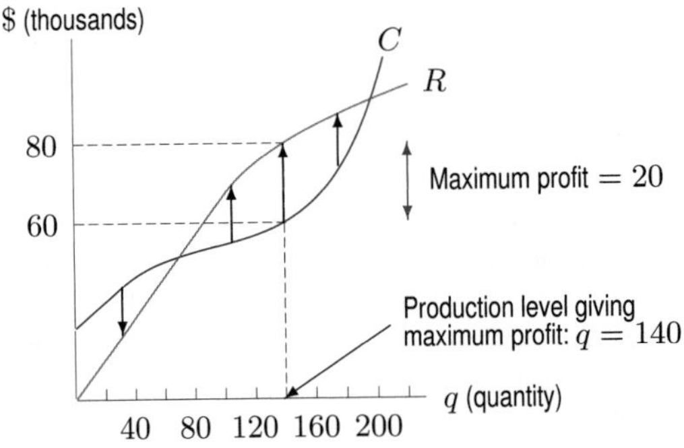

Figure 4.42: Maximum profit at $q = 140$

Solution Since profit is revenue minus cost, the profit is represented by the vertical distance between the cost and revenue curves, marked by the vertical arrows in Figure 4.42. When revenue is below cost, the company is taking a loss; when revenue is above cost, the company is making a profit. The maximum profit must occur between about $q = 70$ and $q = 200$, which is the interval in which the company is making a profit. Profit is maximized when the vertical distance between the curves is largest (and revenue is above cost). This occurs at approximately $q = 140$.

The profit accrued at $q = 140$ is the vertical distance between the curves, so the maximum profit = \$80,000 − \$60,000 = \$20,000.

Maximum Profit Can Occur Where $MR = MC$

We now analyze the marginal costs and marginal revenues near the optimal point. Zooming in on Figure 4.42 around $q = 140$ gives Figure 4.43.

At a production level q_1 to the left of 140 in Figure 4.43, marginal cost is less than marginal revenue. The company would make more money by producing more units, so production should be increased (toward a production level of 140). At any production level q_2 to the right of 140, marginal cost is greater than marginal revenue. The company would lose money by producing more units and would make more money by producing fewer units. Production should be adjusted down toward 140.

What about the marginal revenue and marginal cost at $q = 140$? Since $MC < MR$ to the left of 140, and $MC > MR$ to the right of 140, we expect $MC = MR$ at 140. In this example, profit is maximized at the point where the slopes of the cost and revenue graphs are equal.

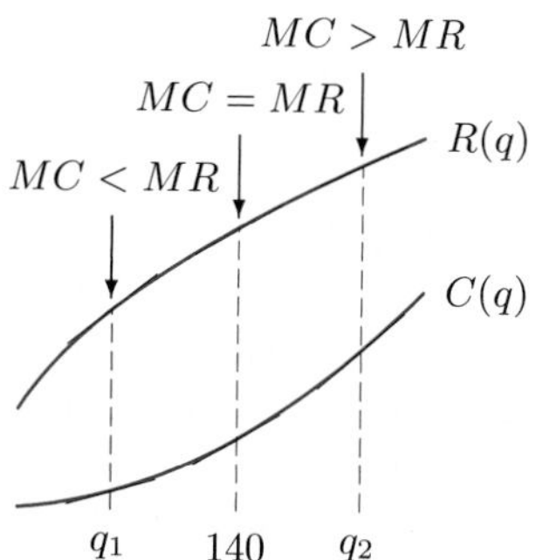

Figure 4.43: Example 1: Maximum profit occurs where $MC = MR$

We can get the same result analytically. Global maxima and minima of a function can only occur at critical points of the function or at the endpoints of the interval. To find critical points of π, look for zeros of the derivative:

$$\pi'(q) = R'(q) - C'(q) = 0.$$

So

$$R'(q) = C'(q),$$

that is, the slopes of the graphs of $R(q)$ and $C(q)$ are equal at q. In economic language,

> The maximum (or minimum) profit can occur where
>
> $$\text{Marginal profit} = 0,$$
>
> that is, where
>
> $$\text{Marginal revenue} = \text{Marginal cost}.$$

Of course, maximum or minimum profit does not *have* to occur where $MR = MC$; either one could occur at an endpoint. Example 2 shows how to visualize maxima and minima of the profit on a graph of marginal revenue and marginal cost.

Example 2 The total revenue and total cost curves for a product are given in Figure 4.44.

(a) Sketch the marginal revenue and marginal cost, MR and MC, on the same axes. Mark the two quantities where marginal revenue equals marginal cost. What is the significance of these two quantities? At which quantity is profit maximized?

(b) Graph the profit function $\pi(q)$.

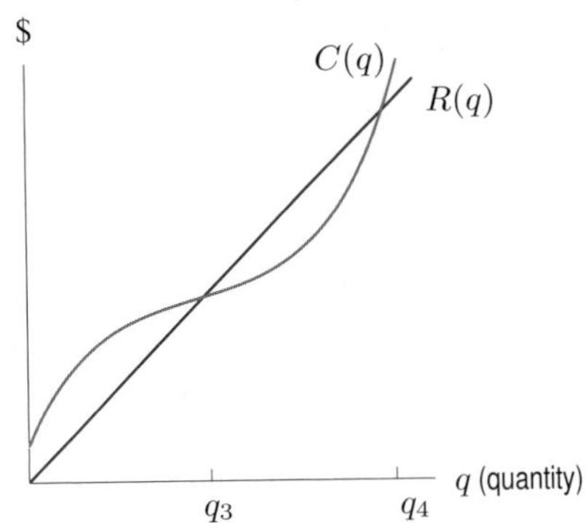

Figure 4.44: Total revenue and total cost

Solution

(a) Since $R(q)$ is a straight line with positive slope, the graph of its derivative, MR, is a horizontal line. (See Figure 4.45.) Since $C(q)$ is always increasing, its derivative, MC, is always positive. As q increases, the cost curve changes from concave down to concave up, so the derivative of the cost function, MC, changes from decreasing to increasing. (See Figure 4.45.) The local minimum on the marginal cost curve corresponds to the inflection point of $C(q)$.

Where is profit maximized? We know that the maximum profit can occur when Marginal revenue = Marginal cost, that is where the curves in Figure 4.45 cross at q_1 and q_2. Do these points give the maximum profit?

We first consider q_1. To the left of q_1, we have $MR < MC$, so $\pi' = MR - MC$ is negative and the profit function is decreasing there. To the right of q_1, we have $MR > MC$, so π' is positive and the profit function is increasing. This behavior, decreasing and then increasing, means that the profit function has a local minimum at q_1. This is certainly not the production level we want.

What happens at q_2? To the left of q_2, we have $MR > MC$, so π' is positive and the profit function is increasing. To the right of q_2, we have $MR < MC$, so π' is negative and the profit function is decreasing. This behavior, increasing and then decreasing, means that the profit function has a local maximum at q_2. The global maximum profit occurs either at the production level q_2 or at an endpoint (the largest and smallest possible production levels). Since the profit is negative at the endpoints (see Figure 4.44), the global maximum occurs at q_2.

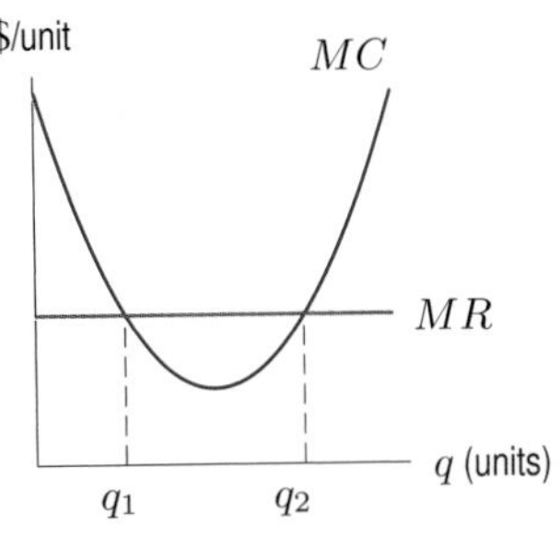

Figure 4.45: Marginal revenue and marginal cost

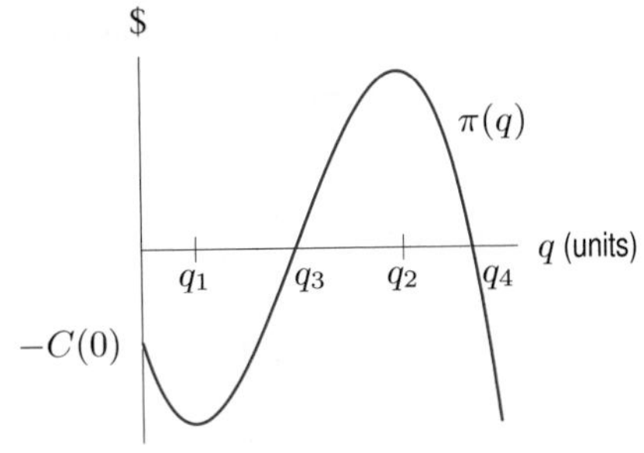

Figure 4.46: Profit function

(b) The graph of the profit function is in Figure 4.46. At the maximum and minimum, the slope of the profit curve is zero:

$$\pi'(q_1) = \pi'(q_2) = 0.$$

Note that since $R(0) = 0$ and $C(0)$ represents the fixed costs of production, we have

$$\pi(0) = R(0) - C(0) = -C(0).$$

Therefore the vertical intercept of the profit function is a negative number, equal in magnitude to the size of the fixed cost.

Example 3 Find the quantity which maximizes profit if the total revenue and total cost (in dollars) are given by

$$R(q) = 5q - 0.003q^2$$
$$C(q) = 300 + 1.1q$$

where q is quantity and $0 \leq q \leq 1000$ units. What production level gives the minimum profit?

Solution We begin by looking for production levels that give Marginal revenue = Marginal cost. Since

$$MR = R'(q) = 5 - 0.006q$$
$$MC = C'(q) = 1.1,$$

$MR = MC$ leads to

$$5 - 0.006q = 1.1$$
$$q = \frac{3.9}{0.006} = 650 \text{ units.}$$

Does this represent a local maximum or minimum of the profit π? To decide, look to the left and right of 650 units.

When $q = 649$, we have $MR = \$1.106$ per unit, which is greater than $MC = \$1.10$ per unit.

Thus, producing one more unit (the 650th) brings in more revenue than it costs, so profit increases.

When $q = 651$, we have $MR = \$1.094$ per unit, which is less than $MC = \$1.10$ per unit.

It is not profitable to produce the 651st unit. We conclude that $q = 650$ gives a local maximum for the profit function π.

To check whether $q = 650$ gives a global maximum, we compare the profit at the endpoints, $q = 0$ and $q = 1000$, with the profit at $q = 650$.

At $q = 0$, the only cost is \$300 (the fixed costs) and there is no revenue, so $\pi(0) = -\$300$.

At $q = 1000$, we have $R(1000) = \$2000$ and $C(1000) = \$1400$, so $\pi(1000) = \$600$.

At $q = 650$, we have $R(650) = \$1982.50$ and $C(650) = \$1015$, so $\pi(650) = \$967.50$.

Therefore, the maximum profit is obtained at a production level of $q = 650$ units. The minimum profit (a loss) occurs when $q = 0$ and there is no production at all.

Maximizing Revenue

For some companies, costs do not depend on the number of items sold. For example, a city bus company with a fixed schedule has the same costs no matter how many people ride the buses. In such a situation, profit is maximized by maximizing revenue.

Example 4 At a price of \$80 for a half-day trip, a white-water rafting company attracts 300 customers. Every \$5 decrease in price attracts an additional 30 customers.

(a) Find the demand equation.
(b) Express revenue as a function of price.
(c) What price should the company charge per trip to maximize revenue?

Solution (a) We first find the equation relating price to demand. If price, p, is 80, the number of trips sold, q, is 300. If p is 75, then q is 330, and so on. See Table 4.1. Because demand changes by a constant (30 people) for every \$5 drop in price, q is a linear function of p. Then

$$\text{Slope} = \frac{300 - 330}{80 - 75} = -\frac{30}{5} = -6 \text{ people/dollar,}$$

so the demand equation is $q = -6p + b$. Since $p = 80$ when $q = 300$, we have

$$\begin{aligned} 300 &= -6 \cdot 80 + b \\ b &= 300 + 6 \cdot 80 = 780. \end{aligned}$$

The demand equation is $q = -6p + 780$.

(b) Since revenue $R = p \cdot q$, revenue as a function of price is

$$R(p) = p(-6p + 780) = -6p^2 + 780p.$$

(c) Figure 4.47 shows this revenue function has a maximum. To find it, we differentiate:

$$\begin{aligned} R'(q) &= -12p + 780 = 0 \\ p &= \frac{780}{12} = 65. \end{aligned}$$

The maximum revenue is achieved when the price is \$65.

Table 4.1 *Demand for rafting trips*

Price, p	Number of trips sold, q
80	300
75	330
70	360
65	390
...	...

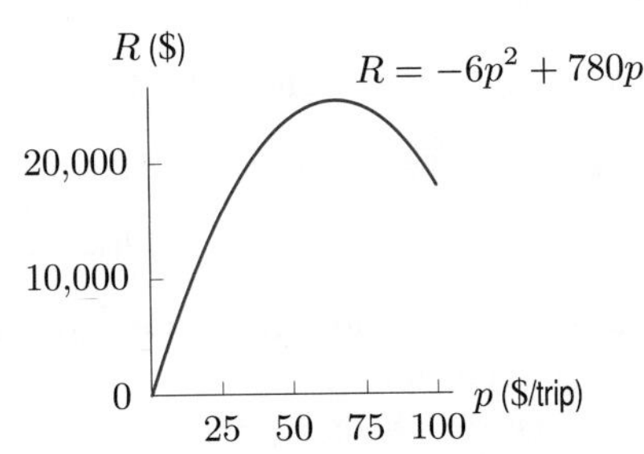

Figure 4.47: Revenue for a rafting company as a function of price

Problems for Section 4.4

1. Figure 4.48 shows cost and revenue. For what production levels is the profit function positive? Negative? Estimate the production at which profit is maximized.

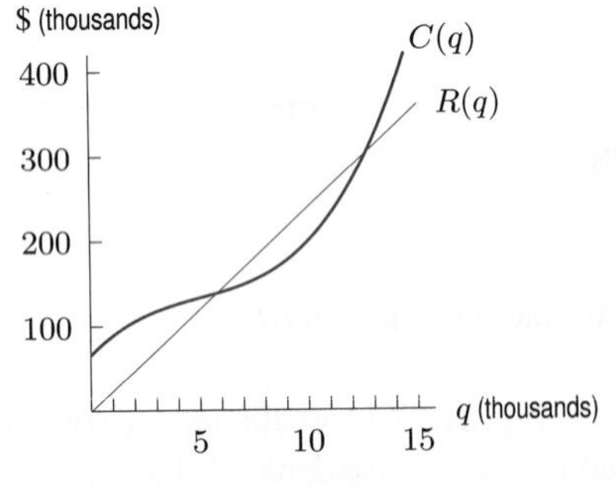

Figure 4.48

2. Using the cost and revenue graphs in Figure 4.49, sketch the following functions. Label the points q_1 and q_2.

(a) Total profit **(b)** Marginal cost
(c) Marginal revenue

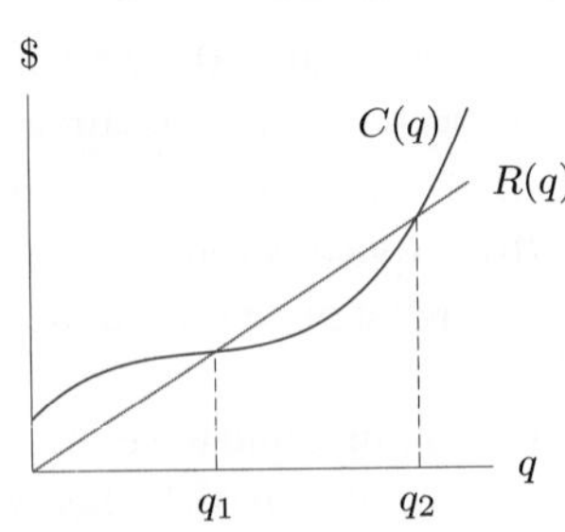

Figure 4.49

3. Table 4.2 shows cost, $C(q)$, and revenue, $R(q)$.

(a) At approximately what production level, q, is profit maximized? Explain your reasoning.
(b) What is the price of the product?
(c) What are the fixed costs?

Table 4.2

q	0	500	1000	1500	2000	2500	3000
$R(q)$	0	1500	3000	4500	6000	7500	9000
$C(q)$	3000	3800	4200	4500	4800	5500	7400

4. A demand function is $p = 400 - 2q$, where q is the quantity of the good sold for price $\$p$.

(a) Find an expression for the total revenue, R, in terms of q.
(b) Differentiate R with respect to q to find the marginal revenue, MR, in terms of q. Calculate the marginal revenue when $q = 10$.
(c) Calculate the change in total revenue when production increases from $q = 10$ to $q = 11$ units. Confirm that a one-unit increase in q gives a reasonable approximation to the exact value of MR obtained in part (b).

5. Let $C(q)$ represent the cost, $R(q)$ the revenue, and $\pi(q)$ the total profit, in dollars, of producing q items.

(a) If $C'(50) = 75$ and $R'(50) = 84$, approximately how much profit is earned by the 51st item?
(b) If $C'(90) = 71$ and $R'(90) = 68$, approximately how much profit is earned by the 91st item?
(c) If $\pi(q)$ is a maximum when $q = 78$, how do you think $C'(78)$ and $R'(78)$ compare? Explain.

6. Figure 4.45 in Section 4.4 shows the points, q_1 and q_2, where marginal revenue equals marginal cost.

(a) On the graph of the corresponding total cost and total revenue functions in Figure 4.50, label the points q_1 and q_2. Using slopes, explain the significance of these points.
(b) Explain in terms of profit why one is a local minimum and one is a local maximum.

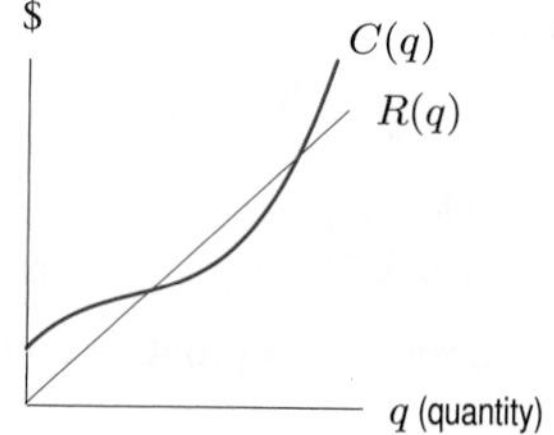

Figure 4.50

7. Table 4.3 shows marginal cost, MC, and marginal revenue, MR.

(a) Use the marginal cost and marginal revenue at a production of $q = 5000$ to determine whether production should be increased or decreased from 5000.
(b) Estimate the production level that maximizes profit.

Table 4.3

q	5000	6000	7000	8000	9000	10000
MR	60	58	56	55	54	53
MC	48	52	54	55	58	63

8. Marginal revenue and marginal cost are given in the following table. Estimate the production levels that could maximize profit. Explain.

q	1000	2000	3000	4000	5000	6000
MR	78	76	74	72	70	68
MC	100	80	70	65	75	90

9. A company estimates that the total revenue, R, in dollars, received from the sale of q items is $R = \ln(1 + 1000q^2)$. Calculate and interpret the marginal revenue if $q = 10$.

10. Figure 4.51 shows cost and revenue for a product.

(a) Estimate the production level that maximizes profit.
(b) Graph marginal revenue and marginal cost for this product on the same axes. Label on this graph the production level that maximizes profit.

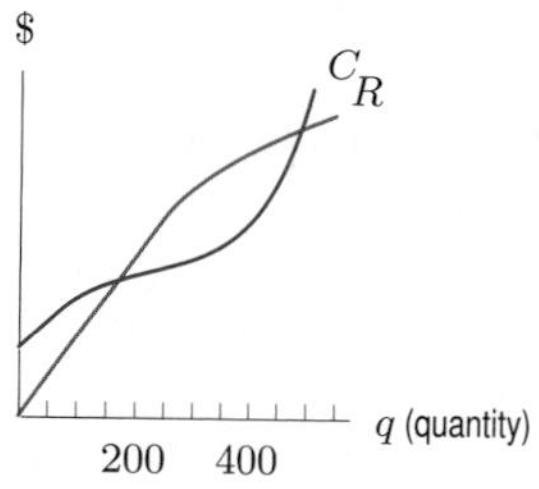

Figure 4.51

11. Figure 4.52 shows graphs of marginal cost and marginal revenue. Estimate the production levels that could maximize profit. Explain your reasoning.

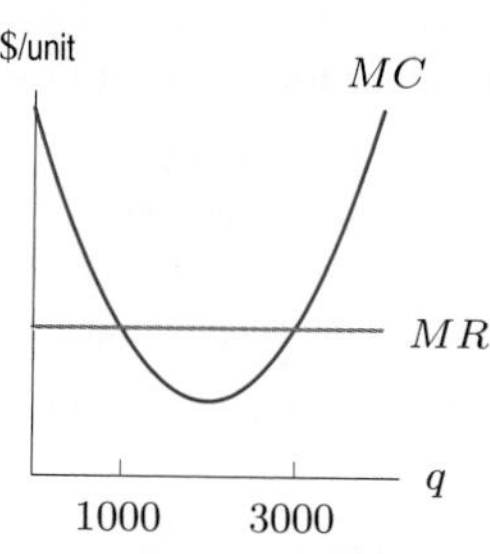

Figure 4.52

12. The marginal cost and marginal revenue of a company are $MC(q) = 0.03q^2 - 1.4q + 34$ and $MR(q) = 30$, where q is the number of items manufactured. To increase profits, should the company increase or decrease production from each of the following levels?

(a) 25 items **(b)** 50 items **(c)** 80 items

13. A manufacturing process has marginal costs given in the table; the item sells for $30 per unit. At how many quantities, q, does the profit appear to be a maximum? In what intervals do these quantities appear to lie?

q	0	10	20	30	40	50	60
MC ($/unit)	34	23	18	19	26	39	58

14. Cost and revenue functions are given in Figure 4.53. Approximately what quantity maximizes profits?

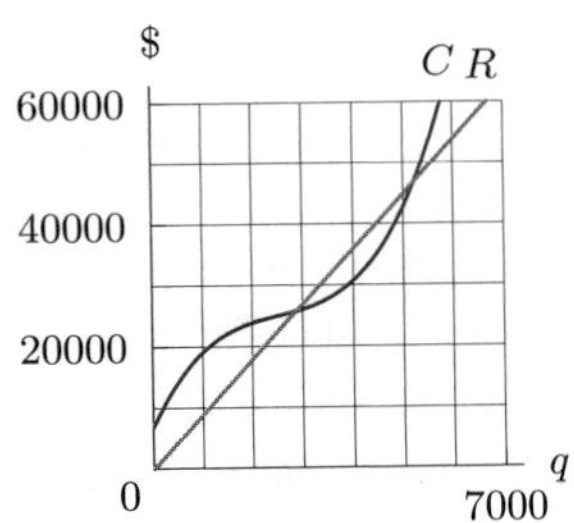

Figure 4.53

15. Cost and revenue functions are given in Figure 4.53.

(a) At a production level of $q = 3000$, is marginal cost or marginal revenue greater? Explain what this tells you about whether production should be increased or decreased.
(b) Answer the same questions for $q = 5000$.

16. When production is 2000, marginal revenue is $4 per unit and marginal cost is $3.25 per unit. Do you expect maximum profit to occur at a production level above or below 2000? Explain.

17. Revenue is given by $R(q) = 450q$ and cost is given by $C(q) = 10{,}000 + 3q^2$. At what quantity is profit maximized? What is the total profit at this production level?

18. The demand equation for a product is $p = 45 - 0.01q$. Write the revenue as a function of q and find the quantity that maximizes revenue. What price corresponds to this quantity? What is the total revenue at this price?

19. Revenue and cost functions for a company are given in Figure 4.54.

(a) Estimate the marginal cost at $q = 400$.
(b) Should the company produce the 500th item? Why?
(c) Estimate the quantity which maximizes profit.

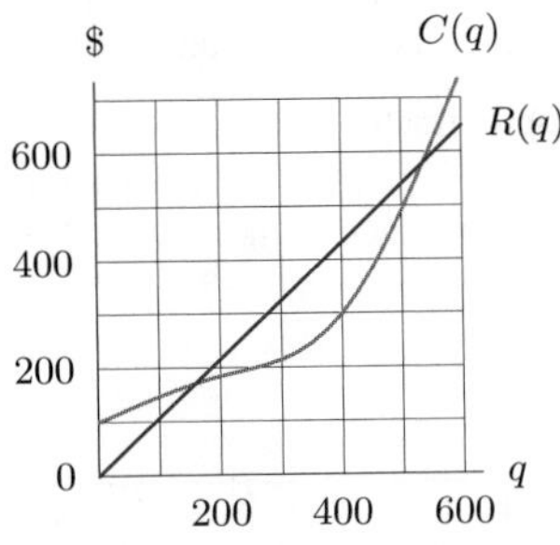

Figure 4.54

20. The following table gives the cost and revenue, in dollars, for different production levels, q.

(a) At approximately what production level is profit maximized?
(b) What price is charged per unit for this product?
(c) What are the fixed costs of production?

q	0	100	200	300	400	500
$R(q)$	0	500	1000	1500	2000	2500
$C(q)$	700	900	1000	1100	1300	1900

21. The demand for tickets to an amusement park is given by $p = 70 - 0.02q$, where p is the price of a ticket in dollars and q is the number of people attending at that price.

(a) What price generates an attendance of 3000 people? What is the total revenue at that price? What is the total revenue if the price is $20?
(b) Write the revenue function as a function of attendance, q, at the amusement park.
(c) What attendance maximizes revenue?
(d) What price should be charged to maximize revenue?
(e) What is the maximum revenue? Can we determine the corresponding profit?

22. An ice cream company finds that at a price of $4.00, demand is 4000 units. For every $0.25 decrease in price, demand increases by 200 units. Find the price and quantity sold that maximize revenue.

23. At a price of $8 per ticket, a musical theater group can fill every seat in the theater, which has a capacity of 1500. For every additional dollar charged, the number of people buying tickets decreases by 75. What ticket price maximizes revenue?

24. The demand equation for a quantity q of a product at price p, in dollars, is $p = -5q + 4000$. Companies producing the product report the cost, C, in dollars, to produce a quantity q is $C = 6q + 5$ dollars.

(a) Express a company's profit, in dollars, as a function of q.
(b) What production level earns the company the largest profit?
(c) What is the largest profit possible?

25. **(a)** Production of an item has fixed costs of \$10,000 and variable costs of \$2 per item. Express the cost, C, of producing q items.
(b) The relationship between price, p, and quantity, q, demanded is linear. Market research shows that 10,100 items are sold when the price is \$5 and 12,872 items are sold when the price is \$4.50. Express q as a function of price p.
(c) Express the profit earned as a function of q.
(d) How many items should the company produce to maximize profit? (Give your answer to the nearest integer.) What is the profit at that production level?

26. A landscape architect plans to enclose a 3000 square-foot rectangular region in a botanical garden. She will use shrubs costing \$45 per foot along three sides and fencing costing \$20 per foot along the fourth side. Find the minimum total cost.

27. You run a small furniture business. You sign a deal with a customer to deliver up to 400 chairs, the exact number to be determined by the customer later. The price will be \$90 per chair up to 300 chairs, and above 300, the price will be reduced by \$0.25 per chair (on the whole order) for every additional chair over 300 ordered. What are the largest and smallest revenues your company can make under this deal?

28. A warehouse selling cement has to decide how often and in what quantities to reorder. It is cheaper, on average, to place large orders, because this reduces the ordering cost per unit. On the other hand, larger orders mean higher storage costs. The warehouse always reorders cement in the same quantity, q. The total weekly cost, C, of ordering and storage is given by

$$C = \frac{a}{q} + bq, \quad \text{where } a, b \text{ are positive constants.}$$

(a) Which of the terms, a/q and bq, represents the ordering cost and which represents the storage cost?
(b) What value of q gives the minimum total cost?

29. A business sells an item at a constant rate of r units per month. It reorders in batches of q units, at a cost of $a+bq$ dollars per order. Storage costs are k dollars per item per month, and, on average, $q/2$ items are in storage, waiting to be sold. [Assume r, a, b, k are positive constants.]

(a) How often does the business reorder?
(b) What is the average monthly cost of reordering?
(c) What is the total monthly cost, C of ordering and storage?
(d) Obtain Wilson's lot size formula, the optimal batch size which minimizes cost.

30. **(a)** A cruise line offers a trip for \$2000 per passenger. If at least 100 passengers sign up, the price is reduced for *all* the passengers by \$10 for every additional passenger (beyond 100) who goes on the trip. The boat can accommodate 250 passengers. What number of passengers maximizes the cruise line's total revenue? What price does each passenger pay then?
(b) The cost to the cruise line for n passengers is $80{,}000+400n$. What is the maximum profit that the cruise line can make on one trip? How many passengers must sign up for the maximum to be reached and what price will each pay?

31. A company manufactures only one product. The quantity, q, of this product produced per month depends on the amount of capital, K, invested (i.e., the number of machines the company owns, the size of its building, and so on) and the amount of labor, L, available each month. We assume that q can be expressed as a *Cobb-Douglas production function*:

$$q = cK^{\alpha}L^{\beta}$$

where c, α, β are positive constants, with $0 < \alpha < 1$ and $0 < \beta < 1$. In this problem we will see how the Russian government could use a Cobb-Douglas function to estimate how many people a newly privatized industry might employ. A company in such an industry has only a small amount of capital available to it and needs to use all of it, so K is fixed. Suppose L is measured in man-hours per month, and that each man-hour costs the company w rubles (a ruble is the unit of Russian currency). Suppose the company has no other costs besides labor, and that each unit of the good can be sold for a fixed price of p rubles. How many man-hours of labor per month should the company use in order to maximize its profit?

32. A company can produce and sell $f(L)$ tons of a product per month using L hours of labor per month. The wage of the workers is w dollars per hour, and the finished product sells for p dollars per ton.

(a) The function $f(L)$ is the company's production function. Give the units of $f(L)$. What is the practical significance of $f(1000) = 400$?
(b) The derivative $f'(L)$ is the company's marginal product of labor. Give the units of $f'(L)$. What is the practical significance of $f'(1000) = 2$?
(c) The real wage of the workers is the quantity of product that can be bought with one hour's wages. Show that the real wage is w/p tons per hour.
(d) Show that the monthly profit of the company is

$$\pi(L) = pf(L) - wL.$$

(e) Show that when operating at maximum profit, the company's marginal product of labor equals the real wage:

$$f'(L) = \frac{w}{p}.$$

4.5 AVERAGE COST

To maximize profit, a company arranges production to equalize marginal cost and marginal revenue. But how do we know if the company makes money? It turns out that whether the maximum profit is positive or negative is determined by the company's average cost of production. Average cost also tells us about the behavior of similar companies in an industry. If average costs are low, more companies will enter the market; if average costs are high, companies will leave the market.

In this section, we see how average cost can be calculated and visualized, and the relationship between average and marginal cost.

What Is Average Cost?

The average cost is the cost per unit of producing a certain quantity; it is the total cost divided by the number of units produced.

> If the cost of producing a quantity q is $C(q)$, then the **average cost**, $a(q)$, of producing a quantity q is given by
> $$a(q) = \frac{C(q)}{q}.$$

Although both are measured in the same units, for example, dollars per item, be careful not to confuse the average cost with the marginal cost (the cost of producing the next item).

Example 1 A salsa company has cost function $C(q) = 0.01q^3 - 0.6q^2 + 13q + 1000$ (in dollars), where q is the number of cases of salsa produced. If 100 cases are produced, find the average cost per case.

Solution The total cost of producing the 100 cases is given by

$$C(100) = 0.01(100^3) - 0.6(100^2) + 13(100) + 1000 = \$6300.$$

We find the average cost per case by dividing by 100, the number of cases produced.

$$\text{Average cost} = \frac{6300}{100} = 63 \text{ dollars/case.}$$

If 100 cases of salsa are produced, the average cost is \$63 per case.

Visualizing Average Cost on the Total Cost Curve

We know that average cost is $a(q) = C(q)/q$. Since we can subtract zero from any number without changing it, we can write

$$a(q) = \frac{C(q)}{q} = \frac{C(q) - 0}{q - 0}.$$

This expression gives the slope of the line joining the points $(0, 0)$ and $(q, C(q))$ on the cost curve. See Figure 4.55.

> $$\begin{array}{c}\text{Average cost}\\ \text{to produce } q \text{ items}\end{array} = \frac{C(q)}{q} = \begin{array}{c}\text{Slope of the line from the origin}\\ \text{to point } (q, C(q)) \text{ on cost curve.}\end{array}$$

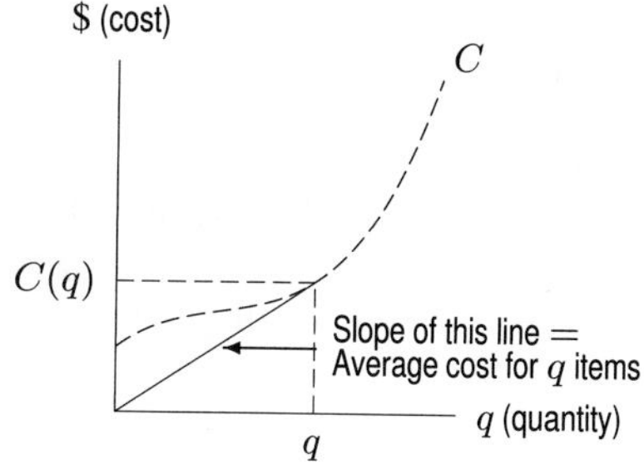

Figure 4.55: Average cost is the slope of the line from the origin to a point on the cost curve

Minimizing Average Cost

We use the graphical representation of average cost to investigate the relationship between average and marginal cost, and to identify the production level which minimizes average cost.

Example 2 A cost function, in dollars, is $C(q) = 1000 + 20q$, where q is the number of units produced. Find and compare the marginal cost to produce the 100th unit and the average cost of producing 100 units. Illustrate your answer on a graph.

Solution The cost function is linear with fixed costs of \$1000 and variable costs of \$20 per unit. Thus,

$$\text{Marginal cost } = C'(q) = 20 \text{ dollars per unit.}$$

This means that after 99 units have been produced, it costs an additional \$20 to produce the next unit. In contrast,

$$\text{Average cost of producing 100 units } = a(100) = \frac{C(100)}{100} = \frac{3000}{100} = 30 \text{ dollars/unit.}$$

Notice that the average cost includes the fixed costs of \$1000 spread over the entire production, whereas marginal cost does not. Thus, the average cost is greater than the marginal cost in this example. See Figure 4.56.

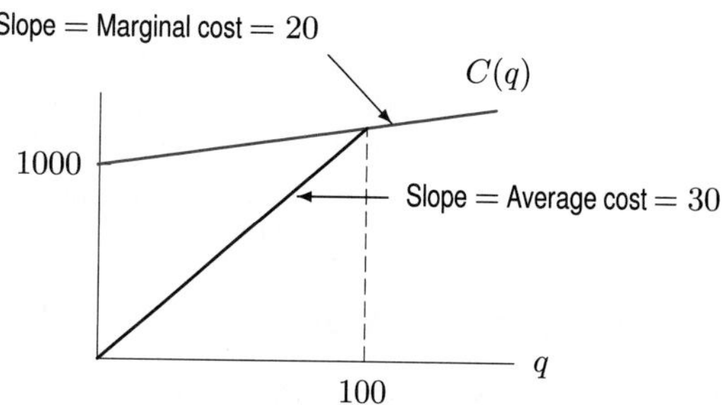

Figure 4.56: Average cost > Marginal cost

Example 3 Mark on the cost graph in Figure 4.57 the quantity at which the average cost is minimized.

Solution In Figure 4.58, the average costs at q_1, q_2, q_3, and q_4 are given by the slopes of the lines from the origin to the curve. These slopes are steep for small q, become less steep as q increases, and then get steeper again. Thus, as q increases, the average cost decreases and then increases, so there is a minimum value. In Figure 4.58 the minimum occurs at the point q_0 where the line from the origin is tangent to the cost curve.

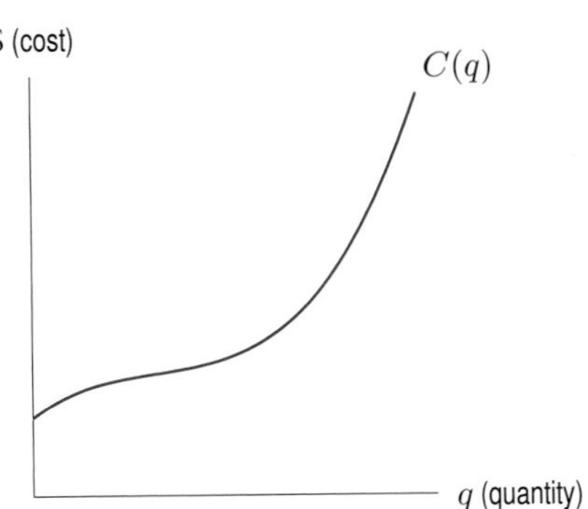

Figure 4.57: A cost function

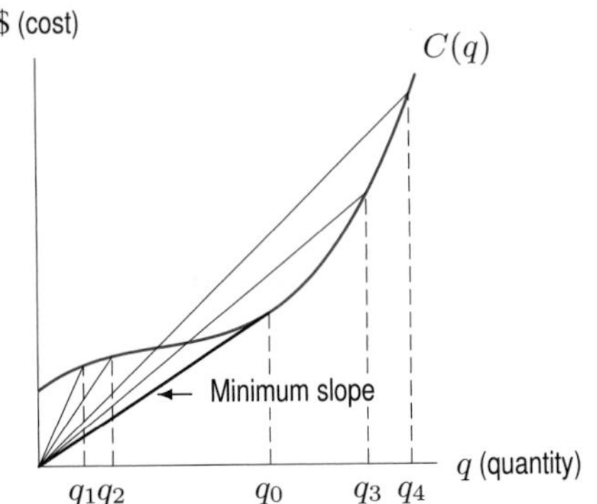

Figure 4.58: Minimum average cost occurs at q_0 where line is tangent to cost curve

In Figure 4.58, notice that average cost is a minimum (at q_0) when average cost equals marginal cost. The next example shows what happens when marginal cost and average cost are not equal.

Example 4 Suppose 100 items are produced at an average cost of \$2 per item. Find the average cost of producing 101 items if the marginal cost to produce the 101st item is: (a) \$1 (b) \$3.

Solution If 100 items are produced at an average cost of \$2 per item, the total cost of producing the items is $100 \cdot \$2 = \$200$.

(a) Since the marginal, or additional, cost to produce the 101st item is \$1, the total cost of producing 101 items is $\$200 + \$1 = \$201$. The average cost to produce these items is $201/101$, or \$1.99 per item. The average cost has gone down.

(b) In this case, the marginal cost to produce the 101st item is \$3. The total cost to produce 101 items is \$203 and the average cost is $203/101$, or \$2.01 per item. The average cost has gone up.

Notice that in Example 4 (a), where it costs less than the average to produce an additional item, average cost decreases as production increases. In Example 4 (b), where it costs more than the average to produce an additional item, average cost increases with production. We summarize:

Relationship Between Average Cost and Marginal Cost

- If marginal cost is less than average cost, then increasing production decreases average cost.
- If marginal cost is greater than average cost, then increasing production increases average cost.
- Marginal cost equals average cost at critical points of average cost.

Example 5 Show analytically that critical points of average cost occur when marginal cost equals average cost.

Solution Since $a(q) = C(q)/q = C(q)q^{-1}$, we use the product rule to find $a'(q)$:

$$a'(q) = C'(q)(q^{-1}) + C(q)(-q^{-2}) = \frac{C'(q)}{q} + \frac{-C(q)}{q^2} = \frac{qC'(q) - C(q)}{q^2}.$$

At critical points we have $a'(q) = 0$, so

$$\frac{qC'(q) - C(q)}{q^2} = 0$$

Therefore, we have

$$\begin{aligned} qC'(q) - C(q) &= 0 \\ qC'(q) &= C(q) \\ C'(q) &= \frac{C(q)}{q}. \end{aligned}$$

In other words, at a critical point:

$$\text{Marginal cost} = \text{Average cost}.$$

Example 6 A total cost function, in thousands of dollars, is given by $C(q) = q^3 - 6q^2 + 15q$, where q is in thousands and $0 \le q \le 5$.

(a) Graph $C(q)$. Estimate visually the quantity at which average cost is minimized.
(b) Graph the average cost function. Use it to estimate the minimum average cost.
(c) Determine analytically the exact value of q at which average cost is minimized.
(d) Graph the marginal cost function on the same axes as the average cost.
(e) Show that at the minimum average cost, Marginal cost $=$ Average cost. Explain how you can see this result on your graph of average and marginal costs.

Solution

(a) A graph of $C(q)$ is in Figure 4.59. Average cost is minimized at the point where a line from the origin to the point on the curve has minimum slope. This occurs where the line is tangent to the curve, which is at approximately $q = 3$, corresponding to a production of 3000 units.
(b) Since average cost is total cost divided by quantity, we have

$$a(q) = \frac{C(q)}{q} = \frac{q^3 - 6q^2 + 15q}{q} = q^2 - 6q + 15.$$

Figure 4.60 suggests that the minimum average cost occurs at $q = 3$.
(c) Average cost is minimized at a critical point of $a(q) = q^2 - 6q + 15$. Differentiating gives

$$\begin{aligned} a'(q) = 2q - 6 &= 0 \\ q &= 3. \end{aligned}$$

The minimum occurs at $q = 3$.
(d) See Figure 4.60. Marginal cost is the derivative of $C(q) = q^3 - 6q^2 + 15q$,

$$MC(q) = 3q^2 - 12q + 15.$$

(e) At $q = 3$, we have

$$\begin{aligned} \text{Marginal cost} &= 3 \cdot 3^2 - 12 \cdot 3 + 15 = 6. \\ \text{Average cost} &= 3^2 - 6 \cdot 3 + 15 = 6. \end{aligned}$$

Thus, marginal and average cost are equal at $q = 3$. This result can be seen in Figure 4.60 since the marginal cost curve cuts the average cost curve at the minimum average cost.

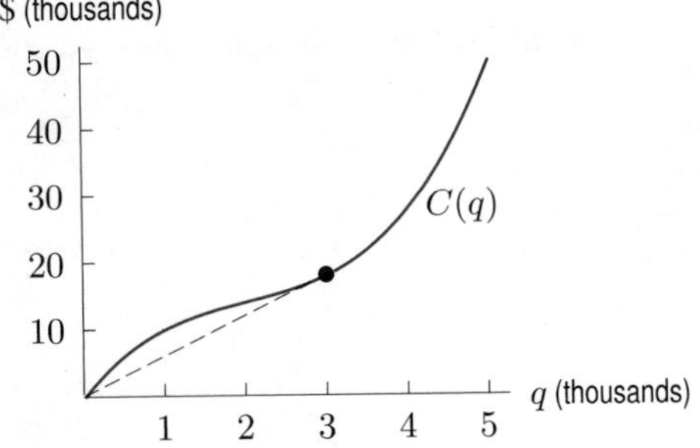

Figure 4.59: Cost function, showing the minimum average cost

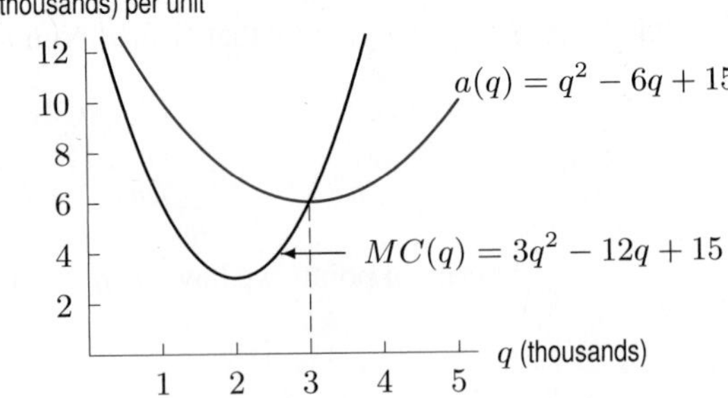

Figure 4.60: Average and marginal cost functions, showing minimum average cost

Problems for Section 4.5

1. For each cost function in Figure 4.61, is there a value of q at which average cost is minimized? If so, approximately where? Explain your answer.

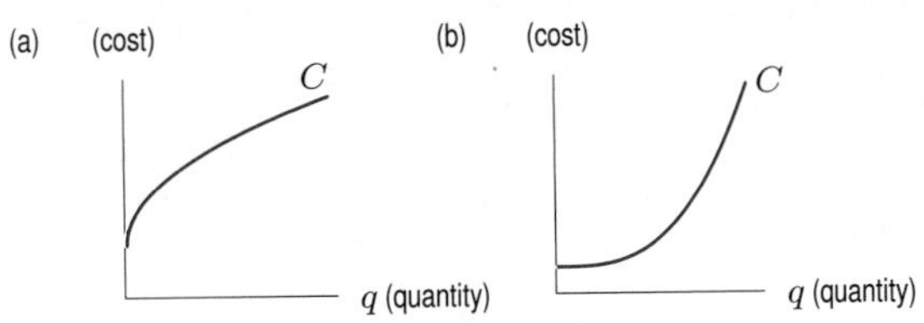

Figure 4.61

2. The graph of a cost function is given in Figure 4.62.

(a) At $q = 25$, estimate the following quantities and represent your answers graphically.

(i) Average cost (ii) Marginal cost

(b) At approximately what value of q is average cost minimized?

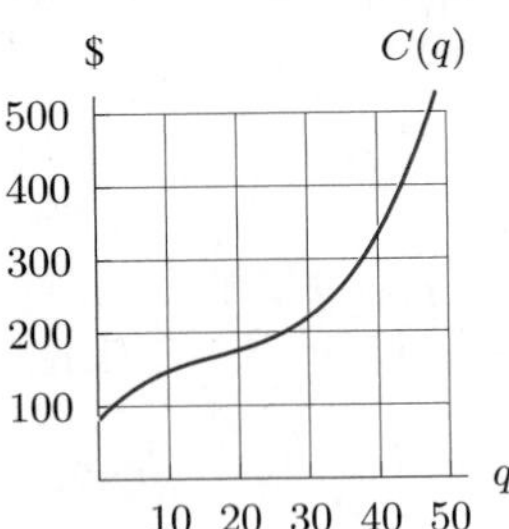

Figure 4.62

3. Figure 4.63 shows cost with $q = 10{,}000$ marked.

(a) Find the average cost when the production level is 10,000 units and interpret it.

(b) Represent your answer to part (a) graphically.

(c) At approximately what production level is average cost minimized?

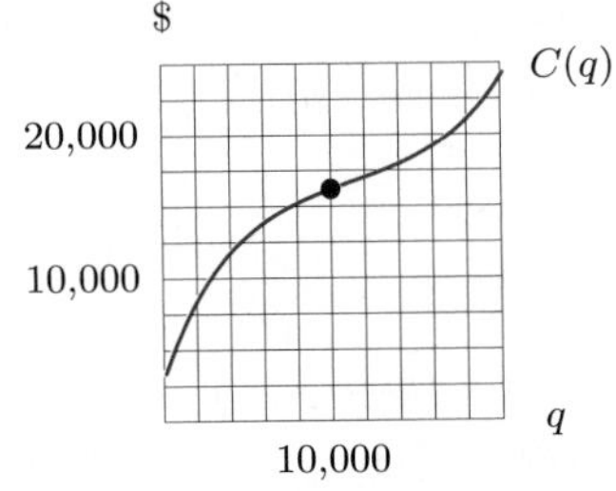

Figure 4.63

4. The cost of producing q items is $C(q) = 2500 + 12q$ dollars.

(a) What is the marginal cost of producing the 100th item? the 1000th item?

(b) What is the average cost of producing 100 items? 1000 items?

5. The cost function is $C(q) = 1000 + 20q$. Find the marginal cost to produce the 200th unit and the average cost of producing 200 units.

6. Graph the average cost function corresponding to the total cost function shown in Figure 4.64.

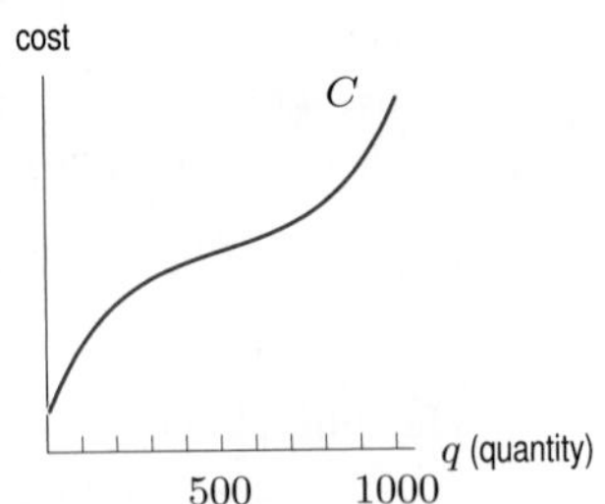

Figure 4.64

7. The total cost of production, in thousands of dollars, is $C(q) = q^3 - 12q^2 + 60q$, where q is in thousands and $0 \leq q \leq 8$.

(a) Graph $C(q)$. Estimate visually the quantity at which average cost is minimized.

(b) Determine analytically the exact value of q at which average cost is minimized.

8. You are the manager of a firm that produces slippers that sell for \$20 a pair. You are producing 1200 pairs of slippers each month, at an average cost of \$2 each. The marginal cost at a production level of 1200 is \$3 per pair.

(a) Are you making or losing money?
(b) Will increasing production increase or decrease your average cost? Your profit?
(c) Would you recommend that production be increased or decreased?

9. The average cost per item to produce q items is given by

$$a(q) = 0.01q^2 - 0.6q + 13, \quad \text{for} \quad q > 0.$$

(a) What is the total cost, $C(q)$, of producing q goods?
(b) What is the minimum marginal cost? What is the practical interpretation of this result?
(c) At what production level is the average cost a minimum? What is the lowest average cost?
(d) Compute the marginal cost at $q = 30$. How does this relate to your answer to part (c)? Explain this relationship both analytically and in words.

10. The marginal cost at a production level of 2000 units of an item is \$10 per unit and the average cost of producing 2000 units is \$15 per unit. If the production level were increased slightly above 2000, would the following quantities increase or decrease, or is it impossible to tell?

(a) Average cost **(b)** Profit

11. An agricultural worker in Uganda is planting clover to increase the number of bees making their home in the region. There are 100 bees in the region naturally, and for every acre put under clover, 20 more bees are found in the region.

(a) Draw a graph of the total number, $N(x)$, of bees as a function of x, the number of acres devoted to clover.
(b) Explain, both geometrically and algebraically, the shape of the graph of:

(i) The marginal rate of increase of the number of bees with acres of clover, $N'(x)$.

(ii) The average number of bees per acre of clover, $N(x)/x$.

12. A developer has recently purchased a laundromat and an adjacent factory. For years, the laundromat has taken pains to keep the smoke from the factory from soiling the air used by its clothes dryers. Now that the developer owns both the laundromat and the factory, she could install filters in the factory's smokestacks to reduce the emission of smoke, instead of merely protecting the laundromat from it. The cost of filters for the factory and the cost of protecting the laundromat against smoke depend on the number of filters used, as shown in the table.

Number of filters	Total cost of filters	Total cost of protecting laundromat from smoke
0	\$0	\$127
1	\$5	\$63
2	\$11	\$31
3	\$18	\$15
4	\$26	\$6
5	\$35	\$3
6	\$45	\$0
7	\$56	\$0

(a) Make a table which shows, for each possible number of filters (0 through 7), the marginal cost of the filter, the average cost of the filters, and the marginal savings in protecting the laundromat from smoke.
(b) Since the developer wishes to minimize the total costs to both her businesses, what should she do? Use the table from part (a) to explain your answer.
(c) What should the developer do if, in addition to the cost of the filters, the filters must be mounted on a rack which costs \$100?
(d) What should the developer do if the rack costs \$50?

13. Figure 4.65 shows the average cost, $a(q) = b + mq$.

(a) Show that $C'(q) = b + 2mq$.
(b) Graph the marginal cost $C'(q)$.

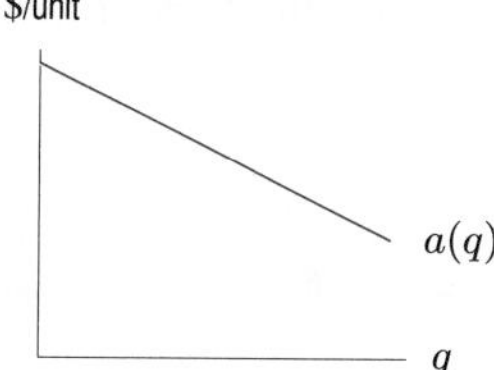

Figure 4.65

14. Show analytically that if marginal cost is less than average cost, then the derivative of average cost with respect to quantity satisfies $a'(q) < 0$.

15. Show analytically that if marginal cost is greater than average cost, then the derivative of average cost with respect to quantity satisfies $a'(q) > 0$.

16. A reasonably realistic model of a firm's costs is given by the *short-run Cobb-Douglas cost curve*

$$C(q) = Kq^{1/a} + F,$$

where a is a positive constant, F is the fixed cost, and K measures the technology available to the firm.

(a) Show that C is concave down if $a > 1$.
(b) Assuming that $a < 1$, find what value of q minimizes the average cost.

4.6 ELASTICITY OF DEMAND

The sensitivity of demand to changes in price varies with the product. For example, a change in the price of light bulbs may not affect the demand for light bulbs much, because people need light bulbs no matter what their price. However, a change in the price of a particular make of car may have a significant effect on the demand for that car, because people can switch to another make.

Elasticity of Demand

We want to find a way to measure this sensitivity of demand to price changes. Our measure should work for products as diverse as light bulbs and cars. The prices of these two items are so different that it makes little sense to talk about absolute changes in price: Changing the price of light bulbs by $\$1$ is a substantial change, whereas changing the price of a car by $\$1$ is not. Instead, we use the percent change in price. How, for example, does a 1% increase in price affect the demand for the product?

Let Δp denote the change in the price p of a product and Δq denote the corresponding change in quantity q demanded. The percent change in price is $\Delta p/p$ and the percent change in quantity demanded is $\Delta q/q$. We assume in this book that Δp and Δq have opposite signs (because increasing the price usually decreases the quantity demanded). Then the effect of a price change on demand is measured by the absolute value of the ratio

$$\left|\frac{\text{Percent change in demand}}{\text{Percent change in price}}\right| = \left|\frac{\Delta q/q}{\Delta p/p}\right| = \left|\frac{\Delta q}{q}\cdot\frac{p}{\Delta p}\right| = \left|\frac{p}{q}\cdot\frac{\Delta q}{\Delta p}\right|$$

For small changes in p, we approximate $\Delta q/\Delta p$ by the derivative dq/dp. We define:

> The **elasticity of demand**[8] for a product, E, is given approximately by
>
> $$E \approx \left|\frac{\Delta q/q}{\Delta p/p}\right|, \quad \text{or exactly by} \quad E = \left|\frac{p}{q}\cdot\frac{dq}{dp}\right|.$$

Increasing the price of an item by 1% causes a drop of approximately $E\%$ in the quantity of goods demanded. For small changes, Δp, in price,

$$\frac{\Delta q}{q} \approx -E\frac{\Delta p}{p}.$$

If $E > 1$, a 1% increase in price causes demand to drop by more than 1%, and we say that demand is *elastic*. If $0 \leq E < 1$, a 1% increase in price causes demand to drop by less than 1%, and we say that demand is *inelastic*. In general, a larger elasticity causes a larger percent change in demand for a given percent change in price.

Example 1 Raising the price of hotel rooms from $\$75$ to $\$80$ per night reduces weekly sales from 100 rooms to 90 rooms.

(a) Approximate the elasticity of demand for rooms at a price of $\$75$.
(b) Should the owner raise the price?

[8] When it is necessary to distinguish it from other elasticities, this quantity is called the elasticity of demand with respect to price, or the price elasticity of demand.

Solution (a) The percent change in the price is

$$\frac{\Delta p}{p} = \frac{5}{75} = 0.067 = 6.7\%$$

and the percent change in demand is

$$\frac{\Delta q}{q} = \frac{-10}{100} = -0.1 = -10\%.$$

The elasticity of demand is approximated by the ratio

$$E \approx \left|\frac{\Delta q/q}{\Delta p/p}\right| = \frac{0.10}{0.067} = 1.5.$$

The elasticity is greater than 1 because the percent change in the demand is greater than the percent change in the price.

(b) At a price of $75 per room,

$$\text{Revenue} = (100 \text{ rooms})(\$75 \text{ per room}) = \$7500 \text{ per week.}$$

At a price of $80 per room,

$$\text{Revenue} = (90 \text{ rooms})(\$80 \text{ per room}) = \$7200 \text{ per week.}$$

A price increase results in loss of revenue, so the price should not be raised.

Example 2 The demand curve for a product is given by $q = 1000 - 2p^2$, where p is the price. Find the elasticity at $p = 10$ and at $p = 15$. Interpret your answers.

Solution We first find the derivative $dq/dp = -4p$. At a price of $p = 10$, we have $dq/dp = -4 \cdot 10 = -40$, and the quantity demanded is $q = 1000 - 2 \cdot 10^2 = 800$. At this price, the elasticity is

$$E = \left|\frac{p}{q} \cdot \frac{dq}{dp}\right| = \left|\frac{10}{800}(-40)\right| = 0.5.$$

The demand is inelastic at a price of $p = 10$: a 1% increase in price results in approximately a 0.5% decrease in demand.

At a price of $15, we have $q = 550$ and $dq/dp = -60$. The elasticity is

$$E = \left|\frac{p}{q} \cdot \frac{dq}{dp}\right| = \left|\frac{15}{550}(-60)\right| = 1.64.$$

The demand is elastic: a 1% increase in price results in approximately a 1.64% decrease in demand.

Revenue and Elasticity of Demand

Elasticity enables us to analyze the effect of a price change on revenue. An increase in price usually leads to a fall in demand. However, the revenue may increase or decrease. The revenue $R = pq$ is the product of two quantities, and as one increases, the other decreases. Elasticity measures the relative significance of these two competing changes.

Example 3 Three hundred units of an item are sold when the price of the item is \$10. When the price of the item is raised by \$1, what is the effect on revenue if the quantity sold drops by

(a) 10 units? (b) 100 units?

Solution Since Revenue = Price · Quantity, when the price is \$10, we have

$$\text{Revenue} = 10 \cdot 300 = \$3000.$$

(a) At a price of \$11, the quantity sold is $300 - 10 = 290$, so

$$\text{Revenue} = 11 \cdot 290 = \$3190.$$

Thus, raising the price has increased revenue.

(b) At a price of \$11, the quantity sold is $300 - 100 = 200$, so

$$\text{Revenue} = 11 \cdot 200 = \$2200.$$

Thus, raising the price has decreased revenue.

Elasticity allows us to predict whether revenue increases or decreases with a price increase.

Example 4 The item in Example 3 (a) is wool whose demand equation is $q = 400 - 10p$. The item in Example 3 (b) is houseplants, whose demand equation is $q = 1300 - 100p$. Find the elasticity of wool and houseplants.

Solution For wool, $q = 400 - 10p$, so $dq/dp = -10$. Thus,

$$E_{\text{Wool}} = \left|\frac{p}{q}\frac{dq}{dp}\right| = \left|\frac{10}{300}(-10)\right| = \frac{1}{3}.$$

For houseplants, $q = 1300 - 100p$, so $dq/dp = -100$. Thus,

$$E_{\text{Houseplants}} = \left|\frac{p}{q}\frac{dq}{dp}\right| = \left|\frac{10}{300}(-100)\right| = \frac{10}{3}.$$

Notice that $E_{\text{Wool}} < 1$ and revenue increases with an increase in price; $E_{\text{Houseplants}} > 1$ and revenue decreases with an increase in price. In the next example we see the relationship between elasticity and maximum revenue.

Example 5 Table 4.4 shows the demand, q, revenue, R, and elasticity, E, for the product in Example 2 at several prices. What price brings in the greatest revenue? What is the elasticity at that price?

Solution Table 4.4 suggests that maximum revenue is achieved at a price of about \$13, and at that price, E is about 1. At prices below \$13, we have $E < 1$, so the reduction in demand caused by a price increase is small; thus, raising the price increases revenue. At prices above \$13, we have $E > 1$, so the increase in demand caused by a price decrease is relatively large; thus lowering the price increases revenue.

Table 4.4 *Revenue and elasticity at different points*

Price p	10	11	12	13	14	15
Demand q	800	758	712	662	608	550
Revenue R	8000	8338	8544	8606	8512	8250
Elasticity E	0.5	0.64	0.81	1.02	1.29	1.64
	Inelastic	Inelastic	Inelastic	Elastic	Elastic	Elastic

Example 6 shows that revenue does have a local maximum when $E = 1$. We summarize as follows:

Relationship Between Elasticity and Revenue

- If $E < 1$, demand is inelastic and revenue is increased by raising the price.
- If $E > 1$, demand is elastic and revenue is increased by lowering the price.
- $E = 1$ occurs at critical points of the revenue function.

Example 6 Show analytically that critical points of the revenue function occur when $E = 1$.

Solution We think of revenue as a function of price. Using the product rule to differentiate $R = pq$, we have

$$\frac{dR}{dp} = \frac{d}{dp}(pq) = p\frac{dq}{dp} + \frac{dp}{dp}q = p\frac{dq}{dp} + q.$$

At a critical point the derivative dR/dp equals zero, so we have

$$\begin{aligned} p\frac{dq}{dp} + q &= 0 \\ p\frac{dq}{dp} &= -q \\ \frac{p}{q}\frac{dq}{dp} &= -1 \\ E &= 1. \end{aligned}$$

Elasticity of Demand for Different Products

Different products generally have different elasticities. See Table 4.5. If there are close substitutes for a product, or if the product is a luxury rather than a necessity, a change in price generally has a large effect on demand, and the demand for the product is elastic. On the other hand, if there are no close substitutes or if the product is a necessity, changes in price have a relatively small effect on demand, and the demand is inelastic. For example, demand for salt, penicillin, eyeglasses, and lightbulbs is inelastic over the usual range of prices for these products.

Table 4.5 *Elasticity of demand (with respect to price) for selected farm products*[9]

Product	Elasticity	Product	Elasticity
Cabbage	0.25	Oranges	0.62
Potatoes	0.27	Cream	0.69
Wool	0.33	Apples	1.27
Peanuts	0.38	Peaches	1.49
Eggs	0.43	Fresh tomatoes	2.22
Milk	0.49	Lettuce	2.58
Butter	0.62	Fresh peas	2.83

[9]Estimated by the US Department of Agriculture and reported in W. Adams & J. Brock, *The Structure of American Industry*, 10th ed (Englewood Cliffs: Prentice Hall, 2000).

Problems for Section 4.6

1. The elasticity of a good is $E = 0.5$. What is the effect on the quantity demanded of:

(a) A 3% price increase? **(b)** A 3% price decrease?

2. The elasticity of a good is $E = 2$. What is the effect on the quantity demanded of:

(a) A 3% price increase? **(b)** A 3% price decrease?

3. What are the units of elasticity if:

(a) Price p is in dollars and quantity q is in tons?
(b) Price p is in yen and quantity q is in liters?
(c) What can you conclude in general?

4. Dwell time, t, is the time in minutes that shoppers spend in a store. Sales, s, is the number of dollars they spend in the store. The elasticity of sales with respect to dwell time is 1.3. Explain what this means in simple language.

5. What is the elasticity for peaches in Table 4.5? Explain what this number tells you about the effect of price increases on the demand for peaches. Is the demand for peaches elastic or inelastic? Is this what you expect? Explain.

6. What is the elasticity for potatoes in Table 4.5? Explain what this number tells you about the effect of price increases on the demand for potatoes. Is the demand for potatoes elastic or inelastic? Is this what you expect? Explain.

7. There are many brands of laundry detergent. Would you expect the elasticity of demand for any particular brand to be high or low? Explain.

8. Would you expect the demand for high-definition television sets to be elastic or inelastic? Explain.

9. There is only one company offering local telephone service in a town. Would you expect the elasticity of demand for telephone service to be high or low? Explain.

10. The demand for a product is given by $q = 200 - 2p^2$. Find the elasticity of demand when the price is \$5. Is the demand inelastic or elastic, or neither?

11. School organizations raise money by selling candy door to door. The table shows p, the price of the candy, and q, the quantity sold at that price.

p	\$1.00	\$1.25	\$1.50	\$1.75	\$2.00	\$2.25	\$2.50
q	2765	2440	1980	1660	1175	800	430

(a) Estimate the elasticity of demand at a price of \$1.00. At this price, is the demand elastic or inelastic?
(b) Estimate the elasticity at each of the prices shown. What do you notice? Give an explanation for why this might be so.
(c) At approximately what price is elasticity equal to 1?
(d) Find the total revenue at each of the prices shown. Confirm that the total revenue appears to be maximized at approximately the price where $E = 1$.

12. The demand for a product is given by $p = 90 - 10q$. Find the elasticity of demand when $p = 50$. If this price rises by 2%, calculate the corresponding percentage change in demand.

13. The demand for yams is given by $q = 5000 - 10p^2$, where q is in pounds of yams and p is the price of a pound of yams.

(a) If the current price of yams is \$2 per pound, how many pounds will be sold?
(b) Is the demand at \$2 elastic or inelastic? Is it more accurate to say "People want yams and will buy them no matter what the price" or "Yams are a luxury item and people will stop buying them if the price gets too high"?

14. The demand for yams is given in Problem 13.

(a) At a price of \$2 per pound, what is the total revenue for the yam farmer?
(b) Write revenue as a function of price, and then find the price that maximizes revenue.
(c) What quantity is sold at the price you found in part (b), and what is the total revenue?
(d) Show that $E = 1$ at the price you found in part (b).

15. It has been estimated that the elasticity of demand for slaves in the American South before the civil war was equal to 0.86 (fairly high) in the cities and equal to 0.05 (very low) in the countryside.[10]

(a) Why might this be?
(b) Where do you think the staunchest defenders of slavery were from, the cities or the countryside?

16. Find the exact price that maximizes revenue for sales of the product in Example 2.

17. If $E = 2$ for all prices p, how can you maximize revenue?

18. If $E = 0.5$ for all prices p, how can you maximize revenue?

19. **(a)** If the demand equation is $pq = k$ for a positive constant k, compute the elasticity of demand.
(b) Explain the answer to part (a) in terms of the revenue function.

20. Show that a demand equation $q = k/p^r$, where r is a positive constant, gives constant elasticity $E = r$.

[10]Donald McCloskey, *The Applied Theory of Price*, p. 134, (New York: Macmillan, 1982).

21. A linear demand function is given in Figure 4.66. Economists compute elasticity of demand E for any quantity q_0 using the formula

$$E = d_1/d_2,$$

where d_1 and d_2 are the vertical distances shown in Figure 4.66.

(a) Explain why this formula works.
(b) Determine the prices, p, at which (i) $E > 1$ (ii) $E < 1$ (iii) $E = 1$

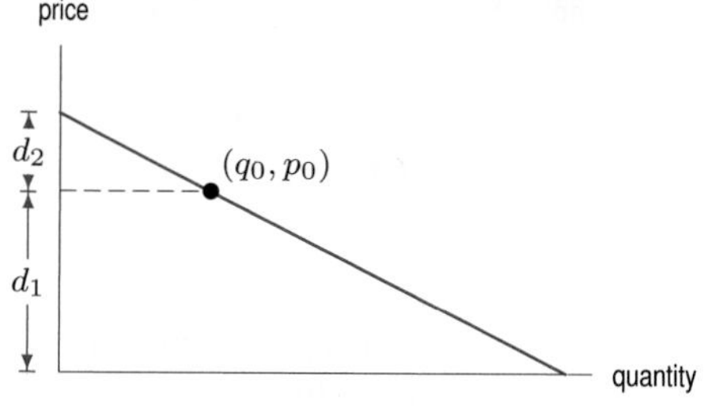

Figure 4.66

22. If p is price and E is the elasticity of demand for a good, show analytically that

$$\text{Marginal revenue} = p(1 - 1/E).$$

23. Suppose cost is proportional to quantity, $C(q) = kq$. Show that a firm earns maximum profit when

$$\frac{\text{Profit}}{\text{Revenue}} = \frac{1}{E}$$

[Hint: Combine the result of Problem 22 with the fact that profit is maximized when $MR = MC$.]

24. Elasticity of cost with respect to quantity is defined as $E_{C,q} = q/C \cdot dC/dq$.

(a) What does this elasticity tell you about sensitivity of cost to quantity produced?
(b) Show that $E_{C,q}$ = Marginal cost/Average cost.

25. If q is the quantity of chicken demanded as a function of the price p of beef, the *cross-price* elasticity of demand for chicken with respect to the price of beef is defined as $E_{\text{cross}} = |p/q \cdot dq/dp|$. What does E_{cross} tell you about the sensitivity of the quantity of chicken bought to changes in the price of beef?

26. The *income* elasticity of demand for a product is defined as $E_{\text{income}} = |I/q \cdot dq/dI|$ where q is the quantity demanded as a function of the income I of the consumer. What does E_{income} tell you about the sensitivity of the quantity of the product purchased to changes in the income of the consumer?

4.7 LOGISTIC GROWTH

In 1923, eighteen koalas were introduced to Kangaroo Island, off the coast of Australia.[11] The koalas thrived on the island and their population grew to about 5000 in 1997. Is it reasonable to expect the population to continue growing exponentially? Since there is only a finite amount of space on the island, the population cannot grow without bound forever. Instead we expect that there is a maximum population that the island can sustain. Population growth with an upper bound can be modeled with a *logistic* or *inhibited growth model.*

Modeling the US Population

Population projections first became important to political philosophers in the late eighteenth century. As concern for scarce resources has grown, so has the interest in accurate population projections. In the US, the population is recorded every ten years by a census. The first such census was in 1790. Table 4.6 contains the census data from 1790 to 2000.

Table 4.6 *US Population,*[12] *in millions, 1790–2000*

Year	Population	Year	Population	Year	Population	Year	Population
1790	3.9	1850	23.1	1910	92.0	1960	179.3
1800	5.3	1860	31.4	1920	105.7	1970	203.3
1810	7.2	1870	38.6	1930	122.8	1980	226.5
1820	9.6	1880	50.2	1940	131.7	1990	248.7
1830	12.9	1890	62.9	1950	150.7	2000	281.4
1840	17.1	1900	76.0				

[11] *Watertown Daily Times*, April 18, 1997.
[12] *The World Almanac and Book of Facts 2005*, pp. 622–623 (New York).

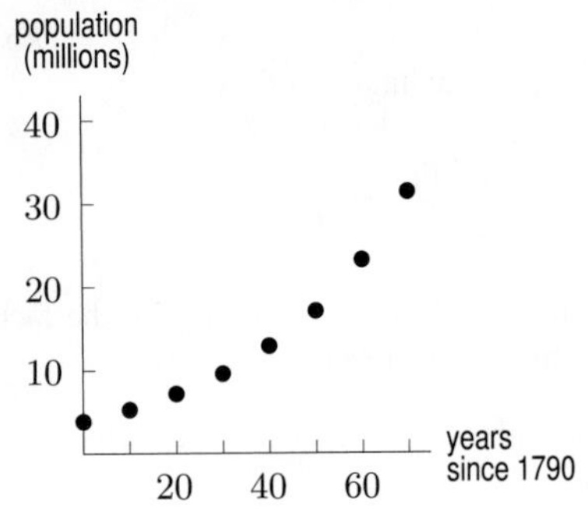

Figure 4.67: US Population, 1790–1860

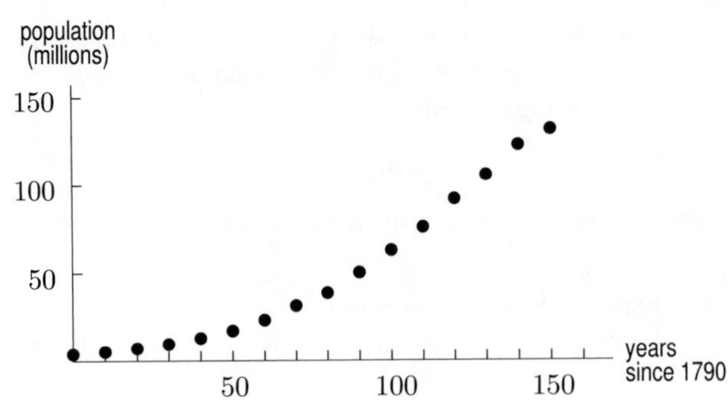

Figure 4.68: US Population, 1790–1940

Figure 4.67 suggests that the population grew exponentially during the years 1790–1860. However, after 1860 the rate of growth began to decrease. See Figure 4.68.

The Years 1790--1860: An Exponential Model

We begin by modeling the US population for the years 1790–1860 using an exponential function. If t is the number of years since 1790 and P is the population in millions, regression gives the exponential function that fits the data as approximately[13]

$$P = 3.9(1.03)^t.$$

Thus, between 1790 and 1860, the US population was growing at an annual rate of about 3%.

The function $P = 3.9(1.03)^t$ is plotted in Figure 4.69 with the data; it fits the data remarkably well. Of course, since we used the data from throughout the 70-year period, we should expect good agreement throughout that period. What is surprising is that if we had used only the populations in 1790 and 1800 to create our exponential function, the predictions would still be very accurate. It is amazing that a person in 1800 could predict the population 60 years later so accurately, especially when one considers all the wars, recessions, epidemics, additions of new territory, and immigration that took place from 1800 to 1860.

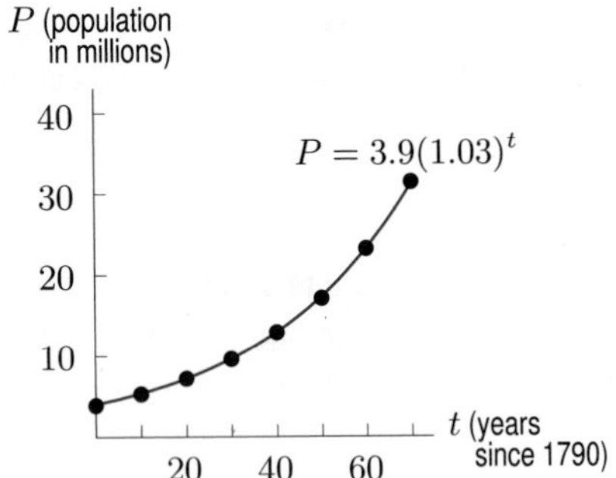

Figure 4.69: An exponential model for the US population, 1790–1860

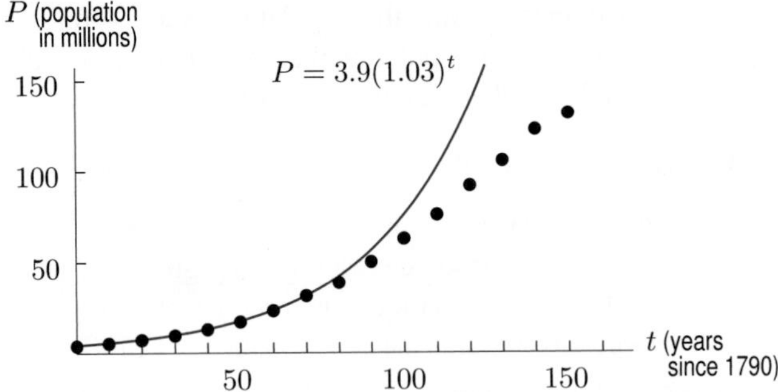

Figure 4.70: The exponential model and the US population, 1790-1940. Not a good fit beyond 1860

The Years 1790--1940: A Logistic Model

How well does the exponential function fit the US population beyond 1860? Figure 4.70 shows a graph of the US population from 1790 until 1940 with the exponential function $P = 3.9(1.03)^t$. The exponential function which fit the data so well for the years 1790–1860 does not fit very well beyond 1860. We must look for another way to model this data.

The graph of the function given by the data in Figure 4.68 is concave up for small values of t,

[13]See Appendix A: Fitting Formulas to Data. Different algorithms may give different formulas.

but then appears to become concave down and to be leveling off. This kind of growth is modeled with a *logistic function*. If t is in years since 1790, the function

$$P = \frac{187}{1 + 47e^{-0.0318t}},$$

which is graphed in Figure 4.71, fits the data well up to 1940. Such a formula is found by logistic regression on a calculator or computer.[14]

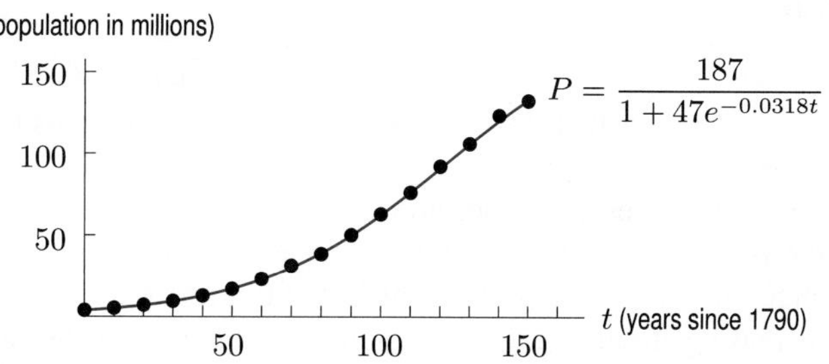

Figure 4.71: A logistic model for US population, 1790–1940

The Logistic Function

A logistic function, such as that used to model the US population, is everywhere increasing. Its graph is concave up at first, then becomes concave down, and levels off at a horizontal asymptote. As we saw in the US population model, a logistic function is approximately exponential for small[15] values of t. A logistic function can be used to model the sales of a new product and the spread of a virus.

> For positive constants L, C, and k, a **logistic function** has the form
>
> $$P = f(t) = \frac{L}{1 + Ce^{-kt}}.$$

The general logistic function has three parameters: L, C, and k. In Example 1, we investigate the effect of two of these parameters on the graph; Problem 5 at the end of the section considers the third.

Example 1 Consider the logistic function $P = \dfrac{L}{1 + 100e^{-kt}}$.

(a) Let $k = 1$. Graph P for several values for L. Explain the effect of the parameter L.

(b) Now let $L = 1$. Graph P for several values for k. Explain the effect of the parameter k.

Solution (a) See Figure 4.72. Notice that the graph levels off at the value L. The parameter L determines the horizontal asymptote and the upper bound for P.

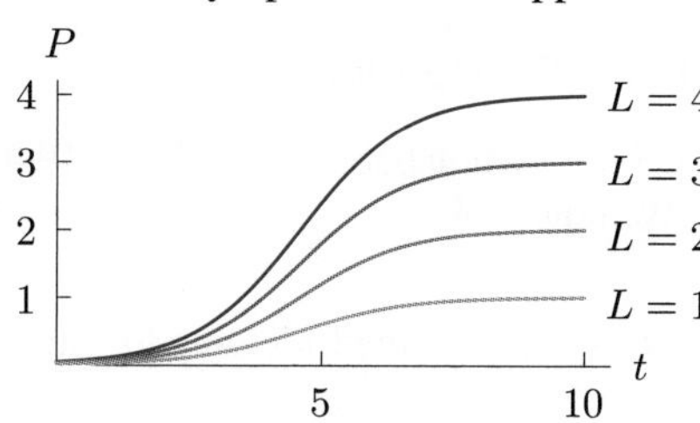

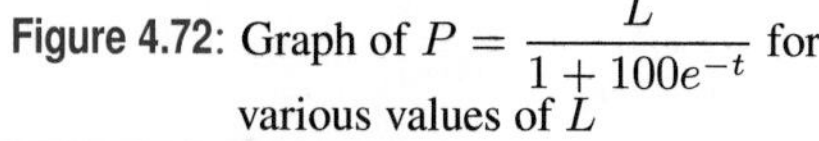

Figure 4.72: Graph of $P = \dfrac{L}{1 + 100e^{-t}}$ for various values of L

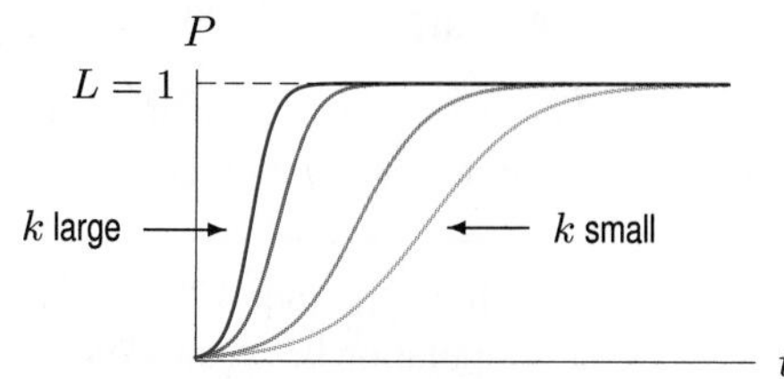

Figure 4.73: Graph of $P = \dfrac{1}{1 + 100e^{-kt}}$ with various values of k

[14]See Appendix A: Fitting Formulas to Data.

[15]Just how small is small enough depends on the values of the parameters C and k.

(b) See Figure 4.73. Notice that as k increases, the curve approaches the asymptote more rapidly. The parameter k affects the steepness of the curve.

The Carrying Capacity and the Point of Diminishing Returns

Example 1 suggests that the parameter L of the logistic function is the value at which P levels off, where

$$P = \frac{L}{1 + Ce^{-kt}}.$$

This value L is called the *carrying capacity* and represents the largest population an environment can support.

One way to estimate the carrying capacity is to find the inflection point. The graph of a logistic curve is concave up at first and then concave down. At the inflection point, where the concavity changes, the slope is largest. To the left of this point, the graph is concave up and the rate of growth is increasing. To the right of this point, the graph is concave down and the rate of growth is diminishing. The inflection point is called the *point of diminishing returns*. Problem 49 in the Review Problems shows that this point is at $P = L/2$. See Figure 4.74. Companies sometimes watch for this concavity change in the sales of a new product and use it to estimate the maximum potential sales.

Properties of the logistic function $P = \dfrac{L}{1 + Ce^{-kt}}$:

- The limiting value L represents the carrying capacity for P.
- The point of diminishing returns is the inflection point where P is growing the fastest. It occurs where $P = L/2$.
- The logistic function is approximately exponential for small values of t, with growth rate k.

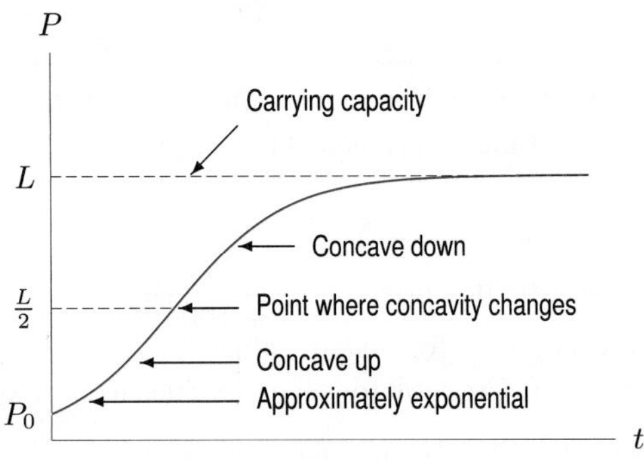

Figure 4.74: Logistic growth

The Years 1790--2000: Another look at the US Population

We used a logistic function to model the US population between 1790 and 1940. How well does this model fit the US population since 1940? We now look at all the population data from 1790 to 2000.

Example 2 If t is in years since 1790 and P is in millions, we used the following logistic function to model the US population between 1790 and 1940:

$$P = \frac{187}{1 + 47e^{-0.0318t}}.$$

According to this function, what is the maximum US population? Is this prediction accurate? How well does this logistic model fit the growth of the US population since 1940?

Table 4.7 *Predicted versus actual US population, in millions, 1940–2000 (logistic model)*

Year	1940	1950	1960	1970	1980	1990	2000
Actual	131.7	150.7	179.3	203.3	226.5	248.7	281.4
Predicted	133.7	145.0	154.4	162.1	168.2	172.9	176.6

Solution Table 4.7 shows the actual US population between 1940 and 2000 and the predicted values using this logistic model. According to the formula for the logistic function, the upper bound for the population is $L = 187$ million. However, Table 4.7 shows that the actual US population was above this figure by 1970. The fit between the logistic function and the actual population is not a good one beyond 1940. See Figure 4.75.

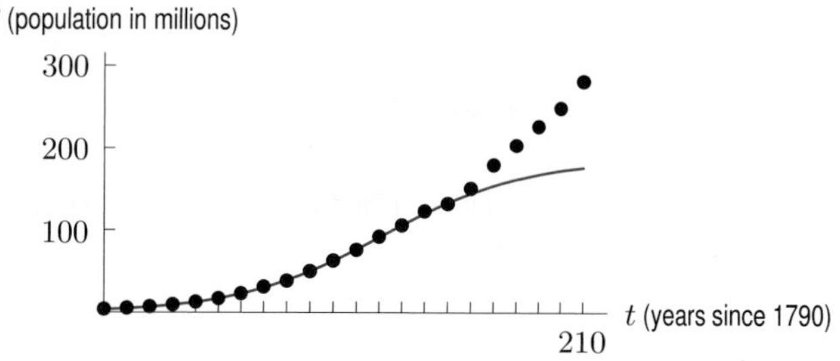

Figure 4.75: The logistic model and the US population, 1790–2000

Despite World War II, which depressed population growth between 1942 and 1945, in the last half of the 1940s the US population surged. The 1950s saw a population growth of 28 million, leaving our logistic model in the dust. This surge in population is referred to as the baby boom.

Once again we have reached a point where our model is no longer useful. This should not lead you to believe that a reasonable mathematical model cannot be found; rather it points out that no model is perfect and that when one model fails, we seek a better one. Just as we abandoned the exponential model in favor of the logistic model for the US population, we could look further.

Sales Predictions

Total sales of a new product often follow a logistic model. For example, when a new compact disc (CD) appears on the market, sales first increase rapidly as word of the CD spreads. Eventually, most of the people who want the CD have already bought it and sales slow down. The graph of total sales against time is concave up at first and then concave down, with the upper bound L equal to the maximum potential sales.

Example 3 Table 4.8 shows the total sales (in thousands) of a new CD since it was introduced.

(a) Find the point where concavity changes in this function. Use it to estimate the maximum potential sales, L.

(b) Using logistic regression, fit a logistic function to this data. What maximum potential sales does this function predict?

Table 4.8 *Total sales of a new CD since its introduction*

t (months)	0	1	2	3	4	5	6	7
P (total sales in 1000s)	0.5	2	8	33	95	258	403	496

Solution

(a) The rate of change of total sales increases until $t = 5$ and decreases after $t = 5$, so the inflection point is at approximately $t = 5$, when $P = 258$. So $L/2 = 258$ and $L = 516$. The maximum potential sales for this CD are estimated to be 516,000.

(b) Logistic regression gives the following function:

$$P = \frac{532}{1 + 869e^{-1.33t}}.$$

Maximum potential sales predicted by this function are $L = 532$, or about 532,000 CDs. See Figure 4.76.

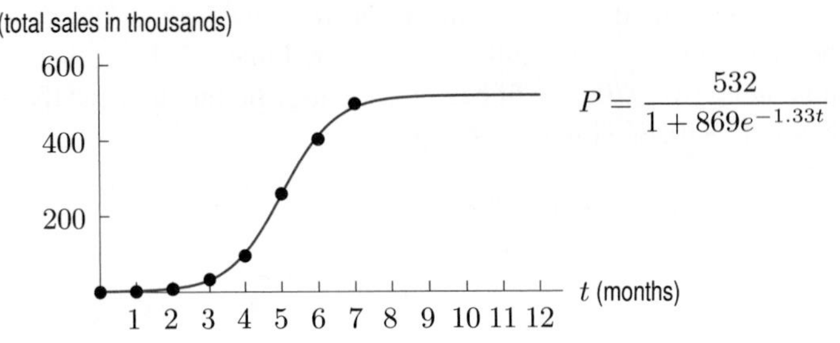

Figure 4.76: Logistic growth: Total sales of a CD

Dose-Response Curves

A *dose-response curve* plots the intensity of physiological response to a drug as a function of the dose administered. As the dose increases, the intensity of the response increases, so a dose-response function is increasing. The intensity of the response is generally scaled as a percentage of the maximum response. The curve cannot go above the maximum response (or 100%), so the curve levels off at a horizontal asymptote. Dose-response curves are generally concave up for low doses and concave down for high doses. A dose-response curve can be modeled by a logistic function with the independent variable being the dose of the drug, not time.

A dose-response curve shows the amount of drug needed to produce the desired effect, as well as the maximum effect attainable and the dose required to obtain it. The slope of the dose-response curve gives information about the therapeutic safety margin of the drug.

Drugs need to be administered in a dose which is large enough to be effective but not so large as to be dangerous. Figure 4.77 shows two different dose-response curves: one with a small slope and one with a large slope. In Figure 4.77(a), there is a broad range of dosages at which the drug is both safe and effective. In Figure 4.77(b), where the slope of the curve is steep, the range of dosages at which the drug is both safe and effective is small. If the slope of the dose-response curve is steep, a small mistake in the dosage can have dangerous results. Administration of such a drug is difficult.

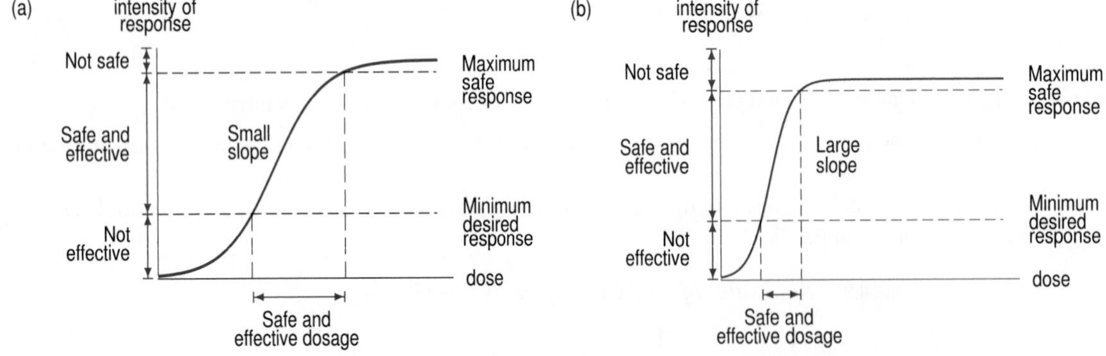

Figure 4.77: What does the slope of the dose-response curve tell us?

Example 4 Figure 4.78 shows dose-response curves for three different drugs used for the same purpose. Discuss the advantages and disadvantages of the three drugs.

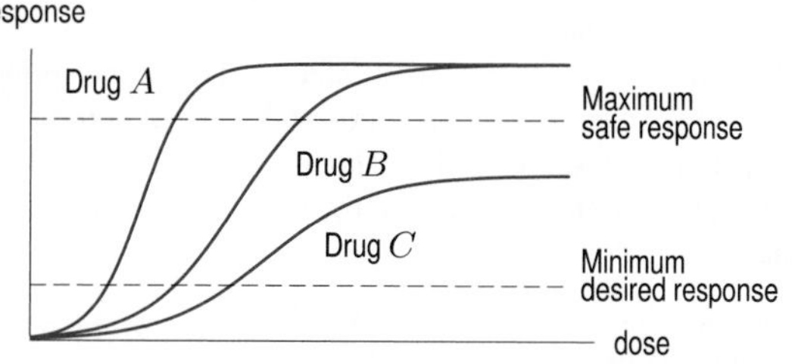

Figure 4.78: What are the advantages and disadvantages of each of these drugs?

Solution Drugs A and B exhibit the same maximum response, while the maximum response of Drug C is significantly less; however all three drugs reach the minimum desired response. The potency of Drugs B and C (the dose required to reach desired effect) is significantly less than the potency of Drug A. (Potency, however, is a relatively unimportant characteristic of a drug, since a less potent drug can simply be given in larger doses.) Drug A has a steeper slope than either of the other two. Both Drugs A and B can exceed the maximum safe response. Thus, Drug C may be the preferred drug despite its lower maximum effect because it is the safest to administer.

Problems for Section 4.7

1. If t is in years since 1990, one model for the population of the world, P, in billions, is

$$P = \frac{40}{1 + 11e^{-0.08t}}.$$

(a) What does this model predict for the maximum sustainable population of the world?
(b) Graph P against t.
(c) According to this model, when will the earth's population reach 20 billion? 39.9 billion?

2. The rate of sales of an automobile anti-theft device are given in the following table.

(a) When is the point of diminishing returns reached?
(b) What are the total sales at this point?
(c) Assuming logistic sales growth, use your answer to part (b) to estimate total potential sales of the device.

Months	1	2	3	4	5	6
Sales per month	140	520	680	750	700	550

3. The following table shows the total sales, in thousands, since a new game was brought to market.

(a) Plot this data and mark on your plot the point of diminishing returns.
(b) Predict total possible sales of this game, using the point of diminishing returns.

Month	0	2	4	6	8	10	12	14
Sales	0	2.3	5.5	9.6	18.2	31.8	42.0	50.8

4. A rumor spreads among a group of 400 people. The number of people, $N(t)$, who have heard the rumor by time t in hours since the rumor started to spread can be approximated by a function of the form

$$N(t) = \frac{400}{1 + 399e^{-0.4t}}.$$

(a) Find $N(0)$ and interpret it.
(b) How many people will have heard the rumor after 2 hours? After 10 hours?
(c) Graph $N(t)$.
(d) Approximately how long will it take until half the people have heard the rumor? Virtually everyone?
(e) Approximately when is the rumor spreading fastest?

5. Investigate the effect of the parameter C on the logistic curve

$$P = \frac{10}{1 + Ce^{-t}}.$$

Substitute several values for C and explain, with a graph and with words, the effect of C on the graph.

6. Write a paragraph explaining why sales of a new product often follow a logistic curve. Explain the benefit to the company of watching for the point of diminishing returns.

7. Figure 4.79 shows the spread of the Code-red computer virus during July 2001. Most of the growth took place starting at midnight on July 19; on July 20, the virus attacked the White House, trying (unsuccessfully) to knock its site off-line. The number of computers infected by the virus is a logistic function of time.

   (a) Estimate the limiting value of $f(t)$ as t increases. What does this limiting value represent in terms of Code-red?
   (b) Estimate the value of t at which $f''(t) = 0$. Estimate the value of n at this time.
   (c) What does the answer to part (b) tell us about Code-red?
   (d) How are the answers to parts (a) and (b) related?

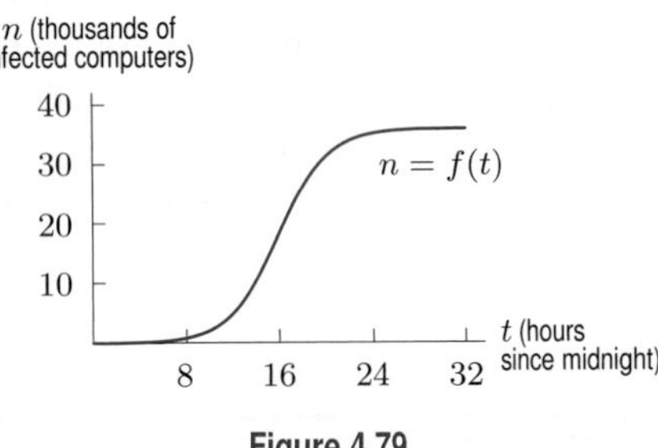

Figure 4.79

8. Find the exact coordinates of the point at which the following curve is steepest:

$$y = \frac{50}{1 + 6e^{-2t}} \quad \text{for } t \geq 0.$$

9. (a) Draw a logistic curve. Label the carrying capacity L and the point of diminishing returns t_0.
   (b) Draw the derivative of the logistic curve. Mark the point t_0 on the horizontal axis.
   (c) A company keeps track of the rate of sales (for example, sales per week) rather than total sales. Explain how the company can tell on a graph of rate of sales when the point of diminishing returns is reached.

10. The Tojolobal Mayan Indian community in Southern Mexico has available a fixed amount of land.[16] The proportion, P, of land in use for farming t years after 1935 is modeled with the logistic function

$$P = \frac{1}{1 + 3e^{-0.0275t}}.$$

   (a) What proportion of the land was in use for farming in 1935?
   (b) What is the long-run prediction of this model?
   (c) When was half the land in use for farming?
   (d) When is the proportion of land used for farming increasing most rapidly?

11. In the spring of 2003, SARS (Severe Acute Respiratory Syndrome) spread rapidly in several Asian countries and Canada. Table 4.9 gives the total number, P, of SARS cases reported in Hong Kong[17] by day t, where $t = 0$ is March 17, 2003.

   (a) Find the average rate of change of P for each interval in Table 4.9.
   (b) In early April 2003, there was fear that the disease would spread at an ever-increasing rate for a long time. What is the earliest date by which epidemiologists had evidence to indicate that the rate of new cases had begun to slow?
   (c) Explain why an exponential model for P is not appropriate.
   (d) It turns out that a logistic model fits the data well. Estimate the value of t at the inflection point. What limiting value of P does this point predict?
   (e) The best-fitting logistic function for this data turns out to be

$$P = \frac{1760}{1 + 17.53e^{-0.1408t}}.$$

   What limiting value of P does this function predict?

Table 4.9 *Total number of SARS cases in Hong Kong by day t (where t = 0 is March 17, 2003)*

t	P	t	P	t	P	t	P
0	95	26	1108	54	1674	75	1739
5	222	33	1358	61	1710	81	1750
12	470	40	1527	68	1724	87	1755
19	800	47	1621				

12. Substitute $t = 0, 10, 20, \ldots, 70$ into the exponential function used in this section to model the US population 1790–1860. Compare the predicted values of the population with the actual values.

13. On page 209, a logistic function was used to model the US population. Use this function to predict the US population in each of the census years from 1790–1940. Compare the predicted and actual values.

[16] Adapted from J. S. Thomas and M. C. Robbins, "The Limits to Growth in a Tojolobal Maya Ejido," *Geoscience and Man* 26, pp. 9–16 (Baton Rouge: Geoscience Publications, 1988).
[17] www.who.int/csr/country/en, accessed July 13, 2003.

14. A curve representing the total number of people, P, infected with a virus often has the shape of a logistic curve of the form

$$P = \frac{L}{1 + Ce^{-kt}},$$

with time t in weeks. Suppose that 10 people originally have the virus and that in the early stages the number of people infected is increasing approximately exponentially, with a continuous growth rate of 1.78. It is estimated that, in the long run, approximately 5000 people will become infected.

(a) What should we use for the parameters k and L?
(b) Use the fact that when $t = 0$, we have $P = 10$, to find C.
(c) Now that you have estimated L, k, and C, what is the logistic function you are using to model the data? Graph this function.
(d) Estimate the length of time until the rate at which people are becoming infected starts to decrease. What is the value of P at this point?

15. If R is percent of maximum response and x is dose in mg, the dose-response curve for a drug is given by

$$R = \frac{100}{1 + 100e^{-0.1x}}.$$

(a) Graph this function.
(b) What dose corresponds to a response of 50% of the maximum? This is the inflection point, at which the response is increasing the fastest.
(c) For this drug, the minimum desired response is 20% and the maximum safe response is 70%. What range of doses is both safe and effective for this drug?

16. Dose-response curves for three different products are given in Figure 4.80.

(a) For the desired response, which drug requires the largest dose? The smallest dose?
(b) Which drug has the largest maximum response? The smallest?
(c) Which drug is the safest to administer? Explain.

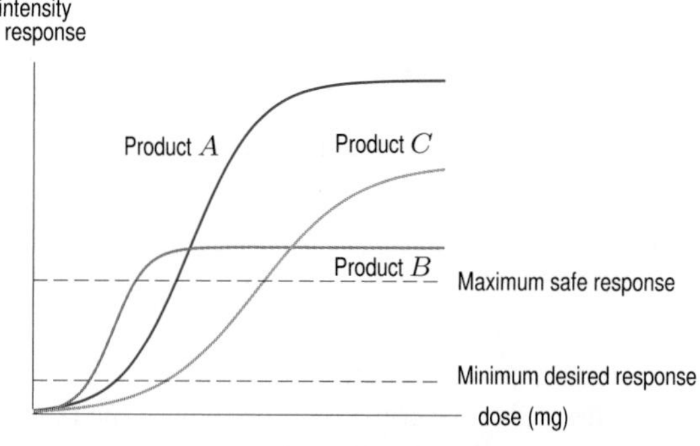

Figure 4.80

17. A dose-response curve is given by $R = f(x)$, where R is percent of maximum response and x is the dose of the drug in mg. The curve has the shape shown in Figure 4.77. The inflection point is at $(15, 50)$ and $f'(15) = 11$.

(a) Explain what $f'(15)$ tells you in terms of dose and response for this drug.
(b) Is $f'(10)$ greater than or less than 11? Is $f'(20)$ greater than or less than 11? Explain.

18. Explain why it is safer to use a drug for which the derivative of the dose-response curve is smaller.

There are two kinds of dose-response curves. One type, discussed in this section, plots the intensity of response against the dose of the drug. We now consider a dose-response curve in which the percentage of subjects showing a specific response is plotted against the dose of the drug. In Problems 19–20, the curve on the left shows the percentage of subjects exhibiting the desired response at the given dose, and the curve on the right shows the percentage of subjects for which the given dose is lethal.

19. In Figure 4.81, what range of doses appears to be both safe and effective for 99% of all patients?

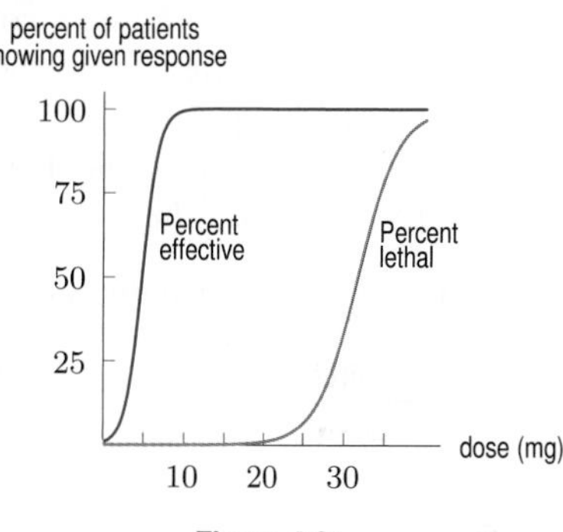

Figure 4.81

20. In Figure 4.82, discuss the possible outcomes and what percent of patients fall in each outcome when 50 mg of the drug is administered.

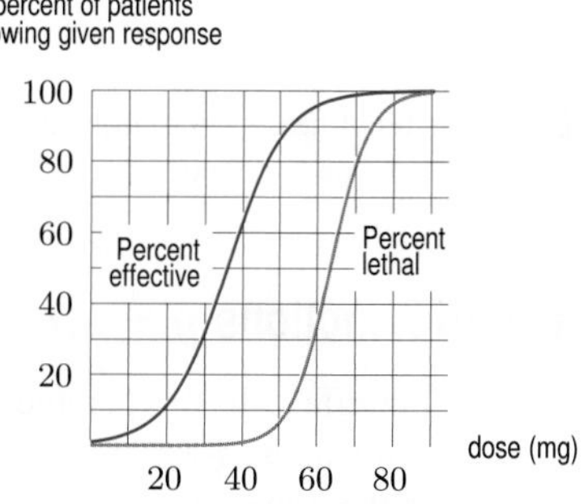

Figure 4.82

21. A population, P, growing logistically is given by

$$P = \frac{L}{1 + Ce^{-kt}}.$$

(a) Show that

$$\frac{L-P}{P} = Ce^{-kt}.$$

(b) Explain why part (a) shows that the ratio of the additional population the environment can support to the existing population decays exponentially.

22. Cell membranes contain ion channels. The fraction, f, of channels that are open is a function of the membrane potential V (the voltage inside the cell minus voltage outside), in millivolts (mV), given by

$$f(V) = \frac{1}{1 + e^{-(V+25)/2}}.$$

(a) Find the values of L, k, and C in the logistic formula for f:

$$f(V) = \frac{L}{1 + Ce^{-kV}}.$$

(b) At what voltages V are 10% , 50% and 90% of the channels open?

4.8 THE SURGE FUNCTION AND DRUG CONCENTRATION

Nicotine in the Blood

When a person smokes a cigarette, the nicotine from the cigarette enters the body through the lungs, is absorbed into the blood, and spreads throughout the body. Most cigarettes contain between 0.5 and 2.0 mg of nicotine; approximately 20% (between 0.1 and 0.4 mg) is actually inhaled and absorbed into the person's bloodstream. As the nicotine leaves the blood, the smoker feels the need for another cigarette. The half-life of nicotine in the bloodstream is about two hours. The lethal dose is considered to be about 60 mg.

The nicotine level in the blood rises as a person smokes, and tapers off when smoking ceases. Table 4.10 shows blood nicotine concentration (in ng/ml) during and after the use of cigarettes. (Smoking occurred during the first ten minutes and the experimental data shown represent average values for ten people.)[18]

The points in Table 4.10 are plotted in Figure 4.83. Functions with this behavior are called *surge functions*. They have equations of the form $y = ate^{-bt}$, where a and b are positive constants.

Table 4.10 *Blood nicotine concentrations during and after the use of cigarettes*

t (minutes)	0	5	10	15	20	25	30	45	60	75	90	105	120
C (ng/ml)	4	12	17	14	13	12	11	9	8	7.5	7	6.5	6

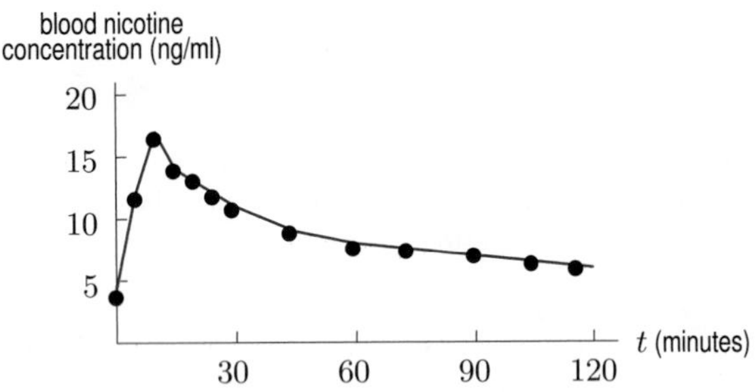

Figure 4.83: Blood nicotine concentrations during and after the use of cigarettes

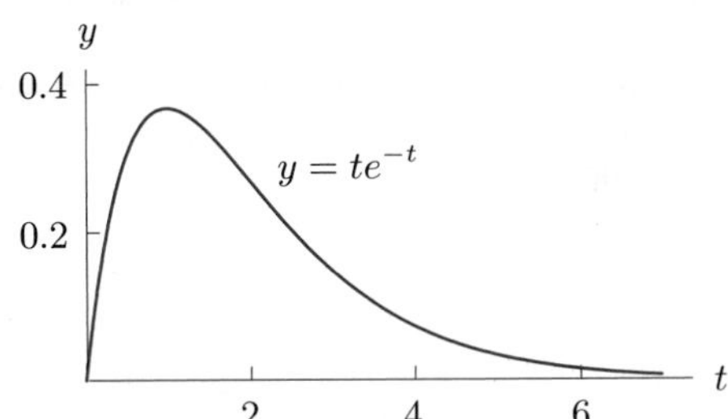

Figure 4.84: One member of the family $y = ate^{-bt}$, with $a = 1$ and $b = 1$

The Family of Functions $y = ate^{-bt}$

What effect do the parameters a and b have on the shape of the graph of $y = ate^{-bt}$? Start by looking at the graph with $a = 1$ and $b = 1$. See Figure 4.84. We consider the effect of the parameter b on the graph of $y = ate^{-bt}$ now; the parameter a is considered in Problem 2 of this section.

[18]Benowitz, Porched, Skeiner, Jacog, "Nicotine Absorption and Cardiovascular Effects with Smokeless Tobacco Use: Comparison with Cigarettes and Nicotine Gum," *Clinical Pharmacology and Therapeutics* 44 (1988): 24.

The Effect of the Parameter b on $y = te^{-bt}$

Graphs of $y = te^{-bt}$ for different positive values of b are shown in Figure 4.85. The general shape of the curve does not change as b changes, but as b decreases, the curve rises for a longer period of time and to a higher value.

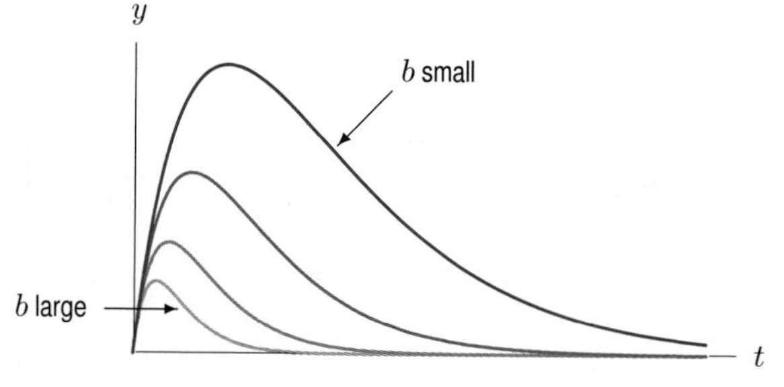

Figure 4.85: Graph of $y = te^{-bt}$, with b varying

Figure 4.86: How does the maximum depend on b?

We see in Figure 4.86 that, when $b = 1$, the maximum occurs at about $t = 1$. When $b = 2$, it occurs at about $t = \frac{1}{2}$, and when $b = 3$, it occurs at about $t = \frac{1}{3}$. The next example shows that the maximum of the function $y = te^{-bt}$ occurs at $t = 1/b$.

Example 1 For $b > 0$, show that the maximum value of $y = te^{-bt}$ occurs at $t = 1/b$ and increases as b decreases.

Solution The maximum occurs at a critical point where $dy/dt = 0$. Differentiating gives

$$\frac{dy}{dt} = 1 \cdot e^{-bt} + t\left(-be^{-bt}\right) = e^{-bt} - bte^{-bt} = e^{-bt}(1 - bt).$$

So $dy/dt = 0$ where

$$\begin{aligned} 1 - bt &= 0 \\ t &= \frac{1}{b} \end{aligned}$$

Substituting $t = 1/b$ shows that at the maximum,

$$y = \frac{1}{b}e^{-b(1/b)} = \frac{e^{-1}}{b}.$$

So, for $b > 0$, as b increases, the maximum value of y decreases and vice versa.

> The **surge function** $y = ate^{-bt}$ increases rapidly and then decreases toward zero with a maximum at $t = 1/b$.

Drug Concentration Curves

When the concentration, C, of a drug in the body is plotted against the time, t, since the drug was administered, the curve generally has the shape shown in Figure 4.87. This is called a *drug concentration curve*, and is modeled using a function of the form $C = ate^{-bt}$. Figure 4.87 shows the peak concentration (the maximum concentration of the drug in the body) and the length of time until peak concentration is reached.

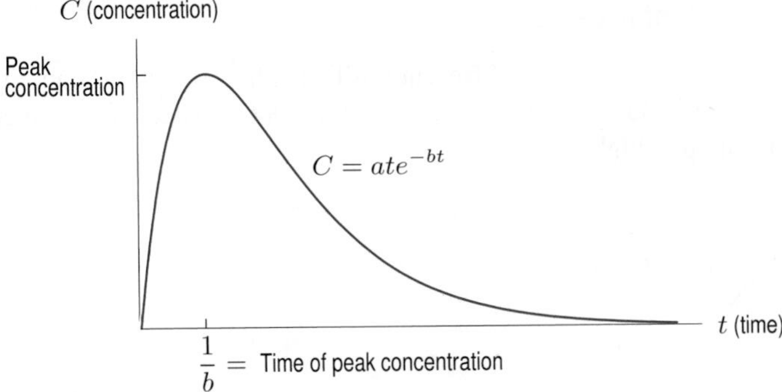

Figure 4.87: Curve showing drug concentration as a function of time

Factors Affecting Drug Absorption

Drug interactions and the age of the patient can affect the drug concentration curve. In Problems 11 and 13, we see that food intake can also affect the rate of absorption of a drug, and (perhaps most surprising) that drug concentration curves can vary markedly between different commercial versions of the same drug.

Example 2 Figure 4.88 shows the drug concentration curves for paracetamol (acetaminophen) alone and for paracetamol taken in conjunction with propantheline. Figure 4.89 shows drug concentration curves for patients known to be slow absorbers of the drug, for paracetamol alone and for paracetamol in conjunction with metoclopramide. Discuss the effects of the additional drugs on peak concentration and the time to reach peak concentration.[19]

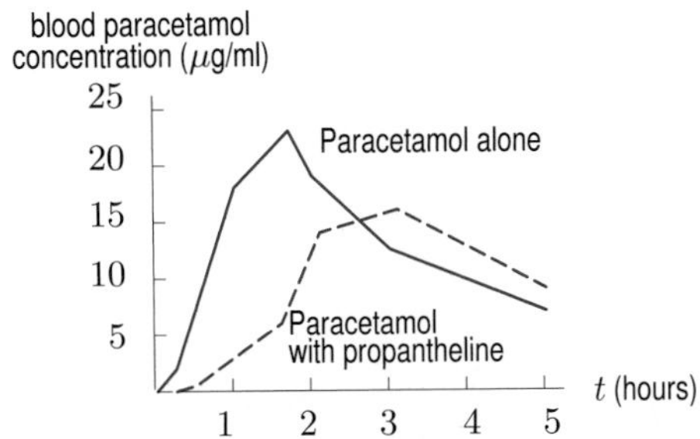

Figure 4.88: Drug concentration curves for paracetamol, normal patients

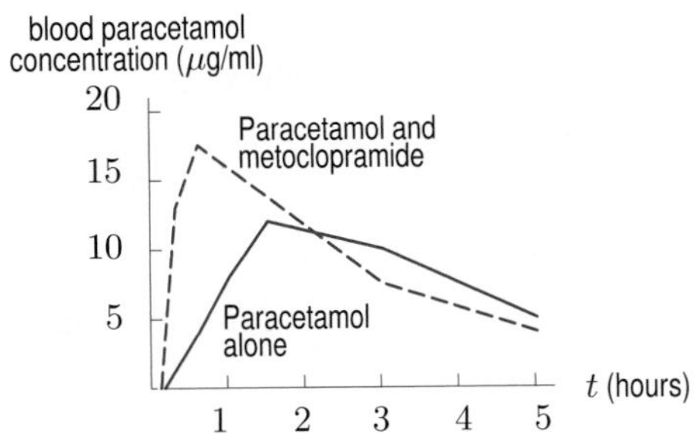

Figure 4.89: Drug concentration curves for paracetamol, patients with slow absorption

Solution Figure 4.88 shows it takes about 1.5 hours for the paracetamol to reach its peak concentration, and that the maximum concentration reached is about 23 μg of paracetamol per ml of blood. However, if propantheline is administered with the paracetamol, it takes much longer to reach the peak concentration (about three hours, or approximately double the time), and the peak concentration is much lower, at about 16 μg/ml.

Comparing the curves for paracetamol alone in Figures 4.88 and 4.89 shows that the time to reach peak concentration is the same (about 1.5 hours), but the maximum concentration is lower for patients with slow absorption. When metoclopramide is given with paracetamol in Figure 4.89, the peak concentration is reached faster and is higher.

---

[19]Graeme S. Avery, ed. *Drug Treatment: Principle and Practice of Clinical Pharmacology and Therapeutics* (Sydney: Adis Press, 1976).

Minimum Effective Concentration

The minimum effective concentration of a drug is the blood concentration necessary to achieve a pharmacological response. The time at which this concentration is reached is referred to as onset; termination occurs when the drug concentration falls below this level. See Figure 4.90.

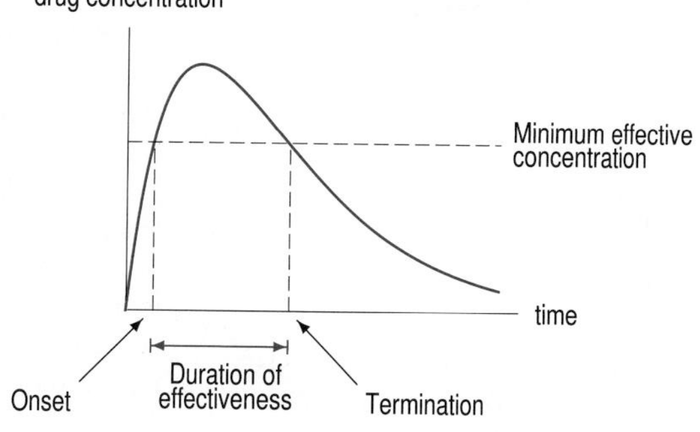

Figure 4.90: When is the drug effective?

Example 3 Depo-Provera was approved for use in the US in 1992 as a contraceptive. Figure 4.91 shows the drug concentration curve for a dose of 150 mg given intramuscularly.[20] The minimum effective concentration is about 4 ng/ml. How often should the drug be administered?

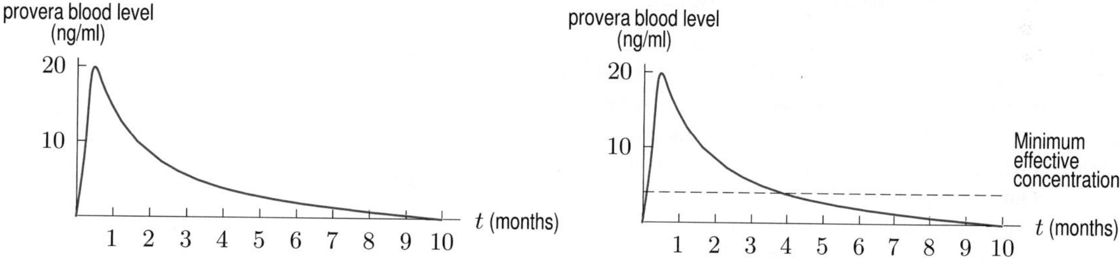

Figure 4.91: Drug concentration curve for Depo-Provera **Figure 4.92**: When should the next dose be administered?

Solution The minimum effective concentration on the drug concentration curve is plotted as a dotted horizontal line at 4 ng/ml. See Figure 4.92. We see that the drug becomes effective almost immediately and ceases to be effective after about four months. Doses should be given about every four months.

Although the dosage interval is four months, notice that it takes ten months after injections are discontinued for Depo-Provera to be entirely eliminated from the body. Fertility during that period is unpredictable.

Problems for Section 4.8

1. If time, t, is in hours and concentration, C, is in ng/ml, the drug concentration curve for a drug is given by

$$C = 12.4te^{-0.2t}.$$

(a) Graph this curve.
(b) How many hours does it take for the drug to reach its peak concentration? What is the concentration at that time?
(c) If the minimum effective concentration is 10 ng/ml, during what time period is the drug effective?
(d) Complications can arise whenever the level of the drug is above 4 ng/ml. How long must a patient wait before being safe from complications?

2. Let $b = 1$, and graph $C = ate^{-bt}$ using different values for a. Explain the effect of the parameter a.

3. Figure 4.93 shows drug concentration curves for anhydrous ampicillin for newborn babies and adults.[21] Discuss the differences between newborns and adults in the absorption of this drug.

[20]Robert M. Julien, *A Primer of Drug Action* (W. H. Freeman and Co, 1995).
[21]*Pediatrics*, 1973, 51, 578.

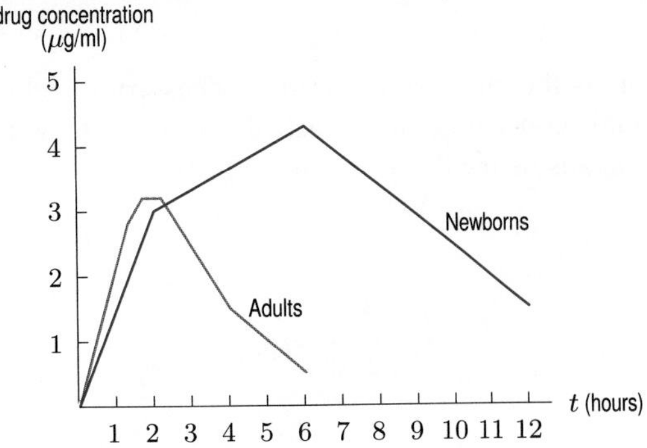

Figure 4.93

4. If t is in hours, the drug concentration curve for a drug is given by $C = 17.2te^{-0.4t}$ ng/ml. The minimum effective concentration is 10 ng/ml.
   (a) If the second dose of the drug is to be administered when the first dose becomes ineffective, when should the second dose be given?
   (b) If you want the onset of effectiveness of the second dose to coincide with termination of effectiveness of the first dose, when should the second dose be given?

5. Absorption of different forms of the antibiotic erythromycin may be increased, decreased, delayed or not affected by food. Figure 4.94 shows the drug concentration levels of erythromycin in healthy, fasting human volunteers who received single oral doses of 500 mg erythromycin tablets, together with either large (250 ml) or small (20 ml) accompanying volumes of water.[22] Discuss the effect of the water on the concentration of erythromycin in the blood. How are the peak concentration and the time to reach peak concentration affected? When does the effect of the volume of water wear off?

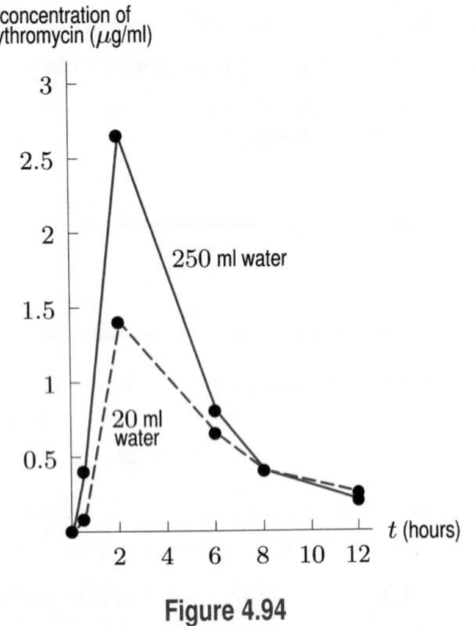

Figure 4.94

6. Hydrocodone bitartrate is a cough suppressant usually administered in a 10 mg oral dose. The peak concentration of the drug in the blood occurs 1.3 hours after consumption and the peak concentration is 23.6 ng/ml. Draw the drug concentration curve for hydrocodone bitartrate.

7. Figure 4.83 shows the concentration of nicotine in the blood during and after smoking a cigarette. Figure 4.95 shows the concentration of nicotine in the blood during and after using chewing tobacco or nicotine gum. (The chewing occurred during the first 30 minutes and the experimental data shown represent the average values for ten patients.)[23] Compare the three nicotine concentration curves (for cigarettes, chewing tobacco and nicotine gum) in terms of peak concentration, the time until peak concentration, and the rate at which the nicotine is eliminated from the bloodstream.

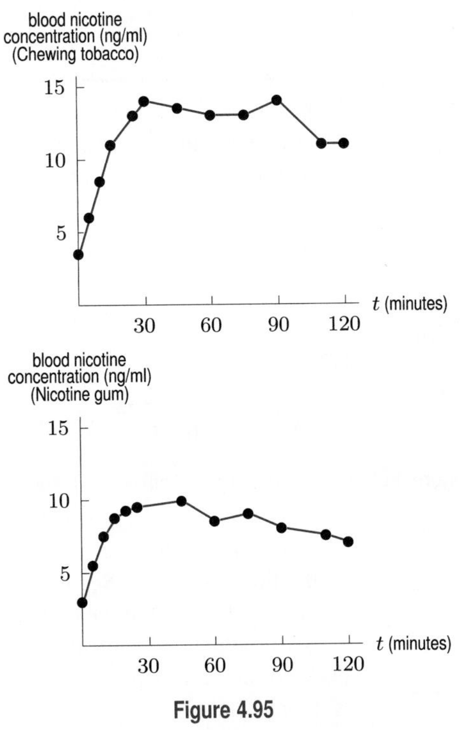

Figure 4.95

8. If t is in minutes since the drug was administered, the concentration, $C(t)$ in ng/ml, of a drug in a patient's bloodstream is given by

$$C(t) = 20te^{-0.03t}.$$

   (a) How long does it take for the drug to reach peak concentration? What is the peak concentration?
   (b) What is the concentration of the drug in the body after 15 minutes? After an hour?
   (c) If the minimum effective concentration is 10 ng/ml, when should the next dose be administered?

[22] J. W. Bridges and L.F. Chasseaud, *Progress in Drug Metabolism* (New York: John Wiley and Sons, 1980).

[23] Benowitz, Porchet, Skeiner, Jacob, "Nicotine Absorption and Cardiovascular Effects with Smokeless Tobacco Use: Comparison with Cigarettes and Nicotine Gum," *Clinical Pharmacology and Therapeutics* 44 (1988): 24.

9. For time $t \geq 0$, the function $C = ate^{-bt}$ with positive constants a and b gives the concentration, C, of a drug in the body. Figure 4.96 shows the maximum concentration reached (in nanograms per milliliter, ng/ml) after a 10 mg dose of the cough medicine hydrocodone bitartrate. Find the values of a and b.

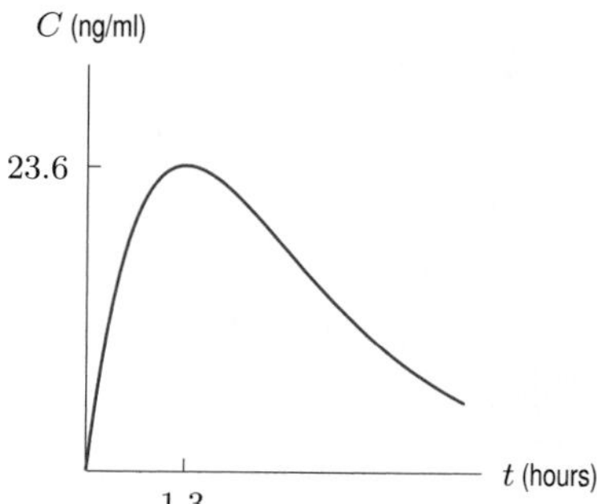

Figure 4.96

10. The method of administering a drug can have a strong influence on the drug concentration curve. Figure 4.97 shows drug concentration curves for penicillin following various routes of administration. Three milligrams per kilogram of body weight were dissolved in water and administered intravenously (IV), intramuscularly (IM), subcutaneously (SC), and orally (PO). The same quantity of penicillin dissolved in oil was administered intramuscularly (P-IM). The minimum effective concentration (MEC) is labeled on the graph.[24]

(a) Which method reaches peak concentration the fastest? The slowest?
(b) Which method has the largest peak concentration? The smallest?
(c) Which method wears off the fastest? The slowest?
(d) Which method has the longest effective duration? The shortest?
(e) When penicillin is administered orally, for approximately what time interval is it effective?

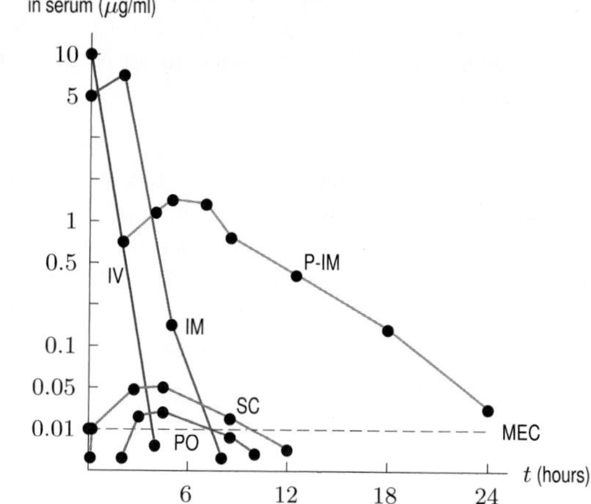

Figure 4.97

11. Figure 4.98 shows the plasma levels of canrenone in a healthy volunteer after a single oral dose of spironolactone given on a fasting stomach and together with a standardized breakfast. (Spironolactone is a diuretic agent that is partially converted into canrenone in the body.)[25] Discuss the effect of food on peak concentration and time to reach peak concentration. Is the effect of the food strongest during the first 8 hours, or after 8 hours?

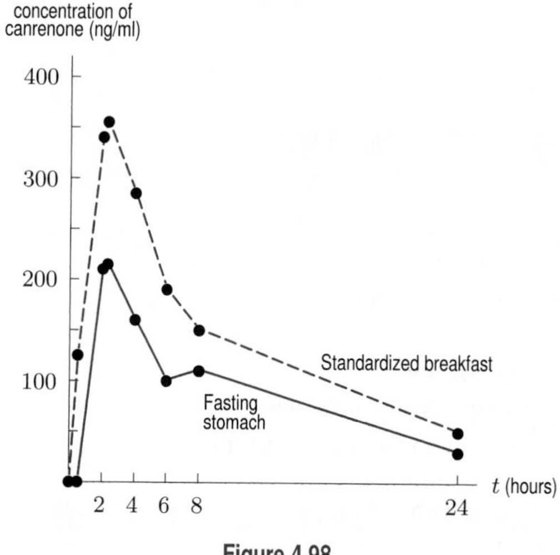

Figure 4.98

12. This problem shows how a surge can be modeled with a difference of exponential decay functions.

(a) Using graphs of e^{-t} and e^{-2t}, explain why the graph of $f(t) = e^{-t} - e^{-2t}$ has the shape of a surge.
(b) Find the critical point and inflection point of f.

[24] J. W. Bridges and L. F. Chasseaud, *Progress in Drug Metabolism* (New York: John Wiley and Sons, 1980).
[25] Welling & Tse, *Pharmacokinetics of Cardiovascular, Central Nervous System, and Antimicrobial Drugs* (The Royal Society of Chemistry, 1985).

13. Figure 4.99 shows drug concentration curves after oral administration of 0.5 mg of four digoxin products. All the tablets met current USP standards of potency, disintegration time, and dissolution rate.[26]

(a) Discuss differences and similarities in the peak concentration and the time to reach peak concentration.
(b) Give possible values for minimum effective concentration and maximum safe concentration that would make Product C or Product D the preferred drug.
(c) Give possible values for minimum effective concentration and maximum safe concentration that would make Product A the preferred drug.

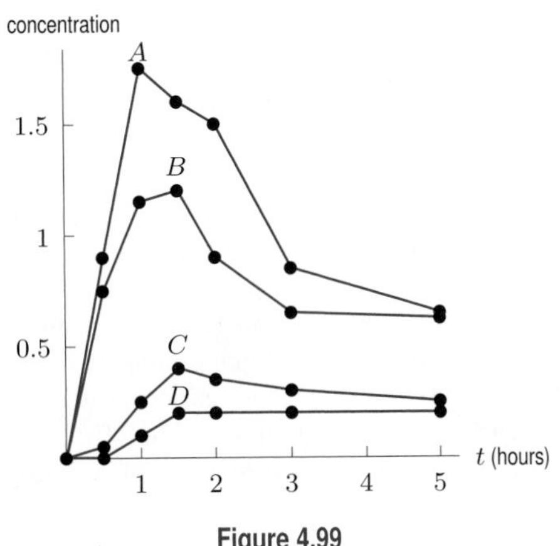

Figure 4.99

14. Figure 4.100 shows a graph of the percentage of drug dissolved against time for four tetracycline products A, B, C, and D. Figure 4.101 shows the drug concentration curves for the same four tetracycline products.[27] Discuss the effect of dissolution rate on peak concentration and time to reach peak concentration.

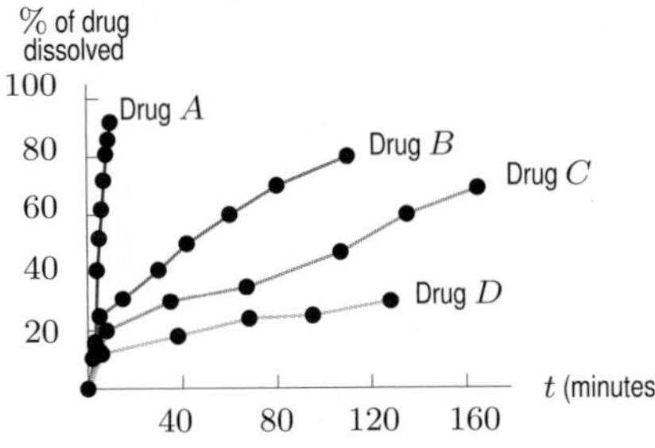

Figure 4.100

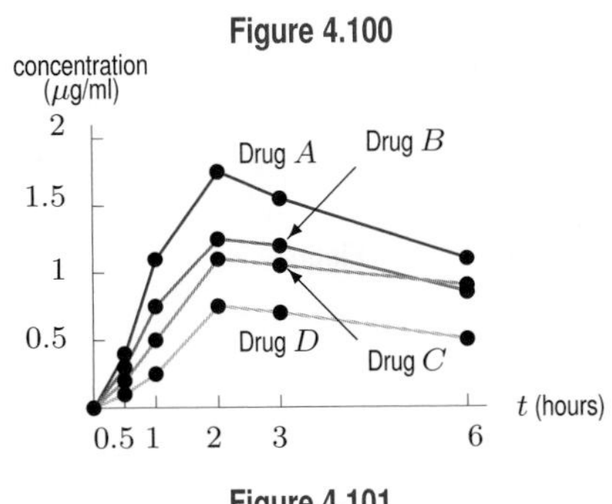

Figure 4.101

CHAPTER SUMMARY

- **Using the first derivative**
  Critical points, local maxima and minima
- **Using the second derivative**
  Inflection points, concavity
- **Optimization**
  Global maxima and minima
- **Maximizing profit and revenue**
- **Average cost**
  Minimizing average cost
- **Elasticity**
- **Families of functions**
  Parameters. The surge function, drug concentration curves. The logistic function, carrying capacity, point of diminishing returns.

REVIEW PROBLEMS FOR CHAPTER FOUR

For Problems 1–2, indicate all critical points on the given graphs. Determine which correspond to local minima, local maxima, global minima, global maxima, or none of these. (Note that the graphs are on closed intervals.)

1.

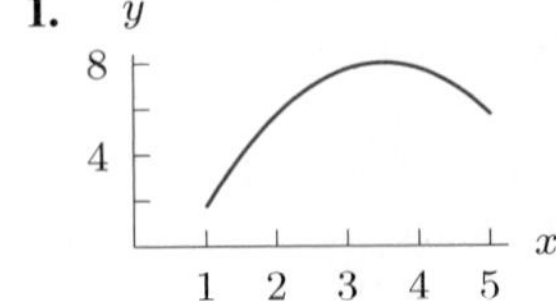

2.

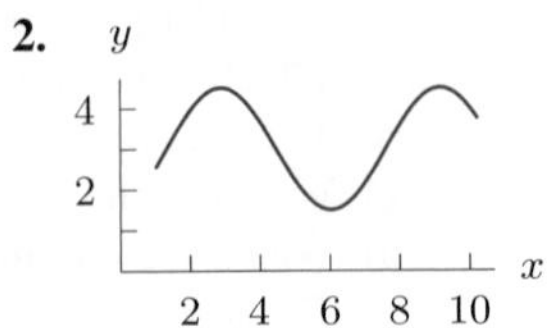

[26] Graeme S. Avery, ed. *Drug Treatment: Principles and Practice of Clinical Pharmacology and Therapeutics* (Sydney: Adis Press, 1976).

[27] J. W. Bridges and L.F. Chasseaud, *Progress in Drug Metabolism* (New York: John Wiley and Sons, 1980).

In Problems 3–4, find the value(s) of x for which:

(a) $f(x)$ has a local maximum or local minimum. Indicate which ones are maxima and which are minima.

(b) $f(x)$ has a global maximum or global minimum.

3. $f(x) = x^{10} - 10x$, and $0 \le x \le 2$

4. $f(x) = x - \ln x$, and $0.1 \le x \le 2$

In Problems 5–7, find the exact global maximum and minimum values of the function.

5. $h(z) = \dfrac{1}{z} + 4z^2$ for $z > 0$

6. $g(t) = \dfrac{1}{t^3 + 1}$ for $t \ge 0$

7. $f(x) = \dfrac{1}{(x-1)^2 + 2}$

8. On July 1, the price of a stock had a critical point. How could the price have been changing during the time around July 1?

9. Let $C = ate^{-bt}$ represent a drug concentration curve.

(a) Discuss the effect on peak concentration and time to reach peak concentration of varying the parameter a while keeping b fixed.

(b) Discuss the effect on peak concentration and time to reach peak concentration of varying the parameter b while keeping a fixed.

(c) Suppose $a = b$, so $C = ate^{-at}$. Discuss the effect on peak concentration and time to reach peak concentration of varying the parameter a.

For the graphs of f' in Problems 10–13, decide:

(a) Over what intervals is f increasing? Decreasing?

(b) Does f have local maxima or minima? If so, which, and where?

10.

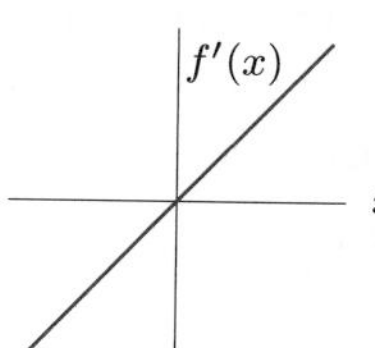

11.

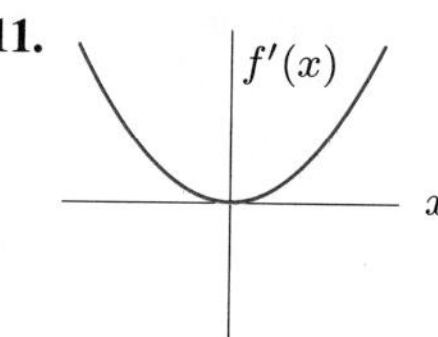

12.

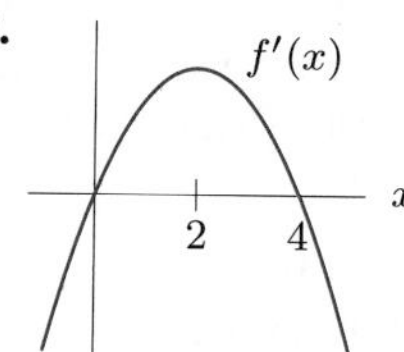

13.

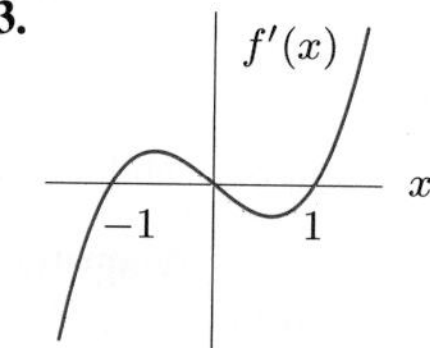

14. The marginal revenue and marginal cost for a certain item are graphed in Figure 4.102. Do the following quantities maximize profit for the company? Explain your answer.

(a) $q = a$ **(b)** $q = b$

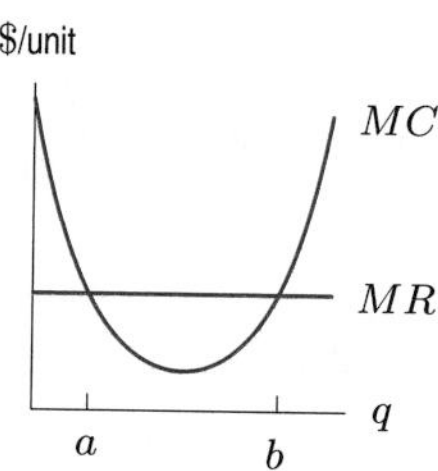

Figure 4.102

Problems 15–18 concern $f(t)$ in Figure 4.103, which gives the length of a human fetus as a function of its age.

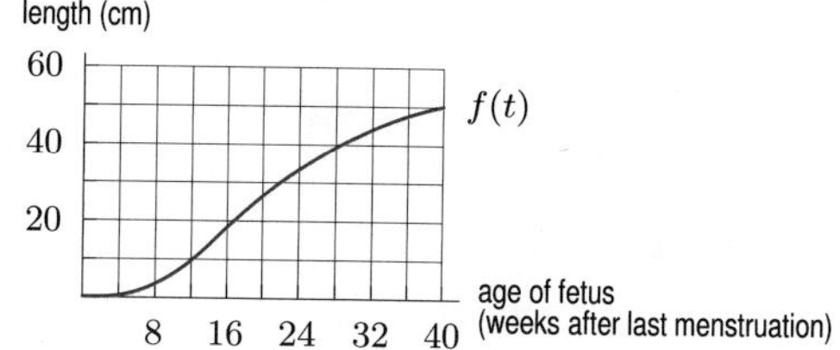

Figure 4.103

15. **(a)** What are the units of $f'(24)$?

(b) What is the biological meaning of $f'(24) = 1.6$?

16. **(a)** Which is greater, $f'(20)$ or $f'(36)$?

(b) What does your answer say about fetal growth?

17. **(a)** At what time does the inflection point occur?

(b) What is the biological significance of this point?

18. Estimate

(a) $f'(20)$ **(b)** $f'(36)$

(c) The average rate of change of length over the 40 weeks shown.

19. Find constants a and b in the function $f(x) = axe^{bx}$ such that $f(\frac{1}{3}) = 1$ and the function has a local maximum at $x = \frac{1}{3}$.

20. Suppose f has a continuous derivative. From the values of $f'(\theta)$ in the following table, estimate the θ values with $1 < \theta < 2.1$ at which $f(\theta)$ has a local maximum or minimum. Identify which is which.

θ	1.0	1.1	1.2	1.3	1.4	1.5
$f'(\theta)$	2.4	0.3	−2.0	−3.5	−3.3	−1.7
θ	1.6	1.7	1.8	1.9	2.0	2.1
$f'(\theta)$	0.8	2.8	3.6	2.8	0.7	−1.6

21. **(a)** Find the derivative of $f(x) = x^5 + x + 7$. What is its sign?
(b) How many real roots does the equation $x^5 + x + 7 = 0$ have? How do you know?
[Hint: How many critical points does this function have?]

22. For the function, f, graphed in Figure 4.104:

(a) Sketch $f'(x)$.
(b) Where does $f'(x)$ change its sign?
(c) Where does $f'(x)$ have local maxima or minima?

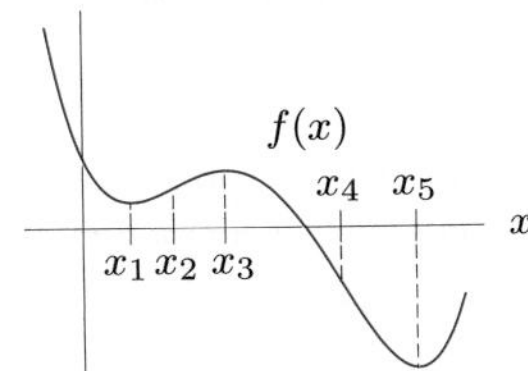

Figure 4.104

23. Using your answer to Problem 22 as a guide, write a short paragraph (using complete sentences) which describes the relationships between the following features of a function f:

- The local maxima and minima of f.
- The points at which the graph of f changes concavity.
- The sign changes of f'.
- The local maxima and minima of f'.

24. The function $y = t(x)$ is positive and continuous with a global maximum at the point $(3, 3)$. Graph $t(x)$ if $t'(x)$ and $t''(x)$ have the same sign for $x < 3$, but opposite signs for $x > 3$.

25. Each of the graphs in Figure 4.105 belongs to one of the following families of functions. In each case, identify which family is most likely:

an exponential function,

a logarithmic function,

a polynomial (What is the degree? Is the leading coefficient positive or negative?),

a periodic function,

a logistic function,

a surge function.

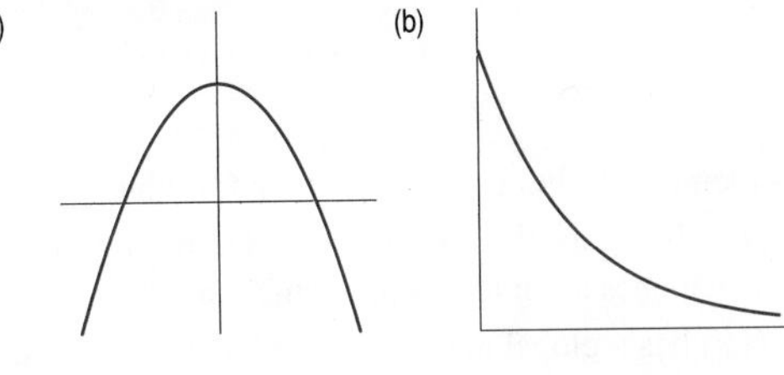

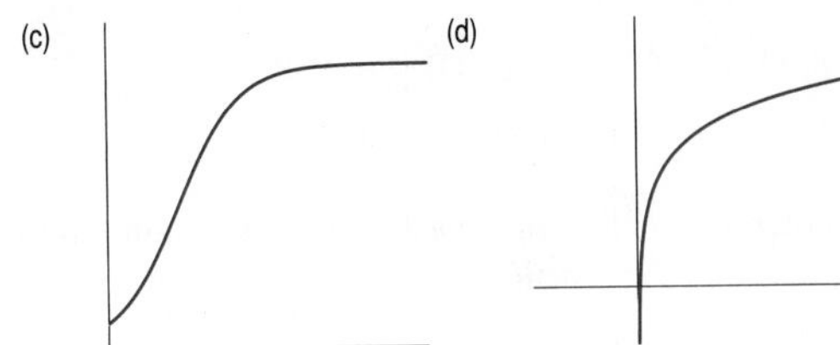

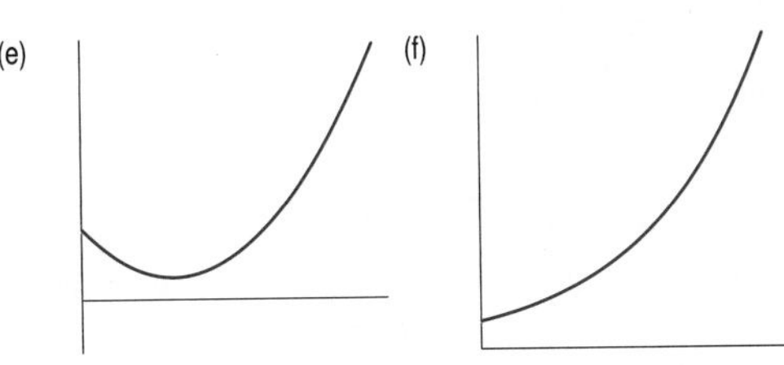

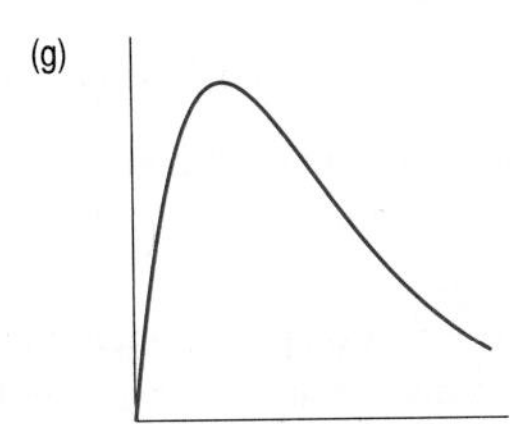

Figure 4.105

26. The total cost of producing q units of a product is given by $C(q) = q^3 - 60q^2 + 1400q + 1000$ for $0 \leq q \leq 50$; the product sells for \$788 per unit. What production level maximizes profit? Find the total cost, total revenue, and total profit at this production level. Graph the cost and revenue functions on the same axes, and label the production level at which profit is maximized, and the corresponding cost, revenue, and profit. [Hint: Costs can go as high as \$46,000.]

27. The total cost $C(q)$ of producing q goods is given by:

$$C(q) = 0.01q^3 - 0.6q^2 + 13q.$$

(a) What is the fixed cost?
(b) What is the maximum profit if each item is sold for \$7? (Assume you sell everything you produce.)
(c) Suppose exactly 34 goods are produced. They all sell when the price is \$7 each, but for each \$1 increase in price, 2 fewer goods are sold. Should the price be raised, and if so by how much?

28. The demand equation for a product is $p = b_1 - a_1 q$ and the cost function is $C(q) = b_2 + a_2 q$, where p is the price of the product and q is the quantity sold. Find the value of q, in terms of the positive constants b_1, a_1, b_2, a_2, that maximizes profit.

29. A manufacturer's cost of producing a product is given in Figure 4.106. The manufacturer can sell the product for a price p each (regardless of the quantity sold), so that the total revenue from selling a quantity q is $R(q) = pq$.

(a) The difference $\pi(q) = R(q) - C(q)$ is the total profit. For which quantity q_0 is the profit a maximum? Mark your answer on a sketch of the graph.

(b) What is the relationship between p and $C'(q_0)$? Explain your result both graphically and analytically. What does this mean in terms of economics? (Note that p is the slope of the line $R(q) = pq$. Note also that $\pi(q)$ has a maximum at $q = q_0$, so $\pi'(q_0) = 0$.)

(c) Graph $C'(q)$ and p (as a horizontal line) on the same axes. Mark q_0 on the q-axis.

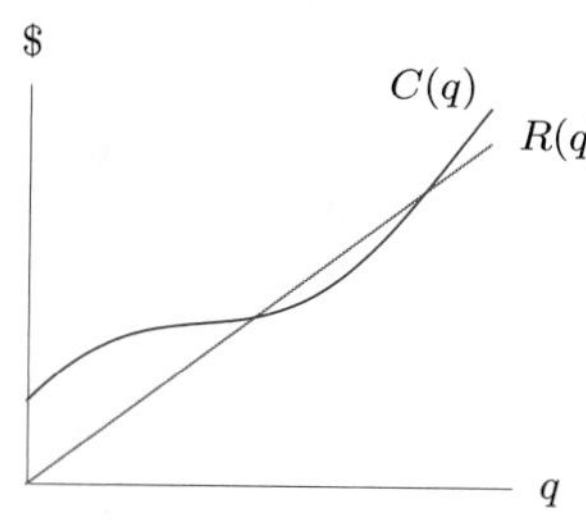

Figure 4.106

30. Let $C(q) = 0.04q^3 - 3q^2 + 75q + 96$ be the total cost of producing q items.

(a) Find the average cost per item as a function of q.
(b) Use a graphing calculator or computer to graph average cost against q.
(c) For what values of q is the average cost per item decreasing? Increasing?
(d) For what value of q is the average cost per item smallest? What is the smallest average cost per item at that point?

31. Graph a cost function where the minimum average cost of \$25 per unit is achieved by producing 15,000 units.

32. Figure 4.107 shows the cost, $C(q)$, and the revenue, $R(q)$, for a quantity q. Label the following points on the graph:

(a) The point F representing the fixed costs.
(b) The point B representing the break-even level of production.
(c) The point M representing the level of production at which marginal cost is a minimum.
(d) The point A representing the level of production at which average cost $a(q) = C(q)/q$ is a minimum.
(e) The point P representing the level of production at which profit is a maximum.

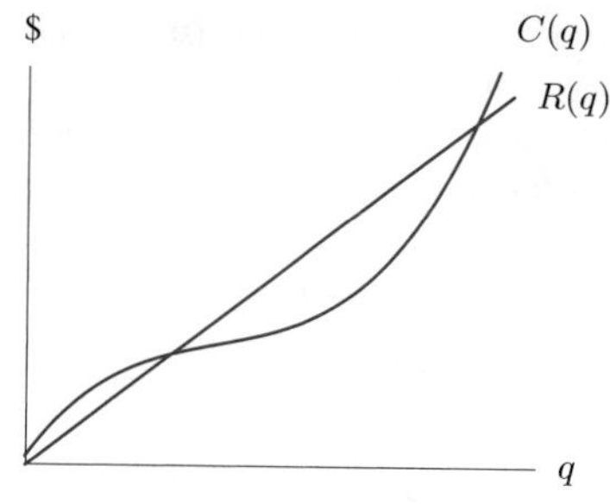

Figure 4.107

In Problems 33–38, cost, $C(q)$, is a positive, increasing, concave down function of quantity produced, q. Which one of the two numbers is the larger?

33. $C'(2)$ and $C'(3)$

34. $C'(5)$ and $\dfrac{C(5) - C(3)}{5 - 3}$

35. $\dfrac{C(100) - C(50)}{50}$ and $\dfrac{C(75) - C(50)}{25}$

36. $\dfrac{C(100) - C(50)}{50}$ and $\dfrac{C(75) - C(25)}{50}$

37. $C'(3)$ and $C(3)/3$

38. $C(10)/10$ and $C(25)/25$

39. The demand for a product is $q = 2000 - 5p$ where q is units sold at a price of p dollars. Find the elasticity if the price is \$20, and interpret your answer in terms of demand.

40. Show analytically that if elasticity of demand satisfies $E > 1$, then the derivative of revenue with respect to price satisfies $dR/dp < 0$.

41. Show analytically that if elasticity of demand satisfies $E < 1$, then the derivative of revenue with respect to price satisfies $dR/dp > 0$.

42. The following table gives the percentage, P, of households with cable television.[28]

Year	1977	1978	1979	1980	1981	1982	1983
P	16.6	17.9	19.4	22.6	28.3	35.0	40.5
Year	1984	1985	1986	1987	1988	1989	1990
P	43.7	46.2	48.1	50.5	53.8	57.1	59.0
Year	1991	1992	1993	1994	1995	1996	1997
P	60.6	61.5	62.5	63.4	65.7	66.7	67.3
Year	1998	1999	2000	2001	2002	2003	
P	67.4	68.0	67.8	69.2	68.9	68.0	

(a) Explain why a logistic model is reasonable for this data.

[28] *The World Almanac and Book of Facts 2005*, p. 310 (New York).

(b) Estimate the point of diminishing returns. What limiting value L does this point predict? Does this limiting value appear to be accurate, given the percentages for 2002 and 2003?

(c) If t is in years since 1977, the best fitting logistic function for this data turns out to be

$$P = \frac{68.8}{1 + 3.486e^{-0.237t}},$$

What limiting value does this function predict?

(d) Explain in terms of percentages of households what the limiting value is telling you. Do you think your answer to part (c) is an accurate prediction? What do you think will ultimately be the percentage of households with cable television?

43. Find the dimensions of the rectangle with perimeter 200 meters that has the largest area.

44. A square-bottomed box with a top has a fixed volume, V. What dimensions minimize the surface area?

45. **(a)** Find the critical points of $p(1-p)^4$.
(b) Classify the critical points as local maxima, local minima, or neither.
(c) What are the maximum and minimum values of $p(1-p)^4$ on $0 \le x \le 1$?

46. A right triangle has one vertex at the origin and one vertex on the curve $y = e^{-x/3}$ for $1 \le x \le 5$. One of the two perpendicular sides is along the x-axis; the other is parallel to the y-axis. Find the maximum and minimum areas for such a triangle.

47. A pigeon is released from a boat (point B in Figure 4.108) floating on a lake. Because of falling air over the cool water, the energy required to fly one meter over the lake is twice the corresponding energy e required for flying over the bank ($e = 3$ joule/meter). To minimize the energy required to fly from B to the loft, L, the pigeon heads to a point P on the bank and then flies along the bank to L. The distance $\overline{AL}$ is 2000 m, and $\overline{AB}$ is 500 m. The angle at A is a right angle.

(a) Express the energy required to fly from B to L via P as a function of the angle θ (the angle BPA).
(b) What is the optimal angle θ?
(c) Does your answer change if $\overline{AL}$, $\overline{AB}$, and e have different numerical values?

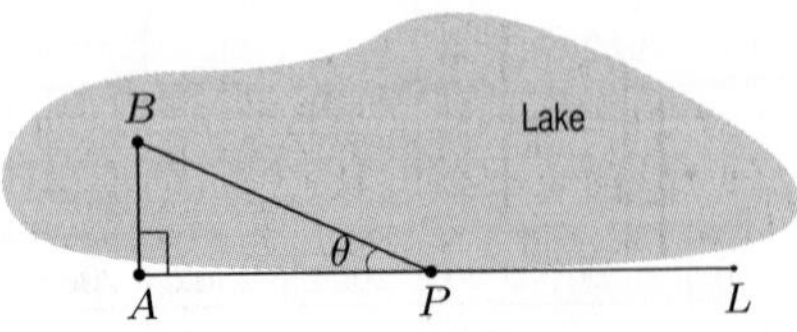

Figure 4.108

48. The bell-shaped curve of statistics has formula

$$p(x) = \frac{1}{\sigma\sqrt{2\pi}} e^{-(x-\mu)^2/(2\sigma^2)}$$

where μ is the mean and σ is the standard deviation.

(a) Where does $p(x)$ have a maximum?
(b) Does $p(x)$ have a point of inflection? If so, where?

49. Consider a population P satisfying the *logistic equation*

$$\frac{dP}{dt} = kP\left(1 - \frac{P}{L}\right).$$

(a) Use the chain rule to find d^2P/dt^2.
(b) Show that the point of diminishing returns, where $d^2P/dt^2 = 0$, occurs where $P = L/2$.

50. Figure 4.109 shows the concentration of bemetizide (a diuretic) in the blood after single oral doses of 25 mg alone, or 25 mg bemetizide and 50 mg triamterene in combination.[29] If the minimum effective concentration in a patient is 40 ng/ml, compare the effect of combining bemetizide with triamterene on peak concentration, time to reach peak concentration, time until onset of effectiveness, and duration of effectiveness. Under what circumstances might it be wise to use the triamterene with the bemetizide?

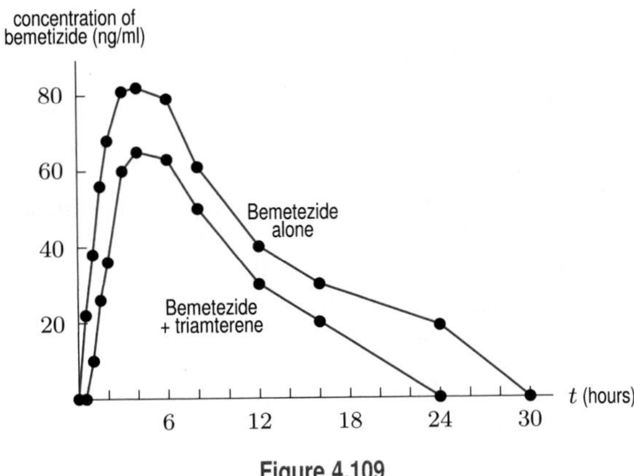

Figure 4.109

51. For $f(x) = \sin(x^2)$ between $x = 0$ and $x = 3$, find the coordinates of all intercepts, critical points, and inflection points to two decimal points.

52. **(a)** Graph $f(x) = x + a\sin x$ for $a = 0.5$ and $a = 3$.
(b) For what values of a is $f(x)$ increasing for all x?

53. **(a)** Graph $f(x) = x^2 + a\sin x$ for $a = 1$ and $a = 20$.
(b) For what values of a is $f(x)$ concave up for all x?

[29] Welling & Tse, *Pharmacokinetics of Cardiovascular, Central Nervous System, and Antimicrobial Drugs* (The Royal Society of Chemistry, 1985).

54. The distance, s, traveled by a cyclist, who starts at 1 pm, is given in Figure 4.110. Time, t, is in hours since noon.

(a) Explain why the quantity s/t is represented by the slope of a line from the origin to the point (t, s) on the graph.
(b) Estimate the time at which the quantity s/t is a maximum.
(c) What is the relationship between the quantity s/t and the instantaneous speed of the cyclist at the time you found in part (b)?

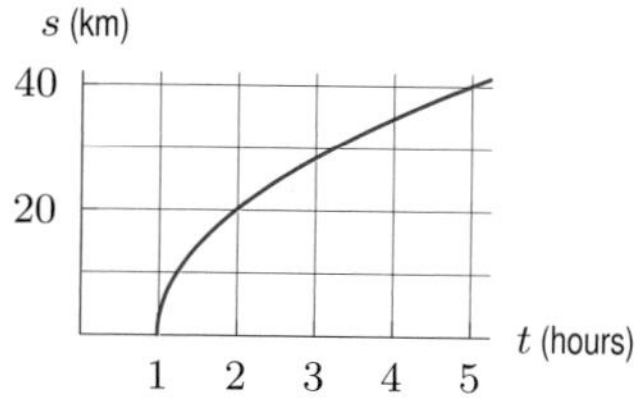

Figure 4.110

55. A bird such as a starling feeds worms to its young. To collect worms, the bird flies to a site where worms are to be found, picks up several in its beak, and flies back to its nest. The *loading curve* in Figure 4.111 shows how the number of worms (the load) a starling collects depends on the time it has been searching for them.[30] The curve is concave down because the bird can pick up worms more efficiently when its beak is empty; when its beak is partly full, the bird becomes much less efficient. The traveling time (from nest to site and back) is represented by the distance PO in Figure 4.111. The bird wants to maximize the rate at which it brings worms to the nest, where

$$\text{Rate worms arrive} = \frac{\text{Load}}{\text{Traveling time} + \text{Searching time}}$$

(a) Draw a line in Figure 4.111 whose slope is this rate.
(b) Using the graph, estimate the load which maximizes this rate.
(c) If the traveling time is increased, does the optimal load increase or decrease? Why?

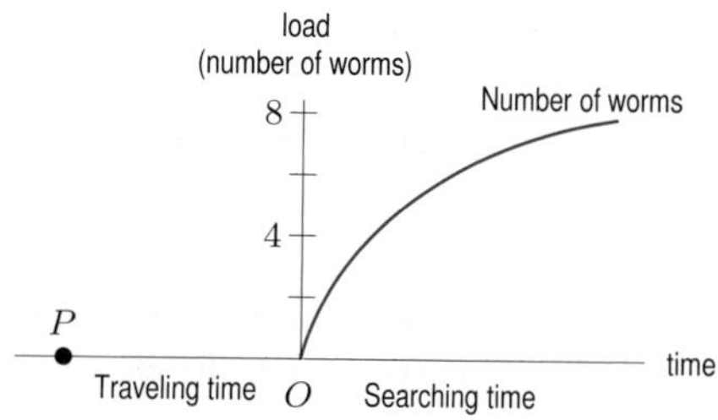

Figure 4.111

56. Table 4.11 shows the total number of cars in a University of Arizona parking lot at 30-minute intervals.[31]

(a) Graph the total number of cars in the parking lot as a function of time. Estimate the capacity of the parking lot, and when it was full.
(b) Construct a table, and then plot a graph, of the rate of arrival of cars as a function of time.
(c) From your graph in part (b), estimate when rush hour occurred.
(d) Explain the relationship between the points on the graphs in parts (a) and (b) where rush hour occurred.

Table 4.11 *Total number of cars, C, at time t*

t	5:00	5:30	6:00	6:30	7:00	7:30	8:00	8:30	9:00
C	4	5	8	18	50	110	170	200	200

57. A line goes through the origin and a point on the curve $y = x^2e^{-3x}$, for $x \geq 0$. Find the maximum slope of such a line. At what x-value does it occur?

58. A rectangle has one side on the x-axis, one side on the y-axis, one vertex at the origin and one on the curve $y = e^{-2x}$ for $x \geq 0$. Find the

(a) Maximum area **(b)** Minimum perimeter

59. A single cell of a bee's honey comb has the shape shown in Figure 4.112. The surface area of this cell is given by

$$A = 6hs + \frac{3}{2}s^2\left(\frac{-\cos\theta}{\sin\theta} + \frac{\sqrt{3}}{\sin\theta}\right)$$

where h, s, θ are as shown in the picture.

(a) Keeping h and s fixed, for what angle, θ, is the surface area a minimum?
(b) Measurements on bee's cells have shown that the angle actually used by bees is about $\theta = 55°$. Comment.

[30] Alex Kacelnick (1984). Reported by J. R. Krebs and N. B. Davis, *An Introduction to Behavioural Ecology* (Oxford: Blackwell, 1987).
[31] Adapted from Nancy Roberts et al., *Introduction to Computer Simulation*, p. 93 (Reading: Addison-Wesley, 1983).

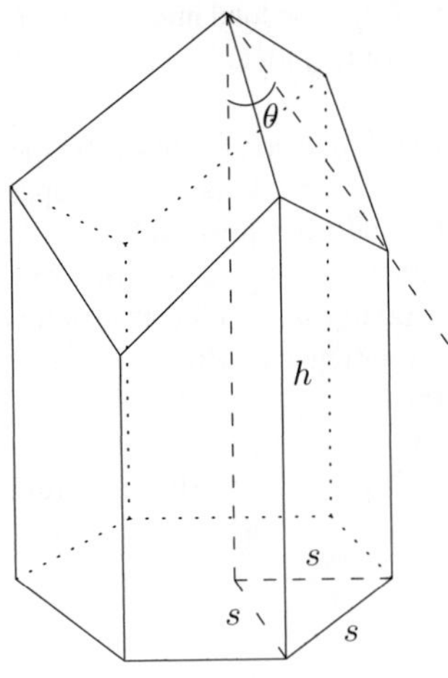

Figure 4.112

60. An organism has size W at time t. For positive constants A, b, and c, the Gompertz growth function gives

$$W = Ae^{-e^{b-ct}}, \quad t \geq 0.$$

(a) Find the intercepts and asymptotes.
(b) Find the critical points and inflection points.
(c) Graph W for various values of A, b, and c.
(d) A certain organism grows fastest when it is about 1/3 of its final size. Would the Gompertz growth function be useful in modeling its growth? Explain.

CHECK YOUR UNDERSTANDING

In Problems 1–80, indicate whether the statement is true or false.

1. The function f has a local maximum at p if $f(p) \leq f(x)$ for points x near p.
2. If $f'(p) = 0$ then p is a critical point of f.
3. If p is a critical point of f then $f'(p) = 0$.
4. If f is increasing at all points to the left of p and decreasing at all points to the right of p then f has a local maximum at p.
5. If $f'(p) = 0$ and $f''(p) > 0$ then f has a local maximum at p.
6. If $f'(p) = 0$ and $f''(p) > 0$ then f has a local minimum at p.
7. If $f''(p) > 0$ then f has a local minimum at p.
8. Every critical point of f is either a local maximum or local minimum of f.
9. A function f must have at least one critical point.
10. If f has a local minimum at $x = p$ then $f'(p) = 0$.
11. A point at which a graph changes concavity is called an inflection point.
12. If $f''(p) = 0$ then p is an inflection point of f.
13. A point p can be both a critical point and an inflection point of a function f.
14. The function $f(x) = x^3$ has an inflection point at $x = 0$.
15. The function $H(x) = x^4$ has an inflection point at $x = 0$.
16. A function f can have one inflection point and no critical points.
17. A function f can have 2 critical points and 3 inflection points.
18. If $f''(x) = x(x+1)$ then f has an inflection point at $x = -1$.
19. If $f''(x) = x(x+1)^2$ then f has an inflection point at $x = -1$.
20. If $f''(x) = e^x(x+1)$ then f has an inflection point at $x = -1$. is an inflection point.
21. A local maximum of f can also be a global maximum of f.
22. A global maximum of f on the interval $1 \leq x \leq 2$ always occurs at a critical point.
23. Every function has a global minimum.
24. If function $y = f(x)$ is increasing on the interval $a \leq x \leq b$, then the global maximum of f on this interval occurs at $x = b$.
25. If a function $y = f(x)$ has $f'(x) < 0$ for all x in the interval $a \leq x \leq b$, then the global maximum of f on this interval occurs at $x = b$.
26. A function $S(x)$ could have a different global maximum on each of the intervals $1 \leq x \leq 2$ and $2 \leq x \leq 3$.
27. The function $k(x) = 1/x$ has a global maximum when $x > 0$.
28. The function f has a global maximum on the interval $-5 \leq x \leq 5$ at p if $f(p) \leq f(x)$ for all $-5 \leq x \leq 5$.
29. The function f has a global minimum on the interval $-5 \leq x \leq 5$ at p if $f(p) \leq f(x)$ for all $-5 \leq x \leq 5$.
30. If $f'(p) = 0$ and $f''(p) > 0$ then p is a global minimum of f.
31. If marginal cost is less than marginal revenue, then increasing quantity sold will increase profit.

32. If marginal cost is greater than marginal revenue, then decreasing quantity sold will increase profit.
33. When marginal revenue equals marginal cost there is maximum profit.
34. If revenue is greater than cost, profit is the vertical distance between the cost and revenue curves.
35. Maximum profit occurs at a critical point of the cost function.
36. Maximum profit can occur when marginal profit is zero.
37. Profit is maximized where the cost and revenue curves cross.
38. Profit is zero where the graphs of the cost and revenue curves cross.
39. If prices are constant, the graph of marginal revenue is a horizontal line.
40. If prices are constant, the graph of revenue is a horizontal line.
41. Average cost is total cost for q items divided by q.
42. Marginal cost and average cost have the same units.
43. Marginal cost is the same thing as average cost.
44. The average cost of q items is the slope of the tangent line to the cost curve at q.
45. If marginal cost is less than average cost, increasing production increases average cost.
46. Marginal cost equals average cost at critical points of marginal cost.
47. If marginal cost is greater than average cost, then increasing production increases average cost.
48. Average cost has a critical point at a quantity where the line from the origin to the cost curve is also tangent to the cost curve.
49. Average cost is a decreasing function of quantity.
50. Marginal and average cost functions are both minimized at the same quantity.
51. The elasticity of demand is given by $E = |q/p \cdot dq/dp|$.
52. If elasticity, E, is greater than one, then demand is inelastic.
53. If elasticity, E, is such that $0 \leq E < 1$ then demand is elastic.
54. Elasticity is a measure of the effect on demand of a change in price.
55. If a product is considered a necessity, the demand is generally elastic.
56. An increase in price always causes an increase in revenue.
57. If elasticity $E > 1$ then revenue increases when price increases.
58. At a critical point of the revenue function, demand is neither elastic nor inelastic.
59. If elasticity $E < 1$ then profit increases with an increase in price.
60. An increase in price always causes an increase in profit.
61. If $P = 1000/(1 + 2e^{-3t})$ then P is a logistic function.
62. If $P = 1000/(1 + 2e^{3t})$ then P is a logistic function.
63. The function $P = 1000/(1 + 2e^{-3t})$ has an inflection point when $t = 500$.
64. The function $P = 1000/(1 + 2e^{-3t})$ has an inflection point when $P = 500$.
65. The logistic function $P = L/(1 + Ce^{-kt})$ approaches L as t increases.
66. If the slope of the dose/response curve is large, a small change in the dose will have a large effect on the response.
67. The carrying capacity of a population growing logistically is the largest population the environment can support.
68. The parameter k in the logistic function $P = L/(1 + Ce^{-kt})$ affects the rate at which the curve approaches its asymptote L.
69. The logistic function $P = L/(1+Ce^{-kt})$ is concave up for $P < L/2$.
70. The logistic function $P = L/(1 + Ce^{-kt})$ is always increasing.
71. The surge function is an exponential decay function.
72. The surge function has one critical point, which is a global maximum.
73. The surge function is always concave down.
74. If minimum effective concentration is positive and less than peak concentration, then the surge function will intersect the minimum effective concentration line at two points.
75. If minimum effective concentration is greater than peak concentration, then the drug will be effective only for the first half of the time interval.
76. The surge function has exactly one inflection point, and it is always at a t-value greater than the t-value of the critical point.
77. The minimum effective concentration of a drug is the blood concentration necessary to achieve a specific pharmacologic response.
78. The function $y = t/(12e^{3t})$ is a surge function.
79. The function $y = t/(12e^{-3t})$ is a surge function.
80. The surge function $y = 5te^{-3t}$ has maximum at $t = 1/3$.

PROJECTS FOR CHAPTER FOUR

1. Average and Marginal Costs

The total cost of producing a quantity q is $C(q)$. The average cost $a(q)$ is given in Figure 4.113. The following rule is used by economists to determine the marginal cost $C'(q_0)$, for any q_0:

- Construct the tangent line t_1 to $a(q)$ at q_0.
- Let t_2 be the line with the same vertical intercept as t_1 but with twice the slope of t_1.

Then $C'(q_0)$ is the vertical distance shown in Figure 4.113. Explain why this rule works.

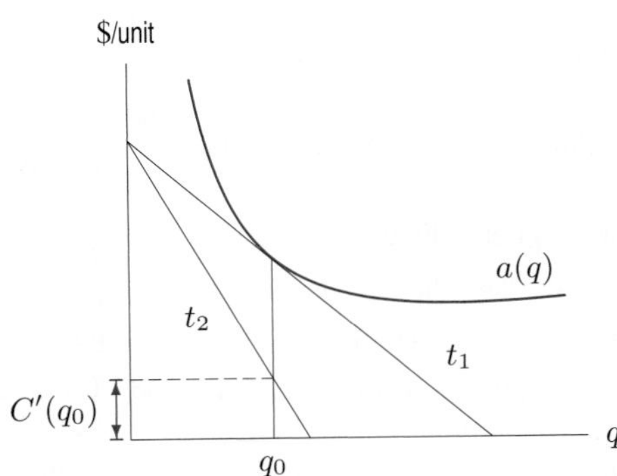

Figure 4.113

2. Firebreaks

The summer of 2000 was devastating for forests in the western US: over 3.5 million acres of trees were lost to fires, making this the worst fire season in 30 years. This project studies a fire management technique called *firebreaks*, which reduce the damage done by forest fires. A firebreak is a strip where trees have been removed in a forest so that a fire started on one side of the strip will not spread to the other side. Having many firebreaks helps confine a fire to a small area. On the other hand, having too many firebreaks involves removing large swaths of trees.[32]

(a) A forest in the shape of a 50 km by 50 km square has firebreaks in rectangular strips 50 km by 0.01 km. The trees between two firebreaks are called a stand of trees. All firebreaks in this forest are parallel to each other and to one edge of the forest, with the first firebreak at the edge of the forest. The firebreaks are evenly spaced throughout the forest. (For example, Figure 4.114 shows four firebreaks.) The total area lost in the case of a fire is the area of the stand of trees in which the fire started plus the area of all the firebreaks.

[32] Adapted from D. Quinney and R. Harding, *Calculus Connections* (New York: John Wiley & Sons, 1996).

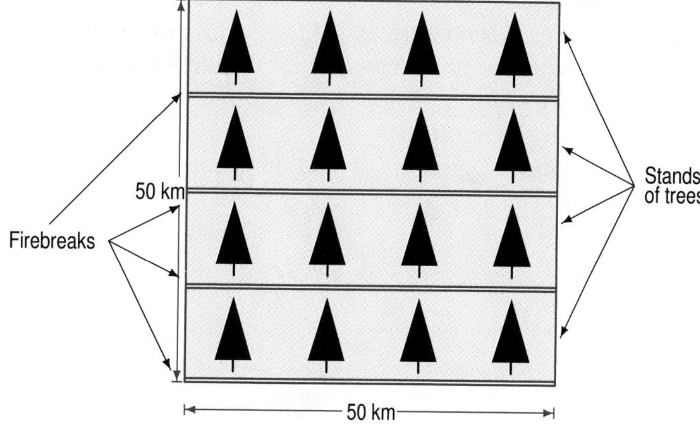

Figure 4.114

(i) Find the number of firebreaks that minimizes the total area lost to the forest in the case of a fire.

(ii) If a firebreak is 50 km by b km, find the optimal number of firebreaks as a function of b. If the width, b, of a firebreak is quadrupled, how does the optimal number of firebreaks change?

(b) Now suppose firebreaks are arranged in two equally spaced sets of parallel lines, as shown in Figure 4.115. The forest is a 50 km by 50 km square, and each firebreak is a rectangular strip 50 km by 0.01 km. Find the number of firebreaks in each direction that minimizes the total area lost to the forest in the case of a fire.

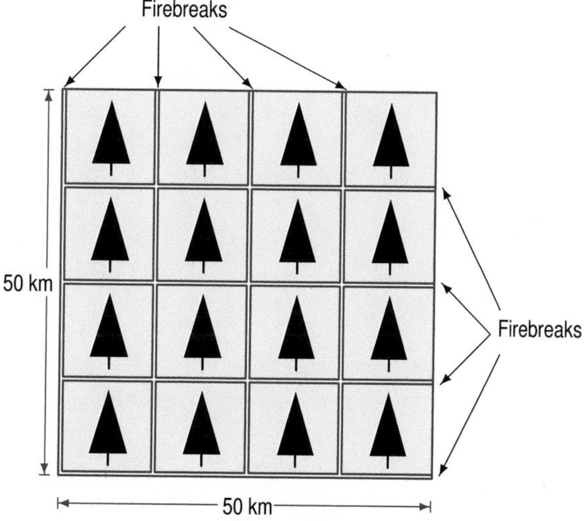

Figure 4.115

3. Production and the Price of Raw Materials

The production function $f(x)$ gives the number of units of an item that a manufacturing company can produce from x units of raw material. The company buys the raw material at price w dollars per unit and sells all it produces at a price of p dollars per unit. The quantity of raw material that maximizes profit is denoted by x^*.

(a) Do you expect the derivative $f'(x)$ to be positive or negative? Justify your answer.

(b) Explain why the formula $\pi(x) = pf(x) - wx$ gives the profit $\pi(x)$ that the company earns as a function of the quantity x of raw materials that it uses.

(c) Evaluate $f'(x^*)$.
(d) Assuming it is nonzero, is $f''(x^*)$ positive or negative?
(e) If the supplier of the raw materials is likely to change the price w, then it is appropriate to treat x^* as a function of w. Find a formula for the derivative dx^*/dw and decide whether it is positive or negative.
(f) If the price w goes up, should the manufacturing company buy more or less of the raw material?

Chapter Five

ACCUMULATED CHANGE: THE DEFINITE INTEGRAL

Contents

5.1 DISTANCE AND ACCUMULATED CHANGE

In Chapter 2, we used the derivative to find the rate of change of a function. Here we see how to go in the other direction. If we know the rate of change, can we find the original function? We start by finding the distance traveled from the velocity.

How Do We Measure Distance Traveled?

The rate of change of distance with respect to time is velocity. If we are given the velocity, can we find the distance traveled? Suppose the velocity was 50 miles per hour throughout a four-hour trip. What is the total distance traveled? Since

$$\text{Distance} = \text{Velocity} \times \text{Time},$$

we have

$$\begin{aligned}\text{Distance traveled} &= (50 \text{ miles/hour}) \times (4 \text{ hours}) \\ &= 200 \text{ miles.}\end{aligned}$$

The graph of velocity against time is the horizontal line in Figure 5.1. Notice that the distance traveled is represented by the shaded area under the graph.

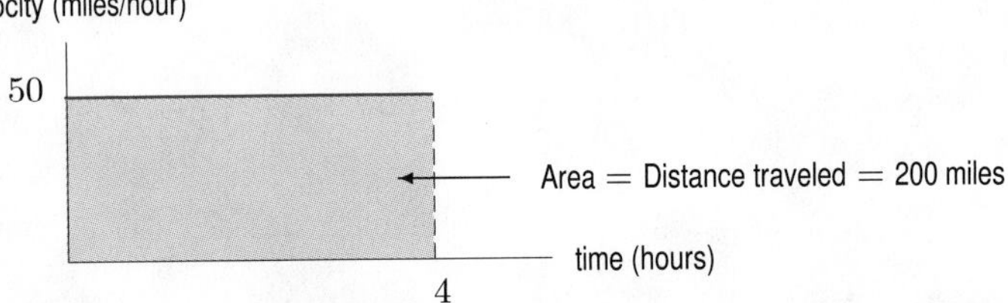

Figure 5.1: Area shaded represents distance traveled in 4 hours at 50 mph

Now let's see what happens if the velocity is not constant.

Example 1 Suppose that you travel 30 miles/hour for 2 hours, then 40 miles/hour for $1/2$ hour, then 20 miles/hour for 4 hours. What is the total distance you traveled?

Solution We compute the distances traveled for each of the three legs of the trip and add them to find the total distance traveled:

$$\begin{aligned}\text{Distance} &= (30 \text{ miles/hour})(2 \text{ hours}) + (40 \text{ miles/hour})(1/2 \text{ hour}) + (20 \text{ miles/hour})(4 \text{ hours}) \\ &= 60 \text{ miles} + 20 \text{ miles} + 80 \text{ miles} \\ &= 160 \text{ miles.}\end{aligned}$$

You travel 160 miles on this trip.

A Thought Experiment: How Far Did the Car Go?

In Example 1, the velocity was constant over intervals. Of course, this is not always the case; we now look at an example where the velocity is continually changing.

Velocity Data Every Two Seconds

Suppose a car is moving with increasing velocity and suppose we measure the car's velocity every two seconds, obtaining the data in Table 5.1:

Table 5.1 *Velocity of car every two seconds*

Time (sec)	0	2	4	6	8	10
Velocity (ft/sec)	20	30	38	44	48	50

How far has the car traveled? Since we don't know how fast the car is moving at every moment, we can't calculate the distance exactly, but we can make an estimate. The velocity is increasing, so the car is going at least 20 ft/sec for the first two seconds. Since Distance = Velocity × Time, the car goes at least $20 \cdot 2 = 40$ feet during the first two seconds. Likewise, it goes at least $30 \cdot 2 = 60$ feet during the next two seconds, and so on. During the ten-second period it goes at least

$$20 \cdot 2 + 30 \cdot 2 + 38 \cdot 2 + 44 \cdot 2 + 48 \cdot 2 = 360 \text{ feet.}$$

Thus, 360 feet is an underestimate of the total distance traveled during the ten seconds.

To get an overestimate, we can reason in a similar way: During the first two seconds, the car's velocity is at most 30 ft/sec, so it moves at most $30 \cdot 2 = 60$ feet. In the next two seconds it moves at most $38 \cdot 2 = 76$ feet, and so on. Therefore, over the ten-second period it moves at most

$$30 \cdot 2 + 38 \cdot 2 + 44 \cdot 2 + 48 \cdot 2 + 50 \cdot 2 = 420 \text{ feet.}$$

Therefore,

$$360 \text{ feet} \leq \text{Total distance traveled} \leq 420 \text{ feet.}$$

There is a difference of 60 feet between the upper and lower estimates.

Velocity Data Every One Second

What if we want a more accurate estimate? We could make more frequent velocity measurements, say every second. The data is in Table 5.2.

As before, we get a lower estimate for each second by using the velocity at the beginning of that second. During the first second the velocity is at least 20 ft/sec, so the car travels at least $20 \cdot 1 = 20$ feet. During the next second the car moves at least 26 feet, and so on. So we say

$$\begin{aligned} \text{New lower estimate} &= 20 \cdot 1 + 26 \cdot 1 + 30 \cdot 1 + 35 \cdot 1 + 38 \cdot 1 \\ &\quad + 42 \cdot 1 + 44 \cdot 1 + 46 \cdot 1 + 48 \cdot 1 + 49 \cdot 1 \\ &= 378 \text{ feet.} \end{aligned}$$

Notice that this is greater than the old lower estimate of 360 feet.

We get a new upper estimate by considering the velocity at the end of each second. During the first second the velocity is at most 26 ft/sec, and so the car moves at most $26 \cdot 1 = 26$ feet; in the next second it moves at most 30 feet, and so on.

$$\begin{aligned} \text{New upper estimate} &= 26 \cdot 1 + 30 \cdot 1 + 35 \cdot 1 + 38 \cdot 1 + 42 \cdot 1 \\ &\quad + 44 \cdot 1 + 46 \cdot 1 + 48 \cdot 1 + 49 \cdot 1 + 50 \cdot 1 \\ &= 408 \text{ feet.} \end{aligned}$$

This is less than the old upper estimate of 420 feet. Now we know that

$$378 \text{ feet} \leq \text{Total distance traveled} \leq 408 \text{ feet.}$$

Notice that the difference between the new upper and lower estimates is now 30 feet, half of what it was before. By halving the interval of measurement, we have halved the difference between the upper and lower estimates.

Table 5.2 *Velocity of car every second*

Time (sec)	0	1	2	3	4	5	6	7	8	9	10
Velocity (ft/sec)	20	26	30	35	38	42	44	46	48	49	50

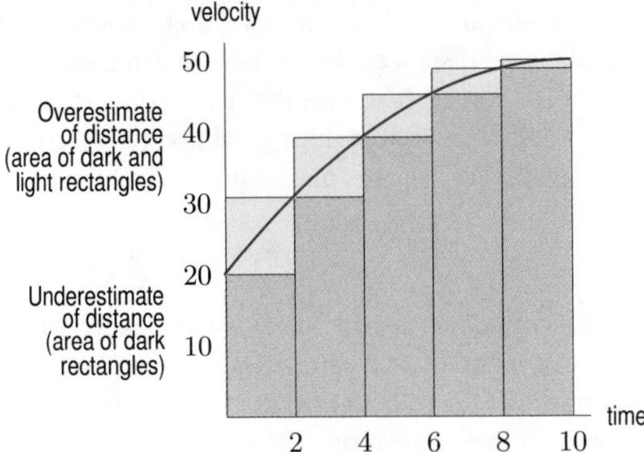

Figure 5.2: Shaded area estimates distance traveled. Velocity measured every 2 seconds

Visualizing Distance on the Velocity Graph

Consider the two-second data in Table 5.1. We can represent both upper and lower estimates on a graph of the velocity against time. The velocity can be graphed by plotting these data and drawing a smooth curve through the data points. (See Figure 5.2.)

We use the fact that for a rectangle, Area $=$ Height $\times$ Width. The area of the first dark rectangle is $20 \cdot 2 = 40$, the lower estimate of the distance moved during the first two seconds. The area of the second dark rectangle is $30 \cdot 2 = 60$, the lower estimate for the distance moved in the next two seconds. The total area of the dark rectangles represents the lower estimate for the total distance moved during the ten seconds.

If the dark and light rectangles are considered together, the first area is $30 \cdot 2 = 60$, the upper estimate for the distance moved in the first two seconds. The second area is $38 \cdot 2 = 76$, the upper estimate for the next two seconds. Continuing this calculation suggests that the upper estimate for the total distance is represented by the sum of the areas of the dark and light rectangles. Therefore, the area of the light rectangles alone represents the difference between the two estimates.

Figure 5.3 shows a graph of the one-second data. The area of the dark rectangles again represents the lower estimate, and the area of the dark and light rectangles together represents the upper estimate. The total area of the light rectangles is smaller in Figure 5.3 than in Figure 5.2, so the underestimate and overestimate are closer for the one-second data than for the two-second data.

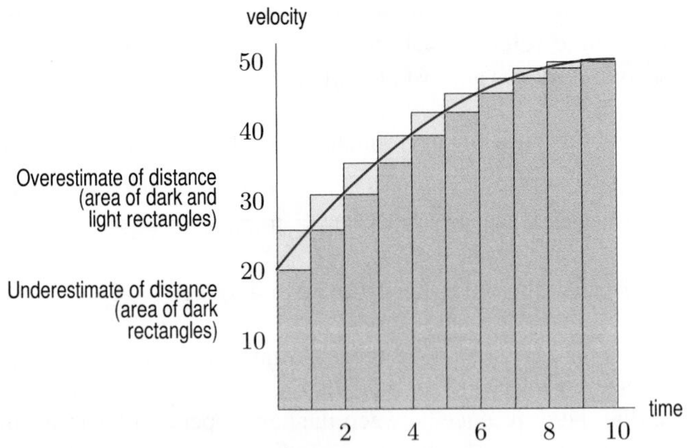

Figure 5.3: Shaded area estimates distance traveled. Velocity measured every second

Visualizing Distance on the Velocity Graph: Area Under Curve

As we make more frequent velocity measurements, the rectangles used to estimate the distance traveled fit the curve more closely. See Figures 5.4 and 5.5. In the limit, as the number of subdivisions increases, we see that the distance traveled is given by the area between the velocity curve and the horizontal axis. See Figure 5.6. In general:

> If the velocity is positive, the total distance traveled is the area under the velocity curve.

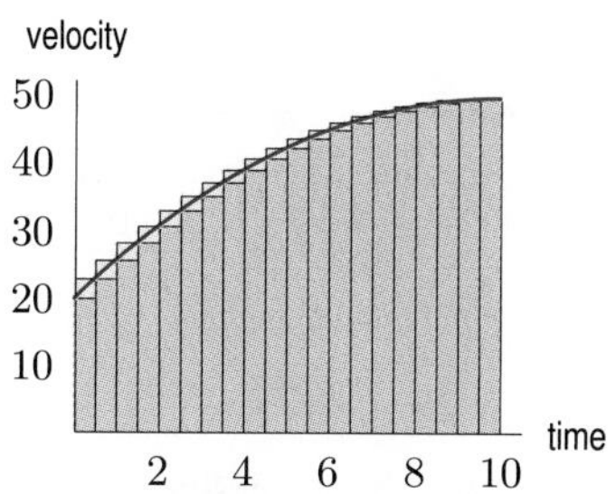

Figure 5.4: Velocity measured every 1/2 second

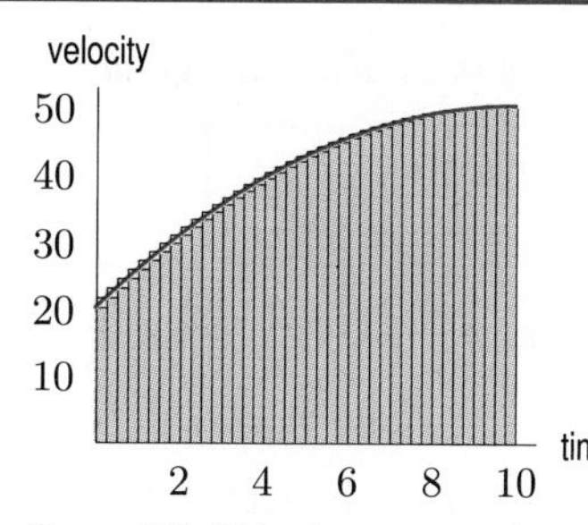

Figure 5.5: Velocity measured every 1/4 second

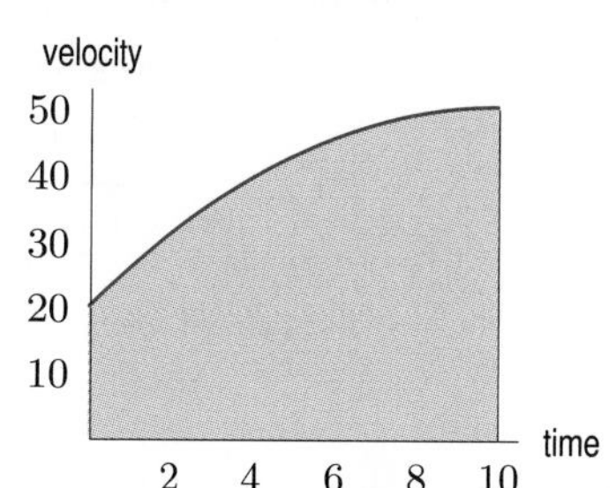

Figure 5.6: Distance traveled is area under curve

Example 2 With time t in seconds, the velocity of a bicycle, in feet per second, is given by $v(t) = 5t$. How far does the bicycle travel in 3 seconds?

Solution The velocity is linear. See Figure 5.7. The distance traveled is the area between the line $v(t) = 5t$ and the t-axis. Since this region is a triangle of height 15 and base 3

$$\text{Distance traveled} = \text{Area of triangle} = \frac{1}{2} \cdot 15 \cdot 3 = 22.5 \text{ feet.}$$

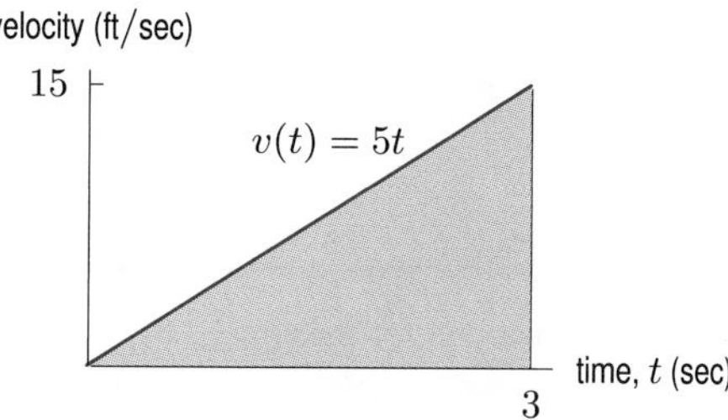

Figure 5.7: Shaded area represents distance traveled

Approximating Total Change from Rate of Change

We have seen how to use the rate of change of distance (the velocity) to calculate the total distance traveled. We can use the same method to find total change from rate of change of other quantities.

Example 3 A city's population grows at the rate of 5000 people/year for 3 years and then grows at the rate of 3000 people/year for the next 4 years. What is the total change in the population of the city during this 7-year period?

Solution The units of people/year remind us that we are given a rate of change of the population (people) with respect to time (years). If the rate of change is constant, we know that

$$\text{Total change in population} = \text{Rate of change per year} \times \text{Number of years.}$$

Thus, the total change in this population is

$$\begin{aligned} \text{Total change} &= (5000 \text{ people/year})(3 \text{ years}) + (3000 \text{ people/year})(4 \text{ years}) \\ &= 15{,}000 \text{ people} + 12{,}000 \text{ people} \\ &= 27{,}000 \text{ people.} \end{aligned}$$

The change in population is 27,000 people. Notice that this does not tell us the population of the city at the end of 7 years; it tells us the change in the population. For example, if the population were initially 100,000, it would be 127,000 at the end of the 7-year period.

Example 4 The rate of sales (in games per week) of a new video game is shown in Table 5.3. Assuming that the rate of sales increased throughout the 20-week period, estimate the total number of games sold during this period.

Table 5.3 *Weekly sales of a video game*

Time (weeks)	0	5	10	15	20
Rate of sales (games per week)	0	585	892	1875	2350

Solution If the rate of sales is constant, we have

$$\text{Total sales} = \text{Rate of sales per week} \times \text{Number of weeks}.$$

How many games were sold during the first five weeks? During this time, sales went from 0 to 585 games per week. If we assume that 585 games were sold every week, we get an overestimate for the sales in the first five weeks of (585 games/week)(5 weeks) $= 2925$ games. Similar overestimates for each of the five-week periods gives an overestimate for the entire 20-week period:

$$\text{Overestimate for total sales} = 585 \cdot 5 + 892 \cdot 5 + 1875 \cdot 5 + 2350 \cdot 5 = 28{,}510 \text{ games}.$$

We underestimate the total sales by taking the lower value for rate of sales during each of the five-week periods:

$$\text{Underestimate for total sales} = 0 \cdot 5 + 585 \cdot 5 + 892 \cdot 5 + 1875 \cdot 5 = 16{,}760 \text{ games}.$$

Thus, the total sales of the game during the 20-week period is between 16,760 and 28,510 games. A good single estimate of total sales is the average of these two numbers:

$$\text{Total sales} \approx \frac{16{,}760 + 28{,}510}{2} = 22{,}635 \text{ games}.$$

Problems for Section 5.1

1. **(a)** Sketch a graph of the velocity function for the trip described in Example 1 on page 234.
   (b) Represent the total distance traveled on this graph.

2. Graph the rate of sales against time for the video game data in Example 4. Represent graphically the overestimate and the underestimate calculated in that example.

3. A car comes to a stop six seconds after the driver applies the brakes. While the brakes are on, the velocities recorded are in Table 5.4.

Table 5.4

Time since brakes applied (sec)	0	2	4	6
Velocity (ft/sec)	88	45	16	0

   (a) Give lower and upper estimates for the distance the car traveled after the brakes were applied.
   (b) On a sketch of velocity against time, show the lower and upper estimates of part (a).

4. A car starts moving at time $t = 0$ and goes faster and faster. Its velocity is shown in the following table. Estimate how far the car travels during the 12 seconds.

t (seconds)	0	3	6	9	12
Velocity (ft/sec)	0	10	25	45	75

5. The velocity of a car is $f(t) = 5t$ meters/sec. Use a graph of $f(t)$ to find the exact distance traveled by the car, in meters, from $t = 0$ to $t = 10$ seconds.

6. Figure 5.8 shows the velocity, v, of an object (in meters/sec). Estimate the total distance the object traveled between $t = 0$ and $t = 6$.

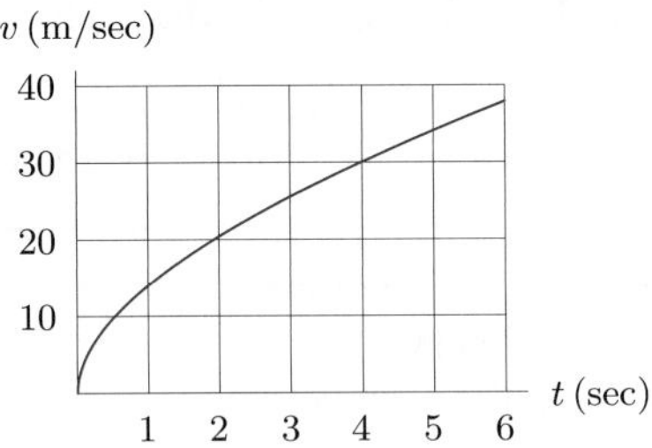

Figure 5.8

7. A car accelerates smoothly from 0 to 60 mph in 10 seconds with the velocity given in Figure 5.9. Estimate how far the car travels during the 10-second period.

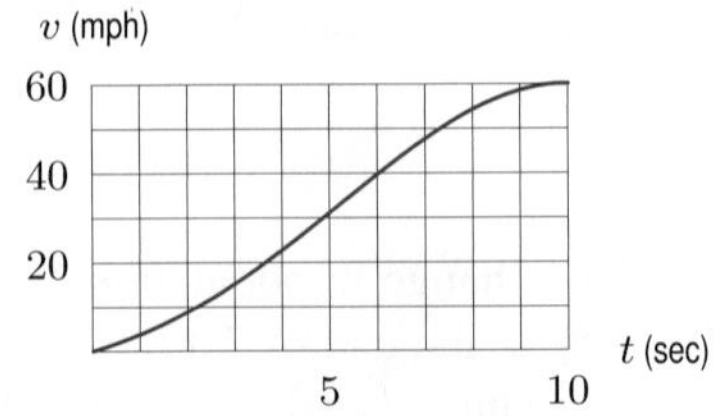

Figure 5.9

8. The following table gives world oil consumption, in billions of barrels per year.[1] Estimate total oil consumption during this 25-year period.

Year	1980	1985	1990	1995	2000	2005
Oil (bn barrels/yr)	22.3	21.3	23.9	24.9	27.0	29.3

9. Filters at a water treatment plant become less effective over time. The rate at which pollution passes through the filters into a nearby lake is given in the following table.

(a) Estimate the total quantity of pollution entering the lake during the 30-day period.
(b) Your answer to part (a) is only an estimate. Give bounds (lower and upper estimates) between which the true quantity of pollution must lie. (Assume the rate of pollution is continually increasing.)

Day	0	6	12	18	24	30
Rate (kg/day)	7	8	10	13	18	35

10. The rate of change of the world's population, in millions of people per year, is given in the following table.

(a) Use this data to estimate the total change in the world's population between 1950 and 2000.
(b) The world population was 2555 million people in 1950 and 6085 million people in 2000. Calculate the true value of the total change in the population. How does this compare with your estimate in part (a)?

Year	1950	1960	1970	1980	1990	2000
Rate of change	37	41	78	77	86	79

11. A village wishes to measure the quantity of water that is piped to a factory during a typical morning. A gauge on the water line gives the flow rate (in cubic meters per hour) at any instant. The flow rate is about 100 m^3/hr at 6 am and increases steadily to about 280 m^3/hr at 9 am. Using only this information, give your best estimate of the total volume of water used by the factory between 6 am and 9 am.

12. Roger runs a marathon. His friend Jeff rides behind him on a bicycle and clocks his speed every 15 minutes. Roger starts out strong, but after an hour and a half he is so exhausted that he has to stop. Jeff's data follow:

Time since start (min)	0	15	30	45	60	75	90
Speed (mph)	12	11	10	10	8	7	0

(a) Assuming that Roger's speed is never increasing, give upper and lower estimates for the distance Roger ran during the first half hour.
(b) Give upper and lower estimates for the distance Roger ran in total during the entire hour and a half.

13. A car initially going 50 ft/sec brakes at a constant rate (constant negative acceleration), coming to a stop in 5 seconds.

(a) Graph the velocity from $t = 0$ to $t = 5$.
(b) How far does the car travel?
(c) How far does the car travel if its initial velocity is doubled, but it brakes at the same constant rate?

14. Figure 5.10 shows the rate of change of a fish population. Estimate the total change in the population during this 12-month period.

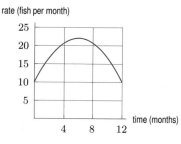

Figure 5.10

15. Two cars start at the same time and travel in the same direction along a straight road. Figure 5.11 gives the velocity, v, of each car as a function of time, t. Which car:

(a) Attains the larger maximum velocity?
(b) Stops first?
(c) Travels farther?

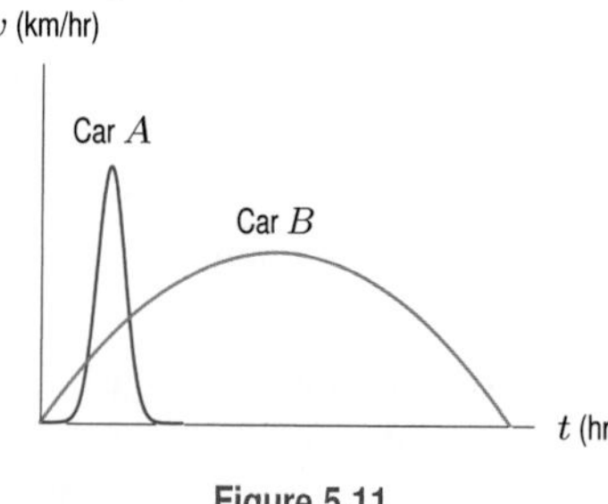

Figure 5.11

[1] www.bp.com/centres/energy/world_stat_rev/oil/reserves.asp. and https://www.cia.gov/library/publications/the-world-factbook/print/xx.html.

16. Two cars travel in the same direction along a straight road. Figure 5.12 shows the velocity, v, of each car at time t. Car B starts 2 hours after car A and car B reaches a maximum velocity of 50 km/hr.

(a) For approximately how long does each car travel?
(b) Estimate car A's maximum velocity.
(c) Approximately how far does each car travel?

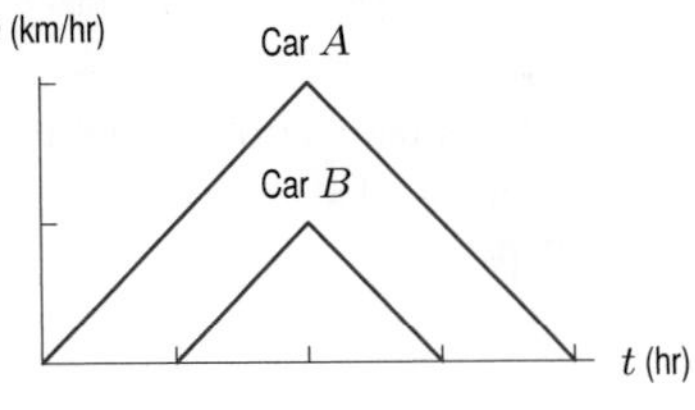

Figure 5.12

17. Your velocity is given by $v(t) = t^2 + 1$ in m/sec, with t in seconds. Estimate the distance, s, traveled between $t = 0$ and $t = 5$. Explain how you arrived at your estimate.

18. An old rowboat has sprung a leak. Water is flowing into the boat at a rate, $r(t)$, given in the following table.

t minutes	0	5	10	15
$r(t)$ liters/min	12	20	24	16

(a) Compute upper and lower estimates for the volume of water that has flowed into the boat during the 15 minutes.
(b) Draw a graph to illustrate the lower estimate.

19. The value of a mutual fund increases at a rate of $R = 500e^{0.04t}$ dollars per year, with t in years since 2010.

(a) Using $t = 0, 2, 4, 6, 8, 10$, make a table of values for R.
(b) Use the table to estimate the total change in the value of the mutual fund between 2010 and 2020.

20. A car speeds up at a constant rate from 10 to 70 mph over a period of half an hour. Its fuel efficiency (in miles per gallon) increases with speed; values are in the table. Make lower and upper estimates of the quantity of fuel used during the half hour.

Speed (mph)	10	20	30	40	50	60	70
Fuel efficiency (mpg)	15	18	21	23	24	25	26

5.2 THE DEFINITE INTEGRAL

In Section 5.1 we saw how to approximate total change given the rate of change. We now see how to make the approximation more accurate.

Improving the Approximation: The Role of n and Δt

To approximate total change, we construct a sum. We use the notation Δt for the size of the t-intervals used. We use n to represent the number of subintervals of length Δt. In the following example, we see how decreasing Δt (and increasing n) improves the accuracy of the approximation.

Example 1 If t is in hours since the start of a 20-hour period, a bacteria population increases at a rate given by

$$f(t) = 3 + 0.1t^2 \text{ millions of bacteria per hour.}$$

Make an underestimate of the total change in the number of bacteria over this period using

(a) $\Delta t = 4$ hours (b) $\Delta t = 2$ hours (c) $\Delta t = 1$ hour

Solution (a) The rate of change is $f(t) = 3 + 0.1t^2$. If we use $\Delta t = 4$, we measure the rate every 4 hours and $n = 20/4 = 5$. See Table 5.5. An underestimate for the population change during the first 4 hours is $(3.0 \text{ million/hour})(4 \text{ hours}) = 12$ million. Combining the contributions from all the subintervals gives the underestimate:

$$\text{Total change} \approx 3.0 \cdot 4 + 4.6 \cdot 4 + 9.4 \cdot 4 + 17.4 \cdot 4 + 28.6 \cdot 4 = 252.0 \text{ million bacteria.}$$

The rate of change is graphed in Figure 5.13 (a); the area of the shaded rectangles represents this underestimate. Notice that $n = 5$ is the number of rectangles in the graph.

Table 5.5 *Rate of change with $\Delta t = 4$ using $f(t) = 3 + 0.1t^2$ million bacteria/hour*

t (hours)	0	4	8	12	16	20
$f(t)$	3.0	4.6	9.4	17.4	28.6	43.0

(b) If we use $\Delta t = 2$, we measure $f(t)$ every 2 hours and $n = 20/2 = 10$. See Table 5.6. The underestimate is

$$\text{Total change} \approx 3.0 \cdot 2 + 3.4 \cdot 2 + 4.6 \cdot 2 + \cdots + 35.4 \cdot 2 = 288.0 \text{ million bacteria.}$$

Figure 5.13 (b) suggests that this estimate is more accurate than the estimate made in part (a).

Table 5.6 *Rate of change with $\Delta t = 2$ using $f(t) = 3 + 0.1t^2$ million bacteria/hour*

t (hours)	0	2	4	6	8	10	12	14	16	18	20
$f(t)$	3.0	3.4	4.6	6.6	9.4	13.0	17.4	22.6	28.6	35.4	43.0

(c) If we use $\Delta t = 1$, then $n = 20$ and a similar calculation shows that we have

$$\text{Total change} \approx 307.0 \text{ million bacteria.}$$

The shaded area in Figure 5.13 (c) represents this estimate; it is the most accurate of the three.

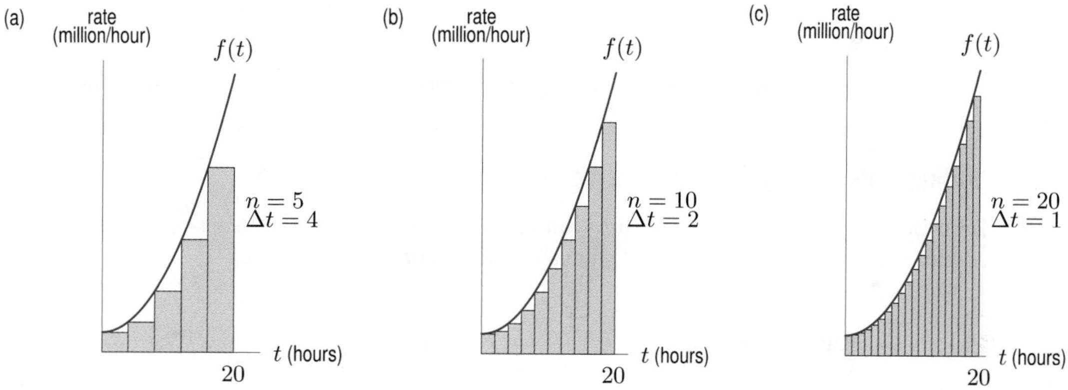

Figure 5.13: More and more accurate estimates of total change from rate of change. In each case, $f(t)$ is the rate of change, and the shaded area approximates total change. Largest n and smallest Δt give the best estimate.

Notice that as n gets larger, the estimate improves and the area of the shaded rectangles approaches the area under the curve.

Left- and Right-Hand Sums

Suppose we have a function $f(t)$ that is continuous for $a \leq t \leq b$. We divide the interval from a to b into n equal subdivisions, each of width Δt, so

$$\Delta t = \frac{b-a}{n}.$$

We let $t_0, t_1, t_2, \ldots, t_n$ be endpoints of the subdivisions, as in Figures 5.14 and 5.15. We construct two sums, similar to the overestimates and underestimates in Section 3.1. For a *left-hand sum*, we use the values of the function from the left end of the interval. For a *right-hand sum*, we use the values of the function from the right end of the interval. We have:

$$\text{Left-hand sum} = f(t_0)\Delta t + f(t_1)\Delta t + \cdots + f(t_{n-1})\Delta t$$

and

$$\text{Right-hand sum} = f(t_1)\Delta t + f(t_2)\Delta t + \cdots + f(t_n)\Delta t.$$

These sums represent the shaded areas in Figures 5.14 and 5.15, provided $f(t) \geq 0$. In Figure 5.14, the first rectangle has width Δt and height $f(t_0)$, since the top of its left edge just touches the curve, and hence it has area $f(t_0)\Delta t$. The second rectangle has width Δt and height $f(t_1)$, and hence has area $f(t_1)\Delta t$, and so on. The sum of all these areas is the left-hand sum. The right-hand sum, shown in Figure 5.15, is constructed in the same way, except that each rectangle touches the curve on its right edge instead of its left.

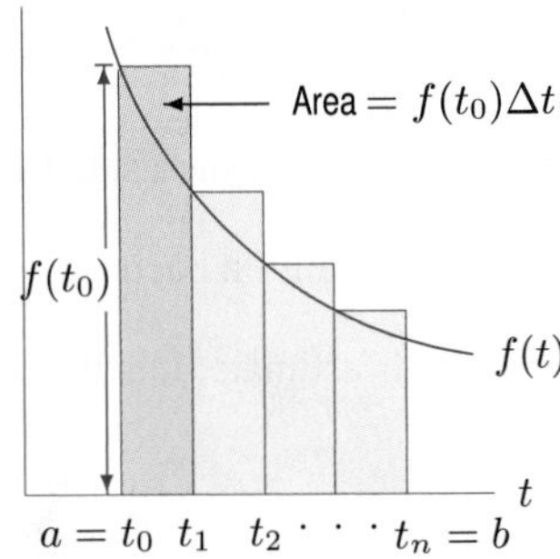

Figure 5.14: Left-hand sum: Area of rectangles

Area = $f(t_1)\Delta t$
$f(t_1)$
$f(t)$
t
$a = t_0$ t_1 t_2 $\cdots$ $t_n = b$

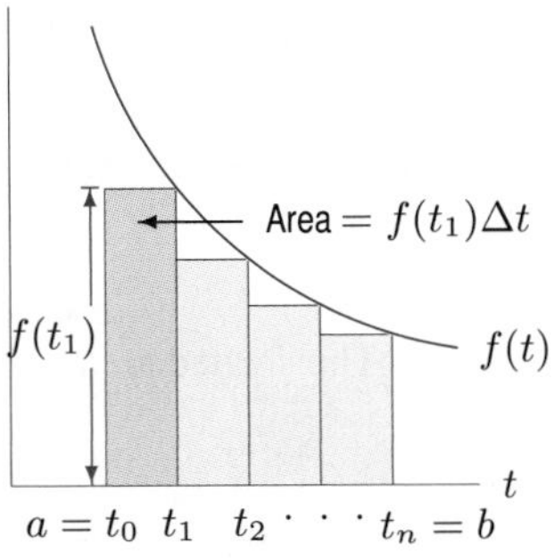

Figure 5.15: Right-hand sum: Area of rectangles

Writing Left- and Right-Hand Sums Using Sigma Notation

Both the left-hand and right-hand sums can be written more compactly using *sigma*, or summation, notation. The symbol $\sum$ is a capital sigma, or Greek letter "S." We write

$$\text{Right-hand sum} = \sum_{i=1}^{n} f(t_i)\Delta t = f(t_1)\Delta t + f(t_2)\Delta t + \cdots + f(t_n)\Delta t.$$

The $\sum$ tells us to add terms of the form $f(t_i)\Delta t$. The "$i = 1$" at the base of the sigma sign tells us to start at $i = 1$, and the "n" at the top tells us to stop at $i = n$.

In the left-hand sum we start at $i = 0$ and stop at $i = n - 1$, so we write

$$\text{Left-hand sum} = \sum_{i=0}^{n-1} f(t_i)\Delta t = f(t_0)\Delta t + f(t_1)\Delta t + \cdots + f(t_{n-1})\Delta t.$$

Taking the Limit to Obtain the Definite Integral

If f is a rate of change of some quantity, then the left-hand sum and the right-hand sum approximate the total change in the quantity. For most functions f, the approximation is improved by increasing the value of n. To find the total change exactly, we take larger and larger values of n and look at the values approached by the left and right sums. This is called taking the *limit* of these sums as n goes to infinity and is written $\lim_{n\to\infty}$. If f is continuous for $a \leq t \leq b$, the limits of the left- and right-hand sums exist and are equal. The *definite integral* is the common limit of these sums.

Suppose f is continuous for $a \leq t \leq b$. The **definite integral** of f from a to b, written

$$\int_a^b f(t)\,dt,$$

is the limit of the left-hand or right-hand sums with n subdivisions of $[a,b]$ as n gets arbitrarily large. In other words, if $t_0, t_1, \ldots t_n$ are the endpoints of the subdivisions,

$$\int_a^b f(t)\,dt = \lim_{n\to\infty}(\text{Left-hand sum}) = \lim_{n\to\infty}\left(\sum_{i=0}^{n-1} f(t_i)\Delta t\right)$$

and

$$\int_a^b f(t)\,dt = \lim_{n\to\infty}(\text{Right-hand sum}) = \lim_{n\to\infty}\left(\sum_{i=1}^{n} f(t_i)\Delta t\right).$$

Each of these sums is called a *Riemann sum*, f is called the *integrand*, and a and b are called the *limits of integration*.

The "$\int$" notation comes from an old-fashioned "S," which stands for "sum" in the same way that $\sum$ does. The "dt" in the integral comes from the factor Δt. Notice that the limits on the $\sum$ symbol are 0 and $n-1$ for the left-hand sum, and 1 and n for the right-hand sum, whereas the limits on the $\int$ sign are a and b.

When $f(t)$ is positive, the left- and right-hand sums are represented by the sums of areas of rectangles, so the definite integral is represented graphically by an area.

Computing a Definite Integral

In practice, we often approximate definite integrals numerically using a calculator or computer. They compute sums for larger and larger values of n, and eventually give a value for the integral. Different calculators and computers may give slightly different estimates, owing to round-off error and the fact that they may use different approximation methods.

Example 2 Compute $\int_1^3 t^2\,dt$ and represent this integral as an area.

Solution Using a calculator, we find

$$\int_1^3 t^2\,dt = 8.667.$$

The integral represents the area between $t=1$ and $t=3$ under the curve $f(t)=t^2$. See Figure 5.16.

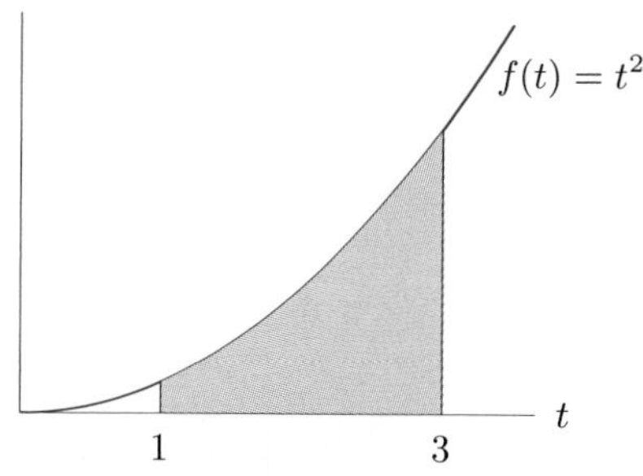

Figure 5.16: Shaded area $= \int_1^3 t^2\,dt$

Estimating a Definite Integral from a Table or Graph

If we have a formula for the integrand, $f(x)$, we can calculate the integral $\int_a^b f(x)\,dx$ using a calculator or computer. If, however, we have only a table of values or a graph of $f(x)$, we can still estimate the integral.

Example 3 Values for a function $f(t)$ are in the following table. Estimate $\displaystyle\int_{20}^{30} f(t)dt$.

t	20	22	24	26	28	30
$f(t)$	5	7	11	18	29	45

Solution Since we have only a table of values, we use left- and right-hand sums to approximate the integral. The values of $f(t)$ are spaced 2 units apart, so $\Delta t = 2$ and $n = (30-20)/2 = 5$. Calculating the left-hand and right-hand sums gives

$$\begin{aligned}\text{Left-hand sum} &= f(20)\cdot 2 + f(22)\cdot 2 + f(24)\cdot 2 + f(26)\cdot 2 + f(28)\cdot 2\\ &= 5\cdot 2 + 7\cdot 2 + 11\cdot 2 + 18\cdot 2 + 29\cdot 2\\ &= 10 + 14 + 22 + 36 + 58\\ &= 140.\end{aligned}$$

$$\begin{aligned}\text{Right-hand sum} &= f(22)\cdot 2 + f(24)\cdot 2 + f(26)\cdot 2 + f(28)\cdot 2 + f(30)\cdot 2\\ &= 7\cdot 2 + 11\cdot 2 + 18\cdot 2 + 29\cdot 2 + 45\cdot 2\\ &= 14 + 22 + 36 + 58 + 90\\ &= 220.\end{aligned}$$

Both left- and right-hand sums approximate the integral. We generally get a better estimate by averaging the two:

$$\int_{20}^{30} f(t)dt \approx \frac{140+220}{2} = 180.$$

Example 4 The function $f(x)$ is graphed in Figure 5.17. Estimate $\displaystyle\int_0^6 f(x)\,dx$.

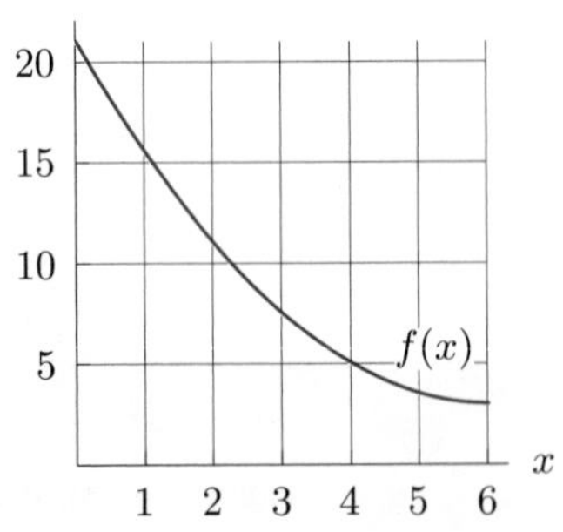

Figure 5.17: Estimate $\int_0^6 f(x)\,dx$

Solution

We approximate the integral using left- and right-hand sums with $n = 3$, so $\Delta x = 2$. Figures 5.18 and 5.19 give

$$\text{Left-hand sum} = f(0) \cdot 2 + f(2) \cdot 2 + f(4) \cdot 2 = 21 \cdot 2 + 11 \cdot 2 + 5 \cdot 2 = 74,$$
$$\text{Right-hand sum} = f(2) \cdot 2 + f(4) \cdot 2 + f(6) \cdot 2 = 11 \cdot 2 + 5 \cdot 2 + 3 \cdot 2 = 38.$$

We estimate the integral by taking the average:

$$\int_0^6 f(x)\, dx \approx \frac{74 + 38}{2} = 56.$$

Alternatively, since the integral equals the area under the curve between $x = 0$ and $x = 6$, we can estimate it by counting grid squares. Each grid square has area $5 \cdot 1 = 5$, and the region under $f(x)$ includes about 10.5 grid squares, so the area is about $10.5 \cdot 5 = 52.5$.

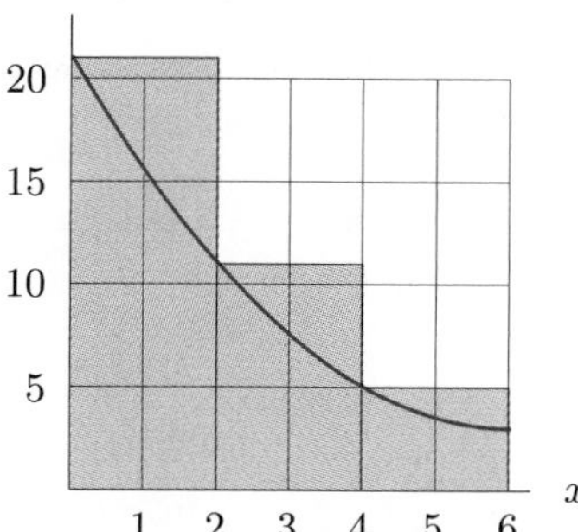

Figure 5.18: Area of shaded region is left-hand sum with $n = 3$

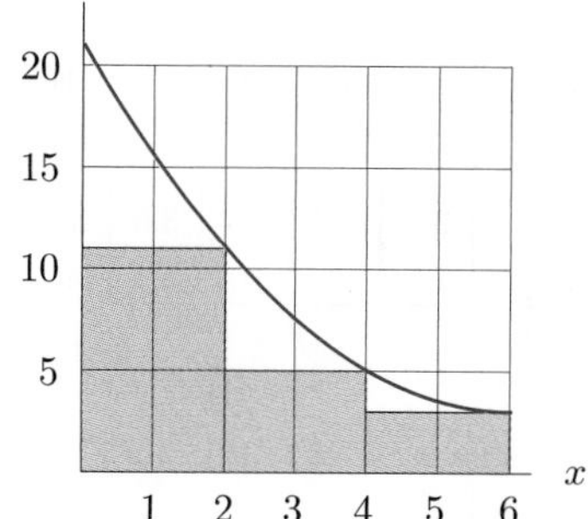

Figure 5.19: Area of shaded region is right-hand sum with $n = 3$

Rough Estimates of a Definite Integral

When calculating an integral using a calculator or computer, it is useful to have a rough idea of the value you expect. This helps detect errors in entering the integral.

Example 5 Three people calculated $\displaystyle\int_1^3 \frac{1}{t}\, dt$ on a calculator and got values 0.023, 11.984, and 1.526. Explain how you can be sure that none of these values is correct.

Solution

Figure 5.20 shows left- and right-hand approximations to $\int_1^3 \frac{1}{t}\, dt$ with $n = 1$. We see that the right-hand sum $2(1/3)$ is an underestimate of $\int_1^3 \frac{1}{t}\, dt$. Since 0.023 is less than $2/3$, this value must be wrong. Similarly, we see that the left-hand sum $2(1)$ is an overestimate of the integral. Since 11.984 is larger than 2, this value is wrong. Since the graph is concave up, the value of the integral is closer to the smaller value of the two sums, $2/3$, than to the larger value, 2. Thus, the integral is less than the average of the two sums, $4/3$. Since $1.526 > 4/3$, this value is wrong too.

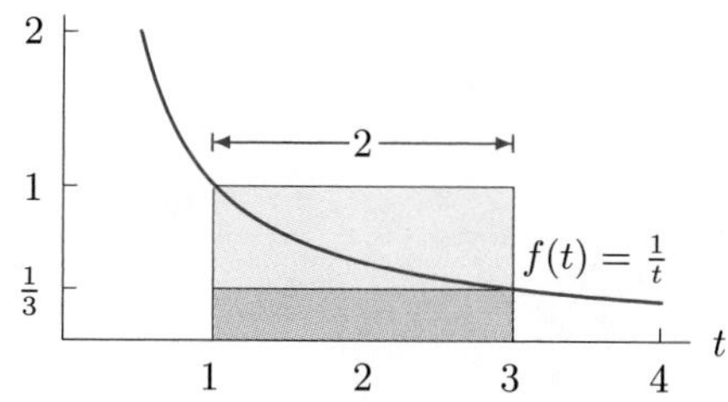

Figure 5.20: Left- and right-hand sums with $n = 1$

Problems for Section 5.2

1. Estimate $\displaystyle\int_0^6 2^x\,dx$ using a left-hand sum with $n = 2$.

2. Estimate $\displaystyle\int_0^{12} \frac{1}{x+1}\,dx$ using a left-hand sum with $n = 3$.

3. Use the following table to estimate $\int_0^{25} f(x)dx$.

x	0	5	10	15	20	25
$f(x)$	100	82	69	60	53	49

4. Use the following table to estimate $\int_3^4 W(t)\,dt$. What are n and Δt?

t	3.0	3.2	3.4	3.6	3.8	4.0
$W(t)$	25	23	20	15	9	2

5. Use the following table to estimate $\int_0^{15} f(x)\,dx$.

x	0	3	6	9	12	15
$f(x)$	50	48	44	36	24	8

6. Use the table to estimate $\int_0^{40} f(x)dx$. What values of n and Δx did you use?

x	0	10	20	30	40
$f(x)$	350	410	435	450	460

7. Using Figure 5.21, draw rectangles representing each of the following Riemann sums for the function f on the interval $0 \le t \le 8$. Calculate the value of each sum.

(a) Left-hand sum with $\Delta t = 4$
(b) Right-hand sum with $\Delta t = 4$
(c) Left-hand sum with $\Delta t = 2$
(d) Right-hand sum with $\Delta t = 2$

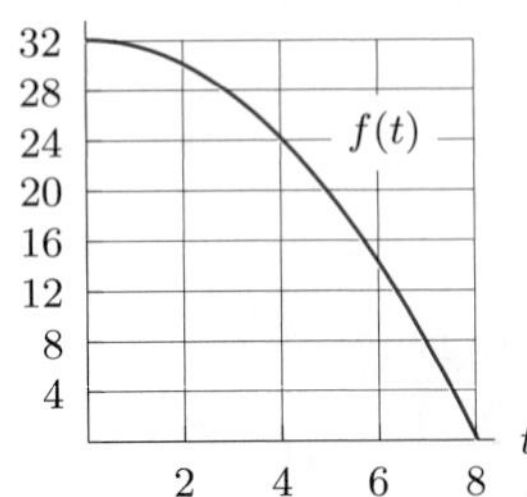

Figure 5.21

8. Use Figure 5.22 to estimate $\int_0^{20} f(x)\,dx$.

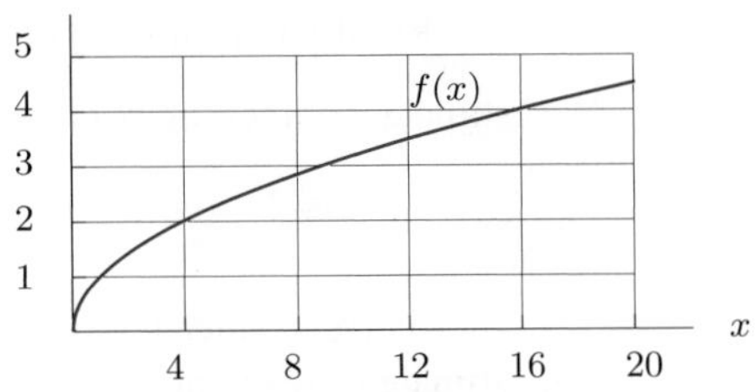

Figure 5.22

9. Use Figure 5.23 to estimate $\int_{-10}^{15} f(x)dx$.

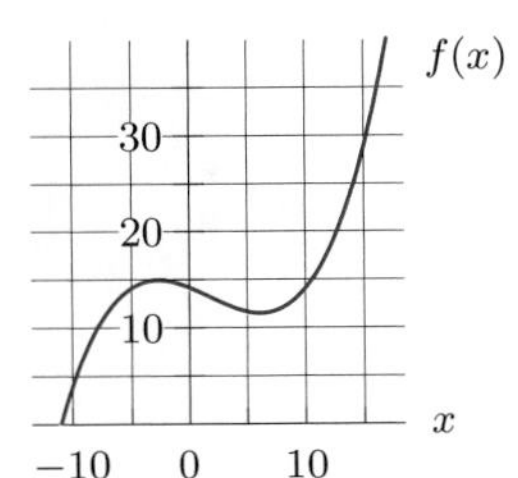

Figure 5.23

Use the graphs in Problems 10–11 to estimate $\int_0^3 f(x)\,dx$.

10.

11.

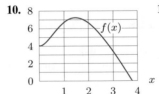

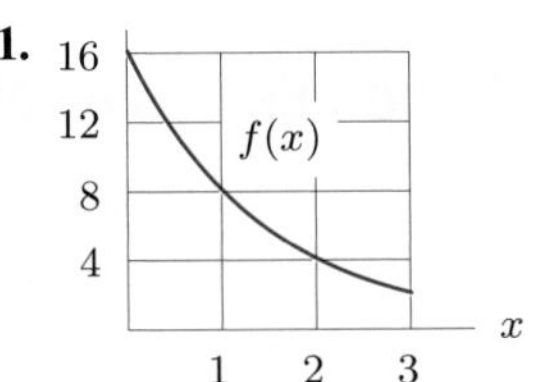

For Problems 12–15:

(a) Use a graph of the integrand to make a rough estimate of the integral. Explain your reasoning.

(b) Use a computer or calculator to find the value of the definite integral.

12. $\displaystyle\int_0^1 x^3\,dx$

13. $\displaystyle\int_0^3 \sqrt{x}\,dx$

14. $\displaystyle\int_0^1 3^t\,dt$

15. $\displaystyle\int_1^2 x^x\,dx$

16. The rate of change of a quantity is given by $f(t) = t^2+1$. Make an underestimate and an overestimate of the total change in the quantity between $t = 0$ and $t = 8$ using

(a) $\Delta t = 4$ **(b)** $\Delta t = 2$ **(c)** $\Delta t = 1$

What is n in each case? Graph $f(t)$ and shade rectangles to represent each of your six answers.

17. **(a)** Use a calculator or computer to find $\int_0^6 (x^2+1)\,dx$. Represent this value as the area under a curve.

(b) Estimate $\int_0^6 (x^2+1)\,dx$ using a left-hand sum with $n = 3$. Represent this sum graphically on a sketch of $f(x) = x^2 + 1$. Is this sum an overestimate or underestimate of the true value found in part (a)?

(c) Estimate $\int_0^6 (x^2+1)\,dx$ using a right-hand sum with $n = 3$. Represent this sum on your sketch. Is this sum an overestimate or underestimate?

18. Using Figure 5.24, find the value of $\int_1^6 f(x)\,dx$.

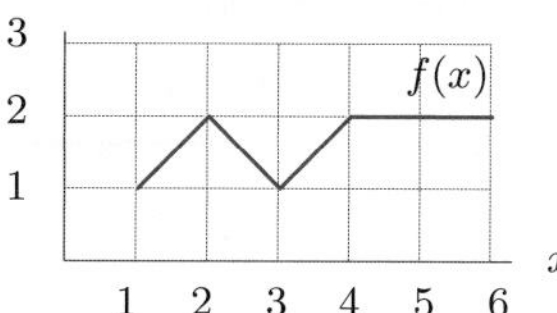

Figure 5.24

19. The graph of a function $f(t)$ is given in Figure 5.25. Which of the following four numbers could be an estimate of $\int_0^1 f(t)dt$ accurate to two decimal places? Explain how you chose your answer.

(a) -98.35 **(b)** 71.84
(c) 100.12 **(d)** 93.47

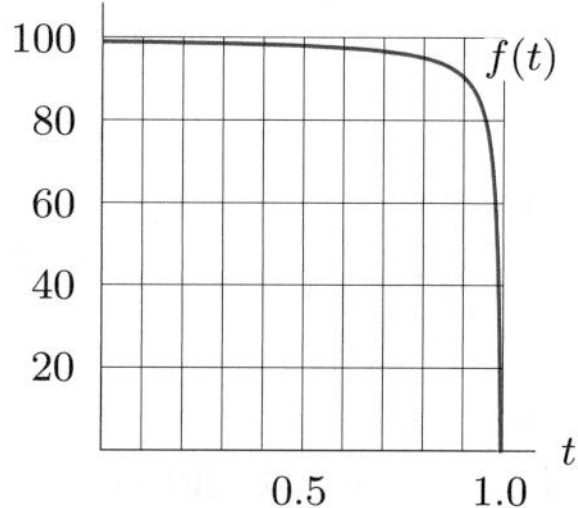

Figure 5.25

In Problems 20–29, use a calculator or computer to evaluate the integral.

20. $\displaystyle\int_0^5 x^2\,dx$

21. $\displaystyle\int_1^5 (3x+1)^2\,dx$

22. $\displaystyle\int_1^4 \frac{1}{\sqrt{1+x^2}}\,dx$

23. $\displaystyle\int_{-1}^1 \frac{1}{e^t}\,dt$

24. $\displaystyle\int_{1.1}^{1.7} 10(0.85)^t\,dt$

25. $\displaystyle\int_1^2 2^x\,dx$

26. $\displaystyle\int_1^2 (1.03)^t\,dt$

27. $\displaystyle\int_1^3 \ln x\,dx$

28. $\displaystyle\int_{1.1}^{1.7} e^t \ln t\,dt$

29. $\displaystyle\int_{-3}^3 e^{-t^2}\,dt$

30. Use the expressions for left and right sums on page 242 and Table 5.7.

(a) If $n = 4$, what is Δt? What are t_0, t_1, t_2, t_3, t_4? What are $f(t_0), f(t_1), f(t_2), f(t_3), f(t_4)$?

(b) Find the left and right sums using $n = 4$.

(c) If $n = 2$, what is Δt? What are t_0, t_1, t_2? What are $f(t_0), f(t_1), f(t_2)$?

(d) Find the left and right sums using $n = 2$.

Table 5.7

t	15	17	19	21	23
$f(t)$	10	13	18	20	30

31. Use the expressions for left and right sums on page 242 and Table 5.8.

(a) If $n = 4$, what is Δt? What are t_0, t_1, t_2, t_3, t_4? What are $f(t_0), f(t_1), f(t_2), f(t_3), f(t_4)$?

(b) Find the left and right sums using $n = 4$.

(c) If $n = 2$, what is Δt? What are t_0, t_1, t_2? What are $f(t_0), f(t_1), f(t_2)$?

(d) Find the left and right sums using $n = 2$.

Table 5.8

t	0	4	8	12	16
$f(t)$	25	23	22	20	17

5.3 THE DEFINITE INTEGRAL AS AREA

The Definite Integral as an Area: When $f(x)$ is Positive

If $f(x)$ is continuous and positive, each term $f(x_0)\Delta x, f(x_1)\Delta x, \ldots$ in a left- or right-hand Riemann sum represents the area of a rectangle. See Figure 5.26. As the width Δx of the rectangles approaches zero, the rectangles fit the curve of the graph more exactly, and the sum of their areas gets closer to the area under the curve shaded in Figure 5.27. In other words:

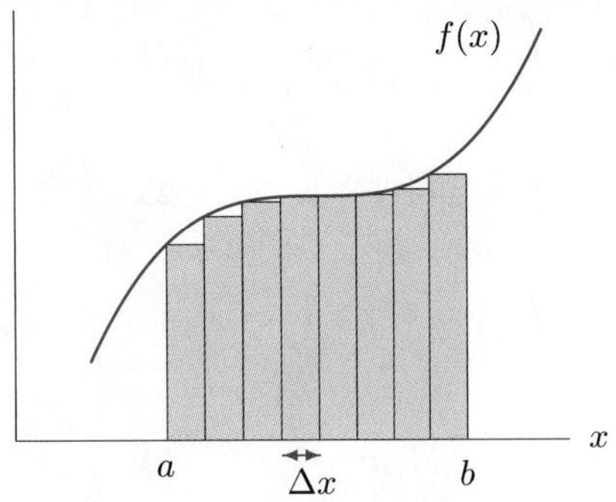

Figure 5.26: Area of rectangles approximating the area under the curve

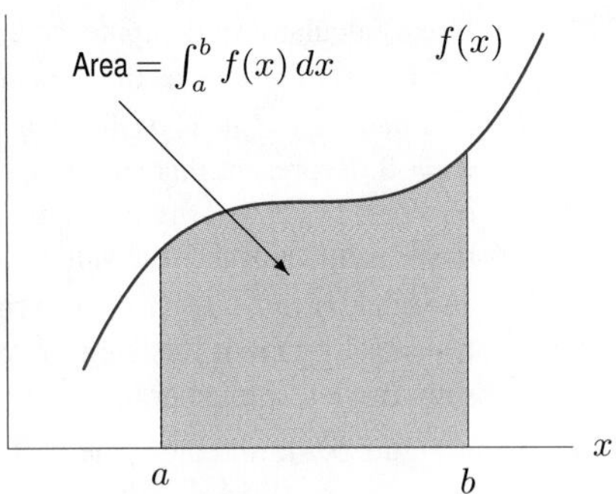

Figure 5.27: Shaded area is the definite integral $\int_a^b f(x)\,dx$

When $f(x)$ is positive and $a < b$:

$$\begin{array}{c}\text{Area under graph of } f \\ \text{between } a \text{ and } b\end{array} = \int_a^b f(x)\,dx.$$

Example 1 Find the area under the graph of $y = 10x(3^{-x})$ between $x = 0$ and $x = 3$.

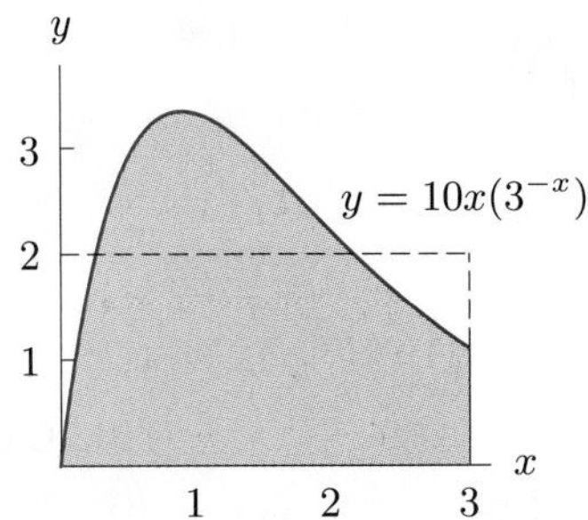

Figure 5.28: Area shaded $= \int_0^3 10x(3^{-x})\,dx$

Solution The area we want is shaded in Figure 5.28. A rough estimate of this area is 6, since it has about the same area as a rectangle of width 3 and height 2. To find the area more accurately, we say

$$\text{Area shaded} = \int_0^3 10x(3^{-x})dx.$$

Using a calculator or computer to evaluate the integral, we obtain

$$\text{Area shaded} = \int_0^3 10x(3^{-x})\,dx = 6.967 \approx 7 \text{ square units.}$$

Relationship Between Definite Integral and Area: When $f(x)$ is Not Positive

We assumed in drawing Figure 5.27 that the graph of $f(x)$ lies above the x-axis. If the graph lies below the x-axis, then each value of $f(x)$ is negative, so each $f(x)\Delta x$ is negative, and the area gets counted negatively. In that case, the definite integral is the negative of the area between the graph of f and the horizontal axis.

Example 2 What is the relation between the definite integral $\int_{-1}^{1} (x^2 - 1)\,dx$ and the area between the parabola $y = x^2 - 1$ and the x-axis?

Solution The parabola lies below the x-axis between $x = -1$ and $x = 1$. (See Figure 5.29.) So,

$$\int_{-1}^{1} (x^2 - 1)\, dx = -\text{Area} = -1.33.$$

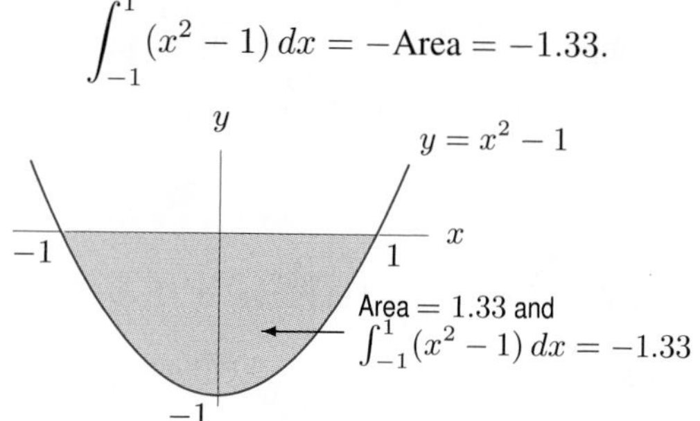

Figure 5.29: Integral $\int_{-1}^{1}(x^2 - 1)\, dx$ is negative of shaded area

Summarizing, assuming $f(x)$ is continuous, we have:

> **When $f(x)$ is positive for some x-values and negative for others**, and $a < b$:
> $\int_a^b f(x)\, dx$ is the sum of the areas above the x-axis, counted positively, and the areas below the x-axis, counted negatively.

In the following example, we break up the integral. The properties that allow us to do this are discussed in the Focus on Theory section at the end of this chapter.

Example 3 Interpret the definite integral $\displaystyle\int_0^4 (x^3 - 7x^2 + 11x)\, dx$ in terms of areas.

Solution Figure 5.30 shows the graph of $f(x) = x^3 - 7x^2 + 11x$ crossing below the x-axis at about $x = 2.38$. The integral is the area above the x-axis, A_1, minus the area below the x-axis, A_2. Computing the integral with a calculator or computer shows

$$\int_0^4 (x^3 - 7x^2 + 11x)\, dx = 2.67.$$

Breaking the integral into two parts and calculating each one separately gives

$$\int_0^{2.38} (x^3 - 7x^2 + 11x)\, dx = 7.72 \quad \text{and} \quad \int_{2.38}^{4} (x^3 - 7x^2 + 11x)\, dx = -5.05,$$

so $A_1 = 7.72$ and $A_2 = 5.05$. Then, as we would expect,

$$\int_0^4 (x^3 - 7x^2 + 11x)\, dx = A_1 - A_2 = 7.72 - 5.05 = 2.67.$$

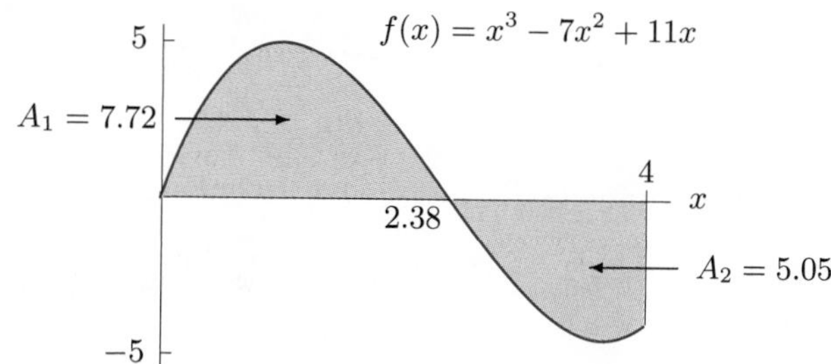

Figure 5.30: Integral $\int_0^4 (x^3 - 7x^2 + 11x)\, dx = A_1 - A_2$

Example 4 Find the total area of the shaded regions in Figure 5.30.

Solution We saw in Example 3 that $A_1 = 7.72$ and $A_2 = 5.05$. Thus we have

$$\text{Total shaded area } = A_1 + A_2 = 7.72 + 5.05 = 12.77.$$

Example 5 For each of the functions graphed in Figure 5.31, decide whether $\int_0^5 f(x)\,dx$ is positive, negative or approximately zero.

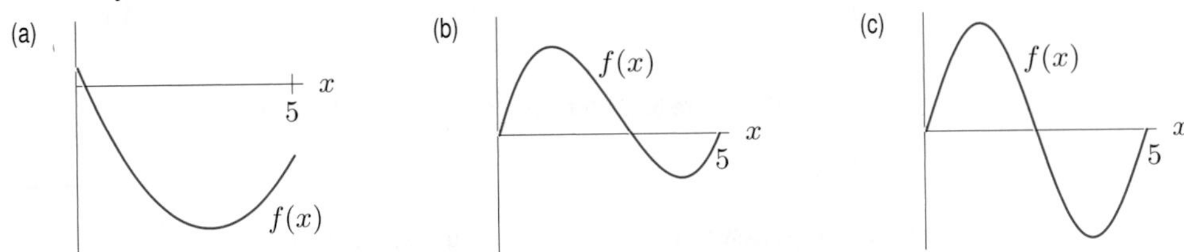

Figure 5.31: Is $\int_0^5 f(x)dx$ positive, negative or zero?

Solution

(a) The graph lies almost entirely below the x-axis, so the integral is negative.
(b) The graph lies partly below the x-axis and partly above the x-axis. However, the area above the x-axis is larger than the area below the x-axis, so the integral is positive.
(c) The graph lies partly below the x-axis and partly above the x-axis. Since the areas above and below the x-axis appear to be approximately equal in size, the integral is approximately zero.

Area Between Two Curves

We can use rectangles to approximate the area between two curves. If $g(x) \leq f(x)$, as in Figure 5.32, the height of a rectangle is $f(x) - g(x)$. The area of the rectangle is $(f(x) - g(x))\Delta x$, and we have the following result:

> If $g(x) \leq f(x)$ for $a \leq x \leq b$:
>
> $$\text{Area between graphs of } f(x) \text{ and } g(x) \text{ for } a \leq x \leq b = \int_a^b (f(x) - g(x))\,dx.$$

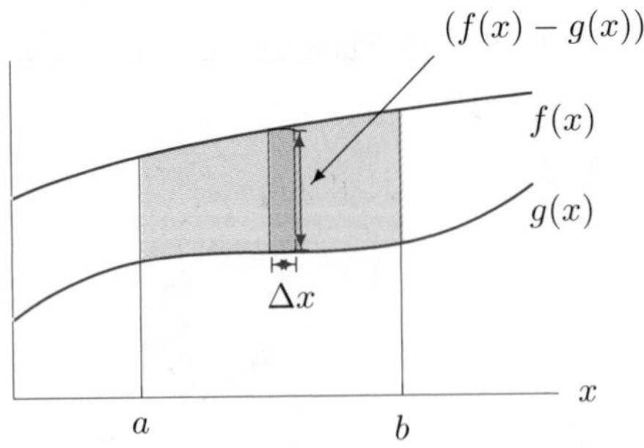

Figure 5.32: Area between two curves $= \int_a^b (f(x) - g(x))\,dx$

Example 6 Graphs of $f(x) = 4x - x^2$ and $g(x) = \frac{1}{2}x^{3/2}$ for $x \geq 0$ are shown in Figure 5.33. Use a definite integral to estimate the area enclosed by the graphs of these two functions.

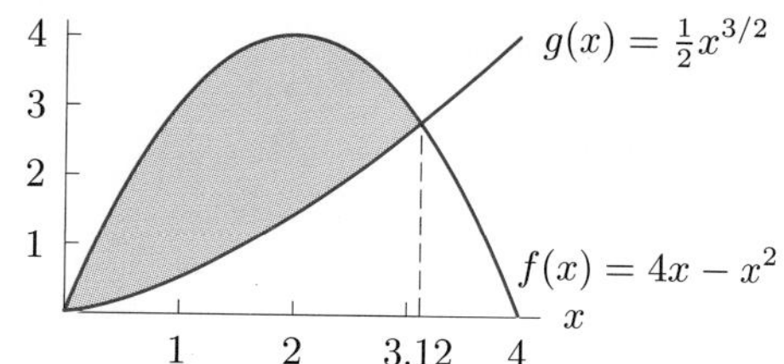

Figure 5.33: Find the area between $f(x) = 4x - x^2$ and $g(x) = \frac{1}{2}x^{3/2}$ using an integral

Solution

The region enclosed by the graphs of the two functions is shaded in Figure 5.33. The two graphs cross at $x = 0$ and at $x \approx 3.12$. Between these values, the graph of $f(x) = 4x - x^2$ lies above the graph of $g(x) = \frac{1}{2}x^{3/2}$. Using a calculator or computer to evaluate the integral, we get

$$\text{Area between graphs} = \int_0^{3.12} \left((4x - x^2) - \tfrac{1}{2}x^{3/2}\right) dx = 5.906.$$

Problems for Section 5.3

1. Find the area under $y = x^3 + 2$ between $x = 0$ and $x = 2$. Sketch this area.

2. Find the area under $P = 100(0.6)^t$ between $t = 0$ and $t = 8$.

3. Find the area between $y = x+5$ and $y = 2x+1$ between $x = 0$ and $x = 2$.

4. Find the area enclosed by $y = 3x$ and $y = x^2$.

5. **(a)** What is the area between the graph of $f(x)$ in Figure 5.34 and the x-axis, between $x = 0$ and $x = 5$?
(b) What is $\int_0^5 f(x)\,dx$?

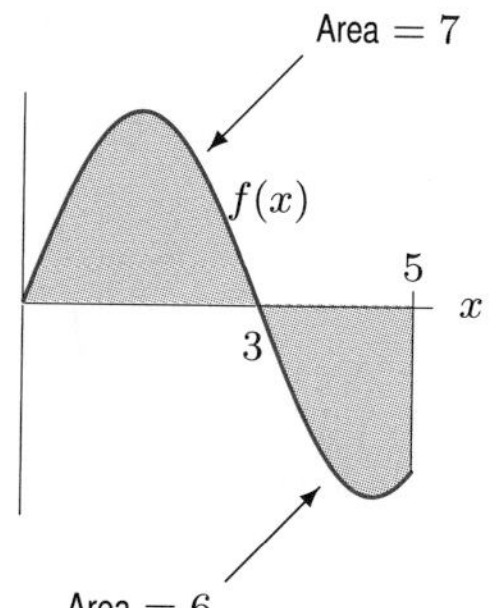

Figure 5.34

In Problems 6–9, decide whether $\int_{-3}^{3} f(x)\,dx$ is positive, negative, or approximately zero.

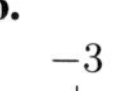

6.

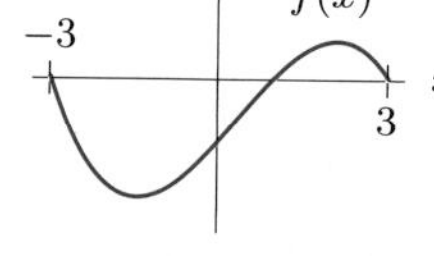

7.

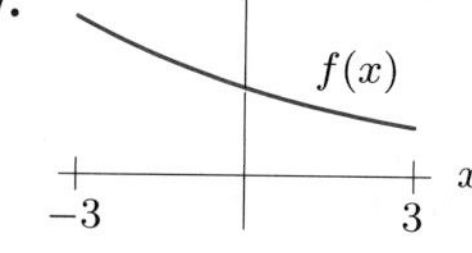

8.

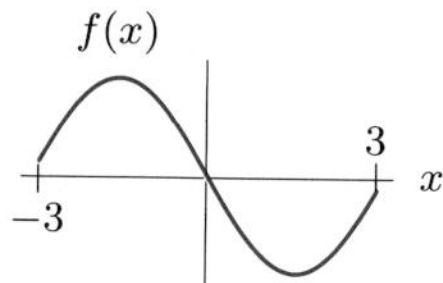

9.

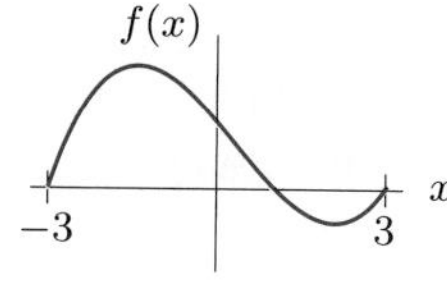

10. **(a)** Estimate (by counting the squares) the total area shaded in Figure 5.35.
(b) Using Figure 5.35, estimate $\int_0^8 f(x)\,dx$.
(c) Why are your answers to parts (a) and (b) different?

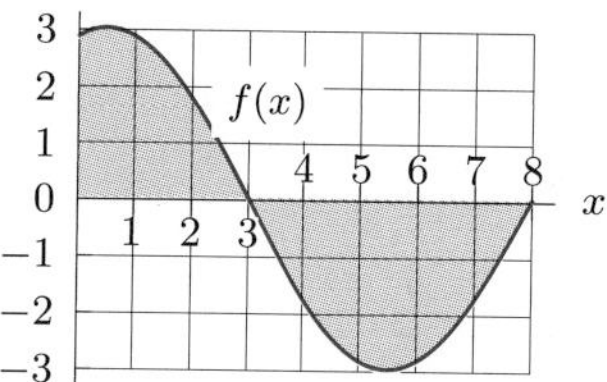

Figure 5.35

11. Using Figure 5.36, estimate $\int_{-3}^{5} f(x)dx$.

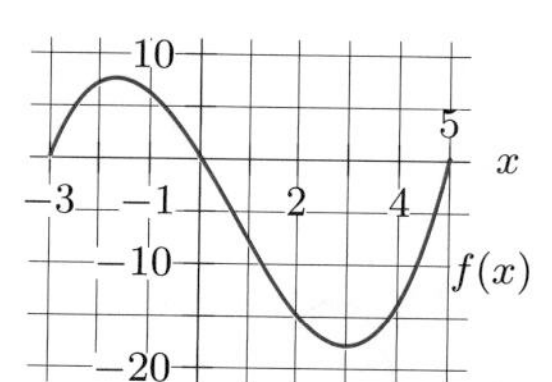

Figure 5.36

12. Given $\int_{-1}^{0} f(x)\,dx = 0.25$ and Figure 5.37, estimate:

(a) $\int_0^1 f(x)\,dx$ **(b)** $\int_{-1}^{1} f(x)\,dx$
(c) The total shaded area.

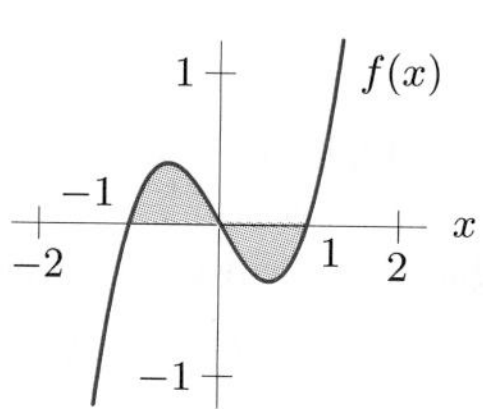

Figure 5.37

13. Given $\int_{-2}^{0} f(x)dx = 4$ and Figure 5.38, estimate:

(a) $\int_{0}^{2} f(x)dx$ **(b)** $\int_{-2}^{2} f(x)dx$

(c) The total shaded area.

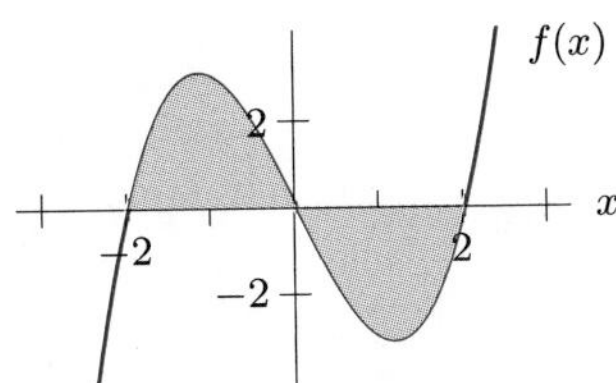

Figure 5.38

In Problems 14–17, match the graph with one of the following possible values for the integral $\int_0^5 f(x)\,dx$:

I. − 10.4 II. − 2.1 III. 5.2 IV. 10.4

14.

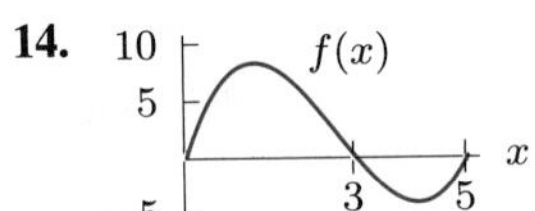

15.

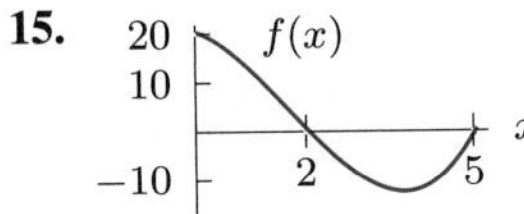

16.

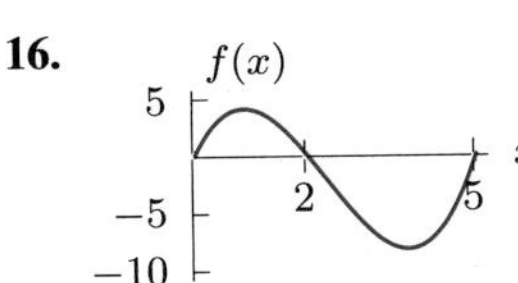

17.

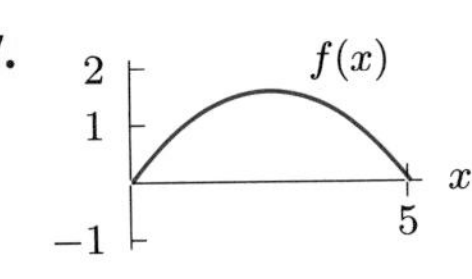

18. Use Figure 5.39 to find the values of

(a) $\int_a^b f(x)\,dx$ **(b)** $\int_b^c f(x)\,dx$

(c) $\int_a^c f(x)\,dx$ **(d)** $\int_a^c |f(x)|\,dx$

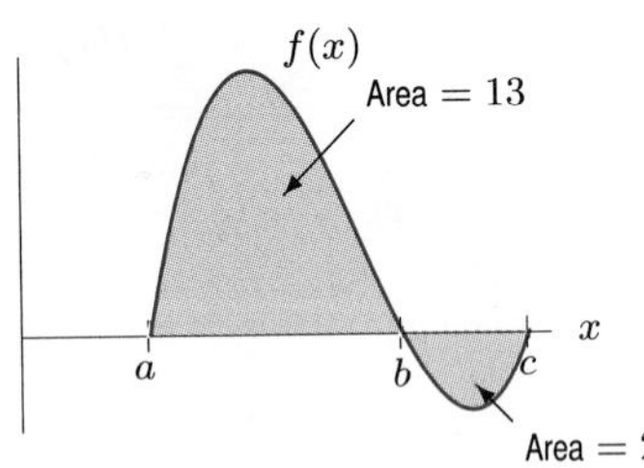

Figure 5.39

19. Using Figure 5.40, list the following integrals in increasing order (from smallest to largest). Which integrals are negative, which are positive? Give reasons.

I. $\int_a^b f(x)\,dx$ II. $\int_a^c f(x)\,dx$ III. $\int_a^e f(x)\,dx$

IV. $\int_b^e f(x)\,dx$ V. $\int_b^c f(x)\,dx$

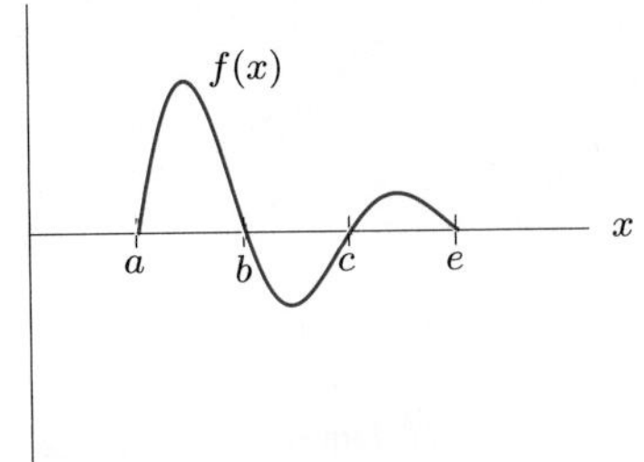

Figure 5.40

20. **(a)** Graph $f(x) = x(x+2)(x-1)$.

(b) Find the total area between the graph and the x-axis between $x = -2$ and $x = 1$.

(c) Find $\int_{-2}^{1} f(x)\,dx$ and interpret it in terms of areas.

21. **(a)** Using Figure 5.41, find $\int_{-3}^{0} f(x)\,dx$.

(b) If the area of the shaded region is A, estimate $\int_{-3}^{4} f(x)\,dx$.

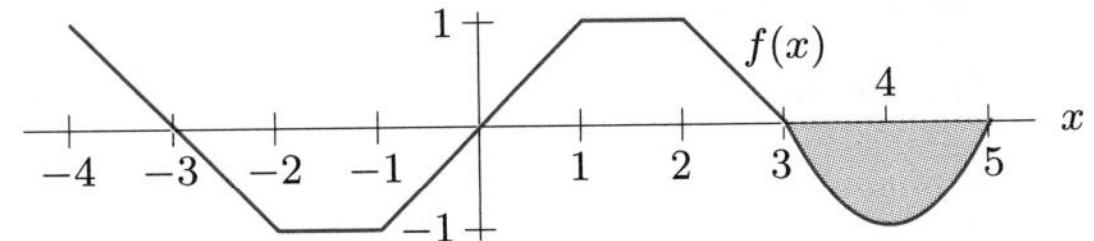

Figure 5.41

22. Use the following table to estimate the area between $f(x)$ and the x-axis on the interval $0 \le x \le 20$.

x	0	5	10	15	20
$f(x)$	15	18	20	16	12

For Problems 23–24, compute the definite integral and interpret the result in terms of areas.

23. $\displaystyle\int_1^4 \frac{x^2-3}{x}\,dx.$ **24.** $\displaystyle\int_1^4 (x - 3\ln x)\,dx.$

25. Compute the definite integral $\int_0^4 \cos\sqrt{x}\,dx$ and interpret the result in terms of areas.

26. Find the area between the graph of $y = x^2 - 2$ and the x-axis, between $x = 0$ and $x = 3$.

In Problems 27–34, use an integral to find the specified area.

27. Under $y = 6x^3 - 2$ for $5 \le x \le 10$.

28. Under $y = 2\cos(t/10)$ for $1 \le t \le 2$.

29. Under $y = 5\ln(2x)$ and above $y = 3$ for $3 \le x \le 5$.

30. Between $y = \sin x + 2$ and $y = 0.5$ for $6 \le x \le 10$.

31. Between $y = \cos x + 7$ and $y = \ln(x-3)$, $5 \le x \le 7$.

32. Above the curve $y = x^4 - 8$ and below the x-axis.

33. Above the curve $y = -e^x + e^{2(x-1)}$ and below the x-axis, for $x \ge 0$.

34. Between $y = \cos t$ and $y = \sin t$ for $0 \le t \le \pi$.

5.4 INTERPRETATIONS OF THE DEFINITE INTEGRAL

The Notation and Units for the Definite Integral

Just as the Leibniz notation dy/dx for the derivative reminds us that the derivative is the limit of a quotient of differences, the notation for the definite integral,

$$\int_a^b f(x)\,dx,$$

reminds us that an integral is a limit of a sum. The integral sign is a misshapen S. Since the terms being added are products of the form "$f(x)$ times a difference in x," we have the following result:

> The unit of measurement for $\int_a^b f(x)\,dx$ is the product of the units for $f(x)$ and the units for x.

For example, if x and $f(x)$ have the same units, then the integral $\int_a^b f(x)\,dx$ is measured in square units, say cm $\times$ cm $=$ cm^2. This is what we would expect, since the integral represents an area.

Similarly, if $f(t)$ is velocity in meters/second and t is time in seconds, then the integral

$$\int_a^b f(t)\,dt$$

has units of (meters/sec) $\times$ (sec) $=$ meters, which is what we expect since the integral represents change in position. We saw in Section 5.1 that total change could be approximated by a Riemann sum formed using the rate of change. In the limit, we have:

> If $f(t)$ is a rate of change of a quantity, then
>
> $$\begin{array}{c}\text{Total change in quantity between}\\ t = a \text{ and } t = b\end{array} = \int_a^b f(t)\,dt$$

The units correspond: If $f(t)$ is a rate of change, with units of quantity/time, then $f(t)\Delta t$ and the definite integral have units of (quantity/time) $\times$ (time) $=$ quantity.

Example 1 A bacteria colony initially has a population of 14 million bacteria. Suppose that t hours later the population is growing at a rate of $f(t) = 2^t$ million bacteria per hour.

(a) Give a definite integral that represents the total change in the bacteria population during the time from $t = 0$ to $t = 2$.

(b) Find the population at time $t = 2$.

Solution (a) Since $f(t) = 2^t$ gives the rate of change of population, we have

$$\begin{array}{c}\text{Change in population between}\\ t = 0 \text{ and } t = 2\end{array} = \int_0^2 2^t\,dt.$$

(b) Using a calculator, we find $\int_0^2 2^t\,dt = 4.328$. The bacteria population was 14 million at time $t = 0$ and increased 4.328 million between $t = 0$ and $t = 2$. Therefore, at time $t = 2$,

$$\text{Population} = 14 + 4.328 = 18.328 \text{ million bacteria.}$$

Example 2 Suppose that $C(t)$ represents the cost per day to heat your home in dollars per day, where t is time measured in days and $t = 0$ corresponds to January 1, 2010. Interpret $\displaystyle\int_0^{90} C(t)\,dt$.

Solution The units for the integral $\int_0^{90} C(t)\,dt$ are (dollars/day) $\times$ (days) $=$ dollars. The integral represents the cost in dollars to heat your house for the first 90 days of 2010, namely the months of January, February, and March.

Example 3 A man starts 50 miles away from his home and takes a trip in his car. He moves on a straight line, and his home lies on this line. His velocity is given in Figure 5.42.

(a) When is the man closest to his home? Approximately how far away is he then?
(b) When is the man farthest from his home? How far away is he then?

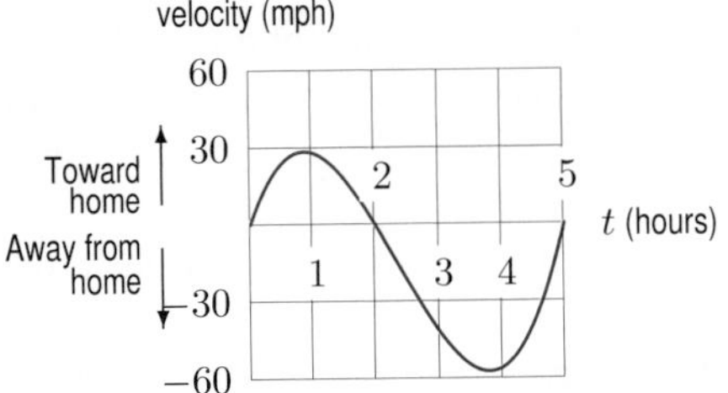

Figure 5.42: Velocity of trip starting 50 miles from home

Solution What happens on this trip? The velocity function is positive the first two hours and negative between $t = 2$ and $t = 5$. So the man moves toward his home during the first two hours, then turns around at $t = 2$ and moves away from his home. The distance he travels is represented by the area between the graph of velocity and the t-axis; since the area below the axis is greater than the area above the axis, we see that he ends up farther away from home than when he started. Thus he is closest to home at $t = 2$ and farthest from home at $t = 5$. We can estimate how far he went in each direction by estimating areas.

(a) The man starts out 50 miles from home. The distance the man travels during the first two hours is the area under the curve between $t = 0$ and $t = 2$. This area corresponds to about one grid square. Since each grid square has area (30 miles/hour)(1 hour) = 30 miles, the man travels about 30 miles toward home. He is closest to home after 2 hours, and he is about 20 miles away at that time.
(b) Between $t = 2$ and $t = 5$, the man moves away from his home. Since this area is equal to about 3.5 grid squares, which is $(3.5)(30) = 105$ miles, he has moved 105 miles farther from home. He was already 20 miles from home, so at $t = 5$ he is about 125 miles from home. He is farthest from home at $t = 5$.

Notice that the man has covered a total distance of $30 + 105 = 135$ miles. However, he went toward his home for 30 miles and away from his home for 105 miles. His *net* change in position is 75 miles.

Example 4 The rates of growth of the populations of two species of plants (measured in new plants per year) are shown in Figure 5.43. Assume that the populations of the two species are equal at time $t = 0$.

(a) Which population is larger after one year? After two years?
(b) How much does the population of species 1 increase during the first two years?

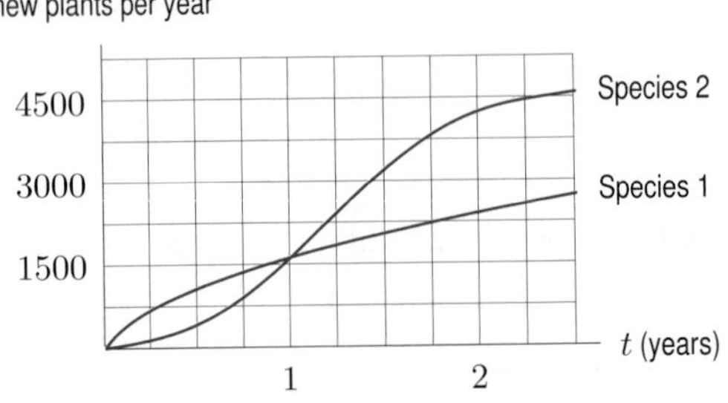

Figure 5.43: Population growth rates for two species of plants

Solution

(a) The rate of growth of the population of species 1 is higher than that of species 2 throughout the first year, so the population of species 1 is larger after one year. After two years, the situation is less clear, since the population of species 1 increased faster for the first year and that of species 2 for the second. However, if $r(t)$ is the rate of growth of a population, we have

$$\text{Total change in population during first two years} = \int_0^2 r(t)dt.$$

This integral is the area under the graph of $r(t)$. For $t = 0$ to $t = 2$, the area under the species 1 graph in Figure 5.43 is smaller than the area under the species 2 graph, so the population of species 2 is larger after two years.

(b) The population change for species 1 is the area of the region under the graph of $r(t)$ between $t = 0$ and $t = 2$ in Figure 5.43. The region consists of about 16.5 grid squares, each of area (750 plants/year)(0.25 year) = 187.5 plants, giving a total of (16.5)(187.5) = 3093.75 plants. The population of species 1 increases by about 3100 plants during the two years.

Bioavailability of Drugs

In pharmacology, the definite integral is used to measure *bioavailability*; that is, the overall presence of a drug in the bloodstream during the course of a treatment. Unit bioavailability represents 1 unit concentration of the drug in the bloodstream for 1 hour. For example, a concentration of 3 μg/cm^3 in the blood for 2 hours has bioavailability of $3 \cdot 2 = 6$ (μg/cm^3)-hours.

Ordinarily the concentration of a drug in the blood is not constant. Typically, the concentration in the blood increases as the drug is absorbed into the bloodstream, and then decreases as the drug is broken down and excreted.[2] (See Figure 5.44.)

Suppose that we want to calculate the bioavailability of a drug that is in the blood with concentration $C(t)\mu\text{g/cm}^3$ at time t for the time period $0 \leq t \leq T$. Over a small interval Δt, we estimate

$$\text{Bioavailability} \approx \text{Concentration} \times \text{Time} = C(t)\Delta t.$$

Summing over all subintervals gives

$$\text{Total bioavailability} \approx \sum C(t)\Delta t.$$

In the limit as $n \to \infty$, where n is the number of intervals of width Δt, the sum becomes an integral. So for $0 \leq t \leq T$, we have

$$\text{Bioavailability} = \int_0^T C(t)dt.$$

That is, the total bioavailability of a drug is equal to the area under the drug concentration curve.

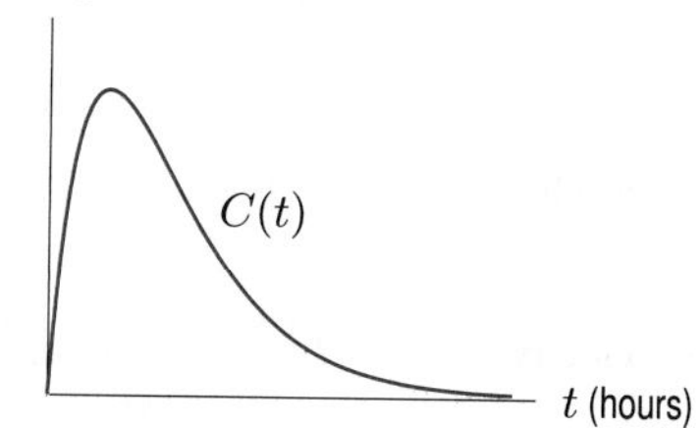

Figure 5.44: Curve showing drug concentration as a function of time

[2] *Drug Treatment*, Graeme S. Avery (Ed.) (Sydney: Adis Press, 1976).

Example 5 Blood concentration curves[3] of two drugs are shown in Figure 5.45. Describe the differences and similarities between the two drugs in terms of peak concentration, speed of absorption into the bloodstream, and total bioavailability.

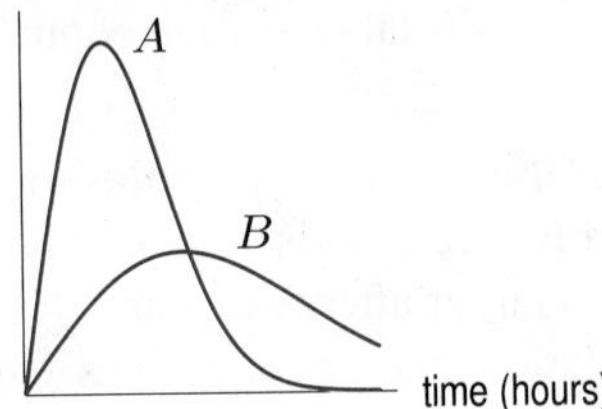

Figure 5.45: Concentration curves of two drugs

Solution Drug A has a peak concentration more than twice as high as that of drug B. Because drug A achieves peak concentration sooner than drug B, drug A appears to be absorbed more rapidly into the blood stream than drug B. Finally, drug A has greater total bioavailability, since the area under the graph of the concentration function for drug A is greater than the area under the graph for drug B.

Problems for Section 5.4

1. The following table gives the emissions, E, of nitrogen oxides in millions of metric tons per year in the US.[4] Let t be the number of years since 1970 and $E = f(t)$.

(a) What are the units and meaning of $\int_0^{30} f(t)dt$?
(b) Estimate $\int_0^{30} f(t)dt$.

Year	1970	1975	1980	1985	1990	1995	2000
E	26.9	26.4	27.1	25.8	25.5	25.0	22.6

2. Annual coal production in the US (in quadrillion BTU per year) is given in the table.[5] Estimate the total amount of coal produced in the US between 1960 and 1990. If $r = f(t)$ is the rate of coal production t years since 1960, write an integral to represent the 1960–1990 coal production.

Year	1960	1965	1970	1975	1980	1985	1990
Rate	10.82	13.06	14.61	14.99	18.60	19.33	22.46

In Problems 3–6, explain in words what the integral represents and give units.

3. $\int_1^3 v(t)\,dt$, where $v(t)$ is velocity in meters/sec and t is time in seconds.

4. $\int_0^6 a(t)\,dt$, where $a(t)$ is acceleration in km/hr^2 and t is time in hours.

5. $\int_{2000}^{2004} f(t)\,dt$, where $f(t)$ is the rate at which the world's population is growing in year t, in billion people per year.

6. $\int_0^5 s(x)\,dx$, where $s(x)$ is rate of change of salinity (salt concentration) in gm/liter per cm in sea water, and where x is depth below the surface of the water in cm.

7. Oil leaks out of a tanker at a rate of $r = f(t)$ gallons per minute, where t is in minutes. Write a definite integral expressing the total quantity of oil which leaks out of the tanker in the first hour.

8. A cup of coffee at 90°C is put into a 20°C room when $t = 0$. The coffee's temperature is changing at a rate of $r(t) = -7(0.9^t)$ °C per minute, with t in minutes. Estimate the coffee's temperature when $t = 10$.

9. After a foreign substance is introduced into the blood, the rate at which antibodies are made is given by

$$r(t) = \frac{t}{t^2+1} \text{ thousands of antibodies per minute,}$$

where time, t, is in minutes. Assuming there are no antibodies present at time $t = 0$, find the total quantity of antibodies in the blood at the end of 4 minutes.

[3] *Drug Treatment*, Graeme S. Avery (Ed.) (Sydney: Adis Press, 1976).
[4] *The World Almanac and Book of Facts 2005*, p. 177 (New York: World Almanac Books).
[5] *World Almanac*, 1995.

10. World annual natural gas[6] consumption, N, in millions of metric tons of oil equivalent, is approximated by $N = 1770 + 53t$, where t is in years since 1990.

(a) How much natural gas was consumed in 1990? In 2010?

(b) Estimate the total amount of natural gas consumed during the 20-year period from 1990 to 2010.

11. Solar photovoltaic (PV) cells are the world's fastest-growing energy source.[7] Annual solar PV production, S, in megawatts, is approximated by $S = 277e^{0.368t}$, where t is in years since 2000. Estimate the total solar PV production between 2000 and 2010.

12. The velocity of a car (in miles per hour) is given by $v(t) = 40t - 10t^2$, where t is in hours.

(a) Write a definite integral for the distance the car travels during the first three hours.

(b) Sketch a graph of velocity against time and represent the distance traveled during the first three hours as an area on your graph.

(c) Use a computer or calculator to find this distance.

13. Your velocity is $v(t) = \ln(t^2 + 1)$ ft/sec for t in seconds, $0 \le t \le 3$. Estimate the distance traveled during this time.

14. Figure 5.46 shows the rate of change of the quantity of water in a water tower, in liters per day, during the month of April. If the tower had 12,000 liters of water in it on April 1, estimate the quantity of water in the tower on April 30.

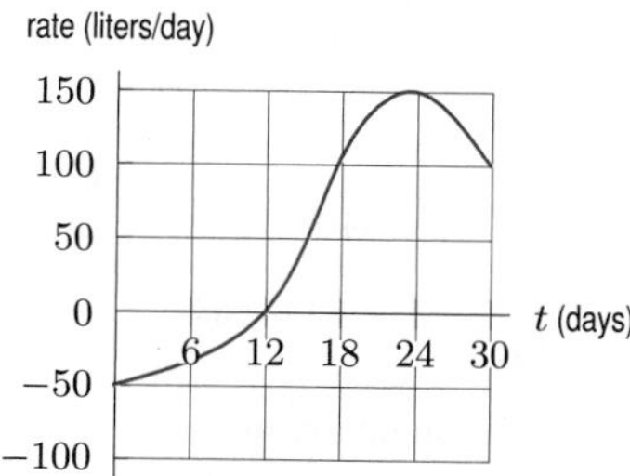

Figure 5.46

15. Figure 5.47 shows the weight growth rate of a human fetus.

(a) What property of a graph of weight as a function of age corresponds to the fact that the function in Figure 5.47 is increasing?

(b) Estimate the weight of a baby born in week 40.

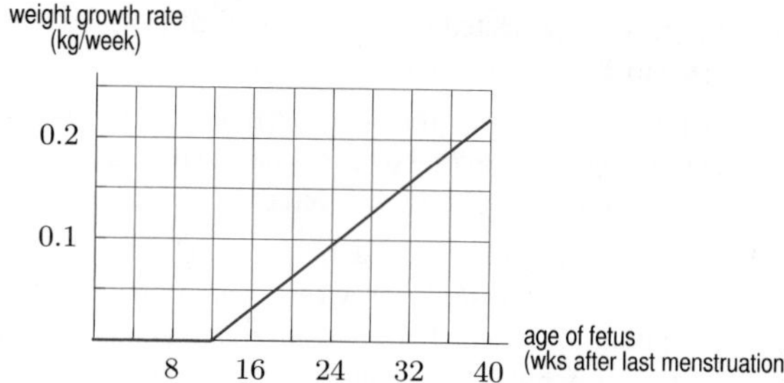

Figure 5.47: Rate of increase of fetal weight

Problems 16–18 concern the future of the US Social Security Trust Fund, out of which pensions are paid. Figure 5.48 shows the rates (billions of dollars per year) at which income, $I(t)$, from taxes and interest is projected to flow into the fund and at which expenditures, $E(t)$, flow out of the fund. Figure 5.49 shows the value of the fund as a function of time.[8]

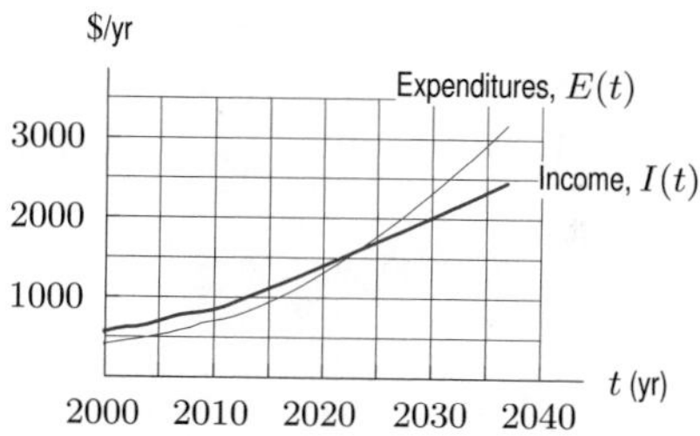

Figure 5.48

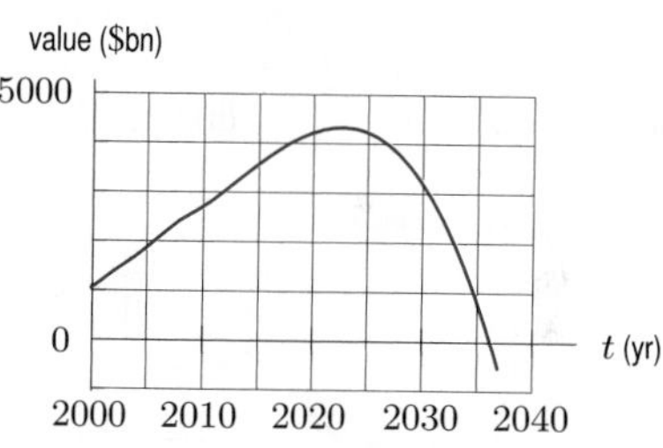

Figure 5.49

16. **(a)** Write each of the following areas in Figure 5.48 from 2000 to 2015 as an integral and explain its significance for the fund.

(i) Under the income curve

(ii) Under the expenditure curve

(iii) Between the income and expenditure curves

(b) Use Figure 5.49 to estimate the area between the two curves from 2000 to 2015.

17. Decide when the value of the fund is projected to be a maximum using

(a) Figure 5.48 **(b)** Figure 5.49

[6] *BP Statistical Review of World Energy 2009*, http://www.bp.com/ (accessed 9/6/2009).
[7] *Vital Signs 2007-2008*, The Worldwatch Institute, W.W. Norton & Company, 2007, p. 38.
[8] The 2009 OASDI Trustees Report, www.ssa.gov/OACT/TR/2009.

18. Express the projected increase in value of the fund from 2000 to 2030 as an integral.

19. A forest fire covers 2000 acres at time $t = 0$. The fire is growing at a rate of $8\sqrt{t}$ acres per hour, where t is in hours. How many acres are covered 24 hours later?

20. Water is pumped out of a holding tank at a rate of $5 - 5e^{-0.12t}$ liters/minute, where t is in minutes since the pump is started. If the holding tank contains 1000 liters of water when the pump is started, how much water does it hold one hour later?

21. Figure 5.50 shows the rate of growth of two trees. If the two trees are the same height at time $t = 0$, which tree is taller after 5 years? After 10 years?

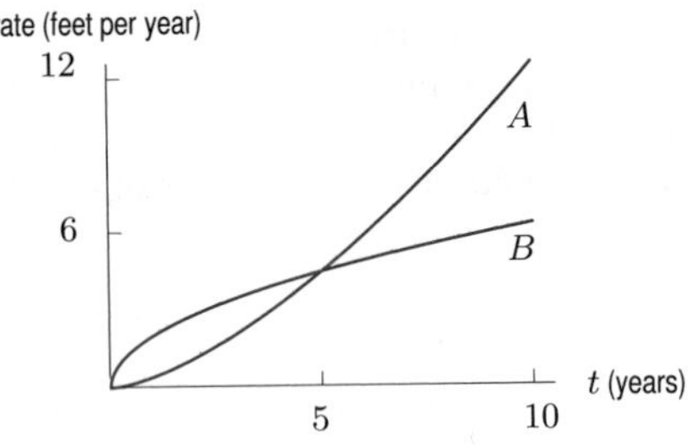

Figure 5.50

22. Figure 5.51 shows the number of sales per month made by two salespeople. Which person has the most total sales after 6 months? After the first year? At approximately what times (if any) have they sold roughly equal total amounts? Approximately how many total sales has each person made at the end of the first year?

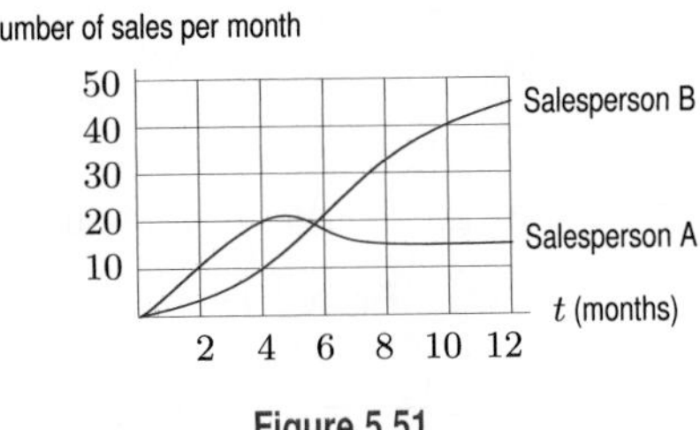

Figure 5.51

23. Height velocity graphs are used by endocrinologists to follow the progress of children with growth deficiencies. Figure 5.52 shows the height velocity curves of an average boy and an average girl between ages 3 and 18.

(a) Which curve is for girls and which is for boys? Explain how you can tell.
(b) About how much does the average boy grow between ages 3 and 10?
(c) The growth spurt associated with adolescence and the onset of puberty occurs between ages 12 and 15 for the average boy and between ages 10 and 12.5 for the average girl. Estimate the height gained by each average child during this growth spurt.
(d) When fully grown, about how much taller is the average man than the average woman? (The average boy and girl are about the same height at age 3.)

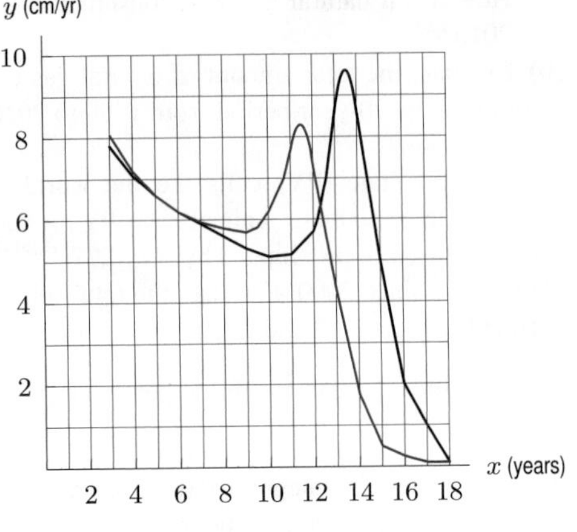

Figure 5.52

24. The birth rate, B, in births per hour, of a bacteria population is given in Figure 5.53. The curve marked D gives the death rate, in deaths per hour, of the same population.

(a) Explain what the shape of each of these graphs tells you about the population.
(b) Use the graphs to find the time at which the net rate of increase of the population is at a maximum.
(c) At time $t = 0$ the population has size N. Sketch the graph of the total number born by time t. Also sketch the graph of the number alive at time t. Estimate the time at which the population is a maximum.

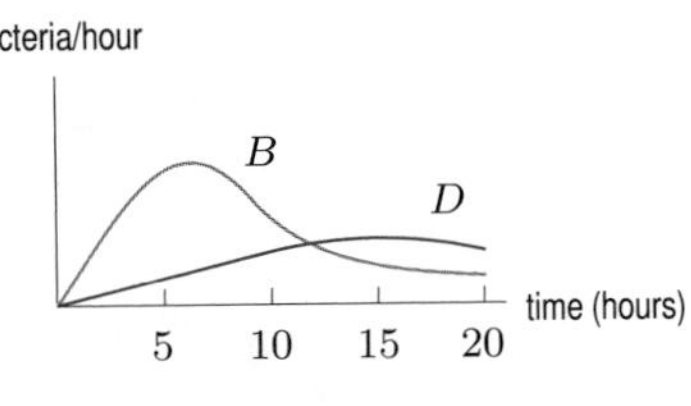

Figure 5.53

25. The rates of consumption of stores of protein and fat in the human body during 8 weeks of starvation are shown in Figure 5.54. Does the body burn more fat or more protein during this period?

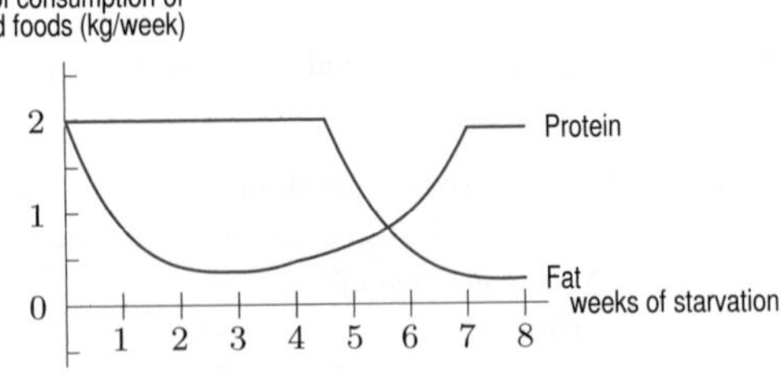

Figure 5.54

A healthy human heart pumps about 5 liters of blood per minute. Problems 26–27 refer to Figure 5.55, which shows the response of the heart to bleeding. The pumping rate drops and then returns to normal if the person recovers fully, or drops to zero if the person dies.

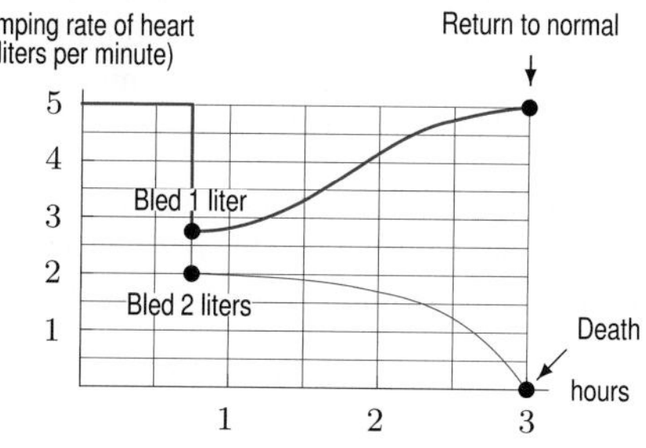

Figure 5.55

26. **(a)** If the body is bled 2 liters, how much blood is pumped during the three hours leading to death?
(b) If $f(t)$ is the pumping rate in liters per minute at time t hours, express your answer to part (a) as a definite integral.
(c) How much more blood would have been pumped during the same time period if there had been no bleeding? Illustrate your answer on the graph.

27. **(a)** If the body is bled 1 liter, how much blood is pumped during the three hours leading to full recovery?
(b) If $g(t)$ is the pumping rate in liters per minute at time t hours, express your answer to part (a) as a definite integral.
(c) How much more blood would have been pumped during the same time period if there had been no bleeding? Show your answer as an area on the graph.

28. The amount of waste a company produces, W, in tons per week, is approximated by $W = 3.75e^{-0.008t}$, where t is in weeks since January 1, 2005. Waste removal for the company costs \$15/ton. How much does the company pay for waste removal during the year 2005?

Problems 29–32 show the velocity, in cm/sec, of a particle moving along the x-axis. Compute the particle's change in position, left (negative) or right (positive), between times $t = 0$ and $t = 5$ seconds.

29.

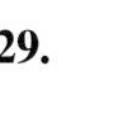

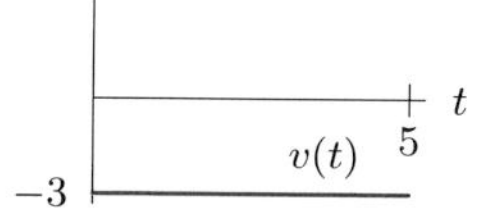

30.

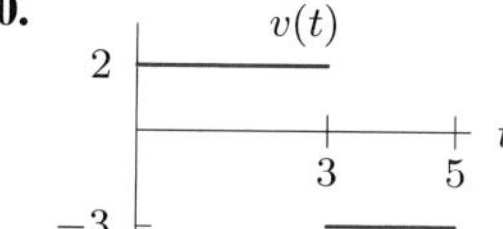

31.

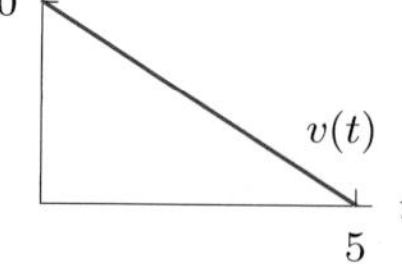

32.

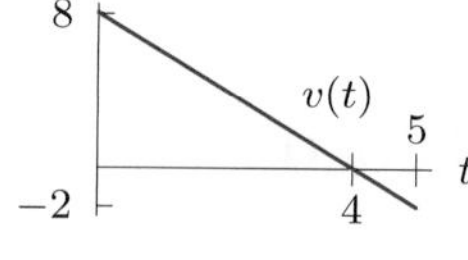

33. Figure 5.56 gives your velocity during a trip starting from home. Positive velocities take you away from home and negative velocities take you toward home. Where are you at the end of the 5 hours? When are you farthest from home? How far away are you at that time?

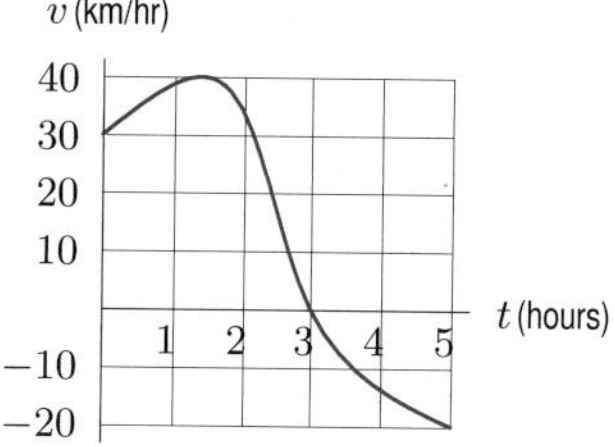

Figure 5.56

34. A bicyclist is pedaling along a straight road for one hour with a velocity v shown in Figure 5.57. She starts out five kilometers from the lake and positive velocities take her toward the lake. [Note: The vertical lines on the graph are at 10 minute (1/6 hour) intervals.]

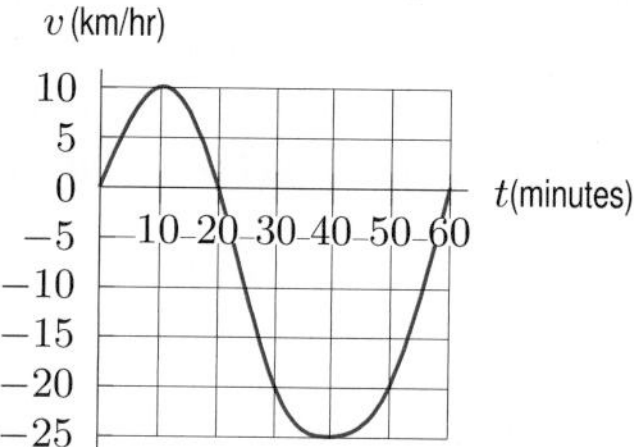

Figure 5.57

(a) Does the cyclist ever turn around? If so, at what time(s)?
(b) When is she going the fastest? How fast is she going then? Toward the lake or away?
(c) When is she closest to the lake? Approximately how close to the lake does she get?
(d) When is she farthest from the lake? Approximately how far from the lake is she then?

35. Figure 5.58 shows plasma concentration curves for two drugs used to slow a rapid heart rate. Compare the two products in terms of level of peak concentration, time until peak concentration, and overall bioavailability.

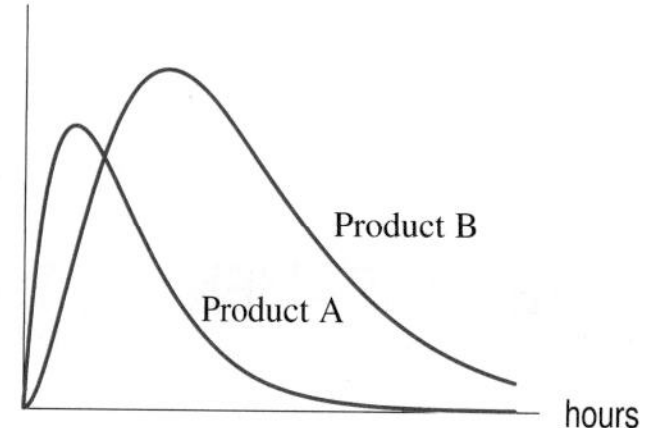

Figure 5.58

36. Figure 5.59 compares the concentration in blood plasma for two pain relievers. Compare the two products in terms of level of peak concentration, time until peak concentration, and overall bioavailability.

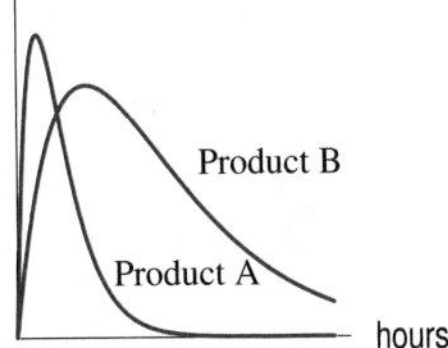

Figure 5.59

37. Draw plasma concentration curves for two drugs A and B if product A has the highest peak concentration, but product B is absorbed more quickly and has greater overall bioavailability.

38. A two-day environmental cleanup started at 9 am on the first day. The number of workers fluctuated as shown in Figure 5.60. If the workers were paid \$10 per hour, how much was the total personnel cost of the cleanup?

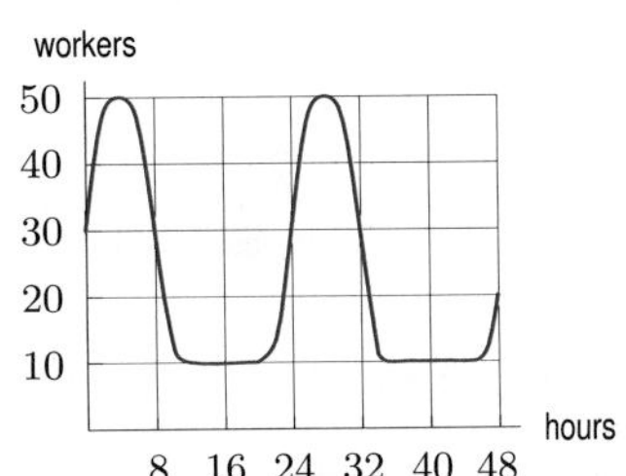

Figure 5.60

39. Suppose in Problem 38 that the workers were paid \$10 per hour for work during the time period 9 am to 5 pm and were paid \$15 per hour for work during the rest of the day. What would the total personnel costs of the clean up have been under these conditions?

40. At the site of a spill of radioactive iodine, radiation levels were four times the maximum acceptable limit, so an evacuation was ordered. If R_0 is the initial radiation level (at $t = 0$) and t is the time in hours, the radiation level $R(t)$, in millirems/hour, is given by

$$R(t) = R_0(0.996)^t.$$

(a) How long does it take for the site to reach the acceptable level of radiation of 0.6 millirems/hour?
(b) How much total radiation (in millirems) has been emitted by that time?

41. If you jump out of an airplane and your parachute fails to open, your downward velocity (in meters per second) t seconds after the jump is approximated by

$$v(t) = 49(1 - (0.8187)^t).$$

(a) Write an expression for the distance you fall in T seconds.
(b) If you jump from 5000 meters above the ground, estimate, using trial and error, how many seconds you fall before hitting the ground.

42. The Montgolfier brothers (Joseph and Etienne) were eighteenth-century pioneers in the field of hot-air ballooning. Had they had the appropriate instruments, they might have left us a record, like that shown in Figure 5.61, of one of their early experiments. The graph shows their vertical velocity, v, with upward as positive.

(a) Over what intervals was the acceleration positive? Negative?
(b) What was the greatest altitude achieved, and at what time?
(c) This particular flight ended on top of a hill. How do you know that it did, and what was the height of the hill above the starting point?

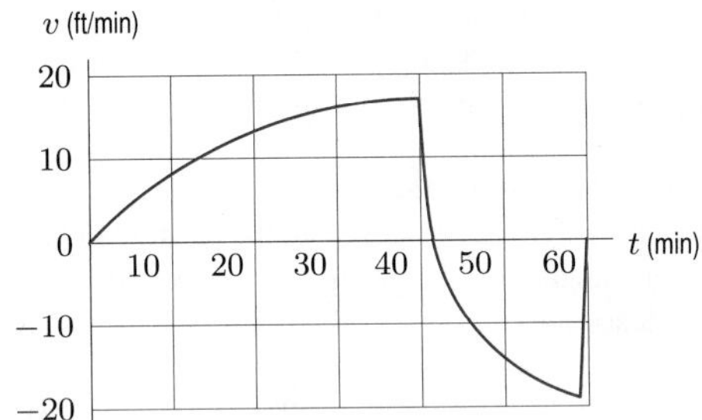

Figure 5.61

5.5 THE FUNDAMENTAL THEOREM OF CALCULUS

In Section 5.4, we saw that the total change of a quantity can be obtained by integrating its rate of change. Since the change in F between a and b is $F(b) - F(a)$ and the rate of change is $F'(t)$ we have the following result:

The Fundamental Theorem of Calculus

If $F'(t)$ is continuous for $a \leq t \leq b$, then

$$\int_a^b F'(t)\,dt = F(b) - F(a).$$

In words:

The definite integral of the derivative of a function gives the total change in the function.

In Section 7.3 we see how to use the Fundamental Theorem to compute a definite integral. The Focus on Theory Section gives another version of the Fundamental Theorem.

Example 1 Figure 5.62 shows $F'(t)$, the rate of change of the value, $F(t)$, of an investment over a 5-month period.

(a) When is the value of the investment increasing in value and when is it decreasing?
(b) Does the investment increase or decrease in value during the 5 months?

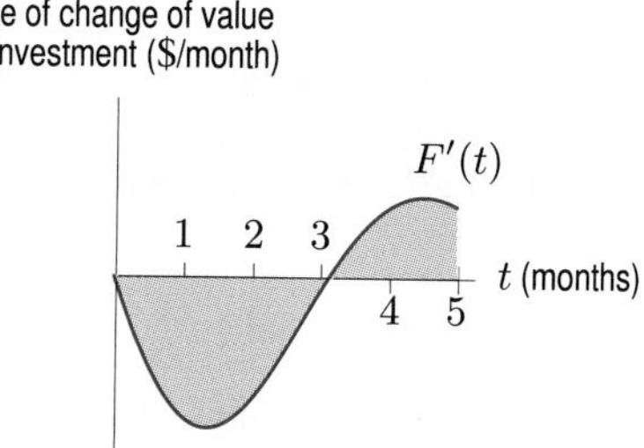

Figure 5.62: Did the investment increase or decrease in value over these 5 months?

Solution

(a) The investment decreased in value during the first 3 months, since the rate of change of value is negative then. The value rose during the last 2 months.
(b) We want to find the total change in the value of the investment between $t = 0$ and $t = 5$. Since the total change is the integral of the rate of change, $F'(t)$, we are looking for

$$\text{Total change in value} = \int_0^5 F'(t)dt.$$

The integral equals the shaded area above the t-axis minus the shaded area below the t-axis. Since in Figure 5.62 the area below the axis is greater than the area above the axis, the integral is negative. The total change in value of the investment during this time is negative, so it decreased in value.

Marginal Cost and Change in Total Cost

Suppose $C(q)$ represents the cost of producing q items. The derivative, $C'(q)$, is the marginal cost. Since marginal cost $C'(q)$ is the rate of change of the cost function with respect to quantity, by the Fundamental Theorem, the integral

$$\int_a^b C'(q)\,dq$$

represents the total change in the cost function between $q = a$ and $q = b$. In other words, the integral gives the amount it costs to increase production from a units to b units.

The cost of producing 0 units is the fixed cost $C(0)$. The area under the marginal cost curve between $q = 0$ and $q = b$ is the total increase in cost between a production of 0 and a production of b. This is called the *total variable cost*. Adding this to the fixed cost gives the total cost to produce b units. In summary,

> If $C'(q)$ is a marginal cost function and $C(0)$ is the fixed cost,
>
> $$\text{Cost to increase production from } a \text{ units to } b \text{ units} = C(b) - C(a) = \int_a^b C'(q)\,dq$$
>
> $$\text{Total variable cost to produce } b \text{ units} = \int_0^b C'(q)\,dq$$
>
> $$\begin{aligned}\text{Total cost of producing } b \text{ units} &= \text{Fixed cost} + \text{Total variable cost} \\ &= C(0) + \int_0^b C'(q)\,dq\end{aligned}$$

Example 2 A marginal cost curve is given in Figure 5.63. If the fixed cost is \$1000, estimate the total cost of producing 250 items.

Solution The total cost of production is Fixed cost + Variable cost. The variable cost of producing 250 items is represented by the area under the marginal cost curve. The area in Figure 5.63 between $q = 0$ and $q = 250$ is about 20 grid squares. Each grid square has area (2 dollars/item)(50 items) = 100 dollars, so

$$\text{Total variable cost} = \int_0^{250} C'(q)\,dq \approx 20(100) = 2000.$$

The total cost to produce 250 items is given by :

$$\begin{aligned}\text{Total cost} &= \text{Fixed cost} + \text{Total variable cost} \\ &\approx \$1000 + \$2000 = \$3000.\end{aligned}$$

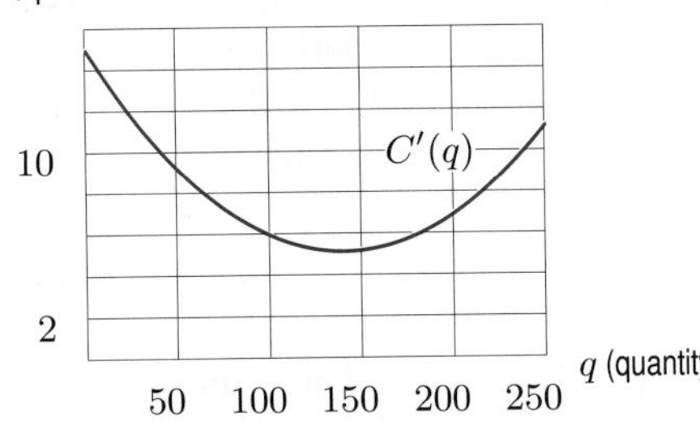

Figure 5.63: A marginal cost curve

Problems for Section 5.5

1. If the marginal cost function $C'(q)$ is measured in dollars per ton, and q gives the quantity in tons, what are the units of measurement for $\int_{800}^{900} C'(q)\,dq$? What does this integral represent?

2. The marginal cost function of a product, in dollars per unit, is $C'(q) = q^2 - 50q + 700$. If fixed costs are \$500, find the total cost to produce 50 items.

3. The total cost in dollars to produce q units of a product is $C(q)$. Fixed costs are \$20,000. The marginal cost is

$$C'(q) = 0.005q^2 - q + 56.$$

   (a) On a graph of $C'(q)$, illustrate graphically the total variable cost of producing 150 units.
   (b) Estimate $C(150)$, the total cost to produce 150 units.
   (c) Find the value of $C'(150)$ and interpret your answer in terms of costs of production.
   (d) Use parts (b) and (c) to estimate $C(151)$.

4. A marginal cost function $C'(q)$ is given in Figure 5.64. If the fixed costs are \$10,000, estimate:

(a) The total cost to produce 30 units.
(b) The additional cost if the company increases production from 30 units to 40 units.
(c) The value of $C'(25)$. Interpret your answer in terms of costs of production.

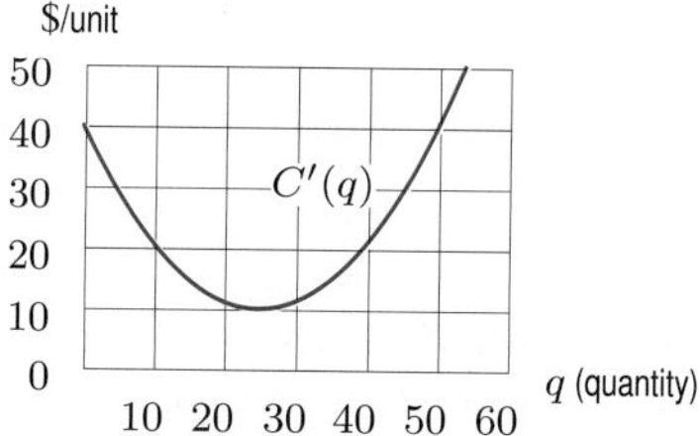

Figure 5.64

5. The population of Tokyo grew at the rate shown in Figure 5.65. Estimate the change in population between 1970 and 1990.

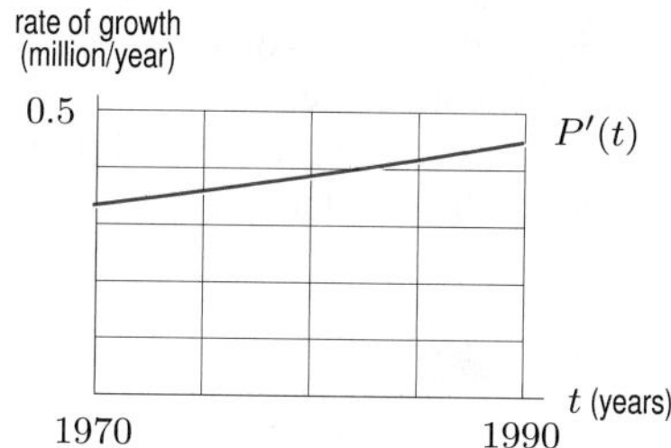

Figure 5.65

6. The marginal cost function for a company is given by

$$C'(q) = q^2 - 16q + 70 \text{ dollars/unit},$$

where q is the quantity produced. If $C(0) = 500$, find the total cost of producing 20 units. What is the fixed cost and what is the total variable cost for this quantity?

7. The marginal cost $C'(q)$ (in dollars per unit) of producing q units is given in the following table.

(a) If fixed cost is \$10,000, estimate the total cost of producing 400 units.
(b) How much would the total cost increase if production were increased one unit, to 401 units?

q	0	100	200	300	400	500	600
$C'(q)$	25	20	18	22	28	35	45

8. The marginal cost function of producing q mountain bikes is

$$C'(q) = \frac{600}{0.3q + 5}.$$

(a) If the fixed cost in producing the bicycles is \$2000, find the total cost to produce 30 bicycles.
(b) If the bikes are sold for \$200 each, what is the profit (or loss) on the first 30 bicycles?
(c) Find the marginal profit on the 31st bicycle.

9. The marginal revenue function on sales of q units of a product is $R'(q) = 200 - 12\sqrt{q}$ dollars per unit.

(a) Graph $R'(q)$.
(b) Estimate the total revenue if sales are 100 units.
(c) What is the marginal revenue at 100 units? Use this value and your answer to part (b) to estimate the total revenue if sales are 101 units.

10. Figure 5.66 shows $P'(t)$, the rate of change of the price of stock in a certain company at time t.

(a) At what time during this five-week period was the stock at its highest value? At its lowest value?
(b) If $P(t)$ represents the price of the stock, arrange the following quantities in increasing order:

$$P(0),\ P(1),\ P(2),\ P(3),\ P(4),\ P(5).$$

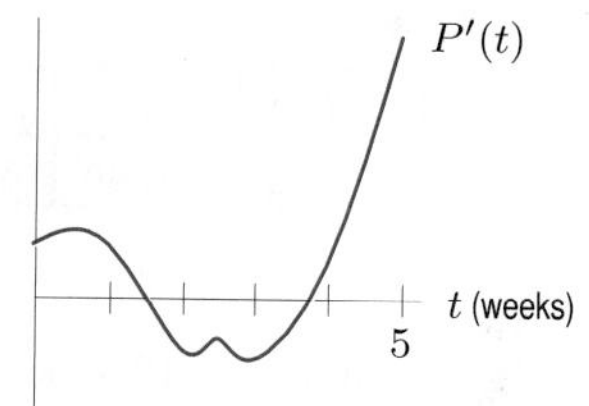

Figure 5.66

11. Ice is forming on a pond at a rate given by

$$\frac{dy}{dt} = \frac{\sqrt{t}}{2} \text{ inches per hour},$$

where y is the thickness of the ice in inches at time t measured in hours since the ice started forming.

(a) Estimate the thickness of the ice after 8 hours.
(b) At what rate is the thickness of the ice increasing after 8 hours?

12. The net worth, $f(t)$, of a company is growing at a rate of $f'(t) = 2000 - 12t^2$ dollars per year, where t is in years since 2005. How is the net worth of the company expected to change between 2005 and 2015? If the company is worth \$40,000 in 2005, what is it worth in 2015?

13. The graph of a derivative $f'(x)$ is shown in Figure 5.67. Fill in the table of values for $f(x)$ given that $f(0) = 2$.

x	0	1	2	3	4	5	6
$f(x)$	2						

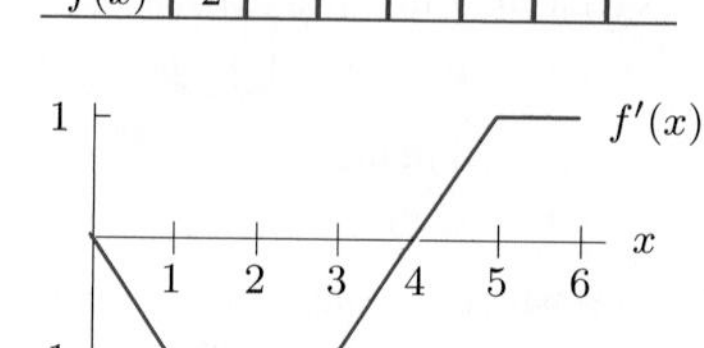

Figure 5.67: Graph of f', not f

CHAPTER SUMMARY

- **Definite integral as limit of right-hand or left-hand sums**
- **Interpretations of the definite integral**
  Total change from rate of change, change in position given velocity, area, bioavailability, total variable cost.
- **Working with the definite integral**
  Estimate definite integral from graph, table of values, or formula.
- **Fundamental Theorem of Calculus**

REVIEW PROBLEMS FOR CHAPTER FIVE

1. The velocity $v(t)$ in Table 5.9 is decreasing, $2 \le t \le 12$. Using $n = 5$ subdivisions to approximate the total distance traveled, find

(a) An upper estimate **(b)** A lower estimate

Table 5.9

t	2	4	6	8	10	12
$v(t)$	44	42	41	40	37	35

2. The velocity $v(t)$ in Table 5.10 is increasing, $0 \le t \le 12$.

(a) Find an upper estimate for the total distance traveled using

(i) $n = 4$ (ii) $n = 2$

(b) Which of the two answers in part (a) is more accurate? Why?

(c) Find a lower estimate of the total distance traveled using $n = 4$.

Table 5.10

t	0	3	6	9	12
$v(t)$	34	37	38	40	45

3. Use the following table to estimate $\int_{10}^{26} f(x)\,dx$.

x	10	14	18	22	26
$f(x)$	100	88	72	50	28

4. If $f(t)$ is measured in miles per hour and t is measured in hours, what are the units of $\int_a^b f(t)\,dt$?

5. If $f(t)$ is measured in meters/second^2 and t is measured in seconds, what are the units of $\int_a^b f(t)\,dt$?

6. If $f(t)$ is measured in dollars per year and t is measured in years, what are the units of $\int_a^b f(t)\,dt$?

7. If $f(x)$ is measured in pounds and x is measured in feet, what are the units of $\int_a^b f(x)\,dx$?

8. As coal deposits are depleted, it becomes necessary to strip-mine larger areas for each ton of coal. Figure 5.68 shows the number of acres of land per million tons of coal that will be defaced during strip-mining as a function of the number of million tons removed, starting from the present day.

(a) Estimate the total number of acres defaced in extracting the next 4 million tons of coal (measured from the present day). Draw four rectangles under the curve, and compute their area.

(b) Reestimate the number of acres defaced using rectangles above the curve.

(c) Use your answers to parts (a) and (b) to get a better estimate of the actual number of acres defaced.

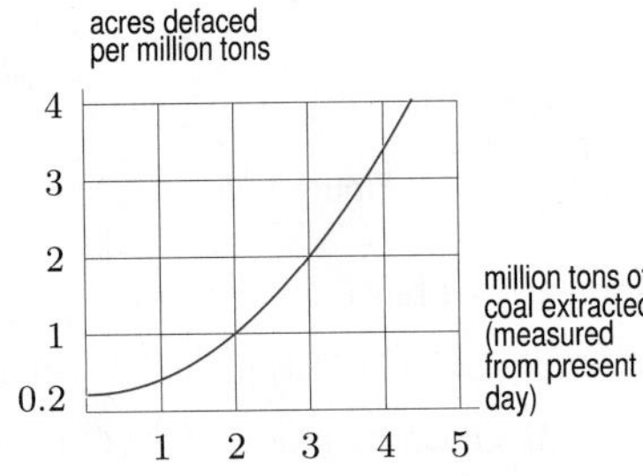

Figure 5.68

For Problems 9–14, use a calculator or computer to evaluate the integral.

9. $\displaystyle\int_0^{10} 2^{-x}\,dx$

10. $\displaystyle\int_1^5 (x^2+1)\,dx$

11. $\displaystyle\int_0^1 \sqrt{1+t^2}\,dt$

12. $\displaystyle\int_{-1}^1 \frac{x^2+1}{x^2-4}\,dx$

13. $\displaystyle\int_2^3 \frac{-1}{(r+1)^2}\,dr$

14. $\displaystyle\int_1^3 \frac{z^2+1}{z}\,dz$

15. Find the area under the graph of $f(x) = x^2 + 2$ between $x = 0$ and $x = 6$.

In Problems 16–19, find the given area.

16. Between $y = x^2$ and $y = x^3$ for $0 \leq x \leq 1$.

17. Between $y = x^{1/2}$ and $y = x^{1/3}$ for $0 \leq x \leq 1$.

18. Between $y = 3x$ and $y = x^2$.

19. Between $y = x$ and $y = \sqrt{x}$.

20. Coal gas is produced at a gasworks. Pollutants in the gas are removed by scrubbers, which become less and less efficient as time goes on. The following measurements, made at the start of each month, show the rate at which pollutants are escaping (in tons/month) in the gas:

Time (months)	0	1	2	3	4	5	6
Rate pollutants escape	5	7	8	10	13	16	20

(a) Make an overestimate and an underestimate of the total quantity of pollutants that escape during the first month.

(b) Make an overestimate and an underestimate of the total quantity of pollutants that escape during the six months.

21. A student is speeding down Route 11 in his fancy red Porsche when his radar system warns him of an obstacle 400 feet ahead. He immediately applies the brakes, starts to slow down, and spots a skunk in the road directly ahead of him. The "black box" in the Porsche records the car's speed every two seconds, producing the following table. The speed decreases throughout the 10 seconds it takes to stop, although not necessarily at a uniform rate.

Time since brakes applied (sec)	0	2	4	6	8	10
Speed (ft/sec)	100	80	50	25	10	0

(a) What is your best estimate of the total distance the student's car traveled before coming to rest?

(b) Which one of the following statements can you justify from the information given?

(i) The car stopped before getting to the skunk.

(ii) The "black box" data is inconclusive. The skunk may or may not have been hit.

(iii) The skunk was hit by the car.

22. The velocity of a particle moving along the x-axis is given by $f(t) = 6 - 2t$ cm/sec. Use a graph of $f(t)$ to find the exact change in position of the particle from time $t = 0$ to $t = 4$ seconds.

23. A baseball thrown directly upward at 96 ft/sec has velocity $v(t) = 96 - 32t$ ft/sec at time t seconds.

(a) Graph the velocity from $t = 0$ to $t = 6$.

(b) When does the baseball reach the peak of its flight? How high does it go?

(c) How high is the baseball at time $t = 5$?

24. A news broadcast in early 1993 said the typical American's annual income is changing at a rate of $r(t) = 40(1.002)^t$ dollars per month, where t is in months from January 1, 1993. How much did the typical American's income change during 1993?

25. Two species of plants have the same populations at time $t = 0$ and the growth rates shown in Figure 5.69.

(a) Which species has a larger population at the end of 5 years? At the end of 10 years?

(b) Which species do you think has the larger population after 20 years? Explain.

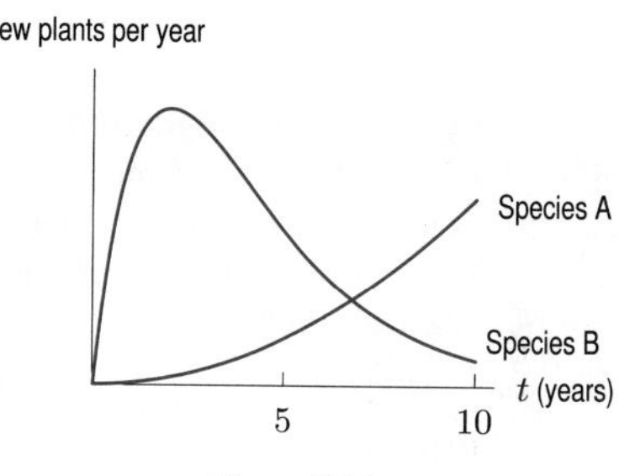

Figure 5.69

26. Figure 5.70 represents your velocity, v, on a bicycle trip along a straight road which starts 10 miles from home. Write a paragraph describing your trip: Do you start out going toward or away from home? How long do you continue in that direction and how far are you from home when you turn around? How many times do you change direction? Do you ever get home? Where are you at the end of the four-hour bike ride?

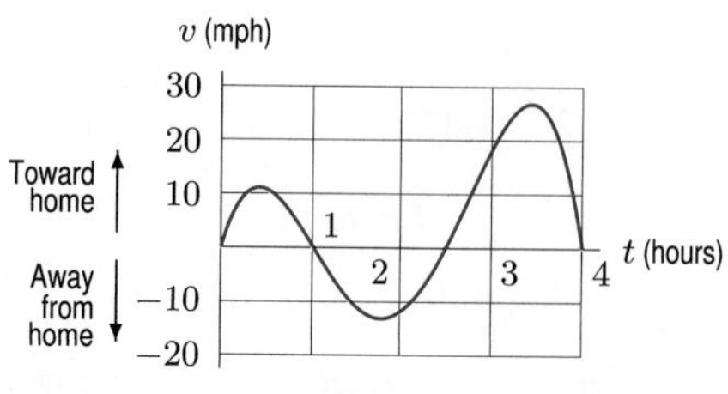

Figure 5.70

27. Figure 5.71 shows the length growth rate of a human fetus.

(a) What feature of a graph of length as a function of age corresponds to the maximum in Figure 5.71?
(b) Estimate the length of a baby born in week 40.

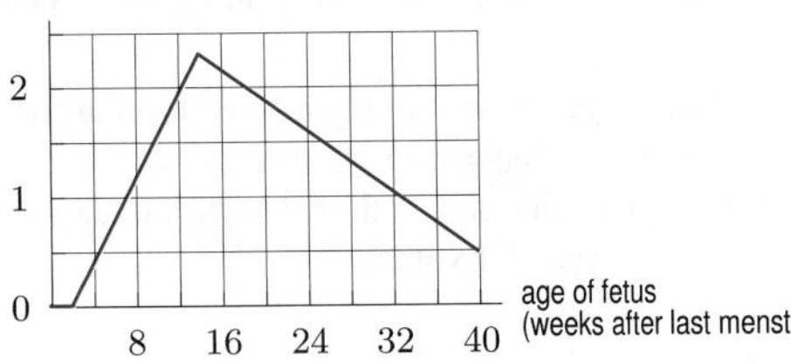

Figure 5.71

28. A bicyclist pedals along a straight road with velocity, v, given in Figure 5.72. She starts 5 miles from a lake; positive velocities take her away from the lake and negative velocities take her toward the lake. When is the cyclist farthest from the lake, and how far away is she then?

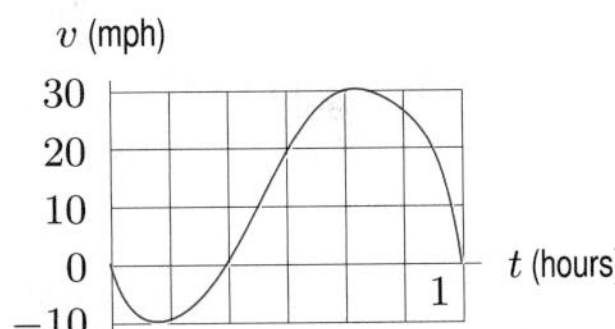

Figure 5.72

29. Using Figure 5.73, decide whether each of the following definite integrals is positive or negative.

(a) $\int_{-5}^{-4} f(x)\,dx$ **(b)** $\int_{-4}^{1} f(x)\,dx$
(c) $\int_{1}^{3} f(x)\,dx$ **(d)** $\int_{-5}^{3} f(x)\,dx$

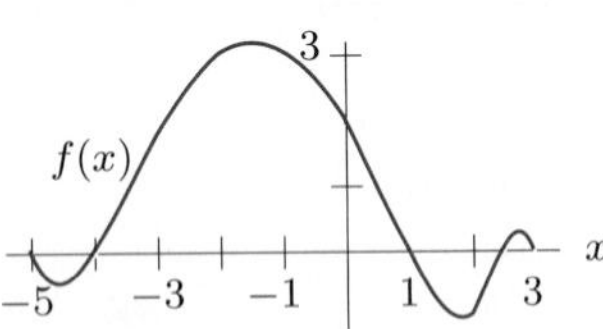

Figure 5.73

30. Using Figure 5.73, arrange the following definite integrals in ascending order:
$\int_{-5}^{-3} f(x)\,dx$, $\int_{-5}^{-1} f(x)\,dx$, $\int_{-5}^{1} f(x)\,dx$, $\int_{-5}^{3} f(x)\,dx$.

31. Use a graph of $y = 2^{-x^2}$ to explain why $\int_{-1}^{1} 2^{-x^2}\,dx$ must be between 0 and 2.

32. Without computation, show that $2 \le \int_0^2 \sqrt{1+x^3}\,dx \le 6$.

33. With t in seconds, the velocity of an object is $v(t) = 10 + 8t - t^2$ m/sec.

(a) Represent the distance traveled during the first 5 seconds as a definite integral and as an area.
(b) Estimate the distance traveled by the object during the first 5 seconds by estimating the area.
(c) Calculate the distance traveled.

34. The world's oil is being consumed at a continuously increasing rate, $f(t)$ (in billions of barrels per year), where t is in years since the start of 1995.

(a) Write a definite integral which represents the total quantity of oil used between the start of 1995 and the start of 2010.
(b) Suppose $r = 32(1.05)^t$. Using a left-hand sum with five subdivisions, find an approximate value for the total quantity of oil used between the start of 1995 and the start of 2010.
(c) Interpret each of the five terms in the sum from part (b) in terms of oil consumption.

35. A car moves along a straight line with velocity, in feet/second, given by

$$v(t) = 6 - 2t \quad \text{for } t \ge 0.$$

(a) Describe the car's motion in words. (When is it moving forward, backward, and so on?)
(b) The car's position is measured from its starting point. When is it farthest forward? Backward?

36. The marginal cost of drilling an oil well depends on the depth at which you are drilling; drilling becomes more expensive, per meter, as you dig deeper into the earth. The fixed costs are 1,000,000 riyals (the riyal is the unit of currency of Saudi Arabia), and, if x is the depth in meters, the marginal costs are

$$C'(x) = 4000 + 10x \quad \text{riyals/meter.}$$

Find the total cost of drilling a 500-meter well.

37. A warehouse charges its customers \$5 per day for every 10 cubic feet of space used for storage. Figure 5.74 records the storage used by one company over a month. How much will the company have to pay?

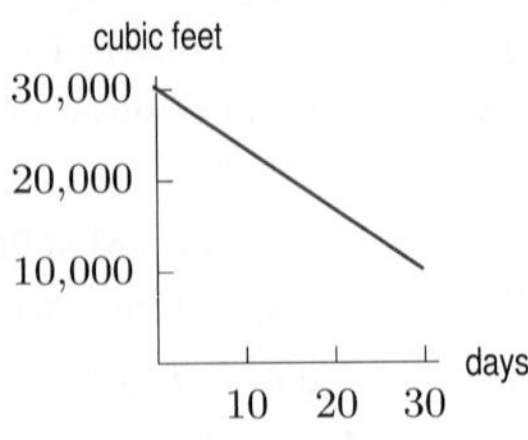

Figure 5.74

38. One of the earliest pollution problems brought to the attention of the Environmental Protection Agency (EPA) was the case of the Sioux Lake in eastern South Dakota. For years a small paper plant located nearby had been discharging waste containing carbon tetrachloride (CCl_4) into the waters of the lake. At the time the EPA learned of the situation, the chemical was entering at a rate of 16 cubic yards/year.

The agency immediately ordered the installation of filters designed to slow (and eventually stop) the flow of CCl_4 from the mill. Implementation of this program took exactly three years, during which the flow of pollutant was steady at 16 cubic yards/year. Once the filters were installed, the flow declined. From the time the filters were installed until the time the flow stopped, the rate of flow was well approximated by

$$\text{Rate (in cubic yards/year)} = t^2 - 14t + 49,$$

where t is time measured in years since the EPA learned of the situation (thus, $t \geq 3$).

(a) Draw a graph showing the rate of CCl_4 flow into the lake as a function of time, beginning at the time the EPA first learned of the situation.
(b) How many years elapsed between the time the EPA learned of the situation and the time the pollution flow stopped entirely?
(c) How much CCl_4 entered the waters during the time shown in the graph in part (a)?

39. (a) Graph $x^3 - 5x^2 + 4x$, marking $x = 1, 2, 3, 4, 5$.
(b) Use your graph and the area interpretation of the definite integral to decide which of the five numbers

$$I_n = \int_0^n (x^3 - 5x^2 + 4x)\,dx \quad \text{for } n = 1, 2, 3, 4, 5$$

is largest. Which is smallest? How many of the numbers are positive? (Don't calculate the integrals.)

40. A mouse moves back and forth in a straight tunnel, attracted to bits of cheddar cheese alternately introduced to and removed from the ends (right and left) of the tunnel. The graph of the mouse's velocity, v, is given in Figure 5.75, with positive velocity corresponding to motion toward the right end. Assuming that the mouse starts ($t = 0$) at the center of the tunnel, use the graph to estimate the time(s) at which:

(a) The mouse changes direction.
(b) The mouse is moving most rapidly to the right; to the left.
(c) The mouse is farthest to the right of center; farthest to the left.
(d) The mouse's speed (i.e., the magnitude of its velocity) is decreasing.
(e) The mouse is at the center of the tunnel.

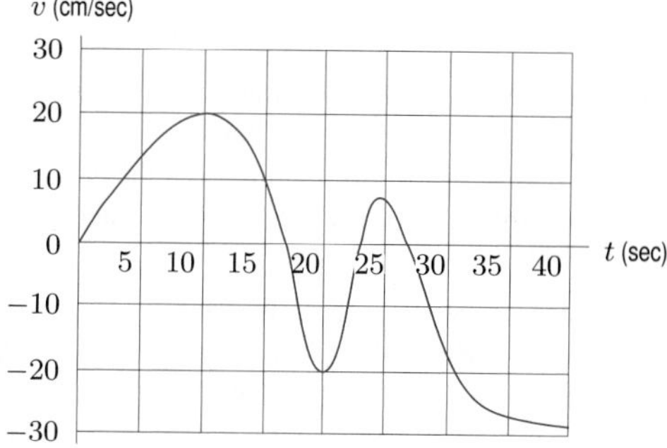

Figure 5.75

41. Pollution is being dumped into a lake at a rate which is increasing at a constant rate from 10 kg/year to 50 kg/year until a total of 270 kg has been dumped. Sketch a graph of the rate at which pollution is being dumped in the lake against time. How long does it take until 270 kg has been dumped?

For Problems 42–44, suppose $F(0) = 0$ and $F'(x) = 4 - x^2$.

42. Calculate $F(b)$ for $b = 0,\ 0.5,\ 1,\ 1.5,\ 2,\ 2.5$.

43. Using a graph of F', decide where F is increasing and where F is decreasing for $0 \leq x \leq 2.5$.

44. Does F have a maximum value for $0 \leq x \leq 2.5$? If so, what is it, and at what value of x does it occur?

CHECK YOUR UNDERSTANDING

In Problems 1–50, indicate whether the statement is true or false.

1. If the velocity is positive, then the total distance traveled is the area under the velocity curve.

2. If velocity is constant and positive, then distance traveled during a time interval is the velocity multiplied by the length of the interval.

3. If velocity is positive and increasing, using the velocity at the beginning of each subinterval gives an overestimate of the distance traveled.

4. A car traveling with increasing velocity (in feet per second) given in the following table travels more than 40 feet between $t = 4$ and $t = 6$ seconds.

t	4	6
$v(t)$	10	20

5. A car traveling with increasing velocity (in feet per second) given in the following table travels less than 40 feet between $t = 4$ and $t = 6$ seconds.

t	4	6
$v(t)$	10	20

6. If water flows out of a tank at an increasing rate starting at 20 gallons per minute at the start of a 10-minute period and ending at 50 gallons per minute at the end of the 10-minute period, then at least 200 gallons have flowed out of the tank.

7. If water flows out of a tank at an increasing rate starting at 20 gallons per minute at the start of a 10-minute period and ending at 50 gallons per minute at the end of the 10-minute period, then at least 500 gallons have flowed out of the tank.

8. At a construction site, money is spent at a continuous, decreasing rate of $r(t)$ dollars per day, where t is in days. If the rates at two particular instants, $t = 3$ and $t = 5$, are given in the table, then at least \$3000 is spent between $t = 3$ and $t = 5$.

t	3	5
$r(t)$	1000	800

9. An object traveling with velocity given by $v(t) = 3t$ feet per second travels exactly 150 feet when $0 \leq t \leq 10$ seconds.

10. The units of total change and rate of change of a quantity are the same.

11. If $f(t)$ is increasing, then the left-hand sum gives an overestimate of $\int_a^b f(t)\,dt$.

12. If $f(t)$ is concave up, then the left-hand sum gives an overestimate of $\int_a^b f(t)\,dt$.

13. A left-hand sum estimate for $\int_3^5 f(t)\,dt$ is 3000, if $f(t)$ is shown in the following table.

t	3	5
$f(t)$	1000	800

14. A right-hand sum estimate for $\int_3^5 f(t)\,dt$ is 1600, if $f(t)$ is shown in the following table.

t	3	5
$f(t)$	1000	800

15. If the number of terms in a Riemann sum increases, the quantity Δt decreases.

16. A 4-term Riemann sum on the interval $4 \leq t \leq 6$ has $\Delta t = 2$.

17. The right-hand sum for $\int_a^b f(t)\,dt$ is the total area of rectangles that are above the graph of $f(t)$.

18. If $f(t) \geq 0$ then $\int_a^b f(t)\,dt$ is the area between the t-axis and the graph of $f(t)$, for $a \leq t \leq b$.

19. If $f(t) = t^2$ then the left-hand sum gives an overestimate for $\int_{-2}^{-1} f(t)\,dt$.

20. The right-hand sum for $\int_5^{25} t^2\,dt$ using $n = 5$ rectangles has $\Delta t = 5$.

21. The integral $\int_0^2 f(x)\,dx$ gives the area between the x-axis and the graph of $f(x)$ between $x = 0$ and $x = 2$.

22. If $\int_0^2 f(x)\,dx = 0$ then $f(x) = 0$ for all $0 \leq x \leq 2$.

23. If $\int_0^2 f(x)\,dx > 0$ then $f(x) > 0$ for all $0 \leq x \leq 2$.

24. If $f(x) > 0$ for all $0 \leq x \leq 2$ then $\int_0^2 f(x)\,dx > 0$.

25. The integral $\int_{-1}^{1} (x^2 - 1)\,dx$ is the negative of the area between the graph of $f(x) = x^2 - 1$ and the x-axis for $-1 \leq x \leq 1$.

26. If $f(x)$ is both positive and negative when $0 \leq x \leq 2$ then $\int_0^2 f(x)\,dx$ is the sum of the areas between the graph and the x-axis for $0 \leq x \leq 2$.

27. The integral $\int_0^3 (1 - x)\,dx$ is the area between the graph of $f(x) = 1 - x$ and the x-axis between $x = 0$ and $x = 3$.

28. The integral $\int_{-1}^{2} e^x\,dx$ is the area between the graph of $f(x) = e^x$ and the x-axis between $x = -1$ and $x = 2$.

29. If $f(x) \geq g(x)$ for all $a \leq x \leq b$ then $\int_a^b f(x) - g(x)\,dx$ gives the area between the graphs of $f(x)$ and $g(x)$ for $a \leq x \leq b$.

30. If the graph of $f(x)$ has more area below the x-axis than above the x-axis when $1 \leq x \leq 10$ then $\int_1^{10} f(x)\,dx$ is negative.

31. If flow rate $r(t)$ has units gallons per hour, and t has units in hours, then $\int_0^{100} r(t)\,dt$ has units of gallons.

32. If expense rate $s(t)$ has units dollars per day, and t has units in days, then $\int_{20}^{35} s(t)\,dt$ has units of days.

33. If acceleration $a(t)$ has units feet/(second)^2, and t has units in seconds, then $\int_{2.1}^{7.2} a(t)\,dt$ has units of feet/second.

34. If $w(t)$ is the number of workers on a building construction site as a function of t, the number of days since the start of construction, then $\int_0^{60} w(t)\,dt$ has units of workers per day.

35. If $C(t)$ is the rate, in dollars per day, for electricity to cool and heat a home on day t, where t is measured in days since January 1, then $\int_0^{365} C(t)\,dt$ has units of dollars.

36. If electricity costs $f(t)$ dollars per day, and t is measured in days, then $\int_0^{30} f(t)\,dt$ gives the total cost of electricity, in dollars, for the 30-day period from $t = 0$ to $t = 30$.

37. If $f(t)$ gives the rate of change of water in a reservoir, in gallons per day, and t is measured in days, then $\int_0^{30} f(t)\,dt$ gives the total volume of water, in gallons, in the reservoir on day $t = 30$.

38. If $f(t)$ gives the rate of change of water in a reservoir, in gallons per day, and t is measured in days, then $\int_0^{30} f(t)\,dt$ gives the total change in the volume of water, in gallons, in the reservoir during the period $t = 0$ to $t = 30$.

39. Bioavailability is the integral of blood concentration as a function of time.

40. If the peak concentration of drug A is greater than the peak concentration of drug B then the bioavailability of drug A is greater than the bioavailability of drug B.

41. The Fundamental Theorem of Calculus says if $F(t)$ is continuous, then $\int_a^b F(t)\,dt = F(b) - F(a)$.

42. The Fundamental Theorem of Calculus says if $g'(t)$ is continuous, then $\int_a^b g'(t)\,dt = g(b) - g(a)$.

43. The Fundamental Theorem of Calculus says if $F'(t)$ is continuous, then $\int_a^b F'(t)\,dt = F'(b) - F'(a)$.

44. If $C(q)$ is the cost to produce q units, then $\int_{100}^{200} C'(q)\,dq$ is the amount it costs to increase production from 100 to 200 units.

45. If $C(q)$ is the cost to produce q units, then $\int_0^{1000} C'(q)\,dq$ is the total amount it costs to produce 1000 units.

46. If the marginal cost function of a product is $C'(q) = 0.03q + 0.1$ dollars, and the fixed costs are \$1500, then the total cost to produce 1000 items is \$15,100.

47. The integral of the marginal cost $C'(q)$ function can be used to find the fixed costs.

48. If $\int_0^5 F'(t)\,dt = 0$, then F is constant on the interval between $t = 0$ and $t = 5$.

49. If $\int_0^5 F'(t)\,dt < 0$, then $F(0) > F(5)$.

50. If $F'(t)$ is constant, then $\int_0^5 F'(t)\,dt = 0$.

PROJECTS FOR CHAPTER FIVE

1. **Carbon Dioxide in Pond Water** Biological activity in a pond is reflected in the rate at which carbon dioxide, CO_2, is added to or withdrawn from the water. Plants take CO_2 out of the water during the day for photosynthesis and put CO_2 into the water at night. Animals put CO_2 into the water all the time as they breathe. Biologists are interested in how the net rate at which CO_2 enters a pond varies during the day. Figure 5.76 shows this rate as a function of time of day.[9] The rate is measured in millimoles (mmol) of CO_2 per liter of water per hour; time is measured in hours past dawn. At dawn, there were 2.600 mmol of CO_2 per liter of water.
   (a) What can be concluded from the fact that the rate is negative during the day and positive at night?
   (b) Some scientists have suggested that plants respire (breathe) at a constant rate at night, and that they photosynthesize at a constant rate during the day. Does Figure 5.76 support this view?
   (c) When was the CO_2 content of the water at its lowest? How low did it go?
   (d) How much CO_2 was released into the water during the 12 hours of darkness? Compare this quantity with the amount of CO_2 withdrawn from the water during the 12 hours of daylight. How can you tell by looking at the graph whether the CO_2 in the pond is in equilibrium?
   (e) Estimate the CO_2 content of the water at three-hour intervals throughout the day. Use your estimates to plot a graph of CO_2 content throughout the day.

[9] Data from R. J. Beyers, *The Pattern of Photosynthesis and Respiration in Laboratory Microsystems* (Mem. 1st Ital. Idrobiol., 1965).

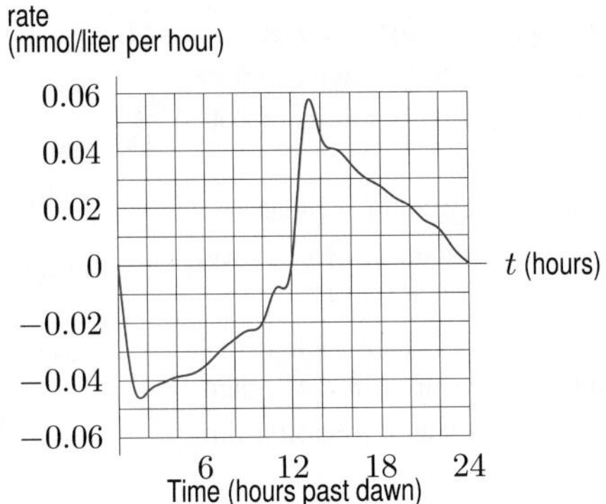

Figure 5.76: Rate at which CO_2 is entering the pond

2. Flooding in the Grand Canyon

The Glen Canyon Dam at the top of the Grand Canyon prevents natural flooding. In 1996, scientists decided an artificial flood was necessary to restore the environmental balance. Water was released through the dam at a controlled rate[10] shown in Figure 5.77. The figure also shows the rate of flow of the last natural flood in 1957.

(a) At what rate was water passing through the dam in 1996 before the artificial flood?
(b) At what rate was water passing down the river in the pre-flood season in 1957?
(c) Estimate the maximum rates of discharge for the 1996 and 1957 floods.
(d) Approximately how long did the 1996 flood last? How long did the 1957 flood last?
(e) Estimate how much additional water passed down the river in 1996 as a result of the artificial flood.
(f) Estimate how much additional water passed down the river in 1957 as a result of the flood.

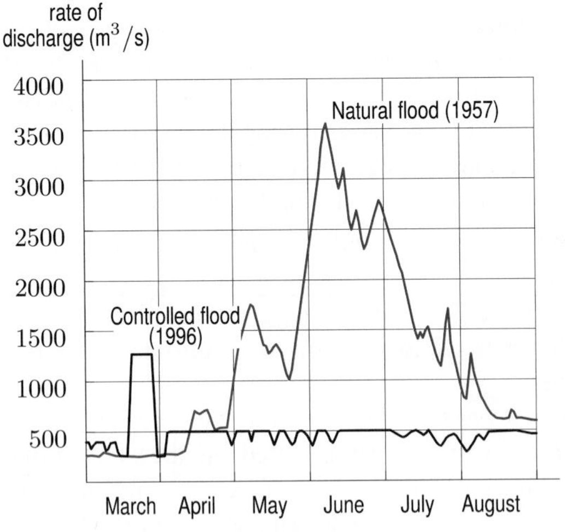

Figure 5.77

[10]Adapted from M. Collier, R. Webb, E. Andrews, "Experimental Flooding in Grand Canyon" in *Scientific American* (January 1997).

FOCUS ON THEORY

THEOREMS ABOUT DEFINITE INTEGRALS

The Second Fundamental Theorem of Calculus

The Fundamental Theorem of Calculus tells us that if we have a function F whose derivative is a continuous function f, then the definite integral of f is given by

$$\int_a^b f(t)\,dt = F(b) - F(a).$$

We now take a different point of view. If a is fixed and the upper limit is x, then the value of the integral is a function of x. We define a new function G on the interval by

$$G(x) = \int_a^x f(t)\,dt.$$

To visualize G, suppose that f is positive and $x > a$. Then $G(x)$ is the area under the graph of f in Figure 5.78. If f is continuous on an interval containing a, then it can be shown that G is defined for all x on that interval.

We now consider the derivative of G. Using the definition of the derivative,

$$G'(x) = \lim_{h\to 0} \frac{G(x+h) - G(x)}{h}.$$

Suppose f and h are positive. Then we can visualize

$$G(x) = \int_a^x f(t)\,dt$$

and

$$G(x+h) = \int_a^{x+h} f(t)\,dt$$

as areas, which leads to representing

$$G(x+h) - G(x) = \int_x^{x+h} f(t)\,dt$$

as a difference of two areas.

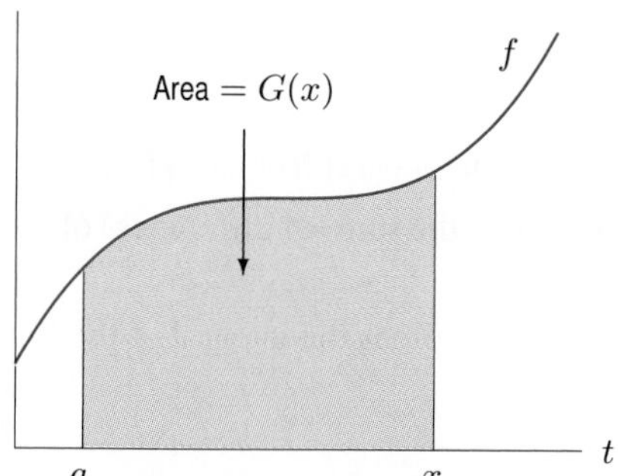

Figure 5.78: Representing $G(x)$ as an area

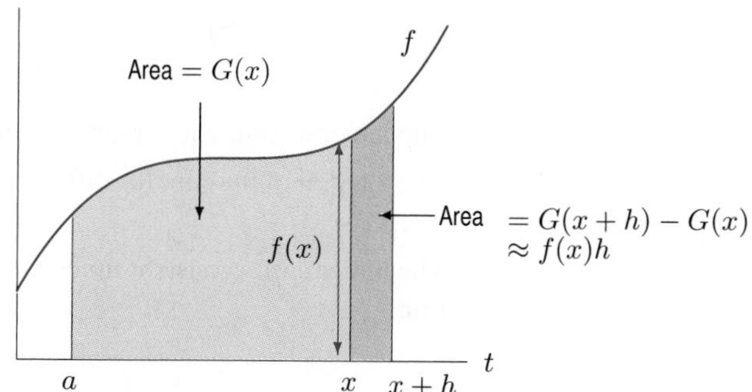

Figure 5.79: $G(x+h) - G(x)$ is the area of a roughly rectangular region

From Figure 5.79, we see that, if h is small, $G(x+h)-G(x)$ is roughly the area of a rectangle of height $f(x)$ and width h (shaded darker in Figure 5.79), so we have

$$G(x+h)-G(x)\approx f(x)h,$$

hence

$$\frac{G(x+h)-G(x)}{h}\approx f(x).$$

The same result holds when h is negative, suggesting that

$$G'(x)=\lim_{h\to 0}\frac{G(x+h)-G(x)}{h}=f(x).$$

This result is another form of the Fundamental Theorem of Calculus. It is usually stated as follows:

Second Fundamental Theorem of Calculus

If f is a continuous function on an interval, and if a is any number in that interval, then the function G defined on the interval by

$$G(x)=\int_a^x f(t)\,dt$$

has derivative f; that is, $G'(x)=f(x)$.

Properties of the Definite Integral

In this chapter, we have used the following properties to break up definite integrals.

Sums and Multiples of Definite Integrals

If a, b, and c are any numbers and f and g are continuous functions, then

1. $\displaystyle\int_a^c f(x)\,dx+\int_c^b f(x)\,dx=\int_a^b f(x)\,dx.$
2. $\displaystyle\int_a^b (f(x)\pm g(x))\,dx=\int_a^b f(x)\,dx\pm\int_a^b g(x)\,dx.$
3. $\displaystyle\int_a^b cf(x)\,dx=c\int_a^b f(x)\,dx.$

In words:

1. The integral from a to c plus the integral from c to b is the integral from a to b.
2. The integral of the sum (or difference) of two functions is the sum (or difference) of their integrals.
3. The integral of a constant times a function is that constant times the integral of the function.

These properties can best be visualized by thinking of the integrals as areas or as the limit of the sum of areas of rectangles.

Problems on the Second Fundamental Theorem of Calculus

For Problems 1–4, find $G'(x)$.

1. $G(x) = \int_a^x t^3\,dt$

2. $G(x) = \int_a^x 3^t\,dt$

3. $G(x) = \int_a^x te^t\,dt$

4. $G(x) = \int_a^x \ln y\,dy$

5. Let $F(b) = \int_0^b 2^x\,dx$.

(a) What is $F(0)$?

(b) Does the value of F increase or decrease as b increases? (Assume $b \geq 0$.)

(c) Estimate $F(1)$, $F(2)$, and $F(3)$.

6. For $x = 0, 0.5, 1.0, 1.5$, and 2.0, make a table of values for $I(x) = \int_0^x \sqrt{t^4+1}\,dt$.

7. Assume that $F'(t) = \sin t \cos t$ and $F(0) = 1$. Find $F(b)$ for $b = 0,\ 0.5,\ 1,\ 1.5,\ 2,\ 2.5$, and 3.

Let $\int_a^b f(x)\,dx = 8$, $\int_a^b (f(x))^2\,dx = 12$, $\int_a^b g(t)\,dt = 2$, and $\int_a^b (g(t))^2\,dt = 3$. Find the integrals in Problems 8–11.

8. $\int_a^b (f(x) + g(x))\,dx$

9. $\int_a^b \left((f(x))^2 - (g(x))^2\right)dx$

10. $\int_a^b (f(x))^2\,dx - (\int_a^b f(x)\,dx)^2$

11. $\int_a^b cf(z)\,dz$

Chapter Six

USING THE DEFINITE INTEGRAL

Contents

6.1 AVERAGE VALUE

In this section we show how to interpret the definite integral as the average value of a function.

The Definite Integral as an Average

We know how to find the average of n numbers: Add them and divide by n. But how do we find the average value of a continuously varying function? Let us consider an example. Suppose $f(t)$ is the temperature at time t, measured in hours since midnight, and that we want to calculate the average temperature over a 24-hour period. One way to start would be to average the temperatures at n equally spaced times, $t_1, t_2, \ldots, t_n$, during the day.

$$\text{Average temperature} \approx \frac{f(t_1) + f(t_2) + \cdots + f(t_n)}{n}.$$

The larger we make n, the better the approximation. We can rewrite this expression as a Riemann sum over the interval $0 \le t \le 24$ if we use the fact that $\Delta t = 24/n$, so $n = 24/\Delta t$:

$$\begin{aligned}\text{Average temperature} &\approx \frac{f(t_1) + f(t_2) + \cdots + f(t_n)}{24/\Delta t} \\ &= \frac{f(t_1)\Delta t + f(t_2)\Delta t + \cdots + f(t_n)\Delta t}{24} \\ &= \frac{1}{24}\sum_{i=1}^{n} f(t_i)\Delta t.\end{aligned}$$

As $n \to \infty$, the Riemann sum tends toward an integral, and the approximation gets better. We expect that

$$\begin{aligned}\text{Average temperature} &= \lim_{n\to\infty} \frac{1}{24}\sum_{i=1}^{n} f(t_i)\Delta t \\ &= \frac{1}{24}\int_0^{24} f(t)\, dt.\end{aligned}$$

Generalizing for any function f, if $a < b$, we have

$$\begin{array}{c}\text{Average value of } f \\ \text{on the interval from } a \text{ to } b\end{array} = \frac{1}{b-a}\int_a^b f(x)\, dx.$$

The units of $f(x)$ are the same as the units of the average value of $f(x)$.

How to Visualize the Average on a Graph

The definition of average value tells us that

$$(\text{Average value of } f) \cdot (b - a) = \int_a^b f(x)\, dx.$$

Let's interpret the integral as the area under the graph of f. If $f(x)$ is positive, then the average value of f is the height of a rectangle whose base is $(b - a)$ and whose area is the same as the area between the graph of f and the x-axis. (See Figure 6.1.)

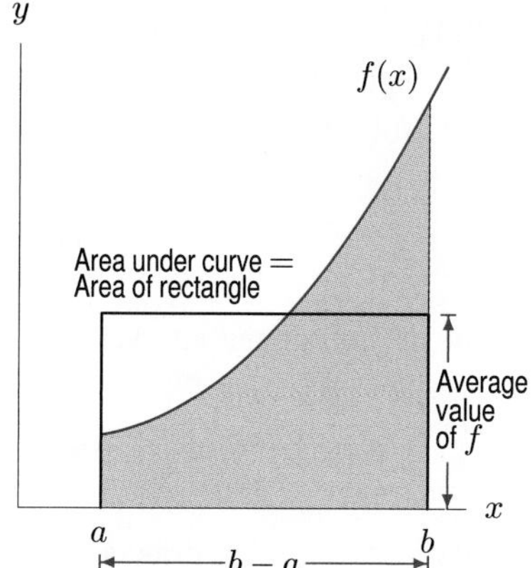

Figure 6.1: Area and average value

Example 1 Suppose that $C(t)$ represents the daily cost of heating your house, in dollars per day, where t is time in days and $t = 0$ corresponds to January 1, 2010. Interpret $\dfrac{1}{90-0}\displaystyle\int_0^{90} C(t)\,dt$.

Solution The units for the integral $\int_0^{90} C(t)\,dt$ are (dollars/day)×(days) = dollars. The integral represents the total cost in dollars to heat your house for the first 90 days of 2010, namely the months of January, February, and March. The expression $\frac{1}{90-0}\int_0^{90} C(t)\,dt$ represents the average cost per day to heat your house during the first 90 days of 2010. It is measured in (1/days) × (dollars) = dollars/day, the same units as $C(t)$.

Example 2 The population of McAllen, Texas can be modeled by the function

$$P = f(t) = 570(1.037)^t,$$

where P is in thousands of people and t is in years since 2000. Use this function to predict the average population of McAllen between the years 2020 and 2040.

Solution We want the average value of $f(t)$ between $t = 20$ and $t = 40$. Using a calculator to evaluate the integral, we get

$$\text{Average population} = \frac{1}{40-20}\int_{20}^{40} f(t)\,dt = \frac{1}{20}(34{,}656.2) = 1732.81.$$

The average population of McAllen between 2020 and 2040 is predicted to be about 1733 thousand people.

Example 3 (a) For the function $f(x)$ graphed in Figure 6.2, evaluate $\displaystyle\int_0^5 f(x)\,dx$.

(b) Find the average value of $f(x)$ on the interval $x = 0$ to $x = 5$. Check your answer graphically.

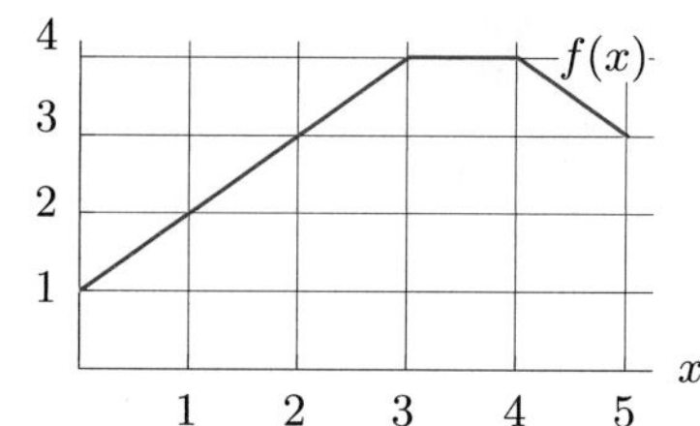

Figure 6.2: Estimate $\int_0^5 f(x)dx$

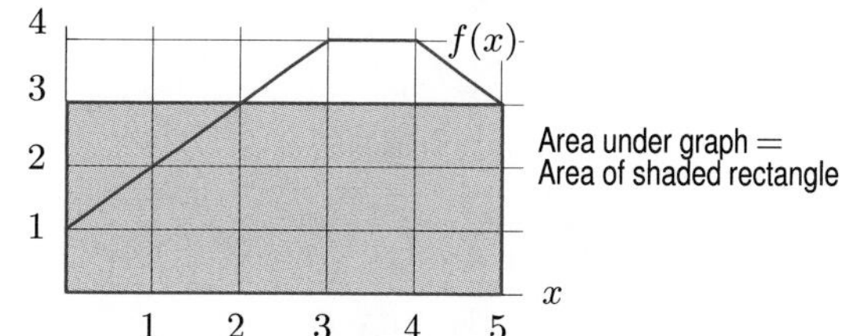

Figure 6.3: Average value of $f(x)$ is 3

Solution (a) Since $f(x) \geq 0$, the definite integral is the area of the region under the graph of $f(x)$ between $x = 0$ and $x = 5$. Figure 6.2 shows that this region consists of 13 full grid squares and 4 half grid squares, each grid square of area 1, for a total area of 15, so

$$\int_0^5 f(x)\,dx = 15.$$

(b) The average value of $f(x)$ on the interval from 0 to 5 is given by

$$\text{Average value} = \frac{1}{5-0}\int_0^5 f(x)\,dx = \frac{1}{5}(15) = 3.$$

To check the answer graphically, draw a horizontal line at $y = 3$ on the graph of $f(x)$. (See Figure 6.3.) Then observe that, between $x = 0$ and $x = 5$, the area under the graph of $f(x)$ is equal to the area of the rectangle with height 3.

Problems for Section 6.1

1. What is the average value of the function f in Figure 6.4 over the interval $1 \leq x \leq 6$?

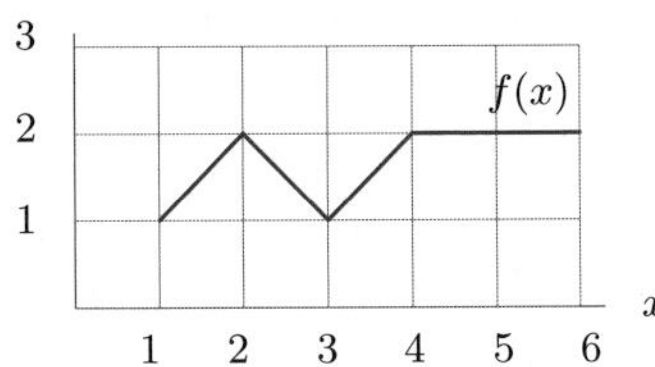

Figure 6.4

2. Use Figure 6.5 to estimate the following:

(a) The integral $\int_0^5 f(x)\,dx$.
(b) The average value of f between $x = 0$ and $x = 5$ by estimating visually the average height.
(c) The average value of f between $x = 0$ and $x = 5$ by using your answer to part (a).

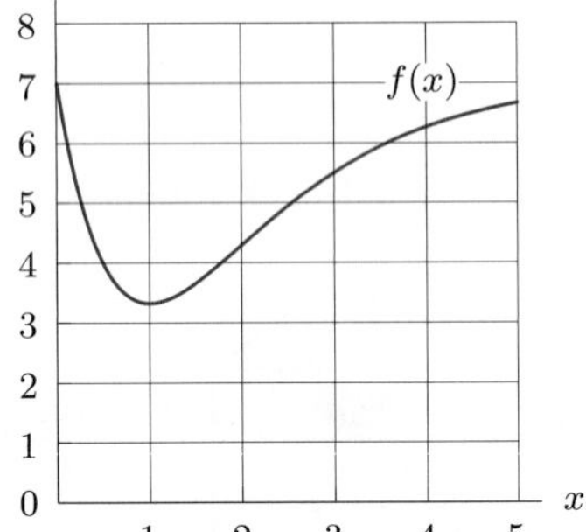

Figure 6.5

3. Find the average value of $g(t) = 1 + t$ over the interval $[0, 2]$

4. Find the average value of the function $f(x) = 5 + 4x - x^2$ between $x = 0$ and $x = 3$.

In Problems 5–6, estimate the average value of the function between $x = 0$ and $x = 7$.

5.

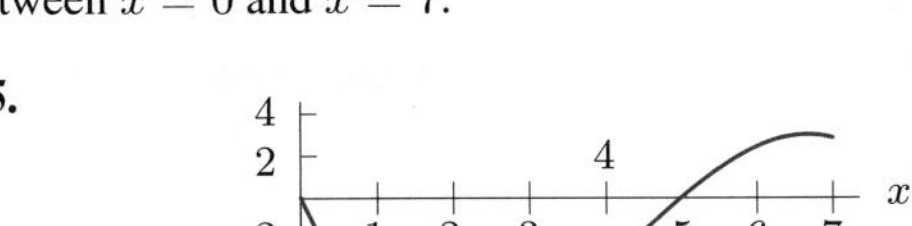
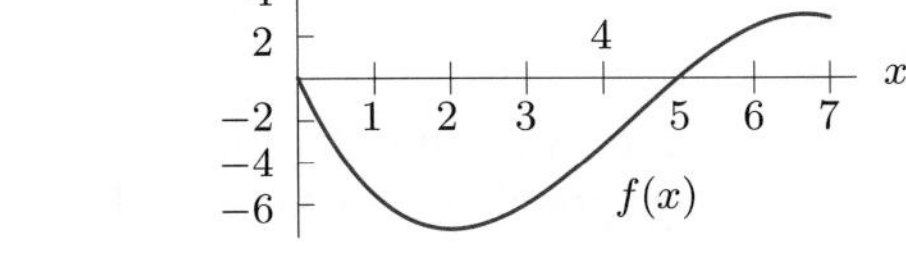

6.

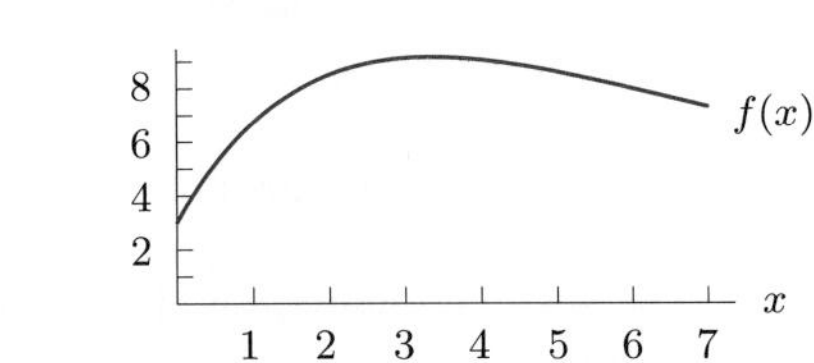

In Problems 7–8, estimate the average value of the function $f(x)$ on the interval from $x = a$ to $x = b$.

7.

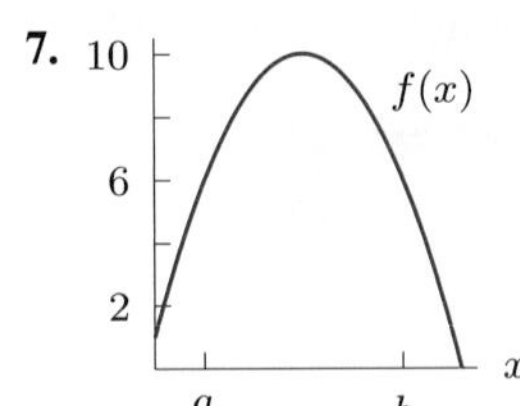

8.

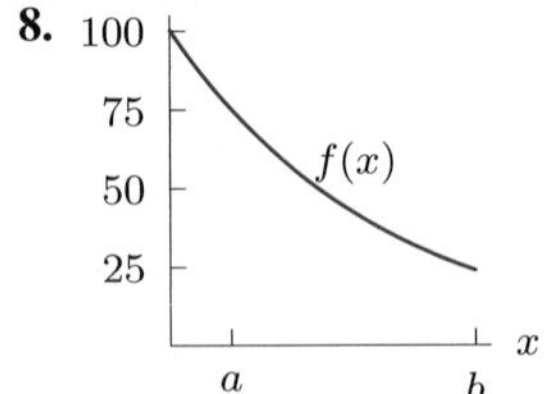

In Problems 9–10 annual income for ages 25 to 85 is given graphically. People sometimes spend less than their income (to save for retirement) or more than their income (taking out a loan). The process of spreading out spending over a lifetime is called consumption smoothing.

(a) Find the average annual income for these years.

(b) Assuming that the person spends at a constant rate equal to their average income, when are they spending less than they earn, and when are they spending more?

9.

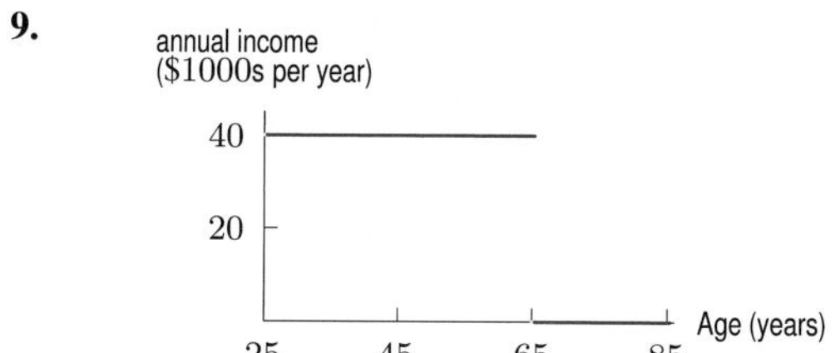

10.

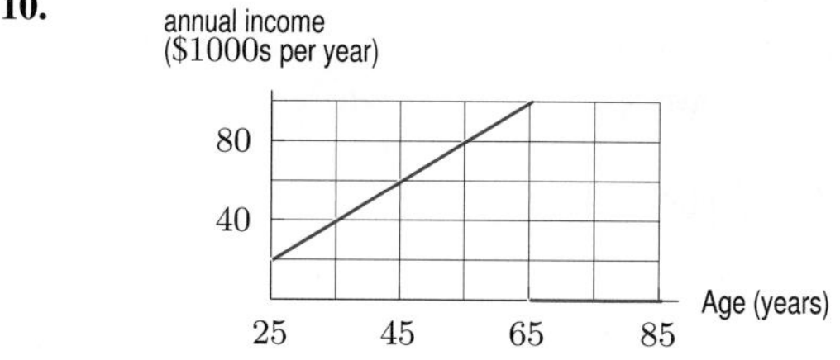

11. The value, V, of a Tiffany lamp, worth \$225 in 1975, increases at 15% per year. Its value in dollars t years after 1975 is given by

$$V = 225(1.15)^t.$$

Find the average value of the lamp over the period 1975–2010.

12. If t is measured in days since June 1, the inventory $I(t)$ for an item in a warehouse is given by

$$I(t) = 5000(0.9)^t.$$

(a) Find the average inventory in the warehouse during the 90 days after June 1.

(b) Graph $I(t)$ and illustrate the average graphically.

Problems 13–14 refer to Figure 6.6, which shows human arterial blood pressure during the course of one heartbeat.

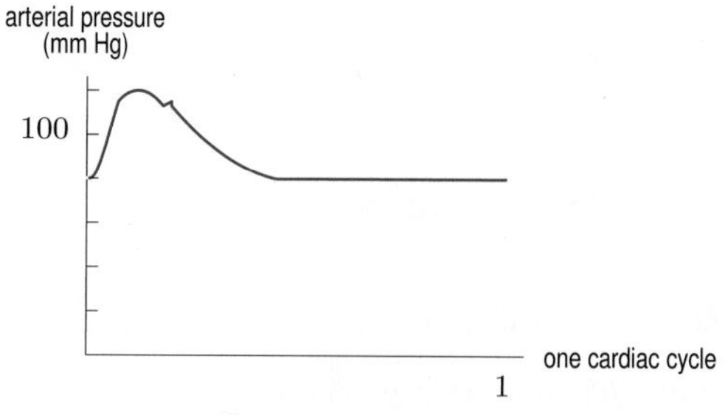

Figure 6.6

13. **(a)** Estimate the maximum blood pressure, called the systolic pressure.

(b) Estimate the minimum blood pressure, called the diastolic pressure.

(c) Calculate the average of the systolic and diastolic pressures.

(d) Is the average arterial pressure over the entire cycle greater than, less than, or equal to the answer for part (c)?

14. Estimate the average arterial blood pressure over one cardiac cycle.

15. Figure 6.7 shows the rate, $f(x)$, in thousands of algae per hour, at which a population of algae is growing, where x is in hours.

(a) Estimate the average value of the rate over the interval $x = -1$ to $x = 3$.

(b) Estimate the total change in the population over the interval $x = -3$ to $x = 3$.

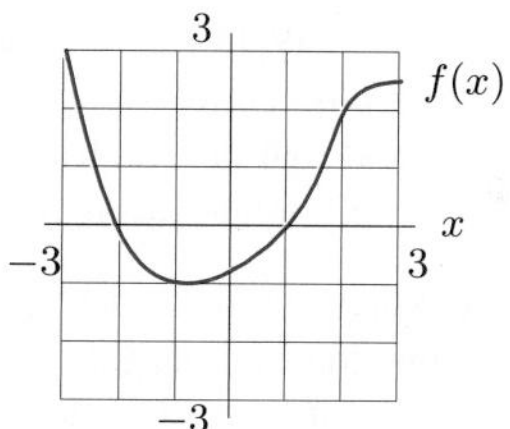

Figure 6.7

16. The population of the world t years after 2000 is predicted to be $P = 6.1e^{0.0125t}$ billion.

(a) What population is predicted in 2010?

(b) What is the predicted average population between 2000 and 2010?

17. The number of hours, H, of daylight in Madrid as a function of date is approximated by the formula

$$H = 12 + 2.4\sin[0.0172(t - 80)],$$

where t is the number of days since the start of the year. Find the average number of hours of daylight in Madrid:

(a) in January **(b)** in June **(c)** over a year

(d) Explain why the relative magnitudes of your answers to parts (a), (b), and (c) are reasonable.

18. A bar of metal is cooling from 1000°C to room temperature, 20°C. The temperature, H, of the bar t minutes after it starts cooling is given, in °C, by

$$H = 20 + 980e^{-0.1t}.$$

(a) Find the temperature of the bar at the end of one hour.

(b) Find the average value of the temperature over the first hour.
(c) Is your answer to part (b) greater or smaller than the average of the temperatures at the beginning and the end of the hour? Explain this in terms of the concavity of the graph of H.

19. The rate of sales (in sales per month) of a company is given, for t in months since January 1, by

$$r(t) = t^4 - 20t^3 + 118t^2 - 180t + 200.$$

(a) Graph the rate of sales per month during the first year ($t = 0$ to $t = 12$). Does it appear that more sales were made during the first half of the year, or during the second half?
(b) Estimate the total sales during the first 6 months of the year and during the last 6 months of the year.
(c) What are the total sales for the entire year?
(d) Find the average sales per month during the year.

20. Throughout much of the 20th century, the yearly consumption of electricity in the US increased exponentially at a continuous rate of 7% per year. Assume this trend continues and that the electrical energy consumed in 1900 was 1.4 million megawatt-hours.

(a) Write an expression for yearly electricity consumption as a function of time, t, in years since 1900.
(b) Find the average yearly electrical consumption throughout the 20th century.
(c) During what year was electrical consumption closest to the average for the century?
(d) Without doing the calculation for part (c), how could you have predicted which half of the century the answer would be in?

21. Using Figure 6.8, list the following numbers from least to greatest:

(a) $f'(1)$
(b) The average value of f on $0 \le x \le 4$
(c) $\int_0^1 f(x)dx$

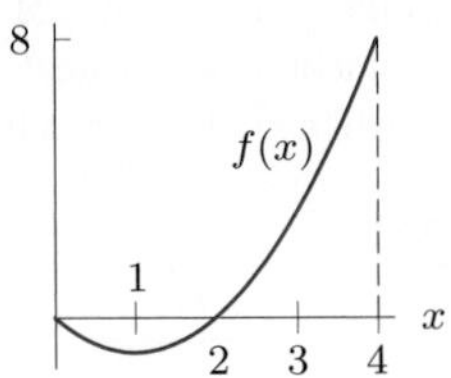

Figure 6.8

22. Using Figure 6.9, list from least to greatest,

(a) $f'(1)$.
(b) The average value of $f(x)$ on $0 \le x \le a$.
(c) The average value of the rate of change of $f(x)$, for $0 \le x \le a$.
(d) $\int_0^a f(x)\,dx$.

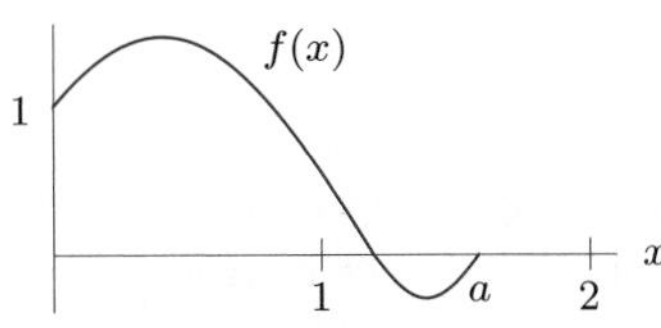

Figure 6.9

6.2 CONSUMER AND PRODUCER SURPLUS

Supply and Demand Curves

As we saw in Chapter 1, the quantity of a certain item produced and sold can be described by the supply and demand curves of the item. The *supply curve* shows what quantity, q, of the item the producers supply at different prices, p. The consumers' behavior is reflected in the *demand curve*, which shows what quantity of goods are bought at various prices. See Figure 6.10.

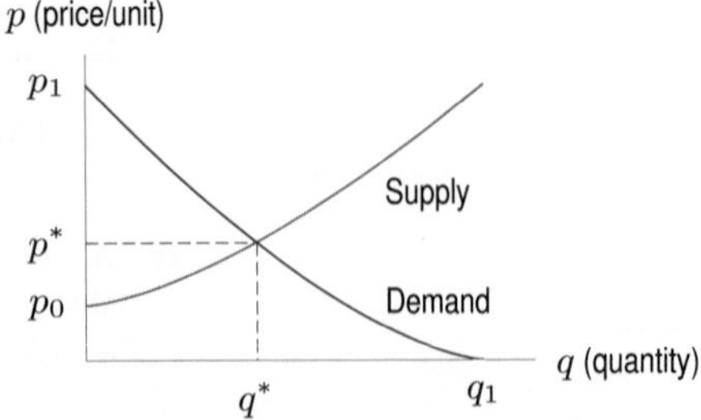

Figure 6.10: Supply and demand curves

It is assumed that the market settles at the *equilibrium price* p^* and *equilibrium quantity* q^* where the graphs cross. At equilibrium, a quantity q^* of an item is produced and sold for a price of p^* each.

Consumer and Producer Surplus

Notice that at equilibrium, a number of consumers have bought the item at a lower price than they would have been willing to pay. (For example, there are some consumers who would have been willing to pay prices up to p_1.) Similarly, there are some suppliers who would have been willing to produce the item at a lower price (down to p_0, in fact). We define the following terms:

- The **consumer surplus** measures the consumers' gain from trade. It is the total amount gained by consumers by buying the item at the current price rather than at the price they would have been willing to pay.
- The **producer surplus** measures the suppliers' gain from trade. It is the total amount gained by producers by selling at the current price, rather than at the price they would have been willing to accept.

In the absence of price controls, the current price is assumed to be the equilibrium price.

Both consumers and producers are richer for having traded. The consumer and producer surplus measure how much richer they are.

Suppose that all consumers buy the good at the maximum price they are willing to pay. Subdivide the interval from 0 to q^* into intervals of length Δq. Figure 6.11 shows that a quantity Δq of items are sold at a price of about p_1, another Δq are sold for a slightly lower price of about p_2, the next Δq for a price of about p_3, and so on. Thus, the consumers' total expenditure is about

$$p_1\Delta q + p_2\Delta q + p_3\Delta q + \cdots = \sum p_i \Delta q.$$

If the demand curve has equation[1] $p = f(q)$, and if all consumers who were willing to pay more than p^* paid as much as they were willing, then as $\Delta q \to 0$, we would have

$$\begin{array}{c}\text{Consumer}\\ \text{expenditure}\end{array} = \int_0^{q^*} f(q)\,dq = \begin{array}{c}\text{Area under demand}\\ \text{curve from 0 to } q^*.\end{array}$$

If all goods are sold at the equilibrium price, the consumers' actual expenditure is only p^*q^*, which is the area of the rectangle between the q-axis and the line $p = p^*$ from $q = 0$ to $q = q^*$. The consumer surplus is the difference between the total consumer expenditure if all consumers pay the maximum they are willing to pay and the actual consumer expenditure if all consumers pay the current price. The consumer surplus is represented by the area in Figure 6.12. Similarly, the producer surplus is represented by the area in Figure 6.13. (See Problems 14 and 15.) Thus:

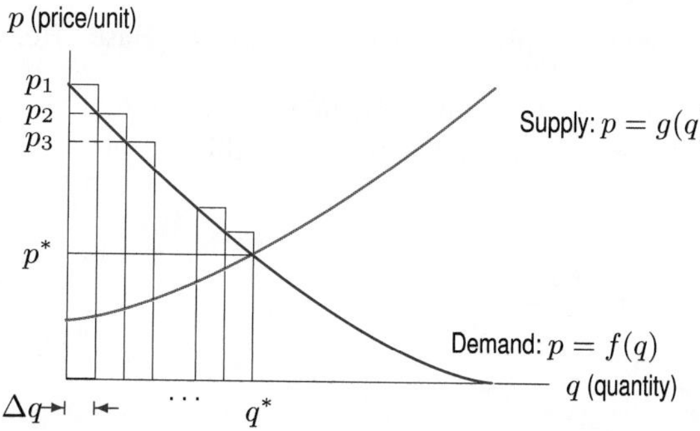

Figure 6.11: Calculation of consumer surplus

[1] Note that here p is written as a function of q.

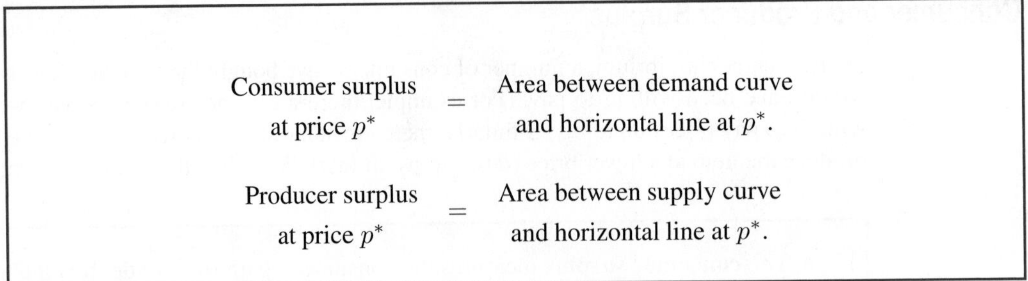

Consumer surplus at price p^* = Area between demand curve and horizontal line at p^*.

Producer surplus at price p^* = Area between supply curve and horizontal line at p^*.

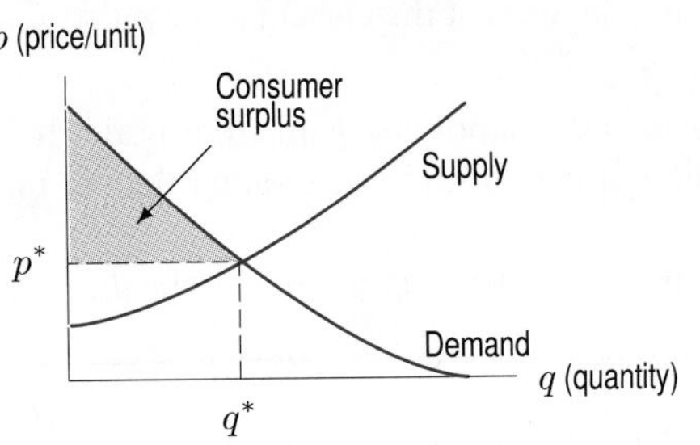

Figure 6.12: Consumer surplus

Figure 6.13: Producer surplus

Example 1 The supply and demand curves for a product are given in Figure 6.14.

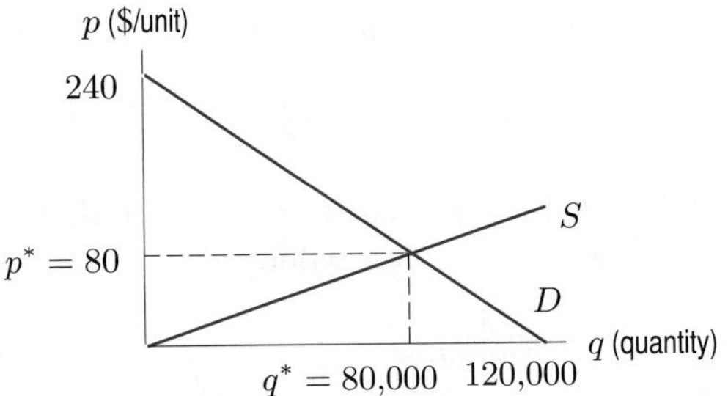

Figure 6.14: Supply and demand curves for a product

(a) What are the equilibrium price and quantity?
(b) At the equilibrium price, calculate and interpret the consumer and producer surplus.

Solution (a) The equilibrium price is $p^* = \$80$ and the equilibrium quantity is $q^* = 80{,}000$ units.
(b) The consumer surplus is the area under the demand curve and above the line $p = 80$. (See Figure 6.15.) We have

$$\text{Consumer surplus} = \text{Area of triangle} = \frac{1}{2}\text{Base} \cdot \text{Height} = \frac{1}{2}80{,}000 \cdot 160 = \$6{,}400{,}000.$$

This tells us that consumers gain \$6,400,000 in buying goods at the equilibrium price instead of at the price they would have been willing to pay.

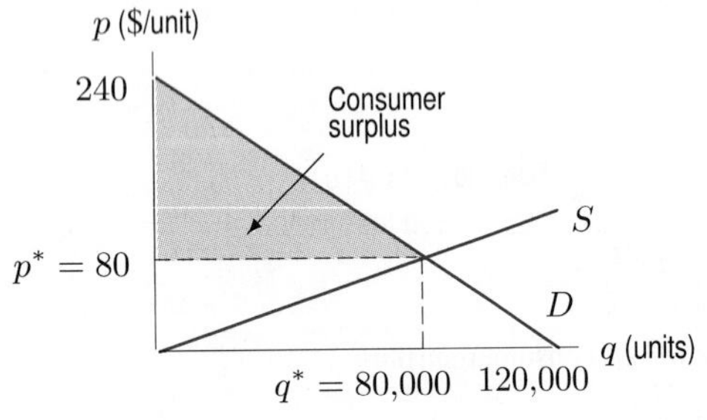

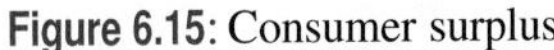

Figure 6.15: Consumer surplus

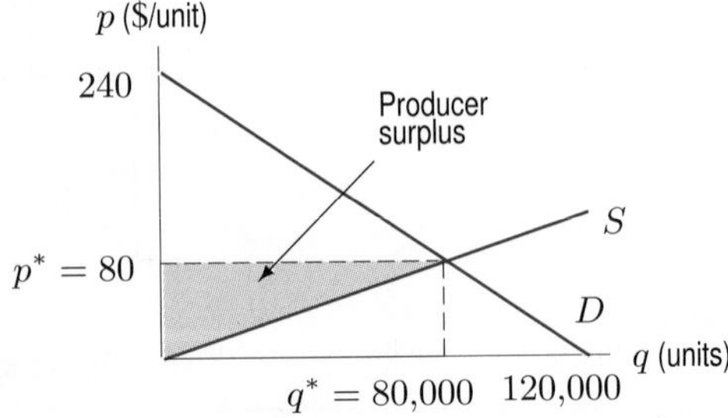

Figure 6.16: Producer surplus

The producer surplus is the area above the supply curve and below the line $p = 80$. (See Figure 6.16.) We have

$$\text{Producer surplus} = \text{Area of triangle} = \frac{1}{2}\text{Base} \cdot \text{Height} = \frac{1}{2} \cdot 80{,}000 \cdot 80 = \$3{,}200{,}000.$$

So, producers gain \$3,200,000 by supplying goods at the equilibrium price instead of the price at which they would have been willing to provide the goods.

Wage and Price Controls

In a free market, the price of a product generally moves to the equilibrium price, unless outside forces keep the price artificially high or artificially low. Rent control, for example, keeps prices below market value, whereas cartel pricing or the minimum wage law raise prices above market value. What happens to consumer and producer surplus at non-equilibrium prices?

Example 2 The dairy industry has cartel pricing: the government has set milk prices artificially high. What effect does raising the price to p^+ from the equilibrium price have on:

(a) Consumer surplus? (b) Producer surplus?

(c) Total gains from trade (that is, Consumer surplus + Producer surplus)?

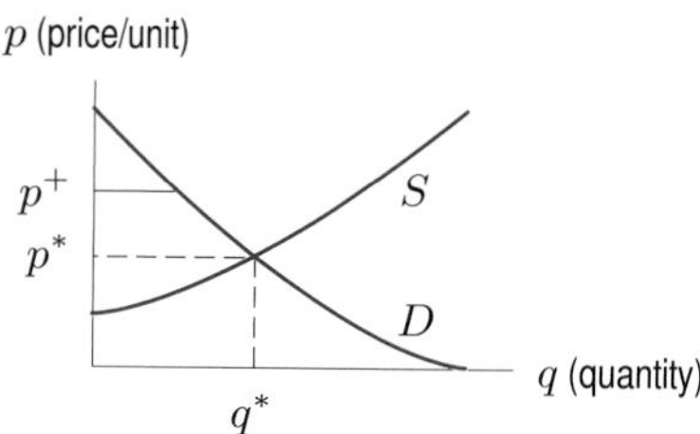

Figure 6.17: What is the effect of the artificially high price, p^+, on consumer and producer surplus? (q^* and p^* are equilibrium values)

Solution (a) A graph of possible supply and demand curves for the milk industry is given in Figure 6.17. Suppose that the price is fixed at p^+, above the equilibrium price. Consumer surplus is the difference between the amount the consumers paid (p^+) and the amount they would have been willing to pay (given on the demand curve). This is the area shaded in Figure 6.18. This consumer surplus is less than the consumer surplus at the equilibrium price, shown in Figure 6.19.

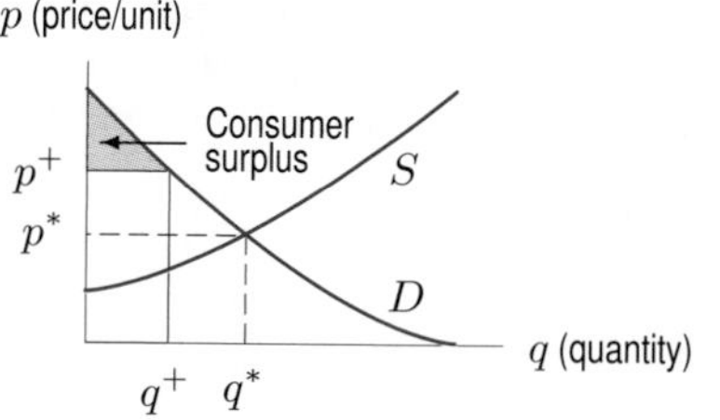

Figure 6.18: Consumer surplus: Artificial price

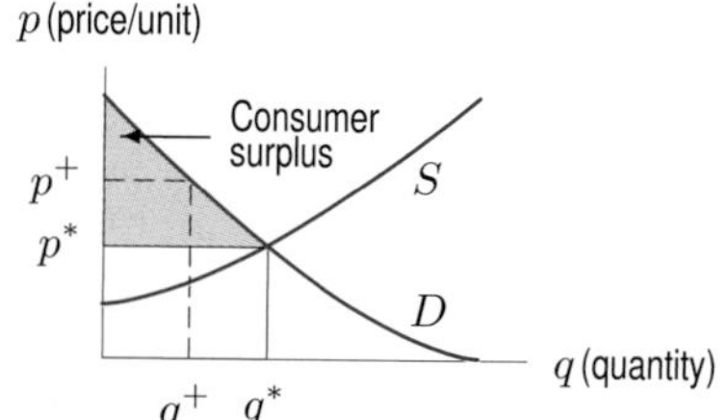

Figure 6.19: Consumer surplus: Equilibrium price

(b) At a price of p^+, the quantity sold, q^+, is less than it would have been at the equilibrium price. The producer surplus is represented by the area between p^+ and the supply curve at this reduced demand. This area is shaded in Figure 6.20. Compare this producer surplus (at the artificially high price) to the producer surplus in Figure 6.21 (at the equilibrium price). In this case, producer surplus appears to be greater at the artificial price than at the equilibrium price. (However, different supply and demand curves might lead to a different answer.)

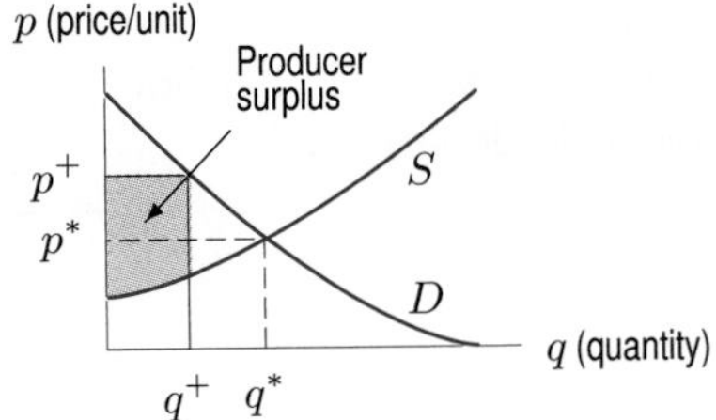

Figure 6.20: Producer surplus: Artificial price

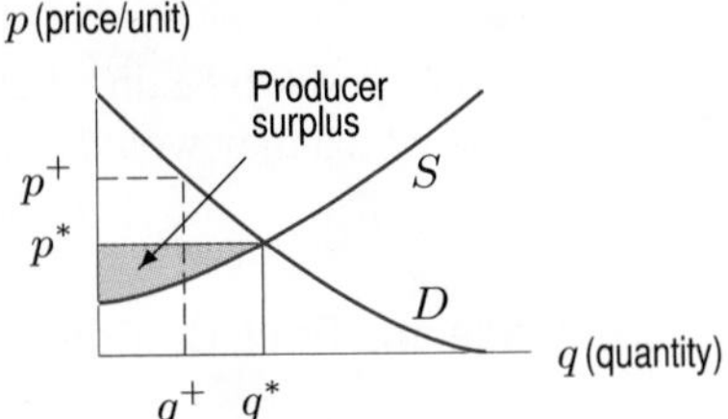

Figure 6.21: Producer surplus: Equilibrium price

(c) The total gains from trade (Consumer surplus + Producer surplus) at the price of p^+ is represented by the area shaded in Figure 6.22. The total gains from trade at the equilibrium price of p^* is represented by the area shaded in Figure 6.23. Under artificial price conditions, the total gains from trade decrease. The total financial effect of the artificially high price on all producers and consumers combined is negative.

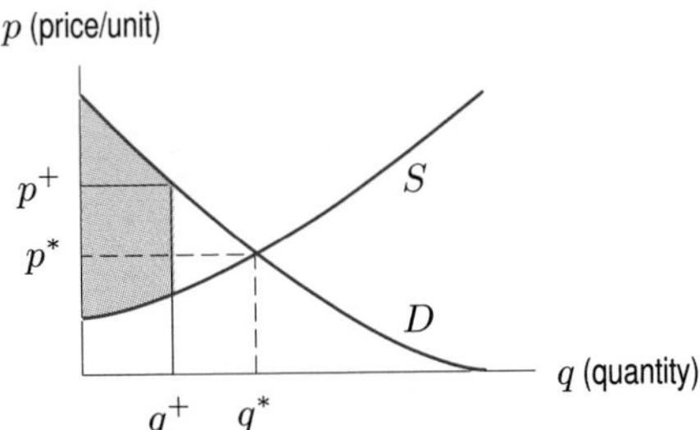

Figure 6.22: Total gains from trade: Artificial price

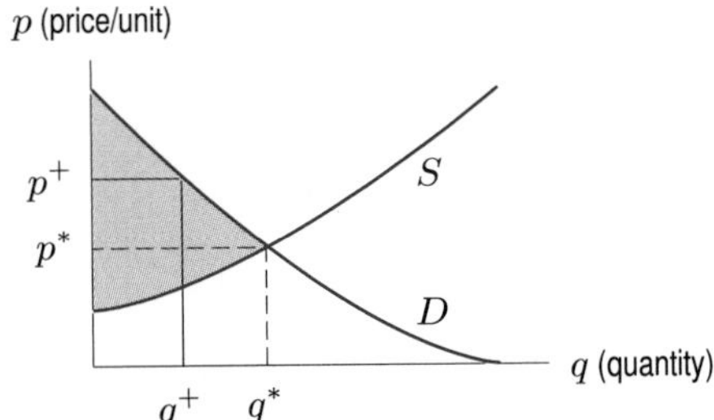

Figure 6.23: Total gains from trade: Equilibrium price

Problems for Section 6.2

1. **(a)** What are the equilibrium price and quantity for the supply and demand curves in Figure 6.24?
   (b) Shade the areas representing the consumer and producer surplus and estimate them.

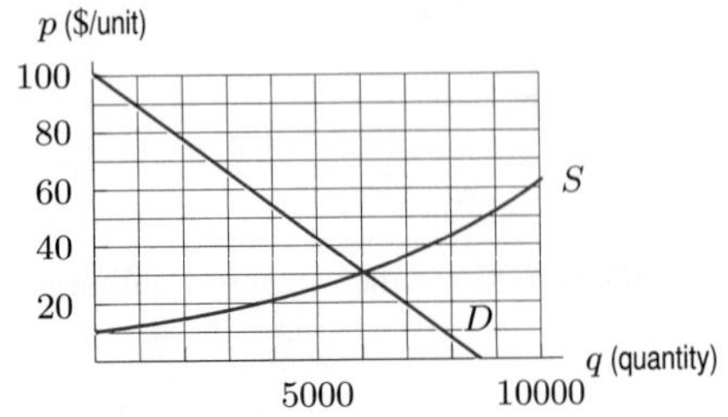

Figure 6.24

2. The supply and demand curves for a product are given in Figure 6.25. Estimate the equilibrium price and quantity and the consumer and producer surplus. Shade areas representing the consumer surplus and the producer surplus.

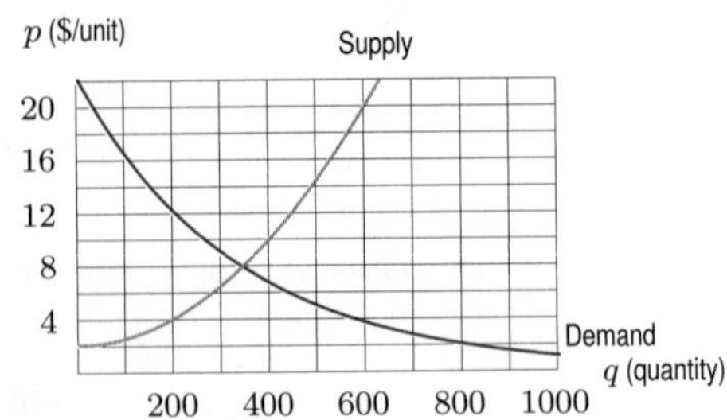

Figure 6.25

3. Find the consumer surplus for the demand curve $p = 100 - 3q^2$ when 5 units are sold.

4. Given the demand curve $p = 35 - q^2$ and the supply curve $p = 3 + q^2$, find the producer surplus when the market is in equilibrium.

5. Find the consumer surplus for the demand curve $p = 100 - 4q$ when $q = 10$.

6. **(a)** Estimate the equilibrium price and quantity for the supply and demand curves in Figure 6.26.
(b) Estimate the consumer and producer surplus.
(c) The price is set artificially low at $p^- = 4$ dollars per unit. Estimate the consumer and producer surplus at this price. Compare your answers to the consumer and producer surplus at the equilibrium price.

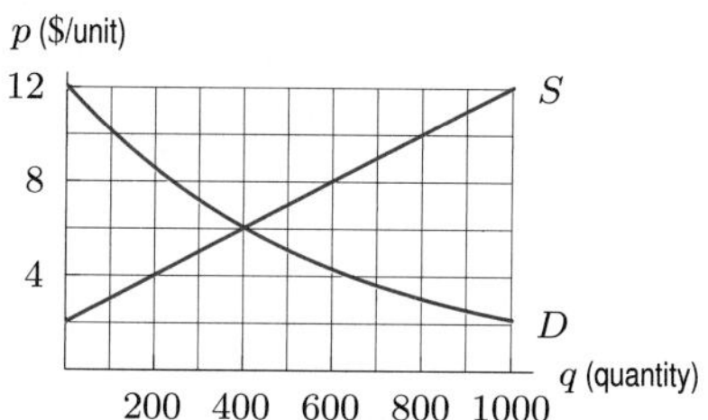

Figure 6.26

7. Supply and demand curves for a product are in Figure 6.27.

(a) Estimate the equilibrium price and quantity.
(b) Estimate the consumer and producer surplus. Shade them.
(c) What are the total gains from trade for this product?

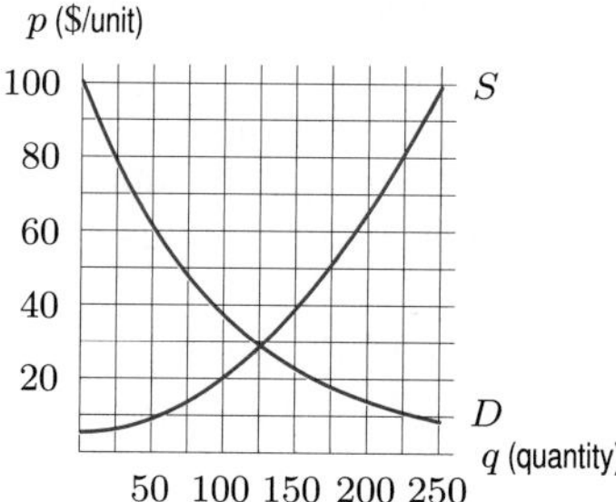

Figure 6.27

8. Supply and demand curves are in Figure 6.27. A price of \$40 is artificially imposed.

(a) At the \$40 price, estimate the consumer surplus, the producer surplus, and the total gains from trade.
(b) Compare your answers in this problem to your answers in Problem 7. Discuss the effect of price controls on the consumer surplus, producer surplus, and gains from trade in this case.

9. The demand curve for a product has equation $p = 20e^{-0.002q}$ and the supply curve has equation $p = 0.02q + 1$ for $0 \le q \le 1000$, where q is quantity and p is price in \$/unit.

(a) Which is higher, the price at which 300 units are supplied or the price at which 300 units are demanded? Find both prices.
(b) Sketch the supply and demand curves. Find the equilibrium price and quantity.
(c) Using the equilibrium price and quantity, calculate and interpret the consumer and producer surplus.

10. Show graphically that the maximum total gains from trade occurs at the equilibrium price. Do this by showing that if outside forces keep the price artificially high or low, the total gains from trade (consumer surplus + producer surplus) are lower than at the equilibrium price.

11. Rent controls on apartments are an example of price controls on a commodity. They keep the price artificially low (below the equilibrium price). Sketch a graph of supply and demand curves, and label on it a price p^- below the equilibrium price. What effect does forcing the price down to p^- have on:

(a) The producer surplus?
(b) The consumer surplus?
(c) The total gains from trade (Consumer surplus + Producer surplus)?

12. Supply and demand data are in Tables 6.1 and 6.2.

(a) Which table shows supply and which shows demand?
(b) Estimate the equilibrium price and quantity.
(c) Estimate the consumer and producer surplus.

Table 6.1

q (quantity)	0	100	200	300	400	500	600
p (\$/unit)	60	50	41	32	25	20	17

Table 6.2

q (quantity)	0	100	200	300	400	500	600
p (\$/unit)	10	14	18	22	25	28	34

13. The total gains from trade (consumer surplus + producer surplus) is largest at the equilibrium price. What about the consumer surplus and producer surplus separately?

(a) Suppose a price is artificially high. Can the consumer surplus at the artificial price be larger than the consumer surplus at the equilibrium price? What about the producer surplus? Sketch possible supply and demand curves to illustrate your answers.
(b) Suppose a price is artificially low. Can the consumer surplus at the artificial price be larger than the consumer surplus at the equilibrium price? What about the producer surplus? Sketch possible supply and demand curves to illustrate your answers.

In Problems 14–16, the supply and demand curves have equations $p = S(q)$ and $p = D(q)$, respectively, with equilibrium at (q^*, p^*).

14. Using Riemann sums, explain the economic significance of $\int_0^{q^*} S(q)\,dq$ to the producers.

15. Using Riemann sums, give an interpretation of producer surplus, $\int_0^{q^*} (p^* - S(q))\,dq$ analogous to the interpretation of consumer surplus.

16. Referring to Figures 6.12 and 6.13 on page 282, mark the regions representing the following quantities and explain their economic meaning:

(a) p^*q^* **(b)** $\int_0^{q^*} D(q)\,dq$

(c) $\int_0^{q^*} S(q)\,dq$ **(d)** $\int_0^{q^*} D(q)\,dq - p^*q^*$

(e) $p^*q^* - \int_0^{q^*} S(q)\,dq$ **(f)** $\int_0^{q^*} (D(q) - S(q))\,dq$

6.3 PRESENT AND FUTURE VALUE

In Chapter 1 on page 54, we introduced the present and future value of a single payment. In this section we see how to calculate the present and future value of a continuous stream of payments.

Income Stream

When we consider payments made to or by an individual, we usually think of *discrete* payments, that is, payments made at specific moments in time. However, we may think of payments made by a company as being *continuous*. The revenues earned by a huge corporation, for example, come in essentially all the time, and therefore they can be represented by a continuous *income stream*. Since the rate at which revenue is earned may vary from time to time, the income stream is described by

$$S(t) \text{ dollars/year.}$$

Notice that $S(t)$ is a *rate* at which payments are made (its units are dollars per year, for example) and that the rate depends on the time, t, usually measured in years from the present.

Present and Future Values of an Income Stream

Just as we can find the present and future values of a single payment, so we can find the present and future values of a stream of payments. As before, the future value represents the total amount of money that you would have if you deposited an income stream into a bank account as you receive it and let it earn interest until that future date. The present value represents the amount of money you would have to deposit today (in an interest-bearing bank account) in order to match what you would get from the income stream by that future date.

When we are working with a continuous income stream, we will assume that interest is compounded continuously. If the interest rate is r, the present value, P, of a deposit, B, made t years in the future is

$$P = Be^{-rt}.$$

Suppose that we want to calculate the present value of the income stream described by a rate of $S(t)$ dollars per year, and that we are interested in the period from now until M years in the future. In order to use what we know about single deposits to calculate the present value of an income stream, we divide the stream into many small deposits, and imagine each deposited at one instant. Dividing the interval $0 \le t \le M$ into subintervals of length Δt:

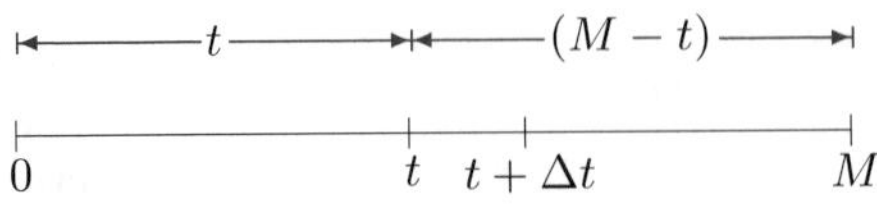

Assuming Δt is small, the rate, $S(t)$, at which deposits are being made does not vary much within one subinterval. Thus, between t and $t + \Delta t$:

$$\begin{aligned}\text{Amount paid} &\approx \text{Rate of deposits} \times \text{Time}\\ &\approx (S(t)\ \text{dollars/year})(\Delta t\ \text{years})\\ &= S(t)\Delta t\ \text{dollars.}\end{aligned}$$

The deposit of $S(t)\Delta t$ is made t years in the future. Thus, assuming a continuous interest rate r,

$$\begin{matrix}\text{Present value of money}\\ \text{deposited in interval } t \text{ to } t+\Delta t\end{matrix} \approx S(t)\Delta t e^{-rt}.$$

Summing over all subintervals gives

$$\text{Total present value} \approx \sum S(t)e^{-rt}\Delta t \text{ dollars.}$$

In the limit as $\Delta t \to 0$, we get the following integral:

$$\text{Present value} = \int_0^M S(t)e^{-rt}dt.$$

As in Section 1.7, the value M years in the future is given by

$$\text{Future value} = \text{Present value} \cdot e^{rM}.$$

Example 1 Find the present and future values of a constant income stream of \$1000 per year over a period of 20 years, assuming an interest rate of 6% compounded continuously.

Solution Using $S(t) = 1000$ and $r = 0.06$, we have

$$\text{Present value} = \int_0^{20} 1000e^{-0.06t}dt = \$11{,}647.$$

We can get the future value, B, from the present value, P, using $B = Pe^{rt}$, so

$$\text{Future value} = 11{,}647e^{0.06(20)} = \$38{,}669.$$

Notice that since money was deposited at a rate of \$1000 a year for 20 years, the total amount deposited was \$20,000. The future value is \$38,669, so the money has almost doubled because of the interest.

Example 2 Suppose you want to have \$50,000 in 8 years' time in a bank account earning 2% interest, compounded continuously.

(a) If you make one lump sum deposit now, how much should you deposit?

(b) If you deposit money continuously throughout the 8-year period, at what rate should you deposit it?

Solution (a) If you deposit a lump sum of \$$P$, then \$$P$ is the present value of \$50,000. So, using $B = Pe^{rt}$ with $B = 50{,}000$ and $r = 0.02$ and $t = 8$:

$$\begin{aligned}50000 &= Pe^{0.02(8)}\\ P &= \frac{50000}{e^{0.02(8)}} = 42{,}607.\end{aligned}$$

If you deposit \$42,607 into the account now, you will have \$50,000 in 8 years' time.

(b) Suppose you deposit money at a constant rate of $\$S$ per year. Then

$$\text{Present value of deposits} = \int_0^8 Se^{-0.02t}\,dt$$

Since S is a constant, we can take it out in front of the integral sign:

$$\text{Present value} = S\int_0^8 e^{-0.02t}\,dt \approx S(7.3928).$$

But the present value of the continuous deposit must be the same as the present value of the lump sum deposit; that is, \$42,607. So

$$42{,}607 \approx S(7.3928)$$
$$S \approx \$5763.$$

To meet your goal of \$50,000, you need to deposit money at a continuous rate of \$5,763 per year, or about \$480 per month.

Problems for Section 6.3

1. Find the present and future values of an income stream of \$3000 per year over a 15-year period, assuming a 6% annual interest rate compounded continuously.

2. Draw a graph, with time in years on the horizontal axis, of what an income stream might look like for a company that sells sunscreen in the northeast United States.

3. (a) Find the present and future value of an income stream of \$6000 per year for a period of 10 years if the interest rate, compounded continuously, is 5%.
   (b) How much of the future value is from the income stream? How much is from interest?

4. Find the present and future values of an income stream of \$12,000 a year for 20 years. The interest rate is 6%, compounded continuously.

5. A small business expects an income stream of \$5000 per year for a four-year period.
   (a) Find the present value of the business if the annual interest rate, compounded continuously, is
   (i) 3% (ii) 10%
   (b) In each case, find the value of the business at the end of the four-year period.

6. A bond is guaranteed to pay $100 + 10t$ dollars per year for 10 years, where t is in years from the present. Find the present value of this income stream, given an interest rate of 5%, compounded continuously.

7. A recently-installed machine earns the company revenue at a continuous rate of $60{,}000t + 45{,}000$ dollars per year during the first six months of operation and at the continuous rate of 75,000 dollars per year after the first six months. The cost of the machine is \$150,000, the interest rate is 7% per year, compounded continuously, and t is time in years since the machine was installed.
   (a) Find the present value of the revenue earned by the machine during the first year of operation.
   (b) Find how long it will take for the machine to pay for itself; that is, how long it will take for the present value of the revenue to equal the cost of the machine?

8. At what constant, continuous rate must money be deposited into an account if the account is to contain \$20,000 in 5 years? The account earns 6% interest compounded continuously.

9. Your company needs \$500,000 in two years' time for renovations and can earn 9% interest on investments.
   (a) What is the present value of the renovations?
   (b) If your company deposits money continuously at a constant rate throughout the two-year period, at what rate should the money be deposited so that you have the \$500,000 when you need it?

10. A company is expected to earn \$50,000 a year, at a continuous rate, for 8 years. You can invest the earnings at an interest rate of 7%, compounded continuously. You have the chance to buy the rights to the earnings of the company now for \$350,000. Should you buy? Explain.

11. Sales of Version 6.0 of a computer software package start out high and decrease exponentially. At time t, in years, the sales are $s(t) = 50e^{-t}$ thousands of dollars per year. After two years, Version 7.0 of the software is released and replaces Version 6.0. You can invest earnings at an interest rate of 6%, compounded continuously. Calculate the total present value of sales of Version 6.0 over the two-year period.

12. Intel Corporation is a leading manufacturer of integrated circuits. In 2004, Intel generated profits at a continuous rate of 7.5 billion dollars per year.[2] Assume the interest rate was 8.5% per year compounded continuously.

    (a) What was the present value of Intel's profits over the 2004 one-year time period?

    (b) What was the value at the end of the year of Intel's profits over the 2004 one-year time period?

13. Harley-Davidson Inc. manufactures motorcycles. During the years following 2003 (the company's 100th anniversary), the company's net revenue can be approximated[3] by $4.6 + 0.4t$ billion dollars per year, where t is time in years since January 1, 2003. Assume this rate holds through January 1, 2013, and assume a continuous interest rate of 3.5% per year.

    (a) What was the net revenue of the Harley-Davidson Company in 2003? What is the projected net revenue in 2013?

    (b) What was the present value, on January 1, 2003, of Harley-Davidson's net revenue for the ten years from January 1, 2003 to January 1, 2013?

    (c) What is the future value, on January 1, 2013, of net revenue for the preceding 10 years?

14. McDonald's Corporation licenses and operates a chain of 31,377 fast-food restaurants throughout the world. Between 2005 and 2008, McDonald's has been generating revenue at continuous rates between 17.9 and 22.8 billion dollars per year.[4] Suppose that McDonald's rate of revenue stays within this range. Use an interest rate of 4.5% per year compounded continuously. Fill in the blanks:

    (a) The present value of McDonald's revenue over a five-year time period is between ____________ and ____________ billion dollars.

    (b) The present value of McDonald's revenue over a twenty-five-year time period is between ____________ and ____________ billion dollars.

15. Your company is considering buying new production machinery. You want to know how long it will take for the machinery to pay for itself; that is, you want to find the length of time over which the present value of the profit generated by the new machinery equals the cost of the machinery. The new machinery costs \$130,000 and earns profit at the continuous rate of \$80,000 per year. Use an interest rate of 8.5% per year compounded continuously.

16. An oil company discovered an oil reserve of 100 million barrels. For time $t > 0$, in years, the company's extraction plan is a linear declining function of time as follows:

$$q(t) = a - bt,$$

    where $q(t)$ is the rate of extraction of oil in millions of barrels per year at time t and $b = 0.1$ and $a = 10$.

    (a) How long does it take to exhaust the entire reserve?

    (b) The oil price is a constant \$20 per barrel, the extraction cost per barrel is a constant \$10, and the market interest rate is 10% per year, compounded continuously. What is the present value of the company's profit?

17. The value of good wine increases with age. Thus, if you are a wine dealer, you have the problem of deciding whether to sell your wine now, at a price of $\$P$ a bottle, or to sell it later at a higher price. Suppose you know that the amount a wine-drinker is willing to pay for a bottle of this wine t years from now is $\$P(1 + 20\sqrt{t})$. Assuming continuous compounding and a prevailing interest rate of 5% per year, when is the best time to sell your wine?

6.4 INTEGRATING RELATIVE GROWTH RATES

Population Growth Rates

In Chapter 5, we saw how to calculate change in a population, P, from its derivative, dP/dt, using the Fundamental Theorem of Calculus. However, population growth rates are often given by the relative rate of change $(1/P)(dP/dt)$, rather than by the derivative. For example, we saw that the population of Nevada is growing at 3.6% per year.

We can use the relative growth rate to find the percentage change in a population. Recall that

$$\text{Relative growth rate} = \frac{1}{P}\frac{dP}{dt} = \frac{d}{dt}(\ln P).$$

By the Fundamental Theorem of Calculus, the integral of the relative growth rate gives the total change in $\ln(P)$:

$$\int_a^b \frac{P'(t)}{P(t)}\,dt = \int_a^b \frac{d}{dt}(\ln P(t))\,dt = \ln(P(b)) - \ln(P(a)) = \ln\left(\frac{P(b)}{P(a)}\right).$$

[2] www.intel.com, accessed May 28, 2005.
[3] 2007 Harley-Davidson Annual Report, accessed from www.harley-davidson.com.
[4] McDonald's Annual Report 2007 accessed at www.mcdonalds.com.

Example 1 The relative rate of growth $P'(t)/P(t)$ of a population $P(t)$ over a 50-year period is given in Figure 6.28. By what factor did the population increase during the period?

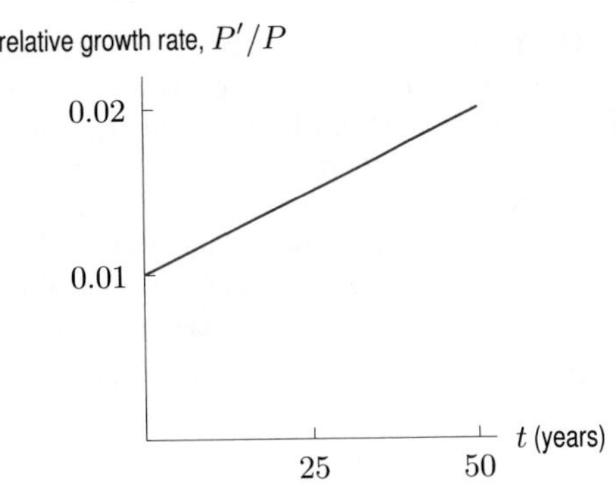

Figure 6.28: The relative growth rate of population

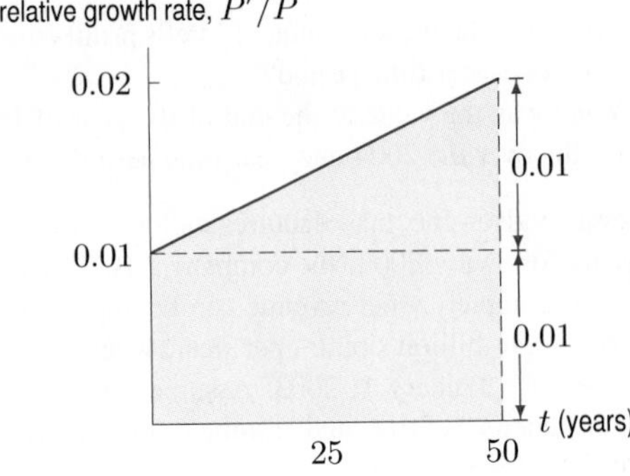

Figure 6.29: Calculating the percentage change in a population from the relative growth rate

Solution We have

$$\ln\left(\frac{P(50)}{P(0)}\right) = \int_0^{50} \frac{P'(t)}{P(t)}\,dt.$$

This integral equals the area under the graph of $P'(t)/P(t)$ between $t = 0$ and $t = 50$. See Figure 6.29. The area of a rectangle and triangle gives

$$\text{Area} = 50(0.01) + \frac{1}{2}\cdot 50(0.01) = 0.75.$$

Thus,

$$\begin{aligned}\ln\left(\frac{P(50)}{P(0)}\right) &= 0.75\\ \frac{P(50)}{P(0)} &= e^{0.75} = 2.1\\ P(50) &= 2.1P(0).\end{aligned}$$

The population more than doubled during the 50 years, increasing by a factor of about 2.1. We cannot determine the amount by which the population increased unless we know how large the population was initially.

If everything else remains constant, the relative growth rate increases if either the relative birth rate increases or the relative death rate decreases. Even if the relative birth rate decreases, we can still see an increase in the relative growth rate if the relative death rate decreases faster. This is the case with the population of the world today. The difference between the birth rate and the death rate is an important variable.

Example 2 Figure 6.30 shows relative birth rates and relative death rates for developed and developing countries.[5]

(a) Which is changing faster, the birth rate or the death rate? What does this tell you about how the populations are changing?

[5] *Food and Population: A Global Concern*, Elaine Murphy, Washington, DC: Population Reference Bureau, Inc., 1984, p. 2.

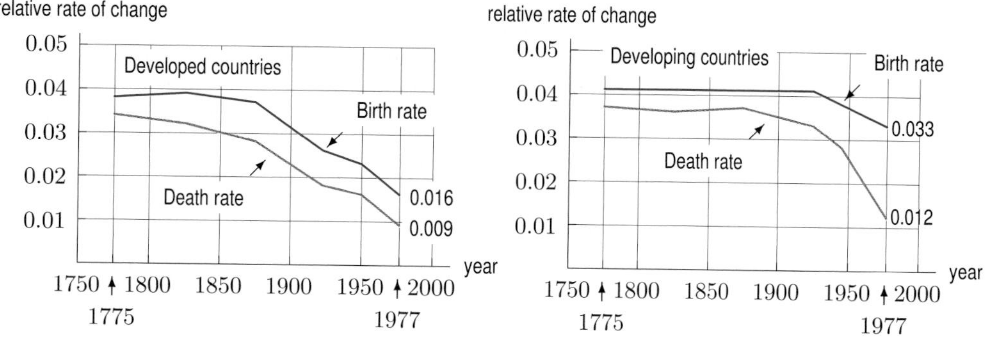

Figure 6.30: Birth and death rates in developed and developing countries, 1775-1977

(b) By what percentage did the population of developing countries increase between 1800 and 1900?

(c) By what percentage did the population of developing countries increase between 1950 and 1977?

Solution

(a) In developed countries, the birth rate is higher than the death rate, so the population is increasing. The birth rate and the death rate are both decreasing, and at approximately the same rate, so the population of developed countries is increasing at a constant relative rate.

In developing countries, the birth rate is higher than the death rate and both have been decreasing since about 1925. In recent years, the death rate has been decreasing faster than the birth rate, so the relative rate of population growth is increasing. The decline in the death rate has contributed significantly to the recent population growth in developing countries.

(b) The relative rate of growth of the population is the difference between the relative birth rate and the relative death rate, so it is represented in Figure 6.30 by the vertical distance between the birth-rate curve and the death-rate curve. The area of the region between the two curves from 1800 to 1900, shown in Figure 6.31, gives the change in $\ln P(t)$. The region has area approximately equal to a rectangle of height 0.005 and width 100, so has area 0.5. We have

$$\ln\left(\frac{P(1900)}{P(1800)}\right) = \int_{1800}^{1900} \frac{P'(t)}{P(t)}\,dt \approx 0.5$$

$$\frac{P(1900)}{P(1800)} \approx e^{0.5} = 1.65$$

During the nineteenth century the population of developing countries increased by about 65%, a factor of 1.65.

(c) The shaded region between the birth rate and death rate curves from 1950 to 1977 in Figure 6.31 consists of approximately 1.5 rectangles, each of which has area $(0.01)(27) = 0.27$. The area of this region is approximately (1.5) (0.27) = 0.405. We have

$$\ln\left(\frac{P(1977)}{P(1950)}\right) = \int_{1950}^{1977} \frac{P'(t)}{P(t)}\,dt \approx 0.405,$$

so

$$\frac{P(1977)}{P(1950)} \approx e^{0.405} = 1.50$$

Between 1950 and 1977, the population of developing countries increased by about 50%, a factor of 1.5.

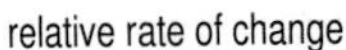

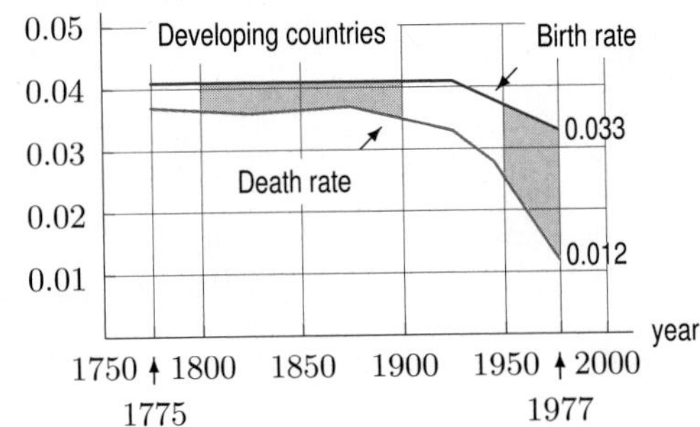

Figure 6.31: Relative growth rate of population = Relative birth rate − Relative death rate

Problems for Section 6.4

1. A town has a population of 1000. Fill in the table assuming that the town's population grows by

(a) 50 people per year **(b)** 5% per year

Year	0	1	2	3	4	...	10
Population	1000					...	

2. Birth and death rates are often reported as births or deaths per thousand members of the population. What is the relative rate of growth of a population with a birth rate of 30 births per 1000 and a death rate of 20 deaths per 1000?

3. The relative growth rate of a population is given in Figure 6.32. By what percentage does the population change over the 10-year period?

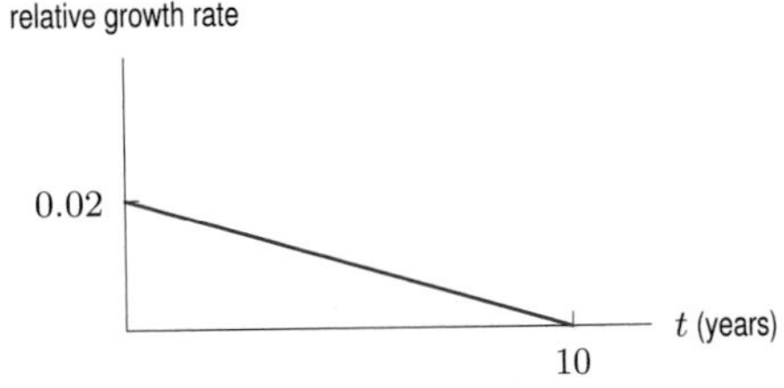

Figure 6.32

4. The article "Job Scene: What's Hot, What's Not in the Next 10 Years," appearing in the *Chicago Tribune* in July 1996, contained the following quote about predicted change in jobs between 1995 and 2005:

- Employment is projected to increase to 144.7 million from 127 million – only **14** percent. The growth rate was **24** percent from 1983 to 1994.
- Jobs in services and retail trades are expected to increase by **16.2** million. Business services, health and education will account for **9.1** million new jobs.
- Manufacturing will lose **1.3** million jobs, a continuation of its decline.
- Jobs for those with master's degrees will grow the most, **28** percent.

(a) The first number in bold is 14. Is this an absolute change, a relative change, an absolute rate of change, or a relative rate of change? Find each of the other three measures of change, corresponding to 14.

(b) Identify each of the numbers in bold as an absolute change, a relative change, an absolute rate of change, or a relative rate of change.

5. Table 6.3 shows the cumulative number of AIDS deaths worldwide.[6] Find the absolute increase in AIDS deaths between 2003 and 2004 and between 2006 and 2007. Find the relative increase between 2003 and 2004 and between 2006 and 2007.

Table 6.3 *Cumulative AIDS deaths worldwide, in millions*

Year	2003	2004	2005	2006	2007
Cases	30.2	33.3	35.5	37.6	39.6

6. A population is 100 at time $t = 0$, with t in years.

(a) If the population has a constant absolute growth rate of 10 people per year, find a formula for the size of the population at time t.

(b) If the population has a constant relative growth rate of 10% per year, find a formula for the size of the population at time t.

(c) Graph both functions on the same axes.

[6] www.unaids.org, May 2009.

7. The size of a bacteria population is 4000. Find a formula for the size, P, of the population t hours later if the population is decreasing by

(a) 100 bacteria per hour **(b)** 5% per hour

In which case does the bacteria population reach 0 first?

8. The relative growth rate of a population $P(t)$ is given in Figure 6.33. By what percentage does the population change over the 8-year period? If the population was 10,000 at time $t = 0$, what is the population 8 years later?

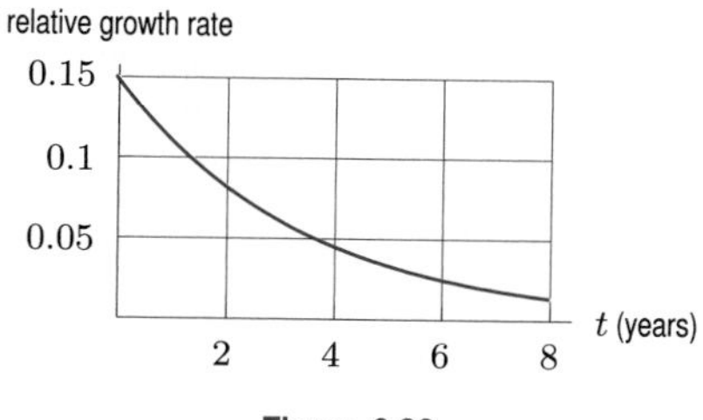

Figure 6.33

In Problems 9–12, a graph of the relative rate of change of a population is given with t in years. By approximately what percentage does the population change over the 10-year period?

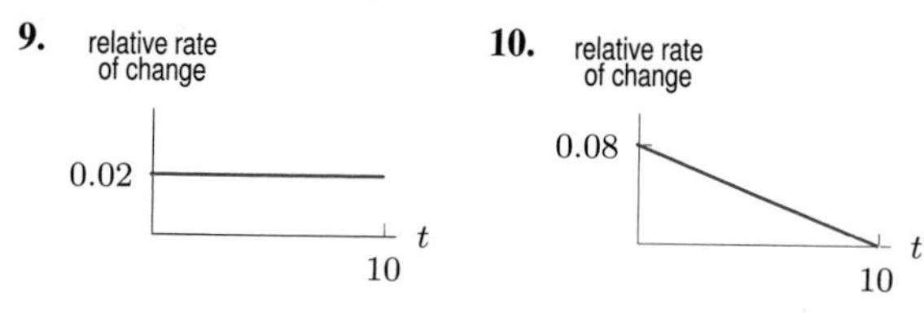

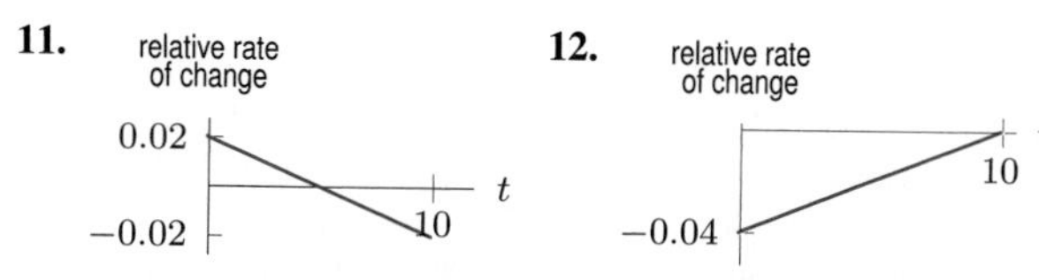

Problems 13–16 show the relative rate of change of f for $0 \leq t \leq 10$. Give the intervals on which f is increasing and on which f is decreasing.

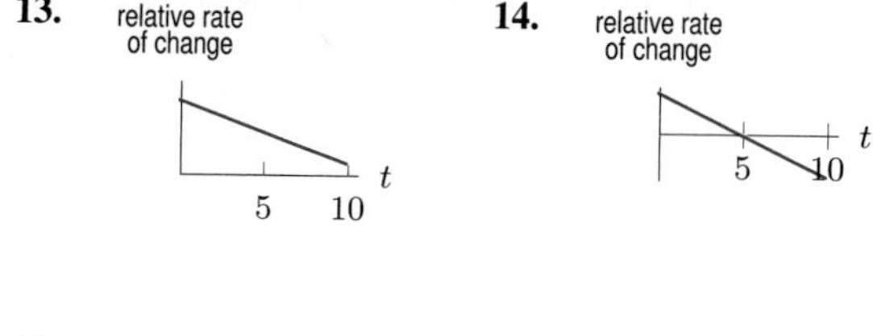

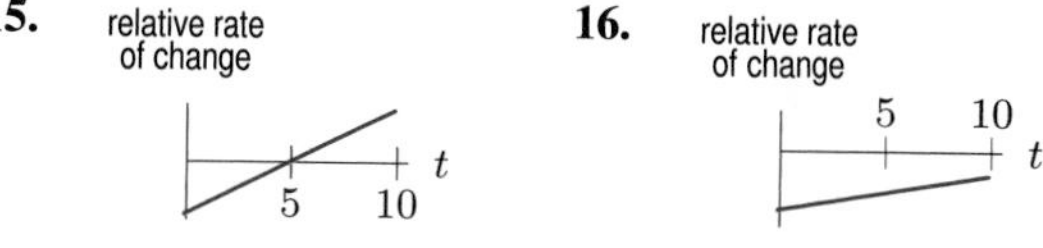

17. The population, P, in millions, of Nicaragua was 5.78 million in 2008 and growing at an annual rate of 1.8%.

(a) Write a formula for P as a function of t, where t is years since 2008.

(b) Find the projected average rate of change (or absolute growth rate) in Nicaragua between 2008 and 2009, and between 2009 and 2010. Explain why your answers are different.

(c) Use your answers to part (b) to confirm that the relative rate of change (or relative growth rate) over both time intervals was 1.8%.

In Problems 18–19, the graph shows relative birth and death rates for a population $P(t)$. Determine whether the population is increasing or decreasing, and find the percentage by which the population changes during the 10-year period.

18.

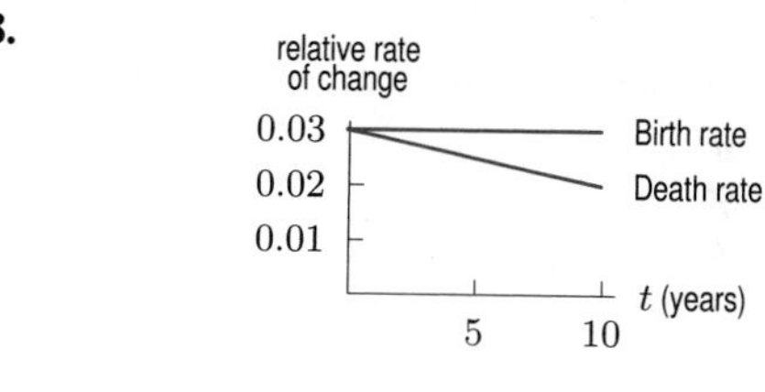

19.

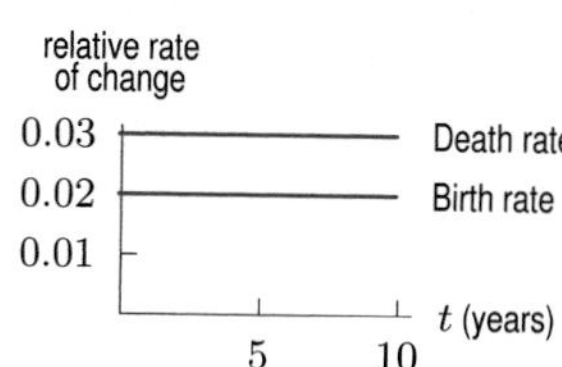

CHAPTER SUMMARY

- **Average value**
- **Consumer and producer surplus**
  Wage and price controls
- **Present and future value**
  Income stream
- **Relative growth rates**

REVIEW PROBLEMS FOR CHAPTER SIX

1. **(a)** Use Figure 6.34 to find $\int_0^6 f(x)\,dx$.
   (b) What is the average value of f on the interval $x = 0$ to $x = 6$?

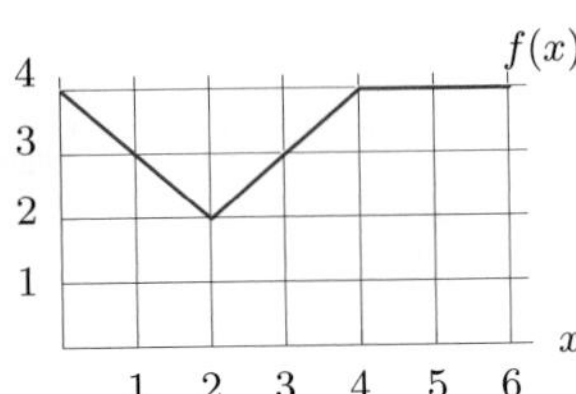

Figure 6.34

2. Find the average value of $g(t) = e^t$ over the interval $0 \le t \le 10$.

3. **(a)** What is the average value of $f(x) = \sqrt{1 - x^2}$ over the interval $0 \le x \le 1$?
   (b) How can you tell whether this average value is more or less than 0.5 without doing any calculations?

4. A service station orders 100 cases of motor oil every 6 months. The number of cases of oil remaining t months after the order arrives is modeled by

$$f(t) = 100e^{-0.5t}.$$

   (a) How many cases are there at the start of the six-month period? How many cases are left at the end of the six-month period?
   (b) Find the average number of cases in inventory over the six-month period.

5. The quantity of a radioactive substance at time t is

$$Q(t) = 4(0.96)^t \text{ grams.}$$

   (a) Find $Q(10)$ and $Q(20)$.
   (b) Find the average of $Q(10)$ and $Q(20)$.
   (c) Find the average value of $Q(t)$ over the interval $10 \le t \le 20$.
   (d) Use the graph of $Q(t)$ to explain the relative sizes of your answers in parts (b) and (c).

In Problems 6–7, estimate the average value of $f(x)$ from $x = a$ to $x = b$.

6. 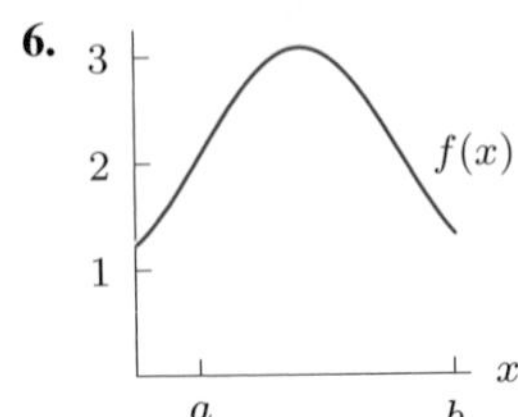

7. 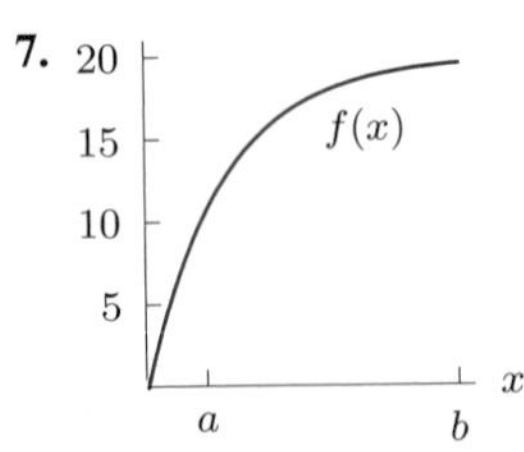

8. The function f in Figure 6.35 is symmetric about the y-axis. Consider the average value of f over the following intervals:

   I. $0 \le x \le 1$ II. $0 \le x \le 2$
   III. $0 \le x \le 5$ IV. $-2 \le x \le 2$

   (a) For which interval is the average value of f least?
   (b) For which interval is the average value of f greatest?
   (c) For which pair of intervals are the average values equal?

9. For the function f in Figure 6.35, write an expression involving one or more definite integrals that denotes:

   (a) The average value of f for $0 \le x \le 5$.
   (b) The average value of $|f|$ for $0 \le x \le 5$.

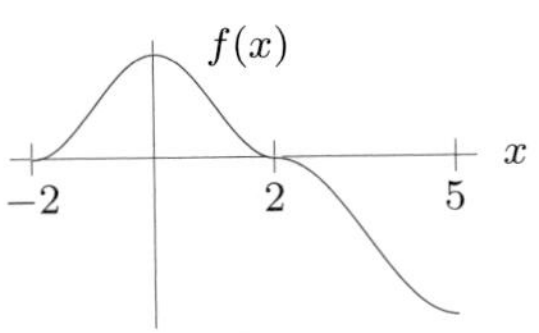

Figure 6.35

10. For a product, the supply curve is $p = 5 + 0.02q$ and the demand curve is $p = 30e^{-0.003q}$, where p is the price and q is the quantity sold at that price. Find:

   (a) The equilibrium price and quantity
   (b) The consumer and producer surplus

11. Sketch possible supply and demand curves where the consumer surplus at the equilibrium price is

   (a) Greater than the producer surplus.
   (b) Less than the producer surplus.

12. In May 1991, *Car and Driver* described a Jaguar that sold for \$980,000. At that price only 50 have been sold. It is estimated that 350 could have been sold if the price had been \$560,000. Assuming that the demand curve is a straight line, and that \$560,000 and 350 are the equilibrium price and quantity, find the consumer surplus at the equilibrium price.

13. For a product, the demand curve is $p = 100e^{-0.008q}$ and the supply curve is $p = 4\sqrt{q} + 10$ for $0 \le q \le 500$, where q is quantity and p is price in dollars per unit.

   (a) At a price of \$50, what quantity are consumers willing to buy and what quantity are producers willing to supply? Will the market push prices up or down?
   (b) Find the equilibrium price and quantity. Does your answer to part (a) support the observation that market forces tend to push prices closer to the equilibrium price?
   (c) At the equilibrium price, calculate and interpret the consumer and producer surplus.

14. Calculate the present value of a continuous revenue stream of $1000 per year for 5 years at an interest rate of 9% per year compounded continuously.

15. **(a)** A bank account earns 10% interest compounded continuously. At what constant, continuous rate must a parent deposit money into such an account in order to save $100,000 in 10 years for a child's college expenses?

(b) If the parent decides instead to deposit a lump sum now in order to attain the goal of $100,000 in 10 years, how much must be deposited now?

16. The Hershey Company is the largest US producer of chocolate. Between 2005 and 2008, Hershey generated net sales at a rate approximated by $4.8 + 0.1t$ billion dollars per year, where t is the time in years since January 1, 2005.[7] Assume this rate continues through the year 2010 and that the interest rate is 2% per year compounded continuously.

(a) Find the value, on January 1, 2005, of Hershey's net sales during the five-year period from from January 1, 2005 to January 1, 2010.

(b) Find the value, on January 1, 2010, of Hershey's net sales during the same five-year period.

17. Determine the constant income stream that needs to be invested over a period of 10 years at an interest rate of 5% per year compounded continuously to provide a present value of $5000.

18. In 1980 West Germany made a loan of 20 billion Deutsche Marks to the Soviet Union, to be used for the construction of a natural gas pipeline connecting Siberia to Western Russia, and continuing to West Germany (Urengoi–Uschgorod–Berlin). Assume that the deal was as follows: In 1985, upon completion of the pipeline, the Soviet Union would deliver natural gas to West Germany, at a constant rate, for all future times. Assuming a constant price of natural gas of 0.10 Deutsche Mark per cubic meter, and assuming West Germany expects 10% annual interest on its investment (compounded continuously), at what rate does the Soviet Union have to deliver the gas, in billions of cubic meters per year? Keep in mind that delivery of gas could not begin until the pipeline was completed. Thus, West Germany received no return on its investment until after five years had passed. (Note: A more complex deal of this type was actually made between the two countries.)

19. Figure 6.36 gives the relative growth rate of a population.

(a) On what interval is the population increasing? By what percentage does the population increase during this interval?

(b) On what interval is the population decreasing? By what percentage does the population decrease during this interval?

(c) By what percentage does the population change during the 15-year period shown?

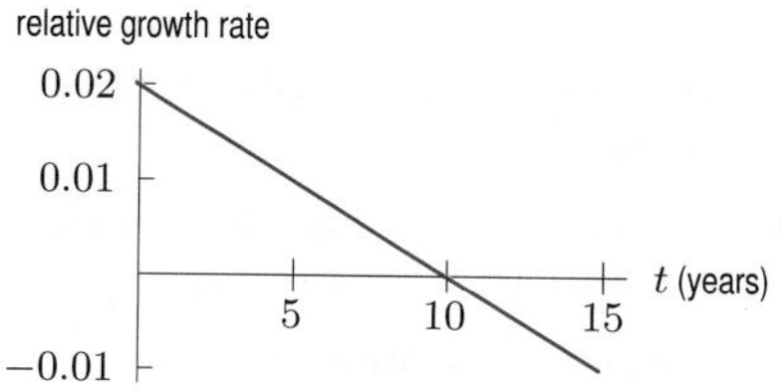

Figure 6.36

20. The number of reported burglary offenses in the US has been mostly decreasing since 1990.[8] If $P(t)$ is the number of reported burglaries as a function of year t, the relative rate of change per year, $P'(t)/P(t)$, is given in the table.

(a) Estimate the integral of the relative rate of change: $\int_{1990}^{2002} \frac{P'(t)}{P(t)}\, dt.$

(b) By what percent did the number of burglaries change during the period 1990–2002?

Year	1990	1991	1992	1993	1994	1995	1996
Rel. rate	−0.03	0.03	−0.06	−0.05	−0.04	−0.04	−0.03
Year	1997	1998	1999	2000	2001	2002	
Rel. rate	−0.02	−0.05	−0.10	−0.02	0.03	0.02	

21. In 1990 humans generated $1.4 \cdot 10^{20}$ joules of energy from petroleum. At the time, it was estimated that all of the earth's petroleum would generate approximately 10^{22} joules. Assuming the use of energy generated by petroleum increases by 2% each year, how long will it be before all of our petroleum resources are used up?

22. In everyday language, exponential growth means very fast growth. In this problem, you will see that any exponentially growing function eventually grows faster than any power function.

(a) Show that the relative growth rate of the function $f(x) = x^n$, for fixed $n > 0$ and for $x > 0$, decreases as x increases.

(b) Assume $k > 0$ is fixed. Explain why, for large x, the relative growth rate of the function $g(x) = e^{kx}$ is larger than the relative growth rate of $f(x)$.

[7] 2008 Annual Report, accessed at www.thehersheycompany.com.
[8] *The World Almanac and Book of Facts 2005*, p. 162 (New York).

CHECK YOUR UNDERSTANDING

In Problems 1–40, indicate whether the statement is true or false.

1. The average value of $f(x)$ on the interval $0 \le x \le 10$ is $\int_0^{10} f(x)\,dx$.
2. If $f(0) = 0$ and $f(10) = 50$, then the average value of f on the interval $0 \le x \le 10$ is between 0 and 50.
3. If f is a continuous increasing function and $f(0) = 0$ and $f(10) = 50$, then the average value of f on the interval $0 \le x \le 10$ is between 0 and 50.
4. The units of the average value of f are the same as the units of f.
5. The average value of f over the interval $0 \le x \le 20$ is twice the average value of f over the interval $0 \le x \le 10$.
6. The average value of $2f(x)$ over the interval $0 \le x \le 10$ is twice the average value of $f(x)$ over the interval $0 \le x \le 10$.
7. If the average value of f over the interval $0 \le x \le 10$ is 0, then $f(x) = 0$ for all $0 \le x \le 10$.
8. If $f(x) > g(x) \ge 0$, then the average value of $f(x)$ for $0 \le x \le 10$ is greater than the average value of $g(x)$ for $0 \le x \le 10$.
9. The average value of f on the interval $5 \le x \le 7$ is one half of $\int_5^7 f(x)\,dx$.
10. The average value of the cost function $C(q)$ for $0 \le q \le 10$ is the same as the average cost for 10 items.
11. The supply curve shows the quantity of an item that a producer supplies at different prices.
12. The demand curve shows the quantity of an item that consumers will purchase at various prices.
13. The equilibrium price p^* is where the demand curve crosses the q-axis.
14. Consumer surplus is the total amount gained by consumers by purchasing items at prices higher than they are willing to pay.
15. The units of consumer surplus are the same as the units of producer surplus.
16. The units of producer surplus are price times quantity.
17. Total gains from trade is the difference between consumer and producer surplus.
18. The area under the demand curve from 0 to the equilibrium quantity q^* is the amount consumers spend at the equilibrium price p^*.
19. Consumer surplus at price p^* is the area between the demand curve and the horizontal line at p^*.
20. Producer surplus at price p^* is the area between the demand curve and the horizontal line at p^*.
21. Assuming a positive interest rate, the present value of an income stream is always less than its future value.
22. The future value of an income stream of \$1000 per year for 5 years is more than \$5000 if the interest rate is 2%.
23. The present value of an income stream of \$1000 per year for 5 years is more than \$5000 if the interest rate is 2%.
24. A single payment at the beginning of the year of \$1000 has the same future value as an income stream of \$1000 per year if we assume a continuous interest rate of 3% for one year for both.
25. If $S(t)$ is an income stream, then $S(t)$ has units of dollars.
26. With a continuous interest rate of r, the future value of a payment of \$3000 today in 5 years is $3000e^{-5r}$.
27. With a continuous interest rate of r, we would have to deposit $3000e^{-5r}$ today to grow to \$3000 in 5 years.
28. If an income stream of 2000 dollars per year grows to \$11,361 in five years, then the amount of interest earned over the five-year period is \$1361.
29. The present value of an income stream of 2000 dollars per year that starts now and pays out over 6 years with a continuous interest rate of 2% is $\int_0^6 2000e^{-2t}\,dt$.
30. The future value of an income stream of 2000 dollars per year that starts now and accumulates over 9 years with a positive interest rate is greater than \$18,000.
31. The relative rate of change of population P with respect to time t is dP/dt.
32. Percent rate of change has the same units as rate of change.
33. If a population P is growing at a continuous rate of 2% per year, then $dP/dt = 0.02$.
34. The relative growth rate of P is the derivative of $\ln(P(t))$.
35. If the percent birth rate is higher than the percent death rate in a country, then the country's population is increasing.
36. If the percent birth rate and the percent death rate in a country are both decreasing, then the country's population is decreasing.
37. The integral of the relative growth rate of a population P gives the total change in P.
38. If the integral of the relative growth rate of a population P over 30 years is 0.5 then the population has decreased by 50% over the 30-year period.
39. If the integral of the relative growth rate of a population is negative on an interval, then the population at the end of the interval is less than the population at the beginning of the interval.
40. If the integral of the relative growth rate of a population is equal to A on an interval, then the population at the end of the interval is e^A times the population at the beginning of the interval.

PROJECTS FOR CHAPTER SIX

1. Distribution of Resources

Whether a resource is distributed evenly among members of a population is often an important political or economic question. How can we measure this? How can we decide if the distribution of wealth in this country is becoming more or less equitable over time? How can we measure which country has the most equitable income distribution? This problem describes a way of making such measurements. Suppose the resource is distributed evenly. Then any 20% of the population will have 20% of the resource. Similarly, any 30% will have 30% of the resource and so on. If, however, the resource is not distributed evenly, the poorest $p\%$ of the population (in terms of this resource) will not have $p\%$ of the goods. Suppose $F(x)$ represents the fraction of the resources owned by the poorest fraction x of the population. Thus $F(0.4) = 0.1$ means that the poorest 40% of the population owns 10% of the resource.

(a) What would F be if the resource were distributed evenly?

(b) What must be true of any such F? What must $F(0)$ and $F(1)$ equal? Is F increasing or decreasing? Is the graph of F concave up or concave down?

(c) Gini's index of inequality, G, is one way to measure how evenly the resource is distributed. It is defined by

$$G = 2\int_0^1 [x - F(x)]\,dx.$$

Show graphically what G represents.

(d) Graphical representations of Gini's index for two countries are given in Figures 6.37 and 6.38. Which country has the more equitable distribution of wealth? Discuss the distribution of wealth in each of the two countries.

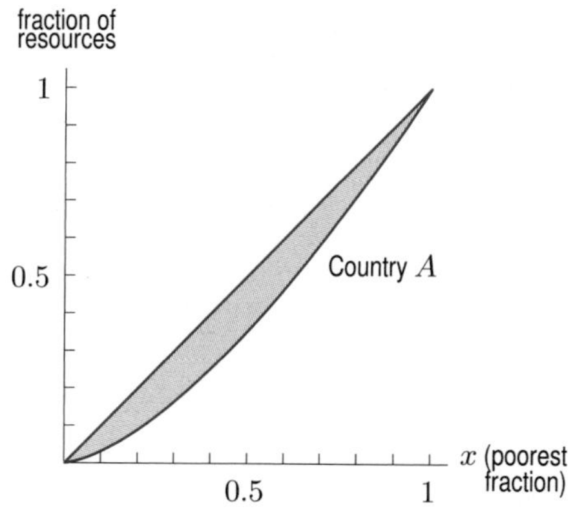

Figure 6.37: Country A

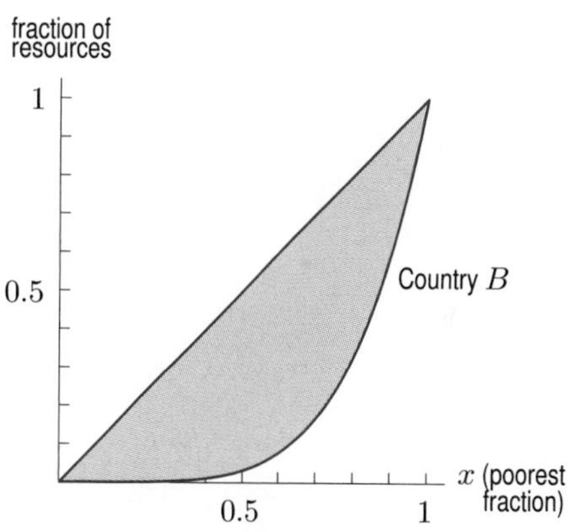

Figure 6.38: Country B

(e) What is the maximum possible value of Gini's index of inequality, G? What is the minimum possible value? Sketch graphs in each case. What is the distribution of resources in each case?

2. Yield from an Apple Orchard

Figure 6.39 is a graph of the annual yield, $y(t)$, in bushels per year, from an orchard t years after planting. The trees take about 10 years to get established, but for the next 20 years they give a substantial yield. After about 30 years, however, age and disease start to take their toll, and the annual yield falls off.[9]

(a) Represent on a sketch of Figure 6.39 the total yield, $F(M)$, up to M years, with $0 \leq M \leq 60$. Write an expression for $F(M)$ in terms of $y(t)$.

[9] From Peter D. Taylor, *Calculus: The Analysis of Functions* (Toronto: Wall & Emerson, Inc., 1992).

(b) Sketch a graph of $F(M)$ against M for $0 \leq M \leq 60$.

(c) Write an expression for the average annual yield, $a(M)$, up to M years.

(d) When should the orchard be cut down and replanted? Assume that we want to maximize average revenue per year, and that fruit prices remain constant, so that this is achieved by maximizing average annual yield. Use the graph of $y(t)$ to estimate the time at which the average annual yield is a maximum. Explain your answer geometrically and symbolically.

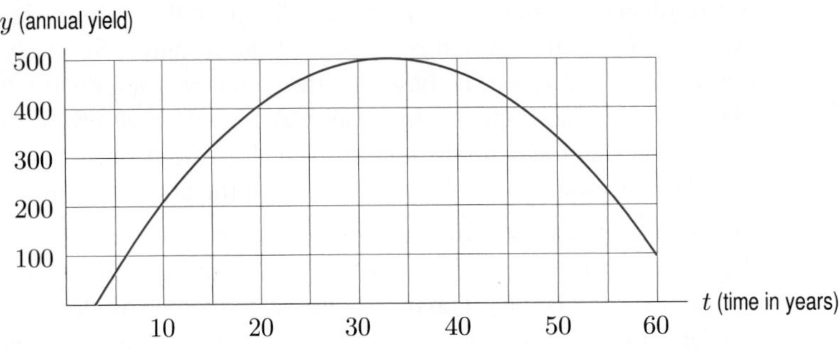

Figure 6.39

Chapter Seven

ANTIDERIVATIVES

Contents

7.1 CONSTRUCTING ANTIDERIVATIVES ANALYTICALLY

What is an Antiderivative?

If the derivative of $F(x)$ is $f(x)$, that is, if $F'(x) = f(x)$, then we call $F(x)$ an *antiderivative* of $f(x)$. For example, the derivative of x^2 is $2x$, so we say that

$$x^2 \text{ is an antiderivative of } 2x.$$

Can you think of another function whose derivative is $2x$? How about $x^2 + 1$? Or $x^2 + 17$? Since, for any constant C,

$$\frac{d}{dx}(x^2 + C) = 2x + 0 = 2x,$$

any function of the form $x^2 + C$ is an antiderivative of $2x$. It can be shown that all antiderivatives of $2x$ are of this form, so we say that

$$x^2 + C \text{ is the family of antiderivatives of } 2x.$$

Once we know one antiderivative $F(x)$ for a function $f(x)$ on an interval, then all other antiderivatives of $f(x)$ are of the form $F(x) + C$.

The Indefinite Integral

We introduce a notation for the family of antiderivatives that looks like a definite integral without the limits. We call $\int f(x)\,dx$ the *indefinite integral* of $f(x)$. If all antiderivatives of $f(x)$ are of the form $F(x) + C$, we write

$$\int f(x)\,dx = F(x) + C.$$

It is important to understand the difference between

$$\int_a^b f(x)\,dx \qquad \text{and} \qquad \int f(x)\,dx.$$

The first is a number and the second is a family of functions. Because the notation is similar, the word "integration" is frequently used for the process of finding antiderivatives as well as of finding definite integrals. The context usually makes clear which is intended.

Finding Formulas for Antiderivatives

Finding antiderivatives of functions is like taking square roots of numbers: if we pick a number at random, such as 7 or 493, we may have trouble figuring out its square root without a calculator. But if we happen to pick a number such as 25 or 64, which we know is a perfect square, then we can easily guess its square root. Similarly, if we pick a function which we recognize as a derivative, then we can find its antiderivative easily.

For example, noticing that $2x$ is the derivative of x^2 tells us that x^2 is an antiderivative of $2x$. If we divide by 2, then we guess that

$$\text{An antiderivative of } x \text{ is } \frac{x^2}{2}.$$

To check this statement, take the derivative of $x^2/2$:

$$\frac{d}{dx}\left(\frac{x^2}{2}\right) = \frac{1}{2} \cdot \frac{d}{dx}x^2 = \frac{1}{2} \cdot 2x = x.$$

What about an antiderivative of x^2? The derivative of x^3 is $3x^2$, so the derivative of $x^3/3$ is $3x^2/3 = x^2$. Thus,

$$\text{An antiderivative of } x^2 \text{ is } \frac{x^3}{3}.$$

Can you see the pattern? It looks like

$$\text{An antiderivative of } x^n \text{ is } \frac{x^{n+1}}{n+1}.$$

(We assume $n \neq -1$, or we would have $x^0/0$, which does not make sense.) It is easy to check this formula by differentiation:

$$\frac{d}{dx}\left(\frac{x^{n+1}}{n+1}\right) = \frac{(n+1)x^n}{n+1} = x^n.$$

Thus, in indefinite integral notation, we see that

$$\int x^n\,dx = \frac{x^{n+1}}{n+1} + C, \quad n \neq -1.$$

Can you think of an antiderivative of the function $f(x) = 5$? We know that the derivative of $5x$ is 5, so $F(x) = 5x$ is an antiderivative of $f(x) = 5$. In general, if k is a constant, the derivative of kx is k, so we have the result:

If k is constant,

$$\int k\,dx = kx + C.$$

Example 1 Find $\int (3x + x^2)\,dx$.

Solution We know that $x^2/2$ is an antiderivative of x and that $x^3/3$ is an antiderivative of x^2, so we expect

$$\int (3x + x^2)\,dx = 3\left(\frac{x^2}{2}\right) + \frac{x^3}{3} + C.$$

Again, check your antiderivatives by differentiation—it's easy to do. Here

$$\frac{d}{dx}\left(\frac{3}{2}x^2 + \frac{x^3}{3} + C\right) = \frac{3}{2}\cdot 2x + \frac{3x^2}{3} = 3x + x^2.$$

The preceding example illustrates that the sum and constant multiplication rules of differentiation work in reverse:

Properties of Antiderivatives: Sums and Constant Multiples

In indefinite integral notation,

1. $\int [f(x) \pm g(x)]\,dx = \int f(x)\,dx \pm \int g(x)\,dx$
2. $\int cf(x)\,dx = c\int f(x)\,dx.$

In words,

1. An antiderivative of the sum (or difference) of two functions is the sum (or difference) of their antiderivatives.
2. An antiderivative of a constant times a function is the constant times an antiderivative of the function.

Example 2 Find antiderivatives of each of the following: (a) x^5 (b) t^8 (c) $12x^3$ (d) $q^3 - 6q^2$

Solution

(a) $\displaystyle\int x^5\,dx = \frac{x^6}{6} + C.$

(b) $\displaystyle\int t^8\,dt = \frac{t^9}{9} + C.$

(c) $\displaystyle\int 12x^3\,dx = 12\left(\frac{x^4}{4}\right) + C = 3x^4 + C.$

(d) $\displaystyle\int q^3 - 6q^2\,dq = \frac{q^4}{4} - 6\left(\frac{q^3}{3}\right) + C = \frac{q^4}{4} - 2q^3 + C.$

To check, differentiate the antiderivative; you should get the original function.

What is the antiderivative of x^n when $n = -1$? In other words, what is an antiderivative of $1/x$? Fortunately, we know a function whose derivative is $1/x$, namely, the natural logarithm. Thus, since

$$\frac{d}{dx}(\ln x) = \frac{1}{x},$$

we know that

$$\int \frac{1}{x}\,dx = \ln x + C, \quad \text{for } x > 0.$$

If $x < 0$, then $\ln x$ is not defined, so it can't be an antiderivative of $1/x$. In this case, we can try $\ln(-x)$:

$$\frac{d}{dx}\ln(-x) = (-1)\frac{1}{-x} = \frac{1}{x}$$

so

$$\int \frac{1}{x}\,dx = \ln(-x) + C, \quad \text{for } x < 0.$$

This means $\ln x$ is an antiderivative of $1/x$ if $x > 0$, and $\ln(-x)$ is an antiderivative of $1/x$ if $x < 0$. Since $|x| = x$ when $x > 0$ and $|x| = -x$ when $x < 0$, we can collapse these two formulas into:

$$\text{An antiderivative of } \frac{1}{x} \text{ is } \ln|x|$$

on any interval that does not contain 0. Therefore

$$\boxed{\int \frac{1}{x}\,dx = \ln|x| + C.}$$

Since the exponential function e^x is its own derivative, it is also its own antiderivative; thus

$$\boxed{\int e^x\,dx = e^x + C.}$$

What about e^{kx}? We know that the derivative of e^{kx} is ke^{kx}, so, for $k \neq 0$, we have

$$\boxed{\int e^{kx}\,dx = \frac{1}{k}e^{kx} + C.}$$

Example 3 Find antiderivatives of each of the following: (a) $8x^3 + \frac{1}{x}$ (b) $12e^{0.2t}$

Solution (a) $\int 8x^3 + \frac{1}{x}\,dx = 8\left(\frac{x^4}{4}\right) + \ln|x| + C = 2x^4 + \ln|x| + C.$

(b) $\int 12e^{0.2t}\,dt = 12\left(\frac{1}{0.2}e^{0.2t}\right) + C = 60e^{0.2t} + C.$

Differentiate your answers to check them.

Antiderivatives of Periodic Functions

The antiderivatives of the sine and cosine are easy to guess. Since

$$\frac{d}{dx}\sin x = \cos x \qquad \text{and} \qquad \frac{d}{dx}\cos x = -\sin x,$$

we get

$$\int \cos x\,dx = \sin x + C \qquad \text{and} \qquad \int \sin x\,dx = -\cos x + C.$$

Since the derivative of $\sin(kx)$ is $k\cos(kx)$ and the derivative of $\cos(kx)$ is $-k\sin(kx)$, we have, for $k \neq 0$,

$$\int \cos(kx)\,dx = \frac{1}{k}\sin(kx) + C \qquad \text{and} \qquad \int \sin(kx)\,dx = -\frac{1}{k}\cos(kx) + C.$$

Example 4 Find $\int(\sin x + 3\cos(5x))\,dx$.

Solution We break the antiderivative into two terms:

$$\int(\sin x + 3\cos(5x))\,dx = \int \sin x\,dx + 3\int \cos(5x)\,dx = -\cos x + \frac{3}{5}\sin(5x) + C.$$

Check by differentiating:

$$\frac{d}{dx}(-\cos x + \frac{3}{5}\sin(5x) + C) = \sin x + 3\cos(5x).$$

Problems for Section 7.1

In Problems 1–26, find an antiderivative.

1. $f(x) = 5$
2. $f(t) = 5t$
3. $g(t) = t^2 + t$
4. $f(x) = x^2$
5. $f(x) = x^4$
6. $g(t) = t^7 + t^3$
7. $g(x) = 6x^3 + 4$
8. $f(q) = 5q^2$
9. $h(y) = 3y^2 - y^3$
10. $k(x) = 10 + 8x^3$
11. $f(x) = 3x^2 + 5$
12. $f(x) = x + x^5 + x^{-5}$
13. $p(x) = x^2 - 6x + 17$
14. $g(z) = \sqrt{z}$
15. $f(x) = 5x - \sqrt{x}$
16. $p(z) = (\sqrt{z})^3$
17. $h(z) = \frac{1}{z}$
18. $p(t) = t^3 - \frac{t^2}{2} - t$
19. $g(z) = \frac{1}{z^3}$
20. $q(y) = y^4 + \frac{1}{y}$

21. $f(x) = x^6 - \frac{1}{7x^6}$

22. $g(x) = \frac{1}{x} + \frac{1}{x^2} + \frac{1}{x^3}$

23. $g(t) = e^{-3t}$

24. $h(t) = \cos t$

25. $g(t) = 5 + \cos t$

26. $g(\theta) = \sin\theta - 2\cos\theta$

In Problems 27–32, find an antiderivative $F(x)$ with $F'(x) = f(x)$ and $F(0) = 0$. Is there only one possible solution?

27. $f(x) = 3$

28. $f(x) = -7x$

29. $f(x) = 2 + 4x + 5x^2$

30. $f(x) = x^2$

31. $f(x) = \sqrt{x}$

32. $f(x) = e^x$

Find the indefinite integrals in Problems 33–62.

33. $\int (5x + 7)\, dx$

34. $\int 9x^2\, dx$

35. $\int 6x^2\, dx$

36. $\int t^{12}\, dt$

37. $\int (x+1)^2\, dx$

38. $\int (x^2 + \frac{1}{x^2})\, dx$

39. $\int (t^2 + 5t + 1)\, dt$

40. $\int 5e^z\, dz$

41. $\int (t^3 + 6t^2)\, dt$

42. $\int (x^5 - 12x^3) dx$

43. $\int 3\sqrt{w}\, dw$

44. $\int (x^2 + 4x - 5) dx$

45. $\int \left(\frac{3}{t} - \frac{2}{t^2}\right) dt$

46. $\int e^{2t}\, dt$

47. $\int \left(x + \frac{1}{\sqrt{x}}\right) dx$

48. $\int (x^3 + 5x^2 + 6) dx$

49. $\int (e^x + 5)\, dx$

50. $\int \left(x^2 + \frac{1}{x}\right) dx$

51. $\int e^{3r}\, dr$

52. $\int \cos\theta\, d\theta$

53. $\int \sin t\, dt$

54. $\int 25e^{-0.04q}\, dq$

55. $\int 100e^{4x}\, dx$

56. $\int (2e^x - 8\cos x)\, dx$

57. $\int (3\cos x - 7\sin x)\, dx$

58. $\int \sin(3x) dx$

59. $\int x\cos(x^2 + 4) dx$

60. $\int 6\cos(3x) dx$

61. $\int (10 + 8\sin(2x)) dx$

62. $\int (12\sin(2x) + 15\cos(5x)) dx$

For Problems 63–66, find an antiderivative $F(x)$ with $F'(x) = f(x)$ and $F(0) = 5$.

63. $f(x) = 6x - 5$

64. $f(x) = x^2 + 1$

65. $f(x) = 8\sin(2x)$

66. $f(x) = 6e^{3x}$

67. A firm's marginal cost function is $MC = 3q^2 + 4q + 6$. Find the total cost function if the fixed costs are 200.

68. The marginal revenue function of a monopolistic producer is $MR = 20 - 4q$.
   (a) Find the total revenue function.
   (b) Find the corresponding demand curve.

7.2 INTEGRATION BY SUBSTITUTION

In Chapter 3, we learned rules to differentiate any function obtained by combining constants, powers of x, $\sin x$, $\cos x$, e^x, and $\ln x$, using addition, multiplication, division, or composition of functions. Such functions are called *elementary*.

In this section, we introduce integration by substitution. However, there is a great difference between looking for derivatives and looking for antiderivatives. Every elementary function has elementary derivatives, but many elementary functions do not have elementary antiderivatives. Some examples are $\sqrt{x^3+1}$, $(\sin x)/x$, and e^{-x^2}. These are ordinary functions that arise naturally, not exotic functions, yet they do not have elementary antiderivatives.

Integration by substitution reverses the chain rule. According to the chain rule,

$$\frac{d}{dx}(f(g(x))) = \underbrace{f'}_{\text{Derivative of outside}}(\overbrace{g(x)}^{\text{Inside}}) \cdot \underbrace{g'(x)}_{\text{Derivative of inside}}.$$

Thus, any function which is the result of differentiating with the chain rule is the product of two factors: the "derivative of the outside" and the "derivative of the inside." If a function has this form, its antiderivative is $f(g(x))$.

Example 1 Use the chain rule to find $f'(x)$ and then write the corresponding antidifferentiation formula.

(a) $f(x) = e^{x^2}$ (b) $f(x) = \frac{1}{6}(x^2+1)^6$ (c) $f(x) = \ln(x^2+4)$

Solution (a) Using the chain rule, we see

$$\frac{d}{dx}\left(e^{x^2}\right) = e^{x^2} \cdot 2x \quad \text{so} \quad \int e^{x^2} \cdot 2x\, dx = e^{x^2} + C.$$

(b) Using the chain rule, we see

$$\frac{d}{dx}\left(\frac{1}{6}(x^2+1)^6\right) = (x^2+1)^5 \cdot 2x \quad \text{so} \quad \int (x^2+1)^5 \cdot 2x\, dx = \frac{1}{6}(x^2+1)^6 + C.$$

(c) Using the chain rule, we see

$$\frac{d}{dx}(\ln(x^2+4)) = \frac{1}{x^2+4} \cdot 2x \quad \text{so} \quad \int \frac{1}{x^2+4} \cdot 2x\, dx = \ln(x^2+4) + C.$$

In Example 1, the derivative of each inside function is $2x$. Notice that the derivative of the inside function is a factor in the integrand in each antidifferentiation formula.

Finding an inside function whose derivative appears as a factor is key to the method of substitution. We formalize this method as follows:

To Make a Substitution in an Integral

Let w be the "inside function" and $dw = w'(x)\, dx = \frac{dw}{dx} dx$. Then express the integrand in terms of w.

Example 2 Make a substitution to find each of the following integrals:

(a) $\int e^{x^2} \cdot 2x\, dx$ (b) $\int (x^2+1)^5 \cdot 2x\, dx$ (c) $\int \frac{1}{x^2+4} \cdot 2x\, dx$

Solution (a) We look for an inside function whose derivative appears as a factor. In this case, the inside function is x^2, with derivative $2x$. We let $w = x^2$. Then $dw = w'(x)\, dx = 2x\, dx$. The original integrand can now be rewritten in terms of w:

$$\int e^{x^2} \cdot 2x\, dx = \int e^w\, dw = e^w + C = e^{x^2} + C.$$

By changing the variable to w, we simplified the integrand. The final step, after antidifferentiating, is to convert back to the original variable, x.

(b) Here, the inside function is x^2+1, with derivative $2x$. We let $w = x^2+1$. Then $dw = w'(x)\, dx = 2x\, dx$. Rewriting the original integral in terms of w, we have

$$\int (x^2+1)^5 \cdot 2x\, dx = \int w^5\, dw = \frac{1}{6}w^6 + C = \frac{1}{6}(x^2+1)^6 + C.$$

Again, by changing the variable to w, we simplified the integrand.

(c) The inside function is x^2+4, so we let $w = x^2+4$. Then $dw = w'(x)\, dx = 2x\, dx$. Substituting, we have

$$\int \frac{1}{x^2+4} \cdot 2x\, dx = \int \frac{1}{w}\, dw = \ln(w) + C = \ln(x^2+4) + C.$$

Notice that the derivative of the inside function must be present in the integral for this method to work. The method works, however, even when the derivative is missing a constant factor, as in the next two examples.

Example 3 Find $\int te^{(t^2+1)}\,dt$.

Solution Here the inside function is t^2+1, with derivative $2t$. Since there is a factor of t in the integrand, we try $w = t^2+1$. Then $dw = w'(t)\,dt = 2t\,dt$. Notice, however, that the original integrand has only $t\,dt$, not $2t\,dt$. We therefore write

$$\frac{1}{2}\,dw = t\,dt$$

and then substitute:

$$\int te^{(t^2+1)}\,dt = \int e^{\overbrace{(t^2+1)}^{w}} \cdot \underbrace{t\,dt}_{\frac{1}{2}dw} = \int e^w\,\frac{1}{2}\,dw = \frac{1}{2}\int e^w\,dw = \frac{1}{2}e^w + C = \frac{1}{2}e^{(t^2+1)} + C.$$

Why didn't we put $\frac{1}{2}\int e^w\,dw = \frac{1}{2}e^w + \frac{1}{2}C$ in the preceding example? Since the constant C is arbitrary, it does not really matter whether we add C or $\frac{1}{2}C$. The convention is always to add C to whatever antiderivative we have calculated.

Example 4 Find $\int x^3\sqrt{x^4+5}\,dx$.

Solution The inside function is x^4+5, with derivative $4x^3$. The integrand has a factor of x^3, and since the only thing missing is a constant factor, we try

$$w = x^4 + 5.$$

Then

$$dw = w'(x)\,dx = 4x^3\,dx,$$

giving

$$\frac{1}{4}dw = x^3\,dx.$$

Thus,

$$\int x^3\sqrt{x^4+5}\,dx = \int \sqrt{w}\,\frac{1}{4}dw = \frac{1}{4}\int w^{1/2}\,dw = \frac{1}{4}\cdot\frac{w^{3/2}}{3/2} + C = \frac{1}{6}(x^4+5)^{3/2} + C.$$

Warning

We saw in the preceding examples that we can apply the substitution method when a *constant* factor is missing from the derivative of the inside function. However, we may not be able to use substitution if anything other than a constant factor is missing. For example, setting $w = x^4+5$ to find

$$\int x^2\sqrt{x^4+5}\,dx$$

does us no good because $x^2\,dx$ is not a constant multiple of $dw = 4x^3\,dx$. In order to use substitution, it helps if the integrand contains the derivative of the inside function, *to within a constant factor*.

Example 5 Find $\displaystyle\int \frac{t^2}{1+t^3}\,dt$.

Solution Observing that the derivative of $1+t^3$ is $3t^2$, we take $w = 1+t^3$, $dw = 3t^2\,dt$, so $\frac{1}{3}\,dw = t^2\,dt$. Thus,

$$\int \frac{t^2}{1+t^3}\,dt = \int \frac{\frac{1}{3}\,dw}{w} = \frac{1}{3}\ln|w| + C = \frac{1}{3}\ln|1+t^3| + C.$$

Since the numerator is $t^2\,dt$, we might have tried $w = t^3$. This substitution leads to the integral $\frac{1}{3}\int 1/(1+w)\,dw$. To evaluate this integral we would have to make a second substitution $u = 1+w$. There is often more than one way to do an integral by substitution.

Using Substitution with Periodic Functions

The method of substitution can be used for integrals involving periodic functions.

Example 6 Find $\displaystyle\int 3x^2\cos(x^3)\,dx$.

Solution We look for an inside function whose derivative appears—in this case x^3. We let $w = x^3$. Then $dw = w'(x)\,dx = 3x^2\,dx$. The original integrand can now be completely rewritten in terms of the new variable w:

$$\int 3x^2\cos(x^3)\,dx = \int \cos\underbrace{(x^3)}_{w}\cdot\underbrace{3x^2\,dx}_{dw} = \int \cos w\,dw = \sin w + C = \sin(x^3) + C.$$

By changing the variable to w, we have simplified the integrand to $\cos w$, which can be antidifferentiated more easily. The final step, after antidifferentiating, is to convert back to the original variable, x.

Example 7 Find $\displaystyle\int e^{\cos\theta}\sin\theta\,d\theta$.

Solution We let $w = \cos\theta$ since its derivative is $-\sin\theta$ and there is a factor of $\sin\theta$ in the integrand. This gives

$$dw = w'(\theta)\,d\theta = -\sin\theta\,d\theta,$$

so

$$-dw = \sin\theta\,d\theta.$$

Thus,

$$\int e^{\cos\theta}\sin\theta\,d\theta = \int e^w\,(-dw) = (-1)\int e^w\,dw = -e^w + C = -e^{\cos\theta} + C.$$

Problems for Section 7.2

Find the integrals in Problems 1–40. Check your answers by differentiation.

1. $\displaystyle\int 3x^2(x^3+1)^4dx$
2. $\displaystyle\int \frac{2x}{x^2+1}dx$
3. $\displaystyle\int (x+10)^3dx$
4. $\displaystyle\int x(x^2+9)^6dx$
5. $\displaystyle\int 2qe^{q^2+1}dq$
6. $\displaystyle\int 5e^{5t+2}dt$
7. $\displaystyle\int te^{t^2}\,dt$
8. $\displaystyle\int e^{-x}\,dx$
9. $\displaystyle\int t^2(t^3-3)^{10}\,dt$
10. $\displaystyle\int x^2(1+2x^3)^2\,dx$
11. $\displaystyle\int x(x^2-4)^{7/2}\,dx$
12. $\displaystyle\int x(x^2+3)^2\,dx$
13. $\displaystyle\int \frac{1}{\sqrt{4-x}}\,dx$
14. $\displaystyle\int \frac{dy}{y+5}$

15. $\int 12x^2\cos(x^3)dx$

16. $\int (2t-7)^{73}\,dt$

17. $\int (x^2+3)^2\,dx$

18. $\int y^2(1+y)^2\,dy$

19. $\int \sin(3-t)\,dt$

20. $\int \sin\theta(\cos\theta+5)^7\,d\theta$

21. $\int \sqrt{\cos 3t}\sin 3t\,dt$

22. $\int \frac{t}{1+3t^2}dt$

23. $\int \sin^6\theta\cos\theta\,d\theta$

24. $\int x^2e^{x^3+1}\,dx$

25. $\int \sin^2 x\cos x dx$

26. $\int \sin^3\alpha\cos\alpha\,d\alpha$

27. $\int x\sin(4x^2)dx$

28. $\int e^{3x-4}dx$

29. $\int xe^{3x^2}\,dx$

30. $\int x\sqrt{3x^2+4}dx$

31. $\int \frac{q}{5q^2+8}dq$

32. $\int \frac{(\ln z)^2}{z}\,dz$

33. $\int \frac{y}{y^2+4}\,dy$

34. $\int \frac{e^t+1}{e^t+t}\,dt$

35. $\int \frac{e^{\sqrt{y}}}{\sqrt{y}}\,dy$

36. $\int \frac{\cos\sqrt{x}}{\sqrt{x}}\,dx$

37. $\int \frac{1+e^x}{\sqrt{x+e^x}}\,dx$

38. $\int \frac{e^t}{e^t+1}dt$

39. $\int \frac{x+1}{x^2+2x+19}dx$

40. $\int \frac{e^x-e^{-x}}{e^x+e^{-x}}\,dx$

41. If appropriate, evaluate the following integrals by substitution. If substitution is not appropriate, say so, and do not evaluate.

(a) $\int x\sin(x^2)\,dx$ **(b)** $\int x^2\sin x\,dx$

(c) $\int \frac{x^2}{1+x^2}\,dx$ **(d)** $\int \frac{x}{(1+x^2)^2}\,dx$

(e) $\int x^3e^{x^2}\,dx$ **(f)** $\int \frac{\sin x}{2+\cos x}\,dx$

42. **(a)** Find $\int(x+5)^2\,dx$ in two ways:
(i) By multiplying out
(ii) By substituting $w=x+5$
(b) Are the results the same? Explain.

43. Find $\int 4x(x^2+1)\,dx$ using two methods:
(a) Do the multiplication first, and then antidifferentiate.
(b) Use the substitution $w=x^2+1$.
(c) Explain how the expressions from parts (a) and (b) are different. Are they both correct?

7.3 USING THE FUNDAMENTAL THEOREM TO FIND DEFINITE INTEGRALS

In the previous section we calculated antiderivatives. In this section we see how antiderivatives are used to calculate definite integrals exactly. This calculation is based on the Fundamental Theorem:

> **Fundamental Theorem of Calculus** If F', the derivative of F, is continuous, then
> $$\int_a^b F'(x)\,dx = F(b)-F(a).$$

So far we have approximated definite integrals using a graph or left- and right-hand sums. The Fundamental Theorem gives us another method of calculating definite integrals. To find $\int_a^b F'(x)\,dx$, we first try to find F, and then calculate $F(b)-F(a)$. This method of computing definite integrals has an important advantage: it gives an exact answer. However, the method works only when we can find a formula for an antiderivative $F(x)$.

Example 1 Compute $\int_1^3 2x\,dx$ numerically and using the Fundamental Theorem.

Solution Using a calculator, we obtain

$$\int_1^3 2x\,dx = 8.000.$$

The Fundamental Theorem allows us to compute the integral exactly. We take $F'(x) = 2x$, so $F(x) = x^2$ and we obtain

$$\int_1^3 2x\,dx = F(3) - F(1) = 3^2 - 1^2 = 8.$$

In Example 1 we used the antiderivative $F(x) = x^2$, but $F(x) = x^2 + C$ works just as well for any constant C, because the constant cancels out when we subtract $F(a)$ from $F(b)$:

$$\int_1^3 2x\,dx = F(3) - F(1) = (3^2 + C) - (1^2 + C) = 8.$$

It is helpful to introduce a shorthand notation for $F(b) - F(a)$: we write

$$F(x)\Big|_a^b = F(b) - F(a).$$

For example:

$$\int_1^3 2x\,dx = x^2\Big|_1^3 = 3^2 - 1^2 = 8.$$

Example 2 Use the Fundamental Theorem to compute the following definite integrals:

(a) $\int_0^2 6x^2\,dx$ (b) $\int_0^2 t^3\,dt$ (c) $\int_1^2 (8x+5)\,dx$ (d) $\int_0^1 8e^{2t}\,dt$

Solution (a) Since $F'(x) = 6x^2$, we take $F(x) = 6(x^3/3) = 2x^3$. So

$$\int_0^2 6x^2 dx = 6\left(\frac{x^3}{3}\right)\Big|_0^2 = 2x^3\Big|_0^2 = 2\cdot 2^3 - 2\cdot 0^3 = 16.$$

(b) Since $F'(t) = t^3$, we take $F(t) = t^4/4$, so

$$\int_0^2 t^3\,dt = F(t)\Big|_0^2 = F(2) - F(0) = \frac{2^4}{4} - \frac{0^4}{4} = \frac{16}{4} - 0 = 4.$$

(c) Since $F'(x) = 8x + 5$, we take $F(x) = 4x^2 + 5x$, giving

$$\int_1^2 (8x+5)dx = (4x^2 + 5x)\Big|_1^2 = (4\cdot 2^2 + 5\cdot 2) - (4\cdot 1^2 + 5\cdot 1)$$
$$= 26 - 9 = 17.$$

(d) Since $F'(t) = 8e^{2t}$, we take $F(t) = (8e^{2t})/2 = 4e^{2t}$, so

$$\int_0^1 8e^{2t} dt = 8\left(\frac{1}{2}e^{2t}\right)\Big|_0^1 = 4e^{2t}\Big|_0^1 = 4e^2 - 4e^0 = 25.556.$$

Example 3 Write a definite integral to represent the area under the graph of $f(t) = e^{0.5t}$ between $t = 0$ and $t = 4$. Use the Fundamental Theorem to calculate the area.

Solution The function is graphed in Figure 7.1. We have

$$\text{Area} = \int_0^4 e^{0.5t}\,dt = 2e^{0.5t}\Big|_0^4 = 2e^{0.5(4)} - 2e^{0.5(0)} = 2e^2 - 2 = 12.778.$$

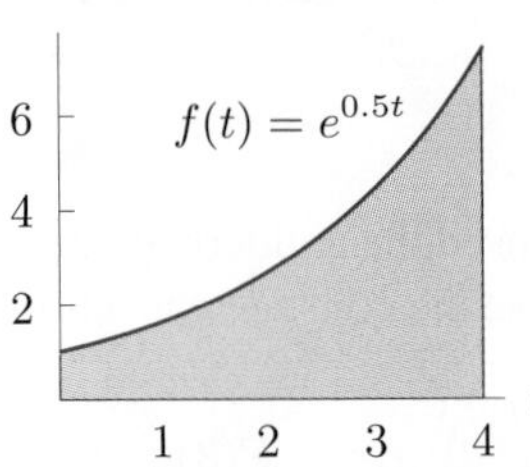

Figure 7.1: Shaded area $= \int_0^4 e^{0.5t}\,dt$

Definite Integrals by Substitution

The following example shows two ways of computing a definite integral by substitution.

Example 4 Compute $\displaystyle\int_0^2 xe^{x^2}\,dx$.

Solution To evaluate this definite integral using the Fundamental Theorem of Calculus, we first need to find an antiderivative of $f(x) = xe^{x^2}$. The inside function is x^2, so we let $w = x^2$. Then $dw = 2x\,dx$, so $\frac{1}{2}\,dw = x\,dx$. Thus,

$$\int xe^{x^2}\,dx = \int e^w \frac{1}{2}\,dw = \frac{1}{2}e^w + C = \frac{1}{2}e^{x^2} + C.$$

Now we find the definite integral:

$$\int_0^2 xe^{x^2}\,dx = \frac{1}{2}e^{x^2}\Big|_0^2 = \frac{1}{2}(e^4 - e^0) = \frac{1}{2}(e^4 - 1).$$

There is another way to look at the same problem. After we established that

$$\int xe^{x^2}\,dx = \frac{1}{2}e^w + C,$$

our next two steps were to replace w by x^2, and then x by 2 and 0. We could have directly replaced the original limits of integration, $x = 0$ and $x = 2$, by the corresponding w limits. Since $w = x^2$, the w limits are $w = 0^2 = 0$ (when $x = 0$) and $w = 2^2 = 4$ (when $x = 2$), so we get

$$\int_{x=0}^{x=2} xe^{x^2}\,dx = \frac{1}{2}\int_{w=0}^{w=4} e^w\,dw = \frac{1}{2}e^w\Big|_0^4 = \frac{1}{2}\left(e^4 - e^0\right) = \frac{1}{2}(e^4 - 1).$$

As we would expect, both methods give the same answer.

To Use Substitution to Find Definite Integrals

Either

- Compute the indefinite integral, expressing an antiderivative in terms of the original variable, and then evaluate the result at the original limits,

or

- Convert the original limits to new limits in terms of the new variable and do not convert the antiderivative back to the original variable.

Improper Integrals

So far, in our discussion of the definite integral $\int_a^b f(x)\,dx$, we have assumed that the interval $a \le x \le b$ is of finite length and the integrand f is continuous. An *improper integral* is a definite integral in which one (or both) of the limits of integration is infinite or the integrand is unbounded. An example of an improper integral is

$$\int_1^\infty \frac{1}{x^2}\,dx$$

This integral represents the area under the graph of $\frac{1}{x^2}$ from $x = 1$ infinitely far to the right. (See Figure 7.2.)

We estimate this area by letting the upper limit of integration get larger and larger. We see that

$$\int_1^{10} \frac{1}{x^2}\,dx = 0.9, \qquad \int_1^{100} \frac{1}{x^2}\,dx = 0.99, \qquad \int_1^{1000} \frac{1}{x^2}\,dx = 0.999,$$

and so on. These calculations suggest that as the upper limit of integration tends to infinity, the area tends to 1. We say that the improper integral $\int_1^\infty \frac{1}{x^2}\,dx$ *converges* to 1. To show that the integral converges to exactly 1 (and not to 1.0001, say), we need to use the Fundamental Theorem of Calculus. (See Problem 38.) It may seem strange that the region shaded in Figure 7.2 (which has infinite length) can have *finite* area. The area is finite because the values of the function $1/x^2$ shrink to zero so fast as $x \to \infty$. In other examples (where the integrand does not shrink to zero so fast), the area represented by an improper integral may not be finite. In that case, we say the improper integral *diverges*. (See Problem 52.)

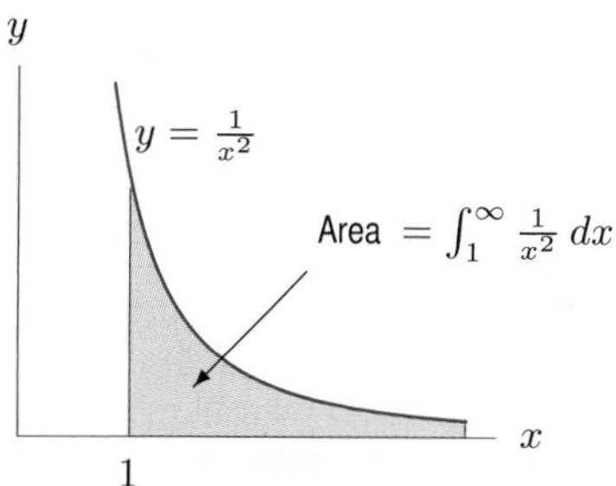

Figure 7.2: Area representation of improper integral

Problems for Section 7.3

Using the Fundamental Theorem, evaluate the definite integrals in Problems 1–20 exactly.

1. $\int_1^3 5\,dx$

2. $\int_0^4 6x\,dx$

3. $\int_1^2 (2x+3)\,dx$

4. $\int_0^2 (3t^2+4t+3)\,dt$

5. $\int_1^2 \frac{1}{t^2}\,dt$

6. $\int_1^4 \frac{1}{\sqrt{x}}\,dx$

7. $\int_0^5 3x^2\,dx$

8. $\int_0^3 t^3\,dt$

9. $\int_1^3 6x^2\,dx$

10. $\int_1^2 5t^3\,dt$

11. $\int_4^9 \sqrt{x}\,dx$

12. $\int_0^1 (y^2+y^4)\,dy$

13. $\int_1^2 \frac{1}{2t}\,dt$

14. $\int_2^5 (x^3-\pi x^2)\,dx$

15. $\int_0^1 e^{-0.2t}\,dt$

16. $\int_0^1 2e^x\,dx$

17. $\int_{-1}^1 \cos t\,dt$

18. $\int_0^{\pi/4} (\sin t+\cos t)\,dt$

19. $\int_0^3 e^{0.05t}\,dt$

20. $\int_0^1 (6q^2+4)\,dq$

21. Use substitution to express each of the following integrals as a multiple of $\int_a^b (1/w)\,dw$ for some a and b. Then evaluate the integrals.

(a) $\displaystyle\int_0^1 \frac{x}{1+x^2}\,dx$ **(b)** $\displaystyle\int_0^{\pi/4} \frac{\sin x}{\cos x}\,dx$

Use integration by substitution and the Fundamental Theorem to evaluate the definite integrals in Problems 22–25.

22. $\displaystyle\int_0^2 x(x^2+1)^2\,dx$ **23.** $\displaystyle\int_0^3 \frac{2x}{x^2+1}\,dx$

24. $\displaystyle\int_0^1 2te^{-t^2}\,dt$ **25.** $\displaystyle\int_0^3 \frac{1}{\sqrt{t+1}}\,dt$

26. Use the Fundamental Theorem to find the area under $f(x) = x^2$ between $x = 1$ and $x = 4$.

27. Write the definite integral for the area under the graph of $f(x) = 6x^2 + 1$ between $x = 0$ and $x = 2$. Use the Fundamental Theorem of Calculus to evaluate it.

28. Use the Fundamental Theorem to find the average value of $f(x) = x^2 + 1$ on the interval $x = 0$ to $x = 10$. Illustrate your answer on a graph of $f(x)$.

29. Use the Fundamental Theorem of Calculus to find the average value of $f(x) = e^{0.5x}$ between $x = 0$ and $x = 3$. Show the average value on a graph of $f(x)$.

30. Find the exact area of the region bounded by the x-axis and the graph of $y = x^3 - x$.

31. Use the Fundamental Theorem to determine the value of b if the area under the graph of $f(x) = 4x$ between $x = 1$ and $x = b$ is equal to 240. Assume $b > 1$.

32. Use the Fundamental Theorem to determine the value of b if the area under the graph of $f(x) = 8x$ between $x = 1$ and $x = b$ is equal to 192. Assume $b > 1$.

33. Use the Fundamental Theorem to determine the value of b if the area under the graph of $f(x) = x^2$ between $x = 0$ and $x = b$ is equal to 100. Assume $b > 0$.

34. Oil is leaking out of a ruptured tanker at the rate of $r(t) = 50e^{-0.02t}$ thousand liters per minute.

(a) At what rate, in liters per minute, is oil leaking out at $t = 0$? At $t = 60$?

(b) How many liters leak out during the first hour?

35. With t in years since 2000, the population, P, of the world in billions can be modeled by $P = 6.1e^{0.012t}$.

(a) What does this model predict for the world population in 2010? In 2020?

(b) Use the Fundamental Theorem to predict the average population of the world between 2000 and 2010.

36. (a) Graph $f(x) = e^{-x^2}$ and shade the area represented by the improper integral $\int_{-\infty}^{\infty} e^{-x^2}\,dx$.

(b) Find $\int_{-a}^{a} e^{-x^2}\,dx$ for $a = 1$, $a = 2$, $a = 3$, $a = 5$.

(c) The improper integral $\int_{-\infty}^{\infty} e^{-x^2}\,dx$ converges to a finite value. Use your answers from part (b) to estimate that value.

37. Graph $y = 1/x^2$ and $y = 1/x^3$ on the same axes. Which do you think is larger: $\int_1^\infty 1/x^2\,dx$ or $\int_1^\infty 1/x^3\,dx$? Why?

38. In this problem, you will show that the following improper integral converges to 1.

$$\int_1^\infty \frac{1}{x^2}\,dx.$$

(a) Use the Fundamental Theorem to find $\int_1^b 1/x^2\,dx$. Your answer will contain b.

(b) Now take the limit as $b \to \infty$. What does this tell you about the improper integral?

39. Decide if the improper integral $\int_0^\infty e^{-2t}\,dt$ converges, and if so, to what value, by the following method.

(a) Evaluate $\int_0^b e^{-2t}\,dt$ for $b = 3, 5, 7, 10$. What do you observe? Make a guess about the convergence of the improper integral.

(b) Find $\int_0^b e^{-2t}\,dt$ using the Fundamental Theorem. Your answer will contain b.

(c) Take a limit as $b \to \infty$. Does your answer confirm your guess?

40. (a) Evaluate $\int_0^b xe^{-x/10}\,dx$ for $b = 10, 50, 100, 200$.

(b) Assuming that it converges, estimate the value of $\int_0^\infty xe^{-x/10}\,dx$.

41. The rate, r, at which people get sick during an epidemic of the flu can be approximated by

$$r = 1000te^{-0.5t},$$

where r is measured in people/day and t is measured in days since the start of the epidemic.

(a) Write an improper integral representing the total number of people that get sick.

(b) Use a graph of r to represent the improper integral from part (a) as an area.

42. Find the exact area below the curve $y = x^3(1-x)$ and above the x-axis.

43. Find the exact area enclosed by the curve $y = x^2(1-x)^2$ and the x-axis.

44. A car moves with velocity, v, at time t in hours by

$$v(t) = \frac{60}{50^t} \quad \text{miles/hour.}$$

(a) Does the car ever stop?

(b) Write an integral representing the total distance traveled for $t \ge 0$.

(c) Do you think the car goes a finite distance for $t \ge 0$? If so, estimate that distance.

45. An island has a carrying capacity of 1 million rabbits. (That is, no more than 1 million rabbits can be supported by the island.) The rabbit population is two at time $t = 1$ day and grows at a rate of $r(t)$ thousand rabbits/day until the carrying capacity is reached. For each of the following formulas for $r(t)$, is the carrying capacity ever reached? Explain your answer.

(a) $r(t) = 1/t^2$ **(b)** $r(t) = t$
(c) $r(t) = 1/\sqrt{t}$

46. **(a)** Between 1995 and 2005, ACME Widgets sold widgets at a continuous rate of $R = R_0 e^{0.15t}$ widgets per year, where t is time in years since January 1, 1995. Suppose they were selling widgets at a rate of 1000 per year on January 1, 1995. How many widgets did they sell between 1995 and 2005? How many did they sell if the rate on January 1, 1995 was 150,000,000 widgets per year?

(b) In the first case (1000 widgets per year on January 1, 1995), how long did it take for half the widgets in the ten-year period to be sold? In the second case (150,000,000 widgets per year on January 1, 1995), when had half the widgets in the ten-year period been sold?

(c) In 2005, ACME advertised that half the widgets it had sold in the previous ten years were still in use. Based on your answer to part (b), how long must a widget last in order to justify this claim?

7.4 INTEGRATION BY PARTS

Now we introduce *integration by parts*, which is a technique for finding integrals based on the product rule. To evaluate

$$\int xe^x \, dx,$$

we look for a function whose derivative is xe^x. The product rule might lead us to guess xe^x, because we know that its derivative has two terms, one of which is xe^x:

$$\frac{d}{dx}(xe^x) = \frac{d}{dx}(x)e^x + x\frac{d}{dx}(e^x) = e^x + xe^x.$$

Of course, our guess is wrong because of the extra e^x. But we can adjust our guess by subtracting e^x; this leads us to try $xe^x - e^x$. Let's check it:

$$\frac{d}{dx}(xe^x - e^x) = \frac{d}{dx}(xe^x) - \frac{d}{dx}(e^x) = e^x + xe^x - e^x = xe^x.$$

It works, so $\int xe^x \, dx = xe^x - e^x + C$.

The General Formula for Integration by Parts

We can formalize this process in the following way. We begin with the product rule:

$$\frac{d}{dx}(uv) = u'v + uv'$$

where u and v are functions of x with derivatives u' and v', respectively. We rewrite this as:

$$uv' = \frac{d}{dx}(uv) - u'v$$

and then integrate both sides:

$$\int uv' \, dx = \int \frac{d}{dx}(uv) \, dx - \int u'v \, dx.$$

Since an antiderivative of $\frac{d}{dx}(uv)$ is just uv, we get the following formula:

Integration by Parts

$$\int uv' \, dx = uv - \int u'v \, dx.$$

This technique is useful when the integrand can be viewed as a product and when the integral on the right-hand side is simpler than that on the left.

Example 1 Use integration by parts to find $\int xe^x\,dx$.

Solution We let $xe^x = (x)\cdot(e^x) = uv'$, and choose $u = x$ and $v' = e^x$. Thus, $u' = 1$ and $v = e^x$, so

$$\int \underbrace{(x)}_{u}\underbrace{(e^x)}_{v'}\,dx = \underbrace{(x)}_{u}\underbrace{(e^x)}_{v} - \int \underbrace{(1)}_{u'}\underbrace{(e^x)}_{v}\,dx = xe^x - e^x + C.$$

Let's look again at Example 1. Notice what would have happened if we took $v = e^x + C_1$. Then

$$\begin{aligned}\int xe^x\,dx &= x(e^x + C_1) - \int (e^x + C_1)\,dx\\ &= xe^x + C_1x - e^x - C_1x + C\\ &= xe^x - e^x + C,\end{aligned}$$

as before. Thus, it is not necessary to include an arbitrary constant in the antiderivative for v; any antiderivative will do.

What would have happened if we had picked u and v' the other way around in Example 1? If $u = e^x$ and $v' = x$, then $u' = e^x$ and $v = x^2/2$. The formula for integration by parts then gives

$$\int xe^x\,dx = \frac{x^2}{2}e^x - \int \frac{x^2}{2}\cdot e^x\,dx,$$

which is true but not helpful, since the new integral on the right seems harder than the original one on the left. To use this method, we must choose u and v' to make the integral on the right no harder to find than the integral on the left.

How to Choose u and v'

- Whatever you let v' be, you need to be able to find v.
- It helps if $u'v$ is simpler (or at least no more complicated) than uv'.

Example 2 Find $\int xe^{3x}\,dx$.

Solution We let $xe^{3x} = (x)\cdot(e^{3x}) = uv'$, and choose $u = x$ and $v' = e^{3x}$. Thus, $u' = 1$ and $v = \frac{1}{3}e^{3x}$. We have

$$\int \underbrace{(x)}_{u}\underbrace{(e^{3x})}_{v'}\,dx = \underbrace{(x)}_{u}\underbrace{(\frac{1}{3}e^{3x})}_{v} - \int \underbrace{(1)}_{u'}\underbrace{(\frac{1}{3}e^{3x})}_{v}\,dx = \frac{1}{3}xe^{3x} - \frac{1}{9}e^{3x} + C.$$

There are some examples which don't look like good candidates for integration by parts because they don't appear to involve products, but for which the method works well. Such examples often involve $\ln x$ or the inverse trigonometric functions. Here is one:

Example 3 Find $\int_2^3 \ln x\,dx$.

Solution This does not look like a product unless we write $\ln x = (1)(\ln x)$. Then we might say $u = 1$ so $u' = 0$, which certainly makes things simpler. But if $v' = \ln x$, what is v? If we knew, we would not need integration by parts. Let's try the other way: if $u = \ln x$, $u' = 1/x$ and if $v' = 1$, $v = x$, so

$$\int_2^3 \underbrace{(\ln x)}_{u}\underbrace{(1)}_{v'}\,dx = \underbrace{(\ln x)}_{u}\underbrace{(x)}_{v}\Big|_2^3 - \int_2^3 \underbrace{\left(\frac{1}{x}\right)}_{u'}\cdot\underbrace{(x)}_{v}\,dx$$

$$= x\ln x\Big|_2^3 - \int_2^3 1\,dx = (x\ln x - x)\Big|_2^3$$

$$= 3\ln 3 - 3 - 2\ln 2 + 2 = 3\ln 3 - 2\ln 2 - 1.$$

Notice that when doing a definite integral by parts, we must remember to put the limits of integration (here 2 and 3) on the uv term (in this case $x\ln x$) as well as on the integral $\int u'v\,dx$.

Example 4 Find $\int x^6 \ln x\,dx$.

Solution We can write $x^6\ln x$ as uv' where $u = \ln x$ and $v' = x^6$. Then $v = \frac{1}{7}x^7$ and $u' = 1/x$, so integration by parts gives us:

$$\int x^6\ln x\,dx = \int(\ln x)x^6\,dx = (\ln x)\left(\frac{1}{7}x^7\right) - \int \frac{1}{7}x^7\cdot\frac{1}{x}\,dx$$

$$= \frac{1}{7}x^7\ln x - \frac{1}{7}\int x^6\,dx$$

$$= \frac{1}{7}x^7\ln x - \frac{1}{49}x^7 + C.$$

In Example 4 we did not choose $v' = \ln x$, because it is not immediately clear what v would be. In fact, we used integration by parts in Example 3 to find the antiderivative of $\ln x$. Also, using $u = \ln x$, as we have done, gives $u'v = x^6/7$, which is simpler to integrate than $uv' = x^6\ln x$. This example shows that u does not have to be the first factor in the integrand (here x^6).

Problems for Section 7.4

Find the integrals in Exercises 1–14.

1. $\int te^{5t}\,dt$

2. $\int pe^{-0.1p}\,dp$

3. $\int (z+1)e^{2z}\,dz$

4. $\int y\ln y\,dy$

5. $\int x^3\ln x\,dx$

6. $\int q^5\ln 5q\,dq$

7. $\int y\sqrt{y+3}\,dy$

8. $\int (t+2)\sqrt{2+3t}\,dt$

9. $\int \frac{z}{e^z}\,dz$

10. $\int \frac{\ln x}{x^2}\,dx$

11. $\int \frac{y}{\sqrt{5-y}}\,dy$

12. $\int \frac{t+7}{\sqrt{5-t}}\,dt$

13. $\int t\sin t\,dt$

14. $\int_3^5 x\cos x\,dx$

In Problems 15–16, use integration by parts twice to evaluate the integral.

15. $\int t^2e^{5t}\,dt$

16. $\int (\ln t)^2\,dt$

Evaluate the integrals in Problems 17–20 both exactly [e.g. $\ln(3\pi)$] and numerically [e.g. $\ln(3\pi)\approx 2.243$].

17. $\int_1^5 \ln t\,dt$

18. $\int_0^{10} ze^{-z}\,dz$

19. $\int_1^3 t\ln t\,dt$

20. $\int_0^5 \ln(1+t)\,dt$

21. For each of the following integrals, indicate whether integration by substitution or integration by parts is more appropriate. Do not evaluate the integrals.

(a) $\displaystyle\int \frac{x^2}{1+x^3}\,dx$ **(b)** $\displaystyle\int xe^{x^2}\,dx$

(c) $\displaystyle\int x^2\ln(x^3+1)\,dx$ **(d)** $\displaystyle\int \frac{1}{\sqrt{3x+1}}\,dx$

(e) $\displaystyle\int x^2\ln x\,dx$ **(f)** $\displaystyle\int \ln x\,dx$

22. Find $\int_1^2 \ln x\,dx$ numerically. Find $\int_1^2 \ln x\,dx$ using antiderivatives. Check that your answers agree.

In Problems 23–25, find the exact area.

23. Under $y = te^{-t}$ for $0 \le t \le 2$.

24. Between $y = \ln x$ and $y = \ln(x^2)$ for $1 \le x \le 2$.

25. Between $f(t) = \ln(t^2 - 1)$ and $g(t) = \ln(t-1)$ for $2 \le t \le 3$.

26. Estimate $\int_0^{10} f(x)g'(x)\,dx$ if $f(x) = x^2$ and g has the values in the following table.

x	0	2	4	6	8	10
$g(x)$	2.3	3.1	4.1	5.5	5.9	6.1

27. The concentration, C, in ng/ml, of a drug in the blood as a function of the time, t, in hours since the drug was administered is given by $C = 15te^{-0.2t}$. The area under the concentration curve is a measure of the overall effect of the drug on the body, called the bioavailability. Find the bioavailability of the drug between $t = 0$ and $t = 3$.

28. During a surge in the demand for electricity, the rate, r, at which energy is used can be approximated by

$$r = te^{-at},$$

where t is the time in hours and a is a positive constant.

(a) Find the total energy, E, used in the first T hours. Give your answer as a function of a.

(b) What happens to E as $T \to \infty$?

29. Derive the formula (called a reduction formula):

$$\int x^n e^x\,dx = x^n e^x - n\int x^{n-1}e^x\,dx.$$

7.5 ANALYZING ANTIDERIVATIVES GRAPHICALLY AND NUMERICALLY

In this section, we use the Fundamental Theorem to approximate values of F when the rate of change, F', and one value of the function, $F(a)$, are known.

Example 1 Suppose $F'(t) = (1.8)^t$ and $F(0) = 2$. Find the value of $F(b)$ for $b = 0, 0.1, 0.2, \ldots, 1.0$.

Solution Apply the Fundamental Theorem with $F'(t) = (1.8)^t$ and $a = 0$ to get values for $F(b)$. Since

$$F(b) - F(0) = \int_0^b F'(t)\,dt = \int_0^b (1.8)^t\,dt$$

and $F(0) = 2$, we have

$$F(b) = 2 + \int_0^b (1.8)^t\,dt.$$

Use a calculator or computer to estimate the definite integral $\int_0^b (1.8)^t\,dt$ for each value of b. For example, when $b = 0.1$, we find that $\int_0^b (1.8)^t\,dt = 0.103$. Thus $F(0.1) = 2.103$. Continuing in this way gives the values in Table 7.1.

Table 7.1 *Approximate values of F*

b	0	0.1	0.2	0.3	0.4	0.5	0.6	0.7	0.8	0.9	1.0
$F(b)$	2	2.103	2.212	2.328	2.451	2.581	2.719	2.866	3.021	3.186	3.361

Notice from the table that the function $F(b)$ is increasing between $b = 0$ and $b = 1$. This is because the derivative $F'(t) = (1.8)^t$ is positive for t between 0 and 1.

Example 2 The graph of the derivative F' of a function F is shown in Figure 7.3. Assuming that $F(20) = 150$, estimate the maximum value attained by F.

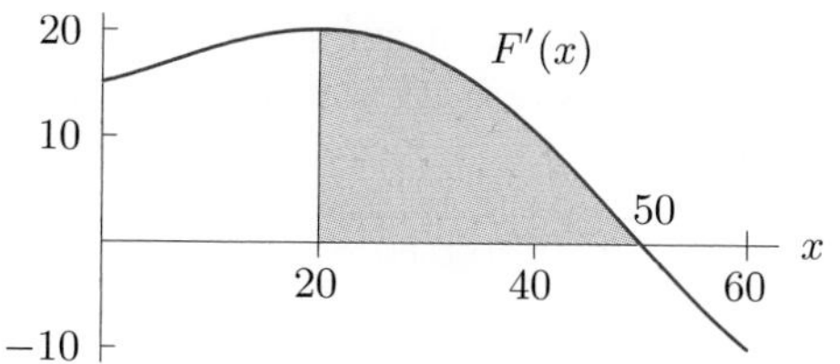

Figure 7.3: Graph of the derivative F' of some function F

Solution We know that $F(x)$ increases for $x < 50$ because the derivative of F is positive for $x < 50$. Similarly, $F(x)$ decreases for $x > 50$ because $F'(x)$ is negative for $x > 50$. Therefore, the graph of F rises until the point at which $x = 50$, and then it begins to fall. So the highest point on the graph of F is at $x = 50$ and the maximum value attained by F is $F(50)$. By the Fundamental Theorem:

$$F(50) - F(20) = \int_{20}^{50} F'(x)\,dx.$$

Since $F(20) = 150$, we have

$$F(50) = F(20) + \int_{20}^{50} F'(x)\,dx = 150 + \int_{20}^{50} F'(x)\,dx.$$

The definite integral is the area of the shaded region under the graph of F', which is roughly a triangle of base 30 and height 20. Therefore, the shaded area is about 300 and the maximum value attained by F is $F(50) \approx 150 + 300 = 450$.

Graphing a Function Given a Graph of its Derivative

Suppose we have the graph of f' and we want to sketch the graph of f. We know that when f' is positive, f is increasing, and when f' is negative, f is decreasing. If we want to know how much f increases or decreases, we compute a definite integral.

Example 3 Figure 7.4 shows the rate of change of the concentration of adrenaline, in micrograms per milliliter per minute, in a person's body. Sketch a graph of the concentration of adrenaline, in micrograms per milliliter, in the body as a function of time, in minutes.

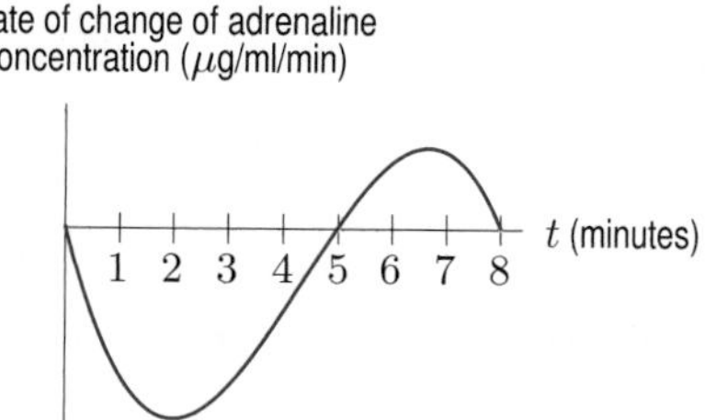

Figure 7.4: Rate of change of adrenaline concentration

Solution Since the initial concentration of the drug is not given, we can start the graph anywhere on the positive vertical axis. The rate of change is negative for $t < 5$ and positive for $t > 5$, so the concentration of adrenaline decreases until $t = 5$ and then increases. Since the area below the t-axis is greater than the area above the t-axis, the concentration of adrenaline decreases more than it increases. Thus, the concentration at $t = 8$ is less than the concentration at $t = 0$. Since the rate of change of concentration is zero at $t = 0, 5$, and 8, the graph of concentration is horizontal at these points. See Figure 7.5.

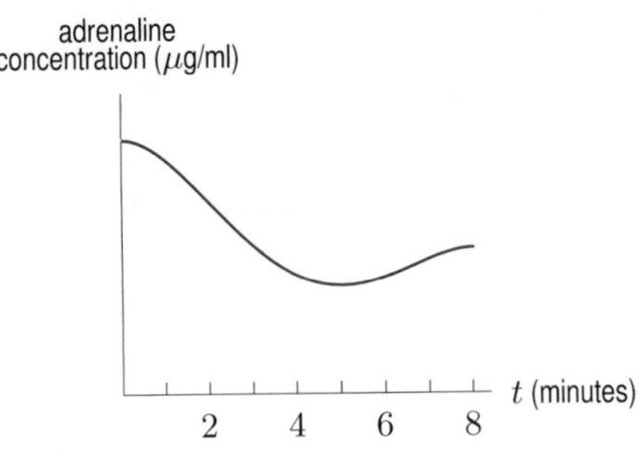

Figure 7.5: Adrenaline concentration

Example 4 Figure 7.6 shows the derivative $f'(x)$ of a function $f(x)$ and the values of some areas. If $f(0) = 10$, sketch a graph of the function $f(x)$. Give the coordinates of the local maxima and minima.

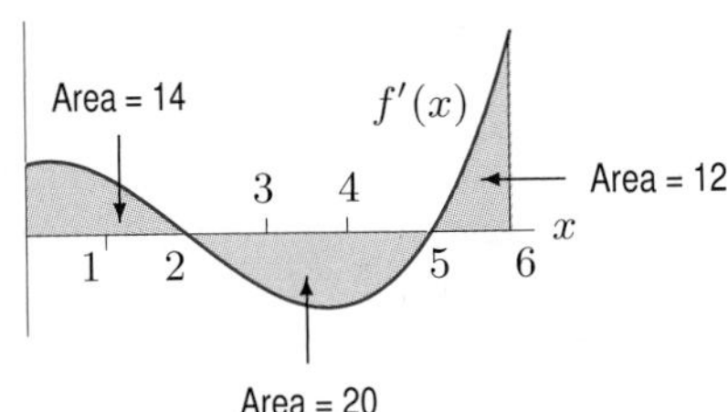

Figure 7.6: The graph of a derivative f'

Solution Figure 7.6 shows that the derivative f' is positive between 0 and 2, negative between 2 and 5, and positive between 5 and 6. Therefore, the function f is increasing between 0 and 2, decreasing between 2 and 5, and increasing between 5 and 6. (See Figure 7.7.) There is a local maximum at $x = 2$ and a local minimum at $x = 5$.

Notice that we can sketch the general shape of the graph of f without knowing any areas. The areas are used to make the graph more precise. We are told that $f(0) = 10$, so we plot the point $(0, 10)$ on the graph of f in Figure 7.8. The Fundamental Theorem and Figure 7.6 show that

$$f(2) - f(0) = \int_0^2 f'(x)\,dx = 14.$$

Therefore, the total change in f between $x = 0$ and $x = 2$ is 14. Since $f(0) = 10$, we have

$$f(2) = 10 + 14 = 24.$$

The point $(2, 24)$ is on the graph of f. See Figure 7.8.

Figure 7.6 shows that the area between $x = 2$ and $x = 5$ is 20. Since this area lies entirely below the x-axis, the Fundamental Theorem gives

$$f(5) - f(2) = \int_2^5 f'(x)\,dx = -20.$$

The total change in f is -20 between $x = 2$ and $x = 5$. Since $f(2) = 24$, we have

$$f(5) = 24 - 20 = 4.$$

Thus, the point $(5,4)$ lies on the graph of f. Finally,

$$f(6) = f(5) + \int_5^6 f'(x)\,dx = 4 + 12 = 16,$$

so the point $(6,16)$ is on the graph of f.

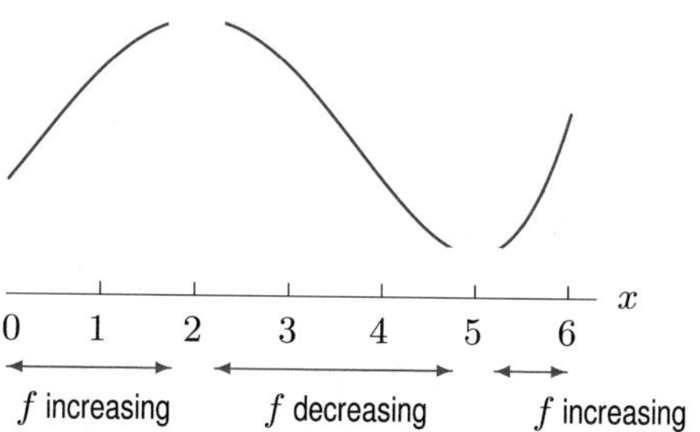

Figure 7.7: The shape of f

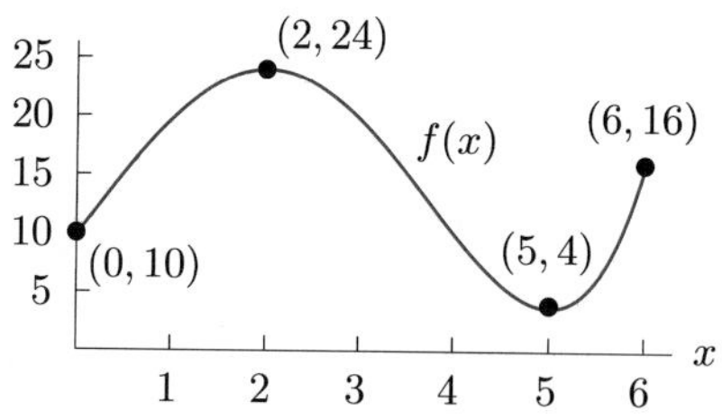

Figure 7.8: The graph of f

In this section we have seen how antiderivatives can by analyzed using the Fundamental Theorem of Calculus in the form

$$F(b) = F(0) + \int_0^b F'(t)\,dt.$$

In Section 8.2 we will see how antiderivatives can be constructed using the Second Fundamental Theorem introduced in Chapter 5's Focus on Theory section. This version of the theorem says that if f is a continuous function on an interval, and if a is any number in that interval, then the function F defined by

$$F(x) = \int_a^x f(t)\,dt$$

is an antiderivative of f; that is $F' = f$.

Problems for Section 7.5

1. The derivative $F'(t)$ is graphed in Figure 7.9. Given that $F(0) = 5$, calculate $F(t)$ for $t = 1, 2, 3, 4, 5$.

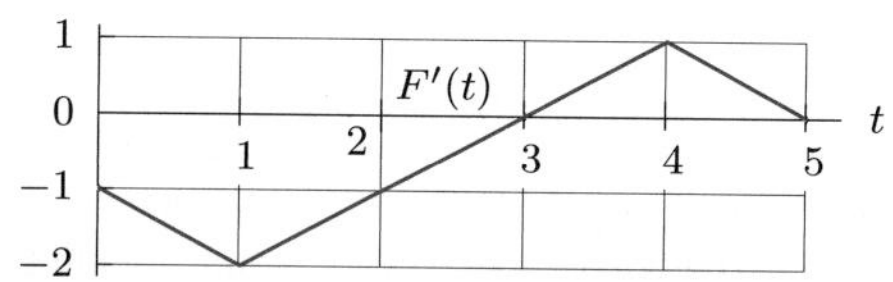

Figure 7.9

2. Figure 7.10 shows the derivative g'. If $g(0) = 0$, graph g. Give (x, y)-coordinates of all local maxima and minima.

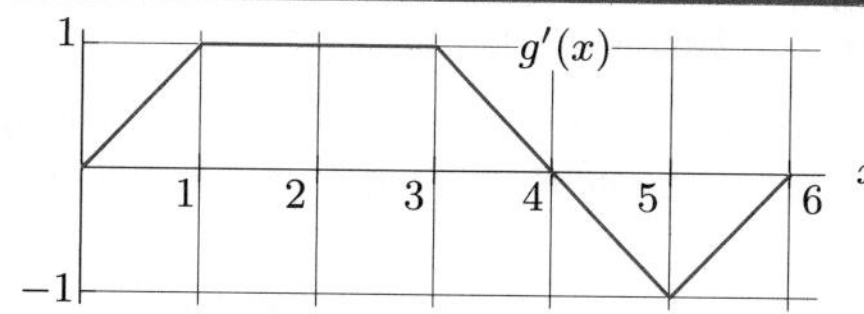

Figure 7.10

3. Figure 7.11 shows f. If $F' = f$ and $F(0) = 0$, find $F(b)$ for $b = 1, 2, 3, 4, 5, 6$.

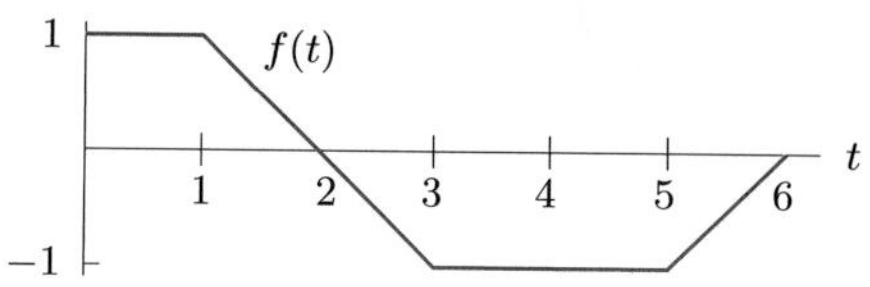

Figure 7.11

4. **(a)** Using Figure 7.12, estimate $\int_0^7 f(x)dx$.
(b) If F is an antiderivative of the same function f and $F(0) = 25$, estimate $F(7)$.

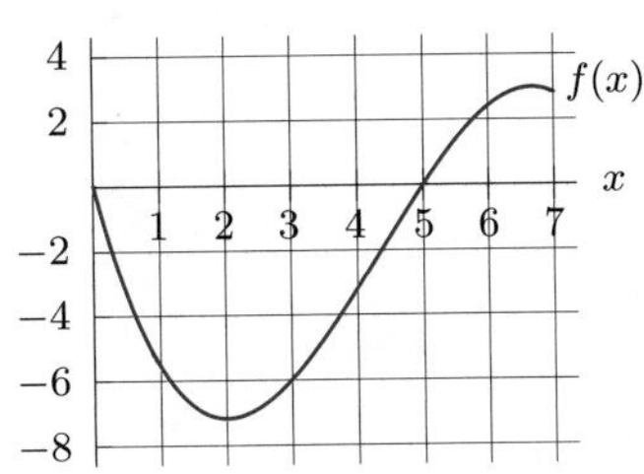

Figure 7.12

In Problems 5–8, sketch two functions F such that $F' = f$. In one case let $F(0) = 0$ and in the other, let $F(0) = 1$.

5.

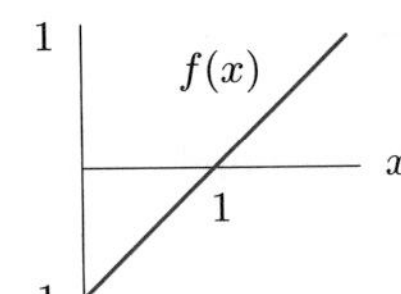

6.

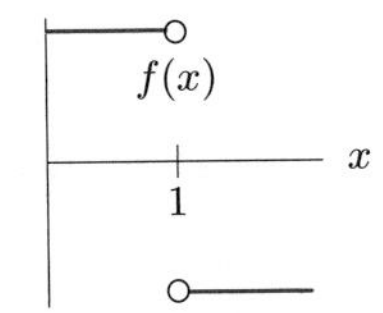

7.

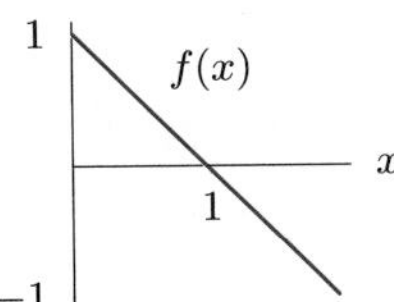

8.

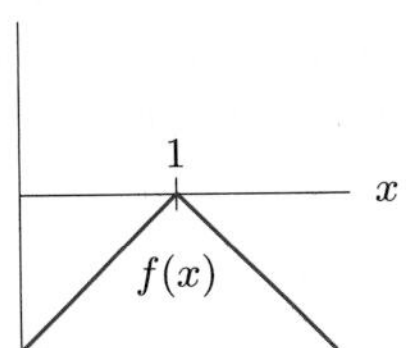

Problems 9–12 show the derivative f' of f.

(a) Where is f increasing and where is f decreasing? What are the x-coordinates of the local maxima and minima of f?

(b) Sketch a possible graph for f. (You don't need a scale on the vertical axis.)

9.

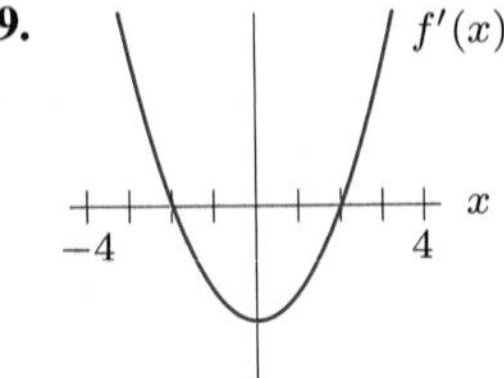

10.

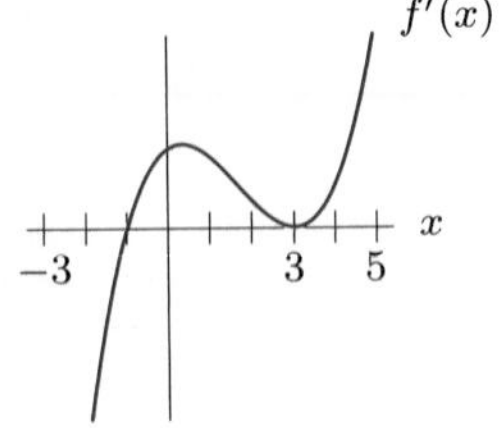

11. **12.**

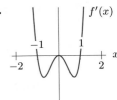

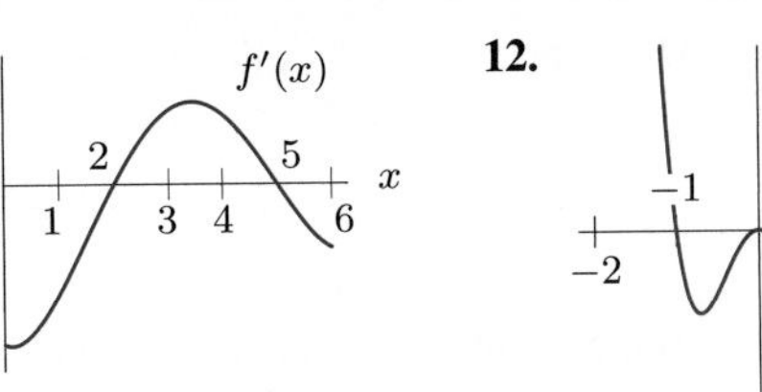

13. Figure 7.13 shows the rate at which photosynthesis is taking place in a leaf. The rate at which the leaf grows is approximately proportional to the rate of photosynthesis. Sketch the size of the leaf against time for 100 days.

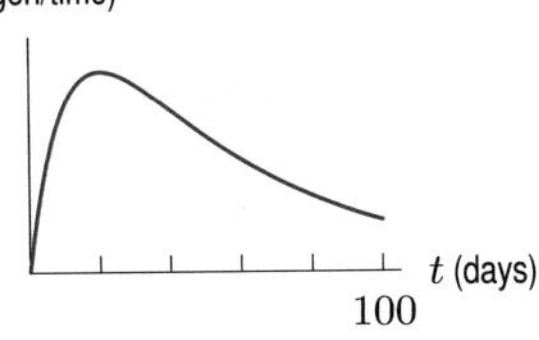

Figure 7.13

14. Figure 7.14 shows the derivative F' of F. Let $F(0) = 0$. Of the four numbers $F(1)$, $F(2)$, $F(3)$, and $F(4)$, which is largest? Which is smallest? How many of these numbers are negative?

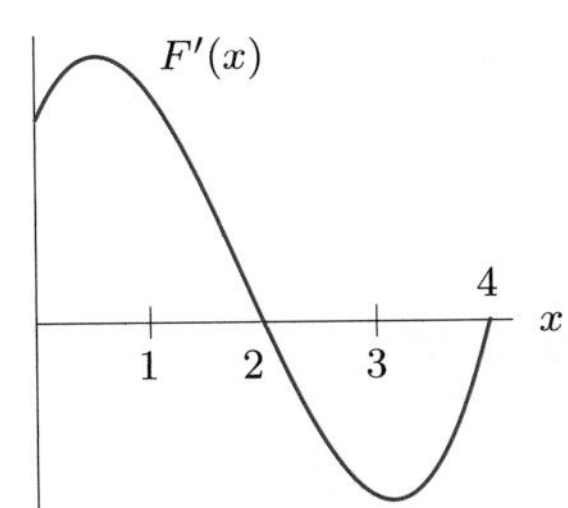

Figure 7.14

15. Urologists are physicians who specialize in the health of the bladder. In a common diagnostic test, urologists monitor the emptying of the bladder using a device that produces two graphs. In one of the graphs the flow rate (in milliliters per second) is measured as a function of time (in seconds). In the other graph, the volume emptied from the bladder is measured (in milliliters) as a function of time (in seconds). See Figure 7.15.

(a) Which graph is the flow rate and which is the volume?

(b) Which one of these graphs is an antiderivative of the other?

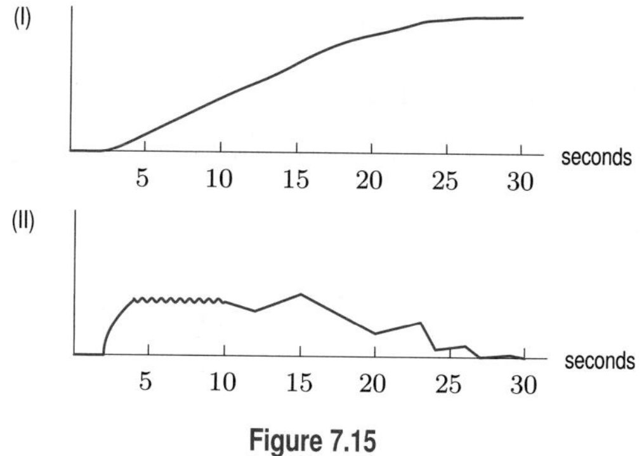

Figure 7.15

16. Use Figure 7.16 and the fact that $F(2) = 3$ to sketch the graph of $F(x)$. Label the values of at least four points.

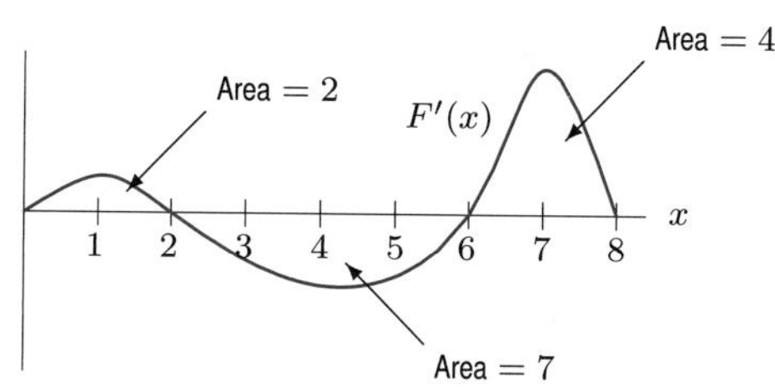

Figure 7.16

17. Figure 7.17 shows the derivative F'. If $F(0) = 14$, graph F. Give (x, y)-coordinates of all local maxima and minima.

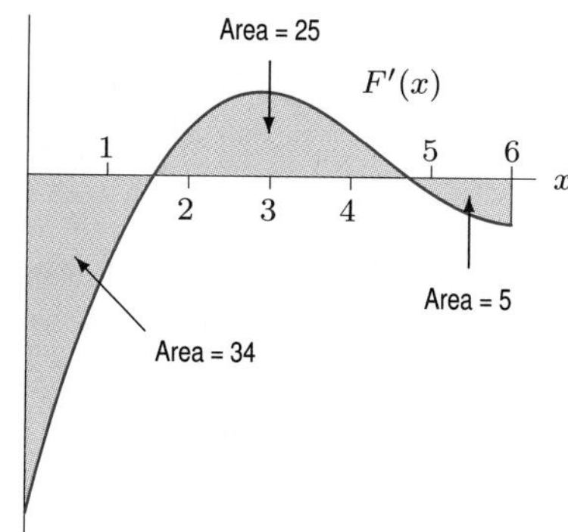

Figure 7.17

18. Figure 7.18 shows the derivative $F'(t)$. If $F(0) = 3$, find the values of $F(2)$, $F(5)$, $F(6)$. Graph $F(t)$.

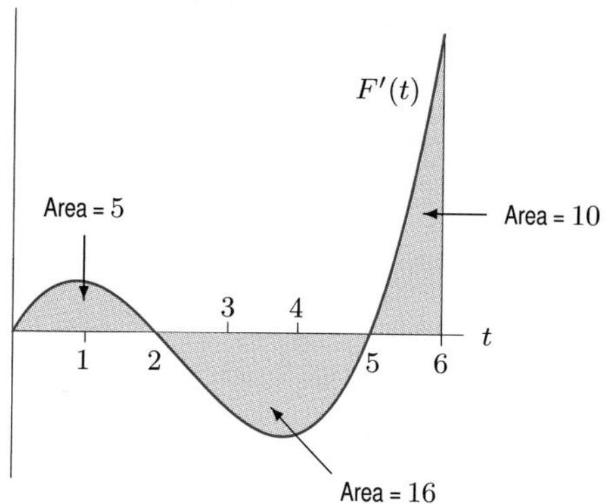

Figure 7.18

19. Using Figure 7.19, sketch a graph of an antiderivative $G(t)$ of $g(t)$ satisfying $G(0) = 5$. Label each critical point of $G(t)$ with its coordinates.

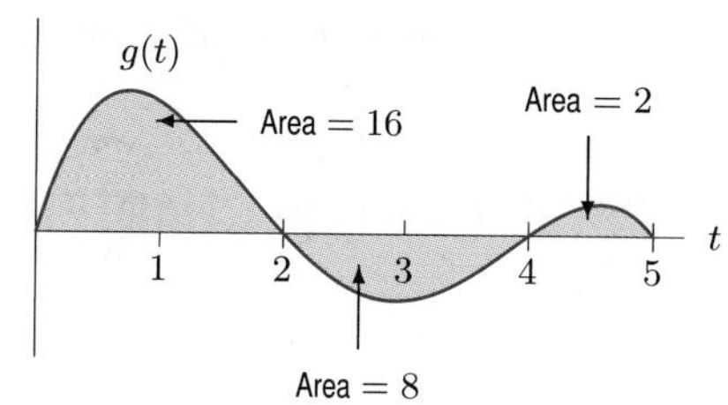

Figure 7.19

In Problems 20–21, a graph of f is given. Let $F'(x) = f(x)$.

(a) What are the critical points of $F(x)$?

(b) Which critical points are local maxima, which are local minima, and which are neither?

(c) Sketch a possible graph of $F(x)$.

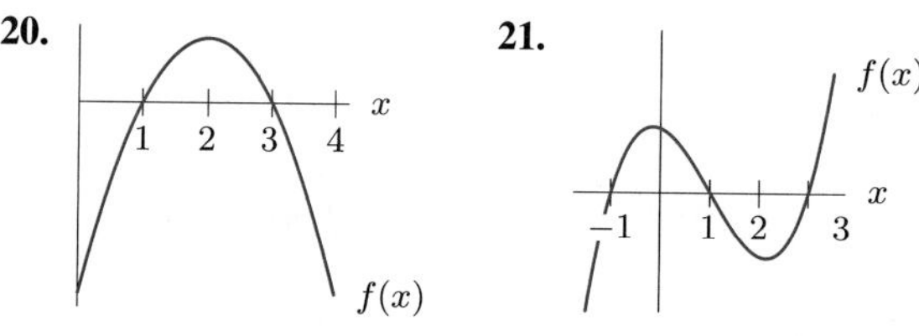

Problems 22–23 concern the graph of f' in Figure 7.20.

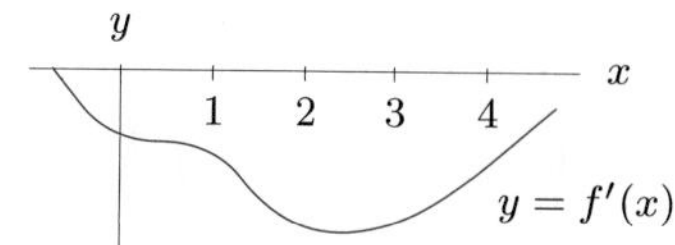

Figure 7.20: Note: Graph of f', not f

22. Which is greater, $f(0)$ or $f(1)$?

23. List the following in increasing order:

$$\frac{f(4) - f(2)}{2}, \quad f(3) - f(2), \quad f(4) - f(3).$$

For Problems 24–27, show the following quantities on Figure 7.21.

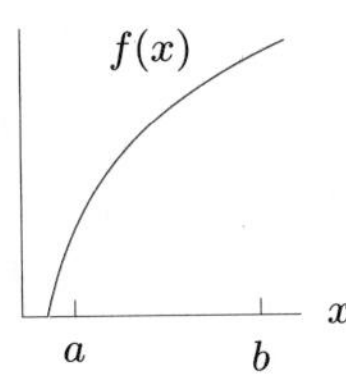

Figure 7.21

24. A length representing $f(b) - f(a)$.

25. A slope representing $\dfrac{f(b) - f(a)}{b - a}$.

26. An area representing $F(b) - F(a)$, where $F' = f$.

27. A length roughly approximating

$$\frac{F(b) - F(a)}{b - a}, \text{ where } F' = f.$$

CHAPTER SUMMARY

- **Computing antiderivatives**
  Powers and polynomials, e^{kx}, $\sin(kx)$, $\cos(kx)$
- Integration by substitution
- Integration by parts
- **Using antiderivatives to compute definite integrals analytically**: Fundamental Theorem of Calculus
- **Using definite integrals to analyze antiderivatives numerically and graphically**
- **Improper integrals**

REVIEW PROBLEMS FOR CHAPTER SEVEN

In Problems 1–10, find an antiderivative.

1. $f(t) = 2t^2 + 3t^3 + 4t^4$

2. $h(t) = 3t^2 + 7t + 1$

3. $f(x) = 6x^2 - 8x + 3$

4. $f(z) = e^z + 3$

5. $p(r) = 2\pi r$

6. $p(y) = \dfrac{1}{y} + y + 1$

7. $r(t) = \dfrac{1}{t^2}$

8. $g(t) = \sin t$

9. $g(x) = (x+1)^3$

10. $f(x) = (2x+1)^3$

Find the indefinite integrals in Problems 11–22.

11. $\displaystyle\int (4t + 7)\, dt$

12. $\displaystyle\int 3x\, dx$

13. $\displaystyle\int (x^3 - x)\, dx$

14. $\displaystyle\int e^{-0.05t}\, dt$

15. $\displaystyle\int \left(\frac{5}{t^2} + \frac{6}{t^3}\right) dt$

16. $\displaystyle\int \left(\frac{x+1}{x}\right) dx$

17. $\displaystyle\int (8t + 3)\, dt$

18. $\displaystyle\int \left(1 + \frac{1}{p}\right) dp$

19. $\displaystyle\int \left(8x^3 + \frac{1}{x}\right) dx$

20. $\displaystyle\int (5\cos x - 3\sin x) dx$

21. $\displaystyle\int \left(\frac{2}{x} + \pi \sin x\right) dx$

22. $\displaystyle\int (4x + 2e^x) dx$

Find the definite integrals in Problems 23–28 using the Fundamental Theorem.

23. $\displaystyle\int_0^2 (12x^2 + 1)\, dx$

24. $\displaystyle\int_{-3}^{-1} \frac{2}{r^3}\, dr$

25. $\displaystyle\int_0^1 \sin\theta\, d\theta$

26. $\displaystyle\int_1^2 \frac{1}{x}\, dx$

27. $\displaystyle\int_1^2 \frac{1}{x^2}\, dx$

28. $\displaystyle\int_0^2 \left(\frac{x^3}{3} + 2x\right) dx$

In Problems 29–31, find an antiderivative $F(x)$ with $F'(x) = f(x)$ and $F(0) = 0$. Is there only one possible solution?

29. $f(x) = 2x$

30. $f(x) = \dfrac{1}{4}x$

31. $\displaystyle\int \frac{2x}{\sqrt{x^2+1}} dx$

In Problems 32–41, integrate by substitution.

32. $\displaystyle\int 2x(x^2+1)^5 dx$

33. $\displaystyle\int xe^{-x^2}\, dx$

34. $\displaystyle\int \frac{4x^3}{x^4+1} dx$

35. $\displaystyle\int \frac{1}{(3x+1)^2} dx$

36. $\displaystyle\int \frac{x}{\sqrt{x^2+4}}\,dx$

37. $\displaystyle\int (5x-7)^{10}\,dx$

38. $\displaystyle\int 100e^{-0.2t}\,dt$

39. $\displaystyle\int x\sqrt{x^2+1}\,dx$

40. $\displaystyle\int x\sin(x^2)\,dx$

41. $\displaystyle\int t\cos(t^2)\,dt$

In Problems 42–43, find the exact area.

42. Under $f(x) = xe^{x^2}$ between $x = 0$ and $x = 2$.

43. Under $f(x) = 1/(x+1)$ between $x = 0$ and $x = 2$.

44. Find the exact average value of $f(x) = 1/(x+1)$ on the interval $x = 0$ to $x = 2$. Sketch a graph showing the function and the average value.

45. If t is in years, and $t = 0$ is January 1, 2005, worldwide energy consumption, r, in quadrillion (10^{15}) BTUs per year, is modeled by

$$r = 462e^{0.019t}.$$

(a) Write a definite integral for the total energy use between the start of 2005 and the start of 2010.

(b) Use the Fundamental Theorem of Calculus to evaluate the integral. Give units with your answer.

46. Use Figure 7.22 and the fact that $P = 2$ when $t = 0$ to find values of P when $t = 1, 2, 3, 4$ and 5.

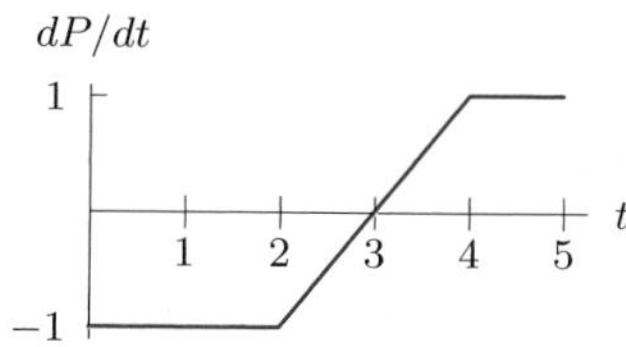

Figure 7.22

Problems 47–48 give a graph of $f'(x)$. Graph $f(x)$. Mark the points $x_1, \ldots, x_4$ on your graph and label local maxima, local minima and points of inflection.

47.

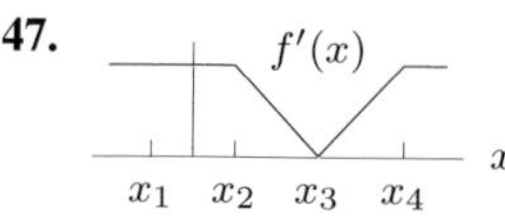

48.

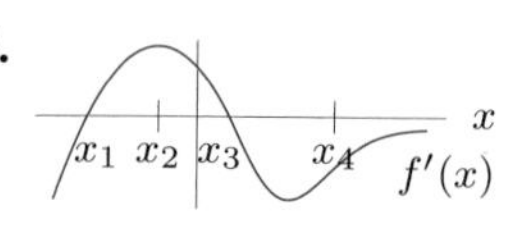

49. Figure 7.23 shows the derivative $F'(x)$. If $F(0) = 5$, find the value of $F(1)$, $F(3)$, and $F(4)$.

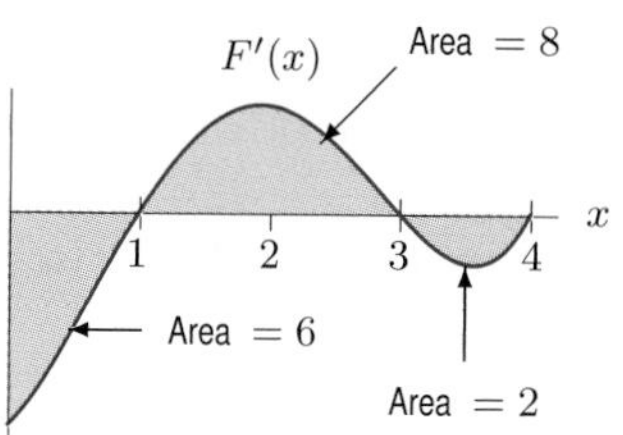

Figure 7.23

50. Suppose $\int_0^2 g(t)\,dt = 5$. Calculate the following:

(a) $\int_0^4 g(t/2)\,dt$ **(b)** $\int_0^2 g(2-t)\,dt$

51. **(a)** Sketch the area represented by the improper integral $\int_0^\infty xe^{-x}\,dx$.

(b) Calculate $\int_0^b xe^{-x}\,dx$ for $b = 5, 10, 20$.

(c) The improper integral in part (a) converges. Use your answers to part (b) to estimate its value.

52. Consider the improper integral

$$\int_1^\infty \frac{1}{\sqrt{x}}\,dx.$$

(a) Use a calculator or computer to find $\int_1^b 1/(\sqrt{x})\,dx$ for $b = 100, 1000, 10{,}000$. What do you notice?

(b) Find $\int_1^b 1/(\sqrt{x})\,dx$ using the Fundamental Theorem of Calculus. Your answer will contain b.

(c) Now take the limit as $b \to \infty$. What does this tell you about the improper integral?

53. At a time t hours after taking a tablet, the rate at which a drug is being eliminated is

$$r(t) = 50\left(e^{-0.1t} - e^{-0.2t}\right) \text{ mg/hr.}$$

Assuming that all the drug is eventually eliminated, calculate the original dose.

Use integration by parts to solve Problems 54–56.

54. $\displaystyle\int x\cos x\,dx$

55. $\displaystyle\int y\sin y\,dy$

56. $\displaystyle\int \ln(x^2)\,dx$

CHECK YOUR UNDERSTANDING

In Problems 1–50, indicate whether the statement is true or false.

1. $F(t) = \dfrac{t^3}{3} + 5$ is an antiderivative of $f(t) = t^2$.

2. $F(x) = \dfrac{x^{-3}}{-3}$ is an antiderivative of $f(x) = x^{-2}$.

3. $F(x) = e^{3x}$ is an antiderivative of $f(x) = e^{3x}$.

4. $\displaystyle\int t^3\, dt = \frac{t^4}{4} + C$.

5. $\displaystyle\int \frac{1}{\sqrt{z}}\, dz = 2\sqrt{z} + C$.

6. $\displaystyle\int e^x\, dx = \frac{e^{x+1}}{x+1} + C$.

7. $\displaystyle\int \ln|t|\, dt = \frac{1}{t} + C$.

8. $\displaystyle\int 2^x\, dx = \frac{1}{\ln 2}2^x + C$.

9. $\displaystyle\int 5\cos x\, dx = 5\sin x + C$.

10. If $F(x)$ and $G(x)$ are both antiderivatives of $h(x)$, then $F(x) - G(x)$ is a constant.

11. The substitution $w = q^3 + 3q^2 - q$ converts the integral $\int (q^3 + 3q^2 - q)^{10}\, dq$ into $\int w^{10}\, dw$.

12. The substitution $w = \ln x$ converts the integral $\displaystyle\int \frac{(\ln x)^2}{x}\, dx$ into $\int w^2\, dw$.

13. The substitution $w = x^2$ converts the integral $\int e^{x^2}\, dx$ into $\int e^w\, dw$.

14. The substitution $w = x^2$ converts the integral $\int xe^{x^2}\, dx$ into $\displaystyle\int \frac{1}{2}e^w\, dw$.

15. The substitution $w = 1 - s$ converts the integral $\displaystyle\int \frac{1}{\sqrt{1-s}}\, ds$ into $\displaystyle\int \frac{1}{\sqrt{w}}\, dw$.

16. The substitution $w = t^2 + 1$ converts the integral $\displaystyle\int \frac{t}{\sqrt{t^2+1}}\, dt$ into $\displaystyle\int \frac{1}{2\sqrt{w}}\, dw$.

17. The substitution $w = e^x + e^{-x}$ converts the integral $\displaystyle\int \frac{e^x - e^{-x}}{e^x + e^{-x}}\, dx$ into $\displaystyle\int \frac{1}{w}\, dw$.

18. The substitution $w = q^3$ converts the integral $\int q^2(q^3 + 5)^{10}\, dq$ into $\displaystyle\int \frac{1}{3}w^{10}\, dw$.

19. The substitution $w = \sin\alpha$ converts the integral $\int \sin^3\alpha\cos\alpha\, d\alpha$ into $\int w^3\, dw$.

20. The substitution $w = \cos x$ converts the integral $\displaystyle\int \frac{\sin x}{\cos x}\, dx$ into $\displaystyle\int \frac{1}{w}\, dw$.

21. $\displaystyle\int_2^3 \frac{1}{x}\, dx = \frac{1}{3} - \frac{1}{2}$.

22. $\displaystyle\int_2^3 \frac{1}{x}\, dx = \ln 3 - \ln 2$.

23. $\displaystyle\int_1^5 2x\, dx = 5^2 - 1^2$.

24. $\displaystyle\int_1^2 3x^2\, dx = 3(2^2) - 3(1^2)$.

25. $\displaystyle\int_0^3 t^4\, dt = \frac{t^5}{5} + C$.

26. $\displaystyle\int_1^2 e^t\, dt = e^2 - e$.

27. The substitution $w = x^2$ converts $\int_0^5 2xe^{x^2}\, dx$ into $\int_0^5 e^w\, dw$.

28. The substitution $w = \ln x$ converts $\int_1^e (\ln x)^3/x\, dx$ into $\int_0^1 w^3\, dw$.

29. If $f(x)$ is any function then $\int_{10}^{20} f(x)\, dx = 10\int_1^2 f(x)\, dx$.

30. The integral $\int_1^2 e^{-kx}\, dx$ is positive for any $k \neq 0$.

31. If a function f is positive on an interval, then its antiderivatives are all increasing on that interval.

32. If a function f is increasing on an interval, then its antiderivatives are all concave up on that interval.

33. For any function F with continuous derivative, $F(5) = F(0) + \int_0^5 F'(t)\, dt$.

34. For any function F with continuous derivative, $F(3) = F(0) + \int_1^3 F'(t)\, dt$.

35. If f' is in Figure 7.24, then $f(4) > f(3)$.

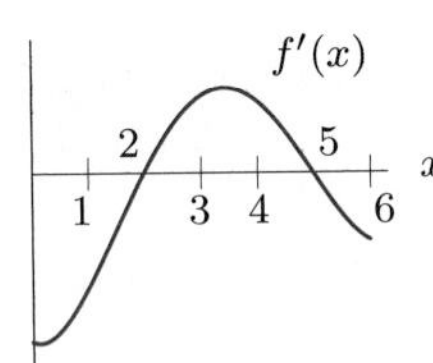

Figure 7.24

36. If f' is in Figure 7.24, then $f(2) > f(1)$.

37. If f' is in Figure 7.24, then $f(3) > f(2)$.

38. If f' is in Figure 7.24, then $f(5) > f(6)$.

39. If f' is in Figure 7.24, then $f(1) > f(0)$.

40. If f' is in Figure 7.24, then $f(1) \approx f(3)$.

41. Setting $u = x^3/3$ and $dv = e^x\,dx$ is a reasonable assignment of the parts for the integral $\int x^2 e^x\,dx$.

42. Setting $u = x$ and $dv = \sqrt{3x+1}\,dx$ is a reasonable assignment of the parts for the integral $\int x\sqrt{3x+1}\,dx$.

43. If $u = x^2$ and $dv = e^{3x}\,dx$ in integration by parts, then $du = 2x\,dx$ and $v = 3e^{3x}$.

44. If $u = x^2$ and $dv = \ln x\,dx$ in integration by parts, then $du = 2x\,dx$ and $v = 1/x$.

45. Integration by parts is an appropriate method to use in evaluating $\int xe^{3x^2}\,dx$.

46. Integration by parts is an appropriate method to use in evaluating $\int xe^{3x}\,dx$.

47. Integration by parts is an appropriate method to use in evaluating $\int \frac{x}{\sqrt{5x+1}}\,dx$.

48. Integration by parts is an appropriate method to use in evaluating $\int \frac{x}{\sqrt{5x^2+1}}\,dx$.

49. Integration by parts is an appropriate method to use in evaluating $\int x^2\sqrt{2x^3+9}\,dx$.

50. Integration by parts is an appropriate method to use in evaluating $\int x^3 \ln x\,dx$.

PROJECTS FOR CHAPTER SEVEN

1. **Quabbin Reservoir** The Quabbin Reservoir in the western part of Massachusetts provides most of Boston's water. The graph in Figure 7.25 represents the flow of water in and out of the Quabbin Reservoir throughout 2007.
   (a) Sketch a graph of the quantity of water in the reservoir, as a function of time.
   (b) When, in the course of 2007, was the quantity of water in the reservoir largest? Smallest? Mark and label these points on the graph you drew in part (a).
   (c) When was the quantity of water increasing most rapidly? Decreasing most rapidly? Mark and label these times on both graphs.
   (d) By July 2008 the quantity of water in the reservoir was about the same as in January 2007. Draw plausible graphs for the flow into and the flow out of the reservoir for the first half of 2008.

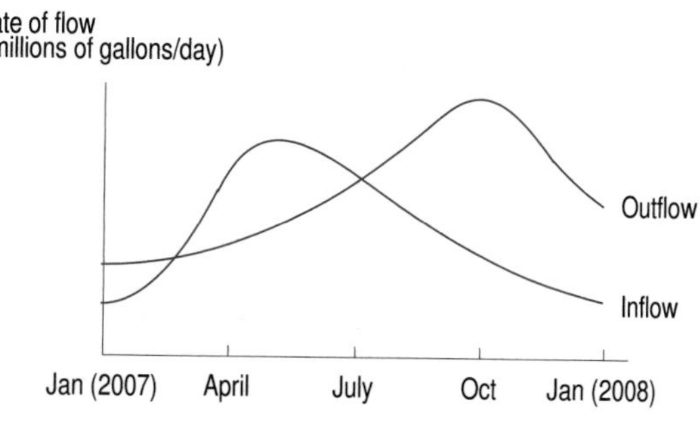

Figure 7.25

FOCUS ON PRACTICE

For Problems 1–48, evaluate the integrals. Assume a, b, A, B, P_0, h, and k are constants.

1. $\int (q^2 + 5q + 2) dq$
2. $\int (u^4 + 5)\, du$
3. $\int (x^2 + 1)\, dx$
4. $\int e^{-3t}\, dt$
5. $\int (6\sqrt{x}) dx$
6. $\int (ax^2 + b)\, dx$
7. $\int (x^3 + 4x + 8)\, dx$
8. $\int 100e^{-0.5t}\, dt$
9. $\int (w^4 - 12w^3 + 6w^2 - 10)\, dw$
10. $\int \left(\frac{4}{x} + \frac{5}{x^2}\right) dx$
11. $\int \frac{dq}{\sqrt{q}}$
12. $\int 3\sin\theta\, d\theta$
13. $\int (p^2 + \frac{5}{p})\, dp$
14. $\int P_0 e^{kt}\, dt$
15. $\int (q^3 + 8q + 15)\, dq$
16. $\int 1000e^{0.075t}\, dt$
17. $\int (5\sin x + 3\cos x)\, dx$
18. $\int (10 + 5\sin x)\, dx$
19. $\int \frac{5}{w}\, dw$
20. $\int \pi r^2 h\, dr$
21. $\int \left(q + \frac{1}{q^3}\right) dq$
22. $\int 15p^2 q^4\, dp$
23. $\int 15p^2 q^4\, dq$
24. $\int (3x^2 + 6e^{2x})\, dx$
25. $\int 5e^{2q}\, dq$
26. $\int \left(p^3 + \frac{1}{p}\right) dp$
27. $\int (Ax^3 + Bx)\, dx$
28. $\int (6\sqrt{x} + 15)\, dx$
29. $\int (x^2 + 8 + e^x)\, dx$
30. $\int 30e^{-0.2t} dt$
31. $\int (t^2 - 6t + 5)\, dt$
32. $\int \left(\frac{a}{x} + \frac{b}{x^2}\right) dx$
33. $\int (Aq + B) dq$
34. $\int \left(\frac{6}{\sqrt{x}} + 8\sqrt{x}\right) dx$
35. $\int (e^{2t} + 5) dt$
36. $\int \sin(3x) dx$
37. $\int 12\cos(4x) dx$
38. $\int \frac{1}{y+2} dy$
39. $\int y(y^2 + 5)^8\, dy$
40. $\int \cos(4x) dx$
41. $\int A\sin(Bt) dt$
42. $\int \sqrt{3x + 1} dx$
43. $\int \frac{e^x}{2 + e^x}\, dx$
44. $\int \sin^6(5\theta)\cos(5\theta)\, d\theta$
45. $\int \frac{\cos x}{\sqrt{1 + \sin x}}\, dx$
46. $\int x\ln x\, dx$
47. $\int xe^x\, dx$
48. $\int_0^{10} ze^{-z}\, dz$

Chapter Eight

PROBABILITY

Contents

8.1 DENSITY FUNCTIONS

Understanding the distribution of various quantities through the population can be important to decision makers. For example, the income distribution gives useful information about the economic structure of a society. In this section we look at the distribution of ages in the US. To allocate funding for education, health care, and social security, the government needs to know how many people are in each age group. We see how to represent such information by a density function.

US Age Distribution

Table 8.1 *Distribution of ages in the US in 2000*

Age group	Percentage of total population
0 – 20	29%
20 – 40	29%
40 – 60	26%
60 – 80	13%
80 – 100	3%

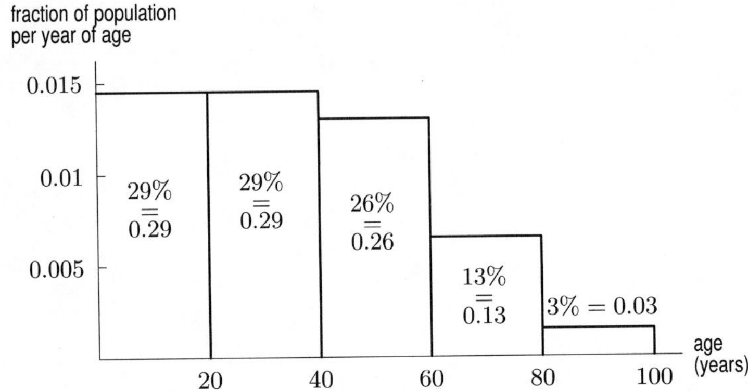

Figure 8.1: How ages were distributed in the US in 2000

Suppose we have the data in Table 8.1 showing how the ages of the US population[1] were distributed in 2000. To represent this information graphically we use a type of *histogram*[2] putting a vertical bar above each age group in such a way that the *area* of each bar represents the percentage in that age group. The total area of all the rectangles is $100\% = 1$. We only consider people who are less than 100 years old.[3] For the 0–20 age group, the base of the rectangle is 20, and we want the area to be 29%, so the height must be $29\%/20 = 1.45\%$. We treat ages as though they were continuously distributed. The category 0–20, for example, contains people who are just one day short of their twentieth birthday. Notice that the vertical axis is measured in percent/year. (See Figure 8.1.)

Example 1 In 2000, estimate what percentage of the US population was:

(a) Between 20 and 60 years old?
(b) Less than 10 years old?
(c) Between 75 and 80 years old?
(d) Between 80 and 85 years old?

Solution

(a) We add the percentages, so $29\% + 26\% = 55\%$.

(b) To find the percentage less than 10 years old, we could assume, for example, that the population was distributed evenly over the 0–20 group. (This means we are assuming that babies were born at a fairly constant rate over the last 20 years, which is probably reasonable.) If we make this assumption, then we can say that the population less than 10 years old was about half that in the 0–20 group, that is, 14.5%. Notice that we get the same result by computing the area of the rectangle from 0 to 10. (See Figure 8.2.)

(c) To find the population between 75 and 80 years old, since 13% of Americans in 2000 were in the 60-80 group, we might apply the same reasoning and say that $\frac{1}{4}(13\%) = 3.25\%$ of the population was in this age group. This result is represented as an area in Figure 8.2. The assumption that the population was evenly distributed is not a good one here; certainly there were more people between the ages of 60 and 65 than between 75 and 80. Thus, the estimate of 3.25% is certainly too high.

[1] www.censusscope.org/us/chart_age.html, accessed May 10, 2005.

[2] There are other types of histograms which have frequency on the vertical axis.

[3] In fact, 0.02% of the population is over 100, but this is too small to be visible on the histogram.

(d) Again using the (faulty) assumption that ages in each group were distributed uniformly, we would find that the percentage between 80 and 85 was $\frac{1}{4}(3\%) = 0.75\%$. (See Figure 8.2.) This estimate is also poor—there were certainly more people in the 80–85 group than, say, the 95–100 group, and so the 0.75% estimate is too low.

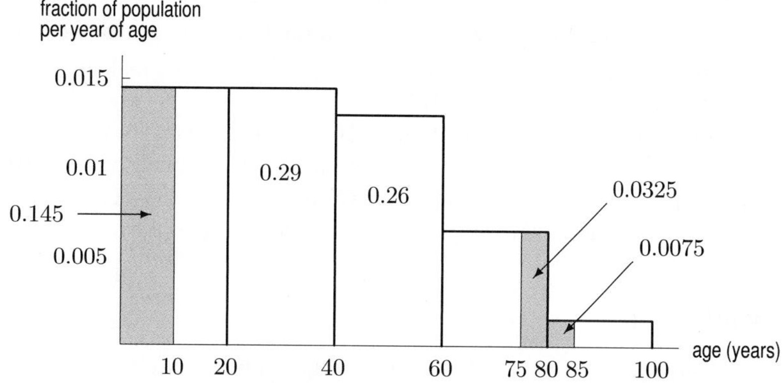

Figure 8.2: Ages in the US in 2000—various subgroups (for Example 1)

Smoothing Out the Histogram

We could get better estimates if we had smaller age groups (each age group in Figure 8.1 is 20 years, which is quite large) or if the histogram were smoother. Suppose we have the more detailed data in Table 8.2, which leads to the new histogram in Figure 8.3.

As we get more detailed information, the upper silhouette of the histogram becomes smoother, but the area of any of the bars still represents the percentage of the population in that age group. Imagine, in the limit, replacing the upper silhouette of the histogram by a smooth curve in such a way that area under the curve above one age group is the same as the area in the corresponding rectangle. The total area under the whole curve is again 100% = 1. (See Figure 8.3.)

The Age Density Function

If t is age in years, we define $p(t)$, the age *density function*, to be a function which "smooths out" the age histogram. This function has the property that

$$\text{Fraction of population between ages } a \text{ and } b = \text{Area under graph of } p \text{ between } a \text{ and } b = \int_a^b p(t)dt.$$

Table 8.2 *Ages in the US in 2000 (more detailed)*

Age group	Percentage of total population
0 – 10	14%
10 – 20	15%
20 – 30	14%
30 – 40	15%
40 – 50	15%
50 – 60	11%
60 – 70	7%
70 – 80	6%
80 – 90	2%
90 – 100	1%

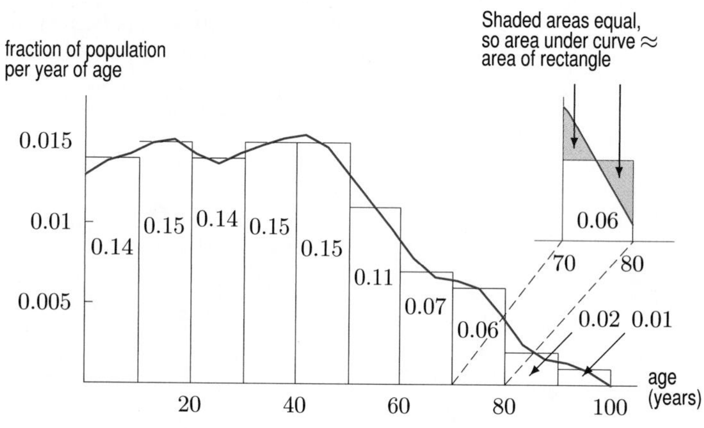

Figure 8.3: Smoothing out the age histogram

If a and b are the smallest and largest possible ages (say, $a = 0$ and $b = 100$), so that the ages of all of the population are between a and b, then

$$\int_a^b p(t)dt = \int_0^{100} p(t)dt = 1.$$

What does the age density function p tell us? Notice that we have not talked about the meaning of $p(t)$ itself, but *only* of the integral $\int_a^b p(t)\,dt$. Let's look at this in a bit more detail. Suppose, for example, that $p(10) = 0.014 = 1.4\%$ per year. This is *not* telling us that 1.4% of the population is precisely 10 years old (where 10 years old means exactly 10, not $10\frac{1}{2}$, not $10\frac{1}{4}$, not 10.1). However, $p(10) = 0.014$ does tell us that for some small interval Δt around 10, the fraction of the population with ages in this interval is approximately $p(10)\,\Delta t = 0.014\,\Delta t$. Notice also that the units of $p(t)$ are $\%$ *per year*, so $p(t)$ must be multiplied by years to give a percentage of the population.

The Density Function

Suppose we are interested in how a certain numerical characteristic, x, is distributed through a population. For example, x might be height or age if the population is people, or might be wattage for a population of light bulbs. Then we define a general density function with the following properties:

The function, $p(x)$, is a **density function** if

Fraction of population for which x is between a and b	$=$	Area under graph of p between a and b	$= \int_a^b p(x)dx.$

$$\int_{-\infty}^{\infty} p(x)\,dx = 1 \quad \text{and} \quad p(x) \geq 0 \quad \text{for all } x.$$

The density function must be nonnegative if its integral always gives a fraction of the population. The fraction of the population with x between $-\infty$ and ∞ is 1 because the entire population has the characteristic x between $-\infty$ and ∞. The function p that was used to smooth out the age histogram satisfies this definition of a density function. Notice that we do not assign a meaning to the value $p(x)$ directly, but rather interpret $p(x)\,\Delta x$ as the fraction of the population with the characteristic in a short interval of length Δx around x.

Example 2 Figure 8.4 gives the density function for the amount of time spent waiting at a doctor's office.

(a) What is the longest time anyone has to wait?
(b) Approximately what fraction of patients wait between 1 and 2 hours?
(c) Approximately what fraction of patients wait less than an hour?

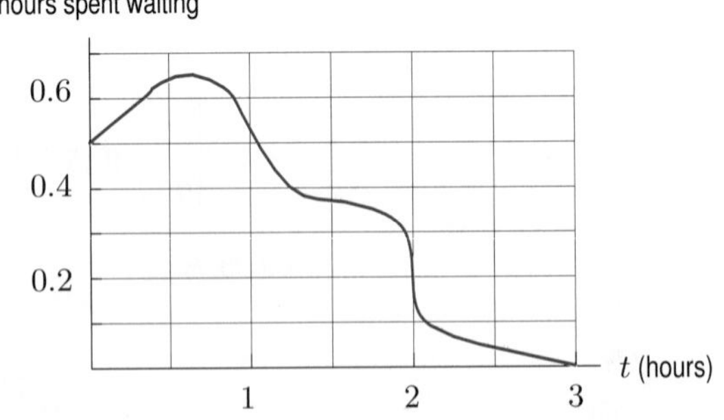

Figure 8.4: Distribution of waiting time at a doctor's office

Solution

(a) The density function is zero for all $t > 3$, so no one waits more than 3 hours. The longest time anyone has to wait is 3 hours.

(b) The fraction of patients who wait between 1 and 2 hours is equal to the area under the density curve between $t = 1$ and $t = 2$. We can estimate this area by counting squares: There are about 7.5 squares in this region, each of area $(0.5)(0.1) = 0.05$. The area is approximately $(7.5)(0.05) = 0.375$. Thus about 37.5% of patients wait between 1 and 2 hours.

(c) This fraction is equal to the area under the density function for $t < 1$. There are about 12 squares in this area, and each has area 0.05 as in part (b), so our estimate for the area is $(12)(0.05) = 0.60$. Therefore, about 60% of patients see the doctor in less than an hour.

Problems for Section 8.1

In Problems 1–4, the distribution of the heights, x, in meters, of trees is represented by the density function $p(x)$. In each case, calculate the fraction of trees which are:

(a) Less than 5 meters high

(b) More than 6 meters high

(c) Between 2 and 5 meters high

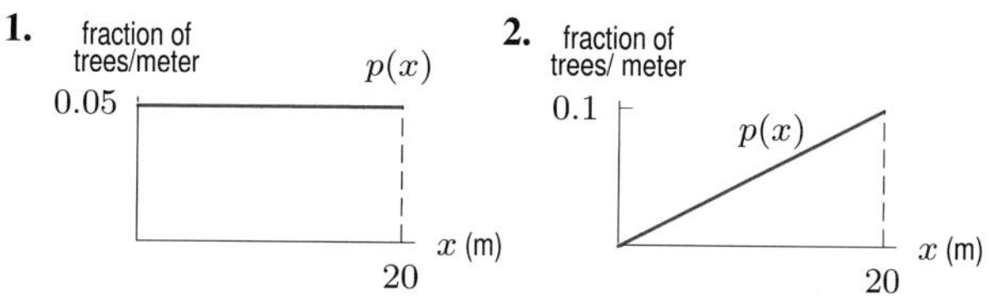

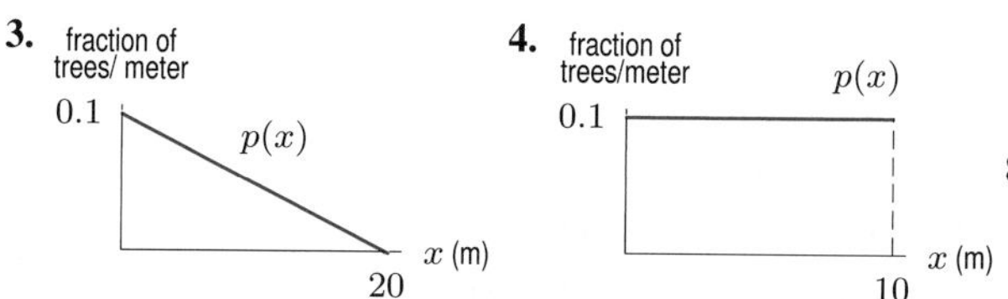

5. Suppose that $p(x)$ is the density function for heights of American men, in inches. What is the meaning of the statement $p(68) = 0.2$?

6. The density function $p(t)$ for the length of the larval stage, in days, for a breed of insect is given in Figure 8.5. What fraction of these insects are in the larval stage for between 10 and 12 days? For less than 8 days? For more than 12 days? In which one-day interval is the length of a larval stage most likely to fall?

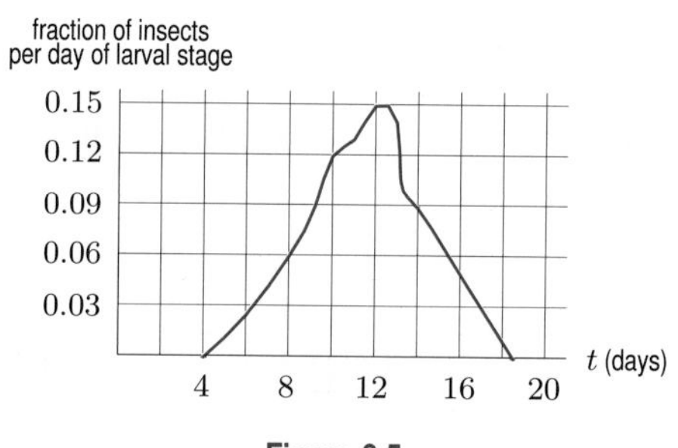

Figure 8.5

7. A machine lasts up to 10 years. Figure 8.6 shows the density function, $p(t)$, for the length of time it lasts.

(a) What is the value of C?

(b) Is a machine more likely to break in its first year or in its tenth year? In its first or second year?

(c) What fraction of the machines lasts 2 years or less? Between 5 and 7 years? Between 3 and 6 years?

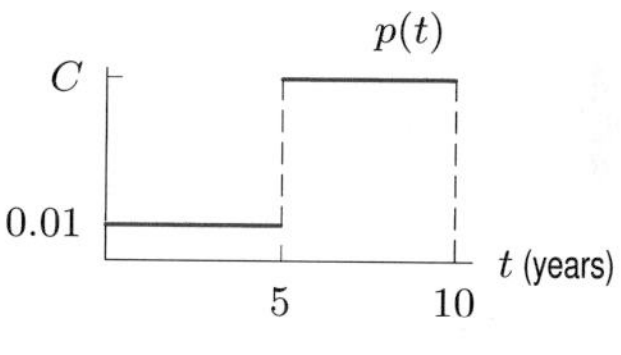

Figure 8.6

8. Figure 8.7 shows the distribution of the number of years of education completed by adults in a population. What does the shape of the graph tell you? Estimate the percentage of adults who have completed less than 10 years of education.

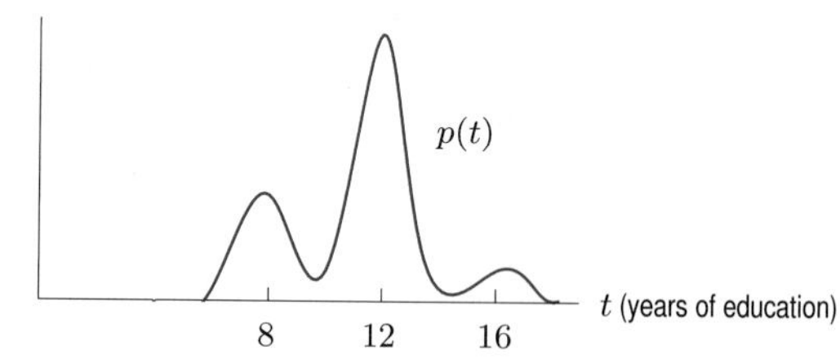

Figure 8.7

In Problems 9–12, given that $p(x)$ is a density function, find the value of a.

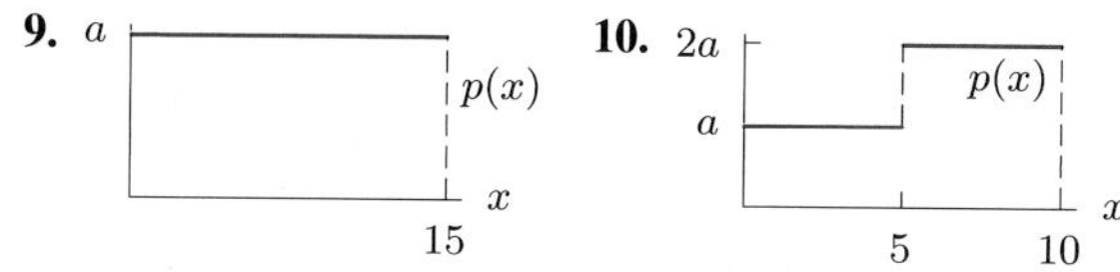

11.

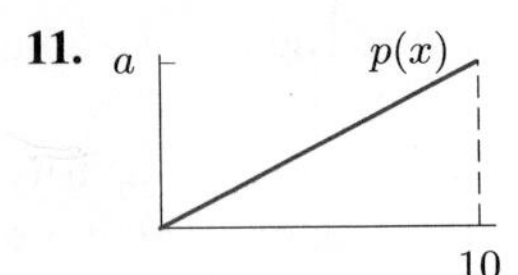

12.

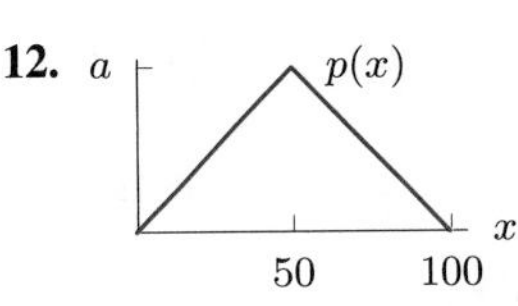

In Problems 13–15, graph a possible density function representing crop yield (in kilograms) from a field under the given circumstance.

13. All yields from 0 to 100 kg are equally likely; the field never yields more than 100 kg.

14. High yields are more likely than low. The maximum yield is 200 kg.

15. A drought makes low yields most common, and there is no yield greater than 30 kg.

16. Which of the following functions makes the most sense as a model for the probability density representing the time (in minutes, starting from $t = 0$) that the next customer walks into a store?

(a) $p(t) = \begin{cases} \cos t & 0 \le t \le 2\pi \\ e^{t-2\pi} & t \ge 2\pi \end{cases}$
(b) $p(t) = 3e^{-3t}$ for $t \ge 0$
(c) $p(t) = e^{-3t}$ for $t \ge 0$
(d) $p(t) = 1/4$ for $0 \le t \le 4$

8.2 CUMULATIVE DISTRIBUTION FUNCTIONS AND PROBABILITY

Section 8.1 introduced density functions which describe the way in which a numerical characteristic is distributed through a population. In this section we study another way to present the same information.

Cumulative Distribution Function for Ages

An alternative way of showing how ages are distributed in the US is by using the *cumulative distribution function* $P(t)$, defined by

$$P(t) = \begin{array}{c}\text{Fraction of population}\\ \text{of age less than } t\end{array} = \int_0^t p(x)dx.$$

Thus, P is the antiderivative of p with $P(0) = 0$, so $P(t)$ is the area under the density curve between 0 and t. See the left-hand part of Figure 8.8.

Notice that the cumulative distribution function is nonnegative and increasing (or at least nondecreasing), since the number of people younger than age t increases as t increases. Another way of seeing this is to notice that $P' = p$, and p is positive (or nonnegative). Thus the cumulative age distribution is a function which starts with $P(0) = 0$ and increases as t increases. We have $P(t) = 0$ for $t < 0$ because, when $t < 0$, there is no one whose age is less than t. The limiting value of P, as $t \to \infty$, is 1 since as t becomes very large (100 say), everyone is younger than age t, so the fraction of people with age less than t tends toward 1.

We want to find the cumulative distribution function for the age density function shown in Figure 8.3. We see that $P(10)$ is equal to 0.14, since Figure 8.3 shows that 14% of the population is between 0 and 10 years of age. Also,

$$P(20) = \begin{array}{c}\text{Fraction of the population}\\ \text{between 0 and 20 years old}\end{array} = 0.14 + 0.15 = 0.29$$

and similarly

$$P(30) = 0.14 + 0.15 + 0.14 = 0.43.$$

Continuing in this way gives the values for $P(t)$ in Table 8.3. These values were used to graph $P(t)$ in the right-hand part of Figure 8.8.

Table 8.3 *Cumulative distribution function, $P(t)$, giving fraction of US population of age less than t years*

t	0	10	20	30	40	50	60	70	80	90	100
$P(t)$	0	0.14	0.29	0.43	0.58	0.73	0.84	0.91	0.97	0.99	1.00

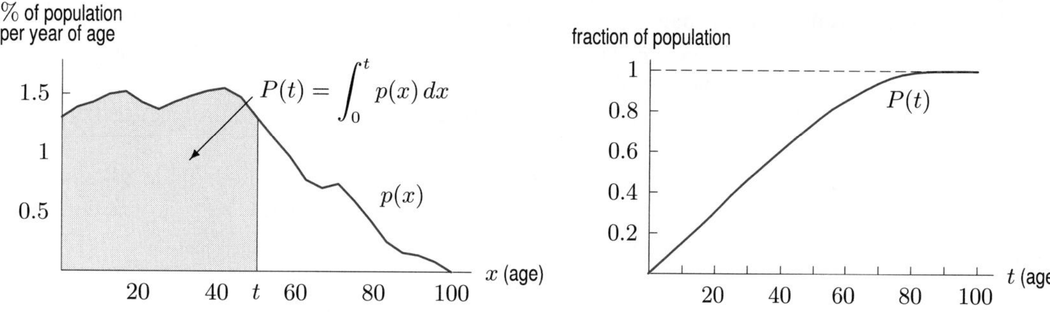

Figure 8.8: Graph of $p(x)$, the age density function, and its relation to $P(t)$, the cumulative age distribution function

Cumulative Distribution Function

A **cumulative distribution function**, $P(t)$, of a density function p, is defined by

$$P(t) = \int_{-\infty}^{t} p(x)\,dx = \text{Fraction of population having values of } x \text{ below } t.$$

Thus, P is an antiderivative of p, that is, $P' = p$.
Any cumulative distribution function has the following properties:

- P is increasing (or nondecreasing).
- $\lim_{t\to\infty} P(t) = 1$ and $\lim_{t\to-\infty} P(t) = 0$.
- Fraction of population having values of x between a and b $= \int_a^b p(x)\,dx = P(b) - P(a)$.

Example 1 The time to conduct a routine maintenance check on a machine has a cumulative distribution function $P(t)$, which gives the fraction of maintenance checks completed in time less than or equal to t minutes. Values of $P(t)$ are given in Table 8.4.

Table 8.4 *Cumulative distribution function for time to conduct maintenance checks*

t (minutes)	0	5	10	15	20	25	30
$P(t)$ (fraction completed)	0	0.03	0.08	0.21	0.38	0.80	0.98

(a) What fraction of maintenance checks are completed in 15 minutes or less?
(b) What fraction of maintenance checks take longer than 30 minutes?
(c) What fraction take between 10 and 15 minutes?
(d) Draw a histogram showing how times for maintenance checks are distributed.
(e) In which of the given 5-minute intervals is the length of a maintenance check most likely to fall?
(f) Give a rough sketch of the density function.
(g) Sketch a graph of the cumulative distribution function.

Solution

(a) The fraction of maintenance checks completed in 15 minutes is $P(15) = 0.21$, or 21%.
(b) Since $P(30) = 0.98$, we see that 98% of maintenance checks take 30 minutes or less. Therefore, only 2% take more than 30 minutes.
(c) Since 8% take 10 minutes or less and 21% take 15 minutes or less, the fraction taking between 10 and 15 minutes is $0.21 - 0.08 = 0.13$, or 13%.
(d) We begin by making a table showing how the times are distributed. Table 8.4 shows that the fraction of checks completed between 0 and 5 minutes is 0.03, and the fraction completed between 5 and 10 minutes is 0.05, and so on. See Table 8.5.

Table 8.5 *Distribution of time to conduct maintenance checks*

t (minutes)	$0-5$	$5-10$	$10-15$	$15-20$	$20-25$	$25-30$	>30
Fraction completed	0.03	0.05	0.13	0.17	0.42	0.18	0.02

The histogram in Figure 8.9 is drawn so that the area of each bar is the fraction of checks completed in the corresponding time period. For instance, the first bar has area 0.03 and width 5 minutes, so its height is $0.03/5 = 0.006$.

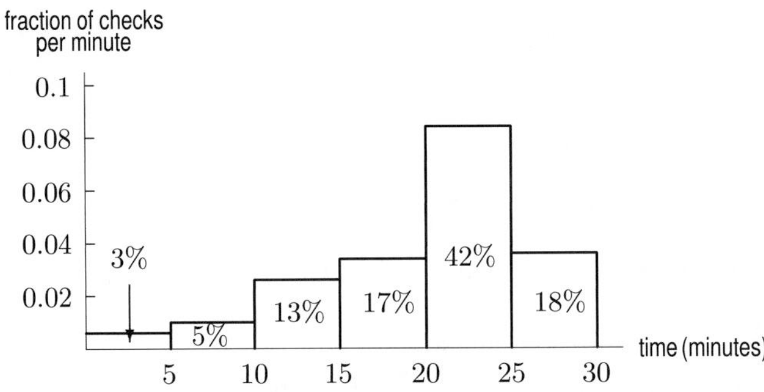

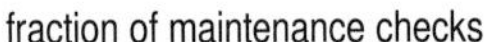

Figure 8.9: Histogram of times for maintenance checks

(e) From Figure 8.9, we see that more of the checks take between 20 and 25 minutes to complete, so this is the most likely length of time.
(f) The density function, $p(t)$, is a smoothed version of the histogram in Figure 8.9. A reasonable sketch is given in Figure 8.10.
(g) A graph of $P(t)$ is given in Figure 8.11. Since $P(t)$ is a cumulative distribution function, $P(t)$ is approaching 1 as t gets large, but is never larger than 1.

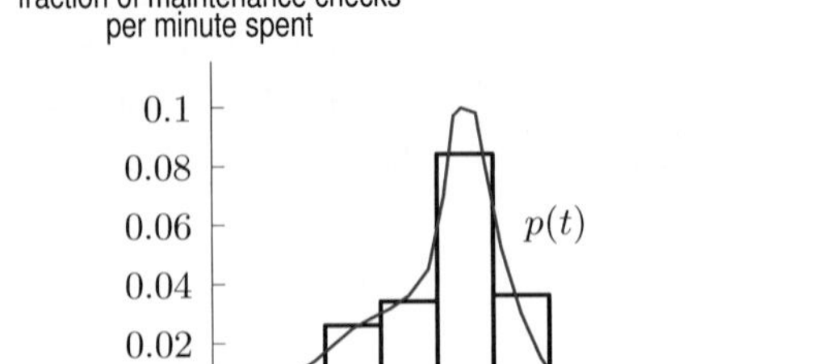

Figure 8.10: Density function for time to conduct maintenance checks

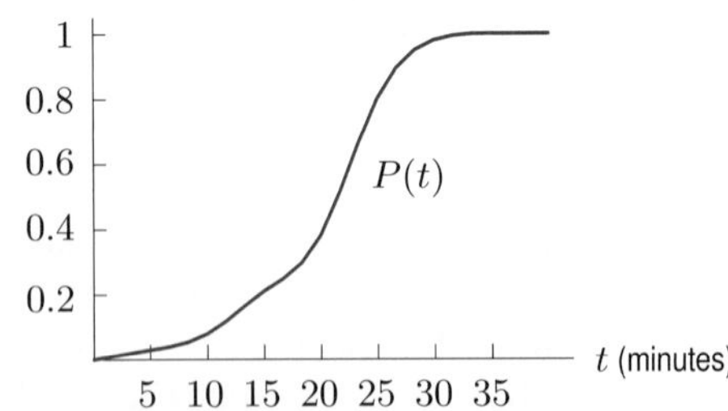

Figure 8.11: Cumulative distribution function for time to conduct maintenance checks

Probability

Suppose we pick a member of the US population at random. What is the probability that we pick a person who is between, say, the ages of 70 and 80? We saw in Table 8.2 on page 329 that 6% of the population is in this age group. We say that the probability, or chance, that the person is between 70 and 80 is 0.06. Using any age density function $p(t)$, we define probabilities as follows:

$$\begin{array}{c}\text{Probability that a person is}\\ \text{between ages } a \text{ and } b\end{array} = \begin{array}{c}\text{Fraction of population}\\ \text{between ages } a \text{ and } b\end{array} = \int_a^b p(t)\,dt.$$

Since the cumulative distribution gives the fraction of the population younger than age t, the cumulative distribution function can also be used to calculate the probability that a randomly selected person is in a given age group.

$$\begin{array}{c}\text{Probability that a person is}\\ \text{younger than age } t\end{array} = \begin{array}{c}\text{Fraction of population}\\ \text{younger than age } t\end{array} = P(t) = \int_0^t p(x)\,dx.$$

In the next example, both a density function and a cumulative distribution function are used to describe the same situation.

Example 2 Suppose you want to analyze the fishing industry in a small town. Each day, the boats bring back at least 2 tons of fish, but never more than 8 tons.

(a) Using the density function describing the daily catch in Figure 8.12, find and graph the corresponding cumulative distribution function and explain its meaning.
(b) What is the probability that the catch is between 5 and 7 tons?

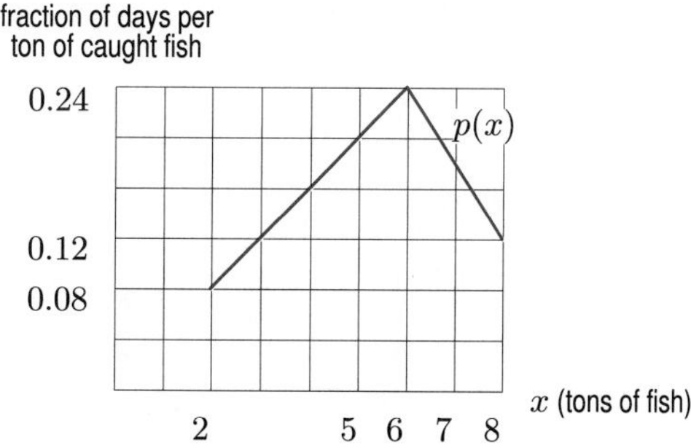

Figure 8.12: Density function of daily catch

Solution (a) The cumulative distribution function $P(t)$ is equal to the fraction of days on which the catch is less than t tons of fish. Since the catch is never less than 2 tons, we have $P(t) = 0$ for $t \leq 2$. Since the catch is always less than 8 tons, we have $P(t) = 1$ for $t \geq 8$. For t in the range $2 < t < 8$ we must evaluate the integral

$$P(t) = \int_{-\infty}^{t} p(x)dx = \int_{2}^{t} p(x)dx.$$

This integral equals the area under the graph of $p(x)$ between $x = 2$ and $x = t$. It can be computed by counting grid squares in Figure 8.12; each square has area 0.04. For example,

$$P(3) = \int_2^3 p(x)dx \approx \text{Area of 2.5 squares} = 2.5(0.04) = 0.10.$$

Table 8.6 contains values of $P(t)$; the graph is shown in Figure 8.13.

Table 8.6 *Estimates for $P(t)$ of daily catch*

t (tons of fish)	$P(t)$ (fraction of fishing days)
2	0
3	0.10
4	0.24
5	0.42
6	0.64
7	0.85
8	1

fraction of days

1

0.8

0.6

0.4

0.2

$P(t)$

2 5 6 7 8 t (tons of fish)

Figure 8.13: Cumulative distribution, $P(t)$, of daily catch

(b) The probability that the catch is between 5 and 7 tons can be found using either the density function p or the cumulative distribution function P. When we use the density function, this probability is represented by the shaded area in Figure 8.14, which is about 10.75 squares, so

$$\begin{array}{c}\text{Probability catch is}\\\text{between 5 and 7 tons}\end{array} = \int_5^7 p(x)\,dx \approx \text{Area of 10.75 squares} = 10.75(0.04) = 0.43.$$

The probability can be found from the cumulative distribution function as follows:

$$\begin{array}{c}\text{Probability catch is}\\\text{between 5 and 7 tons}\end{array} = P(7) - P(5) = 0.85 - 0.42 = 0.43.$$

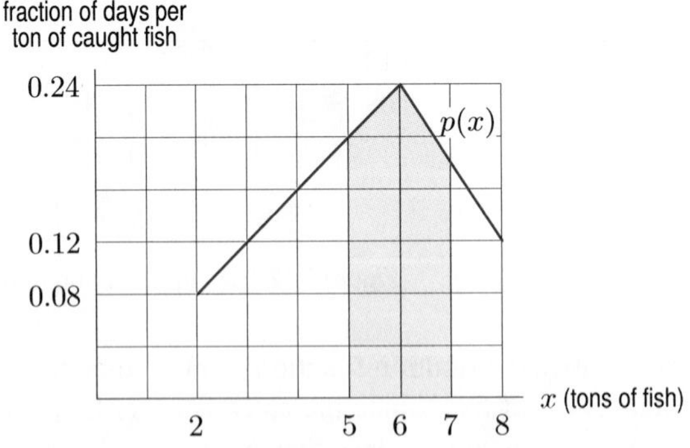

Figure 8.14: Shaded area represents the probability the catch is between 5 and 7 tons

Problems for Section 8.2

1. **(a)** Using the density function in Example 2 on page 330, fill in values for the cumulative distribution function $P(t)$ for the length of time people wait in the doctor's office.

t (hours)	0	1	2	3	4
$P(t)$ (fraction of people waiting)					

(b) Graph $P(t)$.

2. In an agricultural experiment, the quantity of grain from a given size field is measured. The yield can be anything from 0 kg to 50 kg. For each of the following situations, pick the graph that best represents the:
(i) Probability density function
(ii) Cumulative distribution function.

(a) Low yields are more likely than high yields.
(b) All yields are equally likely.
(c) High yields are more likely than low yields.

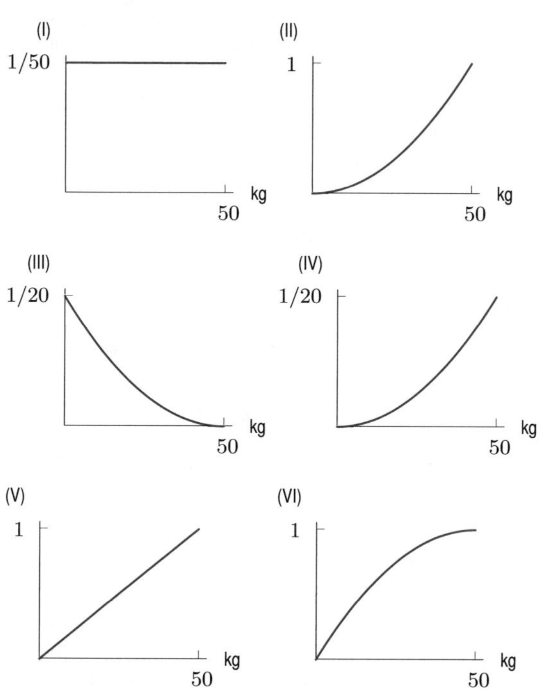

3. A person who travels regularly on the 9:00 am bus from Oakland to San Francisco reports that the bus is almost always a few minutes late but rarely more than five minutes late. The bus is never more than two minutes early, although it is on very rare occasions a little early.

(a) Sketch a density function, $p(t)$, where t is the number of minutes that the bus is late. Shade the region under the graph between $t = 2$ minutes and $t = 4$ minutes. Explain what this region represents.

(b) Now sketch the cumulative distribution function $P(t)$. What measurement(s) on this graph correspond to the area shaded? What do the inflection point(s) on your graph of P correspond to on the graph of p? Interpret the inflection points on the graph of P without referring to the graph of p.

4. The density function and cumulative distribution function of heights of grass plants in a meadow are in Figures 8.15 and 8.16, respectively.

(a) There are two species of grass in the meadow, a short grass and a tall grass. Explain how the graph of the density function reflects this fact.
(b) Explain how the graph of the cumulative distribution function reflects the fact that there are two species of grass in the meadow.
(c) About what percentage of the grasses in the meadow belong to the short grass species?

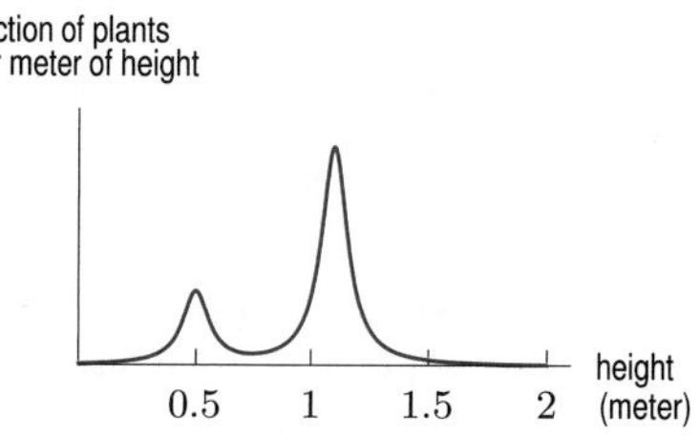

Figure 8.15

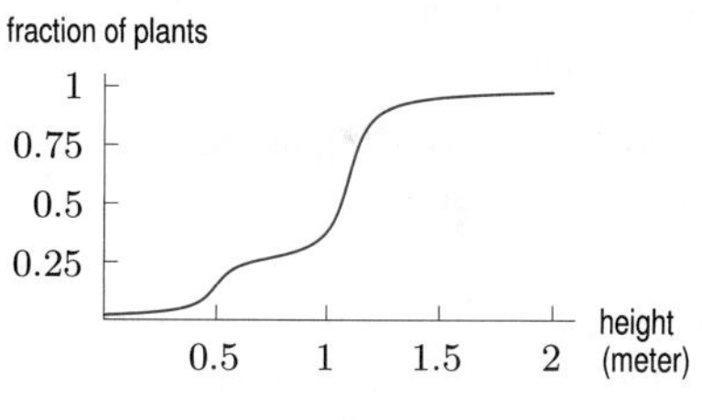

Figure 8.16

5. Show that the area under the fishing density function in Figure 8.12 on page 335 is 1. Why is this to be expected?

6. Figure 8.17 shows a density function and the corresponding cumulative distribution function.[4]

(a) Which curve represents the density function and which represents the cumulative distribution function? Give a reason for your choice.
(b) Put reasonable values on the tick marks on each of the axes.

[4]Adapted from *Calculus*, by David A. Smith and Lawerence C. Moore (Lexington, D.C. Heath, 1994).

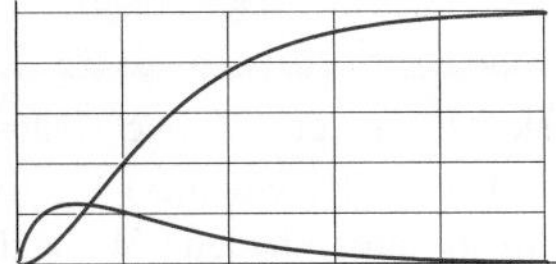

Figure 8.17

7. Students at the University of California were surveyed and asked their grade point average. (The GPA ranges from 0 to 4, where 2 is just passing.) The distribution of GPAs is shown in Figure 8.18.[5]

(a) Roughly what fraction of students are passing?
(b) Roughly what fraction of the students have honor grades (GPAs above 3)?
(c) Why do you think there is a peak around 2?
(d) Sketch the cumulative distribution function.

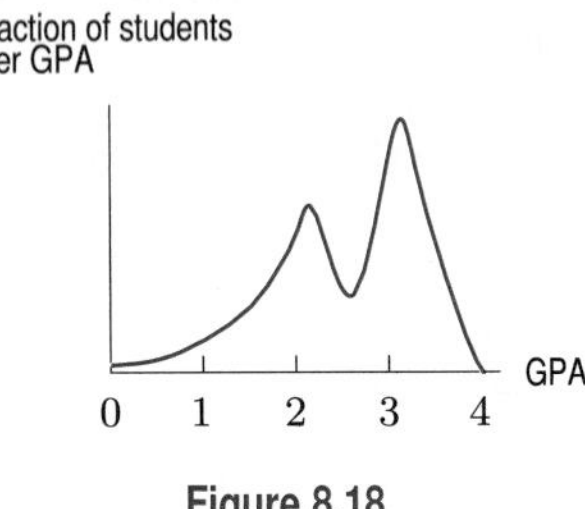

Figure 8.18

8. Suppose $F(x)$ is the cumulative distribution function for heights (in meters) of trees in a forest.

(a) Explain in terms of trees the meaning of the statement $F(7) = 0.6$.
(b) Which is greater, $F(6)$ or $F(7)$? Justify your answer in terms of trees.

9. Figure 8.19 shows $P(t)$, the percentage of inventory of an item that has sold by time t, where t is in days and day 1 is January 1.

(a) When did the first item sell? The last item?
(b) On May 1 (day 121), what percentage of the inventory had been sold?
(c) Approximately what percentage of the inventory sold during May and June (days 121–181)?
(d) What percentage of the inventory remained after half of the year had passed (at day 181)?
(e) Estimate when items went on sale and sold quickly.

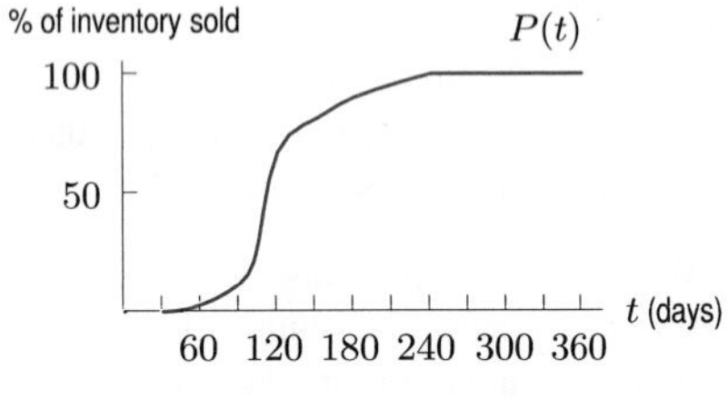

Figure 8.19

10. An experiment is done to determine the effect of two new fertilizers A and B on the growth of a species of peas. The cumulative distribution functions of the heights of the mature peas without treatment and treated with each of A and B are graphed in Figure 8.20.

(a) About what height are most of the unfertilized plants?
(b) Explain in words the effect of the fertilizers A and B on the mature height of the plants.

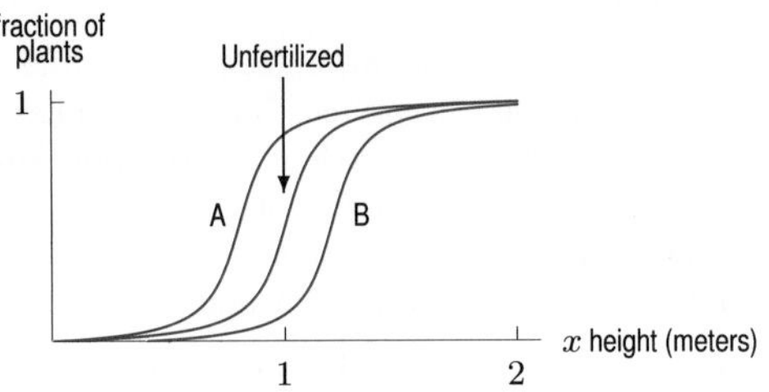

Figure 8.20

For Problems 11–12, let $p(t) = -0.0375t^2 + 0.225t$ be the density function for the shelf life of a brand of banana, with t in weeks and $0 \le t \le 4$. See Figure 8.21.

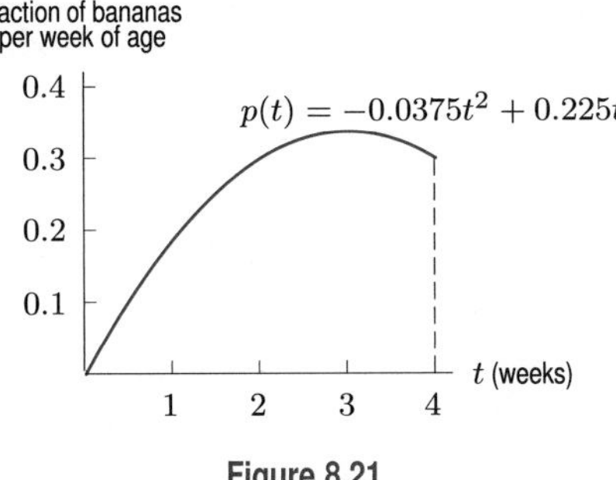

Figure 8.21

11. Find the probability that a banana will last

(a) Between 1 and 2 weeks.
(b) More than 3 weeks.
(c) More than 4 weeks.

12. (a) Sketch the cumulative distribution function for the shelf life of bananas. [Note: The domain of your function should be all real numbers, including to the left of $t = 0$ and to the right of $t = 4$.]
(b) Use the cumulative distribution function to estimate the probability that a banana lasts between 1 and 2 weeks. Check with Problem 11(a).

13. A group of people have received treatment for cancer. Let t be the survival time, the number of years a person lives after the treatment. The density function giving the distribution of t is $p(t) = Ce^{-Ct}$ for some positive constant C. What is the practical meaning of the cumulative distribution function $P(t) = \int_0^t p(x)\,dx$?

[5] Adapted from *Statistics*, by Freedman, Pisani, Purves, and Adikhari (New York: Norton, 1991).

14. The probability of a transistor failing between $t = a$ months and $t = b$ months is given by $c\int_a^b e^{-ct}\,dt$, for some constant c.

(a) If the probability of failure within the first six months is 10%, what is c?

(b) Given the value of c in part (a), what is the probability the transistor fails within the second six months?

15. While taking a walk along the road where you live, you accidentally drop your glove, but you don't know where. The probability density $p(x)$ for having dropped the glove x kilometers from home (along the road) is

$$p(x) = 2e^{-2x} \quad \text{for } x \geq 0.$$

(a) What is the probability that you dropped it within 1 kilometer of home?

(b) At what distance y from home is the probability that you dropped it within y km of home equal to 0.95?

8.3 THE MEDIAN AND THE MEAN

It is often useful to be able to give an "average" value for a distribution. Two measures that are in common use are the *median* and the *mean*.

The Median

A **median** of a quantity x distributed through a population is a value T such that half the population has values of x less than (or equal to) T, and half the population has values of x greater than (or equal to) T. Thus, if p is the density function, a median T satisfies

$$\int_{-\infty}^{T} p(x)\,dx = 0.5.$$

In other words, half the area under the graph of p lies to the left of T. Equivalently, if P is the cumulative distribution function,

$$P(T) = 0.5.$$

Example 1 Let t days be the length of time a pair of jeans remains in a shop before it is sold. The density function of t is graphed in Figure 8.22 and given by

$$p(t) = 0.04 - 0.0008t.$$

(a) What is the longest time a pair of jeans remains unsold?
(b) Would you expect the median time till sale to be less than, equal to, or greater than 25 days?
(c) Find the median time required to sell a pair of jeans.

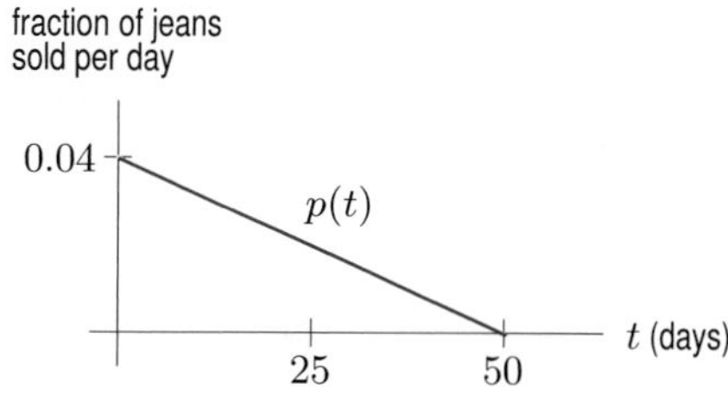

Figure 8.22: Density function for time till sale of a pair of jeans

Solution

(a) The density function is 0 for all times $t > 50$, so all jeans are sold within 50 days.
(b) The area under the graph of the density function in the interval $0 \leq t \leq 25$ is greater than the area under the graph in the interval $25 \leq t \leq 50$. So more than half the jeans are sold before their 25th day in the shop. The median time till sale is less than 25 days.

(c) Let P be the cumulative distribution function. We want to find the value of T such that

$$P(T) = \int_{-\infty}^{T} p(t)\,dt = \int_{0}^{T} p(t)\,dt = 0.5.$$

Using a calculator to evaluate the integrals, we obtain the values for P in Table 8.7.

Table 8.7 *Cumulative distribution for selling time*

T (days)	0	5	10	15	20	25
$P(T)$ (fraction of jeans sold by day T)	0	0.19	0.36	0.51	0.64	0.75

Since about half the jeans are sold within 15 days, the median time to sale is about 15 days. See Figures 8.23 and 8.24. We could also use the Fundamental Theorem of Calculus to find the median exactly. See Problem 19.

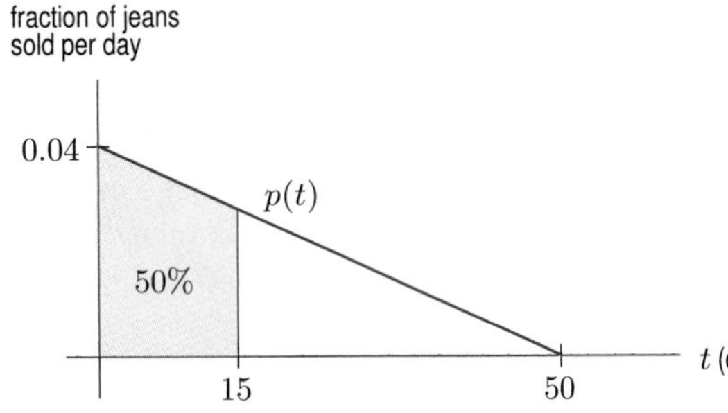

Figure 8.23: Median and density function

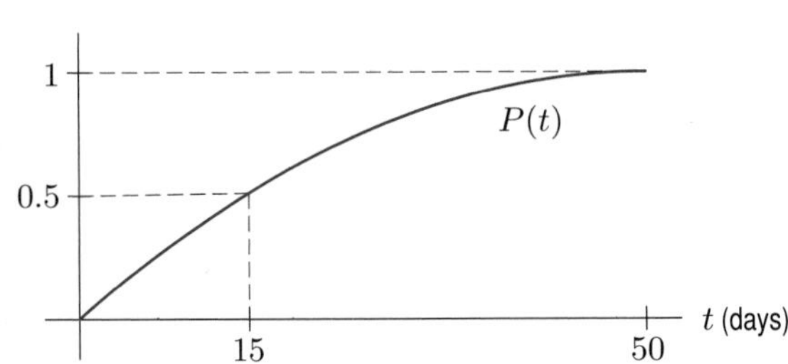

Figure 8.24: Median and cumulative distribution function

The Mean

Another commonly used average value is the *mean*. To find the mean of N numbers, we add the numbers and divide the sum by N. For example, the mean of the numbers 1, 2, 7, and 10 is $(1 + 2 + 7 + 10)/4 = 5$. The mean age of the entire US population is therefore defined as

$$\text{Mean age} = \frac{\sum \text{Ages of all people in the US}}{\text{Total number of people in the US}}.$$

Calculating the sum of all the ages directly would be an enormous task; we approximate the sum by an integral. We consider the people whose age is between t and $t+\Delta t$. How many are there?

The fraction of the population with age between t and $t + \Delta t$ is the area under the graph of p between these points, which is approximated by the area of the rectangle, $p(t)\Delta t$. (See Figure 8.25.) If the total number of people in the population is N, then

$$\begin{matrix}\text{Number of people with age} \\ \text{between } t \text{ and } t+\Delta t\end{matrix} \approx p(t)\Delta t N.$$

The age of each of these people is approximately t, so

$$\begin{matrix}\text{Sum of ages of people} \\ \text{between age } t \text{ and } t+\Delta t\end{matrix} \approx tp(t)\Delta t N.$$

Therefore, adding and factoring out an N gives us

$$\text{Sum of ages of all people} \approx \left(\sum tp(t)\Delta t\right) N.$$

In the limit, as Δt shrinks to 0, the sum becomes an integral. Assuming no one is over 100 years old, we have

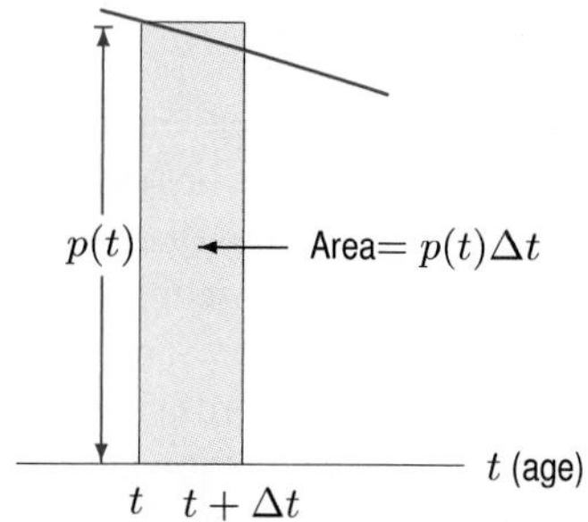

Figure 8.25: Shaded area is percentage of population with age between t and $t+\Delta t$

$$\text{Sum of ages of all people} = \left(\int_0^{100} tp(t)dt\right) N.$$

Since N is the total number of people in the US,

$$\text{Mean age} = \frac{\text{Sum of ages of all people in US}}{N} = \int_0^{100} tp(t)dt.$$

We can give the same argument for any[6] density function $p(x)$.

> If a quantity has density function $p(x)$,
>
> $$\textbf{Mean value} \text{ of the quantity} = \int_{-\infty}^{\infty} xp(x)\,dx.$$

It can be shown that the mean is the point on the horizontal axis where the region under the graph of the density function, if it were made out of cardboard, would balance.

Example 2 Find the mean time for jeans sales, using the density function of Example 1.

Solution The formula for p is $p(t) = 0.04 - 0.0008t$. We compute

$$\text{Mean time} = \int_0^{50} tp(t)\,dt = \int_0^{50} t(0.04 - 0.0008t)\,dt = 16.67 \text{ days}.$$

The mean is represented by the balance point in Figure 8.26. Notice that the mean is different from the median computed in Example 1.

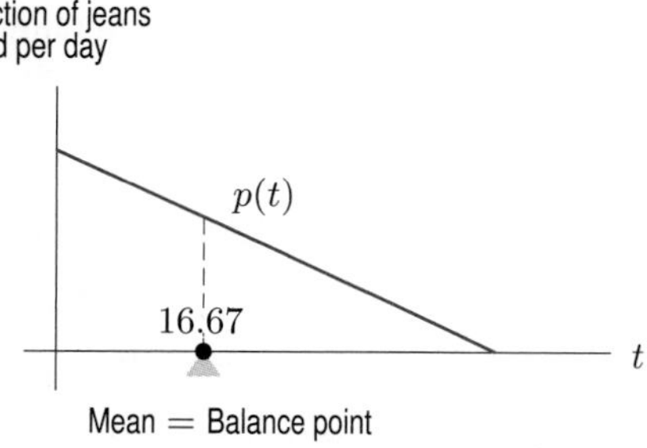

Figure 8.26: Mean sale time for jeans

---

[6]Provided all the relevant improper integrals converge.

Normal Distributions

How much rain do you expect to fall in your home town this year? If you live in Anchorage, Alaska, the answer is something close to 15 inches (including the snow). Of course, you don't expect exactly 15 inches. Some years there are more than 15 inches, and some years there are less. Most years, however, the amount of rainfall is close to 15 inches; only rarely is it well above or well below 15 inches. What does the density function for the rainfall look like? To answer this question, we look at rainfall data over many years. Records show that the distribution of rainfall is well-approximated by a *normal distribution*. The graph of its density function is a bell-shaped curve which peaks at 15 inches and slopes downward approximately symmetrically on either side.

Normal distributions are frequently used to model real phenomena, from grades on an exam to the number of airline passengers on a particular flight. A normal distribution is characterized by its *mean*, μ, and its *standard deviation*, σ. The mean tells us the location of the central peak. The standard deviation tells us how closely the data is clustered around the mean. A small value of σ tells us that the data is close to the mean; a large σ tells us the data is spread out. In the following formula for a normal distribution, the factor of $1/(\sigma\sqrt{2\pi})$ makes the area under the graph equal to 1.

> A **normal distribution** has a density function of the form
>
> $$p(x) = \frac{1}{\sigma\sqrt{2\pi}} e^{-(x-\mu)^2/(2\sigma^2)},$$
>
> where μ is the mean of the distribution and σ is the standard deviation, with $\sigma > 0$.

To model the rainfall in Anchorage, we use a normal distribution with $\mu = 15$ and $\sigma = 1$. (See Figure 8.27.)

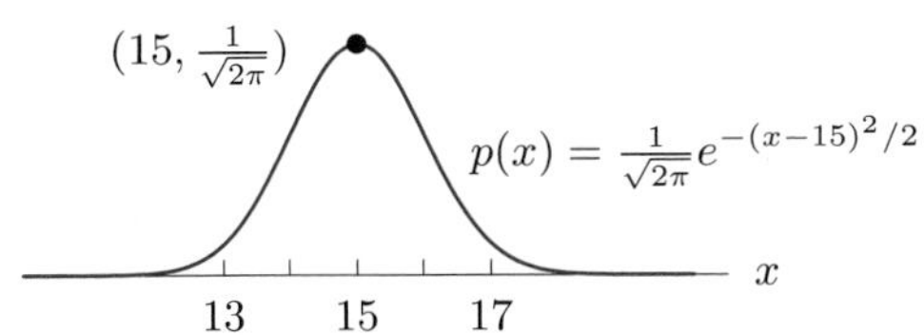

Figure 8.27: Normal distribution with $\mu = 15$ and $\sigma = 1$

Example 3 For Anchorage's rainfall, use the normal distribution with the density function with $\mu = 15$ and $\sigma = 1$ to compute the fraction of the years with rainfall between

(a) 14 and 16 inches, (b) 13 and 17 inches, (c) 12 and 18 inches.

Solution

(a) The fraction of the years with annual rainfall between 14 and 16 inches is $\int_{14}^{16} \frac{1}{\sqrt{2\pi}} e^{-(x-15)^2/2}\,dx$. Since there is no elementary antiderivative for $e^{-(x-15)^2/2}$, we find the integral numerically. Its value is about 0.68.

$$\text{Fraction of years with rainfall between 14 and 16 inches} = \int_{14}^{16} \frac{1}{\sqrt{2\pi}} e^{-(x-15)^2/2}\,dx \approx 0.68.$$

(b) Finding the integral numerically again:

$$\text{Fraction of years with rainfall between 13 and 17 inches} = \int_{13}^{17} \frac{1}{\sqrt{2\pi}} e^{-(x-15)^2/2}\,dx \approx 0.95.$$

(c)

$$\text{Fraction of years with rainfall between 12 and 18 inches} = \int_{12}^{18} \frac{1}{\sqrt{2\pi}} e^{-(x-15)^2/2}\, dx \approx 0.997.$$

Since 0.95 is so close to 1, we expect that most of the time the rainfall will be between 13 and 17 inches a year.

Among the normal distributions, the one having $\mu = 0$, $\sigma = 1$ is called the *standard normal distribution*. Values of the corresponding cumulative distribution function are published in tables.

Problems for Section 8.3

1. Estimate the median daily catch for the fishing data given in Example 2 of Section 8.2.

2. **(a)** Use the cumulative distribution function in Figure 8.28 to estimate the median.

(b) Describe the density function: For what values is it positive? Increasing? Decreasing? Identify all local maxima and minima values.

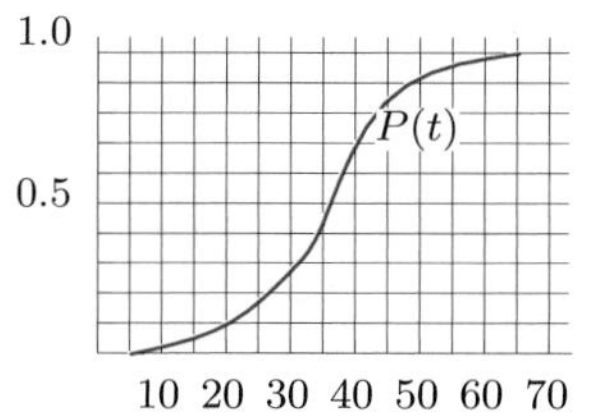

Figure 8.28

3. The speeds of cars on a road are approximately normally distributed with a mean $\mu = 58$ km/hr and standard deviation $\sigma = 4$ km/hr.

(a) What is the probability that a randomly selected car is going between 60 and 65 km/hr?

(b) What fraction of all cars are going slower than 52 km/hr?

4. The distribution of IQ scores can be modeled by a normal distribution with mean 100 and standard deviation 15.

(a) Write the formula for the density function of IQ scores.

(b) Estimate the fraction of the population with IQ between 115 and 120.

For Problems 5–6, let $p(t) = -0.0375t^2 + 0.225t$ be the density function for the shelf life of a brand of banana which lasts up to 4 weeks. Time, t, is measured in weeks and $0 \le t \le 4$.

5. Find the median shelf life of a banana using $p(t)$. Plot the median on a graph of $p(t)$. Does it look like half the area is to the right of the median and half the area is to the left?

6. Find the mean shelf life of a banana using $p(t)$. Plot the mean on a graph of $p(t)$. Does it look like the mean is the place where the density function balances?

7. Suppose that x measures the time (in hours) it takes for a student to complete an exam. All students are done within two hours and the density function for x is

$$p(x) = \begin{cases} x^3/4 & \text{if } 0 < x < 2 \\ 0 & \text{otherwise.} \end{cases}$$

(a) What proportion of students take between 1.5 and 2.0 hours to finish the exam?

(b) What is the mean time for students to complete the exam?

(c) Compute the median of this distribution.

8. Let $p(t) = 0.1e^{-0.1t}$ be the density function for the waiting time at a subway stop, with t in minutes, $0 \le t \le 60$.

(a) Graph $p(t)$. Use the graph to estimate visually the median and the mean.

(b) Calculate the median and the mean. Plot both on the graph of $p(t)$.

(c) Interpret the median and mean in terms of waiting time.

9. Let $P(x)$ be the cumulative distribution function for the household income distribution in the US in 2006. Values of $P(x)$ are in the following table:

Income x (thousand \$)	20	40	60	80	100	150
$P(x)$ (%)	21.7	45.4	63.0	75.8	84.0	94.0

(a) What percent of the households made between \$40,000 and \$60,000? More than \$150,000?

(b) Approximately what was the median income?

(c) Is the statement "More than one-third of households made between \$40,000 and \$80,000" true or false?

CHAPTER SUMMARY

- **Density function**
- **Cumulative distribution function**
- **Probability**
- **Median**
- **Mean**
- **Normal distribution**

REVIEW PROBLEMS FOR CHAPTER EIGHT

1. Match the graphs of the density functions (a), (b), and (c) with the graphs of the cumulative distribution functions I, II, and III.

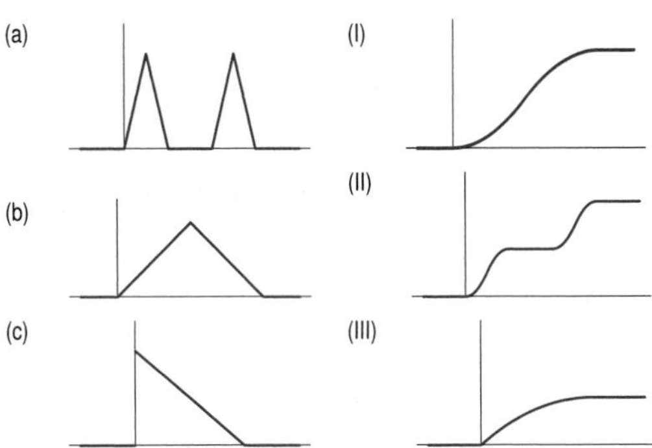

In Problems 2–3, graph a density function representing the given distribution.

2. The age at which a person dies in a society with high infant mortality and in which adults usually die between age 40 and age 60.

3. The heights of the people in an elementary school.

In Problems 4–6, graph a density function and a cumulative distribution function which could represent the distribution of income through a population with the given characteristics.

4. A large middle class.

5. Small middle and upper classes and many poor people.

6. Small middle class, many poor and many rich people.

In Problems 7–10, calculate the value of c if p is a density function.

7.

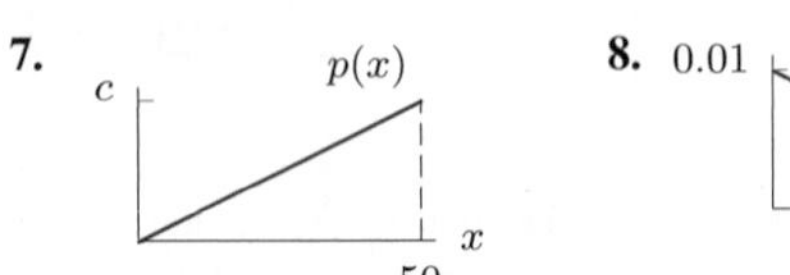

8.

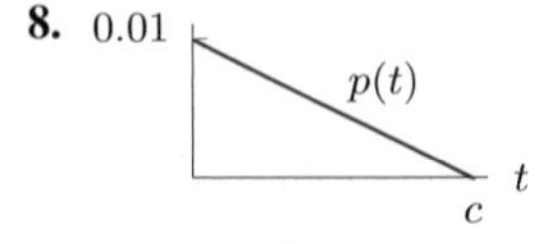

9.

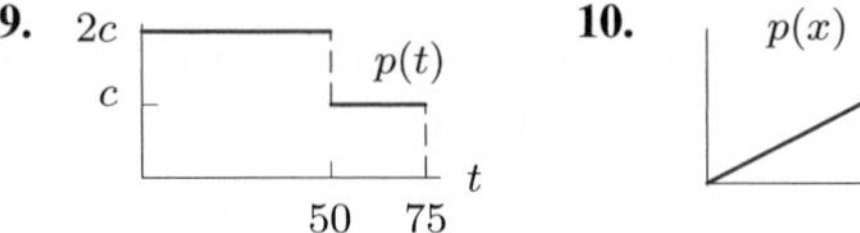

10.

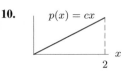

11. An insect has a life-span of no more than one year. Figure 8.29 shows the density function, $p(t)$, for the life-span.

(a) Do more insects die in the first month of their life or the twelfth month of their life?

(b) What fraction of the insects live no more than 6 months?

(c) What fraction of the insects live more than 9 months?

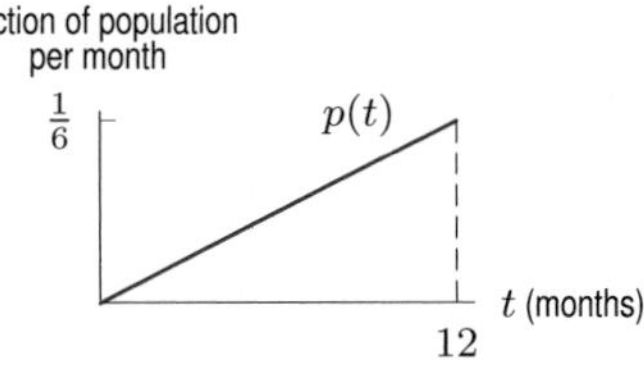

Figure 8.29

12. A large number of people take a standardized test, receiving scores described by the density function p graphed in Figure 8.30. Does the density function imply that most people receive a score near 50? Explain why or why not.

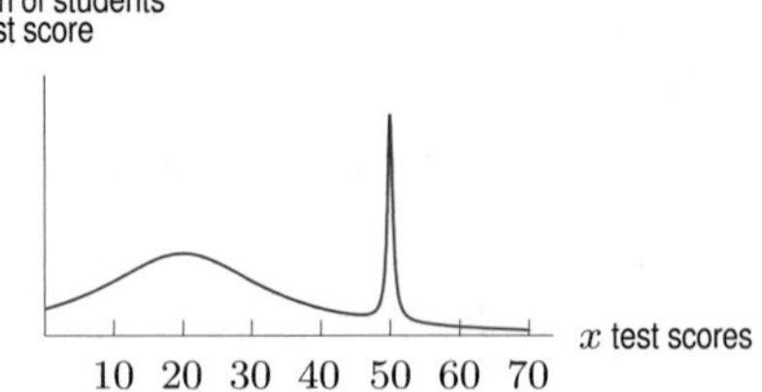

Figure 8.30

13. Figure 8.31[7] shows the distribution of elevation, in miles, across the earth's surface. Positive elevation denotes land above sea level; negative elevation shows land below sea level (i.e., the ocean floor).

(a) Describe in words the elevation of most of the earth's surface.

[7]Adapted from *Statistics*, by Freedman, Pisani, Purves, and Adikhari (New York: Norton).

(b) Approximately what fraction of the earth's surface is below sea level?

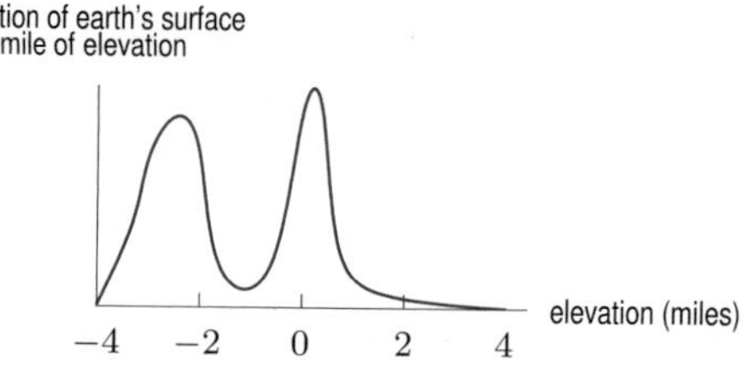

Figure 8.31

14. A congressional committee is investigating a defense contractor whose projects often incur cost overruns. The data in Table 8.8 show y, the fraction of the projects with an overrun of at most $C\%$.

(a) Plot the data with C on the horizontal axis. Is this a density function or a cumulative distribution function? Sketch a curve through these points.
(b) If you think you drew a density function in part (a), sketch the corresponding cumulative distribution function on another set of axes. If you think you drew a cumulative distribution function in part (a), sketch the corresponding density function.
(c) Based on the table, what is the probability that there will be a cost overrun of 50% or more? Between 20% and 50%? Near what percent is the cost overrun most likely to be?

Table 8.8 *Fraction, y, of overruns that are at most $C\%$*

C	−20%	−10%	0%	10%	20%	30%	40%	50%
y	0.01	0.08	0.19	0.32	0.50	0.80	0.94	0.99

15. The density function for radii r (mm) of spherical raindrops during a storm is constant over the range $0 < r < 5$ and zero elsewhere.

(a) Find the density function $f(r)$ for the radii.
(b) Find the cumulative distribution function $F(r)$.

16. Major absorption differences have been reported for different commercial versions of the same drug. One study compared three commercial versions of timed-release theophylline capsules.[8] A theophylline solution was included for comparison. Figure 8.32 shows the cumulative distribution functions $P(t)$, which represent the fraction of the drug absorbed by time t. Which curve represents the solution? Compare absorption rates of the four versions of the drug.

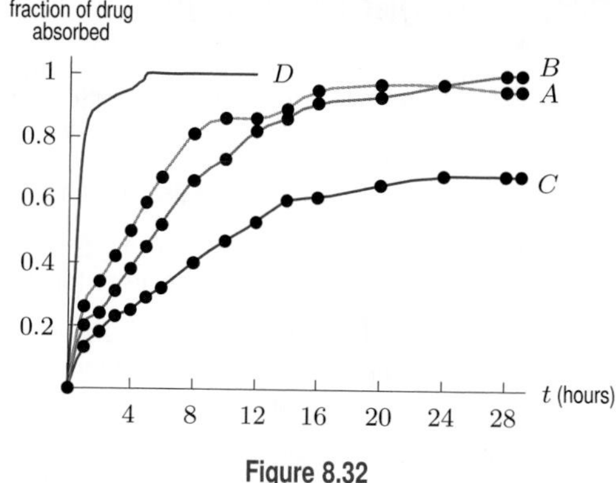

Figure 8.32

17. After measuring the duration of many telephone calls, the telephone company found their data was well-approximated by the density function $p(x) = 0.4e^{-0.4x}$, where x is the duration of a call, in minutes.

(a) What percentage of calls last between 1 and 2 minutes?
(b) What percentage of calls last 1 minute or less?
(c) What percentage of calls last 3 minutes or more?
(d) Find the cumulative distribution function.

18. In southern Switzerland, most rain falls in the spring and fall; summers and winters are relatively dry. Sketch possible graphs for the density function and the cumulative distribution function of the rain distribution over the course of one year. Put the date on the horizontal axis and fraction of the year's rainfall on the vertical axis.

19. Find the median of the density function given by $p(t) = 0.04 - 0.0008t$ for $0 \le t \le 50$ using the Fundamental Theorem of Calculus.

20. In 1950 an experiment was done observing the time gaps between successive cars on the Arroyo Seco Freeway. The data[9] show that, if x is time in seconds and $0 \le x \le 40$, the density function of these time gaps is

$$p(x) = 0.122e^{-0.122x}.$$

Find the median and mean time gap. Interpret them in terms of cars on the freeway.

In Problems 21–25, a quantity x is distributed through a population with probability density function $p(x)$ and cumulative distribution function $P(x)$. Decide if the statements in Problems 21–25 are true or false. Give an explanation for your answer.

21. If $p(10) = 1/2$, then half the population has $x < 10$.
22. If $P(10) = 1/2$, then half the population has $x < 10$.
23. If $p(10) = 1/2$, then the fraction of the population lying between $x = 9.98$ and $x = 10.04$ is about 0.03.
24. If $p(10) = p(20)$, then none of the population has x values lying between 10 and 20.
25. If $P(10) = P(20)$, then none of the population has x values lying between 10 and 20.

[8] *Progress in Drug Metabolism*, Bridges and Chasseaud (eds.) (New York: Wiley, 1980).
[9] Reported by Daniel Furlough and Frank Barnes.

CHECK YOUR UNDERSTANDING

In Problems 1–30, indicate whether the statement is true or false.

1. If $\int_{-\infty}^{\infty} p(x)\,dx = 1$ then $p(x)$ is a density function.

2. The function given by $p(x) = 0.25$ when $0 \le x \le 4$ and $p(x) = 0$ when $x < 0$ or $x > 4$ is a density function.

3. If $p(x)$ is a density function for the age in years of a population, then $\int_0^{10} p(x)\,dx$ is the fraction of the population with ages between 0 and 10 years.

4. If $p(t)$ is a density function for waiting times in minutes at a bank teller, then $\int_{10}^{15} p(x)\,dx$ is the fraction of the people waiting in line for that teller who wait between 10 and 15 minutes.

5. If $p(x)$ is the density function for age in years of the US population, then $\int_0^{70} p(x)\,dx \approx 0.5$.

6. If $p(x)$ is the density function for age in years of a population, then $p(50)$ is the fraction of the population exactly 50 years old.

7. If $p(x)$ is the density function for age in years of a population, and $p(10) = 0.014$, then about 1.4 percent of the population have ages between 9.5 and 10.5 years.

8. If $p(x)$ is a density function, then $\int_0^{\infty} p(x)\,dx = 0.5$.

9. If $p(x)$ is a density function, then $\int_0^1 p(x)\,dx \le \int_0^2 p(x)\,dx$.

10. If $p(x)$ is a density function, then it could never happen that $\int_0^{100} p(x)\,dx = \int_0^{200} p(x)\,dx$.

11. A cumulative distribution function $P(t)$ can never be decreasing.

12. If $P(t)$ is the cumulative distribution function corresponding to the density function $p(t)$, then $p' = P$.

13. If $P(t)$ is a cumulative distribution function for a population, then $P(30)$ is the fraction of the population with values above 30.

14. If $P(t)$ is a cumulative distribution function for a population, then $P(20) - P(10)$ is the fraction of the population with values between 10 and 20.

15. If $P(t)$ is a cumulative distribution function for a population, then $P(30) - P(10) = P(20)$.

16. If $P(t)$ is a cumulative distribution function for age in years of a population and $P(10) = 0.5$, then one half of the population is less than 10 years old.

17. The units of a density function $p(x)$ and its associated cumulative distribution function $P(x)$ are the same.

18. A cumulative distribution function $P(t)$ satisfies $0 \le P(t) \le 1$ for all t.

19. If $P(t)$ is a cumulative distribution function such that $P(10) = 0.05$ and $P(15) = 0.08$, then $P(25) = 0.13$.

20. If $P(t)$ is the cumulative distribution function for a density function $p(x)$, then $P(50) - P(25) = \int_{25}^{50} p(x)\,dx$.

21. If $p(x)$ is the probability density function for a quantity, then the mean value of the quantity is $\int_{-\infty}^{\infty} xp(x)\,dx$.

22. If $P(t)$ is the cumulative distribution function for a quantity, then the mean value of the quantity is given by $\int_{-\infty}^{\infty} tP(t)\,dt$.

23. If $P(t)$ is the cumulative distribution function for a quantity, then the median value T of the quantity is given by $T = P(0.5)$.

24. If $p(x)$ is the density function for a quantity x, then the median T satisfies $\int_{-\infty}^{T} p(x)\,dx = 0.5$.

25. If $p(x)$ is the density function for a quantity x, then the median T satisfies $\int_T^{\infty} p(x)\,dx = 0.5$.

26. If a quantity has density function $p(x)$, then the mean value and median are never equal.

27. The normal distribution with density function $p(x) = (1/\sqrt{2\pi})e^{-x^2/2}$ has mean $\mu = 0$ and standard deviation $\sigma = 1$.

28. The normal distribution with density function $p(x) = (1/\sqrt{2\pi})e^{-(x-5)^2/2}$ has mean $\mu = -5$ and standard deviation $\sigma = 1$.

29. The integral $\int_{-\infty}^{\infty} (1/\sqrt{2\pi})e^{-(x-7)^2/2}\,dx$ equals 1.

30. The mean value of a quantity x distributed through a population is the value T such that half of the population has values x less than or equal to T.

PROJECTS FOR CHAPTER EIGHT

1. Triangular Probability Distribution

Triangular probability distributions, such as the one with density function graphed in Figure 8.33, are used in business to model uncertainty. Such a distribution can be used to model a variable where only three pieces of information are available: a lower bound ($x = a$), a most likely value ($x = c$), and an upper bound ($x = b$).

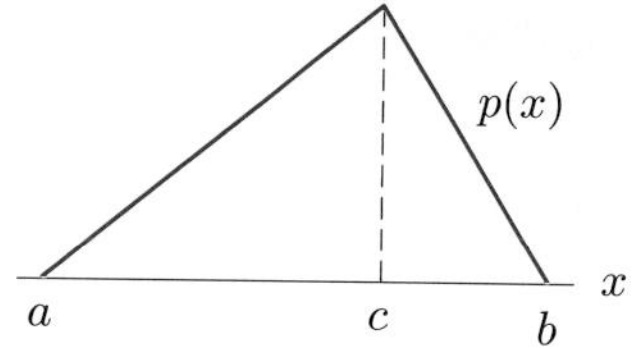

Figure 8.33

Thus, we can write the function $p(x)$ as two linear functions:

$$p(x) = \begin{cases} m_1x + b_1 & a \leq x \leq c \\ m_2x + b_2 & c < x \leq b. \end{cases}$$

(a) Find the value of $p(c)$ geometrically, using the criterion that the probability that x takes on some value between a and b is 1.

Suppose a new product costs between \$6 and \$10 per unit to produce, with a most likely cost of \$9.

(b) Find $p(9)$.
(c) Use the fact that $p(6) = p(10) = 0$ and the value of $p(9)$ you found in part (b) to find m_1, m_2, b_1, and b_2.
(d) What is the probability that the production cost per unit will be less than \$8?
(e) What is the median cost?
(f) Write a formula for the cumulative probability distribution function $P(x)$ for

(i) $6 \leq x \leq 9$, (ii) $9 < x \leq 10$.

Sketch the graph of $P(x)$.

Chapter Nine

FUNCTIONS OF SEVERAL VARIABLES

Contents

9.1 UNDERSTANDING FUNCTIONS OF TWO VARIABLES

In business, science, and politics, outcomes are rarely determined by a single variable. For example, consider an airline's ticket pricing. To avoid flying planes with many empty seats, it sells some tickets at full price and some at a discount. For a particular route, the airline's revenue, R, earned in a given time period is determined by the number of full-price tickets, x, and the number of discount tickets, y, sold. We say that R is a function of x and y, and we write

$$R = f(x, y).$$

This is just like the function notation of one-variable calculus. The variable R is the dependent variable and the variables x and y are the independent variables. The letter f stands for the *function* or rule that gives the value, or output, of R corresponding to given values of x and y. The collection of all possible inputs, (x, y), is called the *domain* of f. We say a function is an *increasing* (*decreasing*) function of one of its variables if it increases (decreases) as that variable increases while the other independent variables are held constant.

A function of two variables can be represented numerically by a table of values, algebraically by a formula, or pictorially by a contour diagram. In this section we give numerical and algebraic examples; contour diagrams are introduced in Section 9.2.

Functions Given Numerically

The revenue, R, (in dollars) from a particular airline route is shown in Table 9.1 as a function of the number of full-price tickets and the number of discount tickets sold.

Table 9.1 *Revenue from ticket sales as a function of x and y*

		Number of full-price tickets, x			
		100	200	300	400
Number of discount tickets, y	200	75,000	110,000	145,000	180,000
	400	115,000	150,000	185,000	220,000
	600	155,000	190,000	225,000	260,000
	800	195,000	230,000	265,000	300,000
	1000	235,000	270,000	305,000	340,000

Values of x are shown across the top, values of y are down the left side, and the corresponding values of $f(x, y)$ are in the table. For example, to find the value of $f(300, 600)$, we look in the column corresponding to $x = 300$ at the row $y = 600$, where we find the number 225,000. Thus,

$$f(300, 600) = 225{,}000.$$

This means that the revenue from 300 full-price tickets and 600 discount tickets is \$225,000. We see in Table 9.1 that f is an increasing function of x and an increasing function of y.

Notice how this differs from the table of values of a one-variable function, where one row or one column is enough to list the values of the function. Here many rows and columns are needed because the function has an output for every pair of values of the independent variables.

Functions Given Algebraically

The function given in Table 9.1 can be represented by a formula. Looking across the rows, we see that each additional 100 full-price tickets sold raises the revenue by \$35,000, so each full-price ticket must cost \$350. Similarly, looking down a column shows that an additional 200 discount tickets sold increases the revenue by \$40,000, so each discount ticket must cost \$200. Thus, the revenue function is given by the formula

$$R = 350x + 200y.$$

Example 1 Give a formula for the function $M = f(B, t)$ where M is the amount of money in a bank account t years after an initial investment of B dollars, if interest accrues at a rate of 5% per year compounded
(a) Annually (b) Continuously.

Solution (a) Annual compounding means that M increases by a factor of 1.05 every year, so

$$M = f(B,t) = B(1.05)^t.$$

(b) Continuous compounding means that M grows according to the function e^{kt}, with $k = 0.05$, so

$$M = f(B,t) = Be^{0.05t}.$$

Example 2 A car rental company charges \$40 a day and 15 cents a mile for its cars.

(a) Write a formula for the cost, C, of renting a car as a function of the number of days, d, and the number of miles driven, m.
(b) If $C = f(d,m)$, find $f(5,300)$ and interpret it.

Solution (a) The total cost in dollars of renting a car is 40 times the numbers of days plus 0.15 times the number of miles, so

$$C = 40d + 0.15m.$$

(b) We have

$$\begin{aligned} f(5,300) &= 40(5) + 0.15(300) \\ &= 200 + 45 \\ &= 245. \end{aligned}$$

We see that $f(5,300) = 245$. This tells us that if we rent a car for 5 days and drive it 300 miles, it costs us \$245.

Strategy to Investigate Functions of Two Variables: Vary One Variable at a Time

We can learn a great deal about a function of two variables by letting one variable vary while holding the other fixed. This gives a function of one variable, called a *cross-section* of the original function.

Concentration of a Drug in the Blood

When a drug is injected into muscle tissue, it diffuses into the bloodstream. The concentration of the drug in the blood increases until it reaches a maximum, and then decreases. The concentration, C (in mg per liter), of the drug in the blood is a function of two variables: x, the amount (in mg) of the drug given in the injection, and t, the time (in hours) since the injection was administered. We are told that

$$C = f(x,t) = te^{-t(5-x)} \qquad \text{for } 0 \le x \le 4 \text{ and } t \ge 0.$$

Example 3 In terms of the drug concentration in the blood, explain the significance of the cross-sections:

(a) $f(4,t)$ (b) $f(x,1)$

Solution (a) Holding x fixed at 4 means that we are considering an injection of 4 mg of the drug; letting t vary means we are watching the effect of this dose as time passes. Thus the function $f(4,t)$ describes the concentration of the drug in the blood resulting from a 4-mg injection as a function of time. Figure 9.1 shows the graph of $f(4,t) = te^{-t}$. Notice that the concentration in the blood from this dose is at a maximum at 1 hour after injection, and that the concentration in the blood eventually approaches zero.

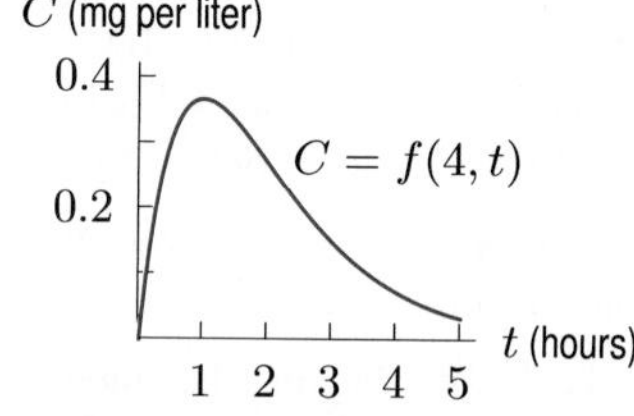

Figure 9.1: The function $f(4,t)$ shows the concentration in the blood resulting from a 4-mg injection

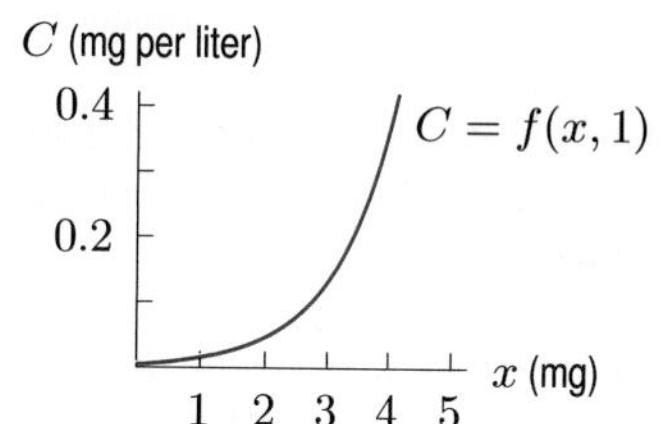

Figure 9.2: The function $f(x,1)$ shows the concentration in the blood 1 hour after the injection

(b) Holding t fixed at 1 means that we are focusing on the blood 1 hour after the injection; letting x vary means we are considering the effect of different doses at that instant. Thus, the function $f(x,1)$ gives the concentration of the drug in the blood 1 hour after injection as a function of the amount injected. Figure 9.2 shows the graph of $f(x,1) = e^{-(5-x)} = e^{x-5}$. Notice that $f(x,1)$ is an increasing function of x. This makes sense: If we administer more of the drug, the concentration in the bloodstream is higher.

Example 4 Continue with $C = f(x,t) = te^{-t(5-x)}$. Graph the cross-sections of $f(a,t)$ for $a = 1, 2, 3$, and 4 on the same axes. Describe how the graph changes for larger values of a and explain what this means in terms of drug concentration in the blood.

Solution The one-variable function $f(a,t)$ represents the effect of an injection of a mg at time t. Figure 9.3 shows the graphs of the four functions $f(1,t) = te^{-4t}$, $f(2,t) = te^{-3t}$, $f(3,t) = te^{-2t}$, and $f(4,t) = te^{-t}$ corresponding to injections of 1, 2, 3, and 4 mg of the drug. The general shape of the graph is the same in every case: The concentration in the blood is zero at the time of injection $t = 0$, then increases to a maximum value, and then decreases toward zero again. We see that if a larger dose of the drug is administered, the peak of the graph is later and higher. This makes sense, since a larger dose will take longer to diffuse fully into the bloodstream and will produce a higher concentration when it does.

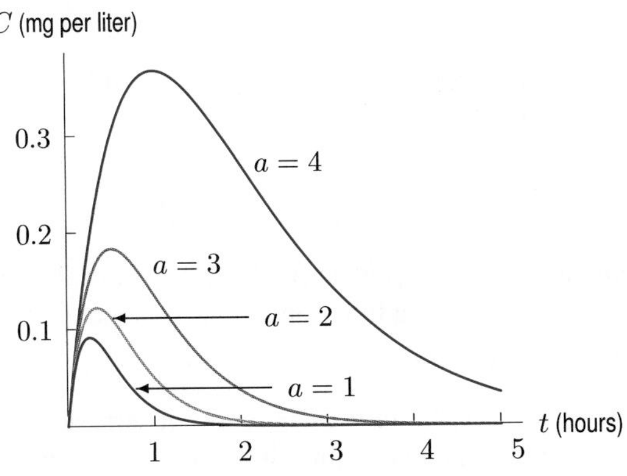

Figure 9.3: Concentration $C = f(a,t)$ of the drug resulting from an a-mg injection

Problems for Section 9.1

Problems 1–2 concern the cost, C, of renting a car from a company which charges \$40 a day and 15 cents a mile, so $C = f(d,m) = 40d + 0.15m$, where d is the number of days, and m is the number of miles.

1. Make a table of values for C, using $d = 1, 2, 3, 4$ and $m = 100, 200, 300, 400$. You should have 16 values in your table.

2. (a) Find $f(3,200)$ and interpret it.
   (b) Explain the significance of $f(3,m)$ in terms of rental car costs. Graph this function, with C as a function of m.
   (c) Explain the significance of $f(d,100)$ in terms of rental car costs. Graph this function, with C as a function of d.

Problems 3–7 refer to Table 9.2, which shows[1] the weekly beef consumption, C, (in lbs) of an average household as a function of p, the price of beef (in \$/lb) and I, annual household income (in \$1000s).

Table 9.2 *Quantity of beef bought (lbs/household/week)*

		p			
		3.00	3.50	4.00	4.50
	20	2.65	2.59	2.51	2.43
	40	4.14	4.05	3.94	3.88
I	60	5.11	5.00	4.97	4.84
	80	5.35	5.29	5.19	5.07
	100	5.79	5.77	5.60	5.53

3. Give tables for beef consumption as a function of p, with I fixed at $I = 20$ and $I = 100$. Give tables for beef consumption as a function of I, with p fixed at $p = 3.00$ and $p = 4.00$. Comment on what you see in the tables.

4. How does beef consumption vary as a function of household income if the price of beef is held constant?

5. Make a table showing the amount of money, M, that the average household spends on beef (in dollars per household per week) as a function of the price of beef and household income.

[1]From Richard G. Lipsey, *An Introduction to Positive Economics*, 3rd Ed. (London: Weidenfeld and Nicolson, 1971).

6. Make a table of the proportion, P, of household income spent on beef per week as a function of price and income. (Note that P is the fraction of income spent on beef.)

7. Express P, the proportion of household income spent on beef per week, in terms of the original function $f(I, p)$ which gave consumption as a function of p and I.

8. Graph the bank-account function f in Example 1 on page 350, holding B fixed at $B = 10, 20, 30$ and letting t vary. Then graph f, holding t fixed at $t = 0, 5, 10$ and letting B vary. Explain what you see.

9. The total sales of a product, S, can be expressed as a function of the price p charged for the product and the amount, a, spent on advertising, so $S = f(p, a)$. Do you expect f to be an increasing or decreasing function of p? Do you expect f to be an increasing or decreasing function of a? Why?

10. The number, n, of new cars sold in a year is a function of the price of new cars, c, and the average price of gas, g.

(a) If c is held constant, is n an increasing or decreasing function of g? Why?

(b) If g is held constant, is n an increasing or decreasing function of c? Why?

11. The heat index is a temperature which tells you how hot it feels as a result of the combination of temperature and humidity. See Table 9.3. Heat exhaustion is likely to occur when the heat index reaches 105°F.

(a) If the temperature is 80°F and the humidity is 50%, how hot does it feel?

(b) At what humidity does 90°F feel like 90°F?

(c) Make a table showing the approximate temperature at which heat exhaustion becomes a danger, as a function of humidity.

(d) Explain why the heat index is sometimes above the actual temperature and sometimes below it.

Table 9.3 *Heat index (°F) as a function of humidity (H%) and temperature (T°F)*

H \ T	70	75	80	85	90	95	100	105	110	115
0	64	69	73	78	83	87	91	95	99	103
10	65	70	75	80	85	90	95	100	105	111
20	66	72	77	82	87	93	99	105	112	120
30	67	73	78	84	90	96	104	113	123	135
40	68	74	79	86	93	101	110	123	137	151
50	69	75	81	88	96	107	120	135	150	
60	70	76	82	90	100	114	132	149		

12. Using Table 9.3, graph heat index as a function of humidity with temperature fixed at 70°F and at 100°F. Explain the features of each graph and the difference between them in common-sense terms.

13. The monthly payments, P dollars, on a mortgage in which A dollars were borrowed at an annual interest rate of r% for t years is given by $P = f(A, r, t)$. Is f an increasing or decreasing function of A? Of r? Of t?

14. You are planning a trip whose principal cost is gasoline.

(a) Make a table showing how the daily fuel cost varies as a function of the price of gasoline (in dollars per gallon) and the number of gallons you buy each day.

(b) If your car goes 30 miles on each gallon of gasoline, make a table showing how your daily fuel cost varies as a function of your daily travel distance and the price of gas.

In Problems 15–16, the fallout, V (in kilograms per square kilometer), from a volcanic explosion depends on the distance, d, from the volcano and the time, t, since the explosion:

$$V = f(d, t) = (\sqrt{t})e^{-d}.$$

15. On the same axes, graph cross-sections of f with $t = 1$, and $t = 2$. As distance from the volcano increases, how does the fallout change? Look at the relationship between the graphs: how does the fallout change as time passes? Explain your answers in terms of volcanoes.

16. On the same axes, graph cross-sections of f with $d = 0$, $d = 1$, and $d = 2$. As time passes since the explosion, how does the fallout change? Look at the relationship between the graphs: how does fallout change as a function of distance? Explain your answers in terms of volcanoes.

17. An airport can be cleared of fog by heating the air. The amount of heat required, $H(T, w)$ (in calories per cubic meter of fog), depends on the temperature of the air, T (in °C), and the wetness of the fog, w (in grams per cubic meter of fog). Figure 9.4 shows several graphs of H against T with w fixed.

(a) Estimate $H(20, 0.3)$ and explain what information it gives us.

(b) Make a table of values for $H(T, w)$. Use $T = 0, 10, 20, 30, 40$, and $w = 0.1, 0.2, 0.3, 0.4$.

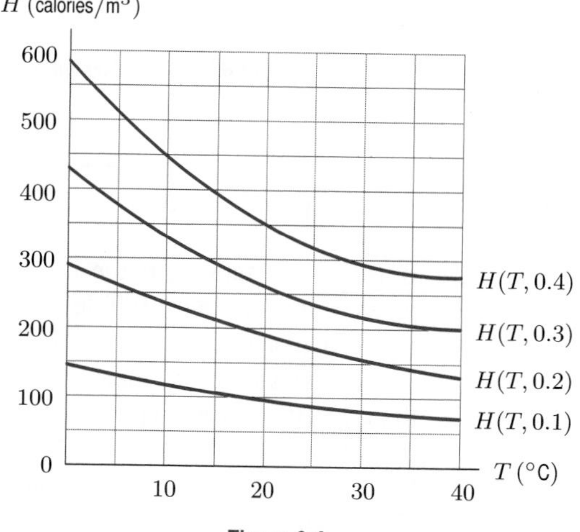

Figure 9.4

9.2 CONTOUR DIAGRAMS

How can we visualize a function of two variables? Just as a function of one variable can be represented by a graph, a function of two variables can be represented by a surface in space or by a *contour diagram* in the plane. Numerical information is more easily obtained from contour diagrams, so we concentrate on their use.

Weather Maps

Figure 9.5 shows a weather map from a newspaper. This contour diagram shows the predicted high temperature, T, in degrees Fahrenheit (°F), throughout the US on that day. The curves on the map, called *isotherms*, separate the country into zones, according to whether T is in the 60s, 70s, 80s, 90s, or 100s. (*Iso* means same and *therm* means heat.) Notice that the isotherm separating the 80s and 90s zones connects all the points where the temperature is predicted to be exactly 90°F.

If the function $T = f(x, y)$ gives the predicted high temperature (in °F) on this particular day as a function of latitude x and longitude y, then the isotherms are graphs of the equations

$$f(x, y) = c$$

where c is a constant. In general, such curves are called *contours*, and a graph showing selected contours of a function is called a contour diagram.

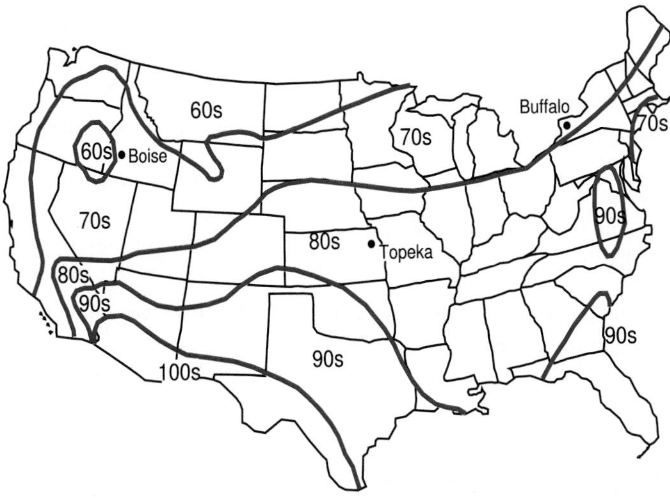

Figure 9.5: Weather map showing predicted high temperatures, T, on a summer day

---

Example 1 Estimate the predicted value of T in Boise, Idaho; Topeka, Kansas; and Buffalo, New York.

Solution Boise and Buffalo are in the 70s region, and Topeka is in the 80s region. Thus, the predicted temperature in Boise and Buffalo is between 70 and 80 while the predicted temperature in Topeka is between 80 and 90.

In fact, we can say more. Although both Boise and Buffalo are in the 70s, Boise is quite close to the $T = 70$ isotherm, whereas Buffalo is quite close to the $T = 80$ isotherm. So we estimate that the temperature will be in the low 70s in Boise and in the high 70s in Buffalo. Topeka is about halfway between the $T = 80$ isotherm and the $T = 90$ isotherm. Thus, we guess that the temperature in Topeka will be in the mid-80s. In fact, the actual high temperatures for that day were 71°F for Boise, 79°F for Buffalo, and 86°F for Topeka.

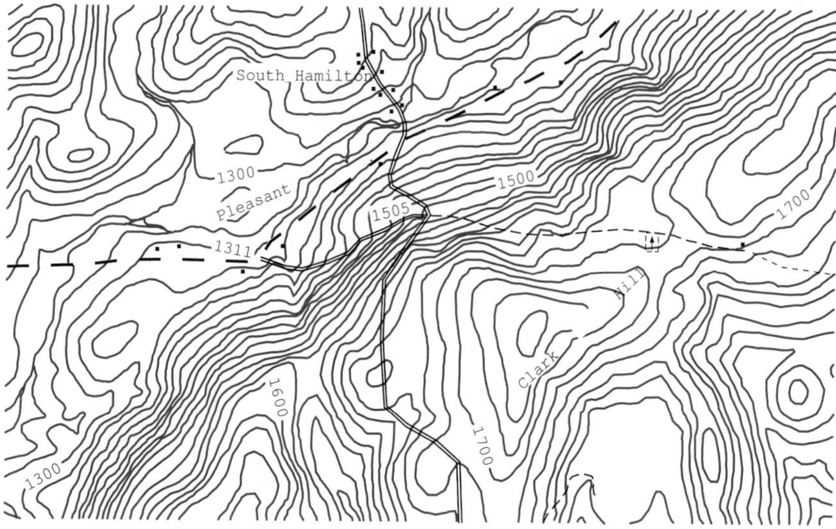

Figure 9.6: A topographical map showing the region around South Hamilton, NY

Topographical Maps

Another common example of a contour diagram is a topographical map like that shown in Figure 9.6. Here, the contours separate regions of lower elevation from regions of higher elevation, and give an overall picture of the nature of the terrain. Such topographical maps are frequently colored green at the lower elevations and brown, red, or even white at the higher elevations.

Example 2 Explain why the topographical map shown in Figure 9.7 corresponds to the surface of the terrain shown in Figure 9.8.

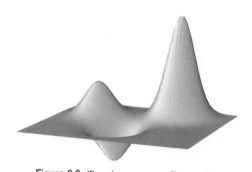

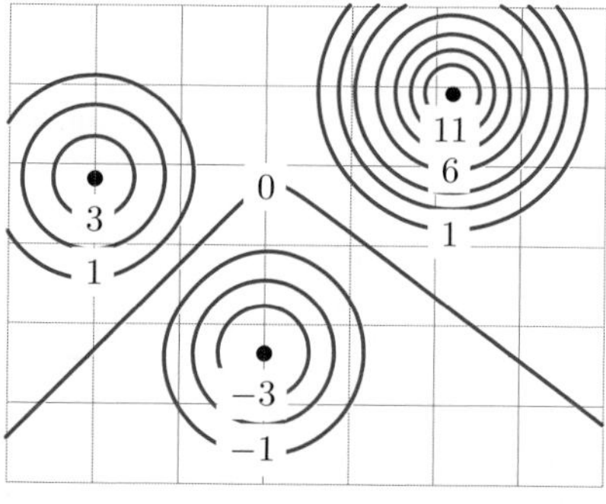

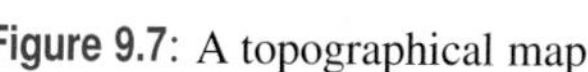

Figure 9.7: A topographical map

Figure 9.8: Terrain corresponding to the topographical map in Figure 9.7

Solution We see from the topographical map in Figure 9.7 that there are two hills, one with height about 12, and the other with height about 4. Most of the terrain is around height 0, and there is one valley with height about -4. This matches the surface of the terrain in Figure 9.8 since there are two hills (one taller than the other) and one valley.

The contours on a topographical map outline the contour or shape of the land. Because every point along the same contour has the same elevation, contours are also called *level curves* or *level sets*. We usually draw contours for equally spaced values of the function. The more closely spaced the contours, the steeper the terrain; the more widely spaced the contours, the flatter the terrain (provided, of course, that the elevation between contours varies by a constant amount). Certain features have distinctive characteristics. A mountain peak is typically surrounded by contours like those in Figure 9.9. A pass in a range of mountains may have contours that look like Figure 9.10. A long valley has parallel contours indicating the rising elevations on both sides of the valley (see Figure 9.11); a long ridge of mountains has the same type of contours, only the elevations decrease on both sides of the ridge. Notice that the elevation numbers on the contours are as important as the curves themselves.

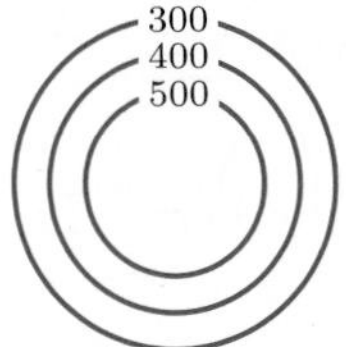

Figure 9.9: Mountain peak

Figure 9.10: Pass between two mountains

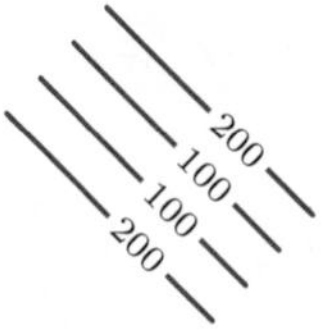

Figure 9.11: Long valley

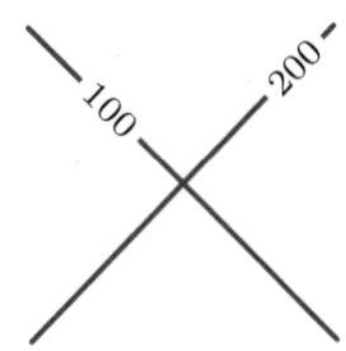

Figure 9.12: Impossible contour lines

There are some things contours cannot do. Two contours corresponding to different elevations cannot cross each other as shown in Figure 9.12. If they did, the point of intersection of the two curves would have two different elevations, which is impossible (assuming the terrain has no overhangs).

Using Contour Diagrams

Consider the effect of different weather conditions on US corn production. What would happen if the average temperature were to increase (due to global warming, for example) or if the rainfall were to decrease (due to a drought)? One way of estimating the effect of these climatic changes is to use Figure 9.13. This map is a contour diagram giving the corn production $C = f(R, T)$ in the US as a function of the total rainfall, R, in inches, and average temperature, T, in degrees Fahrenheit, during the growing season.[2] Suppose at the present time, $R = 15$ inches and $T = 76°$F. Production is measured as a percentage of the present production; thus, the contour through $R = 15, T = 76$ is $C = 100$, that is, $C = f(15, 76) = 100$.

Example 3 Use Figure 9.13 to evaluate $f(18, 78)$ and $f(12, 76)$ and explain the answers in terms of corn production.

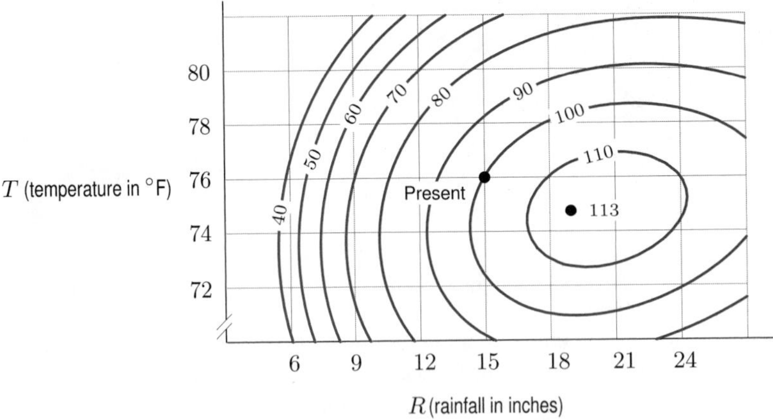

Figure 9.13: Corn production, C, as a function of rainfall and temperature

Solution The point with R-coordinate 18 and T-coordinate 78 is on the contour with value $C = 100$, so $f(18, 78) = 100$. This means that if the annual rainfall were 18 inches and the temperature were 78°F, the country would produce about the same amount of corn as at present, although it would be wetter and warmer than it is now. The point with R-coordinate 12 and T-coordinate 76 is about

[2] Adapted from S. Beaty and R. Healy, *The Future of American Agriculture*, Scientific American, Vol. 248, No. 2, February, 1983.

halfway between the $C = 80$ and $C = 90$ contours, so $f(12, 76) \approx 85$. This means that if the rainfall dropped to 12 inches and the temperature stayed at 76°F, then corn production would drop to about 85% of what it is now.

Example 4 Describe how corn production changes as a function of rainfall if temperature is fixed at the present value in Figure 9.13. Describe how corn production changes as a function of temperature if rainfall is held constant at the present value. Give common-sense explanations for your answers.

Solution To see what happens to corn production if the temperature stays fixed at 76°F but the rainfall changes, look along the horizontal line $T = 76$. Starting from the present and moving left along the line $T = 76$, the values on the contours decrease. In other words, if there is a drought, corn production decreases. Conversely, as rainfall increases, that is, as we move from the present to the right along the line $T = 76$, corn production increases, reaching a maximum of more than 110% when $R = 21$, and then decreases (too much rainfall floods the fields). If, instead, rainfall remains at the present value and temperature increases, we move up the vertical line $R = 15$. Under these circumstances corn production decreases; a 2° increase causes a 10% drop in production. This makes sense since hotter temperatures lead to greater evaporation and hence drier conditions, even with rainfall constant at 15 inches. Similarly, a decrease in temperature leads to a very slight increase in production, reaching a maximum of around 102% when $T = 74$, followed by a decrease (the corn won't grow if it is too cold).

Cobb-Douglas Production Functions

Suppose you are running a small printing business, and decide to expand because you have more orders than you can handle. How should you expand? Should you start a night shift and hire more workers? Should you buy more expensive but faster computers which will enable the current staff to keep up with the work? Or should you do some combination of the two?

Obviously, the way such a decision is made in practice involves many other considerations—such as whether you could get a suitably trained night shift, or whether there are any faster computers available. Nevertheless, you might model the quantity, P, of work produced by your business as a function of two variables: your total number, N, of workers, and the total value, V, of your equipment.

How would you expect such a production function to behave? In general, having more equipment and more workers enables you to produce more. However, increasing equipment without increasing the number of workers will increase production a bit, but not beyond a point. (If equipment is already lying idle, having more of it won't help.) Similarly, increasing the number of workers without increasing equipment will increase production, but not past the point where the equipment is fully utilized, as any new workers would have no equipment available to them.

Example 5 Explain why the contour diagram in Figure 9.14 does not model the behavior expected of the production function, whereas the contour diagram in Figure 9.15 does.

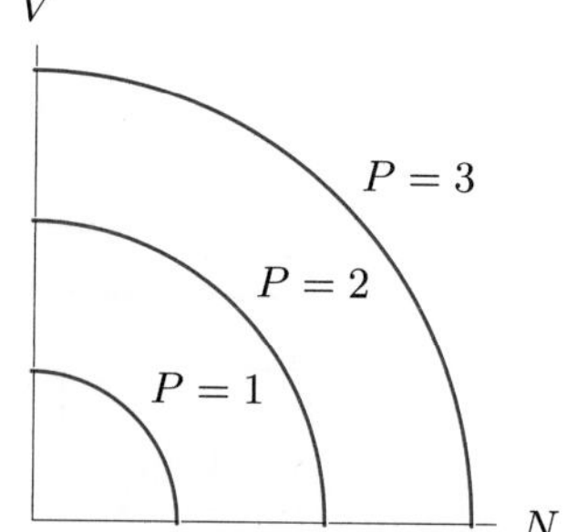

Figure 9.14: Incorrect contours for printing production

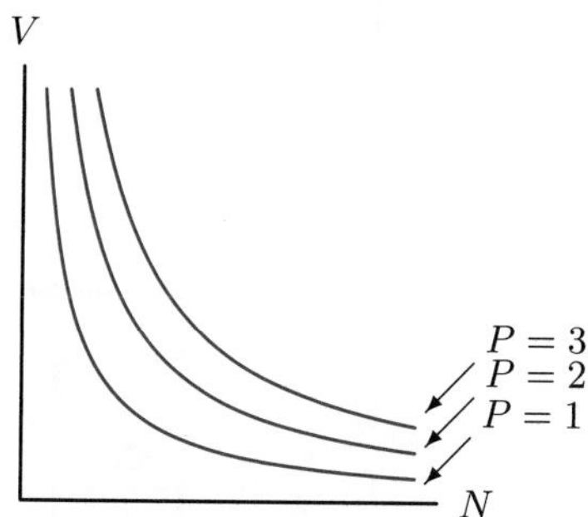

Figure 9.15: Correct contours for printing production

Solution Production P should be an increasing function of N and an increasing function of V. We see that both contour diagrams (in Figure 9.14 and Figure 9.15) satisfy this condition. Which of the contour diagrams has production increasing in the correct way? First look at the contour diagram in Figure 9.14. Fixing V at a particular value and letting N increase means moving to the right on the contour diagram. As we do so, we cross contours with larger and larger P values, meaning that production increases indefinitely. On the other hand, in Figure 9.15, as we move in the same direction we eventually find ourselves moving nearly parallel to the contours, crossing them less and less frequently. Therefore, production increases more and more slowly as N increases while V is held fixed. Similarly, if we hold N fixed and let V increase, the contour diagram in Figure 9.14 shows production increasing at a steady rate, whereas Figure 9.15 shows production increasing, but at a decreasing rate. Thus, Figure 9.15 fits the expected behavior of the production function best.

The Cobb-Douglas Production Model

In 1928, Cobb and Douglas used a simple formula to model the production of the entire US economy in the first quarter of the 20th century. Using government estimates of P, the total yearly production between 1899 and 1922, and of K, the total capital investment over the same period, and of L, the total labor force, they found that P was well approximated by the function:

$$P = 1.01L^{0.75}K^{0.25}.$$

This function turned out to model the US economy surprisingly accurately, both for the period on which it was based, and for some time afterward. The contour diagram of this function is similar to that in Figure 9.15. In general, production is often modeled by a function of the following form:

Cobb-Douglas Production Function

$$P = f(N, V) = cN^{\alpha}V^{\beta}$$

where P is the total quantity produced and c, α, and β are positive constants with $0 < \alpha < 1$ and $0 < \beta < 1$.

Contour Diagrams and Tables

Table 9.4 shows the heat index as a function of temperature and humidity. The heat index is a temperature which tells you how hot it feels as a result of the combination of the two. We can also display this function using a contour diagram. Scales for the two independent variables (temperature and humidity) go on the axes. The heat indices shown range from 64 to 151, so we will draw contours at values of 70, 80, 90, 100, 110, 120, 130, 140, and 150. How do we know where the contour for 70 goes? Table 9.4 shows that, when humidity is 0%, a heat index of 70 occurs between 75°F and 80°F, so the contour will go approximately through the point $(76, 0)$. It also goes through the point $(75, 10)$. Continuing in this way, we can approximate the 70 contour. See Figure 9.16. You can construct all the contours in Figure 9.17 in a similar way.

Table 9.4 *Heat index (°F)*

Humidity (%) \ Temperature (°F)	70	75	80	85	90	95	100	105	110	115
0	64	69	73	78	83	87	91	95	99	103
10	65	70	75	80	85	90	95	100	105	111
20	66	72	77	82	87	93	99	105	112	120
30	67	73	78	84	90	96	104	113	123	135
40	68	74	79	86	93	101	110	123	137	151
50	69	75	81	88	96	107	120	135	150	
60	70	76	82	90	100	114	132	149		

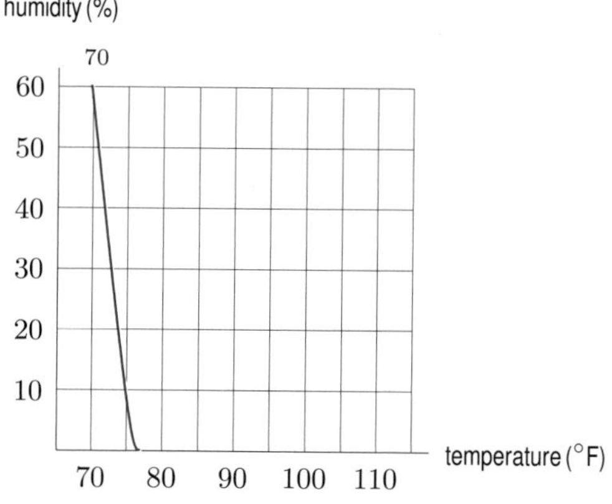

Figure 9.16: The contour for a heat index of 70

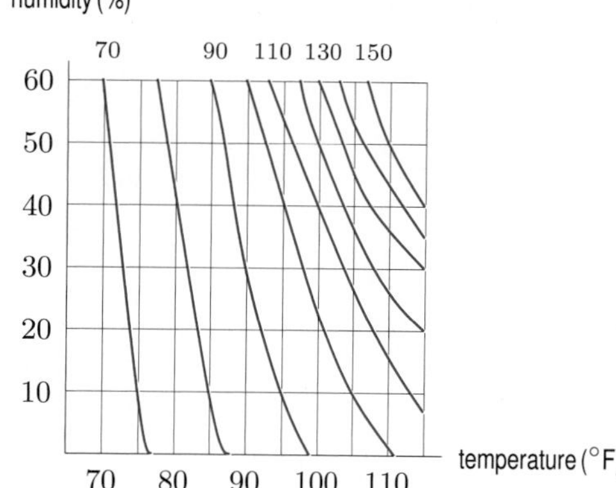

Figure 9.17: Contour diagram for the heat index

Example 6 Heat exhaustion is likely to occur where the heat index is 105 or higher. On the contour diagram in Figure 9.17, shade in the region where heat exhaustion is likely to occur.

Solution The shaded region in Figure 9.18 shows the values of temperature and humidity at which the heat index is above 105.

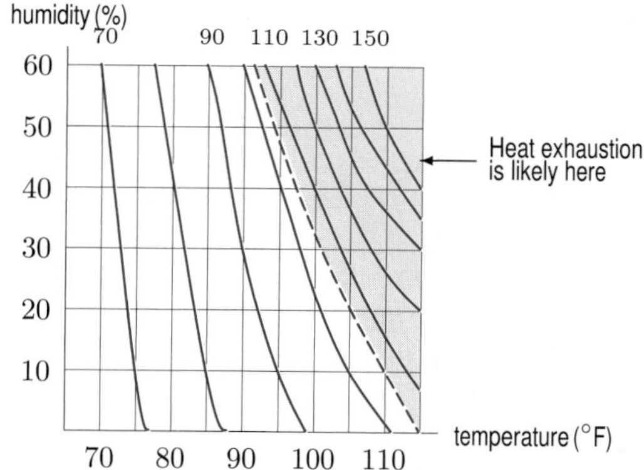

Figure 9.18: Shaded region shows conditions under which heat exhaustion is likely

---

Finding Contours Algebraically

Algebraic equations for the contours of a function f are easy to find if we have a formula for $f(x, y)$. A contour consists of all the points (x, y) where $f(x, y)$ has a constant value, c. Its equation is

$$f(x, y) = c.$$

Example 7 Draw a contour diagram for the airline revenue function $R = 350x + 200y$. Include contours for $R = 4000, 8000, 12000, 16000$.

Solution The contour for $R = 4000$ is given by

$$350x + 200y = 4000.$$

This is the equation of a line with intercepts $x = 4000/350 = 11.43$ and $y = 4000/200 = 20$. (See Figure 9.19.) The contour for $R = 8000$ is given by

$$350x + 200y = 8000.$$

This is the equation of a parallel line with intercepts $x = 8000/350 = 22.86$ and $y = 8000/200 = 40$. The contours for $R = 12000$ and $R = 16000$ are parallel lines drawn similarly. (See Figure 9.19.)

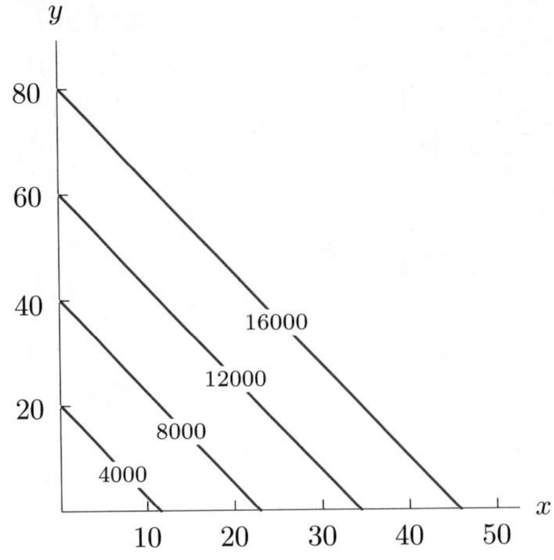

Figure 9.19: A contour diagram for $R = 350x + 200y$

Problems for Section 9.2

1. Figure 9.20 shows contours for the function $z = f(x, y)$. Is z an increasing or a decreasing function of x? Is z an increasing or a decreasing function of y?

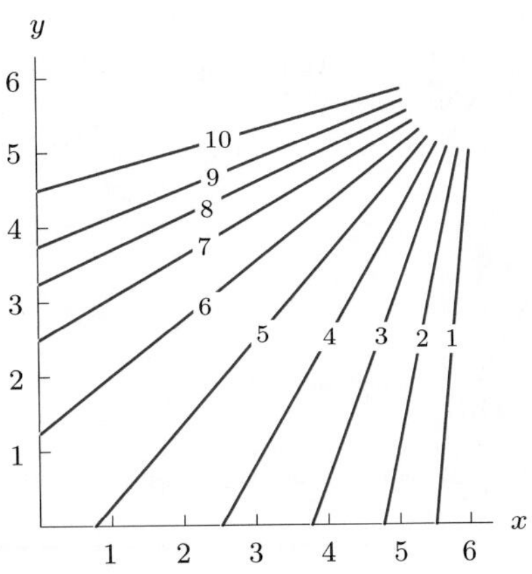

Figure 9.20

2. Figure 9.21 is a contour diagram for the demand for orange juice as a function of the price of orange juice and the price of apple juice. Which axis corresponds to orange juice? Which to apple juice? Explain.

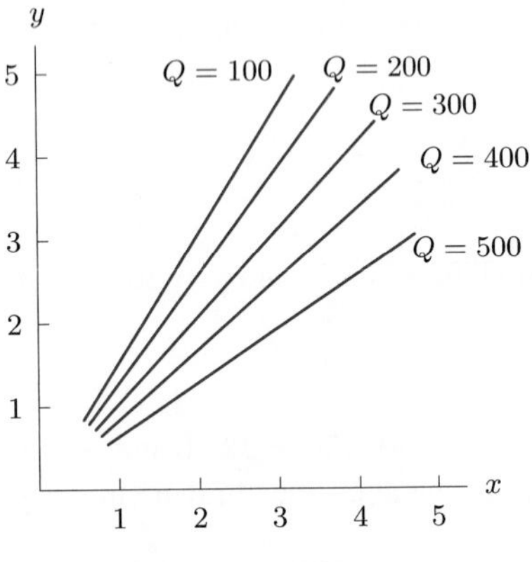

Figure 9.21

3. Figure 9.22 shows contour diagrams of temperature in °C in a room at three different times. Describe the heat flow in the room. What could be causing this?

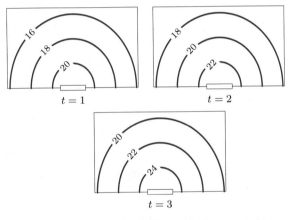

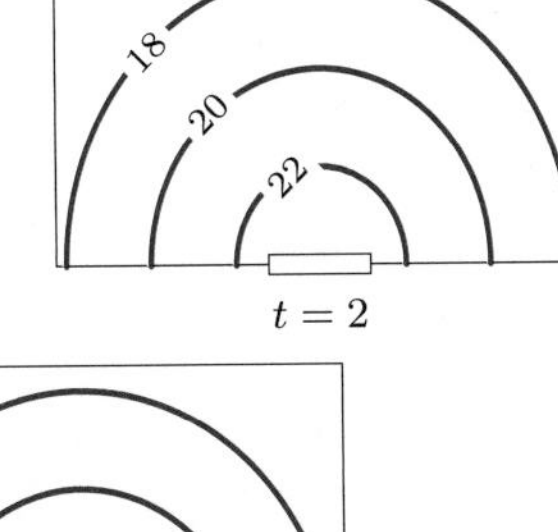

Figure 9.22

4. A topographic map is given in Figure 9.23. How many hills are there? Estimate the x- and y-coordinates of the tops of the hills. Which hill is the highest? A river runs through the valley; in which direction is it flowing?

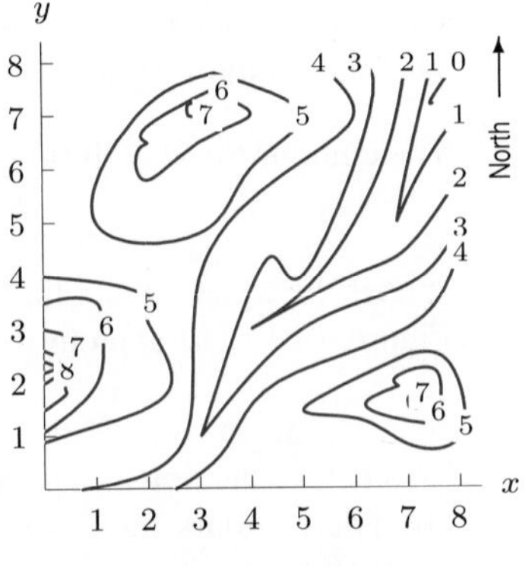

Figure 9.23

5. Draw a contour diagram for the function $C = 40d + 0.15m$. Include contours for $C = 50, 100, 150, 200$.

Problems 6–8 refer to the map in Figure 9.5 on page 354.

6. Give the range of daily high temperatures for:

(a) Pennsylvania **(b)** North Dakota
(c) California

7. Sketch a possible graph of the predicted high temperature T on a line north-south through Topeka.

8. Sketch possible graphs of the predicted high temperature on a north-south line and an east-west line through Boise.

9. Maple syrup production is highest when the nights are cold and the days are warm. Make a possible contour diagram for maple syrup production as a function of the high (daytime) temperature and the low (nighttime) temperature. Label the contours with 10, 20, 30, and 40 (in liters of maple syrup).

10. A manufacturer sells two products, one at a price of \$3000 a unit and the other at a price of \$12,000 a unit. A quantity q_1 of the first product and q_2 of the second product are sold at a total cost of \$4000 to the manufacturer.

(a) Express the manufacturer's profit, π, as a function of q_1 and q_2.
(b) Sketch contours of π for $\pi = 10{,}000$, $\pi = 20{,}000$, and $\pi = 30{,}000$ and the break-even curve $\pi = 0$.

11. Sketch a contour diagram for $z = y - \sin x$. Include at least four labeled contours. Describe the contours in words and how they are spaced.

12. The contour diagram in Figure 9.24 shows your happiness as a function of love and money.

(a) Describe in words your happiness as a function of:
(i) Money, with love fixed.
(ii) Love, with money fixed.
(b) Graph two different cross-sections with love fixed and two different cross-sections with money fixed.

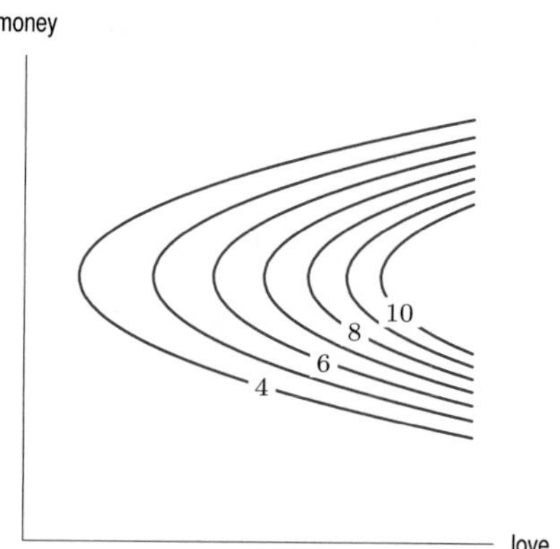

Figure 9.24

13. The concentration, C, of a drug in the blood is given by $C = f(x,t) = te^{-t(5-x)}$, where x is the amount of drug injected (in mg) and t is the number of hours since the injection. The contour diagram of $f(x,t)$ is given in Figure 9.25. Explain the diagram by varying one variable at a time: describe f as a function of x if t is held fixed, and then describe f as a function of t if x is held fixed.

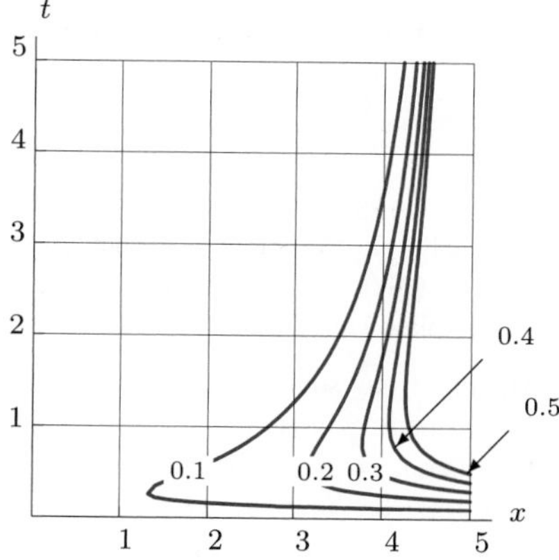

Figure 9.25

14. The cornea is the front surface of the eye. Corneal specialists use a TMS, or Topographical Modeling System, to produce a "map" of the curvature of the eye's surface. A computer analyzes light reflected off the eye and draws level curves joining points of constant curvature. The regions between these curves are colored different colors.

The first two pictures in Figure 9.26 are cross-sections of eyes with constant curvature, the smaller being about 38 units and the larger about 50 units. For contrast, the third eye has varying curvature.

(a) Describe in words how the TMS map of an eye of constant curvature will look.
(b) Draw the TMS map of an eye with the cross-section in Figure 9.27. Assume the eye is circular when viewed from the front, and the cross-section is the same in every direction. Put reasonable numeric labels on your level curves.

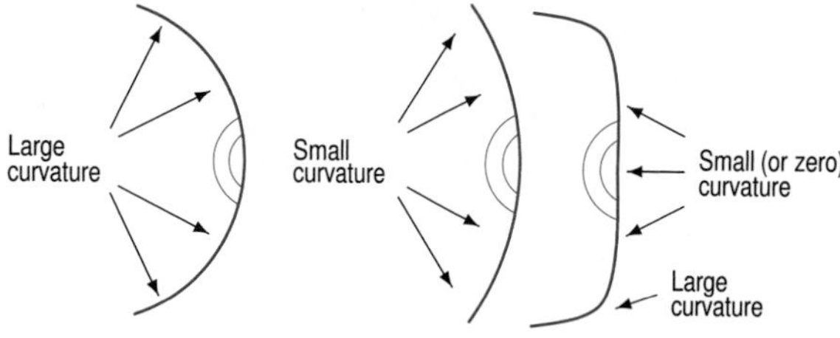

Figure 9.26: Pictures of eyes with different curvature

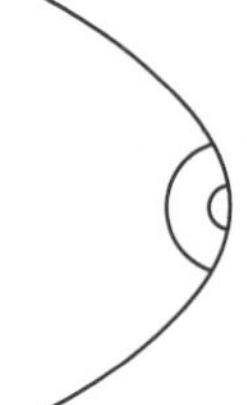

Figure 9.27

In Problems 15–20, sketch a contour diagram for the function with at least four labeled contours. Describe in words the contours and how they are spaced.

15. $f(x, y) = x + y$

16. $f(x, y) = 3x + 3y$

17. $f(x, y) = x + y + 1$

18. $f(x, y) = 2x - y$

19. $f(x, y) = -x - y$

20. $f(x, y) = y - x^2$

21. Figure 9.28 shows contours of the function giving the species density of breeding birds at each point in the US, Canada, and Mexico.[3] Are the following statements true or false? Explain your answers.

(a) Moving from south to north across Canada, the species density increases.

(b) In general, peninsulas (for example, Florida, Baja California, the Yucatan) have lower species densities than the areas around them.

(c) The species density around Miami is over 100.

(d) The greatest rate of change in species density with distance is in Mexico. If this is true, mark the point and direction giving the maximum rate.

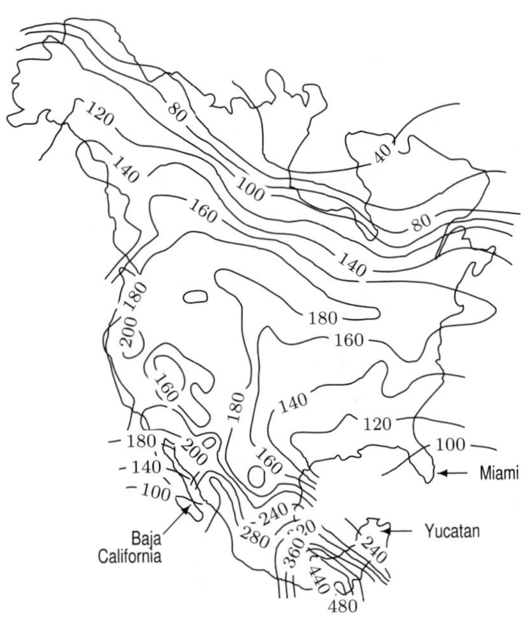

Figure 9.28

22. Each of the contour diagrams in Figure 9.29 shows population density in a certain region of a city. Choose the contour diagram that best corresponds to each of the following situations. Many different matchings are possible. Pick a reasonable one and justify your choice.

(a) The middle contour is a highway.

(b) The middle contour is an open sewage canal.

(c) The middle contour is a railroad line.

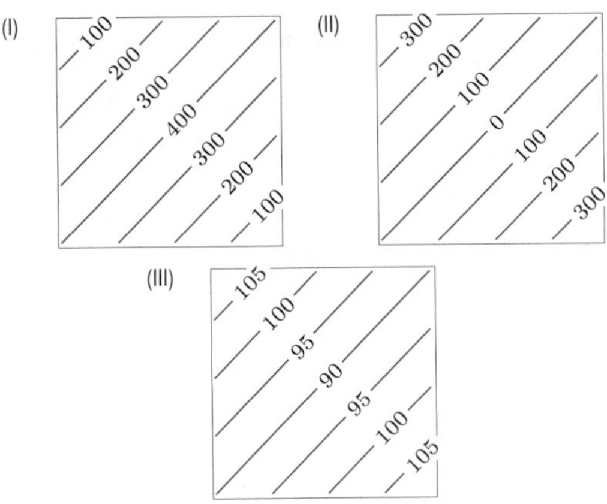

Figure 9.29

23. In a small printing business, $P = 2N^{0.6}V^{0.4}$, where N is the number of workers, V is the value of the equipment, and P is production, in thousands of pages per day.

(a) If this company has a labor force of 300 workers and 200 units worth of equipment, what is production?

(b) If the labor force is doubled (to 600 workers), how does production change?

(c) If the company purchases enough equipment to double the value of its equipment (to 400 units), how does production change?

(d) If both N and V are doubled from the values given in part (a), how does production change?

24. Figure 9.30 shows a contour map of a hill with two paths, A and B.

(a) On which path, A or B, will you have to climb more steeply?

(b) On which path, A or B, will you probably have a better view of the surrounding countryside? (Assume trees do not block your view.)

(c) Alongside which path is there more likely to be a stream?

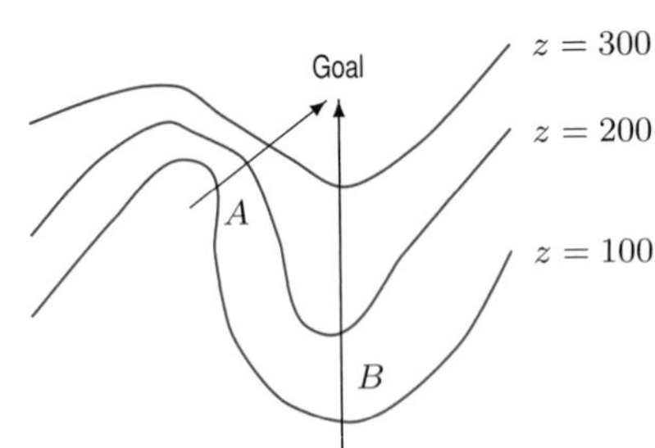

Figure 9.30

[3]From the undergraduate senior thesis of Professor Robert Cook, Director of Harvard's Arnold Arboretum.

25. Match the following descriptions of a company's success with the contour diagrams of success as a function of money and work in Figure 9.31.

(a) Our success is measured in dollars, plain and simple. More hard work won't hurt, but it also won't help.
(b) No matter how much money or hard work we put into the company, we just can't make a go of it.
(c) Although we are not always totally successful, it seems that the amount of money invested does not matter. As long as we put hard work into the company, our success increases.
(d) The company's success is based on both hard work and investment.

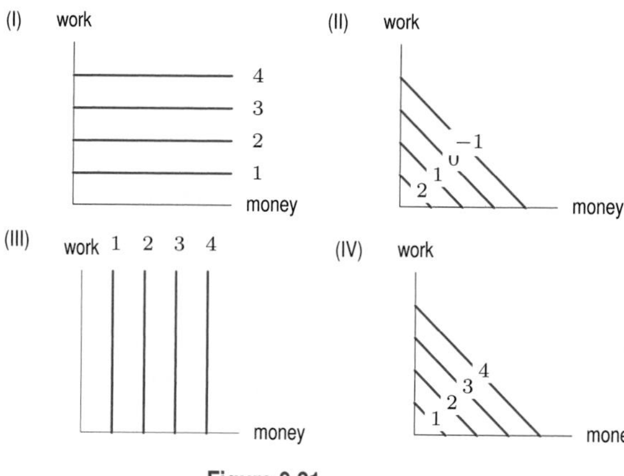

Figure 9.31

26. Figure 9.32 shows cardiac output (in liters per minute) in patients suffering from shock as a function of blood pressure in the central veins (in mm Hg) and the time in hours since the onset of shock.[4]

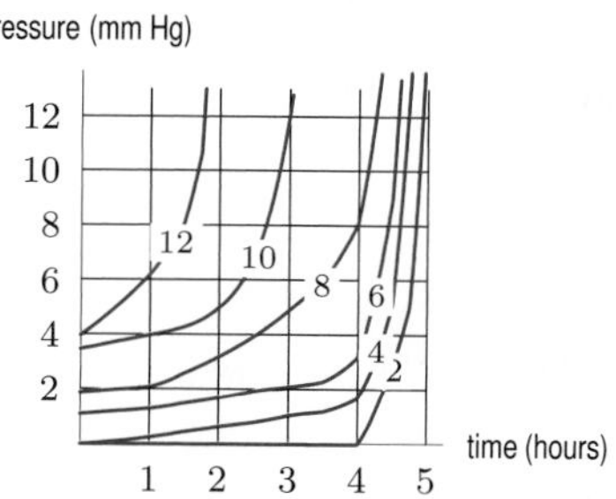

Figure 9.32

(a) In a patient with blood pressure of 4 mm Hg, what is cardiac output when the patient first goes into shock? Estimate cardiac output three hours later. How much time has passed when cardiac output is reduced to 50% of the initial value?
(b) In patients suffering from shock, is cardiac output an increasing or decreasing function of blood pressure?
(c) Is cardiac output an increasing or decreasing function of time, t, where t represents the elapsed time since the patient went into shock?
(d) If blood pressure is 3 mm Hg, explain how cardiac output changes as a function of time. In particular, does it change rapidly or slowly during the first two hours of shock? During hours 2 to 4? During the last hour of the study? Explain why this information is useful to a physician treating a patient for shock.

27. Antibiotics can be toxic in large doses. If repeated doses of an antibiotic are to be given, the rate at which the medicine is excreted through the kidneys should be monitored by a physician. One measure of kidney function is the glomerular filtration rate, or GFR, which measures the amount of material crossing the outer (or glomerular) membrane of the kidney, in milliliters per minute. A normal GFR is about 125 ml/min. Figure 9.33 gives a contour diagram of the percent, P, of a dose of mezlocillin (an antibiotic) excreted, as a function of the patient's GFR and the time, t, in hours since the dose was administered.[5]

(a) In a patient with a GFR of 50, approximately how long will it take for 30% of the dose to be excreted?
(b) In a patient with a GFR of 60, approximately what percent of the dose has been excreted after 5 hours?
(c) Explain how we can tell from the graph that, for a patient with a fixed GFR, the amount excreted changes very little after 12 hours.
(d) Is the percent excreted an increasing or decreasing function of time? Explain why this makes sense.
(e) Is the percent excreted an increasing or decreasing function of GFR? Explain what this means to a physician giving antibiotics to a patient with kidney disease.

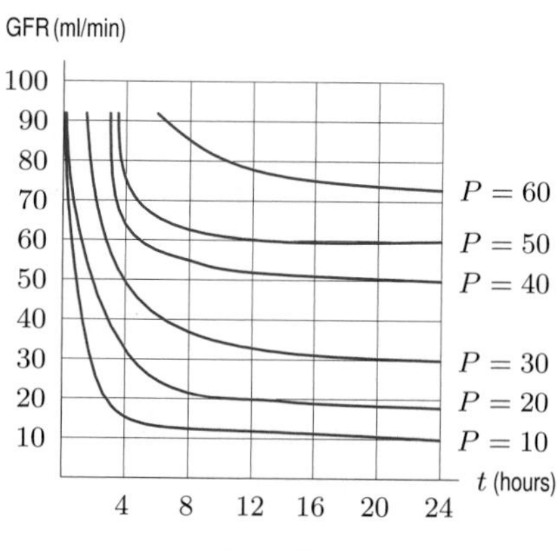

Figure 9.33

[4] Arthur C. Guyton and John E. Hall, *Textbook of Medical Physiology, Ninth Edition*, p. 288 (Philadelphia: W. B. Saunders, 1996).
[5] Peter G. Welling and Francis L. S. Tse, *Pharmacokinetics of Cardiovascular, Central Nervous System, and Antimicrobial Drugs*, The Royal Society of Chemistry, 1985, p. 316.

9.3 PARTIAL DERIVATIVES

In one-variable calculus we saw how the derivative measures the rate of change of a function. We begin by reviewing this idea.

Rate of Change of Airline Revenue

In Section 9.1 we saw a two-variable function which gives an airline's revenue, R, as a function of the number of full price tickets, x, and the number of discount tickets, y, sold:

$$R = f(x, y) = 350x + 200y.$$

If we fix the number of discount tickets at $y = 10$, we have a one-variable function

$$R = f(x, 10) = g(x) = 350x + 2000.$$

The rate of the change of revenue with respect to x is given by the one-variable derivative

$$g'(x) = 350.$$

This tells us that, if y is fixed at 10, then the revenue increases by \$350 for each additional full price ticket sold. We call $g'(x)$ the *partial derivative of* R *with respect to* x at the point $(x, 10)$. If $R = f(x, y)$, we write

$$\frac{\partial R}{\partial x} = f_x(x, 10) = g'(x) = 350.$$

Example 1 Find the rate of change of revenue, R, as y increases with x fixed at $x = 20$.

Solution Substituting $x = 20$ into $R = 350x + 200y$ gives the one-variable function

$$R = h(y) = 350(20) + 200y = 7000 + 200y.$$

The rate of change of R as y increases with x fixed is

$$\frac{\partial R}{\partial y} = f_y(20, y) = h'(y) = 200.$$

We call $\partial R/\partial y = f_y(20, y)$ the *partial derivative of* R *with respect to* y at the point $(20, y)$. The fact that both partial derivatives of R are positive corresponds to the fact that the revenue is increasing as more of either type of ticket is sold.

Definition of the Partial Derivative

For any function $f(x, y)$ we study the influence of x and y separately on the value $f(x, y)$ by keeping one fixed and letting the other vary. The method of the previous example allows us to calculate the rates of change of $f(x, y)$ with respect to x and y. For all points (a, b) at which the limits exist, we make the following definitions:

Partial Derivatives of f with Respect to x and y

The *partial derivative of f with respect to x* at (a, b) is the derivative of f with y constant:

$$f_x(a,b) = \begin{matrix}\text{Rate of change of } f \text{ with } y \text{ fixed} \\ \text{at } b, \text{ at the point } (a,b)\end{matrix} = \lim_{h\to 0} \frac{f(a+h,b)-f(a,b)}{h}.$$

The *partial derivative of f with respect to y* at (a, b) is the derivative of f with x constant:

$$f_y(a,b) = \begin{matrix}\text{Rate of change of } f \text{ with } x \text{ fixed} \\ \text{at } a, \text{ at the point } (a,b)\end{matrix} = \lim_{h\to 0} \frac{f(a,b+h)-f(a,b)}{h}.$$

If we think of a and b as variables, $a = x$ and $b = y$, we have the **partial derivative functions** $f_x(x, y)$ and $f_y(x, y)$.

Just as with ordinary derivatives, there is an alternative notation:

Alternative Notation for Partial Derivatives

If $z = f(x, y)$ we can write

$$f_x(x,y) = \frac{\partial z}{\partial x} \quad \text{and} \quad f_y(x,y) = \frac{\partial z}{\partial y}$$

$$f_x(a,b) = \left.\frac{\partial z}{\partial x}\right|_{(a,b)} \quad \text{and} \quad f_y(a,b) = \left.\frac{\partial z}{\partial y}\right|_{(a,b)}$$

We use the symbol ∂ to distinguish partial derivatives from ordinary derivatives. In cases where the independent variables have names different from x and y, we adjust the notation accordingly. For example, the partial derivatives of $f(u, v)$ are denoted by f_u and f_v.

Estimating Partial Derivatives from a Table

Example 2 An experiment[6] done on rats to measure the toxicity of formaldehyde yielded the data shown in Table 9.5. The values in the table show the percent, P, of rats that survived an exposure with concentration c (in parts per million) after t months, so $P = f(t, c)$. Using Table 9.5, estimate $f_t(18, 6)$ and $f_c(18, 6)$. Interpret your answers in terms of formaldehyde toxicity.

Table 9.5 *Percent, P, of rat population surviving after exposure to formaldehyde vapor*

		Time t (months)												
		0	2	4	6	8	10	12	14	16	18	20	22	24
Conc. c (ppm)	0	100	100	100	100	100	100	100	100	100	100	99	97	95
	2	100	100	100	100	100	100	100	100	99	98	97	95	92
	6	100	100	100	99	99	98	96	96	95	93	90	86	80
	15	100	100	100	99	99	99	99	96	93	82	70	58	36

Solution For $f_t(18, 6)$, we fix c at 6 ppm, and find the rate of change of percent surviving, P, with respect to t. We have

$$f_t(18,6) \approx \frac{\Delta P}{\Delta t} = \frac{f(20,6)-f(18,6)}{20-18} = \frac{90-93}{20-18} \approx -1.5\ \%\text{ per month.}$$

[6] James E. Gibson, *Formaldehyde Toxicity*, p. 125 (Hemisphere Publishing Company, McGraw-Hill, 1983).

This is the rate of change of percent surviving, P, *in the time t direction* at the point $(18, 6)$. The fact that it is negative means that P is decreasing as we read across the $c = 6$ row of the table in the direction of increasing t (that is, horizontally from left to right in Table 9.5). For $f_c(18, 6)$, we fix t at 18, and calculate the rate of change of P as we move in the direction of increasing c (that is, from top to bottom in Table 9.5). We have

$$f_c(18,6) \approx \frac{\Delta P}{\Delta c} = \frac{f(18,15) - f(18,6)}{15-6} = \frac{82-93}{15-6} = -1.22\% \text{ per ppm.}$$

The rate of change of P as c increases is about -1.22% per ppm. This means that as the concentration increases by 1 ppm from 6 ppm, the percent surviving 18 months decreases by about 1.22% per unit increase ppm. The partial derivative is negative because fewer rats survive this long when the concentration of formaldehyde increases. (That is, P goes down as c goes up.)

Using Partial Derivatives to Estimate Values of the Function

Example 3 Use Table 9.5 and partial derivatives to estimate the percent of rats surviving if they are exposed to formaldehyde with a concentration of

(a) 6 ppm for 18.5 months (b) 18 ppm for 24 months (c) 9 ppm for 20.5 months

Solution

(a) Since $t = 18.5$ and $c = 6$, we want to evaluate $P = f(18.5, 6)$. Table 9.5 tells us that $f(18, 6) = 93\%$ and we have just calculated

$$\left.\frac{\partial P}{\partial t}\right|_{(18,6)} = f_t(18,6) = -1.5\% \text{ per month.}$$

This partial derivative tells us that after 18 months of exposure to formaldehyde at a concentration of 6 ppm, P decreases by 1.5% for every additional month of exposure. Therefore after an additional 0.5 month, we have

$$P \approx 93 - 1.5(0.5) = 92.25\%.$$

(b) Now we wish to evaluate $f(24, 18)$. The closest entry to this in Table 9.5 is $f(24, 15) = 36$. We keep t fixed at 24 and increase c from 15 to 18. We estimate the rate of change in P as c changes; this is $\partial P/\partial c$. We see from Table 9.5 that

$$\left.\frac{\partial P}{\partial c}\right|_{(24,15)} \approx \frac{\Delta P}{\Delta c} = \frac{36-80}{15-6} = -4.89\% \text{ per ppm.}$$

The percent surviving 24 months goes down from 36% by about 4.89% for every unit increase in the formaldehyde concentration above 15 ppm. We have:

$$f(24,18) \approx 36 - 4.89(3) = 21.33\%.$$

We estimate that only about 21% of the rats would survive for 24 months if they were exposed to formaldehyde as strong as 18 ppm. Since this figure is an extrapolation from the available data, we should use it with caution.

(c) To estimate $f(20.5, 9)$, we use the closest entry $f(20, 6) = 90$. As we move from $(20, 6)$ to $(20.5, 9)$, the percentage, P, changes both due to the change in t and due to the change in c. We estimate the two partial derivatives at $t = 20$, $c = 6$:

$$\left.\frac{\partial P}{\partial t}\right|_{(20,6)} \approx \frac{\Delta P}{\Delta t} = \frac{86-90}{22-20} = -2\% \text{ per month,}$$

$$\left.\frac{\partial P}{\partial c}\right|_{(20,6)} \approx \frac{\Delta P}{\Delta c} = \frac{70-90}{15-6} = -2.22\% \text{ per month.}$$

The change in P due to a change of $\Delta t = 0.5$ month and $\Delta c = 3$ ppm is

$$\begin{aligned}\Delta P &\approx \text{Change due to } \Delta t + \text{Change due to } \Delta c\\ &= -2(0.5) - 2.22(3)\\ &= -7.66.\end{aligned}$$

So for $t = 20.5$, $c = 9$ we have

$$f(20.5, 9) \approx f(20, 6) - 7.66 = 82.34\%.$$

In Example 3 part (c), we used the relationship between ΔP, Δt, and Δc. In general, the relationship between the change Δf, in function value $f(x, y)$ and the changes Δx and Δy is as follows:

Local Linearity

$$\begin{matrix}\text{Change} \\ \text{in } f\end{matrix} \approx \begin{matrix}\text{Rate of change} \\ \text{in } x\text{-direction}\end{matrix} \cdot \Delta x + \begin{matrix}\text{Rate of change} \\ \text{in } y\text{-direction}\end{matrix} \cdot \Delta y$$

$$\Delta f \approx f_x \cdot \Delta x + f_y \cdot \Delta y$$

Estimating Partial Derivatives from a Contour Diagram

If we move parallel to one of the axes on a contour diagram, the partial derivative is the rate of change of the value of the function on the contours. For example, if the values on the contours are increasing in the direction of positive change, then the partial derivative must be positive.

Example 4 Figure 9.34 shows the contour diagram for the temperature $H(x, t)$ (in °F) in a room as a function of distance x (in feet) from a heater and time t (in minutes) after the heater has been turned on. What are the signs of $H_x(10, 20)$ and $H_t(10, 20)$? Estimate these partial derivatives and explain the answers in practical terms.

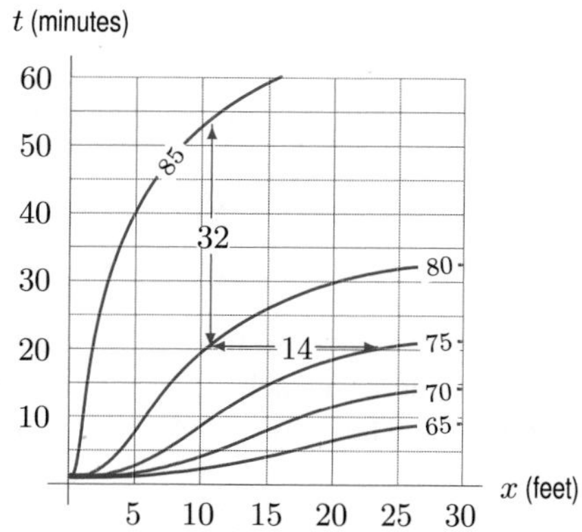

Figure 9.34: Temperature in a heated room

Solution The point $(10, 20)$ is on the $H = 80$ contour. As x increases, we move toward the $H = 75$ contour, so H is decreasing and $H_x(10, 20)$ is negative. This makes sense because as we move further from the heater, the temperature drops. On the other hand, as t increases, we move toward the $H = 85$ contour, so H is increasing and $H_t(10, 20)$ is positive. This also makes sense, because it says that as time passes, the room warms up.

To estimate the partial derivatives, use a difference quotient. Looking at the contour diagram, we see there is a point on the $H = 75$ contour about 14 units to the right of $(10, 20)$. Hence, H decreases by 5 when x increases by 14, so the rate of change of H with respect to x is about $\Delta H/\Delta x = -5/14 \approx -0.36$. Thus, we find

$$H_x(10, 20) \approx -0.36^\circ\text{F/ft}.$$

This means that near the point 10 feet from the heater, after 20 minutes the temperature drops about 1/3 of a degree for each foot we move away from the heater.

To estimate $H_t(10, 20)$, we look again at the contour diagram and notice that the $H = 85$ contour is about 32 units directly above the point $(10, 20)$. So H increases by 5 when t increases by 32. Hence,

$$H_t(10, 20) \approx \frac{\Delta H}{\Delta t} = \frac{5}{32} \approx 0.16^\circ\text{F/min}.$$

This means that after 20 minutes the temperature is going up about 1/6 of a degree each minute at the point 10 ft from the heater.

Using Units to Interpret Partial Derivatives

The units of the independent and dependent variables can often be helpful in explaining the meaning of a partial derivative.

Example 5 Suppose that your weight w in pounds is a function $f(c, n)$ of the number c of calories you consume daily and the number n of minutes you exercise daily. Using the units for w, c and n, interpret in everyday terms the statements

$$\left.\frac{\partial w}{\partial c}\right|_{(2000,15)} = 0.02 \quad \text{and} \quad \left.\frac{\partial w}{\partial n}\right|_{(2000,15)} = -0.025.$$

Solution The units of $\partial w/\partial c$ are pounds per calorie. The statement

$$\left.\frac{\partial w}{\partial c}\right|_{(2000,15)} = 0.02$$

means that if you are presently consuming 2000 calories daily and exercising 15 minutes daily, you will weigh 0.02 pounds more for each extra calorie you consume daily, or about 2 pounds for each extra 100 calories per day. The units of $\partial w/\partial n$ are pounds per minute. The statement

$$\left.\frac{\partial w}{\partial n}\right|_{(2000,15)} = -0.025$$

means that for the same calorie consumption and number of minutes of exercise, you will weigh 0.025 pounds less for each extra minute you exercise daily, or about 1 pound less for each extra 40 minutes per day. So if you eat an extra 100 calories each day and exercise about 80 minutes more each day, your weight should remain roughly steady.

Problems for Section 9.3

1. Using the contour diagram for $f(x,y)$ in Figure 9.35, decide whether each of these partial derivatives is positive, negative, or approximately zero.

(a) $f_x(4,1)$ **(b)** $f_y(4,1)$
(c) $f_x(5,2)$ **(d)** $f_y(5,2)$

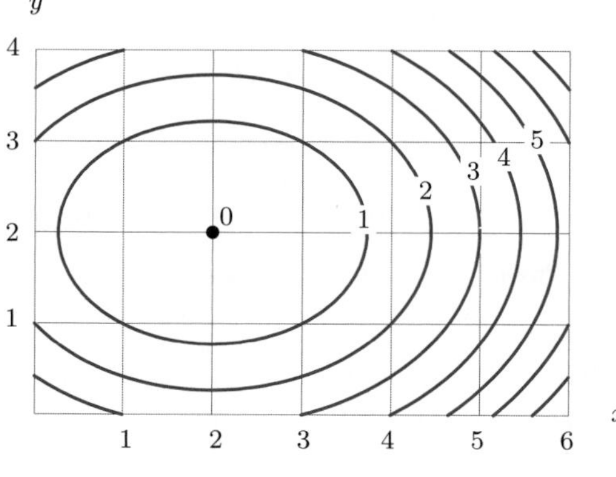

Figure 9.35

2. According to the contour diagram for $f(x,y)$ in Figure 9.35, which is larger: $f_x(3,1)$ or $f_x(5,2)$? Explain.

For Problems 3–4 refer to Table 9.4 on page 358 giving the heat index, I, in °F, as a function $f(H,T)$ of the relative humidity, H, and the temperature, T, in °F. The heat index is a temperature which tells you how hot it feels as a result of the combination of humidity and temperature.

3. Estimate $\partial I/\partial H$ and $\partial I/\partial T$ for typical weather conditions in Tucson in summer ($H = 10$, $T = 100$). What do your answers mean in practical terms for the residents of Tucson?

4. Answer the question in Problem 3 for Boston in summer ($H = 50$, $T = 80$).

5. The demand for coffee, Q, in pounds sold per week, is a function of the price of coffee, c, in dollars per pound and the price of tea, t, in dollars per pound, so $Q = f(c,t)$.

(a) Do you expect f_c to be positive or negative? What about f_t? Explain.

(b) Interpret each of the following statements in terms of the demand for coffee:

$$f(3,2) = 780 \quad f_c(3,2) = -60 \quad f_t(3,2) = 20$$

6. The quantity Q (in pounds) of beef that a certain community buys during a week is a function $Q = f(b,c)$ of the prices of beef, b, and chicken, c, during the week. Do you expect $\partial Q/\partial b$ to be positive or negative? What about $\partial Q/\partial c$?

7. A drug is injected into a patient's blood vessel. The function $c = f(x,t)$ represents the concentration of the drug at a distance x mm in the direction of the blood flow measured from the point of injection and at time t seconds since the injection. What are the units of the following partial derivatives? What are their practical interpretations? What do you expect their signs to be?

(a) $\partial c/\partial x$ **(b)** $\partial c/\partial t$

8. Table 9.6 gives the number of calories burned per minute, $B = f(s,w)$, for someone roller-blading,[7] as a function of the person's weight, w, and speed, s.

(a) Is f_w positive or negative? Is f_s positive or negative? What do your answers tell us about the effect of weight and speed on calories burned per minute?

(b) Estimate $f_w(160,10)$ and $f_s(160,10)$. Interpret your answers.

Table 9.6 *Calories burned per minute*

$w\backslash s$	8 mph	9 mph	10 mph	11 mph
120 lbs	4.2	5.8	7.4	8.9
140 lbs	5.1	6.7	8.3	9.9
160 lbs	6.1	7.7	9.2	10.8
180 lbs	7.0	8.6	10.2	11.7
200 lbs	7.9	9.5	11.1	12.6

9. Estimate $z_x(1,0)$ and $z_x(0,1)$ and $z_y(0,1)$ from the contour diagram for $z(x,y)$ in Figure 9.36.

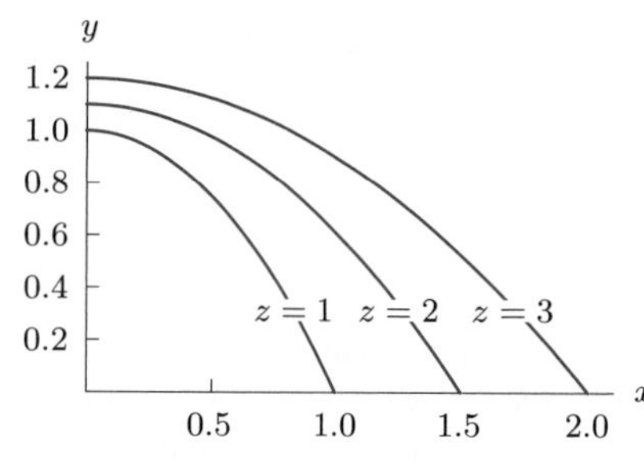

Figure 9.36

10. The monthly mortgage payment in dollars, P, for a house is a function of three variables:

$$P = f(A,r,N),$$

where A is the amount borrowed in dollars, r is the interest rate, and N is the number of years before the mortgage is paid off.

(a) $f(92000, 14, 30) = 1090.08$. What does this tell you, in financial terms?

[7]From the August 28, 1994, issue of *Parade Magazine*.

(b) $\left.\frac{\partial P}{\partial r}\right|_{(92000,14,30)} = 72.82$. What is the financial significance of the number 72.82?

(c) Would you expect $\partial P/\partial A$ to be positive or negative? Why?

(d) Would you expect $\partial P/\partial N$ to be positive or negative? Why?

11. The sales of a product, $S = f(p, a)$, are a function of the price, p, of the product (in dollars per unit) and the amount, a, spent on advertising (in thousands of dollars).

(a) Do you expect f_p to be positive or negative? Why?

(b) Explain the meaning of the statement $f_a(8, 12) = 150$ in terms of sales.

12. Figure 9.37 shows a contour diagram for the monthly payment P as a function of the interest rate, $r\%$, and the amount, L, of a 5-year loan. Estimate $\partial P/\partial r$ and $\partial P/\partial L$ at the point where $r = 8$ and $L = 5000$. Give the units and the financial meaning of your answers.

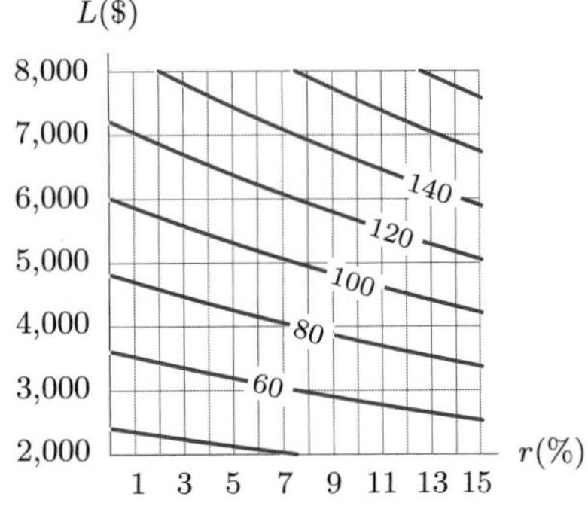

Figure 9.37

13. Figure 9.13 on page 356 gives a contour diagram of corn production as a function of rainfall, R, in inches and temperature, T, in °F. Corn production, C, is measured as a percentage of the present production, and $C = f(R, T)$. Estimate the following quantities. Give units and interpret your answers in terms of corn production:

(a) $f_R(15, 76)$ **(b)** $f_T(15, 76)$

14. Use the diagram from Problem 17 in Section 9.1, to estimate $H_T(T, w)$ for $T = 10, 20, 30$ and $w = 0.1, 0.2, 0.3$. What is the practical meaning of these partial derivatives?

15. People commuting to a city can choose to go either by bus or by train. The number of people who choose either method depends in part upon the price of each. Let $f(P_1, P_2)$ be the number of people who take the bus when P_1 is the price of a bus ride and P_2 is the price of a train ride. What can you say about the signs of $\partial f/\partial P_1$ and $\partial f/\partial P_2$? Explain your answers.

16. In the 1940s the quantity, q, of beer sold each year in Britain was found to depend on I (the aggregate personal income, adjusted for taxes and inflation), p_1 (the average price of beer), and p_2 (the average price of all other goods and services). Would you expect $\partial q/\partial I, \partial q/\partial p_1, \partial q/\partial p_2$ to be positive or negative? Give reasons for your answers.

17. An airline's revenue, R, is a function of the number of full price tickets, x, and the number of discount tickets, y, sold. Values of $R = f(x, y)$ are in Table 9.1 on page 350.

(a) Evaluate $f(200, 400)$, and interpret your answer.

(b) Is $f_x(200, 400)$ positive or negative? Is $f_y(200, 400)$ positive or negative? Explain.

(c) Estimate the partial derivatives in part (b). Give units and interpret your answers in terms of revenue.

18. In Problem 17 the revenue is \$150,000 when 200 full-price tickets and 400 discount tickets are sold; that is, $f(200, 400) = 150{,}000$. Use this fact and the partial derivatives $f_x(200, 400) = 350$ and $f_y(200, 400) = 200$ to estimate the revenue when

(a) $x = 201$ and $y = 400$ **(b)** $x = 200$ and $y = 405$

(c) $x = 203$ and $y = 406$

19. Table 9.5 on page 365 gives the percent of rats surviving, P, as a function of time, t, in months and concentration of formaldehyde, c, in ppm, so $P = f(t, c)$. Use partial derivatives to estimate the percent surviving after 26 months when the concentration is 15.

20. For a function $f(x, y)$, we are given $f(100, 20) = 2750$, and $f_x(100, 20) = 4$, and $f_y(100, 20) = 7$. Estimate $f(105, 21)$.

21. For a function $f(r, s)$, we are given $f(50, 100) = 5.67$, and $f_r(50, 100) = 0.60$, and $f_s(50, 100) = -0.15$. Estimate $f(52, 108)$.

22. The cardiac output, represented by c, is the volume of blood flowing through a person's heart, per unit time. The systemic vascular resistance (SVR), represented by s, is the resistance to blood flowing through veins and arteries. Let p be a person's blood pressure. Then p is a function of c and s, so $p = f(c, s)$.

(a) What does $\partial p/\partial c$ represent?

Suppose now that $p = kcs$, where k is a constant.

(b) Sketch the level curves of p. What do they represent? Label your axes.

(c) For a person with a weak heart, it is desirable to have the heart pumping against less resistance, while maintaining the same blood pressure. Such a person may be given the drug nitroglycerine to decrease the SVR and the drug Dopamine to increase the cardiac output. Represent this on a graph showing level curves. Put a point A on the graph representing the person's state before drugs are given and a point B for after.

(d) Right after a heart attack, a patient's cardiac output drops, thereby causing the blood pressure to drop. A common mistake made by medical residents is to get the patient's blood pressure back to normal by using drugs to increase the SVR, rather than by increasing the cardiac output. On a graph of the level curves of p, put a point D representing the patient before the heart attack, a point E representing the patient right after the heart attack, and a third point F representing the patient after the resident has given the drugs to increase the SVR.

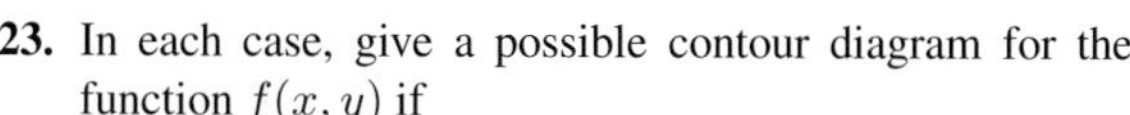

23. In each case, give a possible contour diagram for the function $f(x, y)$ if

(a) $f_x > 0$ and $f_y > 0$ **(b)** $f_x > 0$ and $f_y < 0$
(c) $f_x < 0$ and $f_y > 0$ **(d)** $f_x < 0$ and $f_y < 0$

24. Figure 9.38 shows contours of $f(x, y)$ with values of f on the contours omitted. If $f_x(P) > 0$, find the sign of

(a) $f_y(P)$ **(b)** $f_y(Q)$ **(c)** $f_x(Q)$

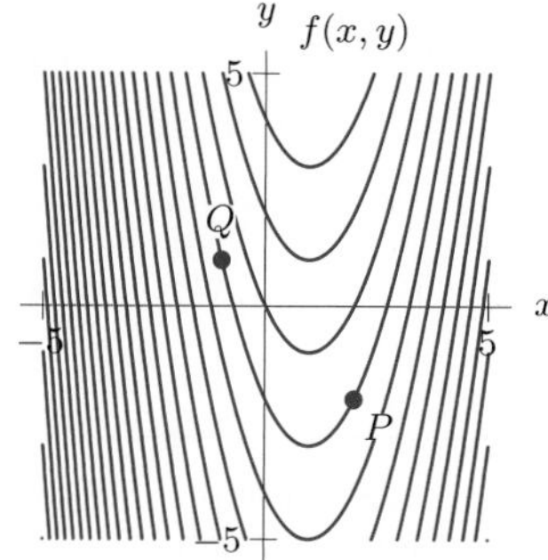

Figure 9.38

9.4 COMPUTING PARTIAL DERIVATIVES ALGEBRAICALLY

The partial derivative $f_x(x, y)$ is the ordinary derivative of the function $f(x, y)$ with respect to x with y fixed, and the partial derivative $f_y(x, y)$ is the ordinary derivative of $f(x, y)$ with respect to y with x fixed. Thus, we can use all the techniques for differentiation from single-variable calculus to find partial derivatives.

Example 1 Let $f(x, y) = x^2 + 5y^2$. Find $f_x(3, 2)$ and $f_y(3, 2)$ algebraically.

Solution We use the fact that $f_x(3, 2)$ is the derivative of $f(x, 2)$ at $x = 3$. To find f_x, we fix y at 2:

$$f(x, 2) = x^2 + 5(2^2) = x^2 + 20.$$

Differentiating with respect to x gives

$$f_x(x, 2) = 2x \qquad \text{so} \qquad f_x(3, 2) = 2(3) = 6.$$

Similarly, $f_y(3, 2)$ is the derivative of $f(3, y)$ at $y = 2$. To find f_y, we fix x at 3:

$$f(3, y) = 3^2 + 5y^2 = 9 + 5y^2.$$

Differentiating with respect to y, we have

$$f_y(3, y) = 10y \qquad \text{so} \quad f_y(3, 2) = 10(2) = 20.$$

Example 2 Let $f(x, y) = x^2 + 5y^2$ as in Example 1. Find f_x and f_y as functions of x and y.

Solution To find f_x, we treat y as a constant. Thus $5y^2$ is a constant and the derivative with respect to x of this term is 0. We have

$$f_x(x, y) = 2x + 0 = 2x.$$

To find f_y, we treat x as a constant and so the derivative of x^2 with respect to y is zero. We have

$$f_y(x, y) = 0 + 10y = 10y.$$

Example 3 Find both partial derivatives of each of the following functions:
(a) $f(x, y) = 3x + e^{-5y}$ (b) $f(x, y) = x^2y$ (c) $f(u, v) = u^2e^{2v}$

Solution

(a) To find f_x, we treat y as a constant, so the term e^{-5y} is a constant, and the derivative of this term is zero. Likewise, to find f_y, we treat x as a constant. We have

$$f_x(x,y) = 3 + 0 = 3 \quad \text{and} \quad f_y(x,y) = 0 + (-5)e^{-5y} = -5e^{-5y}.$$

(b) To find f_x, we treat y as a constant, so the function is treated as a constant times x^2. The derivative of a constant times x^2 is the constant times $2x$, and so we have

$$f_x(x,y) = (2x)y = 2xy \quad \text{Similarly,} \quad f_y(x,y) = (x^2)(1) = x^2.$$

(c) To find f_u, we treat v as a constant, and to find f_v, we treat u as a constant. We have

$$f_u(u,v) = (2u)(e^{2v}) = 2ue^{2v} \quad \text{and} \quad f_v(u,v) = u^2(2e^{2v}) = 2u^2e^{2v}.$$

Example 4 The concentration C of bacteria in the blood (in millions of bacteria/ml) following the injection of an antibiotic is a function of the dose x (in gm) injected and the time t (in hours) since the injection. Suppose we are told that $C = f(x,t) = te^{-xt}$. Evaluate the following quantities and explain what each one means in practical terms: (a) $f_x(1,2)$ (b) $f_t(1,2)$

Solution

(a) To find f_x, we treat t as a constant and differentiate with respect to x, giving

$$f_x(x,t) = -t^2e^{-xt}.$$

Substituting $x = 1, t = 2$ gives

$$f_x(1,2) = -4e^{-2} \approx -0.54.$$

To see what $f_x(1,2)$ means, think about the function $f(x,2)$ of which it is the derivative. The graph of $f(x,2)$ in Figure 9.39 gives the concentration of bacteria as a function of the dose two hours after the injection. The derivative $f_x(1,2)$ is the slope of this graph at the point $x = 1$; it is negative because a larger dose reduces the bacteria population. More precisely, the partial derivative $f_x(1,2)$ gives the rate of change of bacteria concentration with respect to the dose injected, namely a decrease in bacteria concentration of 0.54 million/ml per gram of additional antibiotic injected.

(b) To find f_t, treat x as a constant and differentiate using the product rule:

$$f_t(x,t) = 1 \cdot e^{-xt} - xte^{-xt}.$$

Substituting $x = 1, t = 2$ gives

$$f_t(1,2) = e^{-2} - 2e^{-2} \approx -0.14.$$

To see what $f_t(1,2)$ means, think about the function $f(1,t)$ of which it is the derivative. The graph of $f(1,t)$ in Figure 9.40 gives the concentration of bacteria at time t if the dose of antibiotic is 1 gm. The derivative $f_t(1,2)$ is the slope of the graph at the point $t = 2$; it is negative because after 2 hours the concentration of bacteria is decreasing. More precisely, the partial derivative $f_t(1,2)$ gives the rate at which the bacteria concentration is changing with respect to time, namely a decrease in bacteria concentration of 0.14 million/ml per hour.

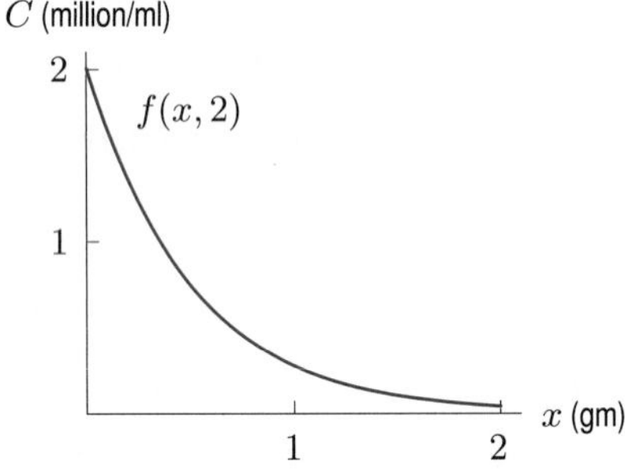

Figure 9.39: Bacteria concentration after 2 hours as a function of the quantity of antibiotic injected

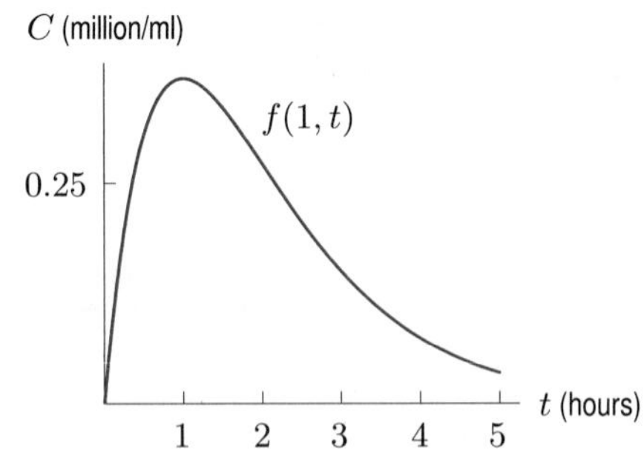

Figure 9.40: Bacteria concentration as a function of time if 1 unit of antibiotic is injected

---

Example 5 Let's consider a small printing business where N is the number of workers, V is the value of the equipment (in units of \$25,000), and P is the production, measured in thousands of pages per day. Suppose the production function for this company is given by

$$P = f(N, V) = 2N^{0.6}V^{0.4}.$$

(a) If this company has a labor force of 100 workers and 200 units' worth of equipment, what is the production output of the company?
(b) Find $f_N(100, 200)$ and $f_V(100, 200)$. Interpret your answers in terms of production.

Solution (a) We have $N = 100$ and $V = 200$, so

$$\text{Production} = 2(100)^{0.6}(200)^{0.4} = 263.9 \text{ thousand pages per day.}$$

(b) To find f_N, we treat V as a constant and differentiate with respect to N:

$$f_N(N, V) = 2(0.6)N^{-0.4}V^{0.4}.$$

Substituting $N = 100$, $V = 200$ gives

$$f_N(100, 200) = 1.2(100^{-0.4})(200^{0.4}) \approx 1.583 \text{ thousand pages/worker.}$$

This tells us that if we have 200 units of equipment and increase the number of workers by 1 from 100 to 101, the production output will go up by about 1.58 units, or 1580 pages per day.

Similarly, to find $f_V(100, 200)$, we treat N as a constant and differentiate with respect to V:

$$f_V(N, V) = 2(0.4)N^{0.6}V^{-0.6}.$$

Substituting $N = 100$, $V = 200$ gives

$$f_V(100, 200) = 0.8(100^{0.6})(200^{-0.6}) \approx 0.53 \text{ thousand pages/unit of equipment.}$$

This tells us that if we have 100 workers and increase the value of the equipment by 1 unit (\$25,000) from 200 units to 201 units, the production goes up by about 0.53 units, or 530 pages per day.

Second-Order Partial Derivatives

Since the partial derivatives of a function are themselves functions, we can usually differentiate them, giving *second-order partial derivatives*. A function $z = f(x, y)$ has two first-order partial derivatives, f_x and f_y, and four second-order partial derivatives.

The Second-Order Partial Derivatives of $z = f(x, y)$

$$\frac{\partial^2 z}{\partial x^2} = f_{xx} = (f_x)_x, \qquad \frac{\partial^2 z}{\partial x \partial y} = f_{yx} = (f_y)_x,$$

$$\frac{\partial^2 z}{\partial y \partial x} = f_{xy} = (f_x)_y, \qquad \frac{\partial^2 z}{\partial y^2} = f_{yy} = (f_y)_y.$$

It is usual to omit the parentheses, writing f_{xy} instead of $(f_x)_y$ and $\frac{\partial^2 z}{\partial y\, \partial x}$ instead of $\frac{\partial}{\partial y}\left(\frac{\partial z}{\partial x}\right)$.

Example 6 Use the values of the function $f(x, y)$ in Table 9.7 to estimate $f_{xy}(1, 2)$ and $f_{yx}(1, 2)$.

Table 9.7 *Values of $f(x, y)$*

y \ x	0.9	1.0	1.1
1.8	4.72	5.83	7.06
2.0	6.48	8.00	9.60
2.2	8.62	10.65	12.88

Solution Since $f_{xy} = (f_x)_y$, we first estimate f_x:

$$f_x(1,2) \approx \frac{f(1.1,2) - f(1,2)}{0.1} = \frac{9.60 - 8.00}{0.1} = 16.0,$$
$$f_x(1,2.2) \approx \frac{f(1.1,2.2) - f(1,2.2)}{0.1} = \frac{12.88 - 10.65}{0.1} = 22.3.$$

Thus,

$$f_{xy}(1,2) \approx \frac{f_x(1,2.2) - f_x(1,2)}{0.2} = \frac{22.3 - 16.0}{0.2} = 31.5.$$

Similarly,

$$f_{yx}(1,2) \approx \frac{f_y(1.1,2) - f_y(1,2)}{0.1} \approx \frac{1}{0.1}\left(\frac{f(1.1,2.2) - f(1.1,2)}{0.2} - \frac{f(1,2.2) - f(1,2)}{0.2}\right)$$
$$= \frac{1}{0.1}\left(\frac{12.88 - 9.60}{0.2} - \frac{10.65 - 8.00}{0.2}\right) = 31.5.$$

Observe that in this example, $f_{xy} = f_{yx}$ at the point $(1, 2)$.

Example 7 Compute the four second-order partial derivatives of $f(x, y) = xy^2 + 3x^2e^y$.

Solution From $f_x(x, y) = y^2 + 6xe^y$ we get

$$f_{xx}(x,y) = \frac{\partial}{\partial x}(y^2 + 6xe^y) = 6e^y \quad \text{and} \quad f_{xy}(x,y) = \frac{\partial}{\partial y}(y^2 + 6xe^y) = 2y + 6xe^y.$$

From $f_y(x, y) = 2xy + 3x^2e^y$ we get

$$f_{yx}(x,y) = \frac{\partial}{\partial x}(2xy + 3x^2e^y) = 2y + 6xe^y \quad \text{and} \quad f_{yy}(x,y) = \frac{\partial}{\partial y}(2xy + 3x^2e^y) = 2x + 3x^2e^y.$$

Observe that $f_{xy} = f_{yx}$ in this example.

The Mixed Partial Derivatives Are Equal

It is not an accident that the estimates for $f_{xy}(1, 2)$ and $f_{yx}(1, 2)$ are equal in Example 6, because the same values of the function are used to calculate each one. The fact that $f_{xy} = f_{yx}$ in Example 7 corroborates the following general result:

> If f_{xy} and f_{yx} are continuous at (a, b), then
> $$f_{xy}(a,b) = f_{yx}(a,b).$$

Most of the functions we will encounter not only have f_{xy} and f_{yx} continuous, but all their higher-order partial derivatives (such as f_{xxy} or f_{xyyy}) will be continuous. We call such functions *smooth*.

Problems for Section 9.4

Find the partial derivatives in Problems 1–13. The variables are restricted to a domain on which the function is defined.

1. f_x and f_y if $f(x, y) = 2x^2 + 3y^2$
2. f_x and f_y if $f(x, y) = 100x^2y$
3. f_x and f_y if $f(x, y) = x^2 + 2xy + y^3$
4. z_x if $z = x^2y + 2x^5y$
5. f_u and f_v if $f(u, v) = u^2 + 5uv + v^2$
6. $\frac{\partial z}{\partial x}$ if $z = x^2e^y$
7. $\frac{\partial Q}{\partial p}$ if $Q = 5a^2p - 3ap^3$
8. f_t if $f(t, a) = 5a^2t^3$
9. f_x and f_y if $f(x, y) = 5x^2y^3 + 8xy^2 - 3x^2$
10. f_x and f_y if $f(x, y) = 10x^2e^{3y}$
11. $\frac{\partial P}{\partial r}$ if $P = 100e^{rt}$
12. $\frac{\partial A}{\partial h}$ if $A = \frac{1}{2}(a + b)h$
13. $\frac{\partial}{\partial m}\left(\frac{1}{2}mv^2\right)$
14. If $f(x, y) = x^3 + 3y^2$, find $f(1, 2)$, $f_x(1, 2)$, $f_y(1, 2)$.
15. If $f(u, v) = 5uv^2$, find $f(3, 1)$, $f_u(3, 1)$, and $f_v(3, 1)$.
16. **(a)** Let $f(x, y) = x^2 + y^2$. Estimate $f_x(2, 1)$ and $f_y(2, 1)$ using the contour diagram for f in Figure 9.41.
    (b) Estimate $f_x(2, 1)$ and $f_y(2, 1)$ from a table of values for f with $x = 1.9, 2, 2.1$ and $y = 0.9, 1, 1.1$.
    (c) Compare your estimates in parts (a) and (b) with the exact values of $f_x(2, 1)$ and $f_y(2, 1)$ found algebraically.

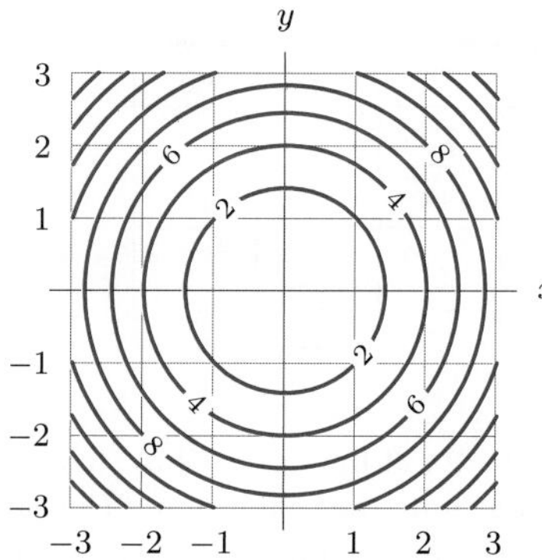

Figure 9.41

17. The amount of money, $\$B$, in a bank account earning interest at a continuous rate, r, depends on the amount deposited, $\$P$, and the time, t, it has been in the bank, where

$$B = Pe^{rt}.$$

Find $\partial B/\partial t$, $\partial B/\partial r$ and $\partial B/\partial P$ and interpret each in financial terms.

18. The cost of renting a car from a certain company is \$40 per day plus 15 cents per mile, and so we have

$$C = 40d + 0.15m.$$

Find $\partial C/\partial d$ and $\partial C/\partial m$. Give units and explain why your answers make sense.

19. A company's production output, P, is given in tons, and is a function of the number of workers, N, and the value of the equipment, V, in units of \$25,000. The production function for the company is

$$P = f(N, V) = 5N^{0.75}V^{0.25}.$$

The company currently employs 80 workers, and has equipment worth \$750,000. What are N and V? Find the values of f, f_N, and f_V at these values of N and V. Give units and explain what each answer means in terms of production.

For Problems 20–31, calculate all four second-order partial derivatives and confirm that the mixed partials are equal.

20. $f(x, y) = x^2y$
21. $f(x, y) = x^2+2xy+y^2$
22. $f(x, y) = xe^y$
23. $f(x, y) = \frac{2x}{y}, \quad y \neq 0$
24. $f = 5 + x^2y^2$
25. $f = e^{xy}$
26. $Q = 5p_1^2p_2^{-1}, \quad p_2 \neq 0$
27. $V = \pi r^2h$
28. $P = 2KL^2$
29. $B = 5xe^{-2t}$
30. $f(x, t) = t^3 - 4x^2t$
31. $f = 100e^{rt}$

32. Is there a function f which has the following partial derivatives? If so what is it? Are there any others?

$$f_x(x, y) = 4x^3y^2 - 3y^4,$$
$$f_y(x, y) = 2x^4y - 12xy^3.$$

33. Show that the Cobb-Douglas function

$$Q = bK^{\alpha}L^{1-\alpha} \text{ where } 0 < \alpha < 1$$

satisfies the equation

$$K\frac{\partial Q}{\partial K} + L\frac{\partial Q}{\partial L} = Q.$$

Problems 34–36 are about the money supply, M, which is the total value of all the cash and checking account balances in an economy. It is determined by the value of all the cash, B, the ratio, c, of cash to checking deposits, and the fraction, r, of checking account deposits that banks hold as cash:

$$M = \frac{c + 1}{c + r}B.$$

(a) Find the partial derivative.
(b) Give its sign.
(c) Explain the significance of the sign in practical terms.

34. $\partial M/\partial B$
35. $\partial M/\partial r$
36. $\partial M/\partial c$

9.5 CRITICAL POINTS AND OPTIMIZATION

To optimize a function means to find the largest or smallest value of the function. If the function represents profit, we may want to find the conditions that maximize profit. On the other hand, if the function represents cost, we may want to find the conditions that minimize cost. In Chapter 4, we saw how to optimize a function of one variable by investigating critical points. In this section, we see how to extend the notions of critical points and local extrema to a function of more than one variable.

Local and Global Maxima and Minima for Functions of Two Variables

Functions of several variables, like functions of one variable, can have *local* and *global extrema* (that is, local and global maxima and minima). A function has a local extremum at a point where it takes on the largest or smallest value in a small region around the point. Global extrema are the largest or smallest value anywhere. For a function f defined on a domain R, we say:

- f has a **local maximum** at P_0 if $f(P_0) \geq f(P)$ for all points P near P_0
- f has a **local minimum** at P_0 if $f(P_0) \leq f(P)$ for all points P near P_0
- f has a **global maximum** at P_0 if $f(P_0) \geq f(P)$ for all points P in R
- f has a **global minimum** at P_0 if $f(P_0) \leq f(P)$ for all points P in R

Example 1 Table 9.8 gives a table of values for a function $f(x, y)$. Estimate the location and value of any global maxima or minima for $0 \leq x \leq 1$ and $0 \leq y \leq 20$.

Table 9.8 *Where are the extreme points of this function $f(x, y)$?*

y \ x	0	0.2	0.4	0.6	0.8	1.0
0	80	84	82	76	71	65
5	86	90	88	73	77	71
10	91	95	93	88	82	76
15	87	91	89	84	78	72
20	82	86	84	79	73	67

Solution The global maximum value of the function appears to be 95 at the point $(0.2, 10)$. Since the table only gives certain values, we cannot be sure that this is exactly the maximum. (The function might have a larger value at, for example, $(0.3, 11)$.) The global minimum value of this function on the points given is 65 at the point $(1, 0)$.

Example 2 Figure 9.42 gives a contour diagram for a function $f(x, y)$. Estimate the location and value of any local maxima or minima. Are any of these global maxima or minima on the square shown?

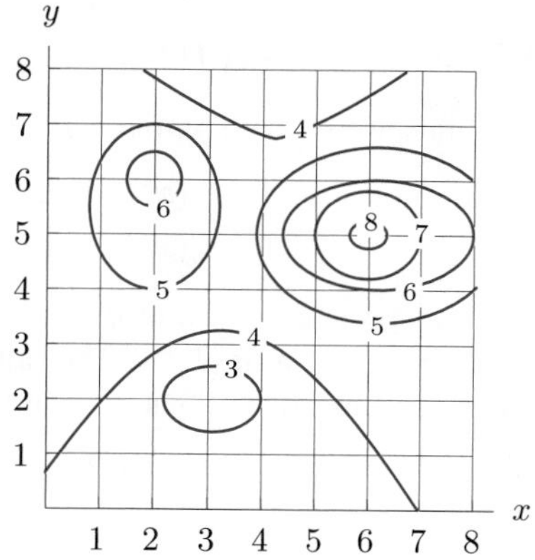

Figure 9.42: Where are the local and global extreme points of this function?

Solution

There is a local maximum of above 8 near the point $(6, 5)$, a local maximum of above 6 near the point $(2, 6)$, and a local minimum of below 3 near the point $(3, 2)$. The value above 8 is the global maximum and the value below 3 is the global minimum on the given domain.

In Example 1 and Example 2, we can estimate the location and value of extreme points, but we do not have enough information to find them exactly. This is usually true when we are given a table of values or a contour diagram. To find local or global extrema exactly, we usually need to have a formula for the function.

Finding a Local Maximum or Minimum Analytically

In one-variable calculus, the local extrema of a function occur at points where the derivative is zero or undefined. How does this generalize to the case of functions of two or more variables? Suppose that a function $f(x, y)$ has a local maximum at a point (x_0, y_0) which is not on the boundary of the domain of f. If the partial derivative $f_x(x_0, y_0)$ were defined and positive, then we could increase f by increasing x. If $f_x(x_0, y_0) < 0$, then we could increase f by decreasing x. Since f has a local maximum at (x_0, y_0), there can be no direction in which f is increasing, so we must have $f_x(x_0, y_0) = 0$. Similarly, if $f_y(x_0, y_0)$ is defined, then $f_y(x_0, y_0) = 0$. The case in which $f(x, y)$ has a local minimum is similar. Therefore, we arrive at the following conclusion:

> If a function $f(x, y)$ has a local maximum or minimum at a point (x_0, y_0) not on the boundary of the domain of f, then either
>
> $$f_x(x_0, y_0) = 0 \quad \text{and} \quad f_y(x_0, y_0) = 0$$
>
> or (at least) one partial derivative is undefined at the point (x_0, y_0). Points where each of the partial derivatives is either zero or undefined are called **critical points**.

As in the single-variable case, the fact that (x_0, y_0) is a critical point for f does not necessarily mean that f has a maximum or a minimum there.

How Do We Find Critical Points?

To find critical points of a function f, we find the points where both partial derivatives of f are zero or undefined.

Example 3 Find and analyze the critical points of $f(x, y) = x^2 - 2x + y^2 - 4y + 5$.

Solution To find the critical points, we set both partial derivatives equal to zero:

$$f_x(x, y) = 2x - 2 = 0,$$
$$f_y(x, y) = 2y - 4 = 0.$$

Solving these equations gives $x = 1$ and $y = 2$. Hence, f has only one critical point, namely $(1, 2)$. What is the behavior of f near $(1, 2)$? The values of the function in Table 9.9 suggest that the function has a local minimum value of 0 at the point $(1, 2)$.

Table 9.9 *Values of $f(x, y)$ near the point* $(1, 2)$

		x				
		0.8	0.9	1.0	1.1	1.2
	1.8	0.08	0.05	0.04	0.05	0.08
	1.9	0.05	0.02	0.01	0.02	0.05
y	2.0	0.04	0.01	0.00	0.01	0.04
	2.1	0.05	0.02	0.01	0.02	0.05
	2.2	0.08	0.05	0.04	0.05	0.08

Example 4 A manufacturing company produces two products which are sold in two separate markets. The company's economists analyze the two markets and determine that the quantities, q_1 and q_2, demanded by consumers and the prices, p_1 and p_2 (in dollars), of each item are related by the equations

$$p_1 = 600 - 0.3q_1 \quad \text{and} \quad p_2 = 500 - 0.2q_2.$$

Thus, if the price for either item increases, the demand for it decreases. The company's total production cost is given by

$$C = 16 + 1.2q_1 + 1.5q_2 + 0.2q_1q_2.$$

If the company wants to maximize its total profits, how much of each product should it produce? What is the maximum profit?[8]

Solution The total revenue R is the sum of the revenues, p_1q_1 and p_2q_2, from each market. Substituting for p_1 and p_2, we get

$$\begin{aligned} R &= p_1q_1 + p_2q_2 \\ &= (600 - 0.3q_1)q_1 + (500 - 0.2q_2)q_2 \\ &= 600q_1 - 0.3q_1^2 + 500q_2 - 0.2q_2^2. \end{aligned}$$

Thus the total profit π is given by

$$\begin{aligned} \pi &= R - C \\ &= 600q_1 - 0.3q_1^2 + 500q_2 - 0.2q_2^2 - (16 + 1.2q_1 + 1.5q_2 + 0.2q_1q_2) \\ &= -16 + 598.8q_1 - 0.3q_1^2 + 498.5q_2 - 0.2q_2^2 - 0.2q_1q_2. \end{aligned}$$

To maximize π, we compute partial derivatives:

$$\frac{\partial \pi}{\partial q_1} = 598.8 - 0.6q_1 - 0.2q_2,$$
$$\frac{\partial \pi}{\partial q_2} = 498.5 - 0.4q_2 - 0.2q_1.$$

[8] Adapted from M. Rosser, *Basic Mathematics for Economists*, p. 316 (New York: Routledge, 1993).

Since the partial derivatives are defined everywhere, the only critical points of π are those where the partial derivatives of π are both equal to zero. Thus, we solve the equations for q_1 and q_2,

$$598.8 - 0.6q_1 - 0.2q_2 = 0,$$
$$498.5 - 0.4q_2 - 0.2q_1 = 0,$$

giving

$$q_1 = 699.1 \approx 699 \quad \text{and} \quad q_2 = 896.7 \approx 897.$$

To see whether this is a maximum, we look at a table of values of profit π around this point. Table 9.10 suggests that profit is greatest at $(699, 897)$. So the company should produce 699 units of the first product priced at \$390.30 per unit, and 897 units of the second product priced at \$320.60 per unit. The maximum profit is then $\pi(699, 897) = \$432{,}797$.

Table 9.10 *Does this profit function have a maximum at* $(699, 897)$*?*

Quantity, q_2	Quantity, q_1: 698	699	700
896	432,796.4	432,796.9	432,796.8
897	432,796.7	432,797.0	432,796.7
898	432,796.6	432,796.7	432,796.2

Is a Critical Point a Local Maximum or a Local Minimum?

We can often see whether a critical point is a local maximum or minimum or neither by looking at a table or contour diagram. The following analytic method may also be useful in distinguishing between local maxima and minima.[9] It is analogous to the Second Derivative Test in Chapter 4.

Second Derivative Test for Functions of Two Variables

Suppose (x_0, y_0) is a critical point where $f_x(x_0, y_0) = f_y(x_0, y_0) = 0$. Let

$$D = f_{xx}(x_0, y_0)f_{yy}(x_0, y_0) - f_{xy}(x_0, y_0)^2.$$

- If $D > 0$ and $f_{xx}(x_0, y_0) > 0$, then f has a local minimum at (x_0, y_0).
- If $D > 0$ and $f_{xx}(x_0, y_0) < 0$, then f has a local maximum at (x_0, y_0).
- If $D < 0$, then f has neither a local maximum or minimum at (x_0, y_0).
- If $D = 0$, the test is inconclusive.

Example 5 Use the second derivative test to confirm that the critical point $q_1 = 699.1$, $q_2 = 896.7$ gives a local maximum of the profit function π of Example 4.

Solution To see whether or not we have found a maximum point, we compute the second-order partial derivatives:

$$\frac{\partial^2 \pi}{\partial q_1^2} = -0.6, \quad \frac{\partial^2 \pi}{\partial q_2^2} = -0.4, \quad \frac{\partial^2 \pi}{\partial q_1 \partial q_2} = -0.2.$$

Since

$$D = \frac{\partial^2 \pi}{\partial q_1^2}\frac{\partial^2 \pi}{\partial q_2^2} - \left(\frac{\partial^2 \pi}{\partial q_1 \partial q_2}\right)^2 = (-0.6)(-0.4) - (-0.2)^2 = 0.2 > 0,$$

the second derivative test implies that we have found a local maximum point.

[9] An explanation of this test can be found, for example, in *Multivariable Calculus* by W. McCallum et al. (New York: John Wiley, 1997).

Problems for Section 9.5

1. Figure 9.43 shows contours of $f(x, y)$. List x- and y-coordinates and the value of the function at any local maximum and local minimum points, and identify which is which. Are any of these local extrema also global extrema on the region shown? If so, which ones?

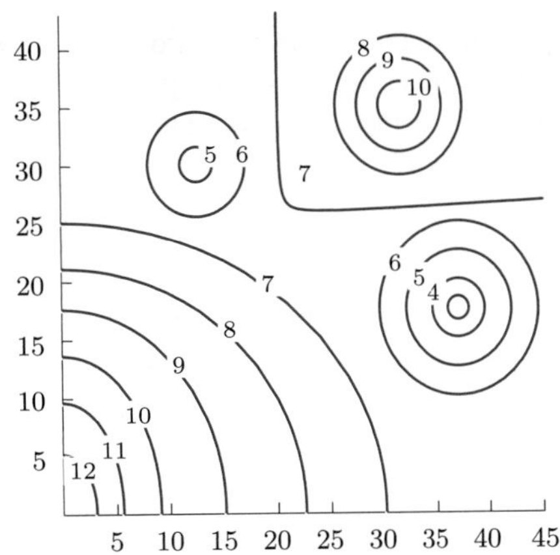

Figure 9.43

2. Figure 9.44 shows contours of $f(x, y)$. List the x- and y-coordinates and the value of the function at any local maximum and local minimum points, and identify which is which. Are any of these local extrema also global extrema on the region shown? If so, which ones?

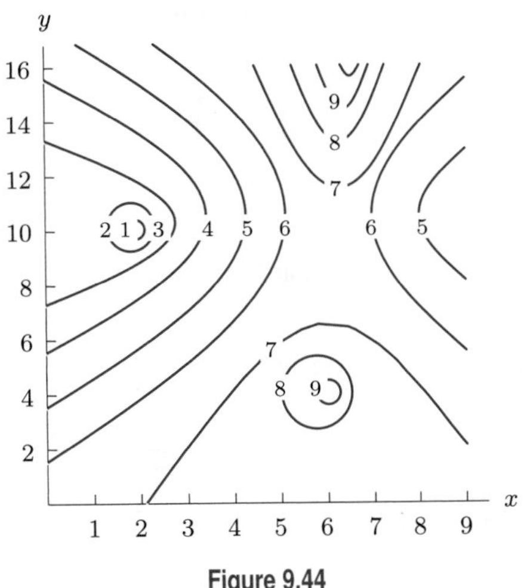

Figure 9.44

In Problems 3–5, estimate the position and approximate value of the global maxima and minima on the region shown.

3.

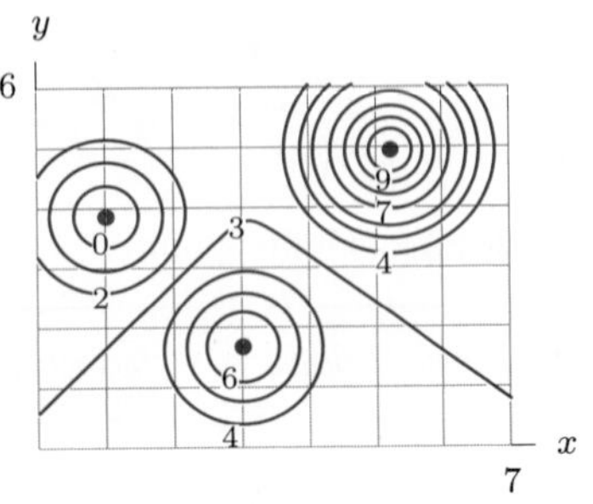

4.

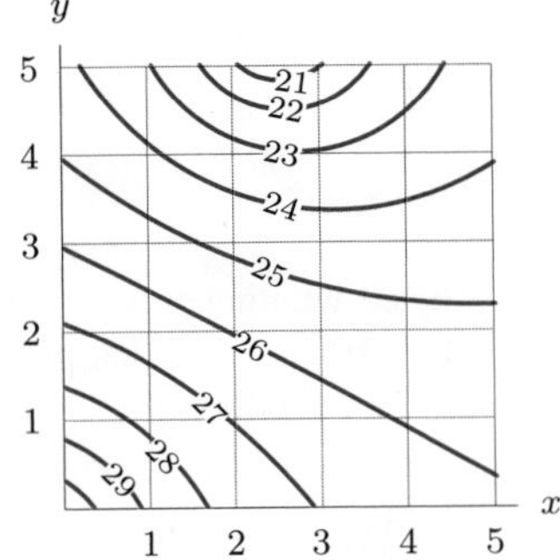

5.

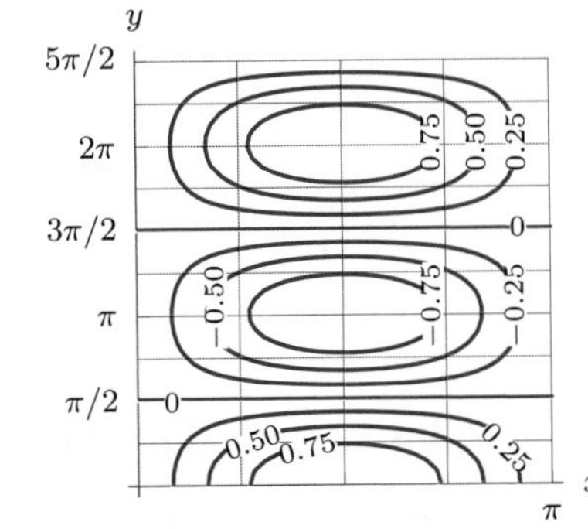

In Problems 6–15, find all the critical points and determine whether each is a local maximum, local minimum, or neither.

6. $f(x, y) = x^2 + 4x + y^2$

7. $f(x, y) = x^2 + xy + 3y$

8. $f(x, y) = x^2 + y^2 + 6x - 10y + 8$

9. $f(x, y) = y^3 - 3xy + 6x$

10. $f(x, y) = x^2 - 2xy + 3y^2 - 8y$

11. $f(x, y) = x^3 - 3x + y^3 - 3y$

12. $f(x, y) = x^3 + y^2 - 3x^2 + 10y + 6$

13. $f(x, y) = x^3 + y^3 - 6y^2 - 3x + 9$

14. $f(x, y) = x^3 + y^3 - 3x^2 - 3y + 10$

15. $f(x, y) = 400 - 3x^2 - 4x + 2xy - 5y^2 + 48y$

16. By looking at the weather map in Figure 9.5 on page 354, find the maximum and minimum daily high temperatures in the states of Mississippi, Alabama, Pennsylvania, New York, California, Arizona, and Massachusetts.

17. For $f(x, y) = A - (x^2 + Bx + y^2 + Cy)$, what values of A, B, and C give f a local maximum value of 15 at the point $(-2, 1)$?

18. A missile has a guidance device which is sensitive to both temperature, t°C, and humidity, h. The range in km over which the missile can be controlled is given by

$$\text{Range} = 27{,}800 - 5t^2 - 6ht - 3h^2 + 400t + 300h.$$

What are the optimal atmospheric conditions for controlling the missile?

19. The quantity of a product demanded by consumers is a function of its price. The quantity of one product demanded may also depend on the price of other products. For example, the demand for tea is affected by the price of coffee; the demand for cars is affected by the price of gas. The quantities demanded, q_1 and q_2, of two products depend on their prices, p_1 and p_2, as follows:

$$q_1 = 150 - 2p_1 - p_2$$

$$q_2 = 200 - p_1 - 3p_2.$$

(a) What does the fact that the coefficients of p_1 and p_2 are negative tell you? Give an example of two products that might be related this way.
(b) If one manufacturer sells both products, how should the prices be set to generate the maximum possible revenue? What is that maximum possible revenue?

20. Two products are manufactured in quantities q_1 and q_2 and sold at prices of p_1 and p_2, respectively. The cost of producing them is given by

$$C = 2q_1^2 + 2q_2^2 + 10.$$

(a) Find the maximum profit that can be made, assuming the prices are fixed.
(b) Find the rate of change of that maximum profit as p_1 increases.

21. A company operates two plants which manufacture the same item and whose total cost functions are

$$C_1 = 8.5 + 0.03q_1^2 \quad \text{and} \quad C_2 = 5.2 + 0.04q_2^2,$$

where q_1 and q_2 are the quantities produced by each plant. The company is a monopoly. The total quantity demanded, $q = q_1 + q_2$, is related to the price, p, by

$$p = 60 - 0.04q.$$

How much should each plant produce in order to maximize the company's profit?[10]

9.6 CONSTRAINED OPTIMIZATION

Many real optimization problems are constrained by external circumstances. For example, a city wanting to build a public transportation system has a limited number of tax dollars available. A nation trying to maintain its balance of trade must spend less on imports than it earns on exports. In this section, we see how to find an optimum value under such constraints.

A Constrained Optimization Problem

Suppose we want to maximize the production of a company under a budget constraint. Suppose production, f, is a function of two variables, x and y, which are quantities of two raw materials, and

$$f(x, y) = x^{2/3}y^{1/3}.$$

If x and y are purchased at prices of p_1 and p_2 dollars per unit, what is the maximum production f that can be obtained with a budget of c dollars?

To increase f without regard to the budget, we simply increase x and y. However, the budget prevents us from increasing x and y beyond a certain point. Exactly how does the budget constrain us? Suppose that x and y each cost \$100 per unit, and suppose that the total budget is \$378,000. The amount spent on x and y together is given by $g(x, y) = 100x + 100y$, and since we can't spend more than the budget allows, we must have:

$$g(x, y) = 100x + 100y \leq 378{,}000.$$

The goal is to maximize the function

$$f(x, y) = x^{2/3}y^{1/3}.$$

Since we expect to exhaust the budget, we have

$$100x + 100y = 378{,}000.$$

[10] Adapted from M. Rosser, *Basic Mathematics for Economists*, p. 318 (New York: Routledge, 1993).

Example 1 A company has production function $f(x, y) = x^{2/3}y^{1/3}$ and budget constraint $100x + 100y = 378{,}000$.

(a) If \$100,000 is spent on x, how much can be spent on y? What is the production in this case?
(b) If \$200,000 is spent on x, how much can be spent on y? What is the production in this case?
(c) Which of the two options above is the better choice for the company? Do you think this is the best of all possible options?

Solution

(a) If the company spends \$100,000 on x, then it has \$278,000 left to spend on y. In this case, we have $100x = 100{,}000$, so $x = 1000$, and $100y = 278{,}000$, so $y = 2780$. Therefore,

$$\text{Production} = f(1000, 2780) = (1000)^{2/3}(2780)^{1/3} = 1406 \text{ units.}$$

(b) If the company spends \$200,000 on x, then it has \$178,000 left to spend on y. Therefore, $x = 2000$ and $y = 1780$, and so

$$\text{Production} = f(2000, 1780) = (2000)^{2/3}(1780)^{1/3} = 1924 \text{ units.}$$

(c) Of these two options, (b) is better since production is larger in this case. This is probably not optimal, since there are many other combinations of x and y that we have not checked.

Graphical Approach: Maximizing Production Subject to a Budget Constraint

How can we find the maximum value of production? We maximize the *objective function*

$$f(x, y) = x^{2/3}y^{1/3}$$

subject to $x \geq 0$ and $y \geq 0$ and the budget constraint

$$g(x, y) = 100x + 100y = 378{,}000.$$

The constraint is represented by the line in Figure 9.45. Any point on or below the line represents a pair of values of x and y that we can afford. A point on the line completely exhausts the budget, while a point below the line represents values of x and y which can be bought without using up the budget. Any point above the line represents a pair of values that we cannot afford.

Figure 9.45 also shows some contours of the production function f. Since we want to maximize f, we want to find the point which lies on the contour with the largest possible f value *and* which lies within the budget. The point we are looking for must lie on the budget constraint because we should spend all the available money. The key observation is this: The maximum occurs at a point P where the budget constraint is tangent to a production contour. (See Figure 9.45.) The reason is

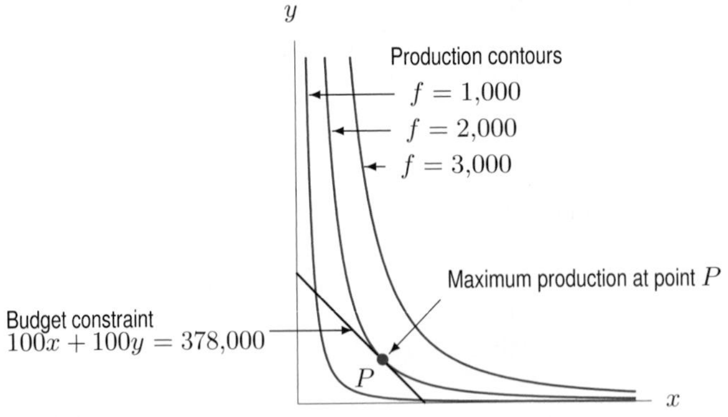

Figure 9.45: At the optimal point P the budget constraint is tangent to a production contour

that if we are on the constraint line to the left of P, moving right on the constraint increases f; if we are on the line to the right of P, moving left increases f. Thus, the maximum value of f on the budget constraint line occurs at the point P.

In general, provided f and g are smooth, we have the following result:

> If $f(x, y)$ has a global maximum or minimum on the constraint $g(x, y) = c$, it occurs at a point where the graph of the constraint is tangent to a contour of f, or at an endpoint of the constraint.[11]

Analytical Approach: The Method of Lagrange Multipliers

Suppose we want to optimize $f(x, y)$ subject to the constraint $g(x, y) = c$. We make the following definition.

> Suppose P_0 is a point satisfying the constraint $g(x, y) = c$.
> - f has a **local maximum** at P_0 **subject to the constraint** if $f(P_0) \geq f(P)$ for all points P near P_0 satisfying the constraint.
> - f has a **global maximum** at P_0 **subject to the constraint** if $f(P_0) \geq f(P)$ for all points P satisfying the constraint.
>
> Local and global minima are defined similarly.

It can be shown[12] that the constraint is tangent to a contour of f at the point which satisfies the equations laid out in the following method.

> **Method of Lagrange Multipliers** To optimize $f(x, y)$ subject to the constraint $g(x, y) = c$, solve the following system of three equations:
>
> $$f_x(x, y) = \lambda g_x(x, y),$$
> $$f_y(x, y) = \lambda g_y(x, y),$$
> $$g(x, y) = c,$$
>
> for the three unknowns x, y, and λ; the number λ is called the *Lagrange multiplier*. If f has a constrained global maximum or minimum, then it occurs at one of the solutions (x_0, y_0) to this system or at an endpoint of the constraint.

Example 2 Maximize $f(x, y) = x^{2/3}y^{1/3}$ subject to $100x + 100y = 378{,}000$ and $x \geq 0$, $y \geq 0$.

Solution Differentiating gives

$$f_x(x, y) = \frac{2}{3}x^{-1/3}y^{1/3} \quad \text{and} \quad f_y(x, y) = \frac{1}{3}x^{2/3}y^{-2/3}$$

[11] If the constraint has endpoints.

[12] See W. McCallum, et al., *Multivariable Calculus* (New York: John Wiley, 2009).

and

$$g_x(x,y) = 100 \quad \text{and} \quad g_y(x,y) = 100,$$

leading to the equations

$$\begin{aligned} \frac{2}{3}x^{-1/3}y^{1/3} &= \lambda(100) \\ \frac{1}{3}x^{2/3}y^{-2/3} &= \lambda(100) \\ 100x + 100y &= 378{,}000. \end{aligned}$$

The first two equations show that we must have

$$\frac{2}{3}x^{-1/3}y^{1/3} = \frac{1}{3}x^{2/3}y^{-2/3}.$$

Using the fact that $x^{-1/3} = 1/x^{1/3}$, we can rewrite this as

$$\frac{2y^{1/3}}{3x^{1/3}} = \frac{x^{2/3}}{3y^{2/3}}.$$

Multiplying through by the denominators gives

$$2y^{1/3}(3y^{2/3}) = x^{2/3}(3x^{1/3}),$$

and simplifying using $y^{1/3} \cdot y^{2/3} = y^1$ gives

$$\begin{aligned} 6y &= 3x \\ 2y &= x. \end{aligned}$$

Since we must also satisfy the constraint $100x + 100y = 378{,}000$, we substitute $x = 2y$ and get

$$\begin{aligned} 100(2y) + 100y &= 378{,}000 \\ 300y &= 378{,}000 \\ y &= 1260. \end{aligned}$$

Since $x = 2y$, we have $x = 2520$. The optimum value occurs at $x = 2520$ and $y = 1260$. For these values,

$$f(2520, 1260) = (2520)^{2/3}(1260)^{1/3} \approx 2000.1.$$

The endpoints of the constraint are the points $(3780, 0)$ and $(0, 3780)$. Since

$$f(3780, 0) = f(0, 3780) = 0,$$

we see that the maximum value of f is approximately 2000 and that it occurs at $x = 2520$ and $y = 1260$.

The Meaning of λ

In the previous example, we never found (or needed) the value of λ. However, λ does have a practical interpretation. In the production problem we maximized

$$f(x,y) = x^{2/3}y^{1/3}$$

subject to the constraint

$$g(x,y) = 100x + 100y = 378{,}000.$$

We solved the equations

$$\frac{2}{3}x^{-1/3}y^{1/3} = 100\lambda,$$
$$\frac{1}{3}x^{2/3}y^{-2/3} = 100\lambda,$$
$$100x + 100y = 378{,}000,$$

to get $x = 2520, y = 1260$. Continuing to find λ gives us

$$\lambda \approx 0.0053.$$

Suppose now we do another, apparently unrelated calculation. Suppose our budget is increased by \$1000, from \$378,000 to \$379,000. The new budget constraint is

$$100x + 100y = 379{,}000.$$

The corresponding solution is at $x = 2527, y = 1263$ and the new maximum value (instead of $f = 2000.1$) is

$$f = (2527)^{2/3}(1263)^{1/3} \approx 2005.4.$$

The additional \$1000 in the budget increased the production level f by 5.3 units. Notice that production increased by $5.3/1000 = 0.0053$ units per dollar, which is our value of λ. The value of λ represents the extra production achieved by increasing the budget by one dollar—in other words, the extra "bang" you get for an extra "buck" of budget.

Solving for λ in either of the equations $f_x = \lambda g_x$ or $f_y = \lambda g_y$ suggests that the Lagrange multiplier is given by the ratio of the changes:

$$\lambda \approx \frac{\Delta f}{\Delta g} = \frac{\text{Change in optimum value of } f}{\text{Change in } g}.$$

These results suggest the following interpretations of the Lagrange multiplier λ:

- The value of λ is approximately the change in the optimum value of f when the value of the constraint is increased by 1 unit.
- The value of λ represents the rate of change of the optimum value of f as the constraint increases.

Example 3 The quantity of goods produced according to the function $f(x, y) = x^{2/3}y^{1/3}$ is maximized subject to the budget constraint $100x + 100y = 378{,}000$. Suppose the budget is increased to allow a small increase in production. What price must the product sell for if it is to be worth the increased budget?

Solution We know that $\lambda = 0.0053$. Therefore, increasing the budget by \$1 increases production by about 0.0053 unit. In order to make the increase in budget profitable, the extra goods produced must sell for more than \$1. If the price is p in dollars, we must have $0.0053p > 1$. Thus, we need $p > 1/0.0053 \approx \$189$.

Example 4 If x and y are the amounts of raw materials used, the quantity, Q, of a product manufactured is

$$Q = xy.$$

Assume that x costs \$20 per unit, y costs \$10 per unit, and the production budget is \$10,000.

(a) How many units of x and y should be purchased in order to maximize production? How many units are produced at that point?
(b) Find the value of λ and interpret it.

Solution

(a) We maximize $f(x,y) = xy$ subject to the constraint $g(x,y) = 20x + 10y = 10{,}000$ and $x \geq 0$, $y \geq 0$. We have the following partial derivatives:

$$f_x = y, \qquad f_y = x, \qquad \text{and} \qquad g_x = 20, \qquad g_y = 10.$$

The method of Lagrange multipliers gives the following equations:

$$\begin{aligned} y &= 20\lambda \\ x &= 10\lambda \\ 20x + 10y &= 10{,}000. \end{aligned}$$

Substituting values of x and y from the first two equations into the third gives

$$\begin{aligned} 20(10\lambda) + 10(20\lambda) &= 10{,}000 \\ 400\lambda &= 10{,}000 \\ \lambda &= 25. \end{aligned}$$

Substituting $\lambda = 25$ in the first two equations above gives $x = 250$ and $y = 500$.

The endpoints of the constraint are the point $(500, 0)$ and $(0, 1000)$. Since

$$f(500, 0) = 0 \quad \text{and} \quad f(0, 1000) = 0,$$

the maximum value of the production function is

$$f(250, 500) = 250 \cdot 500 = 125{,}000 \text{ units}.$$

The company should purchase 250 units of x and 500 units of y, giving 125,000 units of products.

(b) We have $\lambda = 25$. This tells us that if the budget is increased by \$1, we expect production to go up by about 25 units. If the budget goes up by \$1000, maximum production will increase about 25,000 to a total of roughly 150,000 units.

The Lagrangian Function

Constrained optimization problems are frequently solved using a *Lagrangian function*, $\mathcal{L}$. For example, to optimize the function $f(x,y)$ subject to the constraint $g(x,y) = c$, we use the Lagrangian function

$$\mathcal{L}(x, y, \lambda) = f(x,y) - \lambda(g(x,y) - c).$$

To see why the function $\mathcal{L}$ is useful, compute the partial derivatives of $\mathcal{L}$:

$$\begin{aligned} \frac{\partial \mathcal{L}}{\partial x} &= \frac{\partial f}{\partial x} - \lambda \frac{\partial g}{\partial x}, \\ \frac{\partial \mathcal{L}}{\partial y} &= \frac{\partial f}{\partial y} - \lambda \frac{\partial g}{\partial y}, \\ \frac{\partial \mathcal{L}}{\partial \lambda} &= -(g(x,y) - c). \end{aligned}$$

Notice that if (x_0, y_0) gives a maximum or minimum value of $f(x,y)$ subject to the constraint $g(x,y) = c$ and λ_0 is the corresponding Lagrange multiplier, then at the point (x_0, y_0, λ_0), we have

$$\frac{\partial \mathcal{L}}{\partial x} = 0 \quad \text{and} \quad \frac{\partial \mathcal{L}}{\partial y} = 0 \quad \text{and} \quad \frac{\partial \mathcal{L}}{\partial \lambda} = 0.$$

In other words, (x_0, y_0, λ_0) is a critical point for the unconstrained problem of optimization of the Lagrangian, $\mathcal{L}(x, y, \lambda)$.

We can therefore attack constrained optimization problems in two steps. First, write down the Lagrangian function $\mathcal{L}$. Second, find the critical points of $\mathcal{L}$.

Problems for Section 9.6

In Problems 1–10, use Lagrange multipliers to find the maximum or minimum values of $f(x, y)$ subject to the constraint.

1. $f(x, y) = x^2 + 4xy, \quad x + y = 100$

2. $f(x, y) = xy, \quad 5x + 2y = 100$

3. $f(x, y) = x^2 + 3y^2 + 100, \quad 8x + 6y = 88$

4. $f(x, y) = 5xy, \quad x + 3y = 24$

5. $f(x, y) = x + y, \quad x^2 + y^2 = 1$

6. $f(x, y) = x^2 + y^2, \quad 4x - 2y = 15$

7. $f(x, y) = 3x - 2y, \quad x^2 + 2y^2 = 44$

8. $f(x, y) = x^2 + y, \quad x^2 - y^2 = 1$

9. $f(x, y) = xy, \quad 4x^2 + y^2 = 8$

10. $f(x, y) = x^2 + y^2, \quad x^4 + y^4 = 2$

11. Figure 9.46 shows contours of $f(x, y)$ and the constraint $g(x, y) = c$. Approximately what values of x and y maximize $f(x, y)$ subject to the constraint? What is the approximate value of f at this maximum?

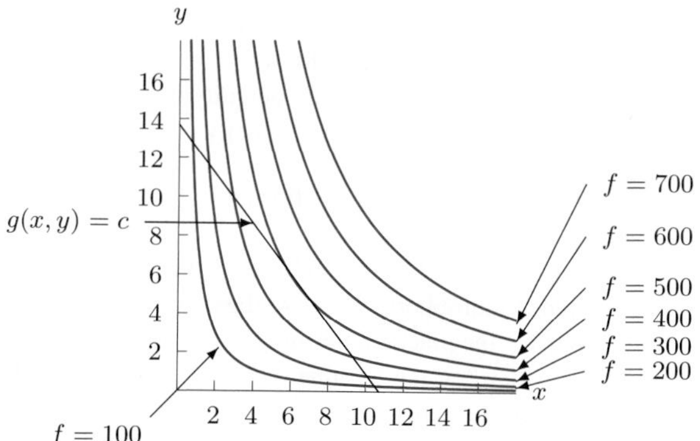

Figure 9.46

12. Figure 9.47 shows contours labeled with values of $f(x, y)$ and a constraint $g(x, y) = c$. Mark the approximate points at which:

(a) f has a maximum

(b) f has a maximum on the constraint $g = c$.

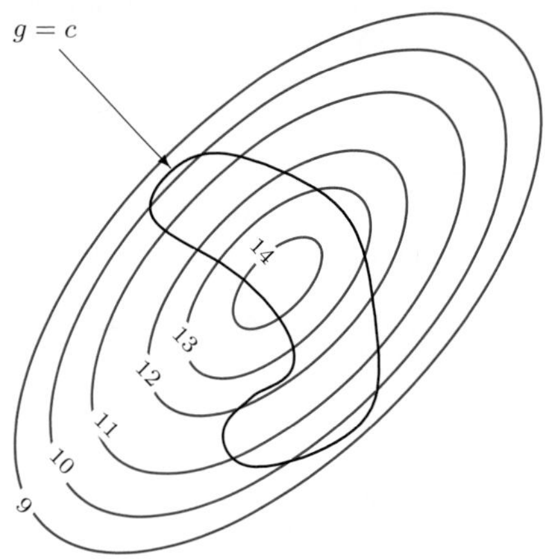

Figure 9.47

13. The quantity, Q, of a good produced depends on the quantities x_1 and x_2 of two raw materials used:

$$Q = x_1^{0.6} x_2^{0.4}.$$

A unit of x_1 costs \$127, and a unit of x_2 costs \$92. We want to minimize the cost, C, of producing 500 units of the good.

(a) What is the objective function?

(b) What is the constraint?

14. The quantity, Q, of a certain product manufactured depends on the quantity of labor, L, and of capital, K, used according to the function

$$Q = 900L^{1/2}K^{2/3}.$$

Labor costs \$100 per unit and capital costs \$200 per unit. What combination of labor and capital should be used to produce $36{,}000$ units of the goods at minimum cost? What is that minimum cost?

15. The Cobb-Douglas production function for a product is

$$P = 5L^{0.8}K^{0.2},$$

where P is the quantity produced, L is the size of the labor force, and K is the amount of total equipment. Each unit of labor costs \$300, each unit of equipment costs \$100, and the total budget is \$15,000.

(a) Make a table of L and K values which exhaust the budget. Find the production level, P, for each.

(b) Use the method of Lagrange multipliers to find the optimal way to spend the budget.

16. A firm manufactures a commodity at two different factories. The total cost of manufacturing depends on the quantities, q_1 and q_2, supplied by each factory, and is expressed by the *joint cost function*,

$$C = f(q_1, q_2) = 2q_1^2 + q_1q_2 + q_2^2 + 500.$$

The company's objective is to produce 200 units, while minimizing production costs. How many units should be supplied by each factory?

17. The quantity, Q, of a product manufactured by a company is given by

$$Q = aK^{0.6}L^{0.4},$$

where a is a positive constant, K is the quantity of capital and L is the quantity of labor used. Capital costs are \$20 per unit, labor costs are \$10 per unit, and the company wants costs for capital and labor combined to be no higher than \$150. Suppose you are asked to consult for the company, and learn that 5 units each of capital and labor are being used.

(a) What do you advise? Should the company use more or less labor? More or less capital? If so, by how much?
(b) Write a one-sentence summary that could be used to sell your advice to the board of directors.

18. For a cost function, $f(x, y)$, the minimum cost for a production of 50 is given by $f(33, 87) = 1200$, with $\lambda = 15$. Estimate the cost if the production quota is:

(a) Raised to 51 **(b)** Lowered to 49

19. A company has the production function $P(x, y)$, which gives the number of units that can be produced for given values of x and y; the cost function $C(x, y)$ gives the cost of production for given values of x and y.

(a) If the company wishes to maximize production at a cost of \$50,000, what is the objective function f? What is the constraint equation? What is the meaning of λ in this situation?
(b) If instead the company wishes to minimize the costs at a fixed production level of 2000 units, what is the objective function f? What is the constraint equation? What is the meaning of λ in this situation?

20. You have set aside 20 hours to work on two class projects. You want to maximize your grade (measured in points), which depends on how you divide your time between the two projects.

(a) What is the objective function for this optimization problem and what are its units?
(b) What is the constraint?
(c) Suppose you solve the problem by the method of Lagrange multipliers. What are the units for λ?
(d) What is the practical meaning of the statement $\lambda = 5$?

21. A steel manufacturer can produce $P(K, L)$ tons of steel using K units of capital and L units of labor, with production costs $C(K, L)$ dollars. With a budget of \$600,000, the maximum production is 2,500,000 tons, using \$400,000 of capital and \$200,000 of labor. The Lagrange multiplier is $\lambda = 3.17$.

(a) What is the objective function?
(b) What is the constraint?
(c) What are the units for λ?
(d) What is the practical meaning of the statement $\lambda = 3.17$?

22. The quantity, q, of a product manufactured depends on the number of workers, W, and the amount of capital invested, K, and is given by the Cobb-Douglas function

$$q = 6W^{3/4}K^{1/4}.$$

In addition, labor costs are \$10 per worker and capital costs are \$20 per unit and the budget is \$3000.

(a) What are the optimum number of workers and the optimum number of units of capital?
(b) Recompute the optimum values of W and K when the budget is increased by \$1. Check that increasing the budget by \$1 allows the production of λ extra units of the product, where λ is the Lagrange multiplier.

23. The terminal velocity (meters/second) that a two-stage rocket achieves is a function of the amount of fuel x_1 and x_2 (measured in liters) loaded into the two stages. You wish to minimize the total quantity of fuel required to achieve a specified terminal velocity, v_0.

(a) What is the objective function and what are its units?
(b) What is the constraint?
(c) Suppose you solve the problem by the method of Lagrange multipliers. What are the units for λ?
(d) What is the practical meaning of the statement $\lambda = 8$ when the terminal velocity of the rocket is 50 meters/second?

24. Each person tries to balance his or her time between leisure and work. The tradeoff is that as you work less your income falls. Therefore each person has *indifference curves* which connect the number of hours of leisure, l, and income, s. If, for example, you are indifferent between 0 hours of leisure and an income of \$1125 a week on the one hand, and 10 hours of leisure and an income of \$750 a week on the other hand, then the points $l = 0$, $s = 1125$, and $l = 10$, $s = 750$ both lie on the same indifference curve. Table 9.11 gives information on three indifference curves, I, II, and III.

Table 9.11

Weekly income			Weekly leisure hours		
I	II	III	I	II	III
1125	1250	1375	0	20	40
750	875	1000	10	30	50
500	625	750	20	40	60
375	500	625	30	50	70
250	375	500	50	70	90

(a) Graph the three indifference curves.
(b) You have 100 hours a week available for work and leisure combined, and you earn \$10/hour. Write an equation in terms of l and s which represents this constraint.
(c) On the same axes, graph this constraint.
(d) Estimate from the graph what combination of leisure hours and income you would choose under these circumstances. Give the corresponding number of hours per week you would work.

25. If x_1 and x_2 are the number of items of two goods bought, a customer's utility is

$$U(x_1, x_2) = 2x_1x_2 + 3x_1.$$

The unit cost is \$1 for the first good and \$3 for the second. Use Lagrange multipliers to find the maximum value of U if the consumer's disposable income is \$100. Estimate the new optimal utility if the consumer's disposable income increases by \$6.

CHAPTER SUMMARY

- **Functions of two variables**
  Represented by: tables, graphs, formulas, cross-sections (one variable fixed), contours (function value fixed).
- **Partial derivatives**
  Definition as a difference quotient, interpreting using units, estimating from a contour diagram or a table, computing from a formula, second-order partial derivatives.
- **Optimization**
  Critical points, local and global maxima and minima.
- **Constrained optimization**
  Geometric interpretation of Lagrange multiplier method, solving Lagrange multiplier problems algebraically, interpreting λ, Lagrangian function.

REVIEW PROBLEMS FOR CHAPTER NINE

1. Use Table 9.12. Is f an increasing or decreasing function of x? Is f an increasing or decreasing function of y?

Table 9.12 *Values of a function $f(x, y)$*

x \ y	0	1	2	3	4	5
0	102	107	114	123	135	150
20	96	101	108	117	129	144
40	90	95	102	111	123	138
60	85	90	97	106	118	133
80	81	86	93	102	114	129

2. The balance, B, in dollars, in a bank account depends on the amount deposited, A dollars, the annual interest rate, $r\%$, and the time, t, in months since the deposit, so $B = f(A, r, t)$.

(a) Is f an increasing or decreasing function of A? Of r? Of t?
(b) Interpret the statement $f(1250, 1, 25) \approx 1276$. Give units.

For each of the functions in Problems 3–4, make a contour plot in the region $-2 < x < 2$ and $-2 < y < 2$. In each case, what is the equation and the shape of the contour lines?

3. $z = 3x - 5y + 1$

4. $z = 2x^2 + y^2$

5. Table 9.13 shows the wind-chill factor as a function of wind speed and temperature. Draw a possible contour diagram for this function. Include contours at wind chills of 20°, 0°, and -20°.

6. The temperature adjusted for wind-chill is a temperature which tells you how cold it feels, as a result of the combination of wind and temperature.[13] See Table 9.13.

(a) If the temperature is 0°F and the wind speed is 15 mph, how cold does it feel?
(b) If the temperature is 35°F, what wind speed makes it feel like 24°F?
(c) If the temperature is 25°F, what wind speed makes it feel like 12°F?
(d) If the wind is blowing at 20 mph, what temperature feels like 0°F?

[13] Data from www.nws.noaa.gov/om/windchill, accessed on May 22, 2009.

Table 9.13 *Temperature adjusted for wind-chill (°F) as a function of wind speed and temperature*

		Temperature (°F)							
		35	30	25	20	15	10	5	0
Wind Speed (mph)	5	31	25	19	13	7	1	−5	−11
	10	27	21	15	9	3	−4	−10	−16
	15	25	19	13	6	0	−7	−13	−19
	20	24	17	11	4	−2	−9	−15	−22
	25	23	16	9	3	−4	−11	−17	−24

7. Using Table 9.13, make tables of the temperature adjusted for wind-chill as a function of wind speed for temperatures of 20°F and 0°F.

8. Using Table 9.13, make tables of the temperature adjusted for wind-chill as a function of temperature for wind speeds of 5 mph and 20 mph.

9. Figure 9.48 is a contour diagram for the sales of a product as a function of the price of the product and the amount spent on advertising. Which axis corresponds to the amount spent on advertising? Explain.

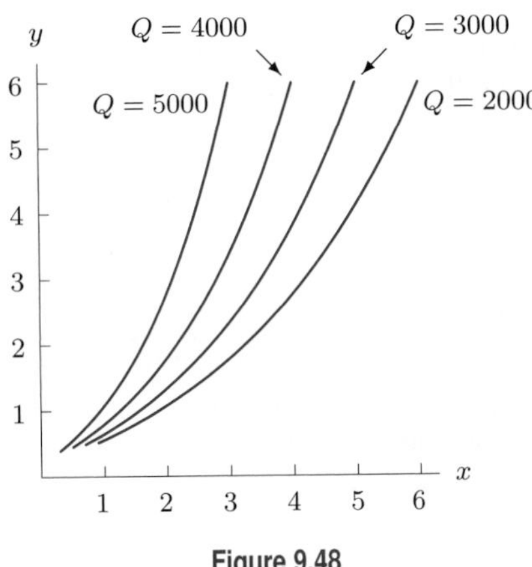

Figure 9.48

10. Each of the contour diagrams in Figure 9.49 shows population density in a certain region. Choose the contour diagram that best corresponds to each of the following situations. Many different matchings are possible. Pick any reasonable one and justify your choice.

(a) The center of the diagram is a city.
(b) The center of the diagram is a lake.
(c) The center of the diagram is a power plant.

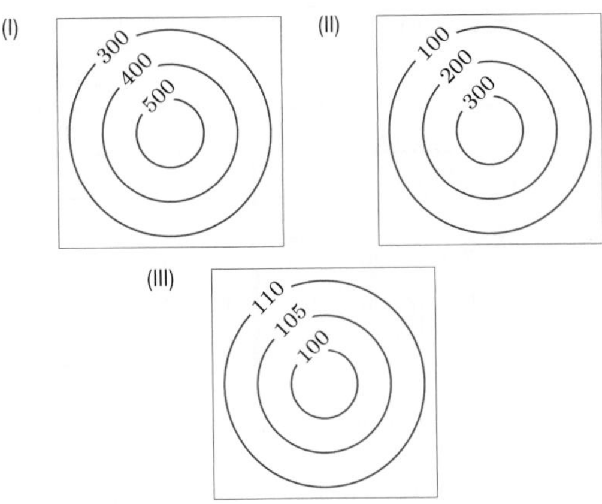

Figure 9.49

11. Figure 9.50 shows the contours of the temperature H in a room near a recently opened window. Label the three contours with reasonable values of H if the house is in the following locations.

(a) Minnesota in winter (where winters are harsh).
(b) San Francisco in winter (where winters are mild).
(c) Houston in summer (where summers are hot).
(d) Oregon in summer (where summers are mild).

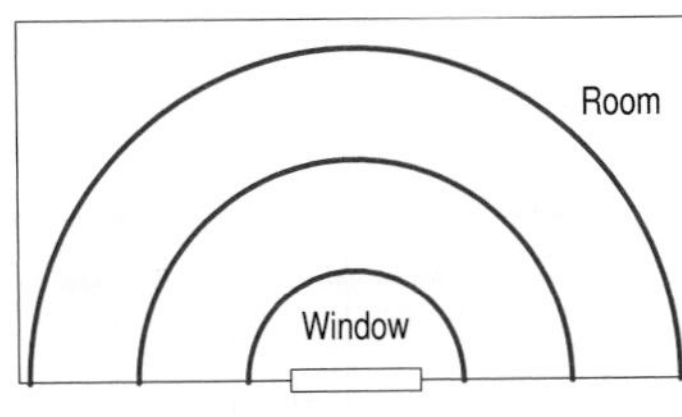

Figure 9.50

12. Figure 9.51 is a contour diagram of the monthly payment on a 5-year car loan as a function of the interest rate and the amount you borrow. The interest rate is 8% and you borrow \$6000 for a used car.

(a) What is your monthly payment?
(b) If interest rates drop to 6%, how much more can you borrow without increasing your monthly payment?
(c) Make a table of how much you can borrow, without increasing your monthly payment, as a function of the interest rate.

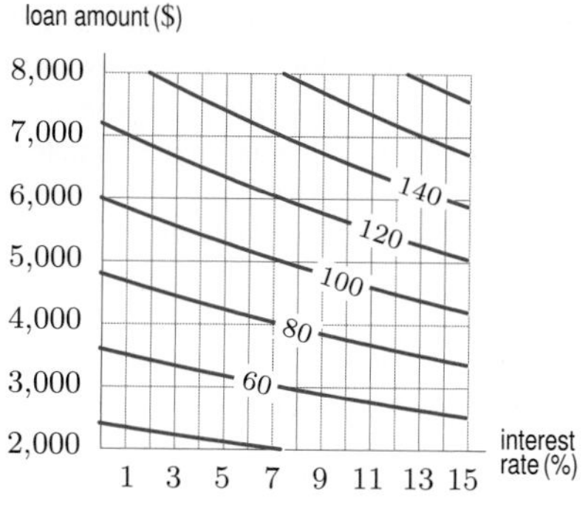

Figure 9.51

13. Match tables (a)–(d) with the contour diagrams (I)–(IV) in Figure 9.52.

(a)

y \ x	-1	0	1
-1	2	1	2
0	1	0	1
1	2	1	2

(b)

y \ x	-1	0	1
-1	0	1	0
0	1	2	1
1	0	1	0

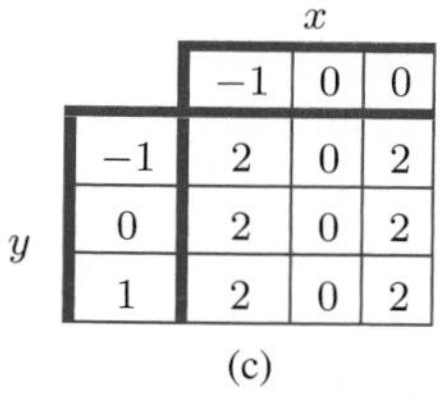

(c)

y \ x	-1	0	0
-1	2	0	2
0	2	0	2
1	2	0	2

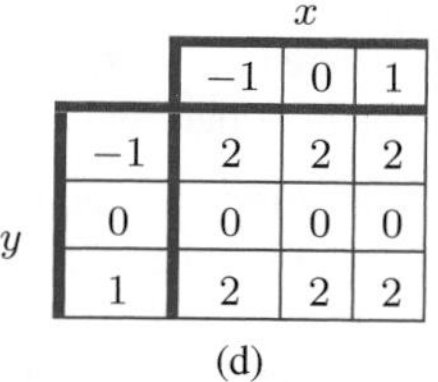

(d)

y \ x	-1	0	1
-1	2	2	2
0	0	0	0
1	2	2	2

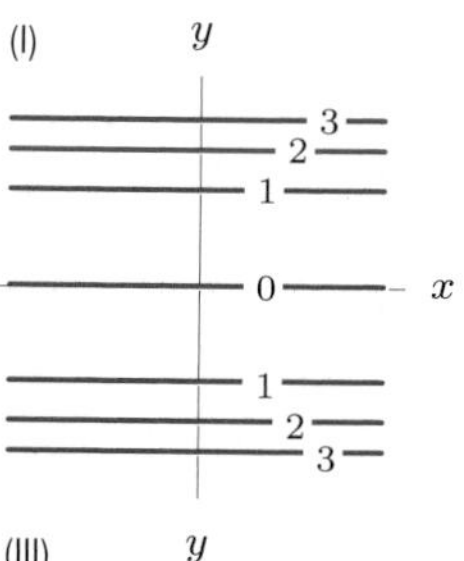

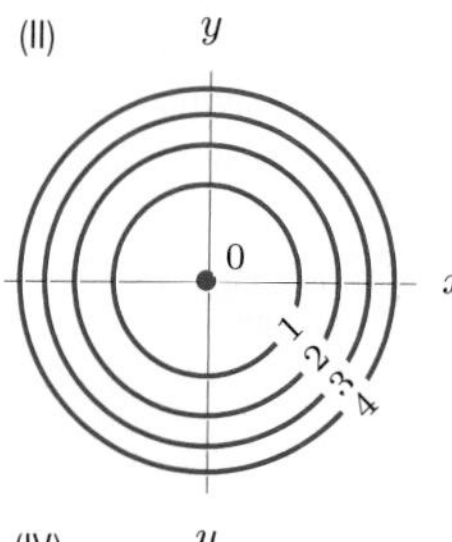

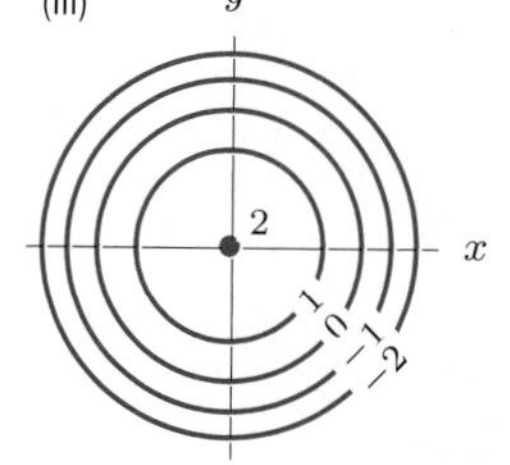

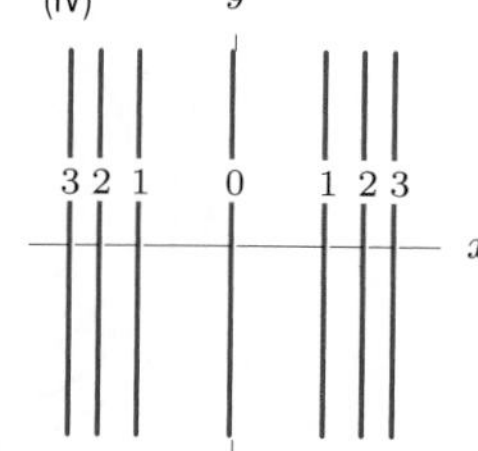

Figure 9.52

14. Figure 9.53 gives contour diagrams for different Cobb-Douglas production functions $F(L, K)$. Match each contour diagram with the correct statement.

(A) Tripling each input triples output.

(B) Quadrupling each input doubles output.

(C) Doubling each input almost triples output.

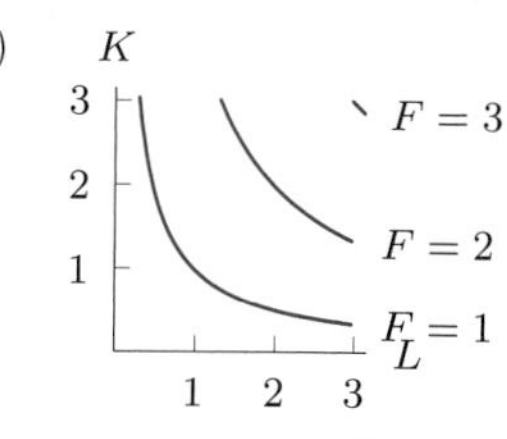

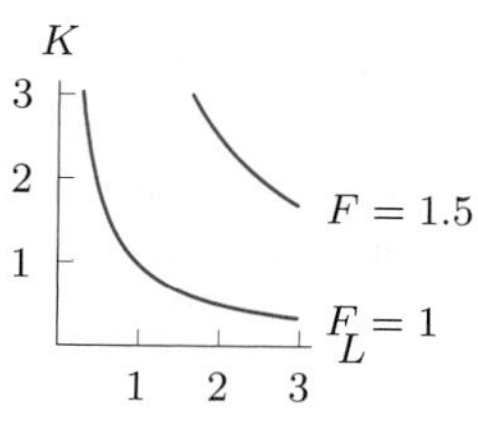

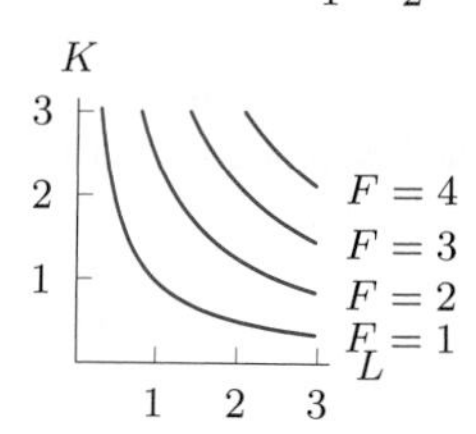

Figure 9.53

15. Figure 9.54 is a contour diagram for $z = f(x, y)$. Is f_x positive or negative? Is f_y positive or negative? Estimate $f(2, 1)$, $f_x(2, 1)$, and $f_y(2, 1)$.

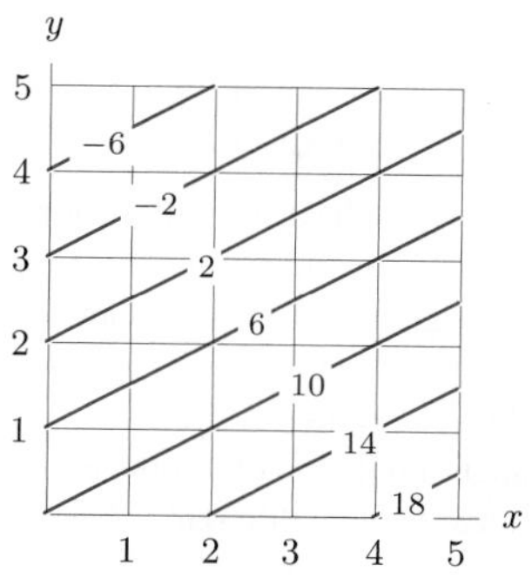

Figure 9.54

16. You borrow $\$A$ at an interest rate of $r\%$ (per month) and pay it off over t months by making monthly payments of $P = g(A, r, t)$ dollars. In financial terms, what do the following statements tell you?

(a) $g(8000, 1, 24) = 376.59$

(b) $\left.\dfrac{\partial g}{\partial A}\right|_{(8000,1,24)} = 0.047$

(c) $\left.\dfrac{\partial g}{\partial r}\right|_{(8000,1,24)} = 44.83$

For Problems 17–19, refer to Table 9.13 on page 390 giving the temperature adjusted for wind-chill, C, in °F, as a function $f(w, T)$ of the wind speed, w, in mph, and the temperature, T, in °F. The temperature adjusted for wind-chill tells you how cold it feels, as a result of the combination of wind and temperature.

17. Estimate $f_w(10, 25)$. What does your answer mean in practical terms?

18. Estimate $f_T(5, 20)$. What does your answer mean in practical terms?

19. From Table 9.13 you can see that when the temperature is 20°F, the temperature adjusted for wind-chill drops by an average of about 0.8°F with every 1 mph increase in wind speed from 5 mph to 10 mph. Which partial derivative is this telling you about?

20. Suppose that x is the price of one brand of gasoline and y is the price of a competing brand. Then q_1, the quantity of the first brand sold in a fixed time period, depends on both x and y, so $q_1 = f(x, y)$. Similarly, if q_2 is the quantity of the second brand sold during the same period, $q_2 = g(x, y)$. What do you expect the signs of the following quantities to be? Explain.

(a) $\partial q_1/\partial x$ and $\partial q_2/\partial y$
(b) $\partial q_1/\partial y$ and $\partial q_2/\partial x$

21. Suppose that x is the average price of a new car and that y is the average price of a gallon of gasoline. Then q_1, the number of new cars bought in a year, depends on both x and y, so $q_1 = f(x, y)$. Similarly, if q_2 is the quantity of gas bought in a year, then $q_2 = g(x, y)$.

(a) What do you expect the signs of $\partial q_1/\partial x$ and $\partial q_2/\partial y$ to be? Explain.
(b) What do you expect the signs of $\partial q_1/\partial y$ and $\partial q_2/\partial x$ to be? Explain.

22. Figure 9.55 shows the density of the fox population P (in foxes per square kilometer) for southern England. Draw two different graphs of the fox population as a function of kilometers north, with kilometers east fixed at two different values, and draw two different graphs of the fox population as a function of kilometers east, with kilometers north fixed at two different values.

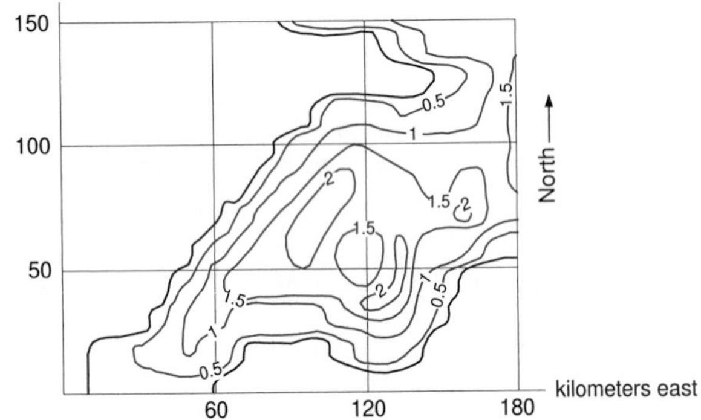

Figure 9.55

23. Figure 9.55 gives a contour diagram for the number n of foxes per square kilometer in southwestern England. Estimate $\partial n/\partial x$ and $\partial n/\partial y$ at the points A, B, and C, where x is kilometers east and y is kilometers north.

Find the partial derivatives in Problems 24–29. The variables are restricted to a domain on which the function is defined.

24. f_x and f_y if $f(x, y) = x^2 + xy + y^2$

25. P_a and P_b if $P = a^2 - 2ab^2$

26. $\dfrac{\partial Q}{\partial p_1}$ and $\dfrac{\partial Q}{\partial p_2}$ if $Q = 50p_1p_2 - p_2^2$

27. $\dfrac{\partial f}{\partial x}$ and $\dfrac{\partial f}{\partial t}$ if $f = 5xe^{-2t}$

28. $\dfrac{\partial P}{\partial K}$ and $\dfrac{\partial P}{\partial L}$ if $P = 10K^{0.7}L^{0.3}$

29. f_x and f_y if $f(x, y) = \sqrt{x^2 + y^2}$

30. A manufacturing company produces two items in quantities q_1 and q_2, respectively. Total production costs are given by

$$\text{Cost} = f(q_1, q_2) = 16 + 1.2q_1 + 1.5q_2 + 0.2q_1q_2.$$

Find $f(500, 1000)$, $f_{q_1}(500, 1000)$, and $f_{q_2}(500, 1000)$. Give units with your answers and interpret each of your answers in terms of production cost.

31. The Cobb-Douglas production function for a product is given by

$$Q = 25K^{0.75}L^{0.25},$$

where Q is the quantity produced for a capital investment of K dollars and a labor investment of L.

(a) Find Q_K and Q_L.
(b) Find the values of Q, Q_K and Q_L given that $K = 60$ and $L = 100$.
(c) Interpret each of the values you found in part (b) in terms of production.

32. Figure 9.56 is a contour diagram of $f(x, y)$. In each of the following cases, list the marked points in the diagram (there may be none or more than one) at which

(a) $f_x < 0$ **(b)** $f_y > 0$
(c) $f_{xx} > 0$ **(d)** $f_{yy} < 0$

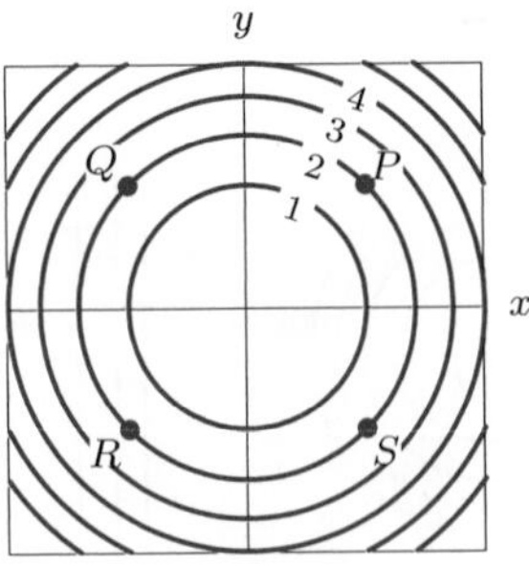

Figure 9.56

33. You are an anthropologist observing a native ritual. Sixteen people arrange themselves with their backs to you along a bench; all but the three on the far left side are seated. The first person on the far left is standing with her hands at her side, the second is standing with his hands raised and the third is standing with her hands at her side. At some unseen signal, the first one sits down, and everyone else copies what his neighbor to the left was doing one second earlier. Every second that passes, this behavior is repeated until all are once again seated.

(a) Draw graphs at several different times showing how the height depends upon the distance along the bench.
(b) Graph the location of the raised hands as a function of time.
(c) What US ritual is most closely related to what you have observed?

34. You are in a stadium doing the wave. This is a ritual in which members of the audience stand up and down in such a way as to create a wave that moves around the stadium. Normally a single wave travels all the way around the stadium, but we assume there is a continuous sequence of waves. Let $h(x,t) = 5 + \cos(0.5x - t)$ be the function describing this stadium wave. The value of $h(x,t)$ gives the height (in feet) of the head of the spectator in seat x at time t seconds. Evaluate $h_x(2,5)$ and $h_t(2,5)$ and interpret each in terms of the wave.

35. Find all critical points of $f(x,y) = x^3 - 3x + y^2$. Make a table of values to determine if each critical point is a local minimum, a local maximum, or neither.

36. Find all critical points of $f(x,y) = x^2 + 3y^2 - 4x + 6y + 10$.

37. A company sells two products which are partial substitutes for each other, such as coffee and tea. If the price of one product rises, then the demand for the other product rises. The quantities demanded, q_1 and q_2, are given as a function of the prices, p_1 and p_2, by

$$q_1 = 517 - 3.5p_1 + 0.8p_2, \quad q_2 = 770 - 4.4p_2 + 1.4p_1.$$

(a) Write total sales revenue as a function of p_1 and p_2.
(b) What prices should the company charge in order to maximize the total sales revenue?[14]

Figure 9.57 shows contours of f. In Problems 38–40 give an approximate maximum or minimum value of f for $0 \le x \le 300$, $0 \le y \le 300$ subject to the given constraint.

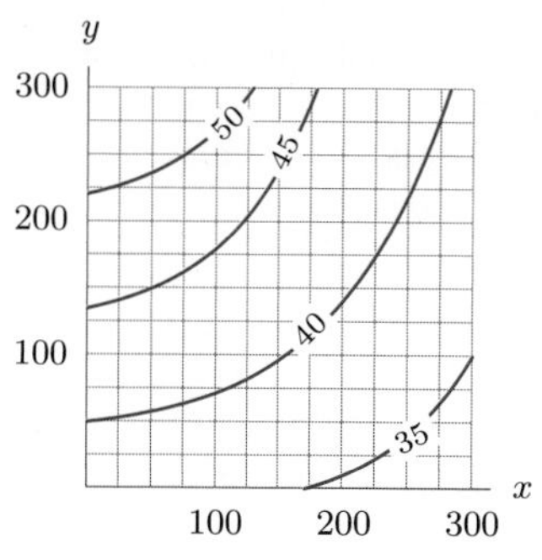

Figure 9.57

38. Minimum, constraint is $y = 100$

39. Maximum, constraint is $y = 100$

40. Maximum, constraint is $y = x$

41. The quantity, Q, of a good produced depends on the quantities x_1 and x_2 of two raw materials used:

$$Q = x_1^{0.3} x_2^{0.7}.$$

A unit of x_1 costs \$10, and a unit of x_2 costs \$25. We want to maximize production with a budget of \$50 thousand for raw materials.

(a) What is the objective function?
(b) What is the constraint?

42. Figure 9.58 shows level curves for production $f(x,y)$ as a function of the quantities x and y of two raw materials utilized. The cost of the materials is $15x + 20y$ thousand dollars. What is the maximum production possible with a budget of 300 thousand dollars? How much of each raw material should be purchased to achieve this maximum?

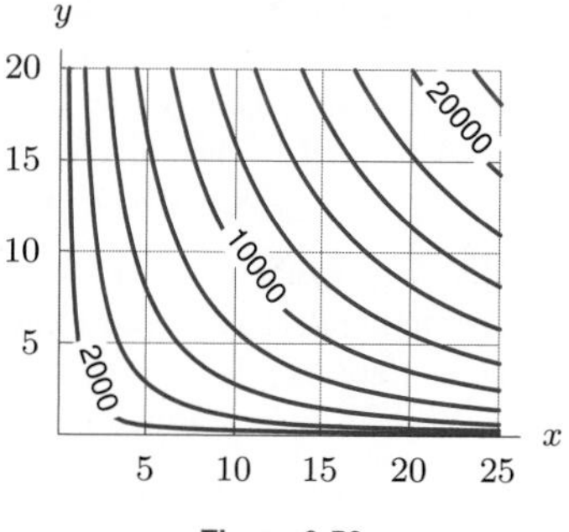

Figure 9.58

43. An automobile manufacturing plant currently employs 1500 workers and has capital investment of 15 million dollars per month. The production function is

$$Q = x^{0.4} y^{0.6},$$

[14] Adapted from M. Rosser, *Basic Mathematics for Economists*, p. 318 (New York: Routledge, 1993).

where Q is the number of cars produced per month, x is the number of workers and y is capital investment. Each worker's salary is $5000 per month and each unit of capital costs $4000 per month.

(a) How many cars is the factory currently assembling each month?

(b) Due to the sluggish economy, the factory decides to decrease production to 2000 cars per month. The factory wants to minimize the cost of producing these 2000 cars. How many workers will need to be laid off? By what amount should monthly investment be decreased?

(c) Give the value of the Lagrange multiplier, λ, and interpret it in terms of the car factory.

44. A company manufactures x units of one item and y units of another. The total cost in dollars, C, of producing these two items is approximated by the function

$$C = 5x^2 + 2xy + 3y^2 + 800.$$

(a) If the production quota for the total number of items (both types combined) is 39, find the minimum production cost.

(b) Estimate the additional production cost or savings if the production quota is raised to 40 or lowered to 38.

45. A monopolistic producer of two goods A and B has a joint total cost function

$$C = 10q_1 + q_1q_2 + 10q_2,$$

where q_1 and q_2 denote the quantities of A and B respectively. The demand curves for the corresponding prices p_1 and p_2 are

$$p_1 = 50 - q_1 + q_2$$
$$p_2 = 30 + 2q_1 - q_2.$$

(a) Find the maximum profit if the firm produces a total of 15.

(b) Estimate the new optimal profit if the production quota increases by one unit.

CHECK YOUR UNDERSTANDING

In Problems 1–60, indicate whether the statement is true or false.

1. If $Q = f(x,t)$ gives the quantity Q of pollutants, in ppm (parts per million), at a distance x kilometers from a waste incinerator at time t hours after incineration ends, we have $f(1.5, 6) = 4.1$. The units for 1.5 are ppm.

2. If $Q = f(x,t)$ gives the quantity Q of pollutants, in ppm (parts per million), at a distance x kilometers from a waste incinerator at time t hours after incineration ends, we have $f(1.5, 6) = 4.1$. The units for 6 are hours.

3. If $Q = f(x,t)$ gives the quantity Q of pollutants, in ppm (parts per million), at a distance x kilometers from a waste incinerator at time t hours after incineration ends, we have $f(1.5, 6) = 4.1$. The units for 4.1 are kilometers.

4. If $Q = f(x,t)$ gives the quantity Q of pollutants, in ppm (parts per million), at a distance x kilometers from a waste incinerator at time t hours after incineration ends, then Q is most likely an increasing function of x.

5. If $Q = f(x,t)$ gives the quantity Q of pollutants, in ppm (parts per million), at a distance x kilometers from a waste incinerator at time t hours after incineration ends, in the statement $f(2, 3) = 5$, the units of the 2 are km.

6. If $f(x,y)$ is a function of two variables, then f is an increasing function of x if f increases when both x increases and y increases.

7. A function $f(x,y)$ can be both an increasing function of x and a decreasing function of y.

8. The function $f(x,y) = x^2 - y$ is a decreasing function of y.

9. If $f(x,y) = e^{xy} - y^2$, then the cross-section $x = 1$ is $f(1,y) = e^y - 1$.

10. If $f(x,y) = e^{xy} - y^2$, then the cross-section $y = 0$ is $f(x,0) = 0$.

11. The function $f(x,y) = y + 3x - 1$ has contours which are lines.

12. The function $f(x,y) = x^2 - y$ has contours which are parabolas.

13. For a given function $f(x,y)$ the two contours $f(x,y) = 1$ and $f(x,y) = 2$ can never intersect.

14. Contours of the function $g(x,y) = 3x + 2y$ are parallel lines.

15. The function $P = 3N^{1/2}V^{1/2}$ is a Cobb-Douglas production function.

16. The function $P = 10N^3V^2$ is a Cobb-Douglas production function.

17. The function $f(x,y)$ has the same value at all points along a specific contour.

18. A contour can consist of a single point.

19. Contours of a Cobb-Douglas production function are decreasing, concave up.

20. Every point in the domain of $g(x,y)$ has a contour that contains it.

21. The partial derivative $f_x(a,b)$ is the rate of change of the function f with respect to x at the point (a,b) with y fixed at b.

22. If $P = f(m,t)$ gives the price P (in dollars) of a used car as a function of its mileage m (in miles) and its age t (in years), then $\partial P/\partial m$ has units miles per year.

23. If $P = f(m,t)$ gives the price P (in dollars) of a used car as a function of its mileage m (in miles) and its age t (in years), then $\partial P/\partial m$ is most likely to be negative.

24. If $W = f(c,t)$ gives the weight W (in pounds) of a person as a function of their daily food intake c (in calories) and daily aerobic exercise time t (in hours), then $\partial W/\partial c$ has units pounds per calorie.

25. If $W = f(c,t)$ gives the weight W (in pounds) of a person as a function of their daily food intake c (in calories) and daily aerobic exercise time t (in hours), then $\partial W/\partial c$ is most likely to be negative.

26. If $W = f(c,t)$ gives the weight W (in pounds) of a person as a function of their daily food intake c (in calories) and daily aerobic exercise time t (in hours), then $\partial W/\partial c$ and $\partial W/\partial t$ most likely have opposite signs.

27. For a function $z = f(x,y)$, assume $f(1,2) = 10$ and $f(1.1,2) = 10.5$ and $f(1,2.1) = 10.8$ and $f(1.1,2.1) = 11.3$. Then $f_x(1,2) \approx 5$.

28. For a function $z = f(x,y)$, assume $f(1,2) = 10$ and $f(1.1,2) = 10.5$ and $f(1,2.1) = 10.8$ and $f(1.1,2.1) = 11.3$. Then $f_y(1,2) \approx 13$.

29. For a function $z = f(x,y)$, assume $f(5,3) = 7$ and $f(5.1,3) = 7.9$ and $f(5,3.1) = 6.4$ and $f(5.1,3.1) = 7.3$. Then $f_x(5,3) \approx 9$.

30. For a function $z = f(x,y)$, assume $f(5,3) = 7$ and $f(5.1,3) = 7.9$ and $f(5,3.1) = 6.4$ and $f(5.1,3.1) = 7.3$. Then $f_y(5,3) \approx 6$.

31. If $f(x,y) = x^2y + 3x$ then $f_x(x,y) = 2xy + 3$.

32. If $f(x,y) = x^2y + 3x$ then $f_y(1,2) = 4$.

33. If $g(u,v) = ue^v$ then $g_u(0,0) = 1$.

34. There exists a function f with $f_x(x,y) = f_y(x,y)$.

35. The function $Q(x,y) = x^3y^2$ is decreasing in the y direction near $(1,2)$.

36. If $P = 2N^{0.6}V^{0.4}$ then $\dfrac{\partial P}{\partial V} = 0.8N^{0.6}V^{-0.6}$.

37. For all functions f it is always true that $f_{xx} = f_{yy}$ if f_{xx} and f_{yy} are continuous.

38. If $f(x,y) = 3x^2e^{2y}$ then $f_y(1,0) < f_x(1,0)$.

39. If $z = p(A,B) = (1/2)(A^2 - B)$ then $\dfrac{\partial z}{\partial A} = A$.

40. If $z = V(r,h) = \pi r^2 h$ then $\dfrac{\partial^2 z}{\partial r \partial h} = 2\pi$.

41. If f is a function with $f_x(1,2) = 0$ then $(1,2)$ is a critical point of f.

42. The point $(1,1)$ is a critical point of $f(x,y) = x^2 + y^2$.

43. The point $(3,2)$ is a critical point of $g(u,v) = (u-3)^2 + (v-2)^2$.

44. The function $f(x,y) = xe^y$ has no critical points.

45. If $(0,0)$ is a critical point of f then f has either a local maximum or local minimum at $(0,0)$.

46. If $D > 0$ and $f_{xx} > 0$ in the second derivative test at the point (a,b) then f has a local minimum at (a,b).

47. To use the second derivative test on a function f at a point (a,b), we must have $f_x(a,b) = 0$ and $f_y(a,b) = 0$.

48. The function $f(x,y) = x^2 - y^2$ has a local minimum at $(0,0)$.

49. The function $f(x,y) = 3xy$ has a neither a local maximum or minimum at $(0,0)$.

50. A local minimum of f can also be a global minimum of f.

51. If f has a local maximum at P_0 subject to the constraint $g(x,y) = c$ then P_0 is a critical point of f.

52. If f has a local maximum at P_0 subject to the constraint $g(x,y) = c$ then P_0 satisfies the equation $g(x,y) = c$.

53. If we wish to maximize production given a fixed budget, then the production function is the constraint equation.

54. If we wish to minimize costs given a fixed production level, then the production equation is the constraint equation.

55. The minimum value of $f(x,y) = x^2 + y^2$ subject to the constraint $x - y = 0$ is $f(0,0) = 0$.

56. The minimum value of $f(x,y) = x^2 + y^2$ subject to the constraint $2x + 3y = 12$ is $f(0,0) = 0$.

57. If the minimum cost is \$50,000 given a fixed production level of 8,000 tons with $\lambda = 120$, then we expect production of 8,001 tons to cost about \$50,120.

58. If the maximum production level is 50,000 tons given a fixed budget of \$80,000 with $\lambda = 120$, then we expect production of \$50,001 tons to cost about \$80,120.

59. The second derivative test can be used to classify a point found by the Lagrange multiplier method as constrained maximum or minimum.

60. If the quantity Q of a good produced depends only on the quantities x and y of two raw materials used to manufacture the good, and there is a total of \$50,000 to spend on the two raw materials, then a budget constraint for Q is $x + y = 50000$.

PROJECTS FOR CHAPTER NINE

1. **A Heater in a Room**
   Figure 9.59 shows the contours of the temperature along one wall of a heated room through one winter day, with time indicated as on a 24-hour clock. The room has a heater located at the left-most corner of the wall and one window in the wall. The heater is controlled by a thermostat about 2 feet from the window.
   (a) Where is the window? **(b)** When is the window open?
   (c) When is the heat on?
   (d) Draw graphs of the temperature along the wall of the room at 6 am, at 11 am, at 3 pm (15 hours) and at 5 pm (17 hours).
   (e) Draw a graph of the temperature as a function of time at the heater, at the window and midway between them.
   (f) The temperature at the window at 5 pm (17 hours) is less than at 11 am. Why do you think this might be?
   (g) To what temperature do you think the thermostat is set? How do you know?
   (h) Where is the thermostat?

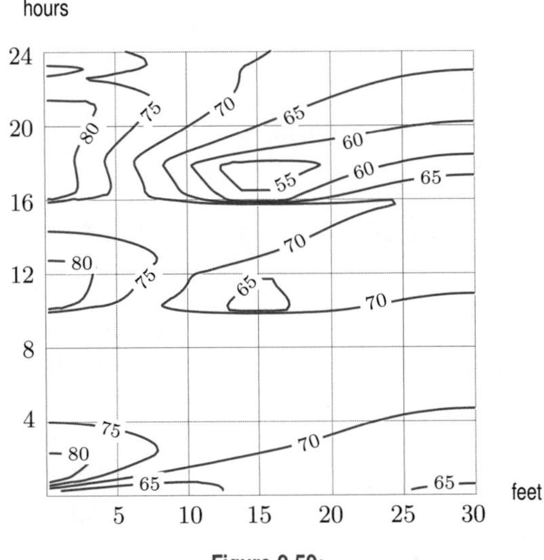

Figure 9.59:

2. **Optimizing Relative Prices for Adults and Children**
   Some items are sold at a discount to senior citizens or children. The reason is that these groups are more sensitive to price, so a discount has greater impact on their purchasing decisions. The seller faces an optimization problem: How large a discount to offer in order to maximize profits? Suppose a theater can sell q_c child tickets and q_a adult tickets at prices p_c and p_a, according to the demand functions:
   $$q_c = rp_c{}^{-4} \quad \text{and} \quad q_a = sp_a{}^{-2},$$
   and has operating costs proportional to the total number of tickets sold. What should be the relative price of children's and adults' tickets?

3. **Maximizing Production and Minimizing Cost: "Duality"**
   A company's production function is $P = 270x_1^{1/3}x_2^{2/3}$ for quantities x_1 and x_2 of two raw materials, costing \$4 per unit and \$27 per unit, respectively.
   (a) How much of each raw material should be used to maximize production if the budget for raw materials is \$324? What is the maximum production achieved, P_0?
   (b) What is the minimum cost at which a production level of P_0 can be achieved? How much of each raw material is used at this minimum?
   (c) Comment on the relationship between your answers to parts (a) and (b).

FOCUS ON THEORY

DERIVING THE FORMULA FOR A REGRESSION LINE

Suppose we want to find the "best fitting" line for some experimental data. In Appendix A, we use a computer or calculator to find the formula for this line. In this section, we derive this formula.

We decide which line fits the data best by using the following criterion. The data is plotted in the plane. The distance from a line to the data points is measured by adding the squares of the vertical distances from each point to the line. The smaller this sum of squares is, the better the line fits the data. The line with the minimum sum of square distances is called the *least-squares line*, or the *regression line*. If the data is nearly linear, the least-squares line will be a good fit; otherwise it may not be. (See Figure 9.60.)

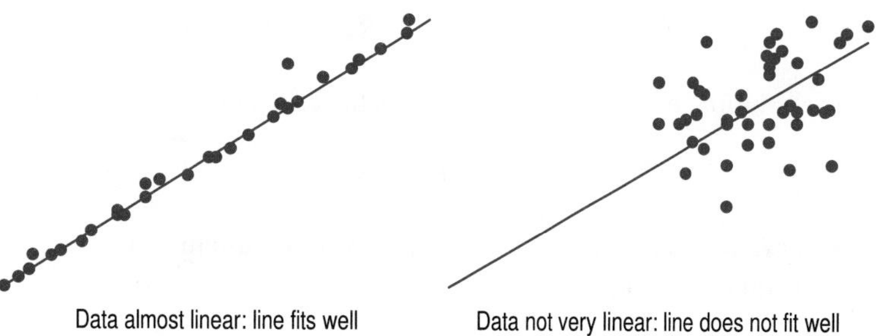

Data almost linear: line fits well
Data not very linear: line does not fit well

Figure 9.60: Fitting lines to data points

Example 1 Find a least-squares line for the following data points: $(1, 1)$, $(2, 1)$, and $(3, 3)$.

Solution Suppose the line has equation $y = b + mx$. If we find b and m then we have found the line. So, for this problem, b and m are the two variables. We want to minimize the function $f(b, m)$ that gives the sum of the three squared vertical distances from the points to the line in Figure 9.61.

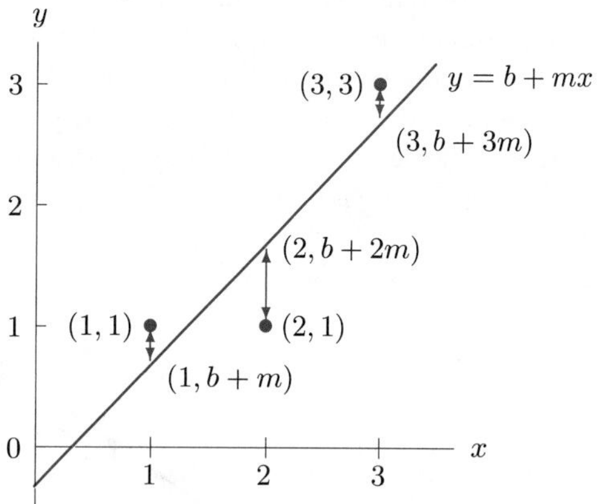

Figure 9.61: The least-squares line minimizes the sum of the squares of these vertical distances

The vertical distance from the point $(1, 1)$ to the line is the difference in the y-coordinates $1 - (b + m)$; similarly for the other points. Thus, the sum of squares is

$$f(b, m) = (1 - (b + m))^2 + (1 - (b + 2m))^2 + (3 - (b + 3m))^2.$$

To minimize f we look for critical points. First we differentiate f with respect to b:

$$\begin{aligned} f_b(b,m) &= -2(1-(b+m)) - 2(1-(b+2m)) - 2(3-(b+3m)) \\ &= -2+2b+2m-2+2b+4m-6+2b+6m \\ &= -10+6b+12m. \end{aligned}$$

Now we differentiate with respect to m:

$$\begin{aligned} f_m(b,m) &= 2(1-(b+m))(-1) + 2(1-(b+2m))(-2) + 2(3-(b+3m))(-3) \\ &= -2+2b+2m-4+4b+8m-18+6b+18m \\ &= -24+12b+28m. \end{aligned}$$

The equations $f_b = 0$ and $f_m = 0$ give a system of two linear equations in two unknowns:

$$\begin{aligned} -10+6b+12m &= 0, \\ -24+12b+28m &= 0. \end{aligned}$$

The solution to this pair of equations is the critical point $b = -1/3$ and $m = 1$. Since

$$D = f_{bb}f_{mm} - (f_{mb})^2 = (6)(28) - 12^2 = 24 \quad \text{and} \quad f_{bb} = 6 > 0,$$

we have found a local minimum. This local minimum is also the global minimum of f. Thus, the least squares line is

$$y = x - \frac{1}{3}.$$

As a check, notice that the line $y = x$ passes through the points $(1,1)$ and $(3,3)$. It is reasonable that introducing the point $(2,1)$ moves the y-intercept down from 0 to $-1/3$.

Derivation of the Formulas for the Regression Line

We use the method of Example 1 to derive the formulas for the least-squares line $y = b + mx$ generated by data points (x_1, y_1), (x_2, y_2), …, (x_n, y_n). Notice that we are looking for the slope and y-intercept, so we think of m and b as the variables.

For each data point (x_i, y_i), the corresponding point directly above the line or below it on the line has the y-coordinate $b + mx_i$. Thus, the squares of the vertical distances from the point to the line is $(y_i - (b + mx_i))^2$. (See Figure 9.62.)

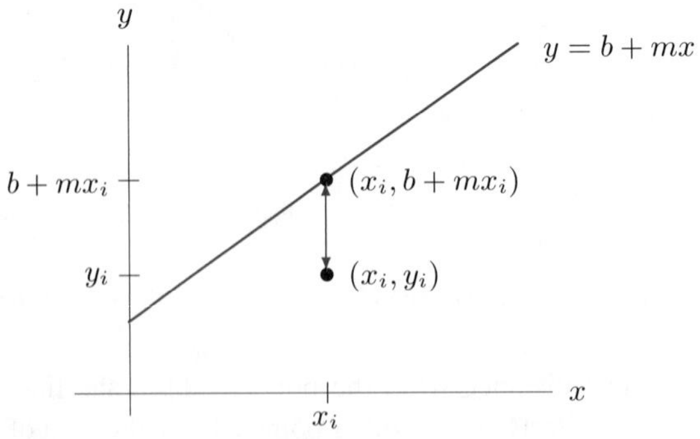

Figure 9.62: The vertical distance from a point to the line

We find the sum of the n squared distances from points to the line, and think of the sum as a function of m and b:

$$f(b,m)=\sum_{i=1}^{n}(y_i-(b+mx_i))^2.$$

To minimize this function, we first find the two partial derivatives, f_b and f_m. We use the chain rule and the properties of sums.

$$\begin{aligned}
f_b(b,m) &= \frac{\partial}{\partial b}\left(\sum_{i=1}^{n}(y_i-(b+mx_i))^2\right)=\sum_{i=1}^{n}\frac{\partial}{\partial b}(y_i-(b+mx_i))^2\\
&=\sum_{i=1}^{n}2(y_i-(b+mx_i))\cdot\frac{\partial}{\partial b}(y_i-(b+mx_i))\\
&=\sum_{i=1}^{n}2(y_i-(b+mx_i))\cdot(-1)\\
&=-2\sum_{i=1}^{n}(y_i-(b+mx_i))
\end{aligned}$$

$$\begin{aligned}
f_m(b,m) &= \frac{\partial}{\partial m}\left(\sum_{i=1}^{n}(y_i-(b+mx_i))^2\right)=\sum_{i=1}^{n}\frac{\partial}{\partial m}(y_i-(b+mx_i))^2\\
&=\sum_{i=1}^{n}2(y_i-(b+mx_i))\cdot\frac{\partial}{\partial m}(y_i-(b+mx_i))\\
&=\sum_{i=1}^{n}2(y_i-(b+mx_i))\cdot(-x_i)\\
&=-2\sum_{i=1}^{n}(y_i-(b+mx_i))\cdot x_i
\end{aligned}$$

We now set the partial derivatives equal to zero and solve for m and b. This is easier than it looks: we simplify the appearance of the equations by temporarily substituting other symbols for the sums: write SY for $\sum y_i$, SX for $\sum x_i$, SXY for $\sum y_i x_i$ and SXX for $\sum x_i^2$. Remember, the x_i and y_i are all constants. We get a pair of simultaneous linear equations in m and b; solving for m and b gives us formulas in terms of SX, SY, SXY, and SXX. We separate $f_b(b,m)$ into three sums as shown:

$$f_b(b,m)=-2\left(\sum_{i=1}^{n}y_i-b\sum_{i=1}^{n}1-m\sum_{i=1}^{n}x_i\right).$$

Similarly, we can separate $f_m(b,m)$ after multiplying through by x_i:

$$f_m(b,m)=-2\left(\sum_{i=1}^{n}y_ix_i-b\sum_{i=1}^{n}x_i-m\sum_{i=1}^{n}x_i^2\right).$$

Rewriting the sums as suggested and setting $\frac{\partial f}{\partial b}$ and $\frac{\partial f}{\partial m}$ equal to zero, we have:

$$\begin{aligned}
0 &= SY-bn-mSX\\
0 &= SYX-bSX-mSXX
\end{aligned}$$

Solving this pair of simultaneous equations, we get the result:

$$\begin{aligned}
b &= ((SXX)\cdot(SY)-(SX)\cdot(SYX))/(n(SXX)-(SX)^2)\\
m &= (n(SYX)-(SX)\cdot(SY))/(n(SXX)-(SX)^2)
\end{aligned}$$

Writing these expressions with summation notation, we arrive at the following result:

The least-squares line for data points (x_1, y_1), (x_2, y_2), $\cdots$, (x_n, y_n) is the line $y = b + mx$ where

$$b = \left(\sum_{i=1}^{n} x_i^2 \sum_{i=1}^{n} y_i - \sum_{i=1}^{n} x_i \sum_{i=1}^{n} y_i x_i\right) \Big/ \left(n \sum_{i=1}^{n} x_i^2 - \left(\sum_{i=1}^{n} x_i\right)^2\right)$$

$$m = \left(n \sum_{i=1}^{n} y_i x_i - \sum_{i=1}^{n} x_i \sum_{i=1}^{n} y_i\right) \Big/ \left(n \sum_{i=1}^{n} x_i^2 - \left(\sum_{i=1}^{n} x_i\right)^2\right).$$

Example 2 Use these formulas to find the best fitting line for the data point $(1, 5)$, $(2, 4)$, $(4, 3)$.

Solution We compute the sums needed in the formulas:

$$\sum_{i=1}^{3} x_i = 1 + 2 + 4 = 7$$

$$\sum_{i=1}^{3} y_i = 5 + 4 + 3 = 12$$

$$\sum_{i=1}^{3} x_i^2 = 1^2 + 2^2 + 4^2 = 1 + 4 + 16 = 21$$

$$\sum_{i=1}^{3} y_i x_i = (5)(1) + (4)(2) + (3)(4) = 5 + 8 + 12 = 25.$$

Since $n = 3$, we have:

$$\begin{aligned} b &= \left(\sum_{i=1}^{3} x_i^2 \sum_{i=1}^{3} y_i - \sum_{i=1}^{3} x_i \sum_{i=1}^{3} y_i x_i\right) \Big/ \left(3 \sum_{i=1}^{3} x_i^2 - \left(\sum_{i=1}^{3} x_i\right)^2\right) \\ &= ((21)(12) - (7)(25)) \,/\, (3(21) - (7^2)) \\ &= 77/14 = 5.5 \end{aligned}$$

and

$$\begin{aligned} m &= \left(3 \sum_{i=1}^{3} y_i x_i - \sum_{i=1}^{3} x_i \sum_{i=1}^{3} y_i\right) \Big/ \left(3 \sum_{i=1}^{3} x_i^2 - \left(\sum_{i=1}^{3} x_i\right)^2\right) \\ &= (3(25) - (7)(12)) \,/\, (3(21) - (7^2)) \\ &= -9/14 = -0.64. \end{aligned}$$

The least-squares line for these three points is

$$y = 5.5 - 0.64x.$$

To check this equation, plot the line and the three points together.

Many calculators have the formulas for the least-squares line built in, so that when you enter the data, out come the values of b and m. At the same time, you get the *correlation coefficient*, which measures how close the data points actually come to fitting the least-squares line.

Problems on Deriving the Formula for Regression Lines

In Problems 1–2, use the method of Example 1 to find the least-squares line. Check by graphing the points with the line.

1. $(-1,2)$, $(0,-1)$, $(1,1)$ **2.** $(0,2)$, $(1,4)$, $(2,5)$

In Problems 3–5, use the formulas for b and m to check that you get the same result as in the problem or example specified.

3. $(-1,2)$, $(0,-1)$, $(1,1)$. See Problem 1.

4. $(0,2)$, $(1,4)$, $(2,5)$. See Problem 2.

5. $(1,1)$, $(2,1)$, $(3,3)$. See Example 1.

In Problems 6–7, we transform nonlinear data so that it looks more linear. For example, suppose the data points (x, y) fit the exponential equation,

$$y = Ce^{ax},$$

where a and C are constants. Taking the natural log of both sides, we get

$$\ln y = ax + \ln C.$$

Thus, $\ln y$ is a linear function of x. To find a and C, we can use least squares for the graph of $\ln y$ against x.

6. The population of the US was about 180 million in 1960, grew to 206 million in 1970, and 226 million in 1980.

(a) Assuming that the population was growing exponentially, use logarithms and the method of least squares to estimate the population in 1990.

(b) According to the national census, the 1990 population was 249 million. What does this say about the assumption of exponential growth?

(c) Predict the population in the year 2010.

7. A biological rule of thumb states that as the area A of an island increases tenfold, the number of animal species, N, living on it doubles. The table contains data for islands in the West Indies. Assume that N is a power function of A.

(a) Use the biological rule of thumb to find

(i) N as a function of A

(ii) $\ln N$ as a function of $\ln A$

(b) Using the data given, tabulate $\ln N$ against $\ln A$ and find the line of best fit. Does your answer agree with the biological rule of thumb?

Island	Area (sq km)	Number of species
Redonda	3	5
Saba	20	9
Montserrat	192	15
Puerto Rico	8858	75
Jamaica	10854	70
Hispaniola	75571	130
Cuba	113715	125

Problems on Deriving the Formula for Regression Lines

Chapter Ten

MATHEMATICAL MODELING USING DIFFERENTIAL EQUATIONS

Contents

10.1 MATHEMATICAL MODELING: SETTING UP A DIFFERENTIAL EQUATION

Sometimes we do not know a key function, but we do have information about its rate of change, or its derivative. Then we may be able to write a new type of equation, called a *differential equation*, from which we can get information about the original function. For example, we may use what we know about the derivative of a population function (its rate of change) to predict the population in the future.

In this section, we use a verbal description to write a differential equation.

Marine Harvesting

We begin by investigating the effect of fishing on a fish population. Suppose that, left alone, a fish population increases at a continuous rate of 20% per year. Suppose that fish are also being harvested (caught) by fishermen at a constant rate of 10 million fish per year. How does the fish population change over time?

Notice that we have been given information about the rate of change, or derivative, of the fish population. Combined with information about the initial population, we can use this to predict the population in the future. We know that

$$\begin{array}{c}\text{Rate of change}\\ \text{of fish population}\end{array} = \begin{array}{c}\text{Rate of increase}\\ \text{due to breeding}\end{array} - \begin{array}{c}\text{Rate fish removed}\\ \text{due to harvesting}\end{array}.$$

Suppose the fish population, in millions, is P and its derivative is dP/dt, where t is time in years. If left alone, the fish population increases at a continuous rate of 20% per year, so we have

$$\begin{aligned}\text{Rate of increase due to breeding} &= 20\% \cdot \text{Current population}\\ &= 0.20P \text{ million fish/year.}\end{aligned}$$

In addition,

$$\text{Rate fish removed by harvesting} = 10 \text{ million fish/year.}$$

Since the rate of change of the fish population is dP/dt, we have

$$\frac{dP}{dt} = 0.20P - 10.$$

This is a differential equation that models how the fish population changes. The unknown quantity in the equation is the function giving P in terms of t.

Net Worth of a Company

A company earns revenue (income) and also makes payroll payments. Assume that revenue is earned continuously, that payroll payments are made continuously, and that the only factors affecting net worth are revenue and payroll. The company's revenue is earned at a continuous annual rate of 5% times its net worth. At the same time, the company's payroll obligations are paid out at a constant rate of 200 million dollars a year.

We use this information to write a differential equation to model the net worth of the company, W, in millions of dollars, as a function of time, t, in years. We know that

$$\begin{array}{c}\text{Rate at which}\\ \text{net worth is changing}\end{array} = \begin{array}{c}\text{Rate revenue}\\ \text{is earned}\end{array} - \begin{array}{c}\text{Rate payroll payments}\\ \text{are made}\end{array}.$$

Since the company's revenue is earned at a rate of 5% of its net worth, we have

$$\text{Rate revenue is earned} = 5\% \cdot \text{Net worth} = 0.05W \text{ million dollars/year.}$$

Since payroll payments are made at a rate of 200 million dollars a year, we have

$$\text{Rate payroll payments are made} = 200 \text{ million dollars/year.}$$

Putting these two together, since the rate at which net worth is changing is dW/dt, we have

$$\frac{dW}{dt} = 0.05W - 200.$$

This is a differential equation that models how the net worth of the company changes. The unknown quantity in the equation is the function giving net worth W as a function of time t.

Pollution in a Lake

If clean water flows into a polluted lake and a stream takes water out, the level of pollution in the lake will decrease (assuming no new pollutants are added).

Example 1 The quantity of pollutant in the lake decreases at a rate proportional to the quantity present. Write a differential equation to model the quantity of pollutant in the lake. Is the constant of proportionality positive or negative? Use the differential equation to explain why the graph of the quantity of pollutant against time is decreasing and concave up, as in Figure 10.1.

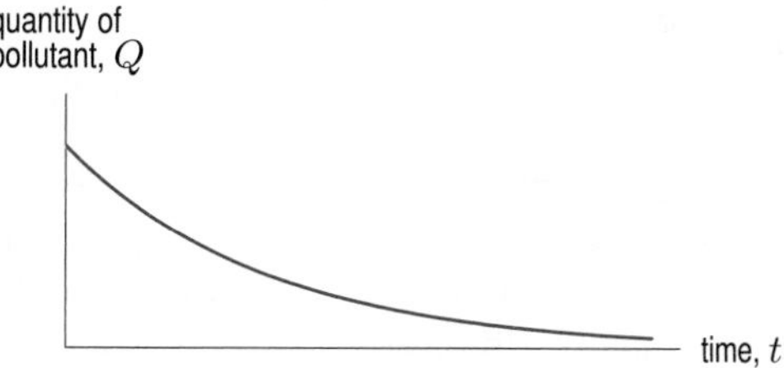

Figure 10.1: Quantity of pollutant in a lake

Solution Let Q denote the quantity of pollutant present in the lake at time t. The rate of change of Q is proportional to Q, so dQ/dt is proportional to Q. Thus, the differential equation is

$$\frac{dQ}{dt} = kQ.$$

Since no new pollutants are being added to the lake, the quantity Q is decreasing over time, so dQ/dt is negative. Thus, the constant of proportionality k is negative.

Why does the differential equation $dQ/dt = kQ$, with k negative, give us the graph shown in Figure 10.1? Since k is negative and Q is positive, we know kQ is negative. Thus, dQ/dt is negative, so the graph of Q against t is decreasing as in Figure 10.1. Why is it concave up? Since Q is getting smaller and k is fixed, as t increases, the product kQ is getting smaller in magnitude, and so the derivative dQ/dt is getting smaller in magnitude. Thus, the graph of Q is more horizontal as t increases. Therefore, the graph is concave up. See Figure 10.1.

The Quantity of a Drug in the Body

In the previous example, the rate at which pollutants leave a lake is proportional to the quantity of pollutants in the lake. This model works for any contaminants flowing in or out of a fluid system with complete mixing. Another example is the quantity of a drug in a person's body.

Example 2 A patient having major surgery is given the antibiotic vancomycin intravenously at a rate of 85 mg per hour. The rate at which the drug is excreted from the body is proportional to the quantity present, with proportionality constant 0.1 if time is in hours. Write a differential equation for the quantity, Q in mg, of vancomycin in the body after t hours.

Solution The quantity of vancomycin, Q, is increasing at a constant rate of 85 mg/hour and is decreasing at a rate of 0.1 times Q. The administration of 85 mg/hour makes a positive contribution to the rate of change dQ/dt. The excretion at a rate of $0.1Q$ makes a negative contribution to dQ/dt. Putting these together, we have

$$\text{Rate of change of a quantity} = \text{Rate in} - \text{Rate out},$$

so

$$\frac{dQ}{dt} = 85 - 0.1Q.$$

The Logistic Model

A population in a confined space grows proportionally to the product of the current population, P, and the difference between the *carrying capacity*, L, and the current population. (The carrying capacity is the maximum population the environment can sustain.) We use this information to write a differential equation for the population P.

The rate of change of P is proportional to the product of P and $L - P$, so

$$\frac{dP}{dt} = kP(L - P), \qquad \text{where } k \text{ is the constant of proportionality.}$$

This is called a *logistic differential equation.* What does it tell us about the graph of P? The derivative dP/dt is the product of k and P and $L - P$, so when P is small, the derivative dP/dt is small and the population grows slowly. As P increases, the derivative dP/dt increases and the population grows more rapidly. However, as P approaches the carrying capacity L, the term $L - P$ is small, and dP/dt is again small and the population grows more slowly. The *logistic growth curve* in Figure 10.2 satisfies these conditions.

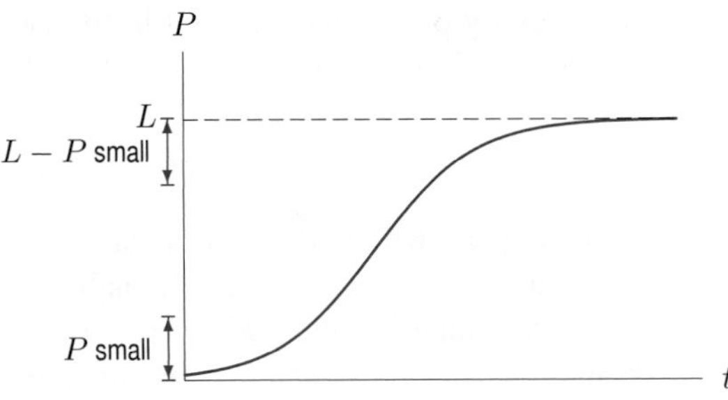

Figure 10.2: The logistic growth curve is a solution to $dP/dt = kP(L - P)$

Problems for Section 10.1

1. Match the graphs in Figure 10.3 with the following descriptions.

(a) The temperature of a glass of ice water left on the kitchen table.

(b) The amount of money in an interest-bearing bank account into which \$50 is deposited.

(c) The speed of a constantly decelerating car.

(d) The temperature of a piece of steel heated in a furnace and left outside to cool.

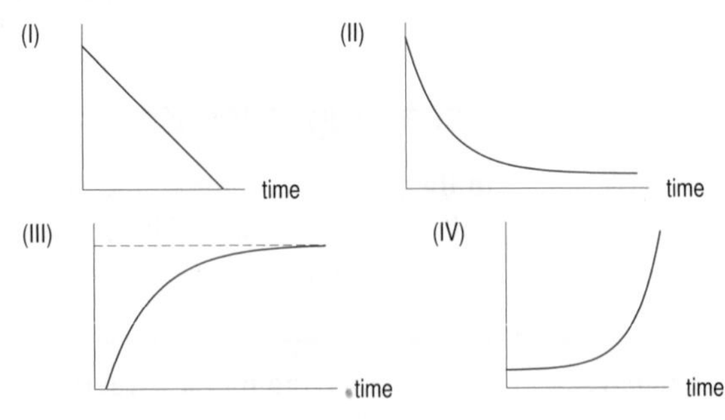

Figure 10.3

2. The graphs in Figure 10.4 represent the temperature, $H(^\circ\text{C})$, of four eggs as a function of time, t, in minutes. Match three of the graphs with the descriptions (a)–(c). Write a similar description for the fourth graph, including an interpretation of any intercepts and asymptotes.

   (a) An egg is taken out of the refrigerator (just above 0°C) and put into boiling water.
   (b) Twenty minutes after the egg in part (a) is taken out of the fridge and put into boiling water, the same thing is done with another egg.
   (c) An egg is taken out of the refrigerator at the same time as the egg in part (a) and left to sit on the kitchen table.

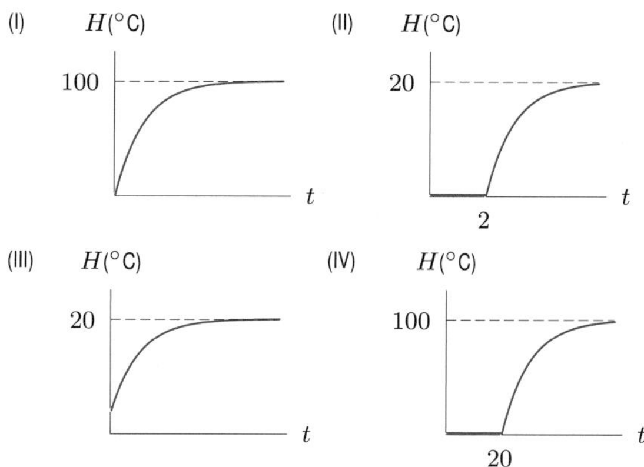

Figure 10.4

3. A population of insects grows at a rate proportional to the size of the population. Write a differential equation for the size of the population, P, as a function of time, t. Is the constant of proportionality positive or negative?

4. Money in a bank account earns interest at a continuous annual rate of 5% times the current balance. Write a differential equation for the balance, B, in the account as a function of time, t, in years.

5. Radioactive substances decay at a rate proportional to the quantity present. Write a differential equation for the quantity, Q, of a radioactive substance present at time t. Is the constant of proportionality positive or negative?

6. A bank account that initially contains \$25,000 earns interest at a continuous rate of 4% per year. Withdrawals are made out of the account at a constant rate of \$2000 per year. Write a differential equation for the balance, B, in the account as a function of the number of years, t.

7. A pollutant spilled on the ground decays at a rate of 8% a day. In addition, clean-up crews remove the pollutant at a rate of 30 gallons a day. Write a differential equation for the amount of pollutant, P, in gallons, left after t days.

8. Morphine is administered to a patient intravenously at a rate of 2.5 mg per hour. About 34.7% of the morphine is metabolized and leaves the body each hour. Write a differential equation for the amount of morphine, M, in milligrams, in the body as a function of time, t, in hours.

9. Alcohol is metabolized and excreted from the body at a rate of about one ounce of alcohol every hour. If some alcohol is consumed, write a differential equation for the amount of alcohol, A (in ounces), remaining in the body as a function of t, the number of hours since the alcohol was consumed.

10. Toxins in pesticides can get into the food chain and accumulate in the body. A person consumes 10 micrograms a day of a toxin, ingested throughout the day. The toxin leaves the body at a continuous rate of 3% every day. Write a differential equation for the amount of toxin, A, in micrograms, in the person's body as a function of the number of days, t.

11. A cup of coffee contains about 100 mg of caffeine. Caffeine is metabolized and leaves the body at a continuous rate of about 17% every hour.

    (a) Write a differential equation for the amount, A, of caffeine in the body as a function of the number of hours, t, since the coffee was consumed.
    (b) Use the differential equation to find dA/dt at the start of the first hour (right after the coffee is consumed). Use your answer to estimate the change in the amount of caffeine during the first hour.

12. A person deposits money into an account at a continuous rate of \$6000 a year, and the account earns interest at a continuous rate of 7% per year.

    (a) Write a differential equation for the balance in the account, B, in dollars, as a function of years, t.
    (b) Use the differential equation to calculate dB/dt if $B = 10{,}000$ and if $B = 100{,}000$. Interpret your answers.

13. A quantity W satisfies the differential equation

$$\frac{dW}{dt} = 5W - 20.$$

    (a) Is W increasing or decreasing at $W = 10$? $W = 2$?
    (b) For what values of W is the rate of change of W equal to zero?

14. A quantity y satisfies the differential equation

$$\frac{dy}{dt} = -0.5y.$$

    Under what conditions is y increasing? Decreasing?

15. An early model of the growth of the Wikipedia assumed that every day a constant number, B, of articles are added by dedicated wikipedians and that other articles are created by the general public at a rate proportional to the number of articles already there. Express this model as a differential equation for $N(t)$, the total number of Wikipedia articles t days after January 1, 2001.

16. A country's infrastructure is its transportation and communication systems, power plants, and other public institutions. The Solow model asserts that the value of national infrastructure K increases due to investment and decreases due to capital depreciation. The rate of increase due to investment is proportional to national income, Y. The rate of decrease due to depreciation is proportional to the value of existing infrastructure. Write a differential equation for K.

10.2 SOLUTIONS OF DIFFERENTIAL EQUATIONS

What does it mean to "solve" a differential equation? A differential equation is an equation involving the derivative of an unknown function. The unknown is not a number but a function. A *solution* to a differential equation is any function that satisfies the differential equation.

In this section, we see how to solve a differential equation numerically and how to check whether or not a function is a solution to a differential equation. In the next section, we see how to visualize a solution.

Another Look at Marine Harvesting

Let's take another look at the fish population discussed in Section 10.1. Left alone, the population increases at a continuous rate of 20% per year. The fish are being harvested at a constant rate of 10 million fish per year. If P is the fish population, in millions, in year t, then we have

$$\frac{dP}{dt} = 0.20P - 10.$$

Solving this differential equation means to find a function giving P in terms of t. Combined with information about the initial population, we can use the equation to predict the population at any time in the future.

Solving the Differential Equation Numerically

Suppose at time $t = 0$, the fish population is 60 million. We can substitute $P = 60$ into the differential equation to compute the derivative, dP/dt:

$$\text{At time } t = 0, \qquad \frac{dP}{dt} = 0.20P - 10 = 0.20(60) - 10 = 12 - 10 = 2.$$

Since at $t = 0$, the fish population is changing at a rate of 2 million fish a year, at the end of the first year, the fish population will have increased by about 2 million fish. So:

$$\text{At } t = 1, \qquad \text{we estimate} \quad P = 60 + 2 = 62.$$

We use this new value of P to estimate dP/dt during the second year:

$$\text{At time } t = 1, \qquad \frac{dP}{dt} = 0.20P - 10 = 12.4 - 10 = 2.4.$$

During the second year, the fish population increased by about 2.4 million fish, so:

$$\text{At } t = 2, \qquad \text{we estimate} \quad P = 62 + 2.4 = 64.4.$$

We use this value of P to estimate the rate of change during the third year, and so on. Continuing in this fashion, we compute the approximate values of P in Table 10.1. This table gives approximate numerical values for P at future times.

Table 10.1 *Approximate values of the fish population as a function of time*

t (years)	0	1	2	3	4	5	...
P (millions)	60	62	64.4	67.28	70.74	74.89	...

A Formula for the Solution to the Differential Equation

A function $P = f(t)$ which satisfies the differential equation

$$\frac{dP}{dt} = 0.20P - 10$$

is called a *solution* of the differential equation. Table 10.1 shows approximate numerical values of a solution. It is sometimes (but not always) possible to find a formula for the solution. In this particular case, there is a formula; it is

$$P = 50 + Ce^{0.20t}, \qquad \text{where } C \text{ is any constant.}$$

We check that this is a solution to the differential equation by substituting it into the left and right sides of the differential equation separately. We find

$$\begin{aligned} \text{Left side} &= \frac{dP}{dt} = 0.20Ce^{0.20t} \\ \text{Right side} &= 0.20P - 10 = 0.20(50 + Ce^{0.20t}) - 10 \\ &= 10 + 0.20Ce^{0.20t} - 10 \\ &= 0.20Ce^{0.20t}. \end{aligned}$$

Since we get the same expression on both sides, we say that $P = 50 + Ce^{0.20t}$ is a solution of this differential equation. Any choice of C works, so the solutions form a family of functions with parameter C. Several members of the family of solutions are graphed in Figure 10.5.

Finding the Arbitrary Constant: Initial Conditions

To find a value for the constant C—in other words, to select a single solution from the family of solutions—we need an additional piece of information, usually the initial population. In this case, we know that $P = 60$ when $t = 0$, so substituting into

$$P = 50 + Ce^{0.20t}$$

gives

$$\begin{aligned} 60 &= 50 + Ce^{0.20(0)} \\ 60 &= 50 + C \cdot 1 \\ C &= 10. \end{aligned}$$

The function $P = 50 + 10e^{0.20t}$ satisfies the differential equation *and* the initial condition that $P = 60$ when $t = 0$.

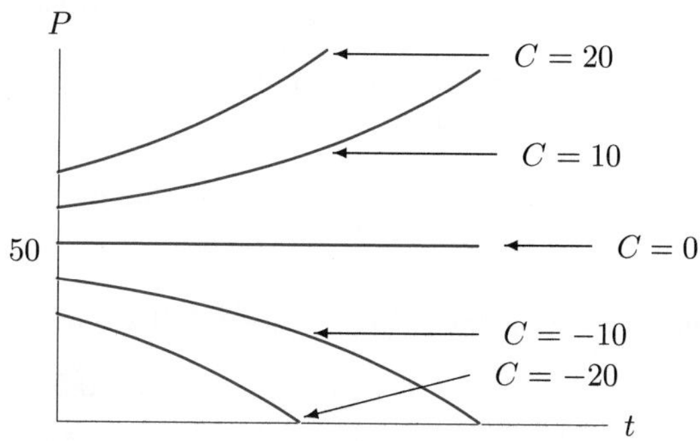

Figure 10.5: Solution curves for $dP/dt = 0.20P - 10$: Members of the family $P = 50 + Ce^{0.20t}$

General Solutions and Particular Solutions

For the differential equation $dP/dt = 0.20P - 10$, it can be shown that every solution is of the form $P = 50 + Ce^{0.20t}$ for some value of C. We say that the *general solution* of the differential equation $dP/dt = 0.20P - 10$ is the family of functions $P = 50 + Ce^{0.20t}$. The solution $P = 50 + 10e^{0.20t}$ that satisfies the differential equation together with the initial condition that $P = 60$ when $t = 0$ is calld a *particular solution*. The differential equation and the initial condition together are called an *initial-value problem.*

Example 1 (a) Check that $P = Ce^{2t}$ is a solution to the differential equation

$$\frac{dP}{dt} = 2P.$$

(b) Find the particular solution satisfying the initial condition $P = 100$ when $t = 0$.

Solution (a) Since $P = Ce^{2t}$ where C is a constant, we find expressions for each side:

$$\text{Left side} = \frac{dP}{dt} = Ce^{2t} \cdot 2 = 2Ce^{2t}$$
$$\text{Right side} = 2P = 2Ce^{2t}.$$

Since the two expressions are equal, $P = Ce^{2t}$ is a solution to the differential equation.

(b) We substitute $P = 100$ and $t = 0$ into the general solution $P = Ce^{2t}$, and solve for C:

$$100 = Ce^{2(0)}$$
$$100 = C \cdot 1$$
$$100 = C.$$

The particular solution for this initial-value problem is $P = 100e^{2t}$.

Example 2 Decide whether or not $y = e^{-2x}$ is a solution of the differential equation $y' - 2y = 0$.

Solution Note that $y' = dy/dx$. Differentiating $y = e^{-2x}$ gives $y' = -2e^{-2x}$. Substituting, we have

$$y' - 2y = -2e^{-2x} - 2e^{-2x} = -4e^{-2x} \neq 0,$$

and so $y = e^{-2x}$ is not a solution to this differential equation.

Example 3 (a) What conditions must be imposed on the constants C and k if $y = Ce^{kt}$ is a solution to the differential equation

$$\frac{dy}{dt} = -0.5y?$$

(b) What additional conditions must be imposed on C and k if $y = Ce^{kt}$ also satisfies the initial condition that $y = 10$ when $t = 0$?

Solution (a) If $y = Ce^{kt}$, then $dy/dt = Cke^{kt}$. Substituting into the equation $dy/dt = -0.5y$ gives

$$Cke^{kt} = -0.5(Ce^{kt}),$$

and therefore, assuming $C \neq 0$, so $Ce^{kt} \neq 0$, we have

$$k = -0.5.$$

So $y = Ce^{-0.5t}$ is a solution to the differential equation. If $C = 0$, then $Ce^{kt} = 0$ is a solution to the differential equation. No conditions are imposed on C.

(b) Since $k = -0.5$, we have $y = Ce^{-0.5t}$. Substituting $y = 10$ when $t = 0$ gives

$$10 = Ce^0$$

so

$$10 = C.$$

So $y = 10e^{-0.5t}$ is a solution to the differential equation together with the initial condition.

Problems for Section 10.2

1. Find the general solution to the differential equation

$$\frac{dy}{dt} = 2t.$$

2. Decide whether or not each of the following is a solution to the differential equation $xy' - 2y = 0$.

(a) $y = x^2$ **(b)** $y = x^3$

3. Check that $y = t^4$ is a solution to the differential equation $t\dfrac{dy}{dt} = 4y$.

In Problems 4–12, use the fact that the derivative gives the slope of a curve to decide which of the graphs (A)–(F) in Figure 10.6 could represent a solution to the differential equation.

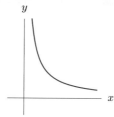

(A)

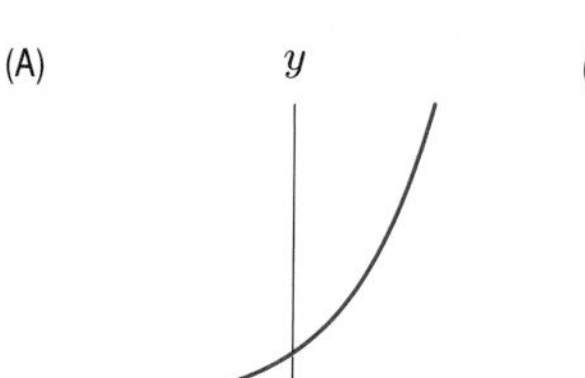

(B) y x

(C)

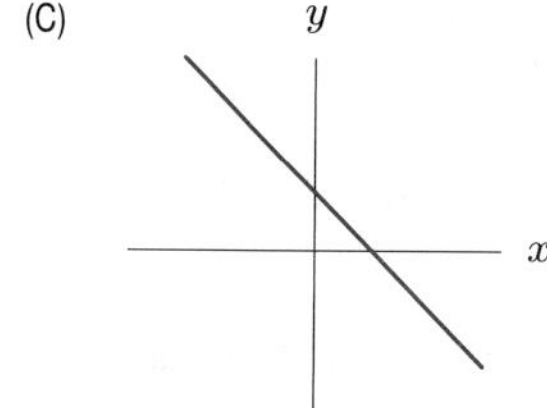

(D)

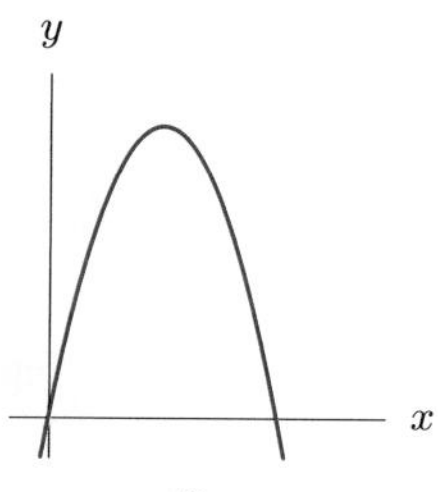

(E)

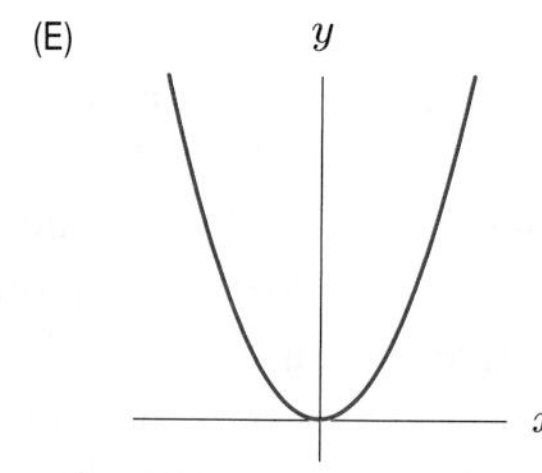

(F)

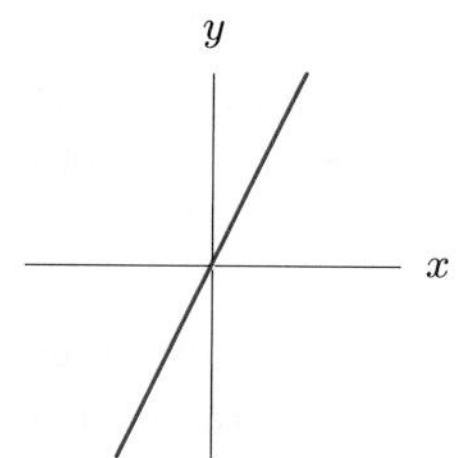

Figure 10.6

4. $\dfrac{dy}{dx} = -1$ **5.** $\dfrac{dy}{dx} = 0.1$ **6.** $\dfrac{dy}{dx} = -y^2$

7. $\dfrac{dy}{dx} = 2x$ **8.** $\dfrac{dy}{dx} = 2$ **9.** $\dfrac{dy}{dx} = y$

10. $\dfrac{dy}{dx} = -\dfrac{1}{x^2}$ **11.** $\dfrac{dy}{dx} = 1 - x$ **12.** $\dfrac{dy}{dx} = 2y$

13. Fill in the missing values in Table 10.2 given that $dy/dt = 0.5t$. Assume the rate of growth, given by dy/dt, is approximately constant over each unit time interval.

Table 10.2

t	0	1	2	3	4
y	8				

14. Fill in the missing values in Table 10.3 given that $dy/dt = 0.5y$. Assume the rate of growth, given by dy/dt, is approximately constant over each unit time interval.

Table 10.3

t	0	1	2	3	4
y	8				

15. Fill in the missing values in Table 10.4 given that $dy/dt = 4 - y$. Assume the rate of growth, given by dy/dt, is approximately constant over each unit time interval.

Table 10.4

t	0	1	2	3	4
y	8				

16. For a certain quantity y, assume that $dy/dt = \sqrt{y}$. Fill in the value of y in Table 10.5. Assume that the rate of growth, dy/dt, is approximately constant over each unit time interval and that the initial value of y is 100.

Table 10.5

t	0	1	2	3	4
y	100				

17. If the initial population of fish is 70 million, use the differential equation $dP/dt = 0.2P - 10$ to estimate the fish population after 1, 2, 3 years.

18. Show that, for any constant P_0, the function $P = P_0 e^t$ satisfies the equation

$$\frac{dP}{dt} = P.$$

19. Suppose $Q = Ce^{kt}$ satisfies the differential equation

$$\frac{dQ}{dt} = -0.03Q.$$

What (if anything) does this tell you about the values of C and k?

20. Is there a value of n which makes $y = x^n$ a solution to the equation $13x(dy/dx) = y$? If so, what value?

21. Find the values of k for which $y = x^2 + k$ is a solution to the differential equation $2y - xy' = 10$.

22. Match solutions and differential equations. (Note: Each equation may have more than one solution, or no solution.)

(a) $\dfrac{dy}{dx} = \dfrac{y}{x}$ (I) $y = x^3$

(b) $\dfrac{dy}{dx} = 3\dfrac{y}{x}$ (II) $y = 3x$

(c) $\dfrac{dy}{dx} = 3x$ (III) $y = e^{3x}$

(d) $\dfrac{dy}{dx} = y$ (IV) $y = 3e^x$

(e) $\dfrac{dy}{dx} = 3y$ (V) $y = x$

10.3 SLOPE FIELDS

In this section, we see how to visualize a differential equation and its solutions. Let's start with the equation

$$\frac{dy}{dx} = y.$$

Any solution to this differential equation has the property that at any point in the plane, the slope of its graph is equal to its y coordinate. (That's what the equation $dy/dx = y$ is telling us!) This means that if the solution goes through the point $(0, 1)$, its slope there is 1; if it goes through a point with $y = 4$ its slope is 4. A solution going through $(0, 2)$ has slope 2 there; at the point where $y = 8$ the slope of this solution is 8. (See Figure 10.7.)

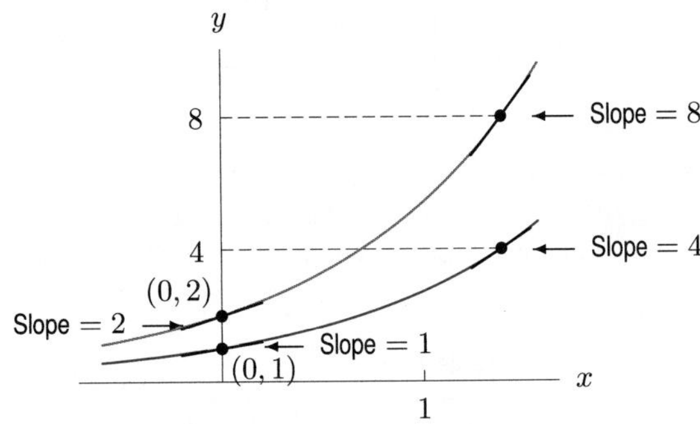

Figure 10.7: Solutions to $\frac{dy}{dx} = y$

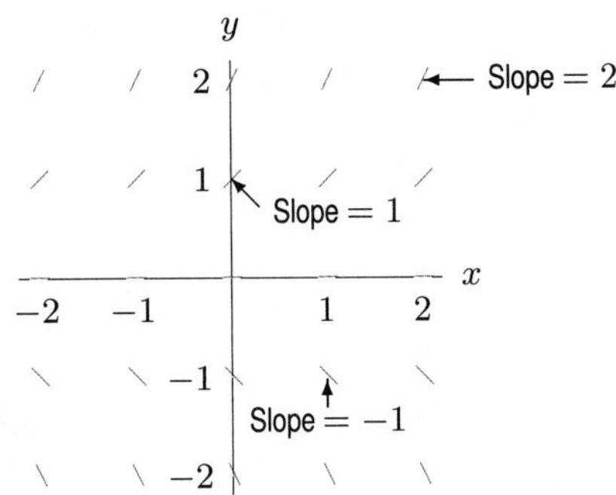

Figure 10.8: Visualizing the slope of y, if $\frac{dy}{dx} = y$

In Figure 10.8 a small line segment is drawn at the marked points showing the slope of the solution curve there. Since $dy/dx = y$, the slope at the point $(1, 2)$ is 2 (the y-coordinate), and so we draw a line segment there with slope 2. We draw a line segment at the point $(0, -1)$ with slope -1, and so on. If we draw many of these line segments, we have the *slope field* for the equation $dy/dx = y$ shown in Figure 10.9. Above the x-axis, the slopes are positive (because y is positive there), and the slopes increase as we move upward (as y increases). Below the x-axis, the slopes are negative, and get more so as we move downward. Notice that on any horizontal line (where y is constant) the slopes are constant. In the slope field you can see the ghost of the solution curve lurking. Start anywhere on the plane and move so that the slope lines are tangent to your path; you will trace out one of the solution curves. Try penciling in some solution curves on Figure 10.9, some above the x-axis and some below. The curves you draw should have the shape of exponential functions. By substituting $y = Ce^x$ into the differential equation, you can check that each curve in the family of exponentials, $y = Ce^x$, is a solution to this differential equation.

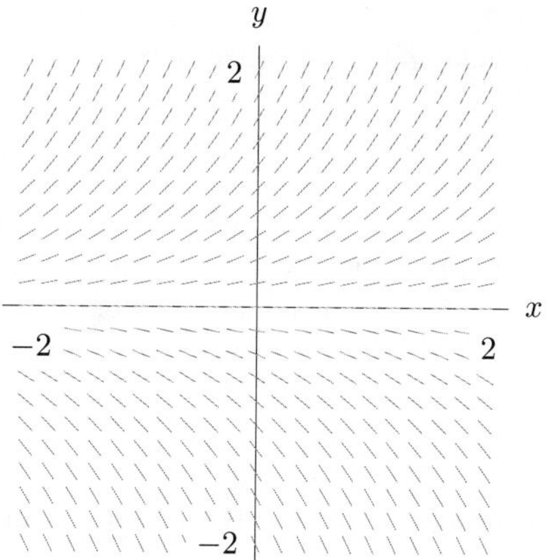

Figure 10.9: Slope field for $\frac{dy}{dx} = y$

In most problems, we are interested in getting the solution curves from the slope field. Think of the slope field as a set of signposts pointing in the direction you should go at each point. Imagine starting anywhere in the plane: look at the slope field at that point and start to move in that direction. After a small step, look at the slope field again, and alter your direction if necessary. Continue to move across the plane in the direction the slope field points, and you'll trace out a solution curve. Notice that the solution curve is not necessarily the graph of a function, and even if it is, we may not have a formula for the function. Geometrically, solving a differential equation means finding the family of solution curves.

Example 1 Figure 10.10 shows the slope field of the differential equation $\dfrac{dy}{dx} = 2x.$

(a) What do you notice about the slope field?
(b) Compare the solution curves in Figure 10.11 with the formula $y = x^2 + C$ for the solutions to this differential equation.

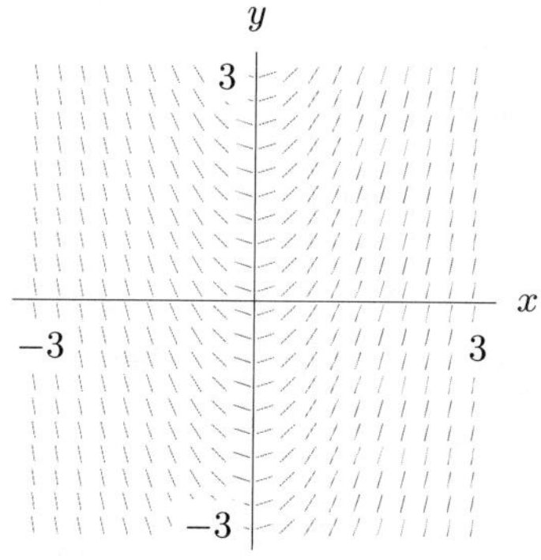

Figure 10.10: Slope field for $\frac{dy}{dx} = 2x$

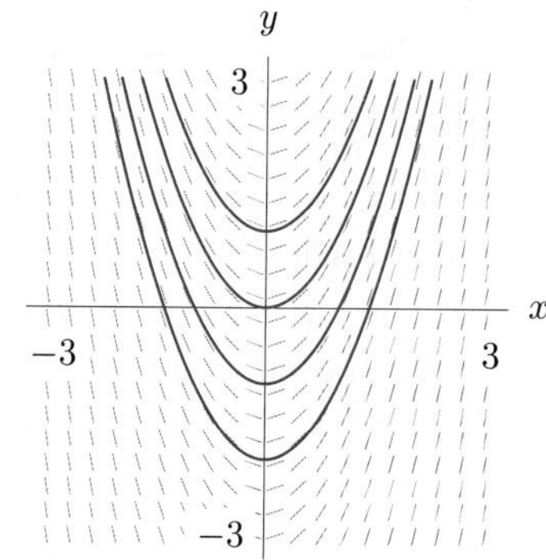

Figure 10.11: Some solutions to $\frac{dy}{dx} = 2x$

Solution

(a) In Figure 10.10, notice that on any vertical line (where x is constant) the slopes are all the same. This is because in this differential equation dy/dx depends on x only. (In the previous example, $dy/dx = y$, the slopes depended on y only.)
(b) The solution curves in Figure 10.11 look like parabolas. It is easy to check by substitution that

$$y = x^2 + C \qquad \text{is a solution to} \qquad \frac{dy}{dx} = 2x,$$

so the parabolas $y = x^2 + C$ are solution curves.

Example 2 Using the slope field, guess the equation of the solution curves of the differential equation

$$\frac{dy}{dx} = -\frac{x}{y}.$$

Solution The slope field is shown in Figure 10.12. Notice that on the y-axis, where x is 0, the slope is 0. On the x-axis, where y is 0, the line segments are vertical and the slope is undefined. At the origin the slope is undefined and there is no line segment.

What do the solution curves of this differential equation look like? The slope field suggests they are circles centered at the origin. We guess that the general solution to this differential equation is

$$x^2 + y^2 = r^2.$$

This solution is derived in the Focus on Theory section at the end of the chapter.

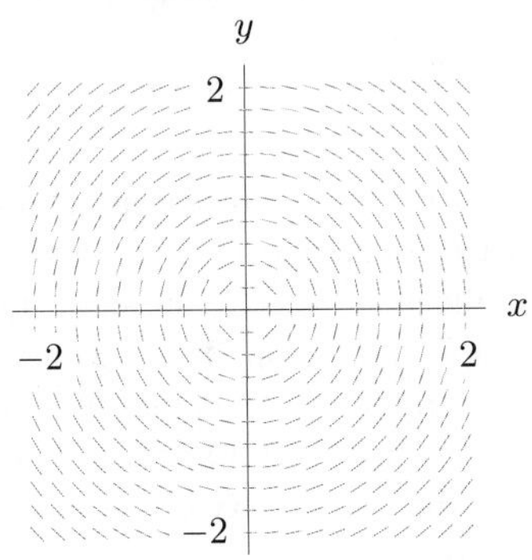

Figure 10.12: Slope field for $\frac{dy}{dx} = -\frac{x}{y}$

The previous example shows that the solutions to differential equations may sometimes be expressed as *implicit functions*. Implicit functions are ones which have not been "solved" for y; in other words, the dependent variable is not expressed as an explicit function of x.

Example 3 The slope fields for $\frac{dy}{dt} = 2 - y$ and $\frac{dy}{dt} = \frac{t}{y}$ are shown in Figure 10.13.

(a) Which slope field corresponds to which differential equation?

(b) Sketch solution curves on each slope field with initial conditions

(i) $y = 1$ when $t = 0$ (ii) $y = 3$ when $t = 0$ (iii) $y = 0$ when $t = 1$

(c) For each solution curve, can you say anything about the long-run behavior of y? In particular, as $t \to \infty$, what happens to the value of y?

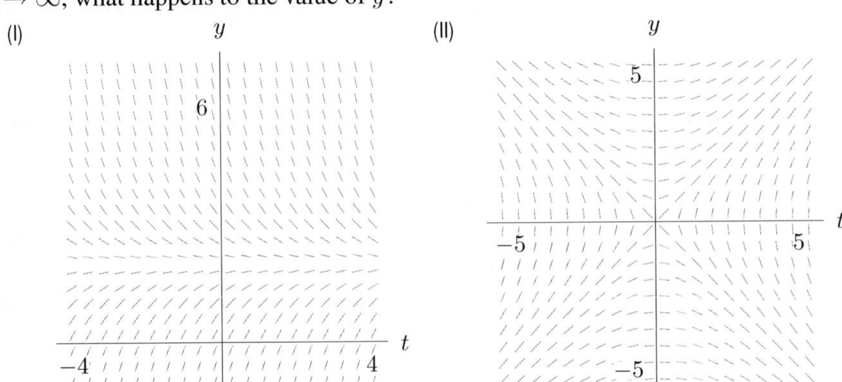

Figure 10.13: Slope fields for $\frac{dy}{dt} = 2 - y$ and $\frac{dy}{dt} = \frac{t}{y}$: Which is which?

Solution

(a) Consider the slopes at different points for the two differential equations. In particular, look at the line $y = 2$ in Figure 10.13. The equation $dy/dt = 2 - y$ has slope 0 all along this line, whereas the line $dy/dt = t/2$ has slope $t/2$. Since slope field (I) looks horizontal at $y = 2$, slope field (I) corresponds to $dy/dt = 2 - y$ and slope field (II) corresponds to $dy/dt = t/y$.

(b) The initial conditions (i) and (ii) give the value of y when t is 0, that is, the y-intercept. To draw the solution curve satisfying the condition (i), draw the solution curve with y-intercept 1. For (ii), draw the solution curve with y-intercept 3. For (iii), the solution goes through the point $(1, 0)$, so draw the solution curve passing through this point. See Figures 10.14 and 10.15.

(c) For $dy/dt = 2 - y$, all solution curves have $y = 2$ as a horizontal asymptote, so $y \to 2$ as $t \to \infty$. For $dy/dt = t/y$ with initial conditions $(0, 1)$ and $(0, 3)$, we see that $y \to \infty$ as $t \to \infty$. The graph has asymptotes which appear to be diagonal lines. In fact, they are $y = t$ and $y = -t$, so $y \to \pm\infty$ as $t \to \infty$.

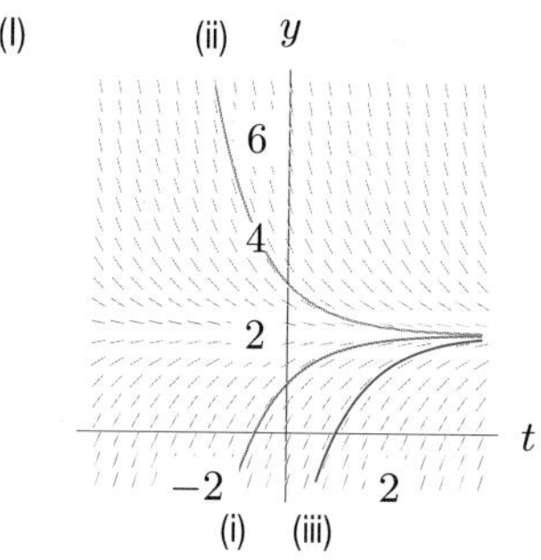

Figure 10.14: Solution curves for $\dfrac{dy}{dt} = 2 - y$

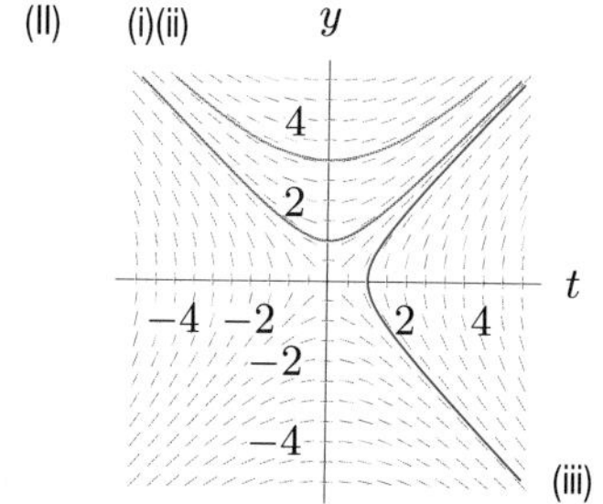

Figure 10.15: Solution curves for $\dfrac{dy}{dt} = \dfrac{t}{y}$

Existence and Uniqueness of Solutions

Since differential equations are used to model many real situations, the question of whether a solution exists and is unique can have great practical importance. If we know how the velocity of a satellite is changing, can we know its velocity for all future time? If we know the initial population of a city, and we know how the population is changing, can we predict the population in the future? Common sense says yes: if we know the initial value of some quantity and we know exactly how it is changing, we should be able to figure out the future value of the quantity.

In the language of differential equations, an initial-value problem (that is, a differential equation and an initial condition) representing a real situation almost always has a unique solution. One way to see this is by looking at the slope field. Imagine starting at the point representing the initial condition. Through that point there will usually be a line segment pointing in the direction the solution curve must go. By following the line segments in the slope field, we trace out the solution curve. Several examples with different starting points are shown in Figure 10.16. In general, at each point there is one line segment and therefore only one direction for the solution curve to go. Thus the solution curve *exists* and is *unique* provided we are given an initial point.

It can be shown that if the slope field is continuous as we move from point to point in the plane, we can be sure that the solution curve exists around every point. Ensuring that each point has only one solution curve through it requires a slightly stronger condition.

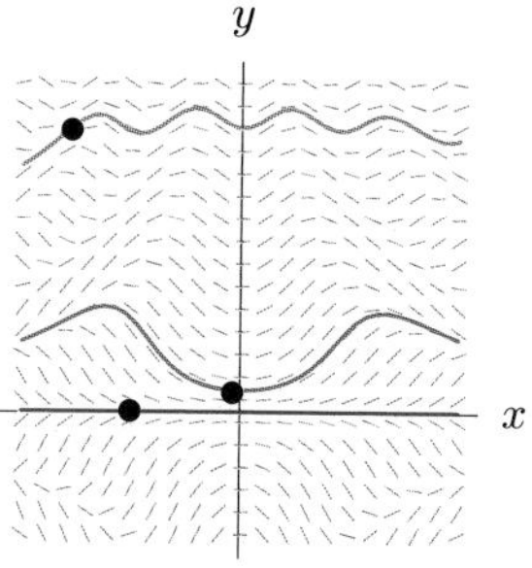

Figure 10.16: There is one and only one solution curve through each point in the plane for this slope field

Problems for Section 10.3

1. Figure 10.17 is a slope field for $dy/dx = y - 10$.

(a) Draw the solution curve for each of the following initial conditions:

(i) $y = 8$ when $x = 0$ (ii) $y = 12$ when $x = 0$
(iii) $y = 10$ when $x = 0$

(b) Since $dy/dx = y - 10$, when $y = 10$, we have $dy/dx = 10 - 10 = 0$. Explain why this matches your answer to part (iii).

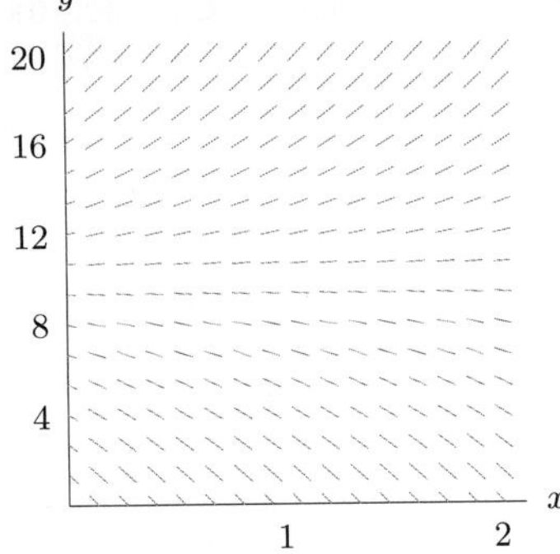

Figure 10.17: Slope field for $dy/dx = y - 10$

2. Sketch three solution curves for each of the slope fields in Figure 10.18.

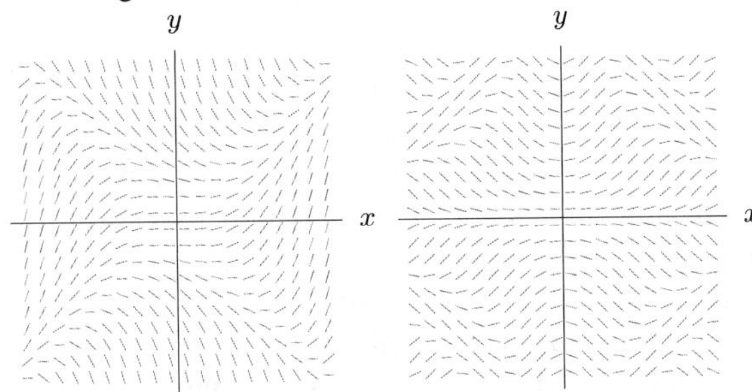

Figure 10.18

3. Figure 10.19 is the slope field for the equation $y' = x+y$.

(a) Sketch the solutions that pass through the points
(i) $(0, 0)$ (ii) $(-3, 1)$ (iii) $(-1, 0)$

(b) From your sketch, guess the equation of the solution passing through $(-1, 0)$.

(c) Check your solution to part (b) by substituting it into the differential equation.

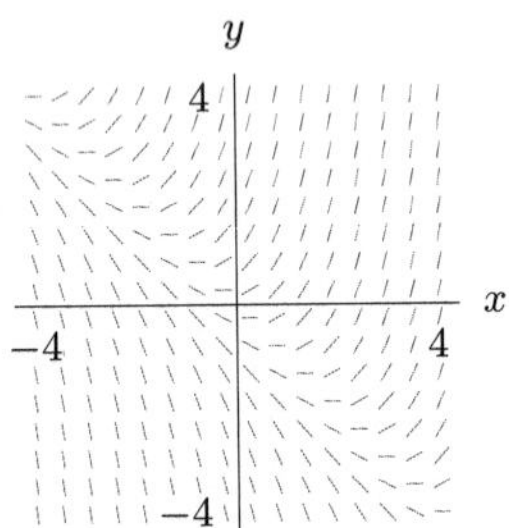

Figure 10.19: Slope field for $y' = x + y$

4. Which one of the following differential equations best fits the slope field shown in Figure 10.20? Explain.

I. $dP/dt = P - 1$ II. $dP/dt = P(P - 1)$
III. $dP/dt = 3P(1 - P)$ IV. $dP/dt = 1/3P(1-P)$

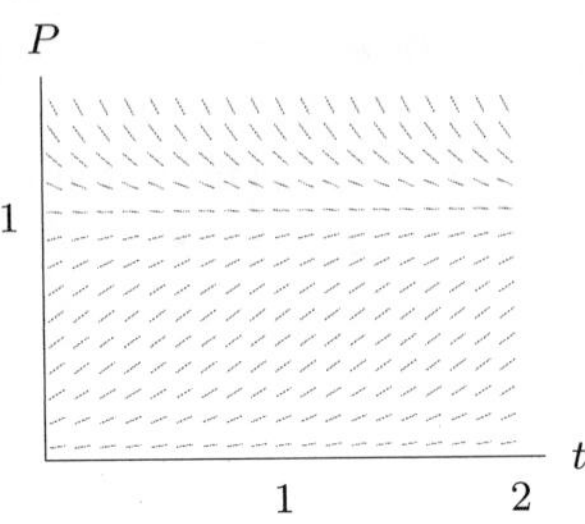

Figure 10.20

5. **(a)** Consider the slope field for $dy/dx = xy$. What is the slope of the line segment at the point $(2, 1)$? At $(0, 2)$? At $(-1, 1)$? At $(2, -2)$?

(b) Sketch part of the slope field by drawing line segments with the slopes calculated in part (a).

6. Match the slope fields in Figure 10.21 with their differential equations:

(a) $y' = -y$ **(b)** $y' = y$ **(c)** $y' = x$
(d) $y' = 1/y$ **(e)** $y' = y^2$

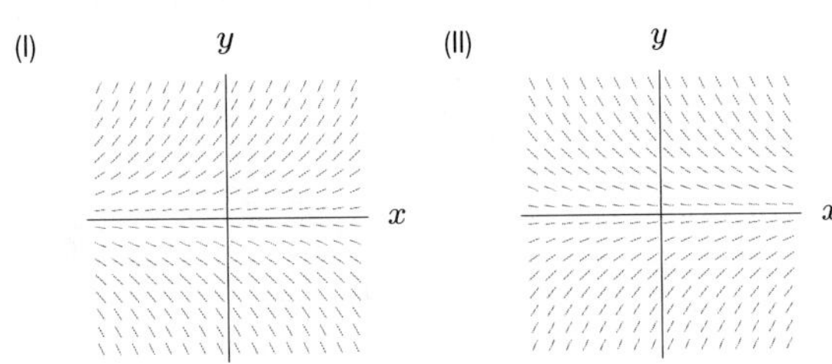

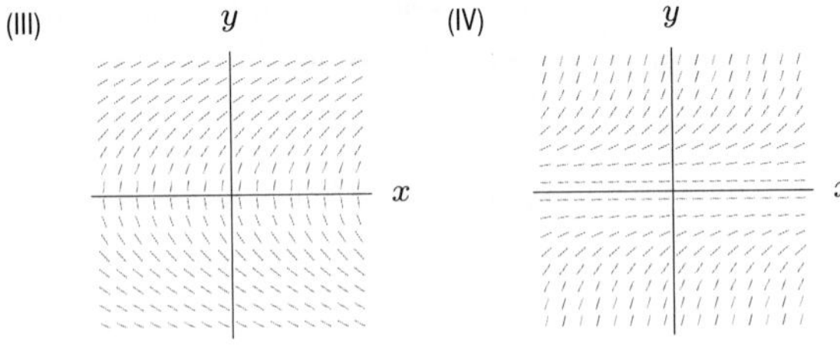

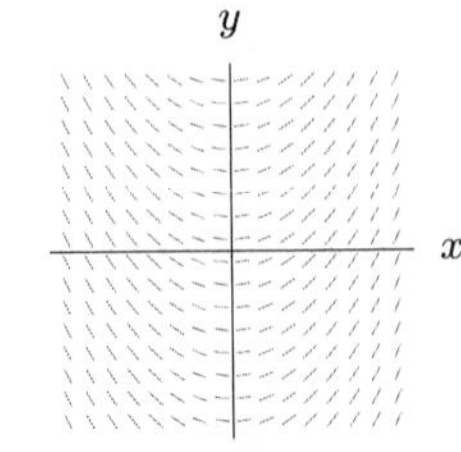

Figure 10.21

7. Match the slope fields in Figure 10.22 with their differential equations:

(a) $y' = 1 + y^2$ **(b)** $y' = x$ **(c)** $y' = \sin x$
(d) $y' = y$ **(e)** $y' = x - y$ **(f)** $y' = 4 - y$

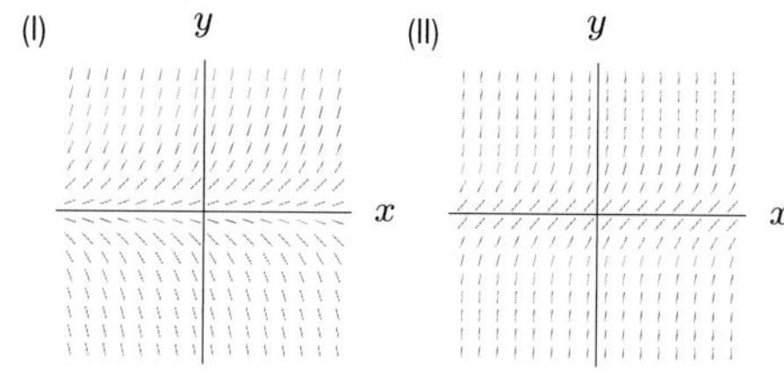

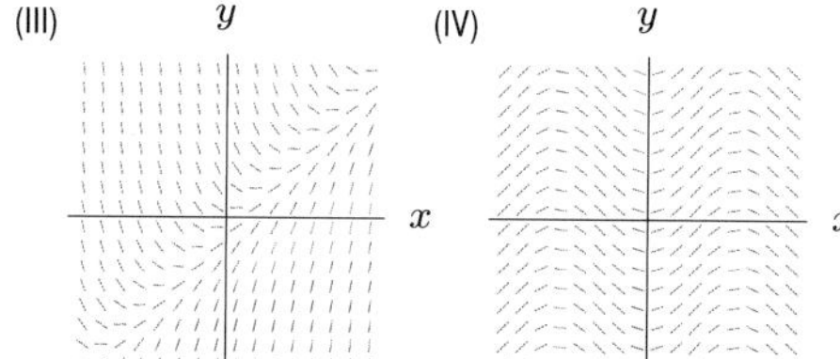

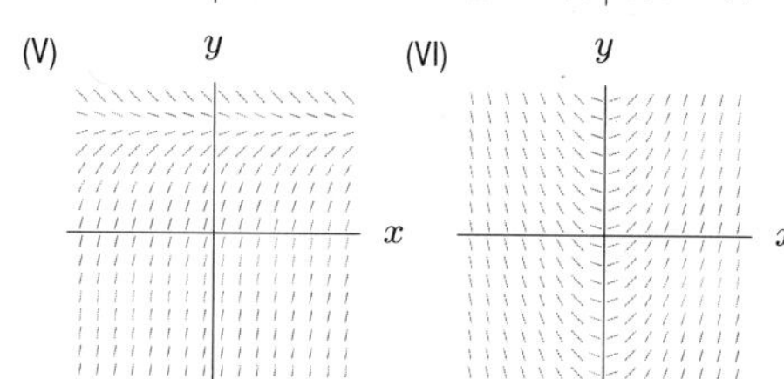

Figure 10.22: Each slope field is graphed for $-5 \leq x \leq 5, -5 \leq y \leq 5$

For Problems 8–13, consider a solution curve for each of the slope fields in Problem 7. Write one or two sentences describing qualitatively the long-run behavior of y. For example, as x increases, does $y \to \infty$, or does y remain finite? You may get different limiting behavior for different starting points. In each case, your answer should discuss how the limiting behavior depends on the starting point.

8. Slope field (I)

9. Slope field (II)

10. Slope field (III)

11. Slope field (IV)

12. Slope field (V)

13. Slope field (VI)

14. The Gompertz equation, which models growth of animal tumors, is $y' = -ay\ln(y/b)$, where a and b are positive constants. Use Figures 10.23 and 10.24 to write a paragraph describing the similarities and/or differences between solutions to the Gompertz equation with $a = 1$ and $b = 2$ and solutions to the equation $y' = y(2 - y)$.

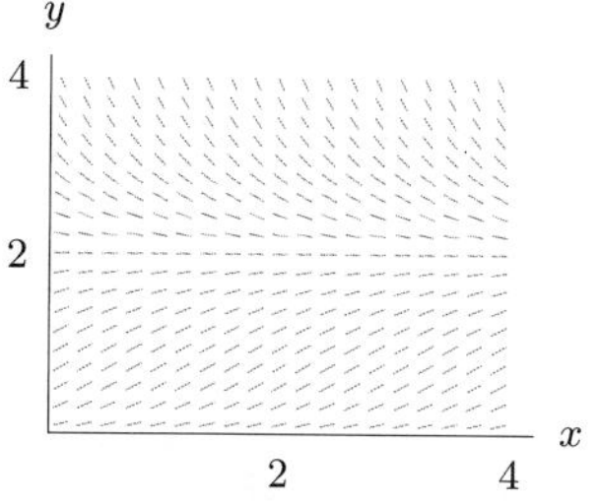

Figure 10.23: Slope field for $y' = -y\ln(y/2)$

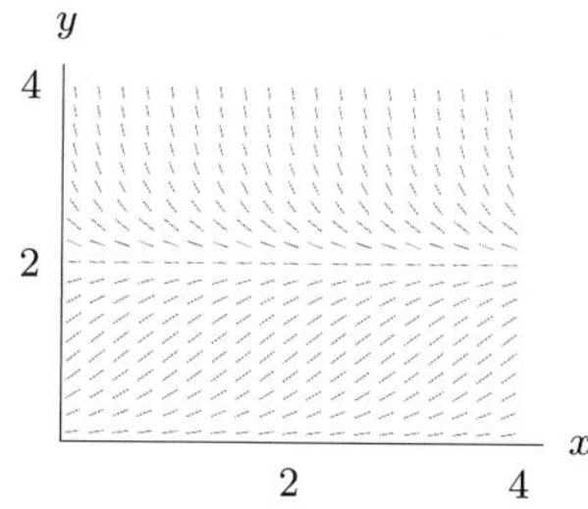

Figure 10.24: Slope field for $y' = y(2 - y)$

10.4 EXPONENTIAL GROWTH AND DECAY

What is a solution to the differential equation

$$\frac{dy}{dt} = y?$$

A solution is a function that is its own derivative. The function $y = e^t$ has this property, so $y = e^t$ is a solution. In fact, any multiple of e^t also has this property. The family of functions $y = Ce^t$ is the general solution to this differential equation. If k is a constant, the differential equation

$$\frac{dy}{dt} = ky,$$

is similar. This differential equation says that the rate of change of y is proportional to y. The constant k is the constant of proportionality. By substituting $y = Ce^{kt}$ into the differential equation, you can check that $y = Ce^{kt}$ is a solution. For another derivation of the solution, see the Focus on Theory section at the end of the chapter. We have the following result:

> The general solution to the differential equation $\frac{dy}{dt} = ky$ is
>
> $$y = Ce^{kt} \qquad \text{for any constant C.}$$
>
> - This is exponential growth for $k > 0$, and exponential decay for $k < 0$.
> - The constant C is the value of y when t is 0.

Graphs of solution curves for some $k > 0$ are in Figure 10.25. For $k < 0$, the graphs are reflected about the y-axis. See Figure 10.26.

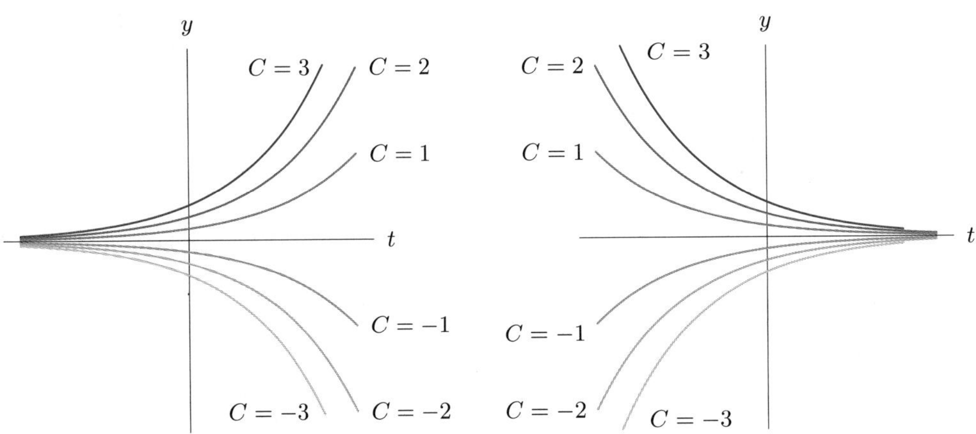

Figure 10.25: Graphs of $y = Ce^{kt}$, which are solutions to $\frac{dy}{dt} = ky$ for some fixed $k > 0$

Figure 10.26: Graphs of $y = Ce^{kt}$, which are solutions to $\frac{dy}{dt} = ky$ for some fixed $k < 0$

Example 1

(a) Find the general solution to each of the following differential equations:

(i) $\frac{dy}{dt} = 0.05y$ (ii) $\frac{dP}{dt} = -0.3P$ (iii) $\frac{dw}{dz} = 2z$ (iv) $\frac{dw}{dz} = 2w$

(b) For differential equation (i), find the particular solution satisfying $y = 50$ when $t = 0$.

Solution

(a) The differential equations given in (i), (ii), and (iv) are all examples of exponential growth or decay, since each is in the form

$$\text{Derivative} = \text{Constant} \cdot \text{Dependent variable.}$$

Notice that differential equation (iii) is not in this form. Example 1 on page 413 showed that the solution to (iii) is $w = z^2 + C$. The general solutions are

(i) $y = Ce^{0.05t}$ (ii) $P = Ce^{-0.3t}$ (iii) $w = z^2 + C$ (iv) $w = Ce^{2z}$

(b) The general solution to (i) is $y = Ce^{0.05t}$. Substituting $y = 50$ and $t = 0$ gives

$$50 = Ce^{0.05(0)}$$
$$50 = C \cdot 1.$$

So $C = 50$, and the particular solution to this initial-value problem is $y = 50e^{0.05t}$.

Population Growth

Consider the population P of a region where there is no immigration or emigration. The rate at which the population is growing is often proportional to the size of the population. This means larger populations grow faster, as we expect since there are more people to have babies. If the population has a continuous growth rate of 2% per unit time, then we know

$$\text{Rate of growth of population} = 2\% \text{ of Current population},$$

so

$$\frac{dP}{dt} = 0.02P.$$

This equation is of the form $dP/dt = kP$ for $k = 0.02$ and has the general solution $P = Ce^{0.02t}$. If the initial population at time $t = 0$ is P_0, then $P_0 = Ce^{0.02(0)} = C$. So $C = P_0$ and we have

$$P = P_0e^{0.02t}.$$

Continuously Compounded Interest

In Chapter 1 we introduced continuous compounding as the limiting case in which interest was added more and more often. Here we approach continuous compounding from a different point of view. We imagine interest being accrued at a rate proportional to the balance at that moment. Thus, the larger the balance, the faster interest is earned and the faster the balance grows.

Example 2 A bank account earns interest continuously at a rate of 5% of the current balance per year. Assume that the initial deposit is \$1000 and that no other deposits or withdrawals are made.

(a) Write a differential equation satisfied by the balance in the account.
(b) Solve the differential equation and graph the solution.

Solution

(a) We are looking for B, the balance in the account in dollars, as a function of t, time in years. Interest is being added continuously to the account at a rate of 5% of the balance at that moment, so

$$\text{Rate at which balance is increasing} = 5\% \text{ of Current balance}.$$

Thus, a differential equation that describes the process is

$$\frac{dB}{dt} = 0.05B.$$

Notice that it does not involve the \$1000, the initial condition, because the initial deposit does not affect the process by which interest is earned.

(b) Since $B_0 = 1000$ is the initial value of B, the solution to this differential equation is

$$B = B_0e^{0.05t} = 1000e^{0.05t}.$$

This function is graphed in Figure 10.27.

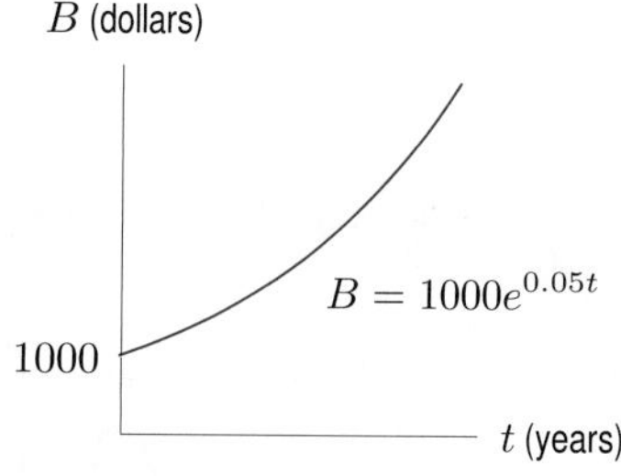

Figure 10.27: Bank balance against time

You may wonder how we can represent an amount of money by a differential equation, since money can only take on discrete values (you can't have fractions of a cent). In fact, the differential equation is only an approximation, but for large amounts of money, it is a pretty good approximation.

Pollution in the Great Lakes

In the 1960s pollution in the Great Lakes became an issue of public concern. We will set up a model for how long it would take the lakes to flush themselves clean, assuming no further pollutants were being dumped in the lake.

Let Q be the total quantity of pollutant in a lake of volume V at time t. Suppose that clean water is flowing into the lake at a constant rate r and that water flows out at the same rate. Assume that the pollutant is evenly spread throughout the lake, and that the clean water coming into the lake immediately mixes with the rest of the water.

How does Q vary with time? First, notice that since pollutants are being taken out of the lake but not added, Q decreases, and the water leaving the lake becomes less polluted, so the rate at which the pollutants leave decreases. This tells us that Q is decreasing and concave up. In addition, the pollutants will never be completely removed from the lake though the quantity remaining will become arbitrarily small. In other words, Q is asymptotic to the t-axis. (See Figure 10.28.)

Setting Up a Differential Equation for the Pollution

To understand how Q changes with time, we write a differential equation for Q. We know that

$$\begin{array}{c}\text{Rate } Q\\ \text{changes}\end{array} = -\left(\begin{array}{c}\text{Rate pollutants}\\ \text{leave in outflow}\end{array}\right)$$

where the negative sign represents the fact that Q is decreasing. At time t, the concentration of pollutants is Q/V and water containing this concentration is leaving at rate r. Thus,

$$\begin{array}{c}\text{Rate pollutants}\\ \text{leave in outflow}\end{array} = \begin{array}{c}\text{Rate of}\\ \text{outflow}\end{array} \times \text{Concentration} = r \cdot \frac{Q}{V}.$$

So the differential equation is

$$\frac{dQ}{dt} = -\frac{r}{V}Q$$

and its general solution is

$$Q = Q_0 e^{-rt/V}.$$

Table 10.6 contains values of r and V for four of the Great Lakes.[1] We use this data to calculate how long it would take for certain fractions of the pollution to be removed from Lake Erie.

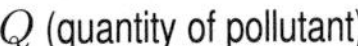

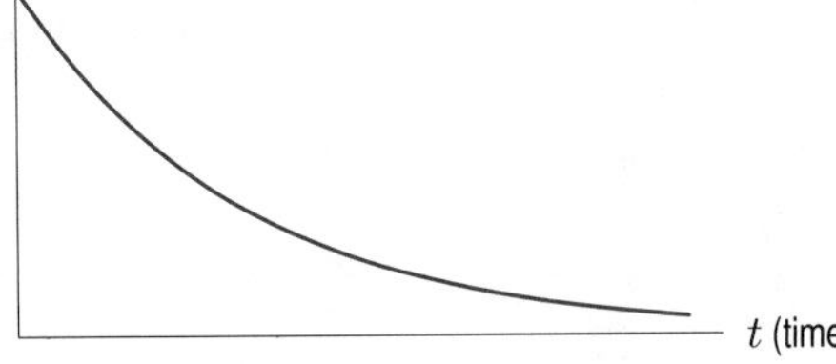

Figure 10.28: Pollutant in lake versus time

Table 10.6 *Volume and outflow in Great Lakes*

	V (km^3)	r (km^3/year)
Superior	12,200	65.2
Michigan	4900	158
Erie	460	175
Ontario	1600	209

Example 3 How long will it take for 90% of the pollution to be removed from Lake Erie? For 99% to be removed?

Solution For Lake Erie, $r/V = 175/460 = 0.38$, so at time t we have

$$Q = Q_0 e^{-0.38t}.$$

When 90% of the pollution has been removed, 10% remains, so $Q = 0.1Q_0$. Substituting gives

$$0.1Q_0 = Q_0 e^{-0.38t}.$$

[1] Data from William E. Boyce and Richard C. DiPrima, *Elementary Differential Equations* (New York: Wiley, 1977).

Canceling Q_0 and solving for t gives

$$t = \frac{-\ln(0.1)}{0.38} \approx 6 \text{ years.}$$

Similarly, when 99% of the pollution has been removed, $Q = 0.01Q_0$, so we solve

$$0.01Q_0 = Q_0e^{-0.38t},$$

giving

$$t = \frac{-\ln(0.01)}{0.38} \approx 12 \text{ years.}$$

The Quantity of a Drug in the Body

As we saw in Section 10.1, the rate at which a drug leaves a patient's body is proportional to the quantity of the drug left in the body. If we let Q represent the quantity of drug left, then

$$\frac{dQ}{dt} = -kQ.$$

The negative sign indicates the quantity of drug in the body is decreasing. The solution to this differential equation is $Q = Q_0e^{-kt}$; the quantity decreases exponentially. The constant k depends on the drug and Q_0 is the amount of drug in the body at time zero. Sometimes physicians convey information about the relative decay rate with a *half life*, which is the time it takes for Q to decrease by a factor of $1/2$.

Example 4 Valproic acid is a drug used to control epilepsy; its half-life in the human body is about 15 hours.

(a) Use the half-life to find the constant k in the differential equation $dQ/dt = -kQ$, where Q represents the quantity of drug in the body t hours after the drug is administered.
(b) At what time will 10% of the original dose remain?

Solution (a) Since the half-life is 15 hours, we know that the quantity remaining $Q = 0.5Q_0$ when $t = 15$. We substitute into the solution to the differential equation, $Q = Q_0e^{-kt}$, and solve for k:

$$\begin{aligned} Q &= Q_0e^{-kt} \\ 0.5Q_0 &= Q_0e^{-k(15)} \\ 0.5 &= e^{-15k} && \text{(Divide through by } Q_0\text{)} \\ \ln 0.5 &= -15k && \text{(Take the natural logarithm of both sides)} \\ k &= \frac{-\ln 0.5}{15} = 0.0462. && \text{(Solve for } k\text{)} \end{aligned}$$

(b) To find the time when 10% of the original dose remains in the body, we substitute $0.10Q_0$ for the quantity remaining, Q, and solve for the time, t.

$$\begin{aligned} 0.10Q_0 &= Q_0e^{-0.0462t} \\ 0.10 &= e^{-0.0462t} \\ \ln 0.10 &= -0.0462t \\ t &= \frac{\ln 0.10}{-0.0462} = 49.84. \end{aligned}$$

There will be 10% of the drug still in the body at $t = 49.84$, or after about 50 hours.

Problems for Section 10.4

Find solutions to the differential equations in Problems 1–6, subject to the given initial condition.

1. $\dfrac{dw}{dr} = 3w, \quad w = 30$ when $r = 0$
2. $\dfrac{dy}{dx} = -0.14y, \quad y = 5.6$ when $x = 0$
3. $\dfrac{dP}{dt} = 0.02P, \quad P(0) = 20$
4. $\dfrac{dp}{dq} = -0.1p, \quad p = 100$ when $q = 5$
5. $\dfrac{dQ}{dt} = \dfrac{Q}{5}, \quad Q = 50$ when $t = 0$
6. $\dfrac{dy}{dx} + \dfrac{y}{3} = 0, \quad y(0) = 10$
7. Money in a bank account grows continuously at an annual rate of r (when the interest rate is 5%, $r = 0.05$, and so on). Suppose $1000 is put into the account in 2000.
   (a) Write a differential equation satisfied by M, the amount of money in the account at time t, measured in years since 2000.
   (b) Solve the differential equation.
   (c) Sketch the solution until the year 2030 for interest rates of 5% and 10%.
8. A deposit of $5000 is made to a bank account paying 1.5% annual interest, compounded continuously.
   (a) Write a differential equation for the balance in the account, B, as a function of time, t, in years.
   (b) Solve the differential equation.
   (c) How much money is in the account in 10 years?
9. A bank account that earns 10% interest compounded continuously has an initial balance of zero. Money is deposited into the account at a continuous rate of $1000 per year.
   (a) Write a differential equation that describes the rate of change of the balance $B = f(t)$.
   (b) Solve the differential equation.
10. The amount of ozone, Q, in the atmosphere is decreasing at a rate proportional to the amount of ozone present. If time t is measured in years, the constant of proportionality is -0.0025. Write a differential equation for Q as a function of t, and give the general solution for the differential equation. If this rate continues, approximately what percent of the ozone in the atmosphere now will decay in the next 20 years?
11. Using the model in the text and the data in Table 10.6 on page 420, find how long it would take for 90% of the pollution to be removed from Lake Michigan and from Lake Ontario, assuming no new pollutants are added. Explain how you can tell which lake will take longer to be purified just by looking at the data in the table.
12. Use the model in the text and the data in Table 10.6 on page 420 to determine which of the Great Lakes would require the longest time and which would require the shortest time for 80% of the pollution to be removed, assuming no new pollutants are being added. Find the ratio of these two times.
13. The rate at which a drug leaves the bloodstream and passes into the urine is proportional to the quantity of the drug in the blood at that time. If an initial dose of Q_0 is injected directly into the blood, 20% is left in the blood after 3 hours.
   (a) Write and solve a differential equation for the quantity, Q, of the drug in the blood after t hours.
   (b) How much of this drug is in a patient's body after 6 hours if the patient is given 100 mg initially?
14. Oil is pumped continuously from a well at a rate proportional to the amount of oil left in the well. Initially there were 1 million barrels of oil in the well; six years later 500,000 barrels remain.
   (a) At what rate was the amount of oil in the well decreasing when there were 600,000 barrels remaining?
   (b) When will there be 50,000 barrels remaining?
15. In some chemical reactions, the rate at which the amount of a substance changes with time is proportional to the amount present. For example, this is the case as δ-glucono-lactone changes into gluconic acid.
   (a) Write a differential equation satisfied by y, the quantity of δ-glucono-lactone present at time t.
   (b) If 100 grams of δ-glucono-lactone is reduced to 54.9 grams in one hour, how many grams will remain after 10 hours?
16. Hydrocodone bitartrate is used as a cough suppressant. After the drug is fully absorbed, the quantity of drug in the body decreases at a rate proportional to the amount left in the body. The half-life of hydrocodone bitartrate in the body is 3.8 hours and the dose is 10 mg.
   (a) Write a differential equation for the quantity, Q, of hydrocodone bitartrate in the body at time t, in hours since the drug was fully absorbed.
   (b) Solve the differential equation given in part (a).
   (c) Use the half-life to find the constant of proportionality, k.
   (d) How much of the 10-mg dose is still in the body after 12 hours?
17. The amount of land in use for growing crops increases as the world's population increases. Suppose $A(t)$ represents the total number of hectares of land in use in year t. (A hectare is about $2\frac{1}{2}$ acres.)
   (a) Explain why it is plausible that $A(t)$ satisfies the equation $A'(t) = kA(t)$. What assumptions are you

making about the world's population and its relation to the amount of land used?

(b) In 1950 about $1 \cdot 10^9$ hectares of land were in use; in 1980 the figure was $2 \cdot 10^9$. If the total amount of land available for growing crops is thought to be $3.2 \cdot 10^9$ hectares, when does this model predict it is exhausted? (Let $t = 0$ in 1950.)

10.5 APPLICATIONS AND MODELING

In the last section, we considered several situations modeled by the differential equation

$$\frac{dy}{dt} = ky.$$

In this section, we consider situations where the rate of change of y is a linear function of y of the form

$$\frac{dy}{dt} = k(y - A), \qquad \text{where } k \text{ and } A \text{ are constants.}$$

The Quantity of a Drug in the Body

A patient is given the drug warfarin, an anticoagulant, intravenously at the rate of 0.5 mg/hour. Warfarin is metabolized and leaves the body at the rate of about 2% per hour. A differential equation for the quantity, Q (in mg), of warfarin in the body after t hours is given by

$$\begin{aligned} \text{Rate of change} &= \text{Rate in} - \text{Rate out} \\ \frac{dQ}{dt} &= 0.5 - 0.02Q. \end{aligned}$$

What does this tell us about the quantity of warfarin in the body for different initial values of Q?

If Q is small, then $0.02Q$ is also small and the rate the drug is excreted is less than the rate at which the drug is entering the body. Since the rate in is greater than the rate out, the rate of change is positive and the quantity of drug in the body is increasing. If Q is large enough that $0.02Q$ is greater than 0.5, then $0.5 - 0.02Q$ is negative, so dQ/dt is negative and the quantity is decreasing.

For small Q, the quantity will increase until the rate in equals the rate out. For large Q, the quantity will decrease until the rate in equals the rate out. What is the value of Q at which the rate in exactly matches the rate out? We have

$$\begin{aligned} \text{Rate in} &= \text{Rate out} \\ 0.5 &= 0.02Q \\ Q &= 25. \end{aligned}$$

If the amount of warfarin in the body is initially 25 mg, then the amount being excreted exactly matches the amount being added. The quantity of drug Q will stay constant at 25 mg. Notice also that when $Q = 25$, the derivative dQ/dt is zero, since

$$\frac{dQ}{dt} = 0.5 - 0.02(25) = 0.5 - 0.5 = 0.$$

If the initial quantity is 25, then the solution is the horizontal line $Q = 25$. This solution is called an *equilibrium solution*.

The slope field for this differential equation is shown in Figure 10.29, with solution curves drawn for $Q_0 = 20$, $Q_0 = 25$, and $Q_0 = 30$. In each case, we see that the quantity of drug in the body is approaching the equilibrium solution of 25 mg. The solution curve with $Q_0 = 30$ should remind you of an exponential decay function. It is, in fact, an exponential decay function that has been shifted up 25 units.

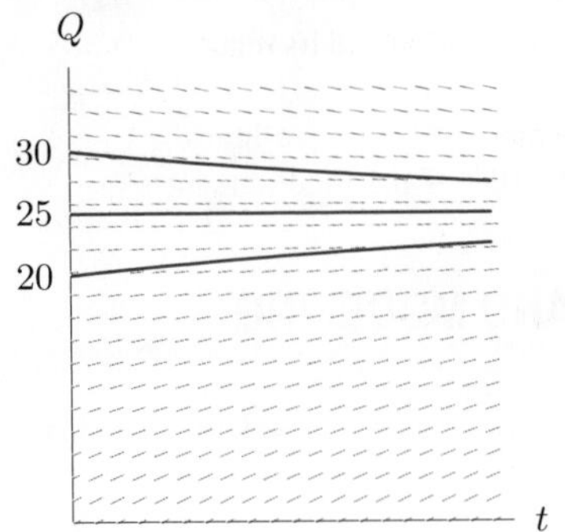

Figure 10.29: Slope field for $dQ/dt = 0.5 - 0.02Q$

Solving the Differential Equation $dy/dt = k(y - A)$

The drug concentration in the previous example satisfies a differential equation of the form

$$\frac{dy}{dt} = k(y - A).$$

Let us find the general solution to this equation. Since A is a constant, $dA/dt = 0$ so that we have

$$\frac{d}{dt}(y - A) = \frac{dy}{dt} - \frac{dA}{dt} = \frac{dy}{dt} - 0 = k(y - A).$$

Thus $y - A$ satisfies an exponential differential equation, so $y - A$ must be of the form

$$y - A = Ce^{kt}.$$

For an alternative derivation of the solution, see the Focus on Theory section at the end of the chapte.

> The general solution to the differential equation
>
> $$\frac{dy}{dt} = k(y - A)$$
>
> is
>
> $$y = A + Ce^{kt}, \qquad \text{for any constant } C.$$

Warning: Notice that, for differential equations of this form, the arbitrary constant C is *not* the initial value of the variable, but rather the initial value of $y - A$.

Example 1 Give the solution to each of the following differential equations:

(a) $\dfrac{dy}{dt} = 0.02(y - 50)$

(b) $\dfrac{dP}{dt} = 5(P - 10), \quad P = 8$ when $t = 0$

(c) $\dfrac{dy}{dt} = 3y - 300$

(d) $\dfrac{dW}{dt} = 500 - 0.1W$

Solution (a) The general solution is $y = 50 + Ce^{0.02t}$.

(b) The general solution is $P = 10 + Ce^{5t}$. Use the initial condition to solve for C:

$$8 = 10 + C(e^0)$$
$$8 = 10 + C$$

So $C = -2$, and the particular solution is $P = 10 - 2e^{5t}$.

(c) First rewrite the right-hand side of the equation in the form $k(y - A)$ by factoring out a 3:

$$\frac{dy}{dt} = 3(y - 100).$$

The general solution to this differential equation is $y = 100 + Ce^{3t}$.

(d) We begin by factoring out the coefficient of W:

$$\frac{dW}{dt} = 500 - 0.1W = -0.1\left(W - \frac{500}{0.1}\right) = -0.1(W - 5000).$$

The general solution to this differential equation is $W = 5000 + Ce^{-0.1t}$.

Example 2 At the start of this section, we gave the following differential equation for the quantity of warfarin in the body:

$$\frac{dQ}{dt} = 0.5 - 0.02Q.$$

Write the general solution to this differential equation. Find particular solutions for $Q_0 = 20$, $Q_0 = 25$, and $Q_0 = 30$.

Solution We first rewrite the differential equation in the form $dQ/dt = k(Q - A)$ by factoring out -0.02:

$$\frac{dQ}{dt} = 0.5 - 0.02Q = -0.02(Q - 25).$$

The general solution to this differential equation is

$$Q = 25 + Ce^{-0.02t}.$$

To find the particular solution when $Q_0 = 20$, we use the initial condition to solve for C:

$$20 = 25 + C(e^0)$$
$$C = -5.$$

The particular solution when $Q_0 = 20$ is $Q = 25 - 5e^{-0.02t}$.

When $Q_0 = 25$, we have $C = 0$ and the particular solution is the horizontal line $Q = 25$. When $Q_0 = 30$, we have $C = 5$ and the particular solution is $Q = 25 + 5e^{-0.02t}$. These three solutions are the three we saw earlier in Figure 10.29.

Example 3 A company's revenue is earned at a continuous annual rate of 5% of its net worth. At the same time, the company's payroll obligations are paid out at a constant rate of 200 million dollars a year. We saw in Section 10.1 that the differential equation governing the net worth, W (in millions of dollars), of this company in year t is given by

$$\text{Rate of change of } W = \text{Rate in} - \text{Rate out}$$
$$\frac{dW}{dt} = 0.05W - 200.$$

(a) Solve the differential equation, assuming an initial net worth of W_0 million dollars.

(b) Sketch the solution for $W_0 = 3000$, 4000 and 5000. For which of these values of W_0 does the company go bankrupt? In which year?

Solution (a) Factor out 0.05 to get

$$\frac{dW}{dt} = 0.05(W - 4000).$$

The general solution is

$$W = 4000 + Ce^{0.05t}.$$

To find C we use the initial condition that $W = W_0$ when $t = 0$.

$$W_0 = 4000 + Ce^0$$
$$W_0 - 4000 = C$$

Substituting this value for C into $W = 4000 + Ce^{0.05t}$ gives

$$W = 4000 + (W_0 - 4000)e^{0.05t}.$$

(b) If $W_0 = 4000$, then $W = 4000$, the equilibrium solution.
If $W_0 = 5000$, then $W = 4000 + 1000e^{0.05t}$.
If $W_0 = 3000$, then $W = 4000 - 1000e^{0.05t}$. The graphs of these functions are in Figure 10.30. Notice that if the net worth starts with W_0 near, but not equal to, \$4000 million, then W moves further away. We see that if $W_0 = 3000$, the value of W goes to 0, and the company goes bankrupt. Solving $W = 0$ gives $t \approx 27.7$, so the company goes bankrupt in its twenty-eighth year.

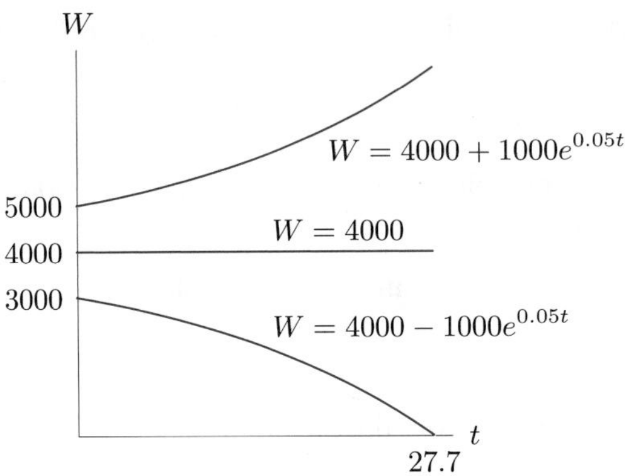

Figure 10.30: Solutions to $\frac{dW}{dt} = 0.05W - 200$

Equilibrium Solutions

Figure 10.29 shows the quantity of warfarin in the body for several different initial quantities. All these curves are solutions to the differential equation

$$\frac{dQ}{dt} = 0.5 - 0.02Q = -0.02(Q - 25),$$

and all the solutions have the form

$$Q = 25 + Ce^{-0.02t}$$

for some C. Notice that $Q \to 25$ as $t \to \infty$ for all solutions because $e^{-0.02t} \to 0$ as $t \to \infty$. In other words, in the long run, the quantity approaches the *equilibrium solution* of $Q = 25$ no matter what the initial quantity.

Notice that the equilibrium solution can be found directly from the differential equation by solving $dQ/dt = 0$:

$$\frac{dQ}{dt} = -0.02(Q - 25) = 0,$$

giving $Q = 25$. Because Q always gets closer and closer to the equilibrium value of 25 as $t \to \infty$, we call $Q = 25$ a *stable* equilibrium for Q.

A different situation is shown in Figure 10.30 with the solutions to the differential equation $dW/dt = 0.05W - 200$. We find the equilibrium by looking at the solution curves or by setting $dW/dt = 0$:

$$\frac{dW}{dt} = 0.05W - 200 = 0.05(W - 4000) = 0,$$

giving $W = 4000$ as the equilibrium solution. This equilibrium solution is called *unstable* because if W starts near, but not equal to, 4000, the net worth W moves further away from 4000 as $t \to \infty$.

- An **equilibrium solution** is constant for all values of the independent variable. The graph is a horizontal line. Equilibrium solutions can be identified by setting the derivative of the function to zero.
- An equilibrium solution is **stable** if a small change in the initial conditions gives a solution which tends toward the equilibrium as the independent variable tends to positive infinity.
- An equilibrium solution is **unstable** if a small change in the initial conditions gives a solution curve which veers away from the equilibrium as the independent variable tends to positive infinity.

In general, a differential equation may have more than one equilibrium solution or no equilibrium solution.

Example 4 Find the equilibrium solution for each of the following differential equations. Determine whether the equilibrium solution is stable or unstable.

(a) $\dfrac{dH}{dt} = -2(H - 20)$ (b) $\dfrac{dB}{dt} = 2(B - 10)$

Solution (a) To find equilibrium solutions, we set $dH/dt = 0$:

$$\frac{dH}{dt} = -2(H - 20) = 0,$$

giving $H = 20$ as the equilibrium solution. The general solution to this differential equation is $H = 20 + Ce^{-2t}$. The solution curves for $H_0 = 10$, $H_0 = 20$, and $H_0 = 30$ are shown in Figure 10.31. We see that the equilibrium solution is stable.

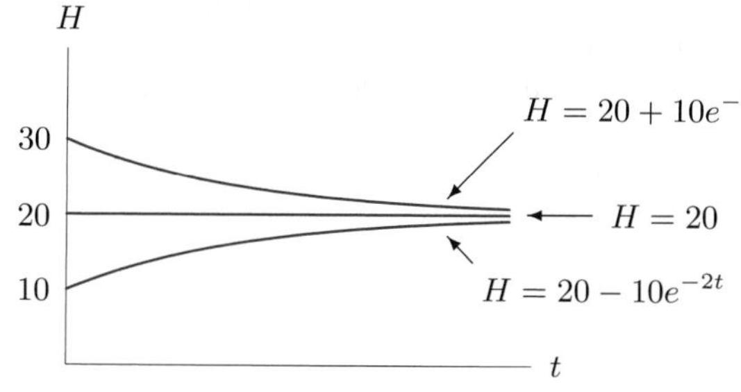

Figure 10.31: $H = 20$ is stable equilibrium

B
10
t
$B = 10 + e^{2t}$
$B = 10$
$B = 10 - e^{2t}$

Figure 10.32: $B = 10$ is unstable equilibrium

(b) To find equilibrium solutions, we set $dB/dt = 0$:

$$\frac{dB}{dt} = 2(B - 10) = 0,$$

giving $B = 10$ as the equilibrium solution. The general solution to this differential equation is $B = 10 + Ce^{2t}$. The solution curves for $B_0 = 9$, $B_0 = 10$, and $B_0 = 11$ are shown in Figure 10.32. We see that the equilibrium solution is unstable.

Newton's Law of Heating and Cooling

Newton proposed that the temperature of a hot object decreases at a rate proportional to the difference between its temperature and that of its surroundings. Similarly, a cold object heats up at a rate proportional to the temperature difference between the object and its surroundings.

For example, a hot cup of coffee standing on a table cools at a rate proportional to the temperature difference between the coffee and the surrounding air. As the coffee cools, the rate at which it cools decreases because the temperature difference between the coffee and the air decreases. In the long run, the rate of cooling tends to zero and the temperature of the coffee approaches room temperature. Figure 10.33 shows the temperature of two cups of coffee against time, one starting at a higher temperature than the other, but both tending toward room temperature in the long run.

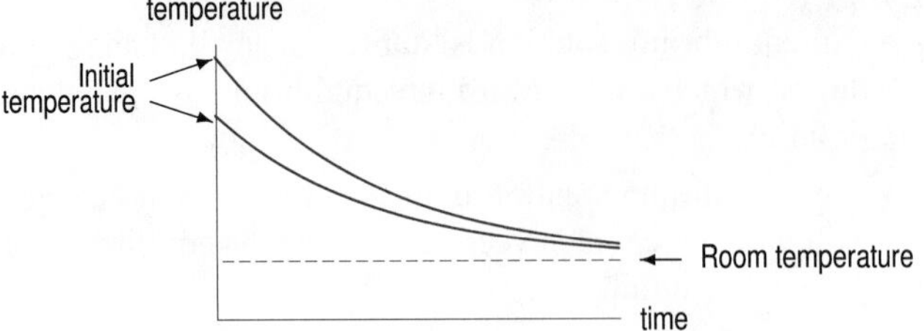

Figure 10.33: Temperature of coffee versus time

Let H be the temperature at time t of a cup of coffee in a 70°F room. Newton's Law says that the rate of change of H is proportional to the temperature difference between the coffee and the room:

$$\text{Rate of change of temperature} = \text{Constant} \cdot \text{Temperature difference.}$$

The rate of change of temperature is dH/dt. The temperature difference between the coffee and the room is $(H - 70)$, so

$$\frac{dH}{dt} = \text{Constant} \cdot (H - 70).$$

What about the sign of the constant? If the coffee starts out hotter than 70° (that is, $H - 70 > 0$), then the temperature of the coffee decreases (i.e., $dH/dt < 0$) and so the constant must be negative:

$$\frac{dH}{dt} = -k(H - 70) \qquad k > 0.$$

What can we learn from this differential equation? Suppose we take $k = 1$. The slope field for this differential equation in Figure 10.34 shows several solution curves. Notice that, as we expect, the temperature of the coffee is approaching the temperature of the room. The general solution to this differential equation is

$$H = 70 + Ce^{-t},$$

where C is an arbitrary constant.

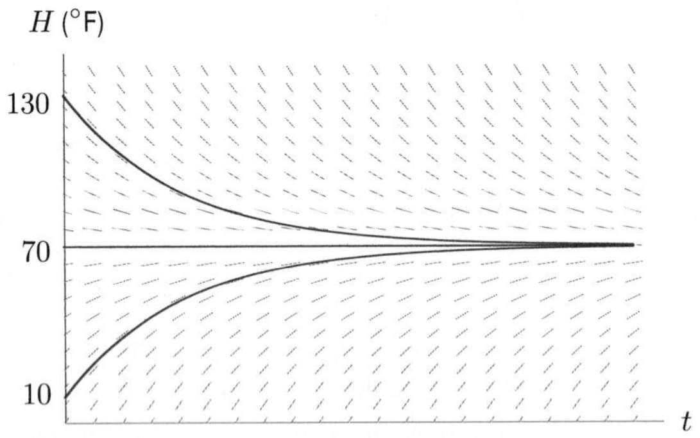

Figure 10.34: Slope field for $\frac{dH}{dt} = -(H - 70)$

Example 5 The body of a murder victim is found at noon in a room with a constant temperature of 20°C. At noon the temperature of the body is 35°C; two hours later the temperature of the body is 33°C.

(a) Find the temperature, H, of the body as a function of t, the time in hours since it was found.
(b) Graph H against t. What happens to the temperature in the long run?
(c) At the time of the murder, the victim's body had the normal body temperature, 37°C. When did the murder occur?

Solution (a) Newton's Law of Cooling says that

$$\text{Rate of change of temperature} = \text{Constant} \cdot \text{Temperature difference}.$$

Since the temperature difference is $H - 20$, we have for some constant k

$$\frac{dH}{dt} = -k(H - 20).$$

The general solution is

$$H = 20 + Ce^{-kt}.$$

To determine C, we use the fact that $H = 35$ at $t = 0$:

$$35 = 20 + C \cdot e^0$$
$$35 = 20 + C$$

So $C = 15$ and we have

$$H = 20 + 15e^{-kt}.$$

To find k, we use the fact that $H = 33$ when $t = 2$:

$$33 = 20 + 15e^{-k(2)}.$$

We isolate the exponential and solve for k:

$$13 = 15e^{-2k}$$
$$\frac{13}{15} = e^{-2k}$$
$$\ln\left(\frac{13}{15}\right) = -2k$$
$$k = -\frac{\ln(13/15)}{2} = 0.072.$$

Therefore, the temperature, H, of the body as a function of time, t, is given by

$$H = 20 + 15e^{-0.072t}.$$

(b) The graph of $H = 20 + 15e^{-0.072t}$ has a vertical intercept of $H = 35$, the initial temperature. The temperature decays exponentially with a horizontal asymptote of $H = 20$. (See Figure 10.35.) "In the long run" means as $t \to \infty$. The graph shows that $H \to 20$ as $t \to \infty$.

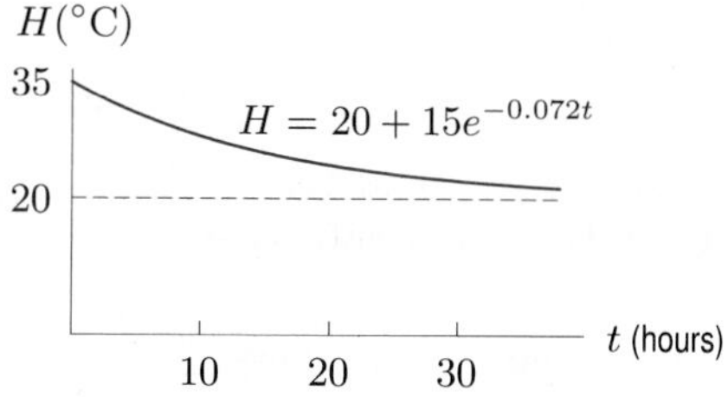

Figure 10.35: Temperature of dead body

(c) We want to know when the temperature was 37°C. We substitute $H = 37$ and solve for t:

$$37 = 20 + 15e^{-0.072t}$$
$$\frac{17}{15} = e^{-0.072t}.$$

Taking natural logs on both sides gives

$$\ln\left(\frac{17}{15}\right) = -0.072t$$

so

$$t = -\frac{\ln(17/15)}{0.072} = -1.74 \text{ hours}.$$

The murder occurred about 1.74 hours before noon, that is, about 10:15 am.

Problems for Section 10.5

Find particular solutions in Problems 1–8.

1. $\dfrac{dH}{dt} = 3(H - 75), \quad H = 0$ when $t = 0$

2. $\dfrac{dy}{dt} = 0.5(y - 200), \quad y = 50$ when $t = 0$

3. $\dfrac{dP}{dt} = P + 4, \quad P = 100$ when $t = 0$

4. $\dfrac{dB}{dt} = 4B - 100, \quad B = 20$ when $t = 0$

5. $\dfrac{dQ}{dt} = 0.3Q - 120, \quad Q = 50$ when $t = 0$

6. $\dfrac{dm}{dt} = 0.1m + 200, \quad m(0) = 1000$

7. $\dfrac{dB}{dt} + 2B = 50, \quad B(1) = 100$

8. $\dfrac{dB}{dt} + 0.1B - 10 = 0 \qquad B(2) = 3$

9. Check that $y = A + Ce^{kt}$ is a solution to the differential equation

$$\frac{dy}{dt} = k(y - A).$$

10. A bank account earns 7% annual interest compounded continuously. You deposit $10,000 in the account, and withdraw money continuously from the account at a rate of $1000 per year.

(a) Write a differential equation for the balance, B, in the account after t years.
(b) What is the equilibrium solution to the differential equation? (This is the amount that must be deposited now for the balance to stay the same over the years.)
(c) Find the solution to the differential equation.
(d) How much is in the account after 5 years?
(e) Graph the solution. What happens to the balance in the long run?

11. A company earns 2% per month on its assets, paid continuously, and its expenses are paid out continuously at a rate of $80,000 per month.

(a) Write a differential equation for the value, V, of the company as a function of time, t, in months.
(b) What is the equilibrium solution for the differential equation? What is the significance of this value for the company?
(c) Solve the differential equation found in part (a).
(d) If the company has assets worth $3 million at time $t = 0$, what are its assets worth one year later?

12. Money in an account earns interest at a continuous rate of 8% per year, and payments are made continuously out of the account at the rate of $5000 a year. The account initially contains $50,000. Write a differential equation for the amount of money in the account, B, in t years. Solve the differential equation. Does the account ever run out of money? If so, when?

13. A bank account earns 5% annual interest, compounded continuously. Money is deposited in a continuous cash flow at a rate of $1200 per year into the account.

(a) Write a differential equation that describes the rate at which the balance $B = f(t)$ is changing.
(b) Solve the differential equation given an initial balance $B_0 = 0$.
(c) Find the balance after 5 years.

14. A patient is given the drug theophylline intravenously at a rate of 43.2 mg/hour to relieve acute asthma. The rate at which the drug leaves the patient's body is proportional to the quantity there, with proportionality constant 0.082 if time, t, is in hours. The patient's body contains none of the drug initially.

(a) Describe in words how you expect the quantity of theophylline in the patient to vary with time.
(b) Write a differential equation satisfied by the quantity of theophylline in the body, $Q(t)$.
(c) Solve the differential equation and graph the solution. What happens to the quantity in the long run?

15. One theory on the speed an employee learns a new task claims that the more the employee already knows, the more slowly he or she learns. Suppose that the rate at which a person learns is equal to the percentage of the task not yet learned. If y is the percentage learned by time t, the percentage not yet learned by that time is $100 - y$, so we can model this situation with the differential equation

$$\frac{dy}{dt} = 100 - y.$$

(a) Find the general solution to this differential equation.
(b) Sketch several solutions.
(c) Find the particular solution if the employee starts learning at time $t = 0$ (so $y = 0$ when $t = 0$).

16. A chain smoker smokes five cigarettes every hour. From each cigarette, 0.4 mg of nicotine is absorbed into the person's bloodstream. Nicotine leaves the body at a rate proportional to the amount present, with constant of proportionality -0.346 if t is in hours.

(a) Write a differential equation for the level of nicotine in the body, N, in mg, as a function of time, t, in hours.
(b) Solve the differential equation from part (a). Initially there is no nicotine in the blood.
(c) The person wakes up at 7 am and begins smoking. How much nicotine is in the blood when the person goes to sleep at 11 pm (16 hours later)?

17. As you know, when a course ends, students start to forget the material they have learned. One model (called the Ebbinghaus model) assumes that the rate at which a student forgets material is proportional to the difference between the material currently remembered and some positive constant, a.

(a) Let $y = f(t)$ be the fraction of the original material remembered t weeks after the course has ended. Set up a differential equation for y. Your equation will contain two constants; the constant a is less than y for all t.
(b) Solve the differential equation.
(c) Describe the practical meaning (in terms of the amount remembered) of the constants in the solution $y = f(t)$.

18. **(a)** What are the equilibrium solutions for the differential equation

$$\frac{dy}{dt} = 0.2(y-3)(y+2)?$$

(b) Use a graphing calculator or computer to sketch a slope field for this differential equation. Use the slope field to determine whether each equilibrium solution is stable or unstable.

19. **(a)** Find the equilibrium solution of the equation

$$\frac{dy}{dt} = 0.5y - 250.$$

(b) Find the general solution of this equation.
(c) Graph several solutions with different initial values.
(d) Is the equilibrium solution stable or unstable?

20. Figure 10.36 gives the slope field for a differential equation. Estimate all equilibrium solutions and indicate whether each is stable or unstable.

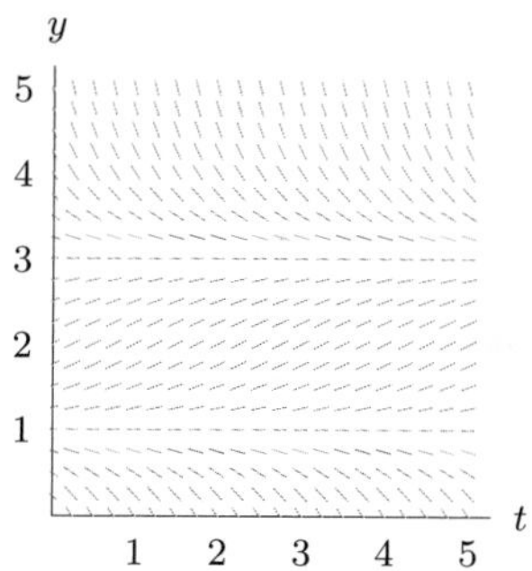

Figure 10.36

21. A yam is put in a 200°C oven and heats up according to the differential equation

$$\frac{dH}{dt} = -k(H-200), \quad \text{for } k \text{ a positive constant.}$$

(a) If the yam is at 20°C when it is put in the oven, solve the differential equation.
(b) Find k using the fact that after 30 minutes the temperature of the yam is 120°C.

22. At 1:00 pm one winter afternoon, there is a power failure at your house in Wisconsin, and your heat does not work without electricity. When the power goes out, it is 68°F in your house. At 10:00 pm, it is 57°F in the house, and you notice that it is 10°F outside.

(a) Assuming that the temperature, T, in your home obeys Newton's Law of Cooling, write the differential equation satisfied by T.
(b) Solve the differential equation to estimate the temperature in the house when you get up at 7:00 am the next morning. Should you worry about your water pipes freezing?
(c) What assumption did you make in part (a) about the temperature outside? Given this (probably incorrect) assumption, would you revise your estimate up or down? Why?

23. A detective finds a murder victim at 9 am. The temperature of the body is measured at 90.3°F. One hour later, the temperature of the body is 89.0°F. The temperature of the room has been maintained at a constant 68°F.

(a) Assuming the temperature, T, of the body obeys Newton's Law of Cooling, write a differential equation for T.
(b) Solve the differential equation to estimate the time the murder occurred.

24. A drug is administered intravenously at a constant rate of r mg/hour and is excreted at a rate proportional to the quantity present, with constant of proportionality $\alpha > 0$.

(a) Solve a differential equation for the quantity, Q, in milligrams, of the drug in the body at time t hours. Assume there is no drug in the body initially. Your answer will contain r and α. Graph Q against t. What is Q_∞, the limiting long-run value of Q?
(b) What effect does doubling r have on Q_∞? What effect does doubling r have on the time to reach half the limiting value, $\frac{1}{2}Q_\infty$?
(c) What effect does doubling α have on Q_∞? On the time to reach $\frac{1}{2}Q_\infty$?

25. Some people write the solution of the initial value problem

$$\frac{dy}{dt} = k(y-A) \qquad y = y_0 \text{ at } t = 0$$

in the form

$$\frac{y-A}{y_0-A} = e^{kt}.$$

Show that this formula gives the correct solution for y, assuming $y_0 \neq A$.

10.6 MODELING THE INTERACTION OF TWO POPULATIONS

So far we have used a differential equation to model the growth of a single quantity. We now consider the growth of two interacting populations, a situation which requires a system of two differential equations. Examples include two species competing for food, one species preying on another, or two species helping each other (symbiosis).

A Predator-Prey Model: Robins and Worms

We model a predator-prey system using what are called the Lotka-Volterra equations. Let's look at a simplified and idealized case in which robins are the predators and worms the prey.[2] Suppose there are r thousand robins and w million worms. If there were no robins, the worms would increase exponentially according to the equation

$$\frac{dw}{dt} = aw \qquad \text{where } a \text{ is a positive constant.}$$

If there were no worms, the robins would have no food and so their population would decrease according to the equation[3]

$$\frac{dr}{dt} = -br \qquad \text{where } b \text{ is a positive constant.}$$

Now imagine the effect of the two populations on one another. Clearly, the presence of the robins is bad for the worms, so

$$\frac{dw}{dt} = aw - \text{Effect of robins on worms.}$$

On the other hand, the robins do better with the worms around, so

$$\frac{dr}{dt} = -br + \text{Effect of worms on robins.}$$

How exactly do the two populations interact? Let's assume the effect of one population on the other is proportional to the number of "encounters." (An encounter is when a robin eats a worm.) The number of encounters is likely to be proportional to the product of the populations because if one population is held fixed, the number of encounters should be directly proportional to the other population. So we assume

$$\frac{dw}{dt} = aw - cwr \qquad \text{and} \qquad \frac{dr}{dt} = -br + kwr,$$

where c and k are positive constants.

To analyze this system of equations, let's look at the specific example with $a = b = c = k = 1$:

$$\frac{dw}{dt} = w - wr \qquad \text{and} \qquad \frac{dr}{dt} = -r + wr.$$

The Phase Plane

To see the growth of the populations, we want graphs of r and w against t. However, it is easier to obtain a graph of r against w first. If we plot a point (w, r) representing the number of worms and robins at any moment, then, as the populations change, the point moves. The wr-plane on which the point moves is called the *phase plane* and the path of the point is called the *phase trajectory*.

To find the phase trajectory, we need a differential equation relating w and r directly. We have the two differential equations

$$\frac{dw}{dt} = w - wr \qquad \text{and} \qquad \frac{dr}{dt} = -r + wr.$$

Thinking of r as a function of w and w as a function of t, the chain rule gives

$$\frac{dr}{dt} = \frac{dr}{dw} \cdot \frac{dw}{dt}.$$

[2] Based on work by Thomas A. McMahon.

[3] This assumption unrealistically predicts that the robin population will decay exponentially, rather than die out in finite time.

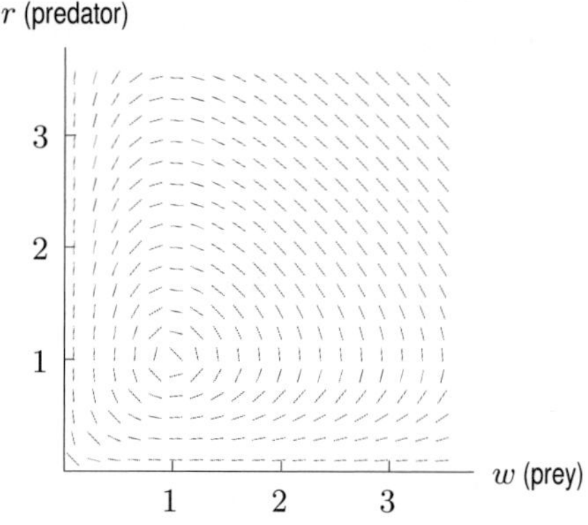

Figure 10.37: Slope field for $\dfrac{dr}{dw} = \dfrac{-r + wr}{w - wr}$

This tells us that

$$\frac{dr}{dw} = \frac{dr/dt}{dw/dt},$$

so we have

$$\frac{dr}{dw} = \frac{-r + wr}{w - wr}.$$

Figure 10.37 shows the slope field of this differential equation in the phase plane.

The Slope Field and Equilibrium Points

We can get an idea of what solutions of this equation look like from the slope field. At the point $(1, 1)$ there is no slope drawn because dr/dw is undefined there since the rates of change of both populations with respect to time are zero:

$$\frac{dw}{dt} = 1 - 1 \cdot 1 = 0, \qquad \text{and} \qquad \frac{dr}{dt} = -1 + 1 \cdot 1 = 0.$$

In terms of worms and robins, this means that if at some moment $w = 1$ and $r = 1$ (that is, there are 1 million worms and 1 thousand robins), then w and r remain constant forever. The point $w = 1$, $r = 1$ is therefore an equilibrium solution. The origin is also an equilibrium point, since if $w = 0$ and $r = 0$, then w and r remain constant. The slope field suggests that there are no other equilibrium points. We check this by solving

$$\frac{dw}{dt} = w - wr = 0 \qquad \text{and} \qquad \frac{dr}{dt} = -r + rw = 0,$$

which yields only $w = 0$, $r = 0$ and $w = 1$, $r = 1$ as solutions.

Trajectories in the wr-Phase Plane

Let's look at the trajectories in the phase plane. A point on a curve represents a pair of populations (w, r) existing at the same time t (though t is not shown on the graph). A short time later, the pair of populations is represented by a nearby point. As time passes, the point traces out a trajectory. It can be shown that the trajectory is a closed curve. See Figure 10.38.

In which direction does the point move on the trajectory? Look at the original pair of differential equations. They tell us how w and r change with time. Imagine, for example, that we are at the point P_0 in Figure 10.39, where $w = 2.2$ and $r = 1$; then

$$\frac{dr}{dt} = -r + wr = -1 + (2.2)(1) = 1.2 > 0.$$

Therefore, r is increasing, so the point is moving in the direction shown by the arrow in Figure 10.39.

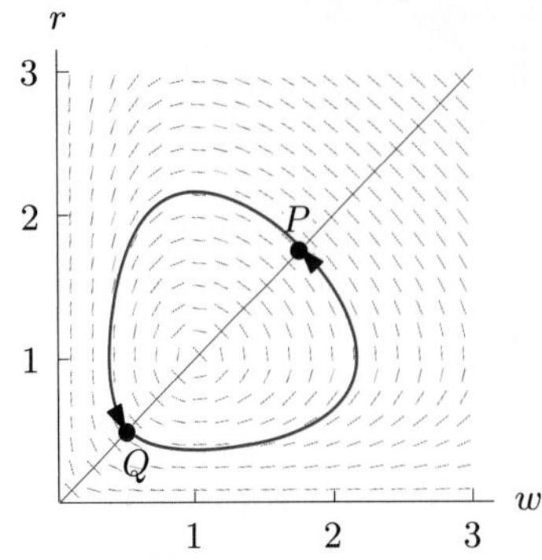

Figure 10.38: Solution curve is closed

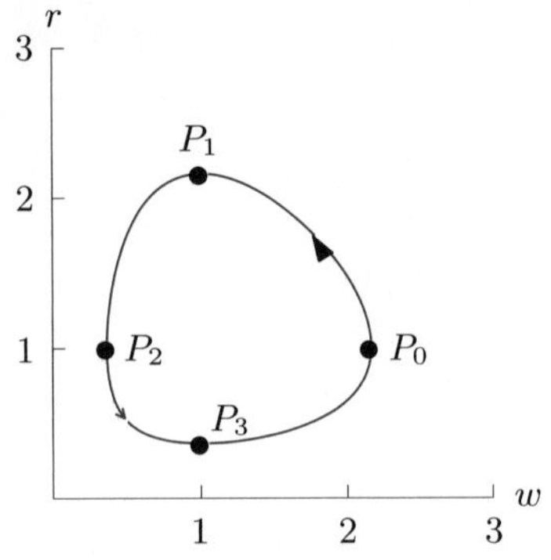

Figure 10.39: A trajectory

Example 1 Suppose that at time $t = 0$, there are 2.2 million worms and 1 thousand robins. Describe how the robin and worm populations change over time.

Solution The trajectory through the point P_0 where $w = 2.2$ and $r = 1$ is shown on the slope field in Figure 10.38 and by itself in Figure 10.39.

Initially there are lots of worms so the robin population does well. The robin population is increasing and the worm population is decreasing until there are about 2.2 thousand robins and 1 million worms (point P_1 in Figure 10.39). At this point, there are too few worms to sustain the robin population; it begins to decrease and the worm population continues to fall as well. The robin population falls dramatically until there are about 1 thousand robins and 0.4 million worms (point P_2 in Figure 10.39). With so few robins, the worm population starts to recover, but the robin population is still decreasing. The worm population increases until there are about 0.4 thousand robins and 1 million worms (P_3 in Figure 10.39). Now there are lots of worms for the small population of robins so both populations increase. The populations return to the starting values (since the trajectory forms a closed curve) and the cycle starts over.

Problem 17 at the end of the section shows how to calculate approximate coordinates of points on the curve.

The Populations as Functions of Time

The shape of a trajectory tells us how the populations vary with time. We use this information to graph each population against time, as in Figure 10.40. The fact that the trajectory is a closed curve means that both populations oscillate periodically. Both populations have the same period, and the worms (the prey) are at their maximum a quarter of a cycle before the robins.

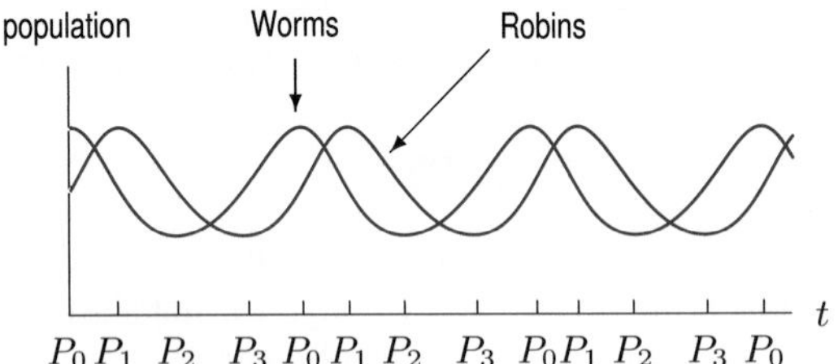

Figure 10.40: Populations of robins (in thousands) and worms (in millions) over time

Lynxes and Hares

A predator-prey system for which there are long-term data is the Canadian lynx and the hare. Both animals were of interest to fur trappers and the records of the Hudson Bay Company shed some light on their populations through much of the 20th century. These records show that both populations oscillated up and down, quite regularly, with a period of about ten years. This is the behavior predicted by Lotka-Volterra equations.

Other Forms of Species Interaction

The methods of this section can be used to model other types of interactions between two species, such as competition and symbiosis.

Example 2 Describe the interactions between two populations x and y modeled by the following systems of differential equations.

(a) $$\frac{dx}{dt} = 0.2x - 0.5xy \qquad \frac{dy}{dt} = 0.6y - 0.8xy$$

(b) $$\frac{dx}{dt} = -2x + 5xy \qquad \frac{dy}{dt} = -y + 0.2xy$$

(c) $$\frac{dx}{dt} = 0.5x \qquad \frac{dy}{dt} = -1.6y + 2xy$$

(d) $$\frac{dx}{dt} = 0.3x - 1.2xy \qquad \frac{dy}{dt} = -0.7y + 2.5xy$$

Solution

(a) If we ignore the interaction terms with xy, we have $dx/dt = 0.2x$ and $dy/dt = 0.6y$, so both populations grow exponentially. Since both interaction terms are negative, each species inhibits the other's growth, such as when deer and elk compete for food.

(b) If we ignore the interaction terms, the populations of both species decrease exponentially. However, both interaction terms are positive, meaning each species benefits from the other, so the relationship is symbiotic. An example is the pollination of plants by insects.

(c) Ignoring interaction, x grows and y decays. But the interaction term means that y benefits from x, in the way birds that build nests benefit from trees.

(d) Without the interaction, x grows and y decays. The interaction terms show that y hurts x while x benefits y. This is a predator-prey model where y is the predator and x is the prey.

Problems for Section 10.6

Problems 1–3 give the rates of growth of two populations, x and y, measured in thousands.

(a) Describe in words what happens to the population of each species in the absence of the other.

(b) Describe in words how the species interact with one another. Give reasons why the populations might behave as described by the equations. Suggest species that might interact in that way.

1. $$\frac{dx}{dt} = 0.01x - 0.05xy \qquad \frac{dy}{dt} = -0.2y + 0.08xy$$

2. $$\frac{dx}{dt} = 0.01x - 0.05xy \qquad \frac{dy}{dt} = 0.2y - 0.08xy$$

3. $$\frac{dx}{dt} = 0.2x \qquad \frac{dy}{dt} = 0.4xy - 0.1y$$

4. The following system of differential equations represents the interaction between two populations, x and y.

$$\frac{dx}{dt} = -3x + 2xy$$
$$\frac{dy}{dt} = -y + 5xy$$

(a) Describe how the species interact. How would each species do in the absence of the other? Are they helpful or harmful to each other?

(b) If $x = 2$ and $y = 1$, does x increase or decrease? Does y increase or decrease? Justify your answers.

(c) Write a differential equation involving dy/dx.

(d) Use a computer or calculator to draw the slope field for the differential equation in part (c).

(e) Draw the trajectory starting at point $x = 2$, $y = 1$ on your slope field, and describe how the populations change as time increases.

Create a system of differential equations to model the situations in Problems 5–7. You may assume that all constants of proportionality are 1.

5. Two businesses are in competition with each other. Both businesses would do well without the other one, but each hurts the other's business. The values of the two businesses are given by x and y.

6. A population of fleas is represented by x, and a population of dogs is represented by y. The fleas need the dogs in order to survive. The dog population, however, is unaffected by the fleas.

7. The concentrations of two chemicals are denoted by x and y, respectively. Alone, each decays at a rate proportional to its concentration. Together, they interact to form a third substance. As the third substance is created, the concentrations of the initial two populations get smaller.

8. Two companies, A and B, are in competition with each other. Let x represent the net worth (in millions of dollars) of Company A, and y represent the net worth (in millions of dollars) of Company B. Four trajectories are given in Figure 10.41. For each trajectory: Describe the initial conditions. Describe what happens initially: Do the companies gain or lose money early on? What happens in the long run?

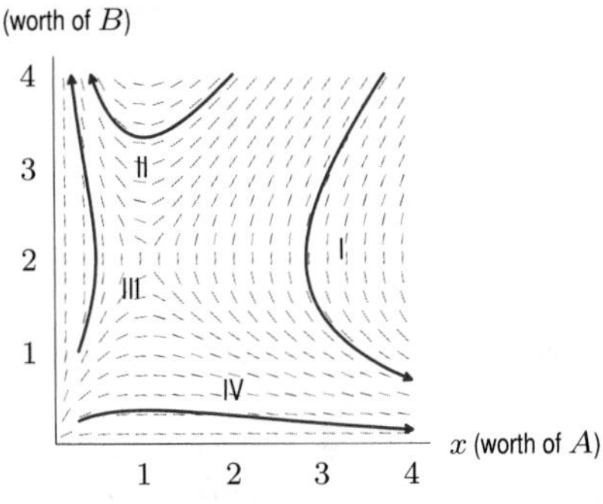

Figure 10.41

For Problems 9–19, let w be the number of worms (in millions) and r the number of robins (in thousands) living on an island. Suppose w and r satisfy the following differential equations, which correspond to the slope field in Figure 10.42.

$$\frac{dw}{dt} = w - wr, \qquad \frac{dr}{dt} = -r + wr.$$

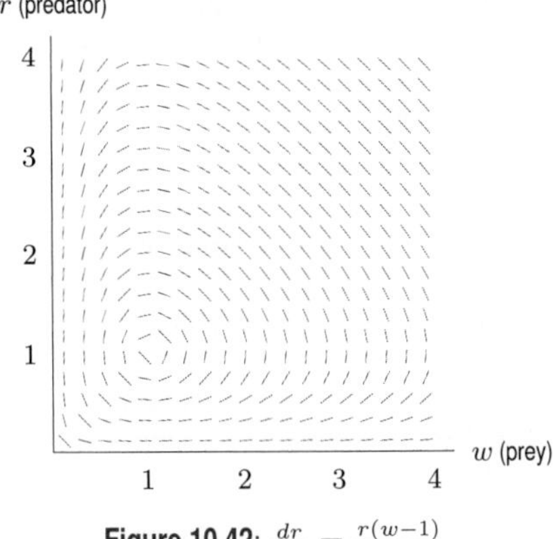

Figure 10.42: $\frac{dr}{dw} = \frac{r(w-1)}{w(1-r)}$

9. Explain why these differential equations are a reasonable model for interaction between the two populations. Why have the signs been chosen this way?

10. Solve these differential equations in the two special cases when there are no robins and when there are no worms living on the island.

11. Describe and explain the symmetry you observe in the slope field. What consequences does this symmetry have for the solution curves?

12. Assume $w = 2$ and $r = 2$ when $t = 0$. Do the numbers of robins and worms increase or decrease at first? What happens in the long run?

13. For the case discussed in Problem 12, estimate the maximum and the minimum values of the robin population. How many worms are there at the time when the robin population reaches its maximum?

14. On the same axes, graph w and r (the worm and the robin populations) against time. Use initial values of 1.5 for w and 1 for r. You may do this without units for t.

15. People on the island like robins so much that they decide to import 200 robins all the way from England, to increase the initial population from $r = 2$ to $r = 2.2$ when $t = 0$. Does this make sense? Why or why not?

16. Assume that $w = 3$ and $r = 1$ when $t = 0$. Do the numbers of robins and worms increase or decrease initially? What happens in the long run?

17. At $t = 0$ there are 2.2 million worms and 1 thousand robins.

(a) Use the differential equations to calculate the derivatives dw/dt and dr/dt at $t = 0$.
(b) Use the initial values and your answer to part (a) to estimate the number of robins and worms at $t = 0.1$.
(c) Using the method of part (a) and (b), estimate the number of robins and worms at $t = 0.2$ and 0.3.

18. **(a)** Assume that there are 3 million worms and 2 thousand robins. Locate the point corresponding to this situation on the slope field given in Figure 10.42. Draw the trajectory through this point.
(b) In which direction does the point move along this trajectory? Put an arrow on the trajectory and justify your answer using the differential equations for dr/dt and dw/dt given in this section.
(c) How large does the robin population get? What is the size of the worm population when the robin population is at its largest?
(d) How large does the worm population get? What is the size of the robin population when the worm population is at its largest?

19. Repeat Problem 18 if initially there are 0.5 million worms and 3 thousand robins.

20. For each system of differential equations in Example 2, determine whether x increases or decreases and whether y increases or decreases when $x = 2$ and $y = 2$.

21. For each system of equations in Example 2, write a differential equation involving dy/dx. Use a computer or calculator to draw the slope field for $x, y > 0$. Then draw the trajectory through the point $x = 3, y = 1$.

10.7 MODELING THE SPREAD OF A DISEASE

Differential equations can be used to predict when an outbreak of a disease becomes so severe that it is called an *epidemic*[4] and to decide what level of vaccination is necessary to prevent an epidemic. Let's consider a specific example.

Flu in a British Boarding School

In January 1978, 763 students returned to a boys' boarding school after their winter vacation. A week later, one boy developed the flu, followed immediately by two more. By the end of the month, nearly half the boys were sick. Most of the school had been affected by the time the epidemic was over in mid-February.[5]

Being able to predict how many people will get sick, and when, is an important step toward controlling an epidemic. This is one of the responsibilities of Britain's Communicable Disease Surveillance Centre and the US's Center for Disease Control and Prevention.

The S-I-R model

We apply one of the most commonly used models for an epidemic, called the S-I-R model, to the boarding school flu example. Imagine the population of the school divided into three groups:

$S =$ the number of *susceptibles*, the people who are not yet sick but who could become sick

$I =$ the number of *infecteds*, the people who are currently sick

$R =$ the number of *recovered*, or *removed*, the people who have been sick and can no longer infect others or be reinfected.

In this model, the number of susceptibles decreases with time, as people become infected. We assume that the rate people become infected is proportional to the number of contacts between susceptible and infected people. We expect the number of contacts between the two groups to be proportional to both S and I. (If S doubles, we expect the number of contacts to double; similarly, if I doubles, we expect the number of contacts to double.) Thus, we assume that the number of contacts is proportional to the product, SI. In other words, we assume that for some constant $a > 0$,

$$\frac{dS}{dt} = -\left(\begin{array}{c}\text{Rate susceptibles} \\ \text{get sick}\end{array}\right) = -aSI.$$

(The negative sign is used because S is decreasing.)

The number of infecteds is changing in two ways: newly sick people are added to the infected group and others are removed. The newly sick people are exactly those people leaving the susceptible group and so accrue at a rate of aSI (with a positive sign this time). People leave the infected group either because they recover (or die), or because they are physically removed from the rest of the group and can no longer infect others. We assume that people are removed at a rate proportional to the number sick, or bI, where b is a positive constant. Thus,

$$\frac{dI}{dt} = \begin{array}{c}\text{Rate susceptibles} \\ \text{get sick}\end{array} - \begin{array}{c}\text{Rate infecteds} \\ \text{get removed}\end{array} = aSI - bI.$$

Assuming that those who have recovered from the disease are no longer susceptible, the recovered group increases at the rate of bI, so

$$\frac{dR}{dt} = bI.$$

[4]Exactly when a disease should be called an epidemic is not always clear. The medical profession generally classifies a disease an epidemic when the frequency is higher than usually expected—leaving open the question of what is usually expected. See, for example, *Epidemiology in Medicine* by C. H. Hennekens and J. Buring (Boston: Little, Brown, 1987).

[5]Data from the Communicable Disease Surveillance Centre (UK); reported in "Influenza in a Boarding School," *British Medical Journal* March 4, 1978, and by J. D. Murray in *Mathematical Biology* (New York: Springer Verlag, 1990).

We are assuming that having the flu confers immunity on a person, that is, that the person cannot get the flu again. (This is true for a given strain of flu, at least in the short run.)

We can use the fact that the total population $S+I+R$ is not changing. (The total population, the total number of boys in the school, did not change during the epidemic; see Problem 2 on page 440.) Thus, once we know S and I, we can calculate R. So we restrict our attention to the two equations

$$\frac{dS}{dt} = -aSI$$
$$\frac{dI}{dt} = aSI - bI.$$

The Constants a and b

The constant a measures how infectious the disease is—that is, how quickly it is transmitted from the infecteds to the susceptibles. In the case of the flu, we know from medical accounts that the epidemic started with one sick boy, with two more becoming sick roughly a day later. Thus, when $I = 1$ and $S = 762$, we have $dS/dt \approx -2$, enabling us to roughly[6] approximate a:

$$a = -\frac{dS/dt}{SI} = \frac{2}{762 \cdot 1} = 0.0026.$$

The constant b represents the rate at which infected people are removed from the infected population. In this case of the flu, boys were generally taken to the infirmary within one or two days of becoming sick. Assuming half the infected population was removed each day, we take $b \approx 0.5$. Thus, our equations are:

$$\frac{dS}{dt} = -0.0026SI$$
$$\frac{dI}{dt} = 0.0026SI - 0.5I.$$

The Phase Plane

As in Section 10.6, we look at trajectories in the phase plane. Thinking of I as a function of S, and S as a function of t, we use the chain rule to get

$$\frac{dI}{dt} = \frac{dI}{dS} \cdot \frac{dS}{dt},$$

so

$$\frac{dI}{dS} = \frac{dI/dt}{dS/dt}.$$

Substituting for dI/dt and dS/dt, we get

$$\frac{dI}{dS} = \frac{0.0026SI - 0.5I}{-0.0026SI}.$$

Assuming I is not zero, this equation simplifies to approximately

$$\frac{dI}{dS} = -1 + \frac{192}{S}.$$

The slope field of this differential equation is shown in Figure 10.43. The trajectory with initial condition $S_0 = 762$, $I_0 = 1$ is shown in Figure 10.44. Time is represented by the arrow showing the direction that a point moves on the trajectory. The disease starts at the point $S_0 = 762$, $I_0 = 1$. At first, more people become infected and fewer are susceptible. In other words, S decreases and I increases. Later, I decreases as S continues to decrease.

[6]The values of a and b are close to those obtained by J. D. Murray in *Mathematical Biology* (New York: Springer Verlag, 1990).

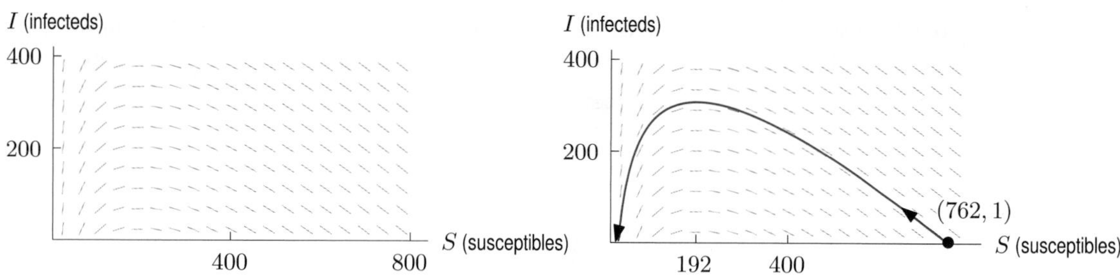

Figure 10.43: Slope field for $dI/dS = -1 + 192/S$

Figure 10.44: Trajectory for $S_0 = 762$, $I_0 = 1$

What does the SI-Phase Plane Tell Us?

To learn how the disease progresses, look at the shape of the curve in Figure 10.44. The value of I first increases, then decreases to zero. This peak value of I occurs when $S \approx 200$. We can determine exactly when the peak value occurs by solving

$$\frac{dI}{dS} = -1 + \frac{192}{S} = 0,$$

which gives

$$S = 192.$$

Notice that the peak value for I always occurs at the same value of S, namely $S = 192$. The graph shows that if a trajectory starts with $S_0 > 192$, then I first increases and then decreases to zero. On the other hand, if $S_0 < 192$, there is no peak, since I decreases right away.

For this example, the value $S = 192$ is called a *threshold population*. If S_0 is around or below 192, there is no epidemic. If S_0 is significantly greater than 192, an epidemic occurs.[7]

The phase diagram makes clear that the maximum value of I is about 300, which is the maximum number infected at any one time. In addition, the point at which the trajectory crosses the S-axis represents the time when the epidemic has passed (since $I = 0$). Thus, the S-intercept shows how many boys never get the flu and, hence, how many do get sick.

Threshold Value

For the general SIR model, we have the following result:

$$\text{Threshold population} = \frac{b}{a}.$$

If S_0, the initial number of susceptibles, is above b/a, there is an epidemic; if S_0 is below b/a, there is no epidemic. See Problem 11.

How Many People Should Be Vaccinated?

Faced with an outbreak of the flu or, as happened on several US campuses in the 1980s, of the measles, many institutions consider a vaccination program. How many students must be vaccinated in order to control an outbreak? To answer this, we can think of vaccination as removing people from the S category (without increasing I), which amounts to moving the initial point on the trajectory to the left, parallel to the S-axis. To avoid an epidemic, the initial value of S_0 should be around or below the threshold value. Therefore, the boarding-school epidemic would have been avoided if all but 192 students had been vaccinated.

Graphs of S and I Against t

On the trajectory in Figure 10.44, the number of susceptible people decreases throughout the epidemic. This makes sense since people are getting sick and then well again, and thus are no longer susceptible to infection. The trajectory also shows that the number of infected people increases and then decreases. Graphs of S and I against time, t, are shown in Figure 10.45.

[7]Here we are using J. D. Murray's definition of an epidemic as an outbreak in which the number of infecteds increases from the initial value, I_0. See *Mathematical Biology* (New York: Springer Verlag, 1990).

To get the scale on the time axis, we would need to use numerical methods. It turns out that the number of infecteds peaked after about 6 days and then dropped. The epidemic ran its course in about 20 days.

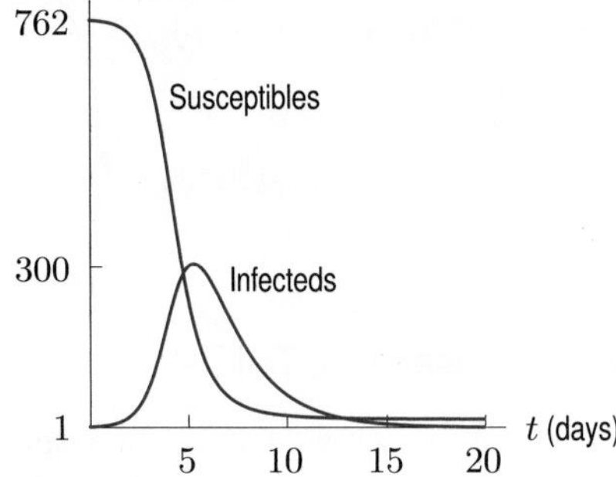

Figure 10.45: Progress of the flu over time

Problems for Section 10.7

1. Let I be the number of infected people and S be the number of susceptible people in an outbreak of a disease. Explain why it is reasonable to model the interaction between these two groups by the differential equations

$$\frac{dS}{dt} = -aSI$$
$$\frac{dI}{dt} = aSI - bI \quad \text{where } a, b \text{ are positive constants.}$$

Why have the signs been chosen this way? Why is the constant a the same in both equations?

2. Show that if S, I, and R satisfy the differential equations in Problem 1, the total population, $S+I+R$, is constant.

3. Explain how you can tell from the graph of the trajectory shown in Figure 10.44 that most people at the British boarding school eventually got sick.

4. **(a)** In a school of 150 students, one of the students has the flu initially. What is I_0? What is S_0?
(b) Use these values of I_0 and S_0 and the equation

$$\frac{dI}{dt} = 0.0026SI - 0.5I$$

to determine whether the number of infected people initially increases or decreases. What does this tell you about the spread of the disease?

5. Repeat Problem 4 for a school with 350 students.

6. **(a)** On the slope field for dI/dS in Figure 10.43 trajectory through the point where $I = 1$ and $S = 400$.
(b) How many susceptible people are there when the number of infected people is at its maximum?

7. Use Figure 10.45 to estimate the maximum number of infecteds. What does this represent? When does it occur?

8. Compare the diseases modeled by each of the following differential equations with the flu model in this section. Match each set of differential equations with one of the following statements. Write a system of differential equations corresponding to each of the unmatched statements.

(I) $\dfrac{dS}{dt} = -0.04SI$, $\quad \dfrac{dI}{dt} = 0.04SI - 0.2I$

(II) $\dfrac{dS}{dt} = -0.002SI$, $\quad \dfrac{dI}{dt} = 0.002SI - 0.3I$

(III) $\dfrac{dS}{dt} = -0.03SI$, $\quad \dfrac{dI}{dt} = 0.03SI$

(a) More infectious; infecteds removed more slowly.
(b) More infectious; infecteds removed more quickly.
(c) Less infectious; infecteds removed more slowly.
(d) Less infectious; infecteds removed more quickly.
(e) Infecteds never removed.

9. For the equations (I) in Problem 8, what is the threshold value of S?

10. For the equations (II) in Problem 8, suppose $S_0 = 100$. Does the disease spread initially? What if $S_0 = 200$?

11. Let S and I satisfy the differential equations in Problem 1. Assume $I \neq 0$.

(a) If $dI/dt = 0$, find S.
(b) Show that I increases if S is greater than the value you found in part (a). Show that I decreases if S is less than the value you found in part (a).
(c) Explain how you know that your answer to part (a) is the threshold value.

12. During World War I, a particularly lethal form of flu killed about 40 million people around the world.[8] The epidemic started in an army camp of 45,000 soldiers outside of Boston, where the first soldier fell sick on September 7, 1918. With time, t, in days since September 7, values of the constants in the SIR model,

[8] "Capturing a Killer Flu Virus," J. Taukenberger, A. Reid, T. Fanning, in *Scientific American*, Vol. 292, No. 1, Jan. 2005.

$$\frac{dS}{dt} = -aSI$$
$$\frac{dI}{dt} = aSI - bI,$$

are estimated to be $a = 0.000267$, $b = 9.865$.

(a) What are the initial values, S_0 and I_0?

(b) Explain how you know that this model predicts an epidemic in this case.

(c) Find the differential equation for dI/dS. Sketch its slope field and estimate the total number of soldiers infected over the course of the disease.

(d) Solve the differential equation for dI/dS analytically. Use the solution to solve approximately for the number of soldiers affected over the course of the disease.

CHAPTER SUMMARY

- **Differential equations terminology**
  Family of solutions, particular solution, initial conditions, stable/unstable equilibrium solutions
- **Estimating values of a solution**
- **Slope fields**
  Visualizing the solution to a differential equation
- **Solving differential equations analytically**
  Solutions to $dy/dt = ky$, and $dy/dt = k(y - A)$
- **Modeling with differential equations**
  Growth and decay, pollution in a lake, quantity of drug in the body, Newton's law of heating and cooling, net worth of a company
- **Systems of differential equations**
  Interaction of two species or businesses, predator-prey model, spread of a disease

REVIEW PROBLEMS FOR CHAPTER TEN

1. Match the graphs in Figure 10.46 with the following descriptions.

(a) The population of a new species introduced onto a tropical island

(b) The temperature of a metal ingot placed in a furnace and then removed

(c) The speed of a car traveling at uniform speed and then braking uniformly

(d) The mass of carbon-14 in a historical specimen

(e) The concentration of tree pollen in the air over the course of a year.

(I) (II) (III) (IV) (V)

Figure 10.46

2. **(a)** Determine which of the following functions is a solution to the differential equation

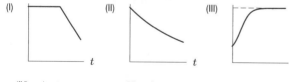

$$x\frac{dy}{dx} = 3y.$$

(i) $y = Cx^2$ (ii) $y = Cx^3$

(iii) $y = x^3 + C$

(b) For any function which is a solution, find C if $y = 40$ when $x = 2$.

3. Is $y = x^3$ a solution to the differential equation $xy' - 3y = 0$? Justify your answer.

4. For a certain quantity y, assume that $dy/dt = -0.20y$. Fill in the values of y in Table 10.7. Assume that the rate of growth given by dy/dt is approximately constant over each unit time interval.

Table 10.7

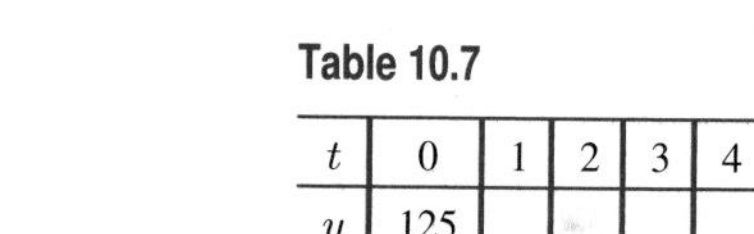

t	0	1	2	3	4
y	125				

5. Slope fields for $dy/dx = 1 + x$ and $dy/dx = 1 + y$ are in Figures 10.47 and 10.48.

(a) Which slope field corresponds to which equation?

(b) On each slope field, draw the solution curve through the origin.

(c) For each slope field, list all equilibrium solutions and indicate whether each is stable or unstable.

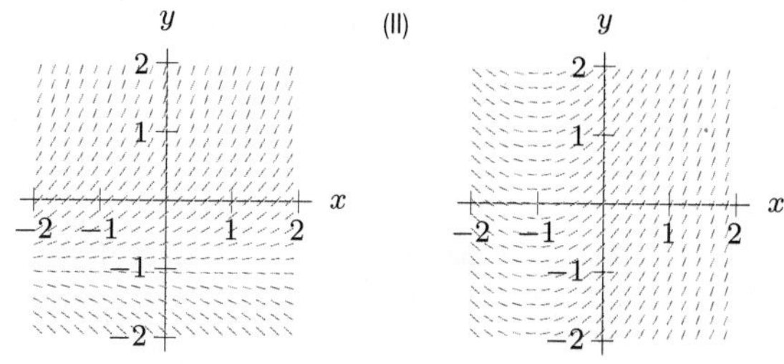

Figure 10.47 Figure 10.48

6. **(a)** Sketch the slope field for the equation $y' = x - y$ in Figure 10.49 at the points indicated.
   (b) Check that $y = x - 1$ is the solution to the differential equation passing through the point $(1, 0)$.

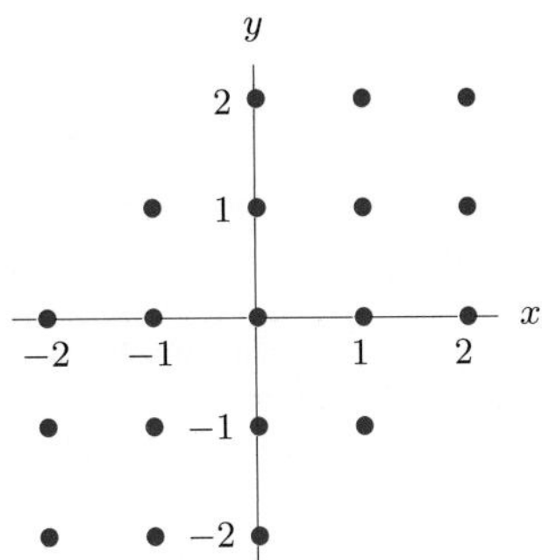

Figure 10.49

7. Which one of the following differential equations best fits the slope field shown in Figure 10.50? Explain.

I. $y' = 1 + y$ II. $y' = 2 - y$

III. $y' = (1 + y)(2 - y)$ IV. $y' = 1 + x$

V. $y' = xy$

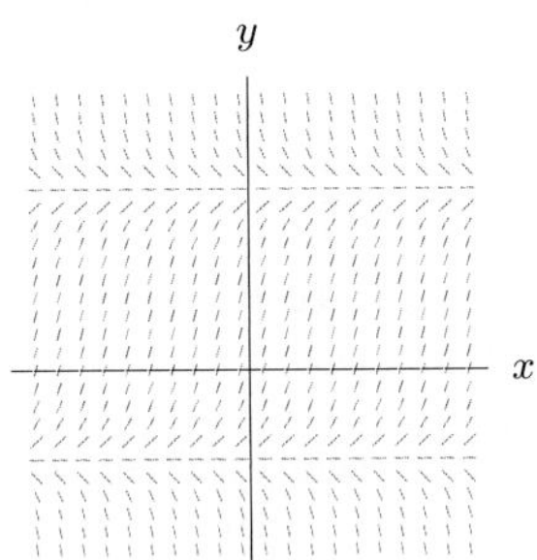

Figure 10.50

8. Match each of the slope field segments in (I)–(VI) with one or more of the differential equations in (a)–(f).

(a) $y' = e^{-x^2}$ **(b)** $y' = \cos y$ **(c)** $y' = \cos(4-y)$

(d) $y' = y(4-y)$ **(e)** $y' = y(3-y)$ **(f)** $y' = x(3-x)$

(I)

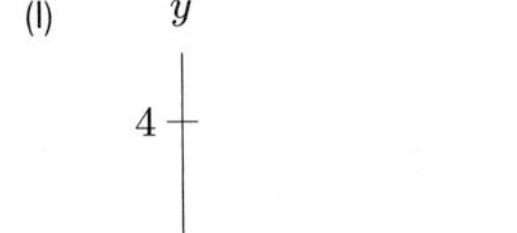

(II)

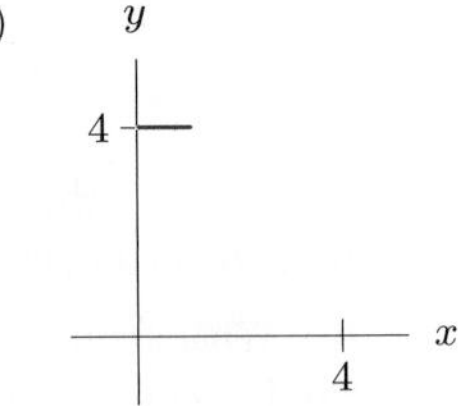

(III)

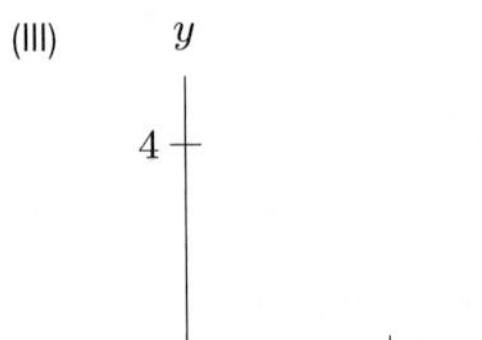

(IV)

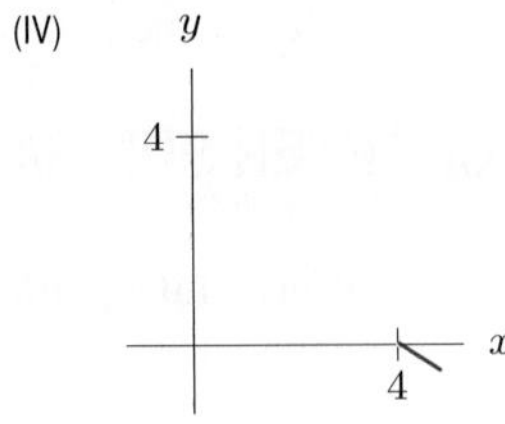

(V)

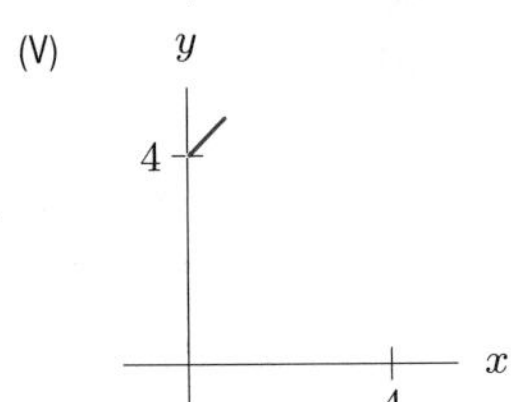

(VI)

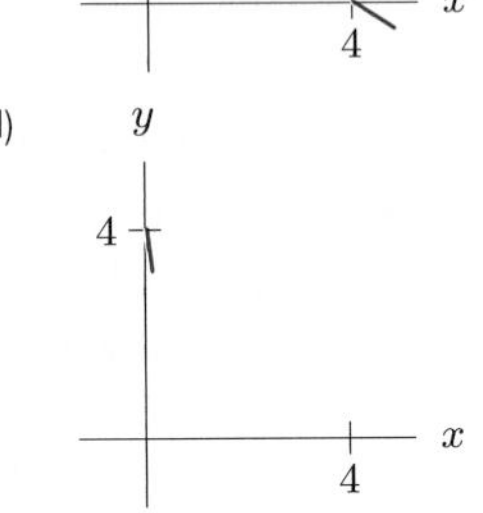

9. A deposit is made to a bank account paying an annual interest rate of 7% compounded continuously. No other deposits or withdrawals are made to the account.
   (a) Write a differential equation satisfied by B, the balance in the account after t years.
   (b) Solve the differential equation given in part (a).
   (c) If the initial deposit is \$5000, give the particular solution satisfying this initial condition.
   (d) How much is in the account after 10 years?

10. Radioactive iodine decays at a continuous rate of about 9% per day. Write a differential equation to model this behavior. Find the general solution.

Solve the differential equations in Problems 11–20.

11. $\dfrac{dP}{dt} = t$ **12.** $\dfrac{dy}{dt} = 5y$

13. $\dfrac{dy}{dt} = 5t$ **14.** $\dfrac{dP}{dt} = 0.03P$

15. $\dfrac{dA}{dt} = -0.07A$ **16.** $\dfrac{1}{Q}\dfrac{dQ}{dt} = 2$

17. $\dfrac{dP}{dt} = 10 - 2P$ **18.** $\dfrac{dy}{dt} = 100 - y$

19. $\dfrac{dy}{dx} = 0.2y - 8$ **20.** $\dfrac{dH}{dt} = 0.5H + 10$

21. Write a differential equation whose solution is the temperature as a function of time of a bottle of orange juice taken out of a 40°F refrigerator and left in a 65°F room. Solve the equation and graph the solution.

22. The rate of growth of a tumor is proportional to the size of the tumor.

(a) Write a differential equation satisfied by S, the size of the tumor, in mm, as a function of time, t.
(b) Find the general solution to the differential equation.
(c) If the tumor is 5 mm across at time $t = 0$, what does that tell you about the solution?
(d) If, in addition, the tumor is 8 mm across at time $t = 3$, what does that tell you about the solution?

23. The radioactive isotope carbon-14 is present in small quantities in all life forms, and it is constantly replenished until the organism dies, after which it decays to stable carbon-12 at a rate proportional to the amount of carbon-14 present, with a half-life of 5730 years. Suppose $C(t)$ is the amount of carbon-14 present at time t.

(a) Find the value of the constant k in the differential equation $C' = -kC$.
(b) In 1988 three teams of scientists found that the Shroud of Turin, which was reputed to be the burial cloth of Jesus, contained 91% of the amount of carbon-14 contained in freshly made cloth of the same material.[9] How old is the Shroud of Turin, according to these data?

24. A bank account earns 5% annual interest compounded continuously. Continuous payments are made out of the account at a rate of \$12,000 per year for 20 years.

(a) Write a differential equation describing the balance $B = f(t)$, where t is in years.
(b) Solve the differential equation given an initial balance of B_0.
(c) What should the initial balance be such that the account has zero balance after precisely 20 years?

25. Warfarin is a drug used as an anticoagulant. After administration of the drug is stopped, the quantity remaining in a patient's body decreases at a rate proportional to the quantity remaining. The half-life of warfarin in the body is 37 hours.

(a) Sketch the quantity, Q, of warfarin in a patient's body as a function of the time, t, since stopping administration of the drug. Mark the 37 hours on your graph.
(b) Write a differential equation satisfied by Q.
(c) How many days does it take for the drug level in the body to be reduced to 25% of the original level?

26. Dead leaves accumulate on the ground in a forest at a rate of 3 grams per square centimeter per year. At the same time, these leaves decompose at a continuous rate of 75% per year. Write a differential equation for the total quantity of dead leaves (per square centimeter) at time t. Sketch a solution showing that the quantity of dead leaves tends toward an equilibrium level. What is that equilibrium level?

[9] *The New York Times*, October 18, 1988

27. Morphine is often used as a pain-relieving drug. The half-life of morphine in the body is 2 hours. Suppose morphine is administered to a patient intravenously at a rate of 2.5 mg per hour, and the rate at which the morphine is eliminated is proportional to the amount present.

(a) Use the half-life to show that, to three decimal places, the constant of proportionality for the rate at which morphine leaves the body (in mg/hour) is $k = -0.347$.
(b) Write a differential equation for the quantity, Q, of morphine in the blood after t hours.
(c) Use the differential equation to find the equilibrium solution. (This is the long-term amount of morphine in the body, once the system has stabilized.)

28. **(a)** Find all equilibrium solutions for the equation

$$\frac{dy}{dx} = 0.5y(y-4)(2+y).$$

(b) With a calculator or computer, draw a slope field for this differential equation. Use it to determine whether each equilibrium solution is stable or unstable.

29. According to a simple physiological model, an athletic adult male needs 20 calories per day per pound of body weight to maintain his weight. If he consumes more or fewer calories than those required to maintain his weight, his weight changes at a rate proportional to the difference between the number of calories consumed and the number needed to maintain his current weight; the constant of proportionality is $1/3500$ pounds per calorie. Suppose that a particular person has a constant caloric intake of I calories per day. Let $W(t)$ be the person's weight in pounds at time t (measured in days).

(a) What differential equation has solution $W(t)$?
(b) Solve this differential equation.
(c) Graph $W(t)$ if the person starts out weighing 160 pounds and consumes 3000 calories a day.

30. **(a)** Graph $f(y) = y - y^2$.
(b) Sketch the slope field of the differential equation

$$\frac{dy}{dx} = y - y^2.$$

(c) Describe how the two graphs are related. In particular, explain how you can determine the equilibrium solutions to the differential equation from the graph of $f(y)$ and how you can tell if the equilibrium solutions are stable.

31. **(a)** What are the equilibrium solutions to the differential equation $y' = f(y)$, where $f(y)$ is graphed in Figure 10.51?
(b) Sketch the slope field for $y' = f(y)$.

(c) For each of the following initial conditions, sketch the solution curve on your slope field:

(i) $y(0) = 0$ (ii) $y(0) = 1$ (iii) $y(0) = 6$
(iv) $y(0) = 8$ (v) $y(0) = 10$ (vi) $y(0) = 16$
(vii) $y(0) = 17$

(d) Which of the equilibrium solutions are stable? Which are unstable?

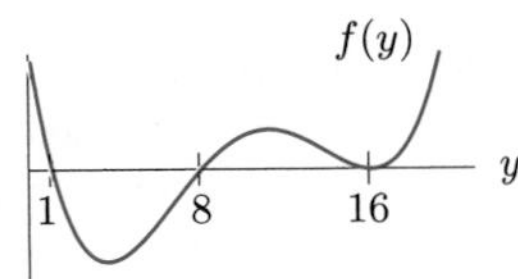

Figure 10.51

For Problems 32–36, suppose x and y are the populations of two different species. Describe in words how each population changes with time.

32. **33.**

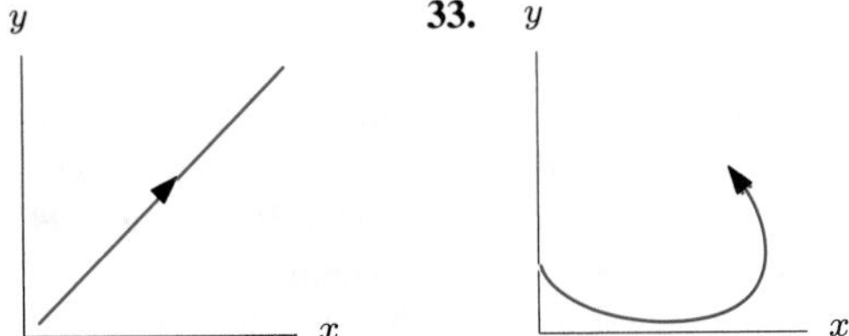

34. **35.**

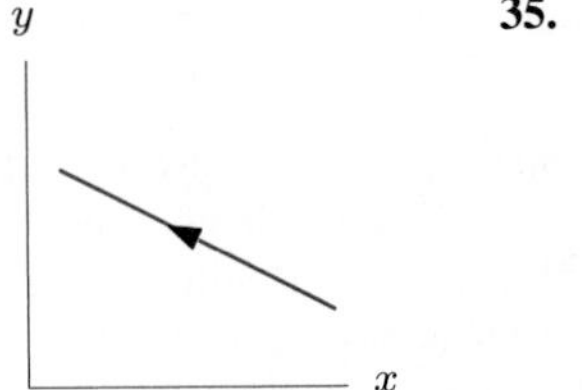

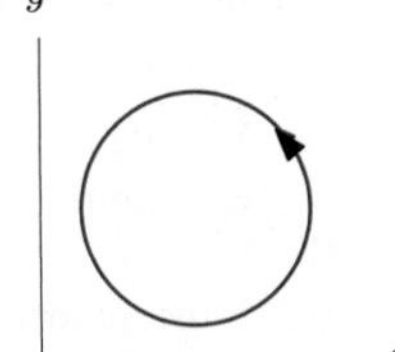

36. A kidney removes toxin from the blood. If a kidney does not function, the toxin can be removed by dialysis. This problem explores a model for $Q_1(t)$, the quantity of toxin in the body outside the blood, and $Q_2(t)$, the quantity of toxin in the blood, where t is the time after dialysis started.

(a) The quantity Q_1 changes for three reasons. First, toxin is created outside the blood at a constant rate, say A. Second, toxin flows into the blood at a rate proportional to the quantity outside the blood. Third, toxin flows out of the blood at a rate proportional to the quantity in the blood. Write a differential equation for Q_1.

(b) The quantity Q_2 changes for three reasons. First, dialysis removes toxin from the blood at a rate proportional to the toxin in the blood. Second and third, the same flows into and out of the blood that change Q_1 also change Q_2. Write a differential equation for Q_2.

CHECK YOUR UNDERSTANDING

In Problems 1–50, indicate whether the statement is true or false.

1. If a quantity Q is increasing at a constant rate of 8 grams per hour and Q is in grams and t is in hours, then the quantity satisfies the differential equation $dQ/dt = 8$.

2. If a population P is decreasing at a continuous rate of 5% per year with t in years, then the population satisfies the differential equation $dP/dt = -5$.

3. If a population P is decreasing at a continuous rate of 5% per year with t in years, then the population satisfies the differential equation $dP/dt = 0.05P$.

4. If the balance B in a bank account earns 3% interest a year compounded continuously, and there are no other deposits to or withdrawals from the account, then the balance satisfies the differential equation $dB/dt = 0.03B$, where t is in years.

5. If the rate at which an investment I (in dollars) grows as a function of time t (in years) is proportional to the size of the investment, then $dI/dt = kI$.

6. If fish in a population are harvested at a rate of 200 tons of fish per year and the fish population would stay stable without the harvesting, then the size of the fish population P in tons satisfies the differential equation $dP/dt = -200P$ where t is in years.

7. If the balance, B, in a bank account is earning interest at a rate of 5 percent per year, compounded continuously, and payments are being made out of the account at a rate of 8000 dollars per year, then the balance B satisfies the differential equation $dB/dt = 0.05B - 8000$ where B is in dollars and t is in years.

8. If the rate at which the quantity Q of pollutants (in tons) in a lake decreases as a function of time (in years) is proportional to Q, and if new pollutants are being dumped into the lake at a rate of 200 tons per year, then $dQ/dt = kQ - 200$.

9. If a drug is entering a patient's body through an intravenous line at a continuous rate of 12 mg per hour and if the drug is being metabolized at a continuous rate of 6.3% per hour, then the quantity, Q, in mg, of the drug in the body at time t hours satisfies the differential equation $dQ/dt = 12 - 0.063Q$.

10. A deposit of \$10,000 is made into a bank account and the account earns interest at a rate of 3.2% per year, compounded continuously. The balance, B, in the account in t years satisfies the differential equation $dB/dt = 10{,}000 + 0.032B$.

11. The differential equation $dP/dt = 3P(10 - P)$ has $P = 10$ as a solution.

12. The differential equation $dP/dt = 3P(10 - P)$ has $P = 0$ as a solution.

13. The differential equation $dP/dt = 3P(10 - P)$ has $P = 5$ as a solution.

14. If $y = Ce^{0.05t}$ is the general solution to a differential equation, then $y = 40e^{0.05t}$ is the particular solution satisfying the initial condition $y(0) = 40$.

15. If $y = 25 + Ce^{0.05t}$ is the general solution to a differential equation, then $y = 25 + 40e^{0.05t}$ is the particular solution satisfying the initial condition $y(0) = 40$.

16. If $y = 25 + Ce^{0.05t}$ is the general solution to a differential equation, then $y = 25 + 15e^{0.05t}$ is the particular solution satisfying the initial condition $y(0) = 40$.

17. If $y(0) = 100$ and $y' = 0.2y$, then $y(1) \approx 20$. Assume the rate of growth is approximately constant over unit intervals.

18. If $y(0) = 100$ and $y' = 0.2y$, then $y(1) \approx 120$. Assume the rate of growth is approximately constant over unit intervals.

19. If $dQ/dt = 5Q - 200$ then when $Q = 10$, the quantity Q will be decreasing.

20. If $dQ/dt = 5Q - 200$ there is a solution of the form $Q(t) = C$ for some constant C.

21. The slope field of the differential equation $dy/dx = 2x$ has slope 5 at the point $(3, 5)$.

22. The slope field of the differential equation $dy/dx = 2x$ has slope 6 at the point $(3, 5)$.

23. The slope field of the differential equation $dy/dx = 3xy$ has slope -6 at the point $(1, -2)$.

24. The slope field of the differential equation $dy/dx = 3xy$ has slope 6 at the point $(2, 2)$.

25. The slope field of the differential equation $dy/dx = 3xy$ has slope 18 at the point $(3, 2)$.

26. The slope field of the differential equation $dy/dx = 2x$ has positive slopes when $y > 0$.

27. The slope field of the differential equation $dy/dx = 2y$ has slope 2 at the points $(a, 1)$ for all a.

28. The slope field of the differential equation $dy/dx = 5(x-3)(y-2)$ has horizontal line segments when $x = 3$.

29. The slope field of the differential equation $dP/dt = 12 - 4P$ has positive slopes when $P > 3$.

30. The lines in a slope field for a differential equation are tangent to solutions of the differential equation.

31. The general solution of the differential equation $dy/dt = ky$ is $y = ke^{Ct}$.

32. The general solution of the differential equation $dQ/dt = 0.25Q$ is $Q = Ce^{0.25t}$.

33. The general solution of the differential equation $dw/dr = 0.3r$ is $w = Ce^{0.3r}$.

34. The function $H = 57e^{0.5t}$ is one solution to the differential equation $dH/dt = 0.5t$.

35. There is exactly one solution of the differential equation $dy/dt = 3y$ which has $y(0) = 5$.

36. The particular solution of $dy/dt = -2y$ satisfying $y = 3$ when $t = 0$ is $y = Ce^{-2t}$.

37. The balance B in a bank account that earns interest continuously at a rate of 3% per year on an initial deposit of \$5000 has differential equation $dB/dt = 5000B$.

38. If $Q(t)$ is the quantity of a drug in a patient's bloodstream at time t, and the rate at which the drug leaves the bloodstream is proportional to the quantity in the bloodstream, then $dQ/dt = -kQ$ where k is some negative constant.

39. A quantity, Q, of dead leaves decomposes at a rate proportional to the quantity present. We can model this with the differential equation $Q = Ce^{kt}$, where k is negative and t represents time.

40. A quantity, Q, of dead leaves decomposes at a rate proportional to the quantity present. We can model this with the differential equation $dQ/dt = kQ$, where k is negative and t represents time.

41. The general solution to the differential equation $dy/dt = 0.3(y - 75)$ is $y = 75 + Ce^{0.3t}$.

42. The general solution to the differential equation $dP/dt = 2P - 100$ is $P = 100 + Ce^{2t}$.

43. The general solution to the differential equation $dQ/dt = 0.5(Q + 20)$ is $Q = 20 + Ce^{0.5t}$.

44. The general solution to the differential equation $dW/dt = 600 - 3W$ is $W = 200 + Ce^{-3t}$.

45. The solution to the differential equation $dA/dt = 0.25(A - 40)$ with initial condition $A(0) = 50$ is $A = 40 + 50e^{0.25t}$.

46. The solution to the differential equation $dQ/dt = 50 - 2Q$ with initial condition $Q(0) = 100$ is $Q = 25 + 75e^{-2t}$.

47. The balance, B, in a bank account earns 4% interest per year, compounded continuously, and payments are made out of the account at a rate of \$12,000 per year. If t is in years, the differential equation to model this situation is $B = 12{,}000 + Ce^{0.04t}$.

48. A drug enters a patient's body intravenously at a continuous rate of 12 mg per hour, and the drug is metabolized at a continuous rate of 18% per hour. If A gives the quantity of drug in the body at hour t, then the differential equation to model this situation is $dA/dt = 12 - 0.18A$.

49. An equilibrium solution for the differential equation $dH/dt = -0.037(H - 225)$ is $H = 225$.

50. The graph of an equilibrium solution for a differential equation is a horizontal line.

In Problems 51–60, indicate whether the statement is true or false. Assume x and y represent the sizes of populations of two interacting species X and Y with system of differential equations as given.

51. Assume $dx/dt = ax + bxy$ and $dy/dt = cy + dxy$. If X would do fine if Y didn't exist, then b must be positive.

52. Assume $dx/dt = ax + bxy$ and $dy/dt = cy + dxy$. If species X eats species Y, then c must be negative.

53. Assume $dx/dt = ax + bxy$ and $dy/dt = cy + dxy$. If species X eats species Y, then d must be negative.

54. Assume $dx/dt = ax + bxy$ and $dy/dt = cy + dxy$. If species X cannot survive without species Y and does fine with species Y, then a must be negative and b must be positive.

55. If $dx/dt = 0.02x - 0.15xy$ and $dy/dt = 0.05y - 0.18xy$, then both populations need the other to survive.

56. If $dx/dt = 0.02x - 0.15xy$ and $dy/dt = 0.05y - 0.18xy$, then both populations would do fine if the other population didn't exist.

57. If $dx/dt = 0.02x - 0.15xy$ and $dy/dt = 0.05y - 0.18xy$, then the two populations have a negative impact on each other.

58. If $dx/dt = -0.12x + 0.07xy$ and $dy/dt = -0.10y + 0.25xy$, then the two populations need each other to survive..

59. Assume $dx/dt = -3x + xy$ and $dy/dt = 2y - 5xy$. If $x = 1$ and $y = 2$, then both populations will decrease in size.

60. Assume $dx/dt = -3x + xy$ and $dy/dt = 2y - 5xy$. If $x = 2$ and $y = 5$, then both populations will decrease in size.

In Problems 61–70, indicate whether the statement is true or false. The problems refer to the $S-I-R$ model, in which the variable S represents the number of people susceptible to becoming sick, the variable I represents the number of people currently infected, and R represents the rest of the population. We have

$$\frac{dS}{dt} = -aSI$$
$$\frac{dI}{dt} = aSI - bI.$$

61. The derivative dS/dt is negative because people are dying from the epidemic.

62. The parameter a in $dS/dt = -aSI$ is the same as the parameter a in $dI/dt = aSI - bI$ because people are moving from one group to the other.

63. The term $-bI$ in $dI/dt = aSI - bI$ is negative because people are moving back to the susceptible group.

64. The term $-bI$ in $dI/dt = aSI - bI$ is negative because people are either recovering or dying or being separated from the rest of the population and are no longer in either the S group or the I group.

65. If Type I flu is much more contagious than Type II flu, then the parameter b will be larger for Type I flu.

66. If Type I flu is much more contagious than Type II flu, then the parameter a will be larger for Type I flu.

67. If Type I flu lasts 10 days and Type II flu lasts 3 days, then the parameter b will be larger for Type I flu.

68. If Type I flu lasts 10 days and Type II flu lasts 3 days, then the parameter b will be smaller for Type I flu.

69. If $a = 0.001$ and $b = 0.3$ and if current numbers are $S = 500$ and $I = 100$, then the number of sick people will increase.

70. If $a = 0.001$ and $b = 0.3$ and if current numbers are $S = 100$ and $I = 500$, then the number of sick people will increase.

PROJECTS FOR CHAPTER TEN

1. Harvesting and Logistic Growth In this project, we look at the effects of *harvesting* a population which is growing logistically. Harvesting could be, for example, fishing or logging. An important question is what level of harvesting leads to a *sustainable yield*. In other words, how much can be harvested without having the population depleted in the long run?

(a) When there is no fishing, a population of fish is governed by the differential equation

$$\frac{dN}{dt} = 2N - 0.01N^2,$$

where N is the number of fish at time t in years. Sketch a graph of dN/dt against N. Mark on your graph the equilibrium values of N.

Notice on your graph that if N is between 0 and 200, then dN/dt is positive and N increases. If N is greater than 200, then dN/dt is negative and N decreases. Check this by sketching a slope field for this differential equation. Use the slope field to sketch solutions showing N against t for various initial values. Describe what you see.

(b) Fish are now removed by fishermen at a continuous rate of 75 fish/year. Let P be the number of fish at time t with harvesting. Explain why P satisfies the differential equation

$$\frac{dP}{dt} = 2P - 0.01P^2 - 75.$$

(c) Sketch dP/dt against P. Find and label the intercepts.

(d) Sketch the slope field for the differential equation for P.

(e) Recall that if dP/dt is positive for some values of P, then P increases for these values, and if dP/dt is negative for some values of P, then P decreases for these values. The value of P, however, never goes past an equilibrium value. Use this information and the graph from part (c) to answer the following questions:

(i) What are the equilibrium values of P?

(ii) For what initial values of P does P increase? At what value does P level off?

(iii) For what initial values of P does P decrease?

(f) Use the slope field in part (d) to sketch graphs of P against t, with the initial values:

(i) $P(0) = 40$ (ii) $P(0) = 50$ (iii) $P(0) = 60$
(iv) $P(0) = 150$ (v) $P(0) = 170$

(g) Using the graphs you drew, decide what the equilibrium values of the populations are and whether or not they are stable.

(h) We now look at the effect of different levels of fishing on a fish population. If fishing takes place at a continuous rate of H fish/year, the fish population P satisfies the differential equation

$$\frac{dP}{dt} = 2P - 0.01P^2 - H.$$

(i) For each of the values $H = 75, 100, 200$, plot dP/dt against P.

(ii) For which of the three values of H that you considered in part (i) is there an initial condition such that the fish population does not die out eventually?

(iii) Looking at your answer to part (ii), decide for what values of H there is an initial value for P such that the population does not die out eventually.

(iv) Recommend a policy to ensure long-term survival of the fish population.

2. Population Genetics

Population genetics is the study of hereditary traits in a population. A specific hereditary trait has two possibilities, one dominant, such as brown eyes, and one recessive, such as blue eyes.[10] Let b denote the gene responsible for the recessive trait and B denote the gene responsible for the dominant trait. Each member of the population has a pair of these genes—either BB (dominant individuals), bb (recessive individuals), or Bb (hybrid individuals). The *gene frequency* of the b gene is the total number of b genes in the population divided by the total number of all genes (b and B) controlling this trait. The gene frequency is essentially constant when there are no mutations or outside influences on the population. In this project, we consider the effect of mutations on the gene frequency.

Let q denote the gene frequency of the b gene. Then q is between 0 and 1 (since it is a fraction of a whole) and, since b and B are the only genes influencing this trait, the gene frequency of the B gene is $1 - q$. Let time t be measured in generations. Every generation, a fraction k_1 of the b genes mutate to become B genes, and a fraction k_2 of the B genes mutate to become b genes.

(a) Explain why the gene frequency q satisfies the differential equation:

$$\frac{dq}{dt} = -k_1q + k_2(1 - q).$$

[10]Adapted from C. C. Li, *Population Genetics* (Chicago: University of Chicago Press, 1995).

(b) If $k_1 = 0.0001$ and $k_2 = 0.0004$, simplify the differential equation for q and solve it. The initial value is q_0. Sketch the solutions with $q_0 = 0.1$ and $q_0 = 0.9$. What is the equilibrium value of q? Explain how you can tell that the gene frequency gets closer to the equilibrium value as generations pass. Explain how you can tell that the equilibrium value is completely determined by the relative mutation rates.

(c) Repeat part (b) if $k_1 = 0.00003$ and $k_2 = 0.00001$.

3. The Spread of SARS

In the spring of 2003, SARS (Severe Acute Respiratory Syndrome) spread rapidly in several Asian countries and Canada. Predicting the course of the disease—how many people would be infected, how long it would last—was important to officials trying to minimize the impact of the disease. This project analyzes the spread of SARS through interaction between infected and susceptible people.

The variables are S, the number of susceptibles, I, the number of infecteds who can infect others, and R, the number removed (this group includes those in quarantine and those who die, as well as those who have recovered and acquired immunity). Time, t, is in days since March 17, 2003, the date the World Health Organization (WHO) started to publish daily SARS reports. On March 17, Hong Kong reported 95 cases. In this model

$$\frac{dS}{dt} = -aSI$$
$$\frac{dI}{dt} = aSI - bI,$$

and $S + I + R = 6.8$ million, the population of Hong Kong in 2003.[11] Estimates based on WHO data give $a = 1.25 \cdot 10^{-8}$.

(a) What are S_0 and I_0, the initial values of S and I?

(b) During March 2003, the value of b was about 0.06. Using a calculator or computer, sketch the slope field for this system of differential equations and the solution trajectory corresponding to the initial conditions. (Use $0 \le S \le 7 \cdot 10^6, 0 \le I \le 0.4 \cdot 10^6$.)

(c) What does your graph tell you about the total number of people infected over the course of the disease if $b = 0.06$? What is the threshold value? What does this value tell you?

(d) During April, as public health officials worked to get the disease under control, people who had been in contact with the disease were quarantined. Explain why quarantining has the effect of raising the value of b.

(e) Using the April value, $b = 0.24$, sketch the slope field. (Use the same value of a and the same window.)

(f) What is the threshold value for $b = 0.24$? What does this tell you? Comment on the quarantine policy.

(g) Comment on the effectiveness of each of the following policies intended to prevent an epidemic and protect a city from an outbreak of SARS in a nearby region.

I Close off the city from contact with the infected region. Shut down roads, airports, trains, and other forms of direct contact.

II Install a quarantine policy. Isolate anyone who has been in contact with a SARS patient or anyone who shows symptoms of SARS.

---

[11] www.census.gov, International Data Base (IDB), accessed June 8, 2004.

FOCUS ON THEORY

SEPARATION OF VARIABLES

We have seen how to sketch solution curves of a differential equation using a slope field. Now we see how to solve certain differential equations analytically, finding an equation for the solution curve.

First, we look at a familiar example, the differential equation

$$\frac{dy}{dx} = -\frac{x}{y},$$

whose solution curves are the circles

$$x^2 + y^2 = C.$$

We can check that these circles are solutions by differentiation; the question now is how they were obtained. The method of *separation of variables* works by putting all the xs on one side of the equation and all the ys on the other, giving

$$y\,dy = -x\,dx.$$

We then integrate each side separately:

$$\int y\,dy = -\int x\,dx,$$

$$\frac{y^2}{2} = -\frac{x^2}{2} + k.$$

This gives the circles we were expecting:

$$x^2 + y^2 = C \qquad \text{where } C = 2k.$$

You might worry about whether it is legitimate to separate the dx and the dy. The reason it can be done is explained at the end of this section.

The Exponential Growth and Decay Equations

We use separation of variables to derive the general solution of the equation

$$\frac{dy}{dt} = ky.$$

Separating variables, we have

$$\frac{1}{y}dy = k\,dt,$$

and integrating,

$$\int \frac{1}{y}\,dy = \int k\,dt,$$

gives

$$\ln|y| = kt + C \quad \text{for some constant } C.$$

Solving for $|y|$ leads to

$$|y| = e^{kt+C} = e^{kt}e^C = Ae^{kt}$$

where $A = e^C$, so A is positive. Thus,

$$y = (\pm A)e^{kt} = Be^{kt}$$

where $B = \pm A$, so B is any nonzero constant. Even though there's no C leading to $B = 0$, we can have $B = 0$ because $y = 0$ is a solution to the differential equation. We lost this solution when we divided through by y at the first step. Thus we have derived the solution used earlier in the chapter:

$$y = Be^{kt} \quad \text{for any constant } B.$$

Example 1 Find all solutions of

$$\frac{dy}{dt} = k(y - A).$$

Solution We separate variables and integrate:

$$\int \frac{1}{y - A}\, dy = \int k\, dt.$$

This gives

$$\ln|y - A| = kt + D,$$

where D is a constant of integration. Solving for y leads to

$$|y - A| = e^{kt+D} = e^{kt}e^{D} = Be^{kt}$$

or

$$y - A = (\pm B)e^{kt} = Ce^{kt}$$
$$y = A + Ce^{kt}.$$

Also, $C = 0$ gives a solution. This is the same result we used earlier.

Example 2 Find and sketch the solution to

$$\frac{dP}{dt} = 2P - 2Pt \qquad \text{satisfying } P = 5 \text{ when } t = 0.$$

Solution Factoring the right-hand side gives

$$\frac{dP}{dt} = P(2 - 2t).$$

Separating variables, we get

$$\int \frac{dP}{P} = \int (2 - 2t)\, dt,$$

so

$$\ln|P| = 2t - t^2 + C.$$

Solving for P leads to

$$|P| = e^{2t - t^2 + C} = e^{C}e^{2t - t^2} = Ae^{2t - t^2}$$

with $A = e^{C}$, so $A > 0$. In addition, $A = 0$ gives a solution. Thus the general solution to the differential equation is

$$P = Be^{2t - t^2} \quad \text{for any } B.$$

To find the value of B, substitute $P = 5$ and $t = 0$ into the general solution, giving

$$5 = Be^{2\cdot 0 - 0^2} = B$$

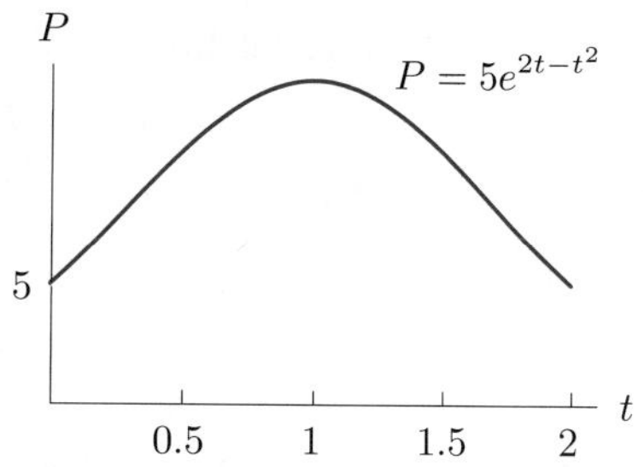

Figure 10.52: Bell-shaped solution curve

so

$$P = 5e^{2t-t^2}.$$

The graph of this function is in Figure 10.52. Since the solution can be rewritten as

$$P = 5e^{1-1+2t-t^2} = 5e^1e^{-1+2t-t^2} = (5e)e^{-(t-1)^2},$$

the graph has the same shape as the graph of $y = e^{-t^2}$, the bell-shaped curve of statistics. Here the maximum, normally at $t = 0$, is shifted one unit to the right to $t = 1$.

Justification for Separation of Variables

Suppose a differential equation can be written in the form

$$\frac{dy}{dx} = g(x)f(y).$$

Provided $f(y) \neq 0$, we write $f(y) = 1/h(y)$ so the right-hand side can be thought of as a fraction,

$$\frac{dy}{dx} = \frac{g(x)}{h(y)}.$$

If we multiply through by $h(y)$ we get

$$h(y)\frac{dy}{dx} = g(x).$$

Thinking of y as a function of x, so $y = y(x)$, and $dy/dx = y'(x)$, we can rewrite the equation as

$$h(y(x)) \cdot y'(x) = g(x).$$

Now integrate both sides with respect to x:

$$\int h(y(x)) \cdot y'(x)\, dx = \int g(x)\, dx.$$

The form of the integral on the left suggests that we use the substitution $y = y(x)$. Since $dy = y'(x)\, dx$, we get

$$\int h(y)\, dy = \int g(x)\, dx.$$

If we can find antiderivatives of h and g, then this gives the equation of the solution curve.

Note that transforming the original differential equation,

$$\frac{dy}{dx} = \frac{g(x)}{h(y)},$$

into

$$\int h(y)\,dy = \int g(x)\,dx$$

looks as though we have treated dy/dx as a fraction, cross-multiplied and then integrated. Although that's not exactly what we have done, you may find this a helpful way of remembering the method. In fact, the dy/dx notation was introduced by Leibniz to allow shortcuts like this (more specifically, to make the chain rule look like cancellation).

Problems on Separation of Variables

Use separation of variables to find the solutions to the differential equations in Problems 1–12, subject to the given initial conditions.

1. $\frac{dP}{dt} = -2P, \quad P(0) = 1$

2. $\frac{dL}{dp} = \frac{L}{2}, \quad L(0) = 100$

3. $P\frac{dP}{dt} = 1, \quad P(0) = 1$

4. $\frac{dm}{ds} = m, \quad m(1) = 2$

5. $2\frac{du}{dt} = u^2, \quad u(0) = 1$

6. $\frac{dz}{dy} = zy, \quad z = 1$ when $y = 0$

7. $\frac{dR}{dy} + R = 1, \quad R(1) = 0.1$

8. $\frac{dy}{dt} = \frac{y}{3+t}, \quad y(0) = 1$

9. $\frac{dz}{dt} = te^z$, through the origin

10. $\frac{dy}{dx} = \frac{5y}{x}, \quad y = 3$ where $x = 1$

11. $\frac{dy}{dt} = y^2(1+t), \quad y = 2$ when $t = 1$

12. $\frac{dz}{dt} = z + zt^2, \quad z = 5$ when $t = 0$

13. Determine which of the following differential equations is separable. Do not solve the equations.

(a) $y' = y$ **(b)** $y' = x + y$
(c) $y' = xy$ **(d)** $y' = \sin(x+y)$
(e) $y' - xy = 0$ **(f)** $y' = y/x$
(g) $y' = \ln(xy)$ **(h)** $y' = (\sin x)(\cos y)$
(i) $y' = (\sin x)(\cos xy)$ **(j)** $y' = x/y$
(k) $y' = 2x$ **(l)** $y' = (x+y)/(x+2y)$

Use separation of variables to solve the differential equations in Problems 14–19. Assume a, b, and k are nonzero constants.

14. $\frac{dP}{dt} = P - a$

15. $\frac{dQ}{dt} = b - Q$

16. $\frac{dP}{dt} = k(P - a)$

17. $\frac{dR}{dt} = aR + b$

18. $\frac{dP}{dt} - aP = b$

19. $\frac{dy}{dt} = ky^2(1+t^2)$

20. **(a)** Find the general solution to the differential equation modeling how a person learns:

$$\frac{dy}{dt} = 100 - y.$$

(b) Plot the slope field of this differential equation and sketch solutions with $y(0) = 25$ and $y(0) = 110$.
(c) For each of the initial conditions in part (b), find the particular solution and add to your sketch.
(d) Which of these two particular solutions could represent how a person learns?

21. **(a)** Sketch the slope field for the differential equation $dy/dx = xy$.
(b) Sketch several solution curves.
(c) Solve the differential equation analytically.

Chapter Eleven

GEOMETRIC SERIES

Contents

11.1 GEOMETRIC SERIES

Repeated Drug Dosage

Malaria is a parasitic infection transmitted by mosquito bites, mainly in tropical areas of the world. The disease has existed since ancient times, and currently there are hundreds of millions of cases each year, with millions of deaths. In the 1640s, the Jesuits in Peru introduced the bark of the cinchona tree to the West as the first treatment for malaria. The drug quinine is the active ingredient in the bark, and it is still used today.

Suppose a person is given a 50-mg dose of quinine at the same time every day for the prevention of malaria. After the first dose, the person has 50 mg of quinine in the body. What about after the second dose? Each day, the person's body metabolizes some of the quinine so that, after one day, 23% of the original amount remains. After the second dose, the amount of quinine in the body is the amount from the second dose (50 mg) plus the remnants of the first dose (that is, $50\cdot 0.23 = 11.5$ mg) for a total of 61.5 mg.

Let Q_n represent the quantity, in mg, of quinine in the body right after the nth dose. Then

$$\begin{aligned}
Q_1 &= \text{First dose} = 50.\\
Q_2 &= \text{Second dose + Remnants of first dose} = 50 + 50(0.23) = 61.5.\\
Q_3 &= \text{Third dose + Remnants of previous doses} = 50 + 61.5(0.23) = 64.145.
\end{aligned}$$

Notice that we can multiply out the expression for Q_3 to show the contributions of the first and second dose separately:

$$\begin{aligned}
Q_3 &= 50 + 61.5(0.23) = 50 + (50 + 50(0.23))(0.23)\\
Q_3 &= 50 + 50(0.23) + 50(0.23)^2,
\end{aligned}$$

so we have

$$Q_3 = \text{Third dose + Remnants of second dose + Remnants of first dose.}$$

The multiplied-out form of Q_3 enables us to guess formulas for later values of Q_n:

$$\begin{aligned}
Q_4 &= 50 + 50(0.23) + 50(0.23)^2 + 50(0.23)^3 = 64.753.\\
Q_5 &= 50 + 50(0.23) + 50(0.23)^2 + 50(0.23)^3 + 50(0.23)^4 = 64.893.\\
Q_6 &= 50 + 50(0.23) + 50(0.23)^2 + 50(0.23)^3 + 50(0.23)^4 + 50(0.23)^5 = 64.925.\\
&\vdots\\
Q_{10} &= 50 + 50(0.23) + 50(0.23)^2 + \cdots + 50(0.23)^8 + 50(0.23)^9 = 64.935.
\end{aligned}$$

The values of Q_6 and Q_{10} suggest that the quantity is stabilizing at around 64.9 mg. See Figure 11.1.

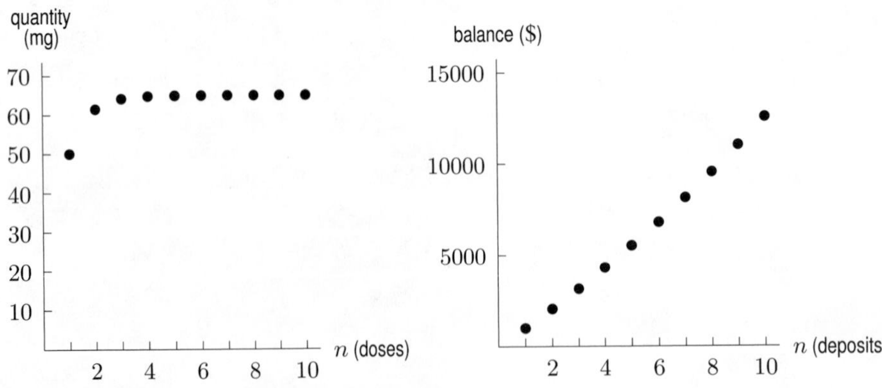

Figure 11.1: Quantity of quinine levels off

Figure 11.2: Bank balance grows without bound

Repeated Deposits into a Savings Account

People who save money often do so by putting a fixed amount aside regularly. Suppose \$1000 is deposited every year in a savings account earning 5% interest a year, compounded annually. Let B_n represent the balance, in dollars, in the account right after the nth deposit. Then

$$\begin{aligned} B_1 &= \text{First deposit} = 1000. \\ B_2 &= \text{Second deposit + Amount from first deposit} = 1000 + 1000(1.05) = 2050. \\ B_3 &= \text{Third deposit + Amount from previous deposits} = 1000 + 2050(1.05) = 3152.5. \end{aligned}$$

As before, we multiply out the expression for B_3 to show the contributions of the first and second deposits separately:

$$\begin{aligned} B_3 &= 1000 + 2050(1.05) = 1000 + (1000 + 1000(1.05))(1.05) \\ B_3 &= 1000 + 1000(1.05) + 1000(1.05)^2 \\ B_3 &= \text{Third deposit + Amount from second deposit + Amount from first deposit.} \end{aligned}$$

The multiplied-out formula for B_3 enables us to guess formulas for B_6 and B_{10}. Evaluating gives

$$B_6 = 1000 + 1000(1.05) + 1000(1.05)^2 + 1000(1.05)^3 + 1000(1.05)^4 + 1000(1.05)^5 = 6801.91.$$

$$B_{10} = 1000 + 1000(1.05) + 1000(1.05)^2 + \cdots + 1000(1.05)^8 + 1000(1.05)^9 = 12{,}577.89.$$

Notice that the balance is growing without bound. See Figure 11.2.

Finite Geometric Series

In the two previous examples, we encountered sums of the form $a+ar+ar^2+ar^3+\cdots+ar^8+ar^9$. Such a sum is called a *finite geometric series.* A geometric series is a sum in which each term is a constant multiple of the preceding one. The first term is a, and the constant multiplier, or common ratio, of successive terms is r.

> A **finite geometric series** with n terms has (for n a positive integer) the form
>
> $$a + ar + ar^2 + ar^3 + \cdots + ar^{n-2} + ar^{n-1}.$$

Sum of a Finite Geometric Series

In the quinine example, suppose we want to find Q_{40}, the quantity in the body after 40 doses:

$$Q_{40} = 50 + 50(0.23) + 50(0.23)^2 + \cdots + 50(0.23)^{38} + 50(0.23)^{39}.$$

To calculate Q_{40}, we could add these 40 terms. Fortunately, there is a better way.

We write S_n for the sum of the first n terms of the series, that is, up to the term ar^{n-1}:

$$S_n = a + ar + ar^2 + ar^3 + \cdots + ar^{n-2} + ar^{n-1}.$$

Multiplying both sides by r gives

$$rS_n = ar + ar^2 + ar^3 + ar^4 + \cdots + ar^{n-1} + ar^n.$$

Now subtract rS_n from S_n, so all the terms except two on the right cancel, giving

$$S_n - rS_n = a - ar^n,$$

so

$$(1 - r)S_n = a(1 - r^n).$$

Provided $r \neq 1$, we can solve for S_n. The result is called a *closed form* for S_n.

The **sum of a finite geometric series** is given by

$$S_n = a + ar + ar^2 + ar^3 + \cdots + ar^{n-1} = \frac{a(1-r^n)}{1-r}, \quad \text{provided } r \neq 1.$$

Note that the value of n in the formula is the number of terms in the sum S_n.

Example 1 In the quinine example, calculate and interpret Q_{40} and Q_{100}.

Solution We saw earlier that

$$Q_{40} = 50 + 50(0.23) + 50(0.23)^2 + \cdots + 50(0.23)^{39}.$$

This is a finite geometric series with $a = 50$ and $r = 0.23$. Using the formula for the sum with $n = 40$, we have

$$Q_{40} = \frac{50(1-(0.23)^{40})}{1-0.23} = 64.935.$$

The amount of quinine in the body right after the 40th dose is 64.935 mg.

Similarly, using $n = 100$, we have

$$Q_{100} = \frac{50(1-(0.23)^{100})}{1-0.23} = 64.935.$$

Right after the 100th dose, the amount of quinine in the body is still 64.935 mg. To three decimal places, the amount appears to have stabilized.

Example 2 In the bank deposit example, calculate and interpret B_{40} and B_{100}.

Solution We have

$$B_{40} = 1000 + 1000(1.05) + 1000(1.05)^2 + \cdots + 1000(1.05)^{39}.$$

This is a finite geometric series with $a = 1000$ and $r = 1.05$. The formula for the sum with $n = 40$ gives

$$B_{40} = \frac{1000(1-(1.05)^{40})}{1-1.05} = 120{,}799.77.$$

The balance in the account right after the 40th deposit is \$120,799.77.

Similarly, using $n = 100$, we have

$$B_{100} = \frac{1000(1-(1.05)^{100})}{1-1.05} = 2{,}610{,}025.16.$$

Right after the 100th deposit, the balance in the account is \$2,610,025.16. Compound interest has increased the \$100,000 investment to over \$2 million.

Infinite Geometric Series

Suppose a finite geometric series has n terms in it. What happens as $n \to \infty$? We get an infinite geometric series that goes on forever.

An **infinite geometric series** has the form

$$a + ar + ar^2 + ar^3 + \cdots + ar^{n-1} + ar^n + \cdots.$$

The "..." at the end of the series tells us that the series is going on forever—it is infinite.

Sum of an Infinite Geometric Series

Given an infinite geometric series

$$a + ar + ar^2 + ar^3 + \cdots,$$

we call the sum of the first n terms a *partial sum*, written S_n. To calculate S_n, we use the formula

$$S_n = \frac{a(1-r^n)}{1-r}.$$

What happens to S_n as $n \to \infty$? It depends on the value of r. If $|r| < 1$, that is, $-1 < r < 1$, then $r^n \to 0$ as $n \to \infty$, so as $n \to \infty$,

$$S_n = \frac{a(1-r^n)}{1-r} \to \frac{a(1-0)}{1-r} = \frac{a}{1-r}.$$

Thus, provided $|r| < 1$, as $n \to \infty$ the partial sums S_n approach a limit of $a/(1-r)$. When this happens, we define the sum of the infinite geometric series to be that limit and say the series *converges* to $a/(1-r)$.

For $|r| < 1$, the **sum of the infinite geometric series** is given by

$$S = a + ar + ar^2 + ar^3 + \cdots + ar^{n-1} + ar^n + \cdots = \frac{a}{1-r}.$$

If, on the other hand, $|r| > 1$, then r^n and the partial sums have no limit as $n \to \infty$ (if $a \neq 0$). In this case, we say the series *diverges*. If $r > 1$, the terms in the series become larger and larger in magnitude, and the partial sums diverge to $+\infty$ if $a > 0$, or to $-\infty$ if $a < 0$. If $r < -1$, the terms become larger in magnitude, the partial sums oscillate as $n \to \infty$, and the series diverges.

What happens if $r = 1$? The series is

$$a + a + a + a + \cdots,$$

so if $a \neq 0$, the partial sums grow without bound, and the series does not converge. If $r = -1$, the series is

$$a - a + a - a + a - \cdots,$$

and, if $a \neq 0$, the partial sums oscillate between a and 0, and the series does not converge.

Example 3 For each of the following infinite series, find the first three partial sums and the sum (if it exists):

(a) $10 + 10(0.75) + 10(0.75)^2 + \cdots$
(b) $250 + 250(1.2) + 250(1.2)^2 + \cdots$

Solution (a) This is an infinite geometric series with $a = 10$ and $r = 0.75$. The first three partial sums are:

$$S_1 = 10.$$
$$S_2 = 10 + 10(0.75) = 10 + 7.5 = 17.5.$$
$$S_3 = 10 + 10(0.75) + 10(0.75)^2 = 10 + 7.5 + 5.625 = 23.125.$$

Since $|r| < 1$, the series converges and the sum is

$$S = \frac{a}{1-r} = \frac{10}{1-0.75} = 40.$$

If we find partial sums for larger and larger n, they get closer and closer to 40. (See Problem 15.)

(b) This is an infinite geometric series with $a = 250$ and $r = 1.2$. The first three partial sums are:

$$S_1 = 250.$$
$$S_2 = 250 + 250(1.2) = 250 + 300 = 550.$$
$$S_3 = 250 + 250(1.2) + 250(1.2)^2 = 250 + 300 + 360 = 910.$$

Since $r > 1$, the series diverges, and the partial sums grow without bound. (See Problem 16.)

Example 4 Suppose 50-mg doses of quinine are taken daily forever. Find the long-run quantities of quinine in the body right after and right before a dose is given.

Solution Since quinine is given forever, from Example 1 we know that the long-run quantity of quinine, right after a dose, is given by

$$Q = 50 + 50(0.23) + 50(0.23)^2 + \cdots.$$

This is an infinite geometric series with $a = 50$ and $r = 0.23$. Since $-1 < r < 1$, the series converges to a finite sum given by

$$Q = \frac{a}{1-r} = \frac{50}{1-0.23} = 64.935.$$

The long-run quantity of quinine in the body right after a dose is 64.935 mg. The quantity levels off to this value in Figure 11.1.

What is the long-run quantity of quinine right before a dose? Since a dose is 50 mg, the quantity of quinine in the body right before a dose is $64.935 - 50 = 14.935$ mg. Thus, in the long run, the quinine level oscillates between 15 mg and 65 mg.

Example 5 Suppose that \$1000 a year is deposited forever into the bank account in Example 2. Does the balance in the account stabilize at a fixed amount? Explain.

Solution Since the deposits are made forever, the account balance right after a deposit is represented by

$$B = 1000 + 1000(1.05) + 1000(1.05)^2 + \cdots.$$

This is an infinite geometric series with $a = 1000$ and $r = 1.05$. Since r is larger than 1, the series diverges. This makes sense, since if you keep depositing \$1000 in an account, your balance grows without bound, even if you don't earn interest. This matches Figure 11.2 and Example 2.

Problems for Section 11.1

1. Find the sum of the following series in two ways: by adding terms and by using the geometric series formula.

$$3 + 3\cdot 2 + 3\cdot 2^2$$

2. Find the sum of the following series in two ways: by adding terms and by using the geometric series formula.

$$50 + 50(0.9) + 50(0.9)^2 + 50(0.9)^3$$

In Problems 3–14, find the sum, if it exists.

3. $5 + 5\cdot 3 + 5\cdot 3^2 + \cdots + 5\cdot 3^{12}$
4. $20 + 20(1.45) + 20(1.45)^2 + \cdots + 20(1.45)^{14}$
5. $100 + 100(0.85) + 100(0.85)^2 + \cdots + 100(0.85)^{10}$
6. $1000 + 1000(1.05) + 1000(1.05)^2 + \cdots$
7. $75 + 75(0.22) + 75(0.22)^2 + \cdots$
8. $500(0.4) + 500(0.4)^2 + 500(0.4)^3 + \cdots$
9. $31500 + 6300 + 1260 + 252 + \cdots$
10. $3 + \frac{3}{2} + \frac{3}{4} + \frac{3}{8} + \cdots + \frac{3}{2^{10}}$
11. $65 + \frac{65}{1.02} + \frac{65}{(1.02)^2} + \cdots + \frac{65}{(1.02)^{18}}$
12. $1000 + 1500 + 2250 + 3375 + 5062.5 + \cdots$
13. $200 + 100 + 50 + 25 + 12.5 + \cdots$
14. $-2 + 1 - \frac{1}{2} + \frac{1}{4} - \frac{1}{8} + \frac{1}{16} - \cdots$
15. In Example 3(a), we found partial sums of the geometric series with $a = 10$ and $r = 0.75$ and showed that the sum of this series is 40. Find the partial sums S_n for $n = 5, 10, 15, 20$. As n gets larger, do the partial sums appear to be approaching 40?
16. In Example 3(b), we found partial sums for the geometric series with $a = 250$ and $r = 1.2$. Find the partial sums S_n for $n = 5, 10, 15, 20$. As n gets larger, do the partial sums appear to grow without bound, as expected if $r > 1$?

17. Every month, \$500 is deposited into an account earning 0.5% interest a month, compounded monthly.

(a) How much is in the account right after the 6th deposit? Right before the 6th deposit?
(b) How much is in the account right after the 12th deposit? Right before the 12th deposit?

18. Each year, a family deposits \$5000 into an account paying 8.12% interest per year, compounded annually. How much is in the account right after the 20th deposit?

19. Each morning, a patient receives a 25 mg injection of an anti-inflammatory drug, and 40% of the drug remains in the body after 24 hours. Find the quantity in the body:

(a) Right after the 3rd injection.
(b) Right after the 6th injection.
(c) In the long run, right after an injection.

20. A smoker inhales 0.4 mg of nicotine from a cigarette. After one hour, 71% of the nicotine remains in the body. If a person smokes one cigarette every hour beginning at 7 am, how much nicotine is in the body right after the 11 pm cigarette?

21. In Example 4, we saw that if 50 mg of quinine is given every 24 hours, the long-run quantity of quinine in the body is about 65 mg right after a dose and about 15 mg right before a dose. The concentration of quinine in the body is measured in milligrams of quinine per kilogram of body weight. To be effective, the average concentration of quinine in the body must be at least 0.4 mg/kg. Concentrations above 3.0 mg/kg are not safe.

(a) Estimate the average quantity of quinine in the body in the long run by averaging the long-run quantities of quinine in the body right after a dose and right before a dose.
(b) Find the average concentration for a person weighing 70 kilograms. Is this treatment safe and effective for such a person?
(c) For what range of weights would this treatment produce a long-run average concentration that is

(i) Too low? (ii) Unsafe?

22. Figure 11.3 shows the quantity of the drug atenolol in the blood as a function of time, with the first dose at time $t = 0$. Atenolol is taken in 50 mg doses once a day to lower blood pressure.

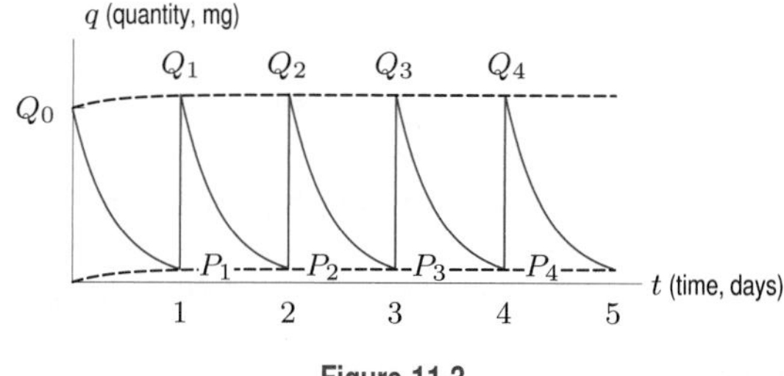

Figure 11.3

(a) If the half-life of atenolol in the blood is 6.3 hours, what percentage of the atenolol present at the start of a 24-hour period is still there at the end?
(b) Find expressions for the quantities $Q_0, Q_1, Q_2, Q_3, \ldots$, and Q_n shown in Figure 11.3. Write the expression for Q_n in closed form.
(c) Find expressions for the quantities $P_1, P_2, P_3, \ldots$, and P_n shown in Figure 11.3. Write the expression for P_n in closed form.

11.2 APPLICATIONS TO BUSINESS AND ECONOMICS

Annuities

An *annuity* is a sequence of equal payments made at regular intervals. We can use the sum of a geometric series to calculate the total value of an annuity.

Example 1 An annuity pays \$5000 every year into an account that earns 7% interest per year, compounded annually. What is the balance in the account right after the 10th deposit?

Solution The 10th deposit contributes \$5000 to the balance. The previous deposit has earned interest for a year, so it contributes \$5000(1.07). The deposit the year before that has earned interest for two years, so it contributes $\$5000(1.07)^2$. Continuing, we see that

$$\text{Balance after } 10^{\text{th}} \text{ deposit} = 5000 + 5000(1.07) + 5000(1.07)^2 + \cdots + 5000(1.07)^9.$$

This sum is a finite geometric series with $a = 5000$ and $r = 1.07$. We use the formula for the sum with $n = 10$:

$$\text{Balance after } 10^{\text{th}} \text{ deposit} = \frac{a(1-r^n)}{1-r} = \frac{5000(1-(1.07)^{10})}{1-1.07} = 69{,}082.24 \text{ dollars.}$$

The balance in the account right after the 10th deposit is \$69,082.24.

Present Value of an Annuity

The *present value of an annuity* is the amount of money that must be deposited today to make a series of fixed payments in the future. How can we compute this present value? We begin by considering a single payment. Suppose a payment of \$1000 is to be made three years in the future from an account paying interest at a rate of 8% per year, compounded annually. The present value is the amount P such that

$$P(1.08)^3 = 1000,$$

so we have

$$\text{Present value} = P = 1000(1.08)^{-3}.$$

To find the present value of four payments of \$1000 at the same 8% interest, one made now, one in one year's time, one in two years, and one in three years, we add their present values:

$$\text{Present value of four payments} = 1000 + 1000(1.08)^{-1} + 1000(1.08)^{-2} + 1000(1.08)^{-3}.$$

This pattern allows us to find the present value of any annuity, as in the following example.

Example 2 An account earns 8% interest per year, compounded annually. Twenty payments of \$10,000 each, made once a year starting now, are to be made out of the account. How much must be deposited in the account now to cover these payments? In other words, what is the present value of this annuity?

Solution The present value of the payment to be made immediately is \$10,000. The present value of next year's payment is $\$10{,}000(1.08)^{-1}$. Since the 20th payment is made 19 years in the future, the present value of the 20th payment is $\$10{,}000(1.08)^{-19}$. The present value, P, of the entire annuity, in dollars, is the sum

$$P = 10{,}000 + 10{,}000(1.08)^{-1} + 10{,}000(1.08)^{-2} + \cdots + 10{,}000(1.08)^{-19}.$$

Rewriting $(1.08)^{-2} = \left((1.08)^{-1}\right)^2$ and $(1.08)^{-3} = \left((1.08)^{-1}\right)^3$, and so on, shows that P is the sum of the finite geometric series

$$P = 10{,}000 + 10{,}000(1.08)^{-1} + 10{,}000((1.08)^{-1})^2 + \cdots + 10{,}000((1.08)^{-1})^{19}.$$

We use the formula for the sum with $a = 10{,}000$ and $r = (1.08)^{-1}$ and $n = 20$, giving

$$\text{Present value} = P = \frac{a(1-r^n)}{1-r} = \frac{10{,}000(1-((1.08)^{-1})^{20})}{1-(1.08)^{-1}} = 106{,}035.99.$$

Thus, \$106,035.99 must be deposited now to cover the payments for this annuity. Notice that the annuity pays out a total of $20 \cdot \$10{,}000 = \$200{,}000$, so the present value is considerably less than the amount eventually paid out.

Example 3 The annuity in Example 2 now makes annual payments of \$10,000 in perpetuity (that is, forever), rather than just twenty times. What is the present value of this annuity?

Solution Since the payments are made forever, the present value is given by the infinite sum:

$$\text{Present value} = 10{,}000 + 10{,}000(1.08)^{-1} + 10{,}000((1.08)^{-1})^2 + 10{,}000((1.08)^{-1})^3 + \cdots.$$

This is an infinite geometric series with $a = 10{,}000$ and $r = (1.08)^{-1} = 0.925926$. Since $-1 < r < 1$, this series converges to a finite sum. We have

$$\text{Present value} = \frac{a}{1-r} = \frac{10{,}000}{1-(1.08)^{-1}} = 135{,}000.$$

The present value of this annuity in perpetuity is \$135,000. Notice that the amount needed to make annual payments forever is only about \$29,000 more than the amount needed to make 20 annual payments. This is the power of compound interest.

The Multiplier Effect

A government decides to give a tax rebate to stimulate the economy. What is the total effect of the rebate on spending? Each individual who receives a tax rebate spends some proportion of the additional income, and this money becomes additional income for a second individual, who spends a proportion of it, providing additional income for a third individual, and so on. The total effect of the rebate on the economy is much larger than the size of the rebate itself; this is called the *multiplier effect.*

Example 4 A government gives tax rebates totaling 3 billion dollars. Everyone who receives money spends 75% of it and saves the other 25%. Find the total additional spending resulting from this tax rebate.

Solution The additional spending refers to all the additional money spent by consumers as a result of this tax rebate. The recipients of the 3 billion dollars spend 75% of what they receive, that is $3(0.75) = 2.25$ billion dollars. The recipients of this 2.25 billion dollars spend 75% of that, or $2.25(0.75) = 1.6875$ billion dollars. The recipients of this money spend 75% of this amount, and so on. Thus,

$$\text{Total additional spending} = 2.25 + 2.25(0.75) + 2.25(0.75)^2 + 2.25(0.75)^3 + \cdots \text{ billion dollars.}$$

(Notice that the initial amount spent was 2.25, not 3 billion dollars.) This is an infinite geometric series with $a = 2.25$ and $r = 0.75$. Since $-1 < r < 1$, this series converges to a finite sum:

$$\text{Total additional spending} = \frac{a}{1-r} = \frac{2.25}{1-0.75} = 9 \text{ billion dollars.}$$

Thus, a 3 billion dollar tax rebate generates 9 billion dollars of additional spending.

Market Stabilization

Each year, a manufacturer produces a fixed number of units of a product and each year a fixed percentage of these units (regardless of age) fail or go out of use. The total number of units in use in the long run is called the *market stabilization point.*

Example 5 The US Mint produces about 7.4 billion pennies a year and about 5% of them are removed from circulation each year.[1] Approximately how many pennies are in circulation?

Solution We can estimate the number of pennies in circulation using geometric series if we assume (for example) that the yearly production takes place at the start of the year and that the 5% are removed at the end of the year. In any year, 7.4 billion pennies are produced, and 7.4(0.95) billion pennies remain from the previous year's production (since 5% went out of circulation). There are $7.4(0.95)^2$ billion pennies remaining from those produced two years before, and so on. If N is the number of pennies in circulation, in billions, then

$$N = 7.4 + 7.4(0.95) + 7.4(0.95)^2 + \cdots.$$

This is an infinite geometric series with $a = 7.4$ and $r = 0.95$. Since $-1 < r < 1$, the series converges and its sum is given by

$$N = \frac{a}{1-r} = \frac{7.4}{1-0.95} = 148.$$

Thus, the market has stabilized with about 148 billion pennies in circulation today. Of the 148 billion pennies in circulation, 5% or $(148)(0.05) = 7.4$ billion are removed each year, which exactly equals the number produced each year.

---

[1] From www.usmint.gov.

Problems for Section 11.2

1. A yearly deposit of \$1000 is made into a bank account that pays 8.5% interest per year, compounded annually. What is the balance in the account right after the 20th deposit? How much of the balance comes from the annual deposits and how much comes from interest?

2. Annual deposits of \$2000 are made into an account paying 6% interest per year, compounded continuously. What is the balance in the account right after and right before the 5th deposit?

3. An annuity earning 0.5% per month, compounded monthly, is to make 36 monthly payments of \$1000 each, starting now. What is the present value of this annuity?

4. An annuity makes annual payments of \$50,000, starting now, from an account paying 7.2% interest per year, compounded annually. Find the present value of the annuity if it makes

   (a) Ten payments **(b)** Payments in perpetuity

5. Twenty annual payments of \$5000 each, with the first payment one year from now, are to be made from an account earning 10% per year, compounded annually. How much must be deposited now to cover the payments?

6. What is the present value of an annuity that pays \$20,000 each year, forever, starting today, from an account that pays 1% interest per year, compounded annually?

7. A deposit of \$100,000 is made into an account paying 8% interest per year, compounded annually. Annual payments of \$10,000 each, starting right after the deposit, are made out of the account. How many payments can be made before the account runs out of money?

8. An employer pays you 1 penny the first day you work and doubles your wages each day after that. Find your total earnings after working 7 days a week for

   (a) One week **(b)** Two weeks
   (c) Three weeks **(d)** Four weeks

9. An employee accepts a job with a starting salary of \$30,000 and a cost-of-living increase of 4% every year for the next 10 years. What is the employee's salary right before the start of the 11th year? What are her total earnings during the first 10 years?

10. Find the market stabilization point for a product if 10,000 new units of the product are manufactured at the start of each year and 25% of the total number of units in use fail at the end of each year.

11. Since 2007, the Bureau of Engraving and Printing has produced about 11 million new \$1 bills a day; worn bills are removed by Federal Reserve banks. There are about 9.2 billion dollar bills currently in circulation. Assuming that a fixed percentage of \$1 bills are removed from circulation each day, use a geometric series to estimate this percentage.[2]

Problems 12–14 are about *bonds*, which are issued by a government to raise money. An individual who buys a \$1000 bond gives the government \$1000 and in return receives a fixed sum of money, called the *coupon*, every six months or every year for the life of the bond. At the time of the last coupon, the individual also gets back the \$1000, or *principal*.

12. What is the present value of a \$1000 bond which pays \$50 a year for 10 years, starting one year from now? Assume the interest rate is 6% per year, compounded annually.

13. What is the present value of a \$1000 bond which pays \$50 a year for 10 years, starting one year from now? Assume the interest rate is 4% per year, compounded annually.

14. **(a)** What is the present value of a \$1000 bond which pays \$50 a year for 10 years, starting one year from now? Assume the interest rate is 5% per year, compounded annually.
    (b) Since \$50 is 5% of \$1000, this bond is called a 5% bond. What does your answer to part (a) tell you about the relationship between the principal and the present value of this bond if the interest rate is 5%?
    (c) If the interest rate is more than 5% per year, compounded annually, which is larger: the principal or the present value of the bond? Why is the bond then described as *trading at a discount*?
    (d) If the interest rate is less than 5% per year, compounded annually, why is the bond described as *trading at a premium*?

15. This problem illustrates how banks create credit and can thereby lend out more money than has been deposited. Suppose that initially \$100 is deposited in a bank. Experience has shown bankers that on average only 8% of the money deposited is withdrawn by the owner at any time. Consequently, bankers feel free to lend out 92% of their deposits. Thus \$92 of the original \$100 is loaned out to other customers (to start a business, for example). This \$92 becomes someone else's income and, sooner or later, is redeposited in the bank. Thus 92% of \$92, or $\$92(0.92) = \$84.64$, is loaned out again and eventually redeposited. Of the \$84.64, the bank again loans out 92%, and so on.

    (a) Find the total amount of money deposited in the bank as a result of these transactions.
    (b) The total amount of money deposited divided by the original deposit is called the *credit multiplier*. Calculate the credit multiplier for this example and explain what this number tells us.

[2] www.dallasnews.com/sharedcontent/dws/bus/stories/DN-obsoletedollarbill_22bus.State.Edition1.c8a2b4.html.

16. To stimulate the economy in 2002, the government gave a tax rebate totaling 40 billion dollars. Find the total additional spending resulting from this tax rebate if everyone who receives money spends

(a) 80% of it **(b)** 90% of it

17. To stimulate the economy in 2008, the government gave a tax rebate totaling 100 billion dollars. Find the total additional spending resulting from this tax rebate if everyone who receives money spends

(a) 80% of it **(b)** 90% of it

18. In April 2009, economists predicted that each dollar in tax cuts would generate \$3 in economic growth. What spending rate was assumed in arriving at this estimated multiplier effect?

19. A person who deposits money in a bank account starts a long process described by the reserve-deposit ratio, r. For every dollar deposited, the bank keeps r dollars and lends $1 - r$ dollars to someone else, who deposits the loan in a bank account. The same fraction of the second deposit is loaned out, to be deposited in turn, and so on. If the initial deposit is N dollars, find the total value of the bank accounts generated by this deposit:

(a) After the second deposit
(b) After the third deposit
(c) If the process continues forever

11.3 APPLICATIONS TO THE NATURAL SCIENCES

Steady-State Drug Levels

A patient is given a drug at regular intervals. In Section 11.1, we saw that in the long run, the quantity of drug in the body varies between a maximum level right after a dose and a minimum level right before a dose. At this *steady state*, the quantity eliminated between doses is equal to one dose. (See Problem 19.)

Example 1 A child with an ear infection is given a 200-mg ampicillin tablet once every 4 hours. About 12% of the drug in the body at the start of a four-hour period is still there at the end of that period. What is the quantity of ampicillin in the body

(a) Right after taking the 3rd tablet? (b) Right after taking the 6th tablet?

(c) At the steady state, right after and right before taking a tablet?

Solution Let Q_n be the quantity of ampicillin, in mg, in the body right after taking the nth tablet. Then

$$Q_n = 200 + 200(0.12) + 200(0.12)^2 + \cdots + 200(0.12)^{n-1}.$$

(a) Using the formula for the sum of a finite geometric series with $a = 200$, $r = 0.12$, and $n = 3$, we have

$$Q_3 = \frac{a(1-r^n)}{1-r} = \frac{200(1-(0.12)^3)}{1-0.12} = 226.88 \text{ mg}.$$

(b) Using $n = 6$, we have

$$Q_6 = \frac{a(1-r^n)}{1-r} = \frac{200(1-(0.12)^6)}{1-0.12} = 227.2720 \text{ mg}.$$

(c) At the steady state, the quantity Q in mg, right after a tablet is taken is the sum of the infinite geometric series

$$Q = 200 + 200(0.12) + 200(0.12)^2 + 200(0.12)^3 + \cdots.$$

Since $r = 0.12$ and $-1 < r < 1$, the series converges to a finite sum. At the steady state

$$\text{Quantity right after a dose} = Q = \frac{a}{1-r} = \frac{200}{1-0.12} = 227.2727 \text{ mg}.$$

The quantity of ampicillin in the body right before a dose is exactly 200 mg less than the quantity right after the dose, so at the steady state

$$\begin{aligned}\text{Quantity before dose} &= \text{Quantity after dose} - \text{Size of one dose}\\ &= 227.2727 - 200\\ &= 27.2727 \text{ mg}.\end{aligned}$$

Problem 4 shows how this relationship can be used to calculate Q, the long-run quantity of ampicillin right after a dose.

Example 2 Valproic acid, a drug used to control epilepsy, has a half-life of 15 hours in the body. If D mg of valproic acid is taken every 12 hours, at the steady state, what quantity of the drug is in the body right after taking a tablet?

Solution After a dose D of valproic acid, the quantity, Q, in the body decays exponentially, so $Q = Db^t$, where t is time in hours. The half-life is 15 hours, so

$$\begin{aligned} 0.5D &= Db^{15} \\ 0.5 &= b^{15} \\ b &= (0.5)^{1/15}. \end{aligned}$$

Right before the next dose at $t = 12$, we have

$$\text{Fraction of drug remaining after 12 hours } = b^{12} = ((0.5)^{1/15})^{12} = (0.5)^{12/15} = (0.5)^{0.8}.$$

Since D mg of valproic acid is given every 12 hours, in the long run

$$\text{Quantity right after dose } = D + D(0.5)^{0.8} + D\left((0.5)^{0.8}\right)^2 + \cdots.$$

This is an infinite geometric series with $r = (0.5)^{0.8} = 0.57435$. Since $-1 < r < 1$, the series converges and its sum is

$$\text{Quantity right after dose } = \frac{D}{1-(0.5)^{0.8}} = 2.35D.$$

Thus, in the long run, the quantity of the drug right after taking a dose is about 2.35 times the dose.

Accumulation of Toxins in the Body

Toxins found in pesticides can get into the food chain and accumulate in people's bodies through the food they eat. We use a geometric series to calculate the total accumulation of toxin in the body.

Example 3 Every day, a person consumes 5 micrograms (μg) of a toxin, which leaves the body at a continuous rate of 2% per day. In the long run, how much toxin is in the body at the end of the day?

Solution Since the toxin leaves the body at a continuous rate of 2% every day, the 5 μg amount consumed one day earlier has decayed to $5e^{-0.02}$, the 5 μg consumed two days earlier has decayed to $5e^{-0.02(2)} = 5(e^{-0.02})^2$, and so on. We assume that the 5 μg consumed during the day has not yet decayed. In the long run, at the end of each day we have, in micrograms,

$$\text{Total accumulation of toxin } = 5 + 5(e^{-0.02}) + 5(e^{-0.02})^2 + 5(e^{-0.02})^3 + \cdots.$$

This is an infinite geometric series with $a = 5$ and $r = e^{-0.02} = 0.9802$. Since $-1 < r < 1$, the series converges and its sum is

$$\text{Total accumulation of toxin } = \frac{a}{1-r} = \frac{5}{1-e^{-0.02}} = 252.5 \text{ micrograms.}$$

In the long run, there are 252.5 micrograms of toxin in the body at the end of the day.

Depletion of Natural Resources

Geometric series can be used to estimate how long a natural resource (such as oil) will last, assuming that usage levels increase at a constant percentage rate.

Example 4 At the end of 2008, world oil reserves were about 1950 billion barrels.[3] During 2008, about 29.3 billion barrels of oil were consumed.[4] Over the past decade, oil consumption has been increasing at about 1% per year.[5] Assuming yearly oil consumption increases at this rate in the future, how long will the reserves last?

[3] www.theoildrum.com/node/5395.
[4] *CIA World Factbook 2008.*
[5] www.eia.doe.gov/emeu/international/oilcomsumption.html.

Solution Under these assumptions, the oil used in 2009, in billions of barrels, is predicted to be $29.3(1.01)$. In 2010, we predict $29.3(1.01)^2$ billion barrels to be used, and $29.3(1.01)^3$ the next year, and so on. Thus, starting with 2009, the total quantity of oil used in n years, Q_n, is

$$Q_n = 29.3(1.01) + 29.3(1.01)^2 + 29.3(1.01)^3 + \cdots + 29.3(1.01)^n \text{ billions of barrels.}$$

This is a finite geometric series with n terms where $a = 29.3(1.01)$ and $r = 1.01$. (Notice that the last term can be written $29.3(1.01)(1.01)^{n-1}$.) The sum is

$$Q_n = \frac{a(1-r^n)}{1-r} = 29.3(1.01)\left(\frac{1-(1.01)^n}{1-1.01}\right) = 2959((1.01)^n - 1) \text{ billions of barrels.}$$

We want to find the value of n for which Q_n reaches the total reserves, 1950. Solving gives

$$\begin{aligned} 2959((1.01)^n - 1) &= 1950 \\ (1.01)^n - 1 &= \frac{1950}{2959} = 0.6590 \\ (1.01)^n &= 1.6590. \end{aligned}$$

Taking logarithms and using $\ln(A^p) = p \ln A$, we have

$$\begin{aligned} n \ln(1.01) &= \ln(1.6590) \\ n &= \frac{\ln(1.6590)}{\ln(1.01)} = 50.9 \text{ years.} \end{aligned}$$

Thus, if present consumption patterns are maintained, the world's oil supply will be exhausted in about 51 years. However, if consumption patterns change, the length of time until the reserves run out can be very different. Problem 2 concerns predictions using a 2.5% yearly increase and a 5.5% yearly decrease, the maximum and minimum figures for the past decade.

Geometric Series and Differential Equations

In this section, we used geometric series to model drug levels; in Chapter 10, we used differential equations to model drug levels. How do we know whether to use a geometric series or a differential equation? The answer depends on whether the drug is given in *discrete* doses (such as a tablet each morning) or *continuously* (such as intravenously).

Example 5 A patient receives 25 mg of a drug each day, and the drug is metabolized and eliminated at a continuous rate of 10% per day. Find the quantity of drug in the patient's body in the long run:

(a) Using a geometric series, assuming the 25-mg dose of the drug is administered in a single injection each morning. (Find the quantity both before and after an injection is given.)
(b) Using a differential equation, assuming the 25-mg dose of the drug is administered continuously throughout the day, using an intravenous drip.

Solution (a) A 25-mg injection is given each day. Since the drug is metabolized at a continuous rate of 10% per day, the quantity remaining a day later is $25e^{-0.1}$ mg. The quantity remaining two days later is $25(e^{-0.1})^2$ mg. In the long run,

$$\text{Quantity after injection} = 25 + 25(e^{-0.1}) + 25(e^{-0.1})^2 + 25(e^{-0.1})^3 + \cdots \text{ mg.}$$

We use the formula for the sum of an infinite geometric series with $a = 25$ and $r = e^{-0.1}$:

$$\text{Quantity after injection} = \frac{a}{1-r} = \frac{25}{1-e^{-0.1}} = 262.7 \text{ mg.}$$

Since each injection is 25 mg, in the long run

$$\text{Quantity before injection} = 262.7 - 25 = 237.7 \text{ mg.}$$

(b) The drug is entering the body at the continuous rate of 25 mg per day and leaving at the continuous rate of 0.1 times the current level in the body. Thus, if Q is the quantity of drug in the body after t days, then

$$\frac{dQ}{dt} = \text{Rate in} - \text{Rate out} = 25 - 0.1Q.$$

In Chapter 10, we saw that Q tends toward the equilibrium solution which occurs when $dQ/dt = 0$. Then

$$\frac{dQ}{dt} = 25 - 0.1Q = 0$$
$$Q = 250 \text{ mg}.$$

When the drug is given continuously, the quantity of the drug in the body levels off at 250 mg.

Problems for Section 11.3

1. In 2008, world oil consumption was 29.3 billion barrels,[6] a decrease of 5.5% from 2007. Assuming that consumption continues to decrease at the same percentage rate, make a table showing yearly consumption between 2008 and 2017, inclusive. Find the total quantity of oil consumed during this decade.

2. As in Example 4, assume that oil reserves at the end of 2008 were 1950 billion barrels and that consumption in 2008 was 29.3 billion barrels. What happens in the long run if oil consumption

(a) Decreases by 5.5% per year
(b) Increases by 2.5% per year

3. Every morning, a patient receives a 50-mg injection of a drug. At the end of a 24-hour period, 60% of the drug remains in the body. What quantity of drug is in the body

(a) Right after the 3rd injection?
(b) Right after the 7th injection?
(c) Right after an injection, at the steady state?

4. This problem gives another way of finding, Q, the long-run ampicillin quantity right after a dose in Example 1. (See page 463.) In the four hours after a dose, 200 mg of ampicillin must be excreted, as the next 200-mg tablet elevates the ampicillin quantity back to Q mg. Use this information to solve for Q.

5. A dose of 120 mg is taken by a patient at the same time every day. In one day, 30% of the drug is excreted.

(a) At the steady state, find the quantity of drug in the body right after a dose.
(b) Check that at the steady state, the quantity excreted in one day is equal to the dose.

6. At the same time every day, a patient takes 50 mg of the antidepressant fluoxetine, whose half-life is 3 days.

(a) What fraction of the dose remains in the body after a 24-hour period?
(b) What is the quantity of fluoxetine in the body right after taking the 7th dose?
(c) In the long run, what is the quantity of fluoxetine in the body right after a dose?

7. A person with chronic pain takes a 30 mg tablet of morphine every 4 hours. The half-life of morphine is 2 hours.

(a) How much morphine is in the body right after and right before taking the 6th tablet?
(b) At the steady state, find the quantity of morphine in the body right after and right before taking a tablet.

8. **(a)** An allergy drug with a half-life of 18 weeks is given in 100-mg doses once a week. At the steady state, find the quantity of the drug in the body right after a dose.
(b) The drug does not become effective until the quantity in the body right after a dose reaches 2000 mg. How many weeks after the first dose does the drug become effective?

9. A cigarette puts 1.2 mg of nicotine into the body. Nicotine leaves the body at a continuous rate of 34.65% per hour, but more than 60 mg can be lethal. If a person smokes a cigarette with each of the following frequencies, find the long-run quantity of nicotine in the body right after a cigarette. Does the nicotine reach the lethal level?

(a) Every hour **(b)** Every half hour
(c) Every 15 minutes **(d)** Every 6 minutes
(e) Every 3 minutes

10. Each day at lunch a person consumes 8 micrograms of a toxin found in a pesticide; the toxin is metabolized at a continuous rate of 0.5% per day. In the long run, how much of this toxin accumulates in the person's body? Give the quantities right after and right before lunch.

11. At the end of 2008, the total reserve of a mineral was 350,000 m^3. In the year 2009, about 5000 m^3 was used. Each year, consumption of the mineral is expected to increase by 8%. Under these assumptions, in how many years will all reserves of the mineral be depleted?

[6] *Statistical Review of World Energy 2008*, www.bp.com.

12. We use 1500 kg of a mineral this year and consumption of the mineral is increasing annually by 4%. The total reserves of the mineral are estimated to be 120,000 kg. Approximately when will the reserves run out?

13. At the end of 2007, natural gas reserves were 180 trillion m^3; during 2007, about 3 trillion m^3 of natural gas were consumed.[7] Estimate how long natural gas reserves will last if consumption increases at 2% per year.

14. Over the past decade, natural gas consumption has been increasing at between 0% and 5% a year. Using the data from Problem 13, estimate how long the natural gas reserves will last assuming the rate of increase is

(a) 0% **(b)** 5%

Problems 15–17 concern how long reserves of the mineral in Problem 11 last if usage patterns change. For example, as reserves get lower, substitutes may be developed.

15. How long will the reserves last if the annual increase in usage is 4%?

16. How long will the reserves last if the annual usage stays constant at 5000 m^3 per year?

17. How long will the reserves last if the usage decreases each year by 4%?

18. **(a)** A dose D of a drug is administered at intervals equal to the half-life. (That is, the second dose is given when half the first dose remains.) At the steady state, find the quantity of drug in the body right after a dose.

(b) If the quantity of a drug in the body after a dose is 300 mg at the steady state and if the interval between doses equals the half-life, what is the dose?

19. A dose, D, of a drug is taken at regular time intervals, and a fraction r remains after one time interval. Show that at the steady state, the quantity of the drug excreted between doses equals the dose.

20. Cephalexin is an antibiotic with a half-life in the body of 0.9 hours, taken in tablets of 250 mg every six hours.

(a) What percentage of the cephalexin in the body at the start of a six-hour period is still there at the end (assuming no tablets are taken during that time)?

(b) Write an expression for Q_1, Q_2, Q_3, Q_4, where Q_n mg is the amount of cephalexin in the body right after the nth tablet is taken.

(c) Express Q_3, Q_4 in closed form and evaluate them.

(d) Write an expression for Q_n and put it in closed form.

(e) If the patient keeps taking the tablets, use your answer to part (d) to find the quantity of cephalexin in the body in the long run, right after taking a tablet.

CHAPTER SUMMARY

- **Geometric series**
  Finite and infinite.
- **Sums of geometric series**
  Partial sums, convergence of infinite series.
- **Applications to business and economics**
  Annuities, present value, multiplier effect, market stabilization.
- **Applications to life sciences**
  Repeated drug doses, accumulation of toxins, depletion of natural resources.

REVIEW PROBLEMS FOR CHAPTER ELEVEN

In Problems 1–8, find the sum, if it exists.

1. $2+2^2+2^3+\cdots+2^{10}$

2. $20+20(1.4)+20(1.4)^2+\cdots+20(1.4)^8$

3. $1000+1000(1.08)+1000(1.08)^2+1000(1.08)^3+\cdots$

4. $500+500(0.6)+500(0.6)^2+\cdots+500(0.6)^{15}$

5. $30+30(0.85)+30(0.85)^2+30(0.85)^3+\cdots$

6. $25+25(0.2)+25(0.2)^2+25(0.2)^3+\cdots$

7. $1+\dfrac{1}{2}+\dfrac{1}{2^2}+\cdots+\dfrac{1}{2^8}$

8. $1+\dfrac{1}{3}+\dfrac{1}{3^2}+\dfrac{1}{3^3}+\cdots$

9. Around January 1, 1993, Barbra Streisand signed a contract with Sony Corporation for \$2 million a year for 10 years. Suppose the first payment was made on the day of signing and that all other payments were made on the first day of the year. Suppose also that all payments were made into a bank account earning 4% a year, compounded annually.

(a) How much money was in the account

(i) On the night of December 31, 1999?

(ii) On the day the last payment was made?

(b) What was the present value of the contract on the day it was signed?

10. A drug is given in daily doses of 100 mg. After 24 hours, 82% of the previous day's dose remains in the body. What is the long-run quantity of drug in the body, right after and right before a dose is given?

[7] www.worldenergyoutlook.org/docs/weo2008/weo2008_es_english.pdf

11. A used car costs $15,000. The repair contract costs $500 at the end of the first year and increases by 20% at the end of each subsequent year. Find the total cost of owning the car for ten years. Include the payment at the end of the tenth year.

12. A donor sets up an endowment to fund an annual scholarship of $10,000. The endowment earns 6% interest per year, compounded annually. Find the amount that must be deposited now if the endowment is to fund one award each year, with one award now and continuing

(a) Until twenty awards have been made
(b) Forever

13. This problem shows how to estimate the cumulative effect of a tax cut on a country's economy. Suppose the government proposes a tax cut totaling $100 million. We assume that all the people who have extra money spend 80% of it and save 20%. Thus, of the extra income generated by the tax cut, $\$100(0.8)$ million $=$ $80 million is spent and becomes extra income to someone else. These people also spend 80% of their additional income, or $\$80(0.8)$ million, and so on. Calculate the total additional spending created by such a tax cut.

14. To stimulate the economy, the government gives a tax rebate totaling 5 billion dollars. Find the total additional spending resulting from this tax rebate if everyone who receives money spends

(a) 80% of it (b) 90% of it

15. A government gives a tax rebate of N dollars to stimulate the economy. Everyone who receives money spends a fixed fraction, k, of the money received, with $0 < k < 1$.

(a) Find a formula (in terms of N and k) for the total additional spending resulting from the tax rebate.
(b) If $k = 0.85$, what is the total additional spending as a multiple of the size, N, of the tax rebate?

16. Before World War I, the British government issued what are called *consols*, which pay the owner or his heirs a fixed amount of money every year forever. (Cartoonists of the time described aristocrats living off such payments as "pickled in consols.") What should a person expect to pay for consols which pay £10 a year forever? Assume the first payment is one year from the date of purchase and that interest remains 4% per year, compounded annually. (£ denotes pounds, the British unit of currency.)

17. A repeating decimal can always be expressed as a fraction. This problem shows how writing a repeating decimal as a geometric series enables you to find the fraction.

(a) Write the repeating decimal 0.232323... as a geometric series using the fact that $0.232323\ldots = 0.23 + 0.0023 + 0.000023 + \cdots$.
(b) Use the formula for the sum of a geometric series to show that $0.232323\ldots = 23/99$.

18. A ball is dropped from a height of 10 feet and bounces. Each bounce is $\frac{3}{4}$ of the height of the bounce before. Thus, after the ball hits the floor for the first time, the ball rises to a height of $10(\frac{3}{4}) = 7.5$ feet, and after it hits the floor for the second time, it rises to a height of $7.5(\frac{3}{4}) = 10(\frac{3}{4})^2 = 5.625$ feet.

(a) Find an expression for the height to which the ball rises after it hits the floor for the nth time.
(b) Find an expression for the total vertical distance the ball has traveled when it hits the floor for the first, second, third, and fourth times.
(c) Find an expression for the total vertical distance the ball has traveled when it hits the floor for the nth time. Express your answer in closed form.

19. One way of valuing a company is to calculate the present value of all its future earnings. A farm expects to sell $1000 worth of Christmas trees once a year forever, with the first sale in the immediate future. What is the present value of this Christmas tree business? The interest rate is 4% per year, compounded continuously.

20. Every year, a company sells 1000 units of a product while 20% of the total number in use fail. Assume sales are at the start of the year and failures are at the end of the year.

(a) Find the market stabilization point for this product.
(b) If the stabilization point is approached very slowly, the number of units in use may not get close to this value because market conditions change first. Make a table for S_n, the number of units in use right after the nth annual sale, for $n = 5, 10, 15, 20$, to see how rapidly this market approaches the stabilization point.

CHECK YOUR UNDERSTANDING

In Problems 1–30, indicate whether the statement is true or false.

1. The sum $1 + 2 + 4 + 8 + 16 + 32$ is a finite geometric series with 6 terms.

2. The sum $1 + 2 + 4 + 8 + 16 + 32 + \cdots + 2^{10}$ is a finite geometric series with 10 terms.

3. The sum $1 + 3 + 5 + 7 + 9 + 11$ is a finite geometric series with 6 terms.

4. The sum $1 - 2 + 4 - 8 + 16 - 32$ is a finite geometric series with 6 terms.

5. The sum of $1 + (1/3) + (1/9) + \cdots + (1/3)^{10}$ is $(1 - (1/3)^{11})/(1 - (1/3))$.

6. The sum of $3 \cdot 1 + 3 \cdot 2 + 3 \cdot 4 + \cdots + 3(2^{20})$ is $3(1 - 2^{20})/(1 - 2)$.

7. The sum of the infinite geometric series $3 + 3^2 + 3^3 + \cdots + 3^n + \cdots$ is $3/(1 - 3)$.

8. The sum of the infinite geometric series $(1/2)+(1/2)^2+(1/2)^3+\cdots+(1/2)^n+\cdots$ is $1/(1-(1/2))$.

9. The sum of the infinite geometric series $(1/3)+(1/3)^2+(1/3)^3+\cdots+(1/3)^n+\cdots$ is $1/2$.

10. The sum of the infinite geometric series $5(1/2)+5(1/2)^2+5(1/2)^3+\cdots+5(1/2)^n+\cdots$ is 5.

11. An annuity is a sequence of equal payments or deposits made at regular intervals.

12. The present value of an annuity is the amount of money deposited today to make a series of fixed payments in the future.

13. The present value of an annuity that makes payments of \$6000 per year for 10 years is less than \$60,000, assuming an annual interest rate of 3%.

14. The present value of a series of constant annual payments made forever is infinite.

15. If annual deposits of \$3000 are made at the beginning of each year into an account paying 2% interest per year, compounded annually, then the account balance after the fourth deposit is $3000(1.02)^4+3000(1.02)^3+3000(1.02)^2+3000(1.02)$ dollars.

16. If annual deposits of \$3000 are made at the beginning of each year into an account paying 2% interest per year, compounded annually, then the account balance after the tenth deposit is $3000(1-(1.02)^{10})/(1-1.02)$ dollars.

17. A deposit of \$735,000 into an account earning 5% compounded annually is sufficient to generate annual payments of \$35,000 in perpetuity, starting now.

18. The present value of a payment 5 years in the future of \$2000, assuming annual interest rate of 3%, is $2000(1.03)^5$ dollars.

19. The present value of 3 annual payments of \$600, starting now, assuming annual interest rate of 4%, is $600+600(1.04)^{-1}+600(1.04)^{-2}$ dollars.

20. The present value of 10 annual payments of \$600, starting now, assuming annual interest rate of 4%, is $600(1-(1.04)^{-10})/(1-(1.04)^{-1})$ dollars.

21. If a person consumes a 25-mg tablet of a drug four times throughout the day, at the end of the day the person will have 100 mg of the drug in the body.

22. If the quantity of a drug in the body has reached the steady-state level for a person taking a drug at regular intervals, then the quantity of drug in the person's body stays constant.

23. A person consuming 3 micrograms of a toxin with breakfast each day, of which 5% leaves the body each day, has 3/(1-0.05) micrograms of toxin in the body right after breakfast, in the long run.

24. If a country used 10 billion barrels of oil last year, and oil consumption increases at 2% annually, then over the next 5 years, the total oil consumption will be $10(1.02)(1-(1.02)^5)/(1-1.02)$ billion barrels.

25. In a person taking a constant dose D mg of medication everyday, the steady-state level is the same before and after each daily dose.

26. In a person taking a constant dose D mg of medication every day, at the steady-state level the quantity of the drug eliminated daily is equal to the daily dose D.

27. If a drug is administered intravenously, then a geometric series is a better model than a differential equation for the quantity of drug in the bloodstream.

28. If a certain drug has a half-life of three hours in the body, then nine hours after a dosage of 160 mg, the quantity in the body drops to 20 mg.

29. If a 50-mg injection of a drug is given once every day, and the drug is metabolized at a continuous rate of 5% per day, then the long-term steady-state quantity in the body after injection is $50/(1-e^{0.05})$.

30. If a drug is administered intravenously at a rate of 50 mg per day, and the drug is metabolized at a continuous rate of 5% per day, then the long-term steady-state quantity in the body is 1000 mg.

PROJECTS FOR CHAPTER ELEVEN

1. Do You Have Any Common Ancestors?

In this project, we estimate the number of ancestors you have and determine whether you have any common ancestors. (A common ancestor is one who appears on two sides of your family tree. For example, if your great-grandmother on your mother's mother's side is also your grandmother on your father's side, then she would be a common ancestor.)

(a) In general, each person has 2 biological parents, 4 biological grandparents, 8 biological great-grandparents, and so on. Write a formula for the number of ancestors you have, going back n generations.

(b) How long is one generation? Estimate the age of typical parents when a baby is born. This is the length of time for a generation. How many generations are included if we go back 100 years? 500 years? 1000 years? 2000 years?

(c) Use your answers to parts (a) and (b) to estimate the number of ancestors you have if we go back 100 years, 500 years, 1000 years, or 2000 years.

(d) In parts (a) and (c), we counted every ancestor separately, so we assumed that you have no common ancestors. Use the fact that the population of the world was about 6 billion people in 1999 and was about 200 million people in the year 1 AD to determine whether this is a reasonable assumption. Explain your reasoning.

2. Harrod-Hicks Model of an Expanding National Economy

In an expanding national economy, the Harrod-Hicks model relates the national income in one year to the national income in the preceding year. If $f(n)$ is the national income in year n, then the model predicts, for some constants k and h with $k > 1$ and $h > 0$, that

$$f(n+1) = kf(n) - h.$$

(a) Let $C = f(0)$. Write $f(1)$, $f(2)$, and $f(3)$ in terms of k, h, and C.

(b) Show that

$$f(1) = kC - h,$$

$$f(2) = k^2C - (1+k)h,$$

$$f(3) = k^3C - (1+k+k^2)h.$$

Use these formulas to guess a formula for $f(n)$.

(c) Use the formula for the sum of a finite geometric series to rewrite the formula for $f(n)$ in closed form.

3. Probability of Winning in Sports

In certain sports, winning a game requires a lead of two points. That is, if the score is tied you have to score two points in a row to win.

(a) For some sports (e.g. tennis), a point is scored every play. Suppose your probability of scoring the next point is always p. Then, your opponent's probability of scoring the next point is always $1 - p$.

(i) What is the probability that you win the next two points?

(ii) What is the probability that you and your opponent split the next two points, that is, that neither of you wins both points?

(iii) What is the probability that you split the next two points but you win the two after that?

(iv) What is the probability that you either win the next two points or split the next two and then win the next two after that?

(v) Give a formula for your probability w of winning a tied game.

(vi) Compute your probability of winning a tied game when $p = 0.5$; when $p = 0.6$; when $p = 0.7$; when $p = 0.4$. Comment on your answers.

(b) In other sports (e.g. volleyball prior to 1999), you can score a point only if it is your turn, with turns alternating until a point is scored. Suppose your probability of scoring a point when it is your turn is p, and your opponent's probability of scoring a point when it is her turn is q.

(i) Find a formula for the probability S that you are the first to score the next point, assuming it is currently your turn.

(ii) Suppose that if you score a point, the next turn is yours. Using your answers to part (a) and your formula for S, compute the probability of winning a tied game (if you need two points in a row to win).

- Assume $p = 0.5$ and $q = 0.5$ and it is your turn.
- Assume $p = 0.6$ and $q = 0.5$ and it is your turn.

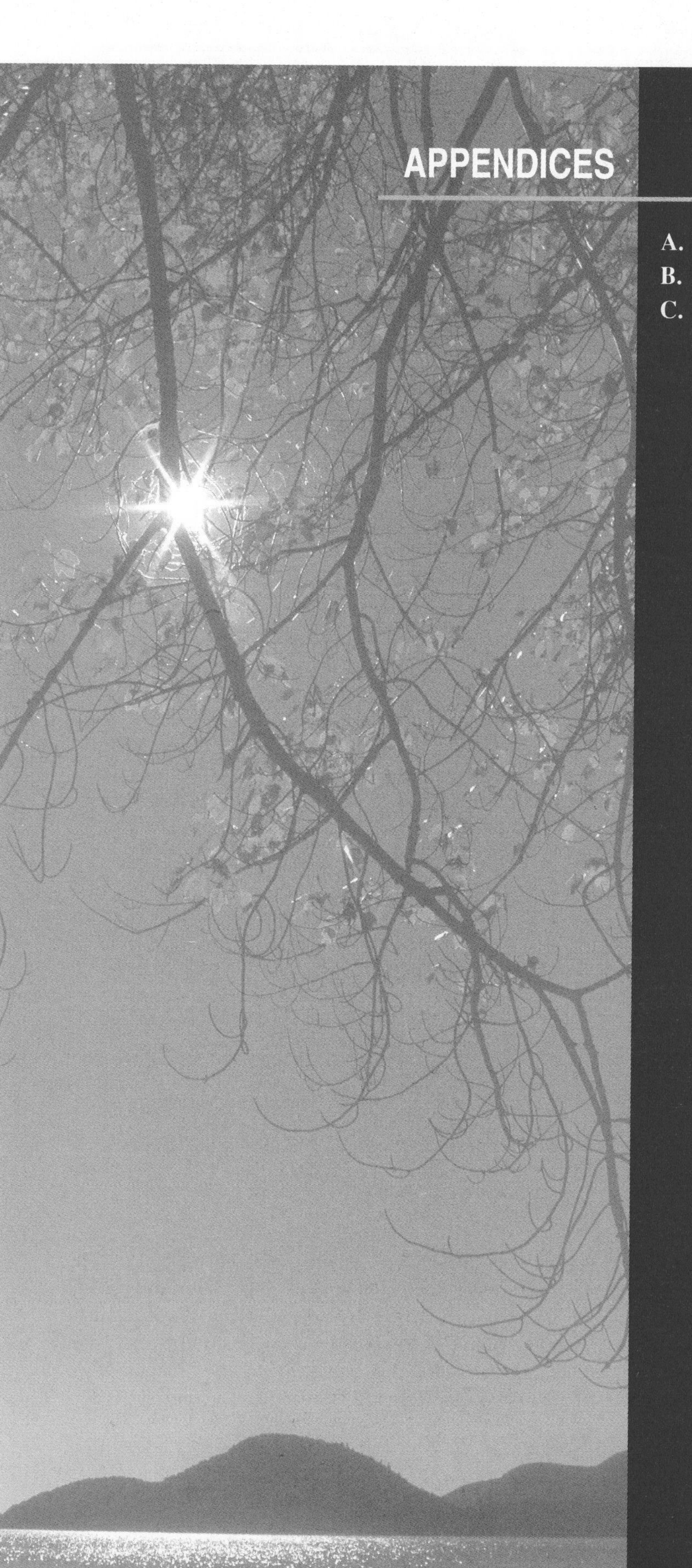

APPENDICES

A FITTING FORMULAS TO DATA

In this section we see how the formulas that are used in a mathematical model can be developed. Some of the formulas we use are exact. However, many formulas we use are approximations, often constructed from data.

Fitting a Linear Function to Data

A company wants to understand the relationship between the amount spent on advertising, a, and total sales, S. The data they collect might look like that found in Table A.1.

Table A.1 *Advertising and sales: Linear relationship*

a (advertising in \$1000s)	3	4	5	6
S (sales in \$1000s)	100	120	140	160

The data in Table A.1 are linear, so a formula fits it exactly. The slope of the line is 20, and we can determine that the vertical intercept is 40, so the line is

$$S = 40 + 20a.$$

Now suppose that the company collected the data in Table A.2. This time the data are not linear. In general, it is difficult to find a formula to fit data exactly. We must be satisfied with a formula that is a good approximation to the data.

Table A.2 *Advertising and sales: Nonlinear relationship*

a (advertising in \$1000s)	3	4	5	6
S (sales in \$1000s)	105	117	141	152

Figure A.1 shows the data in Table A.2. Since the relationship is nearly, though not exactly, linear, it is well approximated by a line. Figure A.2 shows the line $S = 40 + 20a$ and the data.

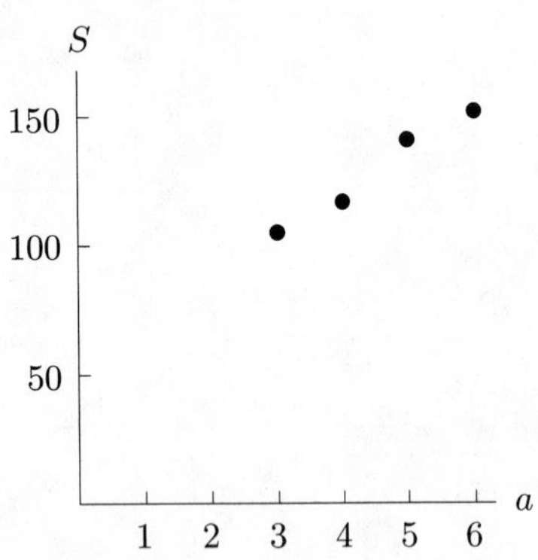

Figure A.1: The sales data from Table A.2

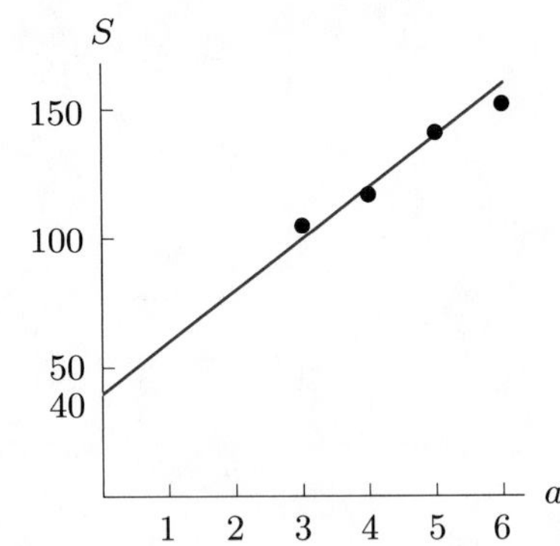

Figure A.2: The line $S = 40 + 20a$ and the data from Table A.2

The Regression Line

Is there a line that fits the data better than the one in Figure A.2? If so, how do we find it? The process of fitting a line to a set of data is called *linear regression* and the line of best fit is called the *regression line.* (Later in the section, we discuss what "best fit" means.) Many calculators and computer programs calculate the regression line from the data points. Alternatively, the regression line can be estimated by plotting the points on paper and fitting a line "by eye." In Chapter 9, we derive the formulas for the regression line. For the data in Table A.2, the regression line is

$$S = 54.5 + 16.5a.$$

This line is graphed with the data in Figure A.3.

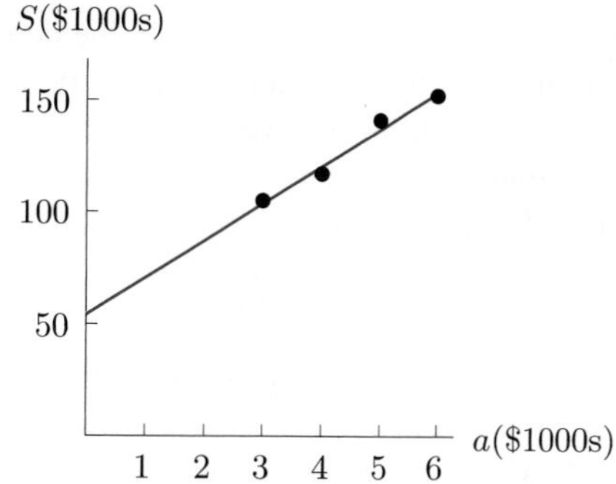

Figure A.3: The regression line $S = 54.5 + 16.5a$ and the data from Table A.2

Using the Regression Line to Make Predictions

We can use the formula for sales as a function of advertising to make predictions. For example, to predict total sales if \$3500 is spent on advertising, substitute $a = 3.5$ into the regression line:

$$S = 54.5 + 16.5(3.5) = 112.25.$$

The regression line predicts sales of \$112,250. To see that this is reasonable, compare it to the entries in Table A.2. When $a = 3$, we have $S = 105$, and when $a = 4$, we have $S = 117$. Predicted sales of $S = 112.25$ when $a = 3.5$ makes sense because it falls between 105 and 117. See Figure A.4. Of course, if we spent \$3500 on advertising, sales would probably not be exactly \$112,250. The regression equation allows us to make predictions, but does not provide exact results.

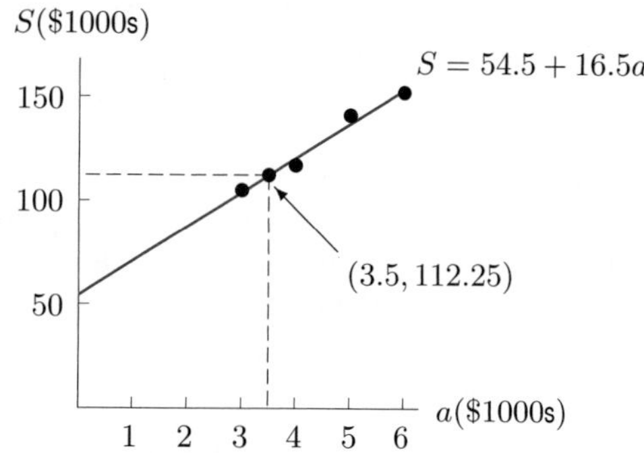

Figure A.4: Predicting sales when spending \$3,500 on advertising

---

Example 1 Predict total sales given advertising expenditures of \$4800 and \$10,000.

Solution When \$4800 is spent on advertising, $a = 4.8$, so

$$S = 54.5 + 16.5(4.8) = 133.7.$$

Sales are predicted to be \$133,700. When \$10,000 is spent on advertising, $a = 10$, so

$$S = 54.5 + 16.5(10) = 219.5.$$

Sales are predicted to be \$219,500.

Consider the two predictions made in Example 1 at $a = 4.8$ and $a = 10$. We have more confidence in the accuracy of the prediction when $a = 4.8$, because we are *interpolating* within an interval we already know something about. The prediction for $a = 10$ is less reliable, because we are *extrapolating* outside the interval defined by the data values in Table A.2. In general, interpolation is safer than extrapolation.

Interpreting the Slope of the Regression Line

The slope of a linear function is the change in the dependent variable divided by the change in the independent variable. For the sales and advertising regression line, the slope is 16.5. This tells us that S increases by about 16.5 whenever a increases by 1. If advertising expenses increase by \$1000, sales increase by about \$16,500. In general, the slope tells us the expected change in the dependent variable for a unit change in the independent variable.

How Regression Works: What "Best Fit" Means

Figure A.5 illustrates how a line is fitted to a set of data. We assume that the value of y is in some way related to the value of x, although other factors could influence y as well. Thus, we assume that we can pick the value of x exactly but that the value of y may be only partially determined by this x-value.

A calculator or computer finds the line that minimizes the sum of the squares of the vertical distances between the data points and the line. See Figure A.5. The regression line is also called a *least-squares line*, or the *line of best fit*.

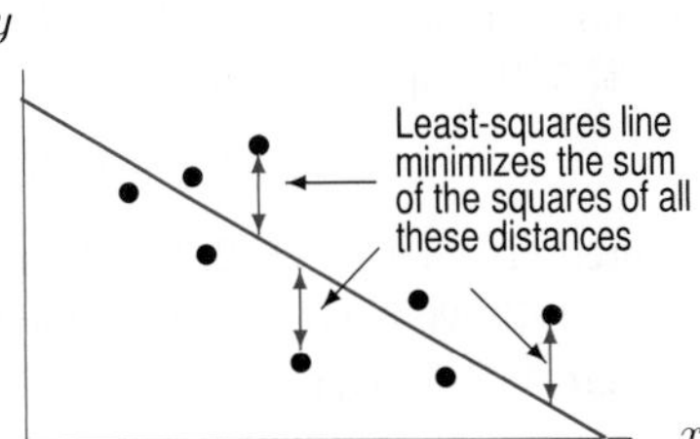

Figure A.5: Data and the corresponding least-squares regression line

Correlation

When a computer or calculator calculates a regression line, it also gives a *correlation coefficient*, r. This number lies between -1 and $+1$ and measures how well the regression line fits the data. If $r = 1$, the data lie exactly on a line of positive slope. If $r = -1$, the data lie exactly on a line of negative slope. If r is close to 0, the data may be completely scattered, or there may be a nonlinear relationship between the variables. (See Figure A.6.)

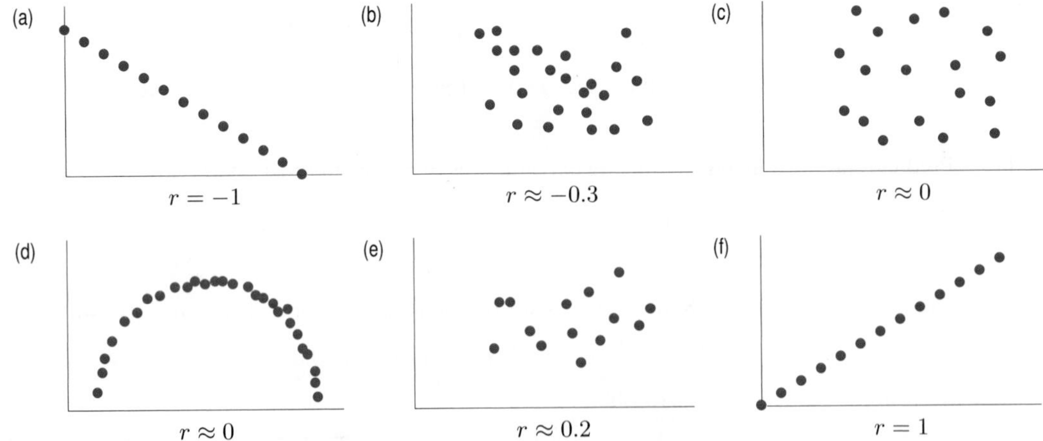

Figure A.6: Various data sets and correlation coefficients

Example 2 The correlation coefficient for the sales data in Table A.2 is $r \approx 0.99$. The fact that r is positive tells us that the regression line has positive slope. The fact that r is close to 1 tells us that the regression line fits the data well.

The Difference Between Relation, Correlation, and Causation

It is important to understand that a high correlation (either positive or negative) between two quantities does *not* imply causation. For example, there is a high correlation between children's reading level and shoe size.[1] However, large feet do not cause a child to read better (or vice versa). Larger feet and improved reading ability are both a consequence of growing older.

Notice also that a correlation of 0 does not imply that there is no relationship between x and y. For example, in Figure A.6(d) there is a relationship between x and y-values, while Figure A.6(c) exhibits no apparent relationship. Both data sets have a correlation coefficient of $r \approx 0$. Thus, a correlation of $r = 0$ usually implies there is no linear relationship between x and y, but this does not mean there is no relationship at all.

Regression When the Relationship Is Not Linear

Table A.3 shows the population of the US (in millions) from 1790 to 1860. These points are plotted in Figure A.7. Do the data look linear? Not really. It appears to make more sense to fit an exponential function than a linear function to this data. Finding the exponential function of best fit is called *exponential regression.* One algorithm used by a calculator or computer gives the exponential function that fits the data as

$$P = 3.9(1.03)^t,$$

where P is the US population in millions and t is years since 1790. Other algorithms may give different answers. See Figure A.8.

Since the base of this exponential function is 1.03, the US population was increasing at the rate of about 3% per year between 1790 and 1860. Is it reasonable to expect the population to continue to increase at this rate? It turns out that this exponential model does not fit the population of the US well beyond 1860. In Section 4.7, we see another function that is used to model the US population.

Table A.3 *US Population in millions, 1790–1860*

Year	1790	1800	1810	1820	1830	1840	1850	1860
Population	3.9	5.3	7.2	9.6	12.9	17.1	23.1	31.4

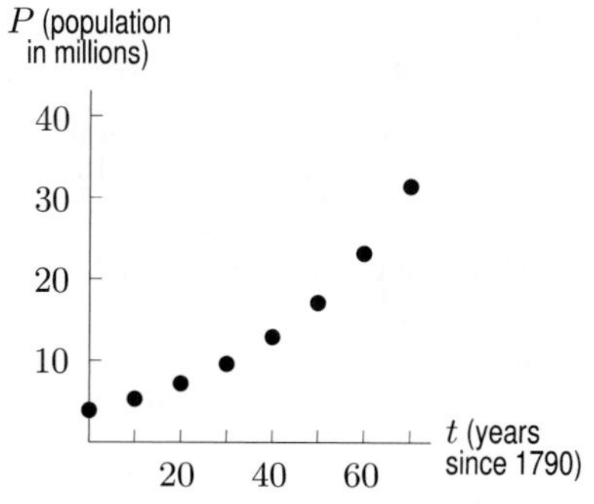

Figure A.7: US Population 1790–1860

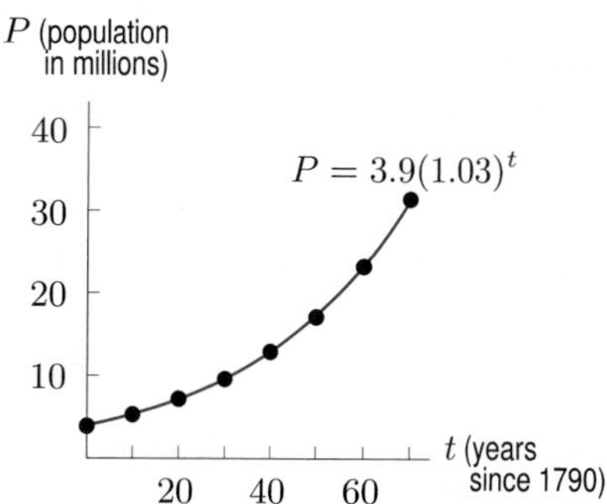

Figure A.8: US population and an exponential regression function

Calculators and computers can do linear regression, exponential regression, logarithmic regression, quadratic regression, and more. To fit a formula to a set of data, the first step is to graph the data and identify the appropriate family of functions.

[1]From *Statistics*, 2nd ed., by David Freedman, Robert Pisani, Roger Purves, Ani Adhikari, p. 142 (New York: W.W.Norton, 1991).

Example 3 The average fuel efficiency (miles per gallon of gasoline) of US automobiles declined until the 1960s and then started to rise as manufacturers made cars more fuel efficient.[2] See Table A.4.

(a) Plot the data. What family of functions should be used to model the data: linear, exponential, logarithmic, power function, or a polynomial? If a polynomial, state the degree and whether the leading coefficient is positive or negative.

(b) Use quadratic regression to fit a quadratic polynomial to the data; graph it with the data.

Table A.4 *What function fits these data?*

Year	1940	1950	1960	1970	1980	1986
Average miles per gallon	14.8	13.9	13.4	13.5	15.5	18.3

Solution

(a) The data are shown in Figure A.9, with time t in years since 1940. Miles per gallon decreases and then increases, so a good function to model the data is a quadratic (degree 2) polynomial. Since the parabola opens up, the leading coefficient is positive.

(b) If $f(t)$ is average miles per gallon, one algorithm for quadratic regression tells us that the quadratic polynomial that fits the data is

$$f(t) = 0.00617t^2 - 0.225t + 15.10.$$

In Figure A.10, we see that this quadratic does fit the data reasonably well.

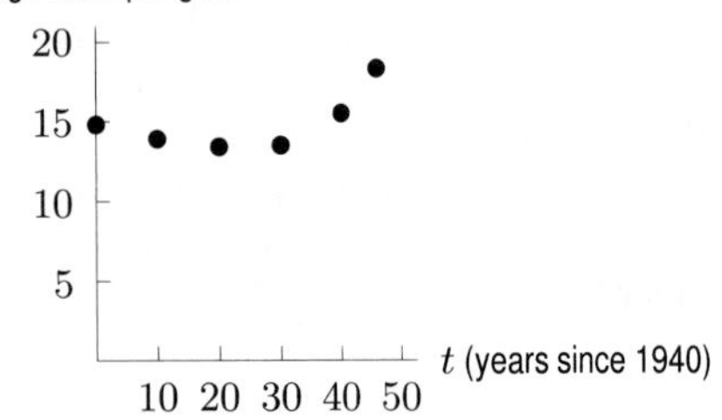

Figure A.9: Data showing fuel efficiency of US automobiles over time

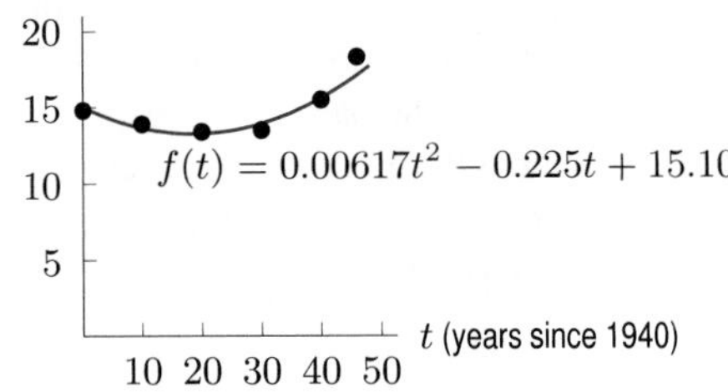

Figure A.10: Data and best quadratic polynomial, found using regression

Problems for Appendix A

1. Table A.5 gives the gross world product, G, which measures global output of goods and services.[3] If t is in years since 1950, the regression line for these data is

$$G = 3.543 + 0.734t.$$

(a) Plot the data and the regression line on the same axes. Does the line fit the data well?

(b) Interpret the slope of the line in terms of gross world product.

(c) Use the regression line to estimate gross world product in 2005 and in 2020. Comment on your confidence in the two predictions.

Table A.5 *G, in trillions of 1999 dollars*

Year	1950	1960	1970	1980	1990	2000
G	6.4	10.0	16.3	23.6	31.9	43.2

2. Table A.6 shows worldwide cigarette production as a function of t, the number of years since 1950.[4]

(a) Find the regression line for this data.

(b) Use the regression line to estimate world cigarette production in the year 2010.

(c) Interpret the slope of the line in terms of cigarette production.

(d) Plot the data and the regression line on the same axes. Does the line fit the data well?

Table A.6 *Cigarette production, P, in billions*

t	0	10	20	30	40	50
P	1686	2150	3112	4388	5419	5564

[2] C. Schaufele and N. Zumoff, *Earth Algebra, Preliminary Version*, p. 91 (New York: Harper Collins, 1993).
[3] The Worldwatch Institute, *Vital Signs* 2001, p. 57 (New York: W.W. Norton, 2001).
[4] The Worldwatch Institute, *Vital Signs* 2001, p. 77 (New York: W.W. Norton, 2001).

3. Table A.7 shows the US Gross National Product (GNP).[5]

 (a) Plot GNP against years since 1970. Does a line fit the data well?
 (b) Find the regression line and graph it with the data.
 (c) Use the regression line to estimate the GNP in 1985 and in 2020. Which estimate do you have more confidence in? Why?

Table A.7 *GNP in 2003 dollars*

Year	1970	1980	1990	2000
GNP (billions)	1045	2824	5838	9856

4. The acidity of a solution is measured by its pH, with lower pH values indicating more acidity. A study of acid rain was undertaken in Colorado between 1975 and 1978, in which the acidity of rain was measured for 150 consecutive weeks. The data followed a generally linear pattern and the regression line was determined to be

$$P = 5.43 - 0.0053t,$$

where P is the pH of the rain and t is the number of weeks into the study.[6]

 (a) Is the pH level increasing or decreasing over the period of the study? What does this tell you about the level of acidity in the rain?
 (b) According to the line, what was the pH at the beginning of the study? At the end of the study ($t = 150$)?
 (c) What is the slope of the regression line? Explain what this slope is telling you about the pH.

5. In a 1977 study[7] of 21 of the best American female runners, researchers measured the average stride rate, S, at different speeds, v. The data are given in Table A.8.

 (a) Find the regression line for these data, using stride rate as the dependent variable.
 (b) Plot the regression line and the data on the same axes. Does the line fit the data well?
 (c) Use the regression line to predict the stride rate when the speed is 18 ft/sec and when the speed is 10 ft/sec. Which prediction do you have more confidence in? Why?

Table A.8 *Stride rate, S, in steps/sec, and speed, v, in ft/sec*

v	15.86	16.88	17.50	18.62	19.97	21.06	22.11
S	3.05	3.12	3.17	3.25	3.36	3.46	3.55

6. Table A.9 shows the atmospheric concentration of carbon dioxide, CO_2 (in parts per million, ppm), at the Mauna Loa Observatory in Hawaii.[8]

 (a) Find the average rate of change of the concentration of carbon dioxide between 1980 and 2000. Give units and interpret your answer in terms of carbon dioxide.
 (b) Plot the data, and find the regression line for carbon dioxide concentration against years since 1980. Use the regression line to predict the concentration of carbon dioxide in the atmosphere in the year 2020.

Table A.9

Year	1980	1985	1990	1995	2000
CO_2	349.6	346.7	354.4	360.8	368.9

7. In Problem 6, carbon dioxide concentration was modeled as a linear function of time. However, if we include data for carbon dioxide concentration from as far back as 1900, the data appear to be more exponential than linear. (They looked linear in Problem 6 because we were only looking at a small piece of the graph.) If C is the CO_2 concentration in ppm and t is in years since 1900, an exponential regression function to fit the data is

$$C = 272.27(1.0026)^t.$$

 (a) What is the annual percent growth rate during this period? Interpret this rate in terms of CO_2 concentration.
 (b) What CO_2 concentration is given by the model for 1900? For 1980? Compare the 1980 estimate to the actual value in Table A.9.

8. **(a)** Fit an exponential function to the population data in Table A.10. Plot the data and the exponential function on the same axes.
 (b) At approximately what percentage rate was the population growing between 1960 and 2000?
 (c) If the population continues to grow at the same percentage rate, what population is projected for 2020?

Table A.10 *US Population 1960-2000*

t, years since 1960	0	10	20	30	40
population (m)	179.3	203.3	226.5	248.7	281.4

[5] *The World Almanac and Book of Facts 2005*, p. 111 (New York).
[6] William M. Lewis and Michael C. Grant, "Acid Precipitation in the Western United States," *Science* 207 (1980), pp. 176-177.
[7] R.C. Nelson, C.M. Brooks, and N.L. Pike, "Biomechanical Comparison of Male and Female Distance Runners." *The Marathon: Physiological, Medical, Epidemiological, and Psychological Studies*, ed. P. Milvy, pp. 793–807 (New York: New York Academy of Sciences, 1977).
[8] www.cmdl.noaa.gov/ccgg/iadv, accessed on February 20, 2005.

9. Table A.11 shows the public debt, D, of the US[9] in billions of dollars, t years after 1998.

(a) Plot the public debt against the number of years since 1998.
(b) Does the data look more linear or more exponential?
(c) Fit an exponential function to the data and graph it with the data.
(d) What annual percentage growth rate does the exponential model show?
(e) Do you expect this model to give accurate predictions beyond 2004? Explain.

Table A.11

t	0	1	2	3	4	5	6
D	5526	5656	5674	5808	6228	6783	7379

10. A company collects the data in Table A.12. Find the regression line and interpret its slope. Sketch the data and the line. What is the correlation coefficient? Why is the value you get reasonable?

Table A.12 *Cost to produce various quantities of a product*

q (quantity in units)	25	50	75	100	125
C (cost in dollars)	500	625	689	742	893

11. Match the r values with scatter plots in Figure A.11.

$$r = -0.98, \quad r = -0.5, \quad r = -0.25,$$

$$r = 0, \quad r = 0.7, \quad r = 1.$$

(a)
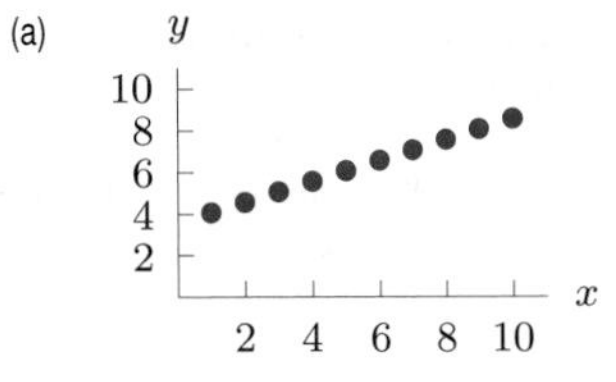
(b)
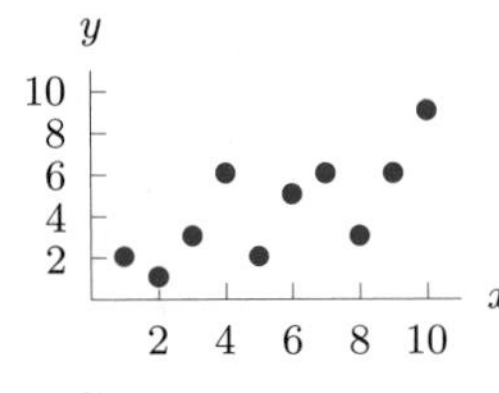
(c)
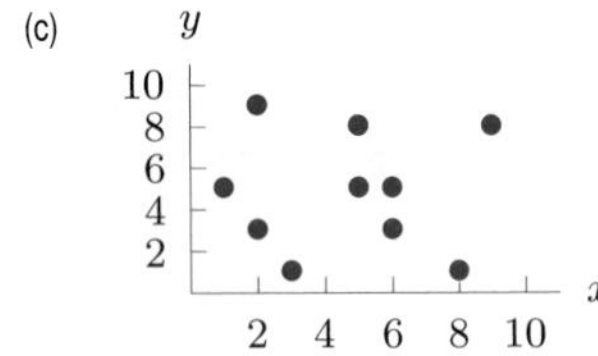
(d)
(e)
(f)
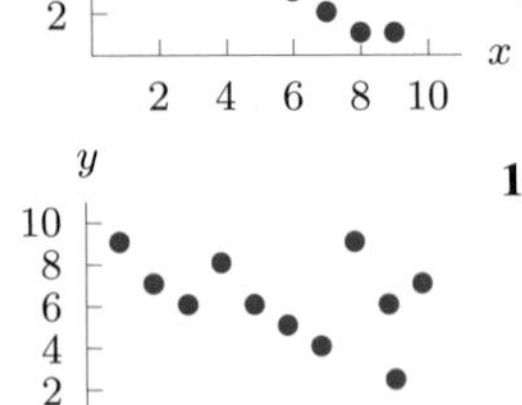

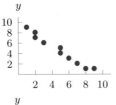

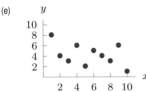

Figure A.11

12. Table A.13 shows the number of cars, N, in millions in the US[10] t years after 1940.

(a) Plot the data, with number of passenger cars as the dependent variable.
(b) Does a linear or exponential model appear to fit the data better?
(c) Use a linear model first: Find the regression line for these data. Graph it with the data. Use the regression line to predict the number of passenger cars in the year 2010 ($t = 70$).
(d) Interpret the slope of the regression line found in part (c) in terms of passenger cars.
(e) Now use an exponential model: Find the exponential regression function for these data. Graph it with the data. Use the exponential function to predict the number of passenger cars in the year 2010 ($t = 70$). Compare your prediction with the prediction obtained from the linear model.
(f) What annual percent growth rate in number of US passenger cars does your exponential model show?

Table A.13 *Number of passenger cars, in millions*

t	0	10	20	30	40	50	60
N	27.5	40.3	61.7	89.2	121.6	133.7	133.6

13. Table A.14 gives the population of the world in billions.

(a) Plot these data. Does a linear or exponential model seem to fit the data best?
(b) Find an exponential regression function.
(c) What annual percent growth rate does the exponential function show?
(d) Predict the population of the world in the year 2020 and in the year 2050. Comment on the relative confidence you have in these two estimates.

Table A.14 *World population in billions*

Year (since 1950)	0	10	20	30	40	50	58
Population (bn)	2.6	3.0	3.7	4.5	5.3	6.1	6.7

14. In 1969, all field goal attempts in the National Football League and American Football League were analyzed. See Table A.15. (The data has been summarized: all attempts between 10 and 19 yards from the goal post are listed as 14.5 yards out, etc.)

(a) Graph the data, with success rate as the dependent variable. Discuss whether a linear or an exponential model fits best.

[9] *The World Almanac and Book of Facts 2005*, p. 119 (New York).
[10] *The World Almanac and Book of Facts 2005*, p. 237 (New York).

(b) Find the linear regression function; graph it with the data. Interpret the slope of the regression line in terms of football.

(c) Find the exponential regression function; graph it with the data. What success rate does this function predict from a distance of 50 yards?

(d) Using the graphs in parts (b) and (c), decide which model seems to fit the data best.

Table A.15 *Successful fraction of field goal attempts*

Distance from goal, x yards	14.5	24.5	34.5	44.5	52.0
Fraction successful, Y	0.90	0.75	0.54	0.29	0.15

15. Table A.16 shows the number of Japanese cars imported into the US.[11]

(a) Plot the number of Japanese cars imported against the number of years since 1964.

(b) Does the data look more linear or more exponential?

(c) Fit an exponential function to the data and graph it with the data.

(d) What annual percentage growth rate does the exponential model show?

(e) Do you expect this model to give accurate predictions beyond 1971? Explain.

Table A.16 *Imported Japanese cars, 1964–1971*

Year since 1964	0	1	2	3	4	5	6	7
Cars (thousands)	16	24	56	70	170	260	381	704

16. Figure A.12 shows oil production in the Middle East.[12] If you were to model this function with a polynomial, what degree would you choose? Would the leading coefficient be positive or negative?

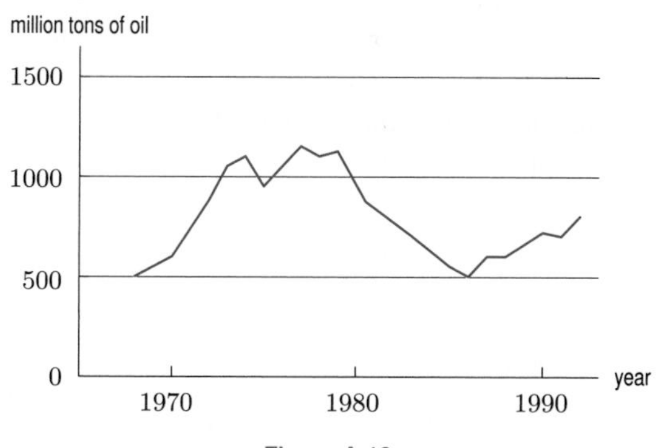

Figure A.12

17. After the oil crisis in 1973, the average fuel efficiency, E, of cars increased until the early 1990s, when it started to decrease again.

(a) Plot the data [13] in Table A.17, using t in years since 1975. If you were to fit a quadratic polynomial to the data, what would be the sign of the leading coefficient?

(b) Fit a quadratic polynomial and plot it with the data.

Table A.17

Year	1975	1980	1985	1990	1995	2000
E, mpg	13.1	19.2	21.3	21.5	21.1	20.7

18. Table A.18 gives the area of rain forest destroyed for agriculture and development.[14]

(a) Plot these data.

(b) Are the data increasing or decreasing? Concave up or concave down? In each case, interpret your answer in terms of rain forest.

(c) Use a calculator or computer to fit a logarithmic function to this data. Plot this function on the axes in part (a).

(d) Use the curve you found in part (c) to predict the area of rain forest destroyed in 2010.

Table A.18 *Destruction of rain forest*

x (year)	1960	1970	1980	1988
y (million hectares)	2.21	3.79	4.92	5.77

In Problems 19–21, tables of data are given.[15]

(a) Use a plot of the data to decide whether a linear, exponential, logarithmic, or quadratic function fits the data best.

(b) Use regression to find a formula for the function you chose in part (a). If the function is linear or exponential, interpret the rate of change or percent rate of change.

(c) Use your function to predict the value of the function in the year 2015.

(d) Plot your function on the same axes as the data, and comment on the fit.

[11] *The World Almanac 1995.*

[12] Lester R. Brown, et al., *Vital Signs*, p. 49 (New York: W. W. Norton and Co., 1994).

[13] *The World Almanac and Book of Facts* (New York, 2005).

[14] C. Schaufele and N. Zumoff, *Earth Algebra, Preliminary Version*, p. 131 (New York: Harper Collins, 1993).

[15] The Worldwatch Institute, *Vital Signs 2007–2008* (New York: W.W. Norton & Company, 2007).

19. *World solar power, S, in megawatts; t in years since 1990*

t	0	1	2	3	4	5	6	7
S	47	55	58	60	69	78	89	126
t	8	9	10	11	12	13	14	15
S	153	201	277	386	547	748	1194	1782

20. *Nuclear warheads, N, in thousands; t in years since 1960*

t	0	5	10	15	20	25	30	35	40	45
N	22	38	39	48	55	65	59	40	33	28

21. *Carbon dioxide, C, in ppm; t in years since 1970*

t	0	5	10	15	20	25	30	35
C	326	331	339	346	354	361	369	380

22. For each graph in Figure A.13, decide whether the best fit for the data appears to be a linear function, an exponential function, or a polynomial.

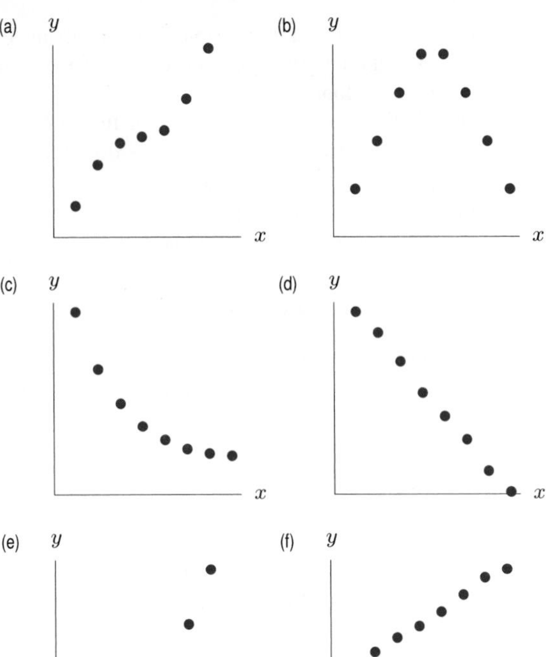

Figure A.13

B COMPOUND INTEREST AND THE NUMBER e

If you have some money, you may decide to invest it to earn interest. The interest can be paid in many different ways—for example, once a year or many times a year. If the interest is paid more frequently than once per year and the interest is not withdrawn, there is a benefit to the investor since the interest earns interest. This effect is called *compounding*. You may have noticed banks offering accounts that differ both in interest rates and in compounding methods. Some offer interest compounded annually, some quarterly, and others daily. Some even offer continuous compounding.

What is the difference between a bank account advertising 8% compounded annually (once per year) and one offering 8% compounded quarterly (four times per year)? In both cases 8% is an annual rate of interest. The expression 8% *compounded annually* means that at the end of each year, 8% of the current balance is added. This is equivalent to multiplying the current balance by 1.08. Thus, if \$100 is deposited, the balance, B, in dollars, will be

$$\begin{aligned} B &= 100(1.08) && \text{after one year,} \\ B &= 100(1.08)^2 && \text{after two years,} \\ B &= 100(1.08)^t && \text{after } t \text{ years.} \end{aligned}$$

The expression 8% *compounded quarterly* means that interest is added four times per year (every three months) and that $\frac{8}{4} = 2\%$ of the current balance is added each time. Thus, if \$100 is deposited, at the end of one year, four compoundings have taken place and the account will contain $\$100(1.02)^4$. Thus, the balance will be

$$\begin{aligned} B &= 100(1.02)^4 && \text{after one year,} \\ B &= 100(1.02)^8 && \text{after two years,} \\ B &= 100(1.02)^{4t} && \text{after } t \text{ years.} \end{aligned}$$

Note that 8% is *not* the rate used for each three-month period; the annual rate is divided into four 2% payments. Calculating the total balance after one year under each method shows that

$$\begin{aligned} \text{Annual compounding:} \quad & B = 100(1.08) = 108.00, \\ \text{Quarterly compounding:} \quad & B = 100(1.02)^4 = 108.24. \end{aligned}$$

Thus, more money is earned from quarterly compounding, because the interest earns interest as the year goes by. In general, the more often interest is compounded, the more money will be earned (although the increase may not be very large).

We can measure the effect of compounding by introducing the notion of *effective annual rate*. Since $\$100$ invested at 8% compounded quarterly grows to $\$108.24$ by the end of one year, we say that the effective annual rate in this case is 8.24%. We now have two interest rates that describe the same investment: the 8% compounded quarterly and the 8.24% effective annual rate. We call the 8% the *nominal rate* (nominal means "in name only"). However, it is the effective rate that tells you exactly how much interest the investment really pays. Thus, to compare two bank accounts, simply compare the effective annual rate. The next time you walk by a bank, look at the advertisements, which should (by law) include both the nominal rate and the effective annual rate.

Using the Effective Annual Yield

Example 1 Which is better: Bank X paying a 7% annual rate compounded monthly or Bank Y offering a 6.9% annual rate compounded daily?

Solution We find the effective annual rate for each bank.

Bank X: There are 12 interest payments in a year, each payment being $0.07/12 = 0.005833$ times the current balance. If the initial deposit were $\$100$, then the balance B would be

$$\begin{aligned} B &= 100(1.005833) \quad \text{after one month,} \\ B &= 100(1.005833)^2 \quad \text{after two months,} \\ B &= 100(1.005833)^t \quad \text{after } t \text{ months.} \end{aligned}$$

To find the effective annual rate, we look at one year, or 12 months, giving $B = 100(1.005833)^{12}$ $= 100(1.072286)$, so the effective annual rate $\approx 7.23\%$.

Bank Y: There are 365 interest payments in a year (assuming it is not a leap year), each being $0.069/365 = 0.000189$ times the current balance. Then the balance is

$$\begin{aligned} B &= 100(1.000189) \quad \text{after one day,} \\ B &= 100(1.000189)^2 \quad \text{after two days,} \\ B &= 100(1.000189)^t \quad \text{after } t \text{ days.} \end{aligned}$$

so at the end of one year we have multiplied the initial deposit by

$$(1.000189)^{365} = 1.071413$$

so the effective annual rate for Bank Y $\approx 7.14\%$.

Comparing effective annual rates for the banks, we see that Bank X is offering a better investment, by a small margin.

Example 2 If $\$1000$ is invested in each bank in Example 1, write an expression for the balance in each bank after t years.

Solution For Bank X, the effective annual rate $\approx 7.23\%$, so after t years the balance, in dollars, will be

$$B = 100\left(1 + \frac{0.07}{12}\right)^{12t} = 1000(1.005833)^{12t} = 1000(1.0723)^t.$$

For Bank Y, the effective annual rate $\approx 7.14\%$, so after t years the balance, in dollars, will be

$$B = 1000\left(1+\frac{0.069}{365}\right)^{365t} = 1000(1.0714)^t.$$

(Again, we are ignoring leap years.)

If interest at an annual rate of r is compounded n times a year, then r/n times the current balance is added n times a year. Therefore, with an initial deposit of P, the balance t years later is

$$B = P\left(1+\frac{r}{n}\right)^{nt}.$$

Note that r is the nominal rate; for example, $r = 0.05$ when the annual rate is 5%.

Increasing the Frequency of Compounding: Continuous Compounding

Let us look at the effect of increasing the frequency of compounding. How much effect does it have?

Example 3 Find the effective annual rate for a 7% annual rate compounded
(a) 1000 times a year. (b) 10,000 times a year.

Solution (a) In one year, a deposit is multiplied by

$$\left(1+\frac{0.07}{1000}\right)^{1000} \approx 1.0725056,$$

giving an effective annual rate of about 7.25056%.

(b) In one year, a deposit is multiplied by

$$\left(1+\frac{0.07}{10{,}000}\right)^{10{,}000} \approx 1.0725079,$$

giving an effective annual yield of about 7.25079%.

Notice that there's not a great deal of difference—7.25056% versus 7.25079%—between compounding 1000 times each year (about three times per day) and 10,000 times each year (about 30 times per day). What happens if we compound more often still? Every minute? Every second? Surprisingly, the effective annual rate does not increase indefinitely, but tends to a finite value. The benefit of increasing the frequency of compounding becomes negligible beyond a certain point.

For example, computing the effective annual rate on a 7% investment compounded n times per year for values of n larger than 100,000 gives

$$\left(1+\frac{0.07}{n}\right)^{n} \approx 1.0725082.$$

So the effective annual rate is about 7.25082%. Even if you take $n = 1{,}000{,}000$ or $n = 10^{10}$, the effective annual rate does not change appreciably. The value 7.25082% is an upper bound that is approached as the frequency of compounding increases.

When the effective annual rate is at this upper bound, we say that the interest is being *compounded continuously*. (The word *continuously* is used because the upper bound is approached by compounding more and more frequently.) Thus, when a 7% nominal annual rate is compounded so frequently that the effective annual rate is 7.25082%, we say that the 7% is compounded *continuously*. This represents the most one can get from a 7% nominal rate.

Where Does the Number e Fit In?

It turns out that e is intimately connected to continuous compounding. To see this, use a calculator to check that $e^{0.07} \approx 1.0725082$, which is the same number we obtained by compounding 7% a large number of times. So you have discovered that for very large n

$$\left(1+\frac{0.07}{n}\right)^n \approx e^{0.07}.$$

As n gets larger, the approximation gets better and better, and we write

$$\lim_{n\to\infty}\left(1+\frac{0.07}{n}\right)^n = e^{0.07},$$

meaning that as n increases, the value of $(1+0.07/n)^n$ approaches $e^{0.07}$.

If P is deposited at an annual rate of 7% compounded continuously, the balance, B, after t years, is given by

$$B = P(e^{0.07})^t = Pe^{0.07t}.$$

> If interest on an initial deposit of P is *compounded continuously* at an annual rate r, the balance t years later can be calculated using the formula
>
> $$B = Pe^{rt}.$$

In working with compound interest, it is important to be clear whether interest rates are nominal rates or effective rates, as well as whether compounding is continuous or not.

Example 4 Find the effective annual rate of a 6% annual rate, compounded continuously.

Solution In one year, an investment of P becomes $Pe^{0.06}$. Using a calculator, we see that

$$Pe^{0.06} = P(1.0618365).$$

So the effective annual rate is about 6.18%.

Example 5 You invest money in a certificate of deposit (CD) for your child's education, and you want it to be worth \$120,000 in 10 years. How much should you invest if the CD pays interest at a 9% annual rate compounded quarterly? Continuously?

Solution Suppose you invest P initially. A 9% annual rate compounded quarterly has an effective annual rate given by $(1+0.09/4)^4 = 1.0930833$, or 9.30833%. So after 10 years you have

$$P(1.0930833)^{10} = 120{,}000.$$

Therefore, you should invest

$$P = \frac{120{,}000}{(1.0930833)^{10}} = \frac{120{,}000}{2.4351885} = 49{,}277.50.$$

On the other hand, if the CD pays 9% per year, compounded continuously, after 10 years you have

$$Pe^{(0.09)10} = 120{,}000.$$

So you would need to invest

$$P = \frac{120{,}000}{e^{(0.09)10}} = \frac{120{,}000}{2.4596031} = 48{,}788.36.$$

Notice that to achieve the same result, continuous compounding requires a smaller initial investment than quarterly compounding. This is to be expected since the effective annual rate is higher for continuous than for quarterly compounding.

Problems for Appendix B

1. A department store issues its own credit card, with an interest rate of 2% per month. Explain why this is not the same as an annual rate of 24%. What is the effective annual rate?

2. A deposit of $10,000 is made into an account paying a nominal yearly interest rate of 8%. Determine the amount in the account in 10 years if the interest is compounded:

   (a) Annually **(b)** Monthly **(c)** Weekly
   (d) Daily **(e)** Continuously

3. A deposit of $50,000 is made into an account paying a nominal yearly interest rate of 6%. Determine the amount in the account in 20 years if the interest is compounded:

   (a) Annually **(b)** Monthly **(c)** Weekly
   (d) Daily **(e)** Continuously

4. Use a graph of $y = (1 + 0.07/x)^x$ to estimate the number that $(1 + 0.07/x)^x$ approaches as $x \to \infty$. Confirm that the value you get is approximately $e^{0.07}$.

5. **(a)** Find $(1 + 0.04/n)^n$ for $n = 10{,}000$, and 100,000, and 1,000,000. Use the results to predict the effective annual rate of a 4% annual rate compounded continuously.
   (b) Confirm your answer by computing $e^{0.04}$.

6. Find the effective annual rate of a 6% annual rate, compounded continuously.

7. What nominal annual interest rate has an effective annual rate of 5% under continuous compounding?

8. What is the effective annual rate, under continuous compounding, for a nominal annual interest rate of 8%?

9. **(a)** Find the effective annual rate for a 5% annual interest rate compounded n times/year if

   (i) $n = 1000$ (ii) $n = 10{,}000$
   (iii) $n = 100{,}000$

   (b) Look at the sequence of answers in part (a), and predict the effective annual rate for a 5% annual rate compounded continuously.
   (c) Compute $e^{0.05}$. How does this confirm your answer to part (b)?

10. A bank account is earning interest at 6% per year compounded continuously.

    (a) By what percentage has the bank balance in the account increased over one year? (This is the effective annual rate.)
    (b) How long does it take the balance to double?
    (c) For a continuous interest rate r, find a formula for the doubling time in terms of r.

11. Explain how you can match the interest rates (a)–(e) with the effective annual rates I–V without calculation.

    (a) 5.5% annual rate, compounded continuously.
    (b) 5.5% annual rate, compounded quarterly.
    (c) 5.5% annual rate, compounded weekly.
    (d) 5% annual rate, compounded yearly.
    (e) 5% annual rate, compounded twice a year.

    I. 5% II. 5.06% III. 5.61%
    IV. 5.651% V. 5.654%

Countries with very high inflation rates often publish monthly rather than yearly inflation figures, because monthly figures are less alarming. Problems 12–13 involve such high rates, which are called *hyperinflation*.

12. In 1989, US inflation was 4.6% a year. In 1989 Argentina had an inflation rate of about 33% a month.

    (a) What is the yearly equivalent of Argentina's 33% monthly rate?
    (b) What is the monthly equivalent of the US 4.6% yearly rate?

13. Between December 1988 and December 1989, Brazil's inflation rate was 1290% a year. (This means that between 1988 and 1989, prices increased by a factor of $1 + 12.90 = 13.90$.)

    (a) What would an article which cost 1000 cruzados (the Brazilian currency unit) in 1988 cost in 1989?
    (b) What was Brazil's monthly inflation rate during this period?

C SPREADSHEET PROJECTS

The following projects require the use of a spreadsheet. They can all be done using only the ideas in Chapter 1. In addition, Project 9 (Verhulst: The Logistic Model) and Project 10 (The Spread of Information) give another perspective on material in Chapters 4 and 10. Project 4 (Comparing Home Mortgages) uses a geometric series but can be done before Chapter 11.

1. MALTHUS: POPULATION OUTSTRIPS FOOD SUPPLY

In this project, we compare exponential and linear growth. We see the eventual dominance of exponential functions over linear functions.

One of the most famous models of population growth was made by Thomas Malthus in the early 19th century. Malthus believed that while human population increased exponentially, its means of subsistence increased linearly. The gloomy conclusion that Malthus drew from this observation was that the population of the earth would inevitably outstrip its means of subsistence, resulting in an inadequate supply of food. (Malthus went on to note that this state of affairs could only be averted by war, famine, epidemic disease, wide-scale sexual restraint, or other such drastic checks on population growth.)

The following table shows part of a spreadsheet showing such as a scenario.[16] The starting population is 1 million, while the available food feeds 2 million people. The population grows at an annual rate of 3% per year and the food production increases by 100,000 per year. These population and food growth rates are in cells on the right of the spreadsheet. The fourth column contains the ratio of available food per person in the population. The spreadsheet includes a safety ratio—so long as the food-to-population ratio is above this figure of 1.5, the fifth column displays "Yes"; whenever the ratio drops below this figure the fifth column displays "No" (as it does by the end of the 21st century).

We see that at first there is plenty of food—the ratio of food to population is 2, which means that there is twice as much food as is necessary to feed the population. For the first few years the ratio increases, but at a certain point it starts to decrease, and eventually the ratio drops below one.

Year	Population	Food supply	Ratio	Above safety ratio?	
1999	1000000	2000000	2.00	Yes	Annual pop growth rate 3.00%
2000	1030000	2100000	2.04	Yes	
2001	1060900	2200000	2.07	Yes	
2002	1092727	2300000	2.10	Yes	Annual food growth rate 100,000
2003	1125509	2400000	2.13	Yes	
2004	1159274	2500000	2.16	Yes	
2005	1194052	2600000	2.18	Yes	Safety ratio 1.5
2006	1229874	2700000	2.20	Yes	
2007	1266770	2800000	2.21	Yes	
2008	1304773	2900000	2.22	Yes	
⋮	⋮	⋮	⋮	⋮	
2098	18658866	11900000	0.64	No	
2099	19218632	12000000	0.62	No	
2100	19795191	12100000	0.61	No	

[16]From Graeme Bird.

1. Set up your spreadsheet to look like the one shown in the table, extending it to the year 2100. Virtually every cell must contain a formula — the exceptions being the six cells containing "1999," "1,000,000," "2,000,000," "3.00%," "100,000," and "1.5."
2. (a) About what year is the food-to-population ratio the highest?
   (b) In which year does this ratio reach 1?
3. There are at least two ways to improve upon the current situation: we can lower the population growth rate, or we can increase the food supply.
   (a) What would the population growth rate have to be lowered to, in order to have the food-to-population ratio not reach 1 until the year 2100? (Keep the food supply increasing at 100,000 per year.)
   (b) What would the food supply rate have to be increased to, in order to achieve this same goal, of the ratio not reaching 1 until the year 2100? (Keep the population growth rate at its original 3%.)
4. Using the original scenario, create each of the following charts (both line and column). Extend the charts to the year 2100, so that the point where the population outstrips the food supply is clearly evident.
   (a) Showing population and food, with the years on the horizontal axis.
   (b) Showing only the ratio, with the years on the horizontal axis.

2. CREDIT CARD DEBT

You have a credit card on which you owe $2000. Your credit card company charges a monthly interest rate of 1.5% and requires a minimum monthly payment of 2.5% of your current balance. (This payment scheme is similar to ones used by many credit card companies, but see Question 8.)

[Note: For Questions 1–2, you will not need a spreadsheet, although you will need a calculator.]

1. If the monthly interest rate is 1.5%, what is the effective annual interest rate?
2. As a rule, the minimum monthly payment required exceeds the interest accrued in a month. (For example, here the minimum monthly payment of 2.5% exceeds the monthly interest charges of 1.5%.) Explain why this should be the case. What would happen to the card balance if the minimum required payment was less than the accrued interest?

Suppose that you decide to pay off your $2000 credit card debt by making only the minimum required payment every month. Assume that you make no further charges to the card, since you're trying to pay it off.

3. Since 2.5% of $2000 is $50, your first monthly payment is $50. Before you do any spreadsheet calculations, guess how long it will take to bring your total balance down from $2000 to less than $50, assuming that you make only the minimum required payment every month. A rough guess is fine; use common sense and explain your reasoning.
4. Over time, your monthly payments, which start at $50, will decrease. Explain why this happens. Does the fact that your monthly payments decrease affect the answer you gave to Question 3?
5. Although you only owe the credit card company $2000, you will end up paying quite a bit more than $2000, due to interest charges. Make your best guess (before making any specific calculations) as to how much, roughly, you will end up having paid the credit card company for your initial $2000 debt.

Set up a spreadsheet showing the number of months since you began paying off your debt, your current balance, the interest due that month, and the payment you make, each in a separate column. Each quantity should be calculated by a formula.

Example: To figure out what formulas you need, recall that your initial balance is $2000, the monthly interest charged is 1.5%, and the minimum required payment is 2.5%. Thus, at the beginning of Month 1, your balance is $2000, since you have paid off nothing yet. Therefore, at the end of Month 1, the interest that you owe is 1.5% of the $2000 balance, or $30. Your minimum payment is 2.5% of the $2000 balance, or $50. Thus, at the beginning of Month 2, your new balance is the old balance of $2000 plus the $30 in interest minus the $50 payment, or $1980. Notice that the figures for Month 2 depend on the figures for Month 1; similarly, the figures for Month 3 depend on Month 2 figures, and so on. Follow this procedure to figure out what formulas you need in each column of your spreadsheet.

Once you have set up a working spreadsheet, answer the following questions.

6. How good was your guess in Question 3? Using your spreadsheet, find out how many months it takes to bring your balance down to less than $50. Was your guess close, or were you surprised by how long it really takes?
7. How good was your guess in Question 5? Using your spreadsheet, figure out exactly how much you pay the credit card company to bring your balance down to less than $50. How does this figure compare to the original debt of $2000?
8. Use your spreadsheet to find out how long it takes to bring your balance down to $0. Or can't you tell? Does there ever come a point when you have exactly paid off your debt? [Hint: Eventually, the minimum monthly payments and the interest charges become unrealistic. In what way are they unrealistic? How do real credit card companies avoid this problem?]
9. Now let's try experimenting with the numbers and see what happens. In each of the following cases, make the appropriate changes to your spreadsheet. Assume that as soon as your balance is under $50, you pay it off in a lump sum.
   (a) If every month you pay $1 more than the minimum required payment, how long does it take to bring your debt down to less than $50? How much do you end up paying to your creditors in total? How much money do you save by using this payment scheme instead of the one in Question 5?
   (b) Your first monthly payment is $50. If you paid $50 every month, instead of the minimum required payment, how long does it take to bring your debt down to less than $50? How much money do you save by using this payment scheme instead of the one in Question 5?
   (c) Recently, many credit card companies have made offers similar to the following: if you transfer your debt from a competitor's card to their card, they will charge you a lower interest rate. Suppose you find a credit card company willing to make this transaction, and that their monthly interest rate is 1%, not 1.5%. Leaving all the other original assumptions unchanged, how long does it take to bring your debt down to less than $50, and how much do you pay your creditors in total? How much money do you save compared to what you would have paid your original card company?
10. Comparing the scheme used in Questions 3–5 with each of the schemes in Question 9, what conclusions can you reach about paying off a credit card debt?

3. CHOOSING A BANK LOAN

A local bank offers the following loan packages. Use a spreadsheet to decide which option is the best. The packages are as follows:

- A loan of $2000, at an annual rate of 9%, payable in 24 monthly installments.
- A loan of $2000, at an annual rate of 10%, payable in 36 monthly installments.
- A loan of $2000, at an annual rate of 9.25%, payable in 52 biweekly installments.

Interest is compounded with the same frequency as payments are made. Notice that the first and last loans have two-year payoff periods; the middle loan is for three years.

1. Use a spreadsheet to decide which loan is cheapest in terms of total payoff to the bank. (See the following hint.)

2. Use a spreadsheet to decide which loan is easiest to afford in terms of lowest monthly payment. (See the following hint.)

Hint: The difficult part of Questions 1 and 2 is figuring out your monthly (or biweekly) payments. There are formulas that give the payment based on the period and amount of the loan and the interest charged, but instead of using them, we will use a spreadsheet. The idea is that you can make an educated guess as to what the payment ought to be, and then use a spreadsheet to check your answer. By looking at the spreadsheet, you can decide whether your guess was too high or too low, and thus improve upon your original guess. It's surprising how quickly you can zero in on the required monthly payment, down to the nearest penny, by this guess-and-check method.

For example, consider the first loan, the two-year \$2000 loan at 9%. Set up a spreadsheet with the initial balance of \$2000, the interest for the first month, which is $(9\%/12) \cdot \$2000 = \$15$, and a guess at the monthly payment. There are lots of ways to make a guess at the monthly payment. One way is to say that if you were to borrow \$2000 for 2 years at 9%, you would owe about $\$2000(1.09)^2 = \$2376$. (Never mind the monthly compounding—this is just a rough approximation.) To pay off this amount in 24 equal monthly payments would require $\$2376/24 = \$99$. So, we guess a monthly payment of \$100. Using this guess, the second month's balance will be

$$(\$2000) + (\$15 \text{ in interest for month } 1) - (\text{Payment of } \$100) = \$1915.$$

Thus, the next month's interest will be $(9\%/12) \cdot \$1915$, and the next month's payment should be the same as the first month's payment, or \$100. Continue this process until 24 months' (two years') worth of payments have been made. You will see that the final balance is negative, meaning you paid the bank more than you really owed. This means that \$100 is too high a monthly payment to pay off your \$2000 loan. (We could have predicted that this was the case when we made our estimate above. Do you see why?) So, since \$100 is too high, you might guess that an \$80 monthly payment would be right. If you do, you'll see that you'd still owe the bank some money after 24 months had passed. This tells you that \$80 is too low a monthly payment, and that the actual payment is somewhere between \$80 and \$100. This procedure can be repeated until the exact monthly payment is reached.

4. COMPARING HOME MORTGAGES

To do this project, first go to any bank and ask for a fact sheet of their most recent *mortgage loan rates*. Banks are happy to provide them.

Obtain rates for a thirty-year loan, a fifteen-year loan, a thirty-year biweekly loan, and a twenty-year loan (if available) for \$100,000 with zero points. (Note: Some loans include points. A point is an additional fee paid to the lender at the time of the loan equal to 1% of the amount borrowed. Typically, you get lower interest rates by paying a point or two. We will only consider loans with zero points.)

The following formula can be used to determine your payment, x:

$$x = \frac{Pr^n(r-1)}{r^n - 1},$$

where P is the amount of the loan—in this case \$100,000—and n is the number of payments. For a thirty-year loan with monthly payments, $n = 360$; for a thirty-year biweekly loan, $n = 780$ (there are 26 payments every year). Finally, r is the interest rate per period plus 1. (For example, if the interest rate is 2%, then $r = 1.02$.) In Question 4, you will derive this formula for x using the following formula for the sum of a geometric series:[17]

$$1 + r + r^2 + \cdots + r^{n-2} + r^{n-1} = \frac{1-r^n}{1-r}.$$

[17]Geometric series are discussed in detail in Chapter 11.

1. Using the information given, as well as the fact sheet you got from the bank, determine which loan (30-year, 30-year biweekly, 20-year or 15-year) is best if you intend to live in your house for the full term of the loan. Assume the best mortgage is the one that ends up costing you the least overall. (The situation in real life can be more complicated when points and taxes are considered.) Although it's possible to work this problem without a spreadsheet, you might want to set one up anyway.
2. Banks usually require that the monthly payments not exceed some stated fraction of the applicant's monthly income. For this reason, it is generally easier to qualify for loans with smaller monthly payments. Thus, it may be that the "best loan"—the one you found in Question 1—is not the "easiest" loan to qualify for. Which of the loans on your fact sheet has the lowest monthly payment? The highest?
3. Suppose that you expect to sell your house for \$145,000 in five years. In this case, which loan should you take? [Hint: The goal here is to maximize profit. Figure out how much money you have paid to the bank after five years, and your remaining debt at that time. When you sell your house, the remaining debt is paid to the bank immediately, so your total profit is (Selling price of house)−(Loan payoff to bank)−(Amount paid to bank during first five years).]
4. Derive the formula for the monthly payment, x. [Hint: Set up a geometric series in terms of x and r to give your loan balance after n months. The loan balance equals 0 when you have paid off your loan; use this fact to solve for x. Simplify the resulting expression (by summing a geometric series) to get the formula given for x.]

5. PRESENT VALUE OF LOTTERY WINNINGS

On Thursday, February 24th, 1993, Bruce Hegarty of Dennis Port, MA, received the first installment of the \$26,680,940 prize he won in the Mass Millions state lottery. Mr. Hegarty was scheduled to receive 19 more such installments on a yearly basis. Each check written by the Lottery Commission is for one twentieth of the total prize, or \$1,334,047. Why doesn't the Lottery Commission pay all of Mr. Hegarty's prize up front, instead of making him wait for twenty years?

1. Compute the present value of the money paid out by the Lottery Commission, assuming annual discount rates (interest rates) of 5%, 10% and 15%. In each case, what percent does the present value represent of the face value of the prize, \$26,680,940?
2. What discount rate would result in a present value of the payments worth only half the face value of the prize?
3. Graph the present value of the payments against the discount rate, ranging from a rate of 0% up to 15%. Describe the graph. What does it tell you about why the Lottery Commission does not pay the prize money up front?

6. COMPARING INVESTMENTS

Consider two investment projects. Project A is built in one year at an initial cost of \$10,000. It then yields the following decreasing stream of benefits over a five-year period: \$5000, \$4000, \$3000, \$2000, \$1000. Project B is built in two years. Initial costs are \$10,000 in the first year and \$5000 in the second year. It then yields yearly profits of \$6000 for the next four years. Which of these investment projects is preferable?

1. Compute the present values of both projects assuming an annual discount rate (interest rate) of 4%. Which project seems preferable? [Hint: Treat expenditures as negative and income as positive.]
2. Compute the present values of both projects assuming an annual discount rate of 16%. Which project seems preferable now?

3. Describe in complete sentences why one of the investment projects is favored by a low discount rate, whereas the other is favored by a high discount rate.
4. The discount rate at which the present value of a project becomes zero is known as the *internal rate of return*. What is the internal rate of return of project A? Of project B? [Hint: Guess different discount rates until you find the one that brings the present value down to $0.]
5. Make a chart of the present value of the two investments against discount rates ranging from 0% to 30%. What features of this chart correspond to the internal rates of return of the two projects?

7. INVESTING FOR THE FUTURE: TUITION PAYMENTS

Parents of two teenagers, ages 13 and 17, deposit a sum of money into an account earning interest at the rate of 7% per year compounded annually. The deposit will be used for a series of eight annual college tuition payments of $10,000 each. Payments out of the account will begin one year after the initial deposit.

1. Use a spreadsheet to model the savings account that the parents opened. At the end of every year, the account earns 7% interest, and then there is a $10,000 withdrawal. Determine what initial deposit provides just enough money to make the eight yearly payments of $10,000. Do this by guessing different values, and seeing which value leaves you with nothing exactly nine years later.
2. Having answered Question 1, use a spreadsheet to compute the present value of eight yearly payments of $10,000 each, beginning one year in the future, at a discount rate of 7%.
3. Compare your answer to Question 1 with your answer to Question 2. Is this a coincidence? Discuss.
4. Suppose the parents have only $50,000 to deposit into the savings account. What annual interest rate must the account earn if the eight payments of $10,000 are to be made? [Hint: Compute the present value of the payments for various discount rates.]

8. NEW OR USED?

You are deciding whether to buy a new or used car (of the same make) and how many years to keep the car. You want to minimize your total costs, which consist of two parts: the loss in value of the car and the repairs. A new car costs $20,000 and loses 20% of its value each year. Repairs are $400 the first year and increase by 25% each subsequent year.

1. Set up a spreadsheet that gives, for each year, the value of the car, its loss in value, its repair costs, and the total cost for that year. The first two lines look like this, rounded to the nearest dollar:

Year	Value	Loss	Repair	Cost
1	20,000	4000	400	4400
2	16,000	3200	500	3700
⋮	⋮	⋮	⋮	⋮

2. Which year has the lowest cost?
3. You intend to keep your car 5 years. Compare your total costs for a new car and for a two-year-old car.
4. How old a car should you buy if you plan to keep it for 5 years?

5. Add two columns to your spreadsheet showing the average yearly cost for second-hand cars of different ages kept for 4 years and 5 years. Which is the best buy?
6. A new car costs \$30,000 and loses 25% of its value each year; repairs start at \$500 and increase at 10% per year. If you buy a seven-year-old car, should you keep it for 4 or 5 years? What is the average yearly cost in each case?
7. A car costs \$30,000 when new. You buy a four-year-old car and keep it for 5 years; repairs are as in Problem 6. Find the rate at which it loses value if the average yearly cost is \$2300.

9. VERHULST: THE LOGISTIC MODEL

The relative growth rate of a population, P, over a time interval, Δt, is given by

$$\text{Relative growth rate} = \frac{1}{P} \cdot \frac{\Delta P}{\Delta t}.$$

In exponential growth, the relative growth rate is a constant. Although exponential growth is often used to model populations, this model predicts that a population will increase without limit, which is unrealistic. In the 1830s, a Belgian mathematician, P. F. Verhulst, suggested the *logistic model*, in which the relative growth rate of a population decreases to 0 linearly as the population increases. Verhulst's model predicts that the population size eventually levels off to a value known as the *carrying capacity*.

To see how Verhulst's logistic model works, assume that a pair of breeding rabbits is introduced onto a small island with no rabbits. At the outset the rabbit population doubles every month. This means that initially the relative growth rate is 100% per month. Eventually, though, as the population grows, the relative growth rate drops down to 0% per month. Suppose that the growth rate reaches 0 when the population reaches 10,000 rabbits. (Thus, 10,000 is the carrying capacity of the island.) Using spreadsheets, we will model the rabbit population over time.

1. Let P be the population and r be the relative growth rate per month. Verhulst assumed that the relative growth rate decreases linearly as population increases. This means that r goes from 100% to 0% as P goes from 0 to 10,000 rabbits. Explain why the following formula for r corresponds to Verhulst's assumptions: $r = 0.0001(10{,}000 - P)$.
2. Use a spreadsheet to model the monthly rabbit population on the island for the first two years (24 months). Graph the rabbit population over time. Describe the behavior of the rabbit population. [Hint: Start with two rabbits, and compute the growth rate using the formula in Question 1. Then, for each month, update the rabbit population as well as the relative growth rate.]
3. Draw a graph comparing your logistic model of the rabbit population to a population growing exponentially at a constant relative growth rate of 100% per month. Both models should start out with two rabbits. Describe the similarities and the differences between the two charts. What advantages does the logistic model have over the exponential model? (You'll have to be careful when setting the chart parameters; otherwise, all you'll be able to see is the exponential population, which climbs so quickly that the logistic one will not be visible at all.)
4. The key to the logistic model is that the relative growth rate is decreasing linearly as the population increases. However, this does not mean that the relative growth rate is decreasing linearly over time. Make a chart of the relative growth rate against time for the first two years. Describe the behavior of the relative growth rate over time.
5. (a) Different assumptions about the growing rabbit population lead to different logistic curves. In Question 1, we assumed that the relative growth rate was 100% initially, dropping to 0% when the population reached 10,000. This led to the formula $r = 0.0001(10000 - P)$. Now assume that the initial relative growth rate is 10% (instead of 100%). What is the new formula relating r and P? (The carrying capacity is still 10,000, so $r = 10\%$ when $P = 0$, and r decreases to 0% as P increases to 10,000.)

(b) Using your new formula for the relative growth rate, r, let's see how different initial populations of rabbits lead to different logistic curves. Model the following scenarios, over a 5-year (60-month) period: a population starting at 100 rabbits, a population starting at 5,000 rabbits, a population starting at 12,500 rabbits, and a population starting at 17,500 rabbits. Place all of your data on the same chart. What happens to the rabbit population when it starts out above the island's rabbit carrying capacity? Why does this make sense?

10. THE SPREAD OF INFORMATION: A COMPARISON OF TWO MODELS

The spread of information through a population is important to policy makers. For example, agricultural ministries use mathematical models to understand the spread of technical innovations or new seed types through their countries.

In this project, you will compare two different models—one of them logistic —for the spread of information. In both cases, assume that the population is 10,000 and that initially only 100 people have the information. Let N be the number of people who have the information at time t.

Model 1: If the information is spread by mass media (TV, radio, newspapers), the absolute rate, $\Delta N/\Delta t$, at which the information is spread is assumed to be proportional to the number of people *not* having the information at that time. If t is in days, the constant of proportionality is 10%. For example, on the first day, the number of people not having the information is $10{,}000 - 100 = 9900$. Since 10% of 9900 is 990, the rate of spread of information is 990 people per day on the first day. This means that on the second day, the number of people not having the information is 8910 and that the rate of spread is 10% of 8910, or 891 people per day, and so on.

Model 2: If instead the information is spread by word of mouth, the absolute rate at which information is spread is assumed to be proportional to the product of the number of people who know and the number of people who do not know. If t is in days, the constant of proportionality is 0.002%. For example, on the first day, the product of the number of people who know and the number of people who do not know is $100 \cdot 9900 = 990{,}000$. Since 0.002% of 990,000 is about 20, the rate of spread of information is 20 people per day on the first day. This means that on the second day, the product of the number of people who know and the number who do not know is $120 \cdot 9880 = 1{,}188{,}600$, giving a rate of spread of 0.002% of 1,188,600 or about 24 people per day, and so on.

1. Using spreadsheets, compare the spread of information throughout the population using both models. Make a chart comparing both models' predictions of the number of people over time who have the information. Describe the similarities and differences between the two models. Why is Model 1 used when mass media are present? Why is Model 2 used when mass media are absent?
2. Which of the two models is logistic? How can you tell? What type of growth does the other model exhibit? How can you tell?
3. By definition, a population exhibits logistic growth if its relative rate of change is a decreasing linear function of the current population. Explain why Model 2 leads to logistic growth although it was defined in terms of absolute growth rates.
4. The solutions from our spreadsheets are only approximations. Discuss why this is the case. [Hint: There's more going on here than rounding error.]

11. THE FLU IN WORLD WAR I

During World War I, a particularly lethal form of flu killed about 40 million people around the world.[18] The epidemic started in an army camp of 45,000 soldiers outside of Boston, where the first soldier fell sick on September 7, 1918. In this problem you will make a spreadsheet for the SIR

[18] "Capturing a Killer Flu Virus," J. Taukenberger, A. Reid, T. Fanning, in *Scientific American*, Vol. 292, No. 1, Jan. 2005.

model of the 1918 flu outbreak. Starting from the initial values S_0 and I_0, for any increment in time Δt, the changes in the number of susceptibles and infecteds are approximated by

$$\Delta S \approx -aSI\Delta t$$
$$\Delta I \approx aSI\Delta t - bI\Delta t.$$

1. Choosing $\Delta t = 0.1$, $a = 0.0003$, $b = 10$, make a spreadsheet whose first few lines look like this:

t	S	I	ΔS	ΔI
0	44999	1	−1.3500	0.3500
0.1	44997.65	1.3500	−1.82240	0.4724
0.2	44995.828	1.8224	...	...

2. How many soldiers got sick on the fifth day? How many were susceptible on this day?
3. Alter the spreadsheet so that it accepts any values of $\Delta t, a, b$ input by the user.
4. Using the values $a = 0.000267, b = 9.865$ for the 1918 epidemic, decrease the value of Δt until a stable estimate is reached for the number of soldiers sick on September 16th. How many soldiers had been infected by this date?
5. Approximately how long did it take for the 1918 epidemic to run its course?

ANSWERS TO ODD-NUMBERED PROBLEMS

Section 1.1

1 (a) (IV)
(b) (II)
(c) (III)

3 Argentina produced 9 million metric tons of wheat in 2002

5

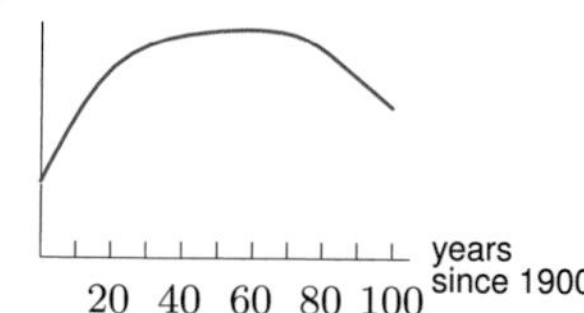

7 $f(5) = 13$

9 $f(5) = 3$

11 $f(5) = 4.1$

13 (b) CFC consumption in 1987
(c) Year CFC consumption is zero

17

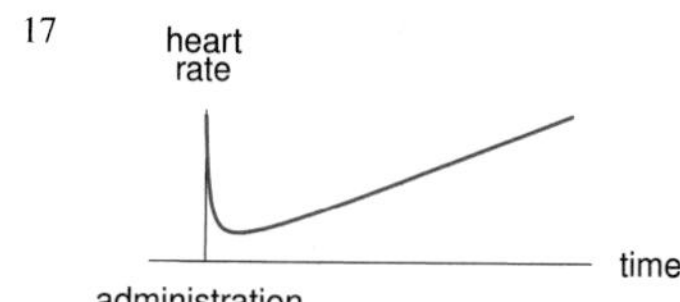

19

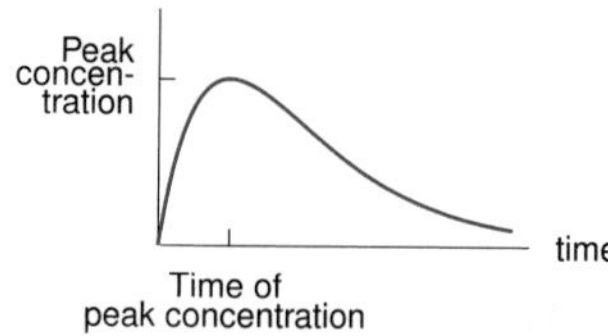

21

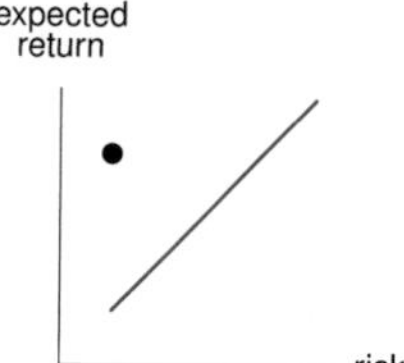

23 (a) (III)
(b) Potato's temperature before put in oven

25

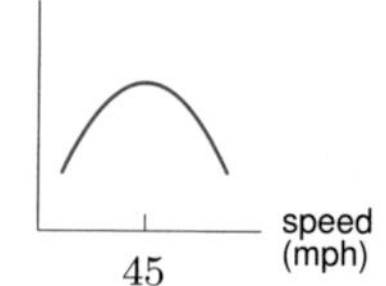

Section 1.2

1 Slope: $-12/7$
Vertical intercept: $2/7$

3 Slope: 2
Vertical intercept: $-2/3$

5 $y = (1/2)x + 2$

7 $y = (1/2)x + 2$

9 (a) l_1
(b) l_3
(c) l_2
(d) l_4

11 (a) $P = 30{,}700 + 850t$
(b) 39,200 people
(c) In 2016

13 (a) $C_1 = 40 + 0.15m$
$C_2 = 50 + 0.10m$
(b)

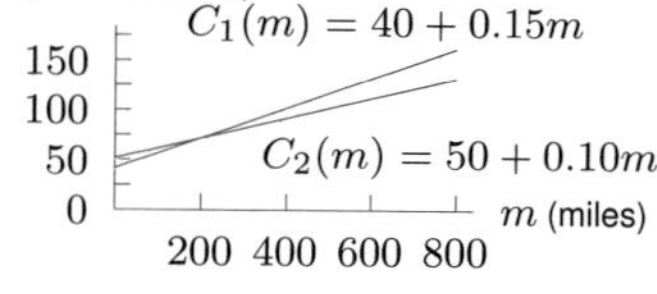

(c) For distances less than 200 miles, C_1 is cheaper.
For distances more than 200 miles, C_2 is cheaper.

15 (a) 1.8 billion dollars/year
(b) 19.1 billion dollars
(c) 28.1 billion dollars
(d) 2011

17 (a) Linear
(b) Linear
(c) Not linear

19 (a) $q = -(1/3)p + 8$
(b) $p = -3q + 24$

21 (a) $P = 11.3 + 0.4t$
(b) 13.7%
(c) 1.4%

23 (b) $P = 100 - 0.5d$
(c) -0.5%/ft
(d) 100%; 200 ft

25 (a) $C = 3.68 + 0.12w$
(b) 0.12 \$/gal
(c) \$3.68

27 (a) $\Delta w/\Delta h$ constant
(b) $w = 5h - 174$; 5 lbs/in
(c) $h = 0.2w + 34.8$; 0.2 in/lb

29 (c)

31 (a) 60, 40 years
(b) (ii)
(c) 6.375 beats/minute more under new formula

33 No

Section 1.3

1 Concave down

3 Concave up

5 Increases by 12.5%

7 Decreases by 6%

9 Decreasing
Concave up

11

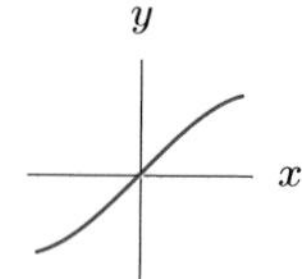
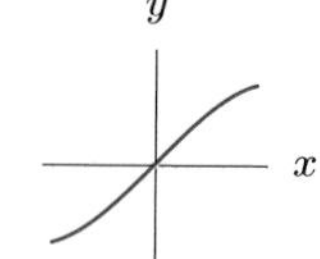

13 -3

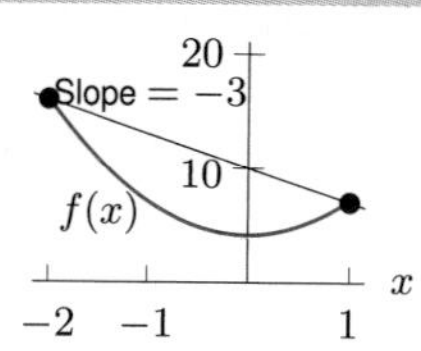

15 (a) 90 million bicycles
(b) 1.8 million bicycles per year

17 (a) 115,000 people/year
(b) 0.07, 0.08, 0.41, 0.06
(c) 115,000 people/year

19 (a) \$18,280 million
(b) \$3656 million per year

21 1 meter/sec

23 $72/7 = 10.286$ cm/sec

25 (a) Negative
(b) Positive
(c) Negative
(d) Negative
(e) Positive

27 1490 thousand people/year
912.9 thousand people/year
1879 thousand people/year

29 (a) $-$\$35 billion dollars
(b) $-$\$7 billion dollars per year
(c) Yes; 2006–2007, 2007–2008

31 (a) Negative
(b) -0.087 mg/hour

33 15.468, 57.654, 135.899, 146.353, 158.549 people/min

35 (a) -11 cm/sec
(b) -5.5 (cm/sec)/kg

37 (a) Concave up; no
(b) 2.6 m/sec

39 Decreasing, concave down

41 (a)

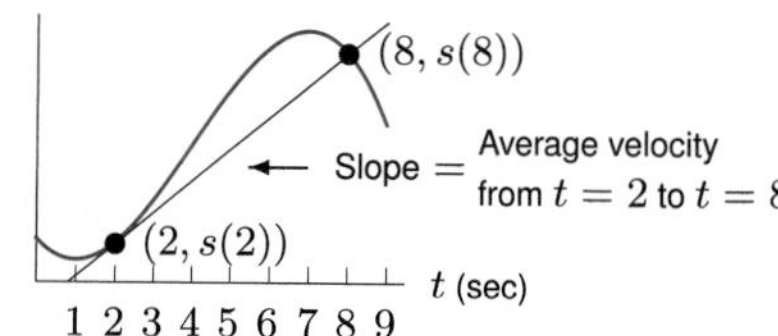

(b) Between $t = 3$ and $t = 6$
(c) Negative

43 The change in 1800-1810

45 The increase from \$100,000 to \$500,000

47 Decrease 12.8%

49

Year	2005	2006	2007	2008
Inflation	4.0%	2.1%	4.3%	0.0%

Section 1.4

1 (a) When more than roughly 335 items are produced and sold
(b) About \$650

3 (a) \$75; \$7.50 per unit
(b) \$150

5 (a) Price \$12, sell 60
(b) Decreasing

7 Vertical intercept: $p = 4$ dollars
Horizontal intercept: $q = 6$ units

9 (a) $C(q) = 5000 + 30q$
$R(q) = 50q$
(b) \$30/unit, \$50/unit
(c)

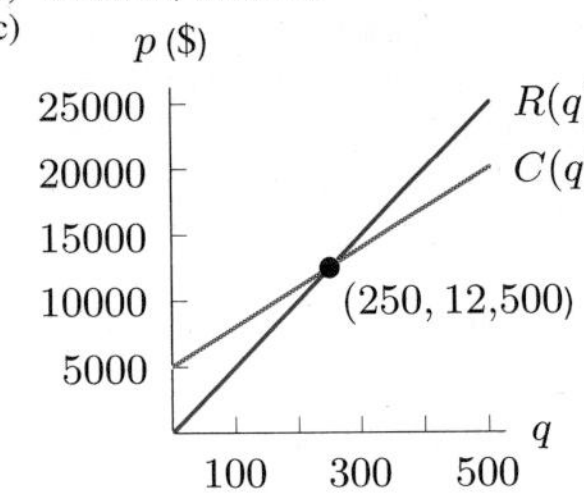

(d) 250 chairs and \$12,500

11 (a) \$4000
(b) \$2
(c) \$10
(d)

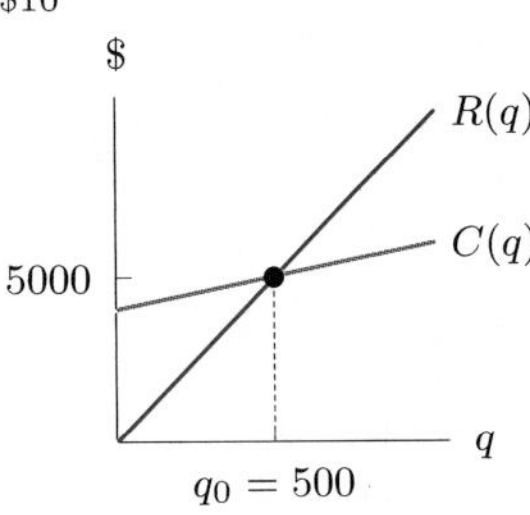

(e) 500

13 (a) When there are are more than 1000 customers
(b)

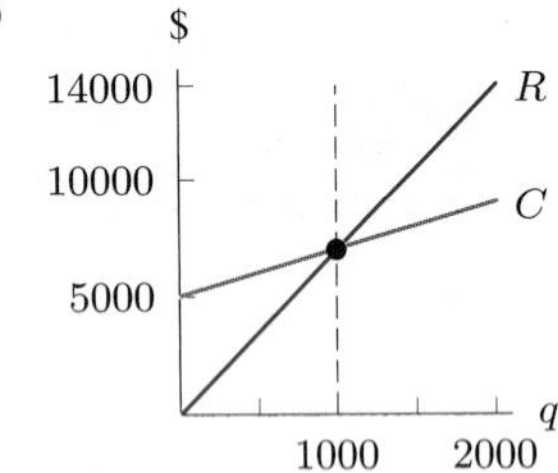

15 (a) $C(q) = 650,000 + 20q$
$R(q) = 70q$
$\pi(q) = 50q - 650,000$
(b) \$20/pair, \$70/pair, \$50/pair
(c) More than 13,000 pairs

17 (a) Between 20 and 60 units
(b) About 40 units

19 (a) $V(t) = -1500t + 15,000$
(b) $V(3) = \$10,500$

21 (a) $V(t) = -2000t + 50,000$
(b)

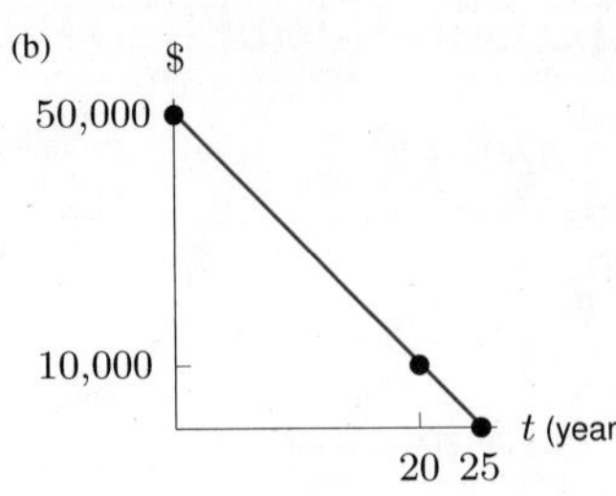

(c) (0 years, \$50,000) and (25 years, \$0)

23 (a) $p = \$10; q = 3000$
(b) Suppliers produce 3500 units; Consumers buy 2500
(c) Suppliers produce 2500 units; Consumers buy 3500

25 (a) $C = 5q + 7000$
$R = 12q$
(b) $q = 1520, \pi(12) = \$3640$
(c) $C = 17,000 - 200p$
$R = 2000p - 40p^2$
$\pi(p) = -40p^2 + 2200p - 17,000$
(d) At \$27.50 per shirt the profit is \$13,250

27 (a) $q = 820 - 20p$
(b) $p = 41 - 0.05q$

29

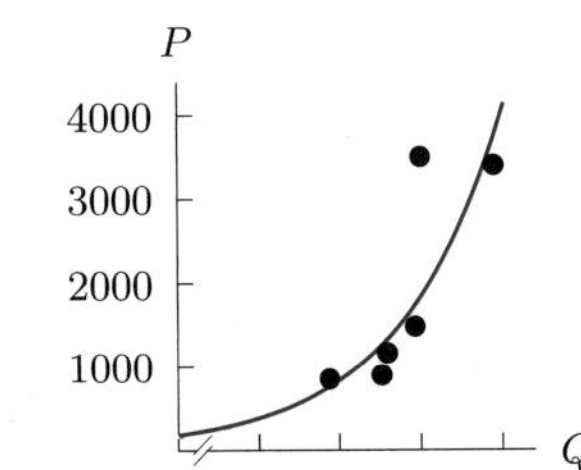

31 (a) $40b + 10s = 1000$
(b)

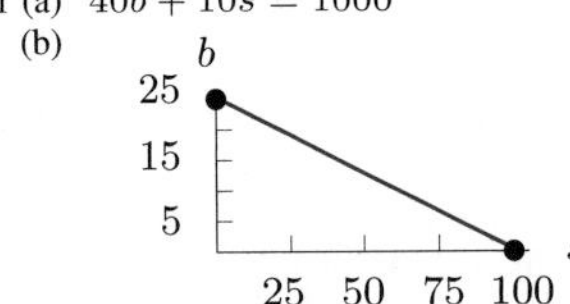

(c) The intercepts are $(0, 25)$ and $(100, 0)$

33 (a)

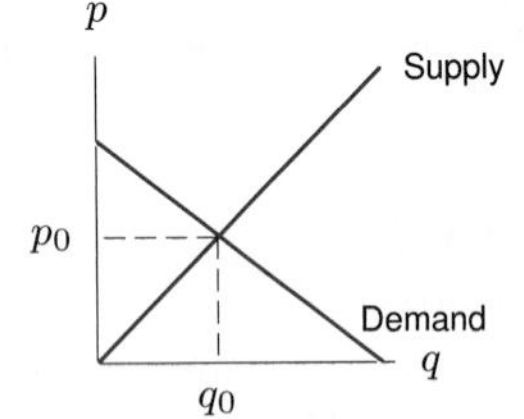

(b) Equilibrium price will increase; equilibrium quantity will decrease
(c) Equilibrium price and quantity will decrease

35 $q = 4p - 28$

37 (a) $p = 100, q = 500$
(b) $p = 102, q = 460$
(c) Consumer pays \$2
Producer pays \$4
(d) \$2760

39 (a) Demand: $q = 100 - 2p$
Supply: $q = 2.85p - 50$
(b) New equilibrium price $p \approx \$30.93$
New equilibrium quantity $q \approx 38.14$ units
(c) Consumer pays \$0.93
Producer pays \$0.62
Total \$1.55
(d) \$59.12

Section 1.5

1 (a) (i), 12%
(b) (ii), 1000
(c) Yes, (iv)

3 (a) II
(b) I
(c) III
(d) V

5 (a) $G = 310(1.03)^t$
(b) $G = 310 + 8t$

7 (a) $Q = 30 - 2t$

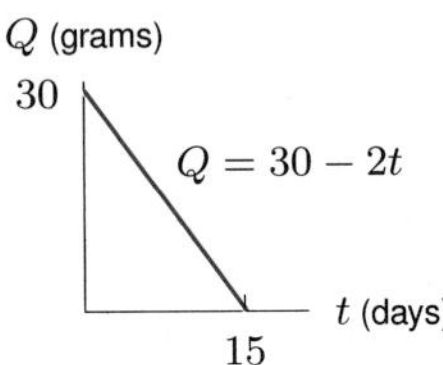

(b) $Q = 30(0.88)^t$

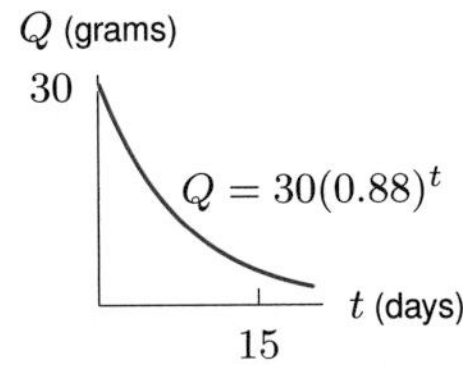

9 (a) $A = 50(0.94)^t$
(b) 11.33 mg
(c) A (mg)

50
5
t (hours)
20 40

(d) About 37 hours

11 CPI $= 211(1.028)^t$

13 (a)

x	0	1	2	3
e^x	1	2.72	7.39	20.09

(b)

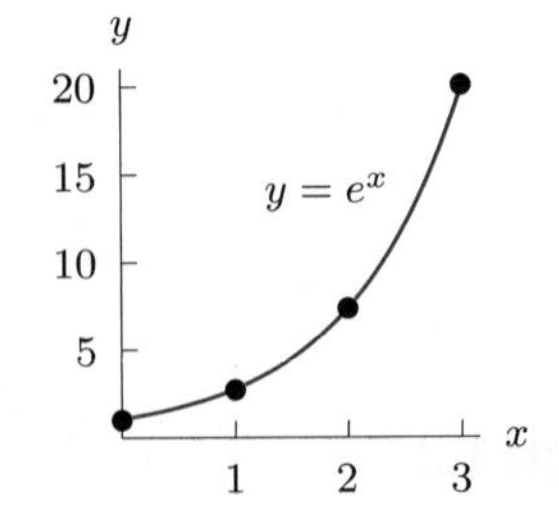

(c)

x	0	1	2	3
e^{-x}	1	0.37	0.14	0.05

(d)

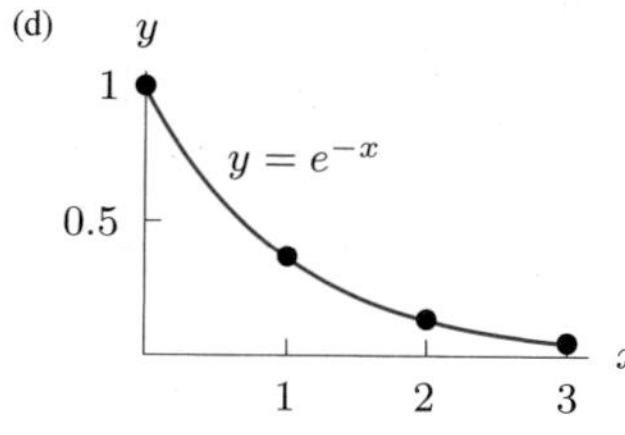

15 $f(x) = 4.30(1.4)^x$

17 $y = 500(1.59)^t$

19 About 6.97 billion; close

21 22.6% per year

23 (a) $W = 40{,}300 + 16{,}178t$
(b) $W = 40{,}300(1.25)^t = 40{,}300e^{0.22t}$
(c)

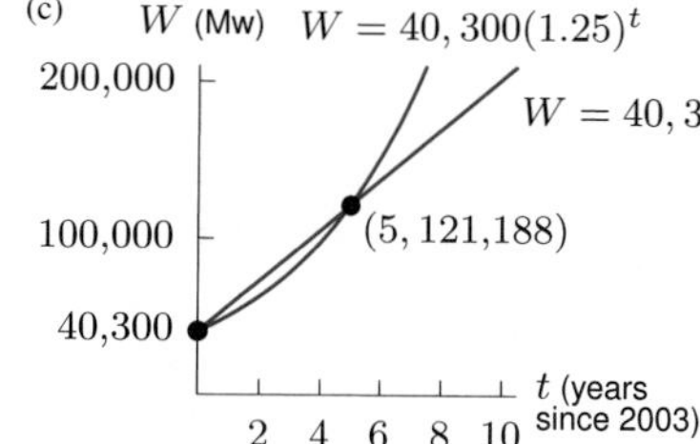

25 (a) Neither
(b) Exponential: $s(t) = 30.12(0.6)^t$
(c) Linear: $g(u) = -1.5u + 27$

27 Min. wage grew 4.69% per year

29 (a) 125%
(b) 9 times

31 $d = 670(1.096)^{h/1000}$

Section 1.6

1 $t = (\ln 7)/(\ln 5) \approx 1.209$

3 $t = (\ln 2)/(\ln 1.02) \approx 35.003$

5 $t = (\ln 5)/(\ln 3) \approx 1.465$

7 $t = \ln 10 \approx 2.3026$

9 $t = (\ln 100)/3 \approx 1.535$

11 $t = 30.54$

13 $t = (\ln B - \ln P)/r$

15 $t = \ln 8 - \ln 5 \approx 0.47$

17 5; 7%

19 15; −6% (continuous)

21 (a) D
(b) C
(c) B

23 $P = 15(1.2840)^t$; growth

25 $P = P_0(1.2214)^t$; growth

27 $P = 15e^{0.4055t}$

29 $P = 174e^{-0.1054t}$

31 $P = 6.4e^{0.01252t}$

33 (a) \$5 million; \$3.704 million dollars
(b) 4.108 years

35 (a) 12%
(b) $P = 25e^{-0.128t}$, 12.8%

37 (a) $P = 5.4(1.034)^t$
(b) $P = 5.4e^{0.0334t}$
(c) Annual = 3.4%
Continuous = 3.3%

39 9.53%

41 2009

Section 1.7

1 (a) $W = 18000e^{0.27t}$
(b) About 2010

3 \$14,918.25

5 About 11.6 years

7 About 10.24 years

9 (a) \$5068.93
(b) \$4878.84

11 (a) $A = 100e^{-0.17t}$
(b) $t \approx 4$ hours

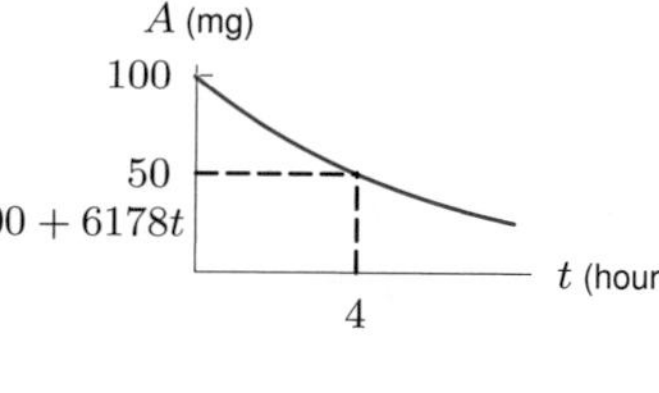

(c) $t = 4.077$ hours

13 A: continuous
B: annual
\$20

15 (a) 47.6%
(b) 23.7%

17 8.45%

19 (a) $P(t) = (0.975)^t$
(b)

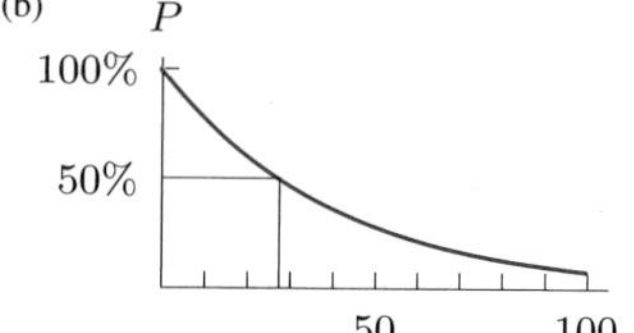

(c) About 27 years
(d) About 8%

21 (a) 4 years
(b) 4 years

23 About 173 hours

25 96.34 years

27 0.0345; 191 million tons

29 (a) (i) About 4.07 billion dollars
(ii) About 7.98 trillion dollars
(b) 1803

31 It is a fake

33 \$35,365.34

35 \$14,522.98

37 (a) Option 1
(b) \$2102.54, \$2051.27, \$2000
(c) \$2000, \$1951.23, \$1902.46

39 (a) Option 1
(b) Option 1: \$10.929 million;
Option 2: \$10.530 million

41 Loan

43 No

Section 1.8

1 (a) $h^2 + 6h + 11$
(b) 11
(c) $h^2 + 6h$

3 (a) 4
(b) 2
(c) $(x+1)^2$
(d) $x^2 + 1$
(e) $t^2(t+1)$

5 (a) e
(b) e^2
(c) e^{x^2}
(d) e^{2x}
(e) $e^t t^2$

7 (a) 9
(b) 20
(c) 25
(d) 11

9 (a) $10x^2 + 3$
(b) $20x^2 + 60x + 45$
(c) $4x + 9$

11 (a) 3
(b) 4
(c) 11
(d) 8
(e) 12

13 (a) $y = 2^u, u = 3x - 1$
(b) $P = \sqrt{u}, u = 5t^2 + 10$
(c) $w = 2\ln u, u = 3r + 4$

15 $2z + 1$

17 $2zh - h^2$

19 0.4

21 −0.9

23 $2(y-1)^3 - (y-1)^2$

25 18

27 Can't be done

29 (a)

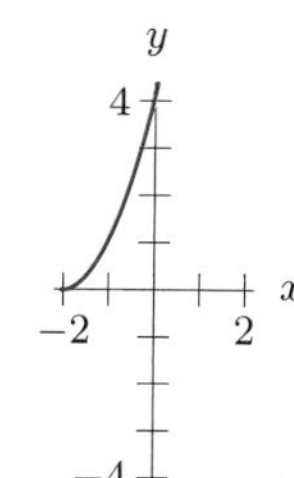

(b)

(c)

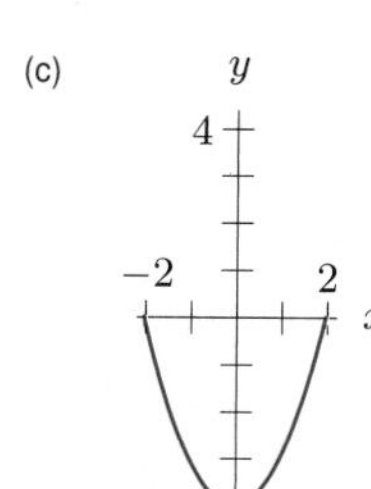

(d)

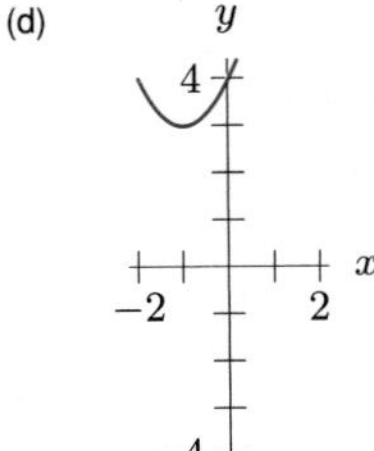

(e)

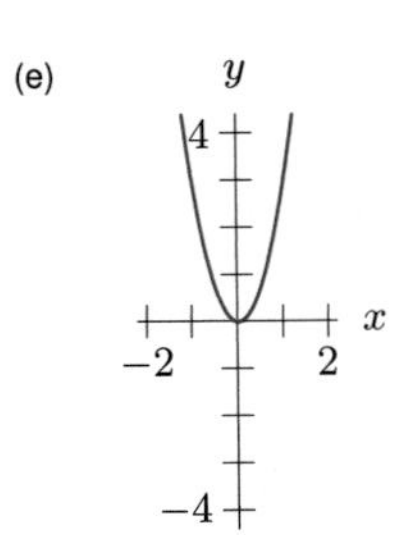

(f)

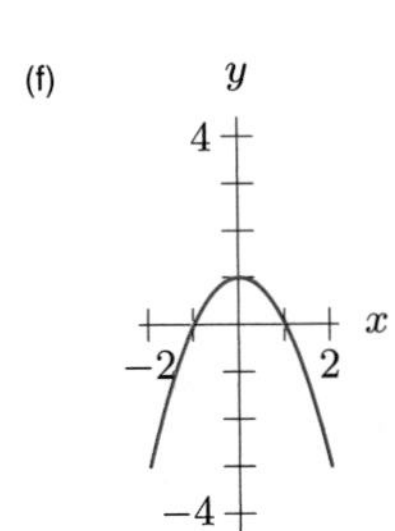

31 (a)

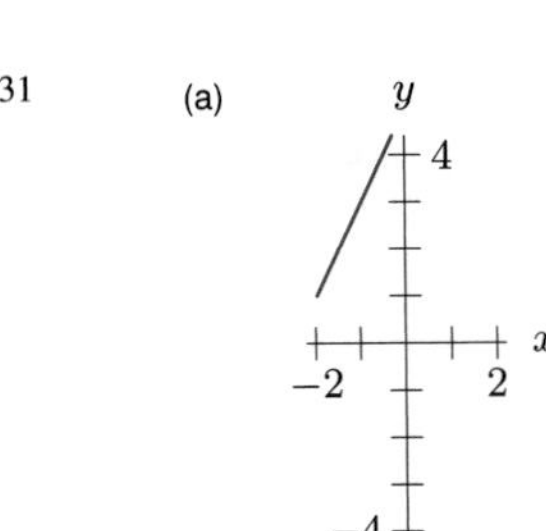

(b)

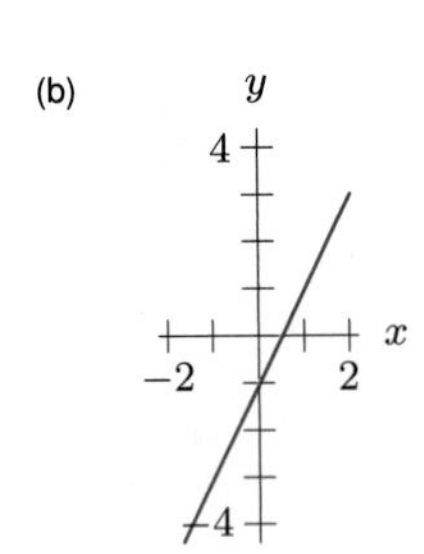

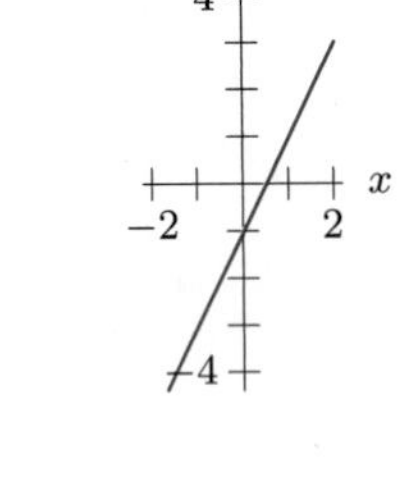

(c)

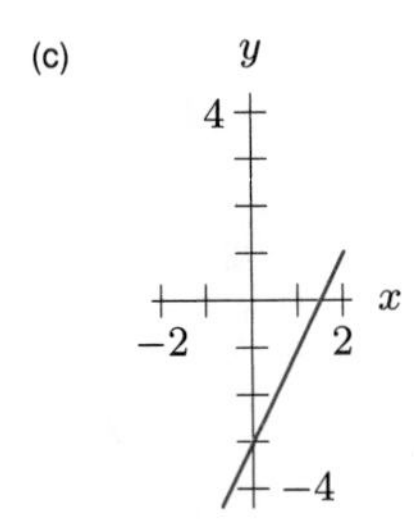

(d)

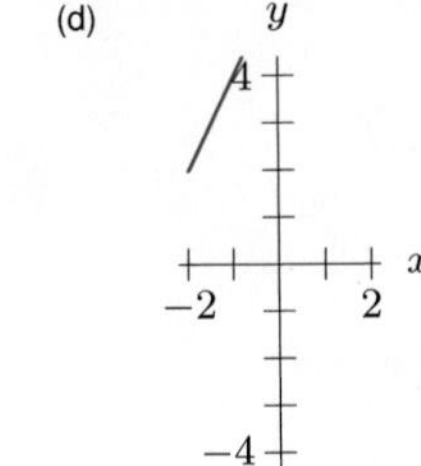

(e)

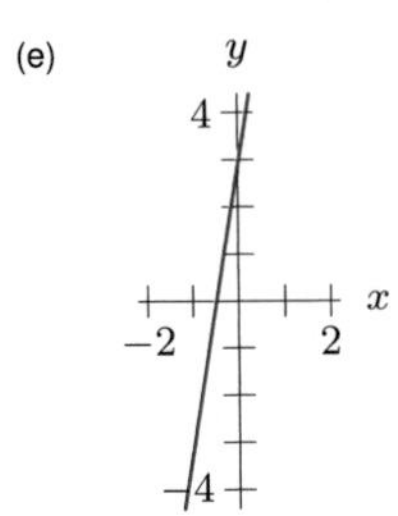

(f)

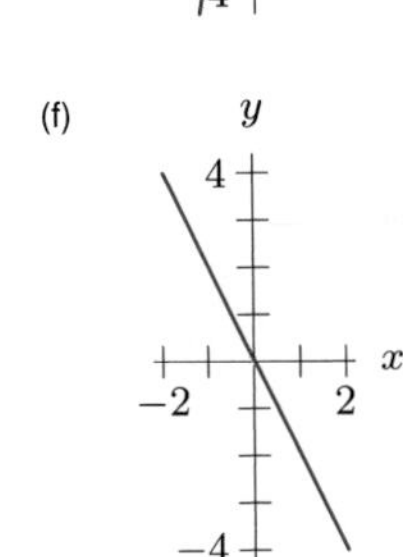

33

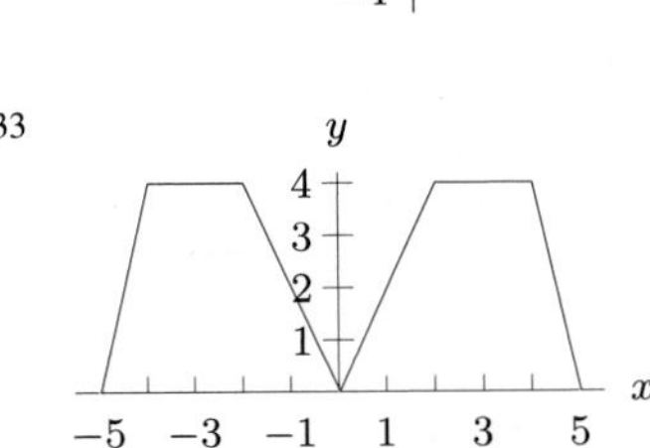

35

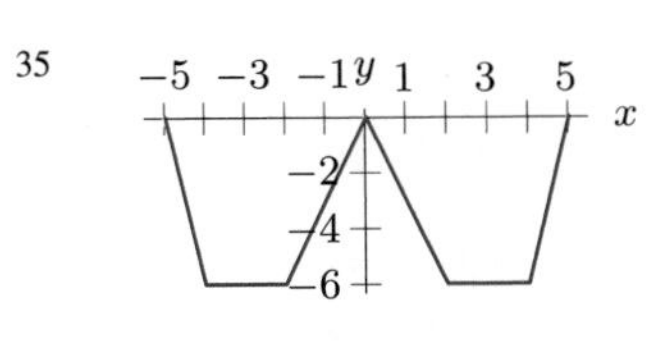

37

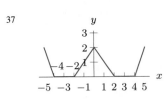

39 **(a)**

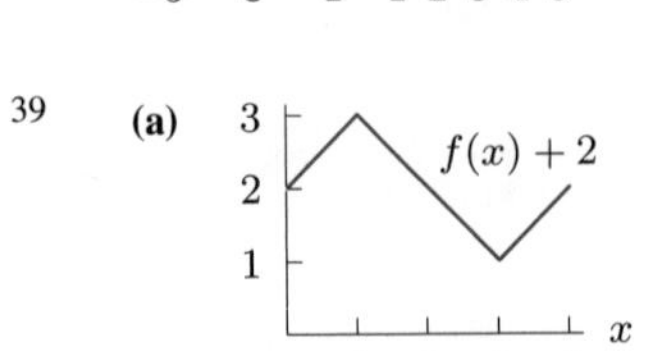

(b)

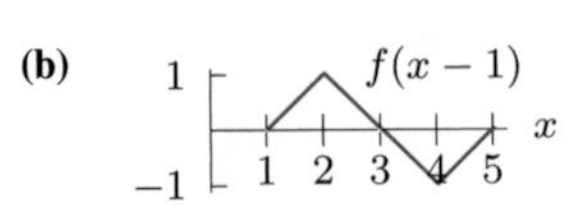

(c)

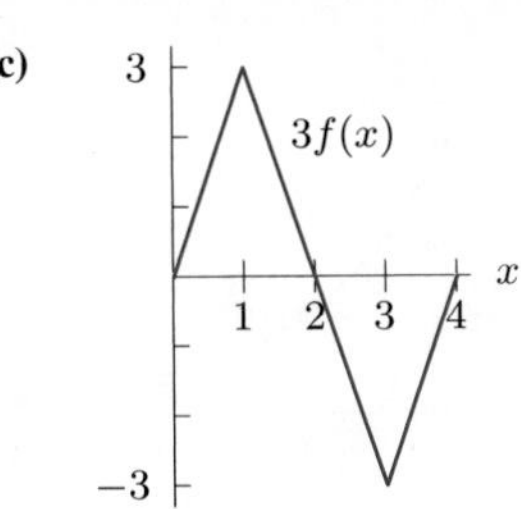

(d)

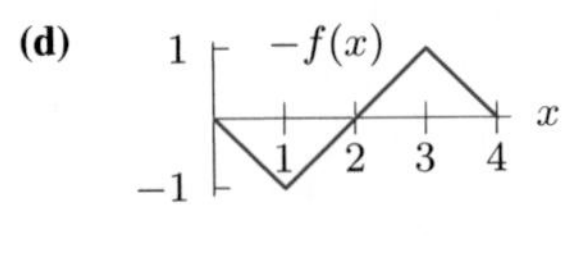

41 **(a)**

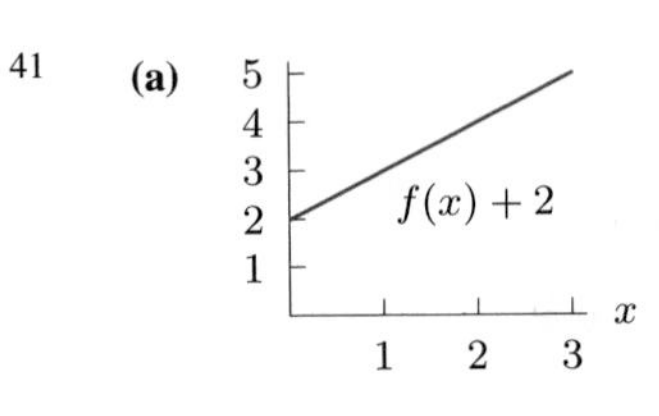

(b)

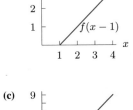

(c)

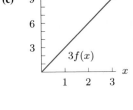

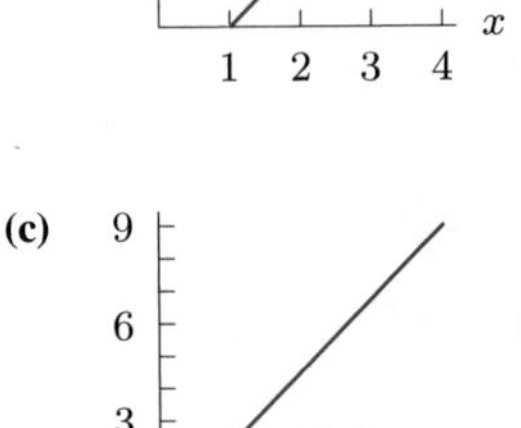

(d)

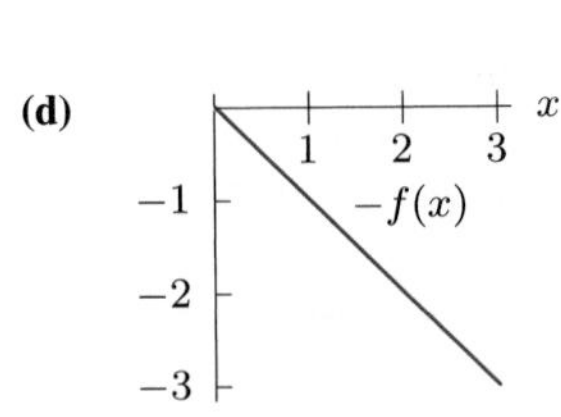

43 (a) $y = 2x^2 + 1$

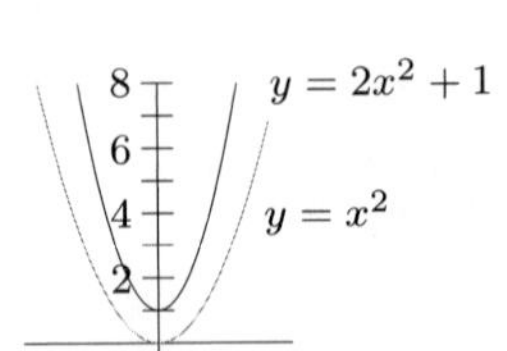

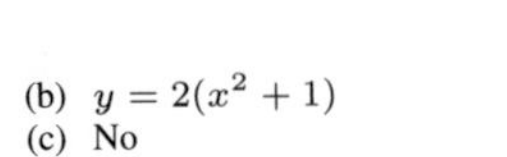

(b) $y = 2(x^2 + 1)$
(c) No

Section 1.9

1 $y = 5x^{1/2}$

3 Not a power function.

5 $y = 9x^{10}$

7 Not a power function

9 $y = 8x^{-1}$

11 Not a power function

13 $S = kh^2$

15 $v = d/t$

17 $N = kA^{1/4}$, with $k > 0$,
Increasing, concave down

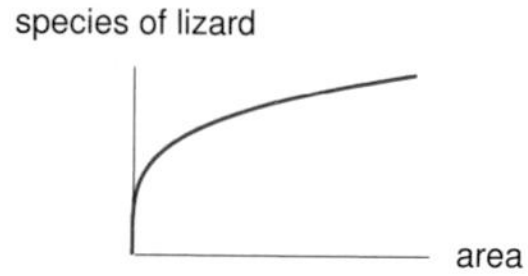

19 (a) $y = (x-2)^3 + 1$
(b) $y = -(x+3)^2 - 2$

21 Yes; $k \approx 0.0087$

23 $N = k/L^2$; small

25 (a) $T = kB^{1/4}$
(b) $k = 17.4$
(c) 50.3 seconds

27 (a) $N = kP^{0.77}$
(b) A has 5.888 times more than B
(c) Town

29 (a) 0.5125
(b) 0.3162
(c) 201,583 dynes/cm^2

31 (a) $C = 115{,}000 - 700p$
$R = 3000p - 20p^2$
(b)

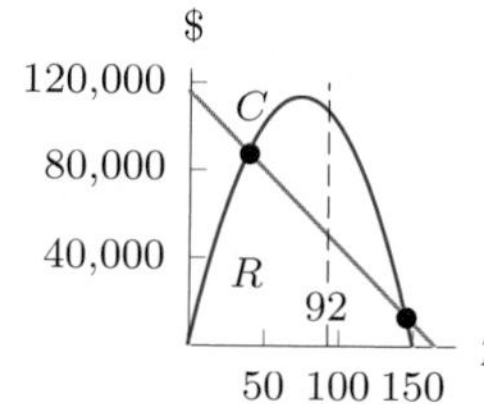

(d) When it charges between \$40 and \$145
(e) About \$92

Section 1.10

1 (b) Max at 7 pm; min at 9 am
(c) Period = one day; amplitude $\approx 2°$C

3

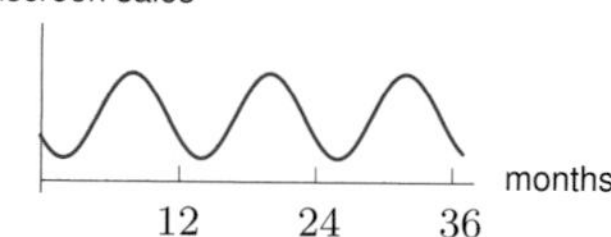

5 Amplitude = 3; Period = π

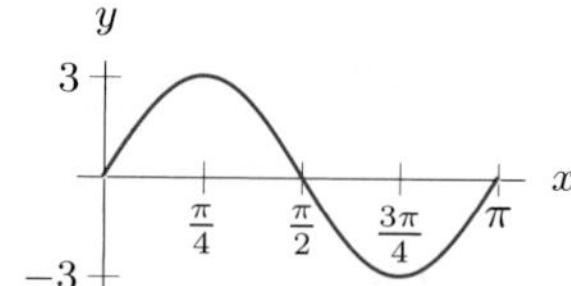

7 Amplitude = 4; Period = π

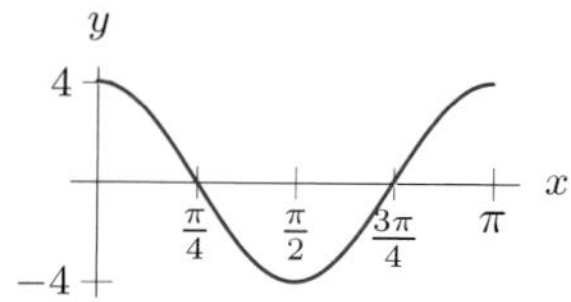

9 Amplitude = 1; Period = π

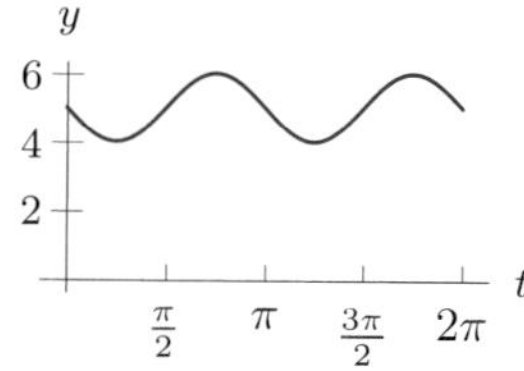

11 (a) 5
(b) 8
(c) $f(x) = 5\cos((\pi/4)x)$

13 $H = -16\cos((\pi/6)t) + 10$

15 $0.35\cos(2\pi t/5.4) + 4$

17 $y = 7\sin(\pi t/5)$

19 $f(x) = 5\cos(x/3)$

21 $f(x) = -4\sin(2x)$

23 $f(x) = -8\cos(x/10)$

25 $f(x) = 5\sin((\pi/3)x)$

27 $f(x) = 3 + 3\sin((\pi/4)x)$

29 Depth $= 7 + 1.5\sin(\pi t/3)$

31 (a) Period is 12; amplitude is 4
(b) $g(34) = 11$; $g(60) = 14$

Chapter 1 Review

1 5 kilometers, 23 minutes

3

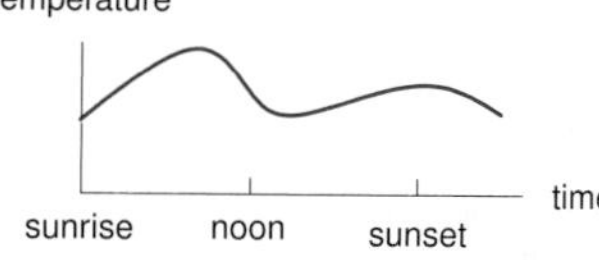

5 (b) 200 bushels
(c) 80 lbs
(d) $0 \le Y \le 550$
(e) Decreasing
(f) Concave down

7

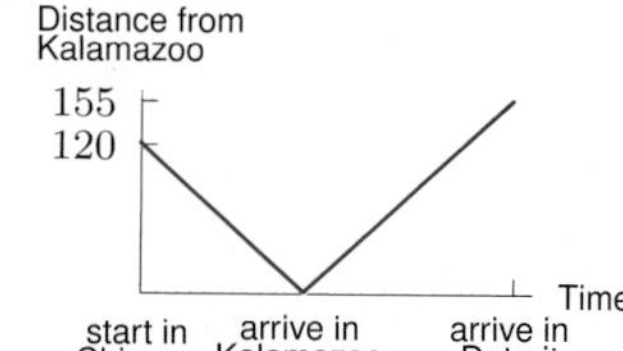

9 $y = 8/3 - x/3$

11 $x = -1$

13 $y = 14x - 45$

15 (a) \$0.025/cubic foot
(b) $c = 15 + 0.025w$
c = cost of water
w = cubic feet of water
(c) 3400 cubic feet

17 $(\ln 3)/2 = 0.549$ mm/sec

19 0 mm/sec

21 0 mm/sec

23 (a)

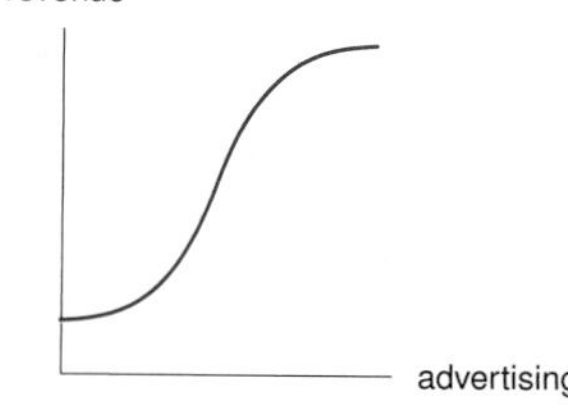

(b)

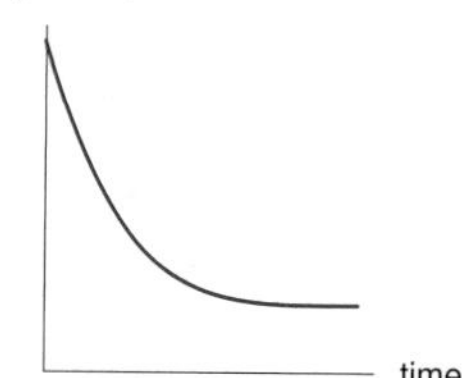

25 (a)

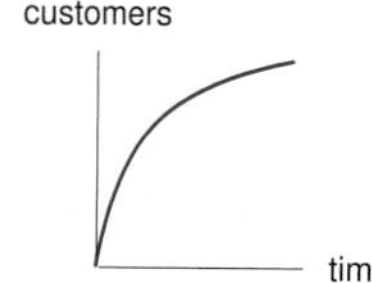

(b) Concave down

27 (a) (i) Positive
(ii) Positive
(iii) Negative
(iv) Positive
(b) (i) $0 \le t \le 5$
(ii) $0 \le t \le 20$
(c) 25 m^3/week

29 (a) \$1000; \$15
(b) It costs the company \$2500 to produce 100 items

31 $y = -(950/7)x + 950$

33 (a) $p = \$250$; $q = 750$
(b) Suppliers produce 875 units;
Consumers buy 625
(c) Suppliers produce 625 units;
Consumers would buy 875

35 $y = (-3/7)x + 3$

37 $y = 3e^{0.2197t}$
or $y = 3(1.2457)^t$

39 $z = 1 - \cos\theta$

41 $f(x)$ is neither,
$g(x) = 30.8 - 3.2x$ is linear,
$h(x) = 15{,}000(0.6)^x$ is exponential

43 $(\log(2/5))/(\log 1.04) = -23.4$

45 $\ln(0.4)/3 = -0.305$

47 (a) 15%
(b) $P = 10(1.162)^t$
(c) 16.2%

(d) Graphs are the same since functions are equal

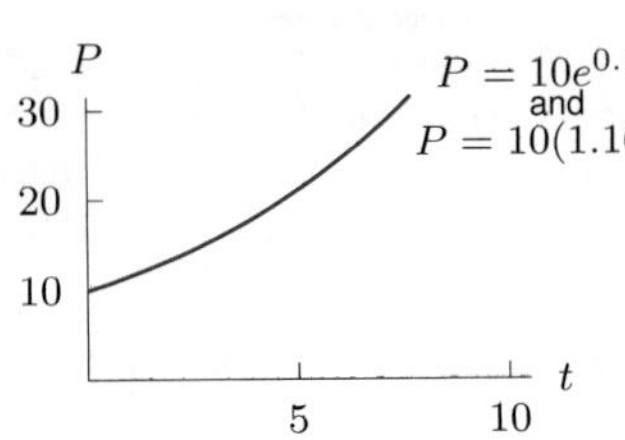

49 (a) 15,678.7 years
(b) 5728.489, or about 5730 years

51 7.925 hours

53 Yes

55 (a) $\ln(2x + 3)$
(b) $2 \ln x + 3$
(c) $4x + 9$

57 

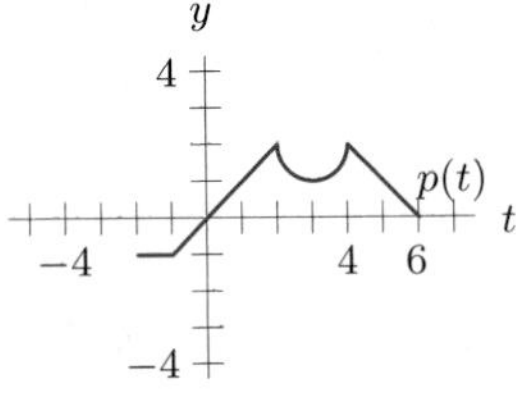

59

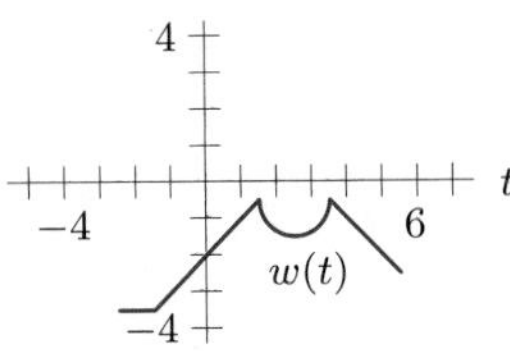

61

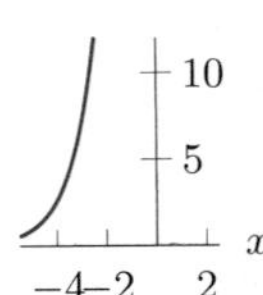

63 (a) A, B positive; C negative
(b) $A + B$
(c) A

65 $y = (x - 2)^2 - 5$

67 (a) $P = k/R$
(b) 300,000; 150,000; 100,000
(c) 6 million; 3 million, 2 million
(d) k is population of largest city

69 $8\pi; 3$

71 (a) Period = 12 months;
Amplitude = 4,500 cases
(b) About 2000 cases and 2000 cases

73 $f(x) = 2\sin(x/4) + 2$

Ch. 1 Understanding

1 False

3 True

5 True

7 True

9 False

11 False

13 True

15 False

17 False

19 False

21 False

23 False

25 True

27 True

29 True

31 True

33 False

35 Possible answer:

$$f(x) = \begin{cases} 1 & x \le 2 \\ x & x > 2 \end{cases}$$

37 Possible answer $f(x) = 1/(x + 7\pi)$

39 Possible answer:
$f(x) = (x - 1)/(x - 2)$

41 $f(x) = x, g(x) = -2x$

43 $f(x) = e^x, g(x) = e^{-2x}$

45 False; $f(x) = x/(x^2 + 1)$

47 False; $y = x + 1$ at points $(1, 2)$ and $(2, 3)$

49 False; $y = 4x + 1$ starting at $x = 1$

51 False

53 True; $f(x) = 0$

55 True

57 True

59 False

61 True

63 False

65 False

67 (a) Follows
(b) Does not follow (although true)
(c) Follows
(d) Does not follow

Section 2.1

1 (a) Positive
(b) Negative

3 (a) (i) 6.3 m/sec
(ii) 6.03 m/sec
(iii) 6.003 m/sec
(b) 6 m/sec

5 (a) 8 ft/sec
(b) 6 ft/sec

7 (a) 63 cubic millimeters
(b) 10.5 cubic millimeters/month
(c) 44.4 cubic millimeters/month

9 $f'(2) \approx 40.268$

11 (a) Positive at C and G
Negative at A and E. Zero at B, D, and F
(b) Largest at G
Most negative at A

13 $f'(d) = 0$, $f'(b) = 0.5$, $f'(c) = 2$, $f'(a) = -0.5$, $f'(e) = -2$

15 (a) The slopes of the two tangent lines at $x = a$ are equal for all a
(b) A vertical shift does not change the slope

17 $P'(0) = 10$

19 (a) $g(2) = 5$
(b) $g'(2) = -0.4$

21 (a) $f(4)$
(b) $f(2) - f(1)$
(c) $(f(2) - f(1))/(2 - 1)$
(d) $f'(1)$

23 300 million people;
2.867 million people/yr

Section 2.2

1 $1.0, 0.3, -0.5, -1$

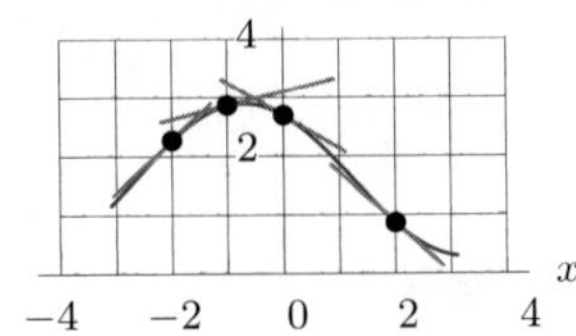

3

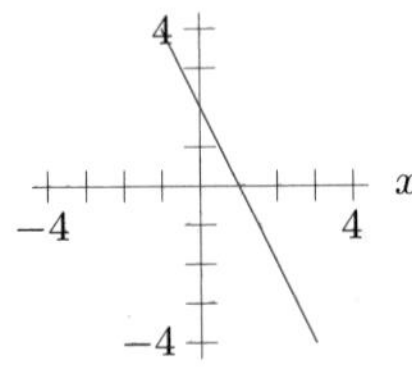

5

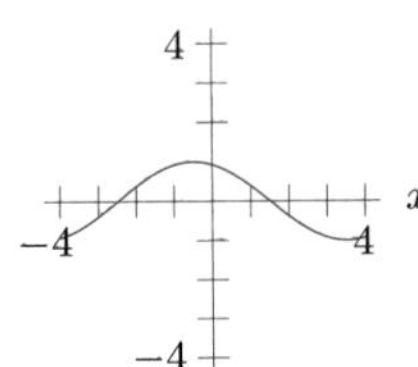

7

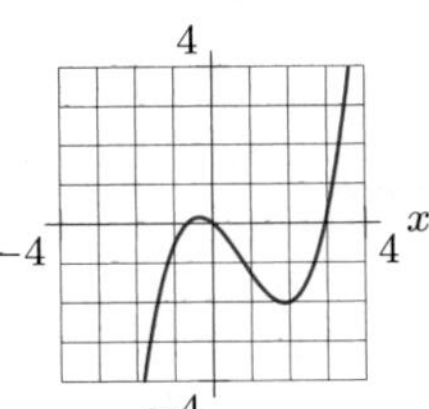

9 $-6, -3, -1.8, -1.2, -1.2$

11

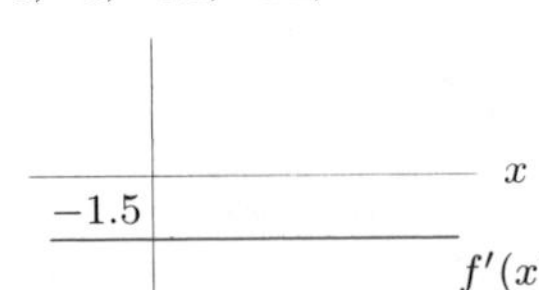

13

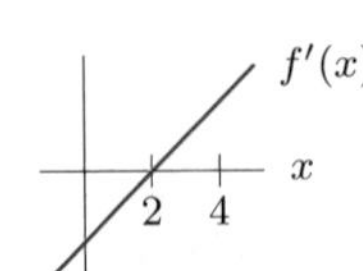

15

20
$f'(x)$
x
−3
3
−20

17 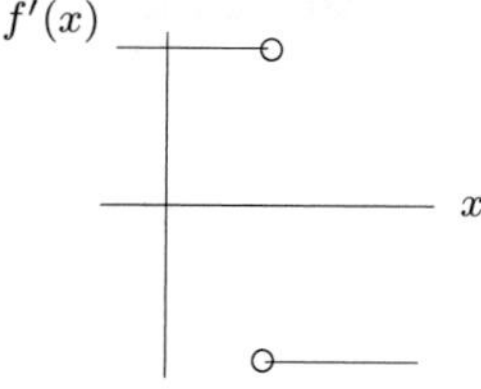

19 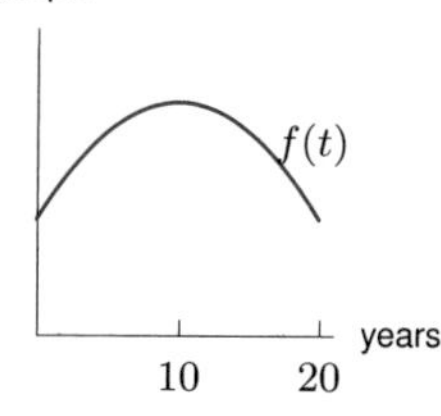

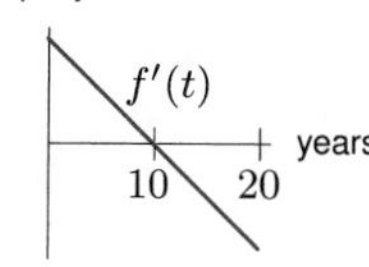

or

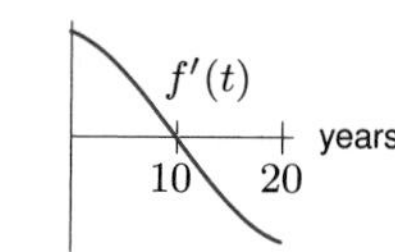

21 VIII

23 II

25 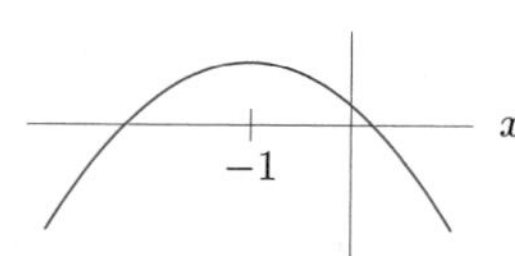

Other answers possible

27 (a) Graph II
(b) Graph I
(c) Graph III

29 $f'(2) = 4$
$f'(3) = 9$
$f'(4) = 16$
The pattern seems to be:
$f'(x) = x^2$.

31 (a) $t = 3$
(b) $t = 9$
(c) $t = 14$
(d) 1 $V'(t)$ 15 18 t 3 6 9 12 -2

Section 2.3

1 dC/dW; dollars per pound

3 dP/dH; dollars per hour

5 (a) 12 pounds, 5 dollars
(b) Positive
(c) 12 pounds, 0.4 dollars/pound, extra pound costs about 40 cents

9 (a) Positive
(b) °F/min

11 (a) Liters per centimeter
(b) About 0.042 liters per centimeter
(c) Cannot expand much more

13 (a) Investing the $1000 at 5% would yield about $1649 after 10 years
(b) Extra percentage point would yield an increase of about $165; dollars/%

15 (a) Consuming 1800 Calories per day results in a weight of 155 pounds; Consuming 2000 Calories per day causes neither weight gain nor loss
(b) Pounds/(Calories/day)

17 (a) Positive
(b) Child weighs 45 pounds at 8 years
(c) lbs/year
(d) The child is growing at a rate of 4 lbs/year at 8 years of age
(e) Decrease

19 $f'(t) \approx 6$ where t is retirement age in years, $f(t)$ is age of onset in weeks

21 (a) kg/week
(b) Growing at 96 gm/wk at week 24

23 (a) Less
(b) Greater

25 About 3.4, about 2.6

27 (a) In 2008: Net sales 5.1 bn dollars; rate increase 0.22 bn dollars/yr
(b) About 5.98 billion dollars

29 (a) Dose for 140 lbs is 120 mg
Dose increases by 3mg/lb
(b) About 135 mg

31 (a) $f(0) = 80$; $f'(0) = 0.50$
(b) $f(10) \approx 85$

33 (a) 1.7 (liters/minute)/hour
(b) About 0.028 liter/minute
(c) $g'(2) = 1.7$

35 (a) $f'(a)$ is always positive
(c) $f'(100) = 2$: more
$f'(100) = 0.5$: less

37 (a) Fat
(b) Protein

39 (a) 2.0 kg/week
(b) 0.6 kg/week
(c) 0.3 kg/week

41 I-fat, II-protein

43 $f(4) = 200$ million users;
$f'(4) \approx 12.5$ million users/month;
Increasing at about 6.25%/month

45 0.50

Section 2.4

1 (a) Negative
(b) Negative
(c) Positive

3 $f'(x) > 0$
$f''(x) > 0$

5 $f'(x) < 0$
$f''(x) = 0$

7 $f'(x) > 0$
$f''(x) < 0$

9 (a) 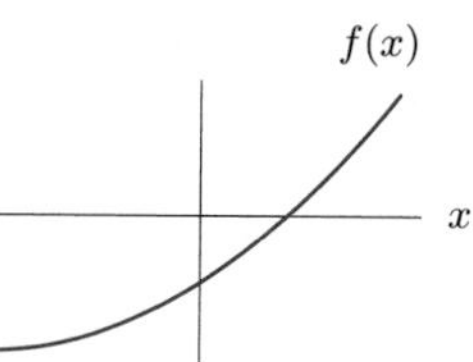

(b) 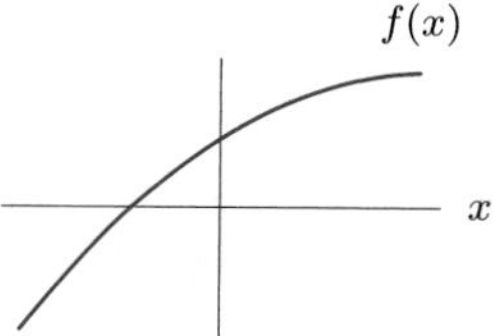

(c) 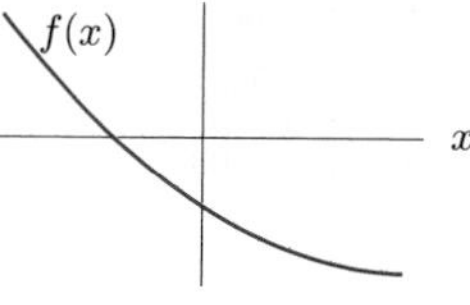

(d) 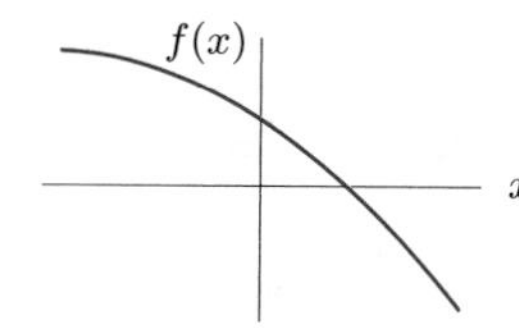

11 $s'(t)$: positive
$s''(t)$: positive or zero

13 A positive second derivative indicates a successful campaign
A negative second derivative indicates an unsuccessful campaign

15 (a) Positive; positive
(b) Number of cars increasing at 3.24 million cars per year in 1975

17 Derivative:
Pos. $-2.3 < t < -0.5$
Neg. $-0.5 < t < 4$
Second derivative:
Pos. $0.5 < t < 4$
Neg. $-2.3 < t < 0.5$

19

Point	f	f'	f''
A	–	0	+
B	+	0	–
C	+	–	–
D	–	+	+

21 (e)

23 22 only possible value

25 (a) 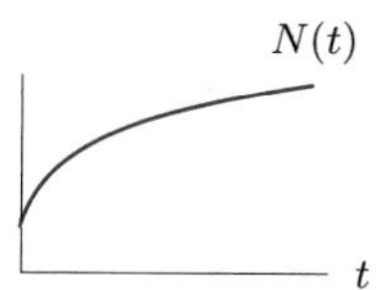

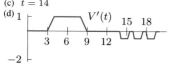

(b) dN/dt is positive.
d^2N/dt^2 is negative.

27 (a)

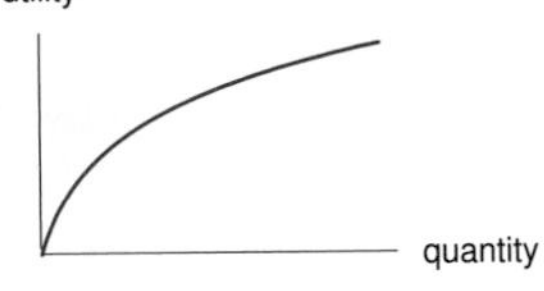

(b) Derivative of utility is positive
2nd derivative of utility is negative

Section 2.5

1 (a) Dollars/barrel
(b) 101 barrels cost about \$3 more than 100 barrels

3 At $q = 5$;
At $q = 40$

5 About \$16.67 (answers may vary)

7 $C'(2000) \approx \$0.37$/ton
The marginal cost is smallest on the interval $2500 \le q \le 3000$.

9 (a) About \$2408
(b) About \$2192

11 (a) About \$4348
(b) \$11 profit
(c) No, company will lose money

13 (a) \$1850 profit
(b) About \$0.40 increase; increase production
(c) About \$0.45 decrease; decrease production

15 (a) Fixed costs
(b) Decreases slowly, then increases

Chapter 2 Review

1 (a) (i) 8.4 m/sec
(ii) 8.04 m/sec
(iii) 8.004 m/sec
(b) 8 m/sec

3 (a) Negative
(b) $f'(1) = -3$

5 Positive: A and D
Negative: C and F
Most positive: A
Most negative: F

7 (a) (i) -1.00801 m/sec
(ii) -0.8504 m/sec
(iii) -0.834 m/sec
(b) -0.83 m/sec

9

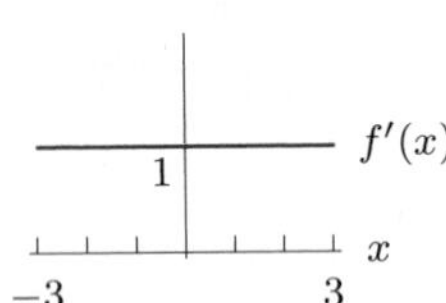

11

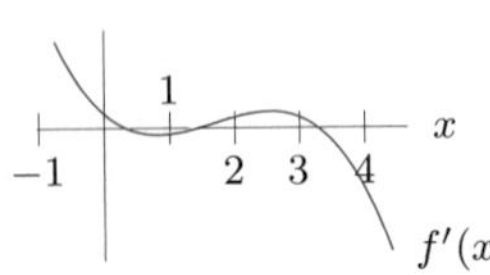

13

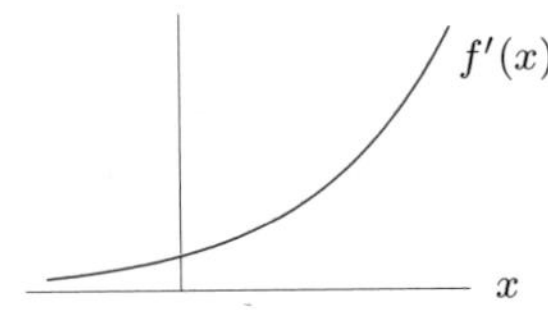

15 (a) $x_1 < x < x_3$
(b) $0 < x < x_1$; $x_3 < x < x_5$

21 $f(21) \approx 65$
$f(19) \approx 71$
$f(25) \approx 53$

23 Wind stronger at 15.1 km than at 15 km

25 About 1.338 billion people in 2009; growing at 8 million people per year

27 (a) $f'(t) > 0$: depth increasing
$f'(t) < 0$: depth decreasing
(b) Depth increasing 20 cm/min
(c) 12 meters/hr

31 (a) Negative
(b) Degrees/min

33 Dollars/year; negative

35 (a)

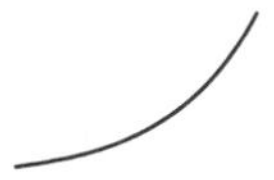

(b)

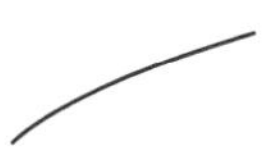

(c)

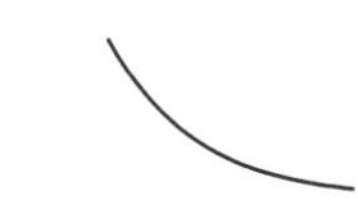

(d)

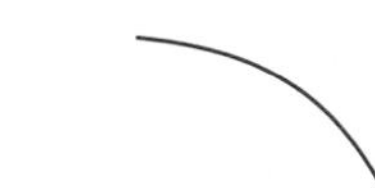

37 (a) Minutes/kilometer
(b) Minutes/kilometer^2

39 (a) x_4, x_5
(b) x_3, x_4
(c) x_3, x_4
(d) x_2, x_3
(e) x_1, x_2, x_5
(f) x_1, x_4, x_5

41 (a) t_3, t_4, t_5
(b) t_2, t_3
(c) t_1, t_2, t_5
(d) t_1, t_2, t_4
(e) t_3, t_4

43 (a)

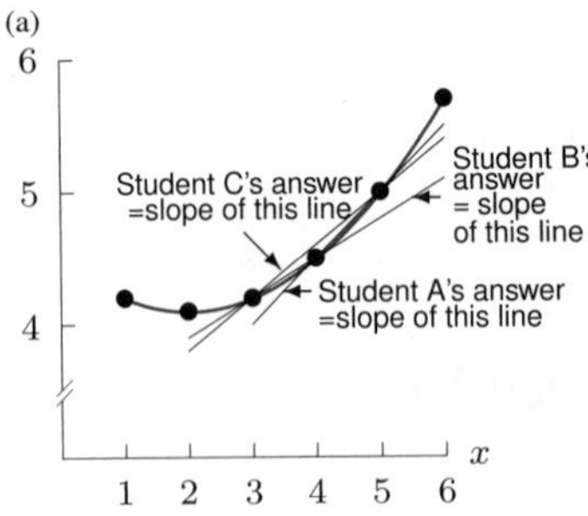

(b) Student C's
(c) $f'(x) = \dfrac{f(x+h) - f(x-h)}{2h}$

Ch. 2 Understanding

1 False
3 True
5 True
7 True
9 False
11 False
13 True
15 False
17 False
19 False
21 False
23 False
25 True
27 True
29 True
31 True
33 False
35 Possible answer:
$$f(x) = \begin{cases} 1 & x \le 2 \\ x & x > 2 \end{cases}$$
37 Possible answer $f(x) = 1/(x + 7\pi)$
39 Possible answer:
$f(x) = (x-1)/(x-2)$
41 $f(x) = x, g(x) = -2x$
43 $f(x) = e^x, g(x) = e^{-2x}$
45 False; $f(x) = x/(x^2+1)$
47 False; $y = x + 1$ at points $(1,2)$ and $(2,3)$
49 False; $y = 4x + 1$ starting at $x = 1$
51 False
53 True; $f(x) = 0$
55 True
57 True
59 False
61 True
63 False
65 False
67 (a) Follows
(b) Does not follow (although true)
(c) Follows
(d) Does not follow

Theory: Limits, Derivatives

1

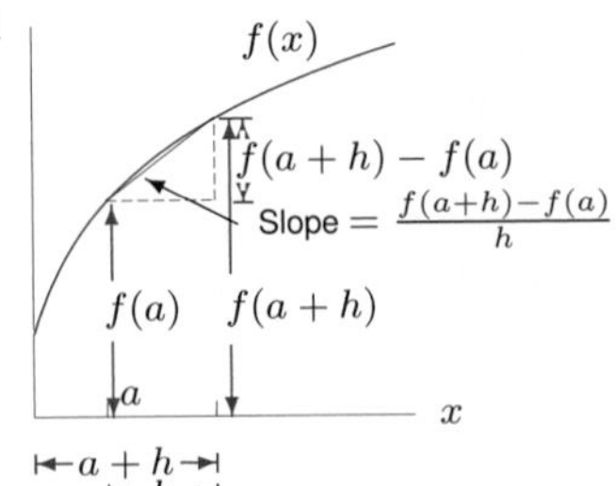

3 1
5 27
7 2.7

9 Yes

11 No; yes

13 Yes

15 Yes

17 No

19 Not continuous

21 Not continuous

23 Not continuous

Section 3.1

1 0

3 $12x^{11}$

5 $\frac{4}{3}x^{1/3}$

7 $12t^3 - 4t$

9 $-4x^{-5}$

11 $2x + 5$

13 $6x + 7$

15 $8.4q - 0.5$

17 $-5t^{-6}$

19 $-(7/2)r^{-9/2}$

21 $-(1/3)\theta^{-4/3}$

23 $15t^4 - \frac{5}{2}t^{-1/2} - 7t^{-2}$

25 $6t - 6/t^{3/2} + 2/t^3$

27 $(3/2)x^{1/2} + (1/2)x^{-1/2}$

29 $2kx$

31 $2aP + 3bP^2$

33 $b/(2\sqrt{t})$

35 $3ab^2$

37 (a) $P'(1)$: Positive;
$P'(3)$: Zero;
$P'(4)$: Negative

8 6 4 2
$P(q) = 6q - q^2$
q
1 2 3 4 5 6

(b) $P'(1) = 4$, $P'(3) = 0$, $P'(4) = -2$

39 (a) $2t - 4$
(b) $f'(1) = -2$, $f'(2) = 0$

41 Height $= 625$ cm,
Changing (eroding) at -30 cm/year

43 $f(10) = 400$ tons;
$f'(10) = 60$ tons per year;
Relative rate $= 15\%$ per year

45 $f'(t) = 6t^2 - 8t + 3$
$f''(t) = 12t - 8$

47 (a) $f(100) = 11.11$ seconds
(b) $f'(100) = 0.05555$ seconds per foot

49 $y = 2x - 1$

51 $y = -2t + 16$

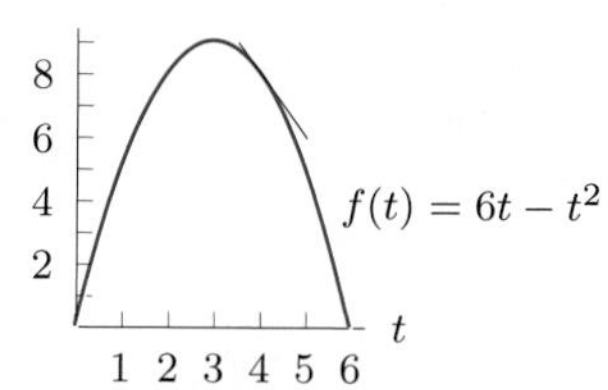

53 (a) $dA/dr = 2\pi r$
(b) Circumference of a circle

55 \$100

57 (a) 770 bushels per acre
(b) 40 bushels per acre per pound of fertilizer
(c) Use more fertilizer

59 (a) $dC/dq = 0.24q^2 + 75$
(b) $C(50) = \$14{,}750$; $C'(50) = \$675$ per item

61 $f'(x) = 3x^2 - 12x - 15$,
$x = -1$ and $x = 5$

63 (a) $R(q) = bq + mq^2$
(b) $R'(q) = b + 2mq$

Section 3.2

1 $2e^x + 2x$

3 $10t + 4e^t$

5 $(\ln 2)2^x - 6x^{-4}$

7 $(\ln 2)2^x + 2(\ln 3)3^x$

9 $3 - 2(\ln 4)4^x$

11 $3e^{3t}$

13 $-4e^{-4t}$

15 $-30e^{-0.6t}$

17 $3000(\ln 1.02)(1.02)^t$

19 Ce^t

21 $Ae^x - 2Bx$

23 $3/q$

25 $2t + 5/t$

27 $2x + 4 - 3/x$

29 $f'(-1) \approx -0.736$
$f'(0) = -2$
$f'(1) \approx -5.437$

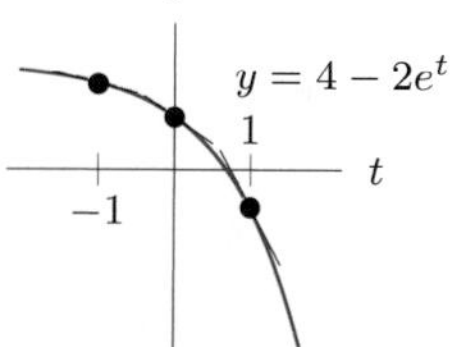

31 $y = -2t + 1$

33 (a) 13,394 fish
(b) 8037 fish/month

35 $f(2) = 6065$, $f'(2) = -1516$

37 $f(5) = \$563.30$;
$f'(5) = \$70$ per week;
Relative rate $= 12.4\%$ per week

39 -444.3 people/year

41 $c = -1/\ln 2$

43 $C(50) \approx 1365$, $C'(50) \approx 18.27$

45 (a) 0.021 micrograms/year
(b) 779.4 years old in 1998

47 (a) $P = 1.166(1.015)^t$
(b) $\frac{dP}{dt} = 1.166(1.015)^t(\ln 1.015)$
$\frac{dP}{dt}|_{t=0} = 0.017$ billion people per year
$\frac{dP}{dt}|_{t=25} = 0.025$ billion people per year

49 (a) $y = x - 1$
(b) 0.1; 1
(c) Yes

Section 3.3

1 $56x(4x^2 + 1)^6$

3 $8q(q^2 + 1)^3$

5 $300t^2(t^3 + 1)^{99}$

7 $3s^2/(2\sqrt{s^3 + 1})$

9 $216q(3q^2 - 5)^2$

11 $25e^{5t+1}$

13 $(e^{\sqrt{s}})/(2\sqrt{s})$

15 $1/(x - 1)$

17 $e^{-x}/(1 - e^{-x})$

19 $25/(5t + 1)$

21 $3/(3t + 2)$

23 $5 + 1/(x + 2)$

25 $0.5/(x(1 + \ln x)^{0.5})$

27 $-x/\sqrt{1 - x^2}$

29 $10/(10t + 5)$

31 5

33 $2/t$

35 1.5

37 $2/t$

39 $y = 3x - 5$

41 $v(t) = 10e^{\frac{t}{2}}$

43 $f(10) = 31.640$ feet;
$f'(10) = 4.741$ ft/sec;
Relative rate $= 15\%$ per second

45 0

47 1/2

49 Approx 1

51 Approx 1.9

Section 3.4

1 $f'(x) = 12x - 1$

3 $e^x(x + 1)$

5 $5e^{x^2} + 10x^2e^{x^2}$

7 $\ln x + 1$

9 $30t + 11$

11 $t + 2t\ln t$

13 $-(5/t^2) - (12/t^3)$

15 $e^{-t^2}(1 - 2t^2)$

17 $2p/(2p + 1) + \ln(2p + 1)$

19 $2we^{w^2}(5w^2 + 8)$

21 $(3t^2 + 5)(t^2 - 7t + 2) + (t^3 + 5t)(2t - 7)$

23 $(1 - x)/e^x$

25 $-2/(1 + t)^2$

27 $(15 + 10y + y^2)/(5 + y)^2$

29 $(ak - bc)/(cx + k)^2$

31 $ae^{-bx} - abxe^{-bx}$

33 $(1 - 2\alpha)e^{-2\alpha}e^{\alpha e^{-2\alpha}}$

35 $y = 0$

37 60.65 mg, 30.33 mg/hr,
41.04 mg, -12.31 mg/hr

39 $(kc)/(k + r)^2$;
Approx change in P per unit increase in r

41 Revenue $R(10) \approx 22{,}466$.
$R'(10) \approx \$449$/dollar.

43 $1/t$

45 $(fg)'/(fg) = (f'/f) + (g'/g)$

Section 3.5

1 $5\cos x$

3 $2t - 5\sin t$

5 $2q + 2\sin q$

7 $3\cos(3x)$

9 $-8t\sin(t^2)$

11 $2x\cos(x^2)$

13 $-4\sin(4\theta)$

15 $2x\cos x - x^2\sin x$

17 $3\theta^2\cos\theta - \theta^3\sin\theta$

19 $(2t\cos t + t^2\sin t)/(\cos t)^2$

21 $y = -x + \pi$

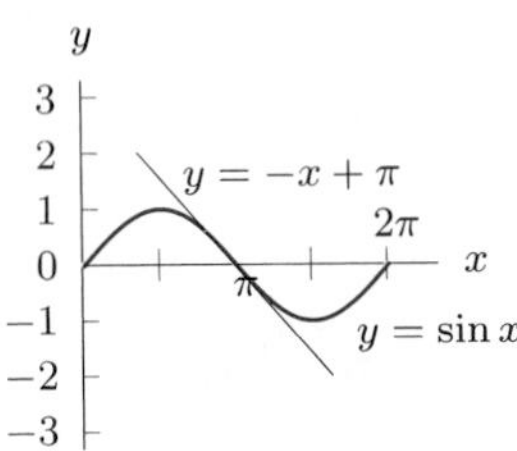

23 Decreasing, concave up

25 (a) max \$2600; min \$1400; April 1

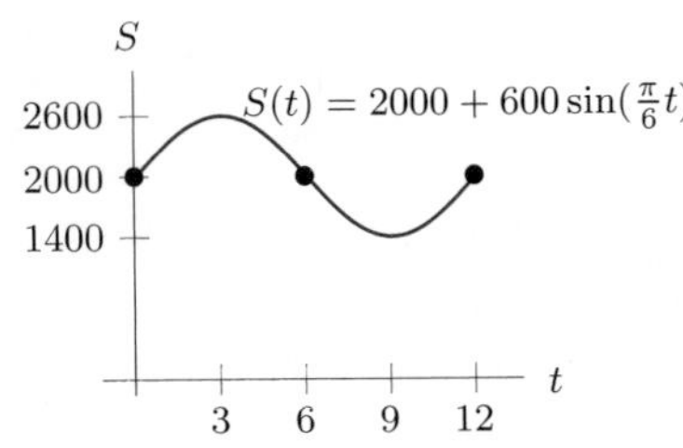

(b) $S(2) \approx 2519.62$; $S'(2) \approx 157.08$

27 (a) Falling, 0.38 m/hr
(b) Rising, 3.76 m/hr
(c) Rising, 0.75 m/hr
(d) Falling, 1.12 m/hr

29 (a) $H'(t) = (-10\pi/3)\sin((\pi/15)t)$
(b) $t = 0, 15, 30$ days; the percentage illuminated is not changing
(c) $H'(t)$ negative for $0 < t < 15$ and positive for $15 < t < 30$

Chapter 3 Review

1 $24t^3$

3 $2e^{2t}$

5 $0.08e^{0.08q}$

7 $e^{3x}(1+3x)$

9 $6(1+3t)e^{(1+3t)^2}$

11 $5 + 3.6e^{1.2t}$

13 $90(5x-1)^2$

15 $10e^x(1+e^x)^9$

17 $x(2\ln x + 1)$

19 $8t + 7\cos t$

21 $(-e^{-t} - 1)/(e^{-t} - t)$

23 $(50x - 25x^2)/(e^x)$

25 $2x\cos x - x^2\sin x$

27 e

29 $(e^x - 2 - e^{-x})/(1 - e^{-x})^2$

31 $xe^x + e^x$

33 $-3x^2\sin(x^3)$

35 $(t^2 + 6t + 13)/(t+3)^2$

37 $((\ln 3)3^x)/3 - (33x^{-3/2})/2$

39 $6y^2 e^{(y^3)} e^{2e^{(y^3)}}$

41 $f'(0) = 0$, $f'(1) = 2$, $f'(2) = 4$, $f'(-1) = -2$

43 $y = -4 - x$

45 30% per year

47 49.7% per year

49 73.7 m/yr

51 (a)

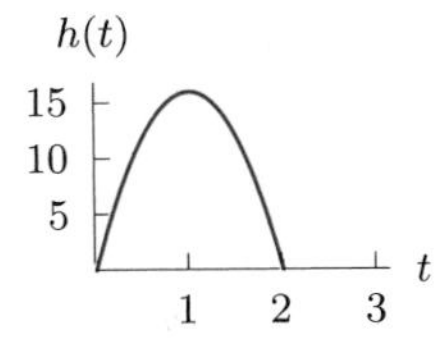

(b) $v(t) = 32 - 32t$

(c) $v(1) = 0$ ft/sec; $h(1) = 16$ ft

53 (a) $f'(0) = -1$
(b) $y = -x$

55 \$596.73/yr

57 (a) $\pi/\sqrt{9.8l}$
(b) Decr

59 (a) $dH/dt = -60e^{-2t}$
(b) $dH/dt < 0$
(c) At $t = 0$

61 (a) \$13,050
(b) $V'(t) = -4.063(0.85)^t$; thousands of dollars/year
(c) $V'(4) = -\$2121$ per year

63 (a) $P(d) = 4.07264 \cdot 10^{-10} d^{3/2}$
(b) Approximately 88 days
(c) $P'(d) = 6.10896 \cdot 10^{-10} d^{1/2}$ days/mile. Farther from the sun, time increases

65 $n = 4$, $a = 3/32$

67 (a) $H(4) = 1$
(b) $H'(4) = 30$
(c) $H(4) = 4$
(d) $H'(4) = 56$
(e) $H'(4) = -1$

69 $b = 1/40$ and $a = 169.36$

71 Approx 0.4

73 Approx 0.7

75 Approx -21.2

77 (a) $x < 1/2$
(b) $x > 1/4$
(c) $x < 0$ or $x > 0$

79 (a) $dy/dt = -(4.4\pi/6)\sin(\pi t/6)$ ft/hr
(b) Occurs at $t = 0$, 6, 12, 18, and 24 hrs

81 (c) $B'(10) \approx -3776.63$

83 If $a \neq e$, two solutions
If $a = e$, one solution

85 (a) 0.04 gal/mile; 0.06 gal/mile
(b) 25 mpg; 16.67 mpg
(d) 1.4 gallons
(e) 2.8 gal/hour; 1.8 gal/hour

87 $331.3 + 0.606T$ m/sec

Ch. 3 Understanding

1 True

3 True

5 True

7 False

9 True

11 False

13 False

15 False; $f(x) = |x|$

17 False; $\cos t + t^2$

19 False; $f(x) = 6, g(x) = 10$

21 False; $f(x) = 5x + 7, g(x) = x + 2$

23 False; $f(x) = x^2, g(x) = x^2 - 1$

25 False; $f(x) = e^{-x}, g(x) = x^2$

27 (a) Not a counterexample
(b) Not a counterexample
(c) Not a counterexample
(d) Counterexample

29 False

31 False

33 Possible answer

$$f(x) = \begin{cases} x & \text{if } 0 \le x < 2 \\ 19 & \text{if } x = 2 \end{cases}$$

Practice: Differentiation

1 $2t + 4t^3$

3 $15x^2 + 14x - 3$

5 $-2/x^3 + 5/(2\sqrt{x})$

7 $10e^{2x} - 2 \cdot 3^x(\ln 3)$

9 $2pe^{p^2} + 10p$

11 $2x\sqrt{x^2+1} + x^3/\sqrt{x^2+1}$

13 $16/(2t+1)$

15 $2^x(\ln 2) + 2x$

17 $6(2q+1)^2$

19 bke^{kt}

21 $2x\ln(2x+1) + 2x^2/(2x+1)$

23 $10\cos(2x)$

25 $15\cos(5t)$

27 $2e^x + 3\cos x$

29 $17 + 12x^{-1/2}$

31 $20x^3 - 2/x^3$

33 $1, x \neq -1$

35 $-3\cos(2-3x)$

37 $6/(5r+2)^2$

39 $ae^{ax}/(e^{ax}+b)$

41 $5(w^4 - 2w)^4(4w^3 - 2)$

43 $(\cos x - \sin x)/(\sin x + \cos x)$

45 $6/w^4 + 3/(2\sqrt{w})$

47 $(2t - ct^2)e^{-ct}$

49 $(\cos\theta)e^{\sin\theta}$

51 $3x^2/a + 2ax/b - c$

53 $2r(r+1)/(2r+1)^2$

55 $2e^t + 2te^t + 1/(2t^{3/2})$

57 $x^2 \ln x$

59 $6x\left(x^2+5\right)^2\left(3x^3-2\right)\left(6x^3+15x-2\right)$

61 $(2abr-ar^4)/(b+r^3)^2$

63 $20w/(a^2-w^2)^3$

Section 4.1

1 One

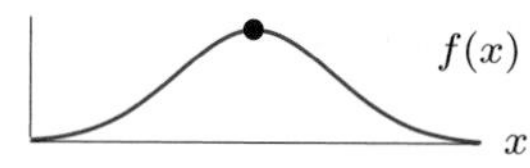

3 Three

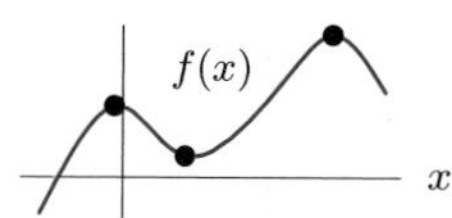

5 (a)

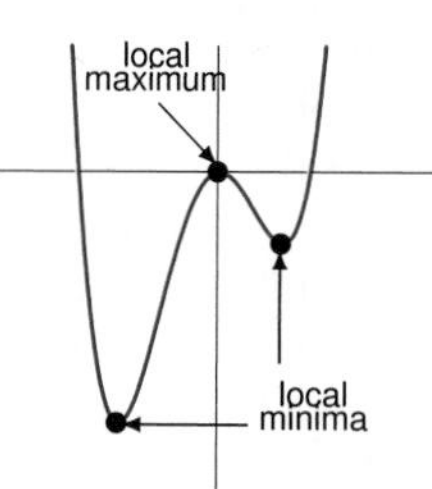

(b)

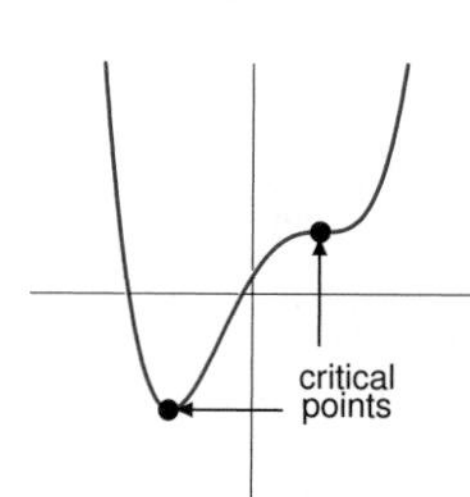

7 (a)

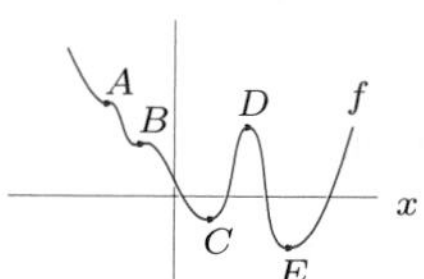

(b)

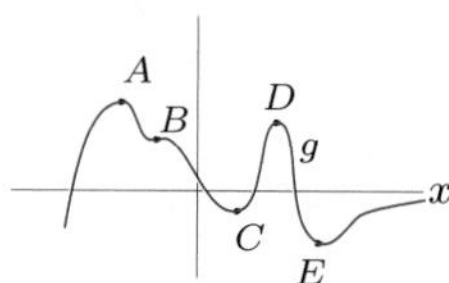

9 A: local max
B: local min
C: neither

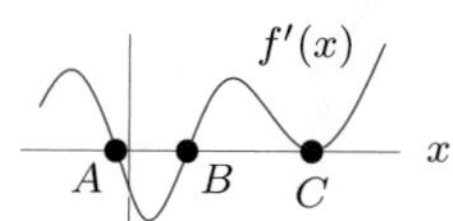

11 Increasing for all x, no critical point

13 Local min: $(2.3, -13.0)$

15 Alternately incr/decr

17

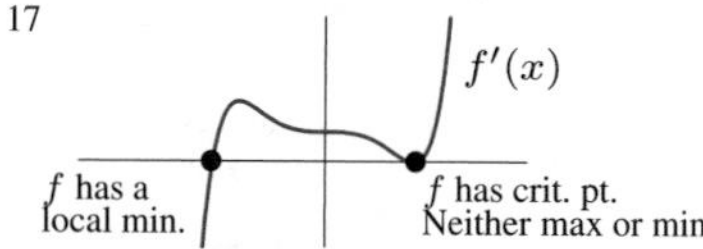

19 $t = 0.5\ln(V/U)$

21 (a) $x \approx 2.5$ (or any $2 < x < 3$)
$x \approx 6.5$ (or any $6 < x < 7$)
$x \approx 9.5$ (or any $9 < x < 10$)
(b) $x \approx 2.5$: local max;
$x \approx 6.5$: local min;
$x \approx 9.5$: local max

23 $x = 0$: not max/min
$x = 3/7$: local max
$x = 1$: local min

25 (a)

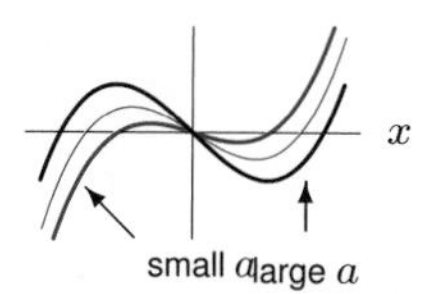

(b) 2 critical points move farther from origin
(c) $x = \pm\sqrt{a/3}$

27 $a = -6$; $b = 14$

29

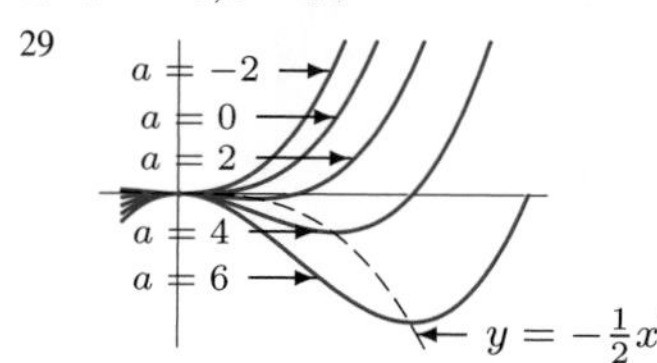

31 $a = -1/3$

33 (a) $x = 0, x = a^2/4$
(b) $a = \sqrt{20}$; Local minimum

35 Domain: All real numbers except $x = b$;
Critical points: $x = 0$, $x = 2b$

37 (a) $f(\theta) = 0$ at $\theta = 0$
(b) $f'(\theta) = 1 - \cos\theta > 0$
for $0 < \theta \leq 1$.
Only zero is at origin

Section 4.2

1 Three

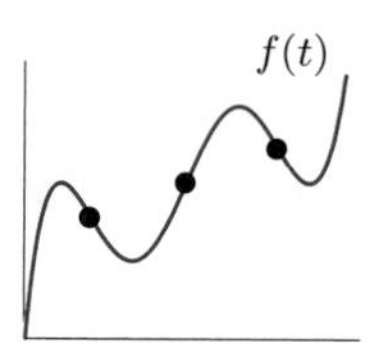

3 One

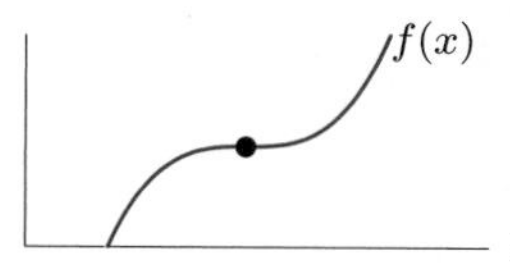

5 (a)

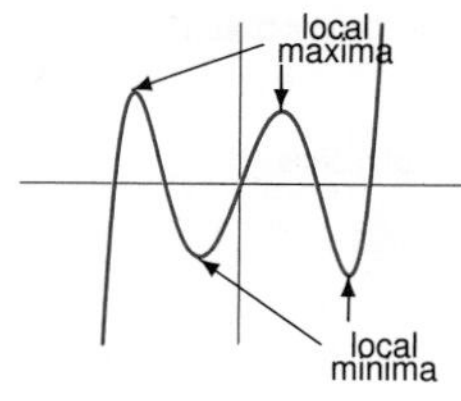

(b) 3

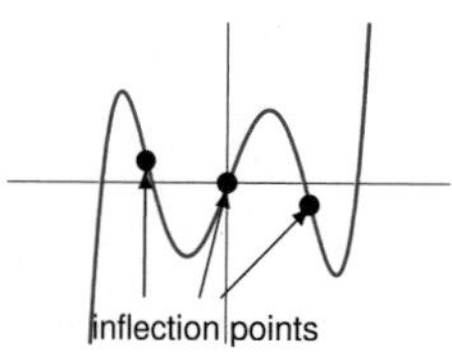

7

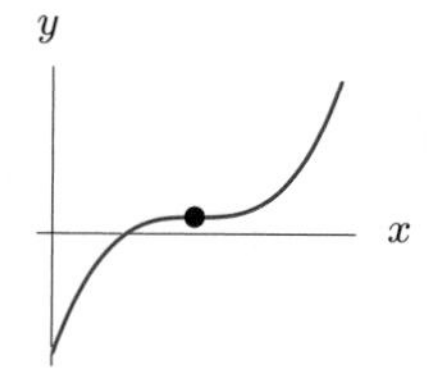

9 (a) 6 pm
(b) Noon; another between noon and 6 pm

11 Critical points: $x = \frac{5}{2}$, local minimum
Inflection points: None

13 Critical points:
$x = -3$ (local max) and $x = 2$ (local min)
Inflection point: $x = -1/2$

15 Critical points: $x = -1$, local min; $x = 0$ local max; $x = 1$, local min
Inflection points: $x = -1/\sqrt{3}$, $x = 1/\sqrt{3}$

17 Critical points:
$x = 0$ (local max) and $x = \pm 2$ (local minima)
Inflection points: $x = \pm 2/\sqrt{3}$

19 Critical points: $x = 0$, local max; $x = 4$, local min
Inflection point: $x = 3$

21 $x = -1, 1/2$

23

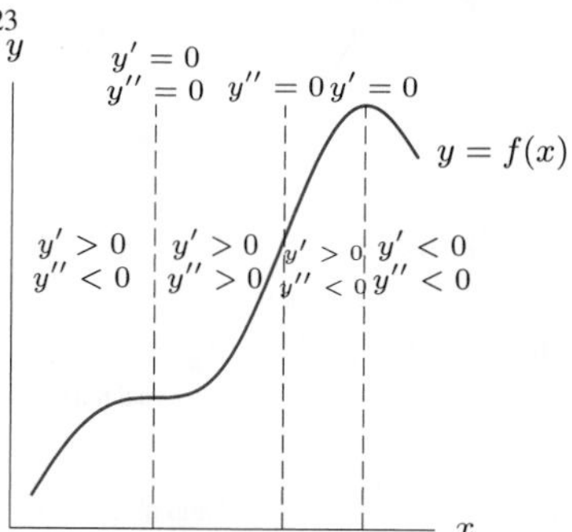

27 (a) Yes, at 2000 rabbits

population of rabbits
2000
1500
1000
500
years since 1774
10 20 30 40

(b) 1787, 1000 rabbits
(c) 1787, 1000 rabbits

29 depth of water

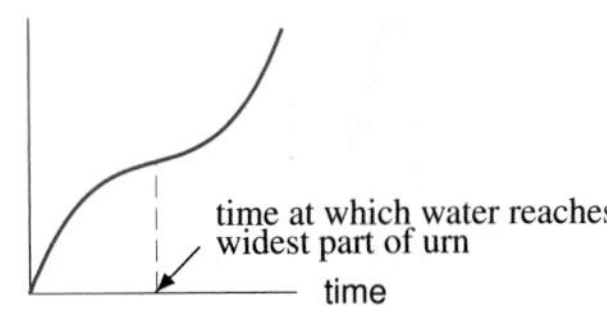

31 H (height)

t (time)
t_1 $2t_1$ t_3

33 $y = x^3 - 3x^2 + 6$

35 (a) $f(x)$

(b)

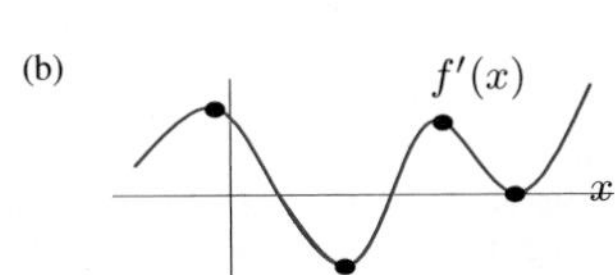

(c)

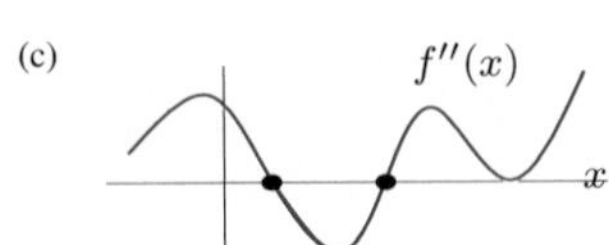

Section 4.3

1

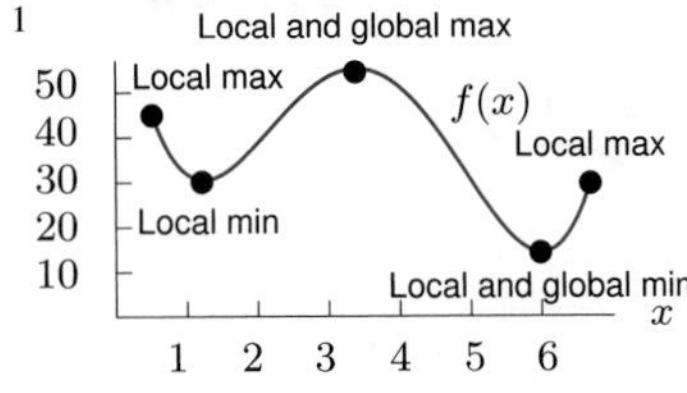

3 (a) (IV)
(b) (I)
(c) (III)
(d) (II)

5

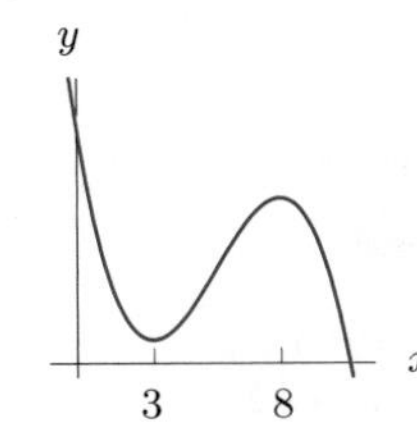

7

y
x

9

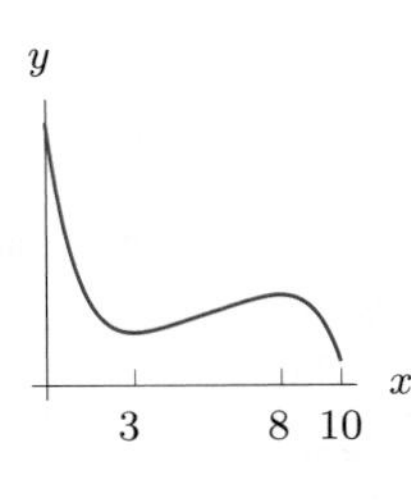

11

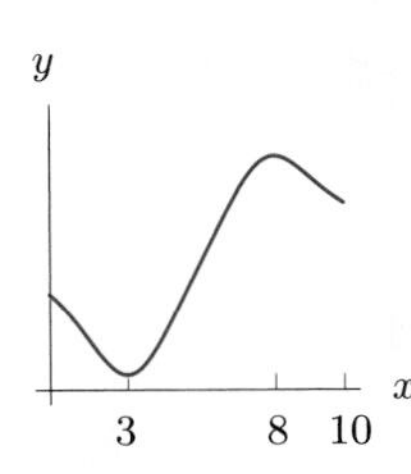

13 44.1 feet

15 (a) $f(0.91)$ is global minimum
$f(3.73)$ is global maximum
(b) $f(-3)$ is global minimum
$f(2)$ is global maximum

17 (a) $D = C$
(b) $D = C/2$

19 (a) $f'(x) = 6x^2 - 18x + 12$,
$f''(x) = 12x - 18$.
(b) $x = 1, 2$
(c) $x = 3/2$
(d) Local minimum: $x = 2$
Local maximum: $x = 1$
Global minimum: $x = -0.5$
Global maximum: $x = 3$
(e)

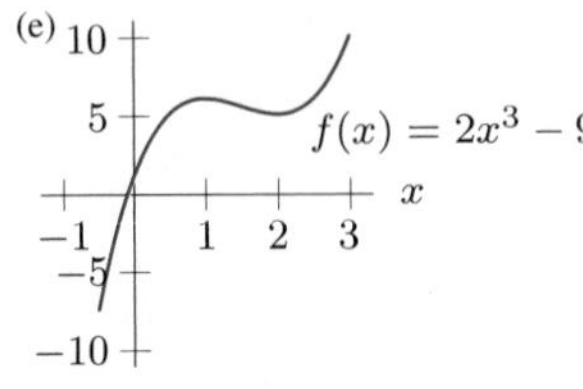

21 (a) $f'(x) = 1 + \cos x$,
$f''(x) = -\sin x$.

(b) $x = \pi$
(c) $x = 0, \pi, 2\pi$
(d) Global minimum: $x = 0$
Global maximum: $x = 2\pi$
(e)

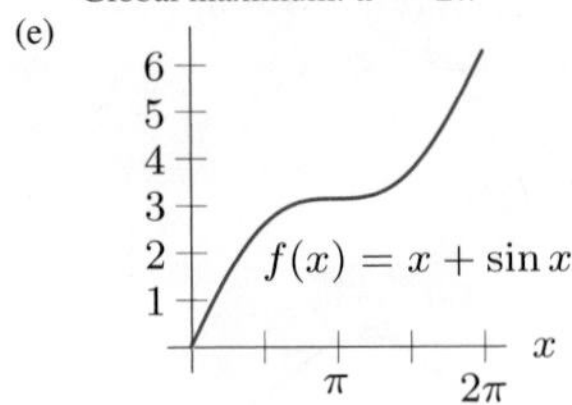

23 Global max $= -1$ at $x = 2$
No global min

25 Global max $= 1/e$ at $t = 1$
No global min

27 Global max $= 1/2$ at $t = 1$
Global min $= -1/2$ at $t = -1$

29 $x = -b/2a$,
Max if $a < 0$, min if $a > 0$

31 (b) Yes, at $x = 0$
(c) Max: $x = -2$, Min: $x = 2$
(d) $5 > g(0) > g(2)$

33 1250 square feet

35 (a) $x + 27/x$ meters
(b) 5.2 meters

37 (a) $y = \begin{cases} 200x & x \leq 200 \\ 600x - x^2 & x > 200 \end{cases}$

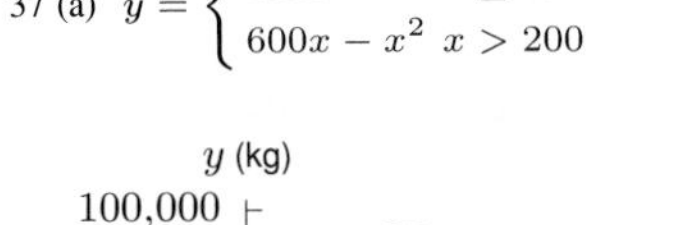

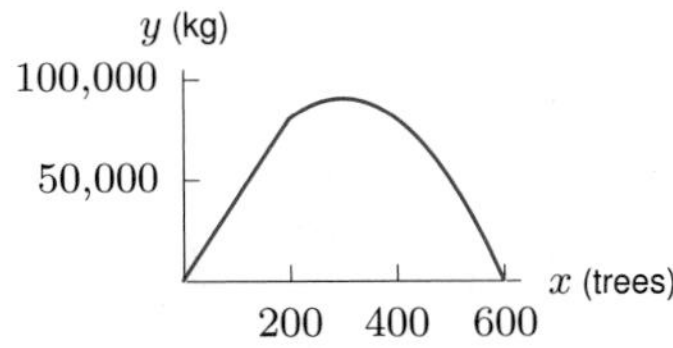

(b) 300 trees/km^2

39 (a) $H = 1/b$, $S = ae^{-1}/b$
(b) a: Increases
b: Decreases

41 (a) 10
(b) 9

43 (a) $k(\ln k - \ln S_0) - k + S_0 + I_0$
(b) Both

45 (a) 120 mm Hg, 80 mm Hg
(b) 0.8 sec
(c)

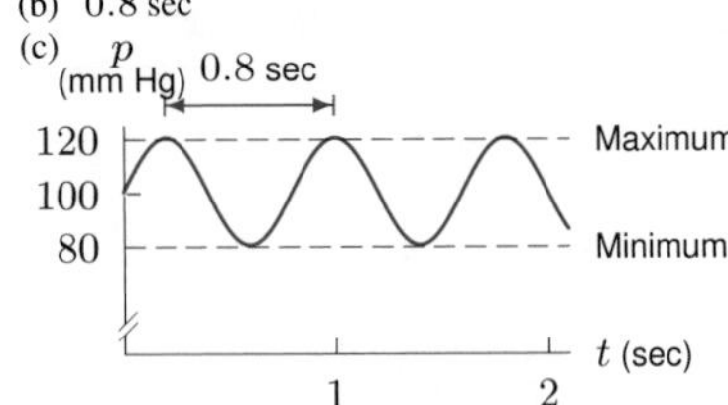

47 (a) $0 \leq y \leq a$

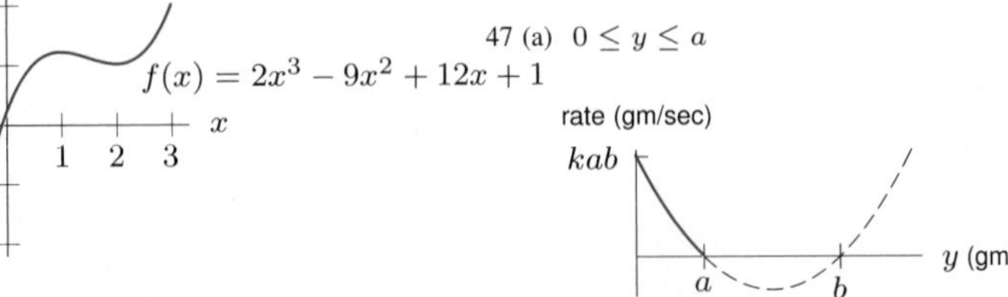

(b) $y = 0$

Section 4.4

1 $5.5 < q < 12.5$ positive;
$0 < q < 5.5$ and $q > 12.5$ negative;
Maximum at $q \approx 9.5$

3 (a) $q = 2500$
(b) \$3 per unit
(c) \$3000

5 (a) \$9
(b) $-\$3$
(c) $C'(78) = R'(78)$

7 (a) Increase production
(b) $q = 8000$

9 \$0.20/item

11 $q = 0$ or $q = 3000$

13 One; between 40 and 50

15 (a) MR; increase production
(b) MC; decrease production

17 Global maximum of \$6875 at $q = 75$

19 (a) Approximately \$1
(b) No
(c) About 400 items

21 (a) \$10; \$30,000; \$50,000
(b) $R(q) = 70q - 0.02q^2$
(c) 1750
(d) \$35
(e) \$61,250

23 \$14.

25 (a) $10{,}000 + 2q$
(b) $q = 37{,}820 - 5544p$
(c) $\pi = -0.00018q^2 + 4.822q - 10{,}000$
(d) $13{,}394$ items, \$22,294

27 Maximum revenue = \$27,225
Minimum = \$0

29 (a) q/r months
(b) $(ra/q) + rb$ dollars
(c) $C = (ra/q) + rb + kq/2$ dollars
(d) $q = \sqrt{2ra/k}$

31 $L = [\beta pcK^{\alpha}/w]^{1/(1-\beta)}$

Section 4.5

1 (a) No
(b) Yes

3 (a) $a(1000) \approx \$1.60$ per unit
(b)

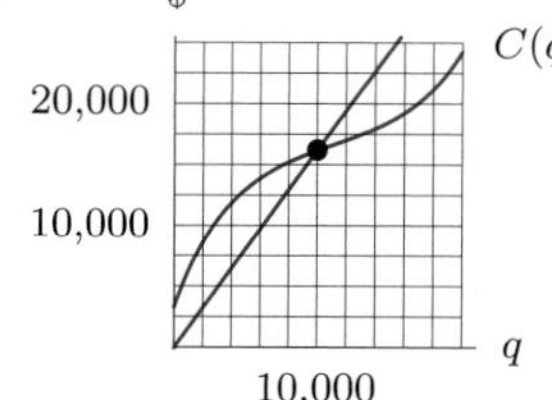

(c) 18,000 units

5 $MC = \$20$; $a(q) = \$25$

7 (a) $q = 6$

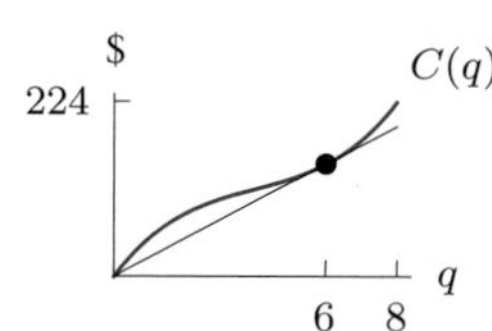

(b) $q = 6$

9 (a) $C(q) = 0.01q^3 - 0.6q^2 + 13q$
(b) \$1
(c) $q = 30$, $a(30) = 4$
(d) Marginal cost is 4

11 (a)

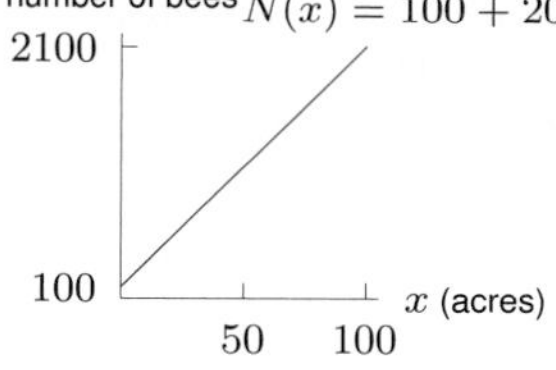

(b) (i) $N'(x) = 20$
(ii) $N(x)/x = (100/x) + 20$

13

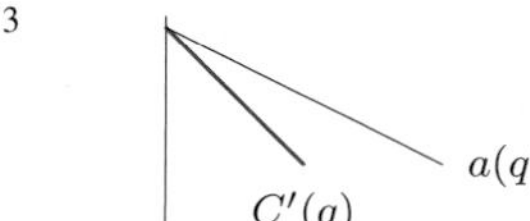

Section 4.6

1 (a) 1.5% decrease
(b) 1.5% increase

5 Elastic

7 High

9 Low

11 (a) $E \approx 0.470$, inelastic
(c) $P = 1.25$ and 1.50

13 (a) $q = 4960$
(b) $E = 0.016$, so demand is inelastic

Section 4.7

1 (a) 40 billion
(b)

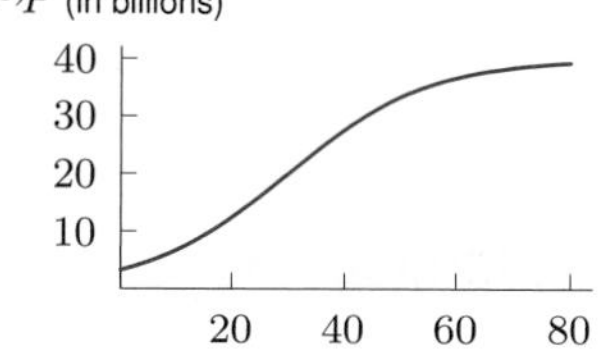

(c) 2020; 2095

3 (a)

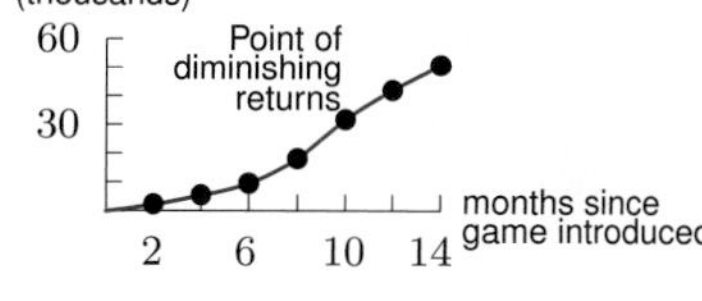

(b) 60,000

7 (a) 36 thousand; total number infected
(b) $t \approx 16$, $n \approx 18$ thousand
(c) Virus spreading fastest
(d) Number infected half total

9 (a) (b)

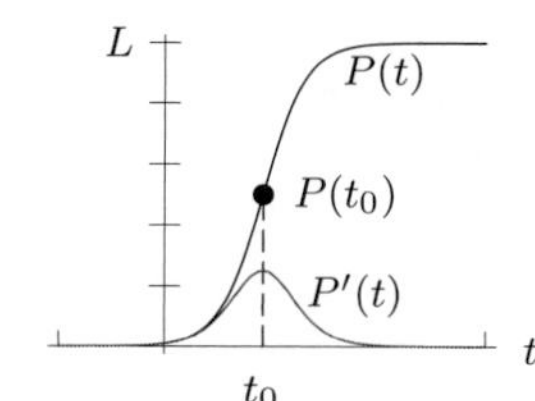

(c) P' maximum

11 (b) April 12, 2003
(d) $t = 19$; 1600 cases
(e) 1760 cases

15 (a)

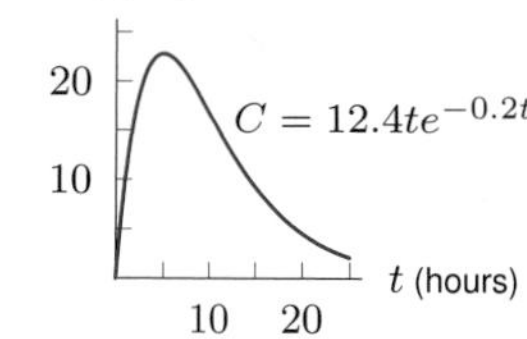

(b) About 46.05
(c) Between 32.12 and 54.52 mg

17 (b) $f'(10) < 11$
$f'(20) < 11$

19 10 mg to 18 mg

Section 4.8

1 (a)

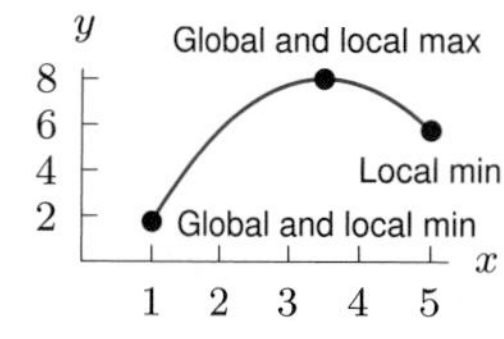

(b) 5 hrs, 22.8 ng/ml
(c) 1 to 14.4 hrs
(d) At least 20.8 hrs

9 $a = 49.3$; $b = 0.769$

13 (b) Min effective ≈ 0.2 Max safe ≈ 1.0
(c) Min effective ≈ 1.2 Max safe ≈ 2.0

Chapter 4 Review

1

Global and local max
Local min
Global and local min

3 (a) $f(1)$ local minimum;
$f(0)$, $f(2)$ local maxima
(b) $f(1)$ global minimum
$f(2)$ global maximum

5 Global min = 3 at $z = 1/2$
No global max

7 Global max = $1/2$ at $x = 1$
No global min

11 (a) Increasing for all x
(b) No maxima or minima

13 (a) Incr: $-1 < x < 0$ and $x > 1$
Decr: $x < -1$ and $0 < x < 1$
(b) Local max: $f(0)$
Local min: $f(-1)$ and $f(1)$

15 (a) cm/week

(b) Growing at 1.6 cm/wk in week 24

17 (a) Week 14
(b) Point of fastest growth

19 $a = 3e, b = -3$

21 (a) $5x^4 + 1$; positive
(b) One

25 (a) Polynomial; negative leading coefficient; degree 2
(b) Exponential.
(c) Logistic
(d) Logarithmic.
(e) Polynomial; positive leading coefficient; degree 2
(f) Exponential.
(g) Surge

27 (a) \$0
(b) \$96.56
(c) Raise the price by \$5

29 (a) $\pi(q)$ max when $R(q) > C(q)$ and R and Q are farthest apart

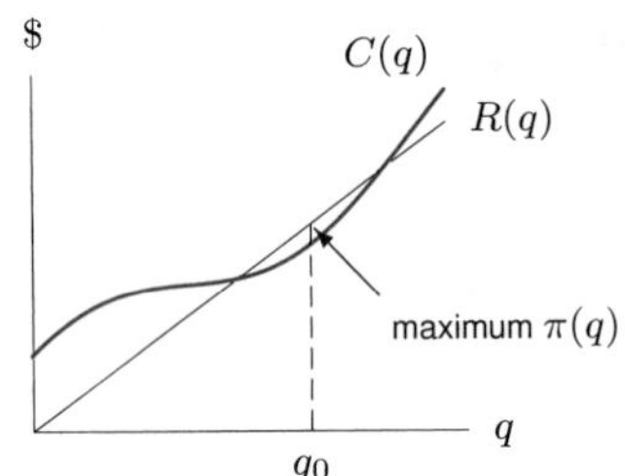

(b) $C'(q_0) = R'(q_0) = p$
(c)

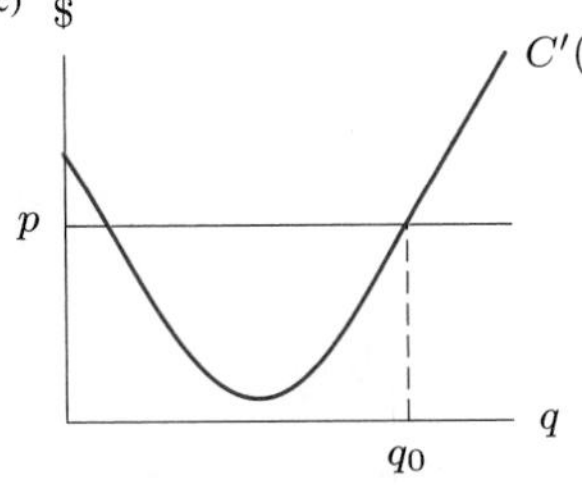

31

33 $C'(2)$

35 $(C(75) - C(50))/25$

37 $C(3)/3$

39 $E = 0.05$, demand is inelastic.

43 50 m by 50 m

45 (a) $1/5, 1$
(b) Local max: $p = 1/5$
Local min: $p = 1$
(c) Max: $256/3125$
Min: 0

47 (a) $E = 500e\left(\dfrac{2-\cos\theta}{\sin\theta}\right) + 2000e$
$\left(\arctan\left(\dfrac{500}{2000}\right) \le \theta \le \pi/2\right)$
(b) $\theta = \pi/3$
(c) Independent of e, but dependent on $\overline{AB}/\overline{AL}$

49 (a) $k(1 - 2P/L) \cdot dP/dt$

51 Intercepts: $(0,0), (1.77,0), (2.51,0)$
Critical Points: $(0,0), (1.25,1), (2.17,-1), (2.80,1)$
Inflection Points: $(0.81,0.61), (1.81,-0.13), (2.52,0.07)$

53 (a)

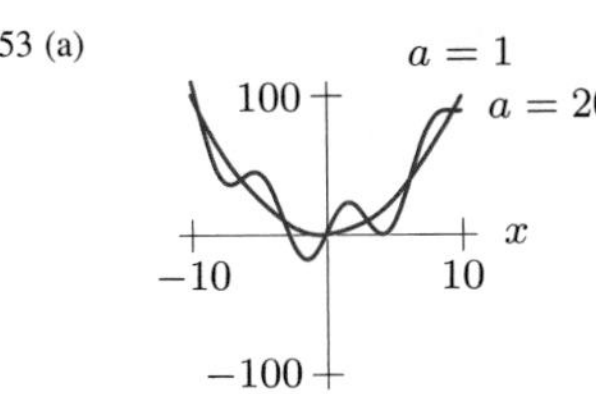

(b) $-2 < a < 2$

55 (a)

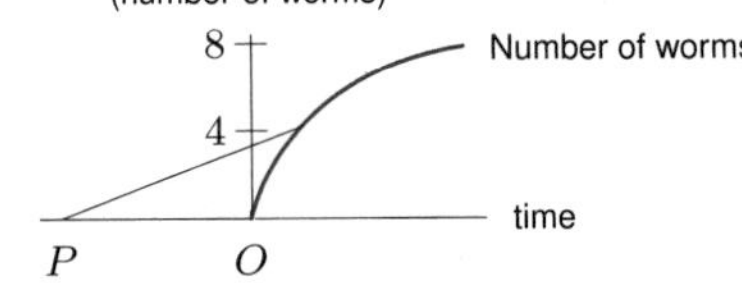

(b) 7 worms
(c) increases

57 Max slope $= 1/(3e)$ at $x = 1/3$

Ch. 4 Understanding

1 True

3 False

5 False

7 False

9 One possibility:
$f(x) = ax^2, a \ne 0$

11 (a) True
(b) False
(c) True
(d) False
(e) True

13 False

15 True

17 True

19 True

21 False

23 False

25 $f(x) = x^2 + 1$

27 $f(x) = -x^2 - 1$

29 Impossible

Section 5.1

1 (a)

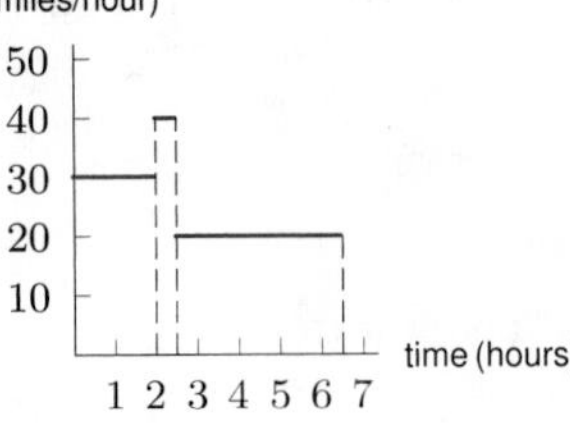

(b)

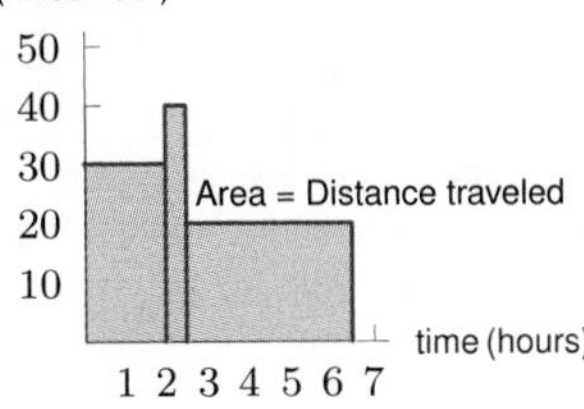

3 (a) Lower estimate $= 122$ ft
Upper estimate $= 298$ ft
(b)

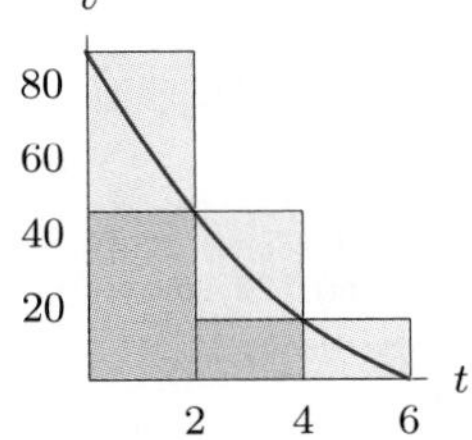

5 250 meters

7 ≈ 455 feet or 0.086 miles

9 (a) About 420 kg
(b) 336 and 504 kg

11 (a) 570 m^3
(b) Every 2 minutes

13 (a)

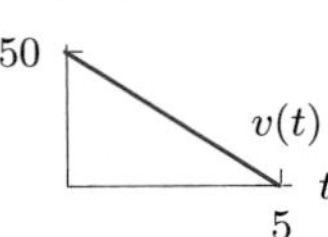

(b) 125 feet
(c) 4 times as far

15 (a) Car A
(b) Car A
(c) Car B

17 60 m (Other answers possible.)

19 (b) \$6151

Section 5.2

1 27

3 1692.5

5 About 543

7 (a) 224

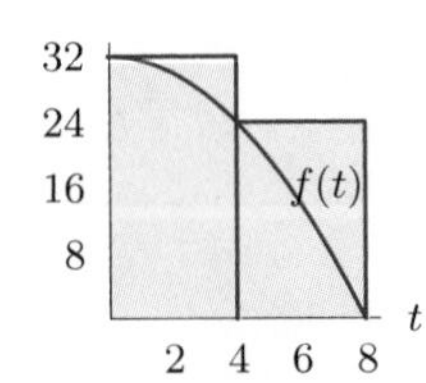

(b) 96

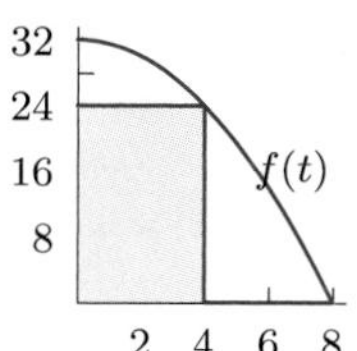

(c) 200

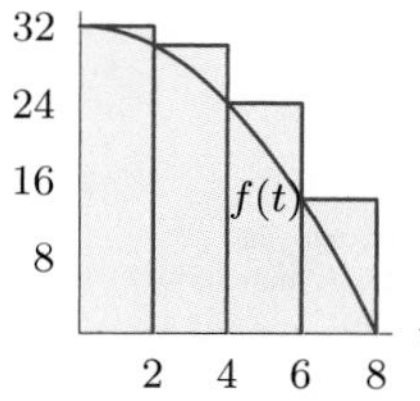

(d) 136

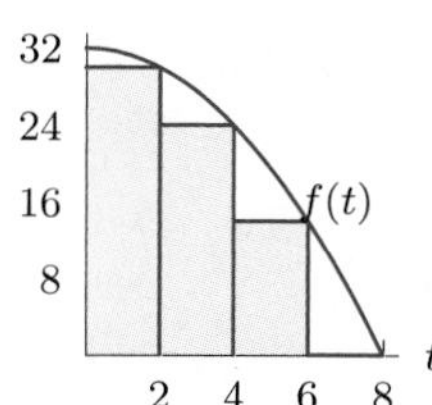

9 350

11 About 20

13 (a) 3.6

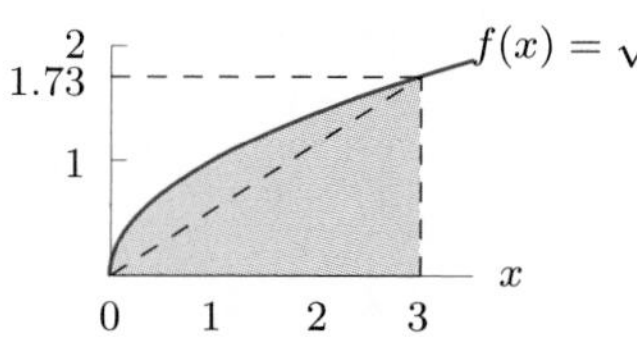

(b) 3.4641

15 (a) 2

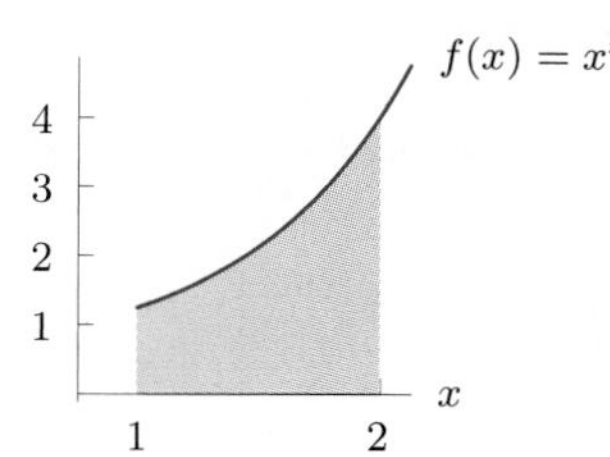

(b) 2.05045

17 (a) 78

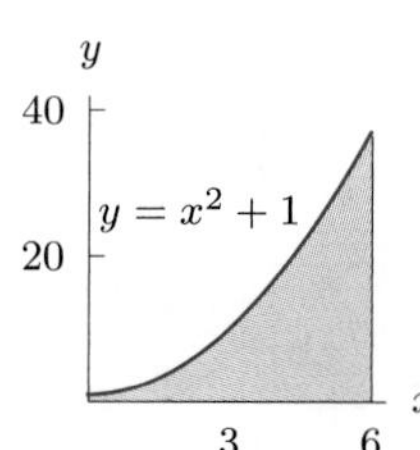

(b) 46; underestimate

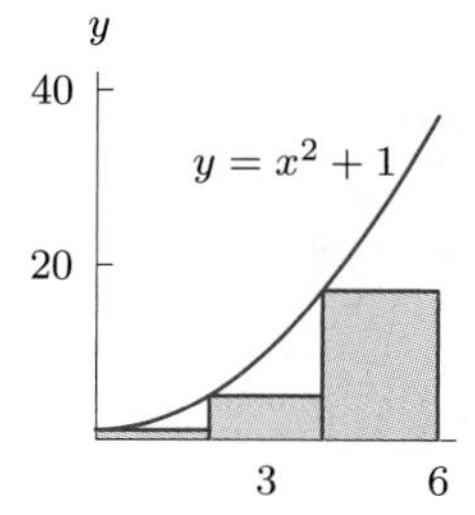

(c) 118; overestimate

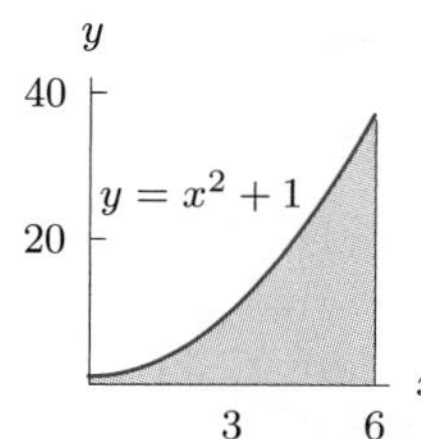

19 93.47

21 448.0

23 2.350

25 2.9

27 1.30

29 1.728, 1.816, 1.772, $n = 140$

31 (a) 4; 0, 4, 8, 12, 16; 25, 23, 22, 20, 17
(b) 360; 328
(c) 8; 0, 8, 16; 25, 22, 17
(d) 376; 312

Section 5.3

1 8

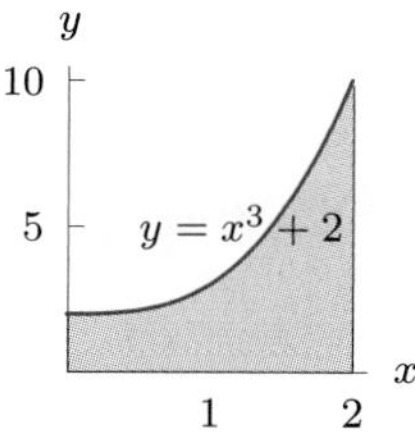

3 $\int_0^2 ((x+5) - (2x+1))\,dx = 6$

5 (a) 13
(b) 1

7 Positive

9 Positive

11 −40

13 (a) −4
(b) 0
(c) 8

15 II

17 III

19 V < IV < II < III < I
I, II, III positive
IV, V negative

21 (a) -2
(b) $-A/2$

23 About 3.34

25 0.80

27 14,052.5

29 14.688

31 13.457

33 2.762

Section 5.4

1 (a) Emissions 1970–2000, m. metric tons
(b) 772.8 million metric tons

3 Change in position; meters

5 Change in world pop; bn people

7 Total amount $= \int_0^{60} f(t)\,dt$.

9 1417 antibodies

11 29,089.813 megawatts

13 3.4 ft

15 (a) Concave up
(b) 3.1 kg

17 (a) 2023, at crossing of curves
(b) 2023, at highest point of curve

19 2627 acres

21 Tree B is taller after 5 years.
Tree A is taller after 10 years.

23 (a) Boys: black curve; girls: colored curve
(b) About 43 cm
(c) Boys: about 23 cm; girls: about 18 cm
(d) About 13 cm taller

25 More fat

27 (a) About 750 liters
(b) $\int_0^3 60g(t)\,dt$
(c) About 150 liters

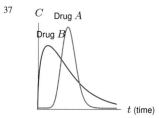

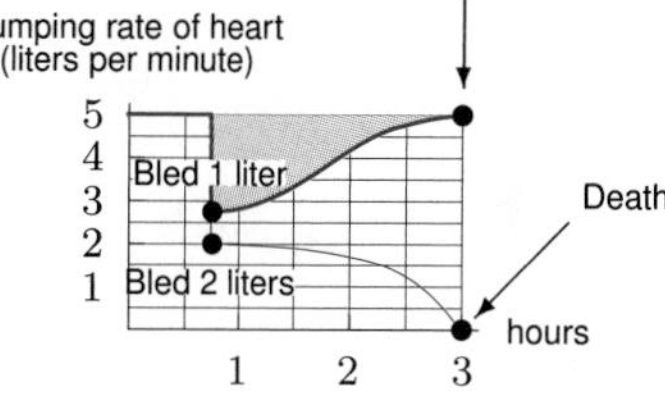

29 15 cm to the left

31 25 cm to the right

33 65 km from home
3 hours
90 km

35 Product B has a greater peak concentration
Product A peaks sooner
Product B has a greater overall bioavailability
Product A should be used

37

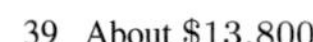

39 About $13,800

41 (a) $\int_0^T 49(1-(0.8187)^t)\,dt$ (meters)
(b) $T \approx 107$ seconds

Section 5.5

1 Dollars; cost of increasing production from 800 tons to 900 tons

3 (a)

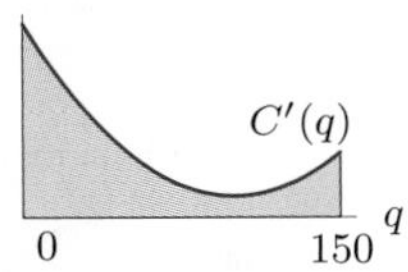

(b) $\$22,775$
(c) $C'(150) = 18.5$
(d) $C(151) \approx \$22,793.50$

5 7.65 million people

7 (a) $\$18,650$
(b) $C'(400) = 28$

9 (a)

200
150
100
50
$R'(q)$
50 100 150
q

(b) $\$12,000$
(c) Marginal revenue is $80/unit
Total revenue is $\$12,080$

11 (a) 7.54 inches after 8 hours
(b) 1.41 inches/hour

Chapter 5 Review

1 (a) 408
(b) 390

3 1096

5 Meters per second

7 Foot-pounds

9 1.44

11 1.15

13 -0.083

15 84

17 0.0833

19 About 0.1667

21 (a) 430 ft
(b) (ii)

23 (a)

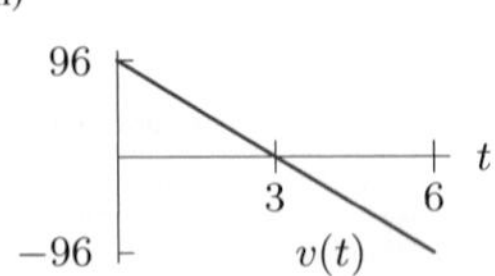

(b) 3 sec, 144 feet
(c) 80 feet

25 (a) Species B for both
(b) Species A

27 (a) Inflection point
(b) About 50 cm

29 (a) Negative
(b) Positive
(c) Negative
(d) Positive

33 (a) $\displaystyle\int_0^5 (10+8t-t^2)\,dt$
(b) 100
(c) 108.33

35 (a) Forward for $t < 3$, backward for $t > 3$
(b) Farthest forward: $t = 3$
Farthest backward:
no upper bound.

37 $\$300,000$

39 (a)

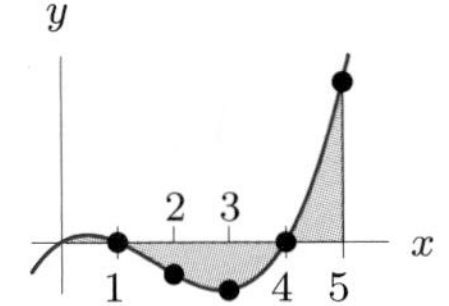

(b) I_1 is largest.
I_4 is smallest.
I_1 is the only positive value.

41 9 years

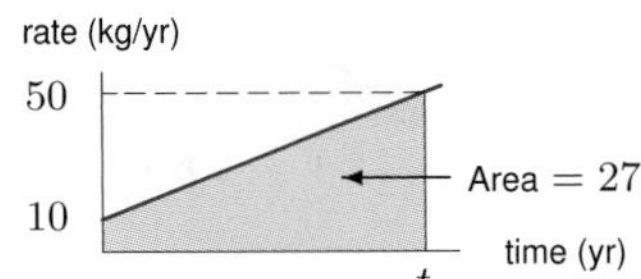

43 $F(x)$ is decreasing for $x < -2$ and $x > 2$;
$F(x)$ is increasing for $-2 < x < 2$

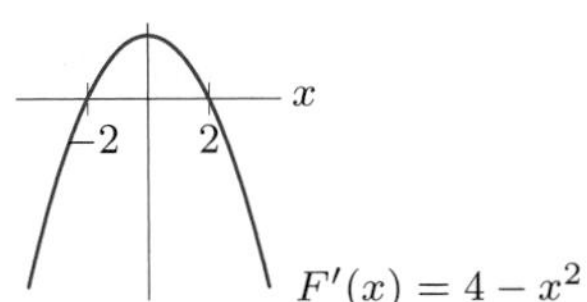

Ch. 5 Understanding

1 False

3 True

5 False

7 False

9 True

11 True

13 False

15 False

17 False

19 True

21 True

23 False

25 False

27

5
$f(x)$
x
0.4
10

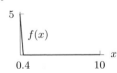

Theory: Second Fund. Thm.

1 x^3

3 xe^x

5 (a) 0
(b) F increases
(c) $F(1) \approx 1.4$, $F(2) \approx 4.3$, $F(3) \approx 10.1$

9 9

11 $8c$

Section 6.1

1 1.7

3 2

5 -3

7 About 8.5

9 (a) $26,667 per year
(b) Less 25–65; more 65–85

11 $6080

13 (a) 120 mm Hg
(b) 80 mm Hg
(c) 100 mm Hg
(d) Less

15 (a) 0.375 thousand/hour
(b) 1.75 thousands

17 (a) 9.9 hours
(b) 14.4 hours
(c) 12.0 hours

19 (a) Second half

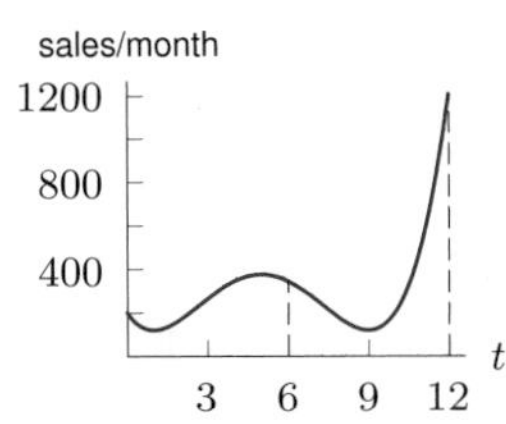

(b) $1531.20, $1963.20
(c) $3494.40
(d) $291.20/month

21 $(c) < (a) < (b)$

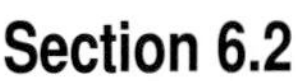

Section 6.2

1 (a) $p^* = \$30$, $q^* = 6000$
(b) Consumer surplus $= \$210,000$;
Producer surplus $\approx \$70,000$

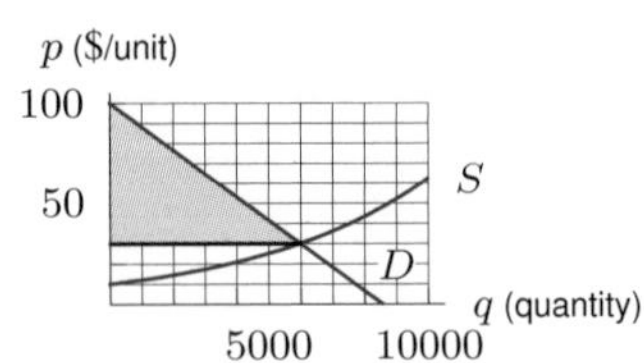

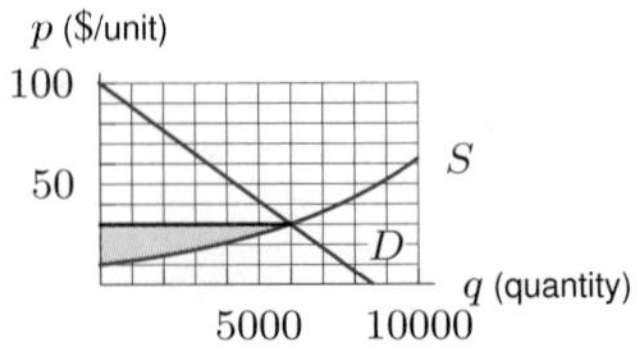

3 250

5 200

7 (a) Equilibrium price is $30
Equilibrium quantity is 125 units
(b) $3500
$2000

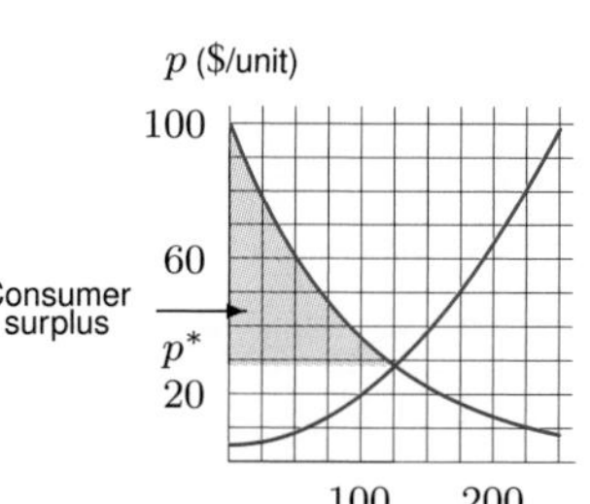

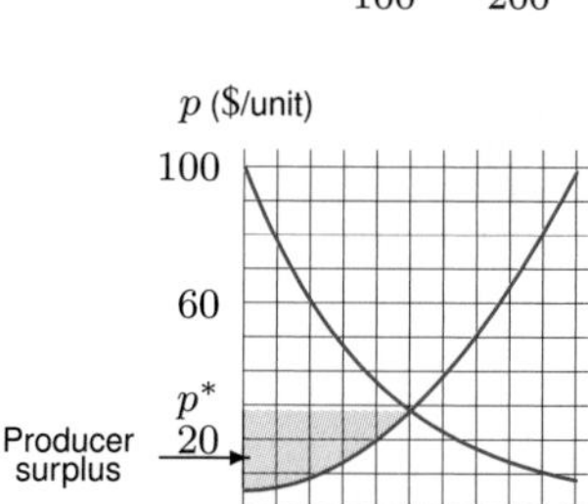

(c) $5500

9 (a) Supplied: $11, demanded: $7
(b) $p^* \approx \$9$
$q^* \approx 400$

(c) $1907
(d) $1600

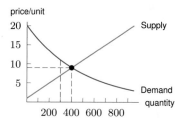

11 (a) Less
(b) Can't tell
(c) Less

13 (a) No, yes

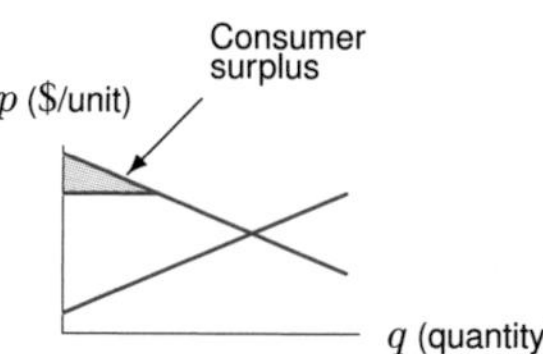

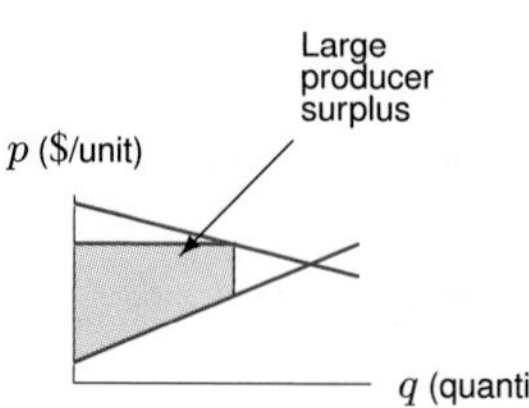

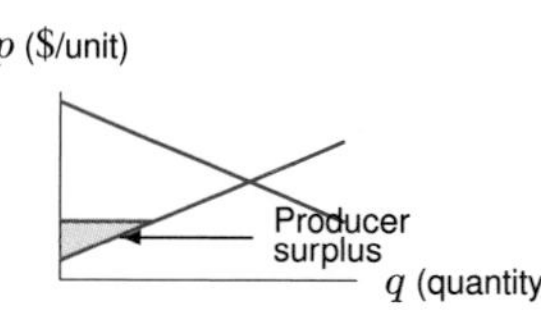

(b) Yes, no

Section 6.3

1 Future value = $72,980.16
Present value = $29,671.52

3 (a) $P = \$47{,}216.32$
$F = \$77{,}846.55$
(b) $60,000; $17,846.55

5 (a) (i) $18,846.59
(ii) $16,484.00
(b) (i) $21,249.47
(ii) $24,591.24

7 (a) $65,022
(b) ≈ 2.27 years

9 (a) $417,635.11
(b) $228,174.64

11 $41,508

13 (a) $4.6 billion; $8.6 billion
(b) $54.7 billion
(c) $77.6 billion

15 About 1.75 years

17 In 10 years

Section 6.4

3 11%

5 Absolute:
2003–2004: 3.1 m
2006–2007: 2.0 m
Relative:
2003–2004: 10.3%
2006–2007: 5.3%

7 (a) $P = 4000 - 100t$
(b) $P = 4000(0.95)^t$
Case (a)

9 22% increase

11 No change

13 Increasing $0 \le t \le 10$

15 Decreasing: $0 < t < 5$
Increasing: $5 < t < 10$

17 (a) $P = 5.78(1.018)^t$
(b) 0.10404 mil/yr
0.10591 mil/yr
(c) 1.8%, 1.8%

19 Decreases by about 9.52%

Chapter 6 Review

1 (a) 20
(b) 10/3

3 (a) 0.79

5 (a) $Q(10) \approx 2.7$,
$Q(20) \approx 1.8$
(b) 2.21
(c) 2.18

7 About 17

9 (a) $(1/5)\int_0^5 f(x)\,dx$
(b) $(1/5)(\int_0^2 f(x)\,dx - \int_2^5 f(x)\,dx)$

11 (a)

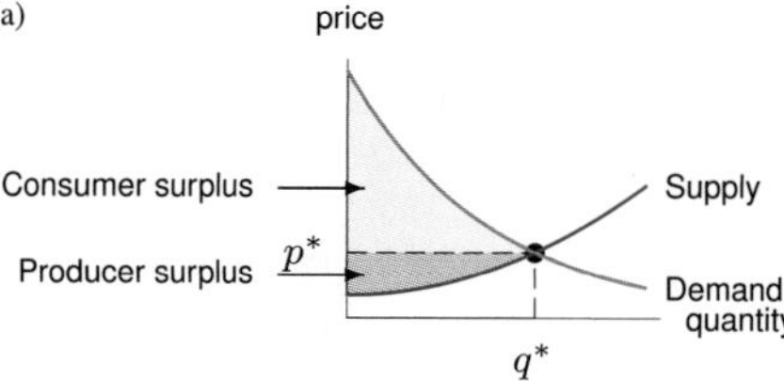

(b)

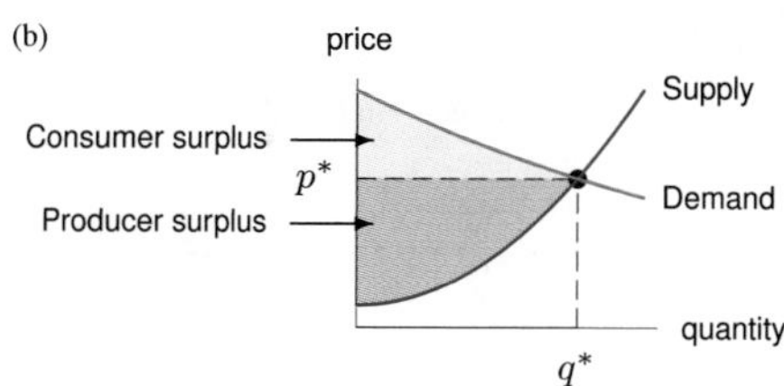

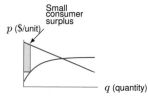

13 (a) Consumer: 87 units
Suppliers: 100 units
Down
(b) $p^* = \$48$
$q^* = 91$ units
(c) Consumer surplus: $2096
Producer surplus: $1143

15 (a) $5820 per year
(b) $36,787.94

17 $635.37 per year

19 (a) $0 \le t \le 10$, 10.5%
(b) $10 \le t \le 15$, 2.5%
(c) 7.8% increase

21 In 45 years; 2035

Ch. 6 Understanding

1 False

3 True

5 False
7 False
9 True
11 True
13 False
15 False
17 False
19 True
21 True
23 False
25 False
27

5

$f(x)$

x

0.4 10

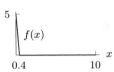

Section 7.1

1 $5x$
3 $t^3/3 + t^2/2$
5 $x^5/5$
7 $3x^4/2 + 4x$
9 $y^3 - y^4/4$
11 $x^3 + 5x$
13 $(x^3/3) - 3x^2 + 17x$
15 $5x^2/2 - 2x^{3/2}/3$
17 $\ln|z|$
19 $-1/2z^2$
21 $F(x) = x^7/7 + x^{-5}/35 + C$
23 $-e^{-3t}/3$
25 $G(t) = 5t + \sin t + C$
27 $F(x) = 3x$
(only possibility)
29 $F(x) = 2x + 2x^2 + (5/3)x^3$
(only possibility)
31 $F(x) = (2/3)x^{3/2}$
(only possibility)
33 $(5/2)x^2 + 7x + C$
35 $2x^3 + C$
37 $(x+1)^3/3 + C$
39 $t^3/3 + 5t^2/2 + t + C$
41 $t^4/4 + 2t^3 + C$
43 $2w^{3/2} + C$
45 $3\ln|t| + \dfrac{2}{t} + C$
47 $x^2/2 + 2x^{1/2} + C$
49 $e^x + 5x + C$
51 $e^{3r}/3 + C$
53 $-\cos t + C$
55 $25e^{4x} + C$
57 $3\sin x + 7\cos x + C$
59 $\frac{1}{2}\sin(x^2+4) + C$
61 $10x - 4\cos(2x) + C$
63 $F(x) = 3x^2 - 5x + 5$
65 $F(x) = -4\cos(2x) + 9$
67 $q^3 + 2q^2 + 6q + 200$

Section 7.2

1 $\frac{1}{5}(x^3+1)^5 + C$
3 $\frac{1}{4}(x+10)^4 + C$
5 $e^{q^2+1} + C$
7 $(1/2)e^{t^2} + C.$
9 $(1/33)(t^3-3)^{11} + C$
11 $(1/9)(x^2-4)^{9/2} + C$
13 $-2\sqrt{4-x} + C$
15 $4\sin(x^3) + C$
17 $(1/5)x^5 + 2x^3 + 9x + C$
19 $\cos(3-t) + C$
21 $-(2/9)(\cos 3t)^{3/2} + C$
23 $(1/7)\sin^7\theta + C$
25 $(\sin x)^3/3 + C$
27 $-\frac{1}{8}\cos(4x^2) + C$
29 $\frac{1}{6}e^{3x^2} + C$
31 $\frac{1}{10}\ln(5q^2+8) + C$
33 $(1/2)\ln(y^2+4) + C$
35 $2e^{\sqrt{y}} + C$
37 $2\sqrt{x+e^x} + C$
39 $(1/2)\ln(x^2+2x+19) + C$
41 (a) Yes; $-0.5\cos(x^2) + C$
(b) No
(c) No
(d) Yes; $-1/(2(1+x^2)) + C$
(e) No
(f) Yes; $-\ln|2+\cos x| + C$
43 (a) $x^4 + 2x^2 + C$
(b) $(x^2+1)^2 + C$
(c) Both correct but differ by a constant

Section 7.3

1 10
3 6
5 1/2
7 125
9 52
11 38/3
13 $(\ln 2)/2 \approx 0.35$
15 $5 - 5e^{-0.2} \approx 0.906$
17 $\sin 1 - \sin(-1) = 2\sin 1$
19 $20(e^{0.15} - 1)$
21 (a) $(\ln 2)/2$
(b) $(\ln 2)/2$
23 $\ln 10$
25 2
27 $\int_0^2 (6x^2+1)\,dx = 18$
29 2.32

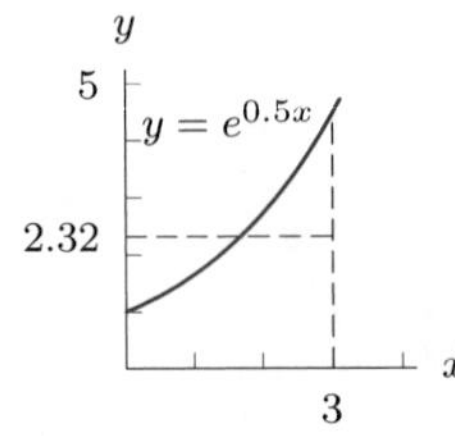

31 11
33 $(300)^{1/3} = 6.694$
35 (a) 6.9 billion, 7.8 billion
(b) 6.5 billion
37 $\int_1^\infty (1/x^2)\,dx$

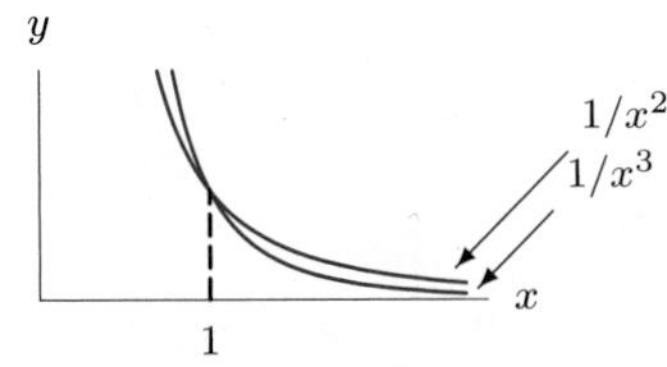

39 (a) $0.4988, 0.49998,$
$0.4999996,$
0.499999998
(b) $(1 - e^{-2b})/2$
(c) Converges to 0.5
41 (a) $\int_0^\infty 1000te^{-0.5t}\,dt$
(b) 

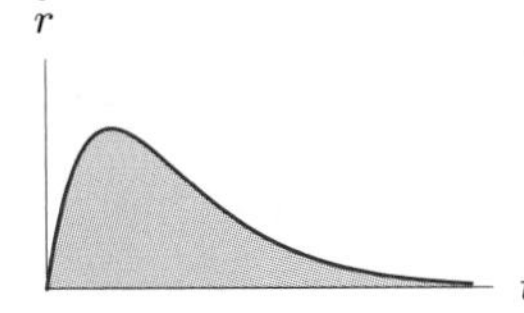

43 1/30
45 (a) No
(b) Yes
(c) Yes

Section 7.4

1 $\frac{1}{5}te^{5t} - \frac{1}{25}e^{5t} + C$
3 $(1/4)(2z+1)e^{2z} + C$
5 $(x^4/4)\ln x - (x^4/16) + C$
7 $(2/3)y(y+3)^{3/2}$
$- (4/15)(y+3)^{5/2} + C$
9 $-(z+1)e^{-z} + C$
11 $-2y(5-y)^{1/2}$
$- (4/3)(5-y)^{3/2} + C$
13 $-t\cos t + \sin t + C$
15 $\frac{1}{5}t^2e^{5t} - \frac{2}{25}te^{5t} + \frac{2}{125}e^{5t} + C$
17 $5\ln 5 - 4 \approx 4.047$
19 $(9/2)\ln 3 - 2 \approx 2.944$
21 (a) Substitution
(b) Substitution
(c) Substitution
(d) Substitution
(e) Parts
(f) Parts
23 $1 - 3e^{-2}$
25 $4\ln 4 - 3\ln 3 - 1$
27 45.71 (ng/ml)-hours
29 Integrate by parts choosing $u = x^n, v' = e^x$

Section 7.5

1 3.5, 2, 1.5, 2, 2.5

3 $F(0) = 0$
$F(1) = 1$
$F(2) = 1.5$
$F(3) = 1$
$F(4) = 0$
$F(5) = -1$
$F(6) = -1.5$

5
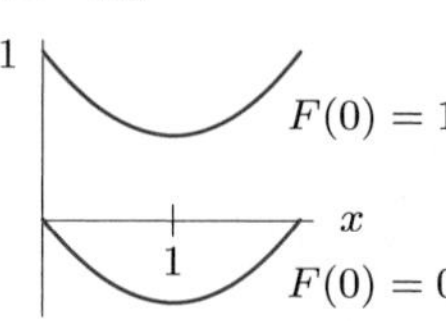

7
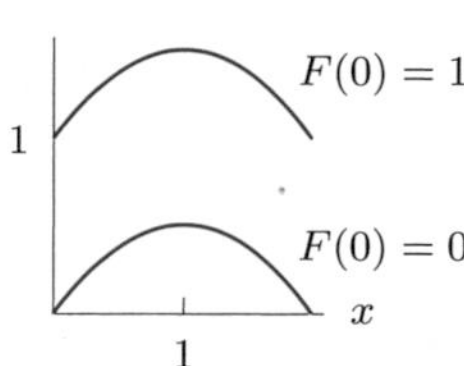

9 (a) Increasing for $x < -2, x > 2$
Decreasing for $-2 < x < 2$
Local maximum at $x = -2$
Local minimum at $x = 2$

(b)
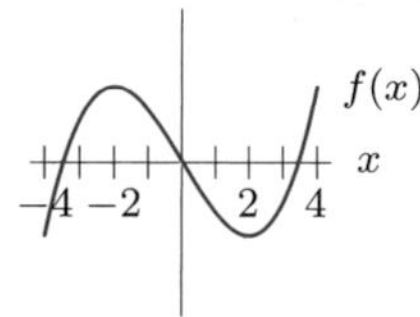

11 (a) $f(x)$ increasing when $2 < x < 5$
$f(x)$ decreasing when $x < 2$ or $x > 5$
f has a local minimum at $x = 2$
f has a local maximum at $x = 5$

(b)
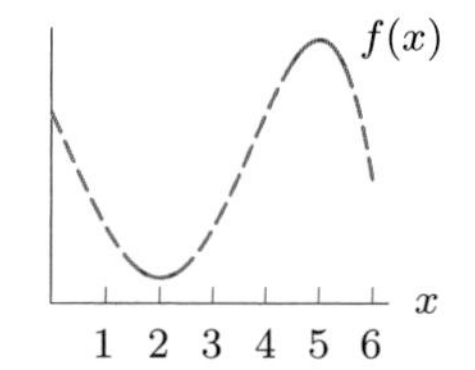

13
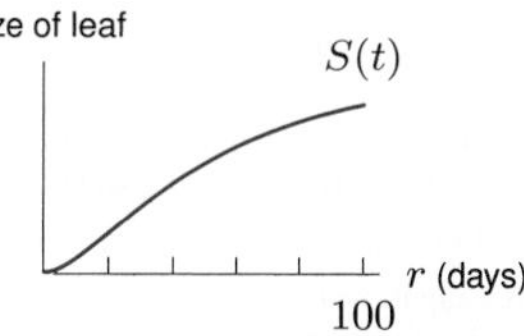

15 (a) (I) volume; (II) flow rate
(b) (I) is an antiderivative of (II)

17 Min: $(1.5, -20)$, max: $(4.67, 5)$

19 Critical points: $(0, 5)$, $(2, 21)$, $(4, 13)$, $(5, 15)$

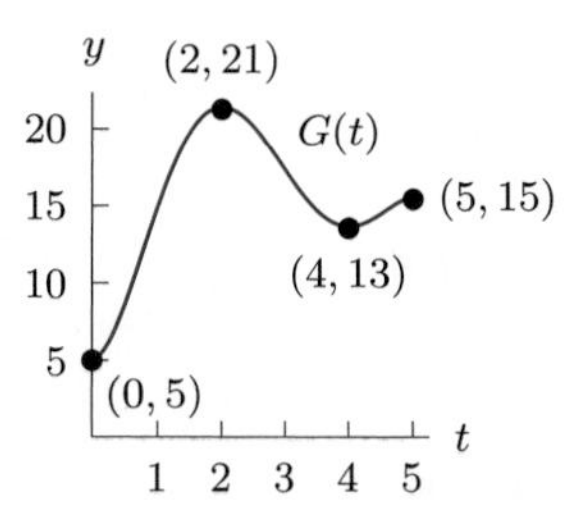

21 (a) $x = -1, x = 1, x = 3$
(b) Local min at $x = -1, x = 3$; local max at $x = 1$
(c)
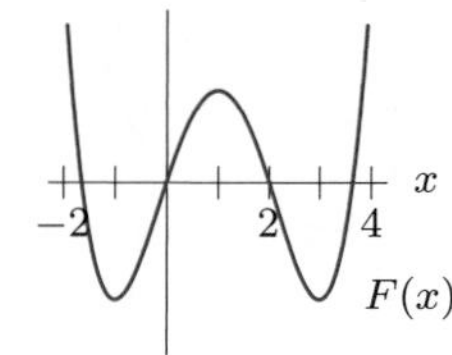

23 $f(3) - f(2)$,
$[f(4) - f(2)]/2$,
$f(4) - f(3)$

25
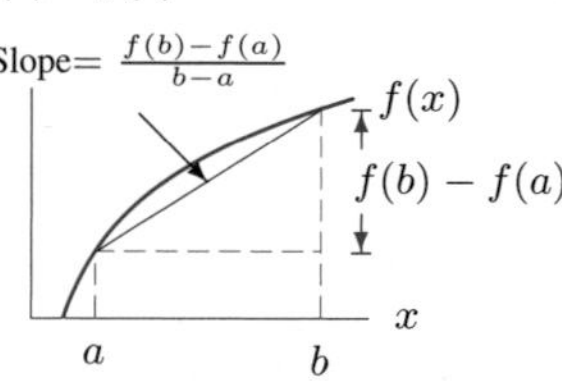

27
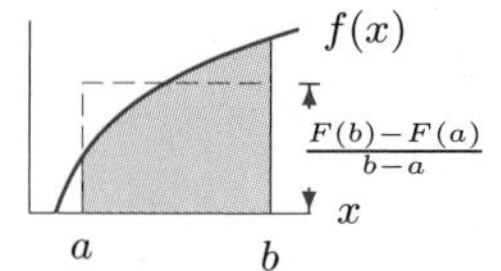

Chapter 7 Review

1 $2t^3/3 + 3t^4/4 + 4t^5/5$

3 $2x^3 - 4x^2 + 3x$

5 $P(r) = \pi r^2 + C$

7 $-1/t$

9 $G(x) = (x+1)^4/4 + C$

11 $2t^2 + 7t + C$

13 $(x^4/4) - (x^2/2) + C$

15 $-5/t - 3/t^2 + C$

17 $4t^2 + 3t + C$

19 $2x^4 + \ln|x| + C$

21 $2\ln|x| - \pi\cos x + C$

23 34

25 $1 - \cos 1 \approx 0.460$

27 $1/2$

29 $F(x) = x^2$
(only possibility)

31 $2\sqrt{x^2+1} + C$

33 $-(1/2)e^{-x^2} + C$

35 $-1/(3(3x+1)) + C$

37 $\frac{1}{55}(5x-7)^{11} + C$

39 $\frac{1}{3}(x^2+1)^{3/2} + C$

41 $0.5\sin(t^2) + C$

43 $\ln 3$

45 (a) $\int_0^5 462e^{0.019t}\,dt$
(b) About 2423 quadrillion BTUs

47
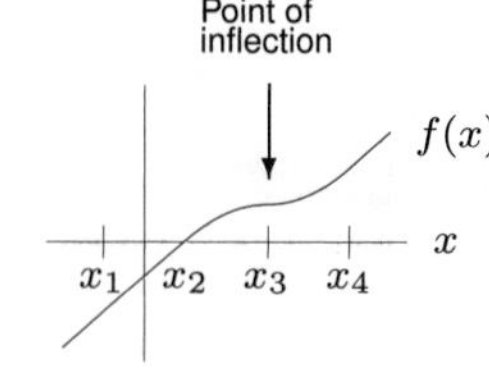

49 $F(1) = -1, F(3) = 7, F(4) = 5$

51 (a)

$f(x) = xe^{-x}$

(b) $0.9596, 0.9995, 0.99999996$
(c) Converges to 1

53 250 mg

55 $-y\cos y + \sin y + C$

Ch. 7 Understanding

1 False

3 True

5 False

7 False

9 True

11 True

13 False

15 False

17 False

19 True

21 True

23 False

25 False

27
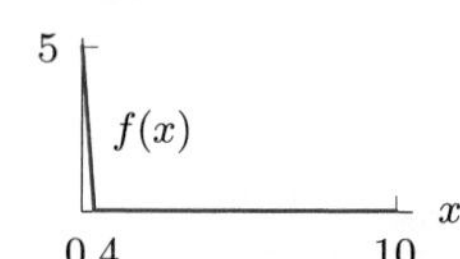

Practice: Integration

1 $q^3/3 + 5q^2/2 + 2q + C$

3 $(x^3/3) + x + C$

5 $4x^{3/2} + C$

7 $(x^4/4) + 2x^2 + 8x + C$

9 $w^5/5 - 3w^4 + 2w^3 - 10w + C$

11 $2q^{1/2} + C$

13 $p^3/3 + 5\ln|p| + C$

15 $q^4/4 + 4q^2 + 15q + C$

17 $-5\cos x + 3\sin x + C$

19 $5\ln|w| + C$

21 $q^2/2 - 1/(2q^2) + C$

23 $3p^2q^5 + C$

25 $2.5e^{2q} + C$

27 $Ax^4/4 + Bx^2/2 + C$

29 $x^3/3 + 8x + e^x + C$

31 $t^3/3 - 3t^2 + 5t + C$

33 $Aq^2/2 + Bq + C$

35 $\frac{1}{2}e^{2t} + 5t + C$

37 $3\sin(4x) + C$

39 $(1/18)(y^2 + 5)^9 + C$

41 $-(A/B)\cos(Bt) + C$

43 $\ln(2 + e^x) + C$

45 $2\sqrt{1 + \sin x} + C$

47 $xe^x - e^x + C$

Section 8.1

1 (a) 0.25
(b) 0.7
(c) 0.15

3 (a) 0.4375
(b) 0.49
(c) 0.2475

7 (a) 0.19
(b) Tenth; both same
(c) 0.02, 0.38, 0.21

9 1/15

11 1/5

13

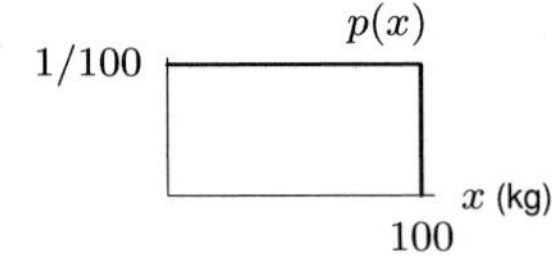

15

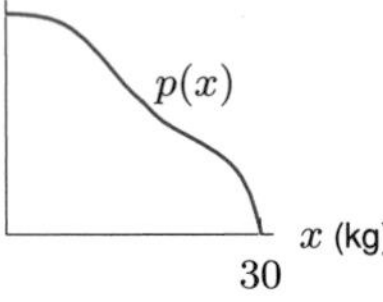

Section 8.2

1 (a)

t	0	1	2	3	4	···
$P(t)$	0	0.60	0.975	1	1	···

(b) fraction of patients

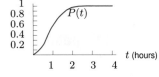

1
0.8
0.6
0.4
0.2
$P(t)$
t (hours)
1 2 3 4

3 (a)

0.25
0.125
$p(t)$
time late (minutes)
−2 −1 1 2 3 4 5

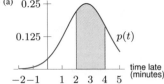

(b)

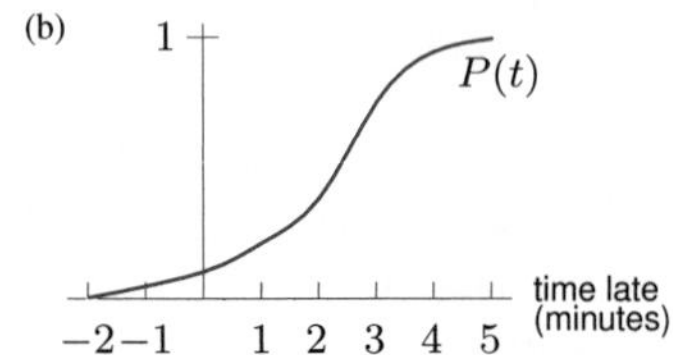

7 (a) 2/3
(b) 1/3
(c) Possibly many work just to pass
(d)

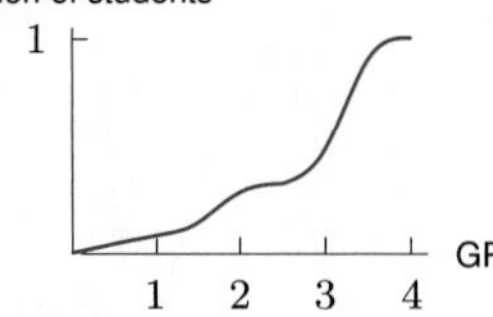

9 (a) First: January 30
Last: August 28
(b) 65%
(c) 25%
(d) 10%
(e) April 10 – April 30

11 (a) 25%
(b) 32.5%
(c) 0

13 Fraction dead at time t

15 (a) $-e^{-2} + 1 \approx 0.865$
(b) $-(\ln 0.05)/2 \approx 1.5$ km

Section 8.3

1 5.35 tons

3 (a) 0.2685
(b) 0.067

5 2.48 weeks

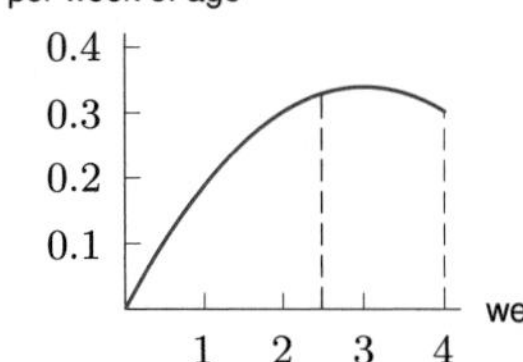

7 (a) 0.684 : 1
(b) 1.6 hours
(c) 1.682 hours

9 (a) 17.6%; 6%
(b) About $45,200
(c) False

Chapter 8 Review

1 (a)-(II), (b)-(I), (c)-(III)

3

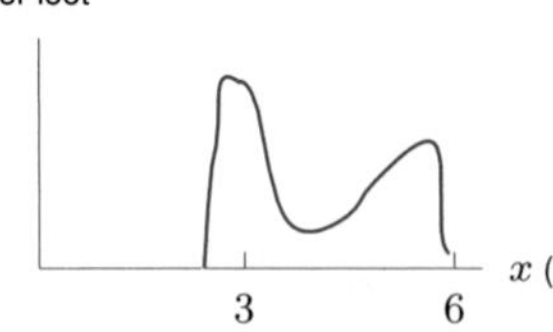

5

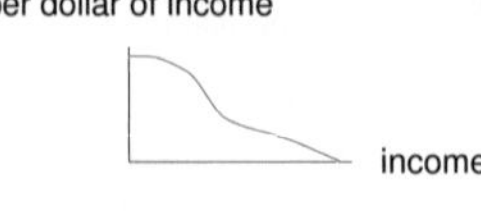

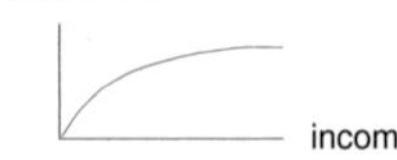

7 0.04

9 0.008

11 (a) Twelfth
(b) 1/4
(c) 7/16

13 (b) About 3/4

15 (a) $f(r) = 0.2\ (0 < r < 5)$
$f(r) = 0\ (5 \le r)$
(b) $F(r) = 0.2r$
$(0 \le r \le 5)$
$F(r) = 1\ (5 < r)$
(c) $G(v) = 0.124r^{1/3}$
$(0 \le v \le 523.6)$
$G(v) = 1\ (523.6 < v)$
(d) $g(v) = 0.0413v^{-2/3}\ (0 < v < 523.6)$
$g(v) = 1\ (523.6 \le v)$

17 (a) 22.1%
(b) 33.0%
(c) 30.1%
(d) $C(h) = 1 - e^{-0.4h}$

19 14.6 days

21 False

23 True

25 True

Ch. 8 Understanding

1 True

3 False

5 False

7 False

9 True

11 True

13 False

15 False

17 False

19 True

21 False

23 False

25 False

27 True

29 False

Section 9.1

3 $f(20, p)$: 2.65, 2.59, 2.51, 2.43
$f(100, p)$: 5.79, 5.77, 5.60, 5.53
$f(I, 3.00)$: 2.65, 4.14, 5.11, 5.35, 5.79
$f(I, 4.00)$ 2.51, 3.94, 4.97, 5.19, 5.60

7 $P = 0.052pf(I, p)/I$

9 Decreasing function of p
Increasing function of a

11 (a) 81°F
(b) 30%

13 Incr of A and r
Decr of t

15

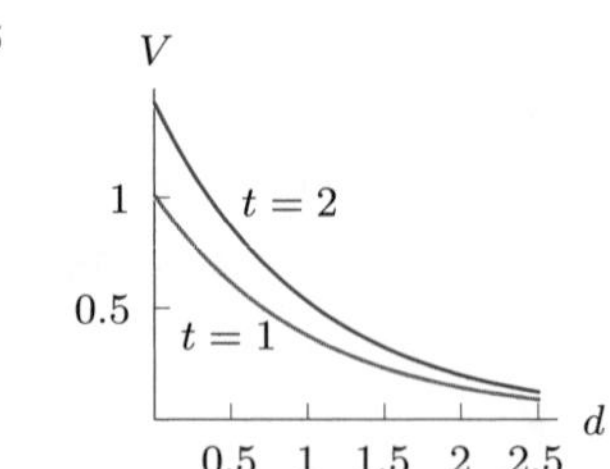

17 (a) 260 cal/m^3

(b)

T (°C) \ w (gm/m^3)	0.1	0.2	0.3	0.4
0	150	290	425	590
10	110	240	330	450
20	100	180	260	350
30	70	150	220	300
40	65	140	200	270

Section 9.2

1 Decreasing function of x
Increasing function of y

3 Heat coming in window

5

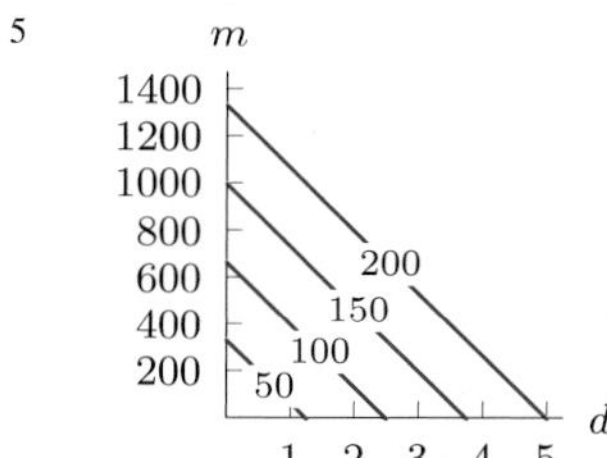

7

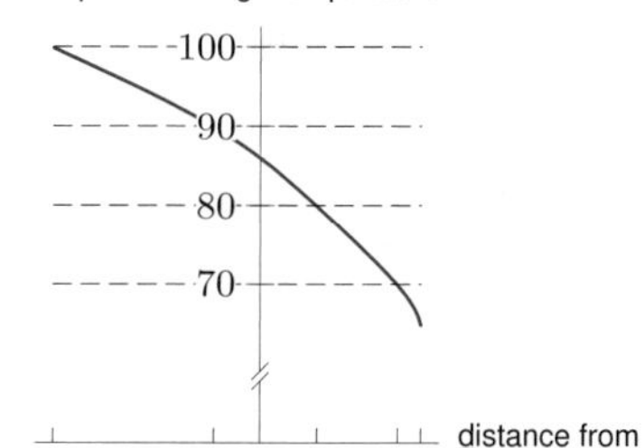

9

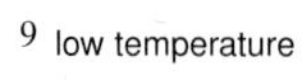

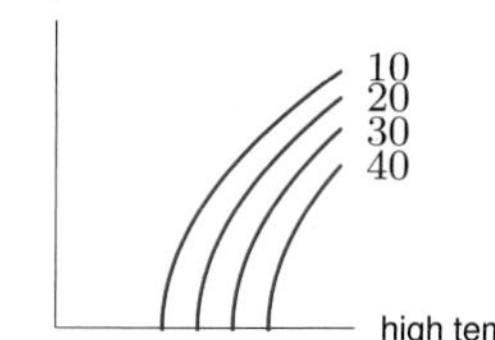

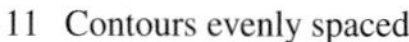

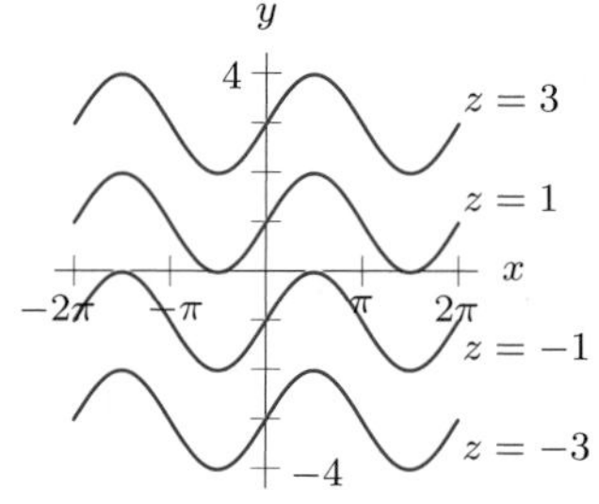

15 Contours evenly spaced

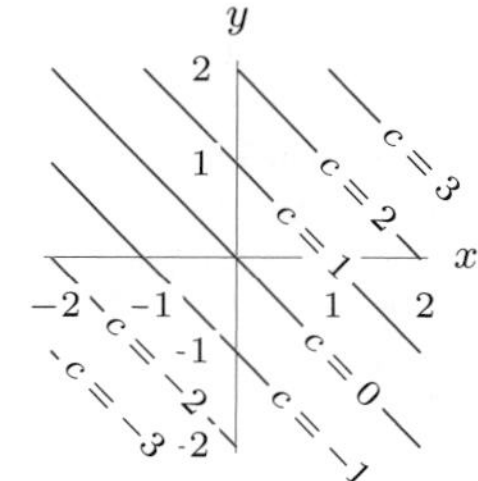

17 Contours evenly spaced

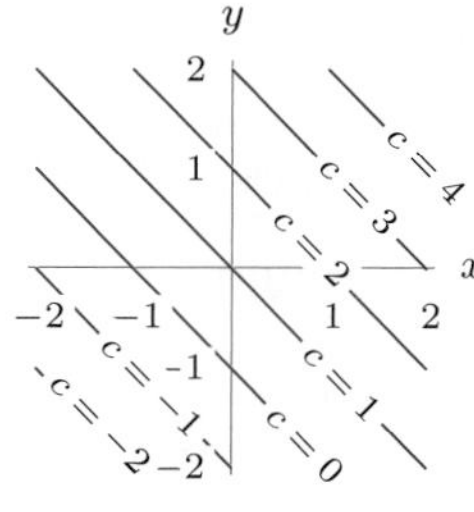
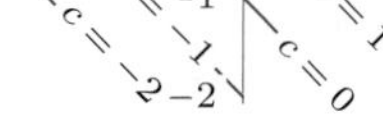
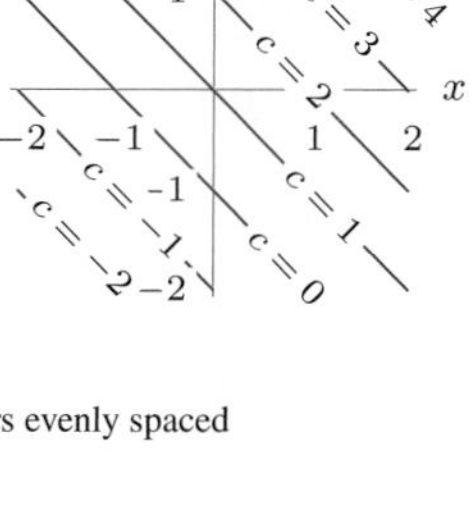

19 Contours evenly spaced

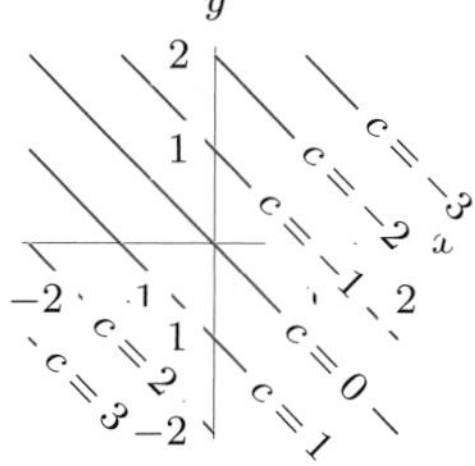

21 (a) False
(b) True
(c) False
(d) True

23 (a) 510.17 thousand pages/day
(b) 773.27 thousand pages/day
(c) 673.17 thousand pages/day
(d) 1020.34 thousand pages/day

25 (a) III
(b) II
(c) I
(d) IV

27 (a) 4 hours
(b) 40%
(c) Contours approx horizontal
(d) Increasing
(e) Increasing

Section 9.3

1 (a) Positive
(b) Negative
(c) Positive
(d) Zero

3 $\frac{\partial I}{\partial H}\Big|_{(10,100)} \approx 0.4$
$\frac{\partial I}{\partial T}\Big|_{(10,100)} \approx 1$

5 (a) f_c is negative
f_t is positive

7 (a) Concentration/distance
Rate of change of concentration with distance
$\partial c/\partial x < 0$

(b) Concentration/time
Rate of change of concentration with time
For small t, $\partial c/\partial t > 0$
For large t, $\partial c/\partial t < 0$

9 $z_x(1,0) \approx 2$
$z_x(0,1) \approx 0$
$z_y(0,1) \approx 10$

11 (a) Negative

13 (a) 3.3 % / in
(b) -5% / °F

15 $\partial f/\partial P_1 < 0$
$\partial f/\partial P_2 > 0$

19 14 %

21 5.67

23 (a)

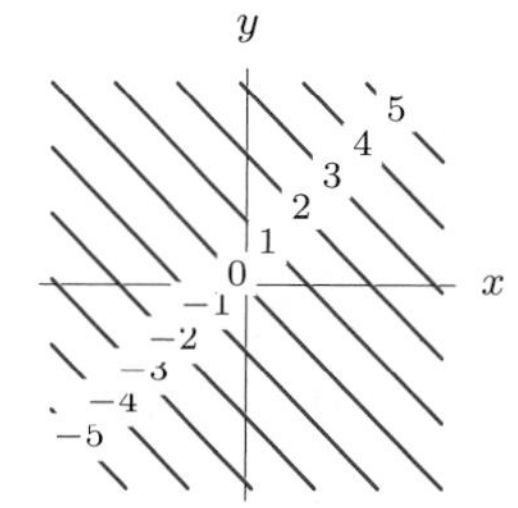

(b)

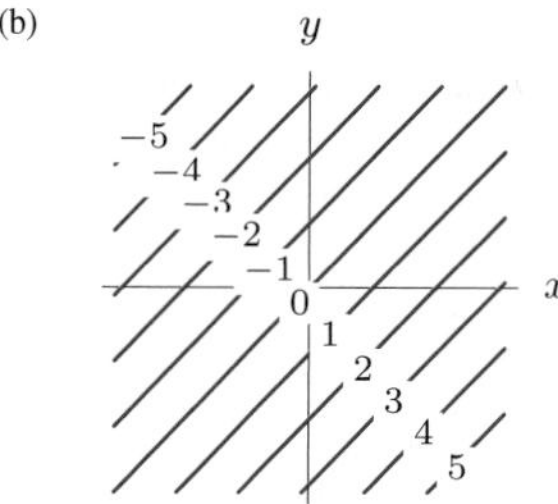

(c)

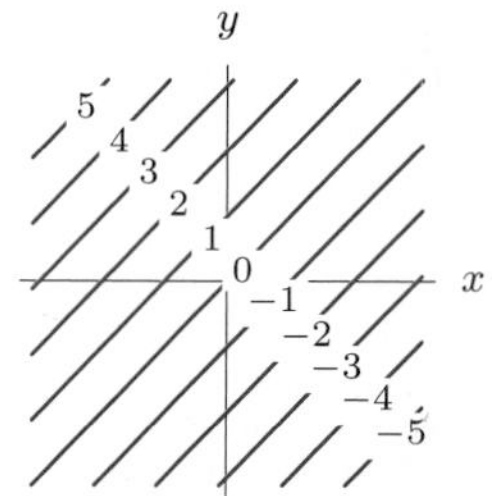

(d)

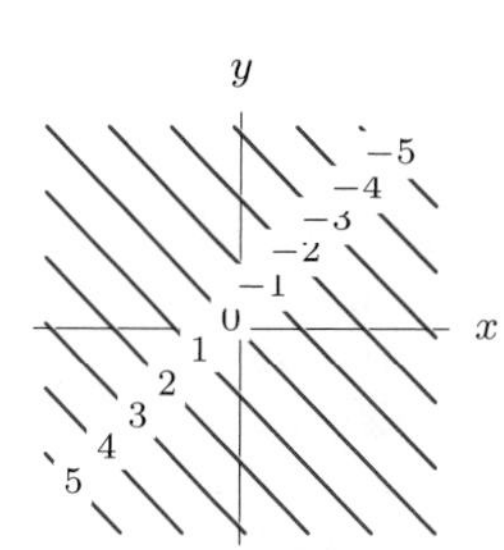

Section 9.4

1 $4x; 6y$

3 $f_x = 2x + 2y$
$f_y = 2x + 3y^2$

5 $2u + 5v; 5u + 2v$

7 $5a^2 - 9ap^2$

9 $f_x = 10xy^3 + 8y^2 - 6x$,
$f_y = 15x^2y^2 + 16xy$

11 $100te^{rt}$

13 $(1/2)v^2$

15 15; 5; 30

17 $Pre^{rt}; Pte^{rt}; e^{rt}$

19 80; 30; 313 tons
2.9 tons per worker
2.6 tons per \$25,000

21 $f_{xx} = 2, f_{xy} = 2$,
$f_{yy} = 2, f_{yx} = 2$

23 $f_{xx} = 0, f_{xy} = -2/y^2$,
$f_{yy} = 4x/y^3, f_{yx} = -2/y^2$

25 $f_{xx} = y^2e^{xy}$,
$f_{xy} = (xy+1)e^{xy}$,
$f_{yy} = x^2e^{xy}$,
$f_{yx} = (xy+1)e^{xy}$

27 $V_{rr} = 2\pi h, V_{hh} = 0$,
$V_{rh} = V_{hr} = 2\pi r$

29 $B_{xx} = 0, B_{tt} = 20xe^{-2t}$,
$B_{xt} = B_{tx} = -10e^{-2t}$

31 $f_{rr} = 100t^2e^{rt}, f_{tt} = 100r^2e^{rt}$,
$f_{tr} = f_{rt} = 100(rt+1)e^{rt}$

35 (a) $-(c+1)B/(c+r)^2$
(b) Negative

Section 9.5

1 $f(0,0) \approx 12.5$ is a local and global maximum
$f(13,30) \approx 4.5$ is a local minimum
$f(37,18) \approx 2.5$ is a local and global minimum
$f(32,34) \approx 10.5$ is a local maximum

3 Max: 11 at $(5.1, 4.9)$
Min: -1 at $(1, 3.9)$

5 Max: 1 at $(\pi/2, 0)$; $(\pi/2, 2\pi)$
Min: -1 at $(\pi/2, \pi)$

7 $(-3, 6)$, neither

9 $(4, 2)$, neither

11 Saddle pts: $(1,-1), (-1,1)$
local max $(-1,-1)$
local min $(1,1)$

13 Local maximum at $(-1, 0)$,
Saddle points at $(1, 0)$ and $(-1, 4)$,
Local minimum at $(1, 4)$

15 Local max: $(1, 5)$

17 $A = 10, B = 4, C = -2$

19 (b) $p_1 = p_2 = 25$
Max revenue is 4375

21 $q_1 = 300, q_2 = 225$.

Section 9.6

1 $f(66.7, 33.3) = 13{,}333$

3 $f(9.26, 2.32) = 201.9$

5 Min $= -\sqrt{2}$, max $= \sqrt{2}$

7 Min $= -22$, max $= 22$

9 Min $= -2$, max $= 2$

11 $x = 6; y = 6; f(6,6) = 400$

13 (a) $C = 127x_1 + 92x_2$
(b) $x_1^{0.6}x_2^{0.4} = 500$

15 (b) $L = 40, K = 30$

17 (a) Reduce K by $1/2$ unit,
increase L by 1 unit.

19 (a) $P(x,y); C(x,y) = 50{,}000$

(b) $C(x,y); P(x,y) = 2000$

21 (a) $P(K, L)$
(b) $C(K, L) = 600{,}000$
(c) Tons/dollar
(d) Extra dollar produces approximately extra 3.17 tons

23 (a) Quantity of fuel, $x_1 + x_2$
(b) Terminal velocity (as function of x_1 and x_2) $= v_0$
(c) Liters per meter/sec
(d) 51 meters/sec requires about 8 more liters than 50 meters/sec

25 1820.04; about 209

Chapter 9 Review

1 Decreasing function of x
Increasing function of y

3 Lines with slope $3/5$, evenly spaced

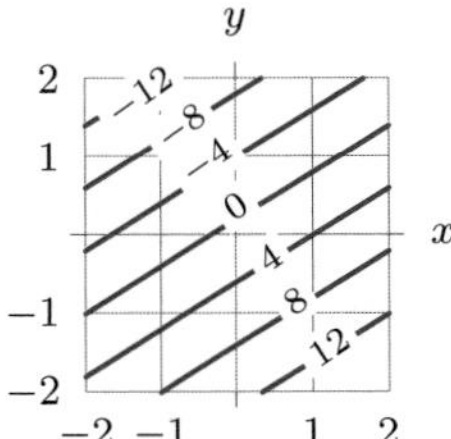

5

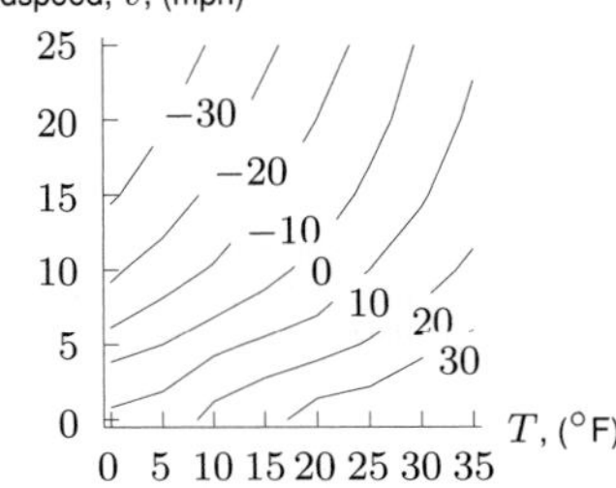

9 x-axis: price
y-axis: advertising

11 Answers in °C:

(a)

10
0
−10

(b)

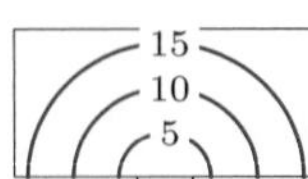

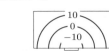

(c)

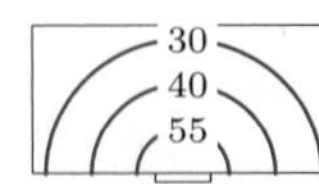

(d)

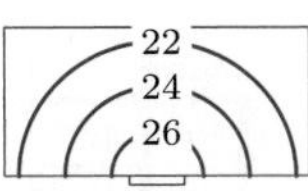

13 Table (a) matches (II)
Table (b) matches (III)
Table (c) matches (IV)
Table (d) matches (I)

15 Positive, Negative, 10, 2, -4

17 $f_w(10, 25) \approx -0.4$°F/mph

19 $f_w(5, 20) \approx -0.8$

21 (a) Both negative
(b) Both negative

23 (A) 0.06, -0.06
(B) 0, -0.05
(C) 0, 0

25 $P_a = 2a - 2b^2, P_b = -4ab$

27 $\dfrac{\partial f}{\partial x} = 5e^{-2t}, \dfrac{\partial f}{\partial t} = -10xe^{-2t}$

29 $f_x = x/\sqrt{x^2+y^2}$
$f_y = y/\sqrt{x^2+y^2}$

31 (a) $Q_K = 18.75K^{-0.25}L^{0.25}$,
$Q_L = 6.25K^{0.75}L^{-0.75}$
(b) $Q = 1704.33$
$Q_K = 21.3$
$Q_L = 4.26$

33 (a)

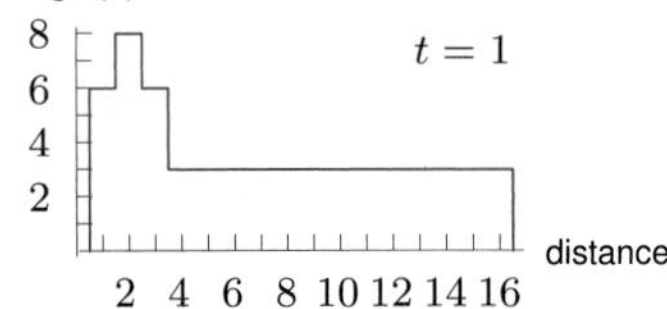

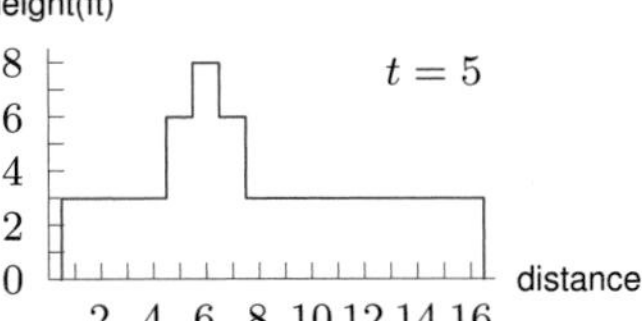

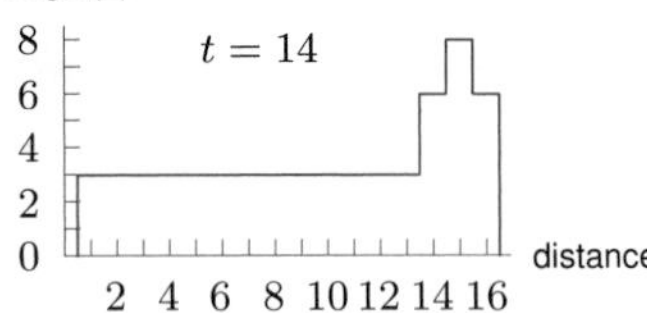

(b)

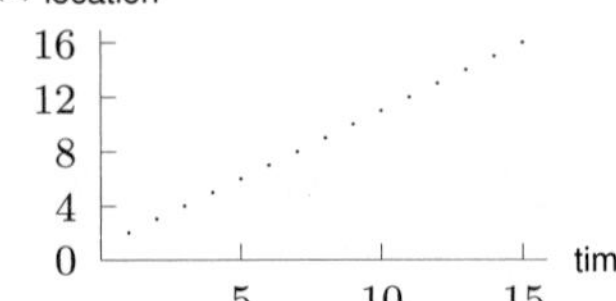

(c) The "wave" at a sports arena

35 $(1, 0), (-1, 0)$; $f(1, 0)$ is a local minimum

37 $p_1 = 110, p_2 = 115$

39 43

41 (a) $Q = x_1^{0.3}x_2^{0.7}$
(b) $10x_1 + 25x_2 = 50{,}000$

43 (a) 2599
(b) 129; $\$4{,}712{,}958$
(c) $\$8572.54$ per car

45 (a) 475 units
(b) 505 units

Ch. 9 Understanding

1 Could not be true
3 Might be true
5 True
7 True
9 False
11 False
13 True
15 True
17 False
19 False
21 True
23 True
25 False
27 True
29 True
31 True
33 False
35 False
37 True
39 False
41 False
43 False
45 True
47 False
49 True
51 True
53 True
55 False
57 True
59 True
61 True
63 False
65 False

Theory: Least Squares

1 $y = 2/3 - (1/2)x$
3 $y = 2/3 - (1/2)x$
5 $y = x - 1/3$
7 (a) (i) Power function
(ii) Linear function
(b) $\ln N = 1.20 + 0.32 \ln A$
Agrees with biological rule

Section 10.1

1 (a) (III)
(b) (IV)
(c) (I)
(d) (II)

3 $dP/dt = kP$, $k > 0$
5 $dQ/dt = kQ$, $k < 0$
7 $dP/dt = -0.08P - 30$
9 $dA/dt = -1$
11 (a) $dA/dt = -0.17A$
(b) -17 mg
13 (a) Increasing, decreasing
(b) $W = 4$
15 $dN/dt = B + kN$

Section 10.2

1 $y = t^2 + C$
5 F
7 E
9 A
11 D
13 8, 8.5, 9.5, 11
15 4, 4, 4, 4
17 74, 78.8, 84.56 million
19 $k = -0.03$ and C is any number, or $C = 0$ and k is any number
21 $k = 5$

Section 10.3

1 (a)

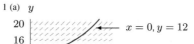

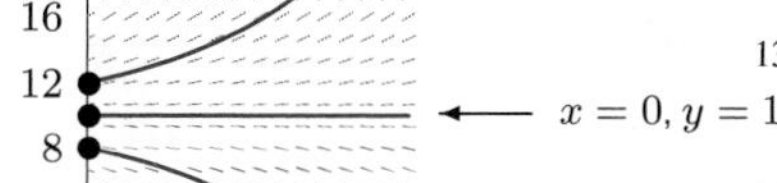

3 (a)

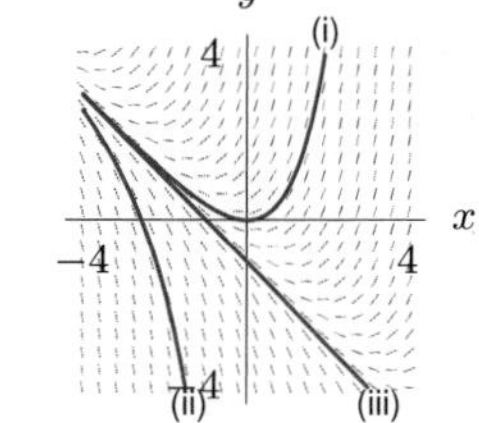

(b) $y = -x - 1$

5 (a) Slopes $= 2, 0, -1, -4$
(b)

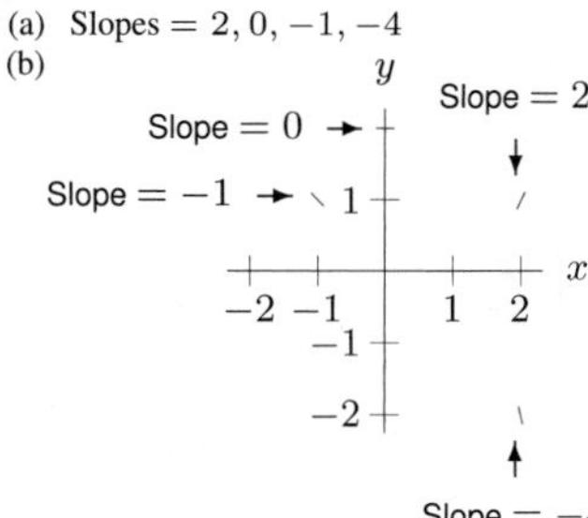

7 (a) II
(b) VI
(c) IV
(d) I
(e) III
(f) V

9 As x increases, $y \to \infty$.
11 As $x \to \infty$, y oscillates within a certain range
13 $y \to \infty$ as $x \to \infty$

Section 10.4

1 $w = 30e^{3r}$
3 $P = 20e^{0.02t}$
5 $Q = 50e^{(1/5)t}$
7 (a) $dM/dt = rM$
(b) $M = 1000e^{rt}$
(c)

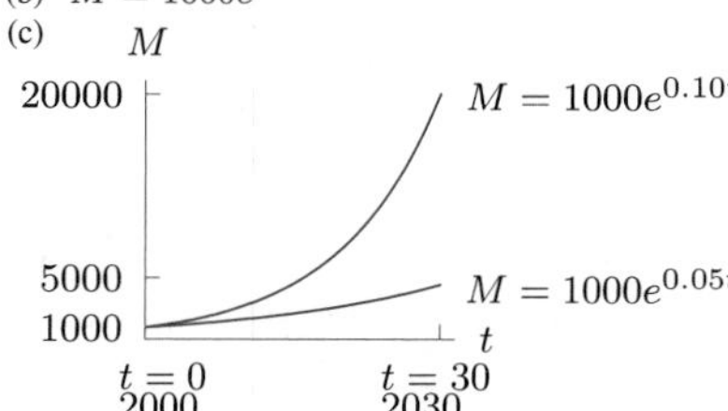

9 (a) $dB/dt = 0.10B + 1000$
(b) $B = 10{,}000e^{0.1t} - 10{,}000$
11 Michigan: 72 years
Ontario: 18 years
13 (a) $dQ/dt = -0.5365Q$
$Q = Q_0e^{-0.5365t}$
(b) 4 mg
15 (a) $dy/dt = ky$
(b) 0.2486 grams
17 (b) 2001

Section 10.5

1 $H = 75 - 75e^{3t}$
3 $P = 104e^t - 4$
5 $Q = 400 - 350e^{0.3t}$
7 $B = 25 + 75e^{2-2t}$
11 (a) $dV/dt = 0.02V - 80{,}000$
(b) $V = \$4{,}000{,}000$
(c) $V = 4{,}000{,}000 + Ce^{0.02t}$
(d) $\$2{,}728{,}751$
13 (a) $dB/dt = 0.05B + 1200$
(b) $B = 24{,}000(e^{0.05t} - 1)$
(c) $\$6816.61$
15 (a) $y = ce^{-t} + 100$
(b)

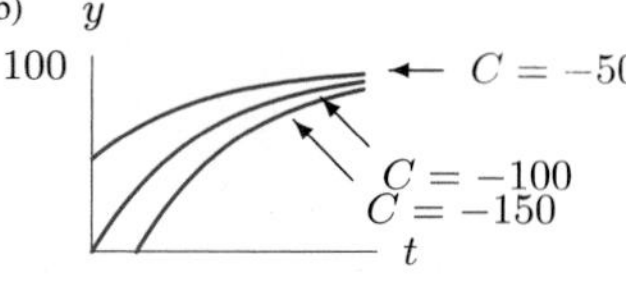

(c) $y = 100 - 100e^{-t}$
17 (a) $dy/dt = -k(y - a)$
(b) $y = (1 - a)e^{-kt} + a$
(c) a: fraction remembered in the long run
k: rate material is forgotten
19 (a) $y = 500$
(b) $y = 500 + Ce^{0.5t}$

(c)

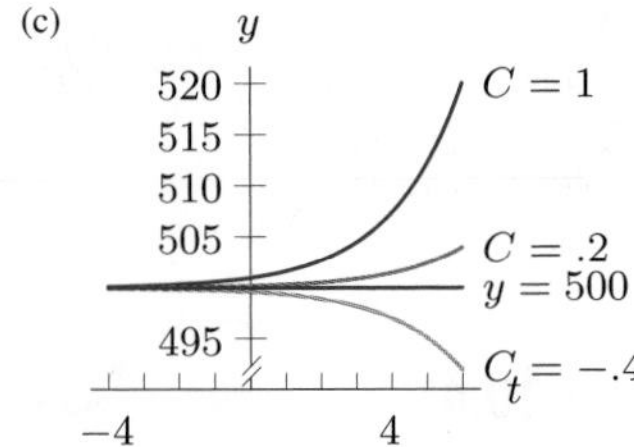

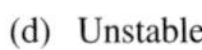

(d) Unstable

21 (a) $H = 200 - 180e^{-kt}$
(b) $k \approx 0.027$ (if t is in minutes)

23 (a) $dT/dt = -k(T - 68)$
(b) $T = 68 + 22.3e^{-0.06t}$;
3:45 am.

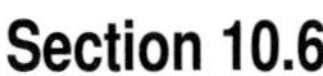

Section 10.6

1 (a) $x \to \infty$ exponentially
$y \to 0$ exponentially
(b) Predator-prey

3 (a) $x \to \infty$ exponentially
$y \to 0$ exponentially

(b) y is helped by the presence of x

5 $dx/dt = x - xy$,
$dy/dt = y - xy$

7 $dx/dt = -x - xy$,
$dy/dt = -y - xy$

11 Symmetric about the line $r = w$;
solutions closed curves

13 Robins:
Max ≈ 2500
Min ≈ 500
When robins are at a max,
the worm population is about 1 million

17 (a) $dw/dt = 0$
$dr/dt = 1.2$
(b) $w \approx 2.2, r \approx 1.1$
(c) At $t = 0.2$:
$w \approx 2.2, r \approx 1.3$
At $t = 0.3$
$w \approx 2.1, r \approx 1.4$

19 (a)

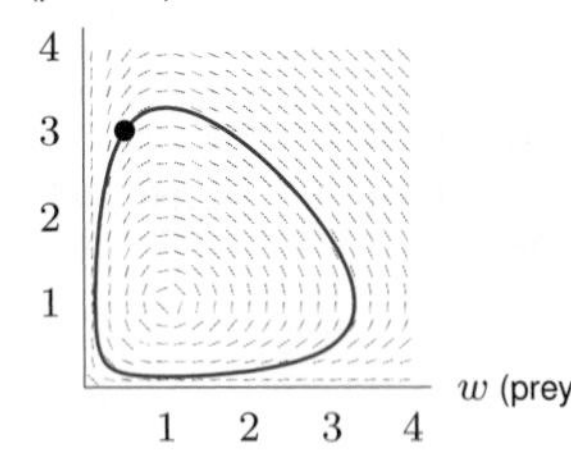

(b) Down and left
(c) $r = 3.3, w = 1$
(d) $w = 3.3, r = 1$

21 (a)

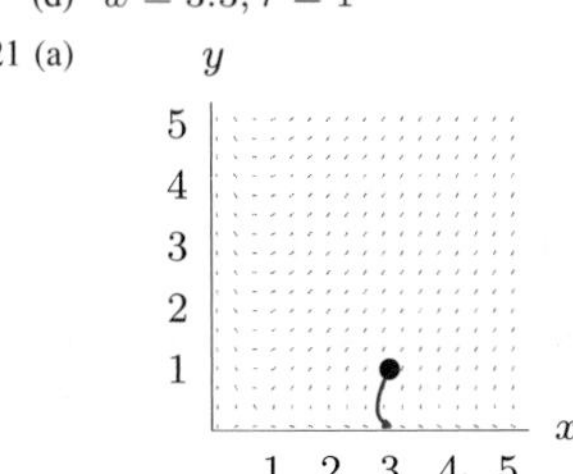

(b)

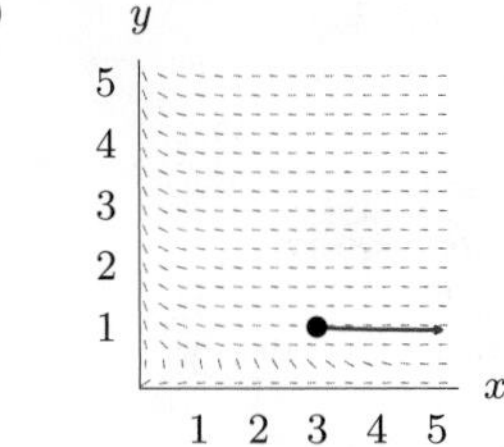

(c)

(d)

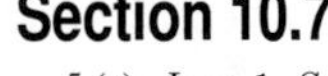

Section 10.7

5 (a) $I_0 = 1, S_0 = 349$
(b) Increases; spreads

7 About 300 boys;
$t \approx 6$ days

9 5

11 (a) b/a

Chapter 10 Review

1 (a) (III)
(b) (V)
(c) (I)
(d) (II)
(e) (IV)

3 Yes

5 (a) I is $y' = 1 + y$;
II is $y' = 1 + x$
(b) I

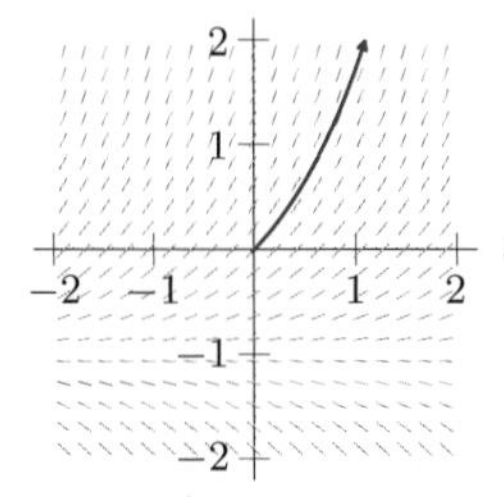

II

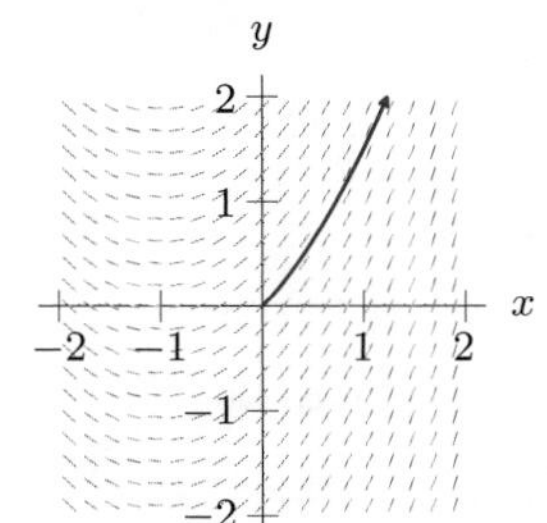

(c) I: $y' = -1$, unstable;
II: None

7 III: $y' = (1 + y)(2 - y)$

9 (a) $dB/dt = 0.07B$
(b) $B = B_0e^{0.07t}$
(c) $B = 5000e^{0.07t}$
(d) $B(10) \approx \$10{,}068.76$

11 $P = (1/2)t^2 + C$

13 $y = (5/2)t^2 + C$

15 $A = Ce^{-0.07t}$

17 $P = Ce^{-2t} + 5$

19 $y = Ce^{0.2x} + 40$

21 $dS/dt = -k(S - 65), k > 0$
$S = 65 - 25e^{-kt}$

23 (a) $k \approx 0.000121$
(b) 779.4 years

25 (a)

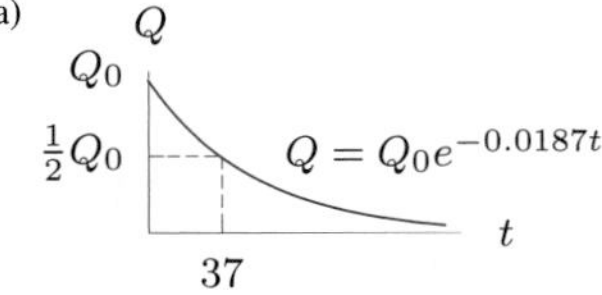

(b) $dQ/dt = -0.0187Q$
(c) 3 days

27 (b) $dQ/dt = -0.347Q + 2.5$
(c) $Q = 7.2$ mg

29 (a) $dW/dt = (1/3500)(I - 20W)$

(b) $W = I/20 + (W_0 - I/20)\,e^{-(1/175)t}$
(c)

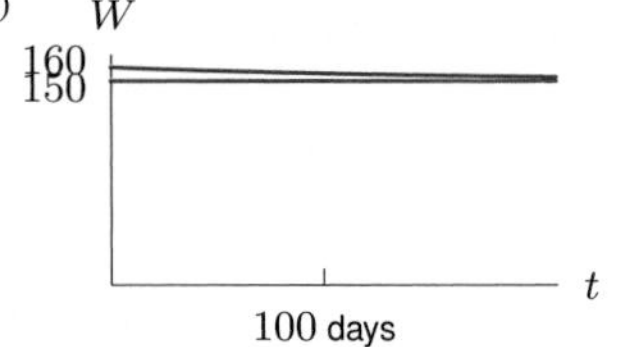

31 (a) $y = 1, y = 8, y = 16$
(d) Stable: $y = 1$
Unstable: $y = 8, y = 16$

33 Initially $x = 0$; y decreases, x increases. Then x increases, y increases. Finally y increases, x decreases

35 Populations oscillate

Ch. 10 Understanding

1 True

3 True

5 True

7 False

9 True

11 False

13 False

15 False; $f(x) = |x|$

17 False; $\cos t + t^2$

19 False; $f(x) = 6, g(x) = 10$

21 False; $f(x) = 5x + 7, g(x) = x + 2$

23 False; $f(x) = x^2, g(x) = x^2 - 1$

25 False; $f(x) = e^{-x}, g(x) = x^2$

27 (a) Not a counterexample
(b) Not a counterexample
(c) Not a counterexample
(d) Counterexample

29 False

31 False

33 Possible answer

$$f(x) = \begin{cases} x & \text{if } 0 \le x < 2 \\ 19 & \text{if } x = 2 \end{cases}$$

Theory: Separation of Vars

1 $P = e^{-2t}$

3 $P = \sqrt{2t+1}$

5 $u = 1/(1 - (1/2)t)$

7 $R = 1 - 0.9e^{1-y}$

9 $z = -\ln(1 - t^2/2)$

11 $y = -2/(t^2 + 2t - 4)$

13 (a) Yes (b) No (c) Yes
(d) No (e) Yes (f) Yes
(g) No (h) Yes (i) No
(j) Yes (k) Yes (l) No

15 $Q = b - Ae^{-t}$

17 $R = -(b/a) + Ae^{at}$

19 $y = -1/\left(k(t + t^3/3) + C\right)$

21 (a)

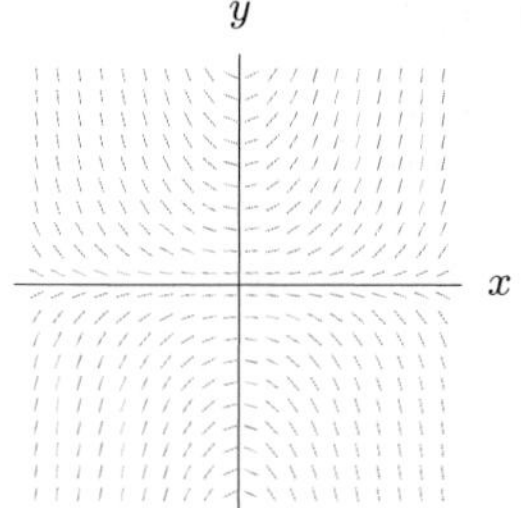

(b)

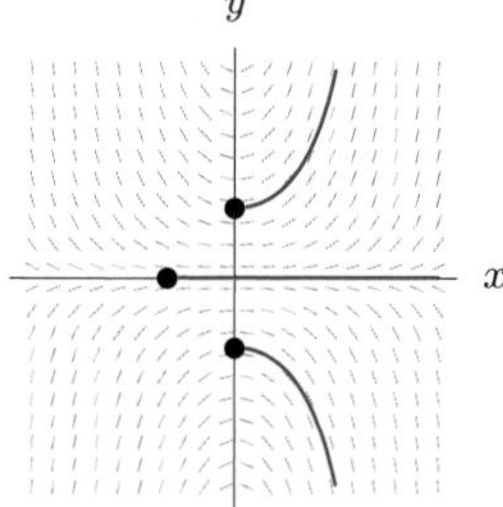

(c) $y(x) = Ae^{x^2/2}$

Section 11.1

1 21

3 3,985,805

5 555.10

7 96.154

9 39,375

11 1039.482

13 400

15 30.51, 37.75, 39.47, 39.87, Yes

17 (a) \$3037.75, \$2537.75
(b) \$6167.78, \$5667.78

19 (a) 39 mg
(b) 41.496 mg
(c) 41.667 mg

21 (a) 40 mg
(b) 0.57 mg/kg, Yes
(c) (i) Greater than 100 kg
(ii) Less than 13.3 kg

Section 11.2

1 Balance = \$48,377.01, \$20,000. from deposits, \$28,377.01 from interest

3 \$33,035.37

5 \$42,567.82

7 17.54 payments

9 \$44,407.33, \$360,183.21

11 0.12%

13 \$1081.11

15 (a) \$1250
(b) 12.50

17 (a) \$400 billion
(b) \$900 billion

19 (a) $N + (1-r)N$ dollars
(b) $N + (1-r)N + (1-r)^2N$ dollars
(c) N/r dollars

Section 11.3

1 230.159 billion barrels

3 (a) 98 mg
(b) 121.5 mg
(c) 125 mg

5 (a) 400 mg
(b) $400(0.30) = 120$ mg

7 (a) 39.99 mg, 9.99 mg
(b) 40 mg, 10 mg

9 (a) 4.10 mg
(b) 7.54 mg
(c) 14.46 mg
(d) 35.24 mg
(e) 69.87 mg

11 24.5 years

13 Until 2046

15 About 34 years

17 Lasts forever

Chapter 11 Review

1 2046

3 Does not exist

5 200

7 1.9961

9 (a) (i) \$16.43 million
(ii) \$24.01 million
(b) \$16.87 million

11 \$27,979.34

13 \$400 million

15 (a) $N(k/(1-k))$
(b) $5.667N$

17 (a) $0.232323\ldots = 0.23 + 0.23(0.01) + 0.23(0.01)^2 + \cdots$
(b) $0.23/(1 - 0.01) = (23)/(99)$

19 \$25,503

Ch. 11 Understanding

1 False

3 True

5 False

7 False

9 False

11 False

13 False

15 False

17 True

19 False

21 False

23 False

25 False

27 False

29 True

31 False

33 False

35 False

37 False

39 True

41 True

43 True

45 True

Appendix A

1 (a)

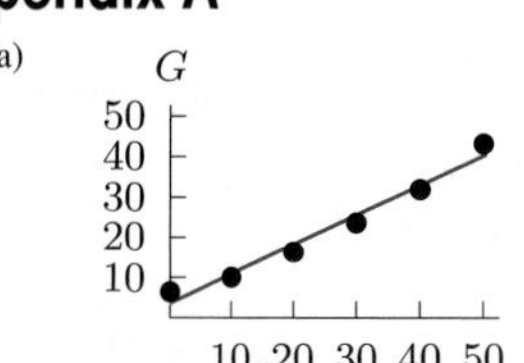

(b) Increasing at a rate of \$734 billion/year
(c) \$43.9 trillion, \$54.9 trillion, More confidence in the 2005 prediction

3 (a)

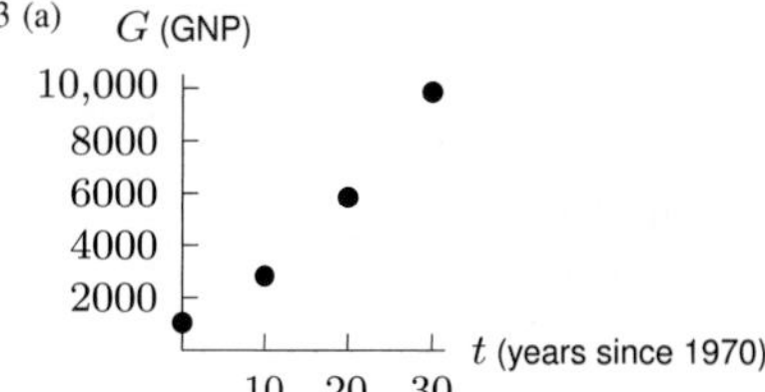

Yes

(b)

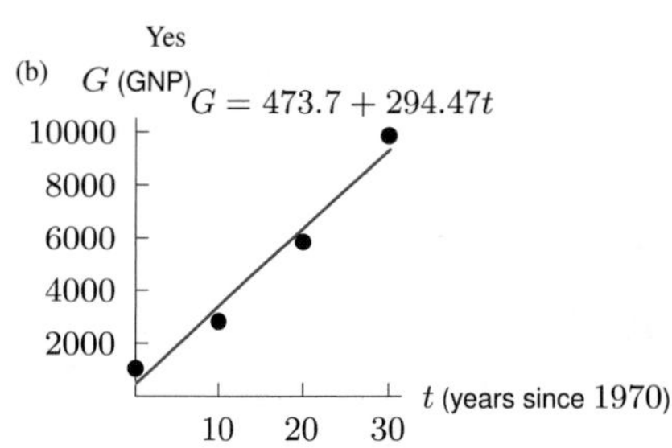

$G = 294.47t + 473.7$

(c) For 1985: 4891
For 2020: 15,197
More confidence in 1985

5 (a) $S = 0.08v + 1.77$
(b)

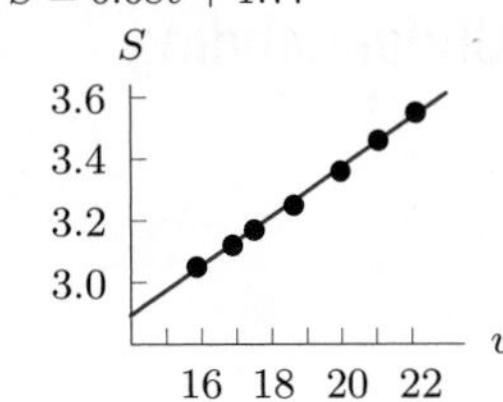

Yes
(c) At $v = 18$ ft/sec, $S = 3.21$
At $v = 10$ ft/sec, $S = 2.57$
$v = 18$ better

7 (a) $0.0026 = 0.26\%$
(b) For 1900, 272.27
For 1980, 335.1

9 (a)

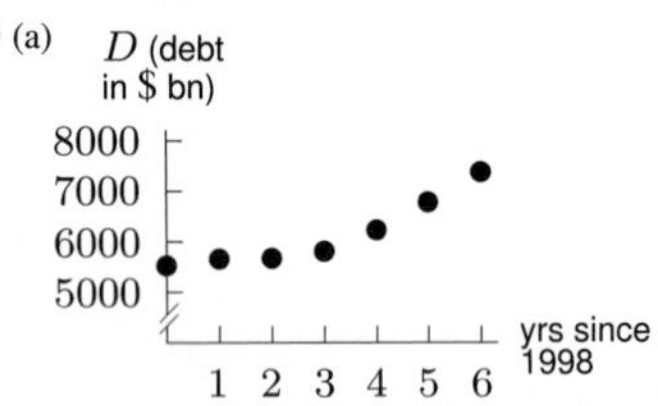

(b) Exponential
(c) $D = 5309(1.048)^t$, answers may vary

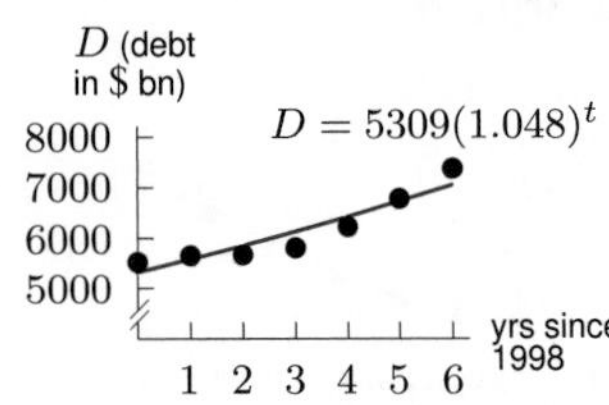

(d) About 4.8%
(e) No

11 (a) $r = 1$
(b) $r = 0.7$
(c) $r = 0$
(d) $r = -0.98$
(e) $r = -0.25$
(f) $r = -0.5$

13 (a) Exponential

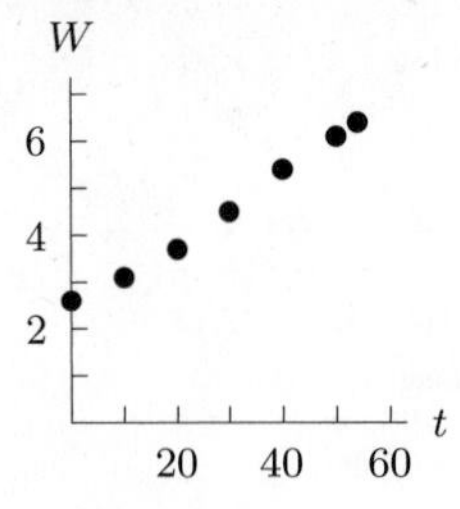

(b) $2.6(1.0165)^t$; answers may vary
(c) 1.65%
(d) At year 2020, 8.175 billion
At year 2050, 13.357 billion
2020 prediction more accurate

15 (a)

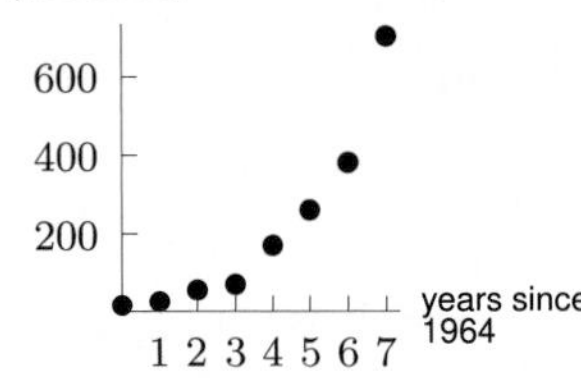

(b) Exponential
(c) $C = 15.9 \cdot (1.725)^t$, answers may vary

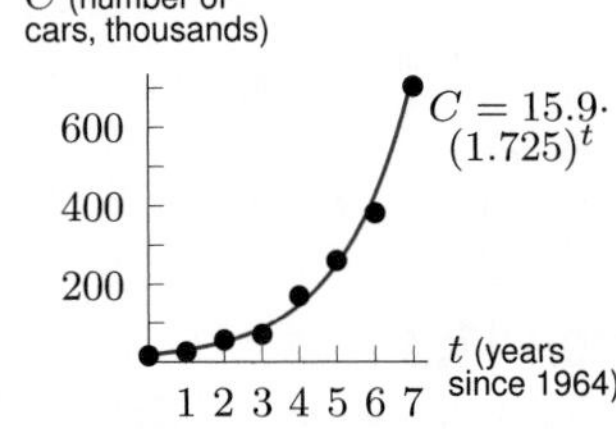

(d) About 73%
(e) No

17 (a) Negative
(b) $f(t) = -0.03t^2 + 1.01t + 13.82$

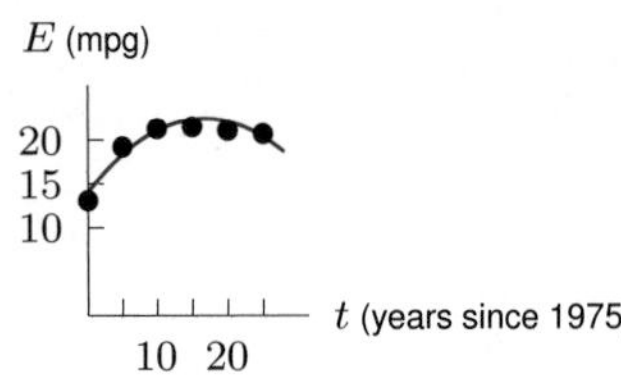

19 (a) Exponential
(b) $S = 29.96(1.30)^t$, answers may vary
Increasing 30%/yr
(c) $21{,}141$ megawatts
(d)

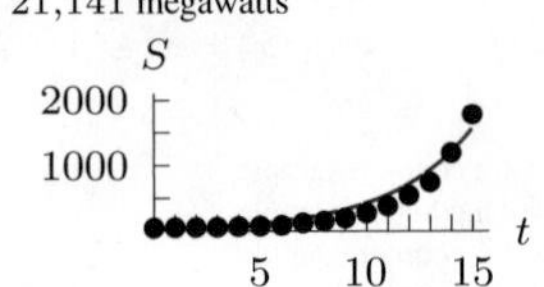

21 (a) Linear
(b) $C = 320 + 1.5t$
Increasing at 1.5 ppm/yr
(c) 387.5 ppm
(d)

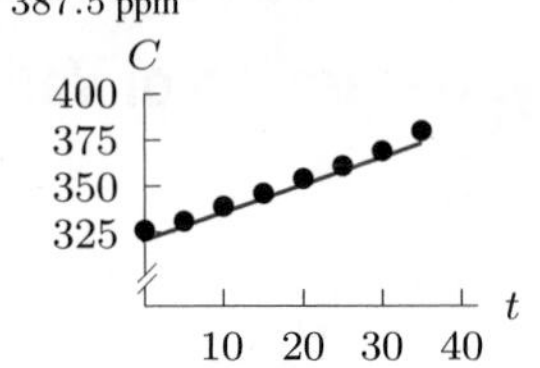

Appendix B

1 27%

3 (a) $\$160{,}356.77$
(b) $\$165{,}510.22$
(c) $\$165{,}891.05$
(d) $\$165{,}989.48$
(e) $\$166{,}005.85$

5 (a) 1.0408107
1.0408108
1.0408108
4% compounded continuously
$\approx 4.08108\%$
(b) $e^{0.04} \approx 1.048108$

7 4.88%

9 (a) (i) $5.126978\ldots\%$
(ii) $5.127096\ldots\%$
(iii) $5.127108\ldots\%$
(b) 5.127%
(c) $e^{0.05} = 1.05127109\ldots$

11 (a) = V, (b) = III, (c) = IV,
(d) = I, (e) = II

13 (a) 13,900 cruzados
(b) 24.52%

PRETEST

The pretest in this section covers skills that are used in this book. Doing it at the start of a course will help you identify areas in algebra where reviewing early on will help you succeed.

Problems for a Pretest

1. What is the equation of the line in Figure P.1?

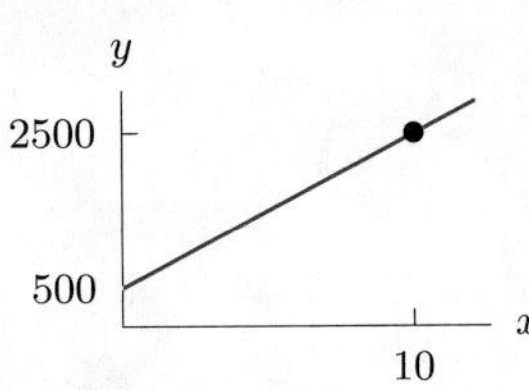

Figure P.1

2. What is the value of a in Figure P.2?

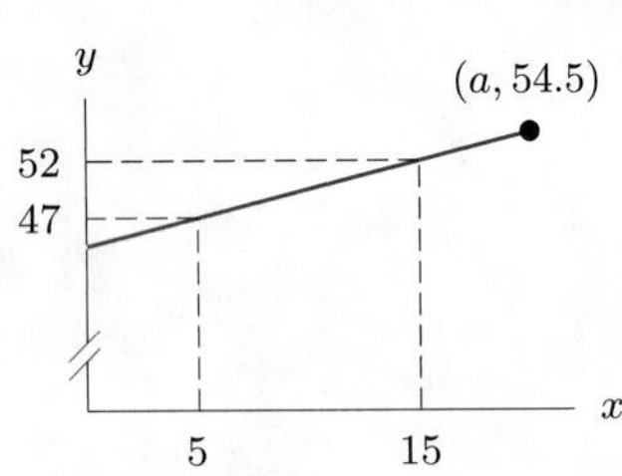

Figure P.2

3. Find a_1 and a_2 from Figure P.3.

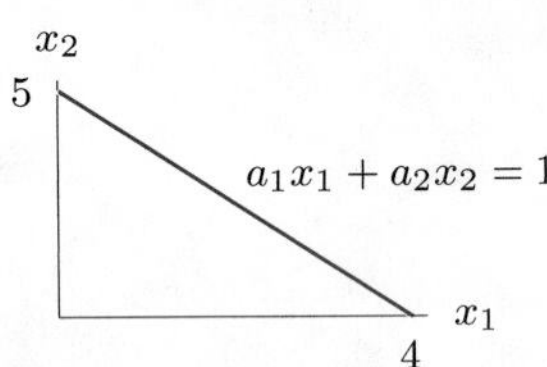

Figure P.3

4. Match each of the four lines in Figure P.4 with one of the slopes 0, 1, 2, −1, −2.

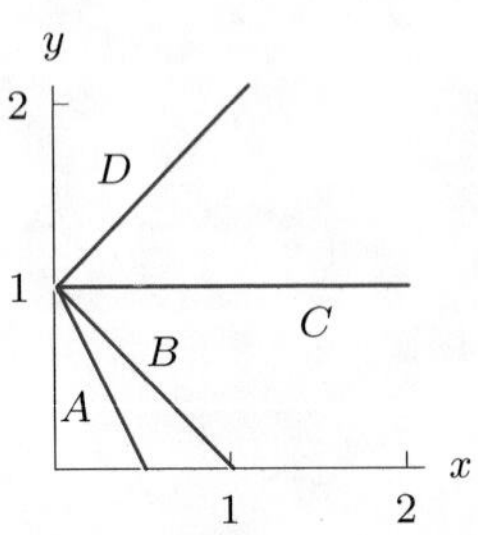

Figure P.4

5. Solve for P_0:

$$P = P_0\left(1 + \frac{r}{n}\right)^t.$$

6. Solve for r:

$$P = \left(1 + \frac{r}{n}\right)^t.$$

7. If $f(t) = 4t + (t+3)^2$, find $f(0)$.

8. If $f(x) = 4x + 28$, solve $f(x) = 0$.

9. Which of the following is equivalent to $16 - x^2 + 6x$?

(a) $7 + (3 - x)^2$
(b) $16 - (x - 3)^2$
(c) $25 - (x - 3)^2$
(d) $52 - (x - 6)^2$
(e) $25 - (x + 3)^2$
(f) None of the above

10. What are the coordinates of the point Q in Figure P.5?

11. What are the coordinates of the point P in Figure P.5?

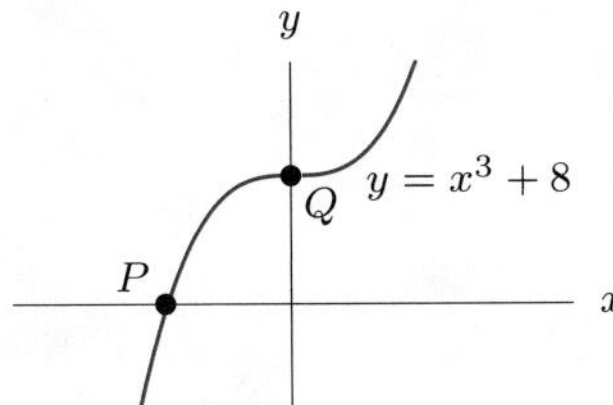

Figure P.5

12. Find $|-10| + |10|$.

13. Which of the following is equivalent to $\dfrac{T}{E} + E$?

(a) $\dfrac{E^2 + T}{E}$
(b) $\dfrac{E}{E^2 + T}$
(c) $E + T$
(d) $\dfrac{T + E}{E + 1}$
(e) $\dfrac{T + E}{E}$

14. Which of the following is equivalent to $\dfrac{1}{y} + \dfrac{1}{u}$?

(a) $\dfrac{1}{uy}$
(b) $\dfrac{1}{u + y}$
(c) $\dfrac{u + y}{uy}$
(d) $\dfrac{u}{y}$
(e) $\dfrac{2}{y + u}$

15. Which of the following is equivalent to $x^{-1}y + y^{-1}x$?

(a) $\dfrac{xy}{x^2+y^2}$
(b) $\dfrac{x^2+y^2}{xy}$
(c) $\dfrac{xy}{x+y}$
(d) $\dfrac{x+y}{xy}$
(e) $\dfrac{y+x}{x+y}$

16. If $\dfrac{\sqrt[3]{t}}{t} = t^a$, what is a?

17. Simplify $(x^2x^5)^4$.

18. Simplify $W^{2/3}W^{3/2}$.

19. Expand and collect like terms: $-5u\left(\dfrac{3}{u} - 2v\right)$.

20. Solve $3p + 4 = 9$ for p.

21. Solve $2x + a = 5(1 - x)$ for x.

22. Solve $2\sqrt{w} - 3 = 9$ for w.

23. Solve $\dfrac{2}{3} = \dfrac{5}{n}$ for n.

24. Solve $Cq + Dq = A$ for q.

25. With $m = 2, x_0 = 3,\ y_0 = 10$, solve $y - y_0 = m(x - x_0)$ for x.

26. Find the value of x when $y = 0$ if $-2x + 9y - 9 = 0$.

27. Find the value of s when $t = s + 1$ if $3s - 8t = 7$.

28. Factor $12x^2 - 6a^2x$.

29. Factor $C^2a^3b - Cab^3$.

30. Which of the following is the factored form of $x^2 + 2x - 15$?

(a) $(x+1)^2 - 16$
(b) $(x-3)(x+5)$
(c) $x(x+2) - 15$
(d) $(x+2)(x-15)$
(e) None of the above

31. What are the zeroes of $(x-2)(x+1)(2x-5)$?

32. What is the y-intercept of $y = (x-2)(x+1)(2x-5)$?

33. If $W^2 - 2W - 8 = 4(W-2)$, find all possible values of W.

34. If $s = d^2 + d + 1$ and $d = g + 1$ express s in terms of g.

35. If $\theta = x^2 - 1$ express $(\theta + 1)^2$ in terms of x.

36. If $b = -2z$ express $b^2 - 2b$ in terms of z.

37. The graph of the equation $a^x = y$ passes through the point $(-3, \frac{1}{8})$. What is a?

38. If $s = 2$ and $t = 0$ is a solution to $as^5 = s^7 + t$, what is a?

39. Using Table P.1, what value of w gives $q = 7$?

Table P.1

w	-4	-1	1	6	10
q	4	2	7	-2	2

40. Using Table P.2, what is the temperature at 6 pm?

Table P.2

Time (hours after midnight)	0	6	12	18
Temperature (°F)	36	48	65	55

41. For some constant k, let $M = kN$. If $M = 0.84$ when $N = 12$, what is M when $N = 6$?

42. What is the area of the shaded rectangle in Figure P.6?

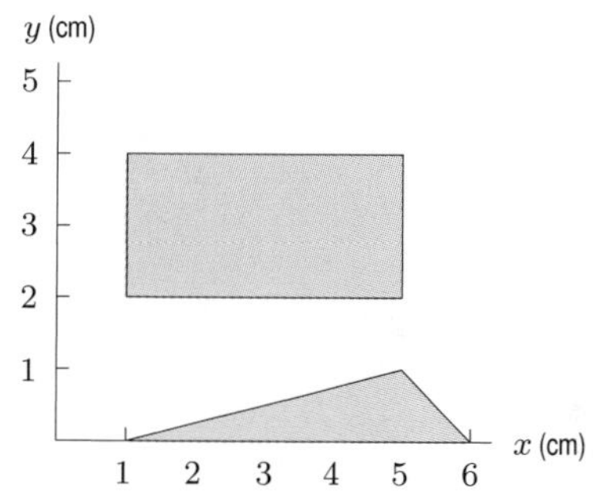

Figure P.6

43. What is the area of the shaded triangle in Figure P.6?

44. A price increases by a factor of 1.042. By what percent has the price increased?

45. A car, initially valued at \$21,000 is now worth 32% less. What is the car's current value?

46. An item priced at \$45 is on sale for 25% off. The customer pays the sale price plus 8% sales tax. How much does the customer pay?

Problems on Trigonometry (Optional)

1. What is the vertical intercept of $y = \cos x$?

2. What are the zeroes of $y = \sin x$ between $x = 0$ and $x = 2\pi$ (inclusive)?

3. How many degrees is 3π radians?

4. What are the coordinates of the highest point on the sine graph in Figure P.7?

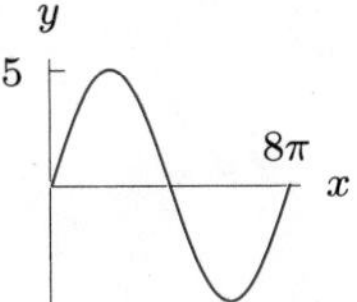

Figure P.7

INDEX

Name: ______________________________ **(Please Print)**

Section: ____________________

Instructions:

1. **DO NOT OPEN THIS EXAM UNTIL YOU ARE INSTRUCTED TO DO SO.**
2. Without fully opening the exam, check that you have pages 1 through 11.
3. Write your name on your exam.
4. Clear your desk of everything but this booklet, your pencils and your calculator. If you need more space to write your solutions, use the backs of the exam pages.
5. Crib sheets (pre-compiled lists of formulas or other information) either written or in a calculator are specifically forbidden. ***Use of a crib sheet of any kind on this exam will result in an automatic zero grade.***
6. The problems on this exam vary in difficulty. You should try to solve these problems in an order that will maximize your score. Solve all the easier problems first, and then go back to the ones that require more thought.
7. Unless otherwise indicated, **SHOW ALL YOUR WORK.** If no work is shown, no credit can be awarded. *Even for calculator solutions, you should include relevant information, like the equation to be solved, the function whose graph is to be sketched, etc.*
8. Unless you are specifically instructed to do otherwise, DO NOT ROUND YOUR ANSWER.
9. You will be given **exactly** 120 minutes for this exam.

I have read and fully understood all of the above instructions:

Signature: ______________________________

Page	**2**	**3**	**4**	**5**	**6**	**7**	**8**	**9**	**10**	**11**	**Total**
Max points	**20**	**24**	**30**	**25**	**8**	**20**	**18**	**15**	**25**	**15**	**200**
Points											

1. (8+4+8=20 points)

a) Let $f(x) = -3x^2 - 4x + 5$, simplify the difference quotient $\dfrac{f(x+h) - f(x)}{h}$ as much as possible.

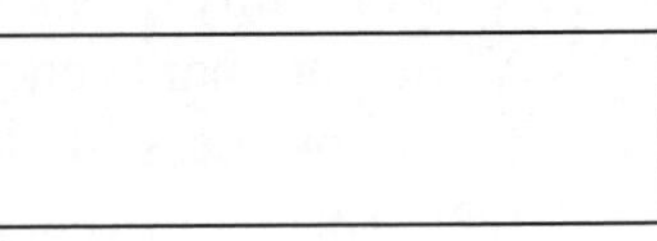

b) Use the limit definition of the derivative, and your answer from part a) to find $f'(x)$. **Note**: NO CREDIT for any other method.

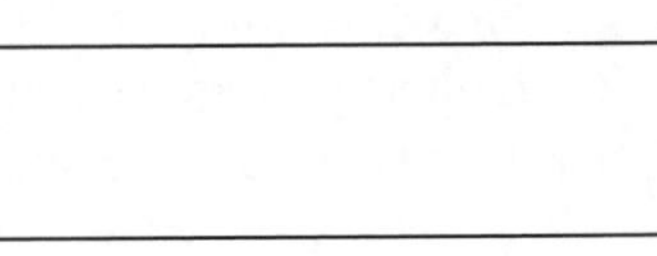

c) Use part b) to find the equation of the tangent line to $y = f(x)$ at $x = 3$.

2. (4+8=12 points) Consider the graph of the function $y = g(x)$ below.

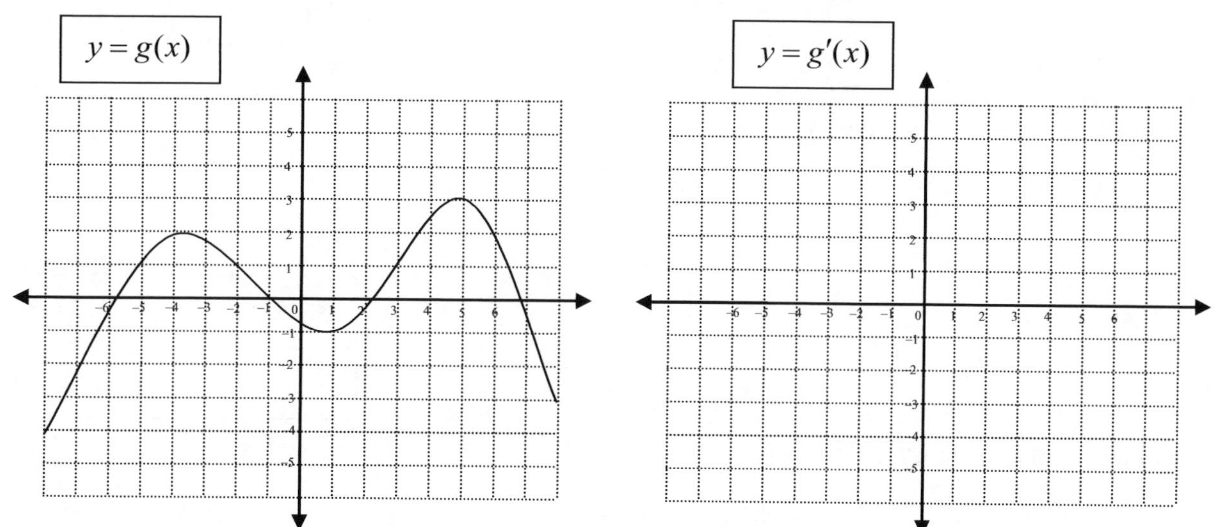

a) Carefully estimate the value of $g'(6)$. Add the corresponding tangent line to the sketch of the graph of $y = g(x)$.

b) Carefully sketch the graph of the derivative function $g'(x)$ on the right.

3. (6+6=12 points) Given $\int_2^8 f(x)dx = -10$, $\int_2^8 g^2(x)dx = 12$, $\int_{-2}^8 g(x)dx = 5$ and $\int_2^8 g(x)dx = 3$

Find the exact value of

a) $\int_2^8 \frac{f(x)}{5} + \frac{3}{4} g^2(x)\,dx$

b) $\left(\int_{-2}^{2} g(x)dx\right)^2$

4. (8+8+8+6=30 points) Evaluate each of the following. *You do NOT need to simplify your answers.*

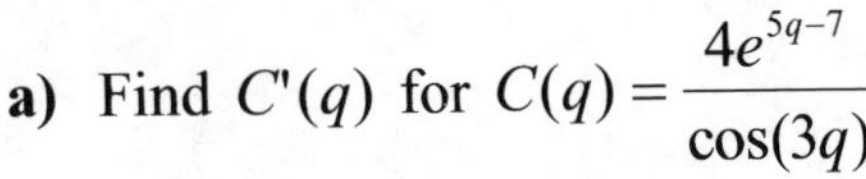

a) Find $C'(q)$ for $C(q) = \dfrac{4e^{5q-7}}{\cos(3q)}$

b) Find $\dfrac{dv}{dt}$ for $v = \ln(2t^3 + 7t) - 16$

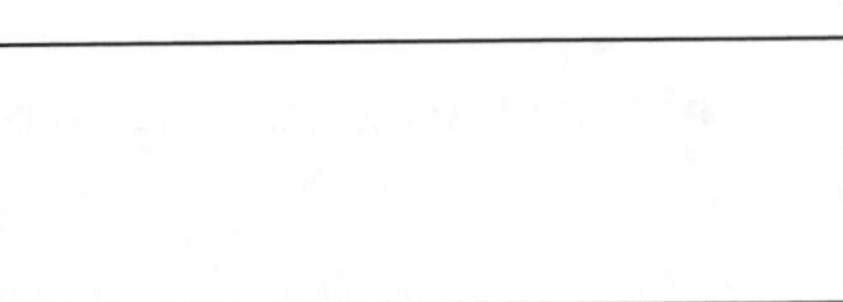

c) Find $P'(x)$ for $P(x) = \left(e^x - \dfrac{1}{x}\right)\sin(2x)$

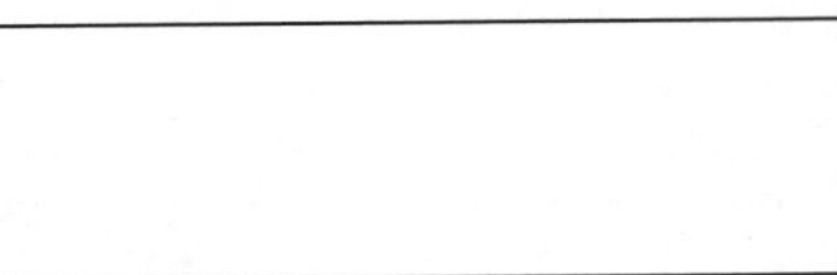

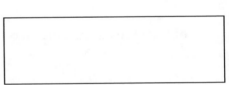

d) Find $\dfrac{dz}{dy}$ for $z = 37(1.2)^y - \pi\ y$

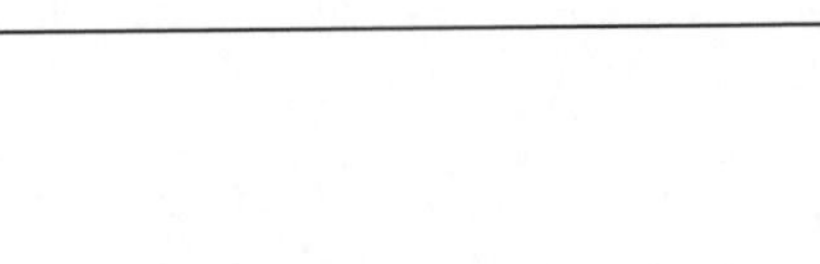

5. (10+2=12 points) The sketch below contains the graph of derivative function $g'(x)$ **(not** $g(x)$**)**. Use the sketch to answer the questions that follow.

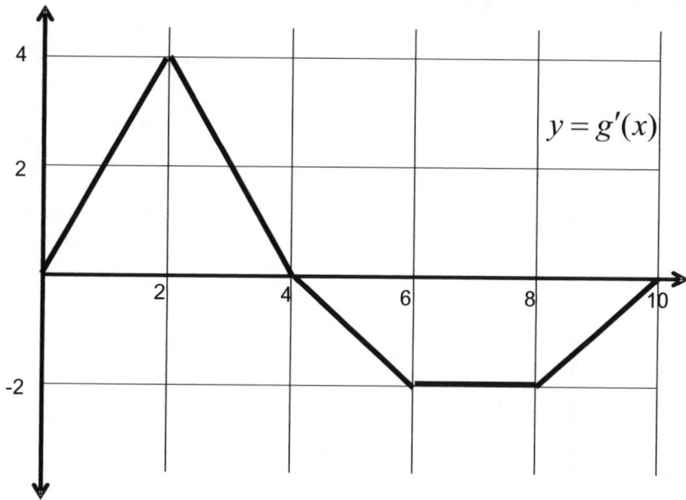

a) Fill in the missing values in the table for $g(x)$ **(not** $g'(x)$**)** given that $g(4) = 7$.

x	0	2	4	6	8	10
$g(x)$			7			

b) Evaluate $\int_2^8 g'(x)dx =$

6. (5+4+4=13 points) Suppose that $G(x) = \int_1^x \frac{\sin\sqrt{t}}{t^2+2}\,dt$. Find:

a) $G'(x) =$ ________________

b) $G(1)$ = ________________

c) $G(4)$ = ________________ (accuracy ±0.0001)

7. (8 points) The region enclosed by $y = 3x^2 + 4x - 11$ and $y = x + 7$ is shown in the sketch below. Write the definite integral used to find the area enclosed by the two curves. ***Write the definite integral only, numerical answers will receive NO credit.***

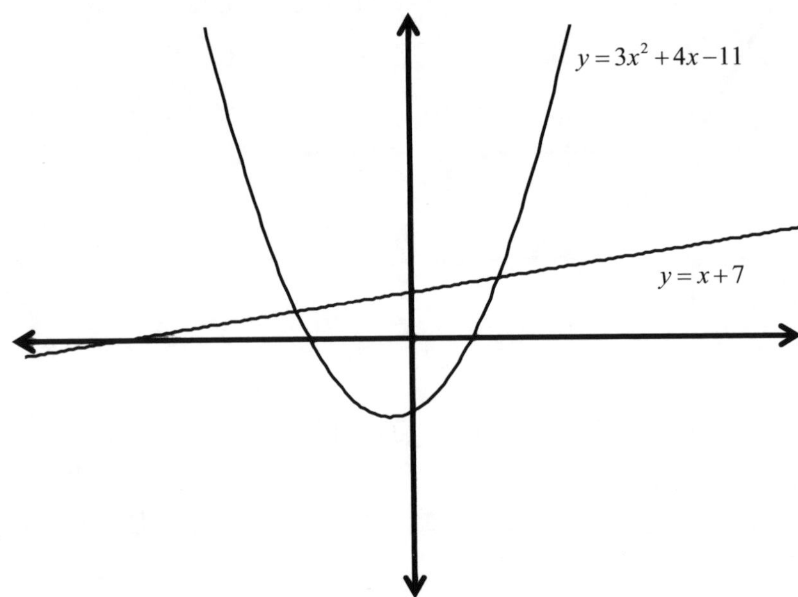

8. (5+5+5+5=20 points) A lab is studying drosophila embryos. The following table gives the number, *N*, of embryos (in thousands) in the lab on January 1, in five-year increments between 1985 and 2005:

Year	*1985*	*1990*	*1995*	*2000*	*2005*
N	*75.27*	*72.12*	*63.19*	*51.27*	*37.43*

Use this table to answer the following:

a) Circle the one correct answer. What type of function is seen in this table?

A) Linear B) Exponential C) Neither

b) Circle the one correct answer. The change in the value of the number of embryos between 1990 and 2000 is:

A) 37.84 B) 24.00

C) 21.15 D) 8.93

E) 11.92 F) None of these

c) Circle the one correct answer. The average rate of change in the number of embryos between 1990 and 2000 is:

A) 2.085 embryos/year B) -2.085 embryos/year

C) -1.892 embryos/year D) 1.892 embryos/year

E) 1.600 embryos/year F) None of these

d) Circle the one correct answer. The instantaneous rate of change in the number of embryos on January 1, 2005 was:

A) -2.768 embryos/year B) -1.892 embryos/year

C) 1.892 embryos/year D) -2.330 embryos/year

E) 2.768 embryos/year F) 2.330 embryos/year

9. (3+5+5+5=18 points) A bear has left his den in search of food. The graph to the right shows his velocity, $v(t)$, in feet per minute. Use this graph to answer the following questions.

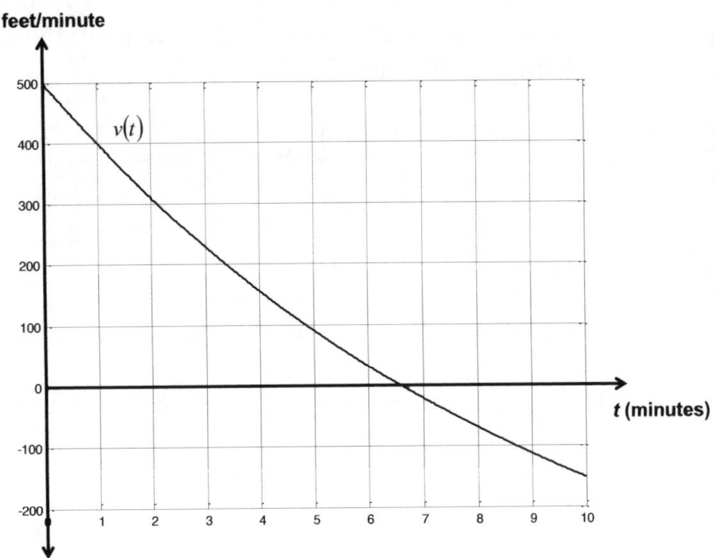

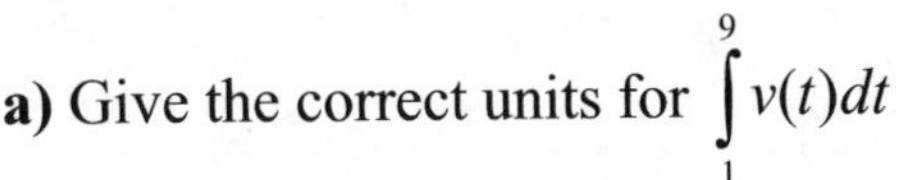

a) Give the correct units for $\int_1^9 v(t)dt$.

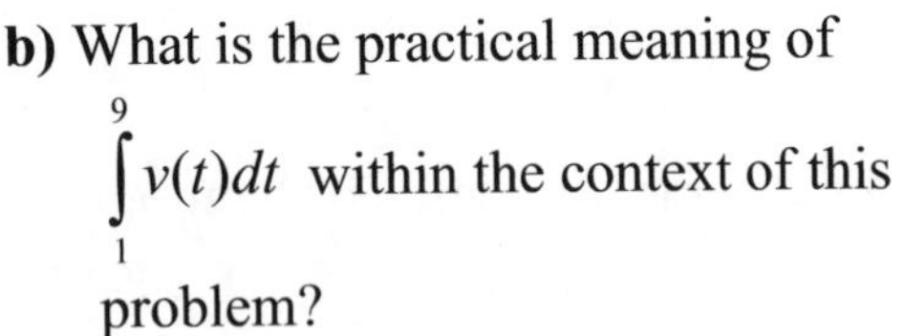

b) What is the practical meaning of $\int_1^9 v(t)dt$ within the context of this problem?

c) Use the sketch to **carefully** shade in the region whose area is given by the **right-hand sum** using $\Delta t = 2$ of the definite integral, $\int_1^9 v(t)dt$.

d) Evaluate the **right-hand sum** using $\Delta t = 2$ that corresponds to the definite integral, $\int_1^9 v(t)dt$.

10. (5+5+5=15 points)

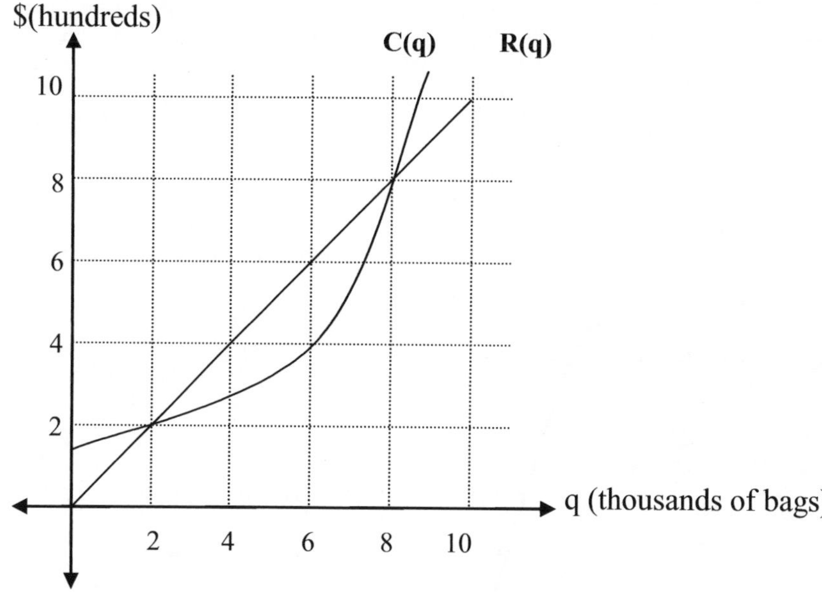

The above graphs are the cost and revenue functions for a candy making company.

a.) Circle the one correct answer. The company makes profit at___ bags of candy.

A) 1,000 B) 4,000 C) 4,000 and 7,000 D) 9,000 E) None of these

b) Circle the one correct answer. The company should NOT make MORE candy when ___ bags of candy have been produced.

A) 2,000 B) 4,000 and 6,000 C) 4,000 D) 8,000 E) None of these

c) Circle the one correct answer. The company reaches its maximum profit when ___ bags of candy are produced.

A) 2,000 and 8,000 B) 4,000 C) 6,000 D) 9,000 E) None of these

11. (5+5+5+5+5=25 points) The sketch below is the graph of $y = f'(x)$ (**NOT** $f(x)$ **).** Use this sketch to answer the following:

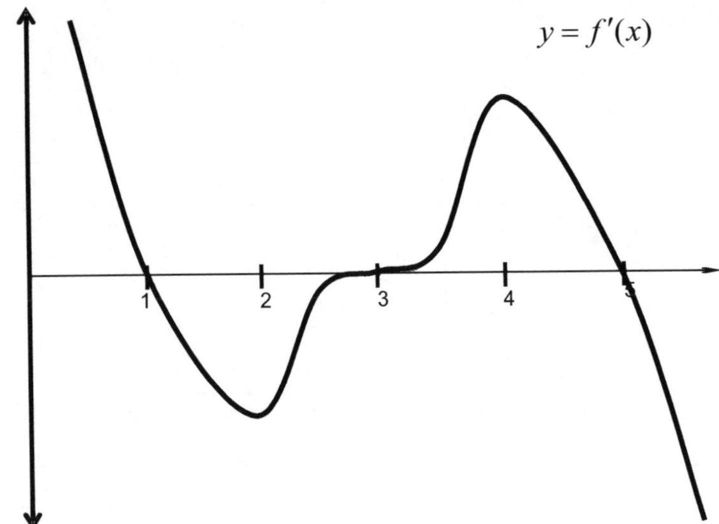

a) Circle the one correct answer. For $4 < x < 5$ the graph of $f(x)$ is:

A) Increasing and concave up
B) Decreasing and concave up
C) Increasing and concave down
D) Decreasing and concave down
E) None of these

b) Circle the one correct answer. Around $x = 2$, the graph of $f(x)$ is:

A) Increasing B) Decreasing C) None of these

c) Circle the one correct answer. The graph of $f(x)$ has a local maximum at $x =$:

A) 4 only B) 3 only C) 1 only D) 1 and 5 E) 1, 3 and 5

d) Circle the one correct answer. $f(x)$ has inflection point at $x =$:

A) 3 only B) 2 and 4 C) 1 and 5 D) 1, 3 and 5 E) None of these

e) Circle the one correct answer. Which of the following is correct?

A) $f(1) < f(2)$ B) $f(2) < f(3)$ C) $f(1) < f(4)$ D) $f(2) < f(5)$ E) None of these

12. (15 points) Sketch the graph of a function $y = f(x)$ that has all of the following properties:

- $f(-1) = -2$
- $f'(x) < 0$ for $x < -2$ or $x > 1$
- $f'(x) > 0$ for $-2 < x < 1$
- $f'(x) = 0$ for $x = -2$ or $x = 1$
- $f''(x) < 0$ for $0 < x < 3$
- $f''(x) > 0$ for $x < 0$ or $x > 3$
- $f''(x) = 0$ for $x = 0$ or $x = 3$

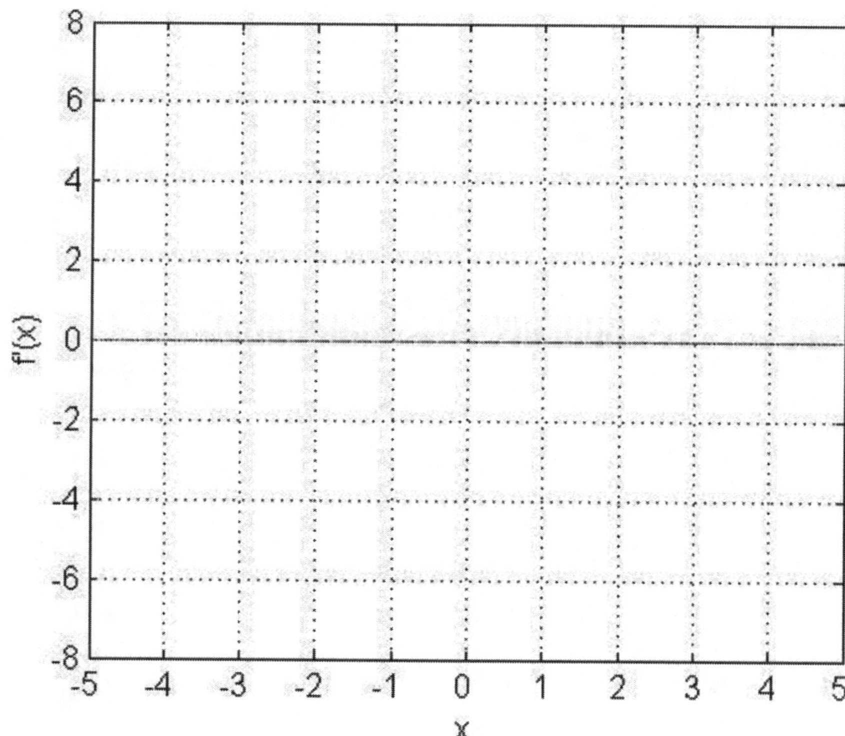